HANDBOOK OF PSYCHOPHYSIOLOGY, THIRD EDITION

The *Handbook of Psychophysiology, Third Edition* is an essential reference for students, researchers, and professionals in the behavioral, cognitive, and biological sciences. Psychophysiological methods, paradigms, and theories offer entry into a biological cosmos that does not stop at skin's edge, and this essential reference is designed as a road map for explorers of this cosmos. The scope and coverage in the *Handbook* have expanded to include both a context for and coverage of the biological bases of cognitive, affective, social, and developmental processes and behavior. In addition to updated coverage of the traditional areas of psychophysiology, coverage of the brain and central nervous system has been expanded to include functional neuroimaging, event-related brain potentials, electrophysiological source dipole localization, lesion methods, and transcranial magnetic stimulation. It also includes a section on cellular and humoral systems with attention to the communication across and interactions among cellular, immunological, endocrinological, and neural processes.

John T. Cacioppo is the Tiffany and Margaret Blake Distinguished Service Professor and the Director of the Center for Cognitive and Social Neuroscience at the University of Chicago. He is the former president of the Society for Psychophysiological Research, president of the Association for Psychological Science, and a recipient of the Society's Award for Distinguished Scientific Contribution and the American Psychological Association's Distinguished Scientific Contribution Award.

Louis G. Tassinary is Professor of Architecture and the Associate Dean for Research in the Department of Architecture at Texas A & M University. He was also the Director of the Environmental Psychophysiology Laboratory at the College of Architecture at Texas A & M University from 1991 to 2001. He has written many articles for journals including *Psychological Science*, *Journal of Environmental Psychology*, *Cognition and Emotion*, and *Journal of Personality and Social Psychology*.

Gary G. Berntson received his Ph.D. in psychology and life sciences from the University of Minnesota, and then completed NSF and USPHS postdoctoral fellowships at Rockefeller University before moving to Ohio State University, where he is currently Professor of Psychology, Psychiatry, and Pediatrics, and a member of the Neuroscience graduate program. He is the Secretary and a member of the Board of Society for Psychophysiological Research.

THIRD EDITION

HANDBOOK OF PSYCHOPHYSIOLOGY

Edited by

John T. Cacioppo
University of Chicago

Louis G. Tassinary
Texas A & M University

Gary G. Berntson
Ohio State University

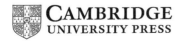

CAMBRIDGE
UNIVERSITY PRESS

CAMBRIDGE UNIVERSITY PRESS
Cambridge, New York, Melbourne, Madrid, Cape Town, Singapore, São Paulo

Cambridge University Press
32 Avenue of the Americas, New York, NY 10013-2473, USA

www.cambridge.org
Information on this title: www.cambridge.org/9780521844710

First published 2007

Printed in the United States of America

A catalog record for this publication is available from the British Library.

Library of Congress Cataloging in Publication Data

Handbook of psychophysiology / edited by John T. Cacioppo, Louis G.
Tassinary, Gary G. Berntson. – 3rd ed.
    p. ;   cm.
Includes bibliographical references and index.
ISBN-13: 978-0-521-84471-0 (hardback)
ISBN-10: 0-521-84471-1 (hardback)
1. Psychophysiology–Handbooks, manuals, etc.   I. Cacioppo, John T.
II. Tassinary, Louis G.   III. Berntson, Gary G.
[DNLM: 1. Psychophysiology.   I. Behavioral Medicine–methods. WL 103
H2363 2007]   I. Title.
QP360.P7515   2007
612.8 – dc22   2006014847

ISBN   978-0-521-84471-0 hardback

Contents

List of Contributors

Ralph Adolphs   *California Institute of Technology*
Gary G. Berntson   *Ohio State University*
Margaret M. Bradley   *University of Florida*
Giovanni Buccino   *Universitá di Parma Italia*
John T. Cacioppo   *University of Chicago*
Rebecca Campo   *University of Utah*
George P. Chrousos   *PREB/NICHD/NIH*
Antonio R. Damasio   *University of Iowa*
Richard J. Davidson *University of Wisconsin-Madison*
Michael E. Dawson   *University of Southern California*
A. Courtney DeVries   *Ohio State University*
Firdaus S. Dhabhar   *Stanford University*
Barry R. Dworkin   *Pennsylvania State University*
J. Christopher Edgar   *University of Illinois, Urbana-Champaign*
Monica Fabiani   *University of Illinois, Urbana-Champaign*
Kara D. Federmeier   *University of Illinois, Urbana-Champaign*
Diane L. Filion   *University of Missouri, Kansas City*
Nathan A. Fox   *University of Maryland*
James H. Geer   *Louisiana State University*
Peter J. Gianaros   *University of Pittsburgh*
Gabrielle Gratton   *University of Illinois, Urbana-Champaign*
Wendy Heller   *University of Illinois, Urbana-Champaign*
Heather A. Henderson   *University of Maryland*
Luis Hernandez   *University of Michigan*
John D. Herrington   *University of Illinois, Urbana-Champaign*
Petr Hlustik   *Palacky University, Olomouc, Czechia*
Julianne Holt-Lunstad   *Brigham Young University*
William G. Iacono   *University of Minnesota*
Erick Jannsen   *Indiana University*
J. Richard Jennings   *University of Pittsburgh*
John Jonides   *University of Michigan*
Gregory A. Kaltsas   *University of Athens*
Philipp Kanske   *Max Planck Institute for Human Cognitive & Brain Sciences*
Jennifer Keller   *Stanford University*
Nicholas Kin   *Ohio State University*
Robert Kluender   *University of California-San Diego*
Kenneth L. Koch   *Wake Forest University*
Michael Koenigs   *University of Iowa*
Arthur F. Kramer   *University of Illinois, Urbana-Champaign*
Marta Kutas   *University of California-San Diego*

Peter J. Lang   *University of Florida*
Max E. Levine   *Wake Forest University*
Martin Lindquist   *Columbia University*
Sara H. Lisanby   *NYS Psychiatric Institute, Columbia University*
Tyler S. Lorig   *Washington and Lee University*
Dave Lozano   *Mindware Technologies*
Bruce Luber   *NYS Psychiatric Institute, Columbia University*
Peter J. Marshall   *Temple University*
Gregory A. Miller   *University of Illinois, Urbana-Champaign*
Eric R. Muth   *Clemson University*
Randy J. Nelson   *Ohio State University*
Laurel C. Newman   *Washington University*
Teresa Nguyen   *NYS Psychiatric Institute, Columbia University*
Howard C. Nusbaum *University of Chicago*
Raja Parasuraman   *George Mason University*
Russ J. Parsons   *Northwest Environmental Psychology*
Angel V. Peterchev   *NYS Psychiatric Institute, Columbia University*
R. T. Pivik   *Arkansas Children's Nutrition Center*
Diego A. Pizzagalli   *Harvard University*
Georg Pongratz   *University Regensburg, Germany*
Michael I. Posner   *University of Orgeon*
Nicole Prause   *Indiana University*
Karen S. Quigley   *New Jersey Medical School*
Maija Reblin   *University of Utah*
M. Rosario Rueda   *Unviersidad de Granada, Spain*
Virginia M. Sanders   *Ohio State University*
Anne M. Schell   *Occidental College*
Louis A. Schmidt   *McMaster University, Ontario, Canada*
Timothy W. Smith   *University of Utah*
Charles T. Snowdon   *University of Wisconsin-Madison*
Ana Solodkin   *University of Chicago*
Michael L. Spezio   *California Institute of Technology*
Alexandra Sporn   *NYS Psychiatric Institute, Columbia University*
Jenny Staab   *University of California-San Diego*
Andrew Steptoe   *University College London*
Robert M. Stern   *Pennsylvania State University*
Esthar M. Sternberg *National Institute of Mental Health*
Michael J. Strube   *Washington University*
Bradley P. Sutton   *University of Illinois, Urbana-Champaign*
Louis G. Tassinary   *Texas A & M University*
Daniel T. Tranel   *University of Iowa*
Bert N. Uchino   *University of Utah*
Eric J. Vanman   *Georgia State University*
Tor D. Wager   *Columbia University*
Toni E. Ziegler   *University of Wisconsin-Madison*

1

Psychophysiological Science: Interdisciplinary Approaches to Classic Questions About the Mind

JOHN T. CACIOPPO, LOUIS G. TASSINARY, AND GARY G. BERNTSON

Psychophysiology is an old idea but a new science. It is a likely assumption that ever since man began to experience himself as an object of his own awareness he has had some intuitive notion that bodily changes were, in some measure, related to his moods, his sentiments, his frustrations, his elations. How to relate these dual aspects of human functioning has been a concern of philosopher-scientists throughout the course of intellectual history. (Greenfield & Sternbach, 1972, p. v)

The first *Handbook of Psychophysiology* was published more than three decades ago (Greenfield & Sternbach, 1972). Coverage in that *Handbook* emphasized the peripheral nervous system, an emphasis that many still identify with the term psychophysiology in accord with the history of psychophysiology. As is the case for physiological and other scientific fields, however, psychophysiology has changed dramatically since the appearance of its first *Handbook*. With the advent of new and powerful probes of the central nervous system (e.g., brain imaging techniques), there is an increased emphasis in the field on investigating the brain and central nervous system as they relate to behavior. Investigations of elementary physiological events in normal thinking, feeling, and interacting individuals are commonplace, and new techniques are providing additional windows through which the neural events underlying psychological processes can be viewed unobtrusively. Instrumentation now makes it possible for investigators to explore the selective activation of discrete parts of the brain during particular psychological operations in normal individuals and patients. Transcranial magnetic stimulation has made it possible to stimulate or temporarily disable a region of the brain to study its role in cognitive operations, and studies of patients with lesions are becoming more precise both in their definition of the lesion and in their specification of behavior.

Preparation of this chapter was supported by National Institute of Aging Program Project Grant No. P01 AG18911. Address correspondence to John T. Cacioppo, Center for Cognitive and Social Neuroscience, 5848 S. University Avenue, Chicago, IL 60637, or by email to *Cacioppo@uchicago.edu*.

Developments in tissue and blood assays, ambulatory recording devices, non-contact recording instruments, and powerful and mobile computing devices make it possible to measure physiological, endocrinological, and immunological responses in naturalistic as well as laboratory settings. New, powerful assays, including DNA genotyping, are now possible using minimally invasive or noninvasive procedures. With recent developments in molecular biology, behavioral genetics is becoming an important new player in the field. However, the views from these windows are clear only because of the deliberate efforts of knowledgeable investigators. Knowledge and principles of physiological mechanisms, biometric and psychometric properties of the measures, statistical representation and analysis of multivariate data, and the structure of scientific inference are important if veridical information is to be extracted from psychophysiological data. These are among the topics covered in depth in this *Handbook*.

The field of psychophysiology has changed dramatically in other ways as well. Psychophysiology used to be divided into distinct territories, typically defined by organ systems (e.g., the heart, eye blinks), with relatively little integration across these systems. The concept of arousal – the peripheral equivalent of the early notions of the reticular activating system in the brain – dominated the field for the better part of the twentieth century and made the selection of measure a matter of preference rather than a theoretical choice because the responses presumably reflected modulations of arousal regardless of the system one was measuring. Although low correlations among such measures were well recognized, the differences across measures were viewed as less interesting and informative at the time than the confluence of these measures.

Advances in our understanding of the neurophysiological basis of these measures have underscored the importance of the unique patterns of peripheral responses that typically emerge across situations and individuals, and the peripheral and central mechanisms that orchestrate these patterns are active areas of inquiry. As part of these inquiries, animal research, molecular studies, and computational modeling are being embraced in the field despite the original definition of psychophysiology in terms of the study of humans rather than nonhuman animals. Moreover, the larger social, cultural, and interpersonal contexts are now recognized as powerful determinants of brain and behavior. Monism has replaced any lingering notions of dualism, as psychological states are more likely to be conceived as represented in and acting through cortical, limbic, and brain stem regions, with influences on autonomic, neuroendocrine, and immune activity, which in turn serve to modulate crucial cellular and molecular processes. Afferent information, in turn, travels from the peripheral to the central nervous system to influence the brain and behavior in social contexts. For instance, interleukin-1β (IL-1β) in the periphery increases in response to the introduction of antigens, and this increase is reflected in the information carried along the vagal afferent nerve to the brain. As a result of these signals from the periphery, IL-1β levels in the brain are increased, producing feelings of illness and fatigue. The notion of embodied cognition has been alive and well in psychophysiology for decades (see review by Cacioppo & Petty, 1981), and the identification of canonical and mirror neurons has renewed interest in this area (Garbarini & Adenzato, 2004).

Rose (2005) noted that there are at least two voluminous scientific literatures on psychological states and physiological events that have not been effectively related to one another: the literature on the CNS mechanisms underlying a variety of psychological processes, and the literature on psychological factors and peripheral biological activities including physical health. These literatures have tended to focus on different psychological processes, but there is an increasing recognition that these two areas of study have much in common. For instance, studies of the brain during exposure to potentially stressful stimuli can be an important tool in studying stress biology and evaluating its impact in various systems (Rose, 2005). Both of these literatures are covered in this *Handbook* and, although much needs to be done to integrate these distinct lines of research, it should be apparent from the chapters in this *Handbook* that this work has begun.

With the dawning of the twenty-first century, recording standards, procedures for signal representation, and powerful techniques for multivariate statistical analyses have been established. Investigators are now as likely to be studying the interrelationships among brain, autonomic, somatic, endocrinologic, immunologic, and/or genetic processes as they are to be studying any of these systems in isolation. Moreover, given that there are many things going on in the brain at any moment in time, only a few of which are relevant to any particular peripheral organ or effect, it is now recognized that the identification of psychological and brain mechanisms that are related to peripheral changes can be advanced significantly by working from the peripheral effects back to central, psychological, and social conditions, just as it can be advanced by the more traditional, complementary approach of manip-

ulating psychological states and observing the subsequent changes in CNS and PNS processes.

Finally, psychophysiology has always had a special appeal in scientific investigations of the mind because it offers tools for mining information about nonconscious and nonreportable states, processes, and events. Psychophysiological studies of attention and cognitive development in neonates, early sensory and attentional processes in schizophrenics, the cognitive operations underlying psychological states, and the study of sleep and dreams in older adults have helped lift the veil from these otherwise difficult-to-gauge behavioral processes.

In sum, psychophysiological research has provided insights into almost every facet of human nature, from the attention and behavior of the neonate to memory and emotions in the elderly. This book is about these insights and advances – what they are, the methods by which they came about, and the conceptualizations that are guiding progress toward future advances in the discipline. Historically, the study of psychophysiological phenomena has been susceptible to "easy generalizations, philosophical pitfalls, and influences from extrascientific quarters" (Harrington, 1987, p. 5). Our objectives in this chapter are to define psychophysiology, briefly review major historical events in the evolution of psychophysiological inference, outline a taxonomy of logical relationships between psychological constructs and physiological events, and specify a scheme for strong inference within each of the specified classes of psychophysiological relationships.

THE CONCEPTUALIZATION OF PSYCHOPHYSIOLOGY

The body is the medium of experience and the instrument of action. Through its actions we shape and organize our experiences and distinguish our perceptions of the outside world from sensations that arise within the body itself. (Miller, 1978, p. 14)

Anatomy, physiology, and psychophysiology are all branches of science organized around bodily systems with the collective aim of elucidating the structure and function of the parts of, and interrelated systems in, the human body in transactions with the environment. Anatomy is the science of body structure and the relationships among structures.

Physiology concerns the study of bodily function or how the parts of the body work. For both of these disciplines, what constitutes a body part varies with the level of bodily organization, going from the molecular to cellular to tissue to organ to body system to the organism. Thus, the anatomy and physiology of the body are intricately interrelated. Neuroscience, in particular, stands at this intersection.

Psychophysiology is intimately related to anatomy and physiology but is also concerned with psychological phenomena – the experience and behavior of organisms in the physical and social environment. The primary distinctions between psychophysiology and behavioral neuroscience are the focus of the former on higher cognitive processes and the interest in relating these higher cognitive processes to the integration of central and peripheral processes. Among the complexity added when moving from physiology to psychophysiology are the capacity by symbolic systems of representation (e.g., language, mathematics) to communicate and to reflect on history and experience; and social and cultural influences on physiological response and behavior. These factors contribute to plasticity, adaptability, and variability in behavior. Psychology and psychophysiology share the goal of explaining human experience and behavior, and physiological constructs and processes are an explicit and integral component of theoretical thinking in psychophysiology. The subject matter of psychophysiology, after all, is an embodied phenomenon.

The technical obstacles confronting early studies, the importance of understanding the physiological systems underlying observations, and the diverse goals and interests of the early investigators in the field fostered a partitioning of the discipline into physiological/measurement areas. The organization of psychophysiology in terms of underlying physiological systems, or what can be called *systemic psychophysiology*, remains important today for theoretical and pedagogical reasons. Physiological systems provide the foundation for human processes and behavior and are often the target of systematic observation. An understanding of the physiological system(s) under study and the bioelectrical principles underlying the perceptual and output responses being measured contribute to the plausible hypotheses, appropriate operationalizations, laboratory safety, discrimination of signal from artifact, acquisition and analysis of the physiological events, legitimate inferences based on the data, and theoretical advancement.

Like anatomy, physiology, and psychology, however, psychophysiology is a broad science organized in terms of a thematic as well as a systemic focus. The organization of psychophysiology in terms of topical areas of research can be called *thematic psychophysiology*. For instance, cognitive psychophysiology concerns the relationship between elements of human information processing and physiological events. Social psychophysiology concerns the study of the cognitive, emotional, and behavioral effects of human association as related to and revealed by physiological measures, interventions, and consequences including the reciprocal relationship between physiological and social systems. Developmental psychophysiology deals with ontological changes in psychophysiological relationships as well as the study of psychological development and aging using physiological measures. Clinical psychophysiology concerns the study of disorders in the organismic-environmental transactions and ranges from the assessment of disorders to interventions and treatments. Environmental psychophysiology elucidates the vagaries of organism-place interdependencies as well as the health consequences of design through unobtrusive physiological measurements. And applied psychophysiology generally deals with the implementation of psychophysiological principles in practice, such as operant training ("biofeedback"), desensitization, relaxation, and the detection of deception.

In each of these areas, the focus of study draws on, but goes beyond, the description of the structure or function of cells or organs, to investigate the organism in transactions with the physical or sociocultural environment. Some of these areas, such as developmental psychophysiology, have counterparts in anatomy and physiology but refer to complementary empirical domains that focus on human experience and behavior. Others, such as social psychophysiology, have a less direct counterpart in anatomy or physiology because the focus begins beyond that of an organism in isolation; yet the influence of social and cultural factors on physiological structures and functions, and their influence as moderators of the effects of physical stimuli on physiological structures and functions, leaves little doubt as to the relevance of these factors for anatomy and physiology as well as for psychophysiology. Meaney and colleagues (Meaney, Bhatnagar, Larocque, McCormick, Shanks, Smythe, Viau, & Plotsky, 1996), for instance, provide evidence that rat pups who are ignored by their mothers develop a more reactive hypothalamic pituitary adrenocortical (HPA) axis than rat pups who are licked and groomed by their mothers.

Because psychophysiology is intimately related to anatomy and physiology, knowledge of the physiological systems and responses under study contribute to both theoretical and methodological aspects of psychophysiological research. However, knowledge of the physiological systems is logically neither necessary nor sufficient to ascribe psychological meaning to physiological responses. The ascription of psychological meaning to physiological responses ultimately resides in factors such as the quality of the experimental design, the psychometric properties of the measures, and the appropriateness of the data analysis and interpretation. For instance, although numerous aspects of the physiological basis of event-related brain potentials remain uncertain, functional relationships within specific paradigms have been established between elementary cognitive operations and components of these potentials by systematically varying one or more of the former and monitoring changes in the latter.

The point is not that either the physiological or the psychological perspective is preeminent, but rather that both are fundamental to psychophysiological inquiries; more specifically, that physiological and psychological levels of organization are complementary. Inattention to the logic underlying psychophysiological inferences simply because one is dealing with observable physiological events is likely to lead either to simple and restricted descriptions of empirical relationships or to erroneous interpretations of these relationships. Similarly, "an aphysiological attitude, such as is evident in some psychophysiological research, is likely to lead to misinterpretation of the empirical relationships that are found between psychophysiological measures and psychological processes or states" (Coles et al., 1986, ix–x). Thus, whether organized in terms of a systemic or a thematic focus, psychophysiology can be conceptualized as a natural extension of anatomy and physiology in the scientific pursuit of understanding human processes and behavior. It is the joint consideration of physiological and functional perspectives, however, that is thought to improve operationalization, measurement, and inference and therefore to enrich research and theory on cognition, emotion, and behavior.

Early definitions of the field of psychophysiology were of two types. One emphasized the operational aspects of the field such as research in which the polygraph was used, research published by workers in the field, and research on physiological responses to behavioral manipulations (e.g., Ax, 1964b). Other early definitions were designed to differentiate psychophysiology from the older and more established field of physiological psychology or psychobiology. Initially, psychophysiology differed from physiological psychology in the use of human in contrast to animals as participants, the manipulation of psychological or behavioral constructs rather than anatomical structures or physiological processes, and the measurement of physiological rather than behavioral responses (Stern, 1964). Although this heritage can still be found, this distinction is often blurred by the fact that psychophysiologists may modify physiology with drugs or conditioning procedures, and psychobiologists often manipulate psychological or behavioral variables and measure physiological outcomes. Contemporary definitions are more likely to emphasize the mapping of the relationships between and mechanisms underlying psychological and physiological events (e.g., Hudgahl, 1995; Stern, Ray, & Quigley, 2001).

A major problem in reaching a consensus has been the need to give the field direction and identity by distinguishing it from other scientific disciplines while not limiting its potential for growth. Operational definitions are unsatisfactory for they do not provide long-term direction for the field. Definitions of psychophysiology as studies in which psychological factors serve as independent variables and physiological responses serve as dependent variables distinguish it from fields such as psychobiology but have been criticized for being too restrictive (Furedy, 1983). For instance, such definitions exclude studies in which physiological events serve as the independent/blocking variable and human experience or behavior serve as the dependent variable (e.g., the sensorimotor behavior associated with manipulations of the physiology via drugs or operant conditioning, or with endogenous changes in cardiovascular or electroencephalographic activity) as well as studies comparing changes in physiological responses across known groups (e.g., the cardiovascular reactivity of offspring of hypertensive vs. normotensive parents).

Moreover, psychophysiology and psychobiology share goals, assumptions, experimental paradigms, and, in some instances, databases, but differ primarily in terms of the analytic focus. In psychophysiology the emphasis is on integrating data from multiple levels of analysis to illuminate psychological functions and mechanisms rather than physiological structures per se. All of these substantive areas have a great deal to contribute to one another, and ideally this complementarity should not be masked in their definition by the need to distinguish these fields. Indeed, the formulation of structure-function relationships is advanced to the extent that "top down" and "bottom up" information can be integrated. The emergence of areas of research in cognitive neuroscience, psychoneuroendocrinology, and psychoneuroimmunology raise additional questions about the scope of psychophysiology.

Anatomy and physiology encompass the fields of neurology, endocrinology, and immunology due both to their common goals and assumptions, and to the embodiment, in a literal sense, of the nervous, endocrine, and immunologic systems within the organism. Relatedly, psychophysiology is based on the assumptions that human perception, thought, emotion, and action are embodied phenomena; and that measures of physical (e.g., neural, hormonal) processes can therefore shed light on the human mind. The level of analysis in psychophysiology is not on isolated components of the body, but rather on organismic-environmental transactions. That is, psychophysiology represents a top-down approach within the neurosciences that complements the bottom-up approach of psychobiology. Thus, psychophysiology can be defined as the scientific study of social, psychological, and behavioral phenomena as related to and revealed through physiological principles and events in functional organisms. Thus, psychophysiology is not categorically different from behavioral neuroscience, but rather there is currently a greater emphasis in psychophysiology on higher cognitive processes and on relating these higher cognitive processes to the integration of central and peripheral processes.

In the following section, we review some of the major historical developments that have influenced contemporary thinking and research in psychophysiology. As might be expected from the discussion thus far, many of these early developments have stemmed from studies of human anatomy and physiology.

HISTORICAL DEVELOPMENTS

Psychophysiology is still quite young as a scientific field. Studies dating back to the turn of the prior century can be found involving the manipulation of a psychological factor and the measurement of one or more physiological responses (e.g., Berger, 1929; Darrow, 1929; Eng, 1925; Jacobson, 1930; Mosso, 1896; Peterson & Jung, 1907; Sechenov, 1878; Tarchanoff, 1890; Wenger, 1941; Wilder, 1931; see also, Woodworth & Schlosberg, 1954), and such studies would now be considered as falling squarely under the rubric of psychophysiology. Chester Darrow (1964), in the inaugural Presidential Address of the Society for Psychophysiological Research, identified Darwin (1872/1873), Vigoroux (1879), James (1884), and Fere (1888) as among the field's earliest pioneers, yet the mixed responses of the scientific community to this pioneering work affected the field for decades (see Daston, 1978).

The first scientific periodical devoted exclusively to psychophysiological research, the Polygraph Newsletter, was not begun until 1955 and was published until 1963 (Ax, 1964a). There was an organizational meeting in 1959 in Cincinnati, a business meeting in 1960 in Chicago, and the first scientific meeting in 1961 in New York City. The first independent meeting of Society for Psychophysiological Research, however, occurred in Denver in 1962, and the Society was incorporated in 1963 at the Detroit meeting. Based on this history, one might surmise that the Society formed in 1959 and began functioning as a scientific society in 1961. The first edition of the journal, *Psychophysiology*, then subtitled "The Journal of Objective Research in the Physiology of Behavior," was published in July, 1964. When precisely psychophysiology emerged as a discipline, therefore, is difficult to specify, but it is usually identified with the first business meeting of the Society for Psychophysiological Research in 1960 or with the publication of the first issue of the journal, *Psychophysiology*, in 1964 (e.g., Fowles, 1975; Greenfield & Sternbach, 1972; Sternbach, 1966).

Although psychophysiology as a formal discipline has been around just over half a century, interest in interrelationships between psychological and physiological events can be traced as far back as the early Egyptians and Greek philosopher-scientists. The Greek philosopher Heraclitus (c. 600 B.C.) referred to the mind as an overwhelming space whose boundaries could never be fully comprehended (Bloom, Lazerson, & Hofstadter, 1985). Plato (c. 400 B.C.) suggested that rational faculties were located in the head; passions were located in the spinal marrow and, indirectly, the heart; and instincts were located below the diaphragm where they influenced the liver. Plato also believed the psyche and body to be fundamentally different; hence, observations of physiological responses provided no grounds for inference about the operation of psyche (Stern, Ray, & Quigley, 2001). Thus, despite the fact that the peripheral and central nervous system, brain, and viscera were known to exist as anatomical entities by the early Greek scientists-philosophers, human nature was dealt with as a incorporeal entity not amenable to empirical study.

In the second century A.D., Galen (c. 130–200) formulated a theory of psychophysiological function that would dominate thought well into the eighteenth century (Brazier, 1961; Wu, 1984). Hydraulics and mechanics were the technology of the times, and aqueducts and sewer systems were the most notable technological achievements during this period. Bloom et al. (1985, p. 13) suggest: "It is hardly by accident, then, that Galen believed the important parts of the brain to lie not in the brain's substance, but in its fluid-filled cavities" (p. 13). Based on his animal dissections and his observations of the variety of fluids that permeated the body, Galen postulated that humors (fluids) were responsible for all sensation, movement, thoughts, and emotion; and that pathologies – physiological or behavioral – were based on humoral disturbances. The role of bodily organs was to produce or process these humors, and the nerves, although recognized as instrumental in thought and action, were assumed to be part of a hydraulic system through which the humors traveled. Galen's views became so deeply entrenched in Western thought that they went practically unchallenged for almost 1500 years (cf. Kottek 1979).

In the sixteenth century, Jean Fernel (1497–1558) published the first textbook on physiology, *De Naturali Parte Medicinae* (1542). According to Brazier (1959), this book was well received, and Fernel revised and expanded the book across numerous editions. The ninth edition of the book was retitled *Medicina*, and the first section was entitled *Physiologia*. Although Fernel's categorization of empirical observations was strongly influenced by Galen's theory, the book "shows dawning recognition of some of the automatic movements which we now know to be reflexly initiated" (Brazier, 1959, p. 2). This represented a marked departure from traditional views that segregated the control of human action and the affairs of the corporeal world.

Studies of human anatomy during this period in history also began to uncover errors in Galen's descriptions (e.g., Vesalius, 1543/1947), opening the way for questions of his methods and of his theory of physiological functioning and symptomatology. Within a century, two additional events occurred that had a profound impact on the nature of inference in psychophysiology. In 1600, William Gilberd (1544–1603) recognized a difference between electricity and magnetism and, more importantly, argued in his book, *De Magnete, Magneticisque Corporibus, et de Magno magnete tellure*, that empirical observations and experiments should replace "the probable guesses and opinions of the ordinary professors of philosophy."

In addition, the reign of authority as the source of answers to questions about the basis of human experience and behavior was challenged by the work of scholars including Galileo, Bacon, and Newton. Galileo (1564–1642) challenged knowledge by authority in matters of science, by which Galileo meant physical sciences and mathematics. He argued that theologians and philosophers had no right to control scientific investigation or theories, and that observation, experiment, and reason along could establish physical truth (Drake, 1967). Galileo was also aware of limitations of sense data. Concerned with the possibility of illusion and misinterpretation, Galileo believed that mathematics alone offered the kind of certainty that could be completely trusted. Galileo did not extend this reasoning beyond the physical sciences, but scientific investigations of the basis of human experience and behavior benefited from his rejection of authority as a source of knowledge about physical reality, his emphasis on the value of skepticism, and his insistence that more could be learned from results that suggested ignorance (disconfirmation) than from results that fit preconceptions (confirmation).

Francis Bacon (1561–1626) took the scientific method a step further in *Novum Organum* (1620/1855), adding induction to observation and adding verification to inference. Bacon was not a scientist, yet he is regarded as a forerunner of the hypothetico-deductive method (Brazier, 1959; Caws, 1967). Subsequent work on the logic of scientific inference (Popper, 1959/1968) led to the now familiar sequence underlying scientific inference: (1) devise alternative hypotheses; (2) devise a crucial experiment, with alternative possible outcomes, each of which will disfavor if not exclude one or more of the hypotheses; (3) execute the experiment to obtain a clean result; and (4) recycle to refine the possibilities that remain. Such a scheme was accepted quickly in the physical sciences, but traditional philosophical and religious views segregating human existence from worldly events slowed its acceptance in the study of human physiology, experience, and behavior (Brazier, 1977; Harrington, 1987; Mecacci, 1979).

William Harvey's (1578–1657) doctoral dissertation, *De Motu Cordis* (1628/1941), represented not only the first major work to use these principles to guide inferences about physiological functioning, but it also disconfirmed Galen's principle that the motion of the blood in the arterial and venous systems ebbed and flowed independent of one another except for some leakage in the heart. Pumps were an important technological development during the seventeenth century, and Harvey perhaps drew on his observations of pumps in positing that blood circulated continuously through a circular system, pushed along by the pumping actions of the heart, and directed through and out of the heart by the one-way valves in each chamber of the heart. Galen, in contrast, had posited that blood could flow in either direction in the veins. To test these competing hypotheses, he tied a tourniquet above the elbow of his arm just tight enough to prevent blood from returning to the heart through the veins but not so tight as to prevent blood from entering the arm through the arteries. The veins swelled below, but not above the tourniquet, implying that the blood could be entering only through the arteries and exiting only through the veins (Miller, 1978). A variation on Harvey's procedure is used in contemporary psychophysiology to gauge blood flow to vascular beds (Williams, 1984).

During this period, which coincided with a burgeoning world of machines, the human eye was conceived as functioning like an optical instrument. Images were conceived as projected onto the sensory nerves of the retina. Movement was thought to reflect the mechanical actions of passive balloon-like structures (muscles) that were inflated or deflated by the nervous fluids or gaseous spirits that traveled through canals in the nerves. And higher mental functions were still considered by many to fall outside the rubric of the physical or biological sciences (Bloom et al., 1985; Brazier, 1959; Harrington, 1987). The writings of Rene Descartes (1596–1650) reflects the presumed division between the mind and body. The actions of animals were viewed as reflexive and mechanistic in

nature, as were most of the actions of humans. But humans alone, Descartes argued, also possess a consciousness of self and of events around them, a consciousness which, like the body, was a thing but, unlike the body, was not a thing governed by material principles or connections. This independent entity called mind, Descartes proposed, resides over volition from the soul's control tower in the pineal gland located at the center of the head:

The soul or mind squeezed the pineal gland this way and that, nudging the animal fluids in the human brain into the pores or valves, 'and according as they enter or even only as they tend to enter more or less into this or that nerve, they have the power of changing the form of the muscle into which the nerve is inserted, and by this means making the limbs move.' (Jaynes, 1973, p. 172, paraphrasing and quoting from Descartes, 1824, p. 347)

Shortly following Descartes' publication of *Traite de l'Homme* (c. 1633), Steno (1638–1686) noted several discrepancies between Descartes' dualistic and largely mechanistic characterization of human processes and the extant evidence about animal and human physiology. For instance, Steno noted that the pineal gland (the purported bridge between the worlds of the human mind and body) existed in animals as well as humans, that the pineal gland did not have the rich nerve supply implied by Descartes' theory, and that the brain was unnecessary to many animal movements (cf. Jaynes, 1973). Giovanni Borelli (1608–1679) disproved the notion that movement was motivated by the inflation of muscles by a gaseous substance in experiments in which he submerged a struggling animal in water, slit its muscles, and looked for the release of bubbles (Brazier, 1959). These observations were published posthumously in 1680, shortly after the suggestion by Francesco Redi that the shock of the electric ray fish was muscular in origin (Basmajian & De Luca, 1985, Ch. 1; Wu, 1984).

Despite the prevalent belief during this period that the scientific study of animal and human behavior could apply only to those structures they shared in common (Bloom et al., 1985; Harrington, 1987), the foundations laid by the great seventeenth-century scientist-philosophers encouraged students of anatomy and physiology in the subsequent century to discount explanatory appeals to the human soul or mind (Brazier, 1959). Consequently, experimental analyses of physiological events and psychological constructs (e.g., sensation, involuntary and voluntary action) expanded and inspired the application of technological advances to the study of psychophysiological questions. For instance, the microscope was employed (unsuccessfully) in the late seventeenth century to examine the prevalent belief that the nerves were small pipes through which nervous fluid flowed.

According to Brazier (1959, 1977), that electricity might be the transmitter of nervous action was initially seen as unlikely because, drawing upon the metaphor of electricity running down a wire, there was believed to be insufficient insulation around the nerves to prevent a dissipation of the electrical signal. Galvani and Volta's (c. 1800) experiments demonstrated that nerves and muscles were indeed electrically excitable, and research by Du Bois-Reymond (1849) established that nerves and muscles were electrically polarized as well as excitable. Based on reaction times, Helmholtz (c. 1850) correctly inferred that nerves and muscles were not like wires because they propagated electrical impulses too slowly. The work that followed ultimately verified that neural signals and muscular actions were electrical in nature, that these electrical signals were the result of biochemical reactions within specialized cells, and that there was indeed some dissipation of these electrical signals through the body fluids that could be detected noninvasively at the surface of the skin. Specific advances during the nineteenth and twentieth centuries in psychophysiological theory and research are discussed in the remainder of this book. However, the stage had been set by these early investigators for the scientific study of psychophysiological relationships.

PSYCHOPHYSIOLOGICAL RELATIONSHIPS AND PSYCHOPHYSIOLOGICAL INFERENCE

We praise the 'lifetime of study,' but in dozens of cases, in every field, what was needed was not a lifetime but rather a few short months or weeks of analytical inductive inference ... We speak piously of taking measurements and making small studies that will 'add another brick to the temple of science.' Most such bricks just lie around the brickyard. (Platt, 1964, p. 351)

The importance of the development of more advanced recording procedures to scientific progress in psychophysiology is clear, as previously unobservable phenomena are rendered observable. Less explicitly studied, but no less important, is the structure of scientific thought about psychophysiological phenomena. For instance, Galen's notions about psychophysiological processes persisted for 1500 years despite the availability for several centuries of procedures for disconfirming his theory in part because the structure of scientific inquiry had not been developed sufficiently.

An important form of psychophysiological inference to evolve from the work of Francis Bacon (1620/1855) and Galileo (Drake, 1967) is the hypothetico-deductive logic outlined above. If the data are consistent with only one of the theoretical hypotheses, then the alternative hypotheses with which the investigator began become less plausible. With conceptual replications to ensure the construct validity, replicability, and generalizability of such a result, a subset of the original hypotheses can be discarded, and the investigator recycles through this sequence. One weakness of this procedure is the myriad sources of variance in psychophysiological investigations and the stochastic nature of physiological events and, consequently, the sometimes poor replicability or generalizability of the results. A second is the intellectual invention and omniscience that is required to specify all relevant alternative hypotheses for the phenomenon of interest. Because neither of these can be overcome with certitude, progress in the short term can be slow and uncertain. Adherence to this sequence provides grounds for strong inference in the long term, however (Platt, 1964).

Physiological responses are often of interest, however, only to the extent that they allow one to index a psychological process, state, or stage. A general analytic framework that has aided the design and interpretation of studies in the area is the subtractive method that has been adapted from studies of mental chronometry. Donders (1868), a Dutch physiologist, proposed that the duration of different stages of mental processing could be determined by subtracting means of simpler tasks that were matched structurally to subsequences of more complex tasks. At the simplest level, experimental design begins with an experimental and a control condition. The experimental condition represents the presence of some factor, and the control condition represents the absence of this factor. The experimental factor might be selected because it is theoretically believed to depend on n information processing stages, and the construction of the control condition is guided to incorporate $n - 1$ information processing stages. This kind of analysis assumes, and depends mathematically on the assumption, that the information processing stages are arranged in strictly serial order with each stage running to completion prior to the initiation of the next.

Nevertheless, the principle underlying the extension of the subtractive design to include physiological (e.g., functional magnetic resonance imaging) measures is twofold: (a) physiological differences between experimental conditions thought to represent n and $n - 1$ processing stages supports the theoretical differentiation of these stages, and (b) the nature of the physiological differentiation of experimental conditions (e.g., the physiological signature of a processing stage) may further support a particular psychological characterization of that information processing stage. According to the subtractive method, the systematic application of the procedure of stage deletion (across conditions of an experimental design) makes it possible to deduce the physiological signature of each of the constituent stages underlying some psychological or behavioral response. For instance, if the experimental task ($n + 1$ stages) is characterized by greater activation of Broca's area than the control task, this is consistent with both the theoretical conception of the experimental and control tasks differing in one (or more) processing stage(s) and the differential processing stage(s) relating to language production.

If using conventional reaction time measures, the psychological significance of timing differences comes primarily from the putative differences between experimental conditions. With biological measures, however, the psychological significance of specific physiological differences (e.g., activation of Broca's area) comes both from the theoretical differences between experimental conditions *and* from the prior scientific literature on the psychological significance of the observed physiological difference. The convergence of these two sources of information makes social neuroscience methods potentially quite powerful even though they tend to be more complicated and nuanced.

It is important to note a critical difference in the properties of the kinds of measures used for response time experiments and for physiological measurements. If we assume that a process takes a certain period of time because it is composed of a series of steps that each takes a measurable time and wherein each must be completed before the next is begun, the decomposition of the total time into the time for each step seems relatively transparent. Note, however, that the conditions under which this kind of analysis fails are precisely those that hold in imaging experiments (Townsend & Ashby, 1983).

When a particular hypothesized stage of information processing is thought to be responsible for the differential impact of two different conditions on behavior, analyses of concomitant physiological activity can be informative, in one of two ways. If the patterns of physiological activity resulting from the isolation of presumably identical stages are dissimilar, the similarity of the stages is challenged even though there may be similarities between the subsequent behavioral outcomes (cf. Cacioppo & Tassinary, 1990). If, on the other hand, similar patterns of physiological activity result from the isolation of stages that are hypothesized to be identical, convergent evidence is obtained that the same fundamental stage is operative. Note that the greater the extant evidence linking the observed physiological event/profile to a specific psychological operation, the greater the value of the convergent evidence. These data do not provide evidence for a strong inference that the stages are the same (Platt, 1964), but instead such a result raises a hypothesis that can be tested empirically in a subsequent study (Cacioppo & Tassinary, 1990).

There are additional issues that should be considered when using a subtractive framework to investigate elementary stages of psychological processes whether using reaction time or physiological (brain) measures. The subtractive method contains the implicit assumption that a stage can be inserted or deleted without changing the nature of the other constituent stages. But this method has long been criticized for ignoring the possibility that manipulating a factor to insert or delete a processing stage might introduce a completely different processing structure (e.g., Townsend & Ashby, 1983). Using multiple operationalizations to insert or delete a stage may be helpful but this still does not insure strong inference. In addition, to construct the set of comparison tasks using the subtractive method one must already have a clearly articulated hypothesis about the sequence of events that transpires between stimulus and overt response. This assumption renders the subtractive method particularly useful in testing an existing theory about the stages constituting a psychological process and in determining whether a given

stage is among the set constituting two separate processes (Cacioppo, Berntson, Lorig, Norris, Rickett, & Nusbaum, 2003). Note, however, that confirmatory evidence can still be questioned by the assertion that the addition or deletion of a particular stage results in an essentially different set of stages or substages, just as is the case with self-report or reaction time measures. If a large corpus of animal and human research links a psychological event to a processing operation, however, the plausibility of the alternative interpretation is greatly diminished.

Whenever a physiological response (or profile) found previously to vary as a function of a psychological processing stage or state is observed, yet another hypothesis is raised – namely, that the same processing stage or state has been detected. A person might be thought to be anxious because they show physiological activation, inattentive because they show diminished activation, happy because they show an attenuated startle response, deceptive because they show activation of the anterior cingulate, and so on. However, one cannot logically conclude that a processing stage or state has definitely been detected simply because a physiological response found previously to vary as a function of a psychological processing stage or state has been observed. (The logical flaw in this form of inference is termed affirmation of the consequent.) We therefore next turn to a general framework for thinking about relationships between psychological concepts and physiological events, and we discuss the rules of evidence for and the limitations to inference in each (see also Cacioppo & Tassinary, 1990; Cacioppo, Tassinary, & Berntson, 2000).

THE PSYCHOLOGICAL AND PHYSIOLOGICAL DOMAINS

A useful way to construe the potential relationships between psychological events and physiological events is to consider these two groups of events as representing independent sets (domains), where a set is defined as a collection of elements who together are considered a whole (Cacioppo & Tassinary, 1990). Psychological events, by which we mean conceptual variables representing functional aspects of embodied processes, are conceived as constituting one set, which we shall call Set Ψ. Physiological (e.g., brain, autonomic, endocrinological) events, by which we mean empirical physical variables, are conceived as constituting another, which we shall call Set Φ. All elements in the set of psychological events are assumed to have some physiological referent – that is, the mind is viewed as having a physical substrate. This framework allows the specification of five general relations that might be said to relate the elements within the domain of psychological events, Ψ, and elements within the domain of physiological events, Φ. These are as follows:

- A one-to-one relation, such that an element in the psychological set is associated with one and only one element in the physiological set, and vice versa.

- A one-to-many relation, meaning that an element in the psychological domain is associated with a subset of elements in the physiological domain.
- A many-to-one relation, meaning that two or more psychological elements are associated with the same physiological element.
- A many-to-many relation, meaning two or more psychological elements are associated with the same (or an overlapping) subset of elements in the physiological domain.
- A null relation, meaning there is no association between an element in the psychological domain and that in the physiological domain.

Of these possible relations, only the first and third allow a formal specification of psychological elements as a function of physiological elements (Cacioppo & Tassinary, 1990). The grounds for theoretical interpretations, therefore, can be strengthened if either (1) a way can be found to specify the relationship between the elements within Ψ and Φ in terms of one-to-one, or at worst, in terms of many-to-one relationships, or (2) hypothetico-deductive logic is employed in the brain imaging studies (Cacioppo, Tassinary, & Berntson, 2000).

Consider that when differences in brain images or physiological events (Φ) are found in contrasts of tasks that are thought to differ only in one or more cognitive functions (Ψ), the data are often interpreted prematurely as showing that Brain Structure (or Event) Φ is associated with Cognitive Function (Ψ). These data are also treated as revealing much the same information that would have been obtained had Brain Structure (or Event) Φ been stimulated or ablated and a consequent change in Cognitive Function Ψ been observed. This form of interpretation reflects the explicit assumption that there is a fundamental localizability of specific cognitive operations, and the implicit assumption that there is an isomorphism between Φ and Ψ (Sarter, Berntson, & Cacioppo, 1996). Interpreting studies of the form $P(\Phi/\Psi)$ (i.e., fMRI studies) as equivalent to studies of the form $P(\Psi/\Phi)$ is misleading unless one is dealing with 1:1 relationships.[1] Fundamentally, this is a premise that needs to be tested rather than treated as an assumption.

It may be useful to illustrate some of these points using a simple physical metaphor in which the bases of a multiply

determined outcome are known. Briefly, let Φ represent the HVAC system, and Ψ the temperature in a house. In the context of psychophysiology, the HVAC system parallels a neural mechanism and the temperature represents the cognitive manifestation of the operation of this mechanism. Although the HVAC system and the temperature are conceptually distinct, the operation of the HVAC system represents both the manipulable cause (see Shadish, Cook, & Campbell, 2002) and a physical basis for the observed temperatures in the house. Thus, $\Psi = f(\Phi)$. A bottom-up approach (i.e., $P(\Psi/\Phi)$) makes clear certain details about the relationship between Ψ and Φ, whereas a top-down approach (i.e., $P(\Phi/\Psi)$) clarifies others. For instance, when the activity of the HVAC system is manipulated (i.e., Φ is stimulated or lesioned), a change in the temperature in the house (Ψ) results. This represents a bottom-up approach to investigating the physical substrates of cognitive phenomena. The fact that manipulating the activity of the HVAC system produces a change in the temperature in the house can be expressed as $P(\Psi/\Phi) > 0$. Note that the $P(\Psi/\Phi)$ need not equal 1 for Φ be a physical substrate of Ψ. This is because, in our illustration, there are other physical mechanisms that can affect the temperature in the house (Ψ), such as the outside temperature (Φ') and the amount of direct sunlight in the house (Φ). That is, there is a lack of complete isomorphism specifiable, at least initially, between the regulated variable (Ψ) and a physical basis (Φ).

In any given context, the temperature in the house may be influenced by any or all of these physical mechanisms. If the outside temperature or the amount of direct sunlight happens to vary when the HVAC system is activated, then the temperature may not covary perfectly with the activation of the HVAC system (i.e., $P(\Psi/\Phi) < 1$) even though the temperature is, at least in part, a function of the operation of the HVAC system (i.e., $P(\Psi/\Phi) > 0$). If the outside temperature and amount of direct sunlight are constant or are perfectly correlated with the activation of the HVAC system, then the temperature in the house and the activity of the HVAC system may covary perfectly (i.e., $P(\Psi/\Phi) = 1$). In the context of psychophysiology, this is analogous to a brain lesion study accounting for some of the variance ($P(\Psi/\Phi) > 0$) or all of the variance ($P(\Psi/\Phi) = 1$) in the cognitive measure in the study. The latter result does not imply the lesioned brain region is a necessary component just as the fact that the temperature in the house covaries perfectly with the activity of the HVAC system does not mean necessarily that there are not other physical mechanisms that may also influence the temperature. Thus, as long as $P(\Psi/\Phi) > 0$, Φ could be considered a predictor (or component) of Ψ; the fact that $P(\Psi/\Phi) = 1$ does not imply that Φ is the only or a necessary cause of Ψ.

The asymmetry between $P(\Psi/\Phi)$ and $P(\Phi/\Psi)$ and the interpretive problems that may result when simply assuming $P(\Psi/\Phi) = P(\Phi/\Psi)$ are also evident in this metaphor. As outlined above, the former term represents variations in temperature in the house given variations in the activity of the HVAC system, whereas $P(\Phi/\Psi)$ represents the activity

---

[1] Research in which psychological or behavioral factors serve as the independent (or blocking) variables and physiological structures or events serve as the dependent variable can be conceptualized as investigating the $P(\Phi/\Psi)$. Research in which physiological structures or events serve as the independent (or blocking) variables and psychological or behavioral factors serve as the dependent variable, in contrast, can be conceptualized as investigating the $P(\Psi/\Phi)$. These conditional probabilities are equal only when the relationship between is Ψ and Φ is 1:1 (Cacioppo & Tassinary, 1990). Accordingly, approaches such as stimulation and ablation studies provide complementary rather than redundant information to studies in which physiological (e.g., fMRI) measures serve as dependent measures. This is because stimulation and ablation studies bear on the relationship $P(\Psi/\Phi)$, whereas studies in which physiological variables serve as dependent measures provide information about $P(\Phi/\Psi)$.

of the heater given variations in the temperature in the house. Although one would expect to find $P(\Phi/\Psi) > 0$ in some contexts, the fact that the temperature in the house is regulated when the HVAC system is activated does not necessarily imply that changes in the temperature in the house will be associated with variations in the activity of the HVAC system. In the context of local changes in temperature distant from the thermostat of the HVAC system, for example, the observed temperature will fluctuate whereas the HVAC system remains inactive (e.g., outside temperature, Φ'; exposure to direct sunlight, Φ). Thus, the finding that $P(\Phi/\Psi) = 0$ does not mean Φ has no role in Ψ, only that Φ has no role in Ψ in that context. In the context of brain imaging studies, areas that are not found to become active as a function of a cognitive operation may nevertheless be part of a physical substrate for that cognitive operation (just as a HVAC system may remain a part of the physical mechanism responsible for the temperature in a house).

The preceding example illustrates why one would not want to exclude a brain area as potentially relevant to a cognitive operation based on the area not being illuminated in a brain image as a function of the cognitive operation. The converse also holds – that is, a brain area that is illuminated as a function of a cognitive operation may or may not contribute meaningfully to the production of the cognitive operation. Consider an LED on a thermostat (which we will call Φ') that illuminates when the HVAC system (Φ) is operating. In this case, the $P(\Phi/\Psi) = P(\Phi'/\Psi) > 0$. That is, the LED represents a physical element that would show the same covariation with the temperature in the house as would the operation of the HVAC system as long as a top-down approach was used. When the complementary bottom-up approach were used, it would become obvious that disconnecting (lesioning) the HVAC system has effects on the temperature in the house whereas disconnecting (or directly activating) the LED has none.

FOUR CATEGORIES OF PSYCHOPHYSIOLOGICAL RELATIONSHIPS

Relations between elements in the psychological and physiological domains should not be *assumed* to hold across situations or individuals. Indeed, elements in the psychological domain are delimited in the subtractive method in part by holding constant other processes that might differentiate the comparison tasks. Such a procedure is no unique to psychophysiology or to the subtractive method, as most psychological and medical tests can involve constructing specific assessment contexts in order to achieve interpretable results. The interpretation of a blood glucose test, for instance, can rest on the assumption that the individual fasted prior to the onset of the test. Only under this circumstance can the amount of glucose measured in the blood across time be used to index the body's ability to regulate the level of blood sugar. The relationship between the physiological data and theoretical construct is said to have a limited range of validity, because the relationship

is clear only in certain well-prescribed assessment contexts. The notion of limited ranges of validity, therefore, raises the possibility that a wide range of complex relationships between psychological and physiological phenomena might be specifiable in simpler, more interpretable forms within specific assessment contexts.

To clarify these issues, it is useful to conceptualize psychophysiological relationships generally in terms of a 2 (One-to-one vs. Many-to-one) × 2 (Situation Specific vs. Cross Situational) taxonomy. The specific families (i.e., categories) of psychophysiological relationships that can be derived from this taxonomy are depicted in Figure 1.1. The criterial attributes for, and theoretical utility in, establishing each of these categories are specified in the three dimensions illustrated in Figure 1.1; causal attributes of the relationships, and whether the relationships are naturally occurring or artificially induced constitute yet other, orthogonal dimensions and are explicitly excluded here for didactic purposes. For instance, the category in Figure 1.1 labeled "concomitant" refers only to the conditions and implications of covariation and is not intended to discriminate between instances in which the psychological factor is causal in the physiological response, vice versa, or a third variable causes both. In the sections that follow, each type of psychophysiological relationship and the nature of the inferences that each suggests are outlined.

Psychophysiological outcomes. In the idealized case, an *outcome* is defined as a many-to-one, situation-specific (context-dependent) relationship between Ψ and Φ. Establishing that a physiological response (i.e., an element in Φ) varies as a function of a psychological change (i.e., an element in Ψ) means one is dealing at the very least with an outcome relationship between these elements. Note that this if often the first attribute of a psychophysiological relationship that is established in laboratory practice. Whether the physiological response follows changes in the psychological event across situations (i.e., has the property of context independence), or whether the response profile follows only changes in the event (i.e., has the property of isomorphism) is not typically addressed initially. Hence, a given psychophysiological relationship may appear to be an outcome but subsequently be identified as being a marker as the question of isomorphism is examined; a relationship that appears to be an outcome may subsequently be reclassified as being a concomitant once the range of validity is examined; and a relationship that appears to be a marker (or concomitant) may emerge as an invariant upon studying the generalizability (or isomorphism) of the relationship. This progression is not problematic in terms of causing erroneous inferences, however, because, as we shall see, any logical inference based on the assumption one is dealing with an outcome relationship holds for marker, concomitant, or invariant psychophysiological relationships, as well.

Despite the outcome serving as the most elemental psychophysiological relationship, it can nevertheless provide

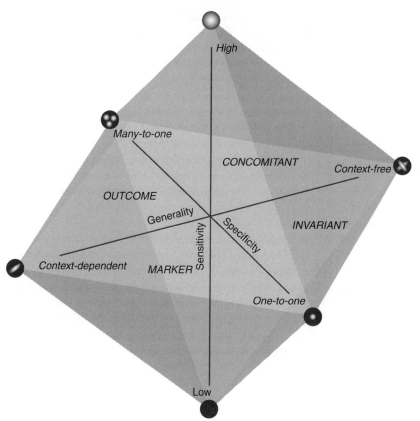

Figure 1.1. Taxonomy of psychophysiological relationships. The dimensions of sensitivity and specificity are related but not synonymous with those used in either signal detection theory or clinical decision analysis. Sensitivity, in this context, refers to likelihood that a physiological response will covary with any psychological element. Specificity, in contrast, refers to the likelihood that that a physiological response will be linked to a particular psychological element or set of elements and simultaneously not linked to another psychological element or set of elements. The horizontal plane bisecting the square bipyramid represents the level of sensitivity necessary to afford maximal differentiation among the psychophysiological relationships.

the basis for strong inferences. Specifically, when two psychological models differ in predictions regarding one or more physiological outcomes, then the logic of the experimental design allows theoretical inferences to be drawn based on psychophysiological outcomes alone. That is, a psychophysiological outcome enables systematic inferences to be drawn about psychological constructs and relationships based on hypothetico-deductive logic. Of course, no single operationalization of the constructs in a crucial experiment is likely to convince the adherents of both theories. If multiple operationalizations of the theoretical constructs result in the same physiological outcome, however, then strong theoretical inferences can be justified.

Importantly, the identification of a physiological response profile that differentiates the psychological element of interest is sufficient to infer the absence of one or more psychological elements, but it does not provide logical grounds to infer anything about the presence of a psychological element. Hence, the identification of psychophysiological outcomes can be valuable in disproving theoretical predictions, but they are problematic as indices of elements in the psychological domain. This caveat is often

noted in discussions of the scientific method and is perhaps equally often violated in scientific practice (Platt, 1964). Skin conductance, for instance, has been a major dependent measure in psychological research because emotional arousal is thought to lead to increased skin conductance. Similarly, EMG activity over the forehead region has been a frequent target measure in relaxation biofeedback because tension has been found to increase EMG activity over this region. As noted in the previous section, however, simply knowing that that manipulating a particular element in the psychological domain leads to a particular response in the physiological domain does not logically enable one to infer anything about the former based on observations of the latter, because one does not know what other antecedents might have led to the observed physiological response. Procedures such as holding constant any variations in the elements in the psychological domain that are not of interest, measuring these elements in addition to those of immediate theoretical interest to determine to which of the observed changes in physiological response are likely to be attributable, and excluding those physiological responses believed to covary with these irrelevant elements all represent attempts to reduce many-to-one relationships to one-to-one relationships (i.e., going from psychophysiological outcomes to psychophysiological markers; see Figure 1.1). Such procedures clearly strengthen the grounds for psychophysiological inference, but they do not assure that all relevant factors have been identified or controlled, nor do they provide a means of quantifying the extent of other influences on psychophysiological responding.

Consider, for example, what can be expected if the probability of a physiological element $\{P(\Phi)\}$ is greater than the probability of the psychological element of interest $\{P(\Psi)\}$. Because this implies that $P(\Psi,\Phi)/P(\Psi) > P(\Psi,\Phi)/P(\Phi)$, it can be seen that the $P(\Phi/\Psi) > P(\Psi/\Phi)$, and, consequently, that research based only on outcome relationships would result in an overestimation of the presence of the psychological element.

We should emphasize that these probabilities are simply a way of thinking more rigorously about psychophysiological relations; one still needs to be cognizant that these relationships (e.g., probabilities) may vary across situations (e.g., assessment contexts). Indeed, comparisons of these probabilities across assessment contexts can provide a means of determining the individual or situational specificity of a psychophysiological relation. Before proceeding to this dimension of the taxonomy outlined in Figure 1.1, however, we elaborate further on psychophysiological relations within a specific assessment context when viewed within the framework of conditional probabilities. In particular, as the $P(\Psi, \Phi)$ approaches 1.0 and the $P(\text{Not-}\Psi, \Phi)$ approaches 0.0 within a specific assessment context, the element in the physiological domain can be described as being an ideal marker of the element in the psychological domain.

Psychophysiological markers. In its idealized form, a psychophysiological *marker* is defined as a one-to-one, situation-specific (i.e., context-dependent) relationship between abstract events Ψ and Φ (see Figure 1.1). The psychophysiological marker relation assumes only that the occurrence of one (usually a physiological response, parameter of a response, or profile of responses) predicts the occurrence of the other (usually a psychological event) within a given context. Thus, markers are characterized by limited ranges of validity. Such a relationship may reflect a natural connection between psychological and physiological elements in a particular measurement situation or it may reflect an artificially induced (e.g., classically conditioned) association between these elements. Importantly, minimal violations of isomorphism between Ψ and Φ within a given assessment context can nevertheless yield a useful (although imperfect) marker when viewed in terms of conditional probabilities.

Markers can vary in their specificity and sensitivity. The more distinctive the form of the physiological response and/or the pattern of associated physiological responses, the greater the likelihood of achieving a one-to-one relationship between the physiological events and psychological construct, and the wider may be the range of validity of the relationship thereby achieved. This is because the utility of an element in Φ to index an element in Ψ is generally strenghthened by the defining the physiological element so as to minimize its occurrence in the absence of the element in the psychological domain.

In terms of sensitivity, a psychophysiological marker may simply signal the occurrence or nonoccurrence of a psychological process or event, possessing no information about the temporal or amplitude properties of the event in a specific assessment context. At the other extreme, a psychophysiological marker may be related in a prescribed assessment context to the psychological event by some well-defined temporal function, such that the measure can be used to delineate the onset and offset of the episode of interest, and/or it may vary in amplitude such that it reflects the intensity of the psychological event.

In sum, markers represent a fundamental relationship between elements in the psychological and physiological domains which enables an inference to be drawn about the nature of the former given measurement of the latter. The major requirements in establishing a response as a marker are to: (1) demonstrate that the presence of the target response reliably predicts the specific construct of interest, (2) demonstrate that the presence of the target response is insensitive to (e.g., uncorrelated with) the presence or absence of other constructs, and (3) specify the boundary conditions for the validity for the relationship. The term "tracer" can be viewed as synonymous with marker, for each refers to a measure so strictly associated with a particular organismic-environmental condition that its presence is indicative of the presence of this condition. The term "indicant," on the other hand, is more generic, including invariants, markers, and concomitants because each allows the prediction of Ψ given Φ. We turn next to a description of concomitants.

Psychophysiological concomitants. A psychophysiological *concomitant* (or correlate), in its idealized form, is defined as a many-to-one, cross-situational (context-independent) association between abstract events Ψ and Φ (see Figure 1.1). That is, the search for psychophysiological concomitants assumes there is a cross-situational covariation between specific elements in the psychological and physiological domains. The assumption of a psychophysiological concomitant is less restrictive than the assumption of invariance in that one-to-one correspondence is not required, although the stronger the association between the elements in the psychological and physiological domains, the more informative tends to be the relationship.

Consider, for instance, the observation that pupillary responses varied as a function of individuals' attitudes toward visually presented stimuli – an observation which was followed by the conclusion that pupillary response was a "correlate" of people's attitudes (Metalis & Hess, 1982). However, evidence of variation in a target physiological response as a function of a manipulated (or naturally varying) psychological event establishes an outcome relation, which is necessary but insufficient for the establishment of a psychophysiological concomitant or correlate.

First, the manipulation of the same psychological element (e.g., attitudes) in another context (e.g., using auditory rather than visual stimuli) may alter or eliminate the covariation between the psychological and physiological elements because the latter is evoked either by a stimulus that had been fortuitously or intentionally correlated with the psychological element in the initial measurement context, or by a noncriterial attribute of the psychological element that does not generalize across situations. For instance, the attitude-pupil size hypothesis has not been supported using nonpictorial (e.g., auditory, tactile) stimuli, where it is possible to control the numerous light-reflex-related variables that can confound studies using pictorial stimuli. It is possible, in several of the studies showing a statistical covariation between attitudes and pupillary response, that the mean luminance of individuals' selected fixations varied inversely with their attitudes toward the visual stimulus.

Second, the manipulation of the same psychological element in another situation may alter or eliminate the covariation between the psychological and physiological elements because the latter is evoked not only by variations in the psychological element but also by variations in one or more additional factors that are introduced in (or are a fundamental constituent of) the new measurement context. Tranel et al. (1985), for instance, demonstrated that the presentation of familiar faces (e.g., famous politicians, actors) evoked larger skin conductance responses (SCRs) than did the presentation of unfamiliar faces. This finding, and the procedure and set of stimuli employed, were subsequently used in a study of patients with prosopagnosia (an inability to recognize visually the faces of persons previously known) to demonstrate that the patients can discriminate autonomically between the familiar and unfamiliar faces despite the absence of any awareness of this knowledge. Thus, the first study established a psychophysiological relationship in a specific measurement context, and the second study capitalized on this relationship. To conclude that a psychophysiological concomitant had been established between familiarity and SCRs, however, would mean that the same relationship would hold across situations and stimuli (i.e., the relationship would be context-independent). Yet ample psychophysiological research has demonstrated the opposite psychophysiological outcome as specified by Tranel et al. (1985) – that is, that novel or unusual (i.e., unfamiliar) stimuli can also evoke larger SCRs than familiar stimuli. Hence, it is safe to conclude that the relation between stimulus familiarity and skin conductance should not be thought of as a psychophysiological concomitant.

Unfortunately, evidence of faulty reasoning based on the premature assumption that one is dealing with a true psychophysiological correlate (or invariant) is all too easy to find:

I find in going through the literature that the psychogalvanic reflex has been elicited by the following varieties of stimuli . . . sensations and perceptions of any sense modality (sight, sounds, taste, etc.), associations (words, thoughts, etc.), mental work or effort, attentive movements or attitudes, imagination and ideas, tickling, painful or nocive stimuli, variations in respiratory movements or rate, suggestion and hypnosis, emotional behavior (fighting, crying, etc.), relating dreams, college examinations, and so forth. . . . Forty investigators hold that it is specific to, or a measure of, emotion of the affective qualities; ten others state that it is not necessarily of an emotional or affective nature; twelve men hold that it is somehow to be identified with conation, volition, or attention, while five hold very definitely that it is nonvoluntary; twenty-one authorities state that it goes with one or another of the mental processes; eight state that it is the concomitant of all sensation and perception; five have called it an indicator of conflict and suppression; while four others have used it as an index of character, personality, or temperament. (Landis, 1930, p. 391)

The hindrances to scientific advances, it would seem, stem not so much from impenetrable psychophysiological relationships as from a failure to recognize the nature of these relationships and their limitations to induction.

As in the case of psychophysiological marker, the empirical establishment of a psychophysiological concomitant logically allows an investigator to make a probability statement about the absence or presence (if not the timing and magnitude) of a particular element in the psychological domain when the target physiological element is observed. It is important to emphasize, however, that the estimate of the strength of the covariation used in such inferences should not come solely from evidence that manipulated or planned variations of an element in Ψ are associated with corresponding changes in an element in Ψ. Measurements of the physiological response each time the psychological element is manipulated or changes can lead to an overestimate of the strength of this relationship and, hence, to erroneous inferences about the psychologic element based on the physiological response. As can be seen in Equations (1) and (2), this overestimation occurs to the extent that there are changes in the physiological response not attributable to variations in the psychological element of interest. Hence, except when one is dealing with an invariant relationship, establishing that the manipulation of a psychological element leads cross-situationally to a particular physiological response or profile of responses is not logically sufficient to infer that the physiological event will be a strong predictor of the psychological element of interest; baserate information about the occurrence of the physiological event across situations must also be considered. This is sometimes done in practice by quantifying the natural covariation between elements in the psychological and physiological domains, and by examining the replicability of the observed covariation across situations.

Psychophysiological invariants. The idealized *invariant* relationship refers to an isomorphic (one-to-one), context-independent (cross-situational) association (see Figure 1.1). To say that there is an invariant relationship, therefore, implies that: (1) a particular element in Φ is present if and only if a specific element in Ψ is present, (2) the specific element in Ψ is present if and only if the corresponding element in Φ is present, and (3) the relation between Ψ and Φ preserves all relevant arithmetical (algebraic) operations. Moreover, only in the case of invariants does $P(\Psi/\Phi) = P(\Phi/\Psi)$, and $P(\text{Not-}\Psi, \Phi) = P(\text{Not-}\Phi, \Psi) = 0$. This means that the logical error of affirmation of the consequent is not a problem in psychophysiological inferences based on an invariant relation. Hence, the establishment of an invariant relationship between a pair of elements from the psychological and the physiological domains provides a strong basis for psychophysiological inference. Unfortunately, invariant relationships are often assumed rather than formally established, and, as we have argued, such an approach leads to erroneous psychophysiological inferences and vacuous theoretical advances.

It has been suggested occasionally that the psychophysiological enterprise is concerned with invariant relationships. As we have seen, the search to establish one-to-one psychophysiological relationships is important. Moreover, as S. S. Stevens (1951) noted:

The scientist is usually looking for invariance whether he knows it or not. Whenever he discovers a functional relation between two variables his next question follows naturally: under what conditions does it hold? In other words, under what transformation is the relation invariant? The quest for invariant relations is essentially the aspiration toward generality, and in psychology, as in physics, the principles that have wide application are those we prize. (p. 20)

It cannot be overemphasized, however, that evidence for invariance should be gathered rather than assumed, and that the utility of psychophysiological analyses does not rest entirely with invariant relationships (Donchin, 1982). Without this recognition, the establishment of any dissociation between the physiological measure and psychological element of interest invalidates not only the purported psychophysiological relationship, but also the utility of a psychophysiological analysis. However, as outlined in the preceding sections of this chapter, and in the chapters that follow, psychophysiology need not be conceptualized as offering only mappings of context-independent, one-to-one relationships to advance our understanding of human processes and behavior.

To summarize, the minimum assumption underlying the psychophysiological enterprise is that psychological and behavioral processes unfold as organismic-environmental transactions and, hence, have physiological manifestations, ramifications, or reflections. Although invariant psychophysiological relationships offer the greatest generality, physiological concomitants, markers, and outcomes also can provide important and sometimes otherwise unattainable information about elements in the psychological domain. These points hold for the neurosciences, as well. In laboratory practice, the initial step is often to establish that variations in a psychological element are associated with a physiological change, thereby establishing that the psychophysiological relationship is, at least, an outcome. Knowledge that changes in an element in the psychological domain is associated with changes in a physiological response/profile neither assures that the response will serve as a marker for the psychological state (because the converse of a statement does not follow logically from the statement), nor that the response is a concomitant or invariant of the psychological state (because the response may occur in only certain situations or individuals, or may occur for a large number of reasons besides changes in the particular psychological state). Nevertheless, both forms of reasoning outlined in this chapter can provide a strong foundation for psychophysiological inferences about behavioral processes.

CONCLUSION

Psychophysiology is based on the dual assumptions that human perception, thought, emotion, and action are embodied and embedded phenomena; and that the measures of the processes of the corporeal brain and body contain information can shed light on the human mind. The level of analysis in psychophysiology is not on isolated components of the body, but rather on organismic-environmental transactions, with reference to both physical and sociocultural environments. Psychophysiology, therefore, like anatomy and physiology, is a branch of science organized around bodily systems whose collective aim is to elucidate the structure and function of the parts of and interrelated systems in the human body in transactions with the environment. Like psychology, however, psychophysiology is concerned with a broader level of inquiry than anatomy and physiology and can be organized in terms of both a thematic as well as a systemic focus. For instance, the social and inferential elements as well as the physical elements of psychophysiology are discussed in the chapters that follow.

The metaphor of the human mind as computer software on a discrete personal computer and the brain the hardware on which this software runs dominated psychology and the cognitive sciences in the latter half of the twentieth century. Interestingly, the notion of a computer disconnected from others is already passé, as mobile computers that are linked through ubiquitous broadband wireless connections have produced remarkable capacities in the form of the Internet. Although access and deposits to the Internet are achieved through the operation of a discrete computer, the study of the software alone of that computer would not reveal its functional capacities given its connectivity and the presence of the Internet. The human brain, of course, has long been mobile and connected to others through broadband telereceptors. A hallmark feature of psychophysiology is the longstanding attention not only to physiological correlates of cognitive or behavioral states but to the elucidation of the structure and function of the parts of and interrelated systems in the human body in transactions with the environment.

The importance of the development of more advanced recording procedures to scientific progress in psychophysiology is clear, as previously unobservable phenomena are rendered tangible. However, advanced recording procedures are not sufficient for progress in the field. The theoretical specification of a psychophysiological relationship necessarily involves reaching into the unknown and, hence, requires intellectual invention and systematic efforts to minimize bias and error. Psychological theorizing based on known physiological and anatomical facts, exploratory research and pilot testing, and classic psychometric approaches can each contribute in important ways here by their generation of testable hypotheses about a psychophysiological relationship. It should be equally clear, however, that the scientific effectiveness of psychophysiological analyses does not derive logically from physiologizing or from the measurement of organismic rather (or in addition to) verbal or chronometric responses. Its great value stems from the stimulation of interesting hypotheses and from the fact that when an experiment agrees with a prediction about orchestrated actions of the organism, a great many alternative hypotheses may be excluded. The study of physiological mechanisms and techniques can sharpen our thinking and reduce the error of our conceptualizations and measurements. Although necessary and important, one should not lose sight of the fact that they are means rather than ends in psychophysiology. Little is gained, for instance, by simply generating an increasingly lengthy list of "correlates" between specific psychological variables and additional psychophysiological measures.

A scientific theory is a description of causal interrelations. Psychophysiological correlations are not causal. Thus in scientific theories, psychophysiological correlations are monstrosities. This does not mean that such correlations have no part in science. They are the instruments by which the psychologist may test his theories. (Gardiner, Metcalf, & Beebe-Center, 1937, p. 385)

To further theoretical thinking, therefore, a taxonomy of psychophysiological relations was outlined, and a scheme for strong inference based on these relationships was suggested. Among the questions the formulation outlined here can help to address are: (1) how does one select the appropriate variable(s) for study, (2) how detailed or refined should be the measurement of the selected variables, (3) how can situational and individual variability in psychophysiological relationships be integrated into theoretical thinking about psychophysiological relationships, and (4) how can physiological measures be used in a rigorous fashion to index psychological factors. The ultimate value of the proposed way of thinking about psychophysiological relationships rests, however, on its effectiveness in guiding psychophysiological inference through the channels of judgmental fallacies, for as Leonardo Da Vinci (c. 1510) noted:

Experience does not ever err, it is only your judgment that errs in promising itself results which are not caused by your experiments.

REFERENCES

Ax, A. F. (1964a). Editorial. *Psychophysiology, 1,* 1–3.

Ax, A. F. (1964b). Goals and methods of psychophysiology. *Psychophysiology, 1,* 8–25.

Barinaga, M. (1997). What makes brain neurons run? *Science, 276,* 196–198.

Basmajian, J. V., & De Luca, C. J. (1985). *Muscles alive: Their functions revealed by electromyography* (5th Edition). Baltimore: Williams & Wilkins.

Berger, H. (1929). Uber das elektrenkephalogramm des menschen (On the electroencephalogram of man). *Archiv fur Psychiatrie und Nervenkrankheiten, 87,* 551–553. Reprinted in English in S. W. Porges & M. G. H. Coles (Eds.), *Psychophysiology.* Stroudsburg, PA: Dowden, Hutchinson, & Ross, Inc.

Bloom, F. E., Lazerson, A., & Hofstadter, L. (1985). *Brain, mind, and behavior.* New York: W. H. Freeman and Company.

Brazier, M. A. (1959). The historical development of neurophysiology. In J. Field (Ed.), *Handbook of physiology. Section I: Neurophysiology. Vol. I* (pp. 1–58). Washington, DC: American Physiological Society.

Brazier, M. A. (1961). *A history of the electrical activity of the brain.* London: Pitman Medical Publishing Co., Ltd.

Brazier, M. A. (1977). *Electrical activity of the nervous system* (4th edition). Baltimore: The Williams & Wilkins Co.

Cacioppo, J. T., Berntson, G. G., Lorig, T. S., Norris, C. J., Rickett, E., & Nusbaum, H. (2003). Just because you're imaging the brain doesn't mean you can stop using your head: A primer and set of first principles. *Journal of Personality and Social Psychology, 85,* 650–661.

Cacioppo, J. T., & Petty, R. E. (1981). Electromyograms as measures of extent and affectivity of information processing. *American Psychologist, 36,* 441–456.

Cacioppo, J. T., & Tassinary, L. G. (1990). Inferring psychological significance from physiological signals. *American Psychologist, 45,* 16–28.

Cacioppo, J. T., Tassinary, L. G., & Berntson, G. G. (2000). *Handbook of psychophysiology, 2nd edition.* New York: Cambridge University Press.

Caws, P. (1967). Scientific method. In P. Edwards (Ed.), *The encyclopedia of philosophy* (pp. 339–343). New York: Macmillan.

Coles, M. G. H., Donchin, E., & Porges, S. W. (1986). *Psychophysiology: Systems, processes, and applications.* New York: Guilford Press.

Darrow, C. W. (1929). Differences in the physiological reactions to sensory and ideational stimuli. *Psychological Bulletin, 26,* 185–201.

Darrow, C. W. (1964). Psychophysiology, yesterday, today and tomorrow. *Psychophysiology, 1,* 4–7.

Darwin, C. (1873). *The expression of the emotions in man and animals.* New York: D. Appleton and Co. (Originally published in 1872.)

Daston, L. J. (1978). British responses to psycho-physiology, 1860–1900. *Isis, 69*(2), 192–208.

Donchin, E. (1982). The relevance of dissociations and the irrelevance of dissociationism: A reply to Schwartz and Pritchard. *Psychophysiology, 19,* 457–463.

Drake, S. (1967). Galileo Galilei. In P. Edwards (Ed.), *The encyclopedia of philosophy* (pp. 262). New York: Macmillan.

Eng, H. (1925). *Experimental investigation into the emotional life of the child compared with that of the adult.* London: Oxford University Press.

Fere, C. (1888/1976). Notes on changes in electrical resistance under the effect of sensory stimulation and emotion. *Comptes Rendus des Seances de la Societe de Biologie, 5,* 217–219. Reprinted in English in S. W. Porges & M. G. H. Coles (Eds.), *Psychophysiology.* Stroudsburg, PA: Dowden, Hutchinson, & Ross, Inc.

Fernel, J. (1542). *De naturali parte medinae.* Paris: Simon de Colies. Cited in Brazier (1959).

Fowles, D. C. (1975). *Clinical applications of psychophysiology.* New York: Columbia University Press.

Garbarini, F., & Adenzato, M. (2004). At the root of embodied cognition: Cognitive science meets neurophysiology. *Brain and Cognition, 56,* 100–106.

Gardiner, H. M., Metcalf, R. C., & Beebe-Center, J. G. (1937). *Feeling and emotion: A history of theories.* New York: American Book Company.

Greenfield, N. S., & Sternbach, R. A. (1972). *Handbook of psychophysiology.* New York: Holt, Rinehart, & Winston, Inc.

Harrington, A. (1987). *Medicine, mind, and the double brain: Study in nineteenth-century thought*. Princeton, NJ: Princeton University Press.

Harvey, W. (1628/1941). *Exercitatio anatomica de motu cordis et sanguinis in animalibus*. Frankfurt: Fitzeri (1628); translated into English by Willius & Keys, Cardiac Classics (1941).

Henle, M., Jaynes, J., & Sullivan, J. J. (1973). *Historical conceptions of psychology*. New York: Springer.

Jacobson, E. (1930). Electrical measurements of neuromuscular states during mental activities: III. Visual imagination and recollection. *American Journal of Physiology, 95*, 694–702.

James, W. (1884). What is an emotion? *Mind, 9*, 188–205.

Jaynes, J. (1973). The problem of animate motion in the seventeenth century. In M. Henle, J. Jaynes, & J. J. Sullivan (Eds.), *Historical conceptions of psychology* (pp. 166–179). New York: Springer.

Kottek, S. S. (1979). The seat of the soul: Contribution to the history of Jewish medieval psycho-physiology (6th to 12th century). *Clio Medica, 13, 3–4*, 219–246.

Landis, C. (1930). Psychology and the psychogalvanic reflex. *Psychological Review, 37*, 381–398.

Littlejohn, J. M. (1899). Lectures on psycho-physiology. Kirksville, MO: E.G. Kinney.

Meaney, M. J., Bhatnagar, S., Larocque, S., McCormick, C. M., Shanks, N., Sharma, S., Smythe, J., Viau, V., & Plotsky, P. M. (1996). Early environment and the development of individual differences in the hypothalamic-pituitary-adrenal stress response. In C. R. Pfeffer (Ed.), *Severe stress and mental disturbance in children* (pp. 85–127). Washington, DC: American Psychiatric Press, Inc.

Mecacci, L. (1979). *Brain and history: The relationship between neurophysiology and psychology in Soviet research*. New York: Brunner/Mazel Publishers.

Metalis, S. A., & Hess, E. H. (1982). Pupillary response/semantic differential scale relationships. *Journal of Research in Personality, 16*, 201–216.

Miller, J. (1978). *The body in question*. New York: Random House.

Mosso, A. (1896). *Fear* (E. Lough & F. Riesow, Translators). New York: Longrans, Green, & Co.

Peterson, F., & Jung, C. G. (1907). Psychophysical investigations with the galvanometer and pneumograph in normal and insane individuals. *Brain, 30*, 153–218.

Platt, J. R. (1964). Strong inference. *Science, 146*, 347–353.

Popper, K. R. (1968). *The logic of scientific discovery*. New York: Harper & Row. (Original work published in 1959.)

Rose, R. M. (2005). Introduction and overview of our model. Paper presented at the National Center for Complementary and Alternative Medicine meeting on Integrating Mechanisms Linking Mind, Brain, and Periphery: Applications in Asthma and Atherosclerosis. Warrenton, VA: 6 July 2005.

Sarter, M., Berntson, G. G., & Cacioppo, J. T. (1996). Brain imaging and cognitive neuroscience: Towards strong inference in attributing function to structure. *American Psychologist, 51*, 13–21.

Sechenov, I. M. (1878). *Elements of thought*. [Originally published in St. Petersburg, 1878. In R. J. Herrnstein & E. G. Boring (Eds.), *A source book in the history of psychology*. Cambridge, MA: Harvard University Press, 1965.]

Shadish, W., Cook, T., & Campbell, D. (2002). Experimental and Quasi-Experimental Designs for Generalized Causal Inference. (pp. 7–9) Boston: Houghton Mifflin.

Stevens, S. S. (1951). *Handbook of experimental psychology*. New York: Wiley.

Stern, J. A. (1964). Toward a definition of psychophysiology. *Psychophysiology, 1*, 90–91.

Stern, R. M., Ray, W. J., & Quigley, K. S. (2001). *Psychophysiological recording, 2nd edition*. New York: Oxford University Press.

Tarchanoff, J. (1890). Galvanic phenomena in the human skin during stimulation of the sensory organs and during various forms of mental activity. *Pflugers Archive fur die gesamte Physiologie des Menschen und der Tiere, 46*, 46–55. Reprinted in English in S. W. Porges & M. G. H. Coles (Eds.), *Psychophysiology*. Stroudsburg, PA: Dowden, Hutchinson, & Ross, Inc.

Townsend, J. T., & Ashby, F. G. (1983). *Stochastic modeling of elementary psychological processes*. Cambridge, UK: Cambridge University Press.

Vesalius, A. (1543/1947). *De humani corporis fabrica*. Basle: Oporinus (1543); translated into English by J. B. de C. M. Saunders & C. D. O'Malley. New York: Schuman (1947).

Vigoroux, R. (1879). Sur le role de la resistance electrique des tissues dans l'electro-diagnostic. *Comptes Rendes Societe de Biologie, 31*, 336–339. Cited in Brazier (1959). New York: Oxford University Press.

Wenger, M. A. (1941). The measurement of individual differences in autonomic balance. *Psychosomatic Medicine, 3*, 427–434.

Wilder, J. (1931/1976). The "law of initial values," a neglected biological law and its significance for research and practice. *Zeitschrift fur die gesamte Neurologie und Psychiatrie, 137*, 317–324. Reprinted in English in S. W. Porges & M. G. H. Coles (Eds.), *Psychophysiology*. Stroudsburg, PA: Dowden, Hutchinson, & Ross, Inc.

Williams, R. B. (1984). Measurement of local blood flow during behavioral experiments: Principles and practice. In A. J. Herd, A. M. Gotto, P. G. Kaufman, & S. M. Weiss (Eds.), *Cardiovascular instrumentation* (pp. 207–217). NIMH (No. 84–1654).

Woodworth, R. S., & Schlosberg, H. (1954). *Experimental psychology*. New York: Holt, Rinehart, & Winston.

Wu, C. H. (1984). Electric fish and the discovery of animal electricity. *American Scientist, 72*, 598–607.

Central Nervous System

SECTION EDITOR: RICHARD J. DAVIDSON

2 Elements of Functional Neuroimaging

TOR D. WAGER, LUIS HERNANDEZ, JOHN JONIDES, AND MARTIN LINDQUIST

There has been explosive interest in the use of brain imaging to study cognitive and affective processes in recent years. Examine Figure 2.1, for example, to see the dramatic rise in numbers of publications using positron emission tomography (PET) and functional Magnetic Resonance Imaging (fMRI) from 1985 to 2004. A recent surge in integrative empirical work that combines data from human performance, neuroimaging, neuropsychology, and psychophysiology provides a more comprehensive, but more complex, view of the human brain-mind than ever before. Because the palette of evidence from which researchers draw is larger, there is an increasing need to for cross-disciplinary integration and education. Our goal in this chapter is to provide an introduction to the growing field of neuroimaging research, including a brief survey of important issues and new directions.

The many aspects of PET and fMRI methodology are organized here into three sections that describe the physical, social, and inferential contexts in which imaging studies are conducted. The first section covers the physical basis of PET and fMRI imaging. This section describes the physics of each technique, what each measures, aspects of data processing, current limits of resolution, and a comparison of the relative advantages and disadvantages of these two techniques. The second section concerns aspects of neuroimaging related to social issues. In this section, we explore the kinds of questions that might be fruitfully addressed using imaging, human factors considerations when designing imaging studies, and a "road map" of an imaging experiment. The third section deals with inference in neuroimaging. It contains a review of types of experimental designs, analysis strategies and statistics, and localization of neuroimaging results in the brain. The statistical part of the section reviews the General Linear Model (GLM; the most commonly used analysis framework), hierarchical and robust extensions to the GLM that are increasingly applied to neuroimaging data, and the most commonly used multivariate analyses. In this section we also address group analyses and multiple comparisons, and pitfalls in the use of the various analysis techniques.

Although we review the physics underlying PET and fMRI here, we would like to emphasize that much of the material in the remainder of the chapter can stand on its own; the reader need not have a thorough grasp of the physics before proceeding to other sections. An outline of the major topics covered is as follows:

I. Physical context
   What PET and fMRI can measure
   PET physics
   MRI physics
   Bold physiology
   Arterial spin labeling (ASL)
   Limitations of PET and fMRI
II. Social and procedural context
   Uses of data from functional neuroimaging
   Human factors in functional neuroimaging
   Data Preprocessing
III. Inferential context
   Forward and reverse inference
   Types of experimental designs
   Techniques for contrasting experimental
      conditions
   The general linear model (GLM) in neuroimaging
   GLM model-building in fMRI
   Extensions of the GLM
   Group analysis
   Statistical Power
   Bayesian inference
   Multivariate analysis
   Thresholding and multiple comparisons

I. PHYSICAL CONTEXT

Imaging methods for human studies include a number of alternatives: fMRI, PET, single positron emission computerized tomography (SPECT), event-related potentials (ERP), electroencephalography (EEG), magnetoencephalography (MEG), and near-infrared spectroscopy. A number of other brain-imaging techniques are available for use in animals using radiolabeling, histological, or optical

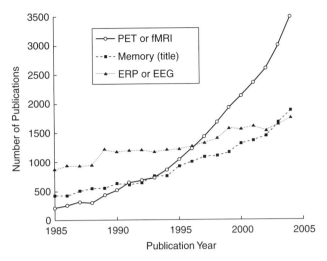

Figure 2.1. Publications by year indexed in Medline for PET and fMRI studies. Neuroimaging studies were identified by inclusively combining the search terms fMRI, PET (but not animal or companion), positron emission tomography, functional magnetic resonance imaging, or brain imaging, limited to human studies. Memory publications were identified using a title search for the word "memory," and ERP/EEG publications were identified by using an inclusive search for these terms.

imaging techniques. Each of these techniques has advantages and disadvantages, and provides a unique perspective on the functions of mind and brain.

We focus chiefly on PET and fMRI because of their popularity and because of their potential for combining with psychological methods to unravel aspects of mind and brain. PET and fMRI offer a balance between spatial resolution and temporal resolution – in contrast to EEG and MEG, which provide millisecond timing information but with uncertain spatial localization. Finally, PET and fMRI can be used to create dynamic (over time) images of the whole brain, including deep subcortical structures whose activity is largely undetectable with EEG and MEG. This last feature offers great potential for synergy with animal research: animal electrophysiology and lesion experiments often focus on isolated brain regions or pathways, whereas imaging can assess global function and interactions across diverse brain systems.

What PET and fMRI can measure

The number of techniques for imaging brain processes with PET and fMRI is growing. Although a thorough discussion of all of these is beyond the scope of this chapter, we provide a brief summary of them here. In the remainder of the chapter, we focus most intensively on measures of regional brain "activation" or "deactivation." We will use these terms to refer to a local increase or decrease, respectively, in signal linked to local blood flow and/or oxygen concentration. Activation and deactivation in PET and fMRI reflect changes in neural activity only indirectly. Table 2.1 shows a summary of the various methods available using PET and fMRI as measurement tools. Following is a brief description of each method. In addition, a summary of the relative advantages and disadvantages of fMRI and PET is provided in Table 2.2.

Structural scans. Although we are largely concerned here with functional studies, we note that MRI by itself can provide detailed anatomical scans of gray and white matter with resolution well below 1 mm^3. This can be useful if one expects structural differences between two populations of individuals, such as schizophrenics versus normal controls (Andreasen et al., 1994), or changes in gross brain structure with practice or some other variable. An example is a recent study that reported larger posterior hippocampi in London taxi drivers who had extensive training in spatial navigation (Maguire et al., 2000).

Anatomical connectivity. Another structural scanning technique is diffusion tensor imaging. This technique allows one to identify white-matter tracts (such as corpus callosum) in the human brain and changes in these structures as a function of some variable, such as age or training. Although not a technique to image brain function, "tractography," most often performed using diffusion tensor imaging (DTI) in MRI, is a technique that allows the investigator to map the white matter tracts that connect regions of the brain and hence determine the physical connectivity network underlying brain activity (Peled, Gudbjartsson, Westin, Kikinis, & Jolesz, 1998). MR images can

Table 2.1. Summary of PET and fMRI methods

What is imaged	PET	fMRI
Brain structure		Structural T1 and T2 scans
Regional brain activation	Blood flow (^{15}O) Glucose metabolism (^{18}FDG) Oxygen consumption	BOLD (T2*) Arterial spin labeling (ASL) FAIR
Anatomical connectivity		Diffusion tensor imaging
Receptor binding and neurochemistry	Benzodiazapines, dopamine, acetylcholine, opioids, other neurochemicals Kinetic modeling	MR spectroscopy
Gene expression	Various radiolabeling compounds	MR spectroscopy with kinetic modeling

Table 2.2. Relative advantages of PET and fMRI

PET	fMRI
Mapping of receptors and other neuroactive agents	Repeated scanning
Direct measurement of glucose metabolism	Single subject analyses possible
No magnetic susceptibility artifacts; better signal around brain sinuses	Higher spatial resolution
Quiet environment for auditory tasks	Higher temporal resolution
Easily combined with ERP and other measurements because there is no magnetic field	Single trial designs; image events within trials
Quantitative baseline possible for measuring resting-state metabolism, comparing scans across days, comparing across long time periods within a session	Estimation of hemodynamic response and separation of stimulus and task set related variables
	Measure dynamic connectivity (correlations) among brain regions
	Lower cost

be made sensitive to the spontaneous diffusion of water. Near a white matter tract, water diffuses most easily along the tract, producing a diffusion tensor (a generalization of a vector) that is large along the axis of the tract and small in the other dimensions. In the published literature, diffusion tensor images are usually labeled with different colors for the x, y, and z components of motion; a solid block of one color indicates fiber tracts running along either the x, y, or z-axis of the image.[1]

DTI can be used to study the structure of fiber tracts in healthy or patient populations, or they can be used in combination with functional imaging studies. For example, a recent implementation of this approach used DTI to define adjacent regions of the anterior cingulate that receive different projections from other brain regions (Johansen-Berg et al., 2004). Subsequent fMRI imaging showed that these adjacent subregions responded to different psychological tasks.

Regional brain activation. Perhaps the most frequent use of both PET and fMRI is the study of metabolic

---

[1] A standard convention, which we adopt throughout this chapter, is to refer to locations in the brain according to their relative position from the anterior commissure. Coordinates are recorded in three dimensions: lateral (negative x values are in the left hemisphere, positive in the right), rostrocaudal (positive is anterior), and dorsal-ventral (positive is superior), referred to as x, y, and z, respectively.

and vascular changes that accompany changes in neural activity. With PET, one may separately measure glucose metabolism, oxygen consumption, and regional cerebral blood flow (rCBF). Each of these techniques allows one to make inferences about the localization of neural activity based on the assumption that neural activity is accompanied by a change in metabolism, in oxygen consumption, or in blood flow.

Functional MRI using the Blood Oxygen Level Dependent method (BOLD) measures the ratio of deoxygenated to deoxygenated hemoglobin in the blood across regions of the brain. The rationale is that (a) more oxygenated blood in an area causes a decrease in BOLD signal, and (b) oxygen consumption is followed by an overcompensatory increase in blood flow, which dilutes the concentration of deoxygenated hemoglobin and produces a relative increase in signal (Hoge et al., 1999); (Kwong et al., 1992); (Kwong et al., 1992). The BOLD effect is a complex interplay between oxygen consumption, blood flow and blood volume, and it is described in more detail in the following section.

Cerebral perfusion can be measured using MRI rapidly and noninvasively by using arterial spin labeling (ASL). These measurements are a more direct, and quantitative measure of brain activity (Duong et al., 2002) but they present some technical challenges that will be discussed in later sections.

Receptor binding. The affinity of particular chemicals for specific types of neurotransmitter receptors offers researchers a leverage point for investigating the functional neurochemistry of the human brain. Radioactive labels are attached to compounds that bind to receptors in the brain. Labeled compounds are injected into the arteries of a subject by either a bolus (a single injection) or continuous infusion of the substance until the brain concentrations reach a steady state. This method can be used to image the density of a specific type of receptor throughout the brain. It can also be used to image the amount of binding to a particular type of receptor that accompanies performance of a task, as it was used in one study of dopamine binding during video game playing (Koepp, 1998).

The most common radioligands and transmitter systems studied are dopamine (particularly D2 receptors) using [11C]raclopride or [123I]iodobenzamide, muscarinic cholinergic receptors using [11C]scopolamine, and benzodiazepines using [11C]flumazenil. In addition, radioactive compounds that bind to serotonin, opioid, and several other receptors have been developed. Because the dynamics of radioligands are complex, a special class of mathematical models, called kinetic models, have been developed to explain the dynamic action of the labels. Kinetic modeling can allow a researcher to estimate how much of the radiolabeled compound is in the vasculature as opposed to in the brain, how much is freely circulating in brain tissue, how much is bound to the specific receptor-type under investigation, and how much is bound to nonspecific sites in the brain. Estimation of these parameters requires a detailed knowledge of the properties of the specific substances used, and how they act in the brain over time.

Having provided a brief summary of these techniques, we shall now concentrate on PET and fMRI as they are used to measure changes in blood flow and oxygenation. In the following sections, we describe the basics of what PET and fMRI measure, and how these measurements are made.

PET physics

Positron Emission Tomography provides a three-dimensional (3-D) image of blood flow, glucose consumption, or neurotransmitter receptor binding by detecting positrons emitted by a radioactive tracer. Positrons are subatomic particles having the same mass but opposite charge as an electron – they are "anti-matter electrons." The most common radioactive tracers are ^{15}O, "oxygen-15," commonly used in blood-flow studies, ^{18}F (fluorine), used in deoxyglucose mapping, and ^{13}C (carbon) or ^{123}I (iodine), used to label raclopride and other receptor agonists and antagonists. The decay rate of such isotopes is quite fast, and their half-lives vary from a couple of minutes to a few hours, which means that a cyclotron must be available nearby in order to synthesize the radioactive tracer minutes before each PET scan.

The tracer is injected into the subject's bloodstream in either a bolus or a constant infusion that produces a steady-state concentration of tracer in the brain. As the tracer decays within the blood vessels and tissue of the brain, positrons are emitted. The positrons collide with nearby electrons (being oppositely charged, they attract), annihilating both particles and emitting two photons that shoot off in opposite directions from one another. The photons are detected by photoreceptive cells positioned in an array around the participant's head. The fact that matched pairs of photons travel in exactly opposite directions and reach the detectors simultaneously are important for the tomographic reconstruction of the 3-D locations where the particles were annihilated. Note that the scanner does not directly detect the positrons themselves; it detects the energy that results from their annihilation.

Depending on the design, most PET scanners are made up of an array of detectors that are arranged in a circle around the patient's head, or in two separate flat arrays that are rotated around the patient's head by a gantry. To detect simultaneously occurring pairs of photons, each pair of detectors on opposite sides of the participant's head must be wired to a "coincidence detector" circuit, as illustrated in Figure 2.2. Small tubes (called "septa" or "collimators") are placed around the detectors to shield them from radiation from the sides and help prevent coincidences due to background radiation.

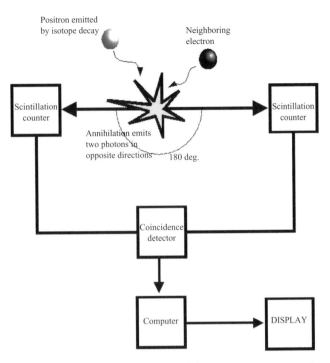

Figure 2.2. A schematic diagram of the main components of a PET scanner.

The injected tracer will be distributed throughout the blood vessels and tissue of the brain (indeed, throughout the rest of the body as well). The goal of *image reconstruction* is to determine the density of radioactive counts, and thus the amount of radioactively labeled substance, in each location within the brain. Here, we describe this process for a single two-dimensional (2-D) slice through the brain. Using mathematical notation, we use the letter **R** to refer to the location in 2-D space within the slice, and the density of tracer in each location as a 2-D function **D(R)**. The goal of reconstruction is to find **D(R)**. Each pair of coincidence detectors counts the number of positrons **P** emitted (plus error) at a particular angle throughout the entire brain slice. Positrons annihilated at a subset of locations **R** will yield coincidence counts on a particular pair of detectors. In mathematical terms, the positron count **P** at each detector is equal to the sum of the positron densities over all locations lying between the detectors:

$$P(\theta) = \sum_r D(r) \cdot \Delta r \qquad (2.1)$$

It's useful to think of P as a 1-D projection, or shadow, of the 2-D densities in the brain slice. The counts at each pair of detectors around the head are a projection at a different angle. For instance, in the image in Figure 2.3A there is a low-intensity gray circle that represents the brain, and a higher density dark circle that represents a tracer-rich area in the brain. The two detectors each contain a projection of the image (imagine a light placed behind the "brain" in Figure 2.3A) at a different angle. A simple way to think of

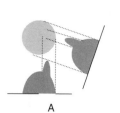
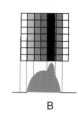
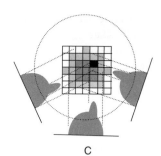

A   B   C

Figure 2.3. PET image reconstruction. The raw data are a set of projections (sums) at different angles, as shown in A. "Backprojecting" the raw data onto the image means adding the numbers of counts in the projection to the pixels that are aligned with each point in the projection, as shown in B. An image can be obtained after the data from all the projections has been added, as shown in C.

reconstruction is to take each detector and assign the number of counts found at that detector to each location **r** that could have produced the counts, as shown for one detector in Figure 2.3B. Summing the reconstructed image over detectors at different angles (Figure 2.3C) yields an estimate of the original densities **D(R)**. As the number of projections is not infinite, and neither is the number of pixels in the image, some severe artifacts will occur in the image, and they must be compensated for by applying different filters to the data. This method is referred to as filtered backprojection.

In practice, this procedure is usually implemented by treating the projections as one-dimensional (1-D) representations of the spatial frequency of the image. Spatial frequencies can be translated into image intensities using the inverse Fourier transform. A Fourier transform is an operation that re-expresses a signal (data collected over time or space) in terms of the power in the signal at different frequencies (spatial or temporal), and it plays an important role in both PET and fMRI data analysis. The inverse Fourier transform, FT^{-1}, expresses frequency-domain signals back in the spatial (or temporal) domain. Thus, the tracer density D(R) can be estimated by taking the inverse 2-D Fourier transform of the count data:

$$D(R) = FT^{-1}\left\{ R \cdot P(\theta) \right\} \qquad (2.2)$$

A more complete explanation of filtered backprojection and other methods can be found in several good texts (Bendriem, 1998; Sandler, 2003).

What do PET counts reflect? The answer depends, of course, on what molecule the label is attached to and where that molecule goes in the brain. Ideally, for [15]O PET, counts reflect the rate of water uptake into tissue. 18-fluorodeoxyglucose (FDG) PET measures glucose uptake, whereas [13]C Raclopride PET measures dopamine binding. However, in practice the observed level of signal depends on a number of factors, including the concentration of the radiolabeled substance in the blood, the blood flow and volume, the binding affinity of the substance to receptors, the presence of other endogenous chemicals that compete with the labeled substance, the rate of dissociation of the substance from receptors, and the rate at which the substance is broken down by endogenous chemicals.

Estimation of all these parameters requires detailed knowledge of the properties of the specific substances and how they act in the brain over time. *Kinetic models* have been developed to estimate how much tracer is contained in different categories, or *compartments*, of blood and tissue. Different forms of kinetic modeling have different numbers of compartments; for example, a two-compartment model estimates how much of the radiolabeled compound is in the vasculature as opposed to in the brain. A three-compartment model used in receptor binding studies estimates tracer quantities in blood, "free" tracer in tissue, and label bound to receptors. Often a reference region with few or no receptors (i.e., the cerebellum for dopamine) is used to model the separation of free from bound tracer; this requires the assumption that none of the signal in the reference region comes from "bound" tracer. A four-compartment model additionally separates tracer bound to receptors of a specific type (called specific binding) from those bound to other receptors (called nonspecific binding).

MRI physics

The raw signals in both NMR and MRI are produced the same way. As we will soon explain in more detail, a sample (e.g., a brain) is placed in a strong magnetic field and radiated with a radiofrequency (RF) electromagnetic field pulse. The nuclei absorb the energy only at a particular frequency, which is dependent on their electromagnetic environment, and then return it at the same frequency. The returned energy is detected by the same antenna that produced the RF field. Pulse sequences, or particular patterns of manipulations of the RF pulse and other magnetic fields, are used to acquire data that can be localized in the 3-D space of the brain.

The human body is made mostly of water, whose two hydrogen atoms are each made up of a single proton and a single electron. Every proton has its own magnetic dipole moment, represented mathematically by a vector in 3-D space. The magnetic moment is the amount of "magnetization" of an object, and it determines how strongly it interacts with magnetic or electric fields (a bar magnet is a dipole, and a very strong one would have a very large dipole moment).

The main magnetic field of an MRI scanner, usually labeled $\mathbf{B_0}$, is extremely powerful – anywhere from 1.5 Tesla (the standard magnet used for clinical scans, 30,000 time stronger than the magnetic field of the earth) to 8 T. To achieve such high magnetic fields requires very high electric currents. Thus, MRI magnets are typically *superconducting* closed loops of wire that carry a large current. The magnet's current is loaded ("ramped") when it is initially installed, and then it is simply allowed to flow along the closed loop perpetually. Due to the superconductive state of the coils, the magnet is always on, although no electricity is being applied to it. The drawback of this is that the magnet requires liquid helium to maintain the superconductive state, and that the perpetual field requires that the operator be constantly vigilant for safety hazards that might arise from inappropriate materials being in the environment of the magnet. Note that the potential for hazard is present even when the rest of the scanner hardware and software is turned off, because the magnetic field is always turned on. The field is most homogenous, or uniform, in the **bore** of the magnet, the hollow core in which the participant's head is situated.

When they are placed in the B_0 field, the precession, or "spins," of a portion of the protons will align with or against the magnetic field. Being aligned with the magnetic field takes less energy than being aligned against it, so a greater number of the spins will be aligned in the direction of the field. The overall net magnetization of the spins in a piece of brain tissue is the *net magnetization vector*. We shall call the net magnetization vector **M**. The larger the magnetic field, the greater the proportion of spins that are aligned, and the easier the magnetization vector is to detect.

The net magnetization vector *precesses* around the axis of the B_0 field, parallel to the long axis of the bore of the magnet. Precession is a movement that looks like a spinning top: The origin of the vector stays fixed, while the end of the vector, describing the net magnetization of the spins in 3-D space, describes a circle around the axis of the B_0 field, as shown in Figure 2.4. One of the most important equations in NMR physics is that describing the rate or angular velocity of precession, also called the *resonance frequency*, ω_0 (pronounced omega-naught):

$$\omega_0 = \gamma B_0 \qquad (2.3)$$

The rate of precession equals the magnetic field B_0, multiplied by a constant, γ (gamma), called the gyromagnetic ratio. The gyromagnetic ratio is specific for the nucleus in question; γ for hydrogen nuclei is 42.58 MHz/Tesla. By introducing systematic local variations in the magnetic field, called *gradients*, the spins precess at different frequencies at different spatial locations. This information is critical to localizing an NMR signal in space. NMR spectroscopy takes advantage of the fact that the number of electrons present, the proximity of other nuclei, and other factors can change the local B_0 field, thus altering ω_0. Certain molecules can be identified by the pattern, or spectrum, of resonance frequencies in a piece of tissue.

The MRI signal is generated by introducing a second magnetic field, which we refer to as B_1. This second field is applied by an antenna and it rotates at the same rate of precession as the magnetization vector. This rate is typi-

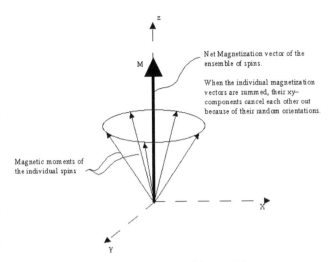

Figure 2.4. The magnetic spin ensemble in MRI.

cally in the radio frequency range, so these pulses are also referred to as "RF pulses." The RF pulse is applied in a direction perpendicular to the main magnetic field.

Physicists typically describe precession by referring to a "rotating frame of reference." This means that the vectors are considered from the point of view of an observer who is rotating along with the B_1 field. To such an observer, the net magnetization vector (**M**) and the RF field (B_1) are stationary and perpendicular to each other, but the rest of the world is spinning. In this frame of reference, the effect of a magnetic field on a magnetic dipole is a rotation of the dipole toward the transverse plane. Thus, by applying the pulse at the frequency ω_0, the pulse tips the net magnetization vector, increasing the "wobble" in the precessing vector. The degree of tipping is called the flip angle. If the flip angle is 90 degrees, as is shown in Figure 2.5, the net magnetization vector will be rotating in a plane transverse

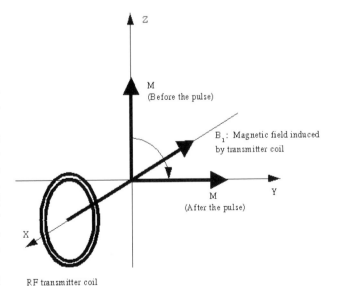

Figure 2.5. Tipping the magnetization vector from the z-axis onto the xy-plane. The duration and strength of the B1 field determine how far the vector is tipped (the "flip angle").

to the direction of $\mathbf{B_0}$. We'll call the $\mathbf{B_0}$ direction $\mathbf{z}$, and the axes of the transverse plane $\mathbf{x}$ and $\mathbf{y}$.

Changes in a magnetic field will induce electrical currents in a wire coil. The antenna used for transmission of the RF pulse is such a coil, and the rotation of $\mathbf{M}$ through the plane of the antenna coil induces a current in the coil. This current induced in the coil is the NMR signal that we observe. The current oscillates at the resonance frequency, and the power (amplitude) of the signal is proportional to the degree of magnetization in the transverse plane.

When the RF pulse is turned off, the magnetization vector will "relax" back to its equilibrium position in line with $\mathbf{B_0}$. This relaxation happens through several mechanisms: "Spin-lattice" relaxation occurs as the spins give away their energy, and they return to their original quantum state. The time this takes is called the T1 relaxation time, and it depends on the density of the microscopic environment of the water protons (hence the protons in hydrogen) in the imaged tissue. This, in turn, will be reflected in differences in brain structure such as gray matter, which has a high water content versus white matter, which has a lower content. Pulse sequences sensitive to differences in T1 relaxation time are called "T1-weighted" images, and they are commonly used for high-resolution structural scans.

Spin-spin relaxation happens along the transverse (i.e., on the x-y plane) component of the magnetization vector. Recall that the magnetization vector that gives rise to the signal is made up of the sum of an ensemble of dipoles that precess at a given rate. Spin-spin relaxation is due to some of the spins rotating faster than others in the transverse plane. When this happens, the ensemble of spins get out of phase with each other and thus decrease magnetic coherence and reduce the net magnetization vector, as illustrated in Figure 2.6. The driving mechanism for this kind of relaxation is collisions between molecules that cause them to get out of phase with each other. The rate at which this happens is called the T2 relaxation rate. Structural images that are sensitive to the differences in T2 relaxation rates among different tissue types can also be acquired; these are called "T2-weighted" images.

Another kind of relaxation is caused by local inhomogeneities in the magnetic field. These variations cause some protons to precess faster than others. Over the course of a few milliseconds, the protons will fall out of phase with each other, and the transverse-plane component of $\mathbf{M}$ will shrink faster than expected due to simple T_2. This change is referred to as T_2^* (pronounced 'T2 star'). A major reason for differences in T_2^* signal over the brain is variation in the local ratio of oxygenated to deoxygenated hemoglobin. A major cause of this variation is differences in regional brain metabolic processes, a signal of interest to neuroscientists. Thus, T_2^* weighted images are a reflection of changes in brain metabolism, and they are the "functional" brain images collected in fMRI BOLD (Blood Oxygen Level Dependent) imaging.

An example of the same slice of tissue imaged with T_1 and T_2 weighting can be seen in Figure 2.7. The images look

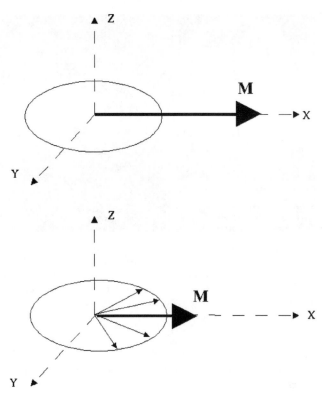

Figure 2.6. The dephasing process occurs because all the spins in the ensemble do not precess at the exact same rate. Some of them get a ahead, and some of them lag behind. The net effect is that they start canceling each other out, shortening the length of the magnetization vector.

strikingly different. Changing the contrast mechanism can be very useful in differentiating brain structures or lesions because some structures will be apparent in some kind of images but not in others. For example, multiple sclerosis lesions are virtually invisible in T_1 weighted images, but appear very brightly in T_2 weighted images.

The differences between T_1, T_2, and T_2^* weighted images lie in the construction of the pulse sequence, the pattern of RF excitations and data collection periods. A thorough discussion of pulse sequences is beyond the scope of this chapter because few neuroscientists or psychologists will ever program one. Rather, this is the province of physicists and bioengineers, and this division of labor is a key indication of how the discipline of neuroimaging is a truly interdisciplinary venture. For a more detailed introduction to types of pulse sequences, we refer the reader to Huettel, Song, & McCarthy (Huettel, 2004).

Now that we have a rough idea of how a signal is produced, let us take a look at how we can extract spatial information from it so that we can form an image. Localization of the signal in 3-D space in the brain is no easy task: it requires producing changes in the signal that vary systematically with location in the x, y, and z direction. MRI and fMRI images are usually acquired slice-by-slice in the z direction; thus, localization in the z direction is handled with *slice selection*, the process of selectively

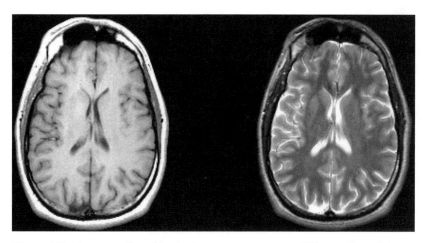

Figure 2.7. The same slice of brain tissue can appear very different, depending on which relaxation mechanism is emphasized as the source of the contrast in the pulse sequence. Using long echo times emphasizes T2 differences between tissues, and shortening the repetition time emphasizes T1 differences in tissue. Left: one slice of a T1 image. Right: the same slice acquired as a T2 image.

exciting one slice of brain tissue at a time. Signal is localized within a slice, in the x and y directions, by *frequency-* and *phase-encoding*, respectively. These are described in the following sections. We mentioned above that the precession frequency of the spins (and thus their resonance frequency) was proportional to the strength of the magnetic field. Now, consider what happens when we apply a *gradient* – another magnetic field in the direction of $\mathbf{B_0}$, except that this field varies linearly in intensity with location along the x-axis (This is called the x-gradient). Because the magnetic field strength varies with position in space, so does the rotational frequency of the magnetization vector, and consequently, the frequency of the detected signal. Hence, the power of the signal collected by the RF antenna at each frequency tells us the power of the signal source at each location along the direction of the applied gradient. This technique is called "frequency encoding." As with PET, the Fourier transform plays a role in reconstructing the image intensities from a frequency encoded signal. In MR image reconstruction, a Fourier transform of the frequency-encoded signal will result in an intensity image. The intensity is the amount of power, or "signal," at each position along the direction of the frequency-encoding gradient.

In reality, things are a bit more complex. Because the spins at different locations along the x-axis are precessing at different rates in the presence of the gradient, their magnetization vectors get out of phase with each other, causing the net transverse magnetization (the overall signal) to decay quickly. The spins can be refocused in two different ways. One could apply a gradient of equal but opposite intensity to undo the phase gain caused by the first gradient, such that the spins will regain their phase coherence and form what's called a "gradient-echo." Alternatively, one could also apply another, "refocusing" RF pulse to rotate the magnetization 180 degrees, and then re-apply the original x gradient so that the spins regain

their phase coherence. This technique is called "spin-echo," and both techniques are illustrated in Figure 2.8. Most BOLD pulse sequences employ the gradient echo technique.

To encode the spatial location along the y-axis, we *briefly* apply a gradient along the y direction prior to applying the frequency encoding gradients. The result of this gradient is a brief change in the spins' precession rate, and they end up a little bit ahead or behind the others depending on where they are along the y-axis. In other words, they gain or lose a little bit of phase relative to the vectors rotating at the resonant frequency, depending on their position along the y-axis and the strength of the applied gradient. This is called phase encoding because the phase gained by the signal is determined by its position in space. This procedure is repeated over a range of gradient amplitudes, so that we obtain a set of signals with a *distribution* of phases along one axis and a distribution of frequencies along the other axis.

It is important (albeit difficult to visualize) to notice that obtaining a distribution of phase gains along the y-direction (phase encoding) is equivalent to frequency encoding, and vice versa. Effectively, there are now two spatial frequency axes, commonly referred to as k_x and k_y. You may find yourself wondering why one doesn't just apply simultaneous frequency encoding gradients along x and y directions. The answer is that doing so would result in a gradient that runs along the diagonal instead because gradients add linearly as vectors.

k_x and k_y data are arranged in "k-space," a 2-D matrix whose rows and columns contain the power in the signal

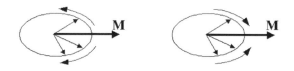

Gradient Echo technique: A gradient in the magnetic field causes the spins to lose phase coherence. Reversal of the gradient causes them to regain it.

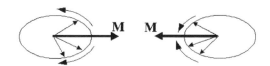

Spin Echo technique: spins are dephased by the gradient. After application of a 180 degree pulse, all the spins are rotated about the y-axis, and the application of the same gradient causes the spins to regain coherence along the negative x-axis.

Figure 2.8. Refocusing of spins in MR imaging by Gradient Echoes and Spin Echoes.

at each frequency. The two-dimensional Fourier transform of the k-space data is an image of the signal contribution from each location in the slice.

Up to this point, we have given a brief description of one of many techniques for generating an MR image. For more in-depth information, we refer the reader to a very approachable text by Elster (1994).

We mentioned earlier that BOLD imaging uses a T_2^*-weighted signal that depends on the oxygenation of hemoglobin. As neural activity increases, so does metabolic demand for oxygen and nutrients. Capillaries in the brain containing oxygen and nutrient-rich blood are separated from brain tissue by a lining of endothelial cells, which are connected to astroglia, a major type of glial cell that provides metabolic and neurochemical-recycling support for neurons. Neural firing signals the extraction of oxygen from hemoglobin in the blood, likely through glial processing pathways (Shulman, Rothman, Behar, & Hyder, 2004; Sibson et al., 1997). As oxygen is extracted from the blood, the hemoglobin becomes paramagnetic – iron atoms are more exposed to the surrounding water – which creates small distortions in the $\mathbf{B_0}$ field that cause the T_2^* effect. Increases in deoxyhemoglobin can lead to a decrease in BOLD signal, often referred to as the "initial dip." The initial decrease in signal (whose existence is controversial) is followed by an increase, due to an over-compensation in blood flow that tips the balance towards oxygenated hemoglobin (and less signal loss due to dephasing). It is this that leads to a higher BOLD signal. Initially, fMRI was performed by injection of contrast agents (such as iron) with paramagnetic properties, but the discovery that the T_2^* relaxation rate of oxygenated hemoglobin was longer than that of deoxygenated hemoglobin led to BOLD imaging as it is currently used with humans, without contrast agents (Kwong et al., 1992; Ogawa, Lee, Kay, & Tank, 1990).

BOLD physiology

How well does BOLD signal reflect increases in neural firing? The answer to this important question is complex, and understanding the physiological basis of the BOLD response is currently a topic of intense research (Buxton & Frank, 1997; Buxton, Uludag, Dubowitz, & Liu, 2004; Vazquez & Noll, 1998; Heeger, 2002). Some relationships among factors that contribute to BOLD signal are summarized in Figure 2.9.

Essentially, the BOLD signal corresponds relatively closely to the local electrical field potential surrounding a group of cells – which is itself likely to reflect changes in post-synaptic activity – under many conditions. Demonstrations by Logothetis and colleagues have shown that high-field BOLD activity closely tracks the position of neural firing and local field potentials in cat visual cortex, even to the locations of specific columns of cells responding to particular line orientations (Logothetis, 2001). However, under other conditions, neural activity and BOLD signal may become decoupled (Disbrow, 2000). Thus, for these

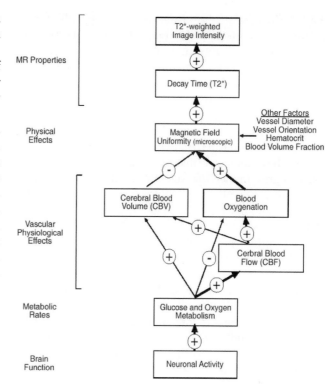

Figure 2.9. Influences on T2*-weighted signal in BOLD fMRI imaging. Courtesy Dr. Doug Noll.

reasons and others, BOLD signal is only likely to reflect a portion of the changes in neural activity in response to a task or psychological state. Many regions may show changes in neural activity that is missed because they do not change the net metabolic demand of the region.

Another important question is whether BOLD signal increases reflect neural excitation or inhibition. Some research supports the idea that much of the glucose and oxygen extraction from the blood is driven by glutamate metabolism, a major (usually) excitatory transmitter in the brain. Shulman and Rothman (Shulman & Rothman, 1998) suggest that increased glucose uptake is controlled by astrocytes, whose end-feet contact the endothelial cells lining the walls of blood vessels. Glutamate, the primary excitatory neurotransmitter in the brain, is released by some 60–90% of the brain's neurons. When glutamate is released into synapses, it is taken up by astrocytes and transformed into glutamine. When glutamate activates the uptake transporters in an astrocyte, it may signal the astrocyte to increase glucose uptake from the blood vessels. Although it remains plausible that some metabolic (and BOLD) increases could be caused by increased *inhibition* of a region, in many tasks where both BOLD studies and neuronal recordings have been made, BOLD increases are found in regions in which many cells increase their activity. This is true in studies of eye movements, task switching, working memory, food reward, pain, and other domains.

Arterial spin labeling (ASL)

Blood Oxygenation Level Dependent (BOLD) fMRI is currently the dominant technique for functional imaging and has produced a wealth of information about the brain's cognitive and affective functions. However, BOLD signal is difficult to quantify in a physically meaningful way because it is a non-linear function of many physiological parameters as well as the scanner's own characteristics (Figure 2.9). An alternative is to measure cerebral perfusion (or cerebral blood flow, CBF), a quantifiable physiological measure that may be more directly related to neuronal metabolism than BOLD. Recent animal imaging studies have indicated that CBF changes are more localized to gray matter than are BOLD changes, consistent with the notion that the BOLD effect is more weighted toward draining veins (Duong et al., 2002; Pfeuffer et al., 2002).

Perfusion imaging, unlike BOLD, may be used to study baseline activity (i.e., the resting state) without comparison to an active state. This type of measurement is particularly desirable for studies concerned with pathological states and/or testing the effects and specificity of different drugs, and in longitudinal studies. Even in non-quantitative studies (relative CBF), it has been shown that the variance of ASL perfusion studies across scanning sessions is dramatically less than that of BOLD, making studies that span days or even months feasible (Wang, Aguirre, Kimberg, & Detre, 2003).

In the pursuit of a practical cerebral perfusion measurement, there has been extensive work toward the development of arterial spin labeling techniques (Alsop & Detre, 1996; Kim, 1995; Wong, Buxton, & Frank, 1997) which employ magnetically labeled arterial water as an endogenous tracer. In typical ASL experiments, two images are collected: one following a tagging period, and the other after a control period during which the tag clears and the system is allowed to return to equilibrium. Subtraction of these two images yields a signal that is proportional to the amount of tag that is in the tissue, and can be used to quantify the perfusion rate.

There are numerous ASL schemes, but they all rely on the same principles and can be categorized as one of two approaches: the label is applied in either a "pulsed" or a "continuous" manner. The pulsed approach is carried out by applying a fast magnetic inversion pulse over a region outside the tissue of interest (e.g., the neck), thus creating a bolus of inverted spins that are allowed to flow into the tissue of interest, where they are detected. The continuous approach, on the other hand, uses a long RF pulse in combination with a magnetic field gradient along the direction of flow that results in the inversion of the spins that flow through the inversion plane. The inversion pulse is usually applied until the tissue of interest is saturated with tagged spins (Williams, Detre, Leigh, & Koretsky, 1992). Whereas the pulsed approach only requires 1–2 seconds for the label to reach its maximum concentration in the tissue, the continuous approach requires approximately 3 seconds before a steady state is reached. However, because of the longer inversion times of the continuous labeling scheme, the amount of tag to be detected is much larger

and thus, the SNR of the method is also larger (Wong, Buxton, & Frank, 1998).

One issue plaguing the BOLD effect technique is that because the BOLD effect is based on sensitivity to local changes in magnetic susceptibility, artifacts due to susceptibility gradients are also greatly exacerbated. These artifacts are especially problematic in areas of the brain that lie near air spaces, such as the roof of the mouth, nose and ear canals, as well as the sinuses. Such air-tissue interfaces create local field gradients that accelerate T_2^* dephasing (Bandettini, Wong, Hinks, Tikofsky, & Hyde, 1992); (Kwong et al., 1992); (Ogawa, Lee, Kay, & Tank, 1990). Arterial spin labeling techniques do not require T_2^* weighting, so one can use standard Spin Echo imaging techniques to collect image data and avoid susceptibility artifacts. Functional imaging studies of the basal forebrain and orbitofrontal cortex would, thus, benefit from such techniques.

BOLD effect imaging remains the dominant technique for fMRI because arterial spin labeling techniques also pose a number of challenges. The techniques suffer from low SNR because less than 10% of the water in a given voxel is contributed by blood (Pawlik, Rackl, & Bing, 1981) and the label decays at a quick rate. This problem can be alleviated by increasing the amount of label that is introduced into the tissue, i.e., using longer RF labeling pulses until the tissue of interest becomes saturated with labeled blood (this approach is referred to as "continuous arterial spin labeling," or CASL). Collecting multi-slice data can also be challenging because the imaging RF pulses can interfere with the inversion label of the arterial water (Silva, Zhang, Williams, & Koretsky, 1995). The technical development of ASL techniques for use in functional MRI is an active field of research, and an increasing number of studies are being carried out with ASL.

Limitations of PET and fMRI

Spatial limitations

There are limitations restricting what both PET and fMRI can measure. Neither technique is good for imaging small subcortical structures or fine-grained analysis of cortical activations. The spatial resolution of PET, on the order of 1–1.5 cc^3, precludes experiments testing for neural activity in focused areas of the brain (e.g., mapping receptive fields of cells in visual cortex). FMRI has a greater spatial resolution, as low as 1 mm^3 but often on the order of 3 mm^3 for most whole-brain functional studies. Careful work in individual participants has demonstrated the imaging of ocular dominance columns in humans (Cheng, 2001).

However, the high potential resolution is limited by several factors. First, fMRI researchers typically smooth (blur) the data before analysis, and some inferential methods (i.e., Gaussian Random Field Theory used in SPM, discussed later) require a high degree of blurring to be valid. Second, making inferences about populations of subjects requires analyzing groups of individuals, each with a different brain. The *normalization* procedures often used to warp individual brains into a common "reference space" introduce spatial imprecision and blurring in the group data. Third, larger activated areas are commonly taken as stronger evidence for activation – an assumption that may be misleading for small anatomical structures! Larger areas of activation often also mean less precise localization. Thus, the effective spatial resolution of both PET and fMRI is likely to be limited not only by the technology itself, but by these other considerations. One impact of spatial limitations and intentional data-blurring is that activation in small structures, particularly compact subcortical nuclei, may be missed entirely or mislocalized. A fruitful approach for those interested in particular subcortical structures is to optimize both the physical acquisition and analysis to detect signal in these regions.

Acquisition artifacts

Artifactual activations (i.e., patterns that appear to be activation arising from non-neural sources) may arise from a number of sources, some unexpected. An early study, for example, found a prominent PET activation related to anticipation of a painful electric shock in the temporal pole (Reiman, Fusselman, Fox, & Raichle, 1989). However, it was discovered some time later that this temporal activation was actually located in the *jaw* – the subjects were clenching their teeth in anticipation of the shock!

Functional MRI signals are especially susceptible to artifacts near air and fluid sinuses and at the edges of the brain. Testing of hypotheses related to activity in brain regions near these sinuses – particularly orbitofrontal cortex, inferior temporal cortex, hypothalamus and basal forebrain, and amygdala – is problematic using fMRI, though a number of groups have used optimized acquisition and analysis schemes to deal with susceptibility. Spiral imaging sequences generally lead to signal loss (dropout) in susceptible regions, causing signal loss, whereas echo planar sequences (EPI) may lead to spatial distortion of the image and mislocalization of signal. The essential problem is that the fluid spaces cause distortions, or inhomogeneities, in the local magnetic field that are different for each participant. Some approaches are to use "z-shimming" during acquisition to make the field more homogenous (Constable & Spencer, 1999), improved reconstruction algorithms (Noll, Fessler, & Sutton, 2005), "unwarping" algorithms that measure EPI distortion by measuring inhomogeneity in the magnetic field and attempting to correct it (Andersson, Hutton, Ashburner, Turner, & Friston, 2001), and use of magnetic inserts in the mouths of participants that act as shims (Wilson & Jezzard, 2003).

Functional MRI also contains more sources of signal variation due to noise than does PET, including a substantial slow drift of the signal in time and higher frequency changes in the signal due to physiological processes accompanying heart rate and respiration (the high frequency noise is especially troublesome for imaging the brainstem). The low-frequency noise component in fMRI can obscure results related to a psychological process of interest and it can produce false positive results, so it is usually removed statistically prior to analysis.

A consequence of slow drift is that it is often practically unfeasible to use fMRI for designs in which a process of interest only happens once or unfolds slowly over time, such as drug highs or the experience of strong emotions (though there are some examples of such studies). The vast majority of fMRI designs use discrete events that can be repeated many times over the course of the experiment – for example, the most common method for studying "emotion" in fMRI is to repeatedly present pictures with emotional content.

Temporal resolution and trial structure

Another important limitation of scanning with PET and fMRI is the temporal resolution of data acquisition. The details of this are discussed in subsequent sections, but it is important to note here that PET and fMRI measure very different things, over different time scales. Because PET computes the amount of radioactivity emitted from a brain region, at least 30 seconds of scanning must pass before a sufficient sample of radioactive counts is collected. This limits the temporal resolution to blocks of time of at least 30 seconds, well longer than the temporal resolution of most cognitive processes. For glucose imaging (FDG) and receptor mapping using radiolabeled ligands, the period of data collection for a single condition is much longer, on the order of 30–40 minutes.

Functional MRI has its own temporal limitation due largely to the latency and duration of the hemodynamic response to a neural event. Typically, changes in blood flow do not reach their peak until several seconds after local neuronal and metabolic activity has occurred. Thus, the locking of neural events to the vascular response is not very tight. Because of this limitation, a promising current direction is the estimation of the onset and peak latency of fMRI responses, and other parameters, averaged over many trials (Menon, Luknowsky, & Gati, 1998). We provide a more thorough discussion of this and related issues in the General Linear Modeling section.

II. SOCIAL AND PROCEDURAL CONTEXT

Uses of data from functional neuroimaging

A fundamental question in neuroimaging research is what one hopes to achieve with the chosen method. We begin our discussion of the social context of neuroimaging with a discussion of the types of questions that neuroimaging is and is suited to answer. Embarking on neuroimaging research requires a solid grasp of what kinds of imaging results would constitute evidence for a psychological or physiological theory, and a grounded understanding of what kinds of results are likely to be obtainable. Following this discussion, we provide a road map of the stages of an fMRI experiment and some of the human factors issues involved in conducting an fMRI study.

Brain mapping: Learning about the brain. Perhaps the most obvious rationale for conducting functional neuroimaging experiments is to correlate structure with function. Through a combination of animal, human patient, neuroimaging, and neurophysiology, we now know that there is substantial localization of many functions in the neural tissue of the brain.

The majority of neuroimaging studies to date may be classified as brain mapping studies, in which investigators are exploring the patterns of activity elicited by a particular psychological process or condition. Brain mapping has been used to investigate virtually every field of study in human psychology and psychiatry, including (for example) attention, perception, memory, learning, emotion, reward, depression and other mood disorders, psychopathy, and Parkinson's and other neurological disorders. Recently, this trend has broadened to include mapping of social processes such as representations of the "self" and of others' intentions, economic principles such as expected utility and risk, and emotional self-regulation. Another approach particularly relevant here is the mapping of brain regions that correspond with changes in the autonomic and endocrine systems as measured by heart rate (Critchley, 2003), electrodermal responses (Critchley, 2000), pupil dilation (Siegle, 2003), and cortisol release (Dedovic, 2005; Oswald, 2005).

Although data are typically analyzed and described in terms of activation changes corresponding to a psychological process region-by-region in the brain (e.g., the "role of the insula in process X"), a more comprehensive view is that psychological processes arise from interactions among distributed networks of neurons. It is quite possible that patterns of *functional connections* among different brain regions may best characterize tasks, and multivariate brain mapping is likely to become more prevalent in the future (Penny, Stephan, Mechelli, & Friston, 2004; Roebroeck, Formisano, & Goebel, 2005; Beckmann, 2005; Calhoun, 2005).

Overall, the sort of behavioral neurology that is provided by studies of functional neuroimaging is quite helpful on several fronts. A detailed mapping of the functions of various brain structures will give us solid evidence about the primitive psychological processes of the brain. It will also provide detailed information for neurosurgical planning. Thus, if there were no other reason to conduct studies that use functional neuroimaging, mapping the brain would be sufficient reason. However, there *are* other reasons as well. Two major ones include psychological inference and prediction of future brain and psychological states.

Psychological inference: Learning about psychology. For reasons that we discuss more extensively in the following section, brain mapping can teach us much about the gross organization of the brain, but it isn't likely in and of itself to be very informative about *psychological mechanisms*. For example, researchers may want to know *how* people make decisions, whether there are *different kinds* of cognitive control processes and how they are organized, or whether there are *distinct mechanisms* for different kinds of memories. Much of cognitive psychology has focused on identifying the component parts of systems such as decision making, attentional control, and memory, among other topics. This has been approached in two major ways: by trying to identify behavioral dissociations in performance between different processes, and by trying to identify the similarities in performance between different processes. The logic of both approaches can also be applied to measures of brain activation.

Studies of dissociations and associations include assessment of two or more tasks studying the same experiment. In a dissociation design, researchers test whether particular brain regions are more active in one condition than in another. A double dissociation occurs when manipulation A affects Task 1 more than Task 2, whereas manipulation B affects Task 2 more than Task 1. In a brain imaging study attempting to establish a double dissociation, investigators might look for two regions, one of which is more active in Task 1 than Task 2, and the other of which is more active in Task 2 than Task 1. Of course, a region need not be limited to one coherent piece of brain tissue; it might well consist of a network of brain areas. Finding a dissociation of this sort is typically considered evidence for separability of the two tasks, in that they each engage component processes differentially.

A recent study in our laboratory illustrates this approach. We sought to discover whether different kinds of shifts of attention activate different brain areas. One kind of attention-shift is required when one must change which of several objects is currently relevant for behavior. For example, an airline pilot may be monitoring the cockpit windshield, and shift attention to the radar display to check for other nearby objects. Another type of attention-shift is between attributes of objects: a pilot may switch attention from the location of objects on the radar to their apparent velocity. In addition to the object and attribute switching described above, the study also manipulated whether attention-switching was performed on items stored in working memory ("internal" representations) or whether they were available on-screen ("external" representations). Figure 2.10 shows results from different types of attention shift in a group of 38 participants.

In a double-dissociation design, investigators might want to know whether there are areas that respond more to object-switching than to attribute-switching, or vice versa. For instance, in Figure 2.10, the region in left inferior frontal gyrus shown in blue responds more to switches between internal than external representations. The extrastriate region shown in yellow, by contrast, responds more to switches of external representations than internal ones. We may conclude from this finding that the two types of attention-switches involve some different processes. There are limitations to this kind of inference, and we discuss them in the following section.

An alternative way to learn about the relationships among different tasks from brain imaging is to examine

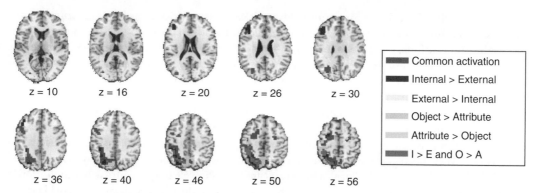

Figure 2.10. Axial slices showing brain regions responsive to different types of switching and their overlap, from Wager et al. (2005). All voxels identified show significant switch costs in at least two switch-no switch contrasts ($p < .05$ corrected in each). Thus, many regions not shown here may also show brain switch costs at less stringent thresholds. Regions colored in red are *common activations* that show no significant differences among costs for different types of switch (at $p < .05$ uncorrected). Other regions show evidence for greater activation in some switch types than others, as indicated in the legend. I, internal; E, external; O, object; A, attribute switch types.

the similarity of activation patterns across tasks. The logic is that the more similar the activation maps are for a pair of tasks or states, the more components the tasks have in common. This logic has been used in studies of individual differences in performance (Miyake, 2000). For example, if math scores and reading scores are highly correlated across individuals, then math and reading are assumed to share some common underlying performance components. In the brain imaging study on attention switching, one might examine the activation patterns for different kinds of task switching and quantify the degree of overlap among them. In this case, the substantial overlap in activations among all four types of attention switching suggests that common mechanisms are shared across all the tasks (red in Figure 2.10). Qualitative analyses of the similarities among activation patterns across tasks are common in the literature. What is critical is to have quantitative analyses of those similarities so that one can determine just how much overlap there is in brain activation between two tasks.

A third approach to use neuroimaging data is to study a psychological process by studying a physiological *marker* for that process. This approach has been taken in the psychophysiological literature – using cardiovascular responses as a marker for discrete or diffuse affective processes – although many researchers in that field are well aware of the problems in equating a physiological process with a psychological one. We discuss issues with this kind of psychological inference more extensively in the following section.

Human factors in functional neuroimaging

Many types of studies are not easily adaptable to the neuroimaging environment. Here, we briefly discuss human factors limitations and some safety issues to consider when embarking on a neuroimaging study. A complete review of safety concerns is beyond the scope of this chapter (see Elster, Link, & Carr, 1994 for more detail), but we cover a few of the basics here.

First, the MR environment is highly magnetic, and the magnetic field in the scanner is always on (barring unusual events that may require a shutdown). The strength of pull of ferromagnetic objects toward the bore of the magnet increases with the *square* of the closeness to the magnet, and the force increases with the mass of the object. Metal objects can fly out of hands or pockets as one moves closer to the bore, and larger objects pose a serious health hazard because they become missiles in the MR environment. Metallic objects in and around the participant's body can become dislodged in the intense magnetic field and cause serious injury or death. Because of the intensity of the magnetic field, participants who have implants that have any chance of being metallic (e.g., pacemakers or any electronic implants) are to be kept out of the magnetic environment. In addition, the presence of metal otherwise in the body (as in metal workers who may have tiny metallic shreds in their eyes) is a strict contraindication for scanning.

Electromagnetic fields can cause heating of tissue if applied with sufficient intensity and over enough time. This is typically not an issue, as most MRI scanners have built-in safeguards to prevent too much RF power deposition into the subject. However, should there be any metal conductors inside the RF coil, they can become quite hot because of induced currents, and they cause burns even at RF power levels that would otherwise be harmless to the participant. This is the same principle that underlies the production of sparks when you put metal objects in the microwave oven. Third, in some rare instances, changes in the magnetic field produced by the gradient coils can induce electric currents in long nerves causing them to depolarize and produce mild twitching. This is referred to as peripheral nerve stimulation (PNS) and occurs only rarely during fast imaging sequences but is more likely at higher field strength.

A safety concern particular to the PET environment is radiation exposure, which is limited by FDA regulations of 5 rem per session or 15 rem annually. NIH guidelines are 3 rem within 13 weeks or 5 rem annually (http://www.cc.nih.gov/ccc/protomechanics/chap_6.html)

In addition to safety precautions, there are other considerations that one must address to protect the integrity of the acquired data. For both PET and fMRI, the participant must remain motionless for the duration of the session, but particularly while imaging data are being collected. PET tolerances for head movement are generally higher, but task-correlated head movement can be a serious confound in either modality. In fMRI, head motion is particularly problematic, as it induces changes in the local magnetic field. Although linear motion-correction algorithms generally do a reasonable job at correcting for gross displacement of the head, they do not correct for the more complex artifacts created with movement. Participants' heads are usually restrained with a vacuum bag (a soft pillow that becomes hard when air is pumped out of it), a forehead strap and foam pads, a bite bar, or some combination of these restraints. Participants who move too much are excluded from analysis.

The restrictiveness of the scanning environment means that it is not generally advisable to use neuroimaging for tasks in which head movement is unavoidable (e.g., studies involving overt speech or pain studies involving sudden-onset electric shocks). Researchers have partially circumvented the problem and collected vocal responses during tasks by pausing data collection during verbalization or including a set of regression predictors to account for motion artifacts (Frackowiak, 1997), but the latter in particular may be only a partial solution.

The enclosed MR environment can also be a problem for individuals with claustrophobia. It is a good idea for groups working with special populations – children and individuals with psychiatric disorders – to familiarize participants in a mock-scanning environment (including an enclosed bore and simulated scanner noise) before they enter the magnet proper.

Functional MRI scanning creates repeated loud tapping and buzzing noises (approximately 100dB at the patient's location), which makes auditory presentation of stimuli more difficult than presentation in other sensory modalities. The noise can be reduced with earplugs and shielded earphones, and so some kinds of auditory studies are possible. However, earphones, like other electrical and electronic devices that may be present in the scanner room, may cause magnetic susceptibility artifacts in the images.

For visual stimulation participants in PET and MRI scanners typically view a visual display either projected by an LCD display onto a screen in the magnet room, on a shielded in-scanner LCD display, or projected onto each eye with fiber optics or LCD screens mounted in goggles. The screen is often projected onto participants' retinas through small mirrors mounted in the head coil (in MRI). The visual angle of presentation is often limited to about 15 degrees. The contrast and display image quality should be assessed before imaging, particularly for tasks that require the viewing of photographs or other fine-grained visual discriminations.

Response devices vary from scanner to scanner, but often the options are limited because in-scanner devices must be adequately RF-shielded. Responses are often limited to pressing buttons, making eye movements (several manufacturers provide scanner-compatible eye trackers), and moving joysticks or trackballs.

In general, any device that has wires or ferromagnetic parts can induce artifacts into the images because they distort the magnetic field. If severe, these artifacts may be visible as stripes or distortions in the structural (T1 or T2) images. However, T_2^* contrast is much more sensitive to artifacts, so distortions may not be visible in the structural scans but present in the functional data. Such artifacts have been observed (in our experience) with electrodermal response (EDR) leads, earphones, joysticks, mice, and keyboards in the scanning room. Some of these were not designed for use in the scanning environment, so there is no surprise that these result in artifacts. However, other commercial products intended to be RF-shielded for fMRI use also may lead to artifacts in images. In general, it is advisable to look carefully at structural and functional scans (and do a complete analysis of a simple paradigm such as visual stimulation) with and without any new piece of equipment in the room.

RF artifacts can also be caused by improper shielding of electrical cables running through the wall from the control room into the scanner room, and even by the use of hair products and makeup that contain ferrous material (not uncommon!). The closer a metallic object is to the patient's head, the greater the potential for artifacts. Jewelry, watches, and credit cards should never be taken into the MR environment (electronics are likely to be destroyed). Small metallic objects far from the participant's head, such as buttons on jeans, haven't presented a problem in our experience.

Another concern is that the neuroimaging environment itself may change performance of the task and other physiological measures. Changes may be due to anxiety about the scanning environment, changes in temperature (many scanner rooms are chilly), changes in posture that induce physiological changes (lying down reduces orthostatic load), practice, a response to the medical context presented by imaging suites, or other variables. It is advisable to test paradigms outside the scanner, and use objective measures of performance and other behaviors whenever possible.

Data preprocessing

Neuroimaging, and particularly fMRI, data undergo substantial processing before data analysis. There are several conditions about the fMRI images that must be met in order to carry out a successful data analysis. Most analyses are based on the assumption that all the voxels in any given image were acquired at the same time. Second, it is assumed that each data point in the time series from a given voxel were collected from that voxel only (i.e., that the participant did not move). Third, it is assumed that the residual variance will be constant over time and have a Gaussian distribution. Additionally, when carrying out analyses across different subjects, we assume that each voxel occupies the same location within the brain for all the subjects in the study. Without any pre-processing, none of these assumptions are entirely true, and the assumptions will introduce errors in the results. Here, we describe preprocessing for an fMRI experiment; other types of neuroimaging will require different steps.

Reconstruction. Images are reconstructed from data in k-space and transformed into image space. Raw and reconstructed data are stored in a variety of formats, but reconstructed images are generally composed of a 3-D matrix of data, containing the signal intensity at each "voxel" or cube of brain tissue sampled in an evenly spaced grid, and a *header* that contains information about the dimensionality, voxel size, and other image parameters. A popular format is Analyze, also known as AVW, which uses a separate header file and image file for each brain volume acquired. Other formats, such as AFNI, are also gaining popularity. A series of images describes the pattern of activity over the course of the experiment. It is also common to store images in a 4-D matrix, where the fourth dimension is time.

Slice timing. Statistical analysis assumes that all the voxels in an image are acquired at the same time. In reality, the data from different slices are shifted in time relative to each other – because most BOLD pulse sequences collect data slice-by-slice, some slices are collected later during the volume acquisition than others. Thus, we need to back calculate what the signal intensity of all the slices would have been at the same moment in the acquisition period. This is done by interpolating the signal intensity at the chosen time point from the same voxel in previous and subsequent acquisitions. A number of interpolation techniques exist, from bilinear to sinc interpolations, with varying degrees of accuracy and speed. Sinc interpolation is the slowest, but generally the most accurate.

Realignment. A major problem in most time-series experiments is movement of the subject's head during acquisition of the time series. When this happens, the image voxels' signal intensity gets "contaminated" by the signal from its neighbors. Thus, one must rotate and translate each individual image to compensate for the subject's movements.

The coordinates of a point in space can be expressed as a vector. It can be shown that the coordinates of a given point in space after any given translation, rotation, or combination of both, can be calculated by multiplying a matrix by the original vector. Such a matrix is called an *affine transformation* matrix. Multiplying all the voxel coordinates of an image by the same matrix will rotate and translate the entire image. Thus, in order to undo the rotation and translation of the head, we begin with a reference image (popular choices are the first image or the mean image) and transform all the other images in the time series to match it. For each image in the times series,

we calculate the elements in a six-parameter affine transformation matrix that corresponds to the displacement (x, y, z) and rotation (roll, pitch, yaw) of the head relative to the reference image. Usually, this is done by a least squares approximation that will minimize the difference between the image to be corrected and the reference. Multiplying by the matrix of best-fitting affine parameters applies the transformation and adjusts the image so that it matches the reference. Realignment corrects adequately for small movements of the head, but it does not correct for the more complex spin-history artifacts created by the motion. The parameters at each time point are saved for later inspection and are often included in the analysis as covariates of no interest.

Smoothing. Currently, many investigators apply a spatial smoothing kernel to the functional data, blurring the image intensities in space. This is ironic, given the push for higher spatial resolutions and smaller voxels – so why does anyone do it? One reason is that in a group analysis, voxels are assumed to occupy the same brain space across individuals. Smoothing can help minimize errors in inter-subject registration and normalization (see the following section). A second reason is that a popular choice for correcting for multiple comparisons, Gaussian Random Field Theory, assumes that the signal over space is a continuous field, and that the images have normally distributed noise. This is not the case in most experiments because the signal is often correlated among different voxels, especially in fMRI experiments. In order to make the noise in the images meet the assumption, the images are convolved with a Gaussian kernel (a 3-D normal probability density function), which gives the noise a more Gaussian distribution. The kernel is often described by the full width of the kernel at half its maximum height ("FWHM") in mm. One estimate of the amount of smoothing required to meet the assumption is a FWHM of 3 times the voxel size (e.g., 9 mm for 3 mm voxels).

Acquiring an image with large voxels and acquiring with small voxels and smoothing an image are not the same thing. The signal-to-noise ratio during acquisition increases as the square of the voxel volume, so acquiring small voxels means that signal is lost that can never be recovered. Thus, it is optimal from a signal-detection point of view to acquire voxels at the desired resolution and *not* smooth the images, using other methods (e.g., the nonparametric methods described in the following section) in the statistical analysis.

Coregistration. Because the high-resolution structural images contain so much more anatomical information than the functional images, it is useful for localization and inter-subject normalization to make sure that the image locations correspond to the same brain regions in both structural and functional images. A problem is that the functional and structural images are collected with different sequences and in different image dimensions. This means that though the images correspond closely, the

Template   OK   Distorted

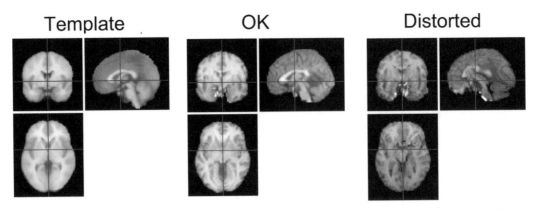

Figure 2.11. Left: the Montreal Neurological Institute average of 152 brains, used here as a spatial normalization template. Center: a subject that turned out OK. Right: a problematic normalization.

intensity values between the two images do not map in a monotonically increasing fashion. For example, the brightness (intensity) of gray, white, and ventricular tissue types may be ordered $W - G - V$ in the T_2^* images, and $V - G - W$ in a T2 image. Minimizing squared errors is inappropriate in this case, but an affine transformation matrix is often estimated by maximizing the *mutual information* among the two images, or the degree that knowing the intensity of one can be used to predict the intensity of the other (Cover, 1991). Often, a single structural image is co-registered to the first or mean functional image. Other schemes co-register a high-resolution structural image to an in-plane structural image (in the same image space as the functional images) acquired immediately before acquisition of the functional images.

Normalization or warping. In order to make quantitative comparisons across subjects, the corresponding brain structures must have the same spatial coordinates in the images. Of course, this is usually not the case because each individual has a uniquely shaped brain. We can however, stretch and compress the images in different directions so that the brain structures are in approximately the same locations. Usually we normalize all the brain images so that they will match a standard *template* (or target) brain (e.g., the Montreal Neurological Institute brain templates).

Whereas the realignment and co-registration procedures perform a *rigid body* rotation, normalization can stretch and shrink different regions of the image to achieve the closest match. The warping is described by a set of cosine basis functions, whose coefficients must be estimated by a least squares error-minimization approach. How closely the algorithm attempts to match the local features of the template depends on the number and spatial frequency of basis functions used. Often, warping that is too flexible (many basis functions) can produce gross distortions in the brain, as local features are matched at the expense of getting the right overall shape, as shown in Figure 2.11. This happens essentially because the problem space is too complex, and the algorithm can settle into a "local minimum"

solution that is not close to the global optimal solution (Frackowiak, 1997).

Following preprocessing, statistical analysis can proceed. The next section describes task design and statistical analysis in more detail. Together, these comprise the inferential context for neuroimaging.

III. INFERENTIAL CONTEXT

The inferential context for neuroimaging studies includes how tasks are designed (including special considerations for neuroimaging studies), how data analysis is conducted, and how results are interpreted in light of other findings – sometimes converging ones from other methodologies. We begin with a discussion of the logic and limitations of psychological inference from brain imaging studies, and we then return to issues of task design and analysis. We believe it is important to begin at the end, so to speak, because limitations in the kinds of inferences that can be made are a major constraint on choices of designs and analyses.

Forward and reverse inference

Once brain mapping has revealed a set of regions that are consistently activated by a task, it is tempting for scientists and lay people alike to believe that this is a brain network that implements the psychological processes involved. Two kinds of inferences emerge from this belief. First, researchers may conclude from a set of data that some brain regions are activated by a task. This is *forward inference*, inference about the brain given a particular psychological manipulation. The second inference is that activation of some regions implies that a particular psychological process has occurred. This is *reverse inference*, inference about psychology given brain activation.

Reverse inference treats a brain region – the anterior cingulate for pain or the caudate for reward – as a marker for a psychological process. That is, if one observes activity in a region, then the corresponding psychological process is assumed to have been engaged. A number of theoretical and practical problems with making reverse inferences about psychology have been described (Sarter, Berntson, & Cacioppo, 1996). However, the temptation to make premature inferences about psychology from brain activations is strong, because the major motivation for conducting research on the brain and behavior is to learn about psychological processes.

Researchers have inferred that romantic love and retribution involve "reward system" activation because these conditions activate the caudate nucleus (Aron et al., 2005; de Quervain et al., 2004), that social rejection is like physical pain because it activates the anterior cingulate (Eisenberger, Lieberman, & Williams, 2003), among countless similar conclusions. The trouble is that both these regions are involved in motor control and cognitive planning and flexibility in a wide range of tasks, including basic shifting of attention, working memory, and inhibition of simple motor responses (Bush, Luu, & Posner, 2000; Kastner & Ungerleider, 2000; Paus, 2001; Wager, Jonides, & Reading, 2004; Wager, Jonides, Smith, & Nichols, 2005). One meta-analytic review concluded that cingulate activity was related most reliably to "task difficulty" In a large range of tasks (Paus, Koski, Caramanos, & Westbury, 1998). Thus, the assumption that one can make reverse inferences in this case is seriously flawed.

These kinds of inferential difficulties are not unique to the brain imaging community. Current issues raised in interpreting brain imaging studies seem eerily similar to the debates over electrical brain stimulation in the 1950s. In a famous case, Jose Delgado claimed that he had identified the aggression centers of the brain (also, incidentally, in the caudate nucleus), and by remote-control stimulation of an implanted electrode could make a raging bull as passive as a gentle lamb. Delgado demonstrated his findings by placing himself in a ring with a Spanish bull and using his device to pacify the animal in mid-charge (Valenstein, 1973). The experiment worked: the bull stopped – but not likely because he was truly pacified. Valenstein (1973) recounts that the electrodes were placed in motor-control regions of the caudate that forced the bull to turn in one direction (and probably confused the animal as well!).

It is useful here to analyze what went wrong in formal terms. What Delgado observed in the previous example is the disruption of aggressive behavior (B), which is "consistent with" the hypothesis that brain circuits for aggression were stimulated (A). That is, there is a high probability of observing B, given the truth of hypothesis A, or $P(B \mid A)$ −>1. But "consistent with" is not good enough. He made an erroneous inference about the probability of hypothesis A given the data B, and concluded that $P(A \mid B)$ is high. According to probability theory, these two statements are not equivalent, but rather $P(A \mid B)$ depends on $P(B \mid A)$, and also on the base rates (prior probabilities) of A and B, as stated by Bayes' Theorem:

$$P(A \mid B) = \frac{P(A \mid B)P(A)}{P(B)} \qquad (2.4)$$

In ignoring what else besides A might have disrupted behavior, they ignored the base rate of B, and reached a false conclusion.

In our brain imaging example, if the base rate of anterior cingulate activation across studies is high – if it's activated in every study – then its activation tells us very little about the engagement of any particular psychological process.

Types of experimental designs

Neuroimaging designs require making tradeoffs. One basic tradeoff is between experimental power and the ability to make strong inferences from results. Some types of designs, such as the simple blocked design, often yield high experimental power, but they provide imprecise information about the particular psychological processes that activate a brain region. Event-related designs allow brain activation to be related more precisely to particular cognitive processes engaged in particular types of trials, but they are often less powerful and require additional assumptions about the underlying hemodynamics of the brain. Researchers may also choose to focus intensively on testing one comparison of interest, maximizing power to detect an effect, or they may test multiple conditions in order to draw inferences about the generality of a brain region's involvement in a class of similar psychological processes. We describe some types of designs and the uses to which they are best suited in the following section.

Blocked designs

Because long intervals of time (30 seconds or more) are required to collect sufficient data in a PET experiment to yield a good image, the standard experimental design used in PET-activation studies is the blocked design. A blocked design is one in which different conditions in the experiment are presented as separate blocks of trials, with each block representing one scan during an experiment. To image a briefly occurring psychological process (e.g., the activation due to attention switching) using a blocked design, one might repeat the process of interest during an experimental block (A) and not during a control block (B). The A – B comparison is a simple *contrast* across experimental conditions; contrasts of various types are used in all kinds of experimental designs. Given the temporal limitation of this technique, PET is not well suited to examining the fine time course of brain activity that may change within seconds or fractions of a second.

The blocked structure of PET designs (and blocked fMRI designs) imposes limitations on the interpretability of results. Activations related to slowly changing factors such as task-set or general motivation are captured well by blocked designs. However, if one wishes to image the neural responses to individual stimuli, blocked designs are not well suited to that goal. In addition, the A – B contrast does not permit the researchers to infer if a region is activated in A but not B, deactivated in B but not A, or shows a combination of both effects. The use of multiple controls and comparison conditions can ameliorate this problem to some degree.

One advantage to a blocked design is that it offers more statistical power to detect a change. Under ideal conditions, blocked designs can be over 6 times as efficient as randomized event-related designs (Wager & Nichols, 2003). Generally, theory and simulations designed to assess experimental power in fMRI designs point to a 16–18 s task/16–18 s control alternating-block design as optimally statistically powerful (Liu, 2004; Skudlarski, Constable, & Gore, 1999; Wager & Nichols, 2003). However, it is worth noting that this is not always true; the relative power of a blocked design depends on whether (a) the target mental process is engaged relatively continuously in A and not at all in B, and (b) imposing a block structure changes the nature of the task. On this latter point, it is easy to imagine that blocking some variable may fundamentally alter the strategy that subjects apply to the task.

Event-related fMRI

To take advantage of the rapid data-acquisition capabilities of fMRI, event-related fMRI designs and analyses have been developed. These designs, when employed judiciously, allow one to estimate the fMRI response evoked by specific stimuli or cognitive events within a trial (Rosen, Buckner, & Dale, 1998). A sample of the MRI signal in the whole brain can be obtained in 2–3 seconds on average (the TR, or repetition time of image acquisition), depending on the way the data are acquired and depending on the required spatial resolution of the voxels that are imaged. The limiting factor in the temporal resolution of fMRI is generally not the speed of data acquisition, but the speed of the underlying evoked hemodynamic response to a neural event (or the hemodynamic response function, HRF), which begins within a second after neural activity occurs and peaks 5–8 seconds after that neural activity has peaked (Aguirre, Zarahn, & D'Esposito, 1998; Friston, Frith, Turner, & Frackowiak, 1995).

Although event-related designs are attractive because of their flexibility and the information they provide about the individual responses, they require more caution in the design and analysis of the experiment. It is quite common to assume an ideal or "canonical" hemodynamic response (HRF) in order to generate linear models for statistical analyses (the fitted curves shown by the dashed lines in Figure 2.12). This procedure requires a realistic model of the shape and timing of the HRF. Notably, the canonical estimates typically used come from studies of brief visual and motor events. In practice, however, the timing and shape of the HRF are quite variable across the brain within an individual and across individuals (Aguirre, Zarahn, & D'Esposito, 1998; Schacter, Buckner, Koutstaal, Dale, & Rosen, 1997). Part of the variability among shapes of the HRF is due to the underlying configuration of the vascular bed, which may cause differences in the HRF across brain regions in the same task for purely physiological reasons. Another source of variability in the shape of the HRF is dif-

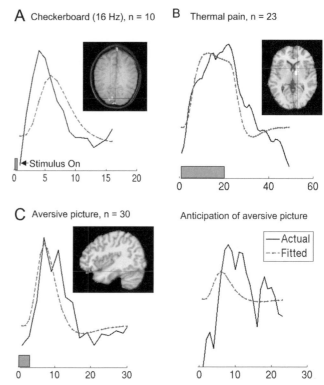

Figure 2.12. Examples of hemodynamic response functions (HRFs) derived from different brain regions in different studies. The brain region for each HRF is shown in the inset panels. The gray boxes at lower left in each panel show the duration of stimulus presentation. Solid lines show group-averaged high-resolution HRF estimates derived using an finite impulse response model. Dashed lines show the fitted responses using the canonical SPM HRF, composed of two gamma functions. The impulse HRF was convolved with a boxcar function equal to the stimulus duration in A and D, providing linear predictions for the response to the epoch. The impulse HRF was fitted to the briefly presented events in B and C.

ferences in the pattern of evoked neural activity in regions performing different functions related to the same task.

Figure 2.12A shows an example of an average response in left visual cortex, identified on an individual basis in 10 participants (scanning time was approximately 60 minutes per participant, with one stimulus every 30 s) (Wager, Vazquez, Hernandez, & Noll, 2005). The figure shows that the HRF peaks earlier than the canonical model, and the magnitude of activation is thus underestimated by about 30% in this group of subjects. Blocked designs are less sensitive to the variability of the HRF because they are dependent on the total activation caused by a *train* of stimulus events (though this depends on the density of psychological activity during the block (Price, Veltman, Ashburner, Josephs, & Friston, 1999)!). For example, Figure 2.12B shows the responses to a 20 s epoch of thermal pain in the right thalamus and caudate, averaged over 23 subjects (Wager et al., 2004). The predicted model of this longer period of stimulation is also based on the canonical HRF. Specifically, the model is generated by convolution of the HRF with a 20-s long step-function representing the stimulation period. The canonical model fits reasonably well in this case.

On the other hand, Figure 2.12C shows a problematic case. The orbitofrontal cortex response to a 3 s presentation of an aversive visual stimulus is somewhat prolonged relative to the model, but the estimated magnitude is reasonably accurate (unpublished data). The right panel, on the other hand, shows the response in the same brain region to anticipation of viewing an aversive picture. In this case, the timing and duration of the cognitive activity are unknown – the activity could occur at the onset of the cue, throughout the anticipation epoch, or with increases proportional to the proximity of the picture. The model fits poorly in this case, illustrating the importance of knowing the onset and duration of the stimulation for linear model analyses.

In a single-trial event-related design, events are spaced far apart in time (every 20–30 s is considered sufficient). FMRI signal can be observed on single trials if the eliciting stimulus is very strong (Duann et al., 2002), permitting the possibility of fitting models at the level of an individual trial (Rissman, Gazzaley, & D'Esposito, 2004). This promising technique enables the testing of relationships between brain activity and trial-level performance measures such as reaction time and emotion ratings for particular stimuli (Phan et al., 2004).

Early studies frequently employed selective averaging of activity following onsets of a particular type (Aguirre, Singh, & D'Esposito, 1999; Buckner et al., 1998)(Menon, Luknowsky, & Gati, 1998)). However, even brief events (e.g., a 125-ms visual checkerboard display) have been shown to affect fMRI signal more than 30 s later (Wager, Vazquez, Hernandez, & Noll, 2005). Because the selective averaging procedure does not take stimulus history into account, it must be used with caution when responses to different events may overlap in time. Because of this, the majority of analyses, including those that estimate the shapes of HRFs, are currently done within the GLM framework (described in the following section).

Reports that the fMRI BOLD response is linear with respect to stimulus history (Boynton, Engel, Glover, & Heeger, 1996) encouraged the use of more rapidly-paced trials (Zarahn, Aguirre, & D'Esposito, 1997), spaced less than 1 s apart in extreme cases (Burock, Buckner, Woldorff, Rosen, & Dale, 1998; Dale & Buckner, 1997). Linearity in this context means that the magnitude and shape of the HRF does not change depending on the preceding stimuli. Studies have found that nonlinear effects in rapid sequences (1 or 2 s) can be quite large (Vazquez & Noll, 1998; Birn, Saad, & Bandettini, 2001; Friston, Mechelli, Turner, & Price, 2000; Wager, Vazquez, Hernandez, & Noll, 2005), but that responses are roughly linear if events are spaced 4–5 s apart (Miezin, Maccotta, Ollinger, Petersen, & Buckner, 2000).

To get an intuition about how rapid designs allow one to discriminate the effects of different conditions, consider this: With a randomized and jittered design, some-times several trials of a single type will occur in a row, and because the hemodynamic response to closely spaced events sums in a roughly linear fashion, the expected response to that trial type will build to a high peak. Introducing longer delays between some trials and shorter ones between others allows peaks and valleys in activation to develop that are specific to particular experimental conditions. Thus, it is critical either to systematically intermix events of different types in a rapid event-related design or to vary (jitter) the inter-stimulus interval (ISI) between trials.

Suppose, for example, you have a rapid sequence with two types of trials – say, attention switch trials (S) and no-switch trials (N) as in task switching experiment described above (Figure 2.10). Randomly intermixing the trials with an ISI of 2 s will allow you to compare responses to S with those to N; that is, you will be able to estimate the difference S − N. However, you will not be able to tell if S and N activate or deactivate relative to some other baseline. If you vary the inter-stimulus intervals randomly between 2 and 16 s, you'll be able to compare S − N (albeit with less power because there will be fewer trials), but you'll also be able to test whether S and N show positive or negative activation responses. This ability comes from the inclusion of inter-trial rest intervals against which to compare S and N, and the relatively unique signature of predicted responses to both S and N afforded by the random variation in ISIs.

The advantages of rapid pacing – including trial pacing comparable to other experiments, reduced boredom, and sometimes increased statistical efficiency – must be weighed against potential problems with nonlinearity, multicolinearity, and model misfitting when very rapid designs are used. A current popular choice is to use jittered designs with inter-stimulus intervals of at least 4 s, with exponentially decreasing frequencies of delays up to 16 s.

Techniques for contrasting experimental conditions

Thus far, we have alluded to a simple kind of contrast between two conditions, the subtraction of a control condition (B) from an experimental one (A). Such contrasts are critical because any task, performed alone, produces activation in huge portions of the brain. To associate changes in brain activation with a particular cognitive process requires that we isolate changes related to that process from changes related to other processes.

The simple contrast discussed above was the first method used to make inferences about psychological processes from neuroimaging data (Petersen, Fox, Posner, Mintun, & Raichle, 1988; Posner, Petersen, Fox, & Raichle, 1988). It is called the subtraction method, the logic of which is this: If one tests two experimental conditions that differ by only one process, then a subtraction of the activations of one condition from those of the other should reveal the brain regions associated with the target process. This subtraction is accomplished one voxel at a time throughout brain regions of interest. Together, the results of the voxel-wise subtractions yield a 3-D matrix of the difference in activation between the two conditions throughout the scanned regions of the brain, or *contrast images*. T-tests can be performed for each voxel to discover where in the brain the difference is reliable. The resulting parametric map of the t-values for each voxel shows the reliability of the difference between the two conditions throughout the brain. Figures of activation maps in publications, such as those shown in Figure 2.10, generally show images of voxels whose t-values or comparable statistics (z or F) exceed a statistical threshold for significance.

Subtraction logic rests on a critical assumption, what has been called the assumption of "pure insertion" (Sternberg, 1969). According to this assumption, changing one process does not change the way other processes are performed. Thus, by this assumption, the process of interest may be "purely" inserted into the sequence of operations without altering any other processes. Although violations of subtraction logic have been demonstrated experimentally (Zarahn, Aguirre, & D'Esposito, 1997), the logic is still widely used because it greatly simplifies the inference-making process. However, if the two tasks studied differ in more than one overt (e.g., visual stimulation) or covert process (e.g., attention, error checking, subvocalization, attention shifts), the results will be ambiguous. With only two tasks or conditions, this is very often the case.

One way to constrain the interpretation of brain activity and strengthen the credibility of subtraction logic is to incrementally vary a parameter of interest across several levels – essentially performing multiple subtractions on a single variable. An example is a study of the Tower of London task (Dagher, Owen, Boecker, & Brooks, 1999), which requires subjects to make a sequence of moves to transfer a stack of colored balls from one post to another in the correct order. The experimenters varied the number of moves incrementally from 1 to 6. Their results showed linear increases in activity in dorsolateral prefrontal cortex across all 6 conditions, suggesting that this area served the planning operations critical for good performance. The contrast tested in this condition is a *linear contrast*. We provide a mathematical explanation of how exactly this and other contrasts are performed in the section on linear modeling. Other contrasts, such as quadratic or monotonic contrasts, can also be specified.

Another extension of subtraction logic is the factorial design. The study of task switching presented in the introduction to this chapter serves as an example. Consider the comparison in this study of two types of switching, each varied independently: switching among objects and switching among attributes of objects. This design is a simple 2 × 2 factorial, with 2 types of trials (switch vs. no switch) crossed with 2 types of judgments (object/attribute). This design permits the testing of three contrasts: (a) a main effect of switch versus no switch; (b) a main effect of task type; and (c) the interaction between the two, which tests whether the switch versus

non-switch difference is larger for one task-type than the other. Factors whose measurements and statistical comparisons are made within subjects, as are those described above, are *within-subjects* factors, and those whose levels contain data from different individuals (e.g., depressed patients vs. controls) are *between-subjects* factors. Within-subjects factors generally offer substantially more power and have fewer confounding issues (e.g., differences in brain structure and HRF shapes) than between-subjects factors.

Factorial designs allow one to investigate the effects of several variables on brain activations. They also permit a more detailed characterization of the range of processes that activate a particular brain region – attention switching in general, or switching more for one task-type than the other. Factorial designs also permit one to discover double dissociations of functions within a single experiment. In our example (Figure 2.10), a factorial design was required in order to infer that a manipulation (e.g., object-switching) affected dorsolateral prefrontal cortex, but a second manipulation (e.g., attribute switching) did not.

Factorial designs also provide some ability to test for brain regions activated in common by a set of related tasks or uniquely by only certain tasks (Fan, Flombaum, McCandliss, Thomas, & Posner, 2003; Wager, Jonides, Smith, & Nichols, 2005; Wager et al., 2005). An important note in this regard is that inferring that an area responds, say, to "task switching in general" requires more than just a significant main effect of switching, but rather a *conjunction* across object and attribute switching. That is, each effect must be independently significant to conclude that both effects were present in a region (T. Nichols, Brett, Andersson, Wager, & Poline, 2005).

Also of great interest to psychologists and neuroscientists is the *specificity* of regional activation to one particular psychological process. An activated region or pattern of activations specific to a process is activated by *only* that process. If such specificity exists, then that pattern may serve as a marker for the psychological process, and reverse inference becomes possible. In general, if such inferences can be made at all, it seems practical to compare across a great many studies using a meta-analysis (Wager, Jonides, & Reading, 2004) – because establishing a marker requires determining which tasks do not activate the region. However, a problem with meta-analyses is their poor spatial resolution compared with individual studies.

One productive line of research attempting to address specificity within individual studies has been pursued by Kanwisher and colleagues in the study of face recognition (Kanwisher, McDermott, & Chun, 1997). In this study and many subsequent ones, they identified an area in the fusiform gyrus that responded to pictures of faces and drawings of faces, but not to houses, scrambled faces, partial faces, facial features, animal faces, and other control stimuli. By presenting a large number of control stimuli of various types, Kanwisher et al. (1997) were able to infer that the brain area they studied, which they called the Fusiform Face Area (FFA), was specific to the perception of faces. They tested both for the types stimuli that elicited an FFA response and for those that did *not* elicit a response. In addition, because this region lies in slightly different locations across different participants, they performed separate "localizer" scans to locate the functionally face-selective region within individual participants.

The general linear model (GLM) in neuroimaging

The techniques described above can be understood mathematically in terms of the GLM framework. GLM is a linear analysis method that subsumes many basic analysis techniques, including t-tests, ANOVA, and multiple regression. In neuroimaging designs, analyses of both blocked and event-related designs are most frequently carried out in the GLM framework, though with some extensions that we describe in the following section. The GLM can be used to estimate whether the brain responds to a single type of event, to compare different types of events, to assess correlations between brain activity and behavioral performance or other psychological variables, and for other tests.

The GLM is appropriate when multiple predictor variables – which together constitute a simplified *model* of the sources of variability in a set of data – are used to explain variability in a single, continuously distributed outcome variable. In a typical neuroimaging experiment, the predictors are related to psychological events, and the outcome variable is signal in a brain voxel or region of interest. In analysis with the "massively univariate" GLM approach commonly used in brain imaging, one performs a separate regression analysis at every voxel in the brain.

In a single-subject fMRI analysis, the GLM assumes that the observed signal time series in a voxel is the sum of the activity evoked by a number of independent processes. Some of these processes are of interest, but others are nuisance contributions to the overall signal (e.g., apparent activation due to movement of the head). Activity evoked by each process is modeled with by constructing a predictor, or estimate of the predicted brain response, for each process. The amplitudes (weights) of the predictors, which reflect the magnitudes of the evoked activity for each process, are unknown. The GLM estimates these magnitudes and determines whether they are significantly different from zero at each voxel in the brain.

By convention, predictors are arranged in columns. The *design matrix*, X, describes the model. It contains a row for each of *n* observations collected (subjects or samples) and a column for each of *k* predictors. The data, *y*, are modeled as a linear combination of the predictors (i.e., a weighted sum) plus error, ε. The GLM framework is described by the equation:

$$y = X\beta + \varepsilon \qquad (2.5)$$

where β is a $k \times 1$ vector containing the predictor weights (also called regression slopes or parameter estimates). The equation is in matrix notation. Thus, X is an $n \times k$ model matrix, y is an $n \times 1$ vector containing the observed data, and ε is an $n \times 1$ vector of unexplained error values. Error

values are assumed to be independent and to follow a normal distribution with mean 0 and standard deviation σ. The β weights in a neuroimaging experiment correspond to the *estimated magnitude of activation* for each psychological condition described in the columns of X.

The model is fit to the data by finding the weights (β) that minimize the squared distance between the vector of fitted values, $X\beta$, and the data. One of the advantages of the GLM is that there is an algebraic solution for the βs that minimizes the squared error:

$$\hat{\beta} = (X^T X)^{-1} X^T y \qquad (2.6)$$

where $\hat{\beta}$ are the estimates of the true regression slopes. In algebraic terms, the GLM projects data (y) in an n-dimensional space (n independent data observations) onto a k-dimensional model subspace (k predictors). The matrix product $(X^T X)^{-1} X^T$ is the matrix of the orthogonal projection onto the reduced-dimensional space of X.

Inference is generally conducted by comparing the $\hat{\beta}$s with their standard errors and using classical inferential procedures to estimate the likelihood of the estimates under the null hypothesis. The standard errors of the estimates are the diagonal elements of the matrix:

$$se(\hat{\beta}) = (X^T X)^{-1} \hat{\sigma} \qquad (2.7)$$

The ratio of betas to their standard errors follows a t-distribution with n – k degrees of freedom. Notably, the error term is composed of two separate terms from different sources. σ is the error variance, and $(X^T X)^{-1}$ depends on the design matrix itself. If the matrix contains high values, the estimates will be less precise, and statistical power will decrease. If X is scaled appropriately, $X^T X$ is the variance-covariance matrix of X. Low values on the diagonal of $X^T X$ (low predictor variability) and high off-diagonal elements (high colinearity) will both cause $(X^T X)^{-1}$, and the variability of the estimates, to grow.

Contrasts

Contrasts across conditions can be easily handled within the GLM framework. Mathematically, a contrast is a linear combination of predictors. The contrast (e.g., A − B in a simple comparison, or A + B − C − D for a main effect in a 2×2 factorial design) is coded as a $k \times 1$ vector of contrast weights, which we denote with the letter c. For example, the contrast weights for a simple subtraction are $c = [1 \ -1]^T$, where T indicates the transpose operator. A single contrast for a linear effect across four conditions might be $c = [-3 \ -1 \ 1 \ 3]^T$. A set of contrasts can be simultaneously tested by concatenating the contrasts into a matrix. Thus, the main effects and interaction contrasts in a 2×2 factorial design can be specified with the following matrix:

$$C = \begin{bmatrix} 1 & 1 & 1 \\ 1 & -1 & -1 \\ -1 & 1 & -1 \\ -1 & -1 & 1 \end{bmatrix};$$

For the contrast to be orthogonal to the intercept, contrast weights must sum to zero. If the weights do not sum to zero, then the contrast values partially reflect overall scanner signal intensity. It is worth going into this level of detail here because contrast weights in statistics packages used with imaging data are often specified by the analyst, rather than being specified automatically as they might be in standard statistical programs such as SPSS or SAS. The true contrast values $C^T \beta$ can be estimated using $C^T \hat{\beta}$, where $\hat{\beta}$ is obtained using Equation (6). The standard errors of each contrast are the diagonals of:

$$se(C^T \hat{\beta}) = C^T (X^T X)^{-1} C \hat{\sigma} \qquad (2.8)$$

Most imaging statistics packages write a series of images to disk containing the betas for each condition throughout the brain, and another set of contrast images containing the values of $C^T \hat{\beta}$ throughout the brain. As the latter images contain estimates of activation differences across conditions, these are typically used in a group analysis. A third set of images contain t-statistics, or the ratio of contrast estimates to their standard errors.

Assumptions

The model-fitting procedure assumes that the effects due to each of the predictors add linearly and do not change over time (i.e., a linear, time-invariant system). The inferential process assumes that the observations are independent, that they all come from the same distribution, and that the residuals are distributed normally and with equal variance across the range of predicted values. All of these assumptions are violated to a degree in at least some brain regions in a typical imaging experiment, which has prompted the development of a number of important extensions. Violations of the assumptions are not merely a theoretical nuisance. They can make the difference between a valid finding and a false positive result, or between finding meaningful activations in the brain and wasting substantial time and money.

Diagnostic tools have been developed for exploring the data, looking for artifacts, and checking a number of assumptions about the data and model (Luo, 2003), and like many tools developed by members of the neuroimaging community, they are freely available on the internet. The quantity of data – for example 100,000 separate regressions on 1000 data points per subject × 20 subjects – and the software and data structures that support its analysis makes it very difficult to examine assumptions and check the data, which makes such diagnostic tools all the more important.

Another active area of research concerns strategies for dealing with some known violations of assumptions, described in the following section. Violations of independence can be handled in a limited way using generalized least squares. Violations of equality and normality can be dealt with by using nonparametric permutation tests to make statistical inferences (Nichols, 2002), or, if they

result from the presence of outliers, by robust regression techniques (Wager, 2005). Free implementations of each of these extensions are available, and we return to a description of them after providing additional background on application of the GLM to imaging experiments.

GLM model-building in fMRI

Perhaps the most challenging task in linear regression analysis is the creation of a *realistic* model of the signal. This model constitutes the matrix X in the general linear model equation. In a neuroimaging study, researchers typically build a model of the predicted brain response to each psychological event-type or condition. A stimulus or psychological *event* that elicits a brief burst of neural activity in an area typically produces a prolonged HRF that peaks 5–6 s later (but may vary across brain regions, as described above!) PET images integrate across many such events, and each brain image (an image containing one data observation at every voxel) reflects overall activity in a particular condition. Thus, much of the remainder of this section does not apply to PET analyses.

Accounting for the delayed hemodynamic response

A popular method of forming a prediction about BOLD activity is to assume that the response to a brief event will follow a canonical shape, such as that shown in Figure 2.12A and the center panel of Figure 2.13, for every event-type and every voxel in the brain. To build the model, researchers start with an "indicator" vector representing the neuronal activity for each condition sampled at the resolution of the fMRI experiment. This vector has zero value except during activation periods, when the signal is assigned a unit value. To form the predicted response in a condition, the indicator vector for that condition is convolved with the assumed HRF, and the result forms a column of the design matrix.

The process, shown in Figure 2.13 for an event-related design with four trial types (A–D), is similar for both blocked and event-related fMRI designs. The left panel shows the indicators, with rows of the plot corresponding to the four conditions. Each of the indicator vectors is convolved with the canonical HRF, shown in the center panel, to yield the predictors shown in the rows of the next panel. The image of the design matrix, a commonly used presentation format in imaging experiments, is shown in the rightmost panel.

If the assumed HRF does not fit, there is at best a drop in power to detect a response. At worst, model misspecification can produce false positive results. Say, for example, the HRF peaks at the expected time in condition B, but later in A. Because the shape is fixed, the amplitude of the fit for B will be greater than A. Without some additional diagnostic tests, one might falsely infer that B activates the brain region more than A.

Comparing groups of individuals (e.g., older versus younger adults, or patients and normal controls) can also

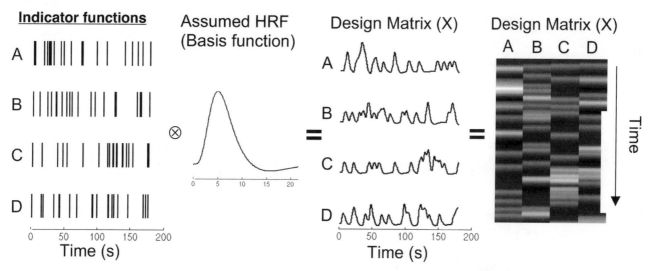

Figure 2.13. Construction of an event-related fMRI design matrix with four event types, using the canonical SPM HRF.

be especially problematic. If one finds differences between Task A and Task B in evoked response magnitude, are those differences caused by differences in neural activity, or by differences in how well subjects' responses fit the canonical, assumed shape? Elderly subjects, for example, have reduced and more variable shapes of their HRFs compared to younger subjects (D'Esposito, Zarahn, Aguirre, & Rypma, 1999).

One approach that has been used to avoid this problem is the measurement of hemodynamic responses in visual and motor cortex for each individual subject (Aguirre, Zarahn, & D'Esposito, 1998). This approach may work for brain regions whose HRF shapes match those in sensorimotor cortex. An alternative approach is to use a more flexible model of the HRF, which we describe in the following section.

Basis sets

In the previous discussion, responses to each psychological event-type or condition are modeled by only one linear regressor, which allows one to estimate only the fitted amplitude of the response. If more than one regressor is used to model each event-type, then the regressors can model different components of the response. The same onsets are convolved with different canonical functions that together can model a range of different HRF shapes. These canonical functions are called basis functions, and the group of basis functions chosen to model the response is called a basis set. Fitting a basis set at each voxel means that the fitted shape of the HRF is allowed to vary across brain regions.

Basis sets vary in the number of parameters estimated per event-type and in the shapes of the basis functions. A flexible basis set will be able to model more different HRF shapes, but generally at the cost of statistical power (more parameters means more variability in parameter estimates). A popular choice is to use a canonical HRF and its derivatives with respect to time and dispersion

(we use TD to denote this hereafter (Friston et al., 2002; Friston, Josephs, Rees, & Turner, 1998). Other choices include basis sets composed of principal components (Aguirre, Zarahn, & D'Esposito, 1998; Woolrich, Behrens, & Smith, 2004), cosine functions (Zarahn, 2002), radial basis functions (Riera et al., 2004), and spectral basis sets (Liao et al., 2002).

One of the most flexible models, a finite impulse response (FIR) basis set, contains one free parameter for every time-point following stimulation in every cognitive event-type that is modeled (Glover, 1999; Goutte, Nielsen, & Hansen, 2000; Ollinger, Shulman, & Corbetta, 2001). Using such a model makes minimal assumptions about the shape of the HRF – in fact, the set of parameter estimates (betas) from this model constitute an estimate of what the shape of the HRF looks like when sampled at the frequency of data collection (the TR).

Figure 2.14 shows fits to some empirical data from our laboratory using three popular basis sets with different degrees of flexibility. The "actual" HRF in these plots (solid lines in the right panels) comes from a region of the right thalamus that responds to viewing aversive emotional pictures. They are estimates using an FIR model with 1 s time bins, so they are the most assumption-free estimates we can obtain of the true response in this region. The SPM2 canonical HRF, composed of two summed gamma functions, is shown in the top-left panel. The image of the basis set is shown in the center panel, and the fit of the basis set to the data is shown in the rightmost panel. As the figure shows, the fit leaves much to be desired, and the height of the response is substantially underestimated, because the actual HRF peaks later and shows a much larger undershoot than the model. The second row of panels shows a plot of the basis set of the SPM2 canonical HRF with its derivatives with respect to time and dispersion (left), the image of the basis set (center), and the fitted response (right). The fit is substantially better, and would probably be adequate in this case to capture the positive-going lobe

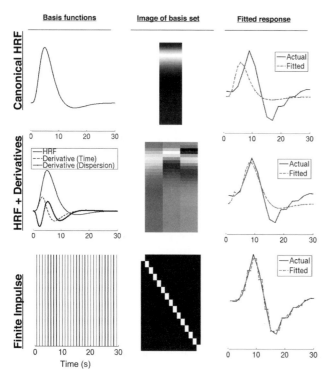

Figure 2.14. Basis functions (left panels), their intensity-mapped images (center), and fitted responses to data for three popular basis sets. Solid lines show group-averaged HRF estimates using a 1-s resolution FIR model. Dashed lines show the fitted response.

of the evoked activation. An FIR model is a linear model too, and the bottom panels show the same results for an FIR model with one estimate every 2 s.

Whatever basis set is used, statistical comparisons across event types must be made. The advantage of assuming a canonical shape is that because beta values represent response amplitudes for different conditions, the differences between betas represent differences in activation across psychological tasks or states. It is thus relatively straightforward to assess contrasts in a subtraction, parametric, or factorial design.

With more flexible basis sets, the parameters for each event-type combine – sometimes in complex ways – to model the HRF, and the betas for one condition cannot simply be subtracted from another. An omnibus F-test in repeated-measures ANOVA can be used to look for parameter × condition interactions (implemented in some neuroimaging statistics packages, such as SPM2), if care is taken to account for the correlations among parameter estimates. However, this approach carries a cost in power and a problem in interpretability: A significant test statistic implies that the conditions differ in some way, but does not specify in what way (amplitude, latency, shape) they are different. For this reason, one-parameter canonical models remain popular despite their problems – but more sophisticated approaches, such as measuring the height and peak/onset delay from estimated HRFs, have been developed and may be implemented in popular packages soon.

Physiological noise and covariates of no interest

In both PET and fMRI designs, additional predictors are typically added to account for known sources of noise in the data. These are covariates of no interest, and they are included to reduce noise and to prevent signal changes related to head movement and physiological (e.g., respiration) artifacts from influencing the contrast estimates. In PET, a common covariate is the global (whole-brain) mean signal value for each subject, included to control for differences in amount of radioactive tracer in circulation.

In fMRI, the signal can drift slowly over time, as shown in Figure 2.15A. These signals were extracted from the ventricles during an fMRI scan, where there is no tissue, and thus no task-related activation. Though there is noise at all frequencies, the noise has greater amplitude at low frequencies, as shown in the spectral plot of the Fourier transform in Figure 2.15B. The Fourier transform of fMRI noise shows an inverse relationship with the noise frequency, and can be approximated by a $1/f$ (1/frequency) function. Also apparent in these data are spikes of high-power at about 0.15 Hz and 0.34 Hz. These frequencies may correspond approximately to average heart rate and respiration rate aliased back into the task frequencies. Aliasing occurs when a true signal (blue in Figure 2.15C) occurs at more than twice the sampling frequency (red circles in Figure 2.15C), and the apparent frequency (e.g., of the red curve) is "reflected" back to a lower value. The power spectra of the original and aliased signals are shown in Figure 2.15D. In fact, much of the autocorrelated noise in fMRI may come from aliased physiological artifacts (Lund, 2005).

Because of slow drift, it is advantageous to filter out low-frequency noise with a *high-pass filter*. This filtering is often performed in the GLM, by adding covariates of no interest (e.g., low-frequency cosines). Such filtering precludes using designs that vary the task condition at low frequencies. To the degree that the task frequencies overlap with the filtered frequencies, the filter will remove the signal of interest from the data! A good practice is to set the lowest period of the cosine functions modeling the drift to twice that of the experimental period. Other types of commonly used covariates of no interest include the estimated movement parameters and their derivatives/squared values, as well as signals from pulse and respiration sensors.

Extensions of the GLM

Autocorrelation and generalized least squares

One issue with the use of the GLM to analyze imaging data is that it assumes that the observations (images) are all independent of one another. In an fMRI time series, the data are correlated across time and space. This means that the activity in a voxel at one time can be partially determined from the preceding activity, and that there are fewer error degrees of freedom than used in the GLM calculations. Such temporal autocorrelation causes apparent p-values from the GLM to be much smaller than they

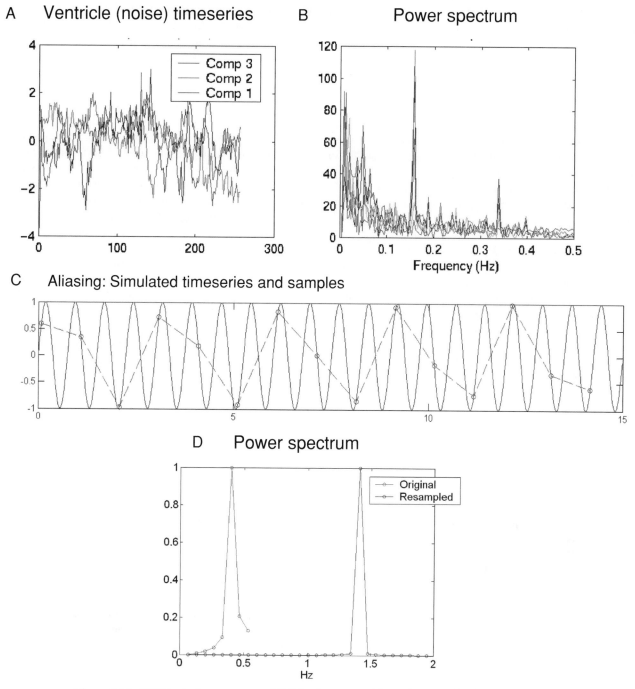

A   Ventricle (noise) timeseries

B   Power spectrum

C   Aliasing: Simulated timeseries and samples

D   Power spectrum

Figure 2.15. (A) Principal components of fMRI noise extracted from the ventricles (fluid spaces) of a single subject. (B) The power spectrum of each component, with frequency on the x-axis and energy on the y-axis. (C) A true signal sampled at a lower temporal resolution (circles), illustrating aliasing. (D) The power spectra of original and estimated signals.

actually are. As a result, inferences about individual subjects cannot be made without correcting for autocorrelation. Group analyses will not be biased by the existence of autocorrelation within individuals, but they will be less powerful than they would be if an appropriate model were used, because the subject-level parameter estimates will be more variable.

There are two basic ways to handle autocorrelation. One way is to estimate the autocorrelation and reduce the degrees of freedom appropriately, for example via the Sattherwaite correction (Neter, 1996). A popular approach using the SPM99 toolbox was to apply temporal smoothing to the data (a low-pass filter, which *introduces* autocorrelation), and then reduce the degrees of freedom based on the applied smoothing. However, a more popular approach recently has been to estimate the autocorrelation and remove it from the data during model fitting. This is called prewhitening because it is an attempt to create "white noise" without temporal structure, and it is statistically efficient (high power) if the autocorrelation is modeled correctly, but it can introduce false positives under certain conditions if the autocorrelation estimates are in error (Friston, 2000).

Prewhitening works by pre-multiplying both sides of the general linear model equation (Eq. 5) by the square root of a filtering matrix W, to create a new design matrix $W^{1/2}X$ and whitened data $W^{1/2}y$. W can stand for 'whitening matrix,' or, as we will see later, more generally for weighting matrix. Just as a properly designed matrix can apply a high-pass or low-pass (smoothing) filter, here the matrix can be used to remove autocorrelation. One way to understand this is to notice that $W^{1/2}X$ is a new linear combination, or weighting, of the predicted values (rows) of X based on the columns of $W^{1/2}$. If the initial predicted responses at each time (in a column of X) are themselves a weighted combination of the current stimulus and past history, then W is designed so that the weights (values) in its rows are the *inverse* of the estimated weights that produced the correlation. Thus, applying $W^{1/2}$ weights the observations so that the autocorrelation is removed. The estimates of the activation magnitudes in this case become:

$$\hat{\beta} = (X^T W X)^{-1} X^T W y \qquad (2.9)$$

This equation describes activation parameter estimation in the generalized least squares (GLS) framework. Several other applications of GLS, including to hierarchical modeling, are described in the following section. The crux of the issue for dealing with autocorrelation is designing the matrix W so that the autocorrelation is removed. A popular approach in SPM2 is to use an AR1 model, which assumes each observation is a weighted combination of the current level of activity plus carryover from the previous time point. This model can account for smooth drift, but not sinusoidal or other oscillating noise structures. Other models allow for influences father back in time (AR2 for two time-points, AR3 for three, and so forth). An approach implemented in VoxBo software is to use an empirically determined autocorrelation function from visual and motor cortex during separate localizer scans to prewhiten the data (Aguirre, 1997). One observation to note is that SPM2 assumes that the autocorrelation (and other parameters such as the covariance and spatial smoothness of the data) is the same everywhere in the brain. FSLs approach implements local (region-by-region) autocorrelation estimates and prewhitening. In principal, if the covariance of the data is given by V, then one should choose $W = V^{-1}$ as the whitening matrix.

We described the W matrix as a weighting matrix above because the form of Equation 9 is not only appropriate for whitening time series data, but it is generally useful whenever cases (observations) should be weighted. Consider the case of the group analysis, in which some subjects' estimates may be much more reliable than others. This may be because the "good" subjects showed consistent task performance, they had strong or regularly shaped HRFs,

the scanner noise was low on the day they were tested, their time series data were more independent of physiological confounds, or for other reasons. In such a case, the $\hat{\beta}$s will be better estimates of the true βs for those subjects, and it is advantageous to weight those cases most highly in the group analysis.

The ability to weight cases based on the intra-subject variance is a primary advantage of using a hierarchical model over the two-level summary statistic approach. Once the intra-subject error terms have been estimated, the individuals with the least certain estimates can be down-weighted in the group analysis. In this case, W is a diagonal matrix whose diagonal elements are $(1/\sigma_G^2 + \sigma^2)$, or the inverse of the sum of intra- and inter-subject variance estimates. The off-diagonals are zero because we assume subjects are independent of one another (the prewhitening matrix has high off-diagonal entries to the degree that the time series is autocorrelated). Group $\hat{\beta}_G$s are estimated using weighted least squares as in Equation 9.

Outliers, artifacts, and robust regression

Statisticians almost universally agree that when performing statistical tests, the data must be examined for outliers and for violations of the statistical assumptions required for inference. Because outliers are far from the group values and the fitting procedure in the GLM minimizes the sum of squared errors, outliers have a disproportionate influence on the group parameter estimates, and they can create violations of the other assumptions. Ideally, the analyst carefully examines the pattern of data and deals with potential outliers on a case-by-case basis.

A major challenge in neuroimaging is that thousands of statistical tests are typically run in parallel, and assumptions are often not checked. Is this a problem? Outliers can cause both null results and false positives, and they may be much more common in imaging data than in many other kinds of data. Simulations performed in our laboratory show that a small proportion of outliers (10% of the sample) can cause a 50% reduction in power over what could be obtained using one of the improved methods described in the following section (Wager, Keller, Lacey, & Jonides, 2005).

Outliers in imaging experiments come from many sources. As mentioned above, some subjects' activation estimates may be more variable than others for a variety of reasons, and some of this variability may be reflected or not in the intra-subject variance. For example, outliers in the individual time series data are regionally specific, very common, and can dramatically influence activation estimates for an individual. These outliers are likely to produce corresponding increases in the variance for that subject. By contrast, errors in the process of normalization, or warping brains into a standard anatomical space, will produce outliers in the group data for a brain region without influencing the intra-subject variance.

Robust regression techniques are a class of statistical tools designed to provide estimates and inferential statistics that are relatively insensitive to the presence of one or more outliers in the data (Huber, 1981; Hubert, 2004; Neter, 1996). They are most appropriate when a large number of regressions are tested and assumptions cannot be evaluated for each individual regression, such as with neuroimaging data. In our work we have compared a number of simple techniques for eliminating or reducing the impact of outliers, focusing mostly on the group analysis level (Wager, Keller, Lacey, & Jonides, 2005). One technique that works well in a variety of situations is iteratively re-weighted least squares (IRLS). It is based on the principle that outliers can be down-weighted rather than dropped altogether, and that outliers can be identified based on how far away they are from the "center of mass" of the data (after accounting for variability explained by the model). The algorithm uses the same weighting scheme used in Equation 9. As with the hierarchical model, the matrix W is a diagonal matrix containing weights for each subject. The regression line and computation of weights based on residual values is iterated until convergence.

Robust regression is a practical tool for group imaging analysis. First, it does not increase the false positive rate under the variety of conditions and types of outliers encountered in imaging studies; and false positive rates are lower than those of the ordinary GLM under some particularly problematic conditions (Wager, Keller, Lacey, & Jonides, 2005). If there are no outliers in a particular brain region, then there is a small cost in power, because the weighting scheme effectively reduces the error degrees of freedom; but the cost is generally relatively minimal compared to the benefits in regions containing outliers. Although running such an analysis on the computers of the 1990s would have been prohibitive in terms of computation time, a consumer-model computer in 2005 can run IRLS on every voxel in the brain in a typical group imaging study in a matter of several hours.

Group analysis

The analysis described so far has been, for fMRI datasets, an analysis of data from a single subject. However, researchers are often interested in making inferences about a population, not just about a single subject or even a set of individual subjects, which requires a group analysis.

There are two main approaches to group analysis that differ in the underlying assumptions that they make and the conclusions that may be drawn from the results of the analysis. The *fixed-effects model* does not model variability across subjects, and the *mixed-effects* (often erroneously referred to as random-effects) *model* provides for inter-subject variability. Only mixed-effects models allow population inference.

Fixed versus mixed effects

Fixed-effects models assume the signal strength is identical in all subjects and the only variation present between subjects is due to measurement error. Early approaches in brain imaging collapsed data across multiple observations within a group of subjects into one large GLM analysis. This approach is a fixed-effects model, because the error variance across subjects is assumed to be fixed rather than modeled as a random variable. The hypothesis tests performed are therefore only about the acquired data and cannot be generalized to a wider population. Early PET analyses seems to have taken a wrong turn early on because of the novelty of the data management problem, but fixed effects analyses are rarely used or considered valid now.

The alternative is to treat the subjects as a random effect, meaning that different subjects may actually respond to the experimental task in a different manner. Mixed effects models assume that the signal strength varies across subjects. In these models there are two sources of variation, the first due to measurement error (as in the fixed-effects model) and the second to differences in the individual's response magnitude. Taking this approach, each subject has a random magnitude that is considered to be drawn from a population with a fixed population mean. By testing observed activation values against estimates of the between-subjects error, can provide a traditional test of significance in a population.

Mechanics of mixed effects and hierarchical models

Both PET and fMRI studies nearly always involve collecting more than one image per subject, and testing for the significance of effects in a group of subjects. The full model can be viewed as being hierarchical in nature, with observations (fMRI signal or PET images) nested within subjects, which are in turn nested within a group, and different random variance components are introduced at each level. In fMRI, typically, separate GLM analyses are conducted on the time series data for each subject at each voxel in the brain to estimate the magnitude of activation evoked by the task. This is called a first-level analysis. These estimates are carried forward and tested for reliability across subjects in a second-level group analysis.

In the *summary statistics* approach, used in SPM99, VoxBo, FSL, AFNI, and often SPM2, a model is fit for each subject. After the effect of interest is defined, a contrast image is constructed for each subject corresponding to this effect. In the second level, a voxel-wise t-test is performed across all of the contrast images. If we have two populations of interest, then a two-sample t-test can be applied at the second level. This approach is simpler than the full hierarchical model, in that it does not explicitly model error at both levels in the second-level analysis. However, it assumes balanced design matrices (e.g., the same design for each subject) and that the within-subject variance is homogeneous across subjects (i.e., no "noisy" subjects). If these assumptions do not hold, a full hierarchical model, discussed in the following section, is more appropriate.

Mathematically, we can describe the second-level analysis in the same way as the first-level GLM discussed earlier. We use X_G to refer to a series of between-subjects predictors. The intercept of this model, which is always included, reflects the mean activity in a population when all other predictors are at zero. If the other predictors are mean-zero, the intercept parameter is the mean activation across subjects. Other predictors in X_G are used to model inter-individual differences (e.g., patients vs. controls, differences in trait anxiety, performance measures, etc.). The vector of the regression slopes (magnitudes) for these effects is β_G, and ε_G is a vector of individual differences not explained by the model. The true activation contrast values for the first-level analysis for each subject are thus a combination of a true population effect plus unexplained individual differences among subjects. The full two-level model can be written:

$$Y = X\beta + \varepsilon$$
$$\beta = X_G\beta_G + \varepsilon_G \qquad (2.10)$$

In particular, note that there are now two sources of noise present in the model, one within subjects and one between subjects.

In the summary statistics approach, we assume that the activation estimates $\hat{\beta}$ are equal to the true values of β. We then run a second GLM, this time with the $\hat{\beta}$s for each subject as the dependent variable and the between-subjects design matrix X_G as predictors. Here the estimate of β_G is dependent on the intermediate estimate $\hat{\beta}$. In the simplest case, a one-sample t-test, $\hat{\beta}$ is an N (subjects) $\times$ 1 vector of estimated activation magnitudes for a condition in one voxel (the group data), X_G is an N $\times$ 1 column of ones (an intercept), and β_G is a single true group activation parameter.

However, in reality $\hat{\beta}$ is not the same as β, because the estimates $\hat{\beta}$ are influenced by the within-subjects (sampling) error as well. To get the full model, we can replace individual subjects' βs (Eq. 5) by a group model consisting of a population parameter β_G plus individual differences ε_G, so that $\beta = X_G\beta_G + \varepsilon_G$. Thus, the full model that relates the predictors to the data for the group of subjects is:

$$y = XX_G\beta_G + X\varepsilon_G + \varepsilon$$
$$= \tilde{X}\beta_G + \gamma \qquad (2.11)$$

where $\tilde{X} = XX_G$ and $\gamma = X\varepsilon_G + \varepsilon$. The error γ is now composed of two parts – individual difference values ε_G that cannot be explained by the model and error values ε based on the sampling error within subjects. Collecting more data per subject can minimize the within-subjects error variance σ^2, (based on ε) but cannot reduce the between-subjects error variance σ_G^2, based on ε_G. Collecting more subjects can reduce the standard error based on ε_G.

If we solve the equation above for β_G, in the full model we get a solution that depends directly on the data y, and not on the intermediate values $\hat{\beta}$. It can be shown that a single-level GLM can be decomposed into an equivalent two-level version if both the $\hat{\beta}$s and their *covariance* are passed down from the first level. Beckmann et al. (Beckmann, Jenkinson, & Smith, 2003) have applied hierarchical modeling to fMRI, and it is implemented in the increasingly popular FILM (fMRIB Improved Linear Model) package as part of the fMRIB Software Library

(FSL; Smith et al., 2004). Hierarchical modeling is also possible in SPM2, though the summary statistics approach is often used in practice (Friston, Stephan, Lund, Morcom, & Kiebel, 2005).

In practice, the relative contribution of the within- and between-subjects error is unknown, and variance components must be estimated. In SPM2 the variance components are estimated using Restricted Maximum Likelihood (ReML) The ReML estimates are calculated using only data from responsive voxels, which are voxels with large F-statistics in a standard pre-analysis of the data, and pooled across those voxels.

Statistical power and sample size

Statistical power rests on having a large activation response (high contrast values) and a low standard error. In a group study, the standard error comes from two sources: variability across subjects (ε_G) and the variability within each subject (ε). At the group level, power can be increased by increasing the sample size, improving methods for selecting comparable brain regions across subjects (e.g., normalization, ROI selection), or testing a more homogenous population (at the cost of generalization to other populations).

What sample size is adequate? This depends on the effect size in the group and scanner noise and signal optimization, and it is different for each task and each brain voxel (Zarahn & Slifstein, 2001); (Desmond & Glover, 2002). Using a large group effect size by conventional standards (Cohen's d = 1) and a simple Bonferroni correction for multiple comparisons (described in the following section) over 30,000 voxels, we can get an idea of what sample size is adequate. As Figure 2.16 shows, the chances of finding a truly activated voxel with n = 10 are virtually zero. With n = 20, power is still less than 10%, but with 30 and 40 subjects, the power increases to. 35 and .7, respectively.

For a given true group effect size and sample size, power depends on the within-subjects standard error, ($se(C^T\hat{\beta})$). As shown in Equation 8, the within-subjects standard error depends on the design matrix (X) and the residual variance, σ. σ can be reduced by optimizing data collection (e.g., pulse sequences and hardware) and in the study design by maximizing the engagement of subjects in the tasks.

However, because the standard error depends on the design matrix (X), power can also be substantially increased by carefully choosing the number, sequence, and spacing of events to minimize the design-related component of the standard error, $C^T(X^TX)^{-1}C$ in Equation 8. Variance in the predicted response and orthogonality in the predicted responses for different events both make a statistically powerful experimental design (Liu, 2004). This is particularly critical in event-related fMRI, where delayed HRFs, overlapping responses, and autocorrelation contribute in complex ways to the overall error. It is possible to build a design in which effects can never be

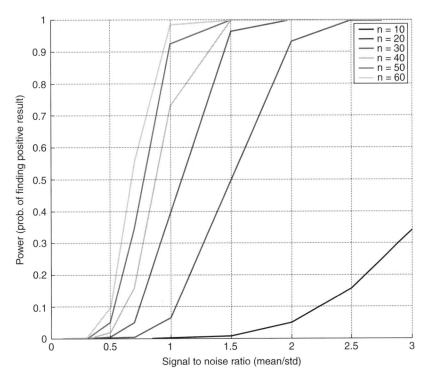

Figure 2.16. Power, or the probability of detecting activation in a truly activated voxel, as a function of effect size (Cohen's d, x-axis) and sample size (lines), using Bonferroni correction for 30,000 voxels. The search area corresponds roughly to a whole-brain search over gray matter only with 3.5 × 3.5 × 5 mm voxel sizes.

detected, even if they actually exist! For this reason, many researchers choose to use computer-aided designs to optimize sequences of trials so that the power to estimate contrasts of interest may be maximized (Buracas & Boynton, 2002; Wager & Nichols, 2003).

Both theory and simulations show that there is a substantial tradeoff in power between *detecting* activation differences between conditions using an assumed HRF shape and estimating the *shape* of evoked activations with a more flexible model (Liu, 2001). This tradeoff is shown in Figure 2.17, in which shape-estimation power is shown on the x-axis and contrast-detection power is shown on the y-axis. The points in the model represent designs with different sequences and timing of events. Blocked designs have the highest detection power, but provide little information about the shape of the response. M-sequences, or sequences that are orthogonal to themselves shifted in time, provide optimal shape estimation power (the nonoptimality in the figure is due to truncation of the m-sequences so they are imperfect), but low detection power (Buracas & Boynton, 2002). Random event-related designs are in between. As the Figure shows, designs optimized with a genetic algorithm (Wager & Nichols, 2003) can produce substantially better results than random designs on both measures.

Bayesian inference

Recently, Bayesian methods have received a great deal of attention in fMRI literature. Bayesian inferential methods are now key components in several major fMRI analysis software packages (e.g., SPM and FSL). Hearkening back to our discussion on inference, we made the

point that P(Activation|Task state), or the probability of observing activation given a task state, is not the same as P(Task|Activation). Bayesian statistics differ from classical statistics in that the unknown true population parameters β are considered to be random variables rather than fixed constants, and what is assessed is $P(\beta \mid y)$, where y is the observed data. According to Bayes's rule (Eq. 4), the probability of activation $P(\beta \mid y)$ is a combination of the likelihood of observing the data and a subjective prior belief about the parameter. This combination is called the posterior distribution, and can be written:

$$P(\beta \mid y) \propto P(y \mid \beta)P(\beta) \qquad (2.12)$$

Here $P(\beta \mid y)$ denotes the posterior, $P(\beta)$ the prior and $P(y \mid \beta)$ the likelihood function. Because these are probability distributions, and β takes on a distribution of values, specifying priors involves specifying multiple parameters of the prior distribution, such as the mean and variance, as well as its distributional form. Note that if we were simply to find the values of $\hat{\beta}$ that maximize the likelihood of the observed data, we would obtain the maximum likelihood estimator (MLE) used in classical inference.

The posterior mean or mode is often used as a parameter estimate, that is, we can estimate β using $\hat{\beta} = E(\beta)$, where E denotes expected value. However, it is often difficult to calculate the exact form of the posterior distribution, and Bayesian inference therefore often requires the numerical evaluation of complicated integrals or sums. Techniques such as Markov-chain Monte-Carlo (MCMC) and Variational Bayes (VB) are used to make relevant numerical calculations about the posterior (Penny et al. 2003, Penny et al. 2004, Woolrich et al. 2005). An excellent overview

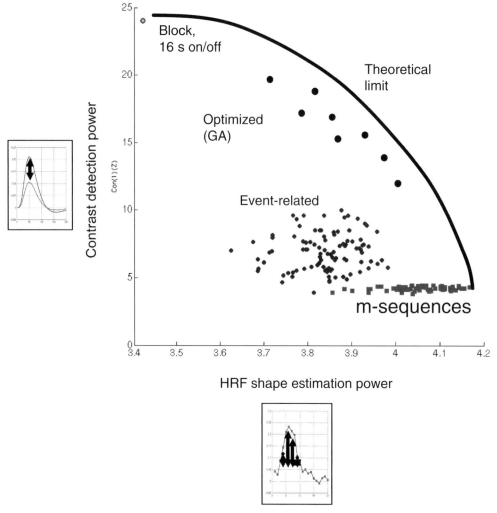

Figure 2.17. The tradeoff between contrast detection and HRF shape estimation power, and the performance of different types of designs on each. Power is expressed here in terms of z-scores in a simulated group analysis (n = 10, effect sizes estimated from visual cortex data in Wager et al., 2005). Yellow circle: an optimal-periodicity block design is shown in yellow. Blue circles: Randomized event-related designs. Red squares: m-sequences. Open circles: genetic algorithm (GA) optimized designs.

of Bayesian statistics can be found in Gelman et al. (2004).

As mentioned above, Bayesian methods require the definition of prior probabilities, and the choice of priors is crucial. Inference is based on a combination of evidence from the observed data and pre-existing beliefs. If strong priors are chosen, the resulting activation maps may reflect prior beliefs more than the story told by the data. If one does not want to impose such beliefs, then it is possible to use *non-informative priors*. This is an approach taken by some neuroimaging applications, for example, FSL, which implements a fully Bayesian approach towards multi-subject analysis with non-informative priors (Woolrich, 2004). For the single-level model this leads to parameter estimates that are equivalent to those obtained using classical inference. Without informative priors, it is unclear whether the Bayesian approach confers an advantage over the classical approach, although the ability to specify priors makes the Bayesian framework more flexible. Another way to choose

prior beliefs is by estimating them from data. This is the empirical Bayes approach. It is a hybrid between classical and Bayesian inference that is used in the SPM2 software (Friston, 2002; Friston, 2002).

Taking a Bayesian approach allows us to calculate the probability that the activation exceeds some specific threshold, given the data (Penny, 2003). Posterior probability maps (PPMs), for example in SPM2, are images depicting these probabilities. In a fully Bayesian framework, there is no hypothesis test and there are no false positives or multiple comparisons problem because one never rejects a null hypothesis. However, if PPM maps are thresholded (e.g., at 0.95) and one wants to infer that some voxels were actually activated by the task, then a hypothesis test is conducted and false positives again become an issue. It is hard to imagine a case where researchers would not want to conclude that some regions were activated by a task, so this theoretical advantage does not translate into a practical advantage.

One place Bayesian methods may be advantageous is in specifying spatial priors on the regression coefficients (Penny, 2005) that incorporate prior knowledge that the evoked responses are both spatially contiguous and locally homogenous.

Multivariate analysis

The massively univariate GLM approach treats each voxel as a separate dependent measure, but it is perhaps more natural to think of brain activity in terms of time-varying processes that are distributed across the brain. Likewise, it seems natural to think of psychological processes as emerging from the *interactions* among a set of brain regions – a concept that is not captured in the univariate approach. Multivariate methods such as those described in the following section generally model the data by decomposing a large dataset (1000 time points × 100,000 voxels × 20 subjects) into a smaller set of *components* and a series of *weights*. The components may be canonical patterns of activity across time and the weights their distribution across brain space, or the other way around.

Such approaches include Principal Components Analysis (PCA), Independent Components Analysis (ICA), Canonical Variate Analysis (CVA), Partial Least Squares (PLS), Factor Analysis, and the Multivariate Linear Model (MLM). They all share the common core idea of decomposition into simpler components that maximize the amount of variability explained by the model. The approaches differ in the criteria used to select and rotate components, and in whether the experimental design is included as part of the data to be modeled.

In practice, an additional important distinction is whether the techniques are used to model the timeseries data within a participant, trials within a participant, or the individual differences in activation across participants. The interpretation of the results is very different depending on which of these types of data is used. Timeseries data can provide evidence on dynamic functional and effective connectivity across time (Mechelli, Penny, Price, Gitelman, & Friston, 2002). Trial-level data can be used to relate brain activity with performance or emotion within subjects (Rissman, Gazzaley, & D'Esposito, 2004). And individual difference data can characterize patterns of individual differences across the brain, that is, the tendency of a particular type of subject to activate a distributed attention network (Habeck et al., 2005; Lin et al., 2003). (As a note of caution, such data is often misinterpreted as reflecting dynamic connectivity).

Though the potential for new information offered by dynamic connectivity makes this type of analysis very appealing, special concerns must be taken to prevent observed patterns from being dominated by timeseries artifacts (Lund, 2001). In addition, for most dynamic connectivity applications, it is critical to provide population-level inference by treating subjects as a random effect, as in the GLM above. Freely available toolboxes exist that can perform this type of analysis – two notable ones are the GIFT package (Calhoun, Adali, & Pekar, 2004) and the tensor-ICA routines in FSL (Beckmann & Smith, 2005).

Another important distinction is between *hypothesis-driven* and *data-driven* approaches. The GLM approach is hypothesis driven, because one seeks to find regions that fit a particular predicted model. Most multivariate approaches (e.g., PCA, ICA, FA) are data-driven, in that they simplify or reduce the data into components without reference to a predictive model (i.e., the design matrix, X). Usually, the multivariate analysis is used to generate components, and then those components are tested for relationships with X (Beckmann & Smith, 2004).

Another approach is to include X in the set of data to be reduced, or to decompose the covariance between the data and the model into components. This approach has the potential to pick out specifically those components that are task-related, but has the potential to capitalize on chance variations in the signal, and thus simulations or permutation methods must be used to control the false positive rate. Partial least squares (McIntosh, Chau, & Protzner, 2004) and semi-blind ICA are examples of this approach (Calhoun, Adali, Stevens, Kiehl, & Pekar, 2005).

Mechanics of multivariate analysis

Each technique described in this section decomposes a matrix of data, Y, into a set of spatial and temporal components. Y is a $[t \times v]$ matrix, with t time points (observations) and v voxels. Each column of Y is the timeseries of one voxel in the brain.

Principal Components Analysis (PCA) decomposes the data by finding linear combinations of timeseries, each a column in matrix U (also of dimension $t \times v$), such that each column of U is uncorrelated with (orthogonal to) every other column of U. The columns of U, called components, are arranged in order of variance explained: the first component explains the most variance possible in Y, the second component explains the maximal amount of remaining variance, and so forth. Together with their spatial maps and variances (described in the following section) these v components perfectly reproduce the data, but most of the total variance is usually captured in just the first few components of U. Thus, the first components are a compressed representation of the data.

Because each component is a weighted sum across timeseries of different voxels, another matrix V (of dimension voxel x component, $[v \times v]$) contains columns of voxel weights used to create each component in U. For example, the first column of V shows how to weight each of the v voxel timeseries in order to capture the most variance in Y, and represents the spatial distribution of the first component. Thus, the columns of U are the temporal components (the canonical timeseries) and those of V are the spatial components (the maps across brain voxels) of these timeseries.

If we think of each voxel as being a variable with its own axis, the weights V describe a rotation of the data Y such that the columns of YV – the new component scores – fall along the axes of greatest covariance across voxels. An algebraic solution for V is given by the eigendecomposition of the covariance matrix of Y, which finds a matrix of eigenvectors V and eigenvalues (weights for V) λ such that $\text{cov}(Y)V = \lambda V$. That is, rotating V by cov(Y) is equivalent to scaling V by scalar weights λ, because V lie along the principal axes of cov(Y). The weights λ are the variances of each component.

In neuroimaging, the components are usually calculated through singular value decomposition (SVD) of the centered (mean-zero) data. SVD is a more general form of PCA that decomposes the data into temporal components U and spatial components V such that:

$$Y = USV^T \qquad (2.13)$$

With centered (mean-zero) data, S is a diagonal matrix (only the diagonal elements are non-zero) whose entries are the singular values, the sums of squared deviations explained by each component. These are related to the eigenvalues such that $\lambda = S^2/(t-1)$. The columns of V are the eigenvectors, as in the eigendecomposition described above, and US are the component scores (components scaled by the amount of variability they explain), equal to YV in the eigendecomposition. A thorough treatment of eigenvectors, eigenvalues, and SVD is provided by Strang (1988).

Once one grasps the central idea of data decomposition into spatial and temporal components, many other techniques can be understood as variations on this theme. Independent Components Analysis (ICA), for example, is a variant of this technique. Rather than maximizing explained variance, the components are chosen to maximize the statistical independence of the components in a more general sense. The components are not required to be orthogonal; rather, the constraint is that the distribution of one component cannot be predicted from the values of the other, and the joint probability P(A,B) of components A and B is equal to P(A)P(B). In the Infomax variant, mutual information between components (a general measure of relationship that is not necessarily linear or monotonic) is minimized (McKeown 1998a). In broad terms, ICA assumes that Y, is a weighted sum of a number of source signals (timeseries), contained in X. The data Y is a linear mixture of these source components described by the weighting or *mixing matrix* of spatial weights M:

$$Y = MX \qquad (2.14)$$

There is no algebraic solution, so iterative search algorithms are used to estimate both M and X. An alternative decomposition is to transpose the data matrix and treat the spatial components as sources and the temporal components as mixing weights. For more details, we refer the reader to (Bell & Sejnowski, 1995; McKeown & Sejnowski, 1998; McKeown et al., 1998; Petersson, Nichols, Poline, & Holmes, 1999b; Petersson, Nichols, Poline, & Holmes, 1999a).

Both PCA and ICA simply reduce the data to a simpler (lower-dimension than that of the v voxels) space by capturing the most prominent variations across the set of voxels. The components may reflect signals of interest or they may be dominated by artifacts, and it is up to the user to determine which are of interest (e.g., task-related). In ICA the order of importance of the independent components cannot be determined. Hence, it is necessary to sift through all of the components to search for ones that are task-related or otherwise of interest. However, both ICA and PCA assume all variability results from signal (noise is not modeled). A popular variant in the social sciences literature is factor analysis, which additionally fits a parameter for the noise (unexplained) variance at each voxel. However, a disadvantage of factor analysis is that the solution is *rotationally indeterminate*, and thus a number of combinations of spatial and temporal components can explain the same variability in the data. Although both ICA and PCA are not rotationally indeterminate, there is some question as to what the "right" rotation is (in PCA it is determined by variance explained). Interpreting thresholded component maps, as is commonly done, depends critically on establishing a rotation that is meaningful and reliable across studies.

These techniques as described so far model only a single subject's data. In a group study there is the additional complexity of making population inference. It is not correct to treat all the data as coming from one super-subject and decomposing the group data matrix, for the same reasons that fixed effects analyses in the GLM are not appropriate. One approach is to decompose the group matrix, and subsequently back-reconstruct or estimate spatial weights for each subject for a component of interest (Calhoun, Adali, Pearlson, & Pekar, 2001). The spatial weights at each voxel across subjects are treated as random variables, and one-sample t-test is conducted to test whether that voxel loaded significantly on that component in the group. Another approach, called *tensor ICA*, is to use a three-way decomposition, using the group data to estimate temporal components and weights for each subject and each voxel (Beckmann & Smith, 2005). The subject weights at each voxel are then tested for significance.

Thresholding and multiple comparisons

As discussed above, the massively univariate approach requires fitting a model at each of many voxels throughout the brain (often 100,000 or more), and constructing maps of the activation statistics and reliability over the brain (statistical parametric maps, or SPMs). In a typical behavioral experiment, test statistics whose p-values are below 0.05 are considered sufficient evidence to reject the null hypothesis, with an acceptable false positive rate (alpha) of 0.05. However, in a neuroimaging experiment, many such tests (e.g., 100,000) are conducted, and a voxel-wise alpha of 0.05 means that 5% of the voxels on average will show false positive results. In our example, that turns out to be 5,000 false positive results. Thus, even if an experiment produces *no true activation*, there is a good chance that without a more conservative correction for multiple comparisons, the activation map will show a number of activated regions, leading to erroneous conclusions.

Many researchers use a more stringent, but arbitrary, threshold of 0.005 or 0.001 to help reduce false positives. The problem with this approach is that the chances of finding at least one false positive is very high, and its exact probability is unknown. It is generally considered desirable to limit the chances of finding a false positive somewhere in the brain to 0.05. This is the family-wise error rate (FWER), the rate at which a statistical test would be expected to produce one or more false positives among a family of tests, under the null hypothesis.

Commonly, researchers impose an additional threshold on extent of activation, requiring k (for example, 5) or more contiguous voxels to be significant at .005 (for example) before considering a region to be significant. This approach does not necessarily control the FWER either. The assumption that the chances of observing 5 contiguous voxels at p < .005 is $.005^5$ (true for independent voxels) is erroneous because imaging data are correlated ("smooth") across space. Without estimating the spatial *smoothness*, one cannot tell what the true probability of observing a contiguous activated cluster of k voxels is under the null hypothesis. Smoothness, number of subjects, and the size of the search volume vary across studies, so the FWER corrected threshold will also be different for different studies.

Another kind of control of the false positive rate is to use the false discovery rate (FDR) control. Imagine that we conduct a study on 100,000 brain voxels at alpha = .001 uncorrected, and we find 300 significant voxels. We expect 100 of them or 33% of our significant discoveries, to be false positives. But which ones they are we cannot tell, and 33% is a substantial proportion. We may want to set a threshold such that only 5% of the significant voxels are expected to be false positives. This is FDR control at the 0.05 level. In this case, we might argue that most of the results are likely to be true activations; however, we will still not be able to tell which voxels are truly activated and which are false positives.

A review of the PET and fMRI literature shows that many investigators use uncorrected thresholds; this is likely because these studies do not have the statistical power to correct for multiple comparisons and still detect a reasonable number (or, indeed, any) of the truly activated areas. This is because as the false positive rate is controlled more conservatively, statistical power decreases. However, from the standpoint of making inferences about regional activation within a study, correcting for multiple comparisons is critical. Without correcting, any of the activations in the study might be simply false, and many such false positive regions are expected. Methods for controlling the FWER and FDR are described briefly in the following section, along with a popular alternative, region-of-interest testing.

FWE correction. The simplest way of controlling the FWER is to use the Bonferroni correction, in which the alpha value is divided by the total number of statistical tests performed (i.e., voxels). However, if there is spatial dependence in the data (as there would be because of spatial smoothing) this is an unnecessarily conservative correction that leads to a decrease in the probability of detecting truly active voxels.

Gaussian Random Field Theory (RFT), used in SPM software, is another approach towards controlling the FWER. If the image is smooth and the number of subjects is relatively high (around 20), RFT is less conservative and provides control closer to the true false positive rate than the Bonferroni method. However, with small samples, RFT is often more conservative than the Bonferroni method. It is acceptable to use the more lenient of the two, as they both control the FWER, which is what SPM currently does. In addition, RFT is used to assess the probability of k contiguous voxels exceeding the threshold under the null hypothesis, leading to a cluster-level correction. Nichols and Hayasaka (T. Nichols & Hayasaka, 2003) provide an excellent review of FWER correction methods, and they find that whereas RFT is overly conservative at the voxel level, it is somewhat too liberal at the cluster level with small sample sizes.

RFT correction begins by estimating the spatial smoothness of the data and the consequent number of independent statistical tests, or *resels* (resolution elements). The number of clusters that should be found solely by chance at a given threshold is known as the Euler characteristic (EC) of the data. The RFT method assumes that the statistic maps are continuous random 3-D fields of values, and so spatial smoothing is often applied (some estimates are three times the voxel dimensions) to satisfy this assumption. In SPM, it also assumes that the smoothness is stationary (does not vary) throughout the brain – an assumption that is often violated.

Both methods described above for controlling the FWER assume that the error values (estimated by the residuals) are normally distributed, and that the variance of the errors is equal across all values of the predictors. Nonparametric methods instead use the data themselves to find the distribution. Using such methods can provide substantial improvements in power and validity, particularly with small sample sizes, and we regard them as the "gold standard" for use in imaging analyses. Thus, these tests can be used to verify the validity of the less computationally expensive parametric approaches.

A popular package for doing non-parametric tests in group analyses, SnPM or Statistical Non-Parametric Mapping (T. E. Nichols & Holmes, 2002), is based on the use of permutation tests. Under the null hypothesis for a one-sample t-test, the signs (+ or −) of the activations are distributed symmetrically around 0. In SnPM, the signs of betas across subjects are permuted, and t-statistics are computed throughout the brain. The maximum t-value from this permuted null hypothesis map is saved, and the simulation is repeated many times (e.g., 10,000) to simulate a distribution of the maximum t-value under the null hypothesis. The 95th percentile of this distribution of maxima is a threshold that provides FWER control at p < .05. Similar permutation tests are available for a variety of types of test, including multiple-condition tests (e.g., ANOVA) and brain-behavior correlations.

FDR control. The false discovery rate (FDR) is a recent development in multiple comparison problems developed by Benjamini and Hochberg (1995). Whereas the FWER controls the probability of any false positives, the FDR controls the proportion of false positives among all rejected tests.

The FDR controlling procedure is adaptive in the sense that the larger the signal, the lower the threshold. If all of the null hypotheses are true, the FDR will be equivalent to the FWER. Any procedure that controls the FWER will also control the FDR. Hence, any procedure that controls the FDR only can be less stringent and lead to a gain in power. A major advantage is that because FDR controlling procedures work only on the p-values and not on the actual test statistics, it can be applied to any valid statistical test.

ROI analysis. Because of the difficulty in preserving both false positive control and power without many subjects, researchers often specify regions-of-interest (ROIs) in which activation is expected before the study is conducted. ROI analyses are conducted variously over the average signal within a region, the peak activation voxel within a region, or – a preferred method – on individually defined anatomical or functional ROIs. Another technique involves testing every voxel within an ROI (e.g., the amygdala) and correcting for the number of voxels in the search volume. This is often referred to as a small-volume correction.

Two important cautions must be mentioned. First, conducting many ROI analyses increases the false positive rate. Although it may be philosophically sound to independently test a small number of areas in which activation is expected, testing many such regions violates the spirit of a priori ROI specification and will lead to an increased false positive rate. Small volume corrections in multiple ROIs also do not preserve the false positive rate across ROIs.

Second, although activated regions can be used as ROIs for subsequent tests, the test used to define the region must be *independent* of the test conducted in that region. Acceptable examples include defining a region based on a main effect and then testing to see of activity in that region is correlated with performance, or using the main effect of (A + B) to define a region and then testing for a difference (A − B). Problematic examples are defining a region activating in older subjects and then testing to see if its activity is reduced in younger subjects or defining a region based on activity in the first run of an experiment and then testing whether it shows less activity in subsequent runs. Both of these are not valid tests because they do not control for regression to the mean.

A final note about uncorrected thresholds. From the standpoint of accumulation of evidence across studies, when testing large samples is impractical, using low thresholds and then using meta-analysis to see which areas are reliably activated makes some sense. Imagine that there are 20 activated regions in a task, and that 50 studies are conducted of the same task. If each study uses FWE correction, the power in each study might be 5%. Each study might be expected to activate 1 of the 20 regions, which one selected at random, and the result would be a literature of 50 papers that show different results, allowing little meaningful aggregation across those studies. Thus, it is a good idea to report results at a reasonable uncorrected threshold (e.g., p < .001 and 10 contiguous voxels) for archival purposes, in addition to reporting corrected results.

ACKNOWLEDGMENTS

We would like to thank Dr. Doug Noll for providing Figure 2.9, and Brent Hughes and Matt Keller for helpful editing.

REFERENCES

Aguirre, G. K., Singh, R., & D'Esposito, M. (1999). Stimulus inversion and the responses of face and object-sensitive cortical areas. *Neuroreport, 10*(1), 189–194.

Aguirre, G. K., Zarahn, E., & D'Esposito, M. (1998). The variability of human, BOLD hemodynamic responses. *Neuroimage, 8*(4), 360–369.

Alsop, D. C., & Detre, J. A. (1996). Reduced transit-time sensitivity in noninvasive magnetic resonance imaging of human cerebral blood flow. *J Cereb Blood Flow Metab, 16*(6), 1236–1249.

Andersson, J. L., Hutton, C., Ashburner, J., Turner, R., & Friston, K. (2001). Modeling geometric deformations in EPI time series. *Neuroimage, 13*(5), 903–919.

Andreasen, N. C., Arndt, S., Swayze, V., 2nd, Cizadlo, T., Flaum, M., O'Leary, D., et al. (1994). Thalamic abnormalities in schizophrenia visualized through magnetic resonance image averaging. *Science, 266*, 294–298.

Aron, A., Fisher, H., Mashek, D. J., Strong, G., Li, H., & Brown, L. L. (2005). Reward, motivation, and emotion systems associated with early-stage intense romantic love. *J Neurophysiol, 94*(1), 327–337.

Bandettini, P. A., Wong, E. C., Hinks, R. S., Tikofsky, R. S., & Hyde, J. S. (1992). Time course EPI of human brain function during task activation. *Magn Reson Med, 25*(2), 390–397.

Beckmann, C. F., & Smith, S. M. (2004). Probabilistic independent component analysis for functional magnetic resonance imaging. *IEEE Trans Med Imaging, 23*(2), 137–152.

Beckmann, C. F., & Smith, S. M. (2005). Tensorial extensions of independent component analysis for multisubject FMRI analysis. *Neuroimage, 25*(1), 294–311.

Bendriem, B., Townsend, D.W. (1998). *The theory and practice of 3D PET*. (Vol. 32). Boston: Dordrecht; Kluwer Academic, 1998.

Birn, R. M., Saad, Z. S., & Bandettini, P. A. (2001). Spatial heterogeneity of the nonlinear dynamics in the FMRI BOLD response. *Neuroimage, 14*(4), 817–826.

Buckner, R. L., Koutstaal, W., Schacter, D. L., Dale, A. M., Rotte, M., & Rosen, B. R. (1998). Functional-anatomic study of episodic retrieval. II. Selective averaging of event-related fMRI trials to test the retrieval success hypothesis. *Neuroimage, 7*(3), 163–175.

Buracas, G. T., & Boynton, G. M. (2002). Efficient design of event-related fMRI experiments using M-sequences. *Neuroimage, 16*(3 Pt 1), 801–813.

Burock, M. A., Buckner, R. L., Woldorff, M. G., Rosen, B. R., & Dale, A. M. (1998). Randomized event-related experimental designs allow for extremely rapid presentation rates using functional MRI. *Neuroreport, 9*(16), 3735–3739.

Bush, G., Luu, P., & Posner, M. I. (2000). Cognitive and emotional influences in anterior cingulate cortex. *Trends in Cognitive Sciences, 4*(6), 215–222. [Record as supplied by publisher].

Buxton, R. B., & Frank, L. R. (1997). A model for the coupling between cerebral blood flow and oxygen metabolism during neural stimulation. *J Cereb Blood Flow Metab, 17*(1), 64–72.

Buxton, R. B., Uludag, K., Dubowitz, D. J., & Liu, T. T. (2004). Modeling the hemodynamic response to brain activation. *Neuroimage, 23 Suppl 1*, S220–233.

Calhoun, V. D., Adali, T., Pearlson, G. D., & Pekar, J. J. (2001). A method for making group inferences from functional MRI data using independent component analysis. *Hum Brain Mapp, 14*(3), 140–151.

Calhoun, V. D., Adali, T., & Pekar, J. J. (2004). A method for comparing group fMRI data using independent component analysis: application to visual, motor and visuomotor tasks. *Magn Reson Imaging, 22*(9), 1181–1191.

Calhoun, V. D., Adali, T., Stevens, M. C., Kiehl, K. A., & Pekar, J. J. (2005). Semi-blind ICA of fMRI: A method for utilizing hypothesis-derived time courses in a spatial ICA analysis. *Neuroimage, 25*(2), 527–538.

Constable, R. T., & Spencer, D. D. (1999). Composite image formation in z-shimmed functional MR imaging. *Magn Reson Med, 42*(1), 110–117.

D'Esposito, M., Zarahn, E., Aguirre, G. K., & Rypma, B. (1999). The effect of normal aging on the coupling of neural activity to the bold hemodynamic response. *Neuroimage, 10*(1), 6–14.

Dagher, A., Owen, A. M., Boecker, H., & Brooks, D. J. (1999). Mapping the network for planning: a correlational PET activation study with the Tower of London task. *Brain, 122*(Pt 10), 1973–1987.

Dale, A. M., & Buckner, R. L. (1997). Selective averaging of rapidly presented individual trials using fMRI. *Human Brain Mapping, 5*, 329–340.

de Quervain, D. J., Fischbacher, U., Treyer, V., Schellhammer, M., Schnyder, U., Buck, A., et al. (2004). The neural basis of altruistic punishment. *Science, 305*(5688), 1254–1258.

Duann, J. R., Jung, T. P., Kuo, W. J., Yeh, T. C., Makeig, S., Hsieh, J. C., et al. (2002). Single-trial variability in event-related BOLD signals. *Neuroimage, 15*(4), 823–835.

Duong, T. Q., Yacoub, E., Adriany, G., Hu, X., Ugurbil, K., Vaughan, J. T., et al. (2002). High-resolution, spin-echo BOLD, and CBF fMRI at 4 and 7 T. *Magn Reson Med, 48*(4), 589–593.

Eisenberger, N. I., Lieberman, M. D., & Williams, K. D. (2003). Does rejection hurt? An FMRI study of social exclusion. *Science, 302*(5643), 290–292.

Elster, A. D. (1994). *Questions and answers in magnetic resonance imaging.* St. Louis, MO: Mosby.

Elster, A. D., Link, K. M., & Carr, J. J. (1994). Patient screening prior to MR imaging: a practical approach synthesized from protocols at 15 U. S. medical centers. *AJR Am J Roentgenol, 162*(1), 195–199.

Fan, J., Flombaum, J. I., McCandliss, B. D., Thomas, K. M., & Posner, M. I. (2003). Cognitive and brain consequences of conflict. *Neuroimage, 18*(1), 42–57.

Frackowiak, R. S. (1997). *Human brain function.* San Diego, CA: Academic Press.

Friston, K. J., Frith, C. D., Turner, R., & Frackowiak, R. S. (1995). Characterizing evoked hemodynamics with fMRI. *Neuroimage, 2*(2), 157–165.

Friston, K. J., Glaser, D. E., Henson, R. N., Kiebel, S., Phillips, C., & Ashburner, J. (2002). Classical and Bayesian inference in neuroimaging: applications. *Neuroimage, 16*(2), 484–512.

Friston, K. J., Josephs, O., Rees, G., & Turner, R. (1998). Nonlinear event-related responses in fMRI. *Magn Reson Med, 39*(1), 41–52.

Friston, K. J., Mechelli, A., Turner, R., & Price, C. J. (2000). Nonlinear responses in fMRI: the Balloon model, Volterra kernels, and other hemodynamics. *Neuroimage, 12*(4), 466–477.

Friston, K. J., Stephan, K. E., Lund, T. E., Morcom, A., & Kiebel, S. (2005). Mixed-effects and fMRI studies. *Neuroimage, 24*(1), 244–252.

Glover, G. H. (1999). Deconvolution of impulse response in event-related BOLD fMRI. *Neuroimage, 9*(4), 416–429.

Goutte, C., Nielsen, F. A., & Hansen, L. K. (2000). Modeling the haemodynamic response in fMRI using smooth FIR filters. *IEEE Trans Med Imaging, 19*(12), 1188–1201.

Habeck, C., Krakauer, J. W., Ghez, C., Sackeim, H. A., Eidelberg, D., Stern, Y., et al. (2005). A new approach to spatial covariance modeling of functional brain imaging data: ordinal trend analysis. *Neural Comput, 17*(7), 1602–1645.

Hoge, R. D., Atkinson, J., Gill, B., Crelier, G. R., Marrett, S., & Pike, G. B. (1999). Investigation of BOLD signal dependence on cerebral blood flow and oxygen consumption: the deoxyhemoglobin dilution model. *Magn Reson Med, 42*(5), 849–863.

Huber, P. J. (1981). *Robust Statistics.* New York: Wiley-Interscience.

Hubert, M., Rosseeuw, P. J., & Val Aelst, S. (2004). Robustness. In B. Sundt & J. Teugels (Eds.), *Encyclopedia of Actuarial Sciences.* New York: Wiley.

Huettel, S. A., et al. (2004). *Functional Magnetic Resonance Imaging.* Sunderland, Mass: Sinauer Associates.

Johansen-Berg, H., Behrens, T. E., Robson, M. D., Drobnjak, I., Rushworth, M. F., Brady, J. M., et al. (2004). Changes in connectivity profiles define functionally distinct regions in human medial frontal cortex. *Proc Natl Acad Sci U S A, 101*(36), 13335–13340.

Kanwisher, N., McDermott, J., & Chun, M. M. (1997). The fusiform face area: A module in human extrastriate cortex specialized for face perception. *J Neuroscience, 17*(11), 4302–4311.

Kastner, S., & Ungerleider, L. G. (2000). Mechanisms of visual attention in the human cortex. *Annu Rev Neurosci, 23*, 315–341.

Kim, S. G. (1995). Quantification of relative cerebral blood flow change by flow-sensitive alternating inversion recovery (FAIR) technique: application to functional mapping. *Magn Reson Med, 34*(3), 293–301.

Koepp, M. J. (1998). Evidence for striatal dopamine release during a video game. *Nature, 393*(21 May), 266–268.

Kwong, K. K., Belliveau, J. W., Chesler, D. A., Goldberg, I. E., Weisskoff, R. M., Poncelet, B. P., et al. (1992). Dynamic magnetic resonance imaging of human brain activity during primary sensory stimulation. *Proc Natl Acad Sci U S A, 89*(12), 5675–5679.

Liao, C. H., Worsley, K. J., Poline, J. B., Aston, J. A., Duncan, G. H., & Evans, A. C. (2002). Estimating the delay of the fMRI response. *Neuroimage, 16*(3 Pt 1), 593–606.

Lin, F. H., McIntosh, A. R., Agnew, J. A., Eden, G. F., Zeffiro, T. A., & Belliveau, J. W. (2003). Multivariate analysis of neuronal interactions in the generalized partial least squares framework: simulations and empirical studies. *Neuroimage, 20*(2), 625–642.

Liu, T. T. (2004). Efficiency, power, and entropy in event-related fMRI with multiple trial types. Part II: design of experiments. *Neuroimage, 21*(1), 401–413.

Lund, T. E. (2001). fcMRI – mapping functional connectivity or correlating cardiac-induced noise? *Magn Reson Med, 46*(3), 628–629.

Maguire, E. A., Gadian, D. G., Johnsrude, I. S., Good, C. D., Ashburner, J., Frackowiak, R. S., et al. (2000). Navigation-related structural change in the hippocampi of taxi drivers. *Proc Natl Acad Sci U S A, 97*(8), 4398–4403.

McIntosh, A. R., Chau, W. K., & Protzner, A. B. (2004). Spatiotemporal analysis of event-related fMRI data using partial least squares. *Neuroimage, 23*(2), 764–775.

Mechelli, A., Penny, W. D., Price, C. J., Gitelman, D. R., & Friston, K. J. (2002). Effective connectivity and intersubject variability: using a multisubject network to test differences and commonalities. *Neuroimage, 17*(3), 1459–1469.

Menon, R. S., Luknowsky, D. C., & Gati, J. S. (1998). Mental chronometry using latency-resolved functional MRI. *Proc Natl Acad Sci U S A, 95*(18), 10902–10907.

Miezin, F. M., Maccotta, L., Ollinger, J. M., Petersen, S. E., & Buckner, R. L. (2000). Characterizing the hemodynamic response: effects of presentation rate, sampling procedure, and the possibility of ordering brain activity based on relative timing. *Neuroimage, 11*(6 Pt 1), 735–759.

Neter, J., Kutner, M. H., Wasserman, W., & Nachtsheim, C. J. (1996). *Applied Linear Statistical Models* (4 ed.): McGraw-Hill/Irwin.

Nichols, T., Brett, M., Andersson, J., Wager, T., & Poline, J. B. (2005). Valid conjunction inference with the minimum statistic. *Neuroimage, 25*(3), 653–660.

Nichols, T., & Hayasaka, S. (2003). Controlling the familywise error rate in functional neuroimaging: a comparative review. *Stat Methods Med Res, 12*(5), 419–446.

Nichols, T. E., & Holmes, A. P. (2002). Nonparametric permutation tests for functional neuroimaging: a primer with examples. *Hum Brain Mapp, 15*(1), 1–25.

Noll, D. C., Fessler, J. A., & Sutton, B. P. (2005). Conjugate phase MRI reconstruction with spatially variant sample density correction. *IEEE Trans Med Imaging, 24*(3), 325–336.

Ogawa, S., Lee, T. M., Kay, A. R., & Tank, D. W. (1990). Brain magnetic resonance imaging with contrast dependent on blood oxygenation. *Proc Natl Acad Sci U S A, 87*(24), 9868–9872.

Ollinger, J. M., Shulman, G. L., & Corbetta, M. (2001). Separating processes within a trial in event-related functional MRI. *Neuroimage, 13*(1), 210–217.

Paus, T. (2001). Primate anterior cingulate cortex: where motor control, drive and cognition interface. *Nat Rev Neurosci, 2*(6), 417–424.

Paus, T., Koski, L., Caramanos, Z., & Westbury, C. (1998). Regional differences in the effects of task difficulty and motor output on blood flow response in the human anterior cingulate cortex: a review of 107 PET activation studies. *Neuroreport, 9*(9), R37–47.

Pawlik, G., Rackl, A., & Bing, R. J. (1981). Quantitative capillary topography and blood flow in the cerebral cortex of cats: an in vivo microscopic study. *Brain Res, 208*(1), 35–58.

Peled, S., Gudbjartsson, H., Westin, C. F., Kikinis, R., & Jolesz, F. A. (1998). Magnetic resonance imaging shows orientation and asymmetry of white matter fiber tracts. *Brain Res, 780*(1), 27–33.

Penny, W. D., Stephan, K. E., Mechelli, A., & Friston, K. J. (2004). Modelling functional integration: a comparison of structural equation and dynamic causal models. *Neuroimage, 23 Suppl 1*, S264–274.

Petersen, S. E., Fox, P. T., Posner, M. I., Mintun, M., & Raichle, M. E. (1988). Positron emission tomographic studies of the cortical anatomy of single-word processing. *Nature, 331*(6157), 585–589.

Pfeuffer, J., Adriany, G., Shmuel, A., Yacoub, E., Van De Moortele, P. F., Hu, X., et al. (2002). Perfusion-based high-resolution functional imaging in the human brain at 7 Tesla. *Magn Reson Med, 47*(5), 903–911.

Phan, K. L., Taylor, S. F., Welsh, R. C., Ho, S. H., Britton, J. C., & Liberzon, I. (2004). Neural correlates of individual ratings of emotional salience: a trial-related fMRI study. *Neuroimage, 21*(2), 768–780.

Posner, M. I., Petersen, S. E., Fox, P. T., & Raichle, M. E. (1988). Localization of cognitive operations in the human brain. *Science, 240*(4859), 1627–1631.

Price, C. J., Veltman, D. J., Ashburner, J., Josephs, O., & Friston, K. J. (1999). The critical relationship between the timing of stimulus presentation and data acquisition in blocked designs with fMRI. *Neuroimage, 10*(1), 36–44.

Reiman, E. M., Fusselman, M. J., Fox, P. T., & Raichle, M. E. (1989). Neuroanatomical correlates of anticipatory anxiety [published erratum appears in Science 1992 Jun 19;256(5064):1696]. *Science, 243*(4894 Pt 1), 1071–1074.

Riera, J. J., Watanabe, J., Kazuki, I., Naoki, M., Aubert, E., Ozaki, T., et al. (2004). A state-space model of the hemodynamic approach: nonlinear filtering of BOLD signals. *Neuroimage, 21*(2), 547–567.

Rissman, J., Gazzaley, A., & D'Esposito, M. (2004). Measuring functional connectivity during distinct stages of a cognitive task. *Neuroimage, 23*(2), 752–763.

Roebroeck, A., Formisano, E., & Goebel, R. (2005). Mapping directed influence over the brain using Granger causality and fMRI. *Neuroimage, 25*(1), 230–242.

Rosen, B. R., Buckner, R. L., & Dale, A. M. (1998). Event-related functional MRI: past, present, and future. *Proc Natl Acad Sci U S A, 95*(3), 773–780.

Sandler, M. P. (2003). *Diagnostic nuclear medicine*. Philadelphia, PA: Lippincott / Williams & Wilkins.

Sarter, M., Berntson, G. G., & Cacioppo, J. T. (1996). Brain imaging and cognitive neuroscience. Toward strong inference in attributing function to structure. *Am Psychol, 51*(1), 13–21.

Schacter, D. L., Buckner, R. L., Koutstaal, W., Dale, A. M., & Rosen, B. R. (1997). Late onset of anterior prefrontal activity during true and false recognition: an event-related fMRI study. *Neuroimage, 6*(4), 259–269.

Shulman, R. G., & Rothman, D. L. (1998). Interpreting functional imaging studies in terms of neurotransmitter cycling. *Proc Natl Acad Sci U S A, 95*(20), 11993–11998.

Shulman, R. G., Rothman, D. L., Behar, K. L., & Hyder, F. (2004). Energetic basis of brain activity: implications for neuroimaging. *Trends Neurosci, 27*(8), 489–495.

Sibson, N. R., Dhankhar, A., Mason, G. F., Behar, K. L., Rothman, D. L., & Shulman, R. G. (1997). In vivo 13C NMR measurements of cerebral glutamine synthesis as evidence for glutamate-glutamine cycling. *Proc Natl Acad Sci U S A, 94*(6), 2699–2704.

Silva, A. C., Zhang, W., Williams, D. S., & Koretsky, A. P. (1995). Multi-slice MRI of rat brain perfusion during amphetamine stimulation using arterial spin labeling. *Magn Reson Med, 33*(2), 209–214.

Skudlarski, P., Constable, R. T., & Gore, J. C. (1999). ROC analysis of statistical methods used in functional MRI: individual subjects. *Neuroimage, 9*(3), 311–329.

Smith, S. M., Jenkinson, M., Woolrich, M. W., Beckmann, C. F., Behrens, T. E., Johansen-Berg, H., et al. (2004). Advances in functional and structural MR image analysis and implementation as FSL. *Neuroimage, 23 Suppl 1*, S208–219.

Sternberg, S. (1969). Memory-scanning: mental processes revealed by reaction-time experiments. *Am Sci, 57*(4), 421–457.

Valenstein, E. (1973). *Brain Control*. New York: John Wiley & Sons.

Vazquez, A. L., & Noll, D. C. (1998). Nonlinear aspects of the BOLD response in functional MRI. *Neuroimage, 7*(2), 108–118.

Wager, T. D., Jonides, J., & Reading, S. (2004). Neuroimaging studies of shifting attention: a meta-analysis. *Neuroimage, 22*(4), 1679–1693.

Wager, T. D., Jonides, J., Smith, E. E., & Nichols, T. E. (2005). Toward a taxonomy of attention shifting: individual differences in fMRI during multiple shift types. *Cogn Affect Behav Neurosci, 5*(2), 127–143.

Wager, T. D., Keller, M. C., Lacey, S. C., & Jonides, J. (2005). Increased sensitivity in neuroimaging analyses using robust regression. *Neuroimage, 26*(1), 99–113.

Wager, T. D., & Nichols, T. E. (2003). Optimization of experimental design in fMRI: a general framework using a genetic algorithm. *Neuroimage, 18*(2), 293–309.

Wager, T. D., Rilling, J. K., Smith, E. E., Sokolik, A., Casey, K. L., Davidson, R. J., et al. (2004). Placebo-induced changes in FMRI in the anticipation and experience of pain. *Science, 303*(5661), 1162–1167.

Wager, T. D., Sylvester, C. Y., Lacey, S. C., Nee, D. E., Franklin, M., & Jonides, J. (2005). Common and unique components of response inhibition revealed by fMRI. *Neuroimage, 27*(2), 323–340.

Wager, T. D., Vazquez, A., Hernandez, L., & Noll, D. C. (2005). Accounting for nonlinear BOLD effects in fMRI: parameter estimates and a model for prediction in rapid event-related studies. *Neuroimage, 25*(1), 206–218.

Wang, J., Aguirre, G. K., Kimberg, D. Y., & Detre, J. A. (2003). Empirical analyses of null-hypothesis perfusion FMRI data at 1.5 and 4 T. *Neuroimage, 19*(4), 1449–1462.

Williams, D. S., Detre, J. A., Leigh, J. S., & Koretsky, A. P. (1992). Magnetic resonance imaging of perfusion using spin inversion of arterial water. *Proc Natl Acad Sci U S A, 89*(1), 212–216.

Wilson, J. L., & Jezzard, P. (2003). Utilization of an intra-oral diamagnetic passive shim in functional MRI of the inferior frontal cortex. *Magn Reson Med, 50*(5), 1089–1094.

Wong, E. C., Buxton, R. B., & Frank, L. R. (1997). Implementation of quantitative perfusion imaging techniques for functional brain mapping using pulsed arterial spin labeling. *NMR Biomed, 10*(4–5), 237–249.

Wong, E. C., Buxton, R. B., & Frank, L. R. (1998). A theoretical and experimental comparison of continuous and pulsed arterial spin labeling techniques for quantitative perfusion imaging. *Magn Reson Med, 40*(3), 348–355.

Woolrich, M. W., Behrens, T. E., & Smith, S. M. (2004). Constrained linear basis sets for HRF modelling using Variational Bayes. *Neuroimage, 21*(4), 1748–1761.

Zarahn, E. (2002). Using larger dimensional signal subspaces to increase sensitivity in fMRI time series analyses. *Hum Brain Mapp, 17*(1), 13–16.

Zarahn, E., Aguirre, G., & D'Esposito, M. (1997). A trial-based experimental design for fMRI. *Neuroimage, 6*(2), 122–138.

Zarahn, E., & Slifstein, M. (2001). A reference effect approach for power analysis in fMRI. *Neuroimage, 14*(3), 768–779.

3 Electroencephalography and High-Density Electrophysiological Source Localization

DIEGO A. PIZZAGALLI

1. INTRODUCTION

In 1924, Hans Berger, a German psychiatrist, performed the first electroencephalographic (EEG) recording in humans (Berger, 1929), a discovery that was initially greeted with great skepticism by the scientific community. By recording from one electrode placed over the forehead and one over the occipital cortex, Berger discovered the existence of rhythmic activity oscillating at approximately 10 Hz, particularly during relaxed wakefulness and in the absence of sensory stimulation or mental activity. In this landmark discovery, Berger described for the first time what would become known as alpha waves. As a result, Berger was among the first to suggest that the periodic fluctuations of the human EEG may be associated with mental processes, including arousal, memory, and consciousness. Over the years, developments in data collection and analyses transformed EEG into one of the prime techniques for studying the human brain. Table 3.1 summarizes selected landmark discoveries and developments that have shaped EEG field throughout the century.

The past two decades in particular have witnessed unparalleled progress in our ability to image human brain function noninvasively. Different imaging techniques are currently available to investigate brain function based on hemodynamic (functional magnetic resonance imaging, fMRI), metabolic (positron emission tomography, PET), or electromagnetic (electroencephalography, EEG; magnetoencephalography, MEG) measurements. In order to investigate spatiotemporal dynamics of brain activity, methods that directly assess neural activity are required. By measuring electrical activity of neuronal assemblies with millisecond temporal resolution, EEG and MEG, unlike hemodynamic techniques, offer the possibility of studying brain function in real time. Unfortunately, as will be discussed in this chapter, the spatial resolution afforded by EEG/MEG is constrained by several factors. The most important of these factors are the distorting effects of the head volume conductor,[1] low signal-to-noise

ratios, and limited spatial sampling due to practical limits on the numbers of electrodes that can be utilized. More importantly, it soon became evident that the neuroelectromagnetic "inverse problem" (the attempt to identify generating sources of measured, scalp-recorded EEG signals) is fundamentally ill-posed. As first described in 1853 by Helmholtz, there are an infinite number of source configurations that can explain a given set of scalp-recorded potentials. Thus, at a first glance, the quest for the development of methods combining millisecond temporal resolution with millimeter spatial resolution appears to be a lost cause. Fortunately, solutions to the inverse problem can be found by postulating physiologically and anatomically sound assumptions about putative EEG sources and by mathematically implementing established laws of electrodynamics.

The main purpose of the present chapter is to review recent advances in the EEG field (event-related potentials, ERPs, will not be discussed here, as they are reviewed elsewhere in this volume). To understand these developments it will first be necessary to detail the physiological basis of the EEG signal. Subsequently, important issues associated with data acquisition, signal processing, and quantitative analyses will be discussed (see Davidson, Jackson, & Larson, 2000; Pivik et al., 1993; Gasser & Molinari, 1996; Nunez et al., 1997; Nuwer et al., 1999; Thakor & Tong, 2004 for more comprehensive reviews of these topics). The largest portion of the chapter will be devoted to reviewing emerging source localization techniques that have been shown to localize EEG activity without postulating a priori assumptions about the number of underlying sources (Baillet et al., 2001; Michel et al., 2004). As we will discuss, perhaps the greatest advancements in the EEG field in the last 5–10 years have been achieved in the development of these localization techniques, in particular when used in concert with high-density EEG recording, realistic head models, and other functional neuroimaging techniques. The picture emerging in light of these achievements reveals that the spatial resolution of the EEG may be substantially higher than previously thought, thus opening exciting and new opportunities for investigating spatiotemporal

---

[1] Volume conduction refers to the process of current flow from the electrical generator to the recording electrode (Fisch, 1999).

Table 3.1. Selected historical landmarks in electroencephalography (adapted from Maurer & Dierks, 1991 and Neidermeyer, 1993)

Year	Name	Description
1875	R. Caton	First tracing in animals of fluctuating potentials that constitute the EEG
1924	H. Berger	First human EEG measurement
1929	H. Berger	First human EEG publication in *Archive für Psychiatrie und Nervenheilkunde*
1932	J. T. Toennies	First ink-writing biological amplifier
1932	G. Dietch	First application of Fourier analyses on human EEG
1934	F. Gibbs	First systematic application of the EEG to epilepsy
1935	A. L. Loomins	First systematic application of the EEG to sleep
1936	W. G. Walter	Discovery of slow (delta) activity in the presence of tumors
1942	K. Motokawa	First EEG brain map
1943	I. Bertrand and R. S. Lacape	First book on EEG modeling
1947		American EEG Society is founded
1947	G. D. Dawson	First demonstration of human evoked potential responses
1949		*Electroencepahlography and Clinical Neurophysiology,* the first EEG journal, is launched
1952	A. Remond and F. A. Offner	First topographic analyses of occipital EEG
1952	M. A. B. Brazier and J. U. Casby	Introduction of auto- and cross-correlation function
1955	A. Remond	Application of topographical EEG analyses
1958	H. Jasper	Introduction of 10–20 system for standardized electrode placement
1960	W. R. Adley	Introduction of Fast Fourier Transformation (start of computerized spectral analyses)
1961	T. M. Itil	Application of EEG analyses for classification of psychopharmacological agents
1963	N. P. Bechtereva	Localization of focal brain lesions by EEG
1965	J. W. Cooley and J. W. Tukey	Introduction of fast Fourier algorithm
1968	D. O. Walter	Introduction of coherence analyses for the human EEG
1970	B. Hjorth	Development of new quantitative methods, including source derivation
1971	D. Lehmann	First multichannel topography of human alpha EEG fields
1973	M. Matousek and I. Petersen	Development of age-corrected EEG spectral parameter for detecting pathology (qEEG)
1977	E. R. John	Introduction of "neurometrics" (standardized qEEG analyses with normative databases)
1978	R. A. Ragot and A. Remond	EEG field mapping
1979	F. H. Duffy	Introduction of brain electrical activity mapping (BEAM)

dynamics of brain mechanisms underlying mental processes and dysfunctions in psychopathology, bringing us closer to fulfillment of Berger's dream that EEG will open a "window to the mind."

2. PHYSIOLOGICAL BASIS OF THE EEG

2.1. EEG generation: I. The role of post-synaptic potentials in cortical pyramidal neurons

In the central nervous system, when a neuron is activated by other neurons through afferent action potentials, excitatory post-synaptic potentials (EPSPs) are triggered at its apical dendrites. When this occurs, the membrane of the apical dendrites becomes depolarized and electronegative, compared to the cell soma (Baillet et al., 2001; Speckmann, Elger, & Altrup, 1993). As a consequence of this transient potential difference, current flows from the nonexcited soma to the excited apical dendritic tree, and a negative polarity emerges at the surface (Speckmann et al., 1993).[2] In the opposite case, with excitation of the soma, the current flow will have inverse direction.

[2] Negative potentials at the surface can arise either due to (a) superficial EPSPs (i.e., excitation at apical dendrites) or (b) deep IPSPs (i.e., inhibition of the soma). Conversely, positive potentials at the surface can arise either due to (a) superficial IPSPs (i.e., inhibition at apical dendrites) or (b) deep EPSPs (i.e., excitation of the soma; Speckmann et al., 1993).

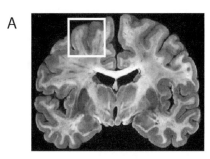

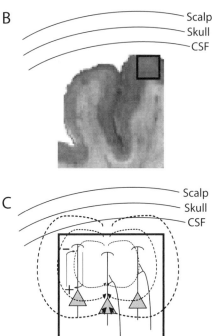

Figure 3.1. Neurophysiological basis of EEG generation. Scalp-recorded EEG oscillations generated by summation of excitatory and inhibitory post-synaptic potentials in cortical pyramidal neurons. (A) A coronal slice of the human brain is shown, with cortical gray matter highlighted in grey color. (B) An expanded view of cerebral gyri and sulci (see inset in A) is shown in relations to the scalp, skull, and cerebral spinal fluid (CSF). (C) A schematic illustration of cortical pyramidal cells within the cortical mantle (see inset in B) is shown. In this example, an excitatory post-synaptic potential (EPSP) is generated at the cell soma; local excitation (+ and −) leads to a tangential current flow (solid lines). The closed loops (dashed lines) represent the summation of extracellular currents produced by the postsynaptic potentials at cortical pyramidal cells, whose dendritic trunks are parallel to each other and perpendicular to the cortical surface. The deep EPSP shown in the example would produce a positive field potential at the cortical surface (Speckmann et al., 1993).

Scalp-recorded EEG oscillations are hypothesized to be generated by the summation of excitatory and inhibitory post-synaptic potentials in cortical pyramidal neurons (Speckmann et al., 1993; Figure 3.1). In the generation of an EEG oscillation, tens of thousands of synchronously activated pyramidal cortical neurons are assumed to be involved. The coherent orientation of their dendritic trunks (parallel to each other and perpendicular to the

cortical surface) allows summation and propagation to the scalp surface (Nunez & Silberstein, 2000). Accordingly, although subcortical contributions to scalp-recorded EEG have been reported (e.g., Llinas, Ribary, Jeanmonod, Kronberg, & Mitra, 1999), cortical macrocolumns are thought to be the main contributors of EEG signals (Fisch, 1999; Baillet et al., 2001).

2.2. EEG generation: II. The role of thalamo-cortical networks

Although mechanisms underlying EEG generation are not fully understood, interactions between thalamic and cortical networks are assumed to play a key role in various rhythmical EEG activities (Steriade, 1993). In animals, neurophysiological evidence has shown that several thalamic, thalamocortical, and cortical neurons display intrinsic oscillatory patterns, which in turn generate rhythmic EEG oscillations. The thalamus, in particular, has been described as a key player in the generation of alpha and beta oscillations. Accordingly, thalamic oscillations in the 7.5–12.5 Hz frequency range have been shown to activate the firing of cortical neurons (Steriade, 1993). The associated depolarization, which mainly occurs in the cortical layer IV, in turn creates a dipolar source with negativity in layer IV and positivity in superficial layers. Placing electrodes at the scalp allows measurement of small but reliable far-field potentials representing the summation of these potential fluctuations. In humans, thalamic contributions to alpha oscillations were investigated in a study integrating positron emission tomography (PET) and EEG recordings (Larson et al., 1998). Cortical alpha power was found to be inversely correlated to glucose metabolism in the thalamus, consistent with the assumption that thalamic activity in response to sensory or cortical input may lead to alpha suppression.

Corticocortical and thalamocortical interactions during information processing have also been postulated in the generation of oscillations at higher frequencies, including the beta band (13–30 Hz). Notably, the thalamus has been also implicated in the generation of delta waves (1–4 Hz), which might arise through interactions between deep cortical layers and the thalamus that are normally inhibited by afferents from the ascending reticular activating system. In addition, the septohippocampal system and various limbic regions (e.g., hippocampus, cingulate cortex) have been implicated in the generation of theta oscillations (Vinogradova, 1995; Bland & Oddie, 1998).

In sum, EEG oscillations appear to be dependent on interactions between the cortex and the thalamus, which both produce intrinsically rhythmical activities. Whereas the thalamus has been critically implicated in the pacing of such rhythmical activities, the cortex provides the coherent output in response to thalamic input and generates the vast majority of oscillations that can be recorded at the scalp (Fisch, 1999).

2.3. EEG generation: III. The role of local-scale and large-scale synchronization

As mentioned above, at any given moment in time, the signal recorded at the scalp is due to spatial summation of current density induced by synchronized post-synaptic potential occurring in large clusters of neurons. Considering that the diameter of EEG electrodes (~10 mm) is several orders of magnitude larger than single neurons (~20 μm) and that the area of an electrode covers approximately 250,000 neurons (Baillet et al., 2001), it is clear that many neurons must be activated synchronously in order to detect an EEG signal at the scalp.

Consistent with this notion, animal studies have described substantial synchronization among neighboring neurons ("local-scale synchronization"; e.g., Llinas, 1988), as well as between neuronal assemblies of distant brain regions ("large-scale synchronization"; e.g., Bressler & Kelso, 2001). Thus, synchronization of oscillations is a key mechanism for neuronal communication between spatially distributed brain networks (see Schnitzler & Gross, 2005 for a recent review). Emerging animal evidence indicates that oscillatory processes might (a) bias input selection, (b) temporally bind neurons into assemblies, and (c) foster synaptic plasticity (Buzsaki & Draguhn, 2004). Intriguingly, higher frequency oscillations (e.g., gamma) appear to originate from smaller neuronal assemblies, whereas low frequency oscillations (e.g., theta) span larger neuronal populations (Buzsaki & Draguhn, 2004). Large-scale neuronal synchronization plays an important role in various cognitive processes that rely on distributed neuronal networks (e.g., language processing; Weiss & Mueller, 2003), and can be studied through EEG coherence analysis, as will be discussed further in Section 5.3.

3. NORMATIVE EEG ACTIVITY

The millisecond temporal resolution of EEG allows scientists to investigate not only fluctuations of EEG activity (i.e., increases/decreases) as a function of task demand or subject samples but also to differentiate between functional inhibitory and excitatory activities. As a general rule, low frequencies (e.g., delta and theta) show large synchronized amplitudes, whereas high EEG frequencies (e.g., beta and gamma) show small amplitudes due to a high degree of desynchronization in the underlying neuronal activity. In adults, the amplitude of normative EEG oscillations lies between 10 and 100 μV (more commonly between 10 and 50 μV; Niedermeyer, 1993). In the following section, a brief review of various EEG bands and their putative functional roles will be presented. For a review of the molecular and physiological basis underlying the generation of various EEG oscillations, the interested reader is referred to Steriade (1993) and Speckmann et al. (1993).

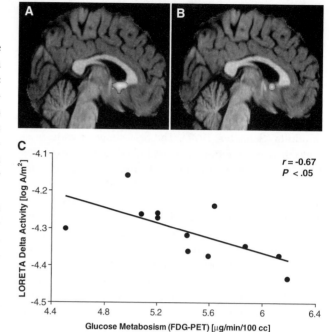

Figure 3.2. Reciprocal relation between delta activity and glucose metabolism. In a recent study integrating concurrently recorded electric (28-channel scalp EEG) and metabolic ([^{18}F]-2-fluoro-2-deoxy-D-glucose positron emission tomography, FDG-PET) measures of brain activity, melancholic depression was characterized by (A) significantly increased delta current density (see yellow-red colors), as assessed with LORETA (see Section 8.2.3.); and (B) significantly decreased glucose metabolism (see blue colors). Statistical maps are thresholded at P < .05 (corrected) and displayed on a representative structural MRI. In psychiatrically healthy subjects, a significant negative correlation between delta current density and glucose metabolism in the subgenual prefrontal cortex emerged (C). Adapted from Pizzagalli et al. (2004) with permission. (See color plate.)

3.1. Delta band (1–4 Hz)

Delta oscillations reflect low-frequency activity (1–4 Hz) typically associated with sleep in healthy humans and neurological pathology. In adults, delta power has been shown to increase in proximity of brain lesions (Gilmore & Brenner, 1981) and tumors (Fernandez-Bouzas et al., 1999), during anesthesia (Reddy, Moorthy, Mattice, Dierdorf, & Deitch, Jr., 1992), and during sleep (Niedermeyer, 1993). Moreover, inverse relationships between delta activity and glucose metabolism have been reported in both pathological (e.g., dementia; Szelies, Mielke, Kessler, & Heiss, 1999) and normal (Pizzagalli et al., 2004) conditions. In our own study, an inverse relationship between delta current density (assessed via an EEG distributed source localization technique) and glucose metabolism (assessed via PET) was found within the subgenual prefrontal cortex (Figure 3.2). Delta is also the predominant activity in infants during the first two years of life. Ontologically, slow delta and theta activity diminish with increasing age, whereas the faster alpha and beta bands increase almost linearly across the life span (e.g., John et al., 1980).

Collectively, these findings suggest that delta activity is mainly an inhibitory rhythm.

3.2. Theta band (4–8 Hz)

Theta activity refers to EEG activity within the 4–8 Hz range, prominently seen during sleep. During wakefulness, two different types of theta activity have been described in adults (Schacter, 1977). The first shows a widespread scalp distribution and has been linked to decreased alertness (drowsiness) and impaired information processing. The second, the so-called frontal midline theta activity, is characterized by a frontal midline distribution and has been associated with focused attention, mental effort, and effective stimulus processing. Recent studies have implicated the anterior cingulate cortex (ACC) as a potential generator of frontal midline theta activity (e.g., Asada, Fukuda, Tsunoda, Yamaguchi, & Tonoike, 1999; Luu, Tucker, Derryberry, Reed, & Poulsen, 2003; Onton, Delorme, & Makeig, 2005). Consistent with these findings, in a recent study integrating electrical (EEG) and metabolic (PET) measurements of brain activity, we found that the ACC (Brodmann area 24/32) was the largest region with significant positive correlations between theta current density and glucose metabolism (Pizzagalli, Oakes, & Davidson, 2003).

Physiologically, the septo-hippocampal system has been strongly implicated in the generation of theta oscillations, although theta has also been recorded in numerous other limbic regions, including the ACC, entorhinal cortex, and the medial septum, among others (Vinogradova, 1995; Bland & Oddie, 1998). In rodents, generation of hippocampal theta activity is crucially dependent on afferents from the medial septum/vertical limb of the diagonal band of Broca complex (MS/vDBB), which is considered the pacemaker of hippocampal theta (Vertes & Kocsis, 1997). Additional evidence suggests that theta can be generated in the cingulate cortex independently of the hippocampal system (e.g., Borst, Leung, & MacFabe, 1987). In light of the observation that these oscillation facilitates transmission between different limbic structures, it has been speculated that theta activity may subserve a gating function on the information processing flow in limbic regions (Vinogradova, 1995).

3.3. Alpha band (8–13 Hz)

The alpha rhythm refers to EEG activity within the 8–13 Hz range. In healthy adults, alpha activity typically has an amplitude between 10 and 45 μV, and can be easily recorded during states of relaxed wakefulness, although large individual differences in amplitudes are not uncommon (Niedermeyer, 1993). Topographically, alpha rhythms show their greatest amplitude over posterior regions, particularly posterior occipito-temporal and parietal regions, and can best be seen during resting periods in which the subjects has his/her eyes closed. In fact, alpha rhythm can

be greatly diminished or abolished by eye opening, sudden alerting, and mental concentration, a phenomenon known as alpha blockage or alpha desynchronization. The alpha rhythm can also be attenuated when alertness decreases to the level of drowsiness; this attenuation is, however, often accompanied by a decrease in frequency.

The physiological role of alpha rhythm remains largely unknown. Traditionally, the posterior distribution of these oscillations and the observation of alpha blockade with eye opening have been interpreted as suggesting that alpha may be associated with visual system functions emerging in the absence of visual input (Fisch, 1999). Indeed, some authors have expanded upon this notion by suggesting that alpha synchronization may represent an electrophysiological correlate of cortical "idling" or cognitive inactivity (e.g., Pfurtscheller, Stancak, Jr., & Neuper, 1996). In recent years, this conjecture has been heavily debated in the literature, particularly in studies investigating evoked EEG activity, in which alpha synchronization has been described during information processing (e.g., Cooper, Croft, Dominey, Burgess, & Gruzelier, 2003; Klimesch, 1999). Further complicating the physiological interpretation of alpha, emerging evidence indicates that different alpha sub-bands may be functionally dissociated, in particular with increasing task demands (Fink, Grabner, Neuper, & Neubauer, 2005). Specifically, in cognitive tasks, lower alpha (e.g., 8–10 Hz) desynchronization (suppression) has been associated with stimulus-unspecific and task-unspecific increases in attentional demands (e.g., Klimesch, 1999). Upper alpha (e.g., 10–12 Hz) desynchronization, on the other hand, appears to be task-specific, and it has been linked to processing of sensory-semantic information, increased semantic memory performance, and stimulus-specific expectancy (Klimesch, 1999).

3.4. Beta band (13–30 Hz)

Traditionally, lower-voltage oscillations within the 13–30 Hz frequency range have been referred to as beta. In adults, beta activity has amplitudes between 10–20 μV, presents mainly a symmetrical fronto-central distribution, and typically replaces alpha rhythm during cognitive activity. Consistent with this view, beta rhythm has been shown to increase with attention (Murthy & Fetz, 1992) and vigilance (Bouyer, Montaron, Vahnee, Albert, & Rougeul, 1987), for example. Collectively, these findings suggest that beta increases generally reflect increased excitatory activity, particularly during diffuse arousal and focused attention (Steriade, 1993).

3.5. Gamma band (36–44 Hz)

Gamma oscillations have been associated with attention, arousal, object recognition, top-down modulation of sensory processes, and, in some cases, perceptual binding (i.e., the brain's ability to integrate various aspects of a stimulus into a coherent whole; Engel, Fries, & Singer, 2001).

Various findings indicate that gamma activity is directly associated with brain activation. First, human intracortical EEG studies have reported increased gamma oscillations during various mental processes, including perception (Rodriguez, Lachaux, Martinerie, Renault, & Varela, 1999) and learning (Miltner, Braun, Arnold, Witte, & Taub, 1999). Second, dose-dependent decreases of gamma activity have been described during anesthesia (Uchida et al., 2000). Third, systematic decreases in gamma activity have been described throughout the sleep-wake cycle (highest during wakefulness, intermediate during REM sleep, and lowest during slow wave sleep; Gross & Gotman, 1999). A recent study from our laboratory using concurrent EEG and PET measurements provided further support for the notion that gamma is a direct indicator of activation because this band had the highest number of positive correlations between current density and glucose metabolism (Oakes et al., 2004).

Although the functional role of gamma oscillations needs to be more fully elucidated, these oscillations are assumed to reflect large-scale integration of and synchrony among widely distributed neurons, particularly in states of diffusely increased vigilance (e.g., Mann & Paulsen, 2005; Steriade, 1993). Physiologically, various mechanisms have been implicated in the generation of gamma oscillations, including: (1) intracortical circuitries, in particular those involving distant brain regions; (2) synaptic interactions among the cortex, thalamus, and limbic structures; and (3) brainstem-thalamic cholinergic activation (Steriade, 1993). Notably, recent animal and human findings have shown that gamma and theta oscillations can be functionally coupled both during activated (task-related) and resting (task-free) states (e.g., Fell et al., 2003; Mann et al., 2005; Schack, Vath, Petsche, Geissler, & Moller, 2002). In general, these studies have shown that gamma bursts occur within periods of the theta phase (Buzsaki, 1996 for review). Consistent with this notion, in a recent 128-channel source localization EEG study (Pizzagalli, Peccoralo, Davidson, & Cohen, 2006), we found significant positive correlations between resting theta and gamma current densities within various subdivisions of the ACC (correlation range: 0.51–0.59).

4. DATA ACQUISITION AND SIGNAL ANALYSIS

In the following sections, a selected discussion will be presented of issues associated with data acquisition and signal processing (for more in-depth reviews, see Davidson et al., 2000; Pivik et al., 1993; Gasser & Molinari, 1996; Nuwer et al., 1999; Thakor et al., 2004).

4.1. Electrodes

4.1.1. Electrode locations and high-density recordings

EEG signals always represent the potential difference between two electrodes, an active electrode and the so-called reference electrode. Accordingly, it is clear that the

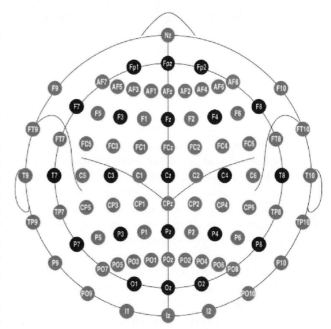

Figure 3.3. Electrode positions and labels in the International 10–20 System. Black circles denote electrode positions and labels from the 10–20 system; gray circles denote additional electrode positions and labels introduced with the 10–10 system. Reprinted from Clinical Neurophysiology, Vol. 112, Oostenveld, R. & Praamstra, P., The five percent electrode system for high-resolution EEG and ERP measurements, pp. 713–719, Copyright (2001), with permission from International Federation of Clinical Neurophysiology.

quality of EEG signals is dependent on the integrity of the electrode-electrolyte-skin interface (for a summary of clinical and experimental electrodes, see Fisch, 1999). Irrespective of their material, EEG electrodes should not attenuate signals between 0.5 and 70 Hz. To allow comparisons among studies it is important to adhere to standardized electrode locations. For many years, the accepted system for electrode placement has been the International 10–20 system proposed by Jasper (1958). The name refers to the fact that electrodes are placed at sites 10% and 20% from four fiduciary points (nasion, inion, left, and right mastoids); this placement schema allows positioning of 19 electrodes homogenously across the scalp. In recent years, this system has been extended to the so-called 10–10 system (American Electroencephalographic Society, 1991) and the 5–5 system (Oostenveld & Praamstra, 2001), in which intermediate positions between those of the 10–20 system have been derived (Figure 3.3).

In recent years, high-resolution EEG systems with numbers of electrodes ranging from 64 up to as many as 256 have been introduced, with the goal of increasing the spatial sampling of the EEG (e.g., Gevins et al., 1994; Tucker, 1993). In one particular dense-array system (Tucker, 1993), scalp abrasion prior to the application of EEG electrodes is not necessary, reducing (a) the electrode application time (e.g., 15-min time for applying a 128-channel EEG net); (b) subject's discomfort; and (c) risk of infections. Instead, these systems are simply soaked in a saline (electrolyte) solution and then applied directly to the head (but see Greischar et al., 2004 for potential issues associated with electrolyte spreading in high-density recordings). The use of high-input impedance (200 MΩ) amplifiers allows the recording of reliable EEG traces with impedances one order of magnitude higher than the traditional 5 KΩ.

Studies using simulated as well as real EEG data have suggested that an electrode distance of 2–3 cm is required to prevent distortions of the scalp potential distribution, and thus allow resolution of spatially focal EEG patterns (e.g., Srinivasan et al., 1998). In addition, recent studies assessing the role of spatial density (i.e., number of electrodes) on *source reconstructions* have clearly shown an improved spatial resolution with high-density recordings. In a simulation study, Lantz, Grave, Spinelli, Seeck, & Michel (2003) reported that the source localization accuracy increased linearly from 25 to 100 electrodes but reached a plateau after 100 electrodes. In the same study, Lantz and coworkers also showed a marked improvement in localization precision of the epileptic sources when increasing electrodes from 31 to 63; again, at least in the case of spatially focal sources in epileptic patients, the improvements in localization accuracy were less dramatic when going from 63 to 123. Similar findings were reported by Luu et al. (2001), who investigated the role of electrode density in the ability to localize scalp abnormalities associated with acute cerebral ischemia. Using sensor downsampling (128, 64, 32, and 19 electrodes), the authors found that only 64 and 128 electrode arrays were capable of resolving spatially localized EEG abnormalities. As in Lantz et al., minimal gain was achieved when moving from 64 to 128 electrodes. Note however that, because Lantz et al. used a source localization technique (EPIFOCUS; Grave de Peralta, Gonzalez, Lantz, Michel, & Landis, 2001) that assumes a single focal source, distributed source localization techniques (see Section 8.2) may benefit from the additional spatial sampling achieved with >100 electrodes. Consistent with this hypothesis, Michel et al. (2004) found that source imaging with 128-channel EEG epileptic spike data led to correct localization (to the order of the affected lobe) in 93.7% of the focal epileptogenic area, as independently assessed through presurgical assessments.

Regardless of the number of electrodes utilized, uniform and homogenous coverage of the scalp is of paramount importance for reliable measurements of the scalp potential field, a critical prerequisite for any source localization technique (Michel et al., 2004). Moreover, measurements of exact 3-D electrode position with a digitizer (if available) may provide important information to account for individual differences in electrode positioning (e.g., Towle et al., 1993). Recently, a solution based on photogrammatic measurements has been developed for quick and accurate measurement of electrode positions in high-density EEG system (Russell, Jeffrey, Poolman, Luu, & Tucker, 2005). In this approach, multiple cameras are used to record the location of individual sensors, allowing for the reconstruc-

tion of the 3-D sensor positions. In sum, both simulation and experimental studies suggest that at least 60 (preferably more) equally distributed electrodes are required for accurate spatial sampling of scalp activities.

4.1.2. Electrode interpolation

The importance of spatial sampling for source localization is associated with the issue of how best to deal with electrodes with corrupted EEG signals due to excessive artifacts or technical malfunction. As mentioned above, source localization strongly relies on the scalp potential distribution, which itself can be distorted by uneven spatial sampling. Consequently, simply omitting corrupted electrodes is not a feasible solution, and interpolation methods are needed. Broadly speaking, two interpolation methods have been utilized: linear (nearest neighbor) and spline interpolation methods (e.g., Perrin, Pernier, Bertrand, & Echallier, 1989). In the first method, corrupted activity is reconstructed through a weighted average using data from neighboring electrodes (the weights are proportional to the Euclidian distance between the electrodes). With the spline interpolation method, information from all sensors is used to represent the overall potential distribution on the entire scalp, and thus to reconstruct the activity at missing channels. Although mathematically simpler, linear interpolations have the disadvantage that (a) edge electrodes cannot be accurately estimated; (b) only a few electrodes are used; and (c) maxima and minima of activity are always located at electrode sites (Maurer & Dierks, 1991). Empirical evidence indicates that non-linear spline interpolation methods achieve greater accuracy (Soufflet et al., 1991).

4.1.3. Recording reference choice

As mentioned in Section 4.1.1, EEG waveforms represent the *differential* voltage between a given electrode and the recording reference. It is therefore clear that the choice of reference completely determines EEG waveforms (Lehmann, 1987; Dien, 1998), an important methodological consideration that all too often is still not recognized in the EEG literature. For example, recording with a vertex (Cz) reference would lead to small EEG deflections in the proximity of Cz due to potential synchronization of firing activities within closely spaced brain regions and volume propagation of the EEG signal. Similarly, recording with mastoid or linked ears montage would lead to rather small waveforms at electrodes positioned over temporal brain regions (Pivik et al., 1993).[3]

Ideally, the reference electrode should be electrically inactive, allowing the measurement of an absolute EEG value. Both cephalic and noncephalic references are never electrically inactive, and thus contribute to recorded EEG signals. Understanding this point is particularly important when deciding the location to the recording reference in

---

[3] Note, however, that information contained in the reference (e.g., Cz) is not permanently lost, but can be recovered by recomputing the EEG data against a different reference electrode.

order to avoid situations in which the reference itself is contaminated by noncephalic activity (e.g., muscle or electrocardiogram artifacts). In these circumstances, because the potential difference is measured between the active and reference electrodes, substantial artifacts would be introduced in all EEG channels.

Due to the fundamental issue of reference-dependency of EEG waveforms, reference-free transformations have been proposed for an unbiased assessment of EEG measures. In particular, the use of an average reference (Lehmann, 1987), radial current flow (Hjorth, 1975), and current source density (Perrin, Bertrand, & Pernier, 1987) have attracted substantial interest. With the average reference approach, at each moment in time, EEG signals are re-derived against the average value across all electrodes. In the Hjorth method, also known as source derivation or Laplacian transformation, the average potential difference between each electrode and the nearest four electrodes is computed.[4] By computing the density of local radial currents, this approach acts as a spatial high pass filter and emphasizes shallow cortical generators. Finally, current source density (also known as surface Laplacian) is computed as the second derivative of the voltage surface; by acting also as a spatial filter, surface Laplacians can be helpful in identifying focal patterns (Nunez & Pilgreen, 1991). Although these reference-free methods have been successfully used in the literature for an unbiased assessment of EEG signals, it is important to stress that they often require a relatively high number of electrodes (e.g., 32 electrodes or more), as well as homogenous electrode distribution across the scalp for reliable estimates (Pivik et al., 1993).

Although the choice of the reference electrode greatly influences *waveform* analyses, it is important to note that the reference choice is completely irrelevant for *any* source localization. In fact, the spatial configuration of the scalp potential distribution is independent of the reference electrode (the reference merely affects the zero line; Lehmann, 1987). As source localization relies on the spatial distribution of the scalp EEG and ERP, different reference montages (e.g., average reference, linked mastoids) lead to identical estimates of intracerebral sources.

4.2. Recording: Filters and sampling rate

The bandwidth of the EEG signal is 0.1–100 Hz in frequency, although most studies focus on frequencies below 30 Hz (or below 50 Hz if gamma activity is investigated). Although a comprehensive review of calibration, filtering, and digitization of EEG signals is beyond the scope of this chapter (see Davidson et al., 2000; Pivik

et al., 1993; Dumermuth & Molinari, 1987 for excellent reviews), some points should be emphasized here. First, the extent to which the digital signal under investigation accurately reflects the physiological (analog) signal completely depends on the sampling rate. As a general rule, the sampling rate should be at least twice the highest frequency present in the signal under investigation. This rule, also known as the *Nyquist Theorem*, prevents the introduction of spurious low-frequency components into the signal, a phenomenon called *aliasing* (Dumermuth & Molinari, 1987). Aliasing occurs when a signal is sampled at a rate that is too low, and introduces irreparable distortion to the digital waveform (Figure 3.4). Two methods can be used to avoid aliasing. First, frequencies higher than half the sampling rate should be removed from the EEG before digitization occurs (e.g., by using an analog or hardware filter). Second, high sampling rates (e.g., four-fold greater than the filter cutoff frequency) could be used. Because the EEG signals of interest are typically between 1 and <60 Hz, a sampling rate of 250 Hz with an analog 0.1–100 Hz filter are appropriate for most EEG studies. If contamination of low frequency artifacts is an issue, the high pass analog filter can be set as high as 1 Hz (Nuwer et al., 1999). Higher sampling rate is required to investigate early sensory ERP components or high-frequency EEG patterns.

4.3. Artifacts

When recorded, the raw EEG signal is virtually always contaminated by various sources of noise and artifacts. In general, biological and non-biological artifacts can be differentiated (see pp. 107–121 in Fisch, 1999 for illustrations of the most common artifacts). The former mainly derive from subjects' movements, muscle activities, blinks, eye movements, heartbeat, and sweating. As will be discussed later, concurrent recording of the electrocardiogram (ECG), electrooculogram (EOG), and electromyogram (EMG) can be very important for a proper detection and removal of these artifacts. Nonbiological artifacts primarily derive from interferences from power lines (50/60 Hz), additional electrical noise, poor subject grounding, and poor electrode contact. One common source of 50/60 Hz noise stems from fluorescent lights. Use of notch filters (50/60 Hz), proper subject grounding, and shielding of the recording system can greatly diminish the influence of nonbiological artifacts. Proper grounding, in particular, can substantially improve the quality of the EEG signals and avoid leakage of current from the EEG system to the subjects.[5] Often, a midforehead electrode is used for this purpose.

Visual and, increasingly more often automatic, offline artifact detection is essential before any EEG analyses, and substantial expertise is required for a proper differentiation of normal and contaminated EEG activity. Drowsiness can introduce a substantial confound in baseline EEG

---

[4] For instance, assume that a researcher wishes to compute the Laplacian transformation at electrode Cz, which has a potential value of 10 μV, and that the four neighboring electrodes Fz, C3, Pz, and C4 have potentials of 3, 5, 12 and 5 μV, respectively. The new source-derivation value for Cz would be 3.75, i.e., [(Cz-Fz) + (Cz-F3) + (Cz-Pz) + (Cz-C4)]/4.

[5] Grounding can be achieved by connecting participants to the ground of the amplifier system.

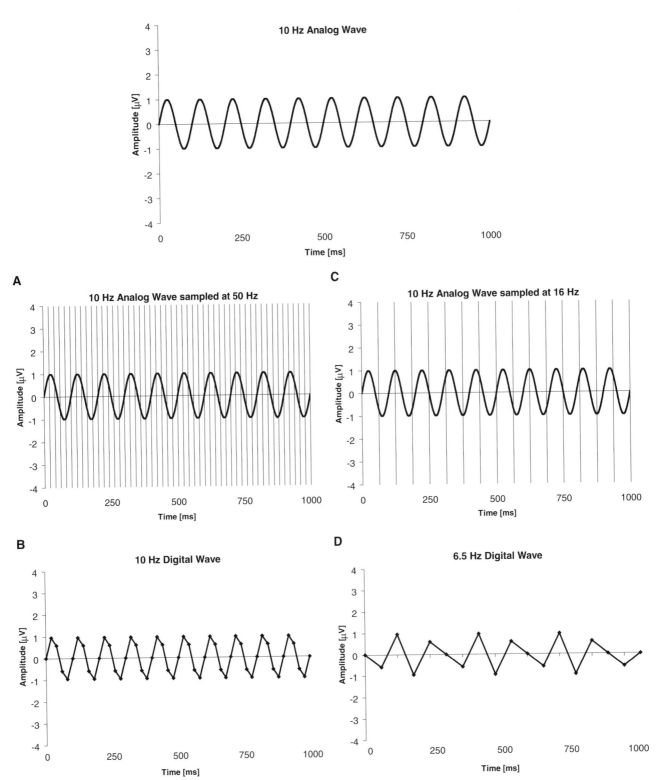

Figure 3.4. Example of aliasing due to insufficient sampling rate. A 10 Hz sine waveform is digitized at two different sampling rates. (A) The sampling rate (50 Hz) is greater than twice the waveform frequency, which results in (B) an appropriate digital representation of the analog signal. (C) The sampling rate (16 Hz) is less than twice the waveform frequency, yielding (D) a false (aliased) representation of the analog signal. Note how undersampling introduces an irreparable lower frequency component in the digital signal. Modified after Fisch (1999).

recording due to a global change in the functional brain state. Typically, EEG slowing over anterior regions, slowing and subsequent decrease of alpha activity, and slow eye movement (particularly horizontal), are associated with subjects' drowsiness. When this pattern is detected, it is recommended to exclude these periods of EEG (Pivik et al., 1993).

Removal of ECG and EOG artifacts is particularly important, because these artifacts overlap in frequency and amplitude with the EEG. In humans, normal ECG is within the 1–1.5 Hz range, suggesting that its second-order harmonics (2–3 Hz) is within the delta range (Thakor et al., 2004). Blinks and eye movements mostly generate activity within the delta and theta range (i.e., <7.5 Hz). Blinks, which typically last 200–400 ms and can generate artifacts with an amplitude up to 800 μV, can however also affect the alpha band (and to a lesser extent the beta band), in particular at anterior sites (Hagemann & Naumann, 2001). For proper detection of ocular artifacts, it is essential to utilize additional channels to record vertical and horizontal eye movements. To record vertical eye movement, two electrodes are affixed below and above one eye; for horizontal movements, two electrodes are affixed at the extremities of an eye. Over the years, several methods have been described in the literature to detect *and* correct both sources of noise (see Croft, Chandler, Barry, Cooper, & Clarke, 2005 for a recent review and comparison of the most widely used EOG correction algorithms).

Artifacts originating from muscle activity can contaminate a broad range of EEG frequencies because the primary energy in EMG signals is between 10 and 200 Hz (Tassinary & Cacioppo, 2000). Due to this overlap with EEG frequencies, occurrence of these artifacts are particularly problematic for EEG analyses. Contamination from muscle activity can be troublesome for studies interested in gamma activity, which can be easily influenced by noncephalic, myogenic sources. Considering the explosion in interest in the functional role of gamma activity in mental processes, it is clear that proper attention must be devoted to the issue of EMG contamination to the gamma band. Due to frequency overlap, removing muscle artifacts through filtering can greatly distort real EEG signals. Accordingly, several authors proposed the use of regression approaches for dealing with this issue (e.g., Allen, Coan, & Nazarian, 2004; Davidson et al., 2000). In this approach, activity in higher frequencies (e.g., 50–70 Hz) is typically taken as a marker of muscle artifact, and its variance is removed using regression analyses or entered as covariate in analyses of variance (ANOVA).

In recent years, the method of independent component analysis (ICA) has been increasingly used for removal of ECG and other artifacts (see Makeig, Bell, Jung, & Sejnowski, 1996 for a tutorial). In view of the fact that artifacts typically do not occur time-locked to a given event or evoked response, ICA is ideally suited to remove such interfering signals. Consistent with this notion, ICA works best when applied to unaveraged (raw) EEG data. In the case of ECG, contaminated EEG is entered into the ICA, which separates the EEG and EOG components. In a subsequent step, the ECG component is set to zero in the coefficient matrix leading to a removal of ECG artifacts. ICA approaches have been also used to remove EOG artifacts (Thakor et al., 2004).

5. QUANTITATIVE SCALP ANALYSES

The introduction of computers has enabled the development of several methods to investigate EEG signals with respect to various parameters, including waveform frequencies, amplitudes, phase, and coherence. Quantitative EEG (qEEG) analyses can be divided into linear and nonlinear approaches. Among the most widely used linear methods to quantify spontaneous or task-related EEG activity are spectral and coherence analyses, which typically assume that the EEG signals are stationary processes.[6] Nonlinear approaches, which often incorporate higher order statistics, information theory, or chaos theory, started to emerge in the 1990s, and have demonstrated their usefulness particularly when applied to transient and irregular EEG patterns (see Thakor et al., 2004 for a review).

5.1. Spectral analyses

Spectral analyses are based on the notion that any oscillatory activity can be characterized by the sum of different sinusoidal waves with distinct frequencies and amplitude (see Figure 3.5 for a simulation). The goal of spectral analyses, which are often performed using the Fast Fourier Transform (FFT), is to estimate the contribution of various frequencies on the measured EEG signal. Commonly, spectral estimates are computed for discrete frequencies (e.g., 8.5–10 Hz for lower alpha). For a given frequency or discrete EEG band, the root-mean-square average amplitude or the power (the square of the amplitude) is used to quantify its contribution to the measured EEG signal. Mathematically, the Fourier coefficients indicate the strength of the signal at a given frequency.

In a typical EEG study, all available artifact-free EEG segments are entered in spectral analyses. When selecting the length of the artifact-free EEG segments, it is important to understand that this variable determines the maximal frequency resolution available for the analyses. Thus, selection of 2-sec segments will provide a 0.5 Hz resolution (i.e., the inverse of 2 sec), allowing to resolve, for example, 10 and 10.5 Hz frequencies. Note, however, that spectral analyses assume that the EEG is a stationary signal. Accordingly, segments entered in FFT analyses cannot be too long because of potential violation of the stationarity assumption (Gasser & Molinari, 1996). When relatively short segments are considered (e.g., <3.5 sec), the

---

[6] In simple terms, stationarity implies that the statistical proprieties of an EEG signal (e.g., mean, variance) do not vary over time.

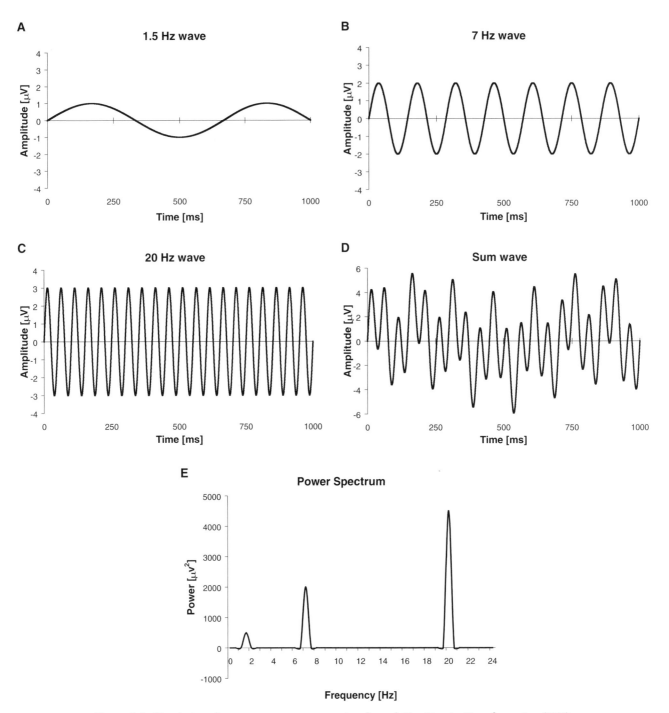

Figure 3.5. Simulation of power spectrum computation through Fast Fourier Transformation (FFT). In (A), (B), and (C), simple sine waves oscillating at 1.5, 7, and 20 Hz are shown. In (D), the sum of these three sine waves is shown. In (E), the results of an FFT analysis of the complex waveform displayed in (D) are shown. Not surprisingly, the spectrum identifies frequency peaks at 1.5, 7, and 20 Hz.

stationarity assumption is typically met in spontaneous EEG recording.

To allow reliable estimation of spectral features and to reduce the impact of second-to-second variability in EEG signals, at least 60 sec of artifact-free data should be used for spectral analyses (Nuwer et al., 1999; Pivik et al., 1993). Further, to avoid introduction ("leakage") of spurious fre-

quencies arising from abrupt changes in EEG signals at the beginning and the end of the EEG segments, a so-called taper transformation should be used. For this purpose, the Hanning (cosine) window has been commonly utilized. This window tapers the beginning and end of the EEG segment to zero, whereas the middle of the segment retains 100% of its amplitude (see Dumermuth & Molinari, 1987 for a review of various windowing approaches). Because the use of windowing reduces the amount of data that can be analyzed within a segment, overlapping segments (e.g., 50%) are often used to restore the amount of data for spectral analyses.

Although we refer to prior reviews for a comprehensive discussion of spectral analyses (e.g., Gasser & Molinari, 1996; Davidson et al., 2000, several important methodological points should be emphasized here. First, an underappreciated issue is that the frequency range for a given oscillatory activity (e.g., alpha activity) can show substantial individual differences. Klimesch (1999) has long advocated the use of individually defined frequency ranges and has shown in several experimental situations that this choice can have substantial effects on the findings. Second, measures of *absolute* or *relative* power can be derived from spectral analyses. Whereas absolute power reflects the amount of a given frequency within the EEG, relative power is calculated as the amount of EEG activity in a given frequency band divided by the total power. In general, absolute power should be preferred because it can be more easily interpreted. Third, when dealing with power data, transformations (e.g., log) are often used before statistical analyses to approximate a Gaussian distribution (Davidson et al., 2000). Finally, ratios or difference scores are often computed between different electrodes in an attempt to draw inferences about differential hemispheric activation. Conceptual and methodological considerations concerning these asymmetry metrics are discussed next (for reviews, see Allen et al., 2004; Coan and Allen, 2004; and Davidson et al., 2000).

5.1.1. Asymmetry metrics

In many experimental situations, psychophysiologists are interested in investigating whether the two brain hemispheres are differentially involved in specific cognitive and affective processes, personality traits, or various forms of psychopathology. Although many metrics have been used to investigate hemispheric differences (Pivik et al., 1993), the alpha power asymmetry index has been among the most commonly used. This index is derived from subtracting the natural logarithm of the left hemisphere power value from the natural logarithm of the right hemisphere power value (ln R − ln L). Because alpha power is considered to be inversely related to brain activation, positive numbers on this index indicate relatively greater right activity, whereas negative numbers denote relatively higher right activity.

The investigation of frontal EEG asymmetry has received particular attention, and over 80 studies have examined its role in emotion, motivation, and psychopathology (for a recent review, see Coan & Allen, 2004). In general, the picture emerging from this literature is that frontal EEG asymmetry is associated with (a) state-dependent emotional reactivity; (b) individual differences in emotional reactivity; and (c) individual differences in risk for a variety of emotion-related disorders (e.g., depression, anxiety). Conceptually, it has been proposed that left prefrontal regions might be implicated in a system that facilitates appetitive behavior and certain forms of affect that are approach-related. Conversely, right prefrontal regions have been implicated in withdrawal-related, negative affect (Davidson, 2004).

From a methodological perspective, the use of asymmetry metrics has several advantages. First, they allow researchers to control for individual differences in skull thickness, a variable that can artificially cause individual differences in scalp power values. Second, asymmetry metrics can increase statistical power by reducing individual differences in overall activity, and limit the number of statistical tests performed. Third, the internal reliability of the alpha power frontal asymmetry index is high, ranging from 0.76 to 0.93 across studies, and the test-retest reliability is acceptable (e.g., 0.69–0.84 across three weeks) (Allen et al., 2004). When asymmetry scores are reported, however, follow-up analyses assessing the unique contribution of each hemisphere to the asymmetry index should be presented. For example, a finding of relatively increased right frontal activity in a given patient population, although an important first step, should be subjected to further analyses to ascertain whether this pattern is due to (1) an increase of right frontal activity; (2) a decrease of left frontal activity; or (3) a combination of the above. From a statistical perspective, a laterality effect can only be claimed if the *Group × Hemisphere* or *Condition × Hemisphere* interaction is significant (Allen et al., 2004; Davidson et al., 2000).

5.2. Time-frequency analyses

From the last section it is clear that spectral analyses can provide important information about the frequency compositions of EEG oscillations. Spectral analyses cannot, however, provide any information about *when in time* such frequency shifts occur. Because the EEG is a dynamic, time-varying, and often non-stationary phenomenon, approaches allowing the investigation of transient changes in the frequency domain appear particularly important. To achieve this goal, various time-frequency analysis methods have been developed, including (a) short-time Fourier Transform (STFT), for computation of an FFT-based time-dependent spectrum (so-called spectrogram); and (b) wavelet analyses, which allow a more adaptive time-frequency approach affording flexible resolution. Wavelet analyses, in particular, have gained popularity in recent years due to their ability to accurately resolve EEG waveforms into specific time and frequency components (see Samar, Bopardikar, Rao, & Swartz, 1999 for a nontechnical tutorial). In this approach, EEG signals are viewed as shifted and scaled versions of a particular mathematical function (the wavelet), rather than a composition of sine waves with varying frequencies as in the FFT.

5.3. Coherence analyses

As summarized in Section 2.3., neurophysiological studies have demonstrated the presence of both local-scale synchronizations (i.e., synchronization among neighboring neurons) as well as large-scale synchronizations (i.e., synchronization among distant regions; e.g., Bressler & Kelso, 2001; Llinas, 1988). In EEG studies, the investigation of large-scale neuronal synchronization appears particularly important in experimental situations hypothesized to recruit distributed neuronal network. In order to quantitatively measure the dynamic functional interactions among EEG signals recorded at different scalp locations, *coherence measures* can be computed (Nunez et al., 1997).

Coherence is a frequency-dependent measure, mathematically obtained by dividing the cross-spectrum between two time series by the root of the two spectra (this computation is similar to a correlation; Schack et al., 2002). Cross-power spectrum is obtained by multiplying the Fourier transform of one signal with the complex conjugate of another signal, thus allowing the quantification of relationships between different EEG signals. Accordingly, coherence can range from 0, indexing the absence of any synchrony, to 1, indicating maximal synchrony between the frequency components of two signals, irrespective of their amplitudes.

Intriguingly, increased synchronization among distant regions has been observed within low-frequency oscillations (e.g., theta), whereas increased local synchronization has been observed for high-frequency oscillations (e.g., gamma; Buzsaki & Draguhn, 2004; von Stein & Sarnthein, 2000). In general, brain regions that are co-activated during a given cognitive process are assumed to show increased coherence ("neuronal synchronization") within specific EEG frequency bands, depending on the nature and difficulty of the task (Weiss & Mueller, 2003). For some authors, such coherence measurements have been interpreted as reflecting cortical interactions or connectivity (e.g., Thatcher, Krause, & Hrybyk, 1986). Consistent with this speculation, increased coherence has been generally observed with increased task complexity and efficient information processing, whereas pathological conditions characterized by dysfunctional networks (e.g., dementia, dyslexia) are characterized by decreased coherence (Leoncani & Comi, 1999; Weiss & Mueller, 2003).

Finally, it is important to note that, although coherence analyses assess the degree of synchronization between different brain regions, they cannot inform us about the *causality* of these interactions or the *direction* and *speed* of the information transferred. Only in recent years, advanced methods for assessing these important aspects of brain function have been described, including the Directed Transfer Function (DTF), the Directed Mutual Information (DMI), and the partial directed coherence (PDC) techniques (Thakor et al., 2004 for a review). In a recent study, Astolfi et al. (2005) presented a promising approach to estimate connectivity by applying structural equation modeling and DTF to cortical signals derived from high-resolution EEG recordings.

5.4. Quantitative EEG (qEEG)

In qEEG studies, also known as "neurometrics" (John et al., 1980), various variables derived from spectral and coherence analyses of multi-channel EEG recordings (e.g., absolute power, relative power, interhemispheric and intrahemispheric coherence, asymmetry scores) are entered into large normative, age-dependent databases in conjunction with demographic and clinical information. Age-regression qEEG equations and Z-scores are then utilized to (1) identify patterns of abnormal EEG patterns associated within specific neurological or psychiatric disorders; and (2) provide supportive evidence for differential diagnoses and treatment decisions (for a recent review, see Hughes & John, 1999). Recent studies have confirmed the ability of qEEG approaches of detecting abnormal EEG patterns in pathological conditions but also some of their limitations, which might in part derive, however, from the fact that clinical conditions are far from being homogenous entities. Thus, whereas abnormal qEEG patterns were found in 83% of 340 psychiatric patients but only in 12% of 67 controls, no EEG abnormality was specific to a given clinical entity, and patients with the same diagnosis often showed different EEG abnormalities (Coutin-Churchman et al., 2003).

5.5. EEG mapping and space-oriented EEG analyses

The advent of multi-channel EEG systems has fostered the development of EEG mapping techniques (Lehmann, 1987; Duffy, Burchfiel, & Lombroso, 1979 for seminal reviews). Conceptually, at a given moment in time, this method considers values at each electrode and through interpolation display the field distribution of brain electric activity. Unlike traditional EEG waveform approaches, EEG mapping considers data in the spatial domain first, and then in the temporal domain, providing a display of the constantly changing spatial distribution of bran activity (see Maurer & Dierks, 1991 for a tutorial). For topographic mapping, at minimum the complete 10–20 system should be used (i.e., >19 electrodes; Nuwer et al., 1999). One of the main advantages of space-oriented EEG analysis is that, at any given time point, activity from all electrodes is considered simultaneously. A second main advantage is that, unlike waveform analyses, space-oriented analysis is independent from the reference electrodes. In fact, the spatial configuration or landscape of a map does not change when a different reference is used. In a manner analogous to a geographical map, the topographical features, such as the location of maximum or minimum potential or the potential gradients, are not affected by the chosen reference that defines the zero line.

Critically, when examining the unfolding of momentary potential distributions over time, one observes that these maps tend to remain relatively constant for some periods of time, and are then abruptly interrupted by the emergence of new landscapes (Lehmann, 1971). Lehmann (1990) called these temporal segments of quasi-stable map landscapes "microstates" and considered them the building blocks of human information processing. Note that different configurations of scalp potentials are assumed to index different functional brain states because (a) different scalp potential distribution must have been generated by different neural sources (Fender, 1987); and (b) different neural sources likely subserve different functions.

Consistent with this assumption that microstates index different functional brain states, studies have shown that different mental processes (Lehmann, Henggeler, Koukkou, & Michel, 1993) or arousal states (Cantero, Atienza, Salas, & Gomez, 1999) are associated with different microstate classes. Further converging evidence comes from the notable observations that different age groups can be characterized by distinctive patterns of changes in microstate durations and preponderance (Koenig et al., 2002). Such age-dependent microstate changes mirror comparable transitional stages classically described by developmental psychologists. Likewise, psychopathological conditions characterized by dysfunctional mental states, such as schizophrenia (e.g., Lehmann et al., 2005) or dementia (e.g., Strik et al., 1997), showed shortened durations for specific microstates. Intriguingly, in a recent study, Lehmann et al. (2005) reported that acute, medication-naïve, first-episode schizophrenic subjects had different "microstate syntax" (i.e., different microstate concatenations and transitions) as well as truncated duration for some microstates, raising the interesting possibility that this disease may be characterized by different concatenations of mental operations and precocious termination of information processing for certain types of mental operations. For methodological details about microstate analyses of EEG data, see Koenig et al. (2002) and Lehmann et al. (2005).

Although EEG mapping represents a powerful and unambiguous approach for scalp EEG data, it is important to stress that this technique does not provide any additional information about the generating sources underlying scalp measurements (Pivik et al., 1993). In Section 8, source localization techniques required for localization of intracerebral sources will be reviewed.

6. SURFACE-SOURCE IMAGING APPROACHES

6.1. Scalp Laplacian mapping

As mentioned in the Introduction, the spatial resolution of scalp EEG is limited by the blurring effects of the head

volume conductor. In fact, the head acts as a low-pass spatial filter, transmitting to the scalp broad, as opposed to focal, spatial patterns of activity (Srinivasan et al., 1998). Scalp Laplacian mapping can be used to restore high-frequency spatial information of brain electric activity that has been distorted by the low-conductivity skull (Hjorth, 1975; Nunez et al., 1997; Perrin et al., 1987). The surface Laplacian approach does not solve the inverse problem (i.e., it is not a 3-D source localization technique); rather it allows source mapping directly over the scalp surface. As reviewed by He (1999), surface Laplacian is thought to represent an approximation of the local current density flowing perpendicularly to the skull into the scalp (for this reason, it has been also called *current source density* or *scalp current density*). A further advantage of surface Laplacian methods is that they are reference-independent.

The scalp Laplacian was first introduced for EEG data by Hjorth (1975), who proposed a difference estimation scheme to calculate local Laplacian by using the potentials at surrounding electrodes (see Footnote 4). Although computationally easy to implement, this so-called local approach was found to have some limitations, including inaccurate estimation for large interelectrode distances and for border electrodes (He, 1999). To overcome these drawbacks, Perrin et al. (1987) introduced a global approach based on the mathematical modeling of the global scalp surface and a curvilinear coordinate system. In their implementation, Perrin and coworkers assumed that the scalp surface can be approximated by a sphere. Later, Babiloni et al. (1996) presented a solution called "realistic Laplacian estimator" that can be applied to any arbitrarily shaped scalp.

6.2. Cortical imaging

To increase the spatial resolution of the EEG, the cortical imaging approach can also be used to deconvolve the low-pass spatial filtering effects of head volume conduction (Gevins et al., 1994). In this approach, biophysical models of the passive conducting features of the head are used to deconvolve a scalp potential distribution into estimation of potentials or current dipole distribution at the superficial cortical surface (for a review, see He, 1999). Gevins and coworkers (1994), for example, presented a deblurring technique based on a realistic biophysical model of the passive conducting properties of the head to estimate the potential distribution at the cortical surface. To this end, a finite element model (see Section 7.1) based on MRI-reconstructed scalp, skull, and cortical surfaces was used. Conceptually, the rationale for this approach stems from the empirical observation that cortical pyramidal cells oriented perpendicularly to the cortical surface mainly contribute to the recorded scalp EEG signal (Speckmann et al., 1993). Note that neither the scalp Laplacian nor the cortical imaging approach are source localization techniques and thus are unable to reconstruct sources in 3-D space. This important topic will be discussed next.

7. THE NEUROELECTROMAGNETIC FORWARD AND INVERSE PROBLEM

The "forward problem" refers to the process of estimating scalp potentials from intracranial current sources (Koles, 1998). If the configurations of intracranial sources and the conductivity proprieties of the tissues are known, then the scalp potential distribution can be calculated using basic physical principles. Therefore, the forward problem can be unambiguously solved. In contrast, the "inverse problem," the estimation of sources underlying scalp-recorded EEG data, is ill-posed. Although recording of the human EEG was first reported by Berger in 1929, it soon became evident that scalp-recorded electromagnetic measurements do not contain sufficient information about the 3-D distribution of the electric neuronal activity. As early as the mid-nineteenth century, Helmoltz (1853) had already described the nonuniqueness of this type of electromagnetic inverse problem: the current distribution inside a conducting volume cannot be uniquely determined by the field and potential information outside it. Thus, scalp-recorded EEG/MEG measurements can be explained by an infinite number of different generating distributions, even with an infinite numbers of recording electrodes (Fender, 1987). To understand this concept, consider that the inverse problem can be mathematically represented as:

$$D = GX + n \qquad (3.1)$$

where D is a vector representing the scalp-recorded potentials, X is an unknown vector representing the generating sources (the current density vector), n is noise, and G is the transfer matrix, which mathematically implements both the electromagnetic (e.g., conductivity values for the brain, skull, and scalp) and geometrical (e.g., shape) features of the solution space considered in the inverse solution ("the head volume conductor model"). The inverse problem refers to finding X given known D. Specifically, the main goal is to minimize the following function:

$$O(X) = ||D - GX||^2 \rightarrow \min \qquad (3.2)$$

In general terms, it is not possible to determine which solution among the infinite possibilities corresponds to the actual solution; consequently, the quest for developing an electromagnetic tomography appears, at first, hopeless. Fortunately, the EEG and MEG follow certain electrophysiological and neuroanatomical constraints, which when combined with the laws of electrodynamics, provide an approximate solution of the inverse problem (Baillet et al., 2001; Michel et al., 2004; Pascual-Marqui, Esslen, Kochi, & Lehmann, 2002). When considering Equation 1, it becomes immediately evident that the localization accuracy of *any* source localization technique is critically dependent on: (1) the head model used to compute the inverse solu-

tion; and (2) the inverse solution itself (Michel et al., 2004). In the following section, these two important aspects will be reviewed, followed by a description of various solutions to the inverse problem currently used in the EEG literature.

7.1. Head volume conductor model

The head volume conductor model plays a critical role in source localization because it determines the way intracerebral sources give rise to the scalp-recorded signal. As indicated above, the head model mathematically implements both the electromagnetic and geometrical properties of the solution space. Over the years, three head models have been used: (1) three-spherical head model (e.g., Ary, Klein, & Fender, 1981); (2) a boundary element model (BEM; e.g., Hamalainen & Sarvas, 1989); and (3) a finite element model (FEM; e.g., Miller & Henriquez, 1990). In terms of complexity and computational burden, the spherical model represents the simplest, the BEM the intermediate, and the FEM the most complex model. BEM and FEM models are typically developed from high-resolution structural MRI scan of individual subjects and can better account for individual anatomical differences, providing therefore more realistic head models.

The three-spherical head model, which has been most frequently used, approximates the head as a set of nested concentric and homogenous spheres, in which the skull, scalp, and brain are modeled as different layers with different conductivity. Typically, standard conductivity values, which have been measured in separate studies from excised tissue, are used for the different compartments, but in recent years attempts to assess conductivities through diffusion tensor MR imaging have begun to emerge (e.g., Tuch, Wedeen, Dale, George, & Belliveau, 1999). In general, spherical models can provide appropriate localization in superior regions of the brain, where the head shape approximates a sphere.

The BEM, in contrast, approximates different compartments of volume conductor models (e.g., skin, skull, cerebral spinal fluid) through closed triangle meshes with different conductivity values and dimension and thus attempts to take into account realistic geometry. Although the BEM clearly represents an improvement and more realistic model than the three-spherical head model, this model assumes homogeneity and isotropy within the head and brain. To cope with this potential issue, FEM models have been developed.

The FEM, unlike other methods, can account for the actual head shape and tissue discontinuities, and accommodate anisotropic tissue[7] in the conductivity model of the head volume, allowing detailed 3-D information on tissue conductivity for each region. This approach models current flow in an inhomogeneous volume by representing the conductor as a complex assemblage of many equally

---

[7] Anisotropy refers to the property of having different values when measured in different directions.

sized cubes or tetrahedron. The use of tetrahedron can accommodate elements that vary in size, thus allow modeling of the head geometry and anisotropy precisely. For several authors, the high computational efficiency of the BEM makes this model a valuable compromise between the oversimplifying sphere head volume model and the computationally intensive FEM model (He, 1999).

8. SOURCE LOCALIZATION TECHNIQUES

Estimating the sources of scalp-recorded electromagnetic activity has attracted considerable interest, and various solutions have been described in the literature. In general these solutions can be divided into two broad categories, *equivalent dipole approaches* and *linear distributed approaches*. The first approach typically assumes that EEG/MEG signals are generated by a relatively small number of discrete and focal sources, which can be modeled as single, fixed, or moving dipoles (e.g., Scherg & Ebersole, 1994). Through an iterative process, locations, orientations, and strength of these equivalent current dipole (ECD) are selected to minimize the difference between the predicted and the actual EEG measurements. The solution derived through this approach strongly relies on the numbers of dipoles; unfortunately, in many experimental situations, the numbers of dipoles cannot be determined a priori (e.g., Phillips, Rugg, & Friston, 2002a).

Distributed approaches, in contrast, consider all possible source locations simultaneously. In addition to the advantage conferred when no a priori assumptions about the numbers of sources are required, distributed approaches typically allow researchers to limit the solution space by means of anatomical and functional constraints. As will be discussed in the next section, anatomical constraints assume that some specific compartments (e.g., gray matter) or regions of the brain (e.g., cortical structures) have a higher likelihood of generating scalp-recorded EEG signals than others, and are thus essential for narrowing the search for a "unique" solution. In the following sections, a non-technical survey of various source localization techniques will be presented (for more technical reviews, see Baillet et al., 2001; Hamalainen & Ilmoniemi, 1994; Grave de Peralta & Gonzalez Andino, 2000; Phillips et al., 2002a; Phillips et al., 2002b; Pascual-Marqui et al., 2002; Trujillo-Barreto et al., 2004).

8.1. Equivalent dipole approaches (Dipole Source Modeling)

The equivalent current dipole (ECD) model is the most basic source localization technique and assumes that scalp EEG potentials are generated by one or few focal sources (for review, see Fuchs, Ford, Sands, & Lew, 2004). A dipole does not reflect the presence of a unique and discrete source but it is rather a mathematically convenient representation (i.e., the center of gravity) of synchronized activation of a large number of pyramidal cells likely extending

larger patches of gray matter (Baillet et al., 2001). In fact, a dipole is assumed to represent a patch of cortical gray matter layer containing approximately 100,000 pyramidal cells oriented in parallel to each other and activated simultaneously (Fuchs et al., 2004). Heuristically, the position of a dipole can provide clues about the extent and configuration of the activated cortical area (Lopes da Silva, 2004): superficial dipoles typically reflect localized cortical activity, whereas deeper dipoles reflect the activity of an extended cortical area.

In this approach, focal sources are modeled by an ECD through six parameters: three location parameters (X, Y, Z), two orientation parameters, and one strength (amplitude) parameter. Depending on the experimental procedures and/or a priori hypotheses, moving, fixed, or rotating dipoles can be used. Using an iterative procedure and nonlinear multidimensional minimization procedures, the inverse problem is solved by attempting to identify dipole parameters that best explain the observed scalp potential measurements (Fuchs et al., 2004). In its simplest terms, initial dipole parameters are selected, the forward solution is computed, and a least-squares comparison between estimated and actual measurements is calculated. This process is continued until the difference between estimated and actual measurements is minimized. Without a priori assumption, one of the main concerns with this approach is that it can get trapped in local minima (Michel et al., 2004). Additionally, depending on the spatial configuration of the underlying sources, a dipole can sometimes be found at physiologically implausible locations, such as within white matter or even outside of the brain.

Over the years, various dipole source models have been developed, including the moving dipole model, rotating dipole model, regional dipole model, fixed (coherent) dipole model, and fixed (multiple signal classification or MUSIC) model (see Fuchs et al., 2004 for a review). Another interesting approach, called EPIFOCUS, has been recently proposed by Grave de Peralta et al. (2001). EPIFOCUS assumes a single focal source, but unlike single dipole modeling, does not assume that this source is spatially restricted to a single point. The *moving dipole model* assumes only one dipole at the time and allows all parameters to vary. The *rotating dipole model* constrains location to a single point but allows orientations and strength to vary. The *fixed dipole model*, in contrast, holds position and orientation constant within a given interval and it estimates the dipole strength for each time point. These subtle differences in these models, which are the ones most frequently used, underscore the need to incorporate prior neuroanatomical and neurophysiological knowledge to guide the selection of the physiologically most plausible model, making source reconstruction a hypothesis-driven process. In general, some caution should be exerted when interpreting dipole modeling solutions because users' interventions and decisions about the number of underlying sources are required in dipole fitting. To cope with this issue, Mosher, Lewis, and Leahy (1992) developed a mathematical approach aimed to estimate the likely number of underlying sources. This method, called multiple signal classification (MUSIC), attempts to decompose the signal to identify underlying components in the time series data (see Mosher & Leahy, 1998 for further improvements).

In recent years, substantial progress has been made to extend the original dipole fitting approach implemented using simplified spherical head models to more realistic geometry head model constructed from single subject's MRI images, in particular using boundary element methods (BEM) or finite element methods (FEM). Not surprisingly, simulation and experimental studies have shown that a more accurate localization can be achieved by using realistic head models (e.g., Fuchs, Wagner, & Kastner, 2001). In a recent study (Cuffin, Schomer, Ives, & Blume, 2001), the best average localization that could be achieved with spherical head model was 10 mm. In addition to improved localization capability, co-registration with MRI images can be used to visualize the dipole location coordinates relative to brain anatomy, facilitating comparisons with other functional imaging modalities. Studies combining electrophysiological and hemodynamic measures have further extended dipole source localization approaches by using PET- or fMRI-identified activation loci to seed the iterative optimization procedure, providing clues about the putative location of sources (e.g., Heinze et al., 1994). As will be discussed in Section 9, the relationship between electrophysiological changes measured by EEG/MEG and hemodynamic changes measured by PET/fMRI is not fully understood (Nunez & Silberstein, 2000), posing some challenges in situations in which fMRI activations are used to choose the *number* and *location* of potential sources. A more promising (and potentially less biased) approach involves independent EEG/MEG source modeling, which is then weighted based on hemodynamic findings to select the most likely solution (e.g., Liu, Belliveau, & Dale, 1998).

In summary, although dipole source modeling has been successfully used to localize spatially restricted and focal sources (e.g., early sensory evoked potentials), its main limitation is that the *exact* number of dipoles often cannot be determined a priori. Further, because intracranial recordings have provided very little support for the notion that only a few sites in the brain are active in generating ERP or spontaneous EEG recording (e.g., Towle et al., 1998), dipole fitting results should be interpreted with caution.

8.1.1. Dipole source modeling for EEG data: FFT-dipole-approximation

As reviewed in Section 5, qEEG approaches have been extensively used in both clinical and experimental settings to investigate the spectral aspects of scalp-recorded EEG signals. For many clinical and experimental researchers, the next step following spectral analysis might be to localize the sources underlying different EEG frequency bands.

Unfortunately, topographic maps of power distributions derived from traditional scalp spectral analyses cannot be used for source localization because (1) these maps represent squared potential values, in which polarity information is lost; and (b) power maps are reference-dependent (Lehmann, 1987). In 1989, Lehmann and Michel published a method, called FFT-Dipole-Approximation, which allows computation of intracerebral, three-dimensional location of single dipole source model in the frequency domain. Conceptually, this approach reduces multi-channel EEG data by focusing on the principal features of the spatial organization of brain activity. In assuming a single, common phase angle for all generator processes, the FFT-Dipole-Approximation approach models multichannel brain electric field data in the frequency domain by a potential distribution map, which contains polarity information and consequently can be used for conventional source modeling.

Analytically, standard frequency analyses via FFT are computed first. Then, for each artifact-free EEG segment, the Fourier coefficients for each electrode are plotted in a sine-cosine diagram, and subsequently projected onto the straight line given by the first principal component of the entries. Note that only assessing the first principal component of standard FFT result implies a single phase-angle modeling (i.e., all phase angles between recording electrodes are either 0° or 180°), which typically explains more than 93% of the variance of the original baseline EEG data (Michel, Lehmann, Henggeler, & Brandeis, 1992). For any user-specified EEG frequency band, the single phase-angle assumption allows the computation of a mean potential distribution map (the FFT Approximation Map), which can then be subjected to standard 3-D equivalent dipole source modeling (Lehmann & Michel, 1989). In a final step, the model source's location coordinates on the anterior-posterior, left-right, and inferior-superior axes and its strength for conventional EEG frequency bands, can be compared between experimental conditions or groups.

The FFT-Dipole-Approximation method has several strengths. First, unlike scalp localization of EEG spectral value, this approach is completely independent from the chosen reference electrode location, and thus does not require any assumptions about an inactive site (Michel et al., 1992). Second, no assumption is needed about the orientation of the generating sources, thus allowing an unbiased approximation of the 3-D spatial organization of brain activity. Physiologically, locations of the model sources describe the center of gravity of all neural elements that are active in the brain during a given recording. Accordingly, different locations of centers of gravity unambiguously imply different geometry (i.e., locations and/or orientations) of the underlying neuronal sources between experimental conditions or groups. The FFT-Dipole-Approximation approach has been successfully used to compute intracerebral sources of various

EEG frequency bands during experimental situations or conditions assumed to involve widely distributed brain systems, including sleep (Tsuno et al., 2002), pathological conditions (e.g., Alzheimer's disease; Huang et al., 2000), and epilepsy (Worrell et al., 2000), among other examples. In situations, in which the assumption of a single oscillating dipole generator is unwarranted or unlikely, results are expected to be less reliable.

8.2. Linear distributed source localization techniques

Considering the intrinsic limitation of dipole modeling, and in particular the fact that it is often difficult to determine a priori the number of underlying sources, it is not surprising that attempts to develop distributed source modeling approaches have received considerable attention. In simple terms, these approaches are based on the estimation of brain electric activity at each point within a 3-D solution space. Each point, in turn, can be considered a dipole. Unlike equivalent dipole models, these "dipoles" have fixed positions (e.g., Pascual-Marqui et al., 1999) and sometimes fixed orientations (e.g., Phillips et al., 2002a; Phillips et al., 2002b), which are determined by anatomical and physiological constraints implemented within the localization algorithms. As these methods are used to estimate the strengths (and in some cases, the orientation) of the source, the equations describing distributed solutions are linear.

Because the number of measurements (electrodes) is typically <100, and the number of unknowns (electrical activity at each point in the solution space) is often on the order of 10,000, it is clear that the inverse problem is greatly underdetermined (Baillet et al., 2001; Michel et al., 2004). Mathematically, so-called regularization methods are needed to limit the range of allowable solutions and identify the "optimal" or "most likely" solution. Regularization methods can be understood as mathematical representations of the physiological/structural assumptions implemented in a given method. In the literature, various regularization methods have been utilized. Some of the most widely used include minimum norm solution (Hamalainen & Ilmoniemi, 1994), maximal smoothness (Pascual-Marqui et al., 1994), structural/functional priors (Phillips et al., 2002a; Phillips et al., 2002b), and fMRI-weighted solution space (Dale et al., 2000). Although some of these methods have received important empirical validation indicating that it is possible to solve the inverse problem, the severe underdetermined nature of the inverse problem leads to the consequence that the solutions have low spatial resolution – their solutions are often blurred. In the following section, a review of distributed source localization techniques is presented. The LORETA algorithm has been used extensively by researchers in the field and by our group (e.g., Pizzagalli et al., 2001; Pizzagalli et al., 2002; Pizzagalli et al., 2003; Pizzagalli et al., 2004;

Pizzagalli et al., 2006). Therefore, a more extended discussion of emerging cross-modal validation as well as limitations of LORETA will be presented in Sections 8.2.3.1 and 8.2.3.3, respectively.

8.2.1. Minimum norm solutions

The MN solution (Hamalainen & Ilmoniemi, 1994) was one of the first linear inverse solutions. In the MN approach, the head model is first mapped onto a 3-D grid, and three mutually perpendicular dipole current sources are placed at each grid point (Koles, 1998). The goal of the MN approach is to estimate the distribution and strengths of these tens of thousands of dipoles. Among the infinite possible, the MN approach selects the one that contains the least energy, that is, minimal overall current density within the brain. Mathematically, the MN solution estimates the 3-D source distribution with the smallest L2-norm solution[8] that fit the actual data.

MN does not incorporate any prior information. In particular, unlike other methods (e.g., Pascual-Marqui et al., 1994; Phillips et al., 2002a; Phillips et al., 2002b), MN solutions do not impose any spatial correlation among sources. However, there is no strong physiological evidence that the solution with the smallest L2-norm is also the most plausible one. In fact, simulation studies have shown that the MN solution typically favors weak and localized activation patterns, and can misplace deep sources onto the outermost cortex (Pascual-Marqui, 1999). Accordingly, MN does not completely fulfill the promise of a 3-D source localization technique. LORETA, as we will see, was the first approach that successfully extended the good localization properties of the 2-D MN solution to 3-D solution space.

8.2.2. Weighted minimum norm solutions

To compensate for the depth dependency of MN solution, in particular the tendency to favor superficial sources, various weighting factors have been suggested. Two solutions are mentioned here. The first, known as the *weighted MN solution*, uses a lead field normalization for compensating for the lower representation of deeper sources (e.g., Jeffs, Leahy, & Singh, 1987). The second, called FOCUSS (Focal Underdetermined System Solution; Gorodnitsky, George, & Rao, 1995), is a nonparametric algorithm for solving the inverse solution, in which the weights are iteratively modified according to the solution estimated in a previous step. Specifically, at each step, the weights of grid points with the lowest current density are reduced, and this process is repeated until the current density at most of the grid points is zero (Koles, 1998). Although these weighted MN approaches gave some promising results for reducing the low spatial resolution (blurring) of all MN solutions and for reducing the depth-dependency of sources

---

[8] In the L2-norm approach, the squared deviation of the data from a given model is minimized using a least-squares method.

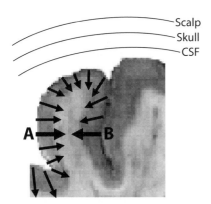

Scalp
Skull
CSF

A → ← B

Figure 3.6. Graphical representation of the LORETA assumptions. The core assumptions of the LORETA algorithm are that (A) neighboring neurons are synchronously activated and display only gradually changing orientations; and (B) the scalp-recorded EEG originates mostly from cortical gray matter. These two assumptions are graphically displayed in the figure. Note that, in this fictive example, activity generated by the dipolar sources A and B would not be detected by scalp EEG; in fact, due to the gyral and sulcal configurations, activity from these opposing dipoles would cancel out.

(Michel et al., 2004), it is important to point out that weighting is selected based on mathematical operations rather than physiological assumptions.

8.2.3. Low-resolution Electromagnetic Tomography (LORETA)

Low-resolution Electromagnetic Tomography (LORETA) (Pascual-Marqui et al., 1994), a form of Laplacian-weighted MN solution, solves the inverse problem by assuming that: (1) neighboring neurons are synchronously activated and display only gradually changing orientations; and (2) the scalp-recorded signal originates mostly from cortical gray matter (Figure 3.6). The first assumption, which is generally consistent with neurophysiological studies in animals (e.g., Haalman & Vaadia, 1997), is mathematically implemented by computing the "smoothest" of all possible activity distributions. Note that the smoothest solution is assumed to be the most plausible one *giving rise to the scalp-recorded EEG signal*. The second assumption constrains the solution space to cortical gray matter (and hippocampi), as defined by a standard brain template. Mathematically, LORETA selects the solution with the smoothest spatial distribution by minimizing the Laplacian (i.e., the second spatial derivatives) of the current sources.

In recent implementations (Pascual-Marqui et al., 1999), LORETA uses a three-shell spherical head model registered to the Talairach brain atlas (available as digitized MRI from the Brain Imaging Centre, Montreal Neurological Institute (MNI); Evans et al., 1993) and EEG electrode coordinates derived from cross-registrations between spherical and realistic head geometry (Towle et al., 1993). The solution space, that is, the 3-D space where the inverse problem is solved, is restricted to corti-

cal gray matter and hippocampi, as defined by a digitized probability atlas provided by the MNI.[9] Under these constraints, the solution space includes 2394 voxels at 7 mm spatial resolution.

For analyses in the frequency domain, LORETA computes current density as the linear, weighted sum of the scalp electrical potentials, and then squares this value for each voxel to yield power of current density in units proportional to amperes per square meter (A/m^2).

In 2002, Pascual-Marqui introduced a variant of the LORETA algorithm, in which localization inferences are based on standardized current density (standardized LORETA, or sLORETA). Conceptually, sLORETA was inspired by work by Dale et al. (2000). Using a two-step process, Dale et al. first estimated current density using the MN solution; subsequently, current density was standardized using its expected standard deviation, which was assumed to fully originate from measurement noise. Although sLORETA uses a slightly different implementation that considers simultaneously two sources of variations (variations of the actual sources and variations due to noisy measurements), its localization inference is also based on standardized values of current density estimates. As a result, unlike LORETA, sLORETA does not introduce Laplacian-based spatial smoothness to solve the inverse problem and does not compute current density but rather statistical scores. In initial simulations, sLORETA was reported to have zero-localization error (Pascual-Marqui, 2002). Independent simulations using (a) a dipolar source, or (b) two spatially well-separated dipolar sources with similar depth replicated that sLORETA had higher localization accuracy than LORETA or MN solutions (Wagner, Fuchs, & Kastner, 2004). However, in the presence of a strong (or superficial) source, a second weak (or deeper) source remained undetectable by all methods, including sLORETA (Wagner et al., 2004). Thus, sLORETA successfully resolved two simultaneously active sources only when their fields were distinct enough and of similar strength.

8.2.3.1. *Cross-modal validation of LORETA.* In initial studies, the physiological validity of LORETA was indirectly evaluated by comparing LORETA solutions with functional imaging findings derived from similar experimental manipulations. For example, physiologically meaningful findings were observed during basic visual, auditory, and motor tasks (e.g., Mulert et al., 2001; Thut et al., 1999), epileptic discharges (e.g., Lantz et al., 1997), and cognitive

[9] Accordingly, LORETA coordinates are in MNI space. Note, however, that the LORETA software uses the Structure-Probability Maps atlas (Lancaster et al., 1997) to label gyri and Brodmann area(s). Because the MNI (used by LORETA) and the Talairach (used by the Structure-Probability Maps atlas) templates do not precisely match, MNI coordinates are temporarily converted to Talairach coordinates (Brett et al., 2002) before the Structure-Probability Maps atlas is utilized. In our publications (e.g., Pizzagalli et al., 2001, 2004) as well as those relying on the LORETA-KEY software, reported coordinates remain in MNI space.

tasks tapping specific brain regions (e.g., Pizzagalli et al., 2002).

In more recent years, important cross-modal validation has come from studies directly combining LORETA with functional fMRI (Mulert et al., 2004; Vitacco, Brandeis, Pascual-Marqui, & Martin, 2002), structural MRI (Worrell et al., 2000), PET (Pizzagalli et al., 2004; but see Gamma et al., 2004), and intracranial recordings (Seeck et al., 1998). In Pizzagalli et al. (2001), theta current density in the rostral anterior cingulate cortex (ACC) was associated with treatment response in major depression; the ACC region implicated in this 28-channel EEG study overlapped with the one implicated in similar studies using PET and fMRI (see Pizzagalli et al., 2006 for a meta-analysis). In Pizzagalli et al. (2004), subjects with the melancholic subtype of depression were characterized by decreased activity within the subgenual PFC, which was manifested as increased inhibitory EEG delta activity and decreased PET glucose metabolism (Figure 3.2A–B). Delta current density and glucose metabolism were significantly and inversely correlated (r = −0.66; Figure 3.2C). In two recent EEG/fMRI studies, LORETA localizations were, on average 16 mm (Mulert et al., 2004) and 14.5 mm (Vitacco et al., 2002) from fMRI activation loci, a discrepancy that is in the range of the spatial resolution of LORETA (1–2 cm). Despite some controversy in the field about the localization capability of LORETA (Grave de Peralta & Andino, 2000) and recent null findings (Gamma et al., 2004), substantial consistency between LORETA findings and other traditional neuroimaging techniques has been reported.

8.2.3.2. Incremental validity of LORETA.

In addition to improving the spatial resolution of EEG data, initial evidence suggests that EEG source localization techniques may allow researchers to uncover information not available in traditional scalp spectral analyses. Two examples from our laboratory are pertinent to this point. In a first study, traditional scalp power and LORETA analyses were applied on the same resting EEG data to investigate putative abnormalities in major depression (Pizzagalli et al., 2002). In the LORETA data, depression severity was significantly correlated (r = 0.60, p < 0.015) with an "intracerebral" frontal asymmetry index that included the inferior and superior frontal gyri, indicating that relatively higher right prefrontal activity was associated with higher depression severity. When identical analyses were performed on the scalp frontal asymmetry index (ln F4 − ln F3), the correlation was not significant.

In a more recent study, we investigated whether resting EEG alpha activity predicted response bias in a separate verbal memory task played under different incentive (monetary) conditions (Pizzagalli, Sherwood, Henriques, & Davidson, 2005). Extending prior scalp frontal EEG asymmetry studies (e.g., Sutton and Davidson, 2000), we found that higher LORETA alpha2 (10.5–12 Hz) current

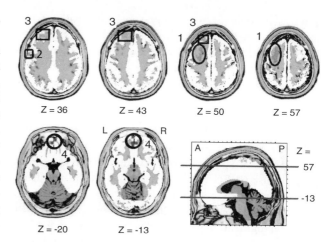

Figure 3.7. Example of LORETA findings highlighting relations between resting intracerebral EEG sources and approach-related behavior. Whole-brain analyses showing voxel-by-voxel correlations between resting alpha2 (10.5–12 Hz) current density and response bias toward reward-related cues for 18 healthy subjects. Six axial brain slices (head seen from above, nose up, L = left, R = right; A = anterior, P = posterior) are shown. Alpha2 current density within both dorsolateral prefrontal regions (clusters #1–3; see green colors) and ventromedial prefrontal regions (cluster #4; see blue colors) was negatively correlated with reward bias, indicating that higher resting activity within these regions was associated with stronger reward bias. Adapted from Pizzagalli et al. (2005). (See color plate.)

density within left dorsolateral regions (Brodmann areas 6, 8, 9, 10, 46) was associated with stronger bias to respond to reward-related cues (Figure 3.7; see clusters #1–3). Notably, left dorsolateral prefrontal resting activity accounted for 54.8% of the variance in reward bias. Whereas this finding fits the hypothesis that frontal EEG asymmetry in favor of the left hemisphere might reflect the propensity to respond with approach-related tendencies (Davidson, 2004), a second important finding emerged: alpha2 current density within ventromedial prefrontal regions (Brodmann areas 10, 11) was also associated with reward bias (Figure 3.7; see cluster #4). This latter finding, which is consistent with functional neuroimaging and animal findings implicating the ventromedial prefrontal cortex in reward monitoring and evaluation of reinforcers, could obviously not have been achieved with scalp EEG data. More generally, findings from this study highlight that source localization techniques can be used to predict complex behavior.

8.2.3.3. Current limitations and future directions of LORETA.

Although the LORETA algorithm has received important cross-modal validation, it is important to highlight three factors that, in most of the studies to date, likely affected the spatial resolution of this method.[10] First, the vast majority of LORETA studies have used a three-shell

---

[10] These methodological limitations are not restricted to the LORETA algorithm but would equally apply to any distributed source localization technique.

spherical head model, which represents only a rather crude approximation of the biophysical problem. As recently demonstrated by Ding, Lai, and He (2005), a more complex head model that better represents the geometry of gray and white matter regions (e.g., FEM) can substantially improve the spatial resolution of LORETA. Second, most of the studies have used a general (average) brain template (Evans et al., 1993). Clearly, use of individual anatomical MRI scans is expected to improve the precision of the solution space. Third, although LORETA studies typically used EEG electrode coordinates derived from cross-registrations between spherical and realistic head geometry (e.g., Towle et al., 1993) and registered to a MRI template, digitization of electrode positions for individual subjects is expected to further improve the spatial resolution of LORETA.

In addition to these issues, which could be addressed in the future, some more conceptual limitations should be mentioned. First, due to the smoothness assumption used to solve the inverse problem, LORETA is incapable of resolving activity from closely spaced sources; in such cases, LORETA will find a smeared, single source located between the original two sources. In fact, in experimental situations in which the generating source is known to be well-represented by a single dipole (e.g., early sensory ERPs), dipole fitting procedures might be preferred, as LORETA will tend to blur the solution (e.g., Fuchs, Wagner, Kohler, & Wischmann, 1999; Moffitt & Grill, 2004). Moreover, despite the fact that LORETA showed the smallest overall localization error in the simulations by Fuchs et al. (1999), these authors found that LORETA tended to overestimate the depth of sources at eccentricities above 70%, likely due to the fact that the 3-D smoothness constraint is difficult to fulfill at the boundary of the solution space. Second, some authors have argued that the electrophysiological and neuroanatomical constraints used by LORETA are somewhat arbitrary. In particular, concerns have been raised about whether the assumption of maximal synchronization between neighboring neuronal populations can be appropriately extended to adjacent voxels (Kincses, Braun, Kaiser, & Elbert, 1999). Third, although sources in LORETA are appropriately constrained to gray matter, their orientation is left undetermined. Phillips et al. (2002a,b) have recently shown that EEG distributed source localization approaches can make better use of anatomical constraints. For example, in their approach, dipole orientation was fixed perpendicular to the interface between gray and white matter, as derived from high-resolution MRI. Fourth, at least in current implementations, LORETA does not accommodate other functional priors (e.g., weighting factors based on independently assessed fMRI activations), which have been recently used to limit the spatial dispersion of distributed source localization techniques (e.g., Phillips et al., 2002a; Phillips et al., 2002b; Dale et al., 2000). Success in addressing these issues is expected to further improve the LORETA localization accuracy.

8.2.4. Variable resolution electromagnetic tomography (VARETA)

Frequency-domain VARETA is a discrete, spline-distributed solution[11] that has been used to estimate sources of EEG frequency bands (Valdes-Sosa, Marti, Garcia, & Casanova, 1996; Bosch-Bayard et al., 2001). Conceptually, it belongs to the family of weighted MN solutions.

As mentioned above, LORETA imposes maximal spatial smoothness; as a consequence, LORETA is able to recover smoothly distributed sources with low localization error, but focal sources are blurred. VARETA, on the other hand, utilizes different amounts of spatial smoothness for different types of generators. This is achieved by a data-driven procedure that estimates the spatial covariance matrix through the scalp cross-spectra, which ultimately selects the amount of spatial smoothness required at each voxel in the brain (Valdes-Sosa et al., 1996). Mathematically, this is done by allowing the regularization parameter to vary according to the location in the solution space. According to the developers, a further key difference between LORETA and their algorithm is that VARETA is able to estimate discrete and distributed sources with equal accuracy (Fernandez-Bouzas et al., 1999). Nonetheless, initial empirical findings seem to contain substantial degree of blurring (e.g., Fernandez et al., 2000; Bosch-Bayard et al., 2001).

In VARETA, current sources are also restricted to gray matter, as defined by a probabilistic brain atlas. Currently, a limited number of studies have used VARETA, although encouraging results have been reported for localizing EEG current density during normative mental processes (e.g., Fernandez et al., 2000) as well as in pathological conditions (e.g., Fernandez-Bouzas et al., 1999). Additional testing from independent laboratories will be important to assess the validity of this promising approach.

8.2.5. Local Auto-Regressive Average (LAURA)

In 2001, Grave de Peralta and colleagues (Grave de Peralta et al., 2001) proposed a distributed linear inverse solution that constrains the minimum norm solution based on biophysical laws. To solve the inverse problem, this technique selects the source configuration that better mirrors the biophysical behavior of electric vector fields. Mathematically, this approach uses a Local Auto-Regressive Average (LAURA) model with coefficients that depend on the distances between solution points in order to mirror the electromagnetic laws that (a) the strength of the source declines with the inverse of the squared distance of the potential field; and (b) the estimated activity at one point depends on the activity at neighboring points. As with other distributed inverse solutions, this method makes no assumptions about the number or location of active sources. Simulation studies show that LAURA is able to resolve multiple simultaneously active sources (Grave de

---

[11] Spline estimates can be understood as the spatially smoothest solutions accounting for the observed data.

Peralta et al., 2001), and promising applications have recently appeared (e.g., Murray et al., 2004).

8.2.6. Bayesian solutions

In recent years, Bayesian approaches have attracted increased attention because they allow incorporation of a priori information into source estimation by means of probability distributions (Phillips et al., 2002a; Phillips et al., 2002b; Trujillo-Barreto et al., 2004). For example, Phillips et al. (2002a,b) described an EEG source localization approach based on the weighted MN solution that incorporates physiological and anatomical constraints derived from other imaging modalities. Their approach rests on three anatomical/physiological assumptions, which are used to reduce the solution space a priori. They assume that sources are: (1) located in gray matter; (2) oriented perpendicularly to the cortical mantle; and (3) locally coherent (i.e., their activity changes smoothly along the cortical mantle). The first assumption can be implemented by constraining the solution space to gray matter, as determined by each subject's structural MRI (e.g., Phillips et al., 2002a). This step can be achieved by segmenting an MRI image into gray matter, white matter, and cerebrospinal fluid and creating a mask containing a gray matter coefficient value ranging from 0 (null probability that a given voxel is in gray matter) to 1 (100% probability). Anatomical information gathered in this first step can also be used to constrain the orientation of a local dipole to fulfill the requirements of the second assumption. Although a description of the mathematical corollaries of these assumptions is beyond the scope of this chapter, it is clear that by determining a priori the orientation of dipoles based on well-grounded anatomical and physiological bases, the inverse problem is reduced from a vectorial problem (orientation and strength are unknown) to a scalar problem (only strength is unknown). The third assumption of locally coherent and synchronized electrical activity can be met by imposing spatial smoothness (Pascual-Marqui et al., 1994), which is mathematically implemented by minimizing differences among neighboring voxels.

In addition to these assumptions, which are essentially identical to the ones implemented by LORETA, Phillips et al. (2002b)'s method allows the use of basis functions to further reduce the solution space in the temporal and spatial domains; in the spatial domain, weighting factors can be introduced a priori based on independent information derived from fMRI, for example. Simulations showed that (1) in the absence of noise and localization priors, the best localization was achieved with a relatively large smoothness constraint; and (2) location priors greatly improved the localization accuracy, even in the presence of noise and with reduced smoothing.

In a recent extension of the Bayesian approach, Trujillo-Barreto et al. (2004) proposed a technique that calculates a "final" solution through averaging of various models, each with different anatomical constraints, which are weighted based on their probability of contributing to the generation of EEG signals. In initial evaluations with simulated and real EEG data, this approach has shown promising findings (Trujillo-Barreto et al., 2004).

8.2.7. Simulation studies comparing different distributed inverse solutions

As evident from the previous section, the past decade has witnessed substantial progress in developing distributed source localization techniques that do not assume a priori the number and location of underlying sources. Although these approaches have similarities and an identical goal (i.e., to solve the underdetermined and ill-posed inverse problem), they often differ in the nature and extent of the anatomical, physiological, and/or statistical assumptions they implement. Ultimately, no matter how sophisticated their mathematical and biophysical implementations are, the validity and reliability of any of these methods should be exclusively evaluated by their ability to provide physiologically meaningful solutions, in particular in relations to other neuroimaging techniques (e.g., fMRI, PET; but see Section 9 for a discussion of challenges relating electrophysiological and hemodynamic measures).

For most of these techniques, however, their reliability and validity have been evaluated by means of artificial data. In these simulation studies, four basic steps are used (Michel et al., 2004): (1) dipole(s) is/are placed at each grid of the solution space; (2) the forward solution is computed to determine the associated scalp potential distribution; (3) sources underlying the scalp potential distribution are estimated using various source localization techniques; and (4) a localization error is computed by comparing the initial and estimated source location. Over the years, several simulations have been published, and a brief summary is reported in the following section.

Pascual-Marqui (1999) compared LORETA, MN, weighted MN, and other linear, distributed inverse solutions. He reported that only LORETA was capable of correct localization with, on average, localization error of 1 voxel resolution, whereas the other methods showed large localization errors, in particular with deep sources. Although LORETA showed the best 3-D localization accuracy, it is important to stress that LORETA tended to underestimate deep sources and that correct localization was achieved with some degree of blurring. Higher localization accuracy for LORETA compared to standard MN solutions has also been reported by Fuchs et al. (1999) and Babiloni et al. (2004a). Fuchs et al.'s (1999) simulations showed, however, that the MN tended to emphasize superficial sources, whereas LORETA tended to suppress them, yielding instead overly deep, blurred solutions for the same sources. In a later simulation, Pascual-Marqui et al. (2002) compared the localization error and spatial dispersion (i.e., resolution) of sLORETA, MN (Hamalainen & Ilmoniemi, 1994), and a new tomographic method described by Dale et al. (2000). Findings showed that sLORETA had smaller localization error and higher spatial resolution, irrespective of the presence or absence of noise and source orientation. Indeed, sLORETA was the only algorithm achieving zero-error localization. Moreover, the spatial blurring of sLORETA was smaller than the one achieved by the method employed by Dale et al. (2000). Recently, Yao and Dewald (2005) compared the performance of moving dipoles, MN solution, and LORETA using simulated EEG data and real ERP data. Compared to the other methods, LORETA had the smallest localization error, as well as the smallest percentage of undetected sources and falsely-detected sources in simulated EEG data. Not unexpectedly, LORETA (as well as the other methods) was unable to separate two discrete sources spaced only by 5 mm. Whereas these simulation studies used the three-spherical head model to solve the inverse solution, Ding et al. (2005) recently evaluated the localization accuracy of LORETA using a realistic geometry head model (BEM). As expected, the LORETA localization error was lower when using the BEM compared to the spherical head model (approximately 10 mm vs. 20–30 mm).

Other simulations, however, have challenged the localization accuracy of LORETA. Grave de Peralta et al. (2001), for example, compared MN, weighted MN, LORETA, and LAURA, and found the best localization accuracy for LAURA, followed by LORETA and the weighted MN solution, which showed similar performances. Similarly, Trujillo-Barreto et al. (2004) compared LORETA with an extension of the Bayesian model incorporating probabilistic maps derived from segmentation of standard brain template within 71 separate brain regions, and found that the latter method gave higher localization accuracy and less spatial distortion (i.e., higher spatial resolution), particularly when subcortical regions were implicated. Better localization accuracy of a Bayesian model incorporating structural and physiological priors compared to LORETA was also reported by Phillips et al. (2002a,b). Indeed, in their simulations, Phillips et al. (2002a,b) showed that the inclusion of a priori location information improved the performance of the distributed minimum norm approach, whereas LORETA tended to oversmooth the solution. In the absence of prior information about location, Phillips's method and LORETA achieved similar localization capabilities.

As correctly pointed out by Michel et al. (2004), these simulation studies are intrinsically limited by the fact that the dipole localization error used to evaluate the "goodness" of any distributed inverse solution is the "most unnatural test for them." In fact, as mentioned above, distributed source localization techniques have been developed to resolve multiple and spatially distributed sources, and thus these simulations cannot predict "how a distributed inverse solution deals with the reciprocal influences of simultaneously active sources (Michel et al., 2004; p. 2205)." Accordingly, real EEG data collected during functionally and anatomically well-characterized experimental tasks (e.g., finger tapping, checkerboard stimula-

tion, N-back working memory task) may provide a better test of various source localization algorithms. Additionally, physiological validation through other neuroimaging techniques would provide converging evidence. As reviewed in Section 4.3.1., encouraging cross-modal validity has started to emerge for the LORETA algorithm, particularly in studies comparing LORETA with functional fMRI (Mulert et al., 2004; Vitacco et al., 2002), structural MRI (Worrell et al., 2000), PET (Pizzagalli et al., 2004), and intracranial recordings (Seeck et al., 1998). Similar cross-modal validity will be necessary for evaluating the localization accuracy of other distributed source localization techniques.

8.2.8. The issue of multiple testing

As with hemodynamic neuroimaging studies, which typically involve statistical comparisons at thousands or tens of thousands of locations in the brain, distributed EEG source localization techniques also face the issue of how best to determine a statistical threshold that will protect against Type I errors due to multiple comparisons. In our own work with LORETA (e.g., Pizzagalli et al., 2001), we have implemented a randomization procedure based on the t_{max} approach to estimate the false-positive rate under the Null Hypothesis of no voxel-wise differences between two given groups or conditions. This approach, which was inspired by statistical solutions developed for neuroimaging data (Arndt et al., 1996; Holmes et al., 1996), relies on permutation procedures. When comparing an experimental and a control group, for example, two randomly selected groups each containing half of the subjects under investigation can be tested at each of the 2394 voxels. At every iteration, the largest absolute t value (from a two-tailed test) can then be stored in a histogram. After 5000 iterations, the t value cutting off the most extreme 5% of the distribution can be identified and used to threshold the data, i.e., to accept or reject the Null Hypothesis.

8.2.9. Summary

The main goal of *any* EEG source imaging technique is to draw reliable conclusions about sources underlying scalp-recorded signals, that is, to solve the inverse problem. Importantly, the choice of the inverse method also depends on the experimental situation. Dipole fitting methods can provide accurate localization in situations of highly focal activations, for example during somatosensory stimulation or epileptic discharges (Michel et al., 2004; Fuchs et al., 2004). In more complex cognitive or pathological conditions that likely recruit widespread neuronal networks, distributed imaging techniques are expected to perform better.

As appropriately emphasized by Michel et al. (2004), it should be beyond the scope of any review to declare a specific source localization algorithm as "the best". Two main reasons justify this position. First, as discussed above, simulation studies based on focal sources may not be the most appropriate test of the localization accuracy of distributed source localization techniques, which may perform substantially better when real EEG data generated by widely distributed neuronal networks are considered. Second, inconsistencies and even contradictions between simulation studies stemming from different laboratories raise some concerns about (1) the mathematical implementations of "competing" localization algorithm (e.g., Pascual-Marqui et al., 2002 for a discussion of this important point); and (2) the selection of test sources that might favor a given algorithm over the others. Clearly, in order to progress in this important field, independent validation studies devoid of experimenter bias or preferences are needed.

9. DIFFICULTIES INTEGRATING ELECTROMAGNETIC AND HEMODYNAMIC VARIABLES

Approaches integrating EEG and PET/fMRI are based on the assumption that brain regions that are electrically more active over time will also show increases in metabolic or hemodynamic activities. Although this assumption is plausible (Logothetis, Pauls, Augath, Trinath, & Oeltermann, 2001), several factors contribute to a difficult comparison between electrophysiological and hemodynamic techniques, making a complete integration conceptually challenging (Nunez & Silberstein, 2000). First, due to the fundamentally different physiological basis of electromagnetic and hemodynamic measures, situations can arise in which the activation period of neurons is too brief to produce a detectable hemodynamic change, whereas it could be easily detected by EEG. Second, scalp EEG signals are highly dependent on synchronization/desynchronization mechanisms, and their relation to glucose or oxygen utilization is unclear (Nunez & Silberstein, 2000). For example, increased neuronal firing and reduced synchrony would produce a small scalp EEG (e.g., alpha blockade after eye opening), a process that would require, however, substantial metabolic supply. Similarly, based on the observation that both excitatory and inhibitory processes require glucose utilization (Ackermann, Finch, Babb, & Engel, 1984), loss of inhibitory synaptic action in pathological conditions (e.g., interictal periods in epileptic patients) would produce large EEG signals but decreased PET metabolic signal. Third, whereas hemodynamic measures are not affected by the spatial arrangement of the activated neurons, scalp EEG cannot detect activity from neuronal assemblies arranged in closed electrical fields (Nunez & Silberstein, 2000). This may explain why in the EEG literature it has been generally very difficult to reliably measure sources originating from the hippocampus, which represents a closed field due to its structural features. Along similar lines, spatial configurations of sources involving opposing dipoles located in sulci would generate activity that cannot be detected by scalp EEG, as the opposing dipoles would cancel each other (see dipolar sources A and B in Figure 3.6).

Consistent with these fundamental limitations, empirical evidence indicates that integration of electromagnetic and hemodynamic measures works extremely well in situations in which the fMRI and EEG/MEG activations correspond (Dale et al., 2000). However, in cases of imperfect or lacking correspondence between the fMRI and MEG/EEG activations, erroneous findings are likely to emerge (Baillet et al., 2001).

10. CONCLUSIONS

The past 20 years have witnessed unprecedented progress in our ability to study human brain function noninvasively. The high temporal resolution of electromagnetic measurements (EEG/MEG) continues to offer a unique window into the dynamics of brain function. In particular, EEG/MEG measures are exquisitely sensitive to spontaneous and induced changes of the functional brain state allowing investigation of brain mechanisms associated with covert internal states, which may not necessarily be accessible to introspection or behavioral observation.

The field of EEG research has perhaps witnessed its largest advances in the critical area of source imaging. A variety of innovative and sophisticated solutions for estimating intracerebral sources are continuing to emerge. In particular, approaches that make no a priori assumptions about the number of underlying sources and incorporate physiologically and anatomically sound priors to mathematically constrain the inverse solution have shown promising results. These improvements have opened exciting new avenues for functional brain imaging with both high temporal and spatial resolution. This is especially relevant for the wide range of experimental situations in which distributed neural networks are implicated.

In conclusion, advances in spatial sampling through high-density recordings, development of more realistic head models through high-resolution MRI, substantial progress in source localization techniques, and integration of different functional neuroimaging techniques have all contributed to improving our ability to investigate spatiotemporal dynamics of brain mechanisms underlying normal and pathological mental processes and states. In fact, the picture emerging from these methodological and conceptual improvements is that the spatial resolution of the EEG may approach that of other neuroimaging approaches, particularly when spatially smoothed fMRI or PET data are considered (e.g., Michel et al., 2004; Babiloni et al., 2004b). In the years to come, critical contributions to our understanding of the human mind can be expected from the EEG field.

ACKNOWLEDGMENTS

Preparation of this chapter was supported by NIMH Research Grant R01MH68376. The author is grateful to Richard Davidson, Alex Shackman, Lawrence Greischar,

Kyle Ratner, and John Potts for their comments on an earlier draft, and to James O'Shea for creating Figures 3.4 and 3.5.

REFERENCES

Ackermann, R. F., Finch, D. M., Babb, T. L., & Engel, J., Jr. (1984). Increased glucose metabolism during long-duration recurrent inhibition of hippocampal pyramidal cells. *Journal of Neuroscience, 4*, 251–264.

Allen, J. J. B., Coan, J. A., & Nazarian, M. (2004) Issues and assumptions on the road from raw signals to metrics of frontal EEG asymmetry in emotion. *Biological Psychology, 67*, 183–218.

American Electroencephalographic Society (1991). Guidelines for standard electrode position nomenclature. *Journal of Clinical Neurophysiology, 8*, 200–202.

Ary, J. P., Klein, S. A., & Fender, D. H. (1981). Location of sources of evoked scalp potentials: corrections for skull and scalp thickness. *IEEE Transactions on Biomedical Engineering, 28*, 447–452.

Arndt, S., Cizadlo, T., Andreasen, N. C., Heckel, D., Gold, S., O'Leary, D. S. (1996). Tests for comparing images based on randomization and permutation methods. *Journal of Cerebral Blood Flow & Metabolism, 16*, 1271–1279.

Asada, H., Fukuda, Y., Tsunoda, S., Yamaguchi, M., & Tonoike, M. (1999). Frontal midline theta rhythms reflect alternative activation of prefrontal cortex and anterior cingulate cortex in humans. *Neuroscience Letters, 274*, 29–32.

Astolfi, L., Cincotti, F., Mattia, D., Babiloni, C., Carducci, F., Basilisco, A. et al. (2005). Assessing cortical functional connectivity by linear inverse estimation and directed transfer function: simulations and application to real data. *Clinical Neurophysiology, 116*, 920–932.

Babiloni, F., Babiloni, C., Carducci, F., Fattorini, L., Onorati, P., & Urbano, A. (1996). Spline Laplacian estimate of EEG potentials over a realistic magnetic resonance-constructed scalp surface model. *Electroencephalography and Clinical Neurophysiology, 98*, 363–373.

Babiloni, F., Babiloni, C., Carducci, F., Romani, G. L., Rossini, P. M., Angelone, L. M., Cincotti, F. (2004a). Multimodal integration of EEG and MEG data: a simulation study with variable signal-to-noise ratio and number of sensors. *Human Brain Mapping, 22*, 52–62.

Babiloni, F., Mattia, D., Babiloni, C., Astolfi, L., Salinari, S., Basilisco, A. et al. (2004b). Multimodal integration of EEG, MEG and fMRI data for the solution of the neuroimage puzzle. *Magnetic Resonance Imaging, 22*, 1471–1476.

Baillet, S., Mosher, J. C., & Leahy, R. M. (2001). Electromagnetic Brain Mapping. *IEEE Signal Processing Magazine, 18*, 14–30.

Berger, H. (1929). Uber das Elektrenkephalogramm des Menschen. *Archiv für Psychiatrie und Nervenkrankheit, 87*, 555–574.

Bland, B. H. & Oddie, S. D. (1998). Anatomical, electrophysiological and pharmacological studies of ascending brainstem hippocampal synchronizing pathways. *Neuroscience and Biobehavioral Reviews, 22*, 259–273.

Borst, J. G., Leung, L. W., & MacFabe, D. F. (1987). Electrical activity of the cingulate cortex. II. Cholinergic modulation. *Brain Research, 407*, 81–93.

Bosch-Bayard, J., Valdes-Sosa, P., Virues-Alba, T., Aubert-Vazquez, E., John, E. R., Harmony, T. et al. (2001). 3D statistical parametric mapping of EEG source spectra by means of variable resolution electromagnetic tomography (VARETA). *Clinical Electroencephalography, 32*, 47–61.

Bouyer, J. J., Montaron, M. F., Vahnee, J. M., Albert, M. P., & Rougeul, A. (1987). Anatomical localization of cortical beta rhythms in cat. *Neuroscience, 22*, 863–869.

Bressler, S. L. & Kelso, J. A. (2001). Cortical coordination dynamics and cognition. *Trends in Cognitive Sciences, 5*, 26–36.

Brett, M., Johnsrude, I. S., & Owen, A. M. (2002). The problem of functional localization in the human brain. *Nature Review Neuroscience, 3*, 243–249.

Buzsaki, G. (1996). The hippocampo-neocortical dialogue. *Cerebral Cortex, 6*, 81–92.

Buzsaki, G. & Draguhn, A. (2004). Neuronal oscillations in cortical networks. *Science, 304, 1926–1929*.

Cantero, J. L., Atienza, M., Salas, R. M., & Gomez, C. M. (1999). Brain spatial microstates of human spontaneous alpha activity in relaxed wakefulness, drowsiness period, and REM sleep. *Brain Topography, 11*, 257–263.

Coan, J. A. & Allen, J. J. B. (2004). Frontal EEG asymmetry as a moderator and mediator of emotion. *Biological Psychology, 67*, 7–50.

Cooper, N. R., Croft, R. J., Dominey, S. J., Burgess, A. P., & Gruzelier, J. H. (2003). Paradox lost? Exploring the role of alpha oscillations during externally vs. internally directed attention and the implications for idling and inhibition hypotheses. *International Journal of Psychophysiology, 47*, 65–74.

Coutin-Churchman, P., Anez, Y., Uzcategui, M., Alvarez, L., Vergara, F., Mendez, L. et al. (2003). Quantitative spectral analysis of EEG in psychiatry revisited: drawing signs out of numbers in a clinical setting. *Clinical Neurophysiology, 114*, 2294–2306.

Croft, R. J., Chandler, J. S., Barry, R. J., Cooper, N. R., & Clarke, A. R. (2005). EOG correction: a comparison of four methods. *Psychophysiology, 42*, 16–24.

Cuffin, B. N., Schomer, D. L., Ives, J. R., & Blume, H. (2001). Experimental tests of EEG source localization accuracy in spherical head models. *Clinical Neurophysiology, 112*, 46–51.

Dale, A. M., Liu, A. K., Fischl, B. R., Buckner, R. L., Belliveau, J. W., Lewine, J. D. et al. (2000). Dynamic statistical parametric mapping: combining fMRI and MEG for high-resolution imaging of cortical activity. *Neuron, 26*, 55–67.

Davidson, R. J., Jackson, D. C., & Larson, C. L. (2000). Human Electroencephalography. In J.T. Cacioppo, L. G. Tassinary, & G. G. Bernston (Eds.), Handbook of Psychophysiology (2nd ed., pp. 27–56). Cambridge: Cambridge University Press.

Dien, J. (1998). Issues in the application of the average reference: Review, critiques, and recommendations. *Behavioral Research Methods, Instruments, and Computers, 30*, 34–43.

Ding, L., Lai, Y., & He, B. (2005). Low resolution brain electromagnetic tomography in a realistic geometry head model: a simulation study. *Physics in Medicine and Biology, 50*, 45–56.

Duffy, F. H., Burchfiel, J. L., & Lombroso, C. T. (1979). Brain electrical activity mapping (BEAM): a method for extending the clinical utility of EEG and evoked potential data. *Annals of Neurology, 5*, 309–321.

Dumermuth, G. & Molinari, L. (1987). Spectral analysis of EEG background activity. In A.S. Gevins & A. Remond (Eds.), *Handbook of Electroencephalography and Clinical Neurophysiology: Methods of Analysis of Brain Electrical and Magnetic Signals* (Revised Series ed., pp. 85–125). Amsterdam: Elsevier.

Engel, A. K., Fries, P., & Singer, W. (2001). Dynamic predictions: oscillations and synchrony in top-down processing. *Nature Reviews Neuroscience, 2*, 704–716.

Evans, A. C., Collins, D. L., Mills, S. R., Brown, E. D., Kelly, R. L., & Peters, T. M. (1993). 3D statistical neuroanatomical models from 305 MRI volumes. *Proceedings IEEE Nuclear Science Symposium and Medical Imaging Conference, 95,* 1813–1817.

Fell, J., Klaver, P., Elfadil, H., Schaller, C., Elger, C. E., & Fernandez, G. (2003). Rhinal-hippocampal theta coherence during declarative memory formation: Interaction with gamma synchronization? *European Journal of Neuroscience, 17,* 1082–1088.

Fender, D. H. (1987). Source localization of brain electrical activity. In A.S. Gevins & A. Remond (Eds.), *Methods of Analysis of Brain Electrical and Magnetic Signals* (pp. 355–403). Amsterdam; New York; Oxford: Elsevier.

Fernandez, T., Harmony, T., Silva-Pereyra, J., Fernandez-Bouzas, A., Gersenowies, J., Galan, L. et al. (2000). Specific EEG frequencies at specific brain areas and performance. *Neuroreport, 11,* 2663–2668.

Fernandez-Bouzas, A., Harmony, T., Bosch, J., Aubert, E., Fernandez, T., Valdes, P. et al. (1999). Sources of abnormal EEG activity in the presence of brain lesions. *Clinical Electroencephalography, 30,* 46–52.

Fink, A., Grabner, R. H., Neuper, C., & Neubauer, A. C. (2005). EEG alpha band dissociation with increasing task demands. *Cognitive Brain Research, 24,* 252–259.

Fisch, B. J. (1999). *Fisch & Spehlmann's EEG Primer: Basic Principles of Digital and Analog EEG.* (3rd (revised) ed.) Amsterdam: Elsevier.

Fuchs, M., Ford, M. R., Sands, S., & Lew, H. L. (2004). Overview of dipole source localization. *Physical Medicine and Rehabilitation Clinics of North America., 15,* 251–262.

Fuchs, M., Wagner, M., & Kastner, J. (2001). Boundary element method volume conductor models for EEG source reconstruction. *Clinical Neurophysiology, 112,* 1400–1407.

Fuchs, M., Wagner, M., Kohler, T., & Wischmann, H. A. (1999). Linear and nonlinear current density reconstructions. *Journal of Clinical Neurophysiology, 16,* 267–295.

Gamma, A., Lehmann, D., Frei, E., Iwata, K., Pascual-Marqui, R. D., & Vollenweider, F. X. (2004). Comparison of simultaneously recorded [H2(15)O]-PET and LORETA during cognitive and pharmacological activation. *Human Brain Mapping, 22,* 83–96.

Gasser, T. & Molinari, L. (1996). The analysis of the EEG. *Statistical Methods in Medical Research, 5,* 67–99.

Gevins, A., Le, J., Martin, N. K., Brickett, P., Desmond, J., & Reutter, B. (1994). High resolution EEG: 124-channel recording, spatial deblurring and MRI integration methods. *Electroencephalography & Clinical Neurophysiology, 90,* 337–358.

Gilmore, P. C. & Brenner, R. P. (1981). Correlation of EEG, computerized tomography, and clinical findings. Study of 100 patients with focal delta activity. *Archives of Neurology, 38,* 371–372.

Gorodnitsky, I. F., George, J. S., & Rao, B. D. (1995). Neuromagnetic source imaging with FOCUSS: a recursive weighted minimum norm algorithm. *Electroencephalography & Clinical Neurophysiology, 95,* 231–251.

Grave de Peralta Menendez R. & Gonzalez Andino, S. L. (2000). Discussing the Capabilities of Laplacian Minimization. *Brain Topography, 13,* 97–104.

Grave de Peralta, M. R., Gonzalez, A. S., Lantz, G., Michel, C. M., & Landis, T. (2001). Noninvasive localization of electromagnetic epileptic activity. I. Method descriptions and simulations. *Brain Topography, 14,* 131–137.

Greischar, L. L., Burghy, C. A., van Reekum, C. M., Jackson, D. C., Pizzagalli, D. A., Mueller, C. et al. (2004). Effects of electrode density and electrolyte spreading in dense array electroencephalographic recording. *Clinical Neurophysiology, 115,* 710–720.

Gross, D. W. & Gotman, J. (1999). Correlation of high-frequency oscillations with the sleep-wake cycle and cognitive activity in humans. *Neuroscience, 94,* 1005–1018.

Haalman, I. & Vaadia, E. (1997). Dynamics of neuronal interactions: Relation to behavior, firing rates, and distance between neurons. *Human Brain Mapping, 5,* 249–253.

Hagemann, D., & Naumann, E. (2001). The effects of ocular artifacts on (lateralized) broadband power in the EEG. *Clinical Neurophysiology, 112,* 215–231.

Hamalainen, M. S. & Ilmoniemi, R. J. (1994). Interpreting magnetic fields of the brain: minimum norm estimates. *Medical & Biological Engineering & Computing, 32,* 35–42.

Hamalainen, M. S. & Sarvas, J. (1989). Realistic conductivity geometry model of the human head for interpretation of neuromagnetic data. *IEEE Transactions on Biomedical Engineering, 36,* 165–171.

He, B. (1999). Brain electric source imaging: Scalp Laplacian mapping and cortical imaging. *Critical Reviews in Biomedical Engineering, 27,* 149–188.

Heinze, H. J., Mangun, G. R., Burchert, W., Hinrichs, H., Scholz, M., Munte, T. F. et al. (1994). Combined spatial and temporal imaging of brain activity during visual selective attention in humans. *Nature, 372,* 543–546.

Helmholtz, H. L. F. (1853). Ueber einige Gesetze der Vertheilung elektrischer Ströme in körperlichen Leitern mit Anwendung aud die thierisch-elektrischen Versuche. *Annalen der Physik und Chemie, 9,* 211–233.

Hjorth, B. (1975). An on-line transformation of EEG scalp potentials into orthogonal source derivations. *Electroencephalography & Clinical Neurophysiology, 39,* 526–530.

Holmes, A. P., Blair, R. C., Watson, J. D. G, & Ford, I (1996). Nonparametric analysis of statistic images from functional mapping experiments. *Journal of Cerebral Blood Flow & Metabolism, 16,* 7–22.

Huang, C., Wahlund, L., Dierks, T., Julin, P., Winblad, B., & Jelic, V. (2000). Discrimination of Alzheimer's disease and mild cognitive impairment by equivalent EEG sources: a cross-sectional and longitudinal study. *Clinical Neurophysiology, 111,* 1961–1967.

Hughes, J. R. & John, E. R. (1999). Conventional and quantitative electroencephalography in psychiatry. *Journal of Neuropsychiatry and Clinical Neurosciences, 11,* 190–208.

Jasper, H. H. (1958). The ten-twenty electrode system of the International Federation. *Electroencephalography & Clinical Neurophysiology, 10,* 371–375.

Jeffs, B., Leahy, R., & Singh, M. (1987). An evaluation of methods for neuromagnetic image reconstruction. *IEEE Transactions on Biomedical Engineering, 34,* 713–723.

John, E. R., Ahn, H., Prichep, L., Trepetin, M., Brown, D., & Kaye, H. (1980). Developmental equations for the electroencephalogram. *Science, 210,* 1255–1258.

Kincses, W. E., Braun, C., Kaiser, S., & Elbert, T. (1999). Modeling extended sources of event-related potentials using anatomical and physiological constraints. *Human Brain Mapping, 8,* 182–193.

Klimesch, W. (1999). EEG alpha and theta oscillations reflect cognitive and memory performance: A review and analysis. *Brain Research Reviews, 29*, 169–195.

Koenig, T., Prichep, L., Lehmann, D., Sosa, P. V., Braeker, E., Kleinlogel, H. et al. (2002). Millisecond by millisecond, year by year: normative EEG microstates and developmental stages. *Neuroimage, 16*, 41–48.

Koles, Z. J. (1998). Trends in EEG source localization. *Electroencephalography & Clinical Neurophysiology, 106*, 127–137.

Lancaster, J. L., Rainey, L. H., Summerlin, J. L., Freitas, C. S., Fox, P. T., Evans, A. C., et al. Automated labeling of the human brain: A preliminary report on the development and evaluation of a forward-transformed method. *Human Brain Mapping, 5*, 238–242.

Lantz, G., Grave de Peralta, R., Spinelli, L., Seeck, M., & Michel, C. M. (2003). Epileptic source localization with high density EEG: how many electrodes are needed? *Clinical Neurophysiology, 114*, 63–69.

Lantz, G., Michel, C. M., Pascual-Marqui, R. D., Spinelli, L., Seeck, M., Seri, S., et al. (1997). Extracranial localization of intracranial interictal epileptiform activity using LORETA (low resolution electromagnetic tomography). *Electroencephalography & Clinical Neurophysiology, 102*, 414–422.

Larson, C. L., Davidson, R. J., Abercrombie, H. C., Ward, R. T., Schaefer, S. M., Jackson, D. C., Holden, J. E., & Perlman, S. B. (1998). Relations between PET-derived measures of thalamic glucose metabolism and EEG alpha power. *Psychophysiology, 35*, 162–169.

Lehmann, D. (1971). Multichannel topography of human alpha EEG fields. *Electroencephalography & Clinical Neurophysiology, 31*, 439–449.

Lehmann, D. (1990). Brain electric microstates and cognition: The atoms of thought. In E.R. John (Ed.), *Machinery of the Mind*. Boston: Birkhäuser, pp. 209–224.

Lehmann, D. (1987). Principles of spatial analysis. In A.S. Gevins & A. Remond (Eds.), *Handbook of Electroencephalography and Clinical Neurophysiology: Methods of Analysis of Brain Electrical and Magnetic Signals* (Revised Series ed., pp. 309–354). Amsterdam: Elsevier.

Lehmann, D., Faber, P. L., Galderisi, S., Herrmann, W. M., Kinoshita, T., Koukkou, M. et al. (2005). EEG microstate duration and syntax in acute, medication-naive, first-episode schizophrenia: a multi-center study. *Psychiatry Research, 138*, 141–156.

Lehmann, D., Henggeler, B., Koukkou, M., & Michel, C. M. (1993). Source localization of brain electric field frequency bands during conscious, spontaneous, visual imagery and abstract thought. *Brain Research: Cognitive Brain Research, 1*, 203–210.

Lehmann, D. & Michel, C. M. (1989). Intracerebral dipole sources of EEG FFT power maps. *Brain Topography, 2*, 155–164.

Leoncani, L. & Comi, G. (1999). EEG coherence in pathological conditions. *Journal of Clinical Neurophysiology, 16*, 548–555.

Liu, A. K., Belliveau, J. W., & Dale, A. M. (1998). Spatiotemporal imaging of human brain activity using functional MRI constrained magnetoencephalography data: Monte Carlo simulations. *Proceedings of the National Academy of Sciences of the United States of America, 95*, 8945–8950.

Llinas, R. R. (1988). The intrinsic electrophysiological properties of mammalian neurons: insights into central nervous system function. *Science, 242*, 1654–1664.

Llinas, R. R., Ribary, U., Jeanmonod, D., Kronberg, E., & Mitra, P. P. (1999). Thalamocortical dysrhythmia: A neurological and neuropsychiatric syndrome characterized by magnetoencephalography. *Proceedings of the National Academy of Sciences of the United States of America, 96*, 15222–15227.

Logothetis, N. K., Pauls, J., Augath, M., Trinath, T., & Oeltermann, A. (2001). Neurophysiological investigation of the basis of the fMRI signal. *Nature, 412*, 150–157.

Lopes da Silva, F. (2004). Functional localization of brain sources using EEG and/or MEG data: volume conductor and source models. *Magnetic Resonance Imaging, 22*, 1533–1538.

Luu, P., Tucker, D. M., Derryberry, D., Reed, M., & Poulsen, C. (2003). Electrophysiological responses to errors and feedback in the process of action regulation. *Psychological Science, 14*, 47–53.

Luu, P., Tucker, D. M., Englander, R., Lockfeld, A., Lutsep, H., & Oken, B. (2001). Localizing acute stroke-related EEG changes: assessing the effects of spatial undersampling. *Journal of Clinical Neurophysiology, 18*, 302–317.

Makeig, S., Bell, A. J., Jung, T. P., & Sejnowski, T. J. (1996). Independent component analysis of electroencephalographic data. *Advances in Neural Information Processing Systems, 8*, 145–151.

Mann, E. O. & Paulsen, O. (2005). Mechanisms underlying gamma ('40 Hz') network oscillations in the hippocampus – a mini-review. *Progress in Biophysics and Molecular Biology, 87*, 67–76.

Maurer, K. & Dierks, T. (1991). *Atlas of Brain Mapping: Topographic Mapping of EEG and Evoked Potentials*. Berlin: Springer-Verlag.

Michel, C. M., Lehmann, D., Henggeler, B., & Brandeis, D. (1992). Localization of the sources of EEG delta, theta, alpha and beta frequency bands using the FFT dipole approximation. *Electroencephalography and Clinical Neurophysiology, 82*, 38–44.

Michel, C. M., Murray, M. M., Lantz, G., Gonzalez, S., Spinelli, L., & Grave, d. P. (2004). EEG source imaging. *Clinical Neurophysiology, 115*, 2195–2222.

Miller, C. E. & Henriquez, C. S. (1990). Finite element analysis of bioelectric phenomena. *Critical Reviews in Biomedical Engineering, 18*, 207–233.

Miltner, W. H., Braun, C., Arnold, M., Witte, H., & Taub, E. (1999). Coherence of gamma-band EEG activity as a basis for associative learning. *Nature, 397*, 434–436.

Moffitt, M. A. & Grill, W. M. (2004). Electrical localization of neural activity in the dorsal horn of the spinal cord: a modeling study. *Annals of Biomedical Engineering, 32*, 1694–1709.

Mosher, J. C. & Leahy, R. M. (1998). Recursive MUSIC: a framework for EEG and MEG source localization. *IEEE Transactions on Biomedical Engineering, 45*, 1342–1354.

Mosher, J. C., Lewis, P. S., & Leahy, R. M. (1992). Multiple dipole modeling and localization from spatio-temporal MEG data. *IEEE Transactions on Biomedical Engineering, 39*, 541–557.

Mulert, C., Gallinat, J., Pascual-Marqui, R., Dorn, H., Frick, K., Schlattmann, P. et al. (2001). Reduced event-related current density in the anterior cingulate cortex in schizophrenia. *Neuroimage, 13*, 589–600.

Mulert, C., Jager, L., Schmitt, R., Bussfeld, P., Pogarell, O., Moller, H. J. et al. (2004). Integration of fMRI and simultaneous EEG: Towards a comprehensive understanding of localization and time-course of brain activity in target detection. *Neuroimage, 22*, 83–94.

Murray, M. M., Michel, C. M., Grave, d. P., Ortigue, S., Brunet, D., Gonzalez, A. S. et al. (2004). Rapid discrimination of visual and multisensory memories revealed by electrical neuroimaging. *Neuroimage, 21*, 125–135.

Murthy, V. N. & Fetz, E. E. (1992). Coherent 25- to 35-Hz oscillations in the sensorimotor cortex of awake behaving monkeys. *Proceedings of the National Academy of Sciences of the United States of America, 89,* 5670–5674.

Niedermeyer, E. (1993). Historical Aspects. In E. Niedermeyer & F. Lopes da Silva (Eds.), *Electroencephalography: Basic principles, clinical applications, and related fields* (3rd ed., pp. 1–14). Baltimore: Williams & Wilkins.

Niedermeyer, E. (1993). Sleep and EEG. In E. Niedermeyer & F. Lopes da Silva (Eds.), *Electroencephalography: Basic Principles, Clinical Applications, and Related Fields* (3rd ed., pp. 153–166). Baltimore: Williams & Wilkins.

Nunez, P. L. & Pilgreen, K. L. (1991). The spline-Laplacian in clinical neurophysiology: a method to improve EEG spatial resolution. *Journal of Clinical Neurophysiology, 8,* 397–413.

Nunez, P. L. & Silberstein, R. B. (2000). On the relationship of synaptic activity to macroscopic measurements: does co-registration of EEG with fMRI make sense? *Brain Topography, 13,* 79–96.

Nunez, P. L., Srinivasan, R., Wijesinghe, R. S., Westdorp, A. F., Tucker, D. M., Silberstein, R. B., & Cadusch, P. J. (1997). EEG coherency. I: Statistics, reference electrode, volume conduction, Laplacians, cortical imaging, and interpretation at multiple scales. *Electroencephalography and Clinical Neurophysiology, 103,* 499–515.

Nuwer, M. R., Lehmann, D., Lopes da Silva, F., Matsuoka, S., Sutherling, W., & Vibert, J. F. (1999). IFCN guidelines for topographic and frequency analysis of EEGs and EPs. The International Federation of Clinical Neurophysiology. *Electroencephalography & Clinical Neurophysiology, 52 (Supplement),* 15–20.

Oakes, T. R., Pizzagalli, D. A., Hendrick, A. M., Horras, K. A., Larson, C. L., Abercrombie, H. C. et al. (2004). Functional coupling of simultaneous electrical and metabolic activity in the human brain. *Human Brain Mapping, 21,* 257–270.

Onton, J., Delorme, A., & Makeig, S. (2005). Frontal midline EEG dynamics during working memory. *NeuroImage, 27,* 341–356.

Oostenveld, R. & Praamstra, P. (2001). The five percent electrode system for high-resolution EEG and ERP measurements. *Clinical Neurophysiology, 112,* 713–719.

Pascual-Marqui, R. D. (1999). Review of methods for solving the EEG inverse problem. *International Journal of Bioelectromagnetism, 1,* 75–86.

Pascual-Marqui, R. D. (2002). Standardized low-resolution brain electromagnetic tomography (sLORETA): technical details. *Methods and Findings in Experimental and Clinical Pharmacology, 24 (Supplement D),* 5–12.

Pascual-Marqui, R. D., Esslen, M., Kochi, K., & Lehmann, D. (2002). Functional imaging with low-resolution brain electromagnetic tomography (LORETA): a review. *Methods and Findings in Experimental and Clinical Pharmacology, 24 (Supplement C),* 91–95.

Pascual-Marqui, R. D., Lehmann, D., Koenig, T., Kochi, K., Merlo, M. C., Hell, D. et al. (1999). Low resolution brain electromagnetic tomography (LORETA) functional imaging in acute, neuroleptic-naive, first-episode, productive schizophrenia. *Psychiatry Research: Neuroimaging, 90,* 169–179.

Pascual-Marqui, R. D., Michel, C. M., & Lehmann, D. (1994). Low resolution electromagnetic tomography: a new method for localizing electrical activity in the brain. *International Journal of Psychophysiology, 18,* 49–65.

Perrin, F., Bertrand, O., & Pernier, J. (1987). Scalp current density mapping: value and estimation from potential data. *IEEE Transactions on Biomedical Engineering, 34,* 283–288.

Perrin, F., Pernier, J., Bertrand, D., & Echallier, J. F. (1989). Spherical splines for scalp potential and current density mapping. *Electroencephalography & Clinical Neurophysiology, 72,* 184–187.

Pfurtscheller, G., Stancak, A., Jr., & Neuper, C. (1996). Event-related synchronization (ERS) in the alpha band – an electrophysiological correlate of cortical idling: A review. *International Journal of Psychophysiology, 24,* 39–46.

Phillips, C., Rugg, M. D., & Friston, K. J. (2002a). Anatomically informed basis functions for EEG source localization: Combining functional and anatomical constraints. *Neuroimage, 16,* 678–695.

Phillips, C., Rugg, M. D., & Friston, K. J. (2002b). Systematic regularization of linear inverse solutions of the EEG source localization problem. *Neuroimage, 17,* 287–301.

Pivik, R. T., Broughton, R. J., Coppola, R., Davidson, R. J., Fox, N., & Nuwer, M. R. (1993). Guidelines for the recording and quantitative analysis of electroencephalographic activity in research contexts. *Psychophysiology, 30,* 547–558.

Pizzagalli, D. A., Lehmann, D., Hendrick, A. M., Regard, M., Pascual-Marqui, R. D., & Davidson, R. J. (2002). Affective judgments of faces modulate early activity (approximately 160 ms) within the fusiform gyri. *Neuroimage, 16,* 663–677.

Pizzagalli, D. A., Nitschke, J. B., Oakes, T. R., Hendrick, A. M., Horras, K. A., Larson, C. L. et al. (2002). Brain electrical tomography in depression: The importance of symptom severity, anxiety and melancholic features. *Biological Psychiatry, 52,* 73–85.

Pizzagalli, D. A., Oakes, T. R., & Davidson, R. J. (2003). Coupling of theta activity and glucose metabolism in the human rostral anterior cingulate cortex: An EEG/PET study of normal and depressed subjects. *Psychophysiology, 40,* 939–949.

Pizzagalli, D. A., Oakes, T. R., Fox, A. S., Chung, M. K., Larson, C. L., Abercrombie, H. C. et al. (2004). Functional but not structural subgenual prefrontal cortex abnormalities in melancholia. *Molecular Psychiatry, 9,* 393–405.

Pizzagalli, D. A., Pascual-Marqui, R. D., Nitschke, J. B., Oakes, T. R., Larson, C. L., Abercrombie, H. C. et al. (2001). Anterior cingulate activity as a predictor of degree of treatment response in major depression: Evidence from brain electrical tomography analysis. *American Journal of Psychiatry, 158,* 405–415.

Pizzagalli, D. A., Peccoralo, L. A., Davidson, R. J., & Cohen, J. D. (2006). Resting anterior cingulate activity and abnormal responses to errors in subjects with elevated depressive symptoms: A 128-channel EEG study. *Human Brain Mapping, 27,* 185–201.

Pizzagalli, D. A., Sherwood, R. J., Henriques, J. B., & Davidson, R. J. (2005). Frontal brain asymmetry and reward responsiveness: A Source-localization study. *Psychological Science, 16,* 805–813.

Reddy, R. V., Moorthy, S. S., Mattice, T., Dierdorf, S. F., & Deitch, R. D., Jr. (1992). An electroencephalographic comparison of effects of propofol and methohexital. *Electroencephalography & Clinical Neurophysiology, 83,* 162–168.

Rodriguez, E., Lachaux, G. N., Martinerie, J., Renault, B., & Varela, F. L. (1999). Perception's shadow: Long distance synchronization of human brain activity. *Nature, 397,* 430–433.

Russell, G. S., Jeffrey, E. K., Poolman, P., Luu, P., & Tucker, D. M. (2005). Geodesic photogrammetry for localizing sensor positions in dense-array EEG. *Clinical Neurophysiology, 116,* 1130–1140.

Samar, V. J., Bopardikar, A., Rao, R., & Swartz, K. (1999). Wavelet analysis of neuroelectric waveforms: A conceptual tutorial. *Brain and Language, 66,* 7–60.

Schack, B., Vath, N., Petsche, H., Geissler, H. G., & Moller, E. (2002). Phase-coupling of theta-gamma EEG rhythms during short-term memory processing. *International Journal of Psychophysiology, 44,* 143–163.

Schacter, D. L. (1977). EEG theta waves and psychological phenomena: A review and analysis. *Biological Psychology, 5,* 47–82.

Scherg, M. & Ebersole, J. S. (1994). Brain source imaging of focal and multifocal epileptiform EEG activity. *Neurophysiologie clinique, 24,* 51–60.

Schnitzler, A. & Gross, J. (2005). Normal and pathological oscillatory communication in the brain. *Nature Reviews Neuroscience, 6,* 285–296.

Seeck, M., Lazeyras, F., Michel, C. M., Blanke, O., Gericke, C. A., Ives, J. et al. (1998). Non-invasive epileptic focus localization using EEG-triggered functional MRI and electromagnetic tomography. *Electroencephalography & Clinical Neurophysiology, 106,* 508–512.

Soufflet, L., Toussaint, M., Luthringer, R., Gresser, J., Minot, R., & Macher, J. P. (1991). A statistical evaluation of the main interpolation methods applied to 3-dimensional EEG mapping. *Electroencephalography & Clinical Neurophysiology, 79,* 393–402.

Speckmann, E., Elger, C. E., & Altrup, U. (1993). Neurophysiologic basis of the EEG. In E. Wyllie (Ed.), *The Treatment of Epilepsy: Principles and Practices* (pp. 185–201). Philadelphia: Lea & Febiger.

Srinivasan, R., Tucker, D. M., & Murias, M. (1998). Estimating the spatial Nyquist of the human EEG. *Behavioral Research Methods, Instruments & Computers, 30,* 8–19.

Steriade, M. (1993). Cellular substrates of brain rhythms. In E. Niedermeyer & F. Lopes da Silva (Eds.), *Electroencephalography: Basic Principles, Clinical Applications, and Related Fields* (3rd ed., pp. 27–62). Baltimore: Williams & Wilkins.

Strik, W. K., Chiaramonti, R., Muscas, G. C., Paganini, M., Mueller, T. J., Fallgatter, A. J. et al. (1997). Decreased EEG microstate duration and anteriorisation of the brain electrical fields in mild and moderate dementia of the Alzheimer type. *Psychiatry Research, 75,* 183–191.

Sutton, S. K., & Davidson, R. J. (2000). Resting anterior brain activity predicts the evaluation of. affective stimuli. *Neuropsychologia, 38,* 1723–1733.

Szelies, B., Mielke, R., Kessler, J., & Heiss, W. D. (1999). EEG power changes are related to regional cerebral glucose metabolism in vascular dementia. *Clinical Neurophysiology, 110,* 615–620.

Tassinary, L. G., & Cacioppo, J. T. (2000). The skeletomuscular system: Surface electromyography. In J. T. Cacioppo, L. G. Tassinary, & G. G. Berntson (Eds.), *Handbook of psychophysiology,* 2nd edition (pp. 163–199). New York: Cambridge University Press.

Thakor, N. V. & Tong, S. (2004). Advances in quantitative electroencephalogram analysis methods. *Annual Review of Biomedical Engineering, 6,* 453–495.

Thatcher, R. W., Krause, P. J., & Hrybyk, M. (1986). Corticocortical associations and EEG coherence: A two-compartment model. *Electroencephalography & Clinical Neurophysiology, 64,* 123–143.

Thut, G., Hauert, C. A., Morand, S., Seeck, M., Landis, T., & Michel, C. (1999). Evidence for interhemispheric motor-level transfer in a simple reaction time task: an EEG study. *Experimental Brain Research, 128,* 256–261.

Towle, V. L., Bolanos, J., Suarez, D., Tan, K., Grzeszczuk, R., Levin, D. N. et al. (1993). The spatial location of EEG electrodes: locating the best-fitting sphere relative to cortical anatomy. *Electroencephalography & Clinical Neurophysiology, 86,* 1–6.

Towle, V. L., Syed, I., Berger, C., Grzeszcuk, R., Milton, J., Erickson, R. K. et al. (1998). Identification of the sensory/motor area and pathologic regions using ECoG coherence. *Electroencephalography & Clinical Neurophysiology, 106,* 30–39.

Trujillo-Barreto, N. J., Aubert-Vazquez, E., & Valdes-Sosa, P. A. (2004). Bayesian model averaging in EEG/MEG imaging. *Neuroimage, 21,* 1300–1319.

Tsuno, N., Shigeta, M., Hyoki, K., Kinoshita, T., Ushijima, S., Faber, P. L. et al. (2002). Spatial organization of EEG activity from alertness to sleep stage 2 in old and younger subjects. *Journal of Sleep Research, 11,* 43–51.

Tuch, D. S., Wedeen, V. J., Dale, A. M., George, J. S., & Belliveau, J. W. (1999). Conductivity mapping of biological tissue using diffusion MRI. *Annals of the New York Academy of Sciences, 888,* 314–316.

Tucker, D. M. (1993). Spatial sampling of head electrical fields: The geodesic sensor net. *Electroencephalography & Clinical Neurophysiology, 87,* 154–163.

Uchida, S., Nakayama, H., Maehara, T., Hirai, N., Arakaki, H., Nakamura, M. et al. (2000). Suppression of gamma activity in the human medial temporal lobe by sevoflurane anesthesia. *Neuroreport, 11,* 39–42.

Valdes-Sosa, P., Marti, F., Garcia, F., and Casanova, R. (1996). Variable Resolution Electric-Magnetic Tomography. In C. Wood (Ed.), *Proceedings of the Tenth International Conference on Biomagnetism.* Santa Fe, New Mexico.

Vertes, R. P. & Kocsis, B. (1997). Brainstem-diencephalo-septohippocampal systems controlling the theta rhythm of the hippocampus. *Neuroscience, 81,* 893–926.

Vinogradova, O. S. (1995). Expression, control, and probable functional significance of the neuronal theta-rhythm. *Progress in Neurobiology, 45,* 523–583.

Vitacco, D., Brandeis, D., Pascual-Marqui, R., & Martin, E. (2002). Correspondence of event-related potential tomography and functional magnetic resonance imaging during language processing. *Human Brain Mapping, 17,* 4–12.

von Stein, A. & Sarnthein, J. (2000). Different frequencies for different scales of cortical integration: from local gamma to long range alpha/theta synchronization. *International Journal of Psychophysiology, 38,* 301–313.

Wagner, M., Fuchs, M., & Kastner, J. (2004). Evaluation of sLORETA in the presence of noise and multiple sources. *Brain Topography, 16,* 277–280.

Weiss, S. & Mueller, H. M. (2003). The contribution of EEG coherence to the investigation of language. *Brain and Language, 85,* 325–343.

Worrell, G. A., Lagerlund, T. D., Sharbrough, F. W., Brinkmann, B. H., Busacker, N. E., Cicora, K. M. et al. (2000). Localization of the epileptic focus by low-resolution electromagnetic tomography in patients with a lesion demonstrated by MRI. *Brain Topography, 12,* 273–282.

Yao, J. & Dewald, J. P. (2005). Evaluation of different cortical source localization methods using simulated and experimental EEG data. *Neuroimage, 25,* 369–382.

4 Event-Related Brain Potentials: Methods, Theory, and Applications

MONICA FABIANI, GABRIELE GRATTON, AND KARA D. FEDERMEIER

1. INTRODUCTION AND HISTORICAL CONTEXT

Ever since Berger (1929) demonstrated that it is possible to record the electrical activity of the brain by placing electrodes on the surface of the scalp, there has been considerable interest in the relationship between these recordings of neurophysiological activity and psychological processes. Although Berger and his followers focused their attention on spontaneous rhythmic oscillations in voltage (i.e., on the electroencephalogram or EEG) more recent research has concentrated on those aspects of the electrical potential that are specifically time-locked to events (i.e., on event-related brain potentials or ERPs). ERPs reflect brain activity from synchronously active populations of neurons that occurs in preparation for or in response to discrete events, be they internal or external to the subject. Conceptually, ERPs are regarded as neural manifestations of specific psychological functions.

The history of ERP research is closely linked with the development of technologies that allow for the extraction of event-related brain activity from the background EEG oscillations, which are usually much larger in amplitude and therefore tend to obscure it (for an extended review see Donchin, 1979). The first of these techniques was based on the photographic superimposition of several time-locked EEG traces (Dawson, 1947; Ciganek, 1964). This method, however, was very cumbersome, and it was soon replaced by the development of several analog signal averagers (see Donchin, 1979). However, it was not until the 1960s and the advent of digital computers (and, thus, of digital signal averaging) that ERP research really took flight.

The last several decades have seen a number of paradigmatic shifts in the focus of this research. In the 1970s and early 1980s, the analysis and interpretation of ERPs was informed by the computer analogy of the human information processing system: ERP components (i.e., peaks and troughs in the waveforms that tend to covary in response to experimental manipulations) could be viewed as subroutines within this system, each indexing some aspect of cognitive processing (Donchin, 1979; 1981). Within this framework, the focus was mostly on the relationship

between specific cognitive processes and ERP activity, without much reference to the possible underlying brain sources of the potentials. Beginning in the 1990s, however, the rapid expansion of non-invasive brain imaging methods (e.g., Toga & Mazziotta, 1996) and recent technological advances that allow for the simultaneous recordings from dense electrode arrays (e.g., Tucker, 1993) have brought forth two further changes (which will be discussed more extensively in Section 2.4): (a) several algorithms have been developed to derive the putative brain sources of scalp-recorded electrical activity; and, (b) several attempts have been made at integrating the recording of ERPs with other brain imaging methods, such as Positron Emission Tomography (PET), functional Magnetic Resonance Imaging (fMRI), magneto-encephalography (MEG) and optical imaging (event-related optical signal, or EROS, and near-infrared spectroscopy, or NIRS). At present, ERPs are one of the most established methods in cognitive neuroscience – and one of the few that provide a direct measure of neural activity – and are considered the "gold standard" for temporal resolution[1] among noninvasive imaging methods.

In Section 2 of this chapter, we will review: (a) the procedures for ERP derivation; (b) what is known about the underlying sources of ERPs and their relationship to physiological function; and (c) the concept of a component and some aspects of component quantification. Later in this chapter, we will focus on the relationship between ERPs and psychological function.

2. THE PHYSICAL CONTEXT

2.1. Deriving event-related potentials

The procedures used to derive ERPs begin with the same amplifiers and filters used to obtain EEG (see Figure 4.1). Electrodes are attached to the scalp at various locations

---

[1] Temporal resolution can be defined as the ability to determine the order of occurrence of two events that are close to each other in time.

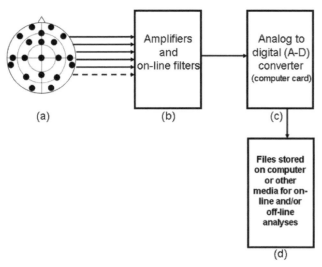

Figure 4.1. Schematic representation of the operations involved in the recording of ERPs. From left to right: (a) Top view of the head, indicating the placements of several electrodes from which EEG is recorded; (b) the EEG signal is then transferred to an amplifying and on-line filtering system; (c) the analog signal is then converted into a digital signal by sampling the potential at a high frequency (usually at least 100 Hz) by an Analog-to-Digital converter (usually a dedicated computer card); (d) the digitally transformed signal is stored on a computer or other media for on-line or off-line analyses, which often include artifact removal and averaging as well a number of other steps.

(at least two leads are needed for measuring a voltage difference) and connected to amplifiers. The recording locations are most often chosen according to the International 10–20 system (Jasper, 1958) or expanded versions of this system (e.g., Nuwer, 1987), to facilitate between-laboratory and between-experiment comparisons. However, given the ever-growing availability of computing power, more and more labs are also using custom-designed dense arrays, often geodesic, to allow for better interpolation and ultimately better characterization of the scalp distributions of the potentials and source modeling. The outputs of the amplifiers are converted to numbers by a device for measuring electrical potentials, an analog-digital converter. The potentials are sampled at a frequency ranging from 100 to 10,000 Hz (cycles per second), depending on the temporal properties of the brain activities of interest, and are then stored in files for subsequent analysis.

The ERP is small (a few microvolts) in comparison to the EEG (about 50 microvolts). Thus, analysis generally begins with procedures to increase the discrimination of the *signal* (the ERP) from the *noise* (background EEG). The most common of these procedures involves *averaging* samples of the EEG that are time-locked to repeated occurrences of a particular event or type of event. The number of samples used in the average is related to the signal-to-noise ratio (see Section 2.6.2). However, in all cases, the samples are selected so that they bear a consistent temporal relationship to the event. Because aspects of the EEG that are not time-locked to the event are assumed to vary randomly from sample to sample, the averaging procedure should

result in a reduction of these noise potentials, rendering the signal, event-related potentials visible.[2] The resulting voltage × time function (see Figure 4.2) contains a number of positive and negative peaks that can then be subjected to a variety of measurement operations (see Section 2.6 and chapters by Jennings et al. and Gratton, this volume).

Because ERPs are always measured as differences in potential between two recording locations, they will also vary as a function of the electrode site at which they are recorded, as well as the reference electrode used. Spatial (topographic) distribution is regarded as an important discriminative characteristic of the ERP (Donchin, 1978; Sutton & Ruchkin, 1984). Therefore, positive and negative peaks in the ERP are generally described in terms of their characteristic scalp distribution, as well as their polarity, and latency.

The labels given to the peaks of an ERP waveform often include descriptors of polarity and latency. According to this logic, P300 refers to a positive deflection with a modal peak latency of 300 ms. A similar labeling system involves a descriptor of polarity (P or N) followed by a number designating the ordinal latency of the component. Within this system, P3 refers to the third positive peak in the waveform. Other descriptors that can be used in labeling peaks make reference to the scalp locations at which the potential is maximal (e.g., frontal P300), or to the psychological or experimental conditions that control the potential (e.g., novelty P3, readiness potential or RP, mismatch negativity, or MMN).

2.2. The exogenous versus endogenous distinction

From a psychological point of view, it has often been convenient to distinguish between different types of ERPs. Traditionally, investigators have identified those ERPs whose characteristics are largely controlled by the physical properties of an external eliciting event. Such evoked potentials are considered to be obligatory (in the sense that if the eliciting stimulus is perceived they will be always be elicited) and are referred to as "sensory" or "exogenous." Examples of these evoked activities are the brainstem potentials. The counterparts of these exogenous activities are ERPs whose characteristics are largely determined by the nature of the interaction between the person and the event. For example, some ERPs vary as a function of the information processing activities required of the subject; others can be elicited in the *absence* of an external eliciting event. These potentials are referred to as "endogenous." Examples of exogenous activities are the P300 and the error-related negativity (ERN; for a discussion of the distinction between exogenous and endogenous potentials, see Donchin, Ritter, and McCallum, 1978).

---

[2] Note that this assumption may not always be valid, as, for example, in the case of variability in the latency and other characteristics of the erp from sample to sample (see Section 2.6.2). Furthermore, the ERP derived by averaging may include potentials that do not originate in the brain but are time-locked to the event (see Section 2.6.1).

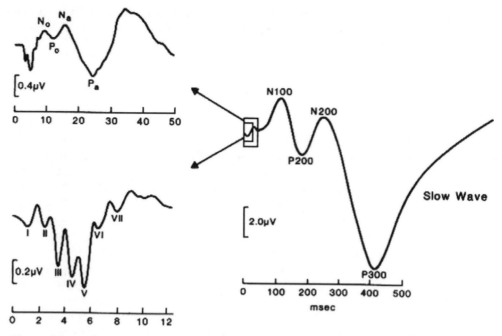

Figure 4.2. A schematic representation of ERP components elicited by auditory, infrequent target stimuli. The three panels represent three different voltage × time functions: the left bottom panel shows the very early sensory components (with a latency of less than 10 ms); the left top panel shows the middle latency sensory components (with a latency of between 10 and 50 ms); and the right panel shows late components (latency exceeding 50 ms). Note the different voltage and time scales used in the three panels, as well as the different nomenclatures used to label the peaks (components). (Adapted with permission of the author from Donchin, 1979, with kind permission of Springer Science and Business media.)

Although the exogenous/endogenous distinction provides a useful method for classifying many ERP components, there are potentials that possess characteristics that are intermediate between these two groups, and are therefore called "mesogenous." The N100 (see Section 4.3.1) is such an example, as it is sensitive to both the physical properties of the stimulus and the nature of the interaction between the subject and the event (e.g., whether the event is to be attended).

2.3. From the brain to the scalp: the generation and physiological basis of ERPs

In this section, we review evidence that relates the scalp-recorded electrical activity to its underlying anatomical and physiological basis (see also Allison, Wood, & McCarthy, 1986; Nunez, 1981). It is generally assumed that ERPs are distant manifestations of the activity of populations of neurons within the brain. This activity can be recorded on the surface of the scalp because the tissue that lies between the source and the scalp acts as a volume-conductor. Because the electrical activity associated with any particular neuron is small, at the scalp it is only possible to record the integrated activity of a large number of neurons. Two requirements must be met for this integration to occur: (a) the neurons must be active synchronously, and (b) the electric fields generated by each particular neuron must be oriented in such a way that their

effects at the scalp cumulate. As a consequence, only a subset of the entire brain electrical activity can be recorded from scalp electrodes.

Two considerations further restrict the likely sources of the scalp-recorded ERP. First, because the ERP represents the synchronous activity of a large number of neurons, it is probably not due to the summation of pre-synaptic potentials (action potentials or spikes), because these potentials have a very high frequency and short duration. In contrast, post-synaptic potentials, having a relatively slower time course, are more likely to be synchronous, and therefore to summate to produce scalp potentials. Thus, it is commonly believed that most scalp-recorded ERPs are the outcomes of summation of post-synaptic potentials of a large number of neurons that are activated (or inhibited) synchronously (see Allison et al., 1986).

A second consideration concerns the orientation of neuronal fields. Because the electric fields associated with the activity of each individual neuron involved must be oriented in such a way as to cumulate at the scalp, only neural structures with a specific spatial organization may generate scalp ERPs. Lorente de Nò (1947) specified the spatial organizations that are required for the distant recording of the electrical activity of a neural structure. He distinguished between two types of configurations: "open fields" and "closed fields." A structure having an open-field organization is characterized by neurons that are ordered so that their dendritic trees are all oriented on one side of the structure, whereas their axons all depart from the other side. In this case, the electric fields generated by the activity of each neuron will all be oriented in the same direction and summate. Only structures with some degree of open-field organization generate potentials that can be recorded at the scalp. Open fields are obtained whenever neurons are organized in layers, as in most of the cortex, parts of the thalamus, the cerebellum, and other structures.

A structure with a closed-field organization is characterized by neurons that are concentrically or randomly organized. In both cases, the electric fields generated by each neuron will be oriented in very different, sometimes opposite, directions, and therefore will cancel each other out. Examples of closed-field organization are given by some midbrain nuclei.

From this analysis it is clear that ERPs represent just a sample of the brain electrical activity associated with a given event. Thus, it is entirely possible that a sizeable portion of the information processing transactions that occur after (or before) the anchor event is "silent" as far as ERPs are concerned. For this reason, some caution should be used in the interpretation of ERP data. For instance, if an experimental manipulation has no effect on the ERP, we cannot conclude that it does not influence brain processes. By the same token, if two experimental manipulations have the same effect on the ERP, it cannot be concluded that they necessarily influence completely identical processes.

2.4. From the scalp to the brain: inferring the sources of ERPs

So far we have examined how particular properties of neuronal phenomena may determine whether they will be recorded at the scalp. We have approached the problem of ERP generation in the "forward" direction – from properties of the generators to predictable scalp observations. In most cases, however, we have only limited information about the neural structure(s) responsible for a specific aspect of the ERP. The typical ERP database consists of observations of voltage differences between scalp electrodes or between scalp electrodes and a reference electrode. To determine which neural structures are responsible for the scalp potentials (i.e., to identify the neural generators of ERPs) we must solve the "inverse problem" – that is, we have to infer the *unique* combination of neural generators whose activity results in the potential observed at the scalp.

In solving this problem, we are confronted with an indefinite number of unknown parameters. In fact, an indefinite number of neural generators may be active simultaneously, and each of them may vary in amplitude, orientation of the electric field, and location inside the head. Because a limited number of observations (the voltage values recorded at different scalp electrodes) is used to estimate an indefinite number of parameters, it is clear that the inverse problem does not have a unique solution (i.e., an infinite number

of different combinations of neuronal generators may produce the same scalp distribution). A further complication is that the head is not a homogeneous medium. Therefore the propagation of an electric field generated by the activity of a given structure is difficult to compute. A particularly important distortion of the electric fields is caused by the skull – a very low conductance medium that reduces and smears electric fields. For all these reasons, we cannot unequivocally determine which structures are responsible for the ERP observed at any point in time, when the only information available is given by the potentials recorded at scalp electrodes.

Notwithstanding these problems, investigators have tried to identify the neural sources of scalp-recorded ERPs using a variety of approaches, involving both noninvasive and invasive techniques. Noninvasive techniques include: (a) scalp recordings from dense electrode arrays combined with interpolated mapping and source analysis algorithms (which involve complex mathematical procedures and are based on a number of assumptions); and (b) combining ERP recordings with other imaging methods that possess higher spatial resolution (e.g., PET, fMRI, MEG, EROS), to help restrict the number of solutions to the inverse problem. Invasive techniques include: (a) recordings from indwelling macro-electrodes (in humans or animals); and (b) lesion data (also in humans or animals).

2.4.1. Dense electrode arrays and source modeling

During the last several years, a number of companies have marketed data acquisition systems for electrophysiology designed to record from a large array of channels (up to 256; e.g., Tucker, 1993). These systems allow investigators to derive detailed maps of brain electrical activity, which can, in principle, reveal differences that are of interest for the study of various experimental conditions and/or subject populations, and may not be visible with sparser electrode montages. Because the skull operates as a low-pass spatial filter, however, one important question concerns the effective optimal spatial sampling for ERP recording. For instance, Srinivasan, Nunez, Tucker, Silberstein, and Cadusch (1996; see also Tucker, 1993) have shown that 256 locations may accurately reproduce the most significant local variations in scalp electrical activity.

The increase in the number of recording locations has facilitated the study of the distribution of ERP activity across the scalp, and, in particular, the construction of accurate maps of surface activity, which are usually based on interpolation procedures (e.g., Perrin, Pernier, Bertrand, Giard, & Echallier, 1987). Another advantage of dense-array recording is the possibility of generating models of the 3-D locations of the brain generators involved in producing the surface ERP activity (i.e., equivalent dipole analysis). Computational approaches to dipole analysis involve generating several alternative hypotheses about the neural structures that may be active at a particular point in time, and that may be responsible for an observed scalp ERP. The distribution of potentials across the scalp that would be generated by each of these structures can then be computed using a forward approach. Finally, the structure whose activity best accounts for the observed scalp distribution can be identified (e.g., Scherg & Von Cramon, 1986; Scherg, Vajsar, & Picton, 1989; see also Gratton, this volume).

The use of large electrode arrays, however, introduces two disadvantages: (a) the probability of channels showing artifacts increases, and (b) the presence of a larger number of channels may reduce the power of the analysis, unless data reduction methods such as Principal Component Analysis, PCA, or Independent Component Analysis, ICA, are used. These issues are discussed more in detail in Gratton (this volume). Thus, the selection of the number of electrode locations to use in a particular study requires an analysis of the related costs and benefits, which may vary from one experiment to another.

2.4.2. Combining ERPs and other imaging methods to infer the sources of ERP activity

The computational approaches highlighted in the previous section make a number of assumptions that cannot always be verified, and require the availability of specific neurophysiological knowledge about candidate underlying structures. In some cases, this knowledge can be based on data obtained with other imaging methods, such as the use of magnetic field recordings (MEG). Magnetic fields generated by brain activity are extremely small in relation to magnetic fields generated by environmental and other bodily sources. Therefore, their measurement is both difficult and expensive. The advantage of measuring magnetic fields is that they are practically insensitive to variations of the conductive media (such as those due to the presence of the skull). It is therefore easier to compute the source of a particular magnetic field than it is to compute the source of the corresponding electric field. An in-depth discussion of the characteristics and problems of MEG is beyond the scope of this chapter and can be found elsewhere (Beatty, Barth, Richer, & Johnson, 1986; Hari, Levanen, & Raij, 2000). We will only note here that using MEG to determine the source of neural components still requires assumptions about the number of neural structures active at a particular moment in time.

In other cases, knowledge about candidate ERP sources can be based on the integration of data from a variety of different imaging methods applied to the same subjects in the same experimental conditions. In this way, one can exploit the differential spatial and temporal resolutions of the different methods (see also Gratton, this volume). For example, several investigators have used data obtained in fMRI studies to "seed" the source modeling of ERP data obtained in the same subjects and paradigm (e.g., Bledowski et al., 2004; Opitz, Mecklinger, Von Cramon, & Kruggel, 1999).

2.4.3. Invasive methods for ERP source localization

Invasive techniques can also be used to identify the sources of ERP components. One such technique involves implant-ing electrodes within the brain of humans or animals. Research on humans has been made possible by the need for recording EEG activity in deep regions of the brain for medical diagnostic purposes (Halgren et al., 1980; Wood et al., 1984; Puce, Allison, & McCarthy, 1999). However, even recording from indwelling electrodes is not completely free from volume conduction issues, which need to be addressed using recordings from very closely spaced electrodes. A clue to the local origin of potentials is given by the presence of polarity inversions at such closely spaced recording locations.

A further problem with human research using indwelling electrodes is that the electrodes are located according to clinical, rather than scientific, criteria, and therefore may fail to map the regions involved in the generation of scalp ERPs. This issue may be partially addressed by research on animals (e.g., Buchwald & Squires, 1983; Csepe, Karmos, & Molnar, 1987; Starr & Farley, 1983; Javitt, Schroeder, Steinschneider, Arezzo, & Vaughan, 1992). However, a problem with animal research is that it is sometimes difficult to determine whether the ERP observed in animals corresponds to that observed in humans, because of fundamental differences in the anatomy and physiology of animal and human brains. Finally, a general problem with depth recording is that it is difficult to know the extent to which the scalp recorded ERP is due to the activity of the structures that have been identified by the indwelling electrodes. This problem can be addressed, at least in part, by lesions studies with animals and humans, showing that lesions in the structure identified as the candidate generator result in the elimination of the scalp potential. Examples of animal lesion studies have been reported by Paller, Zola-Morgan, Squire, and Hillyard (1988) and by Javitt et al. (1992) and examples of studies of lesioned human patients by Alho, Woods, Algazi, Knight, and Näätänen (1994), Knight (e.g., 1984, 1997; see also Knight, Hillyard, Woods, & Neville, 1981; Yamaguchi & Knight, 1992), and Johnson (1988; 1989; 1993).

In summary, although solving the inverse problem does present difficulties, several techniques have been developed for identifying the source of ERP components. Whereas no single method may be able to give definitive answers in all cases, the convergence of several techniques could provide useful information about the neural structures whose activity is manifested at the scalp by the ERP.

2.5. The concept of a component and its alternatives

As noted above, the ERP can be described as a *voltage by time by location* function. We assume that the various voltage fluctuations represented by this function reflect the summed activity of neuronal populations. This neurophysiological activity, in turn, is assumed to correspond to some psychological process or processes. One concept that has evolved in the area of ERP research is that of a "component," which is commonly taken to reflect the tendency of segments of the ERP waveforms to covary in response to specific experimental manipulations. According to this logic, the total ERP is assumed to be an aggregate of a number of ERP components. Components can be defined in three different (but not mutually exclusive) ways (Fabiani, Gratton, Karis, & Donchin, 1987; Näätänen & Picton, 1987). First, components can be defined in terms of the positive and negative peaks (maxima and minima) that are observed in the ERP waveform. Second, components can be defined as aspects of the ERP waveform that are *functionally* associated, that is, which covary across subjects, conditions, and/or locations on the scalp in response to experimental manipulations. Third, components can be defined in terms of those neural structures that generate them. These definitions may converge in some circumstances. However, as Näätänen and Picton (1987) have indicated, a peak in the ERP waveform (for example, the N1) may represent the summation of several functionally and structurally distinct components. It can also be assumed that the same brain structure may contribute to more than one component and that different brain structures may produce activity that is functionally equivalent (e.g., homologous structures in the left and right hemispheres, such as the primary sensory and motor cortices). Thus, the adoption of one or other of these definitions will have important consequences for the interpretation of the component structure of the ERP waveform. A corollary of this discussion is that different measurement procedures will be required depending on which component definition is adopted. These procedures will be reviewed in subsequent sections after a brief discussion of general measurement issues.

Recently, other approaches to the interpretation of the ERP have been developed in which the classic concept of a component is not required. For instance, investigators have used subtraction methods to isolate effects that may subsume several different components, as classically defined. These include, among others, the "repetition effect" (i.e., the differential response observed for items that have been previously seen with respect to new items, see Section 4.4.1.4) and the "attention effect" (i.e., the differential response to items that are attended with respect those that are not, see Section 4.3.1). Note that, by using this approach, the focus is shifted from an interest in describing the functional significance of the ERP component per se (see Section 3.2) to an interest in what the observed ERP can tell us about the way stimuli are processed.

2.6. Quantification of ERP components

In this section, we describe some general measurement issues pertaining the ERP, as well as procedures that have been used to quantify ERP activity. As mentioned earlier, the precise choice of measurement operations will depend, at least in part, on the way in which ERP activity is interpreted. For further information about ERP measurement issues, see Gratton (this volume). In general, ERP measures are quite reliable and adequate to monitor individual differences. For instance, Fabiani et al. (1987) showed that estimates of P300 amplitude can give test-retest reliability of the order of 0.8, comparable to that of many psychological tests.

2.6.1. Artifacts

The potential recorded at the scalp can be influenced by sources of electrical activity that do not arise from the brain, and that therefore are considered spurious or artifactual. Examples of these sources of artifacts include the movement of eyeballs and eyelids, tension of the muscles in the head and neck, and the electrical activity generated by the heart. These artifacts can be dealt with in the following ways. First (and most important), one can set up the recording situation so that artifacts are minimized. This can be accomplished by suitable choice of recording environment, electrode locations, and experimental task. Second, one can simply discard trials that contain artifacts, or, especially in the case of high-density recordings, discard individual artifact-contaminated sites and interpolate. Unfortunately, this procedure may lead to a bias in the selection of the observations and/or subjects. Third, one can use filters (see below) to attenuate artifactual activity. This procedure is most useful when the frequency of the artifactual activity is outside the frequency range of the ERP signals of interest. For example, the frequency of electromyographic activity is higher than that of most endogenous ERP components, and can therefore be attenuated by filtering. Fourth, one can attempt to measure the extent of the artifact and then remove it from the data. This procedure has been used most frequently in the case of ocular artifacts, and a number of correction algorithms have been developed (for reviews see Brunia et al., 1989; Gratton, 1998). The use of correction procedures is particularly useful whenever the number of trials that can be collected is limited, and/or the participants have difficulty in controlling their eye movements (e.g., children or patient populations).

2.6.2. Signal-to-noise ratio

Several procedures have been advocated to increase the signal-to-noise ratio, including filtering, averaging, pattern recognition and use of wavelet analyses (see Coles, Gratton, Kramer, & Miller, 1986; Samar, Bopardikar, Rao, & Swartz, 1999; and Gratton, this volume). Filtering involves the attenuation of noise, whose frequency is different from that of the signal. For example, most endogenous components have frequencies of between 0.5 and 20 Hz. Thus, at the time of recording, or later at the time of analysis, analog or digital filters can be used to attenuate activity outside this frequency range. Great care should be taken in the selection of filters. The amplitude and latency of an ERP component (as well as the general ERP waveform) can be distorted if the bandpass of the filter excludes frequencies

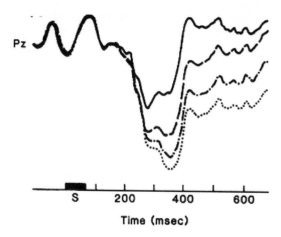

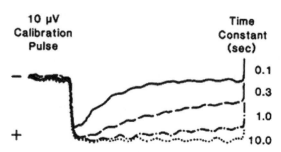

Figure 4.3. ERPs elicited by counted, rare tones (upper panel). The data recorded with four different high-pass filter settings ("time constant") are superimposed. Stimulus occurrence is indicated by an S on the time scale. Calibration pulses (lower panel) are plotted on the same voltage × time scale as the ERPs. Note the reduction in amplitude and deformation of the ERP waveshape produced by progressively shorter time constants, which reduce low frequency activity. (Copyright 1979, Blackwell Publishers. Reprinted with permission of the author and publisher, from Duncan-Johnson & Donchin, 1979.)

of interest (Duncan-Johnson & Donchin, 1979; see Figure 4.3).

Averaging involves the summation of a series of EEG epochs (or trials), each of which is time-locked to the event of interest. These EEG epochs are assumed to be the product of two sources: (a) the ERP, and (b) other voltage fluctuations that are not time-locked to the event. Because, by definition, these other fluctuations are assumed to be random with respect to the event, they should average to zero, leaving the time-locked ERP both visible and measurable. If it is the case that (a) the ERP signals are constant over trials, (b) the noise is random across trials, and (c) the ERP signals are independent of the background noise, then the signal-to-noise ratio will be increased by the square root of the number of trials included in the average.

One of the problems with the averaging procedure is that the three assumptions described in the previous paragraph may not always be satisfied in a typical experiment. In particular, if the latency of the ERP varies from trial to trial (latency jitter) the average ERP waveform will not be representative of the actual ERP of any individual trial. A related issue is that investigators may be interested in

measures of the ERP on individual trials. Thus, a major thrust in ERP methodology has been to derive procedures for single-trial analysis.

Pattern recognition techniques allow the investigator to identify segments of the EEG epoch that contain specific features (e.g., a particular peak pattern, characteristic of a given ERP component). Examples of traditional pattern recognition techniques are cross-correlation, Woody filter (Woody, 1967), and step-wise discriminant analysis (Donchin & Herning, 1975; Horst & Donchin, 1980; Squires & Donchin, 1976). Recently, a number of new pattern recognition procedures have also been applied to ERP analysis, including spatial principal component analysis (spatial PCA; Spencer, Dien, & Donchin, 1999; 2001), independent component analysis (ICA; e.g., Makeig et al., 1997), and wavelets analysis (e.g., Samar et al., 1999). For a more general discussion of pattern recognition techniques, see Glaser and Ruchkin (1976), Fabiani et al. (1987), and Gratton (this volume).

2.6.3. Peak measurement

As indicated above, ERP components can be defined in terms of peaks having characteristic polarities and latency ranges. Thus, a measurement operation that corresponds to this definition involves the assessment of the amplitude of the peak in microvolts, and/or the assessment of its latency in ms (see Figure 4.4). Amplitude is usually measured with reference to either the pre-event voltage level or

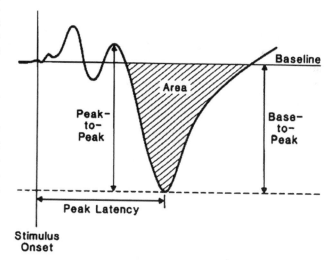

Figure 4.4. Schematic representation of an ERP waveform, indicating different procedures for component quantification. Three types of peak measures are indicated. The peak latency is obtained by measuring the interval (in ms) between the external triggering event and a positive or negative peak in the waveform. The base-to-peak amplitude measure is obtained by computing the voltage difference (in microvolts) between the voltage at the peak point and a baseline level (usually the average pre-stimulus level). The peak-to-peak amplitude measure is obtained by computing the voltage difference (in microvolts) between the voltage at the peak point and the voltage at a previous peak of opposite polarity. The area measure is obtained by integrating the voltage between two timepoints.

baseline (base-to-peak amplitude) or to some other peak in the ERP waveform (peak-to-peak amplitude). Latency is measured with reference to the onset of the event. In some cases, for example when the component under analysis does not have a definite peak, it is customary to measure the integrated activity (area measure) or the average activity (mean-amplitude measure) across a particular latency range. In these cases, the latency of onset or maximum of the effect may also be obtained.

2.6.4. Covariation measures

Components can also be defined in terms of segments of the ERP waveform that covary across subjects, conditions, and scalp locations in response to experimental manipulations. As a consequence, procedures are needed to identify and measure these segments. These procedures often entail measuring the extent to which a particular pattern of variation is represented in a waveform. This can be determined by measuring the covariation (or, sometimes, the correlation) of the waveform (or a segment of it) with an idealized wave, representing the component of interest. The "ideal" wave can be identified using statistical methods, such as PCA (Donchin & Heffley, 1978), discriminant analysis (Donchin & Herning, 1975), ICA (e.g., Makeig et al., 1997), and wavelets analysis (e.g., Samar et al., 1999). Alternatively, the ideal wave can be selected using arbitrary models, such as a cosinusoidal function (e.g., Fabiani et al., 1987; Gratton, Kramer, Coles, & Donchin, 1989). Although these types of analyses may be advantageous in the presence of noise, or when there is substantial component overlap, Fabiani et al. (1987) and Gratton et al. (1989) showed that component recognition using peak procedures may actually be both reliable and valid, provided that data are adequately filtered. Note that similar cross-correlation procedures are used in the analysis of event-related fMRI data (e.g., Dale & Buckner, 1997).

2.6.5. Source activity measures

A third way of defining components is in terms of their underlying sources. According to this definition, we should quantify the activity of these sources to provide latency and amplitude measures of the different components. As we noted earlier (Section 2.4), the relationship between scalp-recorded electrical activity and source activity is difficult to describe and requires a number of assumptions. Recently, important strides have been made in this area, with the development of algorithms for dipole (e.g., BESA, Scherg & Von Cramon, 1986; Scherg et al., 1989) and distributed (e.g., EMSE, Greenblatt, et al., 1997; LORETA, Baillet, & Garnero, 1997; Pascual-Marqui, Michel, & Lehmann, 1994; and minimum norm, Liu, Dale, & Belliveau, 2002) source analyses.

Both of these approaches are based on modeling efforts. Spatio-temporal dipole models fit a small number of individual point-dipoles to data varying over space and time. The location and orientation of the dipoles may be fixed, whereas amplitude and polarity are left free to vary over time. In this way it is possible to represent variations in surface activity in terms of variations of the activity of a few underlying brain structures.

In contrast to dipole models, distributed source models assume that extended segments of the cortex (or even the entire cortex) can be active simultaneously. To express local variations (and, therefore, explain variations in surface distribution) these algorithms allow the relative contribution of individual areas of the cortex to vary over time. These models, although perhaps more realistic, are usually largely under-determined from a statistical point of view (i.e., they include more free parameters than data points). Therefore, external criteria are necessary to constrain the number of possible solutions (e.g., minimum norm, correlation between adjacent data points).

Note that both dipole and distributed modeling efforts can be guided and constrained by anatomical and functional data obtained with other methods, such as MRI, fMRI, and PET (e.g., Bledowski et al., 2004; Opitz, Mecklinger, Von Cramon, & Kruggel, 1999; Liu, Dale, & Belliveau, 2002). These approaches can provide very useful results. However, some caveats should be taken into account when mapping brain signals with very different neurophysiological underpinnings onto each other. In fact, dissociations between hemodynamic and neuronal signals have been observed and may speak to the different nature of the signals (Logothetis et al., 2001; Huettel et al., 2004).

2.6.6. Problems in component measurement

In this section we discuss two specific problems that arise during component measurement. The first problem concerns the commensurability of the measurements of different waveforms. Is a particular component, recorded under a particular set of circumstances, the same as that recorded in another situation? This is especially a problem when we define components as a peak observed at a given latency. For example, if the latency of the peak differs between two experimental conditions, we might be led to conclude that different components are present in the two sets of data. How can we determine whether the same component varies in latency between the two conditions, or, rather, whether two different components are present in the two different conditions? A solution to this problem could be derived from a careful examination of the pattern of results obtained, and from a comparison of these results with what we already know about different ERP components. Of course, this means that we are including a large number of empirical and theoretical arguments in the definition of each ERP component, which, in turn, may differ from one component to another, and from time to time. As a consequence, the definition of a component may include not only polarity and latency, but also distribution across the scalp and sensitivity to experimental manipulations (see, for example Fabiani et al., 1997). Thus, it is clear that a correct interpretation of the component structure of an ERP waveform requires some background information about the components themselves (see Section 2.5). In turn, this indicates that the concept of component is likely to evolve over time (as more knowledge is accumulated) and that revisions of traditional component classifications may some time be necessary.

A second problem in component measurement is that of component overlap. Usually, ERP components do not appear in isolation, but several of them may be active at the same moment in time. This reflects the parallel nature of brain processes. When this occurs, it is difficult to attribute a particular portion of scalp activity to a particular component. Peak and area measures are particularly susceptible to this problem. PCA has been proposed as a tool to separate the contribution of overlapping components (Donchin & Heffley, 1978), but even PCA can, in some cases, misallocate variance across different components (see Wood & McCarthy, 1984). As a result, we may attribute a difference obtained between two particular experimental conditions to the wrong component.

Several procedures have been proposed to solve the problem of component overlap, but none of them seems to have universal validity. In some cases, it can be assumed that only one component varies between two experimental conditions. In this case, the variation of this component can be isolated by subtracting two sets of waveforms and performing the measurement on the resulting "difference waveform." Unfortunately, we cannot always assume that the effect of an experimental variable is so selective. Furthermore, the subtraction procedure implies that only amplitude, and not latency, varies across experimental conditions. Thus, serious interpretation errors may occur when subtracted waveforms are used and latency varies across conditions.

Other approaches are based on using scalp distribution data to decompose overlapping components (Vector Filter, Gratton, Coles, & Donchin, 1989; Gratton et al., 1989; spatial PCA, Spencer et al., 1999; 2001; ICA, Makeig et al., 1997). These procedures involve setting up spatial filters describing the scalp distributions of the components contributing to the data. Note that distributional filters perform the same kind of operations in the spatial domain that frequency filters perform in the frequency domain. Although frequency filters apply different weights to activity in different frequency bands, distributional filters apply different weights to activity from different spatial locations.

3. THE INFERENTIAL CONTEXT

In this section, we review the procedures through which we make inferences about psychological and physiological processes and states from the measurement of ERPs. Previous work by Caccioppo and Tassinary (1990) describes different types of relationships between psychological and physiological variables, which limit the extent to which inferences can be drawn from psychophysiological data, as well as their generalizability. More recent papers (Kutas & Federmeier, 1998; Miller, 1996; Sarter, Berntson, &

Caccioppo, 1996) also discuss existing limitations in making inferences about brain function on the basis of brain imaging data. The general framework described in these papers is assumed in the approach presented here, which is more limited in scope, and is intended as a description of the experimental logic that is often employed in ERP research.

3.1. Experimental logic

If the ERP waveform is interpreted as an aggregate of several components, some theory about the functional significance of each component is useful to the understanding of the meaning of changes that this component will exhibit as a function of specific subject, stimulus, and task contexts. We should emphasize that by "functional significance" we do not necessarily mean a specification of the neurophysiological significance of the component, but rather a specification of the information processing transactions that are manifested by it. In this sense, then, neurophysiological knowledge may be useful, but not necessarily critical, to the psychophysiological enterprise. Of course, neurophysiological knowledge is very important if we wish to use ERPs as a tool to make statements about brain function.

In the case of all ERP components (or effects), the initial phase in the process of establishing functional significance begins with its discovery. A theory about the functional significance of that component/effect is then developed. This is a complex process that involves: (a) studies of the component's "antecedents," where antecedent conditions refer to those experimental manipulations that will produce consistent variations (in amplitude, latency, and in some cases, scalp distribution) in an ERP component or observed effect; (b) establishing the consequences of variation in the latency or amplitude of the component, which can be used to test statements relating to functional significance; and (c) speculations about the psychological and/or neurophysiological function it manifests (e.g., Donchin, 1981).

For cases in which converging evidence about the brain origins of the ERP component or effect of interest are available, these speculations can be corroborated and extended by means of this additional information. One such example is work done by McCarthy and colleagues, who have collected extensive fMRI and intracranial recording data in traditional ERP paradigms (e.g., McCarthy, Nobre, Bentin, & Spencer, 1995; Puce et al., 1999; Huettel & McCarthy, 2004; see also Kiehl et al., 2005; Laurens, Kiehl, & Littel, 2005). Other examples are provided by the simultaneous recording of ERP and fast optical (EROS) data (e.g., DeSoto et al., 2001; Fabiani et al., 2003; 2006; Gratton, Goodman-Wood, & Fabiani, 2001).

In Section 4.4.1, we review examples of this inferential logic as it applies to studies of the P300 component. In the remainder of this section, we will consider the ways in which ERP measures are used to make inferences about psychological processes, and, in some cases, about brain activity. We will review a series of inferential steps that depend to a greater and greater extent on assumptions about the functional significance of the ERP. For the purposes of elucidating the inferential process, we will consider an experiment in which subjects are run in two different conditions.

3.2. Using ERP measures: Psychophysiological inference

3.2.1. Inference 1: Conditions are different

At the most fundamental level, we can ask whether or not the two conditions are associated with different ERP responses. Note that this inference, as well as the next (Section 3.2.2), do not depend on the classification of the ERP into components, but, rather, are based on the evaluation of the waveforms obtained in different conditions. The analytic procedure necessary to answer this question would involve a univariate or multivariate analysis of variance, with *condition* and *measure* (e.g., peak or datapoint within a specified time window) as factors. If such an analysis yields a significant effect of condition or a condition by measure interaction, we can infer that the conditions are different. If we assume that the ERP is an index of brain activity and/or that it reflects some psychological process, then we can infer that the brain activity and associated psychological process are different in the two conditions.

3.2.2. Inference 2: Conditions differ at a particular time

The second level of inference concerns the time at which the two conditions differ. This inference could be made on the basis of post-hoc tests of the significant *condition* by *time* interaction. It would take the form of "processing of stimuli in condition A is different than processing of stimuli in condition B by at least X ms." This kind of inference is frequently made in studies of selective attention, where an important theoretical issue concerns the relative time at which an attended event receives preferential processing. As with the most primitive form of inference, we need only assume that the ERP is a reflection of some non-specified aspect of psychological processing. Note that this same evidence can also be used to infer the time at which some (non-specified) brain structure(s) shows differential processing for two events.

3.2.3. Inference 3: Conditions differ with respect to the latency of some process

For this level of inference, additional assumptions and measurement operations must be made. Here, ERPs are used to study the duration of processes preceding the occurrence of a particular physiological event (such as a component's peak). This requires that we can identify a particular physiological event (or component) across conditions, and that this event varies in latency. Further, we usually assume that the ERP component can only occur *after* a particular psychological process is carried out. Note

that for this inferential level, we must: (a) adopt a procedure to identify the component in question (e.g., by using its polarity, distribution, response properties, etc.); (b) measure its latency; and (c) use an analytic procedure (analysis of variance, *t*-test, etc.) to evaluate the difference between the conditions with respect to the component latency. As a result of this procedure, we make the inference that the conditions differ with respect to the timing of process X.

3.2.4. Inference 4: Conditions differ with respect to the degree to which some process occurs

The notion of component also allows us to use ERPs to infer that a particular process occurs to a greater extent under one condition than under another. In this case, we must assume that a particular ERP component is a manifestation of process X. We must further assume that changes in the magnitude of the component correspond directly to changes in the degree to which the process is invoked. Then, we must devise a suitable measurement procedure to identify and assess the magnitude of the component. Finally, we can proceed with the usual inferential test and determine whether or not the conditions differ with respect to the *degree* of process X. Of course, if precise knowledge were available about the underlying brain sources of a particular ERP activity, statements that are made about the ERP could also apply to the brain structures in question.

4. PSYCHOLOGICAL CONTEXT: SELECTIVE REVIEW OF ERP FINDINGS

In this section, we review a number of findings in the ERP literature. We begin with a discussion of ERPs that are related to the preparation, execution, and evaluation of motor responses. This is followed by a brief overview of sensory and cognitive ERP components that occur after a marker event, with particular emphasis on ERP effects related to attention, memory, and language.

4.1. Response-related potentials

In this section we review research on ERP activity that is typically observed in relationship to movement preparation and generation (readiness potential, or RP, lateralized readiness potential, or LRP, and contingent negative variation, or CNV), or as a reaction to errors (error-related negativity, or ERN).

4.1.1. Movement-related potentials

One class of event-preceding potentials includes those that are apparently related to the preparation for movement. These potentials were first described by Kornhuber and Deecke (1965) who found that a negative potential develops slowly, beginning some 800 ms before the initiation of a voluntary movement (see Figure 4.5). These "Readiness Potentials" (or "Bereitschaftspotentials") were

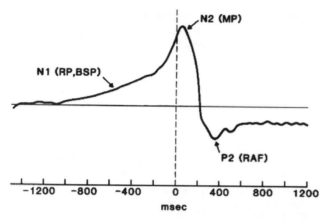

Figure 4.5. Typical movement-related potential (recorded from a central electrode – Cz) preceding a voluntary hand movement. Note that the potential begins about 1 sec before the movement (indicated by the dashed vertical line). The potential can be subdivided into different components as follows: N1 (RP – Readiness Potential, BSP – Bereitschaftspotential); N2 (MP – Motor Potential); and the P2 (RAF – Reafferent Potential). (Copyright 1980, Elsevier Science Publishers. Adapted with permission of the author and publisher from Kutas & Donchin, 1980.)

distinguished from those that followed the movement, the "Reafferent Potentials." In a condition in which a similar, but passive movement was involved, only post-movement potentials were observed. Both readiness and reafferent potentials tend to be maximal at electrodes located over motor areas of the cortex. Furthermore, some components of the potentials are larger at electrode locations *contralateral* to the responding limb (at least for hand and finger movements), as would be expected based on the organization of motor cortex. Indeed, this kind of lateralization has become an important criterion for movement-related potentials.

The investigation of movement-related potentials has developed along several different paths, including (a) the discovery and classification of different components of the movement-related potential (for reviews, see Brunia, Haagh, & Scheirs, 1985, and Deecke et al., 1984), (b) analysis of their neural origin using the scalp topography of ERPs (e.g., Vaughan, Costa, & Ritter, 1972) or magnetic field recordings (e.g., Okada, Williamson, & Kaufman, 1982; Deecke, Weinberg, & Brickett, 1982), (c) analysis of the functional significance of different components (see Brunia et al., 1985, and Deecke et al., 1984, for reviews), and (d) recording of movement-related potentials in special populations (e.g., in mentally retarded children, Karrer & Ivins, 1976, and in Parkinson's patients, Deecke, Englitz, Kornhuber, & Schmidt, 1977). In general, these studies confirm that the potential described by Kornhuber and Deecke is generated, at least in part, by neuronal activity in motor areas of the cortex and is a reflection of processes related to the preparation and execution of movements.

4.1.1.1. *The lateralized readiness potential (LRP).* In the last two decades, movement-related potentials have been

applied to the investigation of human information processing. Studies reviewed in the previous section (Kornhuber & Deecke, 1965) indicated that the readiness potential occurs prior to voluntary movements of the hand and is maximal at central sites, contralateral to the responding hand. In addition, lateralized readiness potentials can also be observed in the foreperiods of warned reaction time tasks, when subjects know in advance which hand to use in response to the imperative stimulus (Kutas & Donchin, 1977).

Based on this evidence, researchers working independently at the Universities of Groningen (De Jong et al., 1988) and Illinois (Coles & Gratton, 1986) concluded that one could exploit the lateralization of the readiness potential in choice reaction time tasks to infer whether and when subjects had preferentially prepared a response (see Gratton et al., 1989; De Jong, Wierda, Mulder, & Mulder, 1988; Gehring, Gratton, Coles, & Donchin, 1992; Gratton, Coles, Sirevaag, Eriksen, & Donchin, 1988; Kutas & Donchin, 1980).

The derivation of the LRP (Coles, 1989) is based on the following steps, which are designed to insure that any observed lateralization can be specifically attributed to motor-related asymmetries rather than to other kinds of asymmetrical brain activity: (a) potentials recorded from electrodes placed over the left and right motor cortices are subtracted. This subtraction is performed separately for the conditions where left-hand movements represent the correct response and those where right-hand movements are correct. In each case, the potential ipsilateral to the side of the correct response is subtracted from the potential contralateral to the side of the correct response, thus eliminating symmetrical activity; (b) the asymmetry values for left- and right-hand movements are then averaged to yield a measure of the average lateralized activity as subjects prepare to move. This average eliminates lateralized activity not related to movement, and yields the LRP.

Measures of the LRP have been used to make three different kinds inferences: (a) To infer whether a response has been preferentially activated or prepared (note that no LRP will be observed if both responses are equally activated); (b) To infer the degree to which a response has been preferentially activated. This inference presupposes that the level of asymmetry as reflected by the LRP is related to the level of differential response activation. In fact, Gratton et al. (1988) showed that the amplitude of the LRP at the time of an overt response was fixed: that is, there appeared to be a threshold level of the LRP which, when crossed, was associated with an overt response (for a similar observation in an animal model see Hanes & Schall, 1996); (c) To infer when a response is preferentially activated. This inference has, perhaps, proved to be the most troublesome, because of the problems associated with the measurement of the onset of the LRP (Smulders, Kenemans, & Kok, 1996).

To use the LRP in the context of research in experimental/cognitive psychology, it is necessary to arrange the experimental design such that the question of interest can be phrased in terms of a question about the *relative* activation of the two responses – responses with the left or right hands. To illustrate the LRP approach, we give two examples of work using the LRP.

The first experiment addressed a question about the nature of information transmission: *Can partial information about a stimulus be transmitted to the response system before the stimulus is completely processed* (e.g., Miller, 1988; Sanders, 1990)? The rationale is as follows. For a stimulus that contains two attributes, compare (a) conditions under which both attributes are mapped to the same (correct) response versus (b) conditions where the attributes are mapped to different (correct and incorrect) responses. If you observe incorrect response activation in the conflict condition, then partial information about the attribute must have been transmitted and processed at some level. Evidence in favor of partial transmission was reported by Gratton et al. (1988; see also Smid et al., 1990, 1991) using a noise compatibility paradigm (Eriksen & Eriksen, 1974). They found that the incorrect response is activated on the conflict trials even though the correct response is executed.

Similar findings were obtained in a Go/No-Go paradigm by Miller and Hackley (1992; see also Osman et al., 1992; Shin, Fabiani, & Gratton, 2004; Heil, Hennighausen, & Ozcan, 1999; van Turrenout, Hagoort, & Brown, 1996). In this case the trick is to map one stimulus attribute to response hand and the other attribute to response decision. If a response is activated when no response is required, then partial information about the attribute associated with response hand must have been transmitted.

In the experiment by Miller and Hackley, the stimuli were letters that had two attributes: size and identity, with size being deliberately made more difficult to determine than identity. Letter size was mapped to the Go/No-Go decision, whereas letter identity was mapped to response hand. Miller and Hackley found that, on Go trials, there was the expected development of an LRP associated with the subject's response on these trials. For No-Go trials, there was also a (smaller) LRP even though the subject showed no sign of any response-related muscular activity. These data indicate that, on No-Go trials, a response was activated, even though that response was never executed. Partial information about letter identity was being transmitted to the response system.

These two examples are illustrative of the kinds of inferences that can be made using the LRP. The LRP has also helped identify the processing locus of particular experimental effects (i.e., whether a given process or effect occurs before or after response activation) and how these effects may vary depending on individual differences (e.g., Low, Miller, & Vierck, 2002). Furthermore, measures of the LRP have provided insights about at which level(s) in the information processing system inhibitory mechanisms can still act to interrupt a response (e.g. De Jong et al., 1990). For further information about these and other issues, the interested reader should consult the following review articles and chapters: Coles, Gratton, and Donchin (1988);

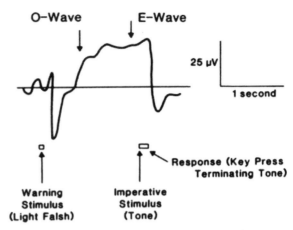

Figure 4.6. Schematic representation of a typical contingent negative variation (CNV) recorded from Cz. The CNV is the negative portion of the wave between the presentation of the warning and imperative stimuli. The early portion of the CNV is labelled "O-wave" (or Orienting wave), whereas the late portion is labelled "E-wave" (or Expectancy wave). (Copyright 1983, Elsevier Science Publishers. Adapted with permission of the author and publisher from Rohrbaugh & Gaillard, 1983.)

Coles, De Jong, Gehring, and Gratton (1991); Coles, Smith, Scheffers, and Otten, 1995; Band & VanBoxtel, 1999).

4.1.1.2. The contingent-negative variation (CNV). The CNV was first described by Walter, Cooper, Aldridge, McCallum, and Winter (1964) as a slow negative wave that occurs during the foreperiod of a reaction time task (see Figure 4.6). A paradigm typically used to study the CNV is the "S1-S2" paradigm, which consists of a warning stimulus (S1) followed, after an interval, by a stimulus requiring a response (imperative stimulus, S2). The CNV tends to be largest over central (vertex) and frontal areas. Researchers investigating its functional significance have manipulated several aspects of the S1-S2 paradigm, including subject's task, discriminability of the imperative stimulus, foreperiod duration, stimulus probability, presence of distractors, and so on. The component has been variously described as related to expectancy, mental priming, association, and attention (for reviews, see Donchin, Ritter, & McCallum, 1978; Rohrbaugh & Gaillard, 1983).

A controversy in research in this area concerns whether the CNV consists of one, or several, functionally distinct, components. A further, but related, question is whether the late portion of the CNV (just prior to the imperative stimulus) reflects more than the process of motor preparation as the subject anticipates making a response to the imperative stimulus. This controversy was raised by Loveless and his co-workers (e.g., Loveless & Sanford, 1974: see also, Connor & Lang, 1969), who argued that the CNV consists of two components, an early orienting wave (the O-wave) and a later expectancy wave (the E-wave). Subsequent research by these investigators led them to argue that the E-wave is a readiness potential and reflects nothing more than motor preparation. Research by Rohrbaugh et al. (1976) and by Gaillard (1978; see also Rohrbaugh & Gaillard, 1983) also supports this interpretation. However, the question of the functional significance of the latter component (the E-wave) remains controversial. Some investigators have claimed that because a late E-wave is evident even in situations in which no overt motor response is required, the E-wave has a significance over and above that of motor preparation. However, it is clear that even though the overt motor response requirement may be removed from these situations, attention to a stimulus necessarily involves some motor activity associated with adjustment of the sensory apparatus. Perhaps the most persuasive arguments for a non-motor role for the late CNV come from a study of Damen and Brunia (1987). These authors found evidence for a motor-independent wave that precedes the delivery of feedback information in a time-estimation task (see also van Boxtel & Brunia, 1994).

4.1.2. The error-related negativity (ERN)

As its name implies, the error-related negativity (ERN) is a negative component of the ERP that occurs when subjects make errors in sensorimotor and similar kinds of tasks. The component was first observed by Falkenstein and colleagues (Falkenstein et al., 1990) but it has been observed in several other laboratories (e.g., Dehaene, Posner, & Tucker, 1994; Gehring et al., 1993).

In the prototypical experiment, subjects perform a choice reaction time task in which they must respond to two different auditory (or visual) stimuli with their left or right hands. When they respond incorrectly, for example by using their left hand to respond to a stimulus requiring a right hand response, a negative potential is observed at the scalp. The ERN peaks at around 150 ms after response onset (defined on the basis of EMG activity) and is maximal at fronto-central scalp sites. Interestingly, the negativity evident in the waveform for the incorrect trials begins to diverge from the waveform associated with correct trials at around the time of the response.

Several different studies have evaluated the functional significance of this component. For example, Gehring et al. (1993; see also Falkenstein et al., 1995) found that the amplitude of the ERN depends on the degree to which experimental instructions stress accuracy over speed. It is larger when accuracy is stressed. Bernstein et al. (1995) found that ERN amplitude also varies with the degree of error (defined on the basis of movement parameters). It is larger when the incorrect response deviates from the correct response in terms of two rather than one parameter. Finally, whereas errors in these tasks are sometimes followed immediately by correct responses, error correction does not appear to be a necessary condition for the appearance of an ERN. In fact, an ERN is observed when subjects respond (incorrectly) to NoGo stimuli, a situation where the errors cannot be corrected by a second motor response (Scheffers et al., 1996).

The ERN is related to a variety of behaviors that, together, can be regarded as remedial actions that are taken to compensate for the fact that an error is being made or has been made. These actions include attempts to inhibit the error, correct the error, or slow down so that the system does not make errors in the future (Gehring et al., 1993; Scheffers et al., 1996).

Evidence for the generality of the process manifested by the ERN has been provided by Miltner, Braun, and Coles (1987). In their experiment, subjects were required to perform a time-interval production task. Shortly after subjects made a response indicating the end of a (perceived) 1-second interval, a feedback stimulus provided information about whether the preceding interval was correct or incorrect. For incorrect feedback stimuli, an ERN-like negative potential was observed. These results suggest that the same error-processing can be engaged by feedback stimuli as by incorrect actions themselves.

Finally, there is evidence to suggest that the ERN is generated by frontal brain structures involving either the supplementary motor area or the anterior cingulate cortex. Equivalent dipole analyses for the ERN observed in choice reaction time tasks (Dehaene et al., 1994; Holroyd, Dien, & Coles, 1998) and for the ERN-like negativity observed to feedback stimuli (Miltner et al., 1997) implicate activity in these neural structures as being responsible for the ERN signal recorded at the scalp.

Involvement of these structures is consistent with the picture that has begun to emerge from the functional studies of the ERN. That picture includes error-monitoring and remedial action processes as essential aspects of the human cognitive system. Whenever humans perform tasks, they must not only set up their cognitive systems to execute the tasks, they must also set up a system to assure that performance on the tasks conforms to task goals. The ERN may be a manifestation of the activity of this system, although it is presently unclear whether it is more closely related to the error-detection process itself or some consequence of error-detection involving an aspect of remedial action (see Coles, Scheffers, & Holroyd, 1998; Falkenstein et al., 1995; Gehring et al., 1995; and Holroyd & Coles, 2002).

Alternative views of the ERN have been proposed by Cohen, Carter, and colleagues (e.g., Botvinik, Cohen, & Carter, 2004) and Luu, Collins, & Tucker (2000). Cohen, Carter, and colleagues propose that the ERN is a manifestation of conflict monitoring – a process they envision as being a part of a general attention system. In support of this idea they point out that activity similar to the ERN can be observed on correct trials in situations of high conflict (correct related negativity, or CRN). Holroyd and Coles (2002) however, argue that these finding may be accounted by a broader definition of error, which takes into account sub-threshold activation of incorrect responses that are more likely to occur on conflict than on no-conflict trials. Interestingly, Bartholow et al. (2005) recently showed that CRN activity can be observed even in no-conflict trials, whenever subjects are led to expect a high-conflict trial and therefore use a conservative response strategy. This suggests that the ERN may be the reflection of a monitoring process that compares the current stimulus with the processing mode currently in use. If the processing mode is likely to lead to an error – or indeed to a high level of response conflict – a remedial action may need to be taken. Luu et al. (2000) take a very different view of the ERN: they interpret it as part of a set of emotional responses related to the detection of errors or conflict. It is difficult to compare this view with the error detection or conflict monitoring views because it represents a very different level of description.

4.2. Sensory components

The presentation of stimuli in the visual, auditory, or somatosensory modality elicits a series of voltage oscillations that can be recorded from scalp electrodes. In practice, sensory potentials can be elicited either by a train of relatively high-frequency stimuli or by transient stimuli. In the former case, the ERP responses to different stimuli overlap in time. The waveforms driven by the periodic stimulation have quite fixed periodic characteristics, and are therefore referred to as "steady-state" responses (see Regan, 1972). In the case of transient stimuli, the responses from different stimuli are separated in time.

Both steady-state and transient potentials appear to be obligatory responses of the nervous system to external stimulation. In fact, the earliest aspects of all sensory potentials (within, say, 100 ms) are invariably elicited whenever the sensory system of interest is intact. In this sense, they are described as "exogenous" potentials. They are thought to represent the activity of the sensory pathways that transmit the signal generated at peripheral receptors to central processing systems. Therefore, these components are modality-specific, that is, they differ both in waveshape and scalp distribution as a function of the sensory modality in which the eliciting stimulus is presented. As would be expected of manifestations of basic sensory processes, sensory components are influenced primarily by stimulus parameters such as intensity, frequency, and so on. For a review of these components, see Hillyard, Picton, and Regan (1978).

For clinical purposes, sensory evoked potentials are used in the diagnosis of neurological diseases (i.e., demyelinating diseases, cerebral tumors and infarctions, etc.). Of particular diagnostic importance are the auditory brainstem potentials (diseases involving the posterior fossa), and the steady-state visual potential (multiple sclerosis). Auditory potentials can also be used to diagnose hearing defects in uncooperative subjects (such as newborn infants). Because most sensory potentials appear to be insensitive to psychological factors, they have not been used extensively in the study of psychological processes.

4.3. The early negativities

Several negative components have been described in the period between 100 and 300 ms after the presentation of an external stimulus. In this section, we will examine two families of negative components that have been associated with selective attention, elementary feature analysis, and auditory sensory memory. Their scalp distribution and morphology vary as a function of the modality of the eliciting stimulus. For these reasons these potentials may be considered "mesogenous" as they lie at the interface between purely exogenous and purely endogenous components.

4.3.1. ERPs and the locus of selective attention

Selective attention refers to the ability of the human information processing system to selectively analyze some stimuli and ignore others. The locus of selective attention within the information processing flow has long been an issue of contention in psychology (e.g., Johnstone & Dark, 1986). Two metaphors have been associated with selective attention, that of filtering (see Broadbent, 1957) and that of resources (see Kahnemann, 1973, Norman & Bobrow, 1975). Filtering theories have focused on the issue of whether filtering occurs at an early, perceptual level (early selection theories, Broadbent, 1957) or at later stages of processing (late selection theories, Deutsch & Deutsch, 1963). According to the resource metaphor, selective attention is a mechanism by which the system allocates more resources to process information coming through a particular attended channel than through other unattended channels. Thus, the primary questions are how many processing activities can be performed simultaneously, and what factors limit the availability of processing resources. These latter questions have mostly been addressed in the context of research on the P300, and will be briefly reviewed in Section 4.4.1. Psychophysiologists in general and ERP researchers in particular have rephrased the question of the locus of selective attention to ask where in the sequence of electrophysiological responses that follow sensory stimulation the effects of attention begin to emerge. The "attention effect" is usually defined as an enhanced response to a stimulus when the subject's attention is directed to some of the stimulus features, as compared with the subject's response when his/her attention is directed elsewhere. For example, the first indications that ERPs could be used to investigate attentional processes came from studies in which the ERP response to attended stimuli was compared with that to unattended stimuli (e.g., Eason et al., 1964; Hillyard, Hink, Schwent, & Picton, 1973). These kinds of studies suggested that attended stimuli are associated with a more negative ERP between 100 and 200 ms. Subsequent research has been concerned with three issues: (a) the use of ERPs to test theories of selective attention; (b) the nature of the attentional effect on ERPs; and, (c) the neurophysiological basis of selective attention effects.

In a typical paradigm (Hillyard et al., 1973), four types of stimuli are presented. The stimuli (e.g., tones) differ along two dimensions (e.g., location and pitch), each having two levels (left vs. right ear and standard vs. deviant pitch). The subject is instructed to attend to stimuli at a particular location and to detect target tones of a deviant pitch (e.g., left ear tones of high pitch). To investigate attention effects,

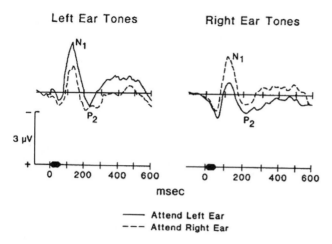

Figure 4.7. The effect of attention on early components of the auditory event-related potential recorded at the vertex electrode (Cz). The left panel shows ERPs for tones presented in the left ear. Note that, the difference between the ERPs to attended tones (solid line) versus those for unattended tones (dashed line) consists of a sustained negative potential. A similar difference can be seen for tones presented to the right ear (see right panel). (Copyright 1981, Elsevier Science Publishers. Adapted with permission of the author and publisher from Knight et al., 1981.)

ERPs to standard tones occurring in the attended channel (location) are compared to those to standard tones in the unattended channel.

Using this paradigm, Hillyard and his colleagues have observed a larger negativity with a peak latency of about 100–150 ms for stimuli presented in the attended channel (see Figure 4.7, which shows data from a similar experiment by Knight, Hillyard, Woods, & Neville, 1981). The moment in time at which the waveforms for attended and unattended stimuli diverge is considered the time at which filtering starts playing a role.

Subsequent studies have shown that, by and large, ERP peaks are influenced by attention manipulations in one of three ways (see Hackley, 1993):

(a) They may be unaffected by the attention manipulation. In this case the ERP activity is considered an automatic response to the stimulation. An ERP response with these properties is often referred to as an "exogenous" component. An example of this type of component is the visual C1 component, believed to arise from primary visual cortical areas (e.g., Di Russo, Martinez, Sereno, Pitzalis, & Hillyard, 2002).

(b) They may be affected by the attention manipulation but occur even when attention is directed somewhere else. In this case the ERP activity can be treated as a "semi-automatic" response, in that it may occur even without attention, but it is larger (or smaller) when attention is deployed to the stimulus. An ERP response with these properties is often labeled a "mesogenous" component. The visual and auditory N100 (or N1) are examples of this type of component (Näätänen & Picton, 1987; Woods, 1995).

(c) They may require attention to occur. In this case, the ERP activity is optional, in that it only occurs when the subject is actively engaged in processing the information provided by the stimulus. An ERP response with these properties is often labeled "endogenous." Perhaps one of the best known of this type of component is the P300, to be discussed in Section 4.4.1.

With respect to the locus of selective attention, the issue then arises of which are the earliest ERP responses (after stimulation) to be influenced by manipulations of attention. A theory advanced by Hernandez-Peon, Scherrer, and Jouvet (1956), called the "peripheral gating hypothesis," proposes that attention influences responses at a very early level within the sensory pathway. In favor of this theory are anatomical observations of centrifugal fibers from the central nervous system directed toward sensory organs (such as the cochlea and the retina). Indeed, Lukas (1980, 1981) reported that the earliest brainstem auditory evoked potentials (BAEPs), with a latency of just a few milliseconds from stimulation, and presumably generated in the cochlea itself or in the early portions of the auditory pathway, were already influenced by attention manipulations. Similar results were reported by Eason et al. (1964) in the visual modality (in this case, using the electroretinogram). However, numerous subsequent attempts to replicate these findings failed, and methodological concerns were raised (for a review, see Hackley, 1993). For this reason, it is now accepted that the earliest auditory evoked potentials that are affected by attention have a latency of approximately 20–25 ms (McCallum, Curry, Cooper, Pocock, & Papakostopoulos, 1983). These are potentials that are likely to be generated in primary auditory cortex (Romani, Williamson, & Kaufman, 1982; Romani, Williamson, Kaufman, & Brenner; 1982; Woldorff et al., 1993) – in which case, selective attention seems to operate when the signal arrives at the cortex. Findings leading to similar conclusions have been obtained for the somatosensory modality (Michie, Bearpark, Crawford, & Glue, 1987).

In the visual modality, however, a different pattern of results emerges. In this case, the earliest responses that are usually attributed to cortical involvement (latency of approximately 50–70 ms) appear unaffected by selective attention manipulations (provided, of course, that eye-movements are not involved – Hansen & Hillyard, 1980; 1984; Mangun, Hillyard, & Luck, 1993). Attention effects occur only later, leading several investigators to speculate that attention effects emerge when the signal is transferred from primary visual cortex to surrounding cortical areas (Mangun et al., 1993; Martinez et al., 1999; 2001; see also Gratton, 1997, for optical imaging evidence of these phenomena). Source modeling efforts (Clark & Hillyard, 1996) and combinations of ERPs with other imaging methods (Heinze et al., 1994; Martinez et al., 1999) have provided support for this hypothesis. Further support has been brought forward recently by optical imaging data showing that early attention effects (latency around 100 ms) are visible in extrastriate (area 19) but not in striate cortex (area 17; Gratton, 1997).

Additional recent studies have also explored the effects of attention on these early visual and auditory components in people that are selected according to specific characteristics. For example, Brumback, Low, Gratton, & Fabiani (2004) reported that individuals selected for having either very high or very low loaded working memory span differ in the amplitude of their auditory N1s and visual P150s in response to stimuli in simple oddball tasks. Similarly, Parasuraman, Greenwood, and Sunderland (2002) have examined the effects of the ApoE-4 allele on attention and brain activity.

Besides their role in studies of selective attention, early negativities such as the auditory N100 have also been used to investigate short-duration forms of memory such as sensory memory. These forms of memory can be analyzed by studying the effects of inter-stimulus interval (ISIs) and stimulus deviance. The effects of stimulus deviance on these early components will be reviewed in Section 4.2.3.1. Here we consider how these early ERP components are affected by ISI. Substantial evidence shows that both visual and auditory N100s are attenuated with repetition at short ISIs (e.g., Gratton et al., 2001; Sussman, Ritter, & Vaughan, 1999; Vaz Pato & Jones, 1999; Yabe, Tervaniemi, Reinikainen, & Näätänen, 1997; Yabe et al., 1998). However, when short, *unattended* trains of stimuli are used, at least for auditory stimuli, the N100 attenuation due to stimulus repetition requires at least 400 ms from the stimulus train onset to reach an effect (Sable et al., 2004). These observations are consistent with seemingly paradoxical effects reported by Budd and Michie (1994) using random ISIs, suggesting that N100 attenuation was less pronounced at ISIs *shorter* than 400 ms.

The Sable et al. (2004) data support the idea that the attenuation of the auditory N100 observed with fast stimulus repetition is not due to refractoriness of the sensory circuit per se, but rather to the engagement of an inhibitory circuit used to shut down the influx of irrelevant information (in a manner reminiscent of the pre-pulse inhibition observed for the blink reflex, or of the inhibition-of-return phenomenon in spatial attention work). Interestingly, several pieces of evidence indicate that these inhibitory events may require an intact prefrontal cortex (Knight & Grabowecky, 1995) and are reduced in old adults (Fabiani et al., 2006; Golob et al., 2001).

4.3.2. The middle-latency cognitive components

So far we have discussed early ERP activity that is influenced by attentional manipulations. However, another set of ERP responses are influenced by the history (or sequence) of stimuli that precede the current eliciting event. Some of this activity appears to occur in an automatic fashion; that is, it occurs in response to both attended and unattended events. The most well-characterized of this type of ERP response is the mismatch

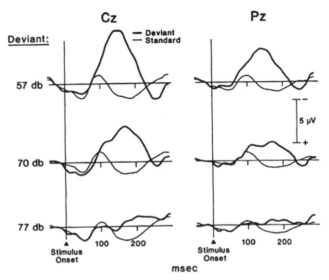

Figure 4.8. The effects of deviance on "mismatch negativity." A standard (80 db) tone was presented on 90% of the trials and a deviant tone (57, 70, or 77 db, in different blocks) was presented on 10% of the trials. The ERP to the standard is indicated by the thin line in each panel; the ERP to the deviant tone is indicated by the thick line. As the degree of mismatch between stimuli increases, the mismatch negativity also increases. (The magnitude of the difference between standard and deviant ERPs increases.) (Copyright 1987, Blackwell Publishers. Adapted with permission of the author and publisher from Näätänen & Picton, 1987.)

negativity or MMN (Näätänen, 1982; Ritter et al., 1995). Because the MMN occurs even in the absence of attention, it has been associated with some form of pre-attentive (or sensory) memory. Other ERP responses – such as the N200s and the P300 – are sensitive to changes in the stimulus sequence, but only occur in response to attended stimuli. These latter components can therefore be considered optional responses, and are associated with post-attentive forms of memory (short-term memory or working memory). In the next two sections we will describe research on the MMN and on the N200s, while research on the frontal (novelty) P3, parietal P300 (or P3b), and slow waves will be reviewed in the section on late positivities.

4.3.2.1. *The MMN.* The MMN was first described by Näätänen, Gaillard, and Mäntysalo (1978; for extended reviews see Näätänen, 1992; Näätänen & Alho, 1995; and Ritter, Deacon, Gomes, Javitt, & Vaughan, 1995). The MMN is typically studied using a passive auditory oddball paradigm. In this paradigm subjects are presented with two auditory stimuli, or classes of stimuli, that occur in a Bernoulli sequence. The probability of one stimulus is generally less than that for the other, but the subject's attention is not devoted to the series of tones, but to another task, such as reading a book or watching a silent movie. To derive the MMN, the average waveform elicited by the standard (frequent) stimuli is subtracted from that of the deviant (rare) stimuli. This subtraction yields a negative component, with an onset-latency as short as 50 ms, and a peak latency of 100–200 ms (see Figure 4.8).

This component is usually largest at frontal and central electrode sites, and inverts in polarity at the mastoids (when the reference electrode is on the nose tip; e.g., Alho, Paavilainen, Reinikainen, Sams, & Näätänen, 1986). This evidence of polarity inversion, as well as intracranial recordings in animals (Csepe et al., 1987; Javitt et al., 1992; Javitt, Steinschneider, Schroeder, Vaughan, & Arezzo, 1994) dipole modeling in humans (Scherg, et al., 1989), and optical recordings in humans (Rinne et al., 1999) suggest that the primary auditory cortex and/or the immediately adjacent areas may be the brain generators of the MMN.

An MMN is elicited whenever the standard and deviant stimuli are discriminable on any of a number of features (such as pitch, intensity, and duration; see Näätänen, 1992 for a review). Its onset latency and amplitude are both dependent on the ease of discriminating the stimuli from one another (i.e., the more discriminable the stimuli, the larger the amplitude of the MMN and the shorter its onset latency – see Figure 4.8). However, it is usually necessary to present a few (2–3) standards in order for a deviant stimulus to elicit an MMN (Cowan, Winkler, Teder, & Näätänen, 1993). In addition, a MMN is elicited with an inter-stimulus interval (ISI) of up to 10 sec between a standard and a deviant stimulus (Böttcher-Gandor, & Ullsperger, 1992). Finally, the amplitude of the MMN is larger for stimuli that differ along more than one dimension, than when they differ on only one dimension (see Ritter et al., 1995).

Recent studies have shown that the MMN is sensitive to high-level, experience-driven discriminations, such as those between native and foreign language phonemes (Näätänen & Alho, 1995), as well as word and grammar processing (Pulvermuller, Shtyrov, Kujala, & Naatanen, 2003; Pulvermuller & Shtyrov, 2004).

Taken together, these characteristics suggest that: (a) the MMN may reflect the operation of a "mismatch detector" (hence the label "mismatch negativity"); (b) because the MMN is obtained even when the subject is not attending the stimuli, it is likely to be related to the automatic and pre-attentive processing of deviant features (cf. Treisman & Gelade, 1980); (c) the MMN may be based on a type of memory that is transient in nature, as an MMN is not recorded after long ISIs; and (d) because the presence of more that one deviant feature affects the amplitude of the MMN, the MMN may reflect the outcome of a comparison in which multiple features can be processed in parallel, including features that are relatively high-level and experience-driven. Thus, it has been suggested that the MMN may be used as an index of the operation of an early, pre-attentive sensory memory (echoic memory; Näätänen, 1992; cf. Cowan, 1995; Ritter et al., 1995).

Some additional evidence, however, suggests that the memory that underlies the MMN may be of longer duration than previously thought (Cowan et al., 1993) and that the sensory memory underlying the MMN and that investigated in behavioral tasks may be different (Ritter et al., 1995; Cowan, 1995). One final problem in using the MMN as an index of sensory memory is that, contrary to behavioral evidence, a visual analog of the MMN has been difficult to obtain (Pazo-Alvarez, Cadaveira, & Amenedo, 2003). However, recent data obtained with optical imaging suggest that early memory effects (with a latency comparable to that of the MMN) can be observed in primary visual cortex and/or adjacent areas (Gratton, 1997; Gratton, Fabiani, Goodman-Wood, & DeSoto, 1998; Fabiani et al., 2003).

4.3.2.2. *The N200s.* The label "N200" (or N2) is used to refer to a family of negative components that are similar in latency, and whose scalp distribution and functional significance vary according to modality and experimental manipulations. For instance, different N200s can be observed for the visual modality (with maximum amplitude at occipital recording sites) and for the auditory modality (with maximum at the central or at frontal recording sites). In many experimental situations, the amplitude of the N200 appears to reflect the detection of some type of mismatch between stimulus features, or between the stimulus and some previously formed template. The N200 differs from the MMN in that the subject's attention is usually engaged, and the "standard template" for the comparison process may be actively generated by the subject.

Squires, Squires, and Hillyard (1975) first described the N200 in a paradigm in which they manipulated stimulus frequency and task relevance independently, and found that the N200 was larger for rare stimuli. Subsequent research has shown that several types of N200 can be described, even within the same modality (e.g., Gehring et al., 1992). Specifically, Gehring et al. (1992) used a two-stimulus visual paradigm in which the first stimulus provided information about the most likely feature to be present in the second stimulus, thus creating expectations for specific stimulus features. They observed a larger N200 (with a frontal distribution) when the features in the second stimulus mismatched with the subject's expectancies created by the first stimulus, than when the stimulus features were consistent with these expectancies. This paradigm differs from the typical MMN paradigm in that "expectancy" for particular features is dissociated from the physical presentation of the stimuli themselves. Therefore, the memory template to which the current stimulus is compared is generated internally, and is not the result of previous presentations of the template itself. In the same paradigm, Gehring et al. also presented stimuli that comprised either homogeneous or heterogeneous features, and observed a larger N200 (with a central distribution) for the heterogeneous than for the homogeneous stimuli.

The N200 has also been used in the investigation of mental chronometry. In particular, Ritter, Simson, Vaughan, and Macht (1982) and Renault (1983) have observed that the latency of this component covaries with reaction time. The high correlation between N200 latency and reaction time may reflect the importance of feature discrimination processes (signaled by the N200) in determining the latency of the overt response. However, the subtraction technique used by Ritter et al. (1982) to derive their measures of N200 must be interpreted with caution, because the latencies of the components in the original waveforms differ. Furthermore, motor potentials, which are characterized by a large negativity, will also covary quite strictly with reaction times. Thus, it is important to disambiguate the N200 component from motor potentials when the former component is used in the study of mental chronometry.

4.4. The late cognitive ERPs: memory and language effects

In this section, we review a sample of the research dealing with two major families of endogenous components, the P300 (and similar late positivities) and the N400 (and other language-related components). For reasons of space we do not discuss in detail other late components, particularly a group of Slow Waves. Currently, the functional significance of the slow waves is largely unknown. However, see Sutton and Ruchkin (1984) and the research on the O-wave (Section 4.1.1.2) for further information.

4.4.1. The P300 and other late positivities

In this section, we focus on studies of the relationship between late positive components (including the P300, the frontal P3 or P3a, and other positive components) and memory. These studies have focused on three types of effects: (a) effects that are associated with deviant, relevant items; (b) effects related to the memorability of items (in memory paradigms involving either direct or indirect memory tests); and (c) effects obtained during the retrieval of items (i.e., at the moment in which the direct or indirect memory test is administered).

4.4.1.1. *Late positivities elicited by deviant stimuli: The "classic" P300.* As mentioned earlier, deviant items in an oddball paradigm elicit early and middle latency negative ERP activity. In addition, if the subject is attending the stimuli, they also elicit various types of late positivities (with a typical latency exceeding 300 ms). The first of these positivities to be identified was the P300 (also labeled P3 or P3b; Sutton, Braren, Zubin, & John, 1965), which is elicited by task relevant oddball stimuli and is maximum at posterior (parietal) scalp locations.

After more than 30 years of research on the P300, there is still no conclusive indication of the brain sources underlying this scalp-recorded activity. The research conducted so far suggests that the P300 may result from the summation of activity from multiple generators, located in widespread cortical and possibly subcortical areas (Knight, Scabini, Woods, & Clayworth, 1989; Johnson, 1988; 1989; 1993; Halgren et al., 1980; McCarthy et al., 1997). There has been some evidence that at least one of these sources may be located in the medial-temporal lobes (Okada, Kaufman, &

Williamson, 1983; Halgren et al., 1980). However, lesion data from animals (Paller et al., 1988) and humans (Johnson, 1988; 1989; 1993) indicate that it is unlikely that the scalp-recorded P300 is entirely generated in this area, as this component can still be recorded in the presence of medial-temporal lesions. In addition, Knight et al. (1989) reported that lesions of the temporo-parietal junction in certain conditions affected the amplitude of the scalp P300. Further, brain imaging studies using variants of the oddball paradigm indicate that target stimuli elicit activity in a widespread network that includes the middle-frontal gyrus, the superior and inferior temporal lobule, and the temporal-parietal junction (Huettel & McCarthy, 2004; Kiehl et al., 2005; Laurens, Kiehl, & Liddle, 2005). All of these areas may contribute to the scalp recorded P300.

In contrast to the uncertainty about its neural origin, extensive information has been accrued on the factors that affect the amplitude and latency of the P300. For example, Duncan-Johnson and Donchin (1977) reported that P300 amplitude is sensitive to stimulus probability, provided that the stimuli are relevant to the subject's task. If the events occur while the subject is performing another task, then even rare events do not elicit the P300 (Figure 4.9; see also Johnson & Donchin, 1978; Gratton et al., 1990). Further research indicated that it is *subjective*, rather than objective, probability that controls the amplitude of the P300 (Squires, Wickens, Squires, & Donchin, 1976). Finally, Polich and Margala (1997) showed that omission of frequent but non-target items does not influence the amplitude of the P300 to the target items.

In addition, the P300 can be elicited by stimuli or stimulus classes in any modality, and the stimuli can be very diverse, as long as the subject is able to classify them unambiguously (Kutas, McCarthy, & Donchin, 1977; Towle, Heuer, & Donchin, 1980; Sutton, Tueting, Zubin, & John, 1967). Finally, in another series of studies, Donchin, Kramer, and Wickens (1986; see also Sirevaag, Kramer, Coles, & Donchin, 1989) demonstrated that the amplitude of the P300 is related to the processing resources demanded by a particular task. In a dual-task situation, P300 amplitude to primary-task events increases with the perceptual/cognitive resource demands, while the P300 response to the concurrent secondary-task decreases.

Research on the latency of the P300 has focused on the identification of those processes that have elapsed prior to its elicitation. Donchin (1979) proposed that P300 latency may reflect stimulus evaluation or categorization time. This idea was supported by the observation that the correlation between P300 latency and reaction time is higher when subjects are given accuracy rather than speed instructions. Furthermore, as categorization becomes more difficult, P300 latency becomes longer (see Figure 4.10: Kutas, McCarthy, & Donchin, 1977). Finally, it appears that the P300 latency is more dependent on the completion of processes of stimulus evaluation and categorization than on those related to the current overt response. Several studies (McCarthy & Donchin, 1981; Magliero,

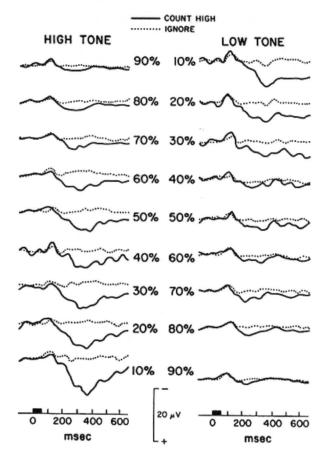

Figure 4.9. Grand-average ERP waveforms at Pz from 10 subjects for counted (high – left column) and uncounted (low – right column) stimuli (tones), with different a priori probabilities. The probability level is indicated by a percentage value beside each waveform. Waveforms from a condition in which the subjects were instructed to ignore the stimuli are are also presented for a comparison. The occurrence of the stimulus is indicated by a black bar on the time scale. Positive voltages are indicated by downward deflections of the waveforms. Note that P300 amplitude is inversely proportional to the probability of the eliciting stimulus ("probability effect"), and, at the same probability level, P300 is larger for counted than uncounted stimuli ("target effect"). (Copyright 1977, Blackwell Publishers. Reprinted with permission of the author and publisher from Duncan-Johnson & Donchin, 1977.)

Bashore, Coles, & Donchin, 1984; Ragot, 1984; Verleger, 1997) demonstrate that manipulations that should affect the duration of response-related processes (i.e., stimulus-response compatibility) have relatively little effect on P300 latency (although a small effect is sometime observed; Ragot, 1984; Verleger, 1997), whereas manipulations of stimulus complexity have a large effect.

These observations led Donchin (1981; Donchin & Coles, 1988a,b) to propose that the P300 may be a manifestation of a process related to the updating of models of the environment or context in working memory. Such an updating will depend on the processing of the current event but will also have implications for the processing of and the response to future events (including the subsequent memory for the event itself). Other theories of

the functional significance of P300 have been offered by Desmedt (1980), Rösler (1983), Verleger (1988), and more recently by Nieuwenhuis, Aston-Jones, and Cohen (2005). Both Desmedt and Verleger proposed that the P300 may be related to the termination or "closure" of processing periods, whereas Rösler proposed that the P300 may reflect controlled processing.

All of these theories provide a good account of the eliciting conditions for the parietal P300. Donchin's context updating hypothesis has also been used to generate predictions about the "future" consequences of the elicitation of a large (or small) P300 at a particular trial. Tests of these predictions have been taken as a validation benchmark for the "context updating" hypothesis. Because other theories did not generate competing hypothesis, it is difficult to determine whether or not they are confirmed by these data. Several data sets have been used to test predictions derived from the context updating model of P300. Klein, Coles, and Donchin (1984) reported that musicians with perfect pitch did not show a P300 in response to rare tones (but only to visual oddball stimuli), as templates of these tones would be available to them without updating. Along similar lines, Brumback, Low, Gratton, and Fabiani (2005)

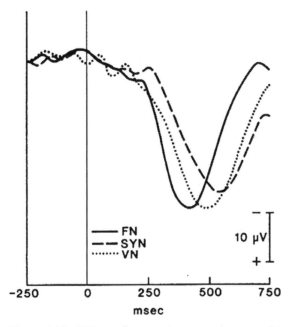

Figure 4.10. ERP waveforms at Pz averaged across subjects for three different semantic categorization tasks. The solid line indicates ERPs obtained during a task in which the subjects had to distinguish between the word DAVID and the word NANCY (the FN condition). The dotted line indicates ERPs obtained during a task in which the subjects had to decide whether a word presented was a male or a female name (the VN condition). The dashed line indicates ERPs obtained during a task in which the subjects had to decide whether a word was or was not a synonym of the word PROD (the SYN condition). These three tasks were considered to involve progressively more difficult discriminations. Note the latency of P300 peak is progressively longer as the discrimination is made more difficult. (Copyright 1977, AAAS. Adapted with permission of the author and publisher from Kutas, McCarthy, & Donchin, 1977.)

hypothesized that individuals with low working memory capacity would need to process changes in a sequence of random but equiprobable stimuli more than high-working memory subjects (as indexed by a larger P300 to sequential changes). This prediction was confirmed (see also Brumback et al., in preparation), suggesting that memory templates of targets stimuli are interfered with by the presence of other stimuli in low-span subjects.

Another data set used to validate the "context updating" hypothesis has been the research on the relationship between the amplitude of P300 elicited by an item and its subsequent memorability. This research will be reviewed in Section 4.4.1.3.

Statements relating to functional significance can be tested by an examination of the predicted consequences of variation in the latency or amplitude of the P300 for the outcome of the interaction between the subject and the environment. For example, if the P300 occurs after the stimulus has been evaluated, then the quality of the subject's response to that event should depend on the timing of that response relative to the occurrence of the P300. Thus, Coles, Gratton, Bashore, Eriksen, and Donchin (1985; see also Donchin, Gratton, Dupree, & Coles, 1988) showed that, for a given response latency, response accuracy was higher the shorter the P300 latency (see Figure 4.11).

The context updating hypothesis predicts further that, to the extent that the subject's future behavior depends on the degree to which an event leads to a change in their model of the environment, that behavior will be related to P300 amplitude. There have been several studies that have demonstrated a relationship between the memorability of an event, assessed at some future time, and the amplitude of the P300 response to the event at the time of initial presentation (see Section 4.4.1.4). As another example, it has been shown that the subject's future strategy as revealed in overt behavior can be predicted from the P300 response to current events (Donchin et al. 1988; Gratton, Coles, & Donchin, 1992). In particular, in a speeded choice reaction time task, the amplitude of the P300 following an error was related to the latency and accuracy of overt responses on subsequent trials.

Other components show characteristics similar to the P300: the Pe component observed in response-locked average on error trials (Falkenstein et al., 1995), and the P600 component observed as a result of syntactic anomalies (Osterhout, 1997). The actual relationship between these components and the P300 is still debated.

4.4.1.2. Late positivities elicited by novel stimuli: The "frontal" P3.
Courchesne, Hillyard, and Galambos (1975), used a modified oddball task in which unrecognizable complex stimuli were unexpectedly interspersed within the oddball sequence. They found that the unexpected novel stimuli elicited a positivity with a latency similar to that of the classic P300, but with a more frontally oriented scalp distribution. Because this initial experiment, a number of additional studies (e.g., Knight, 1987; Friedman, Simpson,

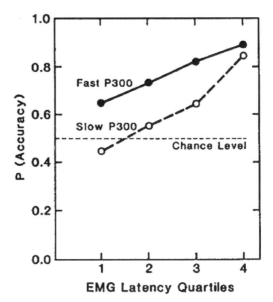

Figure 4.11. Accuracy of reaction time responses given at different latencies ("speed-accuracy functions") for trials with "fast" and "slow" P300. Response latency (defined in terms of the onset of the EMG response) is plotted on the abscissa. The probability that a response would be correct is plotted on the ordinate. Note that the probability of giving a correct response increases as response latency increases. At very short response latencies, responses are at a chance level of accuracy (.5). At long response latencies, responses are usually accurate. The speed/accuracy function for those trials with P300 latency shorter than the median latency ("fast P300" trials) are indicated by solid lines. The speed/accuracy function for those trials with P300 latency longer the median latency ("slow P300" trials) are indicated by dashed lines. Note that, for each response latency, the probability of giving a correct response is higher when the P300 on that trial (reflecting the speed of stimulus processing on that trial) is fast than when it is slow. (Copyright 1985, The American Psychological Association. Reprinted with permission of the publisher from Coles, Gratton, Bashore, Eriksen, & Donchin, 1985.)

& Hamberger, 1993; Yamaguchi & Knight, 1991) have confirmed that a frontally oriented P3 is elicited by deviant stimuli that are exceedingly rare and unexpected within the context, and for which there is no previously formed memory template (novel stimuli). As a consequence, the frontal P300 elicited by these stimuli has also been labeled the "novelty P3."

The relationship between the frontal and parietal P300 has been subject to debate, with some researchers taking the two to be completely different components (see Donchin & Coles, 1988a) and others taking them to be variations of the same component (e.g., Pritchard, 1981). Spencer et al. (1999) have used a combination of spatial and temporal PCA to argue for the independence of the frontal and parietal P300. McCarthy and colleagues (e.g., Kirino, Belger, Goldman-Rakic, & McCarthy, 2000) recorded fMRI during paradigms resembling the novelty oddball task, and found that novel stimuli elicit activation in more ventral frontal areas than the target (and rare) items. Recently, Fabiani and Friedman (1995) have shown that *all* attended deviant items elicit frontal P3s when the stimuli are first presented (i.e., during a practice block). However, with subsequent repetitions of the same stimuli the scalp distribution of the P3 reverts to a parietal maximum as typical for the "classic" P300 in young adult subjects. Interestingly, older adult subjects do not show this scalp distribution change over time, and produce a frontally focused P3 in response to all deviant and novel stimuli (see also Friedman & Simpson, 1994).

Fabiani and Friedman (1995) proposed that the frontal P3 may be elicited by items for which no memory template is available (and "orienting" may be required), and that it diminishes when a template is formed (i.e., with repeated presentations of the same stimuli). Older subjects or subjects with frontal lobe dysfunction may have problems forming and/or maintaining the stimulus template and therefore exhibit a frontal P3 even in response to deviant stimuli that are repeated a number of times. Knight (1984; 1997) found that the frontal portion of the novelty P3 is suppressed in patients with frontal lobe lesions. This, in turn, suggests that the presence of a frontal P3 to subsequent repetitions of deviant items may be associated with frontal lobe dysfunction, as measured by neuropsychological tests (e.g., Wisconsin Card Sorting Test, see Fabiani, Friedman, & Cheng, 1998).

4.4.1.3. *ERP effects associated with subsequent memory.*
The relationship between P300 and memory has been tested in various paradigms. For example, Karis, Fabiani, and Donchin (1984) recorded ERPs to words presented in a series that contained a distinctive word (an "isolate;" cf. von Restorff, 1933). The isolation was achieved by changing the size of the characters in which the word was displayed. As is well documented (von Restorff, 1933; Wallace, 1965), isolated items are better recalled than are comparable non-deviant items (the von Restorff effect). The isolated items, being rare and task-relevant, can be expected to produce large P300s. Thus, it was predicted that the recall variance would be related to the very factors that are known to elicit and control P300 amplitude. Karis et al. (1984) found that the magnitude of the von Restorff effect depends on the mnemonic strategy employed by the subjects. Rote memorizers (i.e., subjects who rehearse the words by repeating them over and over) showed a large von Restorff effect, and poor recall performance, relative to elaborators (i.e., subjects who combine words into complex stories or images in order to improve their recall). For all subjects, isolates elicited larger P300s than nonisolates. For rote memorizers, isolates that were subsequently recalled elicited larger P300s on their initial presentation than did isolates that were not recalled. This relationship between recall and P300 amplitude was not observed in elaborators (see Figure 4.12). It is noteworthy that the amplitude of a frontal-positive slow wave was correlated with subsequent recall in the elaborators, suggesting that this component may be related to the degree of elaborative processing.

Karis et al. (1984) interpreted these data as evidence that all subjects noticed the isolated words and reacted

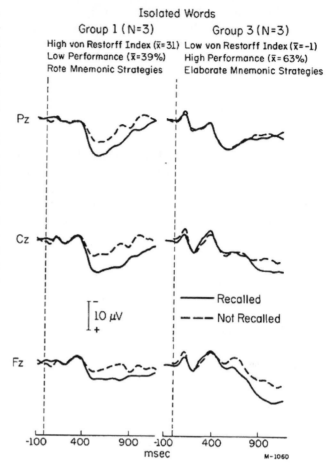

Figure 4.12. ERPs elicited by "isolated" words that were later recalled (solid line) or not-recalled (dashed line). The left column shows ERPs for subjects who used rote mnemonic strategies; the right column shows ERPs for subjects who used elaborative strategies. Note that the amplitude of P300 is related to subsequent recall for the rote memorizers, but not for elaborators. (Copyright 1986, Elsevier Science Publishers. Reprinted with permission of the publisher from Fabiani, Karis, & Donchin, 1986b.)

by updating their memory representations and producing large P300s. However, differences among the subjects emerged when they tried to memorize the stimuli by using different types of rehearsal strategies. When subjects used rote strategies, changes in the stimulus representation, induced by the isolation and manifested by P300, made it easier to recall the word. For the elaborators, whose recall depended on the networks of associations formed as the series were presented, the effects of the initial memory activation and updating manifested by P300 were not noticeable, because they were overshadowed by the more powerful elaborative processing that occurred after the time frame of P300.

The hypothesis that the relationship between P300 amplitude and subsequent recall depends on the mnemonic strategy used by the subject was supported by subsequent studies in which the effects of strategies were investigated by: (a) manipulating instruction on a within-subject basis (Fabiani, Karis, & Donchin, 1990); (b) demonstrating that, in children who do not spontaneously use elaborative strategies, the P300/memory relationship is evident in all subjects in the absence of strategy instructions (Fabiani, Gratton, Chiarenza, & Donchin, 1990); and (c) showing that the P300/memory relationship is clearer in adults in incidental memory paradigms (i.e., when the memory test is unexpected and mnemonic strategies are unlikely to be used; Fabiani, Karis, & Donchin, 1986). Finally, Fabiani and Donchin (1995) investigated the P300/memory relationship in the case in which words are semantically isolated, and also studied the effects of the type of orienting task given during the von Restorff paradigm. They found that both semantic and physically isolated words that were subsequently recalled elicited larger P300s than those that were not, and that the type of orienting task given to the subjects had an effect on whether an isolation effect was obtained or not.

The memory effects that can be observed in the ERP during study are not limited to isolated or rare items. In several recent studies, memory paradigms have been used that do not capitalize on stimuli for which the P300 is expected to be enhanced – that is, paradigms in which neither the distinctiveness nor the probability of occurrence of the stimuli to be memorized are manipulated. A seminal study in this respect is that by Sanquist, Rohrbaugh, Syndulko, and Lindsley (1980), which found that larger amplitude P300s (or late positive components) were elicited, in a same-different judgment task, by stimuli that were correctly recognized in a subsequent recognition test. Johnson, Pfefferbaum, and Kopell (1985) recorded ERPs in a study-test memory paradigm. They reported that the P300 associated with subsequently recognized words was slightly, but not significantly, larger than that elicited by nonrecognized words.

Paller, Kutas, and Mayes (1987) recorded ERPs in an incidental memory paradigm in which the subjects were asked to make either a semantic or a nonsemantic decision, and were subsequently, and unexpectedly, tested for their recognition or recall of the stimuli. They found that ERPs elicited during the decision task were predictive of subsequent memory performance, being more positive for words subsequently recalled or recognized than to words not recalled or recognized. Similarly, Paller, McCarthy, and Wood (1988) recorded ERPs in two semantic judgment tasks, which were followed by a free recall and by a recognition test. ERPs to words later remembered were again more positive than those to words later not remembered, even though the memory effect was smaller for recognition than for recall. Neville, Kutas, Chesney, and Schmidt (1986) recorded ERPs to words that were either congruous or incongruous with a preceding sentence in a task in which subjects were asked to judge whether or not the word was congruent with the sentence. They found that the amplitude of a late positive component (P650) predicted subsequent recognition.

Paller and colleagues called the larger positivity for items later memorized than for items not memorized the *Dm* (or *Difference based on subsequent memory*; Paller et al.,

1987). They used this terminology to stress the possibility that this difference may not be associated with a parietal P300, in part because the scalp distribution of the effect does not correspond exactly to that of the P300. In subsequent studies, Paller and colleagues (Paller, Kutas, Shimamura, & Squire, 1987; Paller, 1990) attempted to determine whether the *Dm* can be observed in indirect (priming) memory tasks as well as direct memory tasks, or whether it is specific to one form of memory. The results were ambiguous: in the first study (Paller et al., 1987) the *Dm* effect was evident for the direct tasks as wells as for the indirect test (stem completion), but in a subsequent study (Paller, 1990) it was only evident for the direct memory tasks. Rugg (1995) summarized a large body of research investigating the relationship between ERPs and the subsequent memory, and concluded that there is an undisputed relationship between a late positivity in the ERPs and the subsequent memory for these items. However, whether or not the "subsequent memory effect" is in fact entirely due to an increased P300 is still subject to debate. It is possible that more than one memory effect may in fact be observable in the ERP, and its nature and scalp distribution may depend on whether or not the memory tasks emphasizes explicit memory instructions and/or the distinctiveness/probability aspects of items. It is important to emphasize that memory is a complex phenomenon that can be influenced by a multitude of variables and that can be probed with a number of different tests. Thus, it is unlikely that a single component of the ERP can be identified as *the* memory component. It is much more likely, and indeed more interesting, that a series of ERP components will prove to be significant in different memory tasks.

Several investigators have recently focused on differences in the scalp distribution of effects as a function of stimulus dimension. For instance, Mecklinger and Müller (1996) presented subjects with a visual recognition paradigm, in which stimuli varied in both position and shape. In different blocks, subjects compared the study and test stimuli on the basis of one of the two dimensions. The interest was in the differences between the potentials elicited by the same stimuli in the two tasks. These changes in the ERP were interpreted as being due to differential use of brain structures for memorization of the shape and position dimensions. The shape task was associated with a posterior (occipital) P200 component, which was not observed for the spatial memory task. In addition, Mecklinger and Muller replicated the P300 and frontal slow wave effects first reported by Karis et al. (1984), although the P300 had a different scalp distribution in the two tasks.

4.4.1.4. ERP effects associated with the repeated presentations of a stimulus.
Since the 1970s, ERPs have been recorded in paradigms testing the recognition of a previously presented item. Some of these early studies employed the Sternberg memory search paradigm, in which the subject is first presented with a short list of items to be memorized (the memory set), and is then

presented with test items (one at a time) and is asked to indicate (using a speeded response) whether or not each item belongs to the memory set. Whereas most of this research focused on variations in the latency of P300 as a function of the number of items in the memory set (e.g., Ford, Pfefferbaum, Tinklenberg, & Kopell, 1982), it was generally observed that positive (yes) responses were associated with larger P300s (or more positive waveforms) than negative (no) responses. This phenomenon was later replicated in studies using a more traditional recognition paradigm (e.g., Karis et al., 1984).

Several investigators have attempted to determine whether the ERPs elicited by test items can be used to validate the so-called *two-process* model of recognition. According to this model, successful recognition may occur either because subjects experience the conscious recollection of having previously seen the test item, or because the item was familiar (although the subject could not recollect explicitly the previous encounter with the test item). The distinction between recollection and familiarity (see Tulving, 1985) has now become a central issue in the investigation of conscious (or explicit) and unconscious (or implicit) processes. A popular paradigm for this research involves using a recognition test that requires subjects to indicate whether they experienced recollection or familiarity when confronted with the test items (i.e., distinguish between REMEMBER and KNOW judgments). Using this paradigm, Smith (1993) observed that a larger P300 (or positivity) was observed for items for which the subjects indicated explicit recollection than for items for which they only experienced familiarity. Items for which a negative response was given elicited the smallest P300s. Smith (1993) interpreted these findings as indicating that the larger positivity is associated with the conscious recollection experience. However, alternative interpretations are possible, including one that assumes that the memory trace is stronger for items that are recollected than for items that are judged familiar. P300 would then be related to the "strength" of the memory trace, rather than to conscious experience. Another explanation was advanced by Spencer, Vila, and Donchin (1994), who suggested that different patterns of results were obtained by different subjects who performed the task in different ways, and that some of the amplitude differences obtained by Smith (1993) may also have been due to latency differences in the averaged waveforms.

Another body of research has focused on the effect of repeating task relevant items in tasks in which memory is not directly tested. As for the recognition paradigm, the repeated items are associated with increased positivity with respect to non-repeated items (e.g., Besson, Kutas, & Van Petten, 1991; Hamberger & Friedman, 1992; Rugg, 1990; for a review see Rugg, 1995). The interpretation of this finding is unclear. Rugg (1995), summarizing a large body of research, suggests that the increased positivity reflects a reduction of the N400 that is obtained after repeated presentations of a particular item (see next sec-

tion), rather than an increase in the amplitude of a positive component. He interprets this reduction in N400 as a manifestation of a context integration process: the first presentation of an item that is "out-of-context" requires processing, which is less required at its subsequent presentations. However, direct tests of this hypothesis have provided ambiguous results (for a discussion, see Rugg, 1995).

In the last few years, investigators have begun to shift their attention from establishing whether the P300 (and other ERP components) are related to various aspects of memory processes to using ERP components to address various types of issues in the memory literature. For instance, several investigators have examined whether the P300 or other ERP components can be used to determine whether subjects have previously encountered a particular stimulus (e.g., Farwell & Donchin, 1991; Johnson & Rosenfeld, 1992). A related question is whether ERPs can be used to separate true recognition from high-confidence false alarms (e.g., Fabiani et al., 2000; Gonsalves & Paller, 2003; Nessler & Mecklinger, 2003) – an issue of interest for understanding illusory memory phenomena (Roediger & McDermott, 2000). In this case, the basic claim is that ERPs can distinguish between different types of memory traces – those left by sensory processes and those associated with semantic processes. ERPs have also been used to separate processes associated with familiarity from those associated with recollection (e.g., Gonsalves & Paller, 2000). Again, the idea is that different types of brain processes underlie these two types of judgments, with familiarity judgments requiring only previous exposure to a particular item and recollection judgments requiring associations between the item and the particular context in which the item was experienced. These associations should in principle require additional processing, with consequent differences in brain activity at the moment of retrieval. A similar type of research has focused on the difference between recognition processing and judgments of order of stimulus presentation (Fabiani et al., 1999) or source memory (e.g., Trott et al., 1997; 1999).

Note that whereas repetitions of verbalizable items are usually associated with increased positivities, this does not appear to be the case for visual material that cannot be verbally categorized. For instance, Gratton, Corballis, and Jain (1997) reported a more negative ERP at parietal locations for old than for new test items in a recognition task using novel line patterns (see also Rugg, Soardi, & Doyle, 1995; Van Petten & Senkfor, 1996). In one experiment, Gratton et al. (1997) used divided-field presentations during the study phase, and foveal presentations during test. They showed an increased temporal negativity during the test phase (when the stimuli were presented centrally) that was systematically contralateral to the side at which the stimuli were presented at study. They interpreted their findings as evidence of a hemispheric organization of visual memory. This finding has been recently expanded to working memory paradigms (Gratton et al., 1998; Fabiani et al., 2003; Shin, Fabiani, & Gratton, 2006), in which lateralized parieto-occipital effects are found to differentiate between items that were presented at study to the left or right of fixation. These lateralized potentials can be considered evidence for the re-activation of sensory memory traces during the retrieval process.

Another example of negative activity (this time larger at right frontal locations) associated with recognition processes has been reported by Friedman (1990). Although the significance of this activity is yet unclear, it is possible that it might be related to retrieval processes. Note that a negativity associated with retrieval processes had also been described by Wijers, Mulder, Okita, and Mulder (1989) in a combined visual/memory search paradigm.

4.4.2. The N400 and other language-related ERP components

In this section we will review a number of ERP components that appear to index various linguistic processes (for a more extended review see Kutas, 1997; this volume). The first of these components to be described is the N400, originally recorded in a sentence reading task by Kutas and Hillyard (1980a). In this paradigm, words are presented serially and the subject is asked to read them silently in order to answer questions about the content of the sentence at the end of the experiment. In two studies reported by Kutas and Hillyard (1980a), 25% of the sentences ended with a semantically incongruous (but syntactically correct) word. These "semantic oddballs" did not elicit a P300 response, as was expected, but rather a centroparietal negativity peaking around 400 ms that came to be known as the N400. The amplitude of this response appeared to be proportional to the degree of incongruity: moderately incongruous words ("he took a sip from the waterfall" had a smaller N400 than strongly incongruous words ("he took a sip from the transmitter"). Kutas and Hillyard (1982) reported that the N400 to incongruous endings was slightly larger and more prolonged over the right than the left hemisphere (see also Kutas, Van Petten, & Besson, 1988). Recent evidence from intracranial recordings suggests that one important source for the N400 may be the parahippocampal anterior fusiform gyrus (McCarthy, Nobre, Bentin, & Spencer, 1995; Nobre, Allison, & McCarthy, 1994; see also Kutas, Hillyard, & Gazzaniga, 1988, for N400 in commissurotomy patients).

The basic incongruity effect reflected by the N400 has been replicated and extended, using variations of the sentence reading paradigm described above. One aim of these studies has been to determine whether the N400 is a specific manifestation of semantic processing, or whether it is elicited, for example, by other kinds of deviance. Kutas and Hillyard (1980b) showed that an N400 is elicited by semantic deviations, whereas a late positive complex (P300) is elicited instead by physical deviations in the same paradigm. In addition, Kutas and Hillyard (1983) inserted a number of semantic and grammatical anomalies in prose passages. They found that large N400s were

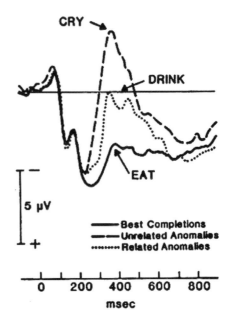

Figure 4.13. The effects of anomalous sentence endings on the N400. The ERPs (from Pz) depicted in the figure were recorded following visual presentation of words that varied in their relationship to the previous words in the sentence. For example, for sentences such as "The pizza was too hot to...", three endings were possible. *Best completion*: "eat"; *Related anomaly*: "drink"; *Unrelated anomaly*: "cry." Note that the N400 component is only present for anomalies, and is larger for unrelated than for related anomalies. (Reproduced with permission of the author and publisher from Kutas & Van Petten, 1988.)

associated with the semantic anomalies embedded in the text, but not with the grammatical errors. Besson and colleagues also found that anomies in music elicited positivities rather than N400 responses (Besson & Macar, 1987; Besson, Faïta, & Requin, 1994). Thus, the N400 seems to be relatively specific to violations of semantic expectations.

However, the N400 does *not* seem to be a semantic "anomaly detector." Instead, Kutas and Hillyard (1984) found that the amplitude of the N400 is closely related to the subject's expectancy of the terminal word (cloze probability), but insensitive to sentential constraints (i.e., to the number of possible alternative endings). Kutas, Lindamood, and Hillyard (1984) also found that anomalous words that were semantically related to the sentence's "best completion" (e.g., "the pizza was too hot to drink") elicited smaller N400s than anomalous words unrelated to the best completion (e.g., "the pizza was too hot to cry;" see also Federmeier and Kutas, 1999). This suggests that degree of semantic relatedness is an important determinant of the N400 (see Figure 4.13), and, indeed, the N400 is also sensitive to semantic relations between words in pairs or in list format (semantic priming effects; e.g., Bentin, McCarthy, and Woods, 1985; Holcomb, 1988). For words out of context or in relatively weak contexts (including early in a sentence, before the context is established), N400 amplitude is also a function of word characteristics, such as frequency (Van Petten and Kutas, 1990; Van Petten and Kutas, 1991), and of repetition (Van Petten et al., 1991).

Rather than being a response to semantic "oddballs," then, the N400 seems to be part of the normal brain response to stimuli that carry meaning, or potentially do so. N400 responses are observed not only during reading, but also in the auditory modality (e.g., McCallum, Farmer, & Pocock, 1984; Connolly, Phillips, Stuart, & Brake, 1992) as well as in American Sign Language (ASL; Neville, 1985), and to nonverbal stimuli such as line drawings, pictures, movies, and faces (Ganis, Kutas, & Sereno, 1996; West & Holcomb, 2002; Sitnikova, Kuperberg, & Holcomb 2003; Barrett & Rugg, 1989). N400s of large amplitude are also observed to pronounceable pseudowords, including those that are not clearly derived from real words (Deacon, Dynowska, Ritter, & Grose-Fifer J., 2004), suggesting that activation of specific meaning information is not necessary for an N400 to be elicited. One interpretation of the N400 is that it reflects search through and/or activation of information stored in long-term memory (see Kutas & Federmeier, 2001 for a review).

Irrespective of its precise functional status, however, N400 has proven an important tool for testing theories and models of semantic activation and integration processes, for single words, sentences, and larger elements of discourse (see Kutas et al., this volume).

Several other ERP components have been observed in response to language processing. For example, a positivity, the P600 (sometimes called the syntactic positive shift, or SPS) is elicited by syntactic anomalies of a variety of types (e.g., Neville et al., 1991; Osterhout & Holcomb 1992); some take this to be within the family of late positivities, sensitive to probability, that includes the P300 (Coulson, King, & Kutas, 1998). A left anterior negativity (LAN) has been associated with other types of structural or referential difficulty, and has been linked by some to working memory (e.g., Kluender & Kutas, 1993). In addition, some slow-developing sentence-wide effects are visible when low-pass filtering is applied to the ERP encompassing an entire sentence (e.g., King & Kutas, 1995). Kutas et al. (this volume) provides more detail.

5. THE SOCIAL AND APPLIED CONTEXT

So far, we have discussed a number of experimental manipulations that affect various ERP components and allow investigators to make inferences about the cognitive significance of the electrical brain activity observed at the scalp. Our brain, however, is also processing emotions and attitudes, and plays a fundamental role in maintaining vital bodily functions (see Kutas & Federmeier, 1998, for an extended discussion of an integrated view of brain function). Thus, it is not surprising that emotional and social factors may also influence the latency and amplitude of ERP components. For example, experimental instructions are an important determinant of endogenous components. In fact, strategy instructions (e.g., Fabiani et al.,

1986), speed-accuracy instructions (e.g., Kutas, McCarthy, & Donchin, 1977), bargaining (e.g., Karis, Druckman, Lissak, & Donchin, 1984), and pay-off manipulations (e.g., Karis, Chesney, & Donchin, 1983) have all been shown to affect the ERP waveform.

As another example, Cacioppo and colleagues have conducted a series of psychophysiological studies of social attitudes, and advocate the use of psychophysiological measures especially in those cases in which subjects do not want to (or are unable to) talk about their attitudes (Cacioppo, Petty, Losch, & Crites, 1994; Cacioppo, Crites, Gardner, & Berntson, 1994; 1995; Cacioppo, Crites, Berntson, & Coles, 1993). Similarly, several investigators have recently used ERPs to investigate stereotypes and racial biases (Bartholow, Dickter, & Sestir, 2006; Amodio et al., 2004; and Ito, Thomson, & Cacioppo, 2004), as well as reactions to incongruous information in person perception (Bartholow et al., 2001, 2003; Bartholow & Dickter, 2007). A review of this social neuroscience perspective can be found in a recent chapter by Cacioppo and colleagues (Cacioppo, Lorig, Nusbaum, & Berntson, 2004).

Several researchers have investigated the effects of emotional stimuli on the ERP. By and large, the data have been interpreted in terms of emotion effects on cognitive processing. For instance, Vanderploeg, Brown, and Marsh (1987) compared the ERP responses to faces and words that did or did not convey emotional meanings, and found that P3 was larger for neutral faces. Kestenbaum and Nelson (1992) compared the ERP elicited by angry and happy faces in seven-year old children and adults, and found different effects of valence on P3 amplitude (see also Stormark, Nordby, & Hugdahl, 1995). Recently, Naumann and colleagues (Diedrich, Naumann, Maier, & Becker, 1997; Naumann, Bartussek, Diedrich, & Laufer, 1992; Naumann et al., 1997) have tried to identify ERP components specifically related to emotion rather than to cognitive processes. Their approach is based on an attempt to manipulate independently the emotional valence and the cognitive demands imposed by the stimuli. However, the results remain ambiguous, and the issue of whether there are ERP components that are specifically related to emotional processes is still open. One candidate seems to be a late, often sustained, right-lateralized posterior positivity that is enhanced for pictures with emotional content and, while modulated by a variety of task-related factors (many similar to those that modulate the P300), seems to be related to the intrinsic motivational significance of these stimuli (e.g., Schupp et al., 2000; Junghoefer, Bradley, Elbert, & Lang, 2001).

There are now a considerable number of studies using ERPs in more applied areas. This includes work in human factors, for which we refer the reader to Kramer (this volume), as well as work on the use of ERPs in "lie detection" and on the effects of alcohol on the ERP. Studies of "lie detection" and ERP use a logic similar to that proposed by Cacioppo et al. (1994) in that stimulus words or phrases relating to a crime may be categorized in one way if the information they represented was unknown to the individual, but in another way if the information was known. The role of the ERPs, then, is to identify the categorization rule being used by the subject, who may otherwise be unwilling to reveal his/her "guilty knowledge." Both the P300 (e.g., Farwell & Donchin, 1991) and the N400 (e.g., Boaz et al., 1991) have been used within this context.

As a final example of a more applied use of ERP research, investigators have been examining the effects of alcohol on P300 and other ERP components (such as the MMN and the O-wave) in the hope of (a) identifying possible biological markers of high risk to develop alcoholism (e.g., Polich & Bloom, 1988; Jaaskelainen, et al., 1996; Eckardt et al., 1996; for reviews, see Jaaskelainen, Näätänen, & Sillanaukee, 1996; Porjesz & Begleiter, 1996); or (b) identifying the acute effects of alcohol on cognitive and social processes, including person perception (Bartholow et al., 2003) and racial stereotypes (Bartholow et al., 2006).

6. SUMMARY AND CONCLUSIONS

In summary, research conducted over the past four decades has established the ERP as one of the main tools available to cognitive neuroscientists. The advantages of ERPs include their exquisite temporal resolution, relatively low cost and portability, and their high level of sensitivity to – and specificity for – aspects of cognitive processing. These qualities have allowed ERPs to be applied to the investigation of a number of theoretical issues that are relevant to cognitive psychology and cognitive neuroscience. Recently, several other neuroimaging techniques have flanked ERPs as tools for investigating the function of the human brain. However, rather than replacing ERPs as a method of choice, it appears that a combination of different approaches (including not only imaging methods but also neuropsychological and neurophysiological data) may provide a more complete description of the mind-brain system than the use of one technique alone.

ACKNOWLEDGMENTS

Preparation of this chapter was supported in part by NIBIB grant #R01 EB002011–08 to Gabriele Gratton and NIA grant #AG21887 to Monica Fabiani. Direct all correspondence to: M. Fabiani, University of Illinois, Beckman Institute, 405 N. Mathews Ave., Urbana, IL 61801. E-mail: mfabiani@uiuc.edu.

REFERENCES

Alho, K., Paavilainen, P., Reinikainen, K., Sams, M., & Näätänen, R. (1986). Separability of different negative components of the event-related potential associated with auditory stimulus processing. *Psychophysiology, 23*(6), 613–23.

Alho, K., Woods, D. L., Algazi, A., Knight, R. T., & Näätänen, R. (1994). Lesions of frontal cortex diminish the auditory mismatch negativity. *Electroencephalography & Clinical Neurophysiology, 91*(5), 353–62.

Allison, T., Wood, C. C., & McCarthy, G. (1986). The central nervous system. In M. G. H. Coles, S. W. Porges, & E. Donchin (Eds.), *Psychophysiology: Systems, processes, and applications* (pp. 5–25). New York: Guilford.

Amodio, D. M., Harmon-Jones, E., Devine, P. G., Curtin, J. J., Hartley, S. L., & Covert, A. E. (2004). Neural signals for the detection of unintentional race bias. *Psychological Science, 15*(2), 88–93.

Baillet, S., & Garnero, L. (1997). A Bayesian approach to introducing anatomo-functional priors in the EEG/MEG inverse problem. *IEEE Transactions on Biomedical Engineering, 44*(5), 374–85.

Band, G. P. H., & van Boxtel, G. J. M. (1999). Inhibitory motor control in stop paradigms: review and reinterpretation of neural mechanisms. *Acta Psychologica, 101*, 179–211.

Barrett, S. E., & Rugg, M. D. (1989). Event-related potentials and the semantic matching of faces. *Neuropsychologia, 27*(7), 913–922.

Bartholow, B. D., & Dickter, C. L. (2007). Social cognitive neuroscience of person perception: A selective review focused on the event-related brain potential. In E. Harmon-Jones & P. Winkielman (Eds.) Social Neuroscience: Integrating biological and psychological explanations of social behavior. New York: Guilford Press.

Bartholow, B. D., Dickter, C. L., & Sestir, M. A. (2006). Stereotype activation and control of race bias: Cognitive control of inhibition and its impairment by alcohol. *Journal of Personality and Social Psychology, 90*, 272–287.

Bartholow, B., Fabiani, M., Gratton, G., & Bettencourt, A. (2001). A psychophysiological analysis of the processing time course of social expectancy violations. *Psychological Science, 12*(3), 197–204.

Bartholow, B. D., Pearson. M., Dickter, C., Sher, K. J., Fabiani, M., & Gratton, G. (2005). Strategic Control and Medial Frontal Negativity in the Event-Related Brain Potential: Beyond Errors and Response Conflict. *Psychophysiology, 42*.

Bartholow, B. D., Pearson, M., Gratton, G., & Fabiani, M. (2003). Effects of alcohol on person perception: A social cognitive neuroscience approach. *Journal of Personality and Social Psychology, 85*(4), 627–638.

Beatty, J., Barth, D. S., Richer, F., & Johnson, R. A. (1986). Neuromagnetometry. In M. G. H. Coles, S. W. Porges, & E. Donchin (Eds.), *Psychophysiology: Systems processes, and applications* (pp. 26–40). New York: Guilford.

Bentin, S., McCarthy, G., & Wood, C. C. (1985). Event-related potentials associated with semantic priming. *Electroencephalography and Clinical Neurophysiology, 60*, 343–355.

Berger, H. (1929). Uber das Elektrenkephalogramm das menchen. *Archiv fur Psychiatrie, 87*, 527–570.

Bernstein, P. S., Scheffers, M. K., & Coles, M. G. H. (1995). (Where did I go wrong? A psychophysiological analysis of error detection. *Journal of Experimental Psychology: Human Perception and Performance, 21*, 1312–1322.

Besson, M., Faita, F., & Requin, J. (1994). Brain waves associated with musical incongruities differ for musicians and non-musicians. *Neuroscience Letters, 168*(1–2), 101–5.

Besson, M., Kutas, M., & Van Petten, C. (1991). ERP signs of semantic congruity and word repetition in sentences. In C. H. M. Brunia, G. Mulder, & M. N. Verbaten (Eds.), *Event-related brain research (EEG Suppl. 42)* (pp. 259–262). Amsterdam: Elsevier.

Besson, M., & Macar, F. (1987). An event-related potential analysis of incongruity in music and other non-linguistic contexts. *Psychophysiology, 24*(1), 14–25.

Bledowski, C., Prvulovic, D., Hoechstetter, K., Scherg, M., Wibral, M., Goebel, R., & Linden, D. E. (2004). Localizing P300 generators in visual target and distractor processing: a combined event-related potential and functional magnetic resonance imaging study. *Journal of Neuroscience, 24*(42), 9353–9360.

Böttcher-Gandor, C., & Ullsperger, P. (1992). Mismatch negativity in event-related potentials to auditory stimuli as a function of varying interstimulus interval. *Psychophysiology, 29*(5), 546–50.

Botvinick, M. M., Cohen, J. D., & Carter, C. S. (2004). Conflict monitoring and anterior cingulate cortex: an update. *Trends in Cognitive Science, 8*(12), 539–546.

Broadbent, D. E. (1957). A mathematical model for human attention and immediate memory. *Psychological Review, 64*, 205–215.

Brumback, C. R., Gratton, G., & Fabiani, M. (in preparation). *Individual differences in working memory capacity of older and younger adults.*

Brumback, C. R., Low, K. A., Gratton, G., & Fabiani, M. (2004). Sensory brain responses predict individual differences in working memory span and fluid intelligence. *NeuroReport, 15*(2), 373–376.

Brumback, C. R., Low, K., Gratton, G., & Fabiani, M. (2005). Putting things into perspective: Differences in working memory span and the integration of information. *Experimental Psycholog, 52*(1), 21–30.

Brunia, C. H. M., Haagh, S. A. V. M., & Scheirs, J. G. M. (1985). Waiting to respond: Electrophysiological measurements in man during preparation for a voluntary movement. In H. Heuer, U. Kleinbeck, & K. H. Schmidt (Eds.), *Motor behavior. Programming, control and acquisition* (pp. 35–78). Berlin: Springer-Verlag.

Brunia, C. H. M., Mocks, J., Van Den Berg-Lenssen, M. M. C., Coelho, M., Coles, M. G. H., Elbert, T., Gasser, T., Gratton, G., Ifeachor, E. C., Jervis, B. W., Lutzenberger, W., Sroka, L., van Blokland-Vogelesang, A. W., van Driel, G., Woestenburg, J. C., Berg, P., McCallum, W. C., Tuan, P. D., Pocock, P. V., & Roth, W. T. (1989). Correcting ocular artifacts: A comparison of several methods. *Journal of Psychophysiology, 3*, 1–50.

Buchwald, J., & Squires, N. (1983). Endogenous auditory potentials in the cat: A P300 model. In C. Woody (Ed.), *Conditioning* (pp. 503–515). New York: Plenum Press.

Budd, T. W., & Michie, P. T. (1994). Facilitation of the N1 peak of the auditory ERP at short stimulus intervals. *Neuroreport, 5*, 2513–2516.

Cacioppo, J. T., Crites, S. L., Berntson, G. G., & Coles, M. G. (1993). If attitudes affect how stimuli are processed, should they not affect the event-related brain potential? *Psychological Science, 4*(2), 108–112.

Cacioppo, J. T., Crites, S. L., Jr., Gardner, W. L., & Bernston, G. G. (1994). Bioelectrical echoes from evaluative categorizations: I. A late positive brain potential that varies as a function of trait negativity and extremity. *Journal of Personality & Social Psychology, 67*(1), 115–25.

Cacioppo, J. T., Lorig, T. S., Nusbaum, H. C., & Berntson, G. G. (2004) Social Neuroscience: Bridging Social and Biological Systems. In C. Sansone, C. C. Morf, & A. T. Panter (Eds.), *The Sage handbook of methods in social psychology* (pp. 383–404). Thousand Oaks, CA: Sage Publications.

Cacioppo, J. T., Petty, R. E., Losch, M. E., & Crites, S. L. (1994). Psychophysiological approaches to attitudes: Detecting affective dispositions when people won't say, can't say, or don't even know. In S. Shavitt & T. C. Brock (Eds.), *Persuasion: Psychological insights and perspectives* (pp. 43–69). Boston: Allyn & Bacon.

Cacioppo, J. T., & Tassinary, L. G. (1990). Inferring psychological significance from physiological signals. *American Psychologist, 45*(1), 16–28.

Ciganek, L. (1964). Excitability cycle of the visual cortex in man. *Annals of the New York Academy of Science, 112*, 241–253.

Clark, V. P., & Hillyard, S. A. (1996). Spatial selective attention affects early extrastriate but not striate components of the visual evoked potential. *Journal of Cognitive Neuroscience, 8*(5), 387–402.

Coles, M. G. H. (1989). Modern mind-brain reading: Psychophysiology, physiology & cognition. *Psychophysiology, 26*, 251–269.

Coles, M. G. H., De Jong, R., Gehring, W. J., & Gratton, G. (1991). Continuous versus discrete information processing: Evidence from movement-related potentials. In C. H. M. Brunia, G. Mulder, & M. N. Verbaten (Eds.), *Event-related brain research (EEG Suppl. 42)*. Amsterdam: Elsevier Science, pp. 260–269.

Coles, M. G. H., & Gratton, G. (1986). Cognitive psychophysiology and the study of states and processes. In G. R. J. Hockey, A. W. K. Gaillard, & M. G. H. Coles (Eds.), *Energetics and human information processing*. Dordrecht, The Netherlands: Martinus Nijhof, pp. 409–424.

Coles, M. G. H., Gratton, G., Bashore, T. R., Eriksen, C. W., & Donchin, E. (1985). A psychophysiological investigation of the continuous flow model of human information processing. *Journal of Experimental Psychology: Human Perception and Performance, 11*, 529–553.

Coles, M. G. H., Gratton, G., & Donchin, E. (1988). Detecting early communication: Using measures of movement-related potentials to illuminate human information processing. In B. Renault, M. Kutas, M. G. H. Coles, & A. W. K. Gaillard (Eds.), *Event-related potential investigations of cognition*. Amsterdam: North-Holland, pp. 69–89.

Coles, M. G. H., Gratton, G., Kramer, A. F., & Miller, G. A. (1986). Principles of signal acquisition and analysis. In M. G. H. Coles, E. Donchin, & S. W. Porges (Eds.), *Psychophysiology: Systems, Processes, and Applications* (pp. 183–221). New York: Guilford.

Coles, M. G. H., Scheffers, M. K., & Holroyd, C. (1998). Berger's dream? The error-related negativity and modern cognitive psychophysiology. In H. Witte, U. Zwiener, B. Schack, & A. Döring (Eds.), *Quantitative and Topological EEG and MEG Analysis*, (pp. 96–102). Jena-Erlangen: Druckhaus Mayer Verlag.

Coles, M. G. H., Smid, H. G. O. M., Scheffers, M. K., & Otten, L. J. (1995). Mental chronometry and the study of human information processing. In M. D. Rugg and M. G. H. Coles (Eds.), *Electrophysiology of mind: Event-related brain potentials and cognition* (pp. 86–131). Oxford, UK: Oxford University Press.

Connor, W. H., & Lang, P. J. (1969). Cortical slow-wave and cardiac rate responses in stimulus orientation and reaction time conditions. *Journal of Experimental Psychology, 82*, 310–320.

Coulson, S., King, J. W., & Kutas, M. (1998). Expect the unexpected: Event-related brain response to morphosyntactic violations. *Language & Cognitive Processes, 13*(1), 21–58.

Courchesne, E., Hillyard, S. A., & Galambos, R. (1975). Stimulus novelty, task relevance and the visual evoked potential in man. *Electroencephalography and Clinical Neurophysiology, 39*, 131–143.

Cowan, N. (1995). Sensory memory and its role in information processing. In G. Karmos, M. Molnar, V. Csepe, I. Czigler, & J. E. Desmedt (Eds.), *Perspectives of event-related potential research (EEG Suppl. 44)* (pp. 21–31). Amsterdam: Elsevier.

Cowan, N., Winkler, I., Teder, W., & Näätänen, R. (1993). Memory prerequisites of mismatch negativity in the auditory event-related potential (ERP). *Journal of Experimental Psychology: Learning, Memory, & Cognition, 19*(4), 909–921.

Csepe, V., Karmos, G., & Molnar, M. (1987). Effects of signal probability on sensory evoked potentials in cats. *International Journal of Neuroscience, 33,* 61–71.

Dale, A. M., & Buckner, R. L. (1997). Selective averaging of rapidly presented individual trials using fMRI. *Human Brain Mapping, 5,* 329–340.

Damen, E. J. P., & Brunia, C. H. M. (1987). Changes in heart rate and slow brain potentials related to motor preparation and stimulus anticipation in a time estimation task. *Psychophysiology, 24,* 700–713.

Dawson, G. D. (1947). Cerebral responses to electrical stimulation of the waking human brain. *Journal of Neurology, Neurosurgery, and Psychiatry, 10,* 134–140.

De Jong, R., Coles, M. G. H., Gratton, G., & Logan, G. L. (1990). In search of the point of no return: The control of response processes. *Journal of Experimental Psychology: Human Perception and Performance, 16,* 164–182.

De Jong, R., Wierda, M., Mulder, G., & Mulder, L. J. M. (1988). Use of partial stimulus information in response processing. *Journal of Experimental Psychology: Human Perception and Performance, 14,* 682–692.

Deacon D., Dynowska, A., Ritter, W., Grose-Fifer, J. (2004). Repetition and semantic priming of nonwords: implications for theories of N400 and word recognition. *Psychophysiology, 41,* 60–74.

Deecke, L., Bashore, T., Brunia, C. H. M., Grunewald-Zuberbier, E., Grunewald, G., & Kristeva, R. (1984). Movement-associated potentials and motor control. In Karrer, R., Cohen, J., & Tueting, P. (Eds.), *Brain and information: Event-related potentials* (pp. 398–428). New York: New York Academy of Science.

Deecke, L., Englitz, H. G., Kornhuber, H. H., & Schmitt, G. (1977). Cerebral potentials preceding voluntary movement in patients with bilateral or unilateral parkinson akinesia. In J. E. Desmedt (Eds.), *Attention, voluntary contraction, and event-related cerebral potentials. Progress in Clinical Neurophysiology,* vol. 1 (pp. 151–163). Basel: Karger.

Deecke, L., Weinberg, H., & Brickett, P. (1982). Magnetic fields of the human brain accompanying voluntary movements. Bereitschaftsmagnetfeld. *Experimental Brain Research, 48,* 144–148.

Dehaene, S., Posner, M. I., & Tucker, D. M. (1994). Commentary: Localization of a neural system for error detection and compensation. *Psychological Science, 5,* 303–305.

Desmedt, J. E. (1980). P300 in serial tasks: An essential post-decision closure mechanism. In H. H. Kornhuber & L. Deecke (Eds.), *Motivation, motor, and sensory processes of the brain. Progress in Brain Research,* vol. 54 (pp. 682–686). Amsterdam: Elsevier-North Holland.

DeSoto, M. C., Fabiani, M., Geary, D. C., & Gratton, G. (2001). When in doubt, do it both ways: Brain evidence of the simultaneous activation of conflicting responses in a spatial Stroop task. *Journal of Cognitive Neuroscience, 13*(4), 523–536.

Deutsch, J. A., & Deutsch, D. (1963). Attention: Some theoretical considerations. *Psychological Review, 70,* 80–90.

Diedrich, O., Naumann, E., Maier, S., & Becker, G. (1997). A frontal positive slow wave in the ERP associated with emotional slides. *Journal of Psychophysiology, 11*(1) 71–84.

Di Russo, F., Martinez, A., Sereno, M. I., Pitzalis, S., & Hillyard, S. A. (2002). Cortical sources of the early components of the visual evoked potential. *Human Brain Mapping, 15,* 95–111.

Donchin, E. (1978). Use of scalp distribution as a dependent variable in event-related potential studies: Excerpts of preconference correspondence. In D. Otto (Ed.), *Multidisciplinary Perspectives in Event-Related Brain Potentials Research* (EPA-600/9-77-043) (pp. 501–510). Washington, DC: U.S. Government Printing Office.

Donchin, E. (1979). Event-related brain potentials: A tool in the study of human information processsing. In H. Begleiter (Ed.), *Evoked potentials and behavior* (pp. 13–75). New York: Plenum Press.

Donchin, E. (1981). Surprise! . . . Surprise? *Psychophysiology, 18,* 493–513.

Donchin, E., & Coles, M. G. H. (1988a). Is the P300 component a manifestation of context updating? *Behavioral and Brain Sciences, 11,* 354–356.

Donchin, E. , & Coles, M. G. H. (1988b). On the conceptual foundations of cognitive psychophysiology: A reply to comments. *Behavioral and Brain Sciences, 11,* 406–417.

Donchin, E., Gratton, G., Dupree, D., & Coles, M. G. H. (1988). After a rash action: Latency and amplitude of the P300 following fast guesses. In G. Galbraith, M. Klietzman, & E. Donchin (Eds.), *Neurophysiology and Psychophysiology: Experimental and Clinical Applications* (pp. 173–188). Hillsdale, NJ: Erlbaum.

Donchin, E., & Heffley, E. (1978). Multivariate analysis of event-related potential data: A tutorial review. In D. Otto (Eds.), *Multidisciplinary perspectives in event-related brain potential research* (pp. 555–572). (EPA-600/9-77-043). Washington, D.C.: U.S. Government Printing Office.

Donchin, E., & Herning, R. I. (1975). A simulation study of the efficacy of Step-Wise Discriminant Analysis in the detection and comparison of event-related potentials. *Electroencephalography and Clinical Neurophysiology, 38,* 51–68.

Donchin, E., Kramer, A. F., & Wickens, C. D. (1986). Applications of event-related brain potentials to problems in engineering psychology. In M. G. H. Coles, E. Donchin, & S. W. Porges (Eds.), *Psychophysiology: Systems, processes, and applications* (pp. 702–718). New York: Guilford Press.

Donchin, E., Ritter, W., & McCallum C. (1978). Cognitive psychophysiology: The endogenous components of the ERP. In E. Callaway, P. Tueting, & S. H. Koslow (Eds.), *Event-related Brain Potentials in Man* (pp. 349–411). New York: Academic Press.

Duncan-Johnson, C. C., & Donchin, E. (1977). On quantifying surprise: The variation of event-related potentials with subjective probability. *Psychophysiology, 14,* 456–467.

Duncan-Johnson, C. C., & Donchin, E. (1979). The time constant in P300 recording. *Psychophysiology, 16,* 53–55.

Eason, R. G., Aiken, L. R., Jr., White, C. T., & Lichtenstein, M. (1964). Activation and behavior: II. Visually evoked cortical potentials in man as indicants of activation level. *Perceptual and Motor Skills, 19,* 875–895.

Eriksen, B. A., & Eriksen, C. W. (1974). Effects of noise letters upon the identification of target letter in a non-search task. *Perception and Psychophysics, 16,* 143–149.

Fabiani, M., & Donchin, E. (1995). Encoding processes and memory organization: A model of the von Restorff effect. *Journal of Experimental Psychology: Learning, Memory and Cognition, 21*(1), 224–240.

Fabiani, M., & Friedman, D. (1995). Changes in brain activity patterns in aging: The novelty oddball. *Psychophysiology, 32,* 579–594.

Fabiani, M., Friedman, D., & Cheng, J. C. (1998). Individual differences in P3 scalp distribution in old subjects, and their relationship to frontal lobe function. *Psychophysiology, 35,* 698–708.

Fabiani, M., Friedman, D., Cheng, J. C., Wee, E., & Trott, C. (1999, abstract). Use it or lose it: effects of aging and education on brain activity in the performance of recency and recognition memory tasks. *Journal of Cognitive Neuroscience Supplement, 83*B, 18.

Fabiani, M., Ho, J., Stinard, A., & Gratton, G. (2003). Multiple visual memory phenomena in a memory search task. *Psychophysiology, 40,* 472–485.

Fabiani, M., Gratton, G., Chiarenza, G. A., & Donchin, E. (1990). A psychophysiological investigation of the von Restorff paradigm in children. *Journal of Psychophysiology, 4,* 15–24.

Fabiani, M., Gratton, G., Karis, D., & Donchin, E. (1987). The definition, identification, and reliability of measurement of the P300 component of the event-related brain potential. In P. K. Ackles, J. R. Jennings, & M. G. H. Coles (Eds.), *Advances in Psychophysiology* (Vol. 1, 1–78). Greenwich, CT: JAI Press, Inc.

Fabiani, M., Karis, D., & Donchin, E. (1986). P300 and recall in an incidental memory paradigm. *Psychophysiology, 23,* 298–308.

Fabiani, M., Karis, D., & Donchin, E. (1990). Effects of mnemonic strategy manipulation in a Von Restorff paradigm. *Electroencephalography & Clinical Neurophysiology, 75*(2), 22–35.

Fabiani, M., Low, K. A., Wee, E., Sable, J. J., & Gratton, G. (2006). Reduced suppression or labile memory? Mechanisms of inefficient filtering of irrelevant information in older adults. *Journal of Cognitive Neuroscience, 18*(4), 637–650.

Fabiani, M., Stadler, M. A., & Wessels, P. M. (2000). True memories but not false ones produce a sensory signature in human lateralized brain potentials. *Journal of Cognitive Neuroscience, 12*(6), 941–949.

Falkenstein, M., Hohnsbein, J., Hoormann, J., & Blanke, L. (1990). Effects of errors in choice reaction tasks on the ERP under focused and divided attention. In C. H. M. Brunia, A. W. K. Gaillard, & A. Kok (Eds.), *Psychophysiological brain research* (pp. 192–195). Tilburg, The Netherlands: Tilburg University Press.

Falkenstein, M., Hohnsbein, J., & Hoormann, J. (1995). Event-related potential correlates of errors in reaction tasks. In G. Karmos, M. Molnar, V. Csepe, I. Czigler, & J. E. Desmedt (Eds.), *Perspectives of event-related potentials research* (EEG Journal Supplement 44) (pp. 280–286). Amsterdam: Elsevier.

Farwell, L. A., & Donchin, E. (1991). The truth will out: Interrogative polygraphy ("lie detection") with event-related brain potentials. *Psychophysiology, 28*(5), 531–547.

Federmeier, K. D., & Kutas, M. (1999). A rose by any other name: Long-term memory structure and sentence processing. *Journal of Memory & Language, 41*(4), 469–495.

Fischler, I., Bloom, P. A., Childers, D. G., Roucos, S. E., & Perry, N. W., Jr. (1983). Brain potentials related to stages of sentence verification. *Psychophysiology, 20,* 400–409.

Fischler, I., Childers, D. G., Achariyapaopan, T., & Perry, N. W., Jr. (1985). Brain potentials during sentence verification: Automatic aspects of comprehension. *Biological Psychology, 21,* 83–105.

Ford, J. M., Pfefferbaum, A., Tinklenberg, J. R., & Kopell, B. S. (1982). Effects of perceptual and cognitive difficulty on P3 and RT in young and old adults. *Electroencephalography & Clinical Neurophysiology, 54*(3), 311–21.

Friedman, D. (1990). ERPs during continuous recognition memory for words. *Biological Psychology, 30,* 61–87.

Friedman, D., & Simpson, G. V. (1994). ERP amplitude and scalp distribution to target and novel events: effects of temporal order in young, middle-aged and older adults. *Brain Research. Cognitive Brain Research, 2*(1), 49–63.

Friedman, D., Simpson, G., & Hamberger, M. (1993). Age-related changes in scalp topography to novel and target stimuli. *Psychophysiology, 30,* 383–396.

Gaillard, A. (1978). *Slow brain potentials preceding task performance.* Doctoral Dissertation. Soesterberg, The Netherlands: Institute for Perception (TNO).

Ganis, G., Kutas, M., & Sereno, M. I. (1996). The search for 'common sense': An electrophysiological study of the comprehension of words and pictures in reading. *Journal of Cognitive Neuroscience, 8,* 89–106.

Gehring, W. J., Coles, M. G. H., Donchin, E., & Meyer, D. E. (1995). A brain potential manifestation of error-related processing. In G. Karmos, M. Molnar, V. Csepe, I. Czigler, & J. E. Desmedt (Eds.), *Perspectives of event-related potentials research* (EEG Journal Supplement 44) (pp. 287–296). Amsterdam: Elsevier.

Gehring, W. J., Gratton, G., Coles, M. G., & Donchin, E. (1992). Probability effects on stimulus evaluation and response processes. *Journal of Experimental Psychology: Human Perception & Performance, 18*(1), 198–216.

Gehring, W. J., Goss, B., Coles, M. G. H., Meyer, D. E., and Donchin, E. (1993). A neural system for error-detection and compensation. *Psychological Science, 4,* 385–390.

Glaser, E. M., & Ruchkin, D. S. (1976). *Principles of neurobiological signal analysis.* New York: Academic Press.

Golob, E. J., Miranda, G. G., Johnson, J. K., & Starr, A. (2001). Sensory cortical interactions in aging, mild cognitive impairment, and Alzheimer's disease. *Neurobiology of Aging, 22,* 755–763.

Gonsalves, B., & Paller, K. A. (2000). Brain potentials associated with recollective processing of spoken words. *Memory & Cognition, 28*(3), 321–330.

Gonsalves, B., & Paller, K. A. (2002). Mistaken memories: Remembering events that never happened. *The Neuroscientist, 8,* 391–395.

Gratton, G. (1997). Attention and probability effects in the human occipital cortex: an optical imaging study. *NeuroReport, 8,* 1749–1753.

Gratton, G. (this volume). *Biosignal processing.* In J. Cacioppo, L. Tassinary, & G. Berntson (Eds.), Handbook of Psychophysiology. New York: Cambridge University Press.

Gratton, G. (1998). Dealing with artifacts: The EOG contamination of event-related brain potential. *Behavior Research Methods, Instruments & Computers, 30,* 44–53.

Gratton, G., Bosco, C. M., Kramer, A. F., Coles, M. G., Wickens, C. D., & Donchin, E. (1990). Event-related brain potentials as indices of information extraction and response priming. *Electroencephalography & Clinical Neurophysiology, 75*(5), 419–32.

Gratton, G., Coles, M. G., & Donchin, E. (1989). A procedure for using multi-electrode information in the analysis of components of the event-related potential: vector filter. *Psychophysiology, 26*(2), 222–32.

Gratton, G., Coles, M. G., & Donchin, E. (1992). Optimizing the use of information: Strategic control of activation of responses. *Journal of Experimental Psychology: General, 121*(4), 480–506.

Gratton, G., Coles, M. G. H., Sirevaag, E. J., Eriksen, C. W., & Donchin, E. (1988). Pre- and post-stimulus activation of response channels: A psychophysiological analysis. *Journal of Experimental Psychology: Human Perception and Performance, 14*, 331–344.

Gratton, G., Corballis, P. M., & Jain, S. (1997). Hemispheric organization of visual memories. *Journal of Cognitive Neuroscience, 9*(1), 92–104.

Gratton, G., Fabiani, M., Goodman-Wood, M. R., & DeSoto, M. C. (1998). Memory-driven processing in human medial occipital cortex: An event-related optical signal (EROS) study. *Psychophysiology, 35*, 348–351.

Gratton, G., Goodman-Wood, M. R., & Fabiani, M. (2001). Comparison of neuronal and hemodynamic measures of the brain response to visual stimulation: an optical imaging study. *Human Brain Mapping, 13*(1), 13–25.

Gratton, G., Kramer, A. F., Coles, M. G., & Donchin, E. (1989). Simulation studies of latency measures of components of the event-related brain potential. *Psychophysiology, 26*(2), 233–248.

Greenblatt, R. E., Nichols, J. D., Voreades, D., & Gao L. (1997). Multimodal, integrated, PC-based functional imaging software. *NeuroImage, 5*, S631 (Abstract).

Hackley, S. A. (1993). An evaluation of the automaticity of sensory processing using event-related potentials and brain-stem reflexes. *Psychophysiology, 30*(5), 415–28.

Halgren, E., Squires, N. K., Wilson, C. L., Rohrbaugh, J. W., Babb, T. L., & Randall, P. H. (1980). Endogenous potentials generated in the human hippocampal formation and amygdala by infrequent events. *Science, 210*, 803–805.

Hamberger, M., & Friedman, D. (1992). Event-related potential correlates of repetition priming and stimulus classification in young, middle-aged and older adults. *Journal of Gerontology: Psychological Sciences, 47*(6), 395–405.

Hanes, D. P., & Schall, J. D. (1996). Neural control of voluntary movement initiation. *Science, 274*(5286), 427–30.

Hansen, J. C., & Hillyard, S. A. (1980). Endogenous brain potentials associated with selective auditory attention. *Electroencephalography and Clinical Neurophysiology, 49*, 277–290.

Hansen, J. C., & Hillyard, S. A. (1984). Effects of stimulation rate and attribute cuing on event-related potentials during selective auditory attention. *Psychophysiology, 21*, 394–405.

Hari, R., Levanen, S., & Raij, T. (2000). Timing of human cortical functions during cognition: role of MEG. *Trends in Cognitive Science, 4*(12), 455–462.

Heil, M., Hennighausen, E., & Ozcan, M. (1999). Central response selection is present during memory scanning, but hand-specific response preparation is absent. *Psychological Research, 62*(4), 289–299.

Heinze, H. J., Mangun, G. R., Burchert, W., Hinrichs, H., Scholz, M., Munte, T. F., Gos, A., Scherg, M., Johannes, S., Hundeshagen, H., & et al. (1994). Combined spatial and temporal imaging of brain activity during visual selective attention in humans. *Nature, 372*(6506), 543–6.

Hernandez-Peon, R., Scherrer, H., Jouvet, M. (1956). Modification of electrical activity in cochlear nucleus during "attention" in unanesthetized cats. *Science, 123*, 331–332.

Hillyard, S. A., Hink, R. F., Schwent, V. L., & Picton, T. W. (1973). Electrical signs of selective attention in the human brain. *Science, 182*, 177–180.

Hillyard, S. A., Picton, T. W., & Regan, D. (1978). Sensation, perception, and attention: Analysis using ERPs. In E. Callaway, P. Tueting, & S. H. Koslow (Eds.), *Event-related brain potentials in man* (pp. 223–321). New York: Academic Press.

Holcomb, P. J. (1988). Automatic and attentional processing: An event-related brain potential analysis of semantic priming. *Brain & Language, 35*(1), 66–85.

Holroyd, C. B., & Coles, M. G. (2002). The neural basis of human error processing: reinforcement learning, dopamine, and the error-related negativity. *Psychological Review, 109*(4), 679–709.

Holroyd, C. B., Dien, J., & Coles, M. G. H. (1998). Error-related scalp potentials elicited by hand and foot movements: Evidence for an output-independent error-processing system in humans. *Neuroscience Letters, 242*, 65–68.

Horst, R. L., & Donchin, E. (1980). Beyond averaging II: Single trial classification of exogenous event-related potentials using Step-Wise Discriminant Analysis. *Electroencephalography and Clinical Neurophysiolgy, 48*, 113–126.

Huettel, S. A., & McCarthy, G. (2004). What is odd in the oddball task? Prefrontal cortex is activated by dynamic changes in response strategy. *Neuropsychologia, 42*(3), 379–386.

Huettel, S. A., McKeown, M. J., Song, A. W, Hart, S., Spencer, D. D., Allison, T., & McCarthy, G. (2004). Linking Hemodynamic and Electrophysiological Measures of Brain Activity: Evidence from Functional MRI and Intracranial Field Potentials. *Cerebral Cortex, 14*, 165–173.

Ito, T. A., Thompson, E., & Cacioppo, J. T. (2004). Tracking the timecourse of social perception: the effects of racial cues on event-related brain potentials. *Personality & Social Psychology Bulletin, 30*(10), 1267–1280.

Jasper, H. H. (1958). The ten-twenty electrode system of the International Federation. *Electroencephalography and Clinical Neurophysiology, 10*, 371–375.

Javitt, D. C., Schroeder, C. E., Steinschneider, M., Arezzo, J. C., & Vaughan, H. G., Jr. (1992). Demonstration of mismatch negativity in the monkey. *Electroencephalography & Clinical Neurophysiology, 83*(1), 87–90.

Javitt, D. C., Steinschneider, M., Schroeder, C. E., Vaughan, H. G., & Arezzo, J. C. (1994). Detection of stimulus deviance within primate primary auditory cortex: Intracortical mechanisms of mismatch negativity (MMN) generation. *Brain Research, 667*(2), 192–200.

Johnson, M. M., & Rosenfeld, J. P. (1992). Oddball-evoked P300-based method of deception detection in the laboratory. II: Utilization of non-selective activation of relevant knowledge. *International Journal of Psychophysiology, 12*(3), 289–306.

Johnson, R., Jr. (1988). Scalp-recorded P300 activity in patients following unilateral temporal lobectomy. *Brain, 111*(Pt 6), 1517–29.

Johnson, R., Jr. (1989). Auditory and visual P300s in temporal lobectomy patients: evidence for modality-dependent generators. *Psychophysiology, 26*(6), 633–50.

Johnson, R., Jr. (1993). On the neural generators of the P300 component of the event-related potential. *Psychophysiology, 30*(1), 90–7.

Johnson, R., Jr., & Donchin, E. (1978). On how P300 amplitude varies with the utility of the eliciting stimuli. *Electroencephalography and Clinical Neurophysiology, 44*, 424–437.

Johnson, R., Jr., Pfefferbaum, A., & Kopell, B. S. (1985). P300 and long-term memory: Latency predicts recognition time. *Psychophysiology, 22*, 498–507.

Johnston, W. A., & Dark, V. J. (1986). Selective attention. *Annual Review of Psychology, 37*, 43–75.

Junghoefer, M., Bradley, M. M., Elbert, T. R., and Lang, P. J. (2001). Fleeting images: A new look at early emotion discrimination. *Psychophysiology, 38*, 175–178.

Kahneman, D. (1973). *Attention and effort*. Englewood Cliffs, NJ: Prentice-Hall.

Karis, D., Druckman, D., Lissak, R., & Donchin, E. (1984). A psychophysiological analysis of bargaining: ERPs and facial expressions. In R. Karrer, J. Cohen, & P. Tueting (Eds.), *Brain and information: Event-related potentials* (pp. 230–235). New York: New York Academy of Sciences.

Karis, D., Fabiani, M., & Donchin, E. (1984). P300 and memory: Individual differences in the von Restorff effect. *Cognitive Psychology, 16*, 177–216.

Karrer, R., & Ivins, J. (1976). Steady potentials accompanying perception and response in mentally retarded and normal children. In R. Karrer (Ed.), *Developmental psychophysiology of mental retardation* (pp. 361–417). Springfield, IL: Thomas.

Kestenbaum, R., & Nelson, C. A. (1992) Neural and behavioral correlates of emotion recognition in children and adults. *Journal of Experimental Child Psychology, 54*(1) 1–18.

Kiehl, K. A., Stevens, M. C., Laurens, K. R., Pearlson, G., Calhoun, V. D., & Liddle, P. F. (2005). An adaptive reflexive processing model of neurocognitive function: supporting evidence from a large scale (n = 100) fMRI study of an auditory oddball task. *Neuroimage, 25*(3), 899–915.

King, J. W., & Kutas, M. (1995). Who did what and when? Using word- and clause-level erps to monitor working memory usage in reading. *Journal of Cognitive Neuroscience, 7*(3), 376–395.

Kirino, E., Belger, A., Goldman-Rakic, P., & McCarthy, G. (2000) Prefrontal activation evoked by infrequent target and novel stimuli in a visual target detection task: an event-related functional magnetic resonance imaging study. *Journal of Neuroscience, 20*(17), 6612–6618.

Klein, M., Coles, M. G. H., & Donchin, E. (1984). People with Absolute Pitch Process Tones without Producing a P300. *Science, 223*(4642), 1306–1309.

Kluender, R., & Kutas, M. (1993). Bridging the gap: Evidence from erps on the processing of unbounded dependencies. *Journal of Cognitive Neuroscience, 5*(2), 196–214.

Knight, R. T. (1984). Decreased response to novel stimuli after prefrontal lesions in man. *Electroencephalography and Clinical Neurophysiology, 59*, 9–20.

Knight, R. T. (1987). Aging decreases auditory event-related potentials to unexpected stimuli in humans. *Neurobiology of Aging, 8*, 109–113.

Knight, R. T. (1997). Distributed cortical network for visual attention. *Journal of Cognitive Neuroscience, 9*(1), 75–91.

Knight, R. T., & Grabowecky, M. (1995). Escape from linear time: Prefrontal cortex and conscious experience. In Gazzaniga, M. (Ed.). *The cognitive neurosciences*. Cambridge: MIT Press, 1357–1371.

Knight, R. T., Hillyard, S. A., Woods, D. L., & Neville, H. J. (1981). The effects of frontal cortex lesions on event-related potentials during auditory selective attention. *Electroencephalography and clinical Neurophysiology, 52*, 571–582.

Knight, R. R., Scabini, D., Woods, D. L., & Clayworth, C. C. (1989). Contributions of temporal-parietal junction to the human auditory P3. *Brain Research, 502*, 109–116.

Kornhuber, H. H., & Deecke, L. (1965). Hirnpotentialanderungen bei Wilkurbewegungen und passiven Bewegungen des Menschen: Bereitschaftpotential und reafferente Potentiale. *Pflugers Archives fur die gesammte Physiologie, 248*, 1–17.

Kounios, J., & Holcomb, P. J. (1992). Structure and process in semantic memory: evidence from event-related brain potentials and reaction times. *Journal of Experimental Psychology: General, 121*(4), 459–79.

Kutas, M. (1997). Views on how the electrical activity that the brain generates reflects the functions of different language structures. *Psychophysiology, 34*(4), 383–398.

Kutas, M., & Donchin, E. (1977). The effect of handedness, of responding hand, and of response force on the contralateral dominance of the readiness potential. In J. Desmedt (Ed), Attention, voluntary contraction and event-related cerebral potentials. *Progress in clinical. neurophysiology*, (Vol. 1). Basel: Karger, pp. 189–210.

Kutas, M., & Donchin, E. (1980). Preparation to respond as manifested by movement-related brain potentials. *Brain Research, 202*, 95–115.

Kutas, M., & Federmeier, K. D. (1998). Minding the body. *Psychophysiology, 35*, 135–150.

Kutas, M., & Federmeier, K. D. (2001). Electrophysiology reveals semantic memory use in language comprehension. *Trends in Cognitive Science, 4*(12), 463–470.

Kutas, M., & Hillyard, S. A. (1980a). Reading senseless sentences: Brain potentials reflect semantic incongruity. *Science, 207*, 203–205.

Kutas, M., & Hillyard, S.A. (1980b). Event-related brain potentials to semantically inappropriate and surprisingly large words. *Biological Psychology, 11*, 99–116.

Kutas, M., & Hillyard, S. A. (1982). The lateral distribution of event-related potentials during sentence processing. *Neuropsychologia, 20*, 579–590.

Kutas, M., & Hillyard, S. A. (1983). Event-related brain potentials to grammatical errors and semantic anomalies. *Memory and Cognition, 11*, 539–550.

Kutas, M., & Hillyard, S. A. (1984). Brain potentials during reading reflect word expectancy and semantic association. *Nature, 307*, 161–163.

Kutas, M., Hillyard, S. A., & Gazzaniga, M. S. (1988). Processing of semantic anomaly by right and left hemispheres of commissurotomy patients. Evidence from event-related brain potentials. *Brain, 111*(Pt 3), 553–76.

Kutas, M., Lindamood, T. E., & Hillyard, S. A. (1984). Word expectancy and event-related brain potentials during sentence processing. In S. Kornblum, & J. Requin (Eds.), *Preparatory states and processes* (pp. 217–237). Hillsdale, NJ: Erlbaum.

Kutas, M., McCarthy, G., & Donchin, E. (1977). Augmenting mental chronometry: The P300 as a measure of stimulus evaluation time. *Science, 197*, 792–795.

Kutas, M., & Van Petten, C. (1988). Event-related brain potential studies of language. In P. K. Ackles, J. R. Jennings, & M. G. H. Coles (Eds.), *Advances in Psychophysiology* (Vol. 3, pp. 139–187). Greenwich, CT: JAI Press Inc.

Kutas, M., Van Petten, C., & Besson, M. (1988). Event-related potential asymmetries during the reading of sentences. *Electroencephalography & Clinical Neurophysiology, 69*(3), 218–233.

Laurens, K. R., Kiehl K.A., & Liddle, P. F. (2005). A supramodal limbic-paralimbic-neocortical network supports goal-directed stimulus processing. *Human Brain Mapping, 24*(1), 35–49.

Liu, A. K., Dale, A. M., & Belliveau, J. W. (2002). Monte Carlo simulation studies of EEG and MEG localization accuracy. *Human Brain Mapping, 16*(1), 47–62.

Logothetis, N. K., Pauls, J., Augath, M., Trinath, T., & Oeltermann, A. (2001). Neurophysiological investigation of the basis of the fMRI signal. *Nature, 412*, 150–157.

Low, K. A., Miller, J., & Vierck, E. (2002). Response slowing in Parkinson's disease: a psychophysiological analysis of premotor and motor processes. *Brain, 125*(Pt 9), 1980–94.

Lorente de Nò, R. (1947). Action potential of the motoneurons of the hypoglossus nucleus. *Journal of Cellular and Comparative Physiology, 29*, 207–287.

Loveless, N. E., & Sanford, A. J. (1974). Slow potential correlates of preparatory set. *Biological Psychology, 1*, 303–314.

Lukas, J. H. (1980). Human auditory attention: the olivocochlear bundle may function as a peripheral filter. *Psychophysiology, 17*(5), 444–52.

Lukas, J. H. (1981). The role of efferent inhibition in human auditory attention: an examination of the auditory brainstem potentials. *International Journal of Neuroscience, 12*(2), 137–145.

Luu, P., Collins, P., & Tucker, D. M. (2000). Mood, personality, and self-monitoring: negative affect and emotionality in relation to frontal lobe mechanisms of error monitoring. *Journal of Exerimental Psychology General, 129*(1), 43–60.

Magliero, A., Bashore, T. R., Coles, M. G. H., & Donchin, E. (1984). On the dependence of P300 latency on stimulus evaluation processes. *Psychophysiology, 21*, 171–186.

Makeig, S., Jung, T. P., Bell, A. J., Ghahremani, D., & Sejnowski, T. J. (1997). Blind separation of auditory event-related brain responses into independent components. *Proceedings of the National Academy of Sciences, USA, 94*(20), 10979–10984.

Mangun, G. R., Hillyard, S. A., & Luck, S. J. (1993). Electrocortical substrates of visual selective attention. In D. Mayer & S. Kornblum (Eds.), *Attention and Performance* (pp. 219–243). Cambridge, MA: MIT Press.

Martinez, A., Anllo-Vento, L., Sereno, M. I., Frank. L.R., Buxton, R. B., Dubowitz, D. J., Wong. E.C., Hinrichs. H., Heinze, H. J., & Hillyard, S. A. (1999). Involvement of striate and extrastriate visual cortical areas in spatial attention. *Nature Neuroscience, 2*, 364–369.

Martinez, A., DiRusso, F., Anllo-Vento, L., Sereno, M. I., Buxton R. B., & Hillyard, S. A. (2001). Putting spatial attention on the map: timing and localization of stimulus selection processes in striate and extrastriate visual areas. *Vision Research, 41*, 1437–1457.

McCallum, W. C., Curry, S. H., Cooper, R., Pocock, P. V., & Papakostopoulos, D. (1983). Brain event-related potentials as indicators of early selective processes in auditory target localization. *Psychophysiology, 20*, 1–17.

McCallum, W. C., Farmer, S. F., & Pocock, P. V. (1984). The effects of physical and semantic incongruities on auditory event-related potentials. *Psychophysiology, 24*, 449–463.

McCarthy, G., & Donchin, E. (1981). A metric for thought: A comparison of P300 latency and reaction time. *Science, 211*, 77–80.

McCarthy, G., Luby, M., Gore, J., & Goldman-Rakic, P. (1997). Infrequent events transiently activate human prefrontal and parietal cortex as measured by functional MRI. *Journal of Neurophysiology, 77*(3), 1630–4.

McCarthy, G., Nobre, A. C., Bentin, S., & Spencer, D. D. (1995). Language-related field potentials in the anterior-medial temporal lobe: I. Intracranial distribution and neural generators. *Journal of Neuroscience, 15*(2), 1080–9.

Mecklinger, A., & Muller, N. (1996). Dissociations in the processing of "what" and "where" information in working memory: An event-related potential analysis. *Journal of Cognitive Neuroscience, 8*(5), 453–473.

Michie, P. T., Bearpark, H. M., Crawford, J. M., & Glue, L. C. T. (1987). The effects of spatial selective attention on the somatosensory event-related potential. *Psychophysiolgy, 24*, 449–463.

Miller, G. A. (1996). How we think about cognition, emotion, and biology in psychopathology. *Psychophysiology, 33*(6), 615–628.

Miller, J. (1988). Discrete and continuous models of human information processing: Theoretical distinctions and empirical results. *Acta Psychologica, 67*, 191–257.

Miller, J. O., & Hackley, S. A. (1992). Electrophysiological evidence for temporal overlap among contingent mental processes. *Journal of Experimental Psychology: General, 121*, 195–209.

Miltner, W. H. R., Braun, C. H., & Coles, M. G. H. (1997). Event-related brain potentials following incorrect feedback in a time-production task: Evidence for a "generic" neural system for error-detection. *Journal of Cognitive Neuroscience, 9*, 787–797.

Näätänen, R. (1982). Processing negativity: An evoked potential reflection of selective attention. *Psychological Bulletin, 92*, 605–640.

Näätänen, R. (1992). *Attention and brain function*. Hillsdale, NJ: Erlbaum.

Näätänen, R., & Alho, K. (1995). Mismatch negativity – a unique measure of sensory processing in audition. *International Journal of Neuroscience, 80*(1–4), 317–337.

Näätänen, R., Gaillard, A. W., & Mantysalo, S. (1978). Early selective-attention effect on evoked potential reinterpreted. *Acta Psychologica, 42*(4), 313–29.

Näätänen, R., & Picton, T. (1987). The N1 wave of the human electric and magnetic response to sound: A review and an analysis of the component structure. *Psychophysiology, 24*, 375–425.

Nessler, D., & Mecklinger, A. (2003). ERP correlates of true and false recognition after different retention delays: stimulus- and response-related processes. *Psychophysiology, 40*(1), 146–159.

Naumann, E., Bartussek, D., Diedrich, O., & Laufer, M. E. (1992). Assessing cognitive and affective information processing functions of the brain by means of the late positive complex of the event-related potential. *Journal of Psychophysiology, 6*(4), 285–298.

Naumann, E., Maier, S., Diedrich, O., Becker, G., et al. (1997). Structural, semantic, and emotion-focused processing of neutral and negative nouns: Event-related potential correlates. *Journal of Psychophysiology, 11*(2), 158–172.

Neville, H. J. (1985). Biological constraints on semantic processing: A comparison of spoken and signed languages. *Psychophysiology, 22*, 576. (Abstract).

Neville, H. J., Kutas, M., Chesney, G., & Schmidt, A. L. (1986). Event-related brain potentials during initial encoding and recognition memory of congruous and incongruous words. *Journal of Memory and Language, 25*, 75–92.

Neville, H. J., Nicol, J. L., Barss, A., Forster, K. I., & Garrett, M. F. (1991). Syntactically based sentence processing classes: Evidence from event-related brain potentials. *Journal of Cognitive Neuroscience, 3*(2), 151–165.

Nieuwenhuis, S., Aston-Jones, G., & Cohen, J.D. (2005). Decision Making, the P3, and the Locus Coeruleus-Norepinephrine System. *Psychological Bulletin, 131*(4), 510–532.

Nobre, A. C., Allison, T., & McCarthy, G. (1994). Word recognition in the human inferior temporal lobe. *Nature, 372*(6503), 260–3.

Norman, D. A., & Bobrow, D. G. (1975). On data-limited and resource-limited processes. *Cognitive Psychology, 7*, 44–64.

Nunez, P. L. (1981). *Electric fields of the brain: The neurophysics of EEG*. London: Oxford University Press.

Nuwer, M. R. (1987). Recording electrode site nomenclature. *Journal of Clinical Neurophysiology, 4*(2), 121–33.

Okada, Y. C., Kaufman, L., & Williamson, S. J. (1983). The hippocampal formation as a source of the slow endogenous potentials. *Electroencephalography and Clinical Neurophysiology, 55*, 416–426.

Okada, Y. C., Williamson, S. J., & Kaufman, L. (1982). Magnetic fields of the human sensory-motor cortex. *International Journal of Neurophysiology, 17*, 33–38.

Opitz, B., Mecklinger, A., Von Cramon, D. Y., & Kruggel, F. (1999). Combining electrophysiological and hemodynamic measures of the auditory oddball. *Psychophysiology, 36*(1), 142–147.

Osman, A., Bashore, T. R., Coles, M. G. H., Donchin, E., & Meyer, D. E. (1992). On the transmission of partial information: Inferences from movement related brain potentials. *Journal of Experimental Psychology: Human Perception and Performance, 18*, 217–232.

Osterhout, L., & Holcomb, P. J. (1992). Event-related brain potentials elicited by syntactic anomaly. *Journal of Memory & Language, 31*(6), 785–806.

Osterhout, L. (1997). On the brain response to syntactic anomalies: manipulations of word position and word class reveal individual differences. *Brain and Language, 59*, 494–522.

Paller, K. A. (1990). Recall and stem-completion priming have different electrophysiological correlates and are differentially modified by directed forgetting. *Journal of Experimental Psychology: Learning, Memory, and Cognition, 16*(6), 1021–1032.

Paller, K. A., Kutas, M., & Mayes, A. R. (1987). Neural correlates of encoding in an incidental learning paradigm. *Electroencephalography & Clinical Neurophysiology, 67*(4), 360–371.

Paller, K. A., Kutas, M., Shimamura, A. P., & Squire, L. R. (1987). Brain responses to concrete and abstract words reflect processes that correlate with later performance on a test of stem-completion priming. *Electroencephalography & Clinical Neurophysiology – Supplement, 40*, 360–5.

Paller, K. A., McCarthy, G., & Wood, C. C. (1988). ERPs predictive of subsequent recall and recognition performance. *Biological Psychology, 26*, 269–276.

Paller, K. A., Zola-Morgan, S., Squire, L. R., & Hillyard, S. A. (1988). P3-like brain waves in normal monkeys and in monkeys with medial temporal lesions. *Behavioral Neuroscience, 102*(5), 714–725.

Parasuraman, R., Greenwood, P. M., & Sunderland, T. (2002). The apolipoprotein E gene, attention, and brain function. *Neuropsychology, 16*(2), 254–274.

Pascual-Marqui, R. D., Michel, C. M., & Lehmann, D. (1994). Low resolution electromagnetic tomography: a new method for localizing electrical activity in the brain. *International Journal of Psychophysiology, 18*(1), 49–65.

Pazo-Alvarez, P., Cadaveira, F., & Amenedo, E. (2003). MMN in the visual modality: a review. *Biological Psychology, 63*(3), 199–236.

Perrin, F., Pernier, J., Bertrand, O., Giard, M. H., & Echallier J. F. (1987). Mapping of scalp potentials by surface spline interpolation. *Electroencephalography & Clinical Neurophysiology, 66*(1), 75–81.

Polich, J., & Margala, C. (1997). P300 and probability: comparison of oddball and single-stimulus paradigms. *International Journal of Psychophysiology, 25*(2), 169–176.

Pritchard, W. S. (1981). Psychophysiology of P300. *Psychological Bulletin, 89*, 506–540.

Puce A, Allison T, McCarthy G. (1999). Electrophysiological studies of human face perception. III: Effects of top-down processing on face-specific potentials. Cereb Cortex. Jul–Aug; 9(5): 445–458.

Pulvermuller, F., & Shtyrov, Y. (2003). Automatic processing of grammar in the human brain as revealed by the mismatch negativity. *Neuroimage, 20*(1), 159–172.

Pulvermuller, F., Shtyrov, Y., Kujala, T., & Näätänen, R. (2004). Word-specific cortical activity as revealed by the mismatch negativity. *Psychophysiology, 41*(1), 106–112.

Pynte, J., Besson, M., Robichon, F. H., & Poli, J. (1996). The time-course of metaphor comprehension: an event-related potential study. *Brain & Language, 55*(3), 293–316.

Ragot, R. (1984). Perceptual and motor space representation: An event-related potential study. *Psychophysiology, 21*, 159–170.

Regan, D. (1972). *Evoked potentials in Psychology, Sensory Physiology, and Clinical Medicine*. New York: Wiley.

Renault, B. (1983). The visual emitted potentials: Clues for information processing. In A. W. K. Gaillard & W. Ritter (Eds.), *Tutorials in event related potential research: Endogenous components* (pp. 159–176). Amsterdam: North-Holland Publishing Company.

Rinne, T., Gratton, G., Fabiani, M., Cowan, N., Maclin, E., Stinard, A., Sinkkonen, J., Alho, K., & Näätänen, R. (1999). Scalp-recorded optical signals make sound processing from the auditory cortex visible. *NeuroImage, 10*, 620–624.

Ritter, W., Deacon, D., Gomes, H., Javitt, D. C., & Vaughan, H. G., Jr. (1995). The mismatch negativity of event-related potentials as a probe of transient auditory memory: a review. *Ear & Hearing, 16*(1), 52–67.

Ritter, W., Simson, R., Vaughan, H. G., Jr., & Macht, M. (1982). Manipulation of event-related potential manifestations of information processing stages. *Science, 218*, 909–911.

Roediger, H. L., & McDermott, K. B. (2000). Distortions of memory. In E. Tulving & F. I. M. Craik (Eds.), *The Oxford handbook of memory* (pp. 149–164). London: Oxford University Press.

Rohrbaugh, J. W., & Gaillard, A. W. K. (1983). Sensory and motor aspects of the contingent negative variation. In A. W. K. Gaillard & W. Ritter (Eds.), *Tutorials in event-related potential research: Endogeneous components* (pp. 269–310). Amsterdam: North-Holland.

Rohrbaugh, J. W., Syndulko, K., & Lindsley, D. B. (1976). Brain components of the contingent negative variation in humans. *Science, 191*, 1055–1057.

Romani, G. L., Williamson, S. J., & Kaufman, L. (1982). Tonotopic organization of the human auditory cortex. *Science, 216*(4552), 1339–40.

Romani, G. L., Williamson, S. J., Kaufman, L., & Brenner, D. (1982). Characterization of the human auditory cortex by the neuromagnetic method. *Experimental Brain Research, 47*(3), 381–93.

Rösler, F. (1983). Endogenous ERPs and cognition: Probes, prospects, and pitfalls in matching pieces of the mind-body problem. In A. W. K. Gaillard & W. Ritter (Eds.), *Tutorials in event-related potential research: Endogenous components* (pp. 9–35). Amsterdam: Elsevier.

Rugg, M. D. (1985). The effects of semantic priming and word repetition on event-related potentials. *Psychophysiology, 22*, 642–647.

Rugg, M. D. (1990). Event-related brain potentials dissociate repetition effects of high- and low-frequency words. *Memory & Cognition, 18*(4), 367–379.

Rugg, M. D. (1995). ERP studies of memory. In M. D. Rugg & M. G. H. Coles (Eds.), *Electrophysiology of mind: Event-related brain potentials and cognition* (Vol. 25, pp. 133–170). Oxford, England: Oxford University Press.

Rugg, M. D., Soardi, M., & Doyle, M. C. (1995). Modulation of event-related potentials by the repetition of drawings of novel objects. *Brain Research. Cognitive Brain Research, 3*(1), 17–24.

Sable, J. J., Low, K. A., Maclin, E. L., Fabiani, M., & Gratton, G. (2004). Latent inhibition mediates N1 attenuation to repeating sounds. *Psychophysiology, 41*, 636–642.

Samar, V. J., Bopardikar, A., Rao, R., & Swartz, K. (1999). Wavelet analysis of neuroelectric waveforms: a conceptual tutorial. *Brain and Language, 66*(1), 7–60.

Sanders, A. F. (1990). Issues and trends in the debate on discrete vs. continuous processing of information. *Acta Psychologica, 74*, 123–167.

Sanquist, T. F., Rohrbaugh, J. W., Syndulko, K., & Lindsley, D. B. (1980). Electrocortical signs of levels of processing: Perceptual analysis and recognition memory. *Psychophysiology, 17*, 568–576.

Sarter, M., Berntson, G. G., & Cacioppo, J. T. (1996). Brain imaging and cognitive neuroscience: Toward strong inference in attributing function to structure. *American Psychologist, 51*(1), 13–21.

Scheffers, M. K., Coles, M. G. H., Bernstein, P., Gehring, W. J., & Donchin, E. (1996). Event-related brain potentials and error-related processing: An analysis of incorrect response to Go and No-go stimuli. *Psychophysiology, 33*, 42–53.

Scherg, M., & Von Cramon, D. (1986). Evoked dipole source potentials of the human auditory cortex. *Electroencephalography & Clinical Neurophysiology, 65*(5), 344–60.

Scherg, M., Vajsar, J., & Picton, T. W. (1989). A source analysis of the late human auditory evoked potentials. *Journal of Cognitive Neuroscience, 1*(4), 336–355.

Schupp, H. T., Cuthbert, B. N., Bradley, M. M., Cacioppo, J. T., Ito, T., and Lang, P. J. (2000). Affective picture processing: The late positive potential is modulated by motivational relevance. *Psychophysiology, 37*, 257–261.

Sirevaag, E. J., Kramer, A. F., Coles, M. G., & Donchin, E. (1989). Resource reciprocity: an event-related brain potentials analysis. *Acta Psychologica, 70*(1), 77–97.

Shin, E., Fabiani, M., & Gratton, G. (2004). Evidence of partial response activation in a memory-search task. *Cognitive Brain Research, 20*, 281–293.

Shin, E., Fabiani, M., & Gratton, G. (2006). *Multiple levels of letter representation in visual working memory. Journal of Cognitive Neuroscience, 18*(5), 844–858.

Sitnikova, T., Kuperberg, G., & Holcomb, P. J. (2003). Semantic integration in videos of real-world events: An electrophysiological investigation. *Psychophysiology, 40*, 160–164.

Smid, H. G. O. M., Lamain, W., Hogeboom, M. M., Mulder, G., & Mulder, L. J. M. (1991). Psychophysiological evidence for continuous information transmission between visual search and response processes. *Journal of Experimental Psychology: Human Perception and Performance, 17*, 696–714.

Smid, H. G. O. M., Mulder, G., & Mulder, L. J. M. (1990). Selective response activation can begin before stimulus recognition is complete: A psychophysiological and error analysis of continuous flow. *Acta Psychologica, 74*, 169–201.

Smith, M. E. (1993). Neurophysiological manifestations of recollective experience during recognition memory judgments. *Journal of Cognitive Neuroscience, 5*(1), 1–13.

Smulders, F. T. Y., Kenemans, J. L., & Kok, A. (1996). Effects of task variables on measures of the mean onset latency of LRP depend on scoring method. *Psychophysiology, 33*, 194–205.

Spencer, K. M., Dien, J., & Donchin, E. (2001). Spatiotemporal analysis of the late ERP responses to deviant stimuli, *Psychophysiology, 38*(2), 343–358.

Spencer, K. M., Dien, J., & Donchin, E. (1999). A componental analysis of the ERP elicited by novel events using a dense electrode array, *Psychophysiology, 36*(3), 409–414.

Spencer, K. M., Vila, E., & Donchin, E. (1994). ERPs and performance measures reveal individual differences in a recollection/familiarity task. *Psychophysiology, 31*, S93 [Abstract].

Squires, K. C., & Donchin, E. (1976). Beyond averaging: The use of discriminant functions to recognize event-related potentials elicited by single auditory stimuli. *Electroencephalography and Clinical Neurophysiology, 41*, 449–459.

Squires, K. C., Squires, N. K., & Hillyard, S. A. (1975). Decision-related cortical potentials during an auditory signal detection task with cued intervals. *Journal of Experimental Psychology: Human Perception and Performance, 1*, 268–279.

Squires, K. C., Wickens, C., Squires, N. K., & Donchin, E. (1976). The effect of stimulus sequence on the waveform of the cortical event-related potential. *Science, 193*, 1142–1146.

Srinivasan, R., Nunez, P. L., Tucker, D. M., Silberstein, R. B., & Cadusch, P. J. (1996). Spatial sampling and filtering of EEG with spline laplacians to estimate cortical potentials. *Brain Topography, 8*(4), 355–66.

Starr, A., & Farley, G. R. (1983). Middle and long latency auditory evoked potentials in cat. II Component distribution and dependence on stimulus factors. *Hearing Research, 10*, 139–152.

Stormark, K. M., Nordby, H., & Hugdahl, K. (1995). Attentional shifts to emotionally charged cues: Behavioural and ERP data. *Cognition & Emotion, 9*(5), 507–523.

Sussman, E., Ritter, W., & Vaughan, H. G., Jr. (1999). An investigation of the auditory streaming effect using event-related brain potentials. *Psychophysiology, 36*, 22–34.

Sutton, S., Braren, M., Zubin, J., & John, E. R. (1965). Evoked potential correlates of stimulus uncertainty. *Science, 150*, 1187–1188.

Sutton, S., & Ruchkin, D. S. (1984). The late positive complex. Advances and new problems. In R. Karrer, J. Cohen, and P. Tueting (Eds.), *Brain and Information: Event-Related Potentials. Annals of the New York Academy of Sciences, Vol. 425* (pp. 1–23).

Sutton, S., Tueting, P., Zubin, J., & John, E. R. (1967). Information delivery and the sensory evoked potentials. *Science, 155*, 1436–1439.

Tervaniemi, M., Lehtokoski, A., Sinkkonen, J., Virtanen, J., Ilmoniemi, R. J., & Näätänen, R. (1999). Test-retest reliability of mismatch negativity for duration, frequency and intensity changes. *Clinical Neurophysiology, 110*, 1388–1393.

Toga, A. W., & Mazziotta, J. C. (Eds.). (1996). *Brain mapping. The methods*. San Diego, CA: Academic Press.

Towle, V. L., Heuer, D., & Donchin, E. (1980). On indexing attention and learning with event-related potentials. *Psychophysiology, 17*, 291. (Abstract)

Treisman, A., & Gelade, G. (1980). A feature integration theory of attention. *Cognitive Psychology, 12*, 97–136.

Trott, C. T., Friedman, D., Ritter, W., & Fabiani, M. (1997). Item and source memory: Differential age effects revealed by event-related potentials. *NeuroReport, 8*, 3373–3378.

Trott, C. T., Friedman, D., Ritter, W., Fabiani, M., & Snodgrass, J. G. (1999). Episodic priming and memory for temporal source: Event-related potentials reveal age-related differences in prefrontal functioning. *Psychology and Aging, 14*, 390–413.

Tucker, D. M. (1993). Spatial sampling of head electrical fields: the geodesic sensor net. *Electroencephalography & Clinical Neurophysiology, 87*(3), 154–63.

Tulving, E. (1985). Memory and consciousness. *Canadian Psychology, 26*, 1–12.

van Boxtel, G. J., & Brunia, C. H. (1994). Motor and non-motor components of the Contingent Negative Variation. *International Journal of Psychophysiology, 17*(3), 269–79.

Vanderploeg, R. D., Brown, W. S., & Marsh, J. T. (1987). Judgments of emotion in words and faces: ERP correlates. *International Journal of Psychophysiology, 5*(3), 193–205.

Van Petten, C. (1995). Words and sentences: event-related brain potential measures. *Psychophysiology, 32*(6), 511–25.

Van Petten, C., & Kutas, M. (1987). Ambiguous words in context: An event-related analysis of the time course of meaning activation. *Journal of Memory and Language, 26*, 188–208.

Van Petten, C., & Kutas, M. (1990). Interactions between sentence context and word frequency in event-related brain potentials. *Memory & Cognition, 18*(4), 380–93.

Van Petten, C., & Kutas, M. (1991). Influences of semantic and syntactic context on open- and closed-class words. *Memory & Cognition, 19*(1), 95–112.

Van Petten, C., Kutas, M., Kluender, R., Mitchiner, M., & McIsaac, H. (1991). Fractionating the word repetition effect with event-related potentials. *Journal of Cognitive Neuroscience, 3*(2), 131–150.

Van Petten, C., & Senkfor, A. J. (1996). Memory for words and novel visual patterns: repetition, recognition, and encoding effects in the event-related brain potential. *Psychophysiology, 33*(5), 491–506.

van Turennout, M., Hagoort, P., & Brown, C. M. (1997). Electrophysiological evidence on the time course of semantic and phonological processes in speech production. *JEP:LMC, 23*(4), 787–806.

Vaz Pato, M., & Jones, S. J. (1999). Cortical processing of complex tone stimuli: Mismatch negativity at the end of a period of rapid pitch modulation. *Cognitive Brain Research, 7*, 295–306.

Vaughan, H. G., Costa, L. D., & Ritter, W. (1972). Topography of the human motor potential. *Electroencephalography and Clinical Neurophysiology, 25*, 1–10.

Verleger, R. (1988). Event-related potentials and memory: A critique of the context updating hypothesis and an alternative interpretation of P3. *Behavioral and Brain Sciences, 11*, 343–356.

Verleger, R. (1997). On the utility of P3 latency as an index of mental chronometry. *Psychophysiology, 34*(2), 131–156.

Von Restorff, H. (1933). Uber die Wirkung von Bereichsbildungen im Spurenfeld. *Psychologische Forschung, 18*, 299–342.

Wallace, W. P. (1965). Review of the historical, empirical, and theoretical status of the von Restorff phenomenon. *Psychological Bulletin, 63*, 410–424.

Walter, W. G., Cooper, R., Aldridge, V. J., McCallum, W. C., & Winter, A. L. (1964). Contingent negative variation: An electrical sign of sensorimotor association and expectancy in the human brain. *Nature, 203*, 380–384.

West, W. C., & Holcomb, P. J. (2002). Event-related potentials during discourse-level semantic integration of complex pictures. *Cognitive Brain Research, 13*(3), 363–375.

Wijers, A. A., Mulder, G., Okita, T., & Mulder, L. J. (1989). Event-related potentials during memory search and selective attention to letter size and conjunctions of letter size and color. *Psychophysiology, 26*(5), 529–47.

Woldorff, M. G., Gallen, C. C., Hampson, S. A., Hillyard, S. A., Pantev, C., Sobel, D., & Bloom, F. E. (1993). Modulation of early sensory processing in human auditory cortex during auditory selective attention. *Proceedings of the National Academy of Sciences of the United States of America, 90*(18), 8722–6.

Wood, C. C., & McCarthy, G. (1984). Principal component analysis of event-related potentials: simulation studies demonstrate misallocation of variance across components. *Electroencephalography and clinical Neurophysiology, 59*, 298–308.

Wood, C. C., McCarthy, G., Squires, N. K., Vaughan, H. G., Woods, D. L., & McCallum, W. C. (1984). Anatomical and physiological substrates of event-related potentials. In R. Karrer, J. Cohen, & P. Tueting (Eds.), *Brain and Information: Event-related Potentials* (pp. 681–721). New York: New York Academy of Sciences.

Woods, D. L. (1995). The component structure of the N1 wave of the human auditory evoked potential. In G. Karmos, M. Molnár, V. Csépe, I. Czigler, & J. E. Desmedt (Eds.), *Perspectives of event-related potentials research (EEG Suppl. 44)* (pp. 102–109). Amsterdam: Elsevier.

Woody, C. D. (1967). Characterization of an adaptive filter for the analysis of variable latency neuroelectrical signals. *Medical and Biological Engineering, 5*, 539–553.

Yabe, H., Tervaniemi, M., Sinkkonen, J., Huotilainen, M., Ilmoniemi, R. J., & Näätänen, R. (1998). Temporal window of integration of auditory information in the human brain. *Psychophysiology, 35*, 615–619.

Yamaguchi, S., & Knight, R. T. (1991). P300 generation by novel somatosensory stimuli. *Electroencephalography and Clinical Neurophysiology, 78*, 50–55.

Yamaguchi, S., & Knight, R. T. (1991). Effects of temporal-parietal lesions on the somatosensory P3 to lower limb stimulation. *Electroencephalography and Clinical Neurophysiology, 84*(2), 139–148.

5 Application of Transcranial Magnetic Stimulation (TMS) in Psychophysiology

BRUCE LUBER, ANGEL V. PETERCHEV, TERESA NGUYEN, ALEXANDRA SPORN, AND SARA H. LISANBY

INTRODUCTION

In the past, much of the research in traditional experimental psychology came down to differences in accuracy and reaction time, and this paucity of measures often led to the inability to choose between competing theories. The promise of psychophysiological experimentation on humans lay in the extra measures it provided, opening a window to the mind by examining brain response. The drawback usually lay in the fact that the physiological evidence discovered was in general correlative: measured changes in brain activity could only suggest psychological relationships. The relatively recently developed technique of transcranial magnetic stimulation, or TMS, offers a way of noninvasively designing psychophysiological experiments that produce causal evidence linking brain with behavior. TMS involves the use of brief magnetic pulses to induce current flow in cortical tissue near the surface of the head, stimulating neurons in a focal region, generating a brief disruption of neural processing typically attributed to temporary, virtual lesions (Pascual-Leone et al., 2000). Actively affecting local cortical processing in this way, within the context of behavioral experimentation and brain imaging, allows causal relationships to be established.

1. THE HISTORICAL CONTEXT FOR PSYCHOLOGICAL INTEREST IN TMS

Historically, the development of magnetic neural stimulation has trailed that of its electrical counterpart. This lag can be explained with the technological challenges of generating the requisite large and rapidly changing magnetic fields, in contrast to the relatively weak currents deployed in electrical stimulation. Faraday's discovery of magnetic induction in 1831 revealed the fundamental physical law that would enable magnetic neural stimulation. Since the work of Galvani and Volta in the 1790s, it had been known that electrical currents can stimulate nerves and muscles. Faraday discovered that a time-varying magnetic field can induce current in conductors. Hence, changing magnetic flux could excite nervous tissue as well. Indeed, in 1896, the French physicist and physician d'Arsonval discovered that subjects experience visual phosphenes (flashes of light) when placed in a strong alternating magnetic field. This finding was subsequently confirmed by other researchers. It was later determined that the phosphenes originated in the retina which has a high sensitivity to electrical currents, and hence a low stimulation threshold. In 1959, Kolin and colleagues demonstrated for the first time that alternating magnetic field can stimulate nerves in addition to the retina, by looping a frog sciatic nerve around the pole of an electromagnet and observing intense contraction of the gastrocnemius muscle. Soon after, Bickford and Fremming used pulsed magnetic field to elicit twitches in intact animals and humans, and asserted that this resulted from eddy currents induced in the vicinity of motor neurons.

In 1981, a team at the University of Sheffield in the United Kingdom led by Barker stimulated superficial nerves with single, short-duration magnetic pulses, and recorded the potentials evoked in nearby muscles. The Sheffield group developed their stimulator further, and in 1985 through the pioneering work of Jalinous, they accomplished transcranial magnetic stimulation of the human motor cortex, resulting in muscle contraction in the subject's hands. A few years earlier, Merton and Morton had demonstrated noninvasive transcranial electrical stimulation of the motor cortex. This technique is painful because it requires high voltages to be applied across the scalp to overcome the high electrical impedance of the skull. On the other hand, the magnetic field flux penetrates the cranium unobstructed, and causes no significant discomfort in the subject. The high impedance of the skull further results in a substantial spread of the current reaching the cortex from scalp electrodes, therefore deteriorating the focality of transcranial electrical stimulation. By contrast, the skull does not defocus the magnetically induced electric field. These aspects of magnetic induction constitute a core advantage in noninvasive brain stimulation. Consequently, despite its relatively recent development, TMS has spawned a wellspring of research and clinical applications. More extensive reviews of the history of TMS can be found in Barker (2002), Walsh and Pascual-Leone (2003), and Geddes (1991).

2. THE ANATOMICAL AND PHYSIOLOGICAL BASIS OF THE SYSTEM AND THE RESPONSES OF INTEREST IN PSYCHOPHYSIOLOGY

2.1. Physical principles

TMS uses the principle of magnetic induction – the one that makes electrical transformers work – to produce transient electric currents in the brain. A coil of wire is placed over the head of the subject, and a large current pulse is delivered to the coil. This results in a brief, but powerful magnetic field generated around the coil. The magnetic field rises from zero to its peak value of over one Tesla in about a tenth of a millisecond. Following Faraday's law of magnetic induction, the changing magnetic flux generates an electric field which, in turn, induces current flow (eddy currents) in the conductive brain tissue. As a consequence of Lenz's law, the eddy currents in the brain under the coil flow in direction opposite to that of the current in the coil. These currents can produce a physiological response by depolarizing neuronal membranes, and thus triggering action potentials.

The TMS-induced electric field and eddy current distribution in the brain depends on a number of factors: the amplitude and shape of the coil-current waveform; the coil size, geometry, and orientation; and the conductivity profile of the head. The complex geometry of the brain, and the heterogeneity and anisotropy of its electrical properties make accurate computations of the electric field difficult. Studies modeling the head as a uniform conducting sphere arrive at two major conclusions (Branston and Tofts, 1991; Heller and van Hulsteyn, 1992). First, only electric fields parallel to the surface can be induced, and hence no radial (normal) field components exist. Second, the electric field maximum is always on the surface of the sphere. Local maxima can still exist inside the brain at the interface between regions with different conductivity, however the global maximum is always on the scalp. This basic fact, combined with the rapid falloff of the electric field strength away from the coil, confines magnetic stimulation to superficial areas of the brain. On the other hand, the rule that no electric field components normal to the scalp exist fails in more realistic models accounting for the brain's irregular geometry, as well as the heterogeneity and anisotropy of its tissue (Miranda et al., 2003; Wagner et al., 2004). These models suggest that the magnitude of the normal electric field component could be a significant fraction of the tangential field magnitude. Another conclusion of these studies is that CSF-filled lesions, such as the ones resulting from brain injury or stroke, can substantially distort the electric field and modify the site of neuronal activation. Further, the induced field in the tissue surrounding such an infraction can be significantly boosted. Therefore,

in both research and clinical settings, care should be exercised when subjects with brain pathologies are stimulated.

2.2. Physiological mechanisms

The electric field induced in the brain by a TMS pulse can depolarize or hyperpolarize the neuronal membranes, affecting the probability of firing of neurons under the coil. This is referred to as direct neuronal activation by TMS. To produce an action potential, the electric field must vary spatially along the length of a nerve fiber, resulting in transmembrane currents (Roth and Basser, 1990; Nilsson et al., 1992). The electric field geometries relative to the nerve fiber, which can induce membrane charges, are termed "activating functions." Transmembrane currents can result in either a straight nerve in a nonuniform field, or a bent or terminated nerve in a uniform field (Amassian et al., 1992; Maccabee et al., 1993; Abdeen and Stuchly, 1994). Because fibers in the cortex tend to be short and bent, TMS excitation is believed to occur at the location of the electric field maximum. By contrast, magnetic stimulation of long straight peripheral nerves takes place at the location of largest spatial derivative of the induced field. In the cortex, direct activation is most likely to occur at the bends and synaptic terminations of axons, whereas direct dendritic activation is considered unlikely at the stimulation levels commonly used (Nagarajan et al., 1993; Abdeen and Stuchly, 1994). Axonal excitation triggers both orthodromic and antidromic actions. Further, TMS can also activate neurons indirectly through transsynaptic interactions. Based on measurements in the hand area of the motor cortex, it has been estimated that the actual site of TMS excitation in the brain lies near the gray-white matter junction, which is located approximately 2 cm from the surface of the scalp (Epstein et al., 1990; Rudiak and Marg, 1994).

2.2.1. Motor cortex

The motor cortex is the most extensively explored part of the brain using TMS. The effect of TMS there can be easily quantified by the elicited motor evoked potentials (MEPs) in small hand muscles. The stimulation level with 50% probability of evoking an MEP with relaxed muscles is referred to as the motor threshold (MT), and the analogous metric with voluntary muscle contraction is called the active MT. The active MT is consistently lower than the MT. Two types of responses are identified in the MEP: direct (D) waves result from direct activation of the corticospinal axon, whereas indirect (I) waves arise from transsynaptic excitation of corticospinal neurons by cortical circuits (Terao and Ugawa, 2002). TMS at the motor threshold predominantly evokes I waves, but at higher intensities it may also evoke a D wave. The first I wave (I1) trails the preceding D wave by about 2 ms, whereas subsequent I waves (I2, I3, . . .) arrive at increments of about 1.5 ms. The exact mechanisms of I-wave generation have not been elucidated (Ziemann and Rothwell, 2000), however, a recent computational model of the thalamocortical motor system (Esser et al., 2005) has revealed a combination of intrinsic neuronal properties and circuit interactions that underlie this phenomenon. The orientation and direction of the current induced by TMS in the motor cortex affects the characteristics of the evoked response, which could be expected from the spatial sensitivity of the activating functions discussed above. Using a figure eight coil and a monophasic stimulus, the lowest threshold for MEPs from the hand area of the cortex is encountered when the induced current is in the posterior-anterior direction across the central sulcus (Brasil-Neto et al., 1992a; Di Lazzaro et al., 2004). This type of stimulation produces predominantly I waves. On the other hand, current induced in the latero-medial direction more easily recruits D waves (Di Lazzaro et al., 2004).

Thus, the application of a single TMS pulse can focally activate circuits in the motor cortex. A single TMS pulse can also produce modulation of cortical excitability over a short period of time, as demonstrated with the paired-pulse paradigm. Paired-pulse techniques use two subsequent TMS pulses, where the second one is used to probe for the excitability changes effected by the first one (Ziemann, 2002). The most common method is to apply first a subthreshold pulse, followed by a suprathreshold one. In normal subjects, delivering the pulse pair with an interval of 1 to 5 ms over the motor cortex results in a decrease of the amplitude of the MEP produced by the second pulse. On the other hand, interstimulus intervals of 10 to 20 ms yields an increase of the MEP amplitude (Kujirai et al., 1993; Ziemann et al., 1996). The MEP size changes are believed to result from intracortical inhibition and facilitation, respectively, via the activation of separate inhibitory and excitatory neuronal circuits in the motor cortex, which, in turn, connect synaptically to the output corticospinal cells (Ziemann, 2002).

While single-pulse TMS can modulate cortical excitability only in the short term, a train of magnetic pulses, referred to as repetitive TMS (rTMS), can produce long-term excitatory or inhibitory effects in neural circuits, which last beyond the stimulation interval. The neural response to rTMS is frequency sensitive. For instance, low-frequency (≤ 1 Hz) stimulation of the motor cortex has an inhibitory effect, whereas high-frequency stimulation (>1 Hz) has an excitatory effect (Chen et al., 1997a; Berardelli et al., 1998; Pascual-Leone et al., 1998). Recently, it has been shown that motor cortex stimulation with theta-burst patterns (brief bursts of 50 Hz delivered at a 5 Hz) results in more intense and longer lasting modulation of motor evoked potentials than that seen with other delivery paradigms (Huang et al., 2005). Remarkably, in this study the stimulation was applied over a short period of 20 to 190 s, yet cortical excitability changes were observed for up to an hour. rTMS is believed to modulate excitability of cortical neurons by changing the effectiveness of synaptic interactions, analogously to electrically induced long-term potentiation (LTP) and depression

(LTD), however the exact mechanisms involved are not yet well understood (Terao and Ugawa, 2002; Huang et al., 2005).

2.2.2. Pulse types

The temporal characteristic of charge transfer to the neuronal membrane is determined by the TMS pulse shape and the membrane time constant. The time constants of neurons in the motor cortex and of peripheral alpha motor axons have been estimated to be around 150 μs (Barker et al., 1991). For efficient stimulation, the induced electric field should have pulsewidth on the order of the membrane time constant. Indeed, most stimulator configurations have magnetic field rise and fall times in the 100 to 200 μs range, yielding electric field pulsewidths in that range.

Available TMS devices usually produce one of three common types of magnetic pulse waveforms: monophasic, biphasic, and polyphasic. In the monophasic pulse, the current rises rapidly to its maximum value in about 100 μs and then slowly decays to zero over about 800 μs. Thus, the current in the coil flows in only one direction, and the corresponding magnetic field is unipolar. By contrast, in the biphasic pulse, the coil current completes a full cycle of a sinusoidal oscillation, with a typical period of around 300 μs. Consequently, the magnetic field swings in both directions with almost equal amplitudes. Finally, the polyphasic pulse consists of a few periods of an exponentially decaying sinusoidal oscillation.

Monophasic pulses are usually used in stimulators in which the pulse repetition rate cannot exceed 1 Hz. On the other hand, biphasic pulses are implemented in rapid-rate stimulators that can produce pulse trains with frequencies of up to 100 Hz. Biphasic and polyphasic pulses accomplish stimulation with a lower peak magnetic field compared to monophasic pulses (Maccabee et al., 1998; Davey and Epstein, 2000; Kammer et al., 2001). However, because they produce electric fields with similar magnitudes in both polarities, oscillatory pulses tend to excite a larger population of neurons compared to monophasic pulses that induce electric fields with one preferential polarity. Further, optimal stimulation is achieved with the positive portion of the monophasic electric field, and, reversely, with the negative half-period of the biphasic electric field. Thus, the optimal coil current direction in biphasic stimulators is the opposite of that in monophasic stimulators. Finally, rTMS with monophasic pulses may produce stronger lasting changes of membrane excitability than biphasic rTMS (Antal et al., 2002; Sommer et al., 2002; Arai et al., 2004), possibly due to polarization effects of the predominantly unipolar induced electric field (Sommer et al., 2002).

2.3. Responses of interest to psychophysiology

The responses of interest to psychophysiology generated by TMS can be grouped into three categories, which roughly follow a historical progression in their development. First are directly observable or phenomenological events caused by direct stimulation of primary motor and sensory cortex, such as finger twitches and phosphenes. Opposite effects can also be produced: behavioral omissions such as visual masking or speech arrest. The second category has to do with measured changes in performance of psychological tasks caused by TMS, for example, changes in reaction time or accuracy. The third category is changes in measured brain activity, such as EEG, PET, and fMRI. A fourth category can be added as well, which has to do with long-lasting neuromodulatory events, such as mood change in depressed persons or learning.

2.3.1. Directly observable or phenomenological events

The most obvious and easy to evoke TMS responses are caused by stimulation of primary motor cortex, and indeed these were the first to be historically observed (Barker et al. 1985). A TMS pulse of sufficient intensity placed at an appropriate scalp location over motor cortex can produce a muscle twitch. These are best measured with electromyography (EMG), in which electrodes are placed on the skin over the targeted muscle. A characteristic voltage change occurs with TMS induced muscle contraction, having a relatively constant onset latency (e.g., between 20–30 ms for the first dorsal interosseus muscle in the hand) and an amplitude related to TMS intensity. With a sufficiently focal coil, topographic mapping of motor cortex can be achieved with TMS (Brasil-Neto et al., 1992b). General cortical excitability is thought to be related to TMS induced motor response, and is typically measured using staircasing methods to obtain a motor threshold. A number of aspects of the EMG-measured response to TMS have been explored. For example, response amplitude caused by a TMS pulse can be facilitated or inhibited by an immediately preceding pulse (Kujirai et al., 1993).

Aside from affecting motor systems, TMS can also generate sensory events, at least in the case of the visual system. In most people, occipital stimulation of enough intensity evokes phosphenes – short-duration unstructured flashes. The flashes tend to be colorless, although slight red or green tinges have been reported with increasing intensity. They are difficult to localize in the visual field, although they can be crudely mapped (Meyer et al., 1991; Kammer et al., 2005). Like motor thresholds, TMS phosphene thresholds can be reliably found using psychophysical staircase methods (Ray et al., 1998; Rauschecker et al., 2004) and may be related to cortical excitability (Stewart et al., 2001). At present, only in the visual modality have TMS evoked sensations been found: no observations of TMS induced sounds or somatic sensations with direct stimulation of primary auditory or somatosensory cortex have been reported.

Besides inducing observable events, TMS can also prevent behavioral or perceptual events from occurring. Such TMS-induced disruption is typically attributed to temporary, virtual lesions in the cortical regions directly stimu-lated (e.g., Pascual-Leone et al., 2000). A straight-forward example in the motor system is speech arrest caused by trains of TMS to left frontal speech production regions (e.g., Pascual-Leone et al., 1991). In the visual system, a single pulse from a magnetic coil placed over the occipital cortex will reduce the visibility of a briefly presented target stimulus to the point where it cannot be identified, if the magnetic pulse is triggered in a time window centered around 80 to 100 ms after the visual presentation (Amassian et al., 1989). The effect of such a pulse has some of the properties of a (temporary) visual field scotoma (Kamitani and Schimojo, 1999).

2.3.2. TMS effects on psychological variables

TMS has been found to produce many subtle effects that can only be measured across many trials using performance variables commonly used in experimental psychology, such as reaction time (RT), accuracy, and discrimination (e.g., d′). For example, quantification of hits, misses, false alarms and correct rejections of visual target presentations while single pulses of TMS were applied to the frontal eye fields (Brodmann area 8) led to a determination that the TMS increased visual discrimination (d′) in a backward masking task (Grosbras and Paus, 2003). Depending on the timing, frequency, and location of TMS application, in various tasks TMS has been shown to speed up or slow down RT, as well as increase or decrease accuracy. For example, trains of 20 Hz rTMS applied over Wernicke's Area immediately prior to a picture presentation sped picture naming RT (Sparing et al., 2001), whereas RT increased in a visual continuous performance task with single pulses of TMS over left dorsolateral prefrontal cortex applied 180 ms after target onset (Mottaghy et al., 2003). Trains of high-frequency rTMS applied to parietal cortex immediately before a mental rotation task increased accuracy (Klimesch et al., 2003), while similar trains presented during a visual working memory task decreased accuracy (Pascual-Leone and Hallett, 1994).

Systematic measurements of performance variables has resulted in an explosion of studies in recent years exploring functional aspects of the entire cerebral cortex, beyond primary motor and sensory areas. In the motor system, such studies include investigations of motor planning (Serrien et al., 2002; Kennerlet et al., 2004), motor imagery (Pulvermuller et al., 2005), consolidation of motor learning (Muellbacher et al., 2002), cognitive and sensory interactions with motor cortex (Bonnard et al., 2003), and eye movement (O'Shea et al., 2004). The large amount of cerebral cortex devoted to it has made the study of visual perception quite amenable to TMS techniques. Many aspects of visual processes have been studied, from binocular (Saint-Amour et al., 2005) and motion discrimination (Matthews et al., 2001) to word recognition (Lavidor and Walsh, 2003), illusory contours (Brighina et al., 2003), and visuospatial processing (Aleman et al., 2002). Beyond motor and sensory systems, TMS effects have also been uncovered in higher order cognitive processing, in areas

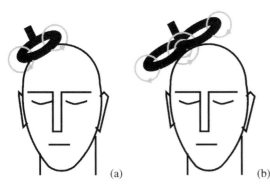
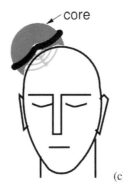

Figure 5.1. Common TMS coil types with corresponding induced electric field shape: *A* circular coil, *B* figure-eight coil, *C* figure eight coil with ferromagnetic core.

such as attention: (Rushworth et al., 2001), task switching (Rushworth et al., 2002), response selection (Hadland et al., 2001), and memory (both short term: Rami et al., 2003; Sandrini et al., 2003, and long term: Rossi et al., 2001), as well as mental imagery (Kosslyn et al., 1999; Sparing et al., 2001; Sparing et al., 2002) and language processing (Shapiro et al., 2001).

2.3.3. TMS induced changes in measured brain activity

While muscle responses and changes in performance measures supply indirect evidence of TMS-induced effects on the brain, in recent years technical improvements in PET, fMRI, and EEG have allowed direct observation of these effects. A closer coupling of TMS and brain imaging allows for a more precise examination of the brain/behavior relationships. It also enables exploration of the connectivity of the stimulated site and other parts of the network it is a part of. For example, 1 Hz TMS stimulation of the motor cortex not only produced activation of that region, but also correlated activation of locations known to be anatomically connected, such as same-hemisphere secondary motor region and supplementary motor area as well as primary and secondary somatosensory regions, and the homologous opposite hemisphere primary motor cortex (Fox et al., 1997). TMS stimulation at 1 Hz of the motor cortex activated the motor network similarly with fMRI, including the expected cortical regions in both hemispheres, and thalamus, basal ganglia, and cerebellum; moreover, this pattern of activation was indistinguishable from that generated by voluntary movement of the same muscles (Denslow et al., 2005). Topographic EEG recording showed the time course of motor network activation, beginning with primary motor cortex directly beneath the coil at 3 ms, with adjacent ipsilateral motor and premotor areas activated over the next 10 ms, and homologous contralateral motor areas active 20 ms post-TMS pulse (Ilmoniemi et al., 1997). The results from all three imaging modalities reflect the expected connectivity of the motor system. This, along with the Denslow et al. finding that TMS connectivity associated with involuntary muscle contractions matched connectivity under "normal" use of those muscles aids in building confidence that less understood networks associated with other behaviors might be successfully mapped using conjoint TMS and imaging techniques. Paus (2002) provides a review of such

explorations in frontal cortex; Paus (2005) reviews some of the advantages and limitations of the method.

3. THE TECHNICAL ISSUES INVOLVED IN DATA ACQUISITION

3.1. Stimulator design

A typical magnetic stimulator consists of five basic components: a charger, an energy-storage capacitor, a discharging circuit, a stimulating coil, and a control circuit (Jalinous, 2002; Ruohonen and Ilmoniemi, 2005). The charger converts AC line voltage to a high DC voltage to charge the energy-storage capacitor. The capacitor can then be connected to the coil through the discharging circuit, yielding a high-current pulse which, in turn, produces a strong transient magnetic field around the coil. Commonplace capacitor voltage, peak coil current, and peak magnetic field are as high as 3000 V, 10,000 A, and 2 T, respectively.

Two basic categories of TMS stimulators are currently available: single-pulse and rapid-rate. Single-pulse stimulators cannot repeat pulses at rates greater than 1 Hz. These stimulators typically produce monophasic pulses. On the other hand, rapid-rate stimulators can generate pulse trains with higher frequencies, reaching 100 Hz in the most advanced models. These stimulators are exclusively used in rTMS applications. They produce biphasic pulses that allow a substantial portion of the energy delivered to the coil to be recycled back to the capacitor for reuse in the subsequent pulse. High-quality, rapid-rate stimulators guarantee the uniformity of the pulse trains, as variability of the individual pulse amplitudes can compromise the safety and the outcome of the procedure. Finally, in paired-pulse paradigms, two magnetic pulses are delivered within as little as 2 ms of each other (Ziemann, 2002). To accomplish such a short interstimulus interval, the outputs of multiple stimulators can be combined within a special device to deliver pulses to a single coil (Jalinous, 2002).

3.2. Coils

Figures 5.1A–C show some TMS coils in common use. The circular TMS coil (Barker et al., 1985) is depicted in Figure 5.1A. Typical circular coils for humans have a 9 cm mean diameter. Pulsing current through the loop produces magnetic flux passing perpendicularly to the plane of the coil. The transient magnetic flux will induce a circular electric field parallel to the plane of the coil, with maximum strength immediately under the wire loop. The circular coil has poor stimulation focality due to the broad, circular electric field maximum obtained. The focality can be somewhat improved by placing only one edge of the coil over the scalp. Roth et al. (1991) calculated the electric fields induced by a number of circular coil configurations in a three-layer spherical head model.

The figure eight coil (Ueno et al., 1988) is shown in Figure 5.1B. In this configuration, two circular coils carry current in opposite directions, and their magnetic fields are constructively combined at the point where the loops meet. The resulting electric field pattern is more focused than that of the circular coil. One measure of focality is the area of tissue with electric field strength of over half the peak value. Thielscher and Kammer (2004) estimated that for a common commercial figure eight coil with a 7 cm mean loop diameter, placed 1.5 cm above a spherical model of the cortex with radius of 8 cm, the focality on the cortical surface is 35 cm². This model also yields electric field strength of 66% and 33% of the surface value, at 0.86 cm and 2.34 cm depth in the cortex, respectively. While these measures of electric field focality are an important metric for characterizing coils, they are only indirectly related to the actual functional focality of TMS. The functional focality depends on a number of parameters, such as the electric field distribution, the orientation of the neural fibers, and the pulse shape. Topographic mapping studies of the human motor cortex, using a figure eight coil with 4.5 cm loop diameter, suggest a practical spatial resolution of TMS of 0.5 cm (Brasil-Neto et al., 1992b).

There exist variations of the figure eight coil, such as the double-cone coil, where the two loops form a 95° angle, and have larger diameters. The double-cone coil can stimulate brain regions located 3–4 cm in depth from the scalp surface, such as the leg area of the motor cortex, but is less focal than the figure eight coil. In general, larger coils tend to provide deeper field penetration, but have poorer focality. For efficient stimulation, it is important that the coil is comparable in size or smaller than the dimensions of the targeted body part (Weissman et al., 1992). For example, scaled-down coils should be used for TMS in children and animals with small crania. Small coils should also be used for peripheral nerve stimulation. For example, figure eight coils with loop diameters down to 2.5 cm are used for animal studies and for peripheral nerve stimulation. The implementation of even smaller coils is constrained by technical limitations.

The coils described above are referred to as air-core coils. A more efficient TMS coil can be implemented by introducing a high-permeability ferromagnetic (iron) core in the figure eight configuration (Figure 5.1C). The iron-core coil (Epstein and Davey, 2002) has larger penetra-

tion depth and induced electric field strength, and higher energy efficiency, compared to air-core coils. These advantages stem from the property of the core to focus the magnetic field to the subject's head. One potential disadvantage of ferromagnetic core materials is that they saturate at field strengths of about 2 T.

A number of practical considerations have to be kept in mind when choosing and deploying TMS coils: Most air-core coils tend to heat up when used with high-energy, high-frequency pulse trains. Commercial coils have built-in thermal sensors that shut the device down if the coil temperature exceeds a safe limit. Special air-cooled and water-cooled coils have been developed for use with high-power trains. Iron-core coils are more efficient and tend to heat up less.

3.3. Safety

In and of themselves, magnetic fields do not pose any discernable risk to humans (National Research Council, 1996). The greatest potential risk in the use of TMS is seizure. Up to 1996, five seizures were reported in neurologically sound, healthy subjects in the early development of rTMS procedures (Wassermann, 1998). These seizures appeared to be the result of excessive stimulator intensity, pulse frequency and train duration and too short inter-train intervals, in various combinations, and resulted in the establishment of safety guidelines for each parameter (Wassermann, 1998). Since the publication of these guidelines, no seizures have been reported in normal participants in TMS studies staying within the suggested safe boundaries.

Higher frequencies of rTMS are most closely associated with seizure risk. Seizures have not been reported when using low frequency TMS (pulses given at a rate of 1 Hz or less, including single-pulse TMS) in healthy subjects. However, single-pulse and paired-pulse TMS have resulted in seizures at rates of up to 2.8% and 3.6%, respectively, in patients with epilepsy (Schrader et al., 2004). Thus, participants should be screened carefully for epilepsy and family history of epilepsy (and neurological status in general), even for low frequency TMS studies.

While quite specific about stimulator intensity, pulse frequency and train duration, the published guidelines were not so clear on length of inter-train intervals. It is now generally accepted that ITI's of greater than or equal to 5 seconds are considered safe for high frequency stimulation (Chen et al., 1997b).

Intensity of TMS used should be tied to the individual's motor threshold. The motor threshold is an estimate of cortical excitability, and is thus thought to be related to seizure susceptibility. However, it should be kept in mind that the motor threshold is only an estimate of general cortical excitability, because it is highly dependent on the distance of the coil to motor cortex, and thus to skull thickness, which is quite variable even in the same individual (McConnell et al., 2001). There is also evidence that cortical reactivity itself varies from region to region (Kahkonen et al., 2004).

Aside from seizure, other adverse effects of TMS include headache and hearing effects. Stimulation over superficial muscles and nerves can result in headaches and local muscle aches, especially with high-frequency TMS. Cramped conditions extended in time within frameless stereotaxic apparatus can also lead to head and body aches. In addition, with TMS animal studies have shown permanent increases in auditory threshold in animals (Counter et al., 1990) and transient increases in humans (Pascual-Leone et al., 1992), leading to the recommendation that all participants wear ear plugs with TMS exposure.

In addition to neurological damage, there are other reasons for exclusion from TMS investigations. Because TMS can heat and move metal, anyone with metallic implants in the head (excluding the mouth) should not participate in TMS studies. Neither should persons with implanted pacemakers or other medical devices, as TMS can disrupt their circuitry. Also, as the effects of TMS on developing bodies are unknown, children and pregnant women should not participate.

4. THE STANDARDS AND METHODS FOR THE QUANTIFICATION AND ANALYSIS OF THESE PHYSIOLOGICAL EVENTS

Investigation of TMS effects on the motor system usually involve measurement of motor evoked potentials (MEPs) using electromyography (EMG). Guidelines for the use of EMG are available elsewhere (e.g., Fridlund and Cacioppo, 1986). Even when not doing motor system research, most TMS studies involve EMG measurement because the choice of stimulator intensity for each participant is governed by his or her motor threshold (MT). As such, EMG recording in TMS will be illustrated within a description of motor threshold procedures.

4.1. Motor threshold

Motor threshold is the minimum stimulus intensity required to produce a reliable MEP in a target muscle (see also Section 2.2.1). In TMS, the MT is the basic unit of dosing and is important in regards to safety. Finding the motor threshold begins with choosing a target muscle, which is usually the abductor pollicis brevis (APB) or first dorsal interosseus (FDI), and attaching recording and ground electrodes. Braiding the electrode wires will reduce artifact. The next step requires hunting for and locating the optimal spot on the scalp that will elicit a reliable MEP. Once the optimal spot is found, the procedure involves positioning the coil in place and finding the motor threshold intensity.

4.1.1. Coil types and coil orientation
With TMS, there are many commonly used coil types (see Section 3.2). Determining which coil type and stimulus location to use mainly depends on what target muscle

is being stimulated (Reid et al., 2002). For distal upper extremity muscles, use a circular coil with vertex localization or a figure eight coil with lateral localization. For proximal upper extremity muscles, use a circular coil with vertex localization. For lower extremity muscles, use either a circular coil or saddle-shaped figure eight coil with localization 2 cm anterior to vertex (Reid et al., 2002).

Excitability of the motor cortex also depends on the direction of the current and the current pulse waveform (Kammer et al., 2001). For monophasic stimulators (e.g., Magstim 200 and Dantec Magpro), the current direction should flow posterior to anterior. Thus, for stimulating the right hemisphere using circular coils centered over the vertex, a clockwise current gives better stimulation, and a counterclockwise current is better for left hemisphere stimulation (this is achieved by turning the coil over, which reverses the current's direction) (Rossini et al., 1994; Reid et al., 2002). If using figure eight coils, placement should be laterally to the vertex, tangentially over the skull/scalp, and perpendicular to the central sulcus (this can be achieved by having the handle of the coil rotated clockwise about 30–45° in the tangential plane) (Kammer et al., 2001; Reid et al., 2002; Awiszus, 2003). For biphasic stimulators (e.g., Magstim Rapid), the most effective current direction is opposite to that for the monophasic stimulators and so, biphasic stimulators are more powerful if their first phase crosses the motor cortex in an anterior to posterior direction (Kammer et al., 2001).

4.1.2. Different methods of threshold-estimation
Though motor threshold is a basic neurophysiological measure of cortical excitability, there are different methods to estimating the motor threshold. The methods vary in such aspects as determining the coil position, defining a reliable response, method of finding the threshold intensity, and number of consecutive stimuli delivered. In estimating the motor threshold, an international committee (IFCN) (Rossini et al., 1994) recommends the following procedure: (1) localize the coil on the frontoparietal region contralateral to the target muscle and move the coil around until the 'hot spot' where the threshold is lowest and the onset latency is shortest is found; (2) increase the stimulus intensity progressively at 5% steps until reaching a level that induces reliable (usually around 100 μV) MEPs in about 50% of 10–20 consecutive stimuli and define this as the excitability threshold. A method recommended by Mills and Nithi (1997) involves placing the coil over a point 5 cm lateral to the vertex on the interaural line for the coil position and averaging the lower threshold (maximum intensity at which 10 stimuli do not produce a response) and upper threshold (minimum intensity at which 10 stimuli all produced a response). In their method, a positive response was any recognizable response of >20% μV amplitude at a latency of 17–30 ms. Another method recommends first finding a spot that elicits the largest response by moving the coil around a few centimeters then decreasing the stimulus intensity by 5% increments until reaching an intensity when fewer than 50% of

six consecutive stimuli elicits a response >20 μV amplitude. The threshold is the lowest intensity when there are at least three of six responses (Reid et al., 2002). (Ascending and descending methods of threshold estimation will yield different results (Reid et al., 2002). A fourth type of threshold-estimation is "adaptive threshold-hunting" (Awiszus, 2003). This procedure estimates threshold continuously throughout the stimulus sequence, where the stimulus strength that is to be used for the next stimulus is calculated from the information obtained from the previous stimuli (Awiszus, 2003). An example of this procedure is the Maximum-Likelihood Strategy using Parameter Estimation by Sequential Testing (MLS-PEST).

4.1.3. Comparison studies of motor threshold

A few studies have compared the different methods of determining the motor threshold. In terms of coil positioning, Conforto et al. (2004) compared the positioning used by Mills and Nithi (1997) (standard position of 5 cm lateral to vertex on the interaural line) to hunting for the optimal position. In this study, the optimal position was found by moving the coil anteroposteriorly and mediolaterally in relation to the standard position in steps of 0.5 cm. They found that the motor threshold was lower at the optimal position than at the standard position. In two studies (Pridmore et al., 1998; Conforto et al., 2004) compared estimating the motor threshold based on visual movement of the hand to a method based on MEP responses. Pridmore and colleagues found that both methods yielded similar results (<10% difference in percentage of total machine output), and, though not significant, the motor threshold obtained by visual movement was often less than one that was obtained by a neurophysiological method. In contrast, Conforto et al. (2004) did find a significant difference in the two methods. The MEP-obtained motor threshold was lower than the motor threshold obtained by the visual movement method. In this study, they also found that performing six instead of ten consecutive trials (i.e., finding reliable responses in 3 out of 6 trials or in 5 out of 10 trials) did not produce differences in motor threshold measurements. Comparison studies (Awiszus, 2003; Mishory et al., 2004) have also examined the efficacy of the different methods of threshold-estimation. Awiszus (2003) compared the IFCN, Mills-Nithi, and MLS-PEST methods and found that the IFCN method was the least accurate and most time consuming whereas the MLS-PEST method was more accurate and less time consuming than the IFCN and Mills-Nithi methods. Mishory et al. (2004) also found the MLS-PEST method to be faster and it used fewer pulses to estimate the motor threshold than a method that was a modification of the IFCN method.

4.2. Experimental issues in TMS

Due to the extremely short duration of TMS pulses, TMS application, particularly in single or paired pulse situations, can be fit into traditional psychological tasks measuring accuracy or RT without change, essentially adding another independent variable for TMS condition. For example, exacting perceptual psychophysical procedures have been used to obtain visual contrast sensitivity thresholds with and without the presence of occipital TMS, in order to provide evidence for the idea that masking effect of TMS is due to an increase in contrast sensitivity most likely caused by the addition of neural noise (Kammer and Nusseck, 1998). In another example, the use of TMS provided evidence that two primary properties of visual motion, speed and direction, can be analyzed independently in the brain (Matthews et al., 2001). In this case, a psychophysical paradigm had already been developed to examine speed and direction discrimination separately in the same set of moving stimuli, using discrimination and bias measures derived from signal detection theory (Matthews and Qian, 1999). Occipital single pulse TMS resulted in large shifts in the bias measure: with TMS, participants became biased to make the choice of slower (as opposed to faster), regardless of the actual speed of the stimulus. Bias in the case of direction discrimination was unaffected by TMS. In effect, TMS altered perceived speed, making stimuli appear to move more slowly, without changing perception of motion direction. This study illustrates one of the best uses of TMS in psychophysiology: employing it within a well-developed experimental paradigm in order to use interruption of brain processes to help decide between theoretical alternatives (in this case, on the independence of speed and direction processing) that have been difficult or impossible to determine with behavioral evidence alone.

On the other hand, a great deal of care must be taken in adapting TMS to this use, as magnetic stimulation has strong superficial effects that can be distracting and disruptive to a finely tuned task paradigm. With TMS, subjects are quite aware that they are part of a physiological as well as a psychological experiment. The pulse creates a sharp clicking noise, quite audible even with earplugs (note: bone transmission of sound as well). There is a somatic sensation in the scalp directly beneath the coil, usually described as a tapping or thumping. Depending on the particular superficial nerves and muscles near the coil, magnetic pulses can produce startling and even painful contractions locally and in the jaws, face, and neck. Study participants must be monitored quite closely, for obvious humane reasons but also to determine the extent the superficial effects of TMS may be interfering with task performance. There is a great degree of intersubject variability both in physical anatomy and in distractibility and pain thresholds, suggesting that pain and discomfort ratings for each scalp location used should be a normal part of the data collected.

It should be noted that not all the superficial effects of TMS are directly observable: some are quite subtle. For example, Pascual-Leone et al. (1994) reported that in a simple RT task, a single TMS pulse to motor cortex immediately before the cue to respond could shorten response time. However, it was later demonstrated that the same simple RT facilitation could be produced by single pulses applied to other parts of the head or neck, and by sham stimulation (Terao et al., 1997). Terao et al. suggested that what was actually being observed was intersensory facilitation (IF), a well-studied effect in which simple RT can be shortened if the cue signal is accompanied by a second stimulation, such as the auditory click of a TMS coil, or the physical sensation TMS causes in skin and superficial muscle.

4.2.1. Pulse timing contrasts

If even unobservable superficial effects can alter task performance, careful choice of control conditions that adequately account for them becomes paramount in a TMS experiment. It is clear that comparing a condition in which there was no TMS with a condition in which there was may not be sufficient. The best comparisons are made between conditions in which TMS occurred during the same task. This has usually been achieved in one of two ways: either by manipulating temporal or spatial aspects of TMS application, or by the use of sham TMS.

One way to compare the effects of TMS is to vary the time pulses are given relative to the timing of the task. One of the clearest examples of this was the first demonstration of the masking of visual stimuli by single magnetic pulses (Amassian et al., 1989). Participants were to identify triplets of letters presented for a few milliseconds in the center of a computer screen. At various times relative to the stimulus presentation, ranging from 0 to 200 ms, a TMS pulse was applied occipitally. Subjects were not able to identify the letters when TMS pulses occurred in a time window centered around 80 to 100 ms after the visual presentation, whereas they had no such difficulty at points outside this window. A physiological explanation is relatively straightforward: the window of visual disruption corresponds to the time when target information initially reaches visual cortex and processing there has begun. Stimulation at time points outside this period has little or no effect on the neural processing underlying letter identification, and performance with stimulation at these outside time points can be used to measure the relative effects of disruption. However, choice of "inactive" time points can be problematic. For example, the single-pulse TMS study of visual motion mentioned previously (Matthews et al., 2001) followed the active/inactive time point strategy. It was initially thought that a condition with pulses 0 ms after stimulus onset could serve as a comparison point, because, as in Amassian et al., these pulses could not affect task-related processing, as they occurred well before visual information reaches visual cortex. Unfortunately, processing in the task was disrupted at this time (as it also had been in a previous TMS study of visual motion: Beckers and Zeki, 1995), and further experimentation was necessary to establish a point 200 ms prior to the onset of the visual stimulus as nondisruptive. In general, because the time course of neural processing underlying performance in a given task is unknown (and is often the goal of the study), the choice of reference time points can

not be determined *a priori* and can only be approached empirically.

4.2.2. Topographic contrasts

Another way to compare the effects of TMS on a task is to stimulate at multiple scalp sites. This is in general done one site at a time, although it is possible to use two coils on the head simultaneously. The most straight forward comparison is between an "active" site (i.e., one where TMS is expected to affect measured behavior) and an "inactive" site. For example, in a visuomotor task in which the participant was to point in a clockwise or counter-clockwise direction by an instructed amount, 20 Hz rTMS to left or right posterior parietal cortex caused RT to be prolonged compared to RT when TMS was applied to the vertex of the head (Bestmann et al., 2002). In this case, TMS to the vertex, which overlies motor leg areas, was not expected to affect task performance and thus was considered an inactive control site. Another approach is a double-dissociation technique, in which sites are chosen where opposite effects are expected to occur with different tasks. In one study for example, a spatial working memory task was disrupted by 1 Hz rTMS to dorsomedial prefrontal cortex but not to ventrolateral prefrontal cortex, while a working memory task using faces as stimuli was disrupted by 1 Hz rTMS to ventrolateral prefrontal cortex but not to dorsomedial prefrontal cortex (Mottaghy et al., 2002). Although comparison of effects across sites is a valid approach, care must be taken in choosing sites that have similar superficial effects, keeping in mind that distracting or painful stimulation can also alter task performance.

4.2.3. Sham TMS contrasts

Use of sham TMS provides another way to observe TMS effects. For example, when 1 Hz rTMS was applied to a left prefrontal site, verb production (but not noun production) was slowed, whereas no such slowing occurred with sham TMS applied at the same location (Shapiro et al., 2001). A valid sham should simulate the ancillary aspects of TMS, such as scalp stimulation and acoustic artifact, as closely as possible to actual TMS but should not result in cortical stimulation. The most common sham conditions angle the coil off the head so that the magnetic field stimulates scalp muscles and produces an acoustic artifact, but presumably does not induce current in the cortex. In this case, the coil should be placed perpendicular to the head, as positions angled less than 90° do result in substantial cortical stimulation (Lisanby et al., 2001). Although use of sham conditions eliminates variation due to different stimulation sites or different times of stimulation used in other comparison methods, it does introduce a new problem in that sham does not feel the same, or, if the coil is visible, does not look the same, as real TMS. This is an especially difficult problem in clinical experimentation, as it can remove the blind from the participant. It also is problematic when observing task performance, as sham stimulation is in general much less distracting. One promising approach is the use of coils that can be electronically switched between the sham and verum condition (Ruohonen et al., 2000). In the figure eight configuration, the currents in the two loops can be switched to flow in the same direction (verum condition) or in opposite directions (sham condition) at the coil center. In the latter case, the electric field under the coil center is reduced to zero, while peripheral field strength is increased: currents are not induced in underlying cortex, but auditory and somatic effects are comparable to actual TMS.

4.3. Spatial targeting

Initially, placement of TMS coils was done by hunting over likely regions where stimulation would create observable effects (e.g., lateral areas near the head's vertex for motor stimulation of the hand) and finding a point of optimal effect. Unfortunately, this method is limited to stimulation of primary motor and sensory areas. Investigators quickly adapted the International 10/20 System for EEG electrode placement for coil placement, as imaging studies have provided some idea of what portions of the cerebral cortex underlie standard electrode sites (e.g., Homan et al., 1987). For example, Harris and Miniussi (2003) wanted to stimulate right and left posterior superior parietal lobe, and marked two points, one halfway between P3 and CP3, and the other halfway between P4 and CP4, as the best estimated scalp locations corresponding to that region in left and right hemispheres. Such use of 10/20 coordinates do provide reasonable estimates of cortical locations to target TMS. However, there is considerable variability between individuals in the relationship between 10/20 scalp sites and the underlying cortex (Homan et al., 1987). A much more reliable (although expensive) method has become available in recent years: using a frameless stereotaxic system involving coregistration of the TMS coil to individual structural high-resolution T1 MRI scans. Hardware/software systems have been developed that offer real-time 3-D display of cortical localization as the TMS coil is moved across the scalp. An infrared camera is used to continuously monitor the location in space of the subject's head and of the TMS coil, via sensors attached to each. Coregistration is achieved by mapping the spatial coordinates of head landmarks (e.g., tip of nose and pre-auricular points), found optically, with their corresponding coordinates in a 3-D reconstruction of the head in MRI space. The coil can then target locations in space that correspond to desired locations in the individual's brain. The position of the coil relative to the participant's head is kept rigid within a subject and coil holder, and minute deviations in position can be monitored and corrected online.

The use of MRI and frameless stereotaxy allows a further step in targeting TMS coils: moving from merely spatial positioning to functional positioning. In this case, sites of activation found in a single individual's fMRI can be targeted, achieving a close complementarity of functional imaging and TMS. This is an important development,

as large individual differences are expected in the locus of specific cortical processes, especially those involved in higher cortical functions. For example, Herwig et al. (2003) scanned subjects while they performed a working memory task. Prefrontal and parietal sites in each subject were selected from the resulting fMRI images by finding the maximally activated voxel in each region. These sites exhibited considerable inter-individual variation, ranging frontally across Brodman Areas 4, 6, 8, 9 and 44, and parietally across areas 7 and 40. Using this information, three seconds of 15 Hz rTMS was applied to those sites and to homologous control sites in the opposite hemisphere, and TMS was found to increase error rates in the task with prefrontal stimulation at the chosen site relative to the control site.

The Herwig et al. study illustrates an ideal experimental context for the use of TMS. A psychological paradigm was utilized whose effects have been parametrically explored since the late 1960s, high resolution physiological activation data were obtained on an individual basis with fMRI, and targeting was achieved with structural MRI and stereotaxic apparatus. The only thing missing was physiological information regarding decisions on when to stimulate, which can be provided by EEG or MEG. Overall, use of TMS in an imaging context in this way allows researchers to investigate links between brain and behavior in a causal way that, with imaging alone, had been only correlative.

The last step in experimental synthesis combining imaging techniques and TMS is to use them simultaneously, such that the physiological effects of employing TMS can be more directly observed, and regional and temporal brain/behavior relationships can be more closely studied, using a "perturb and measure" approach (Paus, 2005). Simultaneous TMS is now possible in the main imaging modalities, as technical problems involving the large magnetic fields of TMS have been overcome. For example, EEG amplifiers are timed to switch on and off with TMS pulses so that they are not swamped by induced currents, allowing high density topographic EEG to be recorded beginning less than a millisecond after a pulse (Ilmoniemi et al., 1997). Similar success has occurred in MRI, where special head and coil holders must be manufactured and the timing of TMS pulses and MRI fields carefully interleaved (Bohning et al., 1997; Bohning et al., 1998) and PET, where TMS pulses even at 40% stimulator intensity can distort the image (Fox et al., 1997; Paus et al., 1997; Paus, 1999).

4.4. Dynamic targeting

The temporal resolution of a TMS pulse is quite high in a psychophysiolgical context, on the order of a millisecond. The duration of its effects on nervous tissue is more problematic. Amplitudes of EMG responses to single pulses applied to motor cortex can diminish markedly when stimuli are not separated by a large enough intertrial interval (at least 5–10 s). Some effects of a session of TMS can last an hour (Grafman, 2000). Thus the time resolution of TMS effects depends on what effects are being measured, and the existence of longer-lasting effects should be factored into design of TMS experiments. However, given the duration of effects seen in such work as TMS masking of visual stimuli, where effects last just a few tens of milliseconds (e.g., Amassian et al., 1989) deciding on when to stimulate can be as important as where to stimulate.

Dynamic targeting of TMS consists of estimating two parameters: the critical time point (or points) during the processing of a task, and the duration of stimulation necessary to achieve an effect. If a single pulse alone can create a behavioral effect, it is the most preferable stimulus, both because that effect can then be linked to processing that occurs over a short span of a few tens of milliseconds, and because a single pulse causes the least behavioral disruption to a task and the least discomfort for the subject. As mentioned previously, single pulses have been used with great success at every level, from stimulation of primary visual cortex, where single pulses at 80 ms post stimulus onset disrupted processes involved in simple visual identification (Amassian et al., 1989; Masur et al., 1993; Miller et al., 1996; Corthout et al., 1999) to stimulation of parietal association cortex, where single pulses at 160 ms post stimulus onset disrupted processes involved in self-recognition (Lou et al., 2004).

Pairs of pulses judiciously timed can also reveal information about the timing of processing (Amassian et al., 1993). For example, in Juan and Walsh (2003) a visual search task was used that had two levels of difficulty: targets that were easy to identify among distractors, and targets that were much harder to distinguish. Pairs of pulses to primary visual cortex between 0 and 120 ms (e.g., occurring at 0 and 100 or 80 and 120 ms) after stimulus onset decreased discriminability for both easy and hard targets, while pulse pairs at 200 and 240 ms did so for the difficult targets. The timing of the behavioral effects suggested that the first visual area is used more extensively with more difficult visual search, and led to some interesting speculations regarding processing in the visual cortical hierarchy.

Single pulses or a pairs of pulses are sometimes not enough to create an effect. As mentioned above, Bestmann et al. (2002) looked at RT in a visuomotor task while TMS was applied to left or right posterior parietal cortex. Initially, they found that single pulses delivered at different times (100, 250, and 800 ms after stimulus onset) did not affect RT. Although this result did not exhaust the list of potential pulse times, it did suggest to the authors that single pulses might not be enough to work in their paradigm, and they tried multiple pulses occurring at 100, 150, 200, and 250 ms (i.e., 4 pulses of 20 Hz rTMS) after the visual stimulus, sacrificing more detailed study of the chronometry of the processes involved in the visuomotor task. The 100–250 ms window was chosen based on peak parietal activation seen with the task using MEG. This duration and frequency of stimulation proved sufficient to increase RT in the task. Further experimentation might indicate whether a short train of pulses is required to alter performance, or whether single pulses (at 150 or 200 ms) or perhaps pairs of pulses would be sufficient. Juan and Walsh (2003) used a different dynamic targeting strategy in the visual search task. They began with 10 Hz trains lasting for 500 ms, and assumed the train would disrupt processing in the first visual area during its course. When the train began with the onset of the visual stimulus, discrimination was disrupted for both easy and hard targets. However, when the train began 100 ms after onset, only discrimination of hard targets was affected. Armed with the knowledge that primary visual cortex participation was only needed up to the first 100 ms for easy targets but longer for more difficult ones, the researchers proceeded to explore the chronometry of the search for hard targets in more detail using paired pulses. Both the Bestmann et al. and the Juan and Walsh studies illustrate heterogeneous approaches to dynamic targeting, alternatively expanding and contracting the range of pulses over time periods likely, according to other studies, to be sensitive to TMS. Until there is a deeper understanding of the interaction of TMS and large populations of cortical neurons, these empirically driven strategies remain a necessary aspect of TMS experimental design.

5. THE RELEVANT THEORIES UNDERLYING PSYCHOLOGICAL INFERENCES BASED ON THESE PHYSIOLOGICAL EVENTS

While the results of a TMS experiment can establish a causal link between brain regions and behavior, much of the theoretical work centers upon how brain regions are affected by TMS to achieve such links. TMS affects the brain by short-term disruption, short-term facilitation, and longer-term modulation of neural processes.

5.1. Short-term disruption

One of the earliest and most straightforward conceptions of TMS action is that in the case where ongoing cortical processing is occurring, TMS can interfere with it. Ordinarily, neurons fire in a coordinated way as they process information, while a TMS pulse results in firing that is most likely random with respect to this coordinated activity: noise is added to the patterned processing, interfering with it. In the visual system, this added neural noise due to TMS has been measured as increases in visual contrast threshold (Kammer and Nusseck, 1998). A TMS pulse of large enough intensity could overwhelm all ordered processing, rendering an area momentarily useless. This state reflects the concept of a temporary "lesion" generated by TMS. Conversely, where minimal processing is occurring in a cortical region, such as in visual cortex with eyes closed or in motor cortex controlling hand muscles when the hand is at rest, the noise created by TMS might make itself evident in the former case as a phosphene, and in the latter case as a muscle twitch. The effects of single and paired pulse TMS on motor cortex have been modeled using a sophisticated computer simulation of 33,000 neurons, both excitatory and inhibitory, arranged according to known anatomy into a multi-layered cortex with over five million intra- and inter-layer synaptic connections (Esser et al., 2005). The cortical outputs of the model cortex after TMS "pulses" accurately reflected such output seen in vivo in animal research. Computer simulations such as this may ultimately supply much needed understanding of the responses by local cortical circuitry to TMS, helping to guide choices of TMS parameters such as intensity, pulse train duration, and time of stimulation.

5.2. Short-term facilitation

Recently, TMS has been found to enhance performance in a number of tasks, including choice reaction time (Evers et al., 2001), picture naming (Topper et al., 1998), mental rotation of 3-D objects (Klimesch et al., 2003), backward masking (Grosbras and Paus, 2003), Stroop (Hayward et al., 2004), recognition memory (Kohler et al., 2004), and analogical reasoning (Boroojerdi et al., 2001). Performance enhancement has been seen in some studies in accuracy measures (Klimesch et al., 2003; Kohler et al., 2004), whereas other studies reported decreases in reaction time (RT) without change in accuracy (Topper et al., 1998; Boroojerdi et al., 2001; Evers et al., 2001; Sparing et al., 2001). Presumably, TMS-induced enhancements in these studies reflect facilitation of neural processing in localized cortical regions, rather than disruption, though this has not been definitively proven.

What might the mechanism be? Two explanations have been proposed, one relying on the disruptive aspects of magnetic stimulation, and the other on possible neural activation. In the former case, processing which normally actually interferes with performance is disturbed by TMS. For example, TMS applied to a superior occipital site resulted in an improvement in performance in a visual search task (Walsh et al., 1999). The task involved searching for a target composed of a conjunction of features also present in a set of distractors (e.g., the target might be a red letter "T" among a set of red "A"s and green "T"s). When one of the features of the search was direction of motion, TMS given over the occipital site, identified as a motion analysis area, delayed response (Walsh et al., 1998). On the other hand, TMS applied to the same site decreased RT when the conjunction target among the moving stimuli was based on form and color rather than motion. This suggests a competition among the various visual cortical areas that process different properties of incoming stimuli in parallel. In the case where information about the movement of the stimuli was irrelevant, disruption of the flow of movement information from the occipital site may have decreased the total processing time necessary. This sort of improvement through subtraction may also have occurred in a study of TMS effects on a Stroop task (Hayward et al., 2004). In that study, TMS applied to anterior cingulate cortex negated the addition to RT caused by Stroop interfer-

ence. This suggested that this region is involved with evaluative processes that are not necessary in this task, such that their disruption allowed overall processing of the stimulus to be faster.

A second mechanism known as "post-tetanic facilitation," posits that TMS delivered just prior to task-related neural processing increases cortical excitability in a way that can enhance performance under some conditions. Direct electrical stimulation of cortical neurons in non-human primates has been shown to enhance task performance. For example, direct stimulation of neurons in the frontal eye fields (FEF; Brodmann's Area 8) during the 100 ms prior to the dimming of a visual target improved its detectability (Moore and Fallah, 2001). Correspondingly, single-pulse TMS to the FEF in humans 12 to 50 ms before a visual target in a backward masking task enhanced its discriminability (Grosbras and Paus, 2003). Trains of TMS pulses can extend facilitatory effects on subsequent neural response. For instance, 5 Hz TMS delivered for four seconds increased cortical excitability in primary motor cortex for 600–900 ms after its offset (Berardelli et al., 1998). Five Hz TMS trains to motor cortex have been shown to produce lasting effects on cortical excitability as measured by electrophysiological response (Peinemann et al., 2000) and with PET imaging (Siebner et al., 2000). In another study, 5 Hz TMS applied to somatosensory cortex immediately before a tactile discrimination task significantly improved performance (Ragert et al., 2003). The mechanism behind such enhancement is unknown. One suggestion is that a local increase in excitability, perhaps produced by a temporary increase in the amplitude of excitatory post-synaptic potentials (e.g., Iriki et al., 1989), may lead to a larger neural response, and thus serve to lower thresholds, increase discriminability, or facilitate EMG amplitudes. Another possibility is that TMS affects the oscillatory dynamics of brain networks, perhaps by generating a resonance with local alpha activity (Klimesch et al., 2003). Studies have shown task performance to be positively correlated with the size of local alpha activity occurring prior to task processing and with the depth of alpha desynchronization after the onset of task-related stimuli (e.g., Neubauer et al., 1995). Klimesch et al. (2003) demonstrated that a train of parietal TMS applied at an individual's peak alpha frequency (about 10 Hz) immediately before a mental rotation task increased both performance accuracy and the depth of alpha desynchronization. This manipulation by TMS of both oscillatory activity and task performance points to the functional relevance of alpha activity.

5.3. Long-term modulation

Experimental effects of TMS are generally short lasting, under some circumstances they have been known to last up to an hour (Grafman, 2000). On the other hand, there is growing evidence that TMS can have much longer lasting effects on the central nervous system, lasting at least over a period of weeks. These effects have been seen in clinical trials investigating the effect of TMS on psychiatric illnesses such as depression, schizophrenia, and OCD. By far the most studies have been of depression.

In depressed patients, the positive effects of rTMS usually last for several weeks (sometimes months) after the course is completed. Treatment typically targets dorsolateral prefrontal cortex (DLPFC). It is accessible to TMS and highly connected with other target structures, such as anterior cingulate regions. The majority of the clinical studies use high-frequency (10–20 Hz) rTMS in the left DLPFC area, the rationale being that activation of that area will lead to lasting changes in the neurocircuitry involved in mood regulation. However, some studies were done with the use of low frequency rTMS to the right prefrontal cortex (Klein et al., 1999; Lisanby et al., 2002; Fitzgerald, 2004; Kauffmann et al., 2004). An argument for using low frequency rTMS to right DLPFC is based on evidence from imaging studies that the left and right hemispheres have opposing roles in mood regulation (Davidson and Hugdahl, 1995). In depression left hypofrontality is accompanied by a relative right-sided overactivation. In addition, for safety reasons, it is better to use low frequency TMS as there is less seizure risk associated with it. A direct comparison between left prefrontal activation and right prefrontal inhibition failed to show any significant difference in efficacy (Fitzgerald et al., 2003; Lisanby, 2003). However, high-frequency right prefrontal rTMS has no antidepressant effect, moreover, in one study it induced tearfulness in some of the depressed subjects (Loo and Mitchell, 2005).

Disregulation of a network that includes prefrontal, cingulate, parietal, and temporal cortical regions as well as parts of the striatum, thalamus, and hypothalamus has been implicated in depression. Most of the available neuroimaging studies of neurocircuitry in depression show decreased blood flow and decreased glucose metabolism in the frontal cortical area (Baxter et al., 1989; Sackeim et al., 1990; Mayberg, 2002; Mayberg, 2003b). Cognitive deficits in depression have been attributed to this so called "hypofrontality." In addition to the deficits in metabolism in frontal cortical areas, depressed patients have increased activity in anterior cingulate cortex, limbic, and subcortical regions (Mayberg, 2003a). Antidepressant pharmacological treatment appears to normalize these deficits (Kennedy et al., 2001), and degree of normalization has been shown to be associated with clinical response (Mayberg et al., 2000). Functional inhibition of the anterior cingulate was found to be associated with treatment response to antidepressants (Drevets et al., 2002; Mayberg, 2002). There is also strong evidence that mood control in humans is lateralized, i.e. left and right hemispheres have different, and even opposing actions. For example, in a study by Tormos, normal volunteers were asked to think either happy or sad thoughts while a single-pulse TMS was applied to their motor cortex on the left or right side. Thinking sad thoughts increased motor potentials evoked by left-hemispheric stimulation, while thinking happy thoughts facilitated motor potentials evoked by right-hemispheric TMS and decreased the amplitude of those evoked by left-hemispheric TMS (Tormos et al., 1997).

It was shown that high-frequency (10–20 Hz) rTMS over the left prefrontal cortex increases cerebral blood flow (CBF) in frontal cortex and related subcortical circuits, while low-frequency rTMS decreases CBF in the same brain structures. Daily rTMS for two weeks of 20-Hz rTMS over the left prefrontal cortex at 100% MT induced persistent increases in rCBF in bilateral frontal, limbic, and paralimbic regions. Low-frequency rTMS produced more circumscribed decreases in the right prefrontal cortex (Speer et al., 2000). In another study, in addition to changes in the right prefrontal cortex, slow rTMS over the right DLPFC was shown to produce significant rCBF increase in the contralateral PFC, contralateral ventral striatum, and ipsilateral anterior cingulate, thus affecting major areas involved in mood regulation (Post et al., 1999; Ohnishi et al., 2004).

One of the possible explanations of the differential effects of high- and low-frequency TMS, and especially rTMS is that it induces lasting changes similar to long-term synaptic potentiation (LTP) and depression (LTD) (Post et al., 1999; Speer et al., 2000). Major depressive disorder is associated with dysregulation of various physiologic systems. These physiologic systems are regulated by the major neurotransmitters implicated in the etiology of mood disorders – norepinephrine, serotonin, and dopamine (Szuba et al., 2000). Brain serotonergic systems have been found to play a central role in depression. Thus, increase of serotonin synaptic availability underlies antidepressant efficacy of most pharmacologic agents. In animal studies, rTMS was shown to produce effects similar to antidepressant treatment in humans. rTMS reduced immobility time in the Forced Swim Test (Sachdev et al., 2002) and enhanced apomorphine-induced stereotypy, similar to electroconvulsive therapy (Lisanby and Belmaker, 2000). In common with several pharmacological antidepressant treatments, chronic rTMS was shown to reduce the sensitivity of post-synaptic 5-HT1A receptors in the hypothalamus (Gur et al., 2004), caused downregulation of 5-HT$_2$ receptors in the frontal cortex (Ben-Shachar et al., 1997; Ben-Shachar et al., 1999), and upregulation of N-methyl-D aspartate (NMDA) receptors in the ventromedial hypothalamus, basolateral amygdala, and parietal cortex (Kole et al., 1999).

6. CONCLUSION

TMS can no longer be characterized as merely a novel technology with great promise. Over the past two decades, as it has successfully been integrated into both behavioral and imaging paradigms, it has developed into a useful investigational tool for psychophysiology. Aside from its clinical promise, it has shown its value in studies encompassing all of experimental psychology, from perception and action, to language and mental imagery, learning, and memory, and attention and executive processing. As magnetic field targeting and physiological models of TMS action become more precise, TMS will continue to evolve into an ever more powerful technique for exploring cortical processing and causal hypotheses linking brain and behavior.

REFERENCES

Abdeen, M. A., and Stuchly, M. A. (1994). Modeling of magnetic field stimulation of bent neurons. *IEEE Transactions on Biomedical Engineering, 41*(11), 1092–1095.

Aleman, A., Schutter, D. L. J. G., Ramsey, N. F., van Honk, J., Kessels, R. P. C., Hoogduin, J. H., Postma, A., Kahn, R. S., and De Haan, E. H. F. (2002). Functional neuroanatomy of top-down visuospatial processing in the human brain: evidence from rTMS. *Cognitive Brain Research, 14*(1), 300–302.

Amassian, V. E., Cracco, R. Q., P. J., M., Cracco, J. B., Rudell, A., and Eberle, L. (1989). Suppression of visual perception by magnetic coil-stimulation of human occipital cortex. *Electroencephalography and Clinical Neurophysiology, 74*(1), 458–462.

Amassian, V. E., Eberle, L., Maccabee, P. J., and Cracco, J. B. (1992). Modelling magnetic coil excitation with a peripheral nerve immersed in a brain-shaped volume conductor: the significance of fiber bending in excitation. *Electroencephalography and Clinical Neurophysiology, 85*(5), 291–301.

Amassian, V. E., Maccabee, P. J., Cracco, R. Q., Cracco, J. B., Rudell, A. P., and Eberle, L. (1993). Measurement of information processing delays in human visual cortex with repetitive magnetic coil stimulation. *Brain Research, 605*(2), 317–321.

Antal, A., Kincses, T. Z., Nitsche, M. A., Bartfai, O., Demmer, I., and Sommer, M. (2002). Pulse configuration-dependent effects of repetitive transcranial magnetic stimulation on visual perception. *NeuroReport, 13*(1), 2229–2233.

Arai, N., Okabe, S., Furubayashi, T., Terao, Y., Yuasa, K., and Ugawa, Y. (2004). Comparison between short train, monophasic and biphasic repetitive transcranial magnetic stimulation (rTMS) of the human motor cortex. *Clinical Neurophysiology, 116*(3), 605–613.

Awiszus, F. (2003). TMS and threshold hunting. *Supplements to EEG Clinical Neurophysiology, 56*(1), 13–23.

Barker, A. T. (2002). The history and basic principles of magnetic nerve stimulation. In A. Pascual-Leone, N. J. Davey, J. Rothwell, E. M. Wassermann and B. K. Puri (Eds.), Handbook of Transcranial Magnetic Stimulation (Vol. 1). New York: Arnold Publishers.

Barker, A. T., Garnham, C. W., and Freeston, I. L. (1991). Magnetic nerve stimulation: the effect of waveform on efficiency, determination of neural membrane time constants and the measurement of stimulator output. *Electroencephalography and Clinical Neurophysiology Supplement, 43*, 227–237.

Barker, A. T., Jalinous, R., and Freeston, I. L. (1985). Non-invasive magnetic stimulation of human motor cortex. *Lancet, 1*(8437), 1106–1107.

Baxter, L. R., Jr., Schwartz, J. M., Phelps, M. E., Mazziotta, J. C., Guze, B. H., Selin, C. E., Gerner, R. H., and Sumida, R. M. (1989). Reduction of prefrontal cortex glucose metabolism common to three types of depression. *Arch Gen Psychiatry, 46*(3), 243–250.

Beckers, G., and Zeki, S. (1995). The consequences of inactivating areas V1 and V5 on visual motion perception. *Brain, 118*(Pt 1), 49–60.

Ben-Shachar, D., Belmaker, R. H., Grisaru, N., and Klein, E. (1997). Transcranial magnetic stimulation induces alterations in brain monoamines. *J Neural Transm, 104*(2–3), 191–197.

Ben-Shachar, D., Gazawi, H., Riboyad-Levin, J., and Klein, E. (1999). Chronic repetitive transcranial magnetic stimulation alters beta-adrenergic and 5-HT2 receptor characteristics in rat brain. *Brain Res, 816*(1), 78–83.

Berardelli, A., Inghilleri, M., Rothwell, J. C., Romeo, S., Curra, A., Gilio, F., Modugno, N., and Manfredi, M. (1998). *Facilitation of muscle evoked responses after repetitive cortical stimulation in man. Experimental Brain Research, 122*(1), 79–84.

Bestmann, S., Thilo, K. V., Sauner, D., Siebner, H. R., and Rothwell, J. C. (2002). Parietal magnetic stimulation delays visuomotor mental rotation at increased processing demands. *Neuroimage, 17*(3), 1512–1520.

Bohning, D. E., Pecheny, A. P., Epstein, C. M., Speer, A. M., Vincent, D. J., Dannels, W., and George, M. S. (1997). Mapping transcranial magnetic stimulation (TMS) fields in vivo with MRI. *Neuroreport, 8*(11), 2535–2538.

Bohning, D. E., Shastri, A., Nahas, Z., Lorberbaum, J. P., Andersen, S. W., Dannels, W. R., Haxthausen, E. U., Vincent, D. J., and George, M. S. (1998). Echopolar BOLD fMRI of brain activation induced by concurrent transcranial magnetic stimulation. *Investigative Radiology, 33*(6), 336–340.

Bonnard, M., Camus, M., de Graaf, J., and Pailhous, J. (2003). Direct evidence for a binding between cognitive and motor functions in humans: a TMS study. *Journal of Cognitive Neuroscience, 15*(1), 1207–1216.

Boroojerdi, B., Phipps, M., Kopylev, L., Wharton, C. M., Cohen, L. G., and Grafman, J. (2001). Enhancing analogic reasoning with rTMS over the left prefrontal cortex. *Neurology, 56*(4), 526–528.

Branston, N. M., and Tofts, P. S. (1991). Analysis of the distribution of currents induced by a changing magnetic field in a volume conductor. *Physics in Medicine and Biology, 36*, 161–168.

Brasil-Neto, J. P., Cohen, L. G., Panissa, M., Nilsson, J., Roth, B. J., and Hallett, M. (1992a). Optimal focal transcranial magnetic activation of the human motor cortex: Effects of coil orientation, shape of the induced current pulse, and stimulus intensity. *Journal of Clinical Neurophysiology, 9*(1), 132–136.

Brasil-Neto, J. P., McShane, L. M., Fuhr, P., Hallett, M., and Cohen, L. G. (1992b). Topographic mapping of the human cortex with magnetic stimulation: factors affecting accuracy and reproducibility. *Electroencephalography and Clinical Neurophysiology, 85*(1), 9–16.

Brighina, F., Ricci, R., and Piazza, A. (2003). Illusory contours and specific regions of human extrastriate cortex: evidence from rTMS. *European Journal of Neuroscience, 17*(1), 2469–2480.

Chen, R., Classen, J., Gerloff, C., Celnik, P., Wassermann, E. M., Hallett, M., and Cohen, L. G. (1997a). Depression of motor cortex excitability by low-frequency transcranial magnetic stimulation. *Neurology, 48*(5), 1398–1403.

Chen, R., Gerloff, C., Classen, J., Wassermann, E. M., Hallett, M., and Cohen, L. G. (1997b). Safety of different inter-train intervals for repetitive transcranial magnetic stimulation and recommendations for safe ranges of stimulation parameters. *Electroencephalography and Clinical Neurophysiology, 105*(6), 415–421.

Conforto, A. B., Z'Graggen, W. J., Kohl, A. S., Rosler, K. M., and Kaelin-Lang, A. (2004). Impact of coil position and electrophysiological monitoring on determination of motor thresholds to transcranial magnetic stimulation. *Clinical Neurophysiology, 115*(1), 812–819.

Corthout, E., Uttl, B., Ziemann, U., Cowey, A., and Hallett, M. (1999). Two periods of processing in the (circum)striate visual cortex as revealed by transcranial magnetic stimulation. *Neuropsychologia, 37*(2), 137–145.

Counter, S. A., Borg, E., Lofqvist, L., and Brismar, T. (1990). Hearing loss from the acoustic artifact of the coil used in extracranial magnetic stimulation. *Neurology, 40*, 1159–1162.

Davey, K., and Epstein, C. M. (2000). Magnetic stimulation coil and circuit design. *IEEE Transactions on Biomedical Engineering, 47*(11), 1493–1499.

Davidson, R. J., and Hugdahl, K. (Eds.). (1995). *Brain Assymmetry*. Cambridge, MA: The MIT Press.

Denslow, S., Bohning, D. E., Bohning, P. A., Lomarev, M. P., and George, M. S. (2005). An increased precision comparison of TMS-induced motor cortex BOLD fMRI response image-guided versus function-guided coil placement. *Cognitive Behavioral Neurology, 18*(2), 119–126.

Di Lazzaro, V., Oliviero, A., Pilato, F., Saturno, E., Dileone, M., Mazzone, P., Insola, A., Tonali, P. A., and Rothwell, J. C. (2004). The physiological basis of transcranial motor cortex stimulation in conscious humans. *Clinical Neurophysiology, 115*(2), 255–266.

Drevets, W. C., Bogers, W., and Raichle, M. E. (2002). Functional anatomical correlates of antidepressant drug treatment assessed using PET measures of regional glucose metabolism. *European Neuropsychopharmacology, 12*(6), 527–544.

Epstein, C. M., and Davey, K. R. (2002). Iron-core coils for transcranial magnetic stimulation. *Journal of Clinical Neurophysiology, 19*(4), 376–381.

Epstein, C. M., Schwartsberg, D. G., Davey, K. R., and Sudderth, D. B. (1990). Localizing the site of magnetic brain stimulation in humans. *Neurology, 40*, 666–670.

Esser, S. K., Hill, S. L., and Tononi, G. (2005). Modeling the effects of transcranial magnetic stimulation on cortical units. *Journal of Neurophysiology, 94*(1), 622–639.

Evers, S., Bockermann, I., and Nyhuis, P. W. (2001). The impact of transcranial magnetic stimulation on cognitive processing: an event-related potential study. *Neuroreport, 12*(13), 2915–2918.

Fitzgerald, P. (2004). Repetitive transcranial magnetic stimulation and electroconvulsive therapy: complementary or competitive therapeutic options in depression? *Australas Psychiatry, 12*(3), 234–238.

Fitzgerald, P. B., Brown, T. L., Marston, N. A., Daskalakis, Z. J., De Castella, A., and Kulkarni, J. (2003). Transcranial magnetic stimulation in the treatment of depression: a double-blind, placebo-controlled trial. *Arch Gen Psychiatry, 60*(10), 1002–1008.

Fox, P., Ingham, R., George, M. S., Mayberg, H., Ingham, J., Roby, J., Martin, C., and Jerabek, P. (1997). Imaging human intracerebral connectivity by PET during TMS. *NeuroReport, 8*(12), 2787–2791.

Fridlund, A. J., and Cacioppo, J. T. (1986). Guidelines for human electromyographic research. *Psychophysiology, 23*(5), 567–589.

Geddes, L. A. (1991). History of magnetic stimulation of the nervous system. *Journal of Clinical Neurophysiology, 8*(1), 3–9.

Grafman, J. (2000). TMS as a primary brain mapping tool. In M. S. George and R. H. Belmaker (Eds.), *Transcranial magnetic stim-

ulation (TMS) in neuropsychiatry* (Vol. 1, pp. 115–140). Washington, DC: American Psychiatric Press, Inc.

Grosbras, M. H., and Paus, T. (2003). Transcranial magnetic stimulation of the human frontal eye field facilitates visual awareness. *European Journal of Neuroscience, 18*(11), 3121–3126.

Gur, E., Lerer, B., van de Kar, L. D., and Newman, M. E. (2004). Chronic rTMS induces subsensitivity of post-synaptic 5-HT1A receptors in rat hypothalamus. *Int J Neuropsychopharmacol, 7*(3), 335–340.

Hadland, K. A., Rushworth, M. F., Passingham, R. E., Jahanshahi, M., and Rothwell, J. C. (2001). Interference with performance of a response selection task that has no working memory component: an rTMS comparison of the dorsolateral prefrontal and medial frontal cortex. *Journal of Cognitive Neuroscience, 13*(1), 1097–1108.

Harris, I. M., and Miniussi, C. (2003). Parietal lobe contribution to mental rotation demonstrated with rTMS. *Journal of Cognitive Neuroscience, 15*(3), 315–323.

Hayward, G., Goodwin, G. M., and Harmer, C. J. (2004). The role of the anterior cingulate cortex in the counting Stroop task. *Experimental Brain Research, 154*(3), 355–358.

Heller, L., and van Hulsteyn, D. B. (1992). Brain stimulation using electromagnetic sources: theoretical aspects. *Biophysical Journal, 63*(1), 129–138.

Herwig, U., Abler, B., Schonfeldt-Lecuona, C., Wunderlich, A., Grothe, J., Spitzer, M., and Walter, H. (2003). Verbal storage in a premotor-parietal network: evidence from fMRI-guided magnetic stimulation. *Neuroimage, 20*(2), 1032–1041.

Homan, R. W., Herman, J., and Purdy, P. (1987). Cerebral location of international 10–20 system electrode placement. *Electroencephalography and Clinical Neurophysiology, 66*(4), 367–382.

Huang, Y. Z., Edwards, M. J., Rounis, E., Bhalia, K. P., and Rothwell, J. C. (2005). Theta burst stimulation of the human motor cortex. *Neuron, 45*, 201–206.

Ilmoniemi, R. J., Virtanen, J., Ruohonen, J., Karhu, J., Aronen, H. J., Naatanen, R., and Katila, T. (1997). Neuronal responses to magnetic stimulation reveal cortical reactivity and connectivity. *Neuroreport, 8*(16), 3537–3540.

Iriki, A., Pavlides, C., Keller, A., and Asanuma, H. (1989). Long-term potentiation in the motor cortex. *Science, 245*(4924), 1385–1387.

Jalinous, R. (2002). Principles of magnetic stimulator design. In A. Pascual-Leone, N. J. Davey, J. Rothwell, E. M. Wassermann and B. K. Puri (Eds.), *Handbook of Transcranial Magnetic Stimulation* (Vol. 1). New York: Arnold Publishers.

Juan, C. H., and Walsh, V. (2003). Feedback to V1: a reverse hierarchy in vision. *Experimental Brain Research, 150*(2).

Kahkonen, S., Wilenius, J., Komssi, S., and Ilmoniemi, R. J. (2004). Distinct differences in cortical reactivity of motor and prefrontal cortices to magnetic stimulation. *Clinical Neurophysiology, 115*(3), 583–588.

Kamitani, Y., and Schimojo, S. (1999). Manifestation of scotomas created by transcranial magnetic stimulation of human visual cortex. *Nature Neuroscience, 2*(1), 767–771.

Kammer, T., Beck, S., Thielscher, A., Laubis-Herrmann, U., and Topka, H. (2001). Motor thresholds in humans: a transcranial magnetic stimulation study comparing different pulse waveforms, current directions and stimulator types. *Clinical Neurophysiology, 112*(1), 250–258.

Kammer, T., and Nusseck, H. G. (1998). Are recognition deficits following occipital lobe TMS explained by raised detection thresholds? *Neuropsychologia, 36*(11), 1161–1166.

Kammer, T., Puls, K., Erb, M., and Grodd, W. (2005). Transcranial magnetic stimulation in the visual system. II. Characterization of induced phosphenes and scotomas. *Experimental Brain Research, 160*(1), 129–140.

Kauffmann, C. D., Cheema, M. A., and Miller, B. E. (2004). Slow right prefrontal transcranial magnetic stimulation as a treatment for medication-resistant depression: a double-blind, placebo-controlled study. *Depress Anxiety, 19*(1), 59–62.

Kennedy, S. H., Evans, K. R., Kruger, S., Mayberg, H. S., Meyer, J. H., McCann, S., Arifuzzman, A. I., Houle, S., and Vaccarino, F. J. (2001). Changes in regional brain glucose metabolism measured with positron emission tomography after paroxetine treatment of major depression. *Am J Psychiatry, 158*(6), 899–905.

Kennerlet, S. W., Sakai, K., and Rushworth, M. F. S. (2004). Organization of action sequences and the role of the pre-SMA. *Journal of Neurophysiology, 91*(1), 978–993.

Klein, E., Kreinin, I., Chistyakov, A., Koren, D., Mecz, L., Marmur, S., Ben-Shachar, D., and Feinsod, M. (1999). Therapeutic efficacy of right prefrontal slow repetitive transcranial magnetic stimulation in major depression: a double-blind controlled study. *Arch Gen Psychiatry, 56*(4), 315–320.

Klimesch, W., Sauseng, P., and Gerloff, C. (2003). Enhancing cognitive performance with repetitive transcranial magnetic stimulation at human individual alpha frequency. *European Journal of Neuroscience, 17*(5), 1129–1133.

Kohler, S., Paus, T., Buckner, R. L., and Milner, B. (2004). Effects of left inferior prefrontal stimulation on episodic memory formation: a two-stage fMRI-rTMS study. *Journal of Cognitive Neuroscience, 16*(2), 178–188.

Kole, M. H., Fuchs, E., Ziemann, U., Paulus, W., and Ebert, U. (1999). Changes in 5-HT1A and NMDA binding sites by a single rapid transcranial magnetic stimulation procedure in rats. *Brain Research, 826*(2), 309–312.

Kosslyn, S. M., Pascual-Leone, A., Felician, O., Camposano, S., Keenan, J. P., Thompson, W. L., Ganis, G., Sukel, K. E., and Alpert, N. M. (1999). The role of area 17 in visual imagery: convergent evidence from PET and rTMS. *Science, 284*(5411), 167–170.

Kujirai, T., Caramia, M. D., Rothwell, J. C., Day, B. L., Thompson, P. D., Ferbert, A., Wroe, S., Asselman, P., and Marsden, C. D. (1993). Corticocortical inhibition in human cortex. *Journal of Physiology in London, 471*(1), 501–519.

Lavidor, M., and Walsh, V. (2003). A magnetic stimulation examination of orthographic neighborhood effects in visual word recognition. *Journal of Cognitive Neuroscience, 15*(1), 354–363.

Lisanby, S. H. (2003). Focal brain stimulation with repetitive transcranial magnetic stimulation (rTMS): implications for the neural circuitry of depression. *Psychol Med, 33*(1), 7–13.

Lisanby, S. H., and Belmaker, R. H. (2000). Animal models of the mechanisms of action of repetitive transcranial magnetic stimulation (RTMS): comparisons with electroconvulsive shock (ECS). *Depress Anxiety, 12*(3), 178–187.

Lisanby, S. H., Gutman, D., Luber, B., Schroeder, C., and Sackeim, H. A. (2001). Sham TMS: intracerebral measurement of the induced electrical field and the induction of motor-evoked potentials. *Biological Psychiatry, 49*(5), 460–463.

Lisanby, S. H., Kinnunen, L. H., and Crupain, M. J. (2002). Applications of TMS to therapy in psychiatry. *J Clin Neurophysiol, 19*(4), 344–360.

Loo, C. K., and Mitchell, P. B. (2005). A review of the efficacy of transcranial magnetic stimulation (TMS) treatment for depression, and current and future strategies to optimize efficacy. *J Affect Disord*.

Lou, H. C., Luber, B., Crupain, M., Keenan, J. P., Nowak, M., Kjaer, T. W., Sackeim, H. A., and Lisanby, S. H. (2004). Parietal cortex and representation of the mental Self. *Proceedings of the National Academy of Sciences United States of America, 101*(17), 6827–6832.

Maccabee, P. J., Amassian, V. E., Eberle, L. P., and Cracco, R. Q. (1993). Magnetic coil stimulation of straight and bent amphibian and mammalian peripheral nerve in vitro: locus of excitation. *Journal of Physiology in London, 460*(1), 210–219.

Maccabee, P. J., Nagarajan, S. S., Amassian, V. E., Durand, D. M., Szabo, A. Z., Ahad, A. B., Cracco, R. Q., Lai, K. S., and Eberle, L. P. (1998). Influence of pulse sequence, polarity and amplitude on magnetic stimulation of human and porcine peripheral nerve. *Journal of Physiology, 513.2*, 571–585.

Masur, H., Papke, K., and Oberwittler, C. (1993). Suppression of visual perception by transcranial magnetic stimulation – experimental findings in healthy subjects and patients with optic neuritis. *Electroencephalography and Clinical Neurophysiology, 86*(4), 259–267.

Matthews, N., Luber, B., Qian, N., and Lisanby, S. (2001). Transcranial magnetic stimulation differentially affects speed and direction judgments. *Experimental Brain Research, 140*(4), 397–406.

Matthews, N., and Qian, N. (1999). Axis-of-motion affects direction discrimination, not speed discrimination. *Vision Research, 39*(13), 2205–2211.

Mayberg, H. S. (2002). Depression, II: localization of pathophysiology. *American Journal of Psychiatry, 159*(1), 1979.

Mayberg, H. S. (2003a). Modulating dysfunctional limbic-cortical circuits in depression: towards development of brain-based algorithms for diagnosis and optimised treatment. *Br Med Bull, 65*, 193–207.

Mayberg, H. S. (2003b). Positron emission tomography imaging in depression: a neural systems perspective. *Neuroimaging Clin N Am, 13*(4), 805–815.

Mayberg, H. S., Brannan, S. K., Tekell, J. L., Silva, J. A., Mahurin, R. K., McGinnis, S., and Jerabek, P. A. (2000). Regional metabolic effects of fluoxetine in major depression: serial changes and relationship to clinical response. *Biol Psychiatry, 48*(8), 830–843.

McConnell, K. A., Nahas, Z., Shastri, A., Lorberbaum, J. P., Kozel, F. A., Bohning, D. E., and George, M. S. (2001). The transcranial magnetic stimulation motor threshold depends on the distance from coil to underlying cortex: a replication in healthy adults comparing two methods of assessing the distance to cortex. *Biological Psychiatry, 49*(5), 454–459.

Meyer, B. U., Diehl, R. R., Steinmetz, H., Britton, T. C., and Benecke, R. (1991). Magnetic stimuli applied over motor cortex and visual cortex: influence of coil position and field polarity on motor responses, phosphenes and eye movements. *Electroencephalography and Clinical Neurophysiology, 43*(1), 121–134.

Miller, M. B., Fendrich, R., Eliassen, J. C., Demirel, S., and Gazzaniga, M. S. (1996). Transcranial magnetic stimulation: delays in visual suppression due to luminance changes. *Neuroreport, 7*(11), 1740–1744.

Mills, K. R., and Nithi, K. A. (1997). Corticomotor threshold to magnetic stimulation: normal values and repeatability. *Muscle Nerve, 20*(1), 570–576.

Miranda, P. C., Hallett, M., and Basser, P. J. (2003). The electric field induced in the brain by magnetic stimulation: a 3-d finite element analysis of the effect of tissue heterogeneity and anisotropy. *IEEE Transactions on Biomedical Engineering 50*(9), 1074–1085.

Mishory, A., Molnar, C., Koola, J., Li, X., Kozel, F. A., Myrick, H., Stroud, Z., Nahas, Z., and George, M. S. (2004). The maximum-likelihood strategy for determining transcranial magnetic stimulation motor threshold, using parameter estimation by sequential testing is faster than conventional methods with similar precision. *Journal of ECT, 20*(1), 160–165.

Moore, T., and Fallah, M. (2001). Control of eye movements and spatial attention. *Proceedings of the National Academy of Sciences United States of America, 98*(3), 1273–1276.

Mottaghy, F. M., Gangitano, M., Horkan, C., Chen, Y., Pascual-Leone, A., and Schlaug, G. (2003). Repetitive TMS temporarily alters brain diffusion. *Neurology, 60*(1), 1539–1541.

Mottaghy, F. M., Gangitano, M., Sparing, R., Krause, B. J., and Pascual-Leone, A. (2002). Segregation of areas related to visual working memory in the prefrontal cortex revealed by rTMS. *Cerebral Cortex, 12*(4), 369–375.

Muellbacher, W., Ziemann, U., Wissel, J., Dang, N., Kofler, M., Facchini, S., Boroojerdi, B., Poewe, W., and Hallett, M. (2002). Early consolidation in human primary motor cortex. *Nature, 415*(6872), 640–644.

Nagarajan, S. S., Durand, D. M., and Warman, E. N. (1993). Effects of induced electrical fields on finite neuronal structures: a simulation study. *IEEE Transactions on Biomedical Engineering, 40*(11), 1175–1188.

National Research Council. (1996). Possible Health Effects of Exposure to Residential Electric and Magnetic Fields. Washington, DC: National Academy Press.

Neubauer, A., Freudenthaler, H. H., and Pfurthscheller, G. (1995). Intelligence and spatiotemporal patterns of event-related desynchronization (ERD). *Intelligence, 20*, 249–266.

Nilsson, J., Panizza, M., Roth, B. J., Basser, P. J., Cohen, L. G., Caruso, G., and Hallett, M. (1992). Determining the site of stimulation during magnetic stimulation of a peripheral nerve. *Electroencephalography and Clinical Neurophysiology, 85*, 253–264.

O'Shea, J., Muggleton, G., Cowey, A., and Walsh, V. (2004). Timing of target discrimination in human frontal eye fields. *Journal of Cognitive Neuroscience, 16*(6), 1060–1067.

Ohnishi, T., Matsuda, H., Imabayashi, E., Okabe, S., Takano, H., Arai, N., and Ugawa, Y. (2004). rCBF changes elicited by rTMS over DLPFC in humans. *Suppl Clin Neurophysiol, 57*, 715–720.

Pascual-Leone, A., Cohen, L. G., Shotland, L. I., Dang, N., Pikus, A., Wassermann, E. M., Brasil-Neto, J. P., Valls-Sole, J., and Hallett, M. (1992). No evidence of hearing loss in humans due to transcranial magnetic stimulation. *Neurology, 41*(647–651).

Pascual-Leone, A., Gates, J. R., and Dhuna, A. (1991). Induction of speech arrest and counting errors with rapid-rate transcranial magnetic stimulation. *Neurology, 41*(5), 697–701.

Pascual-Leone, A., and Hallett, M. (1994). Induction of errors in a delayed response task by repetitive transcranial magnetic stimulation of the dorsolateral prefrontal cortex. *NeuroReport, 5*(1), 2517–2520.

Pascual-Leone, A., Tormos, J. M., Keenan, J. P., Tarazona, F., Canete, C., and Catala, M. D. (1998). Study and modulation of human cortical excitability with transcranial magnetic stimulation. *Journal of Clinical Neurophysiology, 15*(4), 333–343.

Pascual-Leone, A., Valls-Sole, J., Brasil-Neto, J. P., Cohen, L. G., and Hallett, M. (1994). Akinesia in Parkinson's disease. I. Shortening of simple reaction time with focal, single-pulse transcranial magnetic stimulation. *Neurology, 44*(5), 884–891.

Pascual-Leone, A., Walsh, V., and Rothwell, J. (2000). Transcranial magnetic stimulation in cognitive neuroscience – virtual lesion, chronometry, and functional connectivity. *Current Opinion in Neurobiology, 10*(1), 232–237.

Paus, T. (1999). Imaging the brain before, during, and after transcranial magnetic stimulation. *Neuropsychologia, 37*(2), 219–224.

Paus, T. (2002). Combination of transcranial magnetic stimulation of the human frontal cortex: implications for rTMS treatment for depression. *Journal of Psychiatry and Neuroscience, 29*, 268–277.

Paus, T. (2005). Inferring causality in brain images: a perturbation approach. *Philosophical Transactions of the Royal Society B, 360*(1457), 1109–1114.

Paus, T., Jech, R., THompson, C. J., Comeau, R., Peters, T., and Evans, A. C. (1997). Transcranial magnetic stimulation during positron emission tomography: a new method for studying connectivity of the human cerebral cortex. *Journal of Neuroscience, 17*(9), 3178–3184.

Peinemann, A., Lehner, C., Mentschel, C., Munchau, A., Conrad, B., and Siebner, H. R. (2000). Subthreshold 5-Hz repetitive transcranial magnetic stimulation of the human primary motor cortex reduces intracortical paired-pulse inhibition. *Neuroscience Letters, 296*(1), 21–24.

Post, R. M., Kimbrell, T. A., McCann, U. D., Dunn, R. T., Osuch, E. A., Speer, A. M., and Weiss, S. R. (1999). Repetitive transcranial magnetic stimulation as a neuropsychiatric tool: present status and future potential. *J Ect, 15*(1), 39–59.

Pridmore, S., Fernandes Filho, J. A., Nahas, Z., Liberatos, C., and George, M. S. (1998). Motor threshold in transcranial magnetic stimulation: a comparison of a neurophysiological method and a visualization of movement method. *Journal of ECT, 14*(1), 25–27.

Pulvermuller, F., Hauk, O., Nikulin, V., and Ilmoniemi, R. (2005). Functional links between motor and language systems. *European Journal of Neuroscience, 21*(3), 793–797.

Ragert, P., Dinse, H. R., Pleger, B., Wilimzig, C., Frombach, E., Schwenkreis, P., and Tegenthoff, M. (2003). Combination of 5 Hz repetitive transcranial magnetic stimulation (rTMS) and tactile coactivation boosts tactile discrimination in humans. *Neuroscience Letters, 348*(2), 105–108.

Rami, L., Gironell, A., Kulisevsky, J., Garcia-Sanchez, C. M. B., and Estevez-Gonzalez, A. (2003). Effects of repetitive transcranial magnetic stimulation on memory subtypes: a controlled study. *Neuropsychologia, 41*(1), 1877–1883.

Rauschecker, A. M., S., B., Walsh, V., and Thilo, K. V. (2004). Phosphene threshold as a function of contrast of external visual stimuli. *Experimental Brain Research, 157*(1), 124–127.

Ray, P. G., Meador, K. J., Epstein, C. M., Loring, D. W., and Day, L. J. (1998). Magnetic stimulation of the visual cortex: factors influencing the perception of phosphenes. *Journal of Clinical Neurophysiology, 15*(1), 351–357.

Reid, A. E., Chiappa, K. H., and Cros, D. (2002). Motor threshold, facilitation and the silent period in cortical magnetic stimulation. In A. Pascual-Leone, N. J. Davey, J. Rothwell, E. M. Wassermann and B. K. Puri (Eds.), *Handbook of Transcranial Magnetic Stimulation* (Vol. 1, pp. 97–11). New York: Arnold Publishers.

Rossi, S., Cappa, S. F., Babiloni, C., Pasqualetti, P., Miniussi, C., Carducci, F., Babiloni, F., and Rossini, P. M. (2001). Prefrontal cortex in long-term memory: an "interference" approach using magnetic stimulation. *Nature Neuroscience, 4*(1), 948–952.

Rossini, P. M., Barker, A. T., Berardelli, A., Caramia, M. D., Caruso, G., Cracco, R. Q., Dimitrijevic, M. R., Hallett, M., Katayama, Y., Luking, C. H., Maertens de Noordhout, A. L., Marsden, C. D., Murray, N. M. F., Rothwell, J. C., Swash, M., and Tomberg, C. (1994). Non-invasive electrical mad magnetic stimulation of the brain, spinal cord and roots: basic principles and procedures for routine clinical application. Report of an IFCN committee. *Electroencephalography and Clinical Neurophysiology, 91*(1), 79–92.

Roth, B. J., and Basser, P. J. (1990). A Model of the Stimulation of a Nerve Fiber by Electromagnetic Induction. *IEEE Transactions on Biomedical Engineering, 37*(6), 588–597.

Roth, B. J., Saypol, J. M., Hallett, M., and Cohen, L. G. (1991). A theoretical calculation of the electrical field induced in the cortex during magnetic stimulation. *Electroencephalography and Clinical Neurophysiology, 81*(1), 47–56.

Rudiak, D., and Marg, E. (1994). Finding the depth of magnetic brain stimulation: a re-evaluation. *Electroencephalography and Clinical Neurophysiology, 93*(5), 358–371.

Ruohonen, J., and Ilmoniemi, R. J. (2005). Basic Physics and Design of Transcranial Magnetic Stimulation Devices and Coils. In M. Hallett, and S. Chokroverty (Eds.), *Magnetic Stimulation in Clinical Neurophysiology*, Second Edition (pp. 17–30). Philadelphia: Elsevier.

Ruohonen, J., Ollikainen, M., Nikouline, V., Virtanen, J., and Ilmoniemi, R. J. (2000). Coil design for real and sham transcranial magnetic stimulation. *IEEE Transactions on Biomedical Engineering, 47*(2), 145–148.

Rushworth, M. F. S., Hadland, K. A., Paus, T., and Sipila, P. K. (2002). Role of the human medial frontal cortex in task switching: a combined fMRI and TMS study. *Journal of Neurophysiology, 87*(5), 2577–2592.

Rushworth, M. F. S., Paus, T., and Sipila, P. K. (2001). Attention systems and the organization of the human parietal cortex. *Journal of Neuroscience, 21*(14), 5262–5271.

Sachdev, P. S., McBride, R., Loo, C., Mitchell, P. M., Malhi, G. S., and Croker, V. (2002). Effects of different frequencies of transcranial magnetic stimulation (TMS) on the forced swim test model of depression in rats. *Biol Psychiatry, 51*(6), 474–479.

Sackeim, H. A., Prohovnik, I., Moeller, J. R., Brown, R. P., Apter, S., Prudic, J., Devanand, D. P., and Mukherjee, S. (1990). Regional cerebral blood flow in mood disorders. I. Comparison of major depressives and normal controls at rest. *Arch Gen Psychiatry, 47*(1), 60–70.

Saint-Amour, D., Walsh, V., Guillemot, J. P., Lassonde, M., and Lepore, F. (2005). *European Journal of Neuroscience, 21*(4), (1107–1115).

Sandrini, M., Cappa, S. F., Rossi, S., Rossini, P. M., and Miniussi, C. (2003). The role of prefrontal cortex in verbal episodic memory: rTMS evidence. *Journal of Cognitive Neuroscience, 15*(1), 855–861.

Schrader, L. M., Stern, J. M., Koski, L., Nuwer, M. R., and Engel, J., Jr. (2004). Seizure incidence during single- and paired-pulse transcranial magnetic stimulation (TMS) in individuals with epilepsy. *Clinical Neurophysiology, 115*(12), 2728–2737.

Serrien, D. J., Strens, L. H., Oliviero, A., and Brown, P. (2002). Repetitive transcranial magnetic stimulation of the supplementary motor area (SMA) degrades bimanual movement control in humans. *Neuroscience Letters, 328*(2), 89–92.

Shapiro, K. A., Pascual-Leone, A., Mottaghy, F. M., Gangitano, M., and Caramazza, A. (2001). Grammatical distinctions in the left frontal cortex. *Journal of Cognitive Neuroscience, 13*(6), 713–720.

Siebner, H. R., Peller, M., Willoch, F., Minoshima, S., Boecker, H., Auer, C., Drzezga, A., Conrad, B., and Bartenstein, P. (2000). Lasting cortical activation after repetitive TMS of the motor cortex: a glucose metabolic study. *Neurology, 54*(4), 956–963.

Sommer, M., Lang, N., Tergau, F., and Paulus, W. (2002). Neuronal tissue polarization induced by repetitive transcranial magnetic stimulation? *Neuroreport, 13*(6), 809–811.

Sparing, R., Mottaghy, F. M., Ganis, G., Thompson, W. L., Topper, R., Kosslyn, S. M., and Pascual-Leone, A. (2002). Visual cortex excitability increases during visual mental imagery – a TMS study in healthy human subjects. *Brain Research, 938*(1–2), 92–97.

Sparing, R., Mottaghy, F. M., Hungs, M., Brugmann, M., Foltys, H., Huber, W., and Topper, R. (2001). Repetitive transcranial magnetic stimulation effects on language function depend on the stimulation parameters. *Journal of Clinical Neurophysiology, 18*(4), 326–330.

Speer, A. M., Kimbrell, T. A., Wassermann, E. M., J, D. R., Willis, M. W., Herscovitch, P., and Post, R. M. (2000). Opposite effects of high and low frequency rTMS on regional brain activity in depressed patients. *Biol Psychiatry, 48*(12), 1133–1141.

Stewart, L. M., Walsh, V., and Rothwell, J. C. (2001). Motor and phosphene thresholds: a transcranial magnetic stimulation correlation study. *Neuropsychologia, 39*(1), 415–419.

Szuba, M. P., O'Reardon, J. P., and Evans, D. L. (2000). Physiological effects of electroconvulsive therapy and transcranial magnetic stimulation in major depression. *Depress Anxiety, 12*(3), 170–177.

Terao, Y., and Ugawa, Y. (2002). Basic mechanisms of TMS. *Journal of Clinical Neurophysiology, 19*(4), 322–343.

Terao, Y., Ugawa, Y., Suzuki, M., Sakai, K., Hanajima, R., Gemba-Shimizu, K., and Kanazawa, I. (1997). Shortening of simple reation time by peripheral electrical and submotor-threshold magnetic stimulation. *Experimental Brain Research, 115*(3), 541–545.

Thielscher, A., and Kammer, T. (2004). Electrical field properties of two commercial figure-8 coils in TMS: calculation of focality and efficiency. *Clinical Neurophysiology, 115*(7), 1697–1708.

Topper, R., Mottaghy, F. M., Brugmann, M., Noth, J., and Huber, W. (1998). Faciliation of picture naming by focal transcranial magnetic stimulation of Wernicke's area. *Experimental Brain Research, 121*(4), 371–378.

Tormos, J. M., Canete, C., Tarazona, F., Catala, M. D., Pascual-Leone Pascual, A., and Pascual-Leone, A. (1997). Lateralized effects of self-induced sadness and happiness on corticospinal excitability. *Neurology, 49*(2), 487–491.

Ueno, S., Tashiro, T., and Harada, K. (1988). Localized stimulation of neural tissue in the brain by means of a paired configuration of time-varying magnetic fields. *Journal of Applied Physiology, 64*, 5862–5864.

Wagner, T. A., Zahn, M., Grodzinsky, A. J., and Pascual-Leone, A. (2004). Three-dimensional head model stimulation of transcranial magnetic stimulation. *IEEE Transactions on Biomedical Engineering, 51*(9), 1586–1598.

Walsh, V., Ellison, A., Ashbridge, E., and Cowey, A. (1999). The role of the parietal cortex in visual attention – hemispheric asymmetries and the effects of learning: a magnetic stimulation study. *Neuropsychologia, 37*(2), 245–251.

Walsh, V., Ellison, A., Battelli, L., and Cowey, A. (1998). Task-specific impairments and enhancements induced by magnetic stimulation of human visual area V5. *Proceedings Biological Sciences, 265*(1395), 537–543.

Walsh, V., and Pascual-Leone, A. (2003). *Transcranial Magnetic Stimulation: A Neurochronometrics of Mind* (Vol. 1). Boston: MIT Press.

Wassermann, E. M. (1998). Risk and safety of repetitive transcranial magnetic stimulation. *Electroencephalography and Clinical Neurophysiology, 108*(1), 1–16.

Weissman, J. D., Epstein, C. M., and Davey, K. R. (1992). Magnetic brain stimulation and brain size: relevance to animal studies. *Electroencephalography and Clinical Neurophysiology, 85*(3), 215–219.

Ziemann, U. (2002). Paired pulse techniques. In A. Pascual-Leone, N. J. Davey, J. Rothwell, E. M. Wassermann and B. K. Puri (Eds.), *Handbook of Transcranial Magnetic Stimulation* (Vol. 1, pp. 141–159). New York: Arnold Publishers.

Ziemann, U., and Rothwell, J. C. (2000). I-waves in motor cortex. *Journal of Clinical Neurophysiology, 17*(4), 397–405.

Ziemann, U., Rothwell, J. C., and Ridding, M. C. (1996). Interaction between intracortical inhibition and facilitation in human motor cortex. *Journal of Physiology, 496*(3), 873–881.

6 The Lesion Method in Cognitive Neuroscience

MICHAEL KOENIGS, DANIEL T. TRANEL, AND ANTONIO R. DAMASIO

INTRODUCTION: HISTORICAL CONTEXT

Scientific consideration of brain-behavior relationships can be traced to a number of seminal observations beginning more than a century ago (see Benton, 1988, for review). Individual landmark cases have often provided the initial footing for mapping complex cognitive abilities onto discrete brain areas. In the 1860s, Paul Broca (1865) reported on the patient known as "Tan," who developed an inability to produce speech following damage to the left front part of the brain. The discovery led to the suggestion, at the time quite radical, that humans speak with the left side of the brain. A few years later, Carl Wernicke reported a complementary finding: damage to the posterior part of the left hemisphere rendered patients unable to comprehend speech, while leaving speech production relatively unaffected. Integrating these findings, Wernicke formulated a remarkably prescient neurological model of language (Wernicke, 1874), the essence of which is still a leading heuristic in clinical neurology and neuropsychology. About the same time, John Harlow (1868) reported on the case of Phineas Gage, who developed a bizarre, seemingly unbelievable focal impairment in personality and social conduct following an accident in which an iron bar was shot through the front part of his brain, destroying prefrontal cortex bilaterally.

The study of brain-behavior relationships enjoyed another period of remarkable progress following World War II, due in some measure to the ravages of war, which provided a grim service to researchers by producing a large number of suitable subjects for careful experimentation – persons who had sustained focal and stable brain wounds that could be correlated with performances on cognitive tests (Newcombe, 1969). This approach, in fact, which has come to be known as the "lesion method," has remained a methodological workhorse in systems level cognitive neuroscience.

Other developments, centered on key case studies, also helped shape the field. In 1957, Scoville and Milner reported for the first time on the patient known as HM, who developed severe and permanent anterograde amne-

sia (learning impairment) following bilateral resection of the mesial temporal lobes, which was done to control intractable epilepsy. Careful neuropsychological studies of HM yielded a number of key breakthroughs in our understanding of the neural basis of memory, and in particular, focused attention on the role of the mesial temporal region, especially the hippocampus and adjacent cortices, in memory. Studies by Roger Sperry, in collaboration with Joseph Bogen and Michael Gazzaniga (e.g., Sperry, 1968; Gazzaniga, 1987), sparked interest in the dramatic differences between the two hemispheres of the brain. These investigators showed that "split-brain" patients, who had undergone surgical separation of the two hemispheres for control of seizures, retained two more or less separate modes of consciousness, one in the left hemisphere which was language-based and operated in sequential, analytical style, and one in the right hemisphere which was spatially based and operated in gestalt, holistic style. In the modern era, the trend has continued with prototypical cases such as EVR (Eslinger & Damasio, 1985), NA (Squire & Moore, 1979; Teuber et al., 1968), Boswell (Damasio, Eslinger, et al., 1985), and SM (Adolphs & Tranel, 2000).

The emphasis on case studies in neuropsychology prompted understandable concern that findings might not generalize or might not even prove repeatable. Largely, this criticism has been assuaged in modern era studies, in which it has been possible to assemble larger groups of brain-damaged patients and to put various hypotheses to rigorous empirical test. Nonetheless, the attacks of skeptics performed the important function of calling attention to factors such as intelligence, age, gender, and handedness, in neuropsychological research. Other contentious issues in the field include the debate between localizationists and anti-localizationists, the notions of redundancy and equipotentiality, and the ideas of "centers" and "networks" (Geschwind, 1964; Lashley, 1950; see Benton & Tranel, 2000, for review). These debates have been constructive in focusing the field on key issues and in fueling theoretical refinements, and on the practical side, they have facilitated the development of empirically driven rehabilitation programs.

It is worth highlighting some of the themes that have dominated the history of cognitive neuroscience. Consider the age-old debate between localizationists and anti-localizationists, which was firmly joined more than a century ago. The localizationist side was exemplified (some might say caricatured) by the notion of phrenology, a system of brain-behavior relationships articulated by Franz Josef Gall and Johann Spurzheim in the late eighteenth and early nineteenth centuries. Gall and Spurzheim (Spurzheim, 1815) outlined in detail how 27 different cognitive functions and personality traits were subserved by specific brain regions. Phrenology was based on skull saliencies, and bumps on the skull were used as clues about underlying brain specialization. For example, Gall noted that his classmates with superior memory had prominent eyes, and reasoned that this was the result of overdevelopment of underlying brain regions important for memory. The notion of phrenology has been highly controversial since its inception. Not only did the phrenological maps contain a degree of detail about cerebral localization that far outstripped the empirical evidence, but the evidence itself – correlations between skull bumps and mental capacities – bordered on the absurd. Another problem with phrenology was the inclusion of traits such as "God and religion" and "love for one's offspring." Not only was there poor consensus about the meaning of such constructs, but they also had religious connotations that attracted mordacious criticism, especially from those disturbed by the anti-dualistic nature of Gall's position.

The anti-localizationist position was exemplified by investigators such as Pierre Flourens, who argued that all parts of the brain subserved all perceptual, intellectual, and volitional functions equally (Flourens, 1846). Flourens supported his claims with results from ablation experiments, which showed that the crucial factor determining how an organism was affected by brain damage was the extent of tissue removed (size of lesion), and not the location. Complete removal of brain lobes resulted in a complete loss of function; large but incomplete damage created a partial loss of function; but with smaller removals, there was a complete recovery of function. The findings emphasized the notion of redundancy in brain-behavior relationships, a concept that was recapitulated several decades later in Karl Lashley's notion of equipotentiality (e.g., 1929).

In short, localizationists assigned specific functions to specific brain regions, whereas the anti-localizationists insisted that the cerebral hemispheres operated as a unity, without specific specialization of function. This debate has been revisited at regular junctures throughout the twentieth century, often in ways that resembled the polemics of the nineteenth century. For example, discoveries such as those of Broca and Wernicke were countered by experiments such as those of Lashley (e.g., 1929), which demonstrated that all areas of the cerebral cortex were equally important for complex learning and memory. Echoing the ideas of Flourens, Lashley argued that the degree of behavioral impairment following a brain lesion was simply proportional to the amount of brain tissue that had been destroyed, with location being less important or perhaps entirely irrelevant. Lashley emphasized the key ideas of redundancy and equipotentiality.

A somewhat different form of redundancy was postulated by Hughlings Jackson (1870, 1873) in his hierarchical conception of the organization of the nervous system. In Jackson's scheme, sensory and motor functions were represented at each "level," with more complex aspects of function being represented at the highest level of nervous structure. However, the highest level also included nerve fibers from lower levels, making for "multiple representation" of a function at that level. Consequently, a lesion at the highest level left many fibers intact and produced less (or no) impairment in some functions as compared to the same lesion placed at a lower level. "Hence large destroying lesions in the hemisphere will result in no palsy, whereas palsy will follow lesions equally large in the corpus striatum. No fact is better recognized than that a large part of one cerebral hemisphere may be destroyed when there are no obvious symptoms of any kind" (Jackson, 1870, 1873, reprinted in Clarke & O'Malley, 1968). Thus Jackson invoked a redundancy of neural elements to explain the sparing of certain elementary functions following brain injury. Jackson's dictum implied that the behavioral capacities of a brain-lesioned patient were more an expression of the properties of the spared regions of the brain than of the lesioned area. The idea was applied primarily to account for differences in the extent of recovery from motor and speech impairments that were observed between younger and older patients, but in principle it could apply to all individual differences in brain capacity.

Interestingly, the fundamental idea championed by Gall, namely, that specific brain regions are specialized for specific mental functions, has probably turned out to be more right than wrong. In fact, a sort of "neo-phrenology" is very much alive and well today – for instance, one would be hard pressed to distinguish between some claims being made currently, for example, that a religious "center" has been discovered in a particular region of the left temporal lobe (Ramachandran et al., 1997), and some of the ideas elaborated in Gall's phrenological system. We would caution against such extreme claims, but at the same time, there is no question that over the last couple of decades, systems neuroscience has yielded a cascade of breakthroughs supporting remarkably detailed brain-behavior relationships, with a degree of precision that would have been virtually impossible to predict in the era prior to the advent of modern neuroimaging.

THE LESION METHOD

Historical context aside, the lesion method remains a rich and powerful source of knowledge regarding the neural underpinnings of cognition and behavior (A. Damasio & H. Damasio, 1994; H. Damasio & A. Damasio, 2003). The

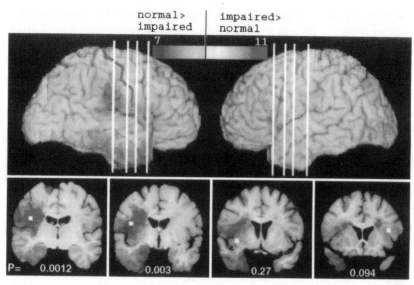

Figure 6.1. Lesion overlap map created with Map-3. In this study 108 subjects performed emotion recognition task. Color (*scale* at *top*) encodes the difference in the density of lesions between the subjects with the lowest and those with the highest scores. Thus, *red regions* correspond to locations at which lesions resulted in impairment more often than not, and *blue regions* correspond to locations at which lesions resulted in normal performance more often than not. *p* values indicating statistical significance are shown in *white* for voxels in four regions (*white squares*) on coronal cuts (*bottom*) that correspond to the *white vertical lines* in the 3-D reconstructions (*top*). (From Adolphs et al., 2000, used with permission.) (See color plate.)

lesion method refers to an approach whereby a focal area of brain damage is correlated with the development of a defect in some aspect of cognition or behavior, and then an inference is made that the damaged brain region is part of the neural substrate for the impaired function. In hypothesis-driven investigations a lesion acts as a *probe* with which the validity of a particular brain-behavior hypothesis can be tested. In humans, obviously, the scientist does not have true control over the lesion, and must rely instead upon the availability of suitable experimental lesions. This does not have to compromise the power of the approach, however, provided it is applied in the context of several important parameters. The following is a brief summary of the lesion method as practiced in our laboratory (see H. Damasio & A. Damasio, 2003).

We believe there are five prerequisites for optimal practice of the lesion method: (1) the availability of detailed structural imaging of the human brain in vivo; (2) a reliable method for neuroanatomical analysis of lesions; (3) a suitable pool of subjects from which to draw, allowing selection of experimental and control subjects in such a way as to remove confounding influences of factors such as age, education, IQ, and socioeconomic status; (4) the availability of methods for reliable cognitive measurements; and (5) testable hypotheses concerning the neural basis for specific cognitive and behavioral functions. So long as these prerequisites are satisfied, the lesion method can produce important new insights into brain-behavior relationships.

Neuroanatomical analysis of brain lesions has been greatly facilitated not only by the availability of fine-grained neuroimaging techniques like magnetic resonance imaging (MRI), but also by the development of analysis techniques that allow precise and reliable mapping of brain lesions. The "template system" developed by Damasio and Damasio (1989) is an example of such a technique. This system has been replaced by an even more powerful approach that is based on a technique known as Brainvox (Frank et al., 1997). Brainvox involves three-dimensional reconstruction of the human brain from high-resolution MRI, permitting the investigator to identify, in vivo, every major gyrus and sulcus of the brain, to slice and reslice the brain in whatever incidence necessary for anatomical analysis, and to define and quantify, in three dimensions, the degree of overlap of brain lesions from various subjects. Three-dimensional maps of lesion overlap can be created with a technique called "Map-3." Map-3 entails the transfer of individual lesions onto a normal reference brain, while taking into account the lesion's relation to sulcal and gyral landmarks. After multiple individual lesions are fitted to the reference brain, the lesions are superimposed to form a lesion overlap map. A region of maximal overlap can then be determined on the basis of the superimposition of individual lesions (Figure 6.1). Using Map-3, lesion commonalities between brain-damaged subjects can be characterized at a level of precision far greater than previously available, allowing rigorous probing of putative brain-behavior relationships. Lesion overlaps can function as either the independent or dependent variable (see H. Damasio et al., 1996; Tranel, Damasio, & Damasio, 1997a, for examples of this approach).

Traditionally, the lesion method was implemented primarily in case studies, and this imposed certain limitations on the findings, especially if they proved difficult to replicate. This weakness has been substantially remedied, however, with more recent work involving large groups of brain damaged subjects, where it has been possible to generate conclusions that are based on subject groups comparable in size to those used in traditional psychological experiments (cf. H. Damasio et al., 1996; Tranel et al., 1994; Tranel, Damasio, & Damasio, 1997a; Saygin et al., 2003; Karnath et al., 2004). Striking case studies will continue to fuel new hypotheses and insights regarding brain-behavior relationships, and the astute clinician/scientist will take advantage of opportunities to explore interesting new leads in individual patients, but the days of relying almost exclusively on single cases are well behind us.

Although significant technological advances have enhanced the practice of the lesion method, a carefully designed and well-controlled cognitive experiment is at the heart of reliable and valid application of any technique to study brain-behavior relationships. Following the tradition of the eminent neuropsychologists who founded the field during the middle part of this century (Benton, 1988; Newcombe, 1969; Teuber, 1968; Weiskrantz, 1968; Zangwill, 1964), modern clinical and experimental neuropsychologists continue to develop and refine a wide variety of cognitive tasks which can be used to measure precisely higher-order functions of the brain such as memory, perception, attention, speech, emotion, and decision making. The specification of detailed methods for conducting neuropsychological evaluation has contributed also (Lezak, 1995; McKenna & Warrington, 1996; Milberg, Hebben, & Kaplan, 1996; Reitan & Wolfson, 1996; Tranel, 1996).

The refinement of neuropsychological assessment and cognitive experimentation follows a long tradition in clinical psychology of careful, standardized measurement of psychological functions. The principal consideration is that the measurements take into account a variety of demographic factors that are common and often potent influences on performance in cognitive tasks, including age, gender, and educational and occupational background. Over the past few decades, the field of clinical neuropsychology has provided wealth of information to deal with this challenge (Benton et al., 1983; Lezak, 1995; Spreen & Strauss, 1990). This information has not only allowed individual case application as required in clinical diagnosis, but has facilitated the power of experimental applications by allowing the removal of unwanted variability in dependent measures.

Despite the historical preeminence of the lesion method in cognitive neuroscience and the more recent advances made in its practical implementation, there remain significant limitations that warrant the development of alternate experimental methods for mapping brain-behavior relationships. First, lesion patients are generally only available to scientists working in close collaboration with a medical center. Critical components of a successful lesion research program include a substantial neurological patient population, structural neuroimaging facilities, standardized neuropsychological assessment of patients, and reliable referral to the research program by clinicians. And, only a limited number of neurological patients are suitable experimental subjects. Subjects must have a clearly demarcated, discrete lesion, with no comorbid or preexisting neurologic or psychiatric condition. Pathologies causing suitable lesions include nonhemorrhagic infarct, herpes simplex encephalitis, and surgical ablation of benign tumors or epileptic foci. However, these pathologies do not sample the brain equally: infarcts most often affect lateral cortical areas and spare medial and basal structures; encephalitis targets the limbic system; tumors tend to arise in convexities; and epileptic foci are usually in temporal lobe. In addition, localizable lesions (often centimeters in diameter) are generally large relative to the functional units of

the brain. A given lesion may encompass multiple cortical and/or subcortical areas. (Hence the necessity of group studies and lesion overlap analysis to disambiguate which area of damage is the cause of observed cognitive defects). Furthermore, cognitive defects could be due to damage to white matter tracts connecting non-lesioned areas, rather than to the loss of adjacent gray matter. In addition, cognitive functions subserved by multiple brain areas may be less susceptible to damage to a single area. That is, a lesion will only reveal if an area is *necessary* for a function; residual ability may be due to incomplete damage or a separate, independent, and still-intact neural system. Lastly, functional and anatomical variability among brains, which can be exaggerated by the presence of a lesion, complicates the comparison of multiple subjects.

FUNCTIONAL NEUROIMAGING

In recent years, functional neuroimaging (and functional magnetic resonance imaging (fMRI) in particular) has emerged as the most widespread method of exploring brain-behavior relationships in cognitive neuroscience. The basis of fMRI is the localized increase in blood flow to the sites of increased neural activity. fMRI allows precise localization of these changes in blood flow during cognitive testing, so activation of a particular brain area can be associated with a particular cognitive function. The merits of this method are evident when contrasted with the lesion method. fMRI is noninvasive and readily accessible to non-medical scientists. Using fMRI, experimenters can visualize areas of brain activation while subjects with *normal* cognitive function perform tasks in the scanner. Thus, investigation of brain-behavior relationships is not limited to a single discrete area of damage. Whereas the lesion method can only identify areas that are necessary for a task, fMRI can theoretically reveal all the brain areas involved in a particular function, including those areas where naturally occurring lesions are rare or function is redundant. Furthermore, fMRI activation maps offer superior spatial localization to the lesion method. Whereas lesions may be many centimeters in diameter and encompass multiple functional modules, fMRI activation loci can be resolved with sub-centimeter accuracy. Future technological developments will only enhance fMRI's capability. Stronger and faster-switching magnets will yield images with better spatial resolution in shorter amounts of imaging time. Combining fMRI data with data from electroencephalogram (EEG) or magnetoencephalogram (MEG), which measure neural activity with millisecond temporal resolution, may yield dynamic brain activation maps that reflect both the timing and location of neural activations.

Despite these benefits, several limitations preclude functional neuroimaging from becoming the sole method of investigating brain-behavior relationships. The generation of an fMRI activation map requires that the brain activity in one state (baseline task) be "subtracted" from the brain activity in another state (activation task). Functional neuroimaging only allows identification of areas that are more active in one state than another. Activations are diminished when the baseline task engages the process of interest, and superfluous activations may result when the activation task engages processes unrelated to the task requirements. Activation maps must be interpreted cautiously, with due consideration of the baseline and activation tasks in the experiment. In no case does an activation map reveal which brain areas are *necessary* or *critical* for a particular task. Furthermore, practical factors limit the range of cognitive abilities and neuroanatomical areas that can be explored with functional neuroimaging. Because the subject is physically confined in the scanner and head motion is the primary cause of data distortion, the subject's behavior is generally limited to a button press response. Due to inhomogeneities in the magnetic field near air/tissue interfaces, it is generally difficult to obtain fMRI data in the orbitofrontal cortex and temporal poles. This signal loss is not a problem in positron emission tomography (PET; another functional neuroimaging technique measuring blood flow in the brain), but PET's utility is limited by the rigidity of the experimental design: tasks must be performed in minute-long blocks and subject participation is restricted by exposure to radioactivity.

Clearly, neither the lesion method nor functional neuroimaging alone stands to address every question of brain-behavior relationship in cognitive neuroscience. Each method entails fundamental and practical limitations, and individual research questions may be best addressed using one method or the other, or a combination of the two. In the following section, we present research from several domains of cognitive function, with particular emphasis on how the lesion method and functional neuroimaging have been employed to varying degrees to answer (and raise) research questions in each domain.

TOPICS IN COGNITIVE NEUROSCIENCE

The following discussion of selected topics in cognitive neuroscience is not intended to be comprehensive, but instead, we have chosen several topics that illustrate the application of the experimental methods described in the previous sections. Specifically, we focus on examples from the domains of memory; decision-making and social conduct; emotion recognition; attention; and cognitive control.

Memory

Memory refers to knowledge that is stored in the brain, and to the processes of acquiring, storing, and retrieving such knowledge. Clearly this is a broad concept, and theorists have partitioned the field along multiple dimensions (e.g., long-term vs. short-term, declarative vs. non-declarative, encoding vs. consolidation vs. recall). Without exhausting the myriad of data relating to the neural bases of the

many proposed memory subtypes, we will illustrate several examples of how the lesion method and functional neuroimaging have been applied to the study of memory.

Long-term declarative memory. As mentioned earlier, the pioneering study on the neural basis of memory was the case report of HM, who suffered a striking anterograde amnesia following bilateral resection of the mesial temporal lobes (hippocampus and adjacent entorhinal, perirhinal, and parahippocampal cortices) (Figure 6.2). Amnesia is an impairment of memory, and it refers specifically to an impairment in the ability to learn new information or to retrieve previously acquired knowledge. The impairment of learning is known as anterograde amnesia, whereas the impairment in retrieving previously acquired knowledge is known as retrograde amnesia, with the demarcation being the point in time at which neurological disease begins. As evidenced by continued study of mesial temporal lesion patients (HM and others), damage to some or all of the mesial temporal structures produces characteristic patterns of amnesia (Cohen & Eichenbaum, 1993; Corkin, 1984; Curran & Schacter, 1997; Damasio, Eslinger, et al., 1985; Mishkin, 1982; Squire, 1992a; Tranel & Damasio, 1995; Zola, 1997). First, there is a consistent (albeit imperfect) correspondence between the side of damage and the type of learning impairment; thus, unilateral lesions tend to produce material-specific amnesia. Specifically, left-sided lesions produce defects primarily in the learning of verbal information (e.g., words, written material), and nonverbal information is largely spared; conversely, right-sided lesions produce defects primarily in the learning of nonverbal material (e.g., complex visual and auditory patterns), and verbal information is largely spared (e.g., Milner, 1972). Second, the mesial temporal region is critical for the acquisition of new information (anterograde memory), but its role in the retrieval of previously learned knowledge (retrograde memory) is minimal. That is, the ability to retrieve information that was acquired prior to the onset of the lesion is usually spared following damage to mesial temporal structures (Cohen & Eichenbaum, 1993; Corkin, 1984; Damasio, Eslinger et al., 1985; O'Connor et al., 1995). Third, structures in the mesial temporal region are crucial for the acquisition of declarative information, that is, knowledge that can be "declared" or brought to mind for conscious inspection, for example facts, words, names, and faces. However, these structures do not appear to be necessary for the acquisition of nondeclarative information, that is, knowledge such as sensorimotor skills (e.g., skiing, dancing) that cannot be declared or brought to mind (Corkin, 1965; Gabrieli et al., 1993; Thompson, 1986; Tranel & Damasio, 1993; Tranel et al., 1994). Fourth, short-term memory (retention on the scale of seconds to minutes) is spared in these patients. In short, patients with damage confined to structures in the mesial temporal region will manifest anterograde amnesia for long-term declarative knowledge, with the material type

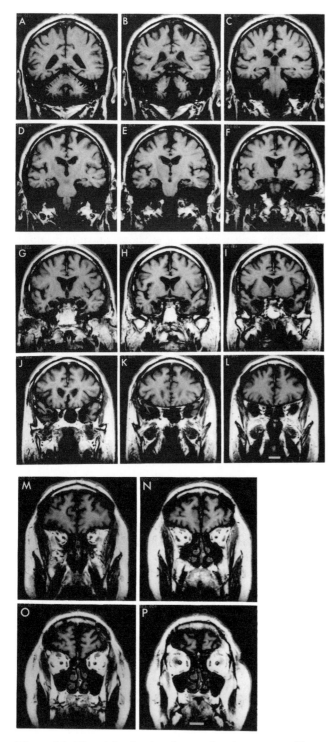

Figure 6.2. T1-weighted series of coronal sections arranged from caudal (*A*) to rostral (*P*) to show the extent of the lesion in H. M. (From Corkin et al., 1997, used with permission.)

(verbal versus nonverbal) influenced by the side of lesion. The precise role of various mesial temporal lobe structures in memory function has not been definitively established through human lesion studies, but there is evidence that damage restricted to hippocampus proper is sufficient to cause an enduring anterograde amnesia (Rempel-Clower et al., 1997; Zola-Morgan et al., 1986).

By contrast, damage to nonmesial portions of the temporal lobe (anterior, inferior, and lateral temporal lobe) is associated with a long-term declarative memory defect encompassing the retrograde compartment (Cermak & O'Connor, 1983; Cohen & Squire, 1981; Kapur, 1993; Kapur et al., 1994; Kopelman, 1992; Markowitsch et al., 1993; Squire & Alvarez, 1995). If the damage spares the mesial temporal region, in fact, the memory defect may be confined to the retrograde compartment (Kapur, 1993; Kapur et al., 1994; Markowitsch et al., 1993; see Hodges, 1995, for review). Frequently, retrograde amnesia affects retrieval of knowledge for unique material more than knowledge for nonunique material. For instance, a patient may have difficulty retrieving detailed information about unique episodes such as the birth of children, the purchase of a home, or facts about public events; however, the patient will remain capable of retrieving nonunique knowledge such as the meanings of words, and the meaning of nonverbal stimuli such as common entities and actions. As in anterograde amnesia, there appears to be a laterality effect regarding the specialization of the left side for verbal material, and parallel specialization of the right side for nonverbal material. Hence, damage to the left anterior temporal region produces an impairment in the retrieval of words for unique entities (proper nouns), without affecting the capacity to retrieve nonverbal conceptual knowledge about those entities (H. Damasio et al., 1996), and damage to the homologous right temporal region will produce an impairment in the retrieval of conceptual knowledge for unique persons, but not an impairment in the retrieval of unique names (Tranel, Damasio, & Damasio, 1997a).

These lesion studies indicated dissociable roles of mesial and non-mesial temporal cortices in long-term declarative memory: encoding and consolidation is associated with hippocampus and adjacent cortices, whereas storage and/or retrieval is associated with anterior, inferior, and lateral temporal cortices. Additional lesion studies of long-term declarative memory have identified two other critical brain areas: basal forebrain and the diencephalon.

The basal forebrain, situated immediately behind the orbital prefrontal cortices, comprises a set of bilateral paramidline gray nuclei which include the septal nuclei, the diagonal band of Broca, the nucleus accumbens, and the substantia innominata. Damage to this region is frequently caused by ruptured aneurysms of the anterior communicating artery or of the anterior cerebral artery. One problem in studying this condition is that most of the affected patients have surgical clips that preclude magnetic resonance imaging, limiting the anatomical analysis that can be performed.

Patients with damage to the basal forebrain manifest a characteristic amnesia that may include deficits in the association of individual features or events, especially with respect to time, as well as a propensity for confabulation, for example, making up fantasy stories about various bizarre adventures that have no basis in fact (Alexander & Freedman, 1984; Damasio, Graff-Radford, et al., 1985;

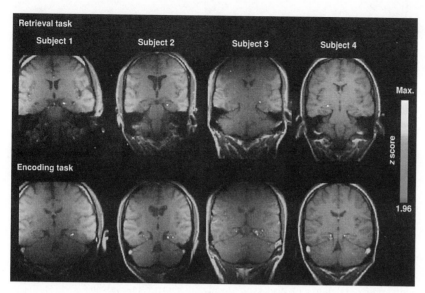

Figure 6.3. Mesial temporal lobe activations during memory encoding and retrieval. The top row shows activations in the subiculum of the hippocampus during the retrieval memory task that were greater for words corresponding to previously seen than unseen line drawings (Subjects 1, 2, and 3) or greater for line drawings corresponding to previously seen than unseen words (Subject 4). The bottom row shows activations in the parahippocampal cortex during the encoding memory task that were greater for novel than for repeated color scenes (Subjects 1, 2, and 3) or greater for novel than for repeated line drawings (Subject 4). (From Gabrieli et al., 1997, used with permission.) (See color plate.)

Deluca & Diamond, 1995). In a direct test of the role of the basal forebrain in the temporal binding of memories, Tranel and Jones (in press) assessed the ability of basal forebrain patients to place various autobiographical memories accurately on a "time-line" of their life. Their performance was compared to patients with mesial temporal lobe damage; patients with damage outside basal forebrain, mesial temporal lobe, and diencephalon; and normal control subjects. Relative to the other groups, basal forebrain patients were significantly impaired in their ability to situate autobiographical memories on a time-line of their lives. It is noteworthy that basal forebrain and mesial temporal lobe patients were comparably impaired in their ability to recall autobiographical events, but only the basal forebrain group exhibited impairment in placing the recalled events in the correct temporal context. These findings highlight a role for the basal forebrain in establishing the temporal relationship of events in memory.

Structures in the diencephalon, particularly the dorosomedial nucleus of the thalamus and the mammillary bodies, have also been shown to play an important role in memory in lesion studies. Damage to these structures produces a severe anterograde amnesia that resembles the amnesia associated with mesial temporal damage. Characteristically, there is a major defect in the acquisition of declarative knowledge, with sparing of learning of nondeclarative information. However, more so than with the amnesia associated with mesial temporal lesions, diencephalic amnesia may involve the retrograde compartment as well. This retrograde amnesia tends to have a "temporal

gradient," so that retrieval of memories acquired closer in time to the onset of the lesion is more severely affected, whereas retrieval of more remote memories is better preserved. Severe alcoholism and stroke are two frequent causes of damage to the diencephalon (Butters & Stuss, 1989; Graff-Radford, Tranel, et al., 1990). The amnesia that develops after prolonged alcoholism is part of a distinctive condition known as Wernicke-Korsakoff syndrome, which has been extensively studied from both neuroanatomical and neuropsychological perspectives (e.g., Victor et al., 1989).

So, in the domain of long-term declarative memory, lesion studies have proven remarkably effective in delineating the critical neural structures. But, significant questions remained unanswered by lesion studies. For example, what are the different contributions of individual mesial temporal lobe structures (e.g., parahippocampal cortex versus hippocampus proper)? Or, are there other cortical areas that are recruited, but not necessary, for memory tasks? Subsequent fMRI studies have yielded answers to some of these questions. Gabrieli et al. (1997) scanned subjects during the encoding and retrieval portions of a memory test. During encoding there was greater activation of posterior mesial temporal lobe (parahippocampal cortex) for novel stimuli than for familiar stimuli, whereas during retrieval there was greater activation of anterior mesial temporal lobe (subiculum of hippocampus) for successfully remembered items. (Figure 6.3). In a similar design using a list of words as stimuli, Wagner et al. (1998) found that left parahippocampal cortex activation during encoding was greater for words that were subsequently recalled successfully, compared to nonremembered words. In addition, Wagner et al. found that activation of an area in left frontal cortex during word encoding also correlated with retrieval success. In a related finding, Kelley et al. (1998) observed that encoding of words produced left-lateralized dorsal frontal activation, whereas encoding of unfamiliar faces produced homologous right-lateralized activation. More recent studies highlight the role of parietal cortex in memory retrieval: activity of posterior parietal cortex has been associated with retrieval success for picture and sound stimuli (Shannon and Buckner, 2004; Konishi et al., 2000; Leube et al., 2003).

Clearly, the current understanding of the neural substrates of long-term declarative memory has benefited from both lesion and functional imaging studies. Although lesion studies laid the foundation in identifying the critical structures, functional imaging studies confirmed, but more importantly, extended the neural model. It is

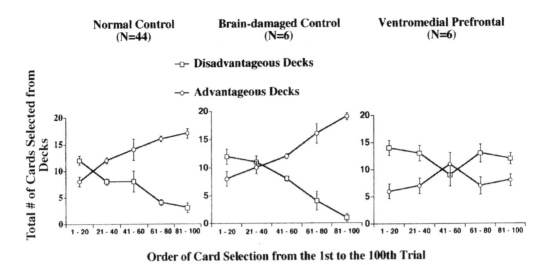

Figure 6.4. (Top) Card selections on the Iowa Gambling Task as a function of group (normal control, brain-damaged control, ventromedial prefrontal damage), deck type (disadvantageous versus advantageous), and trial block. The two control groups gradually shifted their response selections towards the advantageous decks, and this tendency became stronger as the game went on. The ventromedial prefrontal subjects did not make a reliable shift, and continued to opt for the disadvantageous decks even during the latter stages of the game, when controls had almost completely abandoned choosing from the disadvantageous decks. (Bottom) Lesion overlap map of patients with defective IGT performance and "acquired sociopathy." Areas of greater overlap appear darker. (From Tranel, 2002, used with permission)

noteworthy that the majority of findings contributed by each method are nonredundant. As an illustration of this point consider the following four observations: (1) Human lesion studies could not reliably distinguish separate roles of anatomically adjacent structures such as hippocampus and parahippocampal cortex (compare Figures 6.2 and 6.3), (2) Lesion studies could not identify the role of prefrontal and parietal areas in encoding and retrieval, respectively, (3) Functional imaging studies could not distinguish the relative importance (i.e., necessity) of each activated area, and (4) Functional imaging could not identify the unique role of the basal forebrain nuclei in the temporal binding of memories or the involvement of the diencephalon.

Working memory. Whereas lesion studies were a principal methodology for establishing the neural bases of long-term declarative memory, functional imaging has been the primary tool for identifying the substrates of working memory. Working memory refers to a short window of mental processing, on the order of seconds to minutes, during which information is held "on-line" and operations are performed on it – a sort of "mental scratch pad" (Baddeley, 1992). In essence, working memory is a temporary storage and processing system used for problem solving and other cognitive operations that take place over a limited time frame.

Functional imaging studies have robustly implicated the prefrontal cortex, particularly the dorsolateral sector, in the mediation of working memory (Cohen et al., 1997; Courtney et al., 1997; Courtney et al., 1998; Jonides et al., 1993; McCarthy et al., 1994; Smith et al., 1995). As in the case of long-term declarative memory, there is evidence

for left- and right-sided specialization: left prefrontal cortex is preferentially activated during retention of verbal information, whereas right prefrontal cortex is preferentially activated during retention of nonverbal or spatial information (Smith et al., 1996). During maintenance of information in working memory, dorsolateral prefrontal cortex exhibits linearly increasing activation in response to increasing working memory load (Narayanan et al., 2005; Braver et al., 1997) and greater activation of dorsolateral prefrontal cortex during working memory retention is associated with increased accuracy at recall after distraction (Sakai et al., 2002). Although prefrontal activation is the most robust finding in working memory neuroimaging studies, multiple studies have demonstrated the additional activation of parietal cortex (Pessoa et al., 2002; Zahran et al., 1999; Rowe and Passingham, 2001; Cohen et al., 1997).

Lesion studies of working memory are less compelling and straightforward than their neuroimaging counterparts. Studies by Reverberi et al., Bechara et al., and Ferreira et al. illustrate this point. Reverberi et al. (2005) observed working memory impairment in patients with damage restricted to either inferior medial prefrontal cortex or left lateral prefrontal cortex, but not in cases of right lateral prefrontal cortex damage. Bechara et al. (1998) found that patients with posterior ventromedial or right dorsolateral/superior medial prefrontal lesions were impaired on a test of working memory, but patients with damage to anterior ventromedial or left dorsolateral/superior medial prefrontal cortex were not. Ferreira et al. (1998) found that a group of patients with dorsolateral prefrontal damage were impaired relative to normal controls and temporal lobe patients on a working memory test

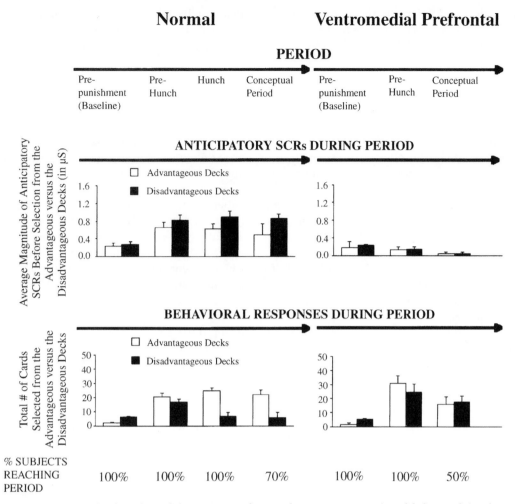

Figure 6.5. Psychophysiological (anticipatory skin conductance responses) and behavioral (card selection) data for control subjects (n = 10) and subjects with ventromedial prefrontal lesions (n = 6), as a function of four "knowledge periods" (see text). Control subjects, even before they knew anything consciously about how the game worked (pre-hunch period), began to generate anticipatory SCRs and shift their selections away from the bad decks. In the controls, anticipatory SCRs, especially to the bad decks, became more pronounced as the game progressed, and the subjects shifted almost exclusively to the good decks. The ventromedial prefrontal subjects never produced anticipatory SCRs, and they also continued to opt more frequently for the bad decks. The pattern occurred even in ventromedial subjects (n=3) who knew at a conscious level (conceptual period) how the game worked, and that some decks were good and some were bad. (From Bechara et al., 1997, used with permission.)

involving the free recall of spatial locations, but not on working memory tests involving the free recall of a temporal sequence or the recognition of spatial locations. In an effort to clarify the contribution of lateral prefrontal cortex to working memory, D'Esposito and Postle (1999) performed a meta-analysis of studies reporting the working memory performance of patients with lesions to the lateral prefrontal cortex. After analyzing the working memory performance of 166 lateral prefrontal patients from 11 studies, D'Esposito and Postle determined there was no significant deficit in working memory performance in these subjects, and therefore concluded that the prefrontal cortex does not make a *necessary* contribution to working memory capacity.

Data from studies of working memory, therefore, represent some lack of convergence between methods. Areas of prefrontal cortex that yield robust, replicable activations in functional neuroimaging studies do not appear to be necessary for working memory because damage to these same areas does not reliably produce an impairment. Such a scenario does not require a denigration of one method in favor of the other (both are capable of producing valid data); rather, it will no doubt spark a host of theoretical refinements and new hypotheses to be investigated with both methods.

Priming. Another subtype of memory is the phenomenon of priming. Here, we would like to briefly describe one experiment that illustrates a creative use of functional neuroimaging to obtain a neural account of a long-known behavioral effect.

"Repetition priming" refers to the observation that repeated exposure to an object facilitates faster processing (e.g., naming, classification) of the object upon subsequent encounters. Interestingly, this form of learning is preserved in anterograde amnesia, indicating that is not dependent on the mesial temporal lobe system (e.g., Cave and Squire, 1992). To investigate the neural correlates of object priming, Buckner et al. (1998) employed a rapid event-related fMRI paradigm in which subjects performed an object classification task ("Does this object move on its own or not?"). Object pictures were presented in the scanner. Prior to scanning, subjects were shown a subset of the objects, so during scanning some objects would be "novel" and others "repeated." Behavioral performance and the brain hemodynamic response were obtained for each object during the task. As expected, classification performance was faster for repeated items, and the classification task (for novel and repeated items) was associated with widespread activations relative to a fixation baseline. Comparison of the hemodynamic responses for novel and repeated items revealed that a subset of areas activated by the object classification task was differentially activated for novel and repeated items, thereby suggesting that the priming-related task facilitation had selective neuroanatomical substrates. Novel and repeated items elicited comparable activations in primary visual cortex (associated with early retinotopic visual processing) and motor areas (associated with response initiation and execution), but a reduction in activation for the repeated items was observed in extrastriate and inferotemporal cortex (associated with higher order visual processing and visual object representation) as well as left doroslateral prefrontal cortex and anterior cingulate cortex (associated with effortful response monitoring and selection). These data suggest that experience-dependent reductions in neural activations associated with object representations are the neuroanatomical correlate of enhanced behavioral performance ("priming") for those objects. The brain-behavior relationship delineated in this study would have been impossible to ascertain using the lesion method. As in the Wagner et al. (1998) study of long-term declarative memory (which showed that parahippocampal activity for individual words during encoding predicted subsequent recall success), only through a functional imaging paradigm that allows comparison of the healthy brain's responses to individual stimuli, could the neural mechanism for repetition priming to be elucidated.

Decision-making and social conduct

As alluded to earlier in the mention of Harlow's seminal case of Phineas Gage, throughout the history of neuropsychology investigators have called attention to the dramatic changes in social behavior that occur in relationship to injuries to the prefrontal region of the brain (e.g., Brickner, 1934; Eslinger & Damasio, 1985; Harlow, 1868; Hebb & Penfield, 1940; Luria, 1969; Stuss & Benson, 1986). As case reports accrued over the past century, it became apparent that the affected patients have a number of features in common (see Damasio & Anderson, 1993): inability to organize future activity and hold gainful employment, diminished capacity to respond to punishment, a tendency to present an unrealistically favorable view of themselves, a tendency to display inappropriate (or absent) emotional reactions, and normal intelligence. Several of these features are highly reminiscent of the personality profile associated with sociopathy, and in fact, we have gone so far as to dub this condition "acquired sociopathy" (Damasio, Tranel, & Damasio, 1990b).

Others have called attention to such characteristics in patients with ventromedial prefrontal cortex (VMPC) damage. For example, Blumer and Benson (1975) noted a personality type that characterized patients with orbital damage (which the authors termed "pseudo-psychopathic"), in which salient features were puerility, a jocular attitude, sexually disinhibited humor, inappropriate and near-total self-indulgence, and complete lack of concern for others. Stuss and Benson (1986) emphasized that such patients demonstrate a remarkable lack of empathy and general lack of concern about others. The patients tend to show callous lack of concern, boastfulness, and unrestrained and tactless behavior. Other descriptors include impulsiveness, facetiousness, and diminished anxiety and concern for the future.

Patients with VMPC lesions and "acquired sociopathy" demonstrate a proclivity to make decisions and engage in behaviors that have negative consequences for their well-being. The patients are usually not destructive and harmful to others in society (a feature that distinguishes the "acquired" form of the disorder from the standard "developmental" form); however, they repeatedly opt for courses of action that are not in their best interest in the long run. They make poor decisions about interpersonal relationships, occupational endeavors, and finances. In short, they act as though they have lost the ability to ponder different courses of action and then select the option that promises the best blend of short- and long-term benefit. What makes this manifestation all the more striking, and what has defied simple explanation ever since the days of Harlow, is the fact that most of the patients retain normal intelligence, conventional memory, language, perception, attention, and so on. In other words, there are no obvious neuropsychological impairments that might account parsimoniously for the erratic behavior.

The rich clinical descriptions outlined above indicate a central role for VMPC in decision-making and social conduct. More systematic laboratory exploration of these patients' deficits suggests a neural mechanism by which VMPC exerts its influence in this cognitive domain. One of the primary experimental paradigms used to investigate decision-making behavior is the Iowa Gambling Task (IGT) (Bechara et al., 1994). The IGT was developed as a laboratory probe to detect and measure the decision-making impairments that are so blatant in the day-to-day lives of VMPC patients. Accordingly, the IGT factors in reward and punishment (winning and losing money) in such a way as to create a conflict between immediate reward and delayed punishment (Bechara, Tranel, & Damasio, 2000). Choices in the task may be risky and uncertain because individual outcomes cannot be calculated. Success on the task depends critically on one's ability to develop "hunches" or "gut feelings" about good and bad decisions in real time.

The IGT consists of four decks of cards named A, B, C, and D. The subject chooses one card at a time from any of the four decks. Each card denotes a net gain or loss of money. The subject is stopped after 100 card selections, but s/he is never aware of when the task will end. The object of the IGT is to maximize profit on a loan of play money. The key manipulation is that the decks are pre-programmed so two decks are "good" in the long run (i.e., continuous selection from these decks results in a net gain of money) and 2 decks are "bad" in the long run (i.e., continuous selection from these decks results in a net loss of money). However, the immediate reward of the bad decks is greater than the good decks, but so is the eventual punishment. So, through variable experiences of reward and punishment with each deck, the subject must formulate a plan of action that is advantageous in the long run (i.e., pick mostly from the good decks). Over the course of the 100 selections, the normal course of behavior is that subjects learn to avoid the bad decks and choose predominantly from the good decks. VMPC patients, on the other hand, continue to select from the bad decks throughout the task. (Figure 6.4) Thus, the IGT captures the real-world defects in decision-making behavior observed in the VMPC patients.

To investigate the pathophysiological basis of the decision-making impairment associated with VMPC damage, Bechara et al. (1996) administered the IGT while recording skin conductance responses (SCRs), a sensitive index of psychosomatic arousal that is reliably elicited by stimuli with emotional or social valence. Both normal subjects and VMPC patients generated SCRs after picking a card and learning they won or lost money. However, as normal subjects progressed through the task they began to generate SCRs prior to the selection of cards, during the time in which subjects consider from which deck to choose. Furthermore, these anticipatory SCRs were larger before picking from a bad deck than picking from a good deck. By contrast, VMPC patients generated no SCRs prior to card selection.

In another instantiation of the IGT, Bechara et al. (1997) recorded SCRs but also intermittently interrupted the subject (every 10 card selections) to ask what the subject knew about the game. Four epochs were defined: (1) "pre-punishment," when the subject had sampled the decks but had not encountered any losses, (2) "pre-hunch," when the subject had encountered losses but had no idea how the decks were different, (3) "hunch," when the subject expressed uncertain guesses about some decks being riskier than others, and (4) "conceptual," when subjects could declare which decks were good and which were bad. Card selection and anticipatory SCRs were compared for the four periods (Figure 6.5). In the pre-punishment period, both VMPC patients and normal subjects selected more from the higher paying bad decks. In the pre-hunch period, normal subjects developed anticipatory SCRs and began selecting more from the good decks. VMPC patients developed no pre-hunch anticipatory SCRs and continued to choose from the bad decks. In the hunch period, normal subjects continued to generate anticipatory SCRs and card selection shifted even more in favor of the good decks. VMPC patients never generated anticipatory SCRs and never reached a hunch period, but 50% reached the conceptual period. Remarkably, despite being able to articulate the relative long-term reward and punishment contingencies of each deck, VMPC patients reaching the conceptual period continued to choose disadvantageously. Conversely, 30% of normal subjects never reached the conceptual period, but still generated anticipatory SCRs and chose advantageously. These data suggest that the critical determinant of successful decision-making is not declarative knowledge, but a somatic signal mediated by VMPC and derived from prior experiences with reward and punishment.

The preceding discussion of acquired sociopathy and defective decision-making was based on neuropsychological studies of patients with *adult-onset, bilateral* VMPC damage. Hence, these studies bear no information on two fundamental considerations of brain-behavior relationships: laterality and development. The following two studies, respectively, discuss acquired sociopathy in these terms. To parse the relative contributions of right and left VMPC damage to acquired sociopathy, Tranel et al. (2002) studied a rare series of patients with focal, unilateral lesions to VMPC. In terms of social conduct (indexed by clinician and family ratings), decision-making (indexed by IGT), and personality (indexed by Iowa Rating Scales of Personality Change; Barrash and Anderson, 1993), the patients with damage restricted to right VMPC approximated the bilateral patients (impaired), whereas patients with damage restricted to left VMPC more closely approximated normal comparison subjects (nonimpaired), indicating that the right VMPC is critically involved in social conduct, decision-making, and personality, whereas the contribution of the left VMPC is less important.

To investigate the role of VMPC in the development of decision-making and social behavior, Anderson and colleagues have assembled the most complete clinical and neuroanatomical descriptions of cases with early-onset (prenatal, infancy, or childhood) VMPC damage, including two cases published in previous articles (Anderson et al., 1999, 2000).[1] These reports indicate that the cluster of antisocial traits common to these two early-onset cases (superficial charm, lying, stealing, manipulative, lack

---

[1] A larger series of cases has now been studied, and comparable results have been obtained; see Anderson, Barrash, Bechara, and Tranel, in press.

of remorse or guilt, shallow affect, lack of empathy, failure to accept responsibility, parasitic, poor behavioral controls, early behavioral problems, lack of realistic long-term goals, irresponsibility, juvenile delinquency, and promiscuity) surpasses that of adult-onset cases in scope and severity. Neuropsychological assessment of the two cases indicates both have intact basic mental abilities (like the adult-onset cases), but significant impairments in executive function, social/moral reasoning, and verbal generation of responses to social situations (unlike adult-onset cases, who are capable of generating appropriate responses to social and moral scenarios when presented in verbal, "off-line" format). As expected, both developmental patients exhibited defective decision-making on the IGT and failed to generate anticipatory SCRs. Even though the reported sample of early-onset damage subjects is small so far, the available data suggest that VMPC is critically involved in the acquisition of social and moral knowledge during development. Adult-onset VMPC patients, who presumably underwent normal social development, retain declarative access to social facts and "off-line" moral reasoning, but they lose access to emotional signals that are necessary to guide appropriate social and decision-making behavior in real-life, real-time situations. Early-onset VMPC patients seem to have never acquired factual social knowledge, nor do they have access to normal "online" emotional signals, resulting in an even greater level of impairment.

As a noteworthy aside, the result of *greater impairment* following *early damage* to VMPC runs contrary to a long-held heuristic of brain-behavior relationships: the Kennard Principle, which holds that functional recovery from brain damage is better when the injury occurs early in life. Lesion studies examining age of onset as an independent variable stand to bear important data regarding the neural bases of the development of specific cognitive abilities.

Clearly, the wealth of clinical, behavioral, psychophysiological, and neuroanatomical data linking VMPC to social conduct and decision-making illustrates the unique capability of the lesion method. Functional imaging studies of social behavior and decision-making processes are challenging for at least two reasons: (1) VMPC, apparently the primary substrate for such abilities, is difficult to image (due to magnetic susceptibility artifact) without sacrificing coverage of more distal regions of cortex, and (2) experimental paradigms involving social interactions or decision-making based on risk, reward, punishment, and uncertainty of future outcomes (like IGT) are often complicated, likely recruiting multiple cognitive systems with difficult-to-model dynamics, thus making an activation map based on subtraction of some other "baseline" task with similar properties difficult to interpret. Although neither challenge is insurmountable (see O'Doherty et al., 2001; Fukui et al., 2005), the lesion method has proven to be the primary experimental tool for elucidating brain-behavior relationships in this domain.

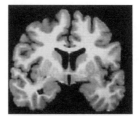

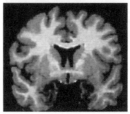

Figure 6.6. MRI of brain with normal amygdala (top) and SM's brain (bottom). Note the restricted, yet complete, damage to the amygdala bilaterally in SM.

Emotion recognition

In contrast to the notable differences in what has been learned about memory and decision-making from lesion versus functional imaging approaches, the neuroanatomical correlates of emotion (particularly fear) recognition have been investigated in lesion and neuroimaging studies in parallel, with remarkably convergent results. Both methods implicate the amygdala as the key structure for the recognition of fearful expressions on faces.

This link has been firmly established in lesion studies, which have shown that bilateral amygdala damage impairs the ability to recognize fearful faces, despite intact perceptual abilities. Undoubtedly, the most informative subject in this respect has been patient SM. As a result of a rare disease, SM suffered brain damage that encompasses all nuclei of the amygdala bilaterally, as well as a small portion of the adjacent entorhinal cortex, yet spares all other subcortical and cortical structures (Figure 6.6), leaving her with essentially normal basic perception, memory, language, and reasoning insofar as these do not involve the processing of emotional material. SM is the most selective case of amygdala damage ever documented in a human subject. Over more than a decade of testing, SM has repeatedly exhibited a selective impairment in the ability to recognize fear from facial expressions, even though she is able to recognize fear from complex visual scenes and tone of voice, and she has normal visual perceptual abilities (Adolphs et al., 1994; Adolphs and Tranel, 2000). Subsequent group studies confirmed the finding that bilateral amygdala damage impairs recognition of facial expressions of fear (Calder et al., 1996; Broks et al., 1998; Adolphs et al., 1999).

Functional imaging research has revealed a complementary and equally robust finding: amygdala activation during the perception of fearful faces (Figure 6.7). Relative to viewing neutral or happy faces, fearful faces elicit amygdala activation during passive viewing (Breiter et al., 1996), subliminal (brief) viewing (Whalen et al., 1998), and during

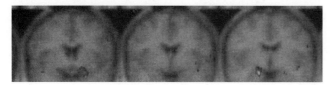

Figure 6.7. Bilateral activation of amygdala in response to subliminal presentation of fearful faces compared to happy faces (From Whalen et al., 1998, used with permission). (See color plate.)

performance of unrelated tasks like gender discrimination (Morris et al., 1998).

Intriguingly, a recent study of SM has indicated a putative mechanism by which amygdala damage impairs the recognition of facial expressions of fear (Adolphs et al., 2005). Using a series of partially occluded faces, Adolphs et al. showed that the eye region is most informative area for identifying fear from faces. Eye-tracking was used to show that SM fails to look at the eye regions of static faces (all faces, not just fearful faces). Thus, her impairment in recognizing fearful faces could be simply explained by the fact that she does not spontaneously look at the region of the face that is particularly useful for identifying fear. Remarkably, a verbal instruction to attend to the eye regions of the faces improved SM's ability to recognize fear to normal levels (Figure 6.8). Absent such an instruction, her performance returned to its previous level of impairment. These data suggest a critical role for the amygdala in the mediation of visual attention, at least for faces.

Outside the domain of facial emotion recognition, functional imaging studies have indicated a broader, multimodal role for the amygdala in the detection of emotional stimuli. Amygdala activation has been reported in response to the sounds of laughter, (Sander and Scheich, 2001), crying, (Sander and Scheich, 2001), and vocal expressions of fear (Phillips et al., 1998), as well as to aversive smells (Zald and Pardo, 1997) and aversive tastes (Zald et al., 1998). Furthermore, both functional imaging (Cahill et al., 1995, 1998) and lesion (Adolphs et al., 1997) studies indicate a role for the amygdala in the enhancement of memory for emotional events. The wealth of lesion and neuroimaging data regarding the amygdala's involvement in emotional processing will no doubt fuel theoretical debate about the primary function of the amygdala and generate hypotheses to be tested with both methods.

Attention

Attention is a broad term in neuropsychology and cognitive neuroscience, with definitions ranging from sustained effort and concentration to visual inspection and saccade modulation. Here, the discussion of attention will be restricted the "spotlight" phenomenon of visual attention: visual information within the spotlight (a circumscribed region of visual space) is processed more quickly or more efficiently than information outside the spotlight. The neural basis of this spatially restricted attentional

effect has been revealed with fMRI, and not with lesion studies. Brefczynski and DeYoe (1999) used a task in which subjects fixated a central marker while spatial attention was directed to a cued target object that was moved to successively greater eccentricities relative to the central fixation. The progressive shift of covert attention to greater eccentricities was associated with a corresponding retinotopic shift of cortical activation, spreading across striate and extrastriate visual cortex (Figure 6.9). In a similar study, Tootell et al. (1998) had subjects continually fixate a central marker while spatial attention was directed to one of four corners of the visual field. Attention to a specific visual field location correlated with greater activity in the retinotopically corresponding location of visual cortex, with the greatest effect in extrastriate areas. These data demonstrate that attention modulation is a "top-down" effect in the brain; retinotopic areas active in visual perception are selectively enhanced when attention is directed to the corresponding location in visual space. Clearly, the lesion method would be unable to reveal this mechanism because damage to the neuroanatomical areas enhanced during attention would impair vision altogether.

Cognitive control

"Cognitive control" refers to the executive allocation of cognitive resources during focused mental effort. Dozens of neuroimaging studies implicate the dorsal anterior cingulate cortex (dACC) as a critical neural substrate for cognitive control (for reviews see van Veen and Carter, 2002; Allman et al., 2001; Duncan and Owen, 2000). dACC is reliably activated during tasks that require response selection from conflicting alternatives, like Go/No-go tasks and the Stroop task. (Pardo et al., 1990; Carter et al., 1995; Carter et al., 2000; Leung et al., 2000) The association

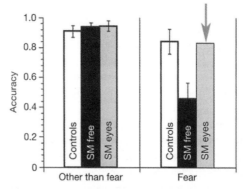

Figure 6.8. Instructed viewing of the eyes improves impaired fear recognition in SM. Accuracy of emotion recognition (± s.e.m.) for ten control subjects (white) and SM. Whereas SM's recognition of fear is impaired when she is allowed to look at the stimuli freely (SM free, black bars), her performance becomes normal relative to control subjects when she is instructed to fixate on the eyes (SM eyes, grey bar, red arrow). The impairment is specific to fear recognition (left panel shows mean recognition accuracy for all emotions other than fear). (From Adolphs et al., 2005, used with permission.)

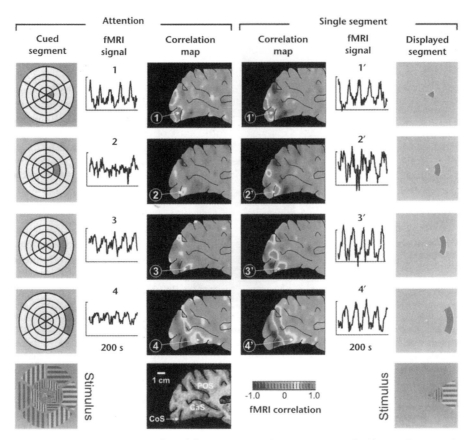

Figure 6.9. Retinotopic attentional modulation compared to activation evoked by cued targets alone. Cued segment (left column) shows schematic sequence of target segments cued for attentional scrutiny. Stimulus (bottom left) is actual target array. FMRI signal (left) shows signal modulation of individual voxels at sites indicated on adjacent correlation maps. Temporal phase shift of the signal at each site identifies the corresponding locus of attention. Correlation maps show sites where timing of modulation was positively correlated (red) or anti-correlated (blue) with the timing of attentional shifts. Displayed segment (right column) shows schematic sequence of single segments presented during otherwise identical control experiment. Composite of single segments shown in stimulus bottom right. FMRI Signal and correlation map on right show results of control experiment. Structural MRI (bottom) is a parasagittal section (13.6 mm left of midline) through occipital lobe in same plane as correlation maps. Sulcal landmarks; CaS, calcarine sulcus; CoS, collateral sulcus; POS; parieto-occipital sulcus. (From Brefczynski and DeYoe, 1999, used with permission) (See color plate.)

between dACC and cognitive control is patently evident from the neuroimaging studies, but the necessity of dACC for cognitive control is a separate question. Fellows and Farah (2005) directly addressed this issue by testing four patients with damage to dACC on the Stroop and go/no go tasks. Surprisingly, the dACC lesion patients, one of whom had bilateral damage, exhibited intact performance on the tasks. So despite the ubiquitous dACC activations observed in neuroimaging studies of cognitive control, a lesion study indicates that this structure is not a critical substrate for cognitive control. This is clearly an area where further work is needed to tease apart the particular roles of different neural structures in more elemental functions such as response selection and conflict monitoring.

Summary

From the tracks of research described above, it is readily apparent that the lesion method and functional neu-

roimaging offer distinct accounts of brain-behavior relationships. In some domains (long-term declarative memory, emotion recognition), imaging and lesion data may be convergent and complementary, but not redundant. In other domains (working memory and cognitive control), lesion studies have served to qualify the conclusions derived from functional imaging studies. In still other areas (priming, attention), functional imaging has provided exclusive insight into brain-behavior relationships, whereas the lesion method has been particularly productive in yet another field (decision-making and social conduct). Regardless of the precise contribution of each method to any individual research topic, it is clear that both methods have engendered inimitable knowledge in the study of brain-behavior relationships. Where these methods converge, theory can solidify and expand into novel branches of inquiry; where discrepancies exist, innovative conjecture and experimentation will soon follow.

CONCLUDING REMARKS

The lesion method has enjoyed a rich and fruitful history in the field of cognitive neuroscience. The lesion method has been, and continues to be, a unique and indispensable tool for investigating brain-behavior relationships. The advent of modern neuroimaging techniques has not only advanced the practice of the lesion method in its own right, but generated an entirely new class of data about the brain's function against which conclusions based on lesion data can be examined. These complementary forms of information have proven synergistic for the discovery of brain-behavior relationships: lesion findings spark neuroimaging hypotheses and vice versa. So long as the link between brain and behavior remains a curiosity worthy of experimentation, the study of brain-damaged patients will retain a central role.

REFERENCES

Adolphs, R., Cahill, L., Schul, R., & Babinsky, R. (1997). Impaired declarative memory for emotional material following bilateral amygdala damage in humans. *Learning & Memory*, 4, 291–300.

Adolphs, R., Damasio, H., Tranel, D., Cooper, G., & Damasio, A. R. (2000). A role for somatosensory cortices in the visual recognition of emotion as revealed by three-dimensional lesion mapping. *Journal of Neuroscience*, 20, 7, 2683–90.

Adolphs, R., Gosselin, F., Buchanan, T. W., Tranel, D., Schyns, P., & Damasio, A. R. (2005). A mechanism for impaired fear recognition after amygdala damage. *Nature*, 433, 68–72.

Adolphs, R., & Tranel, D. (2000). Emotion recognition and the human amygdala. In J. P. Aggleton (Ed.), The amygdala: A functional analysis. New York: Oxford University Press, pp. 587–630.

Adolphs, R., Tranel, D., Damasio, H., & Damasio, A. R. (1994). Impaired recognition of emotion in facial expressions following bilateral damage to the human amygdala. *Nature*, 372, 669–672.

Adolphs, R., Tranel, D., Damasio, H., & Damasio, A. R. (1995). Fear and the human amygdala. *Journal of Neuroscience*, 15, 5879–5891.

Adolphs, R., Tranel, D., Hamann, S., Young, A. W., Calder, A. J., Phelps, E. A., Anderson, A., Lee, G. P., & Damasio, A. R. (1999). Recognition of facial emotion in nine individuals with bilateral amygdala damage. *Neuropsychologia*, 10, 1111–7.

Alexander, M. P., & Freedman, M. (1984). Amnesia after anterior communicating artery rupture. *Neurology*, 34, 752–759.

Anderson, S. W., Bechara, A., Damasio, H., Tranel, D., & Damasio, A. R. (1999). Impairment of social and moral behavior related to early damage in human prefrontal cortex. *Nature Neuroscience*, 2, 11, 1032–7.

Anderson, S. W., Damasio, H., Tranel, D., & Damasio, A. R. (2000). Long-term sequelae of prefrontal cortex damage acquired in early childhood. *Developmental Neuropsychology*, 18, 3, 281–96.

Baddeley, A. D. (1992). Working memory. *Science*, 255, 566–569.

Barrash, J. and Anderson, S. W. (1993), The Iowa Rating Scales of Personality Change University of Iowa Department of Neurology, Iowa City.

Bechara, A., Damasio, A. R., Damasio, H., & Anderson, S. W. (1994). Insensitivity to future consequences following damage to human prefrontal cortex. *Cognition*, 50, 7–12.

Bechara, A., Damasio, H., Tranel, D., & Anderson, S. W. (1998). Dissociation of working memory from decision making within the human prefrontal cortex. *Journal of Neuroscience*, 18, 1, 428–37.

Bechara, A., Damasio, H., Tranel, D., & Damasio, A. R. (1997). Deciding advantageously before knowing the advantageous strategy. *Science*, 275, 1293–1295.

Bechara, A., Tranel, D., & Damasio, H. (2000). Characterization of the decision-making deficit of patients with ventromedial prefrontal cortex lesions. *Brain*, 123, 2189–2202.

Bechara, A., Tranel, D., Damasio, H., & Damasio, A. R. (1996). Failure to respond autonomically to anticipated future outcomes following damage to prefrontal cortex. *Cerebral Cortex*, 6, 215–225.

Benton, A. L. (1988). Neuropsychology: Past, present and future. In F. Boller & J. Grafman (Eds.), *Handbook of neuropsychology*, Vol. 1. New York: Elsevier, pp. 3–27.

Benton, A. L., Hamsher, K., Varney, N. R., & Spreen, O. (1983). Contributions to neuropsychological assessment. New York: Oxford University Press.

Benton, A., & Tranel, D. (2000). Historical notes on reorganization of function and neuroplasticity. In H. S. Levin & J. Grafman (Eds.), *Cerebral reorganization of function after brain damage.* New York: Oxford University Press, pp. 3–23.

Blumer, D., & Benson, D. F. (1975). Personality changes with frontal and temporal lobe lesions. In Benson, D. F., Blumer, D. (Eds.), *Psychiatric aspects of neurologic disease.* New York: Grune & Stratton, pp. 151–169.

Braver, T. S., Cohen, J. D., Nystrom, L. E., Jonides, J., Smith, E. E., & Noll, D. C. (1997). A parametric study of prefrontal cortex involvement in human working memory. *Neuroimage*, 5, 49–62.

Brefczynski, J. A. & DeYoe, E. A., (1999). A physiological correlate of the 'spotlight' of visual attention. *Nature Neuroscience*, 2, 4, 370–4.

Breiter, H. C., Etcoff, N. L., Whalen, P. J., Kennedy, W. A., Rauch, S. L., Buckner, R. L., Strauss, M. M., Hyman, S. E., & Rosen, B. R. (1996). Response and habituation of the human amygdala during visual processing of facial expression. *Neuron*, 17, 875–887.

Brickner, R. M. (1934). An interpretation of frontal lobe function based upon the study of a case of partial bilateral frontal lobectomy. *Research Publication of the Association for Research in Nervous and Mental Disease*, 13, 259–351.

Broca, P. (1865). Sur la faculte du langage articule. *Bull. Soc. Anthropol.*, 6, 337–393.

Broks, P., Young, A. W., Maratos, E. J., Coffey, P. J., Calder, A. J., Isaac, C. L., Mayes, A. R., Hodges, J. R., Montaldi, D., Cezayirli, E., Roberts, N., & Hadley, D. (1998). Face processing impairments after encephalitis: amygdala damage and recognition of fear. *Neuropsychologia*, 36, 1, 59–70.

Butters, N., & Stuss, D. T. (1989). Diencephalic amnesia. InBoller, F., & Grafman, J. (Eds) *Handbook of neuropsychology*, Vol. 3. Amsterdam: Elsevier, pp. 107–148.

Cahill, L., Babinsky, R., Markowitsch, H. J., & McGaugh, J. L. (1995). The amygdala and emotional memory. *Nature*, 377, 295–296.

Cahill, L., Haier, R. J., Fallon, J., Alkire, M. T., Tang, C., Keator, D., Wu, J., & McGaugh, J. L. (1998). Amygdala activity at encoding correlated with long-term, free recall of emotional information. *Proceedings of the National Academy of Science, U.S.A.*, 93, 15, 8016–21.

Calder, A. J., Young, A. W., Rowland, D., Perrett, D. I., Hodges, J. R., & Etcoff, N. L. (1996). Facial emotion recognition after bilateral amygdala damage: differentially severe impairment of fear. *Cognitive Neuropsychology*, 13, 699–745.

Cave, B. C., Squire, L. R. (1992) Intact and long-lasting repetition priming in amnesia. *Journal of Experimental Psychology: Learning, Memory, and Cognition*, 18, 509–20.

Cermak, L. S., & O'Connor, M. (1983). The anterograde and retrograde retrieval ability of a patient with amnesia due to encephalitis. *Neuropsychologia*, 21, 213–234.

Cohen, J. D., Perlstein, W. M., Braver, T. S., Nystrom, L. E., Noll, D. C., Jonides, J., & Smith, E. E. (1997). Temporal dynamics of brain activation during a working memory task. *Nature*, 386, 604–608.

Cohen, N. J., & Eichenbaum, H. (1993). *Memory, amnesia, and the hippocampal system*. Cambridge, MA: The MIT Press.

Cohen, N. J., & Squire, L. R. (1981). Retrograde amnesia and remote memory impairment. *Neuropsychologia*, 19, 337–356.

Corkin, S. (1965). Tactually guided maze learning in man: effects of unilateral cortical excisions and bilateral hippocampal lesions. *Neuropsychologia*, 3, 339–351.

Corkin, S. (1984). Lasting consequences of bilateral medial temporal lobectomy: Clinical course and experimental findings in HM. *Seminars in Neurology*, 4, 249–259.

Corkin, S., Amaral, D. G., Gonzalez, R. G., Johnson, K. A., & Hyman, B. T. (1997). H. M.'s medial temporal lobe lesion: findings from magnetic resonance imaging. *Journal of Neuroscience*, 17, 10, 3964–79.

Courtney, S. M., Ungerleider, L. G., Keil, K., & Haxby, J. V. (1997). Transient and sustained activity in a distributed neural system for working memory. *Nature*, 386, 608–611.

Curran, T., & Schacter, D. L. (1997). Amnesia: Cognitive neuropsychological aspects. In Feinberg, T. E., & Farah, M. J. (Eds), *Behavioral neurology and neuropsychology*. New York: McGraw Hill, pp. 463–471.

Damasio, A. R., & Anderson, S. W. (1993). The frontal lobes. In Heilman, K. M., & Valenstein, E. (Eds.), *Clinical neuropsychology*, 3rd ed. New York: Oxford University Press, pp. 409–460.

Damasio, A. R., Eslinger, P., Damasio, H., VanHoesen, G. W., & Cornell, S. (1985). Multimodal amnesic syndrome following bilateral temporal and basal forebrain damage. *Archives of Neurology*, 42, 252–259.

Damasio, A. R., Graff-Radford, N. R., Eslinger, P. G., Damasio, H., & Kassell, N. (1985). Amnesia following basal forebrain lesions. *Archives of Neurology*, 42, 263–271.

Damasio, H., & Damasio, A. R. (1989). *Lesion analysis in neuropsychology*. New York: Oxford University Press.

Damasio, H., & Damasio, A. R. (2003). The lesion method in behavioral neurology and neuropsychology. In Feinberg, T. E., & Farah, M. J. (Eds), *Behavioral neurology and neuropsychology*, 2nd edition. New York: McGraw Hill, pp 71–83.

Damasio, H., Grabowski, T. J., Tranel, D., Hichwa, R. D., & Damasio, A. R. (1996). A neural basis for lexical retrieval. *Nature*, 380, 499–505.

Deluca, J., & Diamond, B. J. (1995). Aneurysm of the anterior communicating artery: A review of neuroanatomical and neuropsychologic sequelae. *Journal of Clinical and Experimental Neuropsychology*, 17, 100–121.

D'Esposito, M., & Postle, B. R. (1999). The dependence of span and delayed-response performance on prefrontal cortex. *Neuropsychologia*, 11, 1303–15.

Eslinger, P. J., & Damasio, A. R. (1985). Severe disturbance of higher cognition after bilateral frontal lobe ablation: patient EVR. *Neurology*, 35, 1731–1741.

Ferreira, C. T., Verin, M., Pillon, B., Levy, R., Dubois, B., & Agid, Y. (1998). Spatio-temporal working memory and frontal lesions in man. *Cortex*, 1, 83–98.

Flourens, P. (1846). *Phrenology examined* (Charles de Lucena Meigs, trans). Philadelphia: Hogan and Thompson.

Frank, R. J., Damasio, H., & Grabowski, T. J. (1997). Brainvox: An interactive, multimodal visualization and analysis system for neuroanatomical imaging. *NeuroImage*, 5, 13–30.

Fukui, H., Murai, T., Fukuyama, H., Hayashi, T., & Hanakawa, T. (2005). Functional activity related to risk anticipation during performance of the Iowa Gambling Task. *Neuroimage*, 24, 1, 253–9.

Gabrieli, J. D. E., Brewer, J. B., Desmond, J. E., & Glover, G. H. (1997). Separate neural bases of fundamental memory processes in the human medial temporal lobe. *Science*, 276, 264–266.

Gabrieli, J. D. E., Corkin, S., Mickel, S. F., & Growden, J. H. (1993). Intact acquisition and long-term retention of mirror-tracing skill in Alzheimer's disease and in global amnesia. *Behavioral Neuroscience*, 107, 899–910.

Gazzaniga, M. S. (1987). Perceptual and attentional processes following callosal section in human. *Neuropsychologia*, 25, 119–133.

Geschwind, N. (1965). Disconnexion syndromes in animals and man. *Brain*, 88, 237–294, 585–644.

Graff-Radford, N. R., Tranel, D., Van Hoesen, G. W., & Brandt, J. P. (1990). Diencephalic amnesia. *Brain*, 113, 1–25.

Harlow, J. M. (1868). Recovery from the passage of an iron bar through the head. *Publications of the Massachusetts Medical Society*, 2, 327–347.

Hebb, D. O., & Penfield, W. (1940). Human behavior after extensive bilateral removals from the frontal lobes. *Archives of Neurology and Psychiatry*, 44, 421–438.

Hodges, J. R. (1995). Retrograde amnesia. In A.Baddeley, B. A. Wilson, & F. N. Watts (Eds), *Handbook of memory disorders*. New York: John Wiley & Sons. pp. 81–107.

Jackson, J. H. (1870). A study of convulsions. *Transactions, St. Andrews Medical Graduate Association*, 3:162–204. (excerpted in Clarke and O'Malley, 1968).

Jackson, J. H. (1873). On the anatomical and physiological localisation of movement in the brain. *Lancet*, 1:84–85, 162–164, 232–234. (excerpted in Clarke and O'Malley, 1968).

Jonides, J., Smith, E. E., Koeppe, R. A., Awh, E., Minoshima, S., & Mintun, M. A. (1993). Spatial working memory in humans as revealed by PET. *Nature*, 363, 623–625.

Kapur, N. (1993). Focal retrograde amnesia in neurological disease: a critical review. *Cortex*, 29, 217–234.

Kapur, N., Ellison, D., Parkin, A. J., Hunkin, N. M., Burrows, E., Sampson, S. A., & Morrison, E. A. (1994). Bilateral temporal lobe pathology with sparing of medial temporal lobe structures: lesion profile and pattern of memory disorder. *Neuropsychologia*, 32, 23–38.

Karnath, H. O., Fruhmann Berger, M., Kuker, W., & Rorden, C. (2004). The anatomy of spatial neglect based on voxelwise statistical analysis: a study of 140 patients. *Cerebral Cortex*, 10, 1164–72.

Kelley, W. M., Miezin, F. M., McDermott, K. B., Buckner, R. L., Raichle, M. E., Cohen, N. J., Ollinger, J. M., Akbudak, E., Conturo, T. E., Snyder, A. Z., & Petersen, S. E. (1998). Hemispheric specialization in human dorsal frontal cortex and medial temporal lobe for verbal and nonverbal memory encoding. *Neuron*, 20, 5, 927–36.

Konishi, S., Wheeler, M. E., Donaldson, D. I., & Buckner, R. L. (2000). Neural correlates of episodic retrieval success. *Neuroimage*, 12, 3, 276–86.

Kopelman, M. D. (1992). The neuropsychology of remote memory. In Boller, F., & Grafman, J. (Eds), *Handbook of neuropsychology*, Vol. 8. Amsterdam: Elsevier, pp. 215–238.

Lashley, K. S. (1929). *Brain mechanisms and intelligence: A quantitative study of injuries to the brain*. Chicago: University of Chicago Press.

Lashley, K. S. (1950). In search of the engram. *Symposium of the Society for Experimental Biology*, 4, 454–482.

Leube, D. T., Erb, M., Grodd, W., Bartels, M., & Kircher, T. T. (2003). Successful episodic memory retrieval of newly learned faces activates a left fronto-parietal network. *Cognitive Brain Research*, 18, 1, 97–101.

Lezak, M. (1995). *Neuropsychological assessment*, 3rd ed. New York: Oxford University Press.

Luria, A. R. (1969). Frontal lobe syndromes. In Vinken, P. G., & Bruyn, G. W. (Eds.), *Handbook of clinical neurology*, Vol. 2. North Holland, Amsterdam: pp. 725–757.

Markowitsch, H. J., Calabrese, P., Haupts, M., Durwen, H. F., Liess, J., & Gehlen, W. (1993). Searching for the anatomical basis of retrograde amnesia. *Journal of Clinical and Experimental Neuropsychology*, 15, 947–967.

McCarthy, G. (1995). Functional neuroimaging of memory. *The Neuroscientist*, 1, 155–163.

McCarthy, G., Blamire, A. M., Puce, A., Nobre, A. C., Bloch, G., Hyder, F., Goldman-Rakic, P., & Shulman, R. G. (1994). Functional magnetic resonance imaging of human prefrontal cortex activation during a spatial working memory task. *Proceedings of the National Academy of Science*, 91, 8690–8694.

McKenna, P., & Warrington, E. K. (1996). The analytical approach to neuropsychological assessment. In I. Grant & K. M. Adams (Eds.), *Neuropsychological assessment of neuropsychiatric disorders*, 2nd edition. New York: Oxford University Press, pp. 43–57.

Milberg, W. P., Hebben, N., & Kaplan, E. (1996). The Boston process approach to neuropsychological assessment. In I. Grant & K. M. Adams (Eds.), *Neuropsychological assessment of neuropsychiatric disorders*, 2nd edition. New York: Oxford University Press, pp. 58–80.

Milner, B. (1972). Disorders of learning and memory after temporal lobe lesions in man. *Clinical Neurosurgery*, 19, 421–446.

Milner, B., Petrides, M., Smith, M. L. (1985). Frontal lobes and the temporal organization of memory. *Human Neurobiology*, 4, 137–142.

Morris, J. S., Friston, K. J., Buchel, C., Frith, C. D., Young, A. W., Calder, A. J., & Dolan, R. J. (1998). A neuromodulatory role for the human amygdala in processing emotional facial expressions. *Brain*, 121, 47–57.

Narayanan, N. S., Prabhakaran, V., Bunge, S. A., Christoff, K., Fine, E. M., & Gabrieli, J. D. (2005). The role of the prefrontal cortex in the maintenance of verbal working memory: an event-related FMRI analysis. *Neuropsychology*, 2, 223–32.

Newcombe, F. (1969). *Missle wounds of the brain: A study of psychological deficits*. London: Oxford University Press.

O'Connor, M., Verfaellie, M., & Cermak, L. (1995). Clinical differentiation of amnesic subtypes. In A. Baddeley, B. A. Wilson, & F. N. Watts (Eds.), *Handbook of memory disorders*. New York: John Wiley & Sons. Pp. 53–80.

O'Doherty, J., Kringelbach, M. L., Rolls, E. T., Hornak, J., & Andrews, C. (2001). Abstract reward and punishment representations in the human orbitofrontal cortex. *Nature Neuroscience*, 1, 95–102.

Petrides, M., Alivisatos, B., Evans, A. C., & Meyer, E. (1993). Dissociation of human mid-dorsolateral from posterior dorsolateral frontal cortex in memory processing. *Proceedings of the National Academy of Science*, 90, 873–877.

Phillips, M. L., Young, A. W., Scott, S. K., Calder, A. J., Andrew, C., Giampietro, V., Williams, S. C., Bullmore, E. T., Brammer, M., & Gray, J. A. (1998). Neural responses to facial and vocal expressions of fear and disgust. *Proceedings of the Royal Society of London. Series B, Biological Sciences*, 265, 1408, 1809–17.

Raichle, M. E. (1997). Functional imaging in behavioral neurology and neuropsychology. InFeinberg, T. E., & Farah, M. J. (Eds). *Behavioral neurology and neuropsychology*. New York: McGraw Hill, pp. 83–100.

Ramachandran, V. S., Hirstein, W. S., Armel, K. C., Tecoma, E., & Iragui, V. (1997). The neural basis of religious experience. *Society for Neuroscience Abstracts*, 23, 1316.

Reitan, R. M., & Wolfson, D. (1996). Theoretical, methodological, and validational bases of the Halstead-Reitan neuropsychological test battery. In I. Grant & K. M. Adams (Eds.), *Neuropsychological assessment of neuropsychiatric disorders*, 2nd edition. New York: Oxford University Press, pp. 3–42.

Rempel-Clower, N. L., Zola, S. M., Squire, L. R., & Amaral, D. G. (1996). Three cases of enduring memory impairment after bilateral damage limited to the hippocampal formation. *Journal of Neuroscience*, 16, 5233–5255.

Rowe, J. B. & Passingham, R. E. (2001). Working memory for location and time: activity in prefrontal area 46 relates to selection rather than to maintenance in memory. *Neuroimage*, 14, 77–86.

Sakai, K., Rowe, J. B. & Passingham, R. E. (2002). Active maintenance in prefrontal area 46 creates distractor-resistant memory. *Nature Neuroscience*, 5, 479–84.

Sander, K. & Scheich, H. (2001). Auditory perception of laughing and crying activates human amygdala regardless of attentional state. *Cognitive Brain Research*, 2, 181–98.

Saygin, A. P., Dick, F., Wilson, S. M., Dronkers, N. F., & Bates, E. (2003). Neural resources for processing language and environmental sounds: evidence from aphasia. *Brain*, 126, 928–45.

Scott, S. K., Young, A. W., Calder, A. J., Hellawell, D. J., Aggleton, J. P., & Johnson, M. (1997). Impaired auditory recognition of fear and anger following bilateral amygdala lesions. *Nature*, 385, 254–257.

Scoville, W. B., & Milner, B. (1957). Loss of recent memory after bilateral hippocampal lesions. *Journal of Neurology, Neurosurgery, and Psychiatry*, 20, 11–21.

Shannon, B. J. & Buckner, R. L. (2004). Functional-anatomic correlates of memory retrieval that suggest nontraditional processing roles for multiple distinct regions within posterior parietal cortex. *Journal of Neuroscience*, 24, 45, 10084–92.

Smith, E. E., Jonides, J., & Koeppe, R. A. (1996). Dissociating verbal and spatial working memory using PET. *Cerebral Cortex*, 6, 11–20.

Smith, E. E., Jonides, J., Koeppe, R. A., Awh, E., Schumacher, E. H., & Minoshima, S. (1995). Spatial versus object working memory: PET investigations. *Journal of Cognitive Neuroscience*, 7, 337–356.

Sperry, R. W. (1968). The great cerebral commissure. *Scientific American*, 210, 42–52.

Spreen, O., & Strauss, E. (1991). *A compendium of neuropsychological tests: Administration, norms, and commentary*. New York: Oxford University Press.

Spurzheim, J. G. (1815). *The physiognomical system of Drs. Gall and Spurzheim; Founded on an anatomical and physiological examination of the nervous system in general, and of the brain in particular; and indicating the dispositions and manifestations of the mind*. London: Baldwin, Cradock, and Joy.

Squire, L. R. (1992). Memory and hippocampus: a synthesis from findings with rats, monkeys, and humans. *Psychological Review*, 99, 195–231.

Squire, L. R., & Alvarez, P. (1995). Retrograde amnesia and memory consolidation: A neurobiological perspective. *Current Opinion in Neurobiology*, 5, 169–177.

Squire, L. R., & Moore, R. Y. (1979). Dorsal thalamic lesion in a noted case of human memory dysfunction. *Annals of Neurology*, 6, 503–506.

Stuss, D. T., & Benson, D. F. (1986). *The frontal lobes*. New York: Raven Press.

Teuber, H. L. (1968). Alteration of perception and memory in man: reflections on methods. In Weiskrantz, L. (Ed). *Analysis of behavioral change*. New York: Harper & Row. Pp. 274–328.

Teuber, H. L., Milner, B., & Vaughan, H. G. (1968). Persistent anterograde amnesia after stab wound of the basal brain. *Neuropsychologia*, 6, 267–282.

Thompson, R. F. L. (1986). The neurobiology of learning and memory. *Science*, 233, 941–947.

Tranel, D. (1996). The Iowa-Benton school of neuropsychological assessment. In I. Grant & K. M. Adams (Eds.), *Neuropsychological assessment of neuropsychiatric disorders*, 2nd edition. New York: Oxford University Press, pp. 81–101.

Tranel, D. (2002). Emotion, decision making, and the ventromedial prefrontal cortex. In D. T. Stuss and R. T. Knight (Eds.), *Principles of frontal lobe function*. New York: Oxford University Press. Pp. 338–53.

Tranel, D., Bechara, A., & Denburg, N. L. (2002). Asymmetric functional roles of right and left ventromedial prefrontal cortices in social conduct, decision-making, and emotional processing. *Cortex*, 38, 589–612.

Tranel, D., & Damasio, A. R. (1993). The covert learning of affective valence does not require structures in hippocampal system or amygdala. *Journal of Cognitive Neuroscience*, 5, 79–88.

Tranel, D., Damasio, A. R., Damasio, H., & Brandt, J. P. (1994). Sensorimotor skill learning in amnesia: additional evidence for the neural basis of nondeclarative memory. *Learning and Memory*, 1, 165–179.

Tranel, D., & Damasio, H. (1994). Neuroanatomical correlates of electrodermal skin conductance responses. *Psychophysiology*, 31, 427–438.

Tranel, D., & Jones, R. D. (in press). Knowing what and knowing when. *Journal of Clinical and Experimental Neuropsychology*.

Victor, M., Adams, R. D., & Collins, G. H. (1989). *The Wernicke-Korsakoff syndrome and related neurologic disorders due to alcoholism and malnutrition*, 2nd ed. Philadelphia: Davis.

Wagner, A. D., Schacter, D. L., Rotte, M., Koutstaal, W., Maril, A., Dale, A. M., Rosen, B. R., Buckner, R. L. (1998). Building memories: remembering and forgetting of verbal experiences as predicted by brain activity. *Science*, 281, 5380, 1188–91.

Weiskrantz, L. (Ed) (1968). *Analysis of behavioral change*. New York: Harper & Row.

Wernicke, C. (1874). *Der aphasische Symptomencomplex*. Breslau: Cohn und Weigert.

Whalen, P. J., Rauch, S. L., Etcoff, N. L., McInerney, S. C., Lee, M. B., & Jenike, M. A. (1998). Masked presentations of emotional facial expressions modulate amygdala activity without explicit knowledge. *Journal of Neuroscience*, 18, 1, 411–8.

Wilson, F. A. W., O'Scalaidhe, S. P., & Goldman-Rakic, P. S. (1993). Dissociation of object and spatial processing domains in primate prefrontal cortex. *Science*, 260, 1955–1958.

Young, A. W., Aggleton, J. P., Hellawell, D. J., Johnson, M., Broks, P., & Hanley, J. R. (1995). Face processing impairments after amygdalotomy. *Brain*, 118, 15–24.

Zald, D. H., Lee, J. T., Fluegel, K. W., & Pardo, J. V. (1998). Aversive gustatory stimulation activates limbic circuits in humans. *Brain*, 121, 1143–54.

Zald, D. H. & Pardo, J. V. (1997). Emotion, olfaction, and the human amygdala: amygdala activation during aversive olfactory stimulation. *Proceedings of the National Academy of Sciences*, 94, 8, 4119–24.

Zarahn, E., Aguirre, G. K., & D'Esposito, M. (1999). Temporal isolation of the neural correlates of spatial mnemonic processing with fMRI. *Cognitive Brain Research*, 7, 255–68.

Zola-Morgan, S., Squire, L. R., & Amaral, D. G. (1986). Human amnesia and the medial temporal region: enduring memory impairment following a bilateral lesions limited to field CA1 of the hippocampus. *Journal of Neuroscience*, 6, 2950–2967.

Autonomic and Somatic Nervous System

SECTION EDITOR: GARY G. BERNTSON

7 The Electrodermal System

MICHAEL E. DAWSON, ANNE M. SCHELL, AND DIANE L. FILION

PROLOGUE: OVERVIEW

Electrodermal activity (EDA) has been one of the most widely used – some might add "abused" – response systems in the history of psychophysiology. Research involving EDA has been reported in practically all psychology, psychiatry, and psychophysiology research journals. The wide range of journals in which EDA research is published reflects the fact that EDA measures have been applied to a wide variety of questions ranging from basic research examining attention, information processing, and emotion, to more applied clinical research examining predictors and/or correlates of normal and abnormal behavior. The application of EDA measures to a wide variety of issues is due in large part to its relative ease of measurement and quantification combined with its sensitivity to psychological states and processes.

The purpose of this chapter is to provide a tutorial overview of EDA for interested students, researchers, and practitioners who are not specialists in this particular system. We begin with a historical orientation and then discuss the physical, inferential, psychological, and social aspects of EDA.

HISTORICAL BACKGROUND

The discovery of electrodermal activity. The study of psychological effects on the electrical changes in human skin began over 100 years ago in the laboratory of Jean Charcot, the French neurologist famous for his work on hysteria and hypnosis. Vigouroux (1879, 1888), a collaborator of Charcot, measured tonic skin resistance levels from various patient groups as a clinical diagnostic sign. In the same laboratory, Féré (1888) found that by passing a small electrical current across two electrodes placed on the surface of the skin one could measure momentary decreases in skin resistance in response to a variety of stimuli (visual, auditory, gustatory, olfactory, etc.). The basic phenomenon discovered by Féré is that the skin momentarily becomes a better conductor of electricity when external stimuli are presented. Shortly thereafter, the Russian physiologist Tarchanoff (1890) reported that one could measure changes in electrical potential between two electrodes placed on the skin without applying an external current (see Neumann & Blanton, 1970, and Bloch, 1993, for interesting details regarding these initial discoveries). Hence, Féré and Tarchanoff are said to have discovered the two basic methods of recording electrodermal activity in use today. Recording the skin resistance response (or its reciprocal, the skin conductance response) relies on the passage of an external current across the skin and hence is referred to as the *exosomatic* method, whereas recording the skin potential response does not involve an external current and hence is referred to as the *endosomatic* method. The present chapter will focus on the exosomatic method of recording *skin conductance level* (SCL) and *skin conductance response* (SCR) because this clearly is the method of choice among contemporary researchers (Fowles et al., 1981).

Issues in the history of EDA research. Several issues identified in this early research have been sources of considerable speculation and investigation throughout the history of research with this response system. One set of such issues concerns the mechanisms and functions of EDA. In terms of peripheral mechanisms, Vigouroux proposed what became known as the "vascular theory" of EDA (Neumann & Blanton, 1970). The vascular theory associated changes in skin resistance with changes in blood flow. Tarchanoff favored a "secretory theory," which related EDA to sweat gland activity. This theory was supported later by Darrow (1927), who measured EDA and sweat secretion simultaneously and found the two measures to be closely related, although the phasic SCR would begin about one s before moisture would appear on the surface of the skin. Thus, it was concluded that activity of the sweat glands, not sweat on the skin per se, was critical for EDA. (Other lines of evidence indicating that sweat glands are the major contributors to EDA have been reviewed by Fowles, 1986, pp. 74–75.) It was generally known at the time that palmar sweat glands are innervated by the sympathetic chain of the autonomic nervous system, so EDA was said to reflect sympathetic activation. In terms of more central physiological mechanisms, work by early investigators such as Wang and Richter indicated that EDA was complexly determined by both subcortical and cortical areas (for a review of this early research, see Darrow, 1937). Darrow also proposed that "the function of the secretory activity of the palms is primarily to provide a pliable adhesive surface facilitating tactual acuity and grip on objects" (1937, p. 641).

Issues surrounding the proper methods of recording and quantifying EDA also have been important in the history of this response system. Lykken and Venables (1971) noted that EDA has continued to provide useful data "in spite of being frequently abused by measurement techniques which range from the arbitrary to the positively weird" (p. 656). In fact, we would date the beginning of the modern era of EDA research to the early 1970s when Lykken and Venables proposed standardized techniques of recording skin conductance and standardized units of measurement. This was followed shortly by an edited book (Prokasy & Raskin, 1973) devoted entirely to EDA which contained several useful review chapters, including a particularly outstanding chapter by Venables and Christie (1973). Published around the same time were several other excellent reviews (Edelberg, 1972a; Fowles, 1974; Grings 1974). More recent reviews can be found in books by Boucsein (1992) and by Roy et al. (1993), as well as in individual chapters by Andreassi (2000), Fowles (1986), Hugdahl (1995), and Stern, Ray, and Quigley (2001).

Another issue of central importance concerns the psychological significance of EDA. From the beginning, this response system has been closely linked with the psychological concepts of emotion, arousal, and attention. Carl Jung added EDA measurements to his word-association experiments in order to objectively measure the emotional aspects of "hidden complexes." An American friend joined Jung in these experiments and enthusiastically reported that, "Every stimulus accompanied by an emotion produced a deviation of the galvanometer to a degree in direct proportion to the liveliness and actuality of the emotion aroused" (Peterson, 1907, cited by Neumann & Blanton, 1970, p. 470). About half a century later, when the concept of emotion was less in favor, Woodworth and Schlosberg (1954) devoted most of one entire chapter of their classic textbook in experimental psychology to EDA, which they described as "perhaps the most widely used index of activation" (p. 137). They supported this indexing relationship by noting that tonic SCL is generally low during sleep and high in activated states such as rage or mental work. The authors also related phasic SCRs to attention, noting that such responses are sensitive to stimulus novelty, intensity, and significance.

Many of these issues have remained important for contemporary psychophysiologists and are discussed in the remainder of this chapter. In the next section we present a summary of the contemporary perspectives regarding

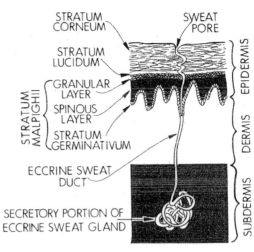

Figure 7.1. Anatomy of the eccrine sweat gland in various layers of skin. (Adapted from Hassett, 1978).

the basic physiological mechanisms and proper recording techniques of EDA.

PHYSICAL CONTEXT

Anatomical and physiological basis. The skin is a selective barrier that serves the function of preventing entry of foreign matter into the body and selectively facilitating passage of materials from the bloodstream to the exterior of the body. It aids in the maintenance of water balance and of constant core body temperature, functions accomplished primarily through vasoconstriction/dilation and through variation in the production of sweat. As pointed out by Edelberg (1972a), it is not surprising that an organ with such vital and dynamic functions constantly receives signals from control centers in the brain, and he suggests that "we can listen in on such signals by taking advantage of the fact that their arrival at the skin is heralded by measurable electrical changes that we call electrodermal activity" (p. 368).

There are two forms of sweat glands in the human body: the apocrine, which have been less studied, and the eccrine, which have been of primary interest to psychophysiologists. The primary function of most eccrine sweat glands is thermoregulation. However, those located on the palmar and plantar surfaces are thought to be more related to grasping behavior than to evaporative cooling (Edelberg, 1972a) and they have been suggested to be more responsive to psychologically significant stimuli than to thermal stimuli. Although all eccrine glands are believed to be involved in psychological sweating, such sweating is usually most evident in these areas primarily because of the high gland density (Shields et al., 1987). The measurement of EDA by psychophysiologists is primarily concerned with psychologically induced sweat gland activity.

Figure 7.1 shows the basic peripheral mechanisms involved in the production of EDA. The extreme outer layer of the skin, the stratum corneum or horny layer, consists of a layer of dead cells that serves to protect the internal organs. Below the stratum corneum lies the stratum lucidum, and just below that is the stratum Malpighii. The eccrine sweat gland itself consists of a coiled compact body that is the secretory portion of the gland, and the sweat duct, the long tube which is the excretory portion of the gland. The sweat duct remains relatively straight in its path through the stratum Malpighii and stratum lucidum, it then spirals through the stratum corneum and opens on the surface of the skin as a small pore (Edelberg, 1972a).

Many models have been suggested to explain how these peripheral mechanisms relate to the electrical activity of the skin and to the transient increases in skin conductance elicited by stimuli. Edelberg (1993) concluded that one can account for the variety of electrodermal phenomena, including changes in tonic SCL and phasic SCR amplitude, with a model based entirely on the sweat glands.

To understand how electrodermal activity is related to the sweat glands, it is useful to think of the sweat ducts (the long tubular portion of the gland that opens onto the skin surface) as a set of variable resistors wired in parallel. Columns of sweat will rise in the ducts in varying amounts and in varying numbers of sweat glands, depending on the degree of activation of the sympathetic nervous system. As sweat fills the ducts, there is a more conductive path through the relatively resistant corneum. The higher the sweat rises, the lower the resistance in that variable resistor. Changes in the level of sweat in the ducts change the values of the variable resistors, and yield observable changes in EDA.

Historically, both the sympathetic and parasympathetic divisions of the autonomic nervous system (ANS) were considered possible mediators of EDA. This is partially because the neurotransmitter involved in the mediation of eccrine sweat gland activity is acetylcholine, which is generally a parasympathetic neurotransmitter, rather than norepinepherine, the neurotransmitter typically associated with peripheral sympathetic activation (Venables & Christie, 1980). It is now generally agreed that human sweat glands have predominantly sympathetic cholinergic innervation from sudomotor fibers originating in the sympathetic chain, although some adrenergic fibers also exist in close proximity (Shields et al., 1987). Convincing evidence for the sympathetic control of EDA has been provided by studies that have measured sympathetic action potentials in peripheral nerves while simultaneously recording EDA. The results have shown that within normal ranges of ambient room temperature and thermoregulatory states of subjects, there is a high correlation between bursts of sympathetic nerve activity and SCRs (Wallin, 1981).

Excitatory and inhibitory influences on the sympathetic nervous system are distributed in various parts of the brain and therefore the neural mechanisms and pathways involved in the central control of EDA are numerous and complex. Boucsein (1992, pp. 30–36) followed the suggestions of Edelberg (1972a) in describing at least two and possibly three relatively independent pathways that lead to the production of SCRs (see Figure 7.2). The *first* and highest level of central EDA control involves contralateral cortical and basal ganglion influences (Sequeira & Roy, 1993). One cortical pathway involves excitatory control by the premotor cortex (Brodmann area 6) descending through the pyramidal tract, and another involves both excitatory and inhibitory influences originating in the frontal cortex. The *second* level of EDA control involves ipsilateral influences from the hypothalamus and limbic system (Sequeira & Roy, 1993). There is considerable evidence of an excitatory hypothalamic descending control of EDA. Limbic influences are complicated, but there is evidence of excitatory influences from the amygdala and inhibitory effects originating from the hippocampus. The *third* and lowest level mechanism is in the reticular formation in the brainstem (see Roy, Sequeira, & Delerm, 1993). Activation of the reticular formation by direct electrical stimulation or sensory stimulation evokes skin potential responses in cats, and presumably skin conductance responses in humans. An inhibitory EDA system has also been located in the bulbar level of the reticular formation.

Most of the evidence regarding the central pathways that control EDA described above was derived from animal studies, usually cats (e.g., Wang, 1964; Roy et al., 1993). More recently however, knowledge of the central control of human EDA, particularly EDA associated with attention and emotional processes, has increased dramatically with advances in neuroimaging technology. Using this technology, two strategies have been used to investigate the neural substrates of EDA: examination of EDA patterns in patients with delineated focal brain lesions (e.g., Asahina et al., 2003; Bechara et al., 1999; Tranel & Damasio, 1994; see review by Tranel, 2000), and examination of the relationship between patterns of brain activation and simultaneously recorded EDA (e.g., Critchley et al., 2000; Fredrikson et al., 1998; Nagai et al., 2004; Patterson, Ungerleider, & Bandettini, 2002; Williams et al., 2000).

Although there is not perfect overlap in the brain areas implicated across these studies, some consistent patterns have emerged. For example, activation of brain areas involved in evaluating stimulus significance, particularly the ventromedial prefrontal cortex, right inferior parietal region, and anterior cingulate, has been found to be associated with elicitation of SCRs. In addition, when the stimulus has emotional significance, the amygdala and orbitofrontal cortex, in addition to the areas mentioned above, are involved. Thermoregulatory sweating is controlled by the hypothalamus, which also integrates patterns of sympathetic activity in emotion, in conjunction with limbic structures.

Physical recording basis. As briefly described earlier, EDA is measured by passing a small current through a pair of

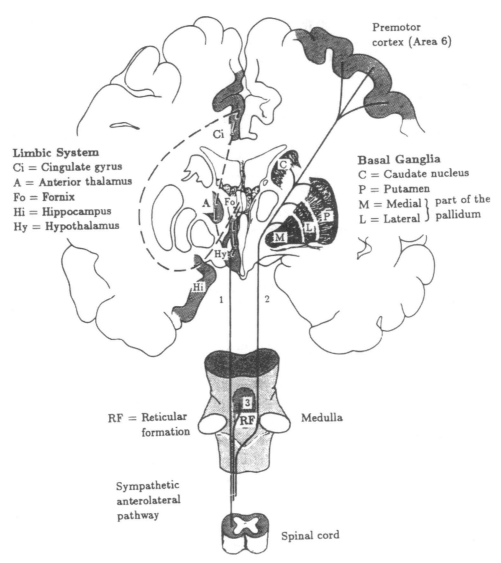

Figure 7.2. Central nervous system determiners of EDA in humans (From Boucsein, 1992).

electrodes placed on the surface of the skin. The principle invoked in the measurement of skin resistance or conductance is that of Ohm's law, which states that skin resistance (R) is equal to the voltage (V) applied between two electrodes placed on the skin surface, divided by the current (I) being passed through the skin. This law can be expressed as $R = V/I$. If the current is held constant then one can measure the voltage between the electrodes, which will vary directly with *skin resistance*. Alternatively, if the voltage is held constant, then one can measure the current flow, which will vary directly with the reciprocal of skin resistance, *skin conductance*. Conductance is expressed in units of Siemens and measures of skin conductance are expressed in units of microSiemens (μS).

Lykken and Venables (1971) argued strongly for the direct measurement of skin conductance with a constant-voltage system rather than measuring skin resistance with a constant current system. A description of constant voltage circuits that allow the direct measurement of skin conductance can be found in Lykken and Venables as well as in Fowles et al. (1981), and most of the physiological recording systems currently on the market include constant voltage systems for the direct recording of skin conductance.

EDA recording systems. Older recording systems, in operation 10 or more years ago, output EDA to a paper record in analog form. Most recording systems today are computer-based systems in which the analog skin conductance signal is digitized and stored on a computer. With such systems, a researcher must select which time points the computer will sample the EDA. Historically, this sampling window has been a few seconds following each presentation of an experimental stimulus. In these cases, EDA at all other time points is lost. Fortunately, with expanding computing capability, it is now generally feasible to sample EDA continuously, to allow an experimenter to flag critical events with a keypress or programmed signal, and to provide a continuous printout of an experimental session. In choosing an EDA recording system one must consider computing capabilities and software issues. For example, some manufacturers offer software packages for the acquisition of EDA, some offer software for the quantification of EDA, and some offer both (a listing of major commercial systems available for the recording and quantification of EDA is available at: *http://www.psychophys.com/company.html*).

In addition to selecting an EDA recording system, special consideration must be given to the choice of recording electrodes, electrode paste, electrode placement, and general environmental considerations. Silver-silver chloride cup electrodes are the type most typically used in skin conductance recording because they minimize the development of bias potentials and polarization. These electrodes can be easily attached to the recording site through the use of double-sided adhesive collars which also serve the purpose of helping to control the size of the skin area that comes in contact with the electrode paste, an important parameter because it is the contact area, not the size of the electrode, that affects the conductance values.

The electrode paste is the conductive medium between the electrodes and the skin. Probably the most important concern in choosing an electrode paste is that it preserve the electrical properties of the response system of interest. Because the measurement of EDA involves a small current passed through the skin, the electrode paste interacts with the tissue over which it is placed. For this reason, the use of a paste which closely resembles sweat in its salinity is recommended (Venables & Christie, 1980). Instructions for making such paste are given in Fowles et al. (1981, p. 235) and Grey and Smith (1984, p. 553). Satisfactory paste is also available commercially. Commercial EKG or EEG gels should not be used because they usually contain near saturation levels of NaCl and have been shown to significantly inflate measures of skin conductance level (Grey & Smith, 1984).

Skin conductance is recorded using two electrodes, both placed on active sites (bipolar recording); hence it does not matter in which direction the current flows between the two electrodes. Skin conductance recordings are typically taken from locations on the palms of the hands, with several acceptable placements. The most common electrode placements are the thenar eminences of the palms, and the volar surface of the medial or distal phalanges of the fingers (see Figure 7.3). It should be noted that although electrodermal activity can be measured from any of these sites, the values obtained are not necessarily comparable. Scerbo et al. (1992) made a direct comparison of EDA recorded from the distal and medial phalange sites simultaneously and found that both the elicited SCR amplitude and SCL were significantly higher from the distal recording site. The greater level of reactivity at the distal site was found to be directly related to a larger number of active sweat glands at that location (Freedman et al., 1994). Therefore, the distal phalange site is recommended unless there are specific reasons for not using the distal site (e.g., recording from children whose fingertips may be too small

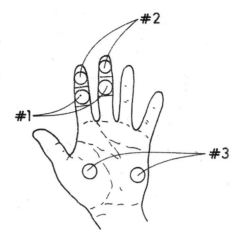

Figure 7.3. Three electrode placements for recording electrodermal activity. Placement #1 involves volar surfaces on medial phalanges, placement #2 involves volar surfaces of distal phalanges, and placement #3 involves thenar and hypothenar eminences of palms.

for stable electrode attachment, presence of cuts or heavy calluses on the fingertips, etc.).

Another recording issue concerns the hand from which to record. Many laboratories use the nondominant hand because it is less likely to have cuts or calluses, and because it leaves the dominant hand free to perform a manual task. However, this begs the question of whether there are significant laterality differences in EDA. Although differences between left and right hand EDA recordings have been reported, the differences reported across studies are often in opposite directions and the interpretations have been ambiguous (see review of early literature by Hugdahl, 1984). It is tempting to speculate that the prior conflicting findings may be because of lack of clear distinctions between emotional and nonemotional tasks (Hugdahl, 1995). EDA in emotional tasks is presumably controlled primarily by the ipsilateral limbic system, whereas EDA in non-emotional tasks may be controlled by the contralateral system (see Figure 7.2). Although research in this area continues (e.g., Brand et al., 2002; 2004; Esen & Esen, 2002; Naveteur et al., 1998; Polagaeva, Egorov, & Pirogov, 1997; Schulter & Papousek, 1998), evidence linking EDA asymmetries to specific patterns of lateralized brain activation is still inconclusive. Taken together, the current literature suggests that sensitive indices of handedness should be included in any study examining bilateral EDA (Schulter & Papousek, 1998), but provides no definitive evidence that EDA recorded from one hand gives consistently different results with respect to the effects of experimental variables than that recorded from the other hand.

Because it is critical in EDA recording that the electrical properties of the response system be preserved, the electrode sites should not receive any special preparation such as cleaning with alcohol or abrasion, which might reduce the natural resistive/conductive properties of the skin. However, because a fall in conductance has been

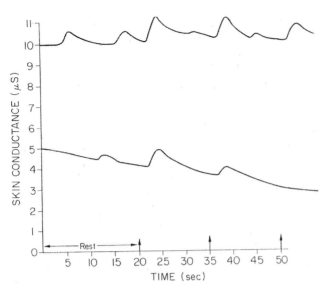

Figure 7.4. Two hypothetical skin conductance recordings during 20 s of rest followed by three repetitions of a simple discrete stimulus. Arrows represent the presentation of a stimulus (From Dawson & Nuechterlein, 1984).

noted following the use of soap and water (Venables & Christie, 1973), and because the length of time since the last wash will be variable across subjects when they arrive at the laboratory, these authors recommended that subjects be asked to wash their hands with a nonabrasive soap prior to having the electrodes attached and that the skin be kept clean and dry.

Ambient temperature and time of day are two environmental factors that should be controlled (e.g., Hot et al., 1999; Venables & Mitchell, 1996). Because EDA is influenced by hydration of the corneum, SCL tends to rise with increases in ambient temperature in the normal room temperature range. Boucsein (1992) recommends a room temperature of 23°C. Likewise, room humidity should be kept as constant as possible. Because diurnal effects may influence EDA, this variable also should be controlled across experimental conditions.

INFERENTIAL CONTEXT

Quantification procedures. Figure 7.4 shows tracings of two hypothetical skin conductance recordings during a 20 s rest period followed by three presentations of a simple discrete stimulus (e.g., a mild tone). Several important aspects of EDA can be seen in Figure 7.4. First, it can be seen that tonic SCL begins at 10 μS in the upper tracing and at 5 μS in the lower tracing. Although tonic SCL can vary widely between different subjects and within the same subject in different psychological states, the typical range is between 2 μS and 20 μS with the types of apparatus and procedures described here. Computing the log of SCL can significantly reduce skew and kurtosis in the SCL data and is recommended by Venables and Christie (1980).

It can also be seen in the lower tracing of Figure 7.4 that the SCL drifts downward from 5 μS to nearly 4 μS

during the rest period. It is common for SCL to gradually decrease while subjects are at rest, rapidly increase when novel stimulation is introduced, and then gradually decrease again after the stimulus is repeated.

Phasic SCRs are only a small fraction of the SCL and have been likened to small waves superimposed on the tidal drifts in SCL (Lykken & Venables, 1971). If the SCR occurs in the absence of an identifiable stimulus, as shown during the rest phase of Figure 7.4, it is referred to as a "spontaneous" or "nonspecific" SCR (NS-SCR). The most widely used measure of NS-SCR activity is their rate per minute, which typically is between 1 and 3/min while the subject is at rest. However, responses can be elicited by deep breaths and bodily movements, so unless these also are recorded, it is impossible to say which responses are truly NS-SCRs.

Presentation of a novel, unexpected, significant, or aversive stimulus will likely elicit an SCR referred to as a "specific" SCR. With the exception of responses elicited by aversive stimuli, these SCRs are generally considered components of the orienting response (OR). As is also the case with NS-SCRs, one must decide on a minimum amplitude change in conductance to count as an elicited SCR. Minimum values between .01 and .05 μS are generally used. Another decision regarding scoring of specific SCRs concerns the latency window during which time a response will be assumed to be elicited by the stimulus. Based on frequency distributions of response latencies to simple stimuli, it is common to use a 1–3 s or 1–4 s latency window. Hence, any SCR that begins between 1 and 3, or between 1 and 4 s, following stimulus onset is considered to be elicited by that stimulus. It is important to select reasonably short latency windows, perhaps even shorter than 1–3 s, so as to reduce the likelihood that NS-SCRs will be counted as elicited SCRs (Levinson, Edelberg, & Bridger, 1984).

An important advance in EDA research during the past decade or two is the development of computerized scoring programs. Scoring software is available from the manufacturers of several EDA recording systems, and customized software or shareware is frequently used as well. One example of shareware is SCRGAUGE by Peter Kohlisch, available in Boucsein (1992). Another shareware with a long history is SCORIT 1980 (Strayer & Williams, 1982), which is a revision of SCORIT (Prokasy, 1974). Interested readers can contact Dr. William C. Williams (*BWilliams@EWU.edu*) for an updated revised version of SCORIT 1980.

Having decided on a minimum response amplitude and a latency window in which a response will be considered a specific stimulus-elicited SCR, one can measure several aspects of the elicited SCR besides its mere occurrence and frequency. Definitions and typical values of the major EDA component measures are given in Table 7.1 and shown graphically in Figure 7.5. The most commonly reported measure is the size of the SCR, which is quantified as the amount of increase in conductance measured from the

Table 7.1. Electrodermal measures, definitions, and typical values

Measure	Definition	Typical Values
Skin conductance level (SCL)	Tonic level of electrical conductivity of skin	2–20 μS
Change in SCL	Gradual changes in SCL measured at two or more points in time	1–3 μS
Frequency of NS-SCRs	Number of SCRs in absence of identifiable eliciting stimulus	1–3 per min
SCR amplitude	Phasic increase in conductance shortly following stimulus onset	0.1–1.0 μS
SCR latency	Temporal interval between stimulus onset and SCR initiation	1–3 s
SCR rise time	Temporal interval between SCR initiation and SCR peak	1–3 s
SCR half recovery time	Temporal interval between SCR peak and point of 50% recovery of SCR amplitude	2–10 s
SCR habituation (trials to habituation)	Number of stimulus presentations before two or three trials with no response	2–8 stimulus presentations
SCR habituation (slope)	Rate of change of ER-SCR amplitude	0.01–0.5 μS per trial

Key: SCL, skin conductance level; SCR, skin conductance response; NS-SCR, nonspecific skin conductance response.

onset of the response to its peak. The size of an elicited SCR typically ranges between .1 and 1.0 μS. The values in Table 7.1 are representative of healthy young adults. Readers interested in the effects of individual differences in age, gender, and ethnicity should consult Boucsein (1992). Although effects of these variables on EDA have been documented and linked to differences in skin physiology, the effects appear to interact with the nature of the eliciting stimuli (e.g., emotional or neutral), recording environment (e.g., season, time of day, etc.), and recording methodology (constant current or constant voltage) (Boucsein, 1992; Venables & Mitchell, 1996). In general, we advise that these individual differences be controlled across experimental conditions.

When a stimulus is repeated several times and an average size of the SCR is to be calculated, one may choose to compute mean SCR amplitude or magnitude. *Magnitude* refers to the mean value computed across all stimulus presentations including those without a measurable response, whereas *amplitude* is the mean value computed across only those trials on which a measurable (nonzero) response

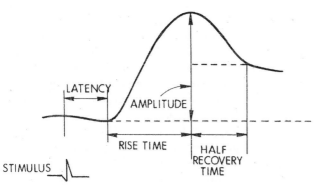

Figure 7.5. Graphical representation of principal EDA components.

occurred (Humphreys, 1943). The magnitude measure is the most commonly used but Prokasy and Kumpfer (1973) argue against its use because it confounds frequency and amplitude, which do not always covary. A magnitude measure can create the impression that the response size is changing when, in fact, it is response frequency that is changing. Hence, these authors recommend separate assessments of frequency and amplitude rather than magnitude. However, it is important to note that a complication with the amplitude measure is that the N used in computing average response size can vary depending on how many measurable responses a subject gives, and the data of subjects without any measurable response must be eliminated. Thus, a subject who responds on each of ten stimulus presentations with a response of .50 μS will have the same mean SCR amplitude as a subject who responds on only the first stimulus presentation with a response of .50 μS, and does not respond thereafter. We concur with Venables and Christie (1980) that there are arguments for and against both amplitude and magnitude and that although no absolute resolution is possible, it is important to keep the difference between the two measures clearly in mind. In some situations it may be reasonable to compute and compare results obtained with SCR frequency, amplitude, and magnitude.

Like SCL, SCR amplitude and magnitude are frequently found to be positively skewed and also leptokurtotic, so a logarithmic transformation is often used to remedy these problems. If measurements are being made of SCR magnitude, so that zero responses are included, then log of (SCR + 1.0) may be calculated, because the logarithm of zero is not defined (Venables & Christie, 1980). Another common practice is to use a square root transformation, $\sqrt{SCR}$, to normalize response amplitude data; this does not require the addition of a constant (Edelberg, 1972a). In some cases the choice of the square root or logarithmic transformation should be guided by considerations of achieving or maintaining the homogeneity of variance across several groups (Ferguson & Takane, 1989). If skew, kurtosis, or homogeneity of variance problems do not exist in a particular set of data, no transformations need be performed.

In addition to response size, one can also measure temporal characteristics of the SCR including onset latency, rise time, and half recovery time. These temporal characteristics of the SCR waveform are not as commonly reported as magnitude, and their relationship to psychophysiological processes is not as well understood at this time. The possibility that SCR recovery time, for example, can provide information independent of other EDA measures and is uniquely responsive to specific psychophysiological processes was suggested by Edelberg (1972b), but was questioned by Bundy and Fitzgerald (1975), and remains unsettled (Fowles, 1986, pp. 84–87; Edelberg, 1993, pp. 14–15). This is not to say that SCR recovery time is without discriminating power; rather, only that its qualitatively different informational properties relative to other EDA components is an open issue.

The usual constellation of EDA components is for high SCL, frequent NS-SCRs, large SCR amplitude, short latency, short rise time, and short recovery time to cluster together. However, the correlations among the EDA components generally are not very high, usually less than .60 (Lockhart & Lieberman, 1979; Venables & Christie, 1980; Schell, Dawson, & Filion, 1988). The size and consistency of these relationships are compatible with the hypothesis that many of the EDA components may represent partially independent sources of information although, as indicated above with SCR recovery time, this is an unsettled hypothesis. The one exception to the modest relationships among EDA components is the consistently high correlation between SCR rise time and recovery time. Based on this relationship, Venables and Christie (1980) suggest that SCR rise time and half recovery time may be essentially redundant measures and, that because recovery time is not always as available as rise time (because of subsequent responses), rise time may be the preferred measure.

A problem with quantifying the SCR components occurs when the response to be scored is elicited immediately after a preceding response that has not had time to fully recover. It is customary to measure the amplitude of each response from its own individual deflection point (Grings & Lockhart, 1965; Edelberg, 1967). However, the amplitude and the temporal characteristics of the second response are distorted by being superimposed on the recovery of the first response. For example, the measurable amplitude of the second response will be smaller given its occurrence following the first response. The amount of distortion of the second response is a function of the size of the first response and the time since the first response (Grings & Schell, 1969). Although there is no perfect solution to the response interference effect when hand-scoring EDA, it can be pointed out that response frequency may

be the least distorted component of the response in this situation. In addition, as mentioned earlier, one advantage of computerized scoring of EDA is the availability of more sophisticated scoring algorithms. In this regard, Lim et al. (1997) applied a multi-parameter curve-fitting algorithm to the scoring of overlapping skin conductance responses and they were able to decompose the overall response complex into meaningful components of the separate responses.

Another problem with quantifying the EDA components concerns the existence of large variability because of extraneous individual differences. Thus, whether an SCL of 8 μS is considered high, moderate, or low will depend upon that specific subject's range of SCLs. For example, one can see in Figure 7.4 that an SCL of 8 μS would be relatively low for the subject depicted in the upper tracing but would be relatively high for the subject depicted in the lower tracing. Similarly, an SCR of .5 μS may be relatively large for one person but relatively small for another. Lykken et al. (1966) proposed an interesting method to correct for this interindividual variance called range correction. The procedure involves computing the possible range for each individual subject and then expressing the subject's momentary value in terms of this range. For example, one may compute a subject's minimum SCL during a rest period and a maximum SCL while the subject blows a balloon to bursting; the subject's present SCL can then be expressed as a proportion of his/her individualized range according to the following formula: (SCL − SCLmin)/(SCLmax − SCLmin). The rationale underlying these procedures is that an individual's range of EDA is due mainly to physiological variables unrelated to psychological processes (e.g., thickness of the corneum). It is the variation within these physiological limits that is normally of psychological interest (Lykken & Venables, 1971).

Although the range correction procedure can reduce error variance and increase the power of statistical tests in some data sets, it also can be problematic in others. For example, range correction would be inappropriate in a situation where two groups being compared had different ranges (Lykken & Venables, 1971). Taking a different approach, Ben-Shakhar (1985) has recommended using within-subject standardized scores to adjust for individual differences because this transformation relies upon the mean, a more stable and reliable statistic than the maximum response. Although these techniques may be useful under some circumstances, most investigators simply compare average values of SCL and SCR across groups, or compare difference scores within a group (e.g., SCL during a task minus SCL during rest).

Another important aspect of elicited SCRs is their decline in amplitude and eventual disappearance with repetition of the eliciting stimulus (SCR habituation). Habituation is a ubiquitous and adaptive phenomenon whereby subjects become less responsive to familiar and nonsignificant stimuli. There are several methods of quantifying habituation of the SCR (Siddle, Stephenson, & Spinks, 1983). One simple method involves counting the number of stimulus repetitions required to reach some predetermined level of habituation (e.g., two or three consecutive trials without measurable SCRs). This "trials-to-habituation" measure is useful and has been widely employed since its use by Sokolov (1963), but it is subject to considerable distortion by the occurrence of a single response. For example, whether an isolated SCR occurs on trial 3 can make the difference between a trials-to-habituation score of "0" (indicative of an atypical nonresponder) and a "3" (indicative of a typical rate of habituation).

Another common measure of habituation is based on the rate of decline of SCR magnitude across trials as assessed by a "trials" main effect or interaction effect within an analysis of variance. However, this measure does not provide information about habituation in individual subjects and moreover can be distorted by differences in initial levels of responding.

A third measure of habituation is based on the regression of SCR magnitude on the log of the trial number (Lader & Wing, 1966; Montague, 1963). The regression approach provides a slope and an intercept score (the latter reflecting initial response amplitude), which are usually highly correlated with each other. Covariance procedures have been used to remove the dependency of slope on intercept, providing what Montague (1963) has called an "absolute rate of habituation." However, this technique rests on the assumptions that slope and intercept reflect different underlying processes and that the treatment effects under investigation do not significantly affect the intercepts (Siddle et al., 1983). Use of the slope measure also assumes that subjects respond on a sufficient number of trials to compute a meaningful slope, which may not be the case for some types of subjects with mild innocuous stimuli. Nevertheless, to the extent that these assumptions can be justified, the slope measure is often preferable because: (1) unlike the analysis of variance approach, individual habituation scores can be derived, (2) unlike the trials-to-habituation measure, isolated SCRs have less of a contaminating effect, (3) unlike trials-to-habituation, the slope measure makes fuller use of the magnitude data, and (4) unlike trials-to-habituation, the slope measure can discriminate between subjects who show varying degrees of habituation but who fail to completely stop responding for two or three consecutive trials.

The temporal stability (test-retest reliability) of EDA measures such as the frequency of NS-SCRs, SCL, responsiveness to stimuli, and habituation have been fairly well investigated in normal healthy adults (see Freixa i Baque, 1983 for a discussion of early studies, and Schell et al., 2002, for a more recent review). Test-retest correlations for periods extending up to one year or more have ranged from approximately .40 to .75 for NS-SCR frequencies, from .40 to .85 for SCL, and from .30 to .80 for number of SCRs elicited by a series of repeated stimuli. Stability

of temporal measures (i.e., latency, rise time, etc.) is typically lower. Schell et al. (2002) found that as measures of overall responsiveness, simple counts of the number of SCRs elicited by a series of stimuli were more reliable than trials-to-habituation measures.

ADVANTAGES AND DISADVANTAGES OF THE USE OF EDA

When one is considering use of EDA as an indicator of some psychological state or process of interest, it is well to remember that in the great majority of situations, changes in electrodermal activity do not occur in isolation. Rather, they occur as part of a complex of responses mediated by the autonomic nervous system.

Experimental treatments that have the effect of increasing SCL and/or NS-SCR rate also are expected to generally increase heart rate level and blood pressure and to produce peripheral vasoconstriction, to mention a few of the more commonly measured autonomic responses (Engel, 1960; see Grings & Dawson, 1978). The response or responses chosen for monitoring by a particular investigator should reflect considerations such as those discussed in the following section.

For some researchers, EDA may be the response system of choice because, unlike most ANS responses, it provides a relatively direct and undiluted representation of sympathetic activity. As has been pointed out above, the neural control of the eccrine sweat glands is entirely under sympathetic control. Therefore, increases in SCL or the SCR are due to increased tonic or phasic sympathetic activation. In contrast, with heart rate as with most ANS functions (pupil diameter, gastric motility, and blood pressure), a change in activity in response to stimuli of psychological significance cannot be unambiguously laid to either sympathetic or parasympathetic activity; it may be due to either one or to a combination of both. Thus, the researcher who wishes an unalloyed measure of sympathetic activity may prefer to monitor EDA, whereas the experimenter who wishes a broader picture of both sympathetic and parasympathetic activity may prefer heart rate, if constraints of instrumentation will allow only one to be recorded. Similarly, if for some reason (perhaps the use of medication with side effects on cholinergic or adrenergic systems) one wishes to monitor a response which is predominately cholinergically mediated at the periphery but which is also influenced by sympathetic activity, then EDA would be the choice.

Another advantage of measuring SCR is that its occurrence is generally quite discriminable. Thus, on a single presentation of a stimulus, one can determine by quick inspection whether or not an SCR has occurred. In contrast, the presence of a heart rate response on single stimulus presentation may be difficult to distinguish from ongoing variability in heart rate that reflects changes in muscle tonus or respiratory sinus arrhythmia.

In addition to decisions made based on neuroanatomical control and basic response characteristics, an investigator may prefer EDA to other response systems because of the nature of the situation in which the subject is assessed. Fowles (1988) argued convincingly that heart rate is influenced primarily by activation of a neurophysiological behavioral activation system that is involved in responding during *appetitive* reward-seeking, to conditioned stimuli associated with reward, and during active avoidance. On the other hand, EDA is influenced primarily by activation of a neurophysiological behavioral *inhibition* system that is involved in responding to punishment, to passive avoidance, or to frustrative nonreward. This latter system is viewed as an anxiety system. Thus, if an investigator is studying the reaction of subjects to a situation or to discrete stimuli that elicit anxiety, but in which no active avoidance response can be made, the electrodermal system should be the physiological system that is most responsive.

For many investigators, an additional advantage of the use of EDA relative to other response systems is that of all forms of ANS activity, individual differences in EDA appear to be most reliably associated with psychopathological states. The correlates of some of these stable EDA differences between individuals are discussed in the following section.

Finally, it is important to note that, in comparison to many other psychophysiological measures, EDA is relatively inexpensive to record. After initial purchase of the recording system, expenses for each subject are trivial, involving electrode collars and paste and the occasional replacement of electrodes. Electrical shielding of the room in which the subject sits which is generally needed for noise-free recording of EEG or event related potentials is unnecessary, and the costs of using EDA as a response measure are minuscule compared to those of hemodynamic techniques such as PET scans or functional MRI. Furthermore, the techniques used to record EDA are completely harmless and risk-free, and thus they can be used with young children and in research designs that require repeated testing at short intervals of time.

There are also potential disadvantages to the use of EDA as a dependent measure. First, EDA is a relatively slow-moving response system. As mentioned previously, the latency of the elicited SCR is between 1.0 and 3.0 s, and tonic shifts in SCL produced by changes in arousal and alertness require approximately the same time to occur. Thus, an investigator who is interested in tracking very rapidly occurring processes, or stages within a complex process, may not find EDA useful. Although the SCR cannot index such rapidly occurring processes as sensory gating or stages of stimulus analysis on a real-time basis, it has been found to be correlated with real-time measures of these processes. For example, Lyytinen, Blomberg, and Näätänen (1992) observed that the parietal P3a was larger when an SCR was elicited by a novel tone than when no SCR was elicited.

Another potential disadvantage is that EDA has multiple causes; the elicited SCR is not specific to a single type of event or situation (as, for instance, the N400 ERP component appears to be specifically influenced by semantic expectancy, Kutas, 1997). However, the multiple influences on EDA may actually be as much an advantage as a disadvantage. As described throughout this chapter, EDA can be used to index a number of processes: activation, attention, and significance or affective intensity of a stimulus. In using EDA as a response measure, one must take care to control experimental conditions – that is, be sure that one is varying only one process that may influence EDA at a time. Such experimental control is essential for all attempts to draw clear inferences from results, whether one is recording EDA, electrocortical activity, or a hemodynamic measure, given the number of processes that may influence these measures as well.

Thus, like any single response system, EDA has distinct advantages and disadvantages. The ideal situation, of course, is one in which the researcher can record more than one response measure. When ANS activity is of primary interest, EDA and heart rate are probably the two most common choices: EDA for its neuroanatomical simplicity, trial-by-trial visibility, and utility as a general arousal/attention indicator and heart rate for its potential differentiation of other psychological and physiological states of interest to the researcher.

PSYCHOLOGICAL AND SOCIAL CONTEXT

In this section, we review the psychological and social factors that have been shown to influence EDA in three types of paradigm: (1) those that involve the presentation of discrete stimuli, (2) those that involve the presentation of continuous stimuli, and (3) those that involve examining the correlates of individual differences in EDA.

Effects of discrete stimuli. Properties of stimuli to which the SCR is sensitive are wide and varied: they include stimulus novelty, surprise, intensity, arousal content, and significance. It might be argued that, because EDA is sensitive to such a wide variety of stimuli, it is not a clearly interpretable measure of any particular psychological process (Landis, 1930). This view is certainly correct in the sense that it is impossible to identify an isolated SCR as an "anxiety" response, or an "anger" response, or an "attentional" response. However, the psychological meaning of an SCR becomes interpretable by taking into account the stimulus condition or experimental paradigm in which the SCR occurred. The better controlled the experimental paradigm, the more conclusive the interpretation. That is, by having only one aspect of the stimulus change across conditions (e.g., task significance) while eliminating other differences (e.g., stimulus novelty, intensity, etc.), then one can more accurately infer the psychological processes mediating the resultant SCR. As we will illustrate in the following discussion, the inference of a specific psychophysiological process requires knowledge of both a well controlled stimulus situation and a carefully measured response.

One discrete stimulus paradigm that relies on the SCR's sensitivity to stimulus significance is the so-called Guilty Knowledge Test (GKT), which is a type of detection of deception test ("lie detection"). The GKT, also sometimes referred to as a "Concealed Knowledge Test," involves recording SCRs (as well as other physiological responses) while presenting subjects with a series of multiple-choice questions (Lykken, 1959). For example, a suspect in a burglary case might be asked to answer "no" to each of the alternatives given for a question concerning details about the burglary. For each question, the correct alternative would be intermixed among other plausible alternatives. The theory behind the technique is that the correct answer to each question will be more psychologically significant to a guilty subject than will the other alternatives, whereas for the innocent subject all of the alternatives would be of equal significance. Therefore, the guilty subject is expected to respond electrodermally more to the correct alternatives, whereas the innocent subject is expected to respond randomly (Lykken, 1959). Lykken (1981) suggested that guilty subjects can be detected nearly 90% of the time and that innocent subjects can be correctly classified nearly 100% of the time with a properly constructed GKT. For a discussion of the differing views of psychophysiological techniques of detecting deception, see Iacono (Chapter 29 in this volume).

Tranel, Fowles, and Damasio (1985) developed another type of discrete stimulus paradigm with which to study the effects of significant stimuli. SCRs were recorded from normal college students while being presented a set of slides depicting faces of famous people (e.g., Ronald Reagan, Bob Hope, etc.) interspersed among a larger number of faces of unfamiliar people. Subjects were instructed simply to sit quietly and look at each slide. The results revealed that the average SCR was much larger to slides of significant faces ($M = 1.26$ μS) than to the nonsignificant faces ($M = .19$ μS).

Although the GKT of Lykken (1959) appears to be quite adequate to detect concealed information (and hence the guilty person), and the paradigm of Tranel et al. (1985) appears adequate to test for recognition of famous faces, one may question whether either paradigm is sufficient to demonstrate the effect of stimulus significance per se on the SCR. It may be argued that both paradigms confounded relative novelty with relative stimulus significance. If guilty subjects dichotomize items into relevant and irrelevant categories in the GKT (Ben-Shakhar, 1977), then the relevant category is presented less often than the irrelevant category and this relative novelty may contribute to the differential SCRs. Likewise, in the studies using slides of famous faces, the significant category of stimuli was presented less often than the nonsignificant category and this difference in relative novelty may have contributed to the differential SCRs. The number of presentations of relevant/significant stimuli should have been equal to that of irrelevant/nonsignificant stimuli in order to unambiguously demonstrate the effect of stimulus signifi-

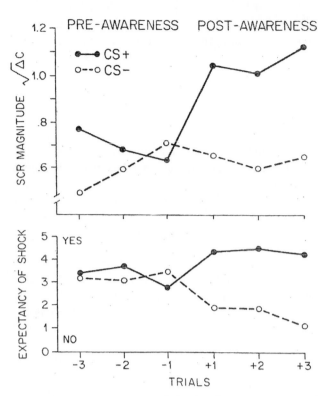

Figure 7.6. Mean SCR magnitude (top) and mean expectancy of shock (bottom) to the reinforced conditioned stimulus (CS+) and the nonreinforced conditioned stimulus (CS−) on three pre-aware and three post-aware trials (Adapted from Dawson & Biferno, 1973).

cance on SCRs. As mentioned earlier in this section, close control over stimulus properties (in this case, novelty and significance) is necessary in order to infer the psychological processes eliciting the SCR. Interestingly, using a modification of the GKT in which relevant and irrelevant items were presented equally often, Verschuere et al. (2004) have found evidence that responses to relevant items remain greater than to irrelevant items. These findings demonstrate the importance of stimulus significance in eliciting SCRs above and beyond novelty.

Another discrete stimulus paradigm in which EDA is commonly measured that highlights the influence of stimulus significance while controlling for stimulus novelty involves discrimination classical conditioning (Grings & Dawson, 1973). For example, Dawson and Biferno (1973) employed a discrimination classical conditioning paradigm in which college student subjects were asked to rate their expectancy of a brief electric shock (unconditioned stimulus, UCS) following each presentation of a CS+ (a conditioned stimulus regularly followed by the shock) and a CS−(a control stimulus never followed by shock). Tones of 800 Hz and 1200 Hz were presented equally often and served as the reinforced CS+ and the nonreinforced CS−, counterbalanced across subjects. Thus, on each conditioning trial, the subject's expectancy of shock and the associated SCR were recorded. The results, shown in Figure 7.6, revealed that subjects tended to respond equally to the reinforced CS+ and to the nonreinforced CS− until they became aware of the contingency between the conditioned stimuli and the shock. There was no evidence of SCR discrimination conditioning prior to the development of awareness; however, once the subject became aware, the CS+ became more significant than the CS−, and there was an abrupt increase in the magnitude of the SCRs elicited by the CS+. Moreover, SCR discrimination conditioning fails to occur when CS-UCS pairings are embedded in distracting tasks that effectively prevent subjects from becoming aware of the critical stimulus relations (see reviews by Dawson & Schell, 1985; Lovibond & Shanks, 2001). These results suggest that awareness of the CS-UCS relation is necessary for human discrimination SCR conditioning.

The conditions under which subjects must be consciously aware of the stimulus significance in order to elicit SCR ORs is a topic of considerable research. For example, SCR discrimination conditioning has been reported to occur without subjects becoming aware of the CS-UCS relationship under special circumstances when "prepared" stimulus relationships are conditioned. The concept of "preparedness" is that certain stimulus associations (e.g., taste with nausea and snakes with pain) are more quickly, easily, and automatically learned than are others (e.g., an arbitrary tone and a shock) and are more resistant to extinction because they have been correlated in our evolutionary past (Seligman, 1970).

Öhman and his colleagues, in an interesting series of studies beginning in the 1970s, extended Seligman's concept to human autonomic conditioning, using types of CSs that have been termed biologically prepared, potentially phobic, or fear-relevant: pictures of spiders, snakes, and angry faces (see Öhman, 1992 for reviews). In the early studies of this series, Öhman and his colleagues demonstrated that SCRs conditioned with fear-relevant CSs and a shock UCS were more resistant to extinction than were SCRs conditioned with neutral CS-UCS relations (pictures of flowers or happy faces as CSs associated with shock). Such SCRs also were more resistant to cognitive manipulations such as extinction instructions informing subjects that the UCS would no longer be delivered (Hugdahl & Öhman, 1977) and were retained past the point of cognitive extinction (no greater expectancy of the UCS after the CS+ than after the CS−) following the presentation of many nonreinforced trials (Schell, Dawson, & Marinkovic, 1991).

In later studies of this series, backward masking was used to prevent awareness of the CS-UCS relation by preventing conscious recognition of the fear-relevant CSs. In this paradigm, visual CSs are presented very briefly (30 ms) and immediately followed by a masking stimulus. These procedures prevent recognition of the CSs in the vast majority of subjects on the vast majority of trials (Öhman, Dimberg, & Esteves, 1989a).

Backwardly masked angry and happy faces have been used as CSs during acquisition (Esteves et al., 1994). In one group, a masked angry face (CS+) was paired with shock, whereas in another group a masked happy face (CS+) was paired with shock. During subsequent extinction, unmasked CSs were presented and conditioned SCRs were elicited to the previously masked angry face CS+, but not to the happy face CS+. Thus, electrodermal conditioning was established "nonconsciously" to a threatening angry face, but not to a friendly smiling face. Conditioning to other masked biologically fear-relevant CSs was replicated in subsequent experiments by Öhman and Soares (1998) using pictures of snakes and spiders rather than angry faces. Studies using functional brain imaging techniques have replicated these SCR results and demonstrated the importance of the amygdala, extended regions of the amygdala complex, and sensory cortex in such conditioning (Morris, Buchel, & Dolan, 2001).

Studies of brain damaged patients also indicate that the amygdala is critical for SCR classical conditioning. For example, Bechara et al. (1995) found that a patient with selective bilateral destruction of the amygdala did show unconditioned SCRs to the unconditioned stimulus but did not show SCR conditioning to the CS, although this patient was aware of the CS-UCS relation. A different patient with bilateral hippocampi damage (but intact amygdala) showed both conditioned and unconditioned SCRs but could not describe the CS-UCS relation. All in all, contrary to the results shown in Figure 7.6, these findings indicate that SCR conditioned responses may be acquired without the subjects' awareness of the CS-UCS relation in some circumstances. The nature of these circumstances (only with biologically prepared fear-relevant stimuli or with certain types of brain damage?) is a topic of ongoing research.

SCRs elicited by discrete nonaversive stimuli are generally considered to be part of the orienting response to novel or significant stimuli. We believe that the data reviewed in this section can be interpreted within this theoretical setting. The task of subjects exposed to the GKT is to deceive or conceal knowledge, and the correct item is more relevant to this task than are incorrect alternative items. Thus, subjects orient more to the task-significant items than the task-nonsignificant items. Verschuere et al. (2004) found greater heart rate deceleration following relevant items than irrelevant items in a GKT which is consistent with the orienting hypothesis. Likewise, faces of famous people may be perceived as more significant than the faces of unfamiliar people, and the signal of an impending shock (CS+) is more significant than the signal of no shock (CS−). Thus, the results observed here are consistent with the notion that the SCR is highly sensitive to stimulus significance, even under certain conditions where the reasons for that significance may not be consciously processed.

There have been several models proposed to account for the elicitation of autonomic ORs such as the SCR (see Siddle et al., 1983, for a review). For example, an influential information processing model has been proposed by

Öhman (1979). This model distinguishes between automatic preattentive processing and controlled capacity-limited processing. Autonomic orienting is elicited when the preattentive mechanisms call for additional controlled processing. According to this model, there are two conditions under which this call is made. First, the call is made and the OR is elicited when the preattentive mechanisms fail to identify the incoming stimulus because there is no matching representation in short-term memory. Thus, the OR is sensitive to stimulus novelty. Second, the call is made and the OR is elicited when the preattentive mechanisms recognize the stimulus as significant. Thus, the OR represents a transition from automatic to controlled processing based on preliminary preattentive analysis of stimulus novelty and stimulus significance. This model allows for the possibility that the OR may be elicited without conscious awareness. Others, however, have suggested that the OR occurs when controlled processing resources are actually allocated to the processing of the stimulus, at least where fear-irrelevant stimuli are concerned (Dawson, Filion, & Schell, 1989; Öhman, 1992).

Other discrete stimuli capable of eliciting SCRs are those with either strong positive or negative affective valence. We orient to stimuli that are significant because they are either very positive or very negative in terms of the emotional response that they elicit. However, unlike responses such as the startle eyeblink, the SCR does not distinguish arousing positive stimuli from equally arousing negative stimuli. Lang, Bradley, Cuthbert, and their colleagues have developed a set of widely used pictures (the International Affective Picture System, IAPS, Lang, Bradley, & Cuthbert, 1998; see Chapter 25, this volume) that are rated for both their arousal–producing quality and valence on a strongly positive to strongly negative scale. SCRs elicited by these pictures have reliably been found to be related to the arousal dimension, with responses increasing in magnitude as arousal rating increased for both positively valenced pictures (greater for erotic pictures than for beautiful flowers) and negatively valenced pictures (greater for striking snakes than for tombstones in a cemetery) (Lang et al., 1993; Cuthbert, Bradley, & Lang, 1996).

Other affective stimuli hypothesized to evoke SCRs are those associated with internal processes involved in making decisions. Damasio (1994) proposed a "somatic marker" hypothesis, the main point of which is that decision-making is influenced by emotional somatic responses. The somatic marker hypothesis has been tested by measuring SCRs during a gambling task (Bechara et al., 1997). In this task subjects select cards from "bad" decks that can yield high immediate financial gain but large long-term losses, or from "good" decks that yield lower immediate gain but a larger long-term gain. After encountering a few losses, normal subjects, as opposed to brain damaged patients, generate SCRs in anticipation of selecting cards from the "bad" deck and begin to avoid selecting cards from that deck. These results were originally interpreted as indicating that SCRs in response to decision-

making processes reflect somatic markers that help the person make advantageous decisions even before conscious knowledge of the rules of the game was available. However, more recent research suggests that, in fact, subjects may have considerable conscious understanding of the game (Maia & McClelland, 2004) and this suggests that the SCR may only indicate when a person has consciously decided to make a risky decision.

In conclusion, in this section we have described some of the discrete stimulus paradigms in which EDA is most often measured and has proven to be most useful. We have emphasized that determining the psychological meaning of any particular SCR is dependent on a well-controlled stimulus situation. In addition, we have described a theoretical model that may be used to account for the SCRs elicited in the paradigms described. Finally, these areas of research examining the SCR to discrete stimuli underscore the point made previously that one advantage of the SCR is that the response can easily be measured on individual presentations of a stimulus. Thus, one may determine whether the response to a "guilty" relevant stimulus in a group of stimuli is greater than that to "innocent" irrelevant stimuli, whether the SCR elicited by a CS+ is greater on the first trial after awareness of the CS-UCS relationship occurs than on the last trial before that awareness occurs, whether the SCR elicited by a fear-relevant CS+ is greater than the SCR elicited by a CS− on the first trial pair following extinction instructions, whether the eliciting stimulus is highly arousing due to affective valence of either a positive or negative nature, and whether arousal states that occur during decision-making guide decisions when risk is involved.

Effects of continuous stimuli. We turn now to an examination of the effects of more chronic, long-lasting stimuli or situations as opposed to the brief, discrete stimuli reviewed above. Chronic stimuli might best be thought of as modulating increases and decreases in tonic arousal. Hence, the most useful electrodermal measures in the context of continuous stimuli are SCL and frequency of NS-SCRs, because they can be measured on an ongoing basis over relatively long periods of time.

One type of continuous stimulus situation that will reliably produce increases in electrodermal activity involves the necessity of performing a task. The anticipation and performance of practically any task will increase both SCL and the frequency of NS-SCRs, at least initially. For example, Lacey et al. (1963) recorded palmar SCL during rest and during the anticipation and performance of eight different tasks. The tasks ranged from those requiring close attention to *external* stimuli, such as listening to an irregularly fluctuating loud white noise, to those requiring close attention to *internal* information processing, such as solving mental arithmetic problems. The impressive finding for present purposes was that SCL increased in each and every one of the task situations. Typically, SCL increased about one μS above resting level during anticipation and then increased another one or two μS during performance of the task. Heart rate, unlike SCL, discriminated between tasks involving attention to external stimuli and tasks requiring attention to internal information processing.

Munro et al. (1988) observed that large increases in SCL and NS-SCR frequency were induced by a different task-significant situation. In this case, college student subjects were tested during a five-minute rest period and then during performance of a continuous vigilance task. The task stimuli consisted of a series of digits presented visually at a rapid rate of one-per-s with exposure duration of 48 ms; the subject's task was to press a button whenever the digit "0" was presented. Both the number of NS-SCRs and SCL initially increased sharply from the resting levels during this demanding task and then gradually declined as the task continued.

The finding that electrodermal activity is reliably elevated during task performance suggests that tonic EDA can be a useful index of a process related to "energy regulation" or "energy mobilization." An information processing interpretation of this finding might be that tasks require an effortful allocation of attentional resources and that this is associated with heightened autonomic activation (Jennings, 1986). A different, but not necessarily mutually exclusive, explanation would invoke the concepts of stress and affect rather than attention and effortful allocation of resources. According to this view, laboratory tasks are challenging stressors, and a reliable physiological response to stressors is increased sympathetic activation, particularly EDA arousal.

Situations in which strong emotions are elicited also increase tonic EDA arousal, as would be expected from the finding discussed above that SCR magnitude is affected by the arousal value of discrete stimuli with emotional valence. In a classic experiment, Ax (1953) created genuine states of fear and anger in his subjects by causing them to feel in danger of a high-voltage shock due to equipment malfunction or by treating them in a rude and inconsiderate fashion. SCL, number of NS-SCRs, and several other measures of sympathetic nervous system activity rose during both the fear and the anger conditions, with the patterns for fear and anger differing to some degree (SCL rose more in fear than in anger, while NS-SCRs and diastolic blood pressure rose more in anger than in fear.) More recently, Levenson, Gross, and their colleagues have used films in a number of studies to elicit emotional states, primarily disgust, lasting for a minute or more (Gross & Levenson, 1993; Gross, 1998). SCL and other measures of sympathetic activation in these studies were higher during the films than during a baseline period, and the rise in SCL was influenced by the emotional regulation strategy that subjects were instructed to use. Subjects instructed to suppress their facial display of emotion, to try to behave as though anyone observing them would not know what they were feeling, showed greater increases in SCL than subjects who simply watched the films or who were instructed to reappraise what they were seeing, to watch the film with a detached, objective, and unemotional attitude.

Social stimulation constitutes another class of continuous stimuli that generally produces increases in EDA arousal. Social situations are ones in which the concepts of stress and affect are most often invoked. For example, early research related EDA recorded during psychotherapeutic interviews to concepts such as "tension" and "anxiety" on the part of both patient and therapist (Boyd & DiMascio, 1954; Dittes, 1957). In one such study, Dittes (1957) measured the frequency of NS-SCRs of a patient during 42 hours of psychotherapy. The results of this study indicated that the frequency of NS-SCRs was inversely related to the judged permissiveness of the therapist, and Dittes concluded that EDA reflects "the anxiety of the patient, or his 'mobilization' against any cue threatening punishment by the therapist" (p. 303).

Schwartz and Shapiro (1973) reviewed several areas of social psychophysiology up to 1970, including those in which EDA was measured during social interactions. These are situations in which intense cognitive and affective reaction may occur, precipitating large changes in EDA and other physiological responses. In a series of social psychophysiological studies conducted since the Schwartz and Shapiro review, EDA was recorded during marital social interactions (Levenson & Gottman, 1983; 1985). The researchers measured SCL (in addition to heart rate, pulse transmission time, and somatic activity) from married couples while they discussed conflict-laden problem areas. It was found that couples from distressed marriages had high "physiological linkage"; that is, there were greater correlations between husbands' and wives' physiological reactions in distressed marriages than those in satisfying marriages during the discussions of problem areas. Moreover, greater physiological arousal, including higher SCL, during the interactions and during baselines was associated with a decline in marital satisfaction over the ensuing three years.

Another series of studies related the effects of stressful social interactions on EDA to relapse among schizophrenia patients. It has been well documented that patients are at increased risk for relapse if their relatives are critical, hostile, or emotionally overinvolved with them at the time of their illness (Brown, Birley, & Wing, 1972; Vaughn & Leff, 1976; Vaughn et al., 1984). The term *expressed emotion* (EE) is used to designate this continuum of affective attitudes ranging from low-EE (less critical) to high-EE (more critical) on the part of the relative.

It has been hypothesized that heightened autonomic arousal may be a mediating factor between the continued exposure to a high-EE relative and the increased risk of symptomatic relapse (Turpin, 1983). According to this notion, living with a high-EE family member produces excessive stress and autonomic hyper-arousal. Autonomic hyper-arousal has been characterized as one of several transient intermediate states that can produce deterioration in the patient's behavior, which in turn can negatively affect people around the patient. Hence, a vicious cycle can be created whereby the increased arousal causes changes in the patient's behavior that have an aggravating effect on the social environment, which then serves to further increase autonomic arousal. Unless such a cycle is broken, (e.g., by removal from that social environment), it can lead to the return of schizophrenia symptoms and a clinical relapse (Dawson, Nuechterlein, & Liberman, 1983; Nuechterlein & Dawson, 1984).

One prediction derived from this model is that patients exposed to high-EE relatives should show heightened sympathetic arousal compared to patients exposed to low-EE relatives. The first study to test this prediction obtained rather clear confirmatory results (Tarrier et al., 1979). These investigators measured the EDA of remitted patients living in the community whose relatives' level of EE had been determined by Vaughn and Leff (1976). Patients were tested for 15 minutes without the key relative and for 15 minutes with the key relative present. The frequency of NS-SCR activity of the patients with high-EE relatives and low-EE relatives did not differ when the relative was absent from the testing room, but if the key relative was present then patients with high-EE relatives exhibited higher rates of NS-SCRs than did patients with low-EE relatives. These results indicate that the presence of high-EE and low-EE relatives have differential effects on EDA which are consistent with the hypothesis that differential autonomic arousal plays a mediating role in the differential relapse rates of the two patient groups. More complete reviews of these studies and their implications can be found in Turpin, Tarrier, and Sturgeon (1988).

Individual differences in EDA. We have discussed the utility of EDA as a dependent variable reflecting situational levels of arousal/activation or attentiveness/responsiveness to individual stimuli. In this section we consider EDA as a relatively stable trait of the individual, as an individual difference variable. Individual differences in EDA are reliably associated with behavioral differences and psychopathological states of some importance, and we will examine some of these.

Individual differences in the rate of NS-SCRs and the rate of SCR habituation have been used to define a trait called "electrodermal lability" (Mundy-Castle & McKiever, 1953; Lacey & Lacey, 1958; Crider, 1993). Electrodermal "labiles" are subjects who show high rates of NS-SCRs and/or slow SCR habituation, whereas electrodermal "stabiles" are those who show few NS-SCRs and/or fast SCR habituation. Electrodermal lability is an individual trait that has been found to be relatively reliable over time, and labiles differ from stabiles with respect to a number of psychophysiological variables, including measures of both electrodermal and cardiovascular responsiveness (Kelsey, 1991; Schell, Dawson, & Filion, 1988). In this section, we review behavioral and psychological differences associated with this individual difference in both normal and abnormal populations.

Electrodermal lability is a trait of interest in psychological research in part because many investigators have reported that labiles outperform stabiles on tasks which require sustained vigilance. When individuals perform a signal detection task that is sustained over time, deterioration across time in the accurate detection of targets is frequently observed, a phenomenon referred to as vigilance decrement (Davies & Parasuraman, 1982). Several experimenters have reported that when vigilance decrement occurs, it is more pronounced among electrodermal stabiles than among labiles. This appears to be particularly true when EDA lability is defined by differences in SCR OR habituation rate (Koelega, 1990). As time on the task goes by, labiles are apparently better able to keep attention focused on the task and to avoid a decline in performance (Crider & Augenbraun, 1975; Hastrup, 1979; Munro et al., 1987; Vossel & Rossman, 1984). With a difficult continuous performance task, Munro et al., for instance, whose study was mentioned above, found that stabiles showed a significant decrement over time in performance, whereas labiles did not. The degree of task-induced sympathetic arousal as measured by increases in NS-SCR rate was negatively correlated across subjects with performance decrement.

Researchers investigating these sorts of behavioral differences between electrodermal stabiles and labiles have concluded that lability reflects the ability to allocate information processing capacity to stimuli that are to be attended (Lacey & Lacey, 1958; Katkin, 1975; Schell et al., 1988). As Katkin (1975, p. 172) concluded, "electrodermal activity is a personality variable that reflects individual differences in higher central processes involved in attending to and processing information." Viewing electrodermal lability in this way suggests that labiles should differ from stabiles in a variety of information processing tasks. Consistent with this view, EDA labile children have been found to generally outperform stabiles on a variety of tasks that require perceptual speed and vigilance (Sakai, Baker, & Dawson, 1992).

In addition to the differences between stabiles and labiles in the normal population, reliable abnormalities in electrodermal lability are associated with diagnosable psychopathology. We will next summarize EDA abnormalities reported in schizophrenia and psychopathy. A more general discussion of psychophysiological abnormalities in these and other psychopathologies can be found in Hicks, Keller, and Miller (Chapter 28, this volume).

In general two types of electrodermal abnormalities have been reported in different subgroups of patients with schizophrenia. First, between 40% and 50% of schizophrenia patients fail to show any SCR orienting responses to mild innocuous tones (termed "nonresponders"), compared to approximately 10% nonresponders in the normal population (see reviews by Bernstein et al., 1982; Dawson & Nuechterlein, 1984; Iacono, Ficken, & Beiser, 1993; Öhman, 1981). The high proportion of electrodermal non-responders in schizophrenia has been a reliable finding across studies. For example, Bernstein et al. (1982) examined a series of 14 related studies in which samples of American, British, and German schizophrenia patients and normal controls were tested using a common methodology and response scoring criteria. The consistent finding was that approximately 50% of the patients were non-responders, compared to only 5 to 10% of controls. (More recent data reported and reviewed by Venables and Mitchell (1996) suggest the percentage of SCR non-responders in normal groups may be closer to 25%.)

The second electrodermal abnormality, found in the "responder" subgroup of patients, is the presence of higher than normal levels of tonic arousal, indicated by high SCLs and a high frequency of NS-SCRS (Dawson & Nuechterlein, 1984; Dawson, Nuechterlein, & Schell 1992a; Öhman, 1981). In effect, the nonresponder group is characterized by hyporesponsivity to stimuli whereas the responder group is characterized by tonic hyperarousal. Both types of abnormalities have been found to be reliable across time. For example, in a group of 56 chronic schizophrenia patients classified as nonresponders on an initial test, 87% remained nonresponders two weeks later and 91% were nonresponders four weeks later (Spohn et al., 1989). In a group of 29 schizophrenia nonresponder outpatients, 62% remained nonresponders one year later (Schell et al., 2002). The tonic measures of SCL and NS-SCRs also remained relatively stable over a one-year period in the schizophrenia outpatients (test-retest rs = .43 and .53 respectively). The latter test-retest correlations, although significant, are in the lower end of the range of correlations found over similar time intervals with normal subjects that were reviewed earlier, possibly because of fluctuating symptoms among the patients.

The hope associated with the identification of responder and nonresponder EDA subgroups is that it will identify meaningful subgroups in terms of different symptomatic types of schizophrenia or different prognoses, or that one or both abnormalities might constitute a vulnerability marker for schizophrenia. Unfortunately, the results relating EDA abnormalities with current symptoms, future prognosis, and vulnerability have not always been consistent. As we point out later, the reasons for these inconsistencies may have to do with different populations of patients and control comparison groups.

Nonresponder and responder subgroups of patients have been reported by some investigators to show different symptomatology at the time of testing, with responders generally displaying more symptoms of excitement, anxiety, manic behavior, and belligerence, whereas nonresponders tend to show more emotional withdrawal, conceptual disorganization, and negative symptoms (e.g., Bernstein et al., 1981; Straube, 1979; Fuentes et al., 1993). Furthermore, SCR hypo-responsivity has been related to a more severe form of illness (Katsanis & Iacono, 1994), poor premorbid adjustment (Öhman et al., 1989), and more psychiatric symptoms overall (positive and negative) (Green, Nuechterlein, & Satz, 1989; Kim et al., 1993). Other investigators, however, have found the hyper-aroused responders to display the greater level of overall symptomatology (Brekke et al., 1997; Dawson et al., 1992b).

Abnormally elevated EDA arousal also has been found particularly during periods of psychotic symptomatology, compared to the same patients during periods of remission (Dawson et al., 1994) (see Figure 7.7). Moreover, heightened EDA arousal has been found to occur within a few weeks prior to an impending psychotic relapse, compared to control periods of stable remission within the same patients (Hazlett et al., 1997). This finding is consistent with a theoretical model that hypothesizes that heightened sympathetic activation is associated with a "transient intermediate state" that precedes psychotic episodes in vulnerable individuals (Nuechterlein & Dawson, 1984). According to this theoretical model, not all such intermediate states will necessarily be followed by psychotic exacerbation or relapse. Rather, these states constitute periods of heightened vulnerability with an increased risk of relapse, with the actual occurrence of relapses or exacerbation being influenced by environmental stressors.

Results regarding prediction of outcome also have been somewhat inconsistent. The predominant finding is that EDA hyperarousal is associated with poor short-term symptomatic prognosis (Brekke, Raine, & Thomson, 1995; Frith et al., 1979; Zahn, Carpenter, & McGlashan, 1981; Dawson et al., 1992b; see review by Dawson & Schell, 2002). However, a minority of studies have reported that EDA hyporesponsivity, not hyperarousal, is associated with poor prognosis. The typical procedure in these short-term studies was to relate EDA recorded during rest and simple orienting tasks from schizophrenia patients initially while in symptomatic states and then relate the EDA measures to subsequent persistence of the symptoms weeks or months later. In a longer-term study (Tarrier & Barrowclough, 1989), the number of NS-SCRs and the regression slopes of SCL measured during interactions with relatives at the time the patients were hospitalized were found to be related to symptomatic relapse over the next two years. The direction of the effect, greater frequency of NS-SCRs and greater rise in SCL among the patients who later relapsed, is consistent with the notion that high EDA arousal is predictive of prognosis. These results are consistent with the hypothesis that patients at high risk of relapse have a predisposition to autonomic hyperarousal to certain environmental or social stimuli.

The studies of prognosis reviewed above relied primarily upon measures of psychotic symptoms or hospital readmission. However, there are some studies that have measured prognosis as functional outcome, such as holding a job or having friends, instead of psychotic symptoms. Öhman et al. (1989b) reported that skin conductance nonresponding and lower levels of tonic EDA activity taken at the beginning of a follow-up period predicted poor social and employment outcome over a two-year period in a subgroup of male schizophrenia patients. Their outcome criteria combined the employment and social-contact outcome

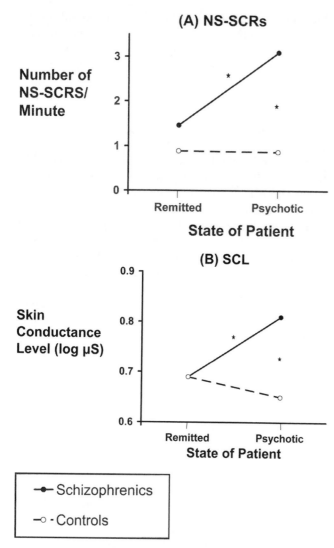

Figure 7.7. (A) Mean number of nonspecific SCRs per minute and (B) mean log SCL obtained from normal controls and patients with schizophrenia when the patients were in remitted and psychotic states. Asterisks indicate significant differences (Adapted from Dawson et al., 1994).

ing mechanisms in ways that exacerbate vulnerabilities in the areas of social competence and coping. These exacerbated cognitive and social deficits may then create a vicious cycle by feedback to the social environment with eventual symptomatic relapse (Dawson, Nuechterlein, & Liberman, 1983; Nuechterlein & Dawson, 1984).

Schell et al. (2005) also raised the possibility that both EDA abnormalities in patients with schizophrenia (nonresponsiveness and hyperarousal) may predict poor outcome. Whether a particular study finds nonresponders or responders to have the poorer outcome may depend upon whether the sample as a whole is more or less responsive or aroused than normal. Many of the studies reviewed above did not include comparison of patients to normal controls, instead selecting their EDA subgroups based solely on the distribution within the patient group. However, interesting differences are present among those that did report comparisons to normal. For example, Öhman et al. (1989), who reported poorer functional outcome among nonresponders, had a sample of patients who were much more likely to be nonresponders and to have lower SCL than normal controls. However, Wieselgren et al. (1994) and Schell et al. (2005), both of whom reported poor outcome associated with the hyperaroused responders, had groups of patients who did not differ from normal on SCR responsivity but did as a whole have higher than normal EDA arousal. Thus, Öhman et al.'s more abnormal non-responders had the poorer outcome, whereas Wieselgren et al.'s and Schell et al.'s more abnormal hyper-aroused responders had the poorer outcome. It may be that either abnormality, hyporesponsivity or hyperarousal with respect to controls, is associated with poor outcome. Hyporesponsiveness may be associated with generally limited cognitive processing capacity, whereas hyperarousal may act to interfere with efficient processing as described above.

Finally, the issue of vulnerability to schizophrenia has been addressed in some EDA studies, again not always with consistent results, by examining first degree relatives of schizophrenia patients, usually the children of schizophrenia patients, who are not manifesting schizophrenic symtomatology. The most common finding in the early research using this methodology was abnormal hyperarousal and/or hyper-reactivity to aversive stimuli in the offspring of schizophrenia patients (see reviews by Dawson & Nuechterlein, 1984; Öhman, 1981). Subsequent research has generally supported this finding. For example, Hollister et al. (1994) found that the young offspring of schizophrenic patients have higher than normal frequency of NS-SCRs, and those who later developed schizophrenia tended to have the highest level of NS-SCRs. Iacono, Ficken, and Beiser (1999) also found a higher than normal rate of NS-SCRs in the responder first-degree relatives of patients with schizophrenia. However, the latter study reported the same abnormality in first degree relatives of patients with major depressive illness, a finding that suggests that electrodermal hyper-arousal may not be a vulnerability marker specific to schizophrenia.

criteria developed by Strauss and Carpenter (1974) into one outcome index. To have a "good" outcome, patients had to simultaneously have at least a minimal social life (meet with friends at least once a month) and had to be employed or enrolled in school at least on a part time basis. Conversely, Wieselgren et al. (1994), using an identical methodology to that used by Öhman et al. (1989b), reported an opposite relation for female schizophrenia patients, with high tonic electrodermal activity predicting poor social and work outcome. More recently Schell et al. (2005) used the same measure of outcome and reported results consistent with Wieselgren et al. That is, high SCL and NS-SCRs (as well as number of SCR ORs) were associated with poor social and occupational outcome and negative symptoms measured one year later. Moreover, this was true for both males and females. These results suggest that hyperarousal and autonomic hyper-reactivity to the environment may interfere with fragile cognitive process-

Abnormalities in tonic EDA and SCR responsiveness have also been reported in other psychopathologies, particularly psychopathy. Psychopaths are usually characterized as low in arousal and deficient in feelings of fear and anxiety, leading to their thrill-seeking and anti-social behavior (Lykken, 1957; Quay, 1965). It would be expected that both of these abnormalities should be reflected in EDA abnormalities, in particular in lower tonic measures of arousal such as SCL and NS-SCRs, and in smaller SCRs given in response to stimuli that would be associated with fear or anxiety in normal individuals. Both such abnormalities have been reported among psychopaths.

Fowles (1993), in a review of EDA during resting conditions, concluded that lower levels of SCL were occasionally found among psychopaths, although effect sizes were small, and less evidence existed for lower NS-SCR levels. Lorber (2004), in a meta-analysis of 95 studies of EDA and HR in psychopathy, concluded that psychopaths were characterized by reduced tonic EDA at rest, although again the effect sizes were small. Clearer differences from normal controls appear in tonic EDA levels as arousal increases, as, for instance, when simple orienting stimuli are presented (Fowles, 1993). Tonic EDA differences between psychopaths and normals clearly maximize when stressful stimuli are present (Fowles, 1993).

In one very well-known study that assessed not only tonic EDA but also response to anxiety-provoking stimuli, Hare (1965) measured SCL in psychopathic and nonpsychopathic prison inmates and college student controls during rest and while they watched the numbers 1–12 presented consecutively on a memory drum at 3 s intervals. A strong electric shock was given as the number 8 was presented. Psychopathic subjects had lower SCL during rest and during the task than the other groups, and psychopathic inmates showed smaller increases in skin conductance from numbers 1 to 8 than did nonpsychopathic inmates, which was interpreted as indicating less fear elicited in the interval prior to anticipated punishment. This finding with the "count-down" procedure has been replicated several times (for reviews, see Fowles, 1993 and Lykken, 1995).

As would be expected from Hare's findings, numerous investigators have reported that psychopaths show impaired SCR conditioning with aversive UCSs (usually electric shocks) (Lykken, 1957; Hare, 1965; for a review, see Fowles, 1993). Psychopaths also exhibit abnormal SCRs to other affective stimuli. Verona et al. (2004) presented positively and negatively affectively valenced and neutral sounds (e.g., laughing baby, crying baby, clucking chicken) from the International Affective Digitized Sounds (IADS; Bradley & Lang, 1999) system to prison inmates assessed with the Psychopathy Checklist – Revised (PCL-R; Hare, 1991). The PCL-R assesses what are generally regarded as two factors of psychopathy, emotional detachment (e.g., egocentricity, shallow affect, and absence of remorse) and antisocial behavior (e.g., frequent trouble with the law, pathological lying, and substance abuse). Inmates scoring high on the emotional detachment factor showed smaller responses to both pleasant and unpleasant sounds than did those who scored low on the factor, indicating that abnormalities in emotional processes in psychopathy extend beyond the realm of fear and anxiety. An interesting study by Blair et al. (1997) presented psychopathic and nonpsychopathic prison inmates with IAPS slides from three categories: nonthreatening (e.g., a book), threatening (e.g., a very angry face), and distress (e.g., a crying child). The two groups did not differ in SCR magnitude to threatening and nonthreatening stimuli, but the psychopaths responded less to the distress cues than nonpsychopaths.

In addition to these abnormalities in EDA seen in adults diagnosed with psychopathy, lower levels of tonic EDA have been reported in adolescents who later exhibited antisocial behavior. Raine, Venables, and Williams (1990) recorded EDA, heart rate (HR), and EEG during rest and several tasks from a sample of unselected 15-year-old schoolboys, and at a 10-year follow-up identified those who during the follow-up period had committed serious criminal offenses. As adolescents, the offenders had a lower rate of resting NS-SCRs, indicating lower arousal levels. The lower resting HR and greater EEG power in low-frequency bands seen in the offender group also were consistent with lower arousal.

It is worth noting that studies of the psychophysiological correlates of psychopathy have typically used only male subjects. Little if anything is known about psychophysiological abnormalities among female psychopaths.

EPILOGUE

EDA is a sensitive peripheral index of sympathetic nervous system activity that has proven to be a useful psychophysiological tool with wide applicability. Social and behavioral scientists have found that tonic EDA is useful to investigate general states of arousal and/or alertness, and that the phasic SCR is useful to study multifaceted attentional processes, as well as individual differences in both the normal and abnormal spectrum. We believe that future research will continue to support the use of EDA in a variety of situations and stimulus conditions.

An important direction for future research involves sharpening the inferential tool characteristics of EDA itself. That is, basic research is needed to address the specific conditions under which specific EDA components reflect specific psychological and physiological processes and mechanisms. For example, under what stimulus conditions does the SCR amplitude component of the orienting response reflect automatic preattentive cognitive processes versus controlled cognitive processes? Likewise, under what test situations do tonic and phasic EDA components reflect different brain systems? We expect that the expanding use of neuroimaging techniques in cognitive and affective neuroscience will elucidate these issues, making EDA an even more interesting and valuable psychophysiological tool.

ACKNOWLEDGMENTS AND DEDICATION

Michael Dawson was supported by a Research Scientist Development Award (K02 MH01086) from the National Institute of Mental Health during preparation of this chapter. We thank the following students for their generous help: Wade R. Elmore, C. Beau Nelson, Albert B. Poje, Anthony Rissling, and Gary L. Thorne. We dedicate this chapter to William W. Grings, one of the pioneers in electrodermal activity who served as mentor to the first two authors, and friend to all three.

REFERENCES

Andreassi, J. L. (2000). *Psychophysiology: Human Behavior and Physiological Response*. Hillsdale, NJ: Lawrence Erlbaum.

Asahina, M., Suzuki, A., Mori, M., Kanesaka, T., & Hattori, T. (2003). Emotional sweating response in a patient with bilateral amygdala damage. *International Journal of Psychophysiology*, 47, 87–93.

Ax, A. (1953). The physiological differentiation between fear and anger in humans. *Psychosomatic Medicine*, 15, 433–442.

Bechara, A., Damasio, H., Tranel, D., & Damasio, A. R. (1997). Deciding advantageously before knowing the advantageous strategy. *Science*, 275, 1293–1295.

Bechara, A., Damasio, A. R., & Lee, G. P. (1999). Different contributions of the human amygdala and ventromedial prefrontal cortex to decision-making. *Journal of Neuroscience*, 19, 5473–5481.

Bechara, A., Tranel, D., Damasio, H., Adolphs, R., Rockland, C., & Damasio, A. R. (1995). Double dissociation of conditioning and declarative knowledge relative to the amygdala and hippocampus in humans. *Science*, 269, 1115–1118.

Ben-Shakhar, G. (1977). A further study of the dichotomization theory of detection of information. *Psychophysiology*, 14, 408–413.

Ben-Shakhar, G. (1985). Standardization within individuals: Simple method to neutralize individual differences in skin conductance. *Psychophysiology*, 22, 292–299.

Bernstein, A., Frith, C., Gruzelier, J., Patterson, T., Straube, E., Venables, P., & Zahn, T. (1982). An analysis of the skin conductance orienting response in samples of American, British, and German schizophrenics. *Biological Psychology*, 14, 155–211.

Bernstein, A. S., Taylor, K. W., Starkey, P., Juni, S., Lubowsky, J., & Paley, H. (1981). Bilateral skin conductance, finger pulse volume, and EEG orienting response to tones of differing intensities in chronic schizophrenics and controls. *Journal of Nervous and Mental Disease*, 169, 513–528.

Blair, R. J. R., Jones, L., Clark, F., & Smith, M. (1997). The psychopathic individual: A lack of responsiveness to distress cues? *Psychophysiology*, 34, 192–198.

Bloch, V. (1993). On the centennial of the discovery of electrodermal activity. In J. C. Roy, W. Boucsein, D. C. Fowles, & J. H. Gruzelier (Eds.), *Progress in Electrodermal Research* (pp. 1–6). New York: Plenum Press.

Boucsein, W. (1992). *Electrodermal Activity*. New York: Plenum Press.

Boyd, R. W., & DiMascio, A. (1954). Social behavior and autonomic physiology (a sociophysiologic study). *Journal of Nervous and Mental Disease*, 120, 207–212.

Bradley, M. M., & Lang, P. J. (1999). International affective digitized sounds (IADS): Stimuli, instruction manual and affective ratings. Technical report no. B-2, Center for Research in Psychophysiology, University of Florida, Gainesville.

Brand, G., Millot, J. L., Saffaux, M., & Morand-Villeneuve, N. (2002). Lateralization in human nasal chemoreception: Differences in bilateral electrodermal responses related to olfactory and trigeminal stimuli. *Behavioral Brain Research*, 133, 205–210.

Brand, G., Millot, J., Jacquot, L. J., Thomas, S., & Wetzel, S. (2004). Left: Right differences in psychophysical and electrodermal measures of olfactory thresholds and their relation to electrodermal indices of hemispheric asymmetries. *Perceptual and Motor Skills*, 98, 759–769.

Brekke, J. S., Raine, A., Ansel, M., Lencz, T., & Bird, L. (1997). Neuropsychological and psychophysiological correlates of psychosocial functioning in schizophrenia. *Schizophrenia Bulletin*, 23, 19–28.

Brekke, J. S., Raine, A., & Thomson, C. (1995). Cognitive and psychophysiological correlates of positive, negative, and disorganized symptoms in the schizophrenia spectrum. *Psychiatry Research*, 57, 241–250.

Brown, G., Birley, J. L. T., & Wing, J. K. (1972). Influence of family life on the course of schizophrenia. *British Journal of Psychiatry*, 121, 241–248.

Bundy, R. S., & Fitzgerald, H. E. (1975). Stimulus specificity of electrodermal recovery time: An examination and reinterpretation of the evidence. *Psychophysiology*, 12, 406–411.

Crider, A. (1993). Electrodermal response lability-stability: Individual difference correlates. In J. C. Roy, W. Boucsein, D. C. Fowles, & J. H. Gruzelier (Eds.), *Progress in Electrodermal Research* (pp. 173–186). New York: Plenum Press.

Crider, A., & Augenbraun, C. (1975). Auditory vigilance correlates of electrodermal response habituation speed. *Psychophysiology*, 12, 36–40.

Critchley, H. D., Elliot, R., Mathias, C. J., & Dolan, R. J. (2000). Neural activity relating to generation and representation of galvanic skin conductance responses: A functional magnetic resonance imaging study. *Journal of Neuroscience*, 20, 3033–3040.

Cuthbert, B. N., Bradley, M. M., & Lang, P. J. (1996). Probing picture perception: Activation and emotion. *Psychophysiology*, 33, 103–111.

Damasio, A. R. (1994). *Descartes' Error: Emotion, Reason, and the Human Brain*. New York: Grosset/Putnam.

Darrow, C. W. (1927). Sensory, secretory, and electrical changes in the skin following bodily excitation. *Journal of Experimental Psychology*, 10, 197–226.

Darrow, C. W. (1937). Neural mechanisms controlling the palmar galvanic skin reflex and palmar sweating. *Archives of Neurology and Psychiatry*, 37, 641–663.

Davies, D. R., & Parasuraman, R. (1982). *The Psychology of Vigilance*. London: Academic Press.

Dawson, M. E., & Biferno, M. A. (1973). Concurrent measurement of awareness and electrodermal classical conditioning. *Journal of Experimental Psychology*, 101, 55–62.

Dawson, M. E., Filion, D. L., & Schell, A. M. (1989). Is elicitation of the autonomic orienting response associated with allocation of processing resources? *Psychophysiology*, 26, 560–572.

Dawson, M. E., & Nuechterlein, K. H. (1984). Psychophysiological dysfunctions in the developmental course of schizophrenic disorders. *Schizophrenia Bulletin*, 10, 204–232.

Dawson, M. E., Nuechterlein, K. H., & Liberman, R. P. (1983). Relapse in schizophrenic disorders: Possible contributing factors and implications for behavior therapy. In M. Rosenbaum, C. M. Franks, & Y. Jaffe (Eds.), *Perspectives on Behavior Therapy in the Eighties* (pp. 265–286). New York: Springer.

Dawson, M. E., Nuechterlein, K. H., & Schell, A. M. (1992a). Electrodermal anomalies in recent-onset schizophrenia: Relationships to symptoms and prognosis. *Schizophrenia Bulletin, 18,* 295–311.

Dawson, M. E., Nuechterlein, K. H., Schell, A. M., Gitlin, M., & Ventura, J. (1994). Autonomic abnormalities in schizophrenia: State or trait indicators? *Archives of General Psychiatry, 51,* 813–824.

Dawson, M. E., Nuechterlein, K. H., Schell, A. M., & Mintz, J. (1992b). Concurrent and predictive electrodermal correlates of symptomatology in recent-onset schizophrenic patients. *Journal of Abnormal Psychology, 101,* 153–164.

Dawson, M. E., & Schell, A. M. (1985). Information processing and human autonomic classical conditioning. In P. K. Ackles, J. R. Jennings, & M. G. H. Coles (Eds.), *Advances in Psychophysiology, Vol. 1* (pp. 89–165). Greenwich, CT: JAI Press.

Dawson, M. E., & Schell, A. M. (2002). What does electrodermal activity tell us about prognosis in the schizophrenia spectrum? *Schizophrenia Research, 54,* 87–93.

Dittes, J. E. (1957). Galvanic skin response as a measure of patient's reaction to therapist's permissiveness. *Journal of Abnormal and Social Psychology, 55,* 295–303.

Edelberg, R. (1967). Electrical properties of the skin. In C. C. Brown (Ed.), *Methods in Psychophysiology* (pp. 1–53). Baltimore: Williams and Wilkens.

Edelberg, R. (1972a). Electrical activity of the skin: Its measurement and uses in psychophysiology. In N. S. Greenfield & R. A. Sternbach (Eds.), *Handbook of Psychophysiology* (pp. 367–418). New York: Holt.

Edelberg, R. (1972b). Electrodermal recovery rate, goal-orientation, and aversion. *Psychophysiology, 9,* 512–520.

Edelberg, R. (1993). Electrodermal mechanisms: A critique of the two-effector hypothesis and a proposed replacement. In J. C. Roy, W. Boucsein, D. C. Fowles, & J. H. Gruzelier (Eds.), *Progress in Electrodermal Research* (pp. 7–29). New York: Plenum Press.

Engel, B. T. (1960). Stimulus-response and individual-response specificity. *Archives of General Psychiatry, 2,* 305–313.

Esen, F., & Esen, H. (2002). Hemispheric modulatory influences on skin resistance response latency: Unilateral stimulation, bilateral recording. *International Journal of Psychophysiology, 112,* 1397–1406.

Esteves, F., Parra, C., Dimberg, U., & Ohman, A. (1994). Nonconscious associative learning: Pavlovian conditioning of skin conductance responses to masked fear-relevant facial stimuli. *Psychophysiology, 31,* 375–385.

Féré, C. (1888). Note on changes in electrical resistance under the effect of sensory stimulation and emotion. *Comptes Rendus des Seances de la Societe de Biologie* Series 9, *5,* 217–219.

Ferguson, G. A. & Takane, Y. (1989). *Statistical Analysis in Psychology and Education (6th edition).* New York: McGraw-Hill.

Fowles, D. C. (1974). Mechanisms of electrodermal activity. In R. F. Thompson & M. M. Patterson (Eds.), *Methods in Physiological Psychology. Part C. Receptor and Effector Processes* (pp. 231–271). New York: Academic Press.

Fowles, D. C. (1986). The eccrine system and electrodermal activity. In M. G. H. Coles, E. Donchin, & S. W. Porges (Eds.), *Psy-*

chophysiology: Systems, Processes, and Applications (pp. 51–96). New York: Guilford Press.

Fowles, D. C. (1993). Electrodermal activity and antisocial behavior: Empirical findings and theoretical issues. In J.-C. Roy, W. Boucsein, D. C. Fowles, & J. H. Gruzelier (Eds.), *Progress in Electrodermal Research* (pp. 223–237). New York: Plenum Press.

Fowles, D. C. (1988). Psychophysiology and psychopathology: A motivational approach. *Psychophysiology, 25,* 373–391.

Fowles, D., Christie, M. J., Edelberg, R., Grings, W. W., Lykken, D. T., & Venables, P. H. (1981). Publication recommendations for electrodermal measurements. *Psychophysiology, 18,* 232–239.

Fredrikson, M., Furmark, T., Olsson, M. T., Fischer, H., Anderson, J., & Langstrom, B. (1998). Functional neuroanatomical correlates of electrodermal activity: A positron emission tomography study. *Psychophysiology, 35,* 179–185.

Freedman, L. W., Scerbo, A. S., Dawson, M. E., Raine, A., McClure, W. O., & Venables, P. H. (1994). The relationship of sweat gland count to electrodermal activity. *Psychophysiology, 31,* 196–200.

Freixa i Baque, E. (1982). Reliability of electrodermal measures: A compilation. *Biological Psychology, 14,* 219–229.

Frith, C. D., Stevens, M., Johnstone, E. C., & Crow, T. J. (1979). Skin conductance responsivity during acute episodes of schizophrenia as a predictor of symptomatic improvement. *Psychological Medicine, 9,* 101–106.

Fuentes, I., Merita, M. G., Miquel, M., & Rojo, J. (1993). Relationships between electrodermal activity and symptomatology in schizophrenia. *Psychopathology, 26,* 47–52.

Green, M. F., Nuechterlein, K. H., & Satz, P. (1989). The relationship of symptomatology and medication to electrodermal activity in schizophrenia. *Psychophysiology, 26,* 148–157.

Grey, S. J., & Smith, B. L. (1984). A comparison between commercially available electrode gels and purpose-made gel, in the measurement of electrodermal activity. *Psychophysiology, 21,* 551–557.

Grings, W. W. (1974). Recording of electrodermal phenomena. In R. F. Thompson & M. M. Patterson (Eds.), *Bioelectric Recording Technique, Part C: Receptor and Effector Processes* (pp. 273–296). New York: Academic Press.

Grings, W. W., & Dawson, M. E. (1973). Complex variables in conditioning. In W. F. Prokasy & D. C. Raskin (Eds.), *Electrodermal Activity in Psychological Research* (pp. 203–254). New York: Academic Press.

Grings, W. W., & Dawson, M. E. (1978). *Emotions and Bodily Responses: A Psychophysiological Approach.* New York: Academic Press.

Grings, W. W., & Lockhart, R. A. (1965). Problems of magnitude measurement with multiple GSRs. *Psychological Reports, 17,* 979–982.

Grings, W. W., & Schell, A. M. (1969). Magnitude of electrodermal response to a standard stimulus as a function of intensity and proximity of a prior stimulus. *Journal of Comparative and Physiological Psychology, 67,* 77–82.

Gross, J. J. (1998). Antecedent- and response-focused emotion regulation: Divergent consequences for experience, expression, and physiology. *Journal of Personality and Social Psychology, 74,* 224–237.

Gross, J. J., & Levenson, R. W. (1993). Emotional suppression: Physiology, self-report, and expressive behavior. *Journal of Personality and Social Psychology, 64,* 970–986.

Hare, R. D. (1991). *The Hare Psychopathy Checklist – Revised.* Toronto: Multi-Health Systems.

Hare, R. D. (1965). Temporal gradient of fear arousal in psychopaths. *Journal of Abnormal Psychology, 70,* 442–445.

Hassett, J. (1978). *A Primer of Psychophysiology.* San Francisco: W. H. Freeman and Company.

Hastrup, J. L (1979). Effects of electrodermal lability and introversion on vigilance decrement. *Psychophysiology, 16,* 302–310.

Hazlett, E. A., Dawson, M. E., Filion, D. L., Schell, A. M., & Nuechterlein, K. H. (1997). Autonomic orienting and the allocation of processing resources in schizophrenia patients and putatively at-risk individuals. *Journal of Abnormal Psychology, 106,* 171–181.

Hazlett, H., Dawson, M. E., Schell, A. M., & Nuechterlein, K. H. (1997). Electrodermal activity as a prodromal sign in schizophrenia. *Biological Psychiatry, 41,* 111–113.

Hollister, J. M., Mednick, S. A., Brennan, P., & Cannon, T. D. (1994). Impaired autonomic nervous system habituation in those at genetic risk for schizophrenia. *Archives of General Psychiatry, 51,* 552–558.

Hot, P., Naveteur, J., Leconte, P., & Sequeira, H. (1999). Diurnal variations of tonic electrodermal activity. *International Journal of Psychophysiology, 33,* 223–230.

Hugdahl, K. (1984). Hemispheric asymmetry and bilateral electrodermal recordings: A review of the evidence. *Psychophysiology, 21,* 371–393.

Hugdahl, K. (1995). *Psychophysiology: The Mind-Body Perspective.* Cambridge, MA: Harvard University Press.

Hugdahl, K., & Öhman, A. (1977). Effects of instruction on acquisition and extinction of electrodermal responses to fear-relevant stimuli. *Journal of Experimental Psychology: Human Learning and Memory, 3,* 608–618.

Humphreys, L. G. (1943). Measures of strength of conditioned eyelid responses. *Journal of General Psychology, 29,* 101–111.

Iacono, W. G., Ficken, J. W., & Beiser, M. (1993). Electrodermal nonresponding in first-episode psychosis as a function of stimulus significance. In J. C. Roy, W. Boucsein, D. C. Fowles, & J. H. Gruzelier (Eds.), *Progress in Electrodermal Activity* (pp. 239–256). New York: Plenum Press.

Iacono, W. G., Ficken, J. W. & Beiser, M. (1999). Electrodermal activation in first-episode psychotic patients and their first-degree relatives. Psychiatry Research, 88, 25–39.

Jennings, J. R. (1986). Bodily changes during attending. In M. G. H. Coles, E. Donchin, & S. W. Porges (Eds.), *Psychophysiology: Systems, Processes, and Applications* (pp. 268–289). New York: Guilford Press.

Katkin, E. S. (1975). Electrodermal lability: A psychophysiological analysis of individual differences in response to stress. In I. G. Sarason, & C. D. Spielberger (Eds.), *Stress and Anxiety, Vol. 2* (pp. 141–176). Washington, DC: Aldine.

Katsanis, J., & Iacono, W. G. (1994). Electrodermal activity and clinical status in chronic schizophrenia. *Journal of Abnormal Psychology, 103,* 777–783.

Kelsey, R. M. (1991). Electrodermal lability and myocardial reactivity to stress. *Psychophysiology, 28,* 619–631.

Kim, D. K., Shin, Y. M., Kim, C. E., Cho, H. S., & Kim, Y. S. (1993). Electrodermal responsiveness, clinical variables, and brain imaging in male chronic schizophrenics. *Biological Psychiatry, 33,* 786–793.

Koelega, H. S. (1990). Vigilance performance: A review of electrodermal predictors. *Perceptual and Motor Skills, 70,* 1011–1029.

Kutas, M. (1997). Views on how the electrical activity that the brain generates reflects the functions of different language structures. *Psychophysiology, 34,* 383–398.

Lacey, J. I., Kagan, J., Lacey, B. C., & Moss, H. A. (1963). The visceral level: Situational determinants and behavioral correlates of autonomic response patterns. In P. H. Knapp (Ed.), *Expression of the Emotions in Man* (pp. 161–196). New York: International Universities Press.

Lacey, J. I. & Lacey, B. C. (1958). Verification and extension of the principle of autonomic response-stereotypy. *American Journal of Psychology, 71,* 50–73.

Lader, M. H., & Wing, L. (1966). *Psychological Measures, Sedative Drugs, and Morbid Anxiety.* London: Oxford University Press.

Landis, C. (1930). Psychology of the psychogalvanic reflex. *Psychological Review, 37,* 381–398.

Lang, P. J., Bradley, M. M., & Cuthbert, B. N. (1998). International affective picture system (IAPS): Technical Manual and Affective Ratings. Center for Research in Psychophysiology, University of Florida, Gainesville.

Lang, P. J., Greenwald, M. K., Bradley, M. M., & Hamm, A. O. (1993). Looking at pictures: Affective, visceral, and behavioral reactions. *Psychophysiology, 30,* 261–173.

Levenson, R. W., & Gottman, J. M. (1983). Marital interaction: Physiological linkage and affective exchange. *Journal of Personality and Social Psychology, 45,* 587–597.

Levenson, R. W., & Gottman, J. M. (1985). Physiological and affective predictors of change in relationship satisfaction. *Journal of Personality and Social Psychology, 49,* 85–94.

Levinson, D. F., Edelberg, R., & Bridger, W. H. (1984). The orienting response in schizophrenia: Proposed resolution of a controversy. *Biological Psychiatry, 19,* 489–507.

Lim, C. L., Rennie, C., Barry, R. J., Bahramali, H., Lazzaro, I., Manor, B., & Gordon, E. (1997). Decomposing skin conductance into tonic phasic components. *International Journal of Psychophysiology, 25,* 97–109.

Lorber, M. F. (2004). Psychophysiology of aggression, psychopathy, and conduct problems: A meta-analysis. *Psychological Bulletin, 130,* 531–552.

Lockhart, R. A., & Lieberman, W. (1979). Information content of the electrodermal orienting response. In H. D. Kimmel, E. H. van Olst, & J. F. Orlebeke (Eds.), *The Orienting Reflex in Humans* (pp. 685–700). Hillsdale, NJ: Lawrence Erlbaum.

Lovibond, P. F., & Shanks, D. R. (2002). The role of awareness in Pavlovian conditioning: Empirical evidence and theoretical implications. *Journal of Experimental Psychology: Animal Behavior Processes, 28,* 3–26.

Lykken, D. T. (1959). The GSR in the detection of guilt. *Journal of Applied Psychology, 43,* 383–388.

Lykken, D. T. (1957). A study of anxiety in the sociopathic personality. *Journal of Abnormal Psychology, 55,* 6–10.

Lykken, D. T. (1995). *The Antisocial Personalities.* Hillsdale, NJ: Lawrence Erlbaum Associates.

Lykken, D. T. (1981). *A Tremor in the Blood.* New York: McGraw-Hill.

Lykken, D. T., Rose, R. J., Luther, B., & Maley, M. (1966). Correcting psychophysiological measures for individual differences in range. *Psychological Bulletin, 66,* 481–484.

Lykken, D. T., & Venables, P. H. (1971). Direct measurement of skin conductance: A proposal for standardization. *Psychophysiology, 8,* 656–672.

Lyytinen, H., Blomberg, A., & Näätänen, R. (1992). Event-related potentials and autonomic responses to a change in unattended auditory stimuli. *Psychophysiology, 29,* 523–534.

Maia, T. V., & McClelland, J. L. (2004). A reexamination of the evidence for the somatic marker hypothesis: What participants really know in the Iowa gambling task. *PNAS, 101,* 16075–16080.

Montague, J. D. (1963). Habituation of the psycho-galvanic reflex during serial tests. *Journal of Psychosomatic Research, 7,* 199–214.

Morris, J. S., Buchel, C., & Dolan, R. J. (2001). Parallel neural responses in amygdala subregions and sensory cortex during implicit fear conditioniry. *NeuroImage,* 13, 1044–1052.

Mundy-Castle, A. C., & McKiever, B. L. (1953). The psychophysiological significance of the galvanic skin response. *Journal of Experimental Psychology, 46,* 15–24.

Munro, L. L., Dawson, M. E., Schell, A. M., & Sakai, L. M. (1987). Electrodermal lability and rapid performance decrement in a degraded stimulus continuous performance task. *Journal of Psychophysiology, 1,* 249–257.

Nagai, Y., Critchley, H. D., Featherstone, E., Trimble, M. R., & Dolan, R. J. (2004). Activity in ventromedial prefrontal cortex covaries with sympathetic skin conductance level: a physiological account of a "default mode" of brain function. *NeuroImage, 22,* 243–251.

Naveteur, J., Godefroy, O., & Sequeira, H. (1998). Electrodermal level asymmetry in a unilateral brain-damaged patient. *International Journal of Psychophysiology, 29,* 237–245.

Nuechterlein, K. H., & Dawson, M. E. (1984). A heuristic vulnerability/stress model of schizophrenic episodes. *Schizophrenia Bulletin, 10,* 300–312.

Neumann, E., & Blanton, R. (1970). The early history of electrodermal research. *Psychophysiology, 6,* 453–475.

Öhman, A. (1979). The orienting response, attention and learning: An information processing perspective. In H. D. Kimmel, E. H. Van Olst, & J. F. Orlebeke (Eds.), *The Orienting Reflex in Humans.* Hillsdale, NJ: Lawrence Erlbaum.

Öhman, A. (1981). Electrodermal activity and vulnerability to schizophrenia: A review. *Biological Psychology, 12,* 87–145.

Öhman, A. (1992). Orienting and attention: Preferred preattentive processing of potentially phobic stimuli. In B. A. Campbell, H. Hayne, & R. Richardson (Eds.), *Attention and Information Processing in Infants and Adults: Perspectives from Human and Animal Research* (pp. 263–295). Hillsdale, NJ: Lawrence Erlbaum.

Öhman, A., Dimberg, U., & Esteves, F. (1989a). Preattentive activation of aversive emotions. In T. Archer & L.-G. Nilsson (Eds.), *Aversion, avoidance, and anxiety* (pp. 169–193). Hillsdale, NJ: Erlbaum.

Öhman, A., Öhlund, L. S., Alm, T., Wieselgren, I. M., Öst, L-G., & Lindstrom, L. H. (1989b). Electrodermal nonresponding, premorbid adjustment, and symptomatology as predictors of long-term social functioning in schizophrenics. *Journal of Abnormal Psychology, 98,* 426–435.

Öhman, A., & Soares, J. J. F. (1998). Emotional conditioning to masked stimuli: Expectancies for aversive outcomes following nonrecognized fear-relevant stimuli. *Journal of Experimental Psychology: General, 127,* 69–82.

Polagava, E. B., Egorov, A. Y., & Pirogov, A. A. (1997). Asymmetry of skin resistance response under activation of the right or left cerebral hemisphere. *Human Physiology, 23,* 531–535.

Patterson, J. C., Ungerleider, L. G., & Bandettini, P. A. (2002). Task-independent functional brain activity correlation with skin conductance changes: An fMRI study. *NeuroImage, 17,* 1797–1806.

Prokasy, W. F. (1974). SCORIT: A computer subroutine for scoring electrodermal responses. *Behavior Research Methods & Instrumentation, 7,* 49–52.

Prokasy, W. F., & Kumpfer, K. L. (1973). Classical conditioning. In W. F. Prokasy & D. C. Raskin (Eds.), *Electrodermal Activity in Psychological Research* (pp. 157–202). New York: Academic Press.

Prokasy, W. F., & Raskin, D. C. (Eds.). (1973). *Electrodermal activity in psychological research.* New York: Academic Press.

Quay, H. C. (1965). Psychopathic personality as pathological stimulation-seeking. *American Journal of Psychiatry, 122,* 180–183.

Raine, A., Venables, P. H., & Williams, M. (1990). Relationships between central and autonomic measures of arousal at age 15 years and criminality at age 24 years. *Archives of General Psychiatry, 47,* 1003–1007.

Roy, J.-C., Sequeira, H., & Delerm, B. (1993). Neural control of electrodermal activity: Spinal and reticular mechanisms. In J. C. Roy, W. Boucsein, D. C. Fowles, & J. H. Gruzelier (Eds.), *Progress in Electrodermal Research* (pp. 73–92). New York: Plenum Press.

Sakai, M. L., Baker, L. A., & Dawson, M. E. (1992). Electrodermal lability: Individual differences affecting perceptual speed and vigilance performance in 9 to 16 year-old children. *Psychophysiology, 29,* 207–217.

Scerbo, A., Freedman, L. W., Raine, A., Dawson, M. E., & Venables, P. H. (1992). A major effect of recording site on measurement of electrodermal activity. *Psychophysiology, 29,* 241–246.

Schell, A. M., Dawson, M. E., & Filion, D. L. (1988). Psychophysiology correlates of electrodermal lability. *Psychophysiology, 25,* 619–632.

Schell, A. M., Dawson, M. E., & Marinkovic, K. (1991). Effects of potentially phobic conditioned stimuli on retention, reconditioning, and extinction of the conditioned skin conductance response. *Psychophysiology, 28,* 140–153.

Schell, A. M., Dawson, M. E., Nuechterlein, K. H., Subotnik, K. L., & Ventura, J. (2002). The temporal stability of electrodermal variables over a one-year period in patients with recent-onset schizophrenia and normal subjects. *Psychophysiology, 39,* 124–132.

Schell, A. M., Dawson, M. E., Rissling, A., Ventura, J., Subotnik, K. L., & Nuechterlein, K. H. (2005). Electrodermal predictors of functional outcome and negative symptoms in recent-onset schizophrenia patients. *Psychophysiology, 42,* 483–492.

Schulter, G., & Papousek, I. (1998). Bilateral electrodermal activity: Relationships to state and trait characteristics of hemisphere asymmetry. *International Journal of Psychophysiology, 31,* 1–12.

Schwartz, G. E., & Shapiro, D. (1973). Social psychophysiology. In W. F. Prokasy & D. C. Raskin (Eds.), *Electrodermal Activity in Psychological Research* (pp. 377–416). New York: Academic Press.

Seligman, M. E. P. (1970). On the generality of the laws of learning. *Psychological Review, 77,* 307–321.

Sequeira, H., & Roy, J.-C. (1993). Cortical and hypothalamo-limbic control of electrodermal responses. In J. C. Roy, W. Boucsein, D. C. Fowles, & J. H. Gruzelier (Eds.), *Progress in Electrodermal Research* (pp. 93–114). New York: Plenum Press.

Shields, S. A., MacDowell, K. A., Fairchild, S. B., & Campbell, M. L. (1987). Is mediation of sweating cholinergic, adrenergic, or both? A comment on the literature. *Psychophysiology, 24,* 312–319.

Siddle, D., Stephenson, D., & Spinks, J. A. (1983). Elicitation and habituation of the orienting response. In D. Siddle (Ed.),

Orienting and Habituation: Perspectives in Human Research (pp. 109–182). Chichester: Wiley and Sons.

Sokolov, E. N. (1963). *Perception and the Conditioned Reflex*. New York: Macmillan.

Spohn, H. E., Coyne, L., Wilson, J. K., & Hayes, K. (1989). Skin-conductance orienting response in chronic schizophrenics: The role of neuroleptics. *Journal of Abnormal Psychology, 98*, 478–486.

Stern, R. M., Ray, W. J., & Quigley, K. S. (2001). *Psychophysiological Recording*. New York: Oxford University Press.

Straube, E. R. (1979). On the meaning of electrodermal nonresponding in Schizophrenia. *Journal of Nervous and Mental Disease, 167*, 601–611.

Strauss, J. S., & Carpenter, W. T. (1974). The prediction of outcome in schizophrenia: II. Relationship between predictor and outcome variables. *Archives of General Psychiatry, 31*, 37–42.

Strayer, D. L., & Williams, W. C. (1982). *SCORIT 1980*. Paper presented at the annual meeting of the Society for Psychophysiological Research, Washington, DC.

Tarchanoff, J. (1890). Galvanic phenomena in the human skin during stimulation of the sensory organs and during various forms of mental activity. *Pflugers Archive fur die Gesamte Physiologie des Menschen und der Tiere, 46*, 46–55.

Tarrier, N., & Barrowclough, C. (1989). Electrodermal activity as a predictor of schizophrenic relapse. *Psychopathology, 22*, 320–324.

Tarrier, N., Vaughn, C., Lader, M. H., & Leff, J. P. (1979). Bodily reactions to people and events in schizophrenics. *Archives of General Psychiatry, 36*, 311–315.

Tranel, D. (2000). Electrodermal activity in cognitive neuroscience: neuroanatomical and neurophysiological correlates. In R. D. Lane & L. Nadel (Eds.), *Cognitive Neuroscience of Emotion* (pp. 192–224). Oxford University Press: New York.

Tranel, D., & Damasio, H. (1994). Neuroanatomical correlates of electrodermal skin conductance responses. *Psychophysiology, 31*, 427–438.

Tranel, D., Fowles, D. C., & Damasio, A. R. (1985). Electrodermal discrimination of familiar and unfamiliar faces: A methodology. *Psychophysiology, 22*, 403–408.

Turpin, G. (1983). Psychophysiology, psychopathology, and the social environment. In A. Gale & J. A. Edwards (Eds.), *Physiological Correlates of Human Behavior* (pp. 265–280). New York: Academic Press.

Turpin, G., Tarrier, N., & Sturgeon, D. (1988). Social psychophysiology and the study of biopsychosocial models of schizophrenia. In H. Wagner (Ed.), *Social Psychophysiology*. Chichester, England: Wiley & Sons.

Vaughn, C., & Leff, J. P. (1976). The influence of family and social factors on the course of psychiatric illness. *British Journal of Psychiatry, 129*, 125–137.

Vaughn, C. E., Snyder, K. S., Jones, S., Freeman, W. B., & Fallon, I. R. H. (1984). Family factors in schizophrenic relapse: A California replication of the British research on expressed emotion. *Archives of General Psychiatry, 41*, 1169–1177.

Venables, P. H., & Christie, M. J. (1973). Mechanisms, instrumentation, recording techniques, and quantification of responses. In W. F. Prokasy & D. C. Raskin (Eds.), *Electrodermal Activity in Psychological Research* (pp. 1–124). New York: Academic Press.

Venables, P. H., & Mitchell, D. A. (1996). The effects of age, sex and time of testing on skin conductance activity. *Biological Psychology, 43*, 87–101.

Venables, P. H., & Christie, M. J. (1980). Electrodermal activity. In I. Martin & P. H. Venables (Eds), *Techniques in Psychophysiology* (pp. 3–67), Chichester UK: Wiley.

Verschuere, B., Crombez, G., De Clercq, A., & Koster, E. H. W. (2004). Autonomic and behavioral responding to concealed information: Differentiating orienting and defensive responses. *Psychophysiology, 41*, 461–466.

Verona, E., Patrick, C. J., Curtin, J., Bradley, M. M., & Lang, P. J. (2004). Psychopathy and physiological responses to emotionally evocative sounds. *Journal of Abnormal Psychology, 113*, 99–108.

Vigouroux, R. (1879). Sur le role de la resistance electrique des tissues dans l'electro-diagnostic. *Comptes Rendus Societe de Biologie, 31*, 336–339.

Vigouroux, R. (1888). The electrical resistance considered as a clinical sign. *Progres Medicale, 3*, 87–89.

Vossel, G., & Rossman, R. (1984). Electrodermal habituation speed and visual monitoring performance. *Psychophysiology, 21*, 97–100.

Wallin, B. G. (1981). Sympathetic nerve activity underlying electrodermal and cardiovascular reactions in man. *Psychophysiology, 18*, 470–476.

Wang, G. H. (1964). *The Neural Control of Sweating*. Madison: University of Wisconsin Press.

Wieselgren, I.-M., Öhlund, L. S., Lindstrom, L. H., & Öhman, A. (1994). Electrodermal activity as a predictor of social functioning in female schizophrenics. *Journal of Abnormal Psychology, 103*, 570–573.

Williams, L. M., Brammer, M. J., Skerrett, D., Lagopolous, J., Rennie, C., Kozek, K., Olivieri, G., Peduto, T., & Gordon, E. (2000). The neural correlates of orienting: An integration of fMRI and skin conductance orienting. *Neuroreport, 11*, 3011–3015.

Woodworth, R. S., & Schlosberg, H. (1954). *Experimental Psychology*. (Rev. Ed.). New York: Holt & Co.

Zahn, T. P., Carpenter, W. T., & McGlashan, T. H. (1981). Autonomic nervous system activity in acute schizophrenia: II. Relationships to short-term prognosis and clinical state. *Archives of General Psychiatry, 38*, 260–266.

8 Cardiovascular Psychophysiology

GARY G. BERNTSON, KAREN S. QUIGLEY, AND DAVE LOZANO

INTRODUCTION

The cardiovascular system is essential for life and has been a central focus of psychophysiological investigation for several reasons. First, at least some its parameters, like heart rate and blood pressure, are readily observed and quantified. Second, the cardiovascular system is a rich and intricate physiological system with multiple regulatory subsystems that are subject to central and peripheral autonomic controls and humoral influences. Consequently, it is highly sensitive to neurobehavioral processes. Finally, the complexity of the cardiovascular system renders it susceptible to a variety of disorders, many of which are impacted by psychological factors such as stress, and hence it assumes special significance in psychosomatic medicine.

The present chapter will provide an overview of the physiology of the cardiovascular system and its central and peripheral autonomic and neuroendocrine controls. It will then consider common psychophysiological measures from the methodological, analytic, and interpretative perspectives. Finally, we will highlight a few current issues and themes in the contemporary literature.

ANATOMY AND PHYSIOLOGY OF THE CARDIOVASCULAR SYSTEM

Overview

The cardiovascular system consists of the heart, a pump, and the vasculature, a distribution system, that together ensure that blood reaches all tissues of the body. The heart provides for a consistent flow of oxygenated blood by sending blood into the lungs (pulmonary circulation) and then to the rest of the body (systemic circulation). Figure 8.1 shows a schematized view of the heart and vasculature to emphasize connections among all the components. Deoxygenated blood from the venous side of the systemic circulation returns via the right atrium and then to the right ventricle of the heart from which it is pumped to the lungs for re-oxygenation. Blood returns from the lungs

by way of the left atrium, then enters the left ventricle from where it is pumped into the aorta, the large vessel from which all oxygenated blood is disseminated to the rest of the body. Blood leaving the aorta passes through ever smaller blood vessels, first entering the large arteries which later branch into smaller arterioles, metarterioles and finally into capillaries. Capillaries are small, thin-walled vessels from which oxygen and other nutrients diffuse into tissues, and into which the tissues release waste products such as carbon dioxide that must eventually be secreted or excreted from the body. After the capillary system, blood passes again into somewhat larger vessels, the venules and finally, the veins that carry blood from the systemic circulation back to the heart. The major veins that drain blood back into the heart, the inferior and superior vena cavae, return blood to the right atrium of the heart, from which blood passes to the right ventricle and again begins its journey through the pulmonary and systemic circulations.

The heart

The crucial pump of the cardiovascular system, the heart, consists of special cardiac muscle with properties different from that of skeletal muscle found elsewhere in the body. Cardiac muscle comes in three forms, atrial, ventricular, and specialized conducting fibers that serve as the electrical conducting system of the heart. The pumping action of the heart is primarily served by the atrial and ventricular muscle fibers. Cardiac muscle cells form a syncytium, so called because the tissue is electrically coupled to permit rapid spread of depolarization across the heart, particularly in a rostral to caudal direction. There are both atrial and ventricular syncytiums connected by an electrical conducting system. In the syncytiums, the boundaries of adjacent muscle cells along the longitudinal axis of the cardiac muscle consist of intercalated discs. These discs are specialized, highly permeable membranes capable of extremely fast spread of depolarization from one cardiac muscle cell to another. This is crucial to the pumping action of the heart where the rostral (atrial) and caudal

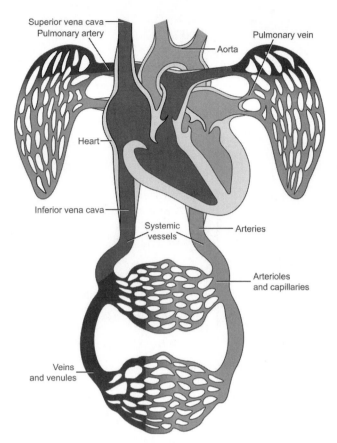

Figure 8.1. Systemic and pulmonary circulation. In keeping with usual depictions of the heart, the right side of the heart is on the left side of the picture. Lighter gray areas indicate oxygenated blood and darker gray areas indicate deoxygenated blood.

(ventricular) portions of the heart each must function as a single pumping unit, and where there must be coordinated action of each chamber.

The atrial and ventricular chambers are electrically connected by way of a conducting system that triggers ventricular contraction shortly after contraction of the atria. The specialized cardiac muscle fibers comprising the conducting system functionally couple the pumping actions of the atria and ventricles. Depolarization of two nodes of electrically active tissue, the sinoatrial (SA) and atrioventricular (AV) nodes, provides the electrical impetus that triggers contraction of the heart. The SA node in the wall of the right atrium just beneath the opening to the superior vena cava serves as the "pacemaker" of the heart. The SA node is the pacemaker because the speed of spontaneous depolarization of this node is typically faster than that of the AV node, and hence generally controls the rate of the beat. A system of internodal fibers forms a conducting system linking the SA and AV nodes. The depolarization wave is conducted away from the AV node and into the ventricles by way of the AV bundle (of His) which branches into the left and right bundles of Purkinje fibers that pass through the septum between the left and right ventricles. This system directs a wave of depolarization from the atria to the ventricles in a controlled

fashion that creates a highly coordinated pumping action with atrial contraction followed shortly by ventricular contraction.

The depolarization of cardiac muscle is different from skeletal muscle in that there is a depolarization spike followed by a sustained depolarization phase or plateau of about 0.2–0.3 seconds before the muscle repolarizes. The presence of the plateau provides a more sustained contraction in cardiac muscle than is typically observed in skeletal muscle. As a result, there is a more effective pumping action by the cardiac muscle because time is needed for blood to travel from the atria to the ventricles before the ventricles contract. The plateau in the depolarization wave of the cardiac muscle occurs because cardiac muscle depolarizes as a result of the opening of fast sodium (Na^+) channels (like those found in skeletal muscle), as well as slow calcium (Ca^{2+}) channels. The combined effect is a sustained depolarization. A similar plateau is seen in the depolarization curve of the Purkinje fibers of the conducting system. However, the velocity of conduction in atrial and ventricular muscle is on average slower (0.3–0.5 m/sec) than in the Purkinje fibers (which vary from 1.5–4.0 m/sec). This faster conduction in the Purkinje fibers permits the depolarization wave to reach all parts of the ventricular muscle quickly.

The cardiac cycle

The events that occur in the heart from one beat to the next beat are collectively referred to as the cardiac cycle (Figure 8.2). The cycle is composed of two main epochs: diastole, during which the heart does not pump and is filling with blood, and systole, during which the heart pumps. The cycle begins with depolarization of the SA node in the right atrium during the latter part of diastole. The wave of depolarization passing through the atrial muscle corresponds to the P wave in the electrical signal generated by the heart (i.e., the electrocardiogram or ECG) as recorded at the body surface (see Figure 8.3, panel A). The P wave is followed shortly thereafter by atrial contraction during which the QRS complex of the ECG appears, reflecting ventricular contraction and demarcating the onset of systole. During ventricular contraction, pressure in the ventricles is high enough to close the atrioventricular (AV) valves between the atria and ventricles. However, after ventricular contraction, as ventricular pressure falls below the atrial pressure, the AV valves open, and blood begins to rapidly fill the ventricles. Initiation of ventricular contraction leads to a large increase in ventricular pressure (more than 100 mmHg in a healthy heart). Once ventricular pressure is higher than the aortic pressure, the aortic valve opens, blood flows into the general circulation, and there is a rapid fall in ventricular volume. Late in the ventricular contraction phase, the ventricles repolarize, a phenomenon seen in the ECG as the T wave, and this initiates relaxation of the ventricles and the onset of diastole.

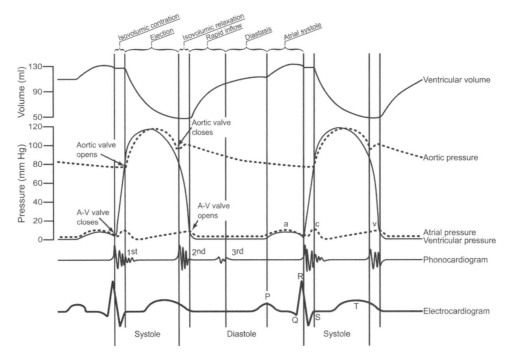

Figure 8.2. The cardiac cycle. Two cardiac cycles are shown for ventricular volume, aortic pressure, atrial pressure, ventricular pressure, the phonocardiogram, and the electrocardiogram (ECG). Phases of the cycle are indicated at the top of the figure above the brackets.

Blood flow, pressure, resistance, and cardiac output

Although Georg Ohm formulated his classic Ohm's law in the context of electrical circuits, the circulatory system adheres to the same basic relations as any other physical system where flow, pressure and resistance are operating. Ohm's Law applied to the circulation reflects the following basic relationships: (a) in order for flow in a vessel to occur, there must be a pressure gradient along the vessel (the homolog to electromotive force), and that (b) the resulting flow (the homolog of electrical current) is a function of the pressure gradient and an inverse function of the vascular resistance to that flow (the homolog of electrical resistance).

These relations are illustrated in Figure 8.4. Here, P_1 is the pressure at the initial portion of the vessel and P_2 is the pressure at the last portion of the vessel. Thus, the

gradient, or pressure differential along this vessel segment is $P_1 - P_2$. Note that as long as P_1 is larger than P_2 then blood will flow through the vessel in the direction indicated. Resistance (R), or the impediment to flow as a result of the vessel wall and the contents flowing in the vessel, occurs along the entire length of the vessel. Resistance can be increased by structural components of the vessel (e.g., bumps along the endothelial surface or bends in the vessel) or by increased viscosity (i.e., thickness) of the blood in the vessel. In this depiction, blood flow rate (Q; usually expressed in liters/min) or the amount of blood that passes a particular point in the circulation in a given time is equal to $P_1 - P_2/R$. Thus, with a constant pressure gradient, when resistance increases, flow decreases. Alternatively, if the pressure gradient is larger, the flow increases (when resistance is the same). One commonly measured aspect of resistance is the total peripheral resistance (TPR) which

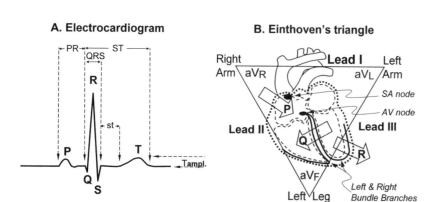

Figure 8.3. The heart and the electrocardiogram. (A) General morphology of the electrocardiographic (ECG) signal showing the P, Q, R, S, & T components, the PR, ST, and QRS intervals, the *st* segment, and the T wave amplitude. (B) The heart, conduction system, and Einthoven's triangle. Open arrow indicates the direction of propagation of electrical activation and the associated component of the ECG.

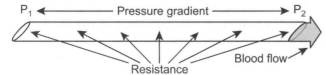

Figure 8.4. Ohm's Law applied to a blood vessel segment. This figure shows pressure differences along a vessel (difference in pressure between P_1 and P_2), resistance to flow in the vessel, and blood flow from the vessel segment. See text for relationships among these parameters.

is the resistance to flow over the entire systemic circulation (measured in dyne · seconds/centimeters[5] or in peripheral resistance units; PRUs). This basic formulation relating resistance, pressure and flow underlies the movement of blood through the circulatory system.

Blood flow rate is also captured in Poiseuille's Law where:

$$Q = \frac{\Delta \text{Pressure} \cdot \pi \cdot \text{Vessel radius}^4}{8 \cdot \text{Vessel length} \cdot \text{Blood viscosity}}$$

This formula illustrates an important aspect of the relationship between the factors that impact on blood flow, namely that changes in vessel diameter have a much greater influence on blood flow than any other factor. Indeed, conductance (or blood flow through a vessel for a given pressure gradient) is the reciprocal of resistance, and is proportional to the vessel diameter[4]. Thus, a very small change in vessel diameter by local, neural and hormonal control of the arterioles results in a relatively large change in blood flow.

Blood pressure is the force exerted by the blood against the vessel walls and is generally measured in units of millimeters of mercury (mmHg). Overall arterial pressure varies between the highest level of pressure seen at systole (systolic blood pressure or SBP) and the lowest level seen in diastole (the diastolic blood pressure or DBP). The difference between the systolic and diastolic pressures is called the pulse pressure (PP). Mean arterial pressure (MAP) is often calculated as: DBP + 1/3 PP (or 2DBP/3 + 1SBP/3) because diastole is about twice as long as systole.

Blood pressure varies across different parts of the circulatory system. When measuring blood pressure, it is important to report the body location from which the pressure is measured (e.g., at the brachial or femoral artery) and for the measurement site to be located at the vertical height of the heart in order to minimize the effects of hydrostatic pressure (the pressure exerted by the fluid in the circulatory system) on the blood pressure measurement. Figure 8.5 shows how blood pressures vary throughout the circulatory system. First note that pressures are high and pulsatile near the aorta where the heart continuously pumps blood into the systemic circulation. As the pressure pulse moves further from the heart, the elastic properties of the large arteries and the control of vessel diameter by smooth muscle in the arterioles damp out much of the pulse in the pressure wave. Because the diameter of the arteriolar vessels is controlled by both intrinsic (local) and extrinsic (autonomic and hormonal) factors, these vessels function essentially as valves controlling the flow of blood into the capillary system. Arterioles are strong walled vessels and their "valvular" function is important because it prevents excessive pressures from reaching the thin walled capillaries where the vessels could be damaged. Systemic pressure falls further as the blood returns from the capillaries, through the small venules and into ever larger veins that eventually return blood to the right atrium. In the normal heart, blood pressure will be at or near zero once blood returns from the largest veins, the inferior and superior vena cavae, to the right atrium. Pressures in the pulmonary circulation are not nearly as high as the systemic circulation, in part due to the short distances the blood must travel through the lungs, relative to the distance traveled in the systemic circulation.

Based on Ohm's Law it would appear that blood pressure would cause a proportional increase in blood flow throughout the body, however, vessels can distend, a fact that complicates the prediction of blood flow with increases in blood pressure. A bolus of blood entering a vessel distends it, and thus the diameter of the vessel does not remain constant. Distensibility is an important feature of veins in particular (which are on average about 8 times more distensible than arteries) because blood is stored in the veins

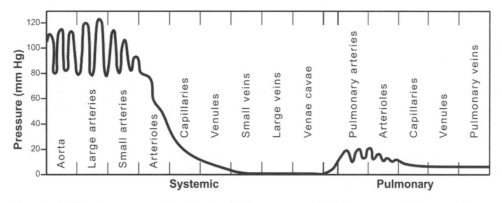

Figure 8.5. Blood pressure variations in the circulatory system. Blood pressure variations are shown for different types of vessels in the systemic and pulmonary circulation.

which form a reservoir from which blood can be marshaled when tissue needs increase. Distensibility of the vessels also helps to damp out pressure pulsations such that by the time blood reaches the capillary beds, the flow of blood is steady and provides a constant supply of nutrients and removal of wastes.

Cardiac output, another critical aspect of circulatory function, is the amount of blood pumped by the left ventricle into the aorta per unit of time (usually expressed as liters/min). Cardiac output can be expressed using another variant of Ohm's Law:

CO = Mean arterial pressure/Total peripheral resistance.

Cardiac output is directly controlled by the venous return, or the amount of blood that returns to the right atrium from the venous system each minute. Indeed the venous return and the cardiac output are usually equal (except when extra blood is stored in the heart or lungs for a few beats). Because the venous return is the sum of the local blood flows in all of the tissues of the body, the cardiac output is thus controlled by all of these local flows. Therefore, it is most appropriate to see the cardiac output as controlled by the local, neural, and hormonal controllers of these local blood flows, rather than as controlled by the heart.

Blood flow regulation

There are important local, intrinsic mechanisms for regulating blood flow to the heart and other tissues, the venous return and the cardiac output. These mechanisms work in concert with the extrinsic mechanisms (autonomic and hormonal) that are discussed in subsequent sections.

The primary intrinsic mechanism controlling blood flow to the heart is the Frank-Starling mechanism. It was observed that when there was greater venous return than was pumped out with the preceding beat, that the heart subsequently pumped more vigorously (i.e., greater contractility) and pumped a greater volume of blood (i.e., stroke volume, or the volume of blood pumped from the left ventricle with each beat of the heart). It was suggested that this phenomenon occurred due to the presence of stretch receptors in the cardiac tissue, which reacted to increased stretch by producing greater contraction of the ventricular muscle. Recent studies have suggested that a key molecular player in the Frank-Starling mechanism is a large, elastic molecule present in the sarcomeres of cardiac muscle, called titin or connectin (Fukuda, & Granzier, 2004). Not only does titin appear to have passive spring-like properties, but it may also be stretch-sensitive and thus play an active role in the Frank-Starling mechanism (Fukuda, Wu, Farman, Irving, & Granzier, 2003). Another intrinsic mechanism controlling the heart beat is that stretch of the right atrial wall produces an increase in the heart rate which in turn increases the stroke volume, although this effect plays a less important role than the Frank-Starling mechanism.

There are also local, tissue-based mechanisms that provide additional blood flow to tissues of the body when there is a local need for greater tissue oxygenation (Guyton and Hall, 2000). These mechanisms act both acutely (several seconds) and over longer periods (minutes to weeks). There are two primary theories about the acute mechanisms by which most initial changes in blood flow are locally regulated. The first is the vasodilator theory according to which blood flow is regulated by the release of vasodilator substances which increase in concentration when oxygen levels fall. Some of the possible vasodilator substances that have been proposed include adenosine (a strong contender), carbon dioxide, lactic acid, potassium ions, and hydrogen ions. The primary concern with this theory has been a problem in demonstrating that enough of these vasodilator substances are produced to account for the degree of vasodilation seen when vessels are deprived of oxygen. A second theory, called the oxygen (or nutrient) demand theory, suggests that the tissue responds to nutrient demand presumably by causing contraction of sphincters located at the entry of blood to capillary beds (i.e., precapillary sphincters) and in small arterioles (i.e., metarterioles). The theory holds that when these sphincters sense increased oxygen, they contract, thus limiting additional flow to those vascular beds with enough oxygen. This theory is based on observations of cyclical opening and closing of the precapillary and metarteriolar sphincters several times over a minute. These studies showed that the time that the sphincters are open is proportional to the amount of oxygen in the tissue. Evidence countering this theory also exists such that in some tissues, vascular smooth muscle will stay contracted even with only very small amounts of oxygen present. Guyton and Hall (2000) suggest that perhaps the mechanisms underlying acute local changes in blood flow are a combination of the mechanisms underlying these two theories.

Following acute changes in blood flow, flow tends to return to the original level through autoregulatory processes. Autoregulation is thought to occur via mechanisms that have been subsumed under one of two different theories: the metabolic theory, and the myogenic theory. The metabolic theory is based on the mechanisms just discussed, (i.e., either release of vasodilator substances or smooth muscle constriction in response to excess oxygen), but now with the effect of resetting blood flow toward the previous level. The myogenic theory, in contrast, suggests that fast stretch of vessel walls leads to smooth muscle constriction. Although this mechanism has been demonstrated in isolated vessels, it is not clear that it would be generally useful throughout the body as any stretch of the vessel wall would lead to vasoconstriction, increased pressure in the vessel, and additional stretch. This vicious cycle would not be effective for the overall functioning of the vascular system.

In combination with these local mechanisms acting predominantly in the smaller vessels (i.e., capillaries and metarterioles), are mechanisms that alter flow in larger vessels. When increased flow enhances shear stress in arterioles and small arteries, the endothelium lining these vessels releases nitric oxide which causes local vasodilation and a concomitant reduction in the shear stress. Thus, local mechanisms are available in most of the vessels that see relatively high pressures and those critical for oxygen delivery to tissues (all arteries except the very large arteries which have little smooth muscle and capillaries). These mechanisms prevent excess pressure in delicate capillaries while maintaining a sufficient supply of nutrient to the tissues.

On a longer time scale, blood flow can increase or decrease when there is a longer term change in need by altering the vascularity of tissue. Vascularity changes are structural resulting either from changing the size and/or number of vessels. A prime example of this mechanism is the increased number of vessels that infiltrate a cancerous tumor that has an ever increasing need for additional blood flow. Together, local mechanisms provide many ways that blood flow can change both acutely and over longer periods to adapt to changing tissue demands.

AUTONOMIC AND HORMONAL CONTROL

Beyond local intrinsic autoregulatory processes are extrinsic regulatory process associated with autonomic and hormonal systems.

Autonomic nervous system

The cardiovascular system is under control of both the sympathetic and parasympathetic branches of the autonomic nervous system. A given organ system is often innervated by both autonomic branches, which typically exert opposing actions. Some organs are not dually innervated, however, and even for dually innervated organs, the autonomic branches may have synergistic rather than opposing effects or may otherwise be asymmetrical in their pattern of innervation or action. These patterns of innervation and effect are important in measuring, interpreting, and conceptualizing cardiovascular psychophysiological relations.

Historically, the peripheral components of the autonomic nervous system were the first to be described and studied, as they were the most distinct and accessible. Central neurons that give rise to the preganglionic axons of the autonomic nervous system are distributed across levels of the spinal cord and brainstem. The preganglionic fibers of the sympathetic system arise from the intermediolateral cell columns of the thoracic and upper lumbar spinal segments (thoracolumbar system). In contrast, the peripheral parasympathetic system arises from the nuclei within the brainstem, 'such as the dorsal motor nucleus and the nucleus ambiguus) and from sacral cord segments (craniosacral system).

With few exceptions, preganglionic axons terminate in peripheral autonomic ganglia, where postganglionic neurons in turn issue projections to the target organs. For the sympathetic system, these ganglia consist of the sympathetic chain ganglia that lie along the vertebrae (also termed paravertebral ganglia) and a few more remote ganglia (e.g., the celiac ganglion). In contrast, the ganglia of the parasympathetic system are more distributed, being located in or around the organ being innervated. Consequently, the postganglionic axons of the parasympathetic system are rather short and the preganglionic fibers are long, whereas the opposite relation holds for the sympathetic system. Because of the heavy interconnections within the sympathetic chain ganglia it was believed historically that the system discharges as a whole, whereas the distinct parasympathetic ganglia allowed for a more organ specific discharge. It is now clear that even the sympathetic system is capable of targeted actions, as microneurographic recordings in conscious subjects have demonstrated a striking specificity in the pattern of sympathetic discharge across organ systems (for review see Valbo, Hagbarth, & Wallin, 2004).

In comparison to the somatic motor system, an obvious question arises as to why the peripheral autonomic nerves are interrupted by a ganglionic synapse. Minimally, this synapse would delay transmission in autonomic efferents. Although conduction velocity is crucial in the somatic motor system, it is perhaps less so for the autonomic system. The emerging picture is that autonomic ganglia may not just passively relay incoming information from preganglionic axons. Rather, autonomic ganglia may represent a first level regulatory system. Parasympathetic cardiac ganglia, for example, have been termed a "heart brain" (Randall, Wurster, Randall, & Xi-Moy, 1996), which is characterized by anatomically and neurochemically distinct sets of interacting neurons that serve to regulate aspects of cardiac function (Gray et al., 2004 a,b; Randall, Wurster, Randall, & Xi-Moy, 1996; Richardson, Grkovic, & Anderson, 2003). The precise functions of these integrative networks within autonomic ganglia have not been fully elucidated and are beyond the scope of the present chapter.

Both sets of preganglionic neurons employ acetylcholine as the primary neurotransmitter, which binds to a nicotinic receptor subtype (N_N) and several muscarinic subtypes on the postganglionic neurons in the peripheral autonomic ganglia of both branches. Nicotinic receptors mediate a direct ion channel effect and muscarinic receptors can also promote activity via intracellular 2nd messenger pathways (for review and recent data see Beker, Weber, Fink, & Adams, 2003). Postganglionic parasympathetic fibers also employ acetylcholine as a primary neurotransmitter, although the receptor sub-types on the target organ are commonly muscarinic (M). In contrast, the postganglionic neurons of the sympathetic system employ norepinephrine as the primary neurotransmitter, which can act on alpha adrenergic (e.g., α_1 in arterioles) or beta adrenergic receptors (e.g., β_1 on the heart). As illustrated in Table 8.1, this pharmacological differentiation allows selective experimental manipulations of the autonomic branches. We will return to this issue later.

Table 8.1. Autonomic pharmacology

Synapse	Receptor	Agonist	Antagonist	Organ systems
Acetylcholine				
Autonomic Ganglia	Nicotinic (N_N)	Nicotine	Pentolinium/ Hexamethonium	broad autonomic
Postganglionic Parasympathetic	Muscarinic	Muscarine/ Pilocarpine	Atropine/ Scopolamine	heart/eccrine glands/sudomotor/ gastrointestinal/ciliary muscle
Norepinephrine				
Postganglionic Sympathetic	α_1	phenylephrine	prazosin	vascular vasoconstrictors
	α_2	clonidine	yohimbine	vascular vasoconstrictors (central antihypertensive actions)
	β_1	isoproterenol	atenolol	heart
	β_2	terbutaline	propranolol	bronchioles, vascular vasodilators, (nonselective) also in heart

There are additional complications and some exceptions to the above schema. Added complexity arises from the fact that many autonomic neurons, in addition to their primary neurotransmitter, express and release a variety of neuropeptides and neuromodulators such as neuropeptide Y, vasoactive intestinal peptide, enkephalins and substance P, which may impact transmitter release and/or receptor action (e.g., see Lindh & Hokfelt, 1990; Richardson, R. J., Grkovic, I., & Anderson, 2003). One rather fascinating exception to the pharmacological differentiation as summarized in Table 8.1 is the sympathetic innervation of eccrine sweat glands, which is cholinergic rather than adrenergic. The postganglionic sympathetic neurons that innervate eccrine glands initially appear to express norepinephrine but undergo a phenotypic switch to cholinergic production on interactions with the target tissue (see Landis, 1996). Subsequently, eccrine gland sweat production is controlled largely by muscarinic receptors, although other receptor types might also be involved (Kurzen, & Schallreuter, 2004; Longmore, Bradshaw, & Szabadi, 1985; see also Dawson, Chapter 7).

Another exception, more apparent than real, is the cholinergic sympathetic innervation of the adrenal medulla. In contrast to the postganglionic cholinergic innervation of eccrine glands, the cholinergic innervation of the adrenal medulla is by preganglionic fibers that bypass the ganglionic synapse. These neurons in fact show the typical cholinergic phenotype for sympathetic preganglionics. Furthermore, the direct innervation of the adrenal gland does not violate the general plan. In contrast to most visceral organs, the adrenal medulla derives embryologically from neural crest cells and is thus homologous with sympathetic ganglia. Also like ganglion cells, the adrenal medulla synthesizes and releases catecholamines – norepinephrine and epinephrine. The major difference is that

these adrenomedullary amines are released humorally into the general circulation where they can act at widespread sites. Epinephrine has a somewhat greater affinity than norepinephrine for α and β_2 receptors and an equal affinity for β_1 receptors. The effects of neural NE release and adrenomedullary NE and EPI release may be distinct, however, as diffusion barriers may reduce effects of circulating catecholamines on synaptic receptors. Of additional relevance are noninnervated α and β receptors on the heart and vasculature, which can only be activated by NE or EPI humorally or by norepinephrine spillover from adjacent synapses.

Heart. The general neuroarchitectural plan of the autonomic innervation of the heart is illustrated in Figure 8.6. Parasympathetic preganglionic projections arising from the nucleus ambiguus and the dorsal motor nucleus of the vagus project to the sinoatrial and posterior atrial ganglia, for the regulation of heart rate (chronotropic control), to the atrioventricular ganglia for the control of conduction (dromotropic control), and to the interventriculo-septal-ganglia for the regulation of myocardial contractility (inotropic control, although this is minimal for the parasympathetic system) (Gray et al., 2004a,b; Johnson et al., 2004; Pirola, & Potter, 1990; Richardson et al., 2003; Sampaio, Mauad, Spyer, & Ford, 2003). The lower central motor neurons that give rise to preganglionic sympathetic cardiac projections reside in the intermediolateral cell columns, mostly in the upper thoracic segments (Ter Horst, Hautvast, De Jongste, & Korf, 1996). These preganglionic neurons project to the stellate and cervical sympathetic ganglia, which in turn issue postganglionic projections to the heart (Anderson, 1998).

The parasympathetic system has a much wider dynamic range of control over cardiac chronotropy than does

Autonomic Innervation

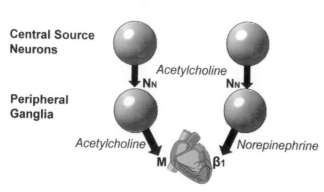

Figure 8.6. General pattern of pharmacology of the autonomic innervations. Abbreviations refer to the relevant postsynaptic receptor populations: N_N – nicotinic cholinergic; M – muscarinic cholinergic; $\beta 1$ – beta1 adrenergic.

the sympathetic system, whereas the sympathetic system has a more predominant effect on the inotropic state. In humans, the dynamic range of sympathetic chronotropic control has been estimated to be about 230 msec, whereas that of the parasympathetic system is about 1710 msec (Berntson, Cacioppo, & Quigley, 1993a). Chronotropic control of heart period is rather linearly related to parasympathetic activity, whereas there is some nonlinearity in the sympathetic branch. When expressed as heart rate, the dynamic range is highly dependent on baseline heart rate, because heart rate is a nonlinear transform of heart period. The typical dynamic range of control of the sympathetic branch, in heart rate over a wide range of baseline values is ~3–55 beats/min and that for the parasympathetic system is ~71–125 beats/min). An additional complexity is that there are interactions between the branches at the level of the sinoatrial node, and these appear to be much greater when the chronotropic state is expressed in heart rate (Berntson, Cacioppo, & Quigley, 1995). Another difference between the sympathetic and parasympathetic innervations of cardiac pacemaker tissue lies in their temporal dynamics. The parasympathetic cholinergic receptor at the sinoatrial node is directly coupled by a G-protein link to a potassium channel through which a hyperpolarizing K+ flux slows the spontaneous depolarization of the pacemaker potential. In contrast, sympathetic noradrenergic receptor action is mediated by a more indirect and slower 2nd messenger signaling pathway. Consequently, the parasympathetic system has a shorter latency of action, a more rapid rise time, and a higher frequency capacity – which is the basis for the selective contribution of vagal control to the high-frequency heart rate variability of respiratory sinus arrhythmia (Berntson, Cacioppo, & Quigley, 1993b; Somsen, Jennings, & Van der Molen, 2004). Vagal activation to a behaviorally relevant event, for example, can alter the

interbeat interval of the very beat within which the event occurs (see Somsen et al., 2004).

In contrast to parasympathetic dominance over heart rate, the sympathetic system dominates the control of cardiac contractility. Although there is parasympathetic innervation of the ventricles (Johnson et al., 2004), stimulation of the parasympathetic system in the absence of sympathetic activation may have relatively little direct effect on contractility beyond a secondary effect of heart rate slowing (Levy, 1984; Takahashi, 2003). Much of the parasympathetic innervation of the ventricles may represent presynaptic terminations on sympathetic synapses, which permits a vagal inhibition of sympathetic inotropic control (Levy, 1984; Takahashi, 2003). Interactions among the sympathetic and parasympathetic cardiac innervations are multiple and complex, and include a nitric oxide mediated parasympathetic inhibition of sympathetic control and neuropeptide Y-mediated sympathetic inhibition of parasympathetic control (Chowdhary, Marsh, Coote, & Townend, 2004; Ren, 1991).

Control of the vasculature. Although the heart is a crucial organ in generating the pressure differentials that contribute to circulation of the blood, the vasculature plays an essential part in the maintenance of blood pressure and the arterio-venous blood pressure difference that underlies the distribution of blood. This contribution is not merely as a passive conduit, but as an active regulator of the circulation and distribution of blood across organ systems. An important aspect of this regulation entails peripheral autoregulatory processes that are sensitive to local tissue conditions.

The autonomic nervous system, especially the sympathetic division, is also an important controller of the vascular smooth muscle. Adrenergic receptors on the smooth muscle serve as vasoconstrictors that regulate vascular tone, vascular resistance, and venous compliance. From the initial distinction between alpha and beta adrenergic receptors, an increasing array of receptor subtypes has been identified (α_1, α_{2A}, α_{2B}, β_1) that have distinct functional roles in cardiovascular control (for review see Guimaraes & Moura, 2001). In the arterial system, the α_1 subtype of adrenoceptors mediates the classical vasoconstrictor actions of both sympathetic innervations and adrenomedullary catecholamines, whereas α_2 receptors are more prevalent in veins where they regulate venous tone and compliance. Several α_2 receptor subtypes are also present as autoreceptors on sympathetic terminals where they serve an inhibitory role in the regulation of NE release (Brede et al., 2004).

In contrast to α-adrenoceptors, the β class of adrenoceptors on smooth muscle mediates adrenergic vasodilation (Guimaraes & Moura, 2001). The β_2 subtype is most common in most vascular beds and mediates, for example, the muscle vasodilation during sympathetic activation associated with exercise. These β_2 adrenoceptors may be particularly driven by humoral adrenomedullary catecholamines. β_2 receptors have also been described as autoreceptors on adrenergic presynaptic terminals. The β_1 subtype has been increasingly recognized as a mediator of vasodilation in certain vascular beds (e.g., the coronary and pulmonary arteries) and a novel β_3 receptor subtype appears to have vasodilatory functions in the mesenteric and other arterial beds.

Water balance. Additional hormonal and organ systems contribute to body water and electrolyte balance and thus play an important role in blood volume, blood pressure, water distribution, and hence cardiovascular regulation (Guthrie & Yucha, 2004). The kidney is the primary route by which fluids are eliminated in normal organisms. The renal tubular system receives a high volume of blood ultrafiltrate (at the renal glomerulus) including water and electrolytes such as sodium and potassium, most of which is ultimately reabsorbed by the renal tubules prior to passing to the urinary bladder for excretion. The hypothalamic-posterior pituitary hormone vasopressin has two important functions in circulation (Guthrie & Yucha, 2004). First it is a potent vasoconstrictor agent, hence its pressor effect, and secondly it promotes water resorption (antidiuretic effect) in the renal tubule system. Vasopressin stimulation is triggered by either osmotic or hypovolemic body water disturbances and its pressor effect serves to compensate for low blood volume, whereas its antidiuretic effect promotes water retention. The absence of vasopressin in *diabetes insipidus* results in a chronic condition of polyuria (frequent urination of large volumes) and polydipsia (frequent drinking).

Another important player in body water balance is the renin-angiotensin system (see Fitzsimons, 1998; Grisk & Rettig, 2004). Renin is a proteolytic enzyme secreted by *juxtaglomerular* cells of the kidney under conditions of low blood pressure and controlled in part by the sympathetic system. Renin converts a blood borne precursor (*angiotensinogen*) to angiotensin I, which is in turn converted to an active peptide hormone, *angiotensin II*, by the action of another enzyme *angiotensin converting enzyme* (ACE). Angiotensin II is notable for its wide range of actions, which include vasoconstriction, stimulation of thirst, and triggering of *aldosterone* release from the adrenal cortex. Aldosterone is an adrenocortical mineralocorticoid that promotes the resorption of sodium from the renal tubules and fosters salt appetite. Collectively, these actions compensate for the loss of body water and electrolytes and expand blood volume. In fact, they are so effective that overactivity in these systems may contribute to hypertension and ACE inhibitors are effective antihypertensive agents (Grisk & Rettig, 2004).

A final humoral system to be briefly mentioned here is the cardiac natriuretic system, which is implicated in water balance, blood volume, and blood pressure regulation (Luchner & Schunkert, 2004). Cardiac natriuretic fac-

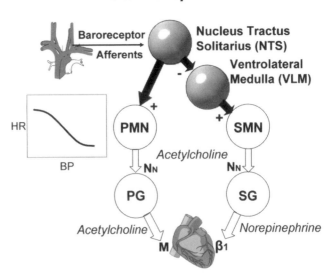

Figure 8.7. General organization of the baroreceptor heart rate reflex. Reflex originates in mechanoreceptors in the heart and the carotid and other great arteries. The NTS excites (+ symbol) the parasympathetic motor neurons (PMN) and inhibits (– symbol) relay neurons to the sympathetic motor neuron pool (SMN). Insert illustrates the relationship between blood pressure (BP) and heart rate (HR). PG and SG depict parasympathetic and sympathetic ganglia, respectively. Other abbreviations are as in Figure 8.6.

tors are released on myocardial stretch and trigger vasodilation, natriuresis (sodium excretion), and inhibition of the sympathetic nervous system and the renin-angiotensin system (Woods, 2004). This natriuretic system is suppressed by a β adrenergic mechanism and may promote vagal control, and illustrates some of the complexities in neural and humoral cardiovascular control.

Central neural control

The cardiovascular system is crucial for survival so it is not surprising that this system is regulated by complex central mechanisms, including lower-level reflex systems as well as higher neurobehavioral mechanisms.

Brainstem reflexes. Among the most well characterized of cardiovascular reflexes are the baroreceptor reflexes, including the baroreceptor heart rate reflex and the baroreceptor vascular reflex (Dampney, Polson, Potts, Hirooka, & Horiuchi, 2003; Ursino & Magosso, 2003; see also Chapter 19, this volume). The baroreceptor heart rate reflex circuit, depicted in Figure 8.7, is comprised of stretch receptor afferents from the carotid and other great arteries to the nucleus tractus solitarius (NTS), the major visceral receiving station in the brainstem. NTS projections can excite activity in parasympathetic source nuclei and via an indirect pathway can inhibit the rostral ventrolateral medulla (VLM) which is a major descending source of tonic drive on the sympathetic output neurons of the intermediolateral cell column. Through this circuit, for example, increasing blood pressure and the associated increase in baroreceptor afferent traffic increases parasympathetic control and decreases sympathetic outflow. These reciprocal changes in the autonomic branches synergistically serve to oppose the pressure perturbation. The increase in parasympathetic and the decrease in sympathetic cardiac chronotropic control both lead to a slowing of heart rate. This, together with the reduced ventricular contractility due to withdrawal of sympathetic inotropic control, leads to a decrease in cardiac output. In addition, the withdrawal of sympathetic vasoconstrictor control results in vasodilation, which further diminishes blood pressure. Conversely, the unloading of baroreceptors during the assumption of an upright posture (orthostatic stress) yields the opposite pattern of autonomic control – an increase in sympathetic and a decrease in parasympathetic outflow, which compensates for the diminished blood pressure associated with the gravitational pooling of the blood in the lower body.

In addition to arterial baroreceptors, there are a variety of cardiopulmonary mechanoreceptors that contribute to reflex regulation of the cardiovascular system. One such reflex, which is often capitalized on in psychophysiology, has its origin in lung stretch receptors (see Berntson, Cacioppo, & Quigley, 1993b). Inspiration results in the activation of these stretch receptors and their afferents, which project to the NTS. Input from stretch receptor afferents results in a reflexive inhibition of parasympathetic cardiac outflow and an excitation of the sympathetic system. As a result, there arise respiratory rhythms in both sympathetic and parasympathetic nerves, as well as in heart rate variability. Because the sympathetic cardiac synapses can not follow the typical respiratory frequencies, however, the respiratory rhythms in heart rate are driven by the parasympathetic system. Consequently, this respiratory sinus arrhythmia is commonly employed as an index of vagal control of the heart. We will return to this issue below.

An additional class of cardiovascular reflexes are the chemoreceptor reflexes (see Ursino & Magosso, 2003). Pure hypoxia (decreased arterial O_2 pressure), for example, triggers a local vasodilation in vital organs. Although this could be considered an adaptive local regulation, if widespread, it could result in a life-threatening hypotension. Chemoreceptors in the carotid bodies and aorta detect this low oxygen pressure and convey an afferent signal to the NTS which results in a reflexive increase in respiratory minute volume. Hypoxia also yields compensatory cardiovascular reflexes, including a sympathetic vasoconstriction of arterioles throughout many organ systems (except for coronary and brain arterioles), which serve to maintain blood pressure and circulation. A concurrent parasympathetic activation results in bradycardia, which may serve to minimize cardiac work in the face of hypoxia and may also enhance cardiac output (by increasing ventricular filling time). Pure hypoxia is rare, however, as hypoxia is generally associated with changes in partial

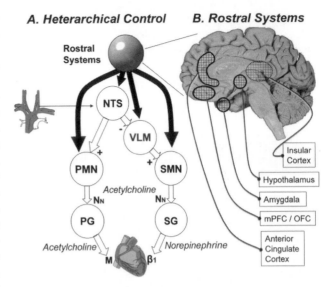

Figure 8.8. Rostral neural systems and heterarchical control. (A) Schematic representation of higher neural control of the autonomic nervous system. The figure illustrates the two general features of heterarchical control: a hierarchical structure together with long ascending (and descending) connections which bypass intermediate levels of organization. (B) Higher neural systems and areas that have been implicated in autonomic control. mPFC – medial prefrontal cortex; OFC – orbitofrontal cortex; other abbreviations are as in Figure 8.7.

pressure of CO_2, which can either increase (hypercapnia, e.g., during asphyxia) or decrease (hypocapnia, e.g., during increased respiration at high altitude). Chemoreceptors are also sensitive to CO_2 pressure (mediated by local pH), with higher levels of hypercapnia yielding progressively greater chemoreceptor activity. This signal has synergistic super-additive effects with hypoxia on chemoreceptor firing.

The cardiovascular reflexes outlined above are far from exhaustive. Rather, they are intended to be illustrative of the powerful reflex control over the cardiovascular system. In psychophysiological contexts, however, higher neuraxial levels may figure more prominently in autonomic regulation.

Higher neural controls. As illustrated in Figure 8.8, higher levels of the neuraxis, including neurobehavioral substrates of the limbic system and other forebrain areas can control, inhibit, or even bypass lower reflex mechanisms in the regulation of autonomic outflows. An example is the stress related suppression of the baroreflex which is mediated by rostral neurobehavioral systems (see Chapter 19, this volume). It is this reflex suppression that allows the concurrent increase in heart rate and blood pressure during stress, in direct conflict with baroreceptor reflexes. As is the case for the somatic nervous system, higher neural autonomic controls are far more flexible and variable than brainstem reflex substrates. Whereas brainstem reflex systems may display a rather fixed, reciprocal pattern of control over the autonomic branches, higher systems are

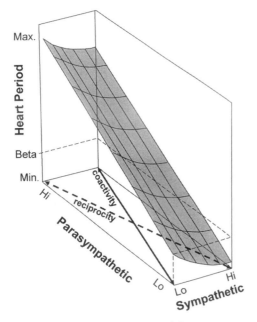

A. Autonomic Continuum

Parasympathetic　　　　　　　Sympathetic.

B. Cardiac Autonomic Space

Figure 8.9. Autonomic space. (A) Continuum model of auto-nomic control, wherein the status of the system can be depicted along a single continuum extending from parasympathetic dom-inance to sympathetic dominance. (B) A more comprehensive model of autonomic control, characterized by an autonomic plane (representing the fact that parasympathetic and sympathetic sys-tems can change reciprocally, coactively, or independently) and an overlying effector surface which illustrates the end organ state (heart period) for any location on the underlying autonomic plane. Beta illustrates the intrinsic heart period in the absence of auto-nomic control.

capable of reciprocal, coactive (coactivation or coinhibi-tion) or independent changes in outflows of the two auto-nomic branches. This has required an expansion from the bipolar model of reciprocal autonomic control to a bivariate autonomic plane and overlying effector surface as depicted in Figure 8.9 (Berntson, Cacioppo, & Quigley, 1991, 1993a; see also Chapter 19, this volume).

There are ample routes by which higher behavioral substrates can impact autonomic cardiovascular regula-tion. Direct monosynaptic projections to brainstem reflex substrates and even to autonomic source nuclei have been described from rostral areas and structures that have been implicated in psychological and behavioral pro-cesses. These include the hypothalamus, amygdala, and prefrontal cortex (see Chapter 19, this volume).

A neuroanatomical tracing study illustrates the rich inte-gration of higher neural systems in autonomic regulation. In this study, pseudorabies virus was injected into distinct areas in the rat heart (Ter Horst, Hautvast, Jongste, & Korf, 1996). Following such injections the viral infection spreads

transneuronally in autonomic nerves, in the retrograde direction back to the central nervous system, where viral labeling can reveal components of multisynaptic networks that regulate autonomic outflow. Among the areas labeled were the NTS and the ventrolateral medulla, as would be expected from Figure 8.8. Higher labeled structures included the raphe nuclei, which give rise to both ascend-ing and descending serotonergic projections, and the A5 cell group, which gives rise to ascending and descend-ing norepinephrine pathways. Additional structures that have been implicated in cognitive and affective processes were also labeled, including the midbrain periaqueductal gray, hypothalamus, amygdala, anterior cingulate gyrus, and the frontal and prefrontal cortex.

A combination of neuroimaging methods and auto-nomic measures is beginning to be applied to questions of rostral autonomic control. Although this integrative effort is in its infancy, initial findings suggest a close correspon-dence between neuroanatomical and neurophysiological studies on the one hand and functional neuroimaging stud-ies of autonomic control on the other. PET and fMRI stud-ies have reported that mental arithmetic, a Stroop-stress paradigm, or emotional contexts engage several forebrain areas that have been implicated in psychological processes and autonomic control, including the cingulate cortex, orbitofrontal cortex, insular cortex, and medial and dor-solateral prefrontal cortex, as well as related areas such as the hypothalamus, amygdala, and cerebellum (Chritch-ley et al., 2005a; Gianaros, May, Siegle, & Jennings, 2005; Gianaros, Van Der Veen, & Jennings, 2004; Lane, Reiman, Ahern, & Thayer, 2001; Matthews, Paulus, Simmons, Nele-sen, & Dimsdale, 2004). Moreover, these studies found that the magnitude of cardiovascular responses (blood pres-sure, heart rate, and heart rate variability) was significantly related to the magnitude of activation in specific brain regions.

With the further development of imaging techniques, this approach will likely be of increasing importance in understanding neurobehavioral systems and their links to autonomic control. Studies using fMRI, for example, have already revealed functional subdivisions even within the anterior cingulate cortex, a complex structure that repre-sents an important interface between cognition and emo-tion. These subdivisions differentially relate to behavioral inhibition (dorsal anterior cingulate) and vagal control (ventral anterior cingulate) in the Stroop task (Matthews, Paulus, Simmons, Nelesen, & Dimsdale, 2004). Brain imaging methods not only hold considerable promise for the elucidation of central autonomic and neurobehav-ioral systems, but also for the clarification of the links between psychological states and processes and cardiovas-cular health outcomes (Critchley et al., 2005b).

Figure 8.8 illustrates some brain areas that have been implicated in both cognitive and affective processes as well as autonomic cardiovascular control. The extensive overlap of these rostral systems likely reflects the close integration between behavioral and autonomic substrates that underlies the neurobiology of psychophysiological relations.

PSYCHOPHYSIOLOGICAL MEASURES: RATIONALE AND PHYSIOLOGICAL BASES

ECG

Electrocardiography (ECG or EKG) has been well developed by the field of medical cardiology (for reviews see Berne & Levy, 2001; Goldberger, 1998). The extremity (limb) leads in clinical electrocardiology can be represented by Einthoven's triangle, as illustrated in Figure 8.3B. These leads consist of the unipolar leads of the right arm (aV_R), left arm (aV_L), and left leg (aV_F) and the bipolar leads I (left arm – right arm), II (left leg – right arm), and III (left leg – left arm), with the right leg serving as ground. These leads are often approximated by electrodes placed on the torso, rather than the limbs. In addition, a series of unipolar precordial chest leads are commonly recognized that extend from the lower peristernal region (V_1) laterally to the left (V_1 through V_5) to the midaxial line on the lateral aspect of the chest (V_6). These multiple leads are important in clinical cardiology as they offer distinct electrical perspectives on the events of the cardiac cycle. For most psychophysiological applications, however, a lead II or comparable configuration (e.g., electrodes at V_6 and the right collar bone or aV_R) work well as they yield a relatively large R-wave.

As depicted in Figure 8.3B, the P wave represents the spread of excitation from the sinoatrial (pacemaker) node through the atria, the QRS complex corresponds to the invasion of the ventricular myocardium, and the T wave reflects the repolarization of the ventricles. The arrows in Figure 8.3B illustrate the electrical vectors during selected events within the cardiac cycle. The QRS complex may manifest in just QR or RS deflections depending on the selected lead and how it "views" the electrical events. For a standard lead II configuration, the Q wave reflects the initial depolarization of the ventricular septum, which is followed by the bulk of the ventricular myocardium (R wave). Although the T wave represents the repolarization phase, it generally has the same polarity as the R wave. This is attributable to regional differences (epicardium vs. endocardium) in electrical properties of the ventricular myocytes, which results in the repolarization wave proceeding in the opposite direction to the depolarization phase (the epicardium depolarizes last, but repolarizes first).

Figure 8.3A also illustrates some time/amplitude parameters that have been employed clinically or experimentally. The PR interval (actually the PQ interval if a Q wave is present) reflects the propagation time through the atria and the atrioventricular (AV) node, by way of the conduction system to the ventricles (dromotropic function).

A PR interval longer than 200 msec suggests a conduction impairment (heart block). Within-subjects variation in the PR interval has sometimes been taken to reflect variations in vagal control of the dromotropic state (it slows conduction), although it is not a reliable measure of vagal control as the sympathetic system also influences conduction time. The QRS interval is typically 100 msec, but a prolonged interval can be seen with a block in one of the bundle branches of the conduction system (see Figure 8.3B). The ST segment corresponds to the peak of the muscle action potential and ventricular ejection, the onset of which is also reflected in the first heart sound corresponding to the opening of the aortic valve. The QT interval represents the time from ventricular excitation to the return to the resting state, it can range from 250–500 msec or so and is dependent on the heart rate (shorter at higher heart rates).

The amplitude of the T wave (see Figure 8.3A) has been proposed as a measure of sympathetic control of the heart, as it is sensitive to sympathetic activation or beta adrenergic drugs, but less so to cholinergic drugs or markers of parasympathetic activity (see Contrada, 1992; Furedy, Heslegrave, & Scher, 1992; Kline, Ginsburg, & Johnston, 1998). This measure has not received general acceptance, however, as it does show some sensitivity to cholinergic manipulations (Annila, Yli-Hankala, & Lindgren, 1994), and shows inherent rate dependent changes (Contrada, 1992; Kline et al., 1998) that are independent of, and can be as large as, autonomic effects (Rashba et al., 2002).

Heart rate/heart period

Heart period, or the time in msec between adjacent heart beats is typically measured between successive R spikes in the ECG given the larger magnitude and sharper inflection of the R spike relative to other ECG components. Traditionally, heart period (in msec) was generally converted to heart rate (in beats/min or bpm), although now both measures are used commonly. Heart period and heart rate are simple reciprocals, and one can convert from one metric to the other by dividing 60000 by the heart rate or heart period value. Heart period values become heart rate (in bpm) and heart rate becomes heart period (in msec).

Previously it was assumed that the choice of cardiac metric or measure was not important, and depending on the experimental question and the nature of the results, that may indeed be true. However, there are times where the metric does matter because heart rate and heart period are not linearly related to each other (Berntson, Cacioppo, & Quigley, 1995). Berntson and colleagues (1995) reviewed literature across several mammalian species, including humans, showing that the relationship between changes in activity of the parasympathetic and sympathetic autonomic branches and heart period are more nearly linear than the relationship between activity in either branch and heart rate. Therefore, a given change in activation of one of the autonomic branches will result in approximately the same change in heart period regardless of the baseline heart period, whereas the same is not true of heart rate. Using data from dogs as an example (from Parker, Celler, Potter, & McCloskey, 1984), an increase in stimulation frequency of 2 Hz of the vagal nerve results in a change of 70–72 msec in heart period regardless of whether the resting (baseline) heart period is 875 msec or 350 msec. However, when the dog's basal heart period is 875 msec (or 68.6 bpm) the change in heart rate with a 2 Hz increment in parasympathetic activation is 5.1 bpm, whereas at a basal heart period of 350 msec, the same 2 Hz change in autonomic input results in a heart rate change of 29.2 bpm. Therefore, the amount of cardiac change reported as a result of an experimental manipulation can differ considerably depending upon the metric chosen to represent change in cardiac function. This is particularly true if the baselines across individuals in a sample are quite different (or different as a function of an experimental factor), or if the amount of change is relatively large. Thus, Berntson and colleagues (1995) recommended that heart period be used as the metric of choice when (a) changes in cardiac function are likely to be a result of autonomic effects (e.g., for many of the short-term cardiac responses seen in the psychophysiology laboratory), and (b) when the changes in cardiac function vary widely as a result of an experimental manipulation or between groups because here the errors due to the nonlinear relationship between autonomic inputs and heart rate can be significant and result in misleading interpretations of the data. The nonlinearity of the effects of autonomic inputs on heart rate also may impact the apparent extent of interactive effects between the two autonomic branches on the heart. The idea that the two branches affect one another and thereby alter the net change in chronotropic control of the heart is termed accentuated antagonism. Although there is no doubt that there are mechanisms by which the two branches interact (see Autonomic and Hormonal Control section), the magnitude of the effects of these interactions may be smaller than has previously been suggested. Studies showing large accentuated antagonism effects have typically used heart rate as the chronotropic metric, whereas the few studies that have used heart period have not seen such large effects. Simulated data also revealed that using the same data to demonstrate interactions between the parasympathetic and sympathetic branches showed much larger apparent interaction effects with heart rate than heart period (Quigley, & Berntson, 1996).

Once the effect of an experimental manipulation is determined using the appropriate cardiac metric, one then can represent cardiac function over a number of beats where the unit of analysis is cardiac time, or over a period of time where the unit of analysis is real time. Heart period permits cardiac function to be reported in either cardiac time or real time, whereas heart rate is represented appropriately only in real time (Berntson et al., 1995; Graham, 1978). To derive heart period or rate in real time, it is important to use a weighted averaging procedure so that the mean reflects the proportion of time that each beat contributes to the overall average.

Heart rate variability

Measures of heart rate variability (HRV) have figured prominently in cardiovascular psychophysiology and there is now an extensive literature on this topic, including two international committee reports on the origins and implications of heart rate variability and methods for quantification (Berntson et al., 1997; Task Force, 1996). Of particular relevance is the fact that high-frequency heart rate variability, in the respiratory frequency range, largely reflects variations in vagal sinoatrial control and has thus been applied as a selective index of parasympathetic cardiac control (see Figure 8.10A). A wide range of measures have been used to assess heart rate variability, including time domain and frequency domain metrics.

Time domain methods include measures of the variance among heart periods, the variance of the differences among heart periods, and geometric methods based on the shape characteristics of heart period distributions (see Task Force, 1996). The simplest of the time domain metrics is the SDNN, which is the standard deviation of the normal beat to normal beat intervals (normal-to-normal or NN). Because the variance of heart periods increases over time, the SDNN is generally derived over fixed time periods, such as 5 min or 24 h. The SDNN has not seen widespread application in the psychophysiological literature, although another time domain measure that is based on the variance of beat-to-beat heart period differences has been used more frequently. This is the square root of the mean squared successive heart period differences or the RMSSD (Root Mean Square Successive Difference) statistic. As this metric is based on the differences between adjacent heart periods it is nominally independent of basal heart period, although heart period level and heart period variability are themselves physiologically correlated. Because the differences between adjacent heart periods sample heart period variability over relatively short periods of time (the duration of a heart period), the RMSSD parses the total variance by filtering out lower frequency variability. Consequently, the RMSSD has been applied as a measure of high-frequency heart period variability and respiratory sinus arrhythmia. Although the RMSSD does effectively filter out low-frequency heart period variance, the properties of this filter, including its cutoff frequency and its frequency-dependent transfer function vary as a function of basal heart period (Berntson, Lozano, & Chen, 2005). A more systematic parsing of heart period variance into specific frequency components can be achieved by frequency domain methods.

Frequency domain (spectral) methods decompose the overall heart period variance into specifiable frequency bands (see Berntson et al., 1997; Task Force, 1996). A common approach is based on the Fourier theorem which

A. Autonomic Origins of Respiratory Sinus Arrhythmia

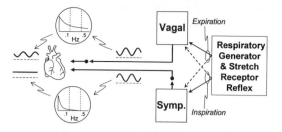

B. Spectral Analysis of Respiratory Sinus Arrhythmia

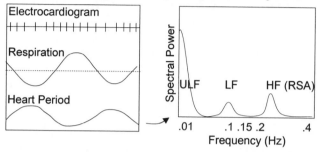

Figure 8.10. Respiratory sinus arrhythmia (RSA). (A) Neurophysiological generators of RSA. Respiratory rhythms are apparent in both sympathetic and parasympathetic nerves, but the different transfer functions (inserts) allow the parasympathetic but not the sympathetic innervations to impart a respiratory rhythm to the beat of the heart. (B) Illustrations of the relation between respiration and heart period, and its quantification by spectral analysis. ULF = ultra-low frequency; LF = low frequency, HF = high frequency.

asserts that any periodic time-varying waveform (in our case, the time varying fluctuations in heart period) can be decomposed into a set of pure sine wave components comprised of a fundamental frequency (f) and a set of harmonics ($2f, 3f, \ldots . nf$). Stated conversely, any periodic time-varying waveform, however complex, can be approximated by the summation of a finite set of pure sinusoids of differing amplitudes.

Computationally, the Fourier transform decomposes the variance of a waveform into its frequency components, and "transforms" the time domain representation of the variance into a frequency domain representation or spectral density function (see Figure 8.10B for illustration). Importantly, the time and frequency domain representations are simply two complementary ways to characterize the same set of variances, with the time domain representation aggregating across frequencies and the frequency domain representation aggregating across time. The former preserves the temporal integrity of the signal at the expense of frequency resolution and the latter preserves the frequency composition of the signal at the expense of temporal resolution. If the spectral density function is integrated (summed) across frequencies, the result will equal the simple statistical variance of the signal in the time domain.

Origin and significance of heart period rhythms. As illustrated in Figure 8.10B, there are several peaks in the spec-

tral density function for heart rate variability, corresponding to one or more physiological processes (Berntson et al., 1997; Eckberg, 2000) Several general frequency bands of heart period variability have been defined in the literature. The high-frequency band (0.15 [or 0.12] to 0.4 Hz in the adult) generally corresponds to respiratory sinus arrhythmia (RSA), which reflects the respiratory gating of autonomic control by afferent input from lung stretch receptors (Berntson et al., 1993a; Eckberg, 2002). Although respiratory rhythms are apparent in the activities of both the sympathetic and parasympathetic cardiac nerves, the low-pass filter properties of the sympathetic sinoatrial synapses effectively smooth out these rhythmical fluctuations into a steady state influence on heart rate. For this reason, respiratory sinus arrhythmia is generally considered to index vagal cardiac control, although there are several caveats in its application (see Berntson et al., 1993a; Berntson et al., 1994, 1997; Cacioppo et al., 1994; Grossman, Karemaker, & Wieling, 1991; Grossman & Kollai, 1993).

Although the high-frequency band may be operationally set at 0.15 (or 0.12) to 0.4 Hz, the respiratory rate in some cases can extend below this band with slow breathing or above this band in infants or with rapid breathing in adults. For children, a commonly used respiratory band is 0.24–1.04 Hz (Quigley & Stifter, 2006). Measures of respiratory sinus arrhythmia will be biased if the breathing rate falls wholly or partially outside the selected band as the power in this frequency will not be captured within the high-frequency variability band. Consequently, it may be desirable to raise the upper band limit to 1.0 Hz with exercise, and to use a higher overall frequency band with infants (e.g., 0.20–1.20 Hz, see Bar-Haim, Marshall, & Fox, 2000). Even when respiration falls within the standard high-frequency band, the transfer function from vagal respiratory rhythms to cardiac respiratory rhythms is not flat, but decreases with increasing frequency. For these reasons it is optimal to obtain respiratory measures to insure that respiratory rates are within the high-frequency band and remain constant from condition to condition (e.g., baseline to task). If respiratory rates do change, this should be recognized and accounted for. The effects of a change in respiratory rate could be statistically controlled by adding respiratory rate as a covariate or by adjusting the estimate of vagal control by the known effects of respiratory frequency (see Berntson et al., 1997).

Respiratory depth can also alter RSA (e.g., see Grossman, Wilhelm, & Spoerle, 2004; Grossman, Karemaker, & Wieling, 1991; Grossman, & Kollai, 1993), although amplitude effects at moderate levels of variation are generally not as large as effects of rate. A paced breathing procedure could be implemented to experimentally control respiration (Grossman, Karemaker, & Wieling, 1991), although paced breathing itself may be stressful (Wilhelm, Grossman, & Coyle, 2004) and may interact with other experimental manipulations. Alternatively, if changes are observed in respiratory depth, this parameter could be entered as a covariate in statistical analyses. A more comprehensive but more complex regression approach entails a transfer function analysis with paced breathing to define adjustment coefficients for respiratory parameters (Wilhelm, Grossman, & Coyle, 2004).

Lower frequency bands of heart period variability have also been defined in the literature. These include the low-frequency band (LF; sometimes termed the mid-frequency band) with a variable bandwidth (e.g., 0.05–0.15 or 0.8 to 0.12) centered around 0.1 Hz (sometimes referred to as the Mayer wave). Even lower frequency bands have been studied in the physiological literature (very-low .003–.05 Hz; ultra low < .003), but have not received much attention in psychophysiology. Variability within any of these bands represents a mixture of sympathetic and parasympathetic rhythms, as sympathetic rhythms can translate into cardiac rhythms at these frequencies. These lower frequency rhythms have received less attention in the psychophysiological literature, although the mid-frequency band has been of some interest and utility in the quantification of mental workload and baroreceptor function (see Boucsein & Backs, 2000; Van Roon, Mulder, Althaus, & Mulder, 2004).

An additional application of the 0.1 Hz rhythm has been in the development of an index of *autonomic balance*, which is said to characterize the relative functional point along a sympathetic-parasympathetic activation continuum (see Malliani, 1999). The index is the ratio of high-frequency variability to low-frequency variability. The general rationale is that variability in the lower band is driven by both branches of the autonomic nervous system so increases in sympathetic control will increase low-frequency variability but not high-frequency variability, and thus reduce the index value. This approach has been severely criticized on physiological grounds (Eckberg, 1997, 1998). One of the problems with this approach is that the low-frequency band is also determined by parasympathetic activity which can confound this index. In addition, the sympathovagal index assumes a reciprocally regulated autonomic continuum, wherein increases in one branch are coupled to decreases in the other. Although this may hold in some cases, such as with orthostatic stress, it does not in others, especially in psychological contexts (Berntson & Cacioppo, 1999).

Quantification. A common approach to quantification of heart period variability is by a Fast Fourier Transform (FFT), which represents a more computationally efficient approach than the full Fourier Transform. This efficiency comes with the restriction that the number of data points must be some power of 2 (e.g., 64, 128, 256, 512), but this does not generally pose a serious limitation. A more complete discussion of analytical approaches can be found in Berntson et al. (1997).

The FFT, as with other spectral methods, quantifies *periodic* components of variability and assumes at least weak stationarity of the signal (constant mean and variance over time). *Aperiodic* components or nonstationar-ities can compromise analysis and interpretation of the data. Although moderate deviations from stationarity may not have large effects on spectral estimates, it is best to avoid these biases. One approach to enhance stationarity is to use short analytical epochs, as nonstationarities tend to increase over time. On the other hand, analytical epochs must be long enough to sample a sufficient number of respiratory cycles (a minimum of 10 cycles is recommended in the Society for Psychophysiological Research Committee Report, Berntson et al., 1997), although these could be aggregated over multiple shorter periods (e.g., 30–60 sec). A simple test is available to confirm stationarity of the data (Weber, Molenaar, & van der Molen, 1992).

Acquisition commonly entails digitization of the ECG signal at a minimum of 500–1000 Hz. Although some information may be derivable at lower frequencies, there is a progressive loss of information as digitization rate is further reduced (Riniolo & Porges, 1997). R waves must then be accurately detected, artifacts removed, and a heart period series derived. Because heart periods vary in duration, this beat series must be converted to a time series by an interpolation algorithm. The sample interval for the time series should provide 2–4 samples/beat (250 msec works with most subjects, although shorter sample times may be desirable with infants). The time series is then detrended with a first order polynomial to remove the mean and any linear trend in the data. The initial and terminal data points should be tapered by a standard hanning window, cosign window or similar function to eliminate starting and ending offsets which can introduce artifacts. The residual series is then submitted to a FFT, yielding an estimate of power ($msec^2/Hz$) distribution across frequencies (see Figure 8.10B) and the power within the frequency bands of interest can be summed (integrated) to yield an estimate of total power ($msec^2$) within those bands. Generally, these total power estimates are natural log transformed to normalize distributions. The power in the high-frequency band represents the quantitative estimate of vagal control of the heart.

Many other approaches to quantification have also been employed. A common alternative approach is autoregressive (AR) modeling, which is another spectral method. In contrast to the FFT, which is considered a descriptive statistic as it includes all data in the analysis, the AR approach views the signal as a combination of deterministic and stochastic components and attempts to model the salient deterministic components while eliminating "noise." In practice, with the applications of filters and other refinements in FFT (see below) these approaches generally give highly similar results. A time domain approach that approximates spectral methods has been developed by Porges and colleagues (see Porges & Bohrer, 1990). After derivation of the time series as outlined above, this approach entails the application of a polynomial filter algorithm to remove frequencies outside the band of interest, and the statistical variance of the residuals is then calculated as an index of RSA. Another time domain approach is the peak-valley method wherein an estimate of RSA is derived from the difference between the longest beats associated with expiration and the shortest beats associated with inspiration (Grossman, van Beek, & Wientjes, 1990). Both of these time domain methods yield values similar to spectral approaches, with each having its advantages and disadvantages. A myriad of additional methods are also available including cross spectral analysis, transfer function analysis, time frequency distributions (smoothed pseudo Wigner-Ville distribution and complex demodulation), and nonlinear dynamical methods to name a few. Space precludes a meaningful coverage of these approaches here, but the interested reader is referred to Monti, Medigue, & Mangin (2002), Pumprla, Howorka, Groves, Chester, & Nolan (2002), and Wilhelm, Grossman, & Roth (1999).

Summary. Patterns of heart rate variability offer important insights into cardiovascular dynamics and their central and peripheral autonomic control. High-frequency heart rate variability is largely attributable to variations in parasympathetic control associated with respiration and is widely used as an index of vagal control of the heart. There are several important caveats in these applications, however. There are many factors that can influence basal levels of RSA, including posture, age, activity, and aerobic fitness to name a few. Consequently, the differences in the magnitude of RSA across subjects or groups may not be a valid metric for differences in vagal control of the heart unless these variables are taken into account. Although within-subjects changes in RSA may be more valid as a marker of changes in vagal control, factors such as posture and activity still need to be considered. Moreover, RSA can be influenced by respiratory rate and to a somewhat lesser extent, respiratory depth, independent of the basal level of vagal control. This has raised a question as to whether the magnitude of RSA is a valid predictor of vagal "tone," or the average basal level of parasympathetic control. To the extent that vagal inhibition is not complete with inspiration, there may be some dissociation between respiratory vagal fluctuations and the basal level of vagal control. Minimally, respiratory parameters should be measured, and should be taken into account if they differ across critical experimental contrasts. The psychological significance of low-frequency heart rate variability is less clear, although as discussed above it may have some utility in assessment of cognitive workload. Although widely used, especially for estimating reflex regulation, the ratio of LF to HF variability as an index of autonomic balance may not have much meaning in psychological contexts unless the predominant mode of response can be shown to be reciprocal.

Blood pressure

Blood pressure can be measured in a number of ways, invasively, using intraarterial pressure transducers, or noninvasively, using auscultatory or oscillometric methods, arterial tonometry, or the volume-clamp method (also called the Peñaz method). The latter two methods are especially useful when the research question calls for beat-to-beat blood pressure. The beat-to-beat methods are also more sensitive to movement, making them more difficult to record with fidelity. Because most psychophysiological laboratories are not equipped to perform invasive measures and provide the participant safeguards needed, we will focus here on the non-invasive measures. It is important to determine for any blood pressure monitoring device that it has met either or both of the Association for the Advancement of Medical Instrumentation (AAMI) or the British Hypertension Society (BHS) standards for accuracy and reproducibility (van Montfrans, 2001).

Auscultatory blood pressure measurement. The auscultatory method takes its name from the fact that auscultation or listening to bodily sounds is the basis of the technique. For arm blood pressure, a cuff is placed on the upper arm, with a stethoscope placed over the brachial artery (if done manually) or a microphone embedded in the cuff (if done with an automated device). When the cuff is inflated to a pressure sufficient to cut off all arterial blood flow (i.e., suprasystolic), no sound is heard. As the pressure in the cuff is slowly bled off, the so-called Korotkoff or K sounds appear. The cuff pressure at which the first sound is heard is taken as the systolic pressure and referred to as the start of phase I. As the pressure in the cuff decreases further, the sounds take on a murmuring quality (phase II) and then become clearer and louder (phase III). Following this, the Korotkoff sounds become muffled (phase IV) and eventually disappear altogether (phase V). In medical practice and typically in the psychophysiology laboratory, the pressure at phase V is considered the diastolic blood pressure, although sometimes Phase IV is used instead. Automated devices are particularly useful in the psychophysiological laboratory so that an experimenter need not be present in the room when a reading is taken, and also because this removes aspects of human error in reading the blood pressure (Shapiro et al., 1996).

Oscillometric blood pressure measurement. The oscillometric method utilizes oscillations in pressure in the cuff to determine systolic, diastolic and mean arterial pressure (Borow & Newberger, 1982; van Montfrans, 2001). With this method, following inflation of the cuff to a pressure above the systolic pressure where oscillations can be measured in the cuff, the cuff is slowly deflated. The systolic pressure is taken as the pressure when the oscillations in the cuff first begin to get larger, the mean arterial pressure is taken as the point when the cuff oscillations are maximal in size, and the diastolic pressure is taken as the point when the cuff pressure oscillations no longer get smaller in amplitude. As van Montfrans (2001) points out, there are issues still to be resolved with this technique, most notably, that specific algorithms used to determine systolic, diastolic, and mean arterial pressure are unlikely to be equally accurate across all individuals thus leading to systematic errors. Especially problematic is the effect of increased arterial stiffness on oscillometric measurements which often is seen in elderly or diabetic subjects. Finally, the algorithms for each oscillometric device are different and proprietary, making it impossible for the researcher to document the algorithms used. Therefore, it is important to report the make and model of the oscillometric device used for any study.

Arterial tonometry. Blood pressure is measured using arterial tonometry (also called arterial applanation tonometry) by placing piezoelectric sensors over an artery that overlies bone (e.g., Colin 7000). Modest pressure is applied to the artery, partially flattening the artery. Multiple sensors are arrayed over the flattened artery and the device then records from the sensor reading the largest arterial pulse wave amplitude. This measure provides a pulse waveform that is calibrated against an oscillometrically derived blood pressure reading from the brachial artery. A common site for tonometric measurements is the radial artery at the wrist. Care must be taken that the sensor is placed correctly over the artery and the technique is sensitive to movement limiting the potential uses of the technique (Kemmotsu, Ueda, Otsuka, Yamamura, Winter, & Eckerle, 1991; Parati et al., 2003).

Volume-clamp or Peñaz method. The volume-clamp method typically uses a cuff on the finger to clamp the vascular volume of the finger at a specific level which is maintained from beat to beat (Parati, et al., 2003; Wesseling, 1990). A photoplethysmographic device (see section on plethysmography below) measures changes in blood volume beneath the sensor, and then using a pneumatic servo-control system, changes are made in the pressure within the finger cuff so that the artery returns to its previous volume. The amount of pressure change in the finger cuff needed to reestablish the volume in the artery is a function of the arterial pressure underlying the cuff. The device using this method that originally saw the widest use was the Finapres, which was withdrawn from the market, although it is still in use in many labs around the world. Newer devices using this technique are currently limited to the Portapres (an ambulatory monitor) and the Finometer (a stationary monitor; Parati et al., 2003).

General measurement issues for blood pressure. We outline here some general aspects of blood pressure measurement. First, because of the regional variations in blood flow, vessel diameter and blood pressure, it is important when measuring blood pressure to report the location from which pressure is measured (e.g., at the brachial or femoral artery). It's also important for the measurement site to be at the same vertical height as the heart to eliminate effects of hydrostatic pressure (i.e., the pressure exerted by the fluid in the circulatory system) on the blood pressure measurement. Another important feature is the size and placement

of the cuff. To determine the appropriate cuff size, the circumference of the upper arm is determined and the cuff width should be at least 40% of arm circumference, and the cuff length at least 80% of the circumference (Bailey & Bauer, 1993). In practice, this is usually accomplished by using standard, small, and large adult cuffs or a pediatric cuff (O'Brien, 1996). Partly because of the limitations of the instrumentation, it is uncommon for cuff occlusions to be made more frequently than once per minute. In addition, more frequent sampling than this may result in unpleasant side effects, and annoyance of the participant (Shapiro et al., 1996). Because of the variability in blood pressure that was noted previously, it is recommended that multiple blood pressure readings taken from a recording epoch be averaged to provide a more stable estimate of the blood pressure for that epoch. For specific recommendations, the reader is referred to Shapiro et al., 1996 and Llabre, Ironson, Spitzer, Gellman, Weidler, & Schneiderman, 1988.

Various participant or environmental factors can make it difficult to accurately interpret blood pressure results. These include recent eating, drinking, smoking, medications or exercise, and not controlling for phase of the menstrual cycle in women, or time of day. Blood pressure is affected by all of these factors and thus, when possible, they should be controlled within a study (Shapiro et al., 1996). Emotional factors also affect blood pressure. A well known example of this is so-called white-coat hypertension, which occurs when readings in a clinical or other evocative setting such as a lab are higher than those in a less evocative setting such as the individual's home.

Other vascular measures

Plethysmography, including venous occlusion plethysmography. Plethysmography is a technique whereby one determines the volume of a structure, either the entire structure (such as in whole body plethysmography) or part of a structure (such as determining blood volume in a body segment like the finger). Volume can be determined using a photoelectric sensor (photoplethysmography), changes in impedance (see section on impedance cardiography for a specific example of this method), or changes in circumference measured with a strain gauge.

The most common photoplethysmographic technique employs a photocell placed over an area of tissue perfused with blood. There are two variations of this method; energy emitted from an infrared source can be measured as it passes through the tissue segment (transillumined) or as it bounces off the tissue (back-scattered). Because electromagnetic radiation in this frequency is scattered by blood, the output of a photodetector is related to the amount of blood within the segment (Jennings, Tahmoush, & Redmond, 1980). In either case, the infrared energy is measured by a photoelectric transducer and recorded as a change in voltage or current. Currently, most photoplethysmographic devices utilize a light-emitting diode (LED) as an emitter and a phototransistor as a detector, which do not alter the underlying skin and blood vessels. If the light is transmitted through the tissue to a photodetector on the other side, only a limited number of sites are convenient (e.g., earlobe, finger), and these are not necessarily sensitive to psychological changes. However, with the back-scattered photoplethysmographic technique, the light source and the photodetector are both located on the same side of the tissue and therefore can be placed almost anywhere on the body. The back-scattered photoplethysmograph is more sensitive to vascular fluctuations occurring close to the skin surface, whereas the transilluminated photoplethysmograph is sensitive to vascular changes in both the skin and deeper tissue. Blood flow also can be measured using a transcutaneous Doppler device which detects acoustic frequency shifts caused by moving red blood cells in underlying tissue (Rose, 2000). Doppler devices share many of the same issues and limitations as photoplethysmographic devices.

Using a strain gauge, one can also measure changes in blood volume of a body segment. The strain gauge is placed around the finger, or other body segment, and changes in resistance or voltage of the strain gauge provide an indirect measurement of blood volume changes. Venous occlusion plethysmography is a special example of the use of strain gauge plethysmography to measure blood volume in limb segments (Wilkinson & Webb, 2001). This technique requires two cuffs, one placed distal to the limb segment of interest, and one placed proximal to the limb segment. The distal cuff is inflated to a pressure above the systolic pressure to prevent blood flow into and out of the distal limb segment. The proximal cuff is inflated to a pressure sufficient to eliminate venous flow from the limb segment, but not preventing arterial flow into the segment. A strain gauge is placed around the limb segment, and the change in limb circumference per unit of time is used to infer the rate of arterial blood flow into the segment. The advantage of this method is that arterial blood flow into an isolated limb segment can be measured independent of other possible sources of blood flow (e.g., venous flow). An obvious limitation of the venous occlusion technique is that measurements cannot be taken continuously, and even at very short intervals, because numbness or pain in the limb can result. Measurements also can be altered by movement of the limb.

Jennings, Tahmoush, and Redmond (1980) reviewed many of the factors that influence vasomotor changes and discussed problems of interpretation using from the indirect measures described here. For example, changes in room temperature from one day to the next during a study alter the measures for reasons unrelated to the experimental situation. Another problem is the wide variation in skin and vessel anatomy (e.g., location of vessels) which make absolute comparisons between subjects impossible. Even within the same subject, difficulty in precise placement of the transducer makes comparisons only relative, especially if the transducer is removed and replaced. Because of differential distributions of muscles and blood vessels in different body areas, it is difficult to compare results between studies when different recording sites are used. Finally, recall that blood flow is a complex function of pressure in the vasculature, the radius of the blood vessels, and the viscosity of the blood, and flow changes may occur via arterial and/or venous flow changes either into or out of the segment of interest. Thus, one must be careful when making interpretations from indirectly measured blood flow changes.

Because of the relative nature of the vasomotor measures described here, experimenters typically examine changes for each participant from a baseline period and compare this to the experimental or task period. The change between baseline and task is generally expressed as a percentage. The magnitude of an individual pulse can be determined by measuring the difference between the lowest point and the peak or an integrating coupler can be used to perform a similar function.

Other non-invasive vascular measures. Several other non-invasive measures of vascular function have been used particularly to assess cardiovascular disease risk. Considered here are only a few of those that do not require medical facilities for their application. Measures such as brachial artery ultrasonography have been used to assess flow-mediated dilation (Corretti et al., 2002). In this technique, suprasystolic cuff pressures are used to occlude all blood flow in the arm for several minutes. Upon release of the cuff pressure, blood flow increases to the occluded limb over and above flow before occlusion (a phenomenon called reactive hyperemia). A small flow-mediated dilation response during reactive hyperemia has been shown to be related to coronary artery disease (Kuvin et al, 2001) and cardiovascular disease risk (Kuvin et al., 2003), the latter case being documented with both brachial artery ultrasonography and peripheral arterial tonometry over a finger. The peripheral arterial tonometry technique is very similar to arterial applanation tonometry used to measure blood pressure, although with peripheral arterial tonometry, the goal is to use the arterial waveform to derive the pulse wave amplitude. This technique has been used to measure other features of vascular physiology including pulse wave velocity and a measure of arterial stiffness called the augmentation index (e.g., Davies & Struthers, 2003; Vuurmans, Boer, & Koomans, 2003).

Pulse transit time, used in calculating pulse wave velocity, was previously used to a considerable extent in psychophysiological assessments, predominantly because it was thought to relate to blood pressure. However, pulse transit time is a function of both cardiac changes (in pre-ejection period) and the stiffness of the peripheral arterial system (Steptoe, Godaert, Ross, & Schreurs, 1983). This means that psychological antecedents which alter pre-ejection period, vascular tone or both can contribute to changes in pulse transit time, and yet the physiological source(s) of these changes will be indeterminate (Shapiro et al., 1996). One approach that may have promise in applying pulse transit time to the measurement of blood pressure, or blood pressure change, is the concurrent monitoring of (e.g., by impedance cardiography), and adjustment for, the cardiac determinants of PTT. A more recent use of pulse transit time has been to detect brief changes in respiratory effort and "microarousals" during sleep, although the physiological basis for these pulse transit time changes remains unclear (Smith, Argod, Pépin, & Lévy, 1999).

Baroreflex measures

The baroreceptor-heart period reflex is important in the short-term control of blood pressure. Estimates of baroreflex function have been proposed using relatively invasive procedures such as pharmacologically induced changes in blood pressure or neck suction to directly activate baroreceptors (for review see Parati, di Rienzo, & Mancia, 2000). However, the focus here will be on non-invasive estimates of baroreflex function derived from spontaneous changes in blood pressure and heart period. Baroreflex sensitivity or gain can be derived using either time domain (e.g., the spontaneous sequence method; Bertinieri, di Rienzo, Cavallazzi, Ferrari, Pedotti, & Mancia, 1985) or frequency domain methods (e.g., spectral methods; DeBoer, Karemaker, & Strackee, 1987). Baroreflex sensitivity estimated from these methods is defined either as the slope of the regression of heart period on systolic blood pressure (ms/mmHg; sequence method), or the gain of the transfer function relating variations in heart period and systolic blood pressure over the frequency range of 0.04 and 0.35 Hz (spectral methods). These estimates of baroreflex sensitivity do not represent identical estimates of sensitivity (Persson et al., 2001). For one, the sequence method utilizes shorter data epochs, namely sequences of 3–6 consecutive R-R intervals where systolic blood pressure increased by more than 1 mmHg over sequential beats and heart period progressively shortened, or where systolic pressure decreased and heart period progressively lengthened. Most sequences that meet these criteria are sequences of 3 interbeat intervals, with progressively fewer sequences observed as the number of interbeat intervals in the sequence increases. Moreover, the 3 interval sequences tend to provide higher estimates of baroreflex sensitivity than the longer sequences (Reyes del Paso, Hernández, & González, 2004), although in most studies, sequences of all lengths are averaged to provide a single baroreflex sensitivity estimate. This finding of differential sensitivity with differing sequence length may be related to the fact that vagal effects on heart period occur much more quickly in response to a pressure change than do sympathetic influences (DeBoer et al., 1987). The spectral methods (using Fast Fourier Transform or autoregressive modeling techniques) are also subject to specific biases. With spectral methods, one typically reports the gain of the transfer function or the square root of the ratio of the spectral powers for the heart period and systolic blood pressure signals, called the α coefficient, over the entire frequency range noted above. However, it has been shown that the highest coherence between heart period and blood pressure occurs in two specific frequency regions, one around 0.1 Hz and the other in the respiratory frequency range (approx. 0.15–0.35 Hz), and there is greater baroreflex influence in the respiratory frequency range than in the lower frequency range (Parati et al., 2000). Also, spectral methods typically do not take into account the phase relationship between heart period and systolic blood pressure. Thus, the estimate is less than optimal because part of the measure is not due to the baroreflex (Parati et al., 2000). Finally, the spectral methods require the use of longer data epochs for calculation than does the sequence method which can be problematic for tracking short-term changes in baroreflex sensitivity. Short-term changes will lead to nonstationarity in the signals, thereby violating a primary assumption of spectral methods. Thus, these two estimates of baroreflex sensitivity derived from spontaneous sequences have different biases, neither being a perfect reflection of the true baroreflex sensitivity, but each of which provides a useful metric under certain circumstances (Persson et al., 2001).

Several studies have demonstrated that psychological events can alter baroreflex sensitivity with mentally stressful events decreasing the gain of the baroreflex (e.g., Reyes del Paso, González, & Hernández, 2004; Steptoe & Sawada, 1989). In addition, respiratory biofeedback using slow paced breathing at approximately 0.1 Hz produced both within session and across session changes in baroreflex gain thereby revealing the influence of respiration on baroreflex sensitivity (Lehrer, et al., 2003).

A relatively new measure has been derived using the spontaneous sequence method called the baroreceptor effectiveness index (BEI; Di Rienzo, Parati, Castiglioni, Tordi, Mancia, & Pedotti, 2001). The BEI provides an estimate of how frequently (over a given period of time), the baroreflex is effective in altering the heart period. The data available to date on this measure show that the BEI is reflective of baroreflex function (the BEI dropped from 0.33 in intact cats to 0.04 after sino-aortic denervation), that the BEI is lower at night than during the day in humans (Di Rienzo et al., 2001), and that a visual attention task produced an increase in the BEI, whereas a mental arithmetic task did not alter BEI (Reyes del Paso, González, & Hernández, 2004). It seems clear that the BEI and baroreceptor sensitivity reflect different aspects of baroreflex function, but the usefulness of the BEI as a physiological indicator is not yet clear.

Impedance cardiography

Impedance cardiography is an important noninvasive method for obtaining more comprehensive information concerning cardiac function than can be derived from heart rate or heart rate variability alone. Impedance cardiography entails the application of a high-frequency,

A. Impedance Cardiography: Electrodes

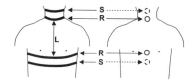

B. Impedance Cardiography: Signals

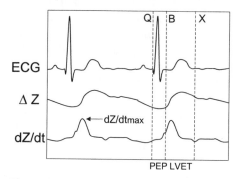

Figure 8.11. Impedance cardiography. (panel A) Typical electrode configurations. Left: standard mylar band electrodes, comprised of outer source (S) electrodes and inner recording (R) electrodes. Right: Qu et al. (1986) spot electrode configuration, consisting of two source electrodes on the dorsum (C4 and T9) and two recording electrodes on the ventrum. L = distance between the inner boundaries of the recording electrodes (for calculation of stroke volume and cardiac output). (panel B) Impedance signals, including the electrocardiogram (ECG) the basal impedance (Z) and the 1st derivative of Z. Q corresponds to the onset (or peak, see text) or the Q wave, B corresponds to the opening of the aortic valve (often indicated by a notch in the dZ/dt signal) and X (onset or peak, see text) corresponds to the closure of the aortic valve. PEP- pre-ejection period; LVET – left ventricular ejection time.

constant-current flow through a set of outer thoracic electrodes and recording of the associated voltage drop across another, inner set of electrodes. Because the current flow is held constant, based on Ohm's Law, the recorded voltage will vary inversely with the resistivity of the thoracic current path. Because the current is alternating, the resistivity to current flow is a function of both the DC resistance and the reactance of the circuit, collectively referred to as impedance. One of Kirchov's Laws stipulates that the distribution of current through parallel resistive paths is inversely proportional to the resistances. The body components with the lowest resistivity are blood and plasma, so the measured thoracic impedance is highly sensitive to changes in the cardiac and aortic distribution and flow of blood during the cardiac cycle (Hoetink, Faes, Visser, & Heethaar, 2004). General methodological guidelines for impedance cardiography are available from a committee report of the Society for Psychophysiological Research (Sherwood et al., 1990).

Instrumentation. In measuring cardiac impedance, four electrodes are typically employed (see Figure 8.11). The outer (source) electrodes provide the constant current sig-

nal path to the subject (typically considered leads 1 and 4). Supply current parameters are not standardized across devices. Current levels generally range from 4 mA down to 0.1 mA, typically at 100 kHz, although lower frequencies have also been used. The inner two electrodes are used to measure voltage, which reflects the changes in impedance due to volumetric alterations in blood distribution and blood flow (recording electrodes, usually leads 2 and 3). The Minnesota Model 403B Impedance Cardiography device (Instrumentation for Medicine, Minneapolis) was one of the earliest and most widely used instrument, although it has now been replaced by the HIC 2000, & 3000 (Bio-Impedance Technology, Inc., Chapel Hill). More recently, impedance measures have been incorporated into ambulatory studies (Hawkley, Burleson, Berntson, & Cacioppo, 2003; Sherwood, McFetridge, & Hutcheson, 1998; Willemsen, De Geus, Klaver, Van Doornen, & Carroll, 1996). Several ambulatory units are now commercially available, including the VU-AMD (Vrije University, Vrije Netherlands), the AIM-8 (Bio-Impedance Technology, Chapel Hill, NC) and the recently introduced MW1000A (Mindware Technologies, Gahanna, OH) that includes a wireless network link.

There are two common electrode configurations used in recording thoracic impedance; band electrodes and spot electrodes. The band electrode consists of a thin, aluminum conductor secured to a Mylar adhesive tape that provides a means of attaching it to the subject. Spot electrodes are small, conductive disks (Ag/AgCl) with adhesive collars (same electrodes as typically used for measuring ECG). The conductive disk is generally covered with an electrode gel using a sponge-like material or imbedded in a conductive medium. Mylar band electrodes represent the standard and have been the most thoroughly validated. Spot electrodes, however, can also yield valid information and are considerably easier to use. The Qu et al. configuration entails two spot electrodes on the back and two on the front as illustrated in Figure 8.11 (Qu, Zhang, Webster, & Tompkins, 1986; see also Sherwood, Royal, Hutcheson, & Turner, 1992). Spot electrodes give generally comparable results to Mylar bands for systolic time intervals, but are less accurate for volumetric measures (stroke volume and cardiac output), especially for between-subject comparisons (Sherwood, Royal, Hutcheson, & Turner, 1992). A variety of other spot electrode placements have also been employed, which can give similar group values, but may yield variable results across individual subjects (Hoetink et al., 2002; Kauppinen, Hyttinen, & Malmivuo, 1998). A "whole-body" impedance approach has also been implemented with limb electrodes, which shows promising results, although it may be less sensitive to some cardiovascular parameters because a large proportion of the basal impedance arises from the limbs (Kauppinen, Koobi, Hyttinen, & Malmivuo, 2000).

The ECG is also required for impedance cardiography, as the Q wave serves as a landmark for the beginning of ventricular electrical activation and the R wave is employed as the fiducial point of alignment for ensemble averaging of signals. Some devices extract the ECG from the impedance recording electrodes, although that does not always provide a very clear signal. Consequently, additional ECG electrodes are also often employed.

The primary dependent variables in impedance cardiography are ECG, Z0 (basal impedance) and dZ/dt (first derivative of Z0). Z0 is a measure of thoracic impedance, in ohms, and reflects the variation in blood volume and distribution over the cardiac cycle. The variations in Z0 over the cardiac cycle are small compared to the overall basal impedance (generally in the range of 10–40 ohms). Consequently, the dZ/dt is either derived electronically or calculated off-line to remove the baseline and to enhance the relevant components of the small variations in the signal. The recorded signal from which these parameters are extracted is a composite of the carrier frequency (100 kHz sine wave), basal impedance (Z0), and ECG. The circuitry in instruments varies from manufacturer to manufacturer, but generally the carrier frequency is demodulated and the Z0 and ECG are routed through low pass filters to remove any remaining high-frequency signals ($>50\,\mathrm{Hz}$). To achieve optimal temporal sensitivity, these signals should be digitized at 1 kHz.

Scoring. Two sets of measures are generally derived from the impedance signal: (a) systolic time intervals such the pre-ejection period (PEP) and the left ventricular ejection time (LVET); and (b) volumetric measures such as stroke volume (SV) and cardiac output (CO). For the measurement of systolic time intervals, two landmarks are determined from dZ/dt, the B and X points. The B point is characterized by a notch or an inflection point near the onset of the rapid upstroke of the dZ/dt waveform, which serves as an index of the point in time when intraventricular pressure becomes higher than aortic pressure, the aortic valve opens, and ventricular ejection commences. The B point can be challenging to localize, especially when a distinct inflection point or notch is not apparent. It corresponds roughly with the peak of the first heart sound of the phonocardiogram, but this acoustic signal is complex and temporally distributed so that it does not serve as a viable marker of ventricular ejection time. Various methods have been used to estimate the B point from the impedance signal in the absence of a clear notch, including identification of the maximum slope or maximum slope change (2nd derivative), or the zero point crossing of the dZ/dt function (see Sherwood et al., 1990). An additional method that shows promise and may be superior to prior approaches is the use of a simple percentage or proportion (about 55%) of the time from the R peak to the peak of the dZ/dt wave (Lozano et al., in preparation).

The X wave peak is the lowest point on the dZ/dt waveform after the peak, and is taken as an index of the time when the aortic valve closes, marking the end of ventricular ejection. The peak (minimum) of the X wave is generally readily identified and has been recommended as the X point (Sherwood et al., 1990). It has been suggested that more accurate volumetric estimates, however, may be obtained by using the X onset point which may more closely correspond to aortic valve closure (for discussion see Brownley, Hurwitz, & Schneiderman, 2000).

Four systolic time interval measures can be derived from these points and the ECG. LVET is the time from the B point to the X point. PEP is generally taken as the time between the Q wave onset and the B point inflection on the dZ/dt waveform, although the onset of the R wave (Q wave peak) has been recommended as a more consistent and identifiable fiducial point (this has been referred to as PEPr; Berntson, Lozano, Chen, & Cacioppo, 2004). PEP and PEPr are measures of contractility that are used to index of sympathetic cardiac control. Additional indices of myocardial contractility include the Heather Index (HI) which is the ratio of the dZ/dt_{max} (ejection velocity) to the Q-dZ/dt peak interval, and the Acceleration Index (ACI) which is the dZ/dt_{max} divided by the B-dZ/dt peak interval. Additional inotropic and autonomic indices have also been derived from impedance signals (Thayer & Uijtdehaage, 2001).

The ejection velocity derived from the peak value of the dZ/dt waveform is used to calculate stroke volume (SV, in milliliters) according to the Kubicek equation (Kubicek et al., 1966):

$$SV = \rho_b\,(L/Z0)^2 \cdot LVET \cdot dZ/dt_{max}$$

where ρ_b is the blood resistivity (often assigned a constant value of 135 ohms/cm, although more accurate estimates may be obtainable by direct measures of this parameter); L is the distance between the recording electrodes; Z0 is the mean thoracic impedance; LVET is as defined above; dZ/dt_{max} is the peak of the dZ/dt function (because it actually reflects a reduced impedance it is sometimes designated dZ/dt_{min}).

From stroke volume and heart rate (HR), cardiac output can be calculated as:

$$CO = SV \cdot HR$$

There have been a variety of alternative formulas offered for the calculation of impedance derived cardiac output estimates, including the Sramek equation, Bernstein's modification of this method, and a more recent proprietary modification of this method (Bernstein, 1986; see also Van De Water et al., 2003). Although some findings suggest that the latter methods may be somewhat superior to the Kubicek formula, the Kubicek equation remains the standard and is most widely used in psychophysiology.

Scoring of impedance cardiography can be accomplished on a beat by beat basis, although the method of ensemble averaging over longer epochs is more efficient and yields highly comparable results (Kelsey et al., 1998). This approach derives an average of both the ECG and dZ/dt waveforms. By ensemble averaging of the signals, random noise and movement artifact that is not synchronized with the R wave is effectively removed, which provides for a more stable representation of cardiac activity. The ensemble method first determines the peak of the R wave of the ECG in the time series. From this point, a composite signal for both ECG and dZ/dt is calculated by averaging the signal from some fixed time before the R wave (typically 100ms) to 500–600 ms after the R peak. From these ensembled waveforms of ECG and dZ/dt, the landmarks for impedance scoring are identified as outlined above for individual cardiac cycles (see Figure 8.11). The duration of the epochs to be ensemble averaged generally ranges from 30 sec to 5 min, based in part on the experimental design and the questions to be addressed. Epochs should be short enough that cardiodynamics are relatively stable, as an average of changing values can be distorted. On the other hand, longer epochs are more efficient for scoring purposes. One minute epochs are satisfactory for most studies, and the results can be further aggregated over longer experimental periods (e.g., as five 1-min epochs over a 5-min stressor). Even longer periods extending over hours may be useable for assessing long term changes in impedance parameters (Riese et al., 2003).

Validity. Under rigorous experimental conditions, impedance-derived estimates of cardiovascular function have been reported to be highly reliable, and to correlate well with parameters determined by echocardiography or invasive techniques such as the Fick (dye dilution) method (Sherwood et al., 1990; Moshkovitz, Kaluski, Milo, Vered, & Cotter, 2004).

Generally, measures of systolic time intervals show greater correlations across methods than do the volumetric measures of stroke volume and cardiac output (Sherwood et al., 1990). Even for volumetric measures, however, a meta-analysis of three decades of validation studies revealed correlations of greater than 0.80 between impedance derived measures and those derived from reference standards, such as echocardiography and the Fick method (Raaijmakers, Faes, Scholten, Goovaerts, & Heethaar, 1999).

The accuracy of impedance estimates is enhanced by rigorous experimental control and the maintenance of constant conditions. Cardiac anomalies, for instance, may impact impedance measures of cardiovascular function. In addition, impedance-derived estimates of stroke volume and cardiac output can be biased by variations in preload or afterload associated with differences in posture or activity, and even vocalization may alter these parameters (Tomaka, Blascovich, & Swart, 1994). These considerations are especially critical for ambulatory studies. Improved volumetric estimates can also be obtained when blood resistivity is estimated from the hematocrit, rather than applying a generic constant (Demeter, Parr, Toth, & Woods, 1993).

With careful attention to experimental design and control, impedance cardiography can offer a range of noninvasive metrics of cardiac performance and autonomic control in psychophysiological contexts.

Cardiac imaging

Psychophysiologists with access to medical facilities are using cardiac imaging techniques that typically fall within the purview of the cardiologist or radiologist. We focus here on techniques that provide non-invasive images, which include echocardiography (either with or without Doppler ultrasound) and magnetic resonance imaging (cardiac MRI). Other common imaging modalities include radionuclide single photon emission computed tomography (SPECT), electron beam computed tomography (CT), and positron emission tomography (PET), which require introducing radioisotopes (Gibbons, & Araoz, 2004). Although these methods will not be considered here, their further development may allow highly specific measures of neurotransmitter release, uptake and receptor action at the level of the heart (Carrio, 2001).

Echocardiography is an ultrasound-based technique that is very commonly available in hospitals, noninvasive, relatively inexpensive, portable, and safe for the subject or patient. Echocardiography is particularly useful in providing quantitative, anatomic information about the heart (Goldin, Ratib, & Aberle, 2000). The disadvantages of echocardiography are that it requires an experienced sonographer to record the images, considerable training to read them, and typically requires breath holding so images are not obscured by lung movements. Originally, echocardiographic images were taken in 2D, and simplifying assumptions were required for calculating measures such as left ventricular volume. Failure of these assumptions introduced large measurement errors across individuals. Echocardiography can also be combined with Doppler ultrasound to determine blood flow. Doppler ultrasound techniques rely on the fact that sounds waves bounced off a moving target change their frequency in direct proportion to the speed of the moving material. From this, blood flow velocities can be calculated and together with echocardiography one can obtain functional and anatomic information about heart function (Fyfe & Parks, 2002). A more recent innovation in echocardiography, known as real-time 3-D echocardiography (RT3DE) appears promising because it requires shorter scanning times (about 4 cardiac cycles) that permit recording during a single breath hold (Weyman, 2005). This technique provides left ventricular volume, mass and ejection fractions that compare well with MRI, which is quickly becoming the gold standard for anatomic measurements (Weyman, 2005). The primary downside of RT3DE is the time required for analyzing the data to make volume calculations, although automated analyses should improve this.

The other primary noninvasive cardiac imaging technique is cardiac MRI. Cardiac MRI relies on the same physical principles as any other MRI used to image the body. In simplified terms, a magnetic field applied around a body part aligns some of the protons (positive charges) on hydrogen ions that are a large component of body tissues and water. When a radio frequency pulse is applied to the magnetic field, these protons change their alignment, and after the pulse, fall back into alignment with the magnetic field. A radio wave produced when the proton falls back into alignment is detected by the MR scanner. The number of protons depends upon the constituents of the tissue, and these different proton densities are translated into different shades of gray or color. Images are acquired in 2-D slices through the tissue and multiple slices are stacked to create a 3-D image. Like echocardiography, MRI is thought to be safe. MRI also has the advantage of not being disrupted by air in the lungs and has a broader field of view than echocardiography (Fyfe & Parks, 2002). MRI has been shown to produce even more accurate estimates of left ventricular mass and volume than echocardiography (Higgins, 2000; Myerson, Bellenger, & Pennell, 2002). Multi-slice images can be presented sequentially in a movie or cine sequence that can show functional aspects of the heart (Goldin et al., 2000). Disadvantages of MRI are that some individuals cannot tolerate the close quarters and noise of an MRI scanner, and that some individuals have internal metallic devices or implants that preclude being able to place them in a strong magnetic field. Together these techniques provide important tools for non-invasive measurements of cardiac anatomy and function.

PSYCHOPHYSIOLOGICAL CONTEXT

A Medline search on the terms "cardiovascular AND psychophysiology" yielded 15,222 hits. Obviously, space precludes a comprehensive overview of the wide range of contemporary lines of investigation in cardiovascular psychophysiology. A few general themes, however, are worth brief mention.

Psychophysiological patterns

Much of the early work in psychophysiology focused on a single response dimension, such as ECG, EMG, or SCR. When more than one measure was taken, it was often to examine replicability across measures or to draw contrasts between the measures and their sensitivity to psychological states. Although there was some early interest in patterns of activity across response domains, it was not until the mid 1900s that the Laceys (Lacey & Lacey, 1962) solidified the construct of autonomic response patterning. Since then, there has been a growing recognition that the psychological and health significance of psychophysiological states may derive more from the profile of activity across response domains, rather than from discrete responses or from simple threshold or sensitivity differences of distinct response domains.

Autonomic branches, psychological states, and cardiac risk stratification. As discussed earlier, the sympathetic and parasympathetic branches are often reciprocally controlled by reflex systems, but higher level neural systems can exert more flexible patterns of control that include reciprocal, coactivational, or independent changes of the autonomic branches. These patterns of response may have distinct functional origins and differing consequences, but may not be apparent by measures of an end organ response (such as a change in heart rate) or by measures of either branch alone. An increase in heart rate, for example, could arise from an increase in sympathetic activity, a decrease in parasympathetic activity, a combination of both, a sympathetically dominated coactivation, or a parasympathetically dominated coinhibition.

These different patterns of autonomic response may arise from distinct neurobehavioral processes. In a conditioning study, Iwata and LeDoux (1988) found comparable heart rate increases to the conditioned stimulus in conditioned and pseudo conditioned groups. This finding raised the possibility that the psychophysiological states associated with these two conditions may not mirror the differences in the psychological significance of the CS. Selective blockades of the autonomic branches, however, revealed a distinct pattern of autonomic response despite the comparable end organ response. The pseudoconditioned CS yielded an independent sympathetic activation that drove the cardiac response. The conditioned CS, in fact, yielded a larger sympathetic activation accompanied by a parasympathetic coactivation, which yielded a comparable overall heart rate response despite different autonomic origins. This psychophysiological differentiation in the pattern of response across the autonomic branches would not have been apparent if only heart rate had been measured. A wide range of autonomic response patterns, including autonomic coactivation (e.g., Gianaros & Quigley, 2001; Bosch et al., 2001), are seen in psychological contexts in humans. An important area for future investigation is the elucidation of the specific determinants of these patterns of response.

Differential patterns of autonomic response may not only reflect distinct functional origins, they may have divergent consequences and health implications. RSA and heart rate variability have been effectively used for risk stratification in cardiac disorders, based on the fact that sympathetic activity can be deleterious, whereas parasympathetic activity may offset those deleterious effects in cardiomyopathies or myocardial infarcts (Gang & Malik, 2002; Schwartz, La Rovere, & Vanoli, 1992; Smith, Kukielka, & Billman, 2005). The importance of broader patterns of autonomic and physiological variables in health and disease is further illustrated by the ongoing development of more comprehensive cardiovascular risk factor profiles, which include multiple interacting dimensions including autonomic, neuroendocrine, and metabolic factors (Rosengren et al., 2004; Wood, 2001).

Loneliness and cardiovascular patterns. Autonomic patterns, rather than differences along single dimensions, also differentiate lonely from nonlonely individuals. Lonely individuals tend to display higher total peripheral resistance (TPR) and lower cardiac output (CO) than do nonlonely people, and they show smaller changes in HR, cardiac contractility, and CO in response to laboratory stressors (Cacioppo et al., 2002; Hawkley, Burleson, Berntson, & Cacioppo, 2003). This pattern is reminiscent of individuals in passive coping contexts and/or making threat-related appraisals (Sherwood, Dolan, & Light, 1990; Tomaka, Blascovich, Kelsey, & Leitten, 1993). The higher TPR of the lonely likely reflect enhanced sympathetic vascular tone, whereas the lower cardiac output and smaller changes in HR and cardiac contractility suggest lower sympathetic cardiac control. These differences are not consistent with simply more or less sympathetic vs. parasympathetic activity, but with probable system-specific patterns of these activities.

The pattern of physiological states and reactivities of lonely individuals may not be limited to the autonomic domain, but may also manifest in neuroendocrine or immune processes as well. It is well established that stressors, such as medical school examinations, can compromise the immune system as evidenced by lower antibody titers to an influenza vaccination (Glaser, Kiecolt-Glaser, Malarkey, & Sheridan, 1998). This stress related deficit in vaccine-induced seroconversion, however, was positively modulated by social embeddedness, suggesting there also may be immunological correlates of loneliness. This possibility was further supported by the finding of diminished wound healing in lonely subjects (see, Cacioppo & Hawkley, 2003). Clearly, an understanding of the psychophysiology of loneliness would not be complete if attention were focused solely on the cardiovascular system or even the autonomic nervous system. Psychophysiological systems are quintessentially interacting systems. Although pragmatics may limit studies to a single or a small number of dimensions, the ultimate understanding of psychophysiological phenomena and their implications for health may require a broader perspective entailing the interactions among multiple psychophysiological systems.

Autonomic, endocrine, and immune interactions

Stressors, especially social stressors can impact immune functions, at least in part by modulating autonomic and/or neuroendocrine process. Social reorganization stress in mice, but not physical stressors such as restraint or shock, has been shown to trigger reactivation of Herpes Simplex virus (Padgett et al., 1998). In addition, introduction of an aggressive intruder, but not physical stressors, can result in notable hyper-inflammatory reactions to foreign antigens which can have lethal consequences (Sheridan, Stark, Avitsur, & Padgett, 2000). This appears to reflect alterations in glucocorticoid functions. Although social stress and physical stress yielded comparable increases in glucocorticoid levels, social stress resulted in the development of glucocorticoid resistance associated with alterations in post-receptor actions (Quan et al., 2003). This resulted in exaggerated immune responses, which were not adequately held in check by glucocorticoids. In this case, the health consequences of social stress were related to altered immune functions, but these immune changes were secondary to an alteration in glucocorticoid processing.

In many cases, the health significance of psychophysiological states may relate to interactions among autonomic, neuroendocrine and immune systems. Exaggerated cardiovascular reactivity to stress has long been recognized as a predictor of atherosclerosis, hypertension and other cardiovascular disorders (Jennings et al., 2004; Matthews, Salomon, Brady, & Allen, 2003). More recent research suggests specific immune links in these relations. Atherosclerosis is now understood to be fundamentally an inflammatory disorder, in which exaggerated immune responses can promote plaque formation, restrict circulation, and foster emboli (see Libby, 2003; Strike & Steptoe, 2004). High heart rate reactions to stressors (especially those driven by sympathetic activation) predict greater immune consequences, and some immune responses to laboratory stressors can be reduced by sympathetic blockade (Bachen et al., 1995; Benschop et al., 1994; Bosch, Berntson, Cacioppo, Dhabhar, & Marucha, 2003; Cacioppo, 1994; Cacioppo et al., 1995). An explicit link between sympathetic reactivity to stress and cardiovascular disease is suggested by the finding that a laboratory speech stressor resulted in sympathetic activation and a correlated mobilization of a subset of T cells and monocytes that express specific cell surface markers (CXCR2, CXCR3, and CCR5; Bosch et al., 2003). The ligands for these markers are chemokines (chemical attractants) that are secreted by activated vascular endothelial cells. Consequently, stress would be expected to promote trafficking of these cells to these areas of activated endothelium and further exaggerate the inflammatory reactions associated with atherosclerosis.

This represents just one example of what are likely multiple and intricate interactions among autonomic, neuroendocrine and immune systems that contribute to health and disease. As the field of psychophysiology develops and becomes more interdisciplinary, it is likely these interactions will assume increasing importance.

REFERENCES

Anderson, C. R. (1998). Identification of cardiovascular pathways in the sympathetic nervous system. *Clinical and Experimental Pharmacology and Physiology, 25*, 449–452.

Annila, P. A., Yli-Hankala, A. M., & Lindgren, L. (1994). The effect of atropine on the T-wave amplitude of ECG during isoflurane anaesthesia. *International Journal of Clinical Monitoring and Computing, 11*, 43–47.

Bailey, R. H., & Bauer, J. H. (1993). A review of common errors in the indirect measurement of blood pressure. *Archives of Internal Medicine, 153*, 2741–2748.

Bar-Haim, Y., Marshall, P. J., Fox, N. A. (2000). Developmental changes in heart period and high-frequency heart period variability from 4 months to 4 years of age. *Developmental Psychobiology, 37*, 44–56.

Beker, F., Weber, M., Fink, R. H., & Adams, D. J. (2003). Muscarinic and nicotinic ACh receptor activation differentially mobilize Ca2+ in rat intracardiac ganglion neurons. *Journal of Neurophysiology, 90*, 1956–1964.

Bachen, E. A., Manuck, S. B., Cohen, S., Muldoon, M. F., Raibel, R., Herbert, T. B., & Rabin, B. S. (1995). Adrenergic blockade ameliorates cellular immune responses to mental stress in humans. *Psychosomatic Medicine, 57*, 366–372.

Benschop, R. J., Nieuwenhuis, E. E. S., Tromp, E. A. M., Godart, G. L. R., Ballieux, R. E., & van Doornen, L. P. J. (1994). Effects of *β*-adrenergic blockade on immunologic and cardiovascular changes induced by mental stress. *Circulation, 89*, 762–769.

Berntson, G. G., Bigger, J. T., Eckberg, D. L., Grossman, P., Kaufmann, P. G., Malik, M., Nagaraja, H. N., Porges, S. W., Saul, J. P., Stone, P. H., & van der Molen, M. W. (1997). Heart rate variability: Origins, methods, and interpretive caveats. *Psychophysiology, 34*, 623–648.

Berntson, G. G., & Cacioppo, J. T. (1999). Heart rate variability: A neuroscientific perspective for further studies. *Cardiac Electrophysiology Review, 3*, 279–282.

Berntson, G. G., Cacioppo, J. T., Binkley, P. F., Uchino, B. N., Quigley, K. S., & Fieldstone, A. (1994). Autonomic cardiac control: III. Psychological stress and cardiac response in autonomic space as revealed by pharmacological blockades. *Psychophysiology, 31*, 599–608.

Berntson, G. G., Cacioppo, J. T., & Quigley, K. S. (1991). Autonomic Determinism: The modes of autonomic control, the doctrine of autonomic space, and the laws of autonomic constraint. *Psychological Review, 98*, 459–487.

Berntson, G. G., Cacioppo, J. T., & Quigley, K. S. (1993a). Cardiac psychophysiology and autonomic space in humans: Empirical perspectives and conceptual implications. *Psychological Bulletin, 114*, 296–322.

Berntson, G. G., Cacioppo, J. T., & Quigley, K. S. (1993b). Respiratory sinus arrhythmia: Autonomic origins, physiological mechanisms, and psychophysiological implications. *Psychophysiology, 30*, 183–196.

Berntson, G. G., Cacioppo, J. T., & Quigley, K. S. (1995). The metrics of cardiac chronotropism: Biometric perspectives. *Psychophysiology, 32*, 162–171.

Berntson, G. G., Lozano, D. L., & Chen, Y.-J. (2005). Filter properties of the root mean square successive difference (RMSSD) statistic in heart rate. *Psychophysiology, 42*, 246–252.

Berntson, G. G., Lozano, D. L., Chen, Y.-J, & Cacioppo, J. T. (2004). Where to Q in PEP: Reliability and validity. *Psychophysiology, 41*, 333–337.

Bernstein, D. P. (1986). A new stroke volume equation for thoracic electrical bioimpedance: Theory and rationale. *Critical Care Medicine, 14*, 904–909.

Bertinieri, G., di Rienzo, M., Cavallazzi, A., Ferrari, A. U., Pedotti, A., & Mancia, G. (1985). A new approach to analysis of the arterial baroreflex. *Journal of Hypertension, 3*(suppl 3), S79–S81.

Borow, K. M., & Newberger, J. W. (1982). Noninvasive estimation of central aortic pressure using the oscillometric method for analyzing systemic artery pulsatile blood flow: Comparative study of indirect systolic, diastolic and mean brachial artery pressure with simultaneous direct ascending aortic pressure measurements. *American Heart Journal, 103*, 879–886.

Bosch, J. A., Berntson, G. G., Cacioppo, J. T., Dhabhar, F. S., & Marucha, P. T. (2003). Acute stress evokes a selective mobilization of T cells that differ in chemokine receptor expression: A potential pathway linking immunologic reactivity to cardiovascular disease. *Brain, Behavior, & Immunity, 17*, 251–259.

Bosch, J. A., de Geus, E. J., Kelder, A., Veerman, E. C., Hoogstraten, J., & Amerongen, A. V. (2001). Differential effects of active versus passive coping on secretory immunity. *Psychophysiology, 38*, 836–846.

Boucsein, W., & Backs, R. W. (2000). Engineering psychophysiology as a discipline: Historical and theoretical aspects. In R. W. Backs, & W. Boucsein (Eds.), *Engineering Psychophysiology: Issues and applications* (pp. 3–30). London: Lawrence Erlbaum Associates.

Brede, M., Philipp, M., Knaus, A., Muthig, V., & Hein, L. (2004). Alpha2-adrenergic receptor subtypes – novel functions uncovered in gene-targeted mouse models. *Biology of the Cell, 96*, 343–348.

Cacioppo, J. T. (1994). Social neuroscience: Autonomic, neuroendocrine, and immune responses to stress. *Psychophysiology, 31*, 113–128.

Cacioppo, J. T., Berntson, G. G., Binkley, P. F., Quigley, K. S., Uchino, B. N., & Fieldstone, A. (1994). Autonomic cardiac control. II. Basal response, noninvasive indices, and autonomic space as revealed by autonomic blockades. *Psychophysiology, 31*, 586–598.

Cacioppo, J. T., Malarkey, W. B., Kiecolt-Glaser, J. K., Uchino, B. N., Sgoutas-Emch, S. A., Sheridan, J. F., Berntson, G. G., & Glaser, R. (1995). Heterogeneity in neuroendocrine and immune responses to brief psychological stressors as a function of autonomic cardiac activation. *Psychosomatic Medicine, 57*, 154–164.

Cacioppo, J. T., & Hawkley, L. C. (2003). Social isolation and health, with an emphasis on underlying mechanisms. *Perspectives in Biology and Medicine, 46*(3 Suppl), S39–52.

Cacioppo, J. T., Hawkley, L. C., Crawford, L. E., Ernst, J. M., Burleson, M. H., Kowalski, R. B., Malarkey, W. B., VanCauter, E., & Berntson, G. G. (2002). Loneliness and health: Potential mechanisms. *Psychosomatic Medicine, 64*, 407–417.

Carrio, I. (2001). Cardiac neurotransmission imaging. *Journal of Nuclear Medicine, 42*, 1062–1076.

Chowdhary, S., Marsh, A. M., Coote, J. H., & Townend, J. N. (2004). Nitric oxide and cardiac muscarinic control in humans. *Hypertension, 43*, 1023–1028.

Contrada, R. J. (1992). T-wave amplitude: On the meaning of a psychophysiological index. *Biological Psychology, 33*, 249–258.

Corretti, M. C., Anderson, T. J., Benjamin, E. J., Celermajer, D., Charbonneau, F., Creager, M. A., Deanfield, J., Drexler, H., Gerhard-Herman, M., Herrington, D., Vallance, P., Vita, J., & Vogel, R. (2002). Guidelines for the ultrasound assessment of endothelial-dependent flow-mediated vasodilation of the brachial artery. *Journal of the American College of Cardiology, 39*, 257–265.

Critchley, H. D., Rotshtein, P., Nagai, Y., O'doherty, J., Mathias, C. J., Dolan, R. J. (2005a). Activity in the human brain predicting differential heart rate responses to emotional facial expressions. *Neuroimage, 24*, 751–762.

Critchley, H. D., Taggart, P., Sutton, P. M., Holdright, D. R., Batchvarov, V., Hnatkova, K., Malik, M., & Dolan, R. J. (2005b). Mental stress and sudden cardiac death: Asymmetric midbrain activity as a linking mechanism. *Brain, 128*, 75–85.

Dampney, R. A., Polson, J. W., Potts, P. D., Hirooka, Y., & Horiuchi, J. (2003). Functional organization of brain pathways subserving the baroreceptor reflex: Studies in conscious animals using immediate early gene expression. *Cellular and Molecular Neurobiology, 23,* 597–616.

Davies, J. I., & Struthers, A. D. (2003). Pulse wave analysis and pulse wave velocity: A critical review of their strengths and weaknesses. *Journal of Hypertension, 21,* 463–472.

DeBoer, R. W., Karemaker, J. M., & Strackee, J. (1987). Hemodynamic fluctuations and baroreflex sensitivity in humans: A beat-to-beat model. *American Journal of Physiology, 253,* 680–689.

Demeter, R. J., Parr, K. L., Toth, P. D., & Woods, J. R. (1993). Use of noninvasive bioelectric impedance to predict cardiac output in open heart recovery. *Biological Psychology, 36,* 23–32.

Di Rienzo, M., Parati, G., Castiglioni, P., Tordi, R., Mancia, G., & Pedotti, A. (2001). Baroreflex effectiveness index: An additional measure of baroreflex control of heart rate in daily life. *American Journal of Physiology, 280,* R744–R751.

Eckberg, D. L. (1997). Sympathovagal balance: A critical appraisal. *Circulation, 96,* 3224–3232.

Eckberg, D. L. (1998). Sympathovagal balance: A critical appraisal. Reply. *Circulation, 98,* 2643–2644.

Eckberg, D. L. (2000). Physiological basis for human autonomic rhythms. *Annals of Medicine, 32,* 341–349.

Eckberg, D. L. (2003). The human respiratory gate. *Journal of Physiology, 548,* 339–352.

Fitzsimons, J. T. (1998). Angiotensin, thirst, and sodium appetite. *Physiological Review, 78,* 583–686.

Fukuda, N., & Granzier, H. (2004). Role of the giant elastic protein titin in the Frank-Starling mechanism of the heart. *Current Vascular Pharmacology, 2,* 135–139.

Fukuda, N., Wu, Y. Farman, G. Irving, T. C., & Granzier, H. (2003). Titin isoform variance and length dependence of activation in skinned bovine cardiac muscle. *Journal of Physiology, 553,* 147–154.

Furedy, J. J., Heslegrave, R. J., & Scher, H. (1992). T-wave amplitude utility revisited: Some physiological and psychophysiological considerations. *Biological Psychology, 33,* 241–248.

Fyfe, D. A., & Parks, W. J. (2002). Noninvasive diagnostics in congenital heart disease: Echocardiography and magnetic resonance imaging. *Critical Care Nursing Quarterly, 25,* 26–36.

Gang, Y., & Malik, M. (2002). Heart rate variability in critical care medicine. *Current Opinion in Critical Care, 8,* 371–375.

Gianaros, P. J., May, J. C., Siegle, G. J., & Jennings, J. R. (2005). Is there a functional neural correlate of individual differences in cardiovascular reactivity? *Psychosomatic Medicine, 67,* 31–39.

Gianaros, P. J., Van Der Veen, F. M., & Jennings, J. R. (2004). Regional cerebral blood flow correlates with heart period and high-frequency heart period variability during working-memory tasks: Implications for the cortical and subcortical regulation of cardiac autonomic activity. *Psychophysiology, 41,* 521–530.

Gibbons, R. J., & Araoz, P. A. (2004). The year in cardiac imaging. *Journal of the American College of Cardiology, 44,* 1937–1944.

Glaser, R., Kiecolt-Glaser, J. K., Malarkey, W. B., & Sheridan, J. F. (1998). The influence of psychological stress on the immune response to vaccines. *Annals of the New York Academy of Sciences, 840,* 649–655.

Goldberger, A. L. (1998). *Clinical Electrocardiography: A Simplified Approach.* New York: C. V. Mosby.

Goldin, J. G., Ratib, O., & Aberle, D. R. (2000). Contemporary cardiac imaging: An overview. *Journal of Thoracic Imaging, 15,* 218–229.

Gray, A. L., Johnson, T. A., Ardell, J. L., & Massari, V. J. (2004a). Parasympathetic control of the heart. II. A novel interganglionic intrinsic cardiac circuit mediates neural control of heart rate. *Journal of Applied Physiology, 96,* 2273–2278.

Gray, A. L., Johnson, T. A., Lauenstein, J. M., Newton, S. S., Ardell, J. L., & Massari, V. J. (2004b). Parasympathetic control of the heart. III. Neuropeptide Y-immunoreactive nerve terminals synapse on three populations of negative chronotropic vagal preganglionic neurons. *Journal of Applied Physiology, 96,* 2279–2287.

Grisk, O., & Rettig, R. (2004). Interactions between the sympathetic nervous system and the kidneys in arterial hypertension. *Cardiovascular Research, 61,* 238–246.

Grossman, P., Karemaker, J., & Wieling, W. (1991). Prediction of tonic parasympathetic cardiac control using respiratory sinus arrhythmia: The need for respiratory control. *Psychophysiology, 28,* 201–216.

Grossman, P., & Kollai, M. (1993). Respiratory sinus arrhythmia, cardiac vagal tone, and respiration: Within- and between-individual relations. *Psychophysiology, 30,* 486–495.

Grossman, P., van Beek, J., & Wientjes, C. (1990). A comparison of three quantification methods for estimation of respiratory sinus arrhythmia. *Psychophysiology, 27,* 702–714.

Grossman, P., Wilhelm, F. H., & Spoerle, M. (2004). Respiratory sinus arrhythmia, cardiac vagal control, and daily activity. *American Journal of Physiology: Heart, & Circulatory Physiology, 287,* H728–H734.

Guimaraes, S., & Moura, D. (2001). Vascular adrenoceptors: An update. *Pharmacological Review, 53,* 319–356.

Guthrie, D., & Yucha, C. (2004). Urinary concentration and dilution. *Nephrolology Nursing Journal, 31,* 297–303.

Guyton, A. C., & Hall, J. E. (2000). *Textbook of Medical Physiology* (10th ed.). Philadelphia: W.B. Saunders Co.

Hakim, K., Fischer, M., Gunnicker, M., Poenicke, K., Zerkowski, H. R., & Brodde, O. E. (1997). Functional role of beta2-adrenoceptors in the transplanted human heart. *Journal of Cardiovascular Pharmacology, 30,* 811–816.

Hawkley, L. C., Burleson, M. H., Berntson, G. G., & Cacioppo, J. T. (2003). Loneliness in everyday life: Cardiovascular activity, psychosocial context, and health behaviors. *Journal of Personality and Social Psychology, 85,* 105–120.

Higgins, C. B. (2000). Cardiac imaging. *Radiology, 217,* 4–10.

Hoetink, A. E., Faes, T. J., Schuur, E. H., Gorkink, R., Goovaerts, H. G., Meijer, J. H., Heethaar, R. M. (2002). Comparing spot electrode arrangements for electric impedance cardiography. *Physiological Measurement, 23,* 457–467.

Hoetink, A. E., Faes, T. J., Visser, K. R., & Heethaar, R. M. (2004). On the flow dependency of the electrical conductivity of blood. *IEEE Transactions on Biomedical Engineering, 51,* 1251–1261.

Iwata, J., & LeDoux, J. E. (1988). Dissociation of associative and nonassociative concomitants of classical fear conditioning in the freely behaving rat. *Behavioral Neuroscience, 102,* 66–76.

Jennings, J. R., Kamarck, T. W., Everson-Rose, S. A., Kaplan, G. A, Manuck,. S. B., & Salonen, J. T. (2004). Exaggerated blood pressure responses during mental stress are prospectively related to enhanced carotid atherosclerosis in middle-aged Finnish men. *Circulation, 110,* 2198–2203.

Jennings, J. R., Tahmoush, A. J., & Redmond, D. P. (1980). Noninvasive measurement of peripheral vascular activity. In I. Martin, & P. H. Venables (Eds.), *Techniques in psychophysiology* (pp. 69–137). New York: John Wiley & Sons.

Johnson, T. A., Gray, A. L., Lauenstein, J. M., Newton, S. S., & Massari, V. J. (2004). Parasympathetic control of the heart. I. An interventriculo-septal ganglion is the major source of the vagal intracardiac innervation of the ventricles. *Journal of Applied Physiology, 96,* 2265–2272.

Joyner, M. J., & Dietz, N. M. (2003). Sympathetic vasodilation in human muscle. *Acta Physiologica Scandinavica, 177,* 329–336.

Kauppinen, P. K., Hyttinen, J. A., & Malmivuo, J., A. (1998). Sensitivity distributions of impedance cardiography using band and spot electrodes analyzed by a three-dimensional computer model. *Annals of Biomedical Engineering, 26,* 694–702.

Kauppinen, P. K., Koobi, T., Hyttinen, J., & Malmivuo, J. (2000). Segmental composition of whole-body impedance cardiogram estimated by computer simulations and clinical experiments. *Clinical Physiology, 20,* 106–113.

Kelsey, R. M., Reiff, S., Wiens, S., Schneider, T. R., Mezzacappa, E. S., & Guethlein, W. (1998). The ensemble-averaged impedance cardiogram: An evaluation of scoring methods and interrater reliability. *Psychophysiology, 35,* 337–340.

Kemmotsu, O., Ueda, M., Otsuka, H., Yamamura, T., Winter, D. C., & Eckerle, J. S. (1991). Arterial tonometry for noninvasive, continuous blood pressure monitoring during anesthesia. *Anesthesiology, 75,* 333–340.

Kline, K. P., Ginsburg, G. P., & Johnston, J. R. (1998). T-wave amplitude: Relationships to phasic RSA and heart period changes. *International Journal of Psychophysiology, 29,* 291–301.

Kubicek, W. G., Karnegis, J. N., Patterson, R. P., Witsoe, D. A., & Mattson, R. H. (1966). Development and evaluation of an impedance cardiac output system. *Aerospace Medicine, 37,* 1208–1212.

Kurzen, H., & Schallreuter, K. U. (2004). Novel aspects in cutaneous biology of acetylcholine synthesis and acetylcholine receptors. *Experimental Dermatology, 13* (Suppl 4), 27–30.

Kuvin, J. T., Patel, A. R., Sliney, K. A., Pandian, N. G., Rand, W. M., Udelson, J. E., & Karas, R. H. (2001). Peripheral vascular endothelial function testing as a noninvasive indicator of coronary artery disease. *Journal of the American College of Cardiology, 38,* 1843–1849.

Kuvin, J. T., Patel, A. R., Sliney, K. A., Pandian, N. G., Sheffy, J., Schnall, R. P., Karas, R. H., & Udelson, J. E. (2003). Assessment of peripheral vascular endothelial function with finger arterial pulse wave amplitude. *American Heart Journal, 146,* 168–174.

Lacey, J. I., & Lacey, B. C. (1962). The law of initial value in the longitudinal study of autonomic constitution: Reproducibility of autonomic responses and response patterns over a four-year interval. *Annals of the New York Academy of Sciences, 98,* 1257–1290.

Landis, S. C. (1996.) The development of cholinergic sympathetic neurons: A role for neuropoietic cytokines? *Perspectives in Developmental Neurobiology, 4,* 53–63.

Lane, R. D., Reiman, E. M., Ahern, G. L., & Thayer, J. F. (2001). Activity in medial prefrontal cortex correlates with vagal component of heart rate variability during emotion. *Brain and Cognition, 47,* 97–100.

Lehrer, P. M., Vaschillo, E., Vaschillo, B., Lu, S-E., Eckberg, D. L., Edelberg, R., Shih, W. J., Lin, Y., Kuusela, T. A., Tahvanainen, K. U.O., & Hamer, R. M. (2003). Heart rate variability biofeedback increases baroreflex gain and peak expiratory flow. *Psychosomatic Medicine, 65,* 796–805.

Levy, M. N. (1984). Cardiac sympathetic-parasympathetic interactions. *Federation Proceedings, 43,* 2598–2602.

Libby, P. (2003). Vascular biology of atherosclerosis: Overview and state of the art. *American Journal of Cardiology, 91,* 3A–6A.

Lindh, B., & Hokfelt, T. (1990). Structural and functional aspects of acetylcholine peptide coexistence in the autonomic nervous system. *Progress in Brain Research, 84,* 175–191.

Llabre, M. M., Ironson, G. H., Spitzer, S. B., Gellman, M. D., Weidler, D. J., & Schneiderman, N. (1988). How many blood pressure measurements are enough?: An application of generalizability theory to the study of blood pressure reliability. *Psychophysiology, 25,* 97–106.

Longmore, J., Bradshaw, C. M., & Szabadi, E. (1985). Effects of locally and systemically administered cholinoceptor antagonists on the secretory response of human eccrine sweat glands to carbachol. *British Journal of Clinical Pharmacology, 20,* 1–7.

Luchner, A., & Schunkert, H. (2004). Interactions between the sympathetic nervous system and the cardiac natriuretic peptide system. *Cardiovascular Research, 63,* 443–449.

Malliani, A. (1999). The pattern of sympathovagal balance explored in the frequency domain. *News in Physiological Sciences, 14,* 111–117.

Matthews, K. A., Salomon, K., Brady, S. S., & Allen, M. T. (2003). Cardiovascular reactivity to stress predicts future blood pressure in adolescence. *Psychosomatic Medicine, 65,* 410–415.

Matthews, S. C., Paulus, M. P., Simmons, A. N., Nelesen, R. A., Dimsdale, J. E. (2004). Functional subdivisions within anterior cingulate cortex and their relationship to autonomic nervous system function. *Neuroimage, 22,* 1151–1156.

Monti, A., Medigue, C., & Mangin, L. (2002). Instantaneous parameter estimation in cardiovascular time series by harmonic and time-frequency analysis. *IEEE Transactions in Biomedical Engineering, 49,* 1547–1556.

Moshkovitz, Y., Kaluski, E., Milo, O., Vered, Z., & Cotter G. (2004). Recent developments in cardiac output determination by bioimpedance: Comparison with invasive cardiac output and potential cardiovascular applications. *Current Opinion in Cardiology, 19,* 229–237.

Myerson, S. G., Bellenger, N. G., & Pennell, D. J. (2002). Assessment of left ventricular mass by cardiovascular magnetic resonance. *Hypertension, 39,* 750–755.

O'Brien, E. (1996). Review: A century of confusion: Which bladder for accurate blood pressure measurement? *Journal of Human Hypertension, 10,* 565–572.

Padgett, D. A., Sheridan, J. F., Dorne, J., Berntson, G. G., Candelora, J., & Glaser, R. (1998). Social stress and the reactivation of latent herpes simplex virus-type 1. *Proceedings of the National Academy of Sciences, 95,* 7231–7235.

Parati, G., Di Rienzo, M., & Mancia, G. (2000). How to measure baroreflex sensitivity: From the cardiovascular laboratory to daily life. *Journal of Hypertension, 18,* 7–19.

Parati, G., Ongaro, G., Bilo, G., Glavina, F., Castiglioni, P., Di Rienzo, M., & Mancia, G. (2003). Non-invasive beat-to-beat blood pressure monitoring: New developments. *Blood Pressure Monitoring, 8,* 31–36.

Persson, P. B., Di Rienzo, M., Castiglioni, P., Cerutti, C., Pagani, M., Honzikova, N., Akselrod, S., & Parati, G. (2001). Time versus frequency domain techniques for assessing baroreflex sensitivity. *Journal of Hypertension, 19,* 1699–1705.

Pirola, F. T., & Potter, E. K. (1990). Vagal action on atrioventricular conduction and its inhibition by sympathetic stimulation and neuropeptide Y in anaesthetised dogs. *Journal of the Autonomic Nervous System, 31,* 1–12.

Porges, S. W., & Bohrer, R. E. (1990). Analysis of periodic processes in psychophysiological research. In J. T. Cacioppo, & L. G. Tassinary (Eds.), *Principles of psychophysiology: Physical, social and inferential elements* (pp. 708–753). New York: Cambridge University Press.

Pumprla, J., Howorka, K., Groves, D., Chester, M., & Nolan, J. (2002). Functional assessment of heart rate variability: Physiological basis and practical applications. *International Journal of Cardiology, 84,* 1–14.

Qu, M. H., Zhang, Y. J., Webster, J. G., & Tompkins, W. J. (1986). Motion artifact from spot and band electrodes during impedance cardiography. *IEEE Transactions in Biomedical Engineering, 33,* 1029–1036.

Quan, N., Avitsur, R., Stark, J. L., He, L., Lai, W., Dhabhar, F., & Sheridan, J. F. (2003). Molecular mechanisms of glucocorticoid resistance in splenocytes of socially stressed male mice. *Journal of Neuroimmunology, 137,* 51–58.

Quigley, K. S., & Stifter, C. A. (2006). A comparative validation of sympathetic reactivity in children and adults. *Psychophysiology 43,* 357–365.

Raaijmakers, E., Faes, T. J., Scholten, R. J., Goovaerts, H. G., & Heethaar, R. M. (1999). A meta-analysis of published studies concerning the validity of thoracic impedance cardiography. *Annals of the New York Academy of Sciences, 873,* 121–127.

Randall, W., Wurster, R. Randall, D., & Xi-Moy, S. (1996). From cardioaccelerator and inhibitory nerves to a "heart brain": An evolution of concepts. In Shepard J. T., & Vatner, S. F. (Eds.), *Nervous control of the heart.* Amsterdam: Harwood Academic Publishers.

Rashba, E. J., Cooklin, M., MacMurdy, K., Kavesh, N., Kirk, M., Sarang, S., Peters, R. W., Shorofsky, S. R., & Gold, M. R. (2002). Effects of selective autonomic blockade on T-wave alternans in humans. *Circulation, 105,* 837–842.

Ren, L. M., Furukawa, Y., Karasawa, Y., Murakami, M., Takei, M., Narita, M., & Chiba, S. (1991). Differential inhibition of neuropeptide Y on the chronotropic and inotropic responses to sympathetic and parasympathetic stimulation in the isolated, perfused dog atrium. *Journal of Pharmacology and Experimental Therapeutics, 259,* 38–43.

Reyes del Paso, G. A., González, I., & Hernández, J. A. (2004). Baroreceptor sensitivity and effectiveness varies differentially as a function of cognitive-attentional demands. *Biological Psychology, 67,* 385–395.

Reyes del Paso, G. A., Hernández, J. A., & González, I. (2004). Differential analysis in the time domain of the baroreceptor cardiac reflex sensitivity as a function of sequence length. *Psychophysiology, 41,* 483–488.

Richardson, R. J., Grkovic, I., & Anderson, C. R. (2003). Immunohistochemical analysis of intracardiac ganglia of the rat heart. *Cell and Tissue Research, 314,* 337–350.

Riese, H., Groot, P. F., van den Berg, M., Kupper, N. H., Magnee, E. H., Rohaan, E. J., Vrijkotte, T. G., Willemsen, G., & de Geus, E. J. (2003). Large-scale ensemble averaging of ambulatory impedance cardiograms. *Behavioral Research Methods, Instruments and Computers, 35,* 467–477.

Riniolo, T., & Porges, S. W. (1997). Inferential and descriptive influences on measures of respiratory sinus arrhythmia: Sampling rate, R-wave trigger accuracy, and variance estimates. *Psychophysiology, 34,* 613–621.

Rose, S. C. (2000). Noninvasive vascular laboratory for evaluation of peripheral arterial occlusive disease: Part I – Hemodynamic principles and tools of the trade. *Journal of Vascular and Interventional Radiology, 11,* 1107–1114.

Rosengren, A., Hawken, S., Ounpuu, S., Sliwa, K., Zubaid, M., Almahmeed, W. A., Blackett, K. N., Sitthi-amorn, C., Sato, H., & Yusuf, S. (2004). Association of psychosocial risk factors with risk of acute myocardial infarction in 11119 cases and 13648 controls from 52 countries (the INTERHEART study): Case-control study. *Lancet, 364,* 953–62.

Sampaio, K. N., Mauad, H., Spyer, K. M., & Ford, T. W. (2003). Differential chronotropic and dromotropic responses to focal stimulation of cardiac vagal ganglia in the rat. *Experimental Physiology, 88,* 315–327.

Schwartz, P. J., La Rovere, M. T., & Vanoli, E. (1992). Autonomic nervous system and sudden cardiac death. Experimental basis and clinical observations for post-myocardial infarction risk stratification. *Circulation, 85,* I77–191.

Shapiro, D., Jamner, L. D., Lane, J. D., Light, K. C., Myrtek, M., Sawada, Y., & Steptoe, A. (1996). Blood pressure publication guidelines. *Psychophysiology, 33,* 1–12.

Sheridan, J. F., Stark, J. L., Avitsur, R., & Padgett, D. A. (2000). Social disruption, immunity, and susceptibility to viral infection. Role of glucocorticoid insensitivity and NGF. *Annals of the New York Academy of Sciences, 917,* 894–905.

Sherwood, A., McFetridge, J., & Hutcheson, J. S. (1998) Ambulatory impedance cardiography: a feasibility study. *Journal of Applied Physiology, 85,* 2365–2369.

Sherwood, A., Allen, M. T., Fahrenberg, J., Kelsey, R. M., Lovallo, W. R., & van Doornen, L. J. (1990). Methodological guidelines for impedance cardiography. *Psychophysiology, 27,* 1–23.

Sherwood, A., Royal, S. A., Hutcheson, J. S., & Turner, J. R. (1992). Comparison of impedance cardiographic measurements using band and spot electrodes. *Psychophysiology, 29,* 734–741.

Smith, R. P., Argod, J., Pépin, J.-L., & Lévy, P. A. (1999). Pulse transit time: An appraisal of potential clinical applications. *Thorax, 54,* 452–458.

Smith, L. L., Kukielka, M., & Billman, G. E. (2005). Heart rate recovery after exercise: A predictor of ventricular fibrillation susceptibility after myocardial infarction. *American Journal of Physiology: Heart and Circulatory Physiology,* H1763–1769.

Somsen, R. J., Jennings, J. R., & Van der Molen, M. W. (2004). The cardiac cycle time effect revisited: Temporal dynamics of the central-vagal modulation of heart rate in human reaction time tasks. *Psychophysiology, 41,* 941–953.

Steptoe, A., Godaert, G., Ross, A., & Schreurs, P. (1983). The cardiac and vascular components of pulse transmission time: A computer analysis of systolic time intervals. *Psychophysiology, 20,* 251–259.

Steptoe, A., & Sawada, Y. (1989). Assessment of baroreceptor reflex function during mental stress and relaxation. *Psychophysiology, 26,* 140–1147.

Strike, P. C., & Steptoe, A. (2004). Psychosocial factors in the development of coronary artery disease. *Progress in Cardiovascular Disease, 46,* 337–347.

Takahashi, H., Maehara, K., Onuki, N., Saito, T., & Maruyama, Y. (2003). Decreased contractility of the left ventricle is induced by the neurotransmitter acetylcholine, but not by vagal stimulation in rats. *Japanese Heart Journal, 44,* 257–270.

Task Force of the European Society of Cardiology and the North American Society of Pacing and Electrophysiology. (1996). Heart rate variability: Standards of measurement, physiological interpretation, and clinical use. *Circulation, 93,* 1043–1065.

Ter Horst, G. J., Hautvast, R. W., De Jongste, M. J., & Korf, J. (1996). Neuroanatomy of cardiac activity-regulating circuitry: A transneuronal retrograde viral labelling study in the rat. *European Journal of Neuroscience, 8*, 2029–2041.

Thayer, J. F., & Uijtdehaage, S. H. (2001). Derivation of chronotropic indices of autonomic nervous system activity using impedance cardiography. *Biomedical Sciences Instrumentation, 37*, 331–336.

Tomaka, J., Blascovich, J., & Swart, L. (1994). Effects of vocalization on cardiovascular and electrodermal responses during mental arithmetic. *International Journal of Psychophysiology, 18*, 23–33.

Ursino, M., & Magosso, E. (2003). Short-term autonomic control of cardiovascular function: A mini-review with the help of mathematical models. *Journal of Integrative Neuroscience, 2*, 219–247.

Vallbo, A. B., Hagbarth, K. E., & Wallin, B. G. (2004). Microneurography: How the technique developed and its role in the investigation of the sympathetic nervous system. *Journal of Applied Physiology, 96*, 1262–1269.

Van De Water, J. M., Miller, T. W., Vogel, R. L., Mount, B. E., & Dalton, M. L. (2003). Impedance cardiography: The next vital sign technology? *Chest, 123*, 2028–2033.

Van Roon, A. M., Mulder, L. J., Althaus, M., & Mulder, G. (2004). Introducing a baroreflex model for studying cardiovascular effects of mental workload. *Psychophysiology, 41*, 961–981.

Vilches, J. J., Navarro, X., & Verdu, E. (1995). Functional sudomotor responses to cholinergic agonists and antagonists in the mouse. *Journal of the Autonomic Nervous System, 55*, 105–111.

van Montfrans, G. A. (2001). Oscillometric blood pressure measurements: Progress and problems. *Blood Pressure Monitoring, 6*, 287–290.

Vuurmans, T. J. L., Boer, P., & Koomans, H. A. (2003). Effects of endothelin-1 and endothelin-1 receptor blockade on cardiac output, aortic pressure, and pulse wave velocity in humans. *Hypertension, 41*, 1253–1258.

Weber, E. J., Molenaar, P. C., & van der Molen, M. W. (1992). A nonstationarity test for the spectral analysis of physiological time series with an application to respiratory sinus arrhythmia. *Psychophysiology, 29*, 55–65.

Wesseling, K. H. (1990). Finapres, continuous noninvasive finger arterial pressure based on the method of Peñaz. In W. Meyer-Sabellek, M. Anlauf, R. Gotzen & L. Steinfeld (Eds.), *Blood pressure measurement* (pp. 161–172). Darmstadt: Steinkopff.

Weyman, A. E. (2005). The year in echocardiography. *Journal of the American College of Cardiology, 45*, 448–455.

Wilhelm, F. H., Grossman, P., & Roth, W. T. (1999). Analysis of cardiovascular regulation. *Biomedical Sciences and Instrumentation, 35*, 135–140.

Wilhelm, F. H., Grossman, P., & Coyle, M. A. (2004). Improving estimation of cardiac vagal tone during spontaneous breathing using a paced breathing calibration. *Biomedical Sciences Instrumentation, 40*, 317–324.

Wilkinson, I. B., & Webb, D. J. (2001). Venous occlusion plethysmography in cardiovascular research: Methodology and clinical applications. *British Journal of Clinical Pharmacology, 52*, 631–646.

Willemsen, G. H., De Geus, E. J., Klaver, C. H., Van Doornen, L. J., & Carroll, D. (1996). Ambulatory monitoring of the impedance cardiogram. *Psychophysiology, 33*, 184–193.

Wood, D. (2001). Established and emerging cardiovascular risk factors. *American Heart Journal, 141*, 49–57.

Woods, R. L. (2004). Cardioprotective functions of atrial natriuretic peptide and B-type natriuretic peptide: A brief review. *Clinical and Experimental Pharmacology and Physiology, 31*, 791–794.

9 Gastrointestinal Response

ROBERT M. STERN, KENNETH L. KOCH, MAX E. LEVINE, AND ERIC R. MUTH

PROLOGUE

Overview

Questions about the interaction between brain and the gastrointestinal (GI) system have interested investigators at least as far back as 1833, when Beaumont described his experiments on a fistulated patient, Alexis St. Martin. In the case of St. Martin, his fistula, or external opening into the stomach, was created by an accidental gunshot wound. Beaumont reported that upsetting emotions suppressed gastric secretion and delayed gastric emptying in his subject. Between 1840 and 1870 several physiologists created fistulas in dogs, based on Beaumont's work, and found that an intact vagus was needed for normal brain-gut interaction. This was an important finding because it indicates that one pathway by which the brain and gut communicate is via the vagus nerve or parasympathetic nervous system. Today we use the term cephalic-vagal reflex to refer to, for example, the anticipatory stomach contractions that occur when thinking about an appetizing meal. More about the cephalic-vagal reflex will follow in a later section of this chapter, but we should keep in mind that brain-gut interaction is a two-way street. That is, not only does brain activity affect GI activity, but GI activity also affects the activity in the brain. An example of the latter, which will be discussed in some detail later in this chapter, is the effect of changes in stomach activity on the sensation of nausea.

During the first half of the twentieth century, gastrointestinal scientists and clinicians were deeply committed to an interactive brain-gut view of gastrointestinal functioning and, therefore, had a lot to say to psychophysiologists. Wolf and Wolff (1943) wrote a fascinating book about their experiences over many years with their fistulated subject Tom. Their basic findings were that when Tom was fearful or depressed his gastric activity decreased, but when he was angry or hostile his gastric activity increased. During this same period, Cannon studied the effects of various emotions on GI activity and published several books on the topic including *Digestion and Health* (1936), which contains chapters on the nature of appetite and hunger, and indigestion from pain, worry and excitement. Alvarez, perhaps the best-known gastroenterologist of the century, in his writings, both scientific and popular, always stressed the interaction of psychological and physiological factors in GI functioning. His book *Nervousness, Indigestion, and Pain* (1943) is highly recommended reading for psychophysiologists.

During the second half of the twentieth-century gastroenterologists developed many new techniques for measuring the activity of the GI system and adhered, in general, to a medical model. Unlike Alvarez, who said "... to understand a man's stomach, one must understand the man," gastroenterologists relied more and more on the results of laboratory tests of the GI system and ignored the "man." This meant that there was little interaction between gastroenterologists and psychophysiologists, or psychologists of any type, and because most of the new tests of GI activity were invasive, most psychophysiologists could not make use of them outside of a medical center. Fortunately, the pendulum has swung back during the past few years and as one indication, an interdisciplinary group of scientists and clinicians trained in gastroenterology, psychophysiology, epidemiology, and clinical psychology have formed an association called the Functional Brain-Gut Research Group.

As a consequence of the paucity of interaction between gastroenterologists and psychophysiologists until recently, the authors know of no psychophysiological studies of absorption, and psychophysiologists have conducted few studies of gastric acid secretion. However, several studies of motor activity, particularly in the stomach, have been conducted. In this chapter we review psychophysiological studies that have measured gastric motor activity; the major emphasis will be on the motor activity of the stomach as measured with a noninvasive technique first used by Alvarez in 1921, the electrogastrogram or EGG. Brief information about two additional noninvasive measures of motor activity appears at the end of this chapter. These measures are (1) gastric emptying time and (2) oral-cecal transit time.

Electrogastrography refers to the recording of electro-gastrograms (EGGs). Electrogastrograms reflect gastric myoelectrical activity as it is recorded from the abdominal surface with electrodes placed on the skin. EGGs are more or less sinusoidal waves recurring at a rate of 3 cycles per minute (cpm) in healthy humans. This predominant frequency is usually discernable by visual inspection of the signal, but computer analysis is essential for quantitative study of EGG recordings.

The stomach is also the source of abnormally fast or slow – usually dysrhythmic – myoelectrical signals, the tachygastrias and bradygastrias. Acute or chronic shifts from normal 3 cpm EGG signals to the gastric dysrhythmias are associated with a variety of clinical symptoms, particularly nausea. In contrast to the level of research on abnormalities in frequency, such as the gastric dysrhythmias, there has been little study about the amplitude, duration, wave form and wave propagation characteristics of the EGG.

HISTORICAL BACKGROUND

In the mid-1950s, R.C. Davis, one of the founders of the Society for Psychophysiological Research, began a series of exploratory studies with the EGG. Davis, like Alvarez, was primarily interested in the interaction of psychological and physiological factors on gastric functioning. Davis published two papers before his untimely death in 1961, papers that stimulated several other investigators to begin doing EGG research. In a 1957 paper (Davis, Garafolo, & Gault, 1957), Davis and his co-workers described their attempt to validate the EGG using simultaneous recordings from needle electrodes, a mine detector that picked up the movements of a steel ball in the subject's GI tract, and the EGG. They used needle electrodes that were insulated except at the tip so that they could rule out cutaneous tissue as the source of the EGG signal.

In a 1959 paper (Davis, Garafolo, & Kveim, 1959), Davis and his co-workers described their continuing validation of the EGG using swallowed balloons, and their studies of the effects of eating on the EGG. They reported that the activity of the stomach is at its lowest point when the stomach is empty, a controversial finding in light of the reports of so-called hunger contractions by Cannon and Carlson (Cannon & Washburn, 1912; Carlson, 1916). After recording the EGG from many fasted subjects both with and without a balloon in the stomach, Davis concluded that hunger contractions are rare and are usually stimulated by the introduction of a balloon into the stomach. This is a good example of one of the advantages of using psychophysiological methods, that is, noninvasive recording techniques that do not interfere with the behavior being studied. All other methods of recording stomach activity either require putting something inside the stomach – which stimulates it to contract – or are dangerous to use for extended periods, such as X-rays or fluoroscopy. For more information about the history of EGG see Chapter 1 in Koch and Stern (2004).

PHYSIOLOGICAL BASES OF GASTRIC MOTOR ACTIVITY AND ELECTROGASTROGRAPHY

The GI system extends from the mouth to the rectum and includes the mouth, esophagus, stomach, small intestine, large intestine, and rectum. The three functions of the GI system are movement of food through the alimentary tract, secretion of substances that aid in digestion or protect the alimentary tract, and absorption of the digestive end products. The GI tract may be considered to be a series of muscular tubes that perform region-specific digestive functions, that is, transit of food from esophagus to stomach, mixing and emptying of ingested foods from the stomach into the duodenum, and absorption of micronutrients from the small intestine. Other specialized tubes (i.e., the cecum; ascending, transverse, and descending colon; and rectum) conserve water, electrolytes, and nutrients and evacuate wastes. These functions require exquisite control and integration of relevant neural, muscular, mucosal, and hormonal systems within the GI tract.

Gastric anatomy

In most healthy humans the stomach lies in the upper quadrant of the abdomen, although there is a wide range of variability in its shape and form (see Figure 9.1). As is shown in Figure 9.1, the esophagus enters the stomach in the fundic region; the antrum is connected to the first portion of the duodenum, the duodenal bulb, via the pylorus.

As can be seen at the top of Figure 9.1, the stomach has three major regions: the fundus, body, and antrum. The middle of the figure shows the three layers of the stomach: outermost is the serosa; innermost is the mucosa, which secretes acid and pepsin; and the thickest layer is the muscular portion, which has three layers, an outer longitudinal layer, an inner circular layer, and in some areas an oblique layer. The bottom of the figure shows the relationship among the circular muscle layer, the myenteric neurons, and the interstitial cells of Cajal (ICC). The ICC are the origin of the electrical rhythmicity that is recorded as the gastric pacesetter potential. For additional information about the ICC and their relationship to gastric electrical rhythmicity see Chapter 2 in Koch and Stern (2004).

The muscular wall of the stomach contains extensive neural elements, both extrinsic and intrinsic. Extrinsic nerves are pre- and postganglionic parasympathetic fibers from the vagus nerve and postganglionic neurons from the sympathetic splanchnic nerves. These extrinsic neural circuits are closely integrated with the intrinsic nervous system of the stomach and of all regions of the GI tract, the enteric nervous system.

The enteric nervous system is a collection of nerve cell bodies in plexi located between the circular and longitudinal muscle layers, that is, the myenteric plexus (Auerbach's plexus) and submucosal plexus (see Figure 9.1). The myenteric and submucosal plexi are the largest, but

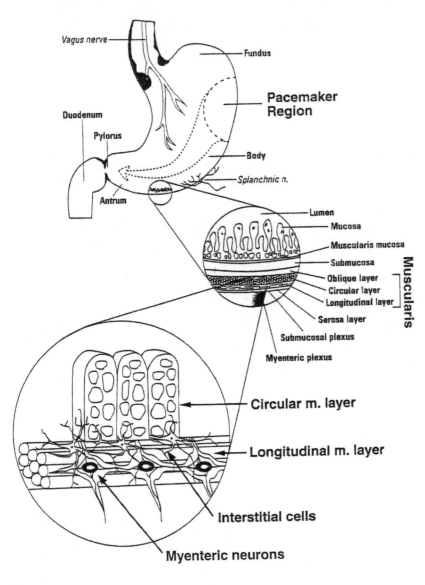

Figure 9.1. Anatomical regions of the stomach. The upper figure shows the fundus, body, and antrum of the stomach. The pacemaker region is the origin of gastric pacesetter potential activity. The cutout of the gastric wall shown in the middle portion of the figure depicts the lumen of the stomach, the mucosa, and the muscularis of the stomach wall. The main muscle layers of the stomach are the longitudinal and circular muscle layers, with some contribution by the oblique muscle layer. In the lower portion of the figure, the relationships among the circular muscle layer, the interstitial cells of Cajal, and the myenteric neurons of Auerbach's plexus are shown. The interstitial cells of Cajal synapse with the circular muscle layer as well as the myenteric neurons. The interstitial cells of Cajal are the origin of the electrical rhythmicity that is recorded as the gastric pacesetter potentials. The gastric pacesetter potentials coordinate the frequency and the propagation of the circular smooth muscle contractions. (Reprinted with permission from Koch & Stern (2004).)

seven discrete plexi have been identified. Postganglionic parasympathetic neurons, internuncial neurons, and sensory neurons are present within the plexi. Many different types of enteric neurons have been identified by immunohistochemical methods (Furness & Costa, 1980). It has been estimated that there are 10^9 neurons in the enteric nervous system, a number similar to that in the spinal cord. Fibers from the sympathetic neurons synapse on myenteric plexus neurons and innervate the circular muscle layer. Thus, the muscular layers of the stomach, particularly the circular muscle layer, have rich neural integration that allows for fine control of muscular contraction required for normal digestive function. The interested reader may refer to review articles on neural control of gastric motility (Wood, 2002).

Gastric physiology

Postprandial gastric physiology. The major physiological activities of the stomach are to receive ingested foodstuffs and to mix the foodstuffs into suspensions until they are appropriate for emptying and further digestion in the small intestine.

Normal reception of ingested food requires the gastric fundus to relax and to accommodate the particular ingested volume. These muscular activities of the stomach are termed receptive relaxation and accommodation and are accomplished via vagal efferent activity (Roman & Gonella, 1987). Moreover, because nearly 90% of vagal fibers are sensory, it is assumed that sensory vagal traffic modulates ongoing vagal efferent activity.

After ingestion, solid foods are moved from the gastric fundus into the gastric body and antrum for mixing and emptying. This period is called the lag phase because it precedes actual emptying of the nutrient suspensions from the stomach into the duodenum (Lavigne, Wiley, Meyer, Martin, & MacGregor, 1978; Meyer, MacGregor, Gueller, Martin, & Cavalieri, 1976). In contrast to solids, nonnutrient liquids such as water have no lag phase. Before emptying, solids are normally mixed and reduced to 0.1–1 mm diameter particles and suspended in gastric juice (Meyer, Ohashi, Jehn, & Thompson, 1981).

The stomach accomplishes the work of mixing and emptying through a series of smooth rhythmic contractions at the rate of 3 cycles per minute (cpm). This phase in the digestive process, known as peristalsis, commences in the gastric body and moves through this region into the antrum where the waves dissipate in the prepyloric region. As a result of these wavelike contractions, small food particles already in suspension are carried through the open pyloric sphincter into the duodenum (Meyer et al., 1981; Meyer, Gu, Dressman, & Amidon, 1986). The pylorus and the duodenum may contract to create resistance to gastric emptying or may relax to promote gastroduodenal synchrony and enhance gastric emptying (Meyer, 1987). The hydrodynamics of the suspension itself may determine which particles are emptied and their rate of emptying (Meyer et al., 1986).

Control of the mixing and emptying of gastric content is complex. In addition to physical properties of the gastric contents and the various neural-muscular responses, the release of gastrointestinal hormones (e.g., gastrin, secretin, cholecystokinin, enteroglucagon, gastric inhibitory polypeptide, somatostatin, vasoactive intestinal polypeptide, and motilin, to name a few of the more than 20 GI hormones and candidate hormones) is believed to modulate the contractile responses of the stomach and to affect overall gastric emptying rates. However, specific actions of most GI hormones on gastric motility in humans remain to be determined.

The rate at which foodstuffs are emptied from the stomach is dependent on many factors including the volume of ingested material, caloric density (i.e., fat, protein, or carbohydrate), osmolality, temperature, acidity, and viscosity. These factors are adjusted by chemo- and mechanoreceptors in the stomach and duodenum and the variety of hormones released by the specific foodstuffs (Meyer, 1987).

Emptying of liquids is thought to be controlled by fundic tone. That is, after the ingestion of a liquid such as water, fundic pressure is greater than duodenal pressure. The pressure gradient between fundus and duodenum provides the force necessary to empty the liquid from the stomach (Meyer, 1987). Other studies indicate that the antrum has a more active role in the emptying of liquids (Camilleri, Malagelada, Brown, Becker, & Zinsmeister, 1985; Stemper, & Cooke, 1975).

Gastric physiology during fasting. During the interdigestive state (e.g., an overnight fast), the stomach completes its digestive function and participates in a stereotyped periodic sequence of contractile events termed the interdigestive complex. The complex is divided into three phases: Phase I is a period of quiescence lasting approximately 20 min; Phase II is a period of irregular contractile activity of the body and antrum lasting about 80–90 min; and Phase III is a 5–10 min period of regular and intense 3-cpm contractions of the gastric body and antrum. The antral contractions are peristaltic, moving into the duodenum and subsequently through the small bowel. Phase III activity occurs approximately every 90–110 min in humans during prolonged fasts and has been associated with bursts of pancreatic and biliary secretions and elevations in plasma motilin levels (Code & Marlett, 1975; Lee, Chey, Tai, & Yajima, 1978; Meyer, 1987; Schlegel & Code, 1975; Vantrappen et al., 1979).

From a physiological viewpoint, Phase III contractions have been shown to empty fibrous meal residue from the stomach (Schlegel & Code, 1975). The Phase III contractions may serve a similar function in the small intestine and have been termed the "intestinal housekeeper."

Relationship between gastric neuromuscular activity and gastric myoelectric activity

For a general discussion of myoelectrical and contractile activity of the GI system see Sarna (2002). The gastric contractions that occur at 3 cpm during the mixing and emptying of meals are the result of coordinated electromechanical coupling of circular layer smooth muscle cells. A description of the electrical and mechanical events within the smooth muscle that underlie the mechanical work performed by the stomach follows.

Gastric slow waves. Gastric slow waves are the electrical events that control gastric contractions, and recent studies have shown that the electrical slow waves are generated by the interstitial cells of Cajal (ICC). The slow waves result from spontaneous depolarization of the ICCs in the region of the juncture of the fundus and body on the greater curvature. From this region, the pacemaker area, the depolarization wave front moves circumferentially and distally toward the distal antrum. The normal slow-wave frequency in humans is 3 cpm (Abell & Malagelada, 1985; Couturier, Roze, Paologgi, & Debray, 1972; Hamilton, Bellahsene, Reichelderfer, Webster, & Bass, 1986; Hinder & Kelly, 1977; Kwong, Brown, Whittaker, & Duthie, 1970). The slow wave does not move into the fundic area, which is electrically silent. The slow wave is a spontaneous, sodium-mediated, and omnipresent event that is associated with very low-amplitude contractile activity (Morgan, Schmalz, & Szurszewski, 1978; You & Chey, 1984).

The slow wave coordinates the frequency and propagation velocity of gastric contractions in the corpus antrum. That is, the slow wave brings the circular muscle layer near the point of depolarization and, if physical, neural, and/or hormonal signals are appropriate for contraction, the depolarization threshold is reached and circular muscle contraction occurs. Because circular muscle contractions are linked with the slow wave, the circular muscle contractions occur at the slow-wave frequency (3 cpm in humans) and the contractions propagate at the slow-wave velocity (0.8–4 cm/s). For these reasons the slow waves have also been called pacesetter potentials and electrical control activity (Meyer, 1987; Roman & Gonella, 1987).

Slow waves are considered to originate in the ICCs, but extrinsic neural input may modulate the rhythmicity of depolarization. For example, after vagotomy in dogs and humans, the slow-wave frequency may be disrupted for weeks (Kelly, Code, & Elveback, 1969; Stoddard, Smallwood, & Duthie, 1981).

Gastric spike potentials. The electrical events underlying circular smooth muscle contractions are plateau and spike potentials. Depolarizations of the circular muscle, in contrast to the longitudinal muscle, are very fast (i.e., spikes). The spikes may or may not occur on plateau potentials, which are associated with the slow wave. The spikes reflect fluxes of calcium passing through the circular muscle membrane. Contractions of the circular muscle may increase tone and/or intraluminal pressure, particularly if they form concentric ring contractions. Such strong contractions may be recorded with strain gauges, intraluminal pressure transducers, or perfused catheters. However, gastric contractions that are not concentric and lumen-occluding may not be recorded by intraluminal devices but will be recorded by strain gauges positioned on the muscle itself (You & Chey, 1984).

In summary, gastric slow waves, generated by the ICC, are present at all times and control the frequency and propagation velocity of spike potentials (i.e., circular muscle contractions) when the latter are elicited by the appropriate stimuli. Gastric slow waves and spike potentials are the myoelectric components of gastric contractions. The gastric contractions perform the work of mixing and emptying foodstuffs. Slow waves and spike potentials from the stomach may be recorded from electrodes sewn to the serosa or from electrodes applied to the gastric mucosa. Because slow waves occur within a conducting medium (i.e., the body), they are also recorded with fidelity from electrodes positioned on the skin – the EGG (Abell & Malagelada, 1985; Brown, Smallwood, Duthie, & Stoddard, 1975; Familoni, Bowes, Kingma, & Cole 1987; Hamilton et al., 1986). Figure 9.2 shows gastric myoelectric activity recorded from serosal and cutaneous electrodes during motor quiescence (A) and during gastric peristalsis (B).

Physiological basis of the EGG

Important anatomical and functional relationships exist among the circular smooth muscle layer, the myenteric neurons, and the interstitial cells of Cajal (ICCs) (see Figure 9.1, bottom). As indicated above, the ICCs are the pacemaker cells, the cells that spontaneously depolarize and repolarize and set the myoelectrical rhythmicity of the stomach and other areas of the gastrointestinal tract (Thunberg, 1989; Huisinga, 2001). The interstitial cells are electrically coupled with the circular muscle cells. Low amplitude rhythmic circular contractions occur at the pacemaker rhythm (Kim et al., 2002). Rhythmicity and contractility of the circular muscle layer are modulated by ongoing excitatory and inhibitory activity of myenteric neurons that synapse with the interstitial cells. The interstitial cells have a variety of other receptors. Electrocon-

tractile activities of the gastric smooth muscle are modified by neuronal and hormonal inputs appropriate for fasting and specific postprandial conditions. Control of rhythmicity may be modulated by a variety of stimuli that affect the interstitial cells and is a focus of intense investigation.

As stated earlier, human gastric slow wave or pacesetter potential activity generated by the ICCs occurs at a rate of 3 cpm (e.g., Koch, 2002). Pacesetter potential activity is illustrated in Figure 9.2. Electrodes sewn onto the serosa of the stomach record the depolarization and repolarization waves of the pacesetter potentials. The electrical wave front travels around the circumference of the stomach at a fast rate of speed and migrates slowly toward the antrum at an increasing velocity. As a slow wave disappears in the distal antrum, another slow wave originates in the pacemaker area and begins to migrate toward the antrum approximately every 20 seconds. When there is little smooth muscle contractility (Phase I or phase II of the interdigestive state, described above), these electrical events reflect depolarization and repolarization of the ICCs and some small degree of contractility of the circular muscle cells.

From an in vivo electrical viewpoint, the fasting pacesetter potential activity is relatively weak compared with the gastric myoelectrical activity during the postprandial period, when luminal contents and other stimuli augment gastric neuromuscular activity (Lin & Hasler, 1995; Lacy, Koch, & Crowell, 2002). Figure 9.3 shows a conceptualization of the human gastric pacesetter potential as an "electrical halo" migrating around the stomach very quickly and moving distally through the antrum in approximately 20 seconds resulting in the normal gastric electrical frequency of 3 cpm. It is this moving electrical wave front that is recorded in the electrogastrogram (EGG), the gastric myoelectrical activity recorded from electrodes placed onto the surface of the epigastrium.

Additional gastric myoelectrical activity occurs when stronger circular muscle contraction occurs; for example, when vagal efferent activity and release of acetylcholine from the postganglionic cholinergic neurons are elicited in response to ingestion of a meal. In this postprandial situation, plateau potentials and action potentials occur during circular muscle contraction. If more action potentials or greater amplitude and duration of the plateau potentials occur, then stronger circular muscle contractions occur. Migrating circular muscle contractions may result in gentle peristaltic waves or strong lumen-obliterating contractions. Figure 9.2B shows the relationship between the pacesetter potential that is linked to the action potential or plateau potential activity and the formation of a circular muscle contraction that migrates from proximal to distal stomach. Thus, the action potential and/or the plateau potential, linked to the migrating pacesetter potential, forms the myoelectrical basis for the gastric peristaltic contractions that ultimately mix and triturate intraluminal contents. When conditions are appropriate, peristaltic contractions empty 2- to 4-ml aliquots of chyme from the stomach into the duodenum to accomplish the

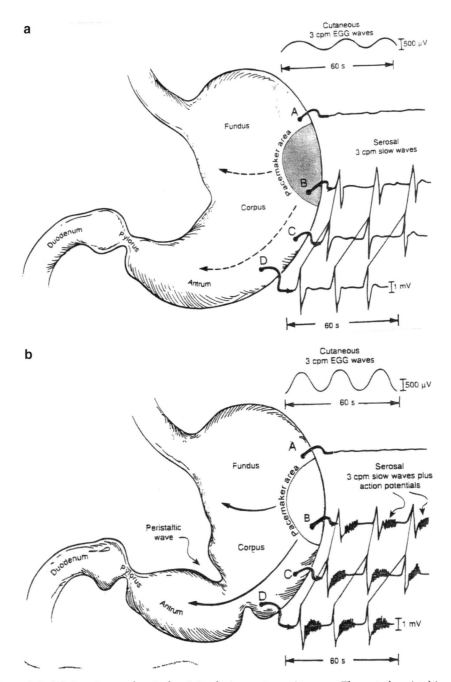

Figure 9.2. (A) Gastric myoelectrical activity during motor quiescence. The antral peristaltic contractions that produce flow of gastric content are controlled by gastric electrical slow waves. The fundus does not have pacemaker activity as shown by electrode A. Pacesetter potentials begin in the pacemaker area located in the proximal gastric body along the greater curve as shown by the gray area. Slow waves spread circumferentially and distally from the pacemaker region and migrate through the antrum (as shown by serosal electrodes, B, C, D). The slow wave migration ends at the pylorus. As the slow wave dissolves in the terminal antrum, another slow wave begins to migrate distally from the pacemaker region. Thus, as shown in the figure, three slow waves will propagate from proximal to distal stomach every 60 seconds, i.e., 3 cpm slow waves. As shown in A, the cutaneous electrogastrogram (EGG) reflects the dipole created by the migrating slow wave, which occurs every 20 seconds. **(B)** Gastric myoelectrical activity during gastric peristalsis. Action potentials occur during gastric circular muscle contraction; the action potentials are linked to the gastric slow waves or pacesetter potentials as shown in the extracellular recordings from the serosal electrodes (B, C, and D). As the slow wave linked with action potentials migrates distally along the gastric body and antrum, one gastric peristaltic wave occurs, and one EGG wave is recorded, as measured from the surface electrodes. Thus, gastric peristalses normally occur at a rate of 3 cpm. During gastric peristaltic contractions, the EGG amplitude is generally increased (compare with Figure 9.2(A). (Reprinted with permission from Stern, Koch, and Muth (2000).)

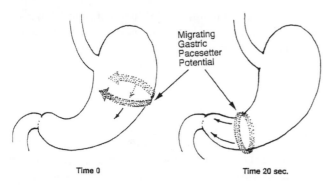

Figure 9.3. Propagation of the gastric pacesetter potential is illustrated as a faint electrical "halo." The depolarization-repolarization electrical wavefront migrates from the pacemaker region of the corpus (time 0) through the corpus to the distal antrum (time 20 seconds). These pacesetter potentials occur at approximately 3 cpm. (Reprinted with permission from Koch and Stern (2004).)

neuromuscular work of gastric emptying. Because of the increased gastric myoelectrical activity, the EGG signal during the postprandial peristaltic contractions is generally higher in amplitude in healthy subjects compared with the fasting EGG (Figure 9.2B).

Figure 9.4 illustrates a stronger "electrical halo" formed in the postprandial period when the additional gastric myoelectrical activity of the plateau potentials or spike potentials is linked to the migrating gastric pacesetter potential. Compared with the fasted condition, shown in Figure 9.3, greater myoelectrical activity occurs at the normal 3-cpm frequency during regular peristaltic contractions. The additional intensity of gastric myoelectrical activity is present because action potentials or plateau potentials are now linked to the ongoing gastric pacesetter potential activity. Furthermore, the electrocontractile complex (the peristaltic wave) travels circumferentially as well as distally, thus forming the stronger depolarization–repolarization wave front (i.e., stronger "halo") shown moving through the corpus to the distal antrum where the contraction dissipates. Thus, as stated above, compared with fasting, the amplitude of the EGG wave is generally greater in the postprandial condition depending on the specific meal ingested. The distance of the electrodes from the stomach may also affect amplitude of the EGG signal. These basic gastric myoelectrical activities form the physiological basis for understanding both fasting and postprandial EGG patterns recorded in healthy individuals.

RECORDING AND ANALYSIS OF THE EGG

Recording the EGG

Subjects are instructed what and when to eat prior to an EGG recording session because the contents of the stomach will affect the EGG. For most studies, subjects are instructed to fast for at least 4 hours prior to the experimental session. In other studies subjects are asked to fast overnight and consume one piece of toast and 4 ounces of

juice 2 hours prior to coming to the lab. This standard 200 Kcal meal ensures a consistent baseline EGG. An attempt should be made to reduce apprehension and to ensure the subject that he/she cannot get shocked. To reduce possible embarrassment and potential liability, female experimenters should either apply the electrodes or be present when EGG electrodes are applied to female subjects.

High-quality, fresh, disposable electrodes, such as those used for recording the EKG, are recommended for recording the EGG. Electrodes are placed on the skin surface of the epigastrium over the general area of the antrum of the stomach. EGGs are obtained with electrodes arranged for bipolar recordings. A reference electrode is positioned on the right side of the subject's abdomen. One active electrode should be placed approximately 10 cm cephalad from the umbilicus and 6cm to the subject's left. It is important to place this electrode below, and not on, the lowest rib to avoid respiratory signals. The second active electrode should be placed approximately 4 cm above the umbilicus (midway between the umbilicus and xiphoid) on the midline of the abdomen. The reference electrode is placed 10 to 15 cm to the right of the midline electrode, usually along the midclavicular line and 2 to 3 cm below the lowest anterior rib on the right side. The recording sites selected depend on the nature of the EGG signal desired. From our experience, the electrode locations just described provide the largest possible amplitude and least artifact in EGGs from most people. The exact placement of the electrodes is not important if the frequency of the EGG signal is what is of interest. For a discussion of the advantages and disadvantages of different electrode placements for EGG recording, see Smout et al. (1994) and Mirizzi and Scafoglieri (1983).

We have sometimes recorded from two or three abdominal sites simultaneously and chosen the more artifact-free EGG signal for analysis and interpretation (Stern et al., 1985). Chen and colleagues (Chen et al., 1996) have recorded multichannel EGGs, using four active electrodes

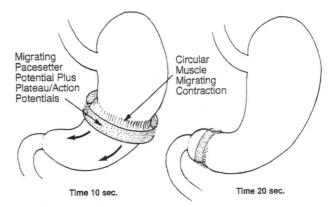

Figure 9.4. The migration of the pacesetter potential plus plateau or action potential activity is illustrated as a stronger, moving electrical "halo" compared with the noncontractile state (compare with Figure 9.3). The movement of the electrocontractile complex across the stomach is shown at 10 and 20 seconds. (Reprinted with permission from Koch and Stern (2004).)

and a common reference electrode, and reported detecting gastric slow wave propagation. They also reported quantifying the degree of slow wave coupling in normal controls and in patient groups such as individuals with systemic sclerosis (McNearney et al., 2002). In general, single-channel EGG recording is sufficient for detecting gastric dysrhythmias.

The EGG can be recorded from the wrists, but the amplitude will be low compared with recordings from the abdomen because electrodes located on wrists are far from the source of the signal, that is, the gastric pacemaker in the corpus antrum (Stern & Stacher, 1982). On the other hand, wrist electrodes are recommended when recording from obese patients, to minimize the fat layer under the electrodes, which acts as an insulator and decreases the amplitude of the EGG signal. For more details about the procedure for recording EGG, see Chapter 4 in Koch and Stern (2004).

Analyzing the EGG

Spectral analysis. Spectral analysis typically uses the Fast Fourier transform (FFT) to convert a signal in the time domain into the frequency domain. The output of a spectral analysis is the squared magnitude of the Fourier transform and is typically graphed as a curve showing the strength, or power, of the frequencies into which the original signal can be decomposed. Although power has a very specific meaning in mathematics and physics, we may think of it as an index of the amplitude of the sine waves of a particular frequency that would be required in order to recreate the EGG record. In the analysis of EGG recordings we are usually interested in the power within the following four frequency bands: 0–2.25, 2.5–3.5, 3.75–9.75, and 10.0–15.0 cpm. The exact cut-offs for these bands vary in the literature. This is due to the fact that the frequency resolution (bin-width) of the FFT is equal to the sampling rate divided by the number of samples in a window. Hence, varying sampling rates and window size will produce slightly different bandwidths based on the spectral resolution in the frequency domain. The first frequency band represents the often found but poorly understood ultra slow rhythm referred to as bradygastria. The second encompasses the normal electrical rhythm of the healthy human gastric antrum (3 cpm). The third includes frequencies commonly associated with nausea and is referred to as tachygastria. The fourth frequency may include duodenal pacesetter potentials and/or respiratory signals.

Spectral analysis is currently the most commonly used method of analyzing the EGG (see Smallwood & Brown, 1983) and the method favored by the authors. Van der Schee, Smout, and Grashuis (1982) have described an extension of this method that makes use of running spectral analysis to depict EGG data. Running spectral analysis, with overlapping power spectra displayed as a function of time, yields both frequency and time information. The more conventional spectral analysis provides power only as a function of frequency, not time. With running spectral analysis, frequency, power, and time can be depicted two-dimensionally either with a pseudo 3-D display or with a gray-scale plot. Figures 9.5 and 9.6 show examples of pseudo 3-D displays. A description of the procedure used to go from raw EGG data to a pseudo 3-D display can be found in Chapter 5 in Koch and Stern (2004).

The first step in any quantification procedure is to insure that quality data are being analyzed (Kingma, 1989). Because of the relatively slow electrical changes that are associated with EGG, only a very electrically stable electrode can be used; silver-silver chloride (Ag/AgCl) electrodes are recommended. The optimal recording sites will depend on the nature of the signal desired: for example, the largest possible amplitude; lowest artifact from EKG, respiration and subject movement; and position of the subject's internal organs, particularly the antrum of the stomach and the diaphragm (Mirizzi & Scafoglieri, 1983). The amplifying and recording system should filter out signals below 0.5 cpm and above 15 cpm. With these filter settings one can record ultra slow rhythms (0.5–2.0) but still eliminate shifts in baseline due to DC potentials. Frequencies higher than 15 cpm are filtered out to avoid domination of the gastric signal by EKG. Respiration can also obscure the EGG, when its frequency range falls near that of tachygastria or duodenal signals. Rather than remove respiration signals with analog filters at the time of the recording, it is preferable to remove it later with more precise and flexible digital filters or by using a separate respiration tracing to visually select and exclude data that contain respiration artifact.

In order to produce a running spectral analysis, one overlaps consecutive data segments by, for example, 75%. In other words, segment one includes minutes 1–4, segment two includes minutes 2–5, and so on. Thus, one minute of new information is provided in each consecutive power spectrum. These overlapping power spectra can be plotted in a pseudo-3-D fashion to allow easy viewing of changes in power at various frequencies as a function of time (see Figures 9.5 and 9.6).

Although such running spectral analyses do provide a useful way to view frequency and power changes over time, it is important to note that transient changes in the EGG may go unnoticed if they are small. If such transient changes are large enough they will appear but only as a gradual change with the peak in spectral density appearing in the pseudo 3-D display several minutes after it occurred in real time. Thus, running spectral analysis may not be appropriate for experiments in which very short duration stimulus induced changes are expected. For such cases adaptive spectral analysis methods are recommended (Lin & Chen, 1994; Chen, Stewart, & McCallum, 1993; Chen & McCallum, 1991; and Chen, Vandewalle, Sansen, Vantrappen, & Janssens, 1990).

Similarly, spectral analysis is useful only when the EGG signal contains a significant amount of cyclical activity. This is usually the case for 3 cpm activity. However,

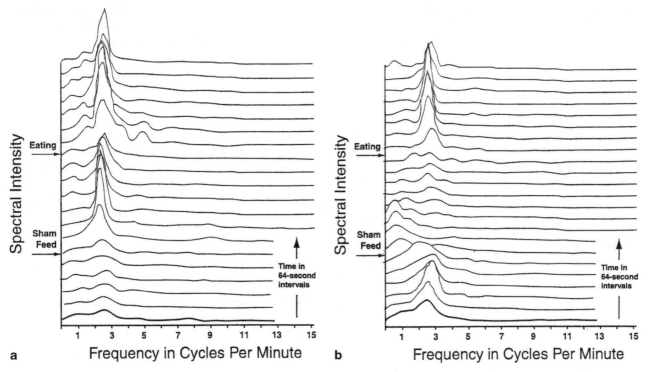

Figure 9.5. **(A)** Running spectral analysis of the EGG of a subject who reported that the experience of sham feeding was not disgusting. Note the low level of activity at approximately 2.5 cpm before sham feeding and the increase in power during sham feeding and during eating. **(B)** Running spectral analysis of the EGG from a subject who reported that the experience of sham feeding was disgusting. This subject showed power at approximately 2.8 cpm before sham feeding and a decrease during sham feed. The subject showed the typical increase in power during eating. (Reprinted with permission from Stern, Koch, and Muth (2000).)

some gastric phenomena occur intermittently and may not appear in a spectral plot. For most studies examining only the 3 cpm activity, this is not a problem because any segment of normal EGG is likely to contain a strong cyclical component. However, for phenomena such as tachygastria the issue is less clear. We have experienced no difficulty in quantifying this phenomenon through spectral analysis. When bursts of tachygastria are seen during motion sickness, they are typically one or more minutes in duration and are seen quite clearly in running spectral plots of 4-min epochs (Stern, Koch, Stewart, & Lindblad, 1987). However, there may indeed be more appropriate methods of analysis for quantification of very brief duration, intermittent phenomena lasting less than one minute (see for example, Hölzl et al., 1985; Lin & Chen, 1994; and Moraes et al., 2003).

Once spectral power estimates have been calculated, data reduction is usually performed. The best method for reducing the EGG frequency and power data from an FFT is still unsettled. In most cases it will depend on the question to be answered and several methods have merit. No matter what analysis method is used, it is critical that quality raw recordings are obtained with high signal-to-noise ratio. In addition, data from healthy subjects during normal psychophysiological states should be recorded for comparison purposes.

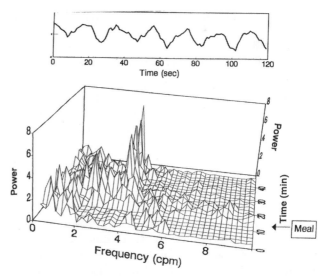

Figure 9.6. A representative raw electrogastrographic tracing (top) and spectral analysis plot (bottom) are shown for a pregnant woman with nausea before and after ingestion of a liquid protein-predominant meal. Postprandial raw signal exhibits a normal-appearing near-sinusoidal oscillation with a period of ~20 s. Spectral analysis reveals extensive dysrhythmic activity during fasting with peaks in both bradygastric and tachygastric frequency ranges. After meal ingestion, signal stabilizes with development of normal 3-cycles-per-minute (cpm) activity. (Reprinted with permission from Jednak et al. (1999).)

SPECIFIC MEASURES OF EGG ACTIVITY

1. *Percentage distribution of electrogastrographic power in the four frequency bands of interest.* The percentage distribution of EGG power in the four relevant frequency bands is the measure that the authors have found most useful in more than 25 years of experience in recording and analyzing EGGs in studies involving patients and healthy research participants (e.g., Stern, Koch, & Muth, 2000; Koch, 2002). The percentage distribution of total EGG power is calculated for each of the frequency bands of interest: bradygastria, normal 3 cpm, tachygastria, and duodenal/respiration. The power estimates for a given frequency range (e.g., the 1–2.5 bradygastria range) are obtained from the spectral analysis. The sum of the bradygastria power for a given time period is divided by the power for the entire frequency range (1–15 cpm) for the same time period and multiplied by 100%. Thus, the percentage distribution of all of the power from 1 to 15 cpm is determined for each of the four relevant frequency ranges: bradygastria, normal, tachygastria, and duodenal/respiration. The percentage of EGG power in the different frequency bands is altered by provocative stimuli such as the stress of doing mental arithmetic, the water load test, a caloric meal, or drug therapy. This measure should not be confused with percentage of time with the dominant frequency in the normal (or other) frequency bands, which is described next.

2. *Percentage of time with the dominant frequency in the normal (or other) frequency band* – This measure calculates the percentage of time (within a defined period) that the dominant EGG frequency (the specific frequency with the greatest power as determined by computer analysis) lies within a certain range of frequencies, such as 2–4 cpm (Chen & McCallum, 1994). An adaptive filter analysis of the EGG is first computed using 1 or 2 minutes of EGG data to construct each power spectrum. A spectrum is considered normal if the dominant (highest) peak lies in the 2- to 4-cpm range. The percentage of time that the highest peak is in the 2- to 4-cpm range is determined visually. Thus, if eight 1-minute spectra had the highest peak in the 2- to 4-cpm range in a 10-minute period, then the percentage of time the dominant frequency was in the normal range would be 80%. A limitation of this measure is that it ignores much of the data present in the EGG signal and focuses solely on the time that the dominant frequency is or is not within the frequency range of interest. For example, a 2-minute EGG signal with six 20-second sine waves or a 2-minute EGG signal with one large 20-second sine wave and a variety of other low amplitude waves spread out in frequencies other than 2 to 4 cpm would be labeled normal. This is why the percentage of time measure produces higher percentages of normal activity compared with the percentage distribution of EGG power, the technique described previously. Recall that the percentage distribution of EGG power compares the 3 cpm activity present in the EGG signal with the activity in all frequencies from 1 to 15 cpm for a given period of time. Compared with that method, the percentage of time with the dominant frequency in the normal frequency band includes only a small, select portion of the total EGG data. Therefore, investigators who use this measure may arrive at erroneous conclusions about the effects of a drug or other therapy on EGG because of the selective nature of the data that are included in this measure. In addition, the percentage of time with the dominant frequency in the normal range is usually derived from an adaptative spectral analysis, not a Fourier spectral analysis, and therefore does not always accurately present the relative amplitude of the different frequencies that comprise the EGG signal.

3. *Power ratio* – The EGG activity in the frequency band of interest after a test or therapy is compared with EGG activity in that same frequency band during the baseline period. For example, a clinician might calculate the ratio of power in the normal range before and after treatment with a particular drug used to reduce nausea and use the ratio as a measure of improvement. However, an increase in EGG activity in all frequency bands may occur and would make interpretation of the specific ratio difficult.

4. *Dominant frequency and stability of the dominant frequency* – The dominant frequency is determined visually by identifying the frequency with the greatest power in the FTT or RSA during a specific time period. Frequencies can change even in healthy subjects. Note that a frequency dip to 1 to 2 cpm occurs briefly after a meal. Smout, Jebbink, and Samsom (1994) calculated various measures of stability of the dominant frequency and concluded that there is little evidence that either dominant frequency or the stability of the dominant frequency is physiologically related to gastric function.

Analysis of EGG recordings is based on the recording of high-quality EGG signals, review of the signal to identify any artifacts, and use of validated software for quantitative analysis of the EGG signal (for possible pitfalls see Ver Hagen et al., 1998. For greater details about the analysis of EGG recordings see Chapter 5 in Koch and Stern (2004).

INFERENTIAL CONTEXT

Validation of the EGG

EGG and gastric myoelectric activity. Nelsen and Kohatsu (1968) simultaneously recorded the electrical activity from electrodes implanted on the serosal surface of the stomach and EGGs from 13 patients. They found an excellent correspondence between the frequency of the signals obtained from the EGG and the internal electrodes. They did not compare the amplitudes of the signals. A comparison of EGG and serosal recordings from dogs by Smout, van der

Schee, and Grashuis (1980b) indicated a perfect correspondence between the frequency of the signals.

In an effort to study the relationship of the EGG to internal electrical activity of the stomach without involving surgery, several investigators have compared the EGG to simultaneously recorded mucosal signals. The mucosal signals are obtained from swallowed electrodes (i.e., electrodes inside the stomach). Hamilton et al. (1986) compared EGG and mucosal signals from 20 human subjects during fasting, after ingesting milk, and in one case, during a period of spontaneous dysrhythmia. They summarized their findings as follows:

We did find that the surface recordings were of similar visual form as those obtained directly from the mucosa simultaneously. In addition, frequency analysis determined that the two simultaneously obtained signals were of the same frequency. Finally when the rare arrhythmic events occurred, they were detected in both the mucosal and cutaneous signals. Therefore, the signal obtained from the skin does seem to accurately reflect the BER as measured directly from the stomach mucosa. (p. 37)

Abell and Malagelada (1985) used magnetic force to maintain internal electrodes in opposition with the gastric wall and compared signals obtained from the mucosal electrodes with those obtained from the EGG. They also reported that frequency analysis showed very good correspondence between the internal and EGG signals. Mintchev, Otto and Bowes (1997) made simultaneous serosal and EGG recordings from dogs in whom they had created dysrhythmias by surgical means. They reported that the EGG could be used to detect severely abnormal gastric myoelectric activity 93% of the time, and mild abnormalities 74% of the time.

EGG and gastric motor activity

Until the mid-1960s investigators who used the EGG assumed that they were recording from the surface of the skin, voltage changes that were due to the contractions of the smooth muscle of the stomach; that is, they assumed a one-to-one relationship between the EGG and contractions of the stomach. However, in 1968 Nelsen and Kohatsu presented a different view of the source of the EGG signal. They stated that the EGG was a function of gastric slow-wave activity, or pacesetter potentials. Nelsen and Kohatsu and others have claimed that the surface-recorded EGG reflects the waxing and waning of pacesetter potentials of the stomach but not gastric contractions. However, they did present evidence that indicated that when contractions do occur, they are time locked to the slow wave and, therefore, to the EGG.

Beginning in 1975, Smallwood and his colleagues published a number of studies (e.g., Smallwood, 1978; Smallwood & Brown, 1983) in which they examined the frequency of the EGG and made numerous advances in techniques for analysis of the EGG signal. In some studies (e.g., Brown et al., 1975) they compared the EGG signal with intragastric pressure recordings. Their findings were the same as those of Nelsen and Kohatsu (1968). When contractions occurred, they occurred at the same frequency as the EGG signals; and whereas the EGG showed 3 cpm almost continuously for most subjects, contractions as recorded with intragastric pressure instruments did not.

It should be noted that the simultaneous presence of 3-cpm EGG and the absence of changes in intragastric pressure does not necessarily indicate that the EGG is unrelated to contractions as Nelsen and Kohatsu (1968), Brown et al. (1975), and others have suggested. The possibility exists that the EGG is a more sensitive measure of gastric contractile activity than the pressure-sensitive probes. That is, the EGG may reflect increases in electrical activity (i.e., spike activity) during low-level contractile events that do not alter gastric intraluminal pressure. In fact, Vantrappen, Hostein, Janssens, Vanderweerd, and De Wever (1983) indicated that low-amplitude 5-cpm motor activity is always present in the dog. In addition, You and Chey (1984) have shown that in dogs the 5-cpm pacesetter potentials correlated well with low-amplitude contractions recorded by strain gauges sewn to serosa but correlated poorly with intraluminal pressure changes.

From 1980 to present, published reports have appeared that not only suggest that the EGG provides information about frequency of contractions but also, indeed, that the amplitude of the EGG is related to the degree of contractile activity (Smout, 1980; Smout, van der Schee, & Grashuis 1980a; Smout et al., 1980b). One of the major contributions of Smout and his colleagues was to point out that the amplitude of the EGG increases when a contraction occurs. They concluded that the pacesetter potential and the second potential, which is related to contractions, are reflected in the EGG. Abell, Tucker, and Malagelada (1985) conducted a study in which they compared the EGG signal from healthy human subjects with the electrical signal recorded from the mucosal surface of the stomach, and intraluminal pressure. They summarized their findings as follows: "Antral phasic pressure activity, when present, was accompanied by an increase in amplitude and/or a change in shape of both the internal and external EGG" (p. 86).

Koch and Stern (1985) reported a perfect correlation of EGG waves and peristaltic antral contractions observed during simultaneous EGG-fluoroscopy recordings in four healthy subjects. Hamilton et al. (1986) reported that fluoroscopy revealed contractions in the antrum that correlated with three- and fourfold increases in amplitude of the EGG. The relationship of the amplitude of EGG waves to contractions is complex and not totally understood at this time. However, in addition to the studies mentioned, there is considerable indirect evidence linking amplitude changes in the EGG with strength of contractile activity. For example, in situations where increased contractile activity would be expected (e.g., eating, after swallowing barium), EGG amplitude increases (Hamilton et al., 1986; Jones & Jones, 1985; Koch, Stewart, & Stern, 1987). And in patients with diabetic gastroparesis, where one would expect weak contractile activity, Hamilton et al. (1986) found no increase in the amplitude of EGG after eating.

EGG amplitude alone cannot be used to infer reliably the presence or absence of GI contractions. It is possible that with improved methods of measuring contractile activity, we shall find that all myoelectric activity is accompanied by some contractile activity (see Morgan et al., 1978; Vantrappen et al., 1983; You & Chey, l984) and that the amplitude of the EGG is related to its intensity or strength. A significant question then becomes: Can the amplitude of the EGG be used to determine whether the accompanying gastric contractile activity is of sufficient strength to do the motor work of the stomach (i.e., mixing and propelling)?

Several investigators (e.g., Bruley, Mizrahi, & Dubois, l991; Dubois & Mizrahi, l994) have examined the possibility of using the EGG as an indirect measure of gastric emptying. Chiloiro, Riezzo, Guerra, Reddy, and Giorgio (1994) simultaneously recorded gastric emptying using ultrasound and the power in the normal 3 cpm EGG from healthy subjects. The correlations ranged from 0.68 to 0.96. Other investigators (e.g., Chen, Richards, & McCallum, l993) have demonstrated a negative relationship between the presence of dysrhythmias in the EGG and gastric emptying. And Bortolotti, Sarti, Barara, and Brunelli (1990) have demonstrated the presence of tachygastria in patients suffering from idiopathic gastroparesis, that is patients with severely delayed gastric emptying with no known cause.

In summary, the frequency of the EGG is identical to the frequency of gastric pacesetter potentials recorded from the mucosal or serosal surface of the stomach. There is, however, less general agreement as to the interpretation of the amplitude of the EGG. Indirect evidence from several studies has demonstrated that amplitude increases during an increase in contractile activity, but the amplitude of the EGG alone cannot be used to determine the presence or absence of contractions.

Applications of EGG recording

Some of the applications of EGG recording that have been described in the psychological literature that will be described below include eating, sham feeding, stress and anxiety, motion sickness and nausea, and monitoring the effects of gastric electrical stimulation.

Eating

A number of investigators have reported effects of nutrient meals on EGG patterns. Yogurt or pancake meals increase the amplitude of the 3 cpm EGG wave as one would expect, because the presence of food in the stomach is the natural stimulus for it to contract (Geldof et al., 1986). Initially, the increase in amplitude occurs at a slower frequency, 2.2–2.5 cpm, a so-called frequency dip; after approximately 10–15 minutes, the EGG frequency gradually shifts back to the 3 cpm range. Smout, van der Schee, and Grashuis (1980b) and Jones and Jones (1985) have reported finding similar increases in the amplitude of the 3 cpm EGG following eating. Ingestion of whole milk has also been shown to increase the amplitude of 3 cpm EGG waves (Hamilton et al., 1986). A technetium-labeled omelet meal evokes a complex series of events including increased 3 cpm waves in the first 15 minutes after ingestion, followed by an increase in the 1–2 cpm EGG activity during the linear phase of gastric emptying (Koch, Stern, Bingaman, & Eggli, 1991). Uijtdehaage, Stern, and Koch (1992) reported that eating a small breakfast not only increased the power of normal 3 cpm EGG, but also increased respiratory sinus arrhythmia, a measure of parasympathetic nervous system activity, and inhibited motion sickness symptoms. Nonnutrient meals such as water loads also stimulate 3 cpm waves of increased amplitude and a brief frequency dip (Koch & Stern, l993; Koch, Hong, & Xu, 2000). Koch et al. (1993) reported successfully recording the EGG from premature and term infants. Riezzo et al. (2003) reported that breast-fed newborn healthy babies show adult-like normal 3 cpm gastric activity after nursing, but formula-fed newborns do not.

Chen, Davenport, and McCallum (1993) investigated the effect of a fat preload on gastric myoelectric activity in healthy humans using EGG. They reported that fat preload significantly decreased the postprandial 3 cpm EGG amplitude, implying a decrease in gastric contractility. In a related study, Chen, Lin, Parolisi, and McCallum (1995) looked at the effect of cholecystokinin (CCK) on postprandial gastric myoelectric activity. It is generally accepted that CCK released endogenously by a meal delays gastric emptying and inhibits additional eating. Chen et al. (1995) found that CCK given at a physiological concentration significantly decreased postprandial EGG amplitude, as did a fat preload, but did not affect the frequency or regularity of the EGG.

Do patients with anorexia nervosa or unexplained nausea and vomiting respond with an increase in the amplitude of their 3 cpm EGG following the eating of pleasant food? Abell, Lucas, Brown, and Malagelada (1985) have reported that several of their anorexic subjects failed to show an increase in amplitude of their 3 cpm EGG following eating and some showed tachygastria (4–9 cpm). Geldof, van der Schee, Blankenstein, and Grashuis (1983) found that 49% of their patients with unexplained nausea and vomiting showed tachygastria and the absence of the normal increase in amplitude of the EGG after eating. Diamanti et al. (2003) found that adolescent patients with bulimia displayed abnormal gastric activity, but patients with anorexia did not. The authors suggest that one possible explanation is the fact that the anorectic patients used in this study had a shorter disorder duration than the bulimic patients. Ogawa et al. (2004) recorded the EGG from 36 eating disorder patients following the water load test. The percentage of normal 3 cpm gastric activity was significantly less for the eating disorder patients

(44%) than controls (74%). The authors state the following pointing out the difficulty of determining which came first, the abnormal gastric activity or the eating disorder:

In conclusion it is suggested that longstanding abnormal eating in patients with eating disorders may induce disturbances to gastric motor function, resulting in abnormal, eating-related behavior, a form of a symptomatic vicious circle. The EGG may be a promising method for determining the pathophysiology of eating disorders and for developing effective therapeutic approaches. (p. 301)

Sham feeding

Stern, Crawford, Stewart, Vasey, and Koch (1989) used a sham feeding procedure to examine the cephalic-vagal reflex, a response that was mentioned in the introduction to this chapter. Previous research by several authors had shown that food or even the presence of non-nutritive substances in the stomach stimulate an increase in the amplitude of the 3 cpm EGG. The question asked by Stern et al. was whether the sight, smell, and taste of food would do the same thing to the EGG. Following a 15-min baseline period, subjects were required to chew and expectorate a hotdog and roll. After another baseline period, subjects were given a second hotdog to eat normally. The effect on the EGG of eating the hotdog was as expected, a large increase in the amplitude of the 3 cpm EGG wave that lasted several minutes. The effect on the EGG of sham feeding was an equally large but short-lasting increase in the amplitude of the EGG as can be seen in Figure 9.5A. Figure 9.5A depicts the data for one subject in the form of a running spectral analysis. EGG frequency is plotted on the X axis, time is plotted on the Y axis going from the bottom to the top of the figure, and power or spectral intensity is the third dimension. It was of interest to note that two subjects who reported after the session that the experience of chewing and expectorating the hotdog was disgusting showed a decrease rather than an increase in the amplitude of their EGG during sham feeding (see Figure 9.5B).

Following this serendipitous finding, we (Stern, Jokerst, Levine, & Koch, 2001) conducted another study in which one group of subjects was given pleasant food, a cooked hot dog, to chew and spit, and a second group was given an unpleasant food, an uncooked tofu dog, to chew and spit. The hot dog group showed a significant increase in 3 cpm activity and the tofu group did not. This result supported our initial finding that the cephalic-vagal reflex, as measured by the power in the EGG 3 cpm, depends on the subjective palatability of the food. We think that this is a good example of the sensitivity of the EGG to cognitive processing.

Stress and anxiety

The GI system may be conceptualized as a buffer between an individual and his/her environment. When extra energy is needed for fight or flight, the GI system slows down or shuts down. Anxieties and worries also slow down the GI system. In terms of the activity of the autonomic nervous system – one of the pathways for communication between the brain and the GI system – fight, flight, anxiety, and worry are all usually associated with an increase in activity in the sympathetic branch (SNS) of the autonomic nervous system. And numerous studies have shown that an increase in activity in SNS activity decreases stomach activity. Increases in activity in the parasympathetic branch (PNS) of the autonomic nervous system increase normal stomach activity. The cephalic-vagal reflex, described above, is an example of this relationship. A complication, however, is that not a lot is known about the changes in PNS activity that are associated with different psychological states for different people, or the relationship between SNS and PNS activity. For a discussion of this most important issue see Berntson, Cacioppo, Binkley, Uchino, Quigley, and Fieldstone (1994). As can be seen in the examples that follow, in a particular stress situation, some individuals might show an increase in SNS and little change in PNS, or even an increase in PNS activity, whereas in a different stress situation some individuals might show an increase in SNS activity and a decrease in PNS activity. Note that the normal functioning of the GI system is not crucial for momentary survival, as is the case with the cardiovascular system. Wide swings in functioning of the GI system have been documented, and these extreme responses may be perceived by some individuals as GI symptoms.

As stated earlier in this chapter, the area of brain-gut interaction has a long history, going back to Beaumont (1833), but a short past in that little work has followed up on the very early studies. In the case of autonomic-GI interactions, a relatively recent study has set the stage for applying EGG findings to clinical work (Muth, Koch, & Stern, 2000). This study examined the EGG and ANS activity in people suffering from functional dyspepsia. Functional dyspepsia is a gastrointestinal disorder characterized by a symptom cluster that often includes nausea, pain, bloating and/or early satiety after eating, with no organic findings that explain the symptoms (e.g., the presence of an ulcer). A comparison of gastric emptying, gastric myoelectrical activity, symptoms, and psychological factors separated participants into two groups: SNS reactive and PNS rigid. The SNS reactive had more ANS variability, higher sympathetic activity, more cardiac reactivity, and higher scores of neuroticism. The PNS rigid group had more PNS activity, lower ANS variability, and more abnormal EGG tests that indicated gastric myoelectrical abnormalities. These findings seem to point to a brain-gut explanation to the symptoms in these patients. In one sub-group it appears that psychological causes may be at the root of the problem and the individuals are perhaps hypersensitive or vigilant to conditions when the GI system is functioning at the extreme; and these extremes may get internalized as symptoms for these patients. In the other sub-group, it appears that autonomic dysfunction may cause symptoms by affecting the electrical activity of the stomach directly as indexed by the EGG. Research needs to be done to explore further these hypotheses, but this research is an example of the use of EGG to gain a better understanding of how stress affects the GI system.

Stressors can be classified as either primary physiological or primary psychological in nature. Changes in the EGG have been examined in relationship to both types of stressors. Physiological stressors seem to yield relatively consistent effects on the EGG, but psychological stressors some times do not.

Muth, Thayer, Stern, Friedman, and Drake (1998) studied the effect on the EGG of two tasks, reaction time/shock avoidance, and cold face stress. As expected, the RT task produced shorter cardiac IBIs than baseline, and placing a cool bag of water on the face produced longer IBIs than baseline. These manipulation checks supported the experimenters' assumption that the RT task would increase SNS activity whereas the cold face stress would increase PNS. Analyses of the EGG data indicated that there was significantly greater normal 3 cpm activity during the cold face stress than during the RT task. And there was greater tachygastria during RT than during the cold face stress. These findings are in agreement with the results of motion sickness studies (see below) that have shown that increased PNS activity increases 3 cpm EGG activity and decreases symptoms of motion sickness. On the other hand, subjects who experience motion sickness show an increase in SNS activity, a decrease in PNS activity, and tachygastria (e.g., Stern & Koch, 1994) as well as delays in oral-cecal transit time (Muth, Stern, & Koch, 1996).

Stern, Vasey, Hu, and Koch (1991) examined the effects of another stressor, the cold pressor test on EGG activity. The procedure used was similar to that used by Thompson, Richelson, and Malagelada (1982), who reported a significant decrease in gastric emptying as a response to cold stress. In our experiment, subjects who had recently eaten were asked to put their hand into a container of ice water (4°C) for 1 min, take it out for 15 s, put it back for 1 min, and so on, for a total of 20 min. The results were similar to those reported by Stewart (unpublished) for the effects of the Stroop stress test and are what would be predicted by the gastric emptying results of Thompson et al. (1982). There was a significant attenuation of EGG 3 cpm activity starting at the point in time when the subject put his/her hand into the ice water. Tachygastria was not seen as a response to the cold pressor test, a procedure that induces pain but not nausea.

The results of two additional studies reporting the effects of psychological stressors on the EGG have been inconsistent. Baldaro et al. (2001), who used viewing an unpleasant film as a stressor, and Riezzo et al. (1996), who used the Stroop color-word test as a stressor, failed to find a difference in EGG activity between their stressor group and a control group. In the absence of detailed information about the EGG equipment and analysis programs used in these studies, we assume that the lack of a significant difference in the EGG was a function of the nature of the psychological stressors used in these two studies.

Gianaros et al. (2001) in a two-part study, presented subjects with two laboratory stressors: speech preparation and isometric handgrip and measured ANS and EGG responses. As expected the stressful tasks produced tachygastria, and increases in SNS activity and decreases in PNS activity. In the second part of the study, the same subjects were exposed to a rotating optokinetic drum. The results demonstrated that the extent of decrease in PNS activity to the laboratory stressors in the first part of the study predicted motion sickness susceptibility. Further these data show that both physiological and psychological stressors can affect stomach electrical activity and the EGG.

We consider the EGG to be a valuable noninvasive instrument to study the effects of stress on the GI system, especially considering the fact that the measure itself evokes no stress, and does not interfere with the activity of the stomach. A better understanding of the effects of stress on the GI system could result from the use of the EGG to study brain-stomach relationships in functional GI disorders such as functional dyspepsia, as described above.

Motion sickness and nausea

During the past 25 years, we have been using a rotating optokinetic drum to produce nausea and other symptoms of motion sickness in healthy subjects and recording EGG and other physiological measures. In the first experiment that attempted to relate changes in gastric myoelectric activity to the development of symptoms of motion sickness, Stern, Koch, Leibowitz, Lindblad, Shupert, and Stewart (1985) obtained EGGs from 21 healthy human subjects who were seated within an optokinetic drum, the rotation of which produced vection (illusory self-motion). Fourteen subjects developed symptoms of motion sickness during vection, and in each the EGG frequency shifted from the normal 3 cpm, to 4–9 cpm, tachygastria. In six of seven asymptomatic subjects, the 3-cpm EGG pattern was unchanged during vection. It was concluded that the sensory mismatch created by the illusory self-motion produced tachygastria and symptoms of motion sickness in susceptible subjects. In a follow-up study (Stern, Koch, Stewart, & Lindblad, 1987), 15 healthy subjects were exposed to the rotation of the same drum. Ten subjects showed a shift of the dominant frequency of their EGG from normal to tachygastria, during drum rotation and reported symptoms of motion sickness. A comparison of running spectral analyses and symptom reports revealed a close correspondence over time between tachygastria and the development of symptoms of motion sickness.

It is important to note that during tachygastria, gastric motility decreases or even completely shuts down, and one of the most common symptoms of motion sickness is nausea. It is of interest to note that Wolf (1943) showed many years ago that stressful situations, including putting cold water in one ear, swinging, rotation of the head, situations involving fear, inhibited gastric contractile activity, and provoked nausea. The advantage of our current use of the EGG in similar studies is that it is noninvasive; Wolf's subjects had a balloon positioned in their stomach to record gastric pressure changes. Wolf grappled with a problem inherent in all studies that relate some bodily change to a sensation, in his case the relationship of inhibited gastric motor activity to the sensation of nausea. To what extent is the altered bodily change essential to the occurrence of the sensation? In a series of ingenious experiments, unfortunately with only three subjects, Wolf gave his subjects a combination of two drugs that prevented the inhibition of gastric motor activity, exposed the subjects to the stress situations that had previously provoked nausea, and found that no nausea was reported. Wolf (1943) concluded as follows: "The fact that nausea may be prevented, despite strong nauseating stimuli, by controlling with drugs the pattern of gastric motility indicates that gastric relaxation and hypomotility are essential to the occurrence of nausea" (p. 882).

In our labs, 50% percent of healthy European-American and African-American subjects and 80–90% of Asian and Asian-American subjects developed tachygastria and got motion sick while sitting inside a rotating optokinetic drum. We have been studying this differential susceptibility to motion sickness for over 25 years and published a review article summarizing our results (Stern & Koch, 1996).

In a study not of the nausea of motion sickness, but rather of the nausea of the first trimester of pregnancy, Jednak et al. (1999) reported that a high protein meal decreased nausea significantly better than a high carbohydrate meal (see Figure 9.6). Levine et al (2004) followed this study with a motion sickness study and demonstrated that a high protein meal consumed prior to exposure to a rotating drum decreased tachygastria and the symptoms of motion sickness.

To summarize our findings with regard to the relationship of EGG activity to nausea, any manipulation that increases PNS and normal 3 cpm EGG activity, such as eating, deep breathing, gastric electrical stimulation, or biofeedback, decreases nausea.

Monitoring the effects of gastric electrical stimulation (GES)

An exciting new area of GI research involves gastric electrical stimulation to either strengthen normal 3 cpm activity in, for example, gastroparetic patients refractory to medical treatment, or to disrupt normal gastric activity in an effort to reduce appetite in obese patients. In either model EGG recording is essential to determine if the stimulation is having the desired effect on the stomach. The two areas that require considerable additional research are as follows: (a) the characteristics of the electrical signal, and the time of stimulation (e.g., continuous, when fed, when the

patient shows gastric dysrhythmias); and (b) diagnostic criteria that indicate which patients will benefit from GES, and the characteristics of the electrical signal for optimal improvement of the symptoms of different patients.

The following quote from a noted gastroenterologist that appeared in the *American Journal of Gastroenterology* sums up our opinion of the status of GES in 2004:

… neural electrical gastric stimulation, consists of a microprocessor-controlled sequential activation of a series of annular electrodes which encircle the distal two thirds of the stomach and induce propagated contractions causing a forceful emptying of the gastric contents. This method is the most promising, but it has so far only been tested in animals and would need to be tested in patients with gastroparesis before it can be used as a solution for this disease. (Bortolotti, 2002, p. 1874)

OTHER NONINVASIVE GASTROINTESTINAL MEASURES OF INTEREST TO PSYCHOPHYSIOLOGISTS

The goal of this section is to introduce briefly two additional measures of GI activity, gastric emptying time and oral-cecal transit time. Both of these measures of GI motor activity can be measured noninvasively and complement the electrical-based EGG measure.

Gastric emptying

The two most common indicators of gastric emptying are the lag phase, referred to as T_{lag}, and the half emptying time, referred to as $T_{1/2}$. The lag phase of gastric emptying is the amount of time it takes for food to begin to empty from the stomach to the small intestine. The half emptying time is the amount of time it takes for half of the test meal to empty from the stomach. Both of these measures include the time it takes for the meal to get from the mouth to the stomach, which is usually considered negligible and ignored. The classic method of measuring gastric emptying involves having the subject ingest radio-isotope-labeled scrambled eggs and using a procedure called scintigraphy tracking the meal. However, a breath test method (Ghoos et al., 1993) has been developed for deriving gastric emptying data, and commercial devices are beginning to appear on the market that are relatively easy to use by a nonmedical person to derive these measures.

The breath test method of measuring gastric emptying involves having an individual ingest a test meal, such as 100 mg of sodium octanoate (also known as caprylic acid), that is not broken down and absorbed in the stomach, but rather in the small intestine (see Figure 9.7). The sodium octanoate is modified such that instead of containing carbon-12 or radio-active carbon-14, it contains carbon-13. As the labeled meal passes from the stomach into the small intestine, the sodium octanoate is broken down by the small intestine. The carbon-13 is then absorbed in the bloodstream as carbon dioxide, eventually

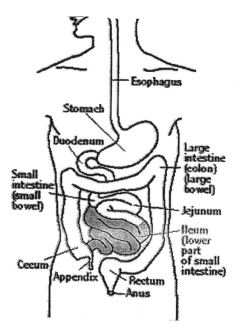

Figure 9.7. This figure shows the general anatomy of the gastrointestinal (GI) tract. The duodenum is the beginning of the small intestine where sodium-octanoate is broken down and absorbed. Oral-cecal transit time is the time it takes for a meal to path from the mouth to the junction between the large and small intestine called the cecum.

flows to the lungs and is exhaled in the breath. An infrared spectrometer is then used to compare the ratio of carbon-12 to carbon-13 in the exhaled breath. As the ratio changes in the favor of more carbon-13 it is an indicator that the test meal is being emptied from the stomach. Procedures have been developed to derive T_{lag} and $T_{1/2}$ times from the breath samples over time (Ghoos et al., 1993). Several companies have incorporated these procedures into relatively easy to use, albeit expensive, devices. However, this procedure can be performed providing you have an adequate breath collection system and a way to sample the carbon-12/carbon-13 ratio with an infrared spectrometer which is often available in a university chemistry laboratory.

Oral-cecal transit time

Oral-cecal transit time (OCTT) refers to the time it takes for a meal to travel from the mouth to the junction between the small and large intestine called the cecum (see Figure 9.7). Breath testing procedures for deriving OCTT are well established (Sciarretta et al., 1994; Read et al., 1984). The procedure is very similar to the breath testing for gastric emptying. In the case of OCTT, a nonabsorbable carbohydrate such as 10 g lactulose is added to a test meal and ingested. The lactulose passes through the stomach and small intestine and is not broken down until it passes into the large intestine. The digestion process releases hydrogen into the blood stream that reaches and exhaled by the lungs. By measuring breath hydrogen production using a gas chromatograph, OCTT is indicated as the time from meal ingestion to a peak in breath hydrogen. Again, sev-

eral companies produce commercial devices specifically for measuring breath hydrogen as part of breath testing procedures. However, as with the gastric emptying tests, if one has access to a gas chromatograph and adequate breath collection devices, it is possible to perform this test without further specialized equipment.

It is important to note that if both gastric emptying measures and OCTT are collected simultaneously on the same test meal, a third measure can be derived. That measure is small bowel transit time (SBTT). SBTT is the time for the meal to travel through the small intestine. It can be derived by subtracting T_{lag} from OCTT.

Research in the authors' laboratories has shown that both psychological stressors (Muth, Koch, Stern, and Thayer, 1999) and physiological stressors (Muth, Stern, and Koch, 1996) can affect these GI measures. It is currently unknown if different stressors affect the GI system differently and if different parts of the GI system (i.e., stomach and small intestine) respond to stress differently. Psychophysiologists can now do research in the area of stress effects on the GI system using the noninvasive EGG method coupled with other noninvasive measures of GI neuromuscular activity.

EPILOGUE

Unanswered questions

Why do many people complain of GI symptoms when they are under stress? We take a functionalist position on this question and, as we stated earlier, think that the GI system acts as a buffer or special response system between the organism and the environment. When extra energy is needed for fighting with or fleeing from a saber-toothed tiger, for example, the GI system shuts down. In our labs and in others, the EGG has been used to document and quantify the shutting down of the stomach. Two distinct patterns of EGG activity have been identified which are associated with a decrease in normal neuromuscular activity of the stomach: a flat line (the absence of cyclic myoelectrical activity), and tachygastria. We know that tachygastria is associated with the experience of nausea, but we don't know much about the association of the absence of cyclic activity in the EGG and GI symptoms. This is an unexplored area. Perhaps symptoms are only experienced after the passage of a certain period of time. Or, perhaps unpleasant symptoms are only experienced if one eats while one's stomach is shut down.

We know that eating or thinking about eating pleasant food increases the amplitude of normal 3 cpm activity in the EGG of healthy subjects. Disgusting food does not have this effect. These studies raise important methodological questions that have not been systematically studied. For example, how fast does gastric myoelectric activity, as measured with EGG, change? That is, can we expect to see a measurable change in the EGG following the presentation of a brief discrete stimulus? Or, how long would a given stimulus have to be presented before we would expect to see a change in the EGG? In general, we think of the GI system as being slow responding compared to other biological systems because momentary adjustments in activity are not essential to survival, but data on this issue are lacking. And how should one interpret abnormal EGGs recorded from a patient with an eating disorder? Is the abnormal EGG just a result of abnormal eating, or is it contributing to the behavior? We don't know. It is possible that in some cases abnormal gastric activity was a part of the individual's pathology, but as time passed, the abnormal eating caused the gastric activity to worsen and a vicious cycle was created.

Future directions

The EGG, because of its noninvasive nature, will continue to aid basic researchers in their quest for additional information about gastric myoelectric activity, gastric neuromuscular activity, and their relationship in normal and pathophysiological conditions.

Applied research using the EGG by gastroenterologists is increasing rapidly largely due to the ease and reliability of its use in detecting gastric dysrhythmias and the recently established relationship between gastric dysrhythmias and upper GI disorders including delayed gastric emptying, nausea, and dyspepsia. Pharmaceutical companies have supported much of this research, and we anticipate that this will continue. Many disorders, such as diabetic gastroparesis, are marked by abnormal EGG recordings, and studies of the degree to which EGG normalization accompanies improvement in symptoms are likely to provide new insights into the complex relationship between gastric myoelectric activity and the pathophysiology of these disorders.

A related exciting new area that requires EGG recording in order to assess results of therapeutic interventions is gastric electrical stimulation of the stomach (GES). As described above, studies are currently in progress using GES to both strengthen normal 3 cpm activity in patients with nausea and/or delayed gastric emptying, and to disrupt normal 3 cpm activity in obese patients in an effort to decrease appetite. Another area of research that we are engaged in is biofeedback of EGG for individuals with gastric dysrhythmias in an effort to restore normal 3 cpm activity, and thereby, relieve nausea. In a recent study (Stern et al., 2004), we demonstrated that healthy people can increase their normal 3 cpm activity with biofeedback. Future studies should explore both the sub-group(s) of nausea patients who might benefit from the procedure, and the most efficacious procedure.

EGG recording may also prove to be of value in the study of eating disorders. A potential application of our finding, described above, that sham feeding of disgusting food is not accompanied by an increase in normal 3 cpm EGG activity is to use the EGG response to the sham feeding of pleasant food to track the progress during therapy of individuals with eating disorders. Assuming that subjects with certain types of eating disorders cognitively appraise eating as less than pleasant, we would expect them, therefore, not to show an increase in EGG 3 cpm activity during sham feeding. Quantification of the cephalic-vagal reflex, as measured by the EGG 3 cpm activity, might provide a more valid measure of recovery than weight gain or the judgment of the therapist.

The increase in the use of the EGG by gastroenterologists has brought with it refinements in both hardware and software, including ambulatory units that have flown on NASA Shuttle flights. We predict that with the availability of this new equipment additional psychophysiologists will soon be using the EGG as an noninvasive window into the complex brain-stomach relationship that was first brought to the attention of GI researchers and clinicians by Beaumont's description of changes in the stomach activity of his fistulated subject in 1833.

REFERENCES

Abell, T. L., Lucas, A., R., Brown, M. L., & Malagelada, J. R. (1985). Gastric electrical dysrhythmias in anorexia nervosa (AN). *Gastroenterology, 88A,* 1300.

Abell, T. L., & Malagelada, J. R. (1985). Glucagon-evoked gastri-dysrhythmias in humans shown by an improved electrogastrographic technique. *Gastroenterology, 88,* 1932–1940.

Abell, T. L., Tucker, R., & Malagelada, J. R. (1985). Simultaneous gastric electro-manometry in man. In R. M. Stern, & K. L. Koch (Eds.), *Electrogastrography* (pp. 78–88). New York: Praeger.

Alvarez, W. C. (1922). The electrogastrogram and what it shows. *Journal of the American Medical Association, 78,* 1116–1119.

Alvarez, W. C. (1943). *Nervousness, indigestion, and pain.* New York: Hoeber.

Baldaro, B., Mazzetti, M., Codispoti, M., Tuozzi, G., Bolzani, R., & Trombini, G. (2001). Autonomic reactivity during viewing of an unpleasant film. *Perceptual Motor Skills, 93,* 797–805.

Beaumont, W. (1833/1959). *Experiments and observations on the gastric juice and the physiology of indigestion.* New York: Dover.

Berntson, G. G., Cacioppo, J. T., Binkley, P. F., Uchino, B. N., Quigley, K. S., & Fieldstone, A. (1994). Autonomic cardiac control. III. Psychological stress and cardiac response in autonomic space as revealed by pharmacological blockades. *Psychophysiology, 31,* 599–608.

Bortolotti, M., Sarti, P., Barara, L., & Brunelli, F. (1990). Gastric myoelectrical activity in patients with chronic idiopathic gastroparesis. *Journal of Gastrointestinal Motility, 2,* 104–108.

Bortolotti, M. (2002). The electrical way to cure gastroparesis. *American Journal of Gastroenterology, 97,* 1874–1883.

Brown, B. H., Smallwood, R. H., Duthie, H. L., & Stoddard, C. J. (1975). Intestinal smooth muscle electrical potentials recorded from surfaces electrodes. *Medical Biological Engineering, 13,* 97–103.

Bruley des Varannes, S., Mizrahi, M., Curran, P., Kandasamy, A., & Dubois, A. (1991). Relation between postprandial gastric emptying and cutaneous electrogastrogram in primates. *American Journal Physiology, 261,* G248–G225.

Camilleri, M., Malagelada, J. R., Brown, M. L., Becker, G., & Zinsmeister, A. R. (1985). Relation between antral motility and gastric emptying of solids and liquids in humans. *American Journal of Physiology, 249,* G580–G585.

Cannon, W. B., & Washburn, A. L. (1912). An explanation of hunger. *American Journal of Physiology, 29,* 441–454.

Cannon, W. B. (1936). *Digestion and health.* New York: Norton.

Carlson, A. J. (1916). *The control of hunger in health and disease.* Chicago: University of Chicago Press.

Chen, J., Vandewalle, J., Sansen, W., Vantrappen G., & Janssens, J. (1990). Adaptive spectral analysis of cutaneous electrical signals using autoregressive moving average modeling. *Med Biol Eng Comput, 28,* 531–536.

Chen J., & McCallum, R. W. (1991). Electrogastrogram: Measurement, analysis and prospective applications. *Med Biol Eng Comput, 29,* 339–350.

Chen, J., Stewart, W. R., & McCallum, R. W. (1993). Adaptive spectral analysis of episodic rhythmic variations in gastric myoelectric potentials. *IEEE Trans Biomed Eng, 40,* 128–135.

Chen, J. D. Z., Davenport, K., & McCallum, R. W. (1993). Effects of fat preload on gastric myoelectrical activity in normal humans. *J. Gastrointest Mot, 5,* 281.

Chen, J., Richards, R., & McCallum, R. W. (1993). Frequency components of the electrogastrogram and their correlations with gastrointestinal motility. *Med Biol Eng Comput, 31,* 60–67.

Chen, J. D. Z., Lin, Z. Y., Parolisi, S., & McCallum, R. W. (1995). Inhibitory effects of cholecystokinin on postprandial gastric myoelectric activity. *Digestive Diseases and Sciences. 40,* 2614–2622.

Chen, J. D. Z., Zou, X. P., Lin, X. M., et al. (1996). Detection of slow wave propagation from the cutaneous electrogastrogram. *American Journal of Physiology, 277,* G4124–G430.

Chiloiro, M., Riezzo, G., Guerra, V., Reddy, S. N., & Girgio, I. (1994). The cutaneous electrogastrogram reflects postprandial gastric emptying in humans. In J. Z. Chen, & R. W. McCallum (Eds.), *Electrogastrography: Principles and applications* (pp. 293–306). New York: Raven Press.

Code, C. F., & Marlett, J. A. (1975). The interdigestive myo-electric complex of the stomach and small bowel of dogs. *Journal of Physiology, 246,* 289–309.

Couturier, D., Roze, C., Paologgi, J., & Debray, C. (1972). Electrical activity of the normal human stomach: A comparative study of recordings obtained from serosal and mucosal sites. *Digestive Diseases and Sciences, 17,* 969–976.

Davis, R. C., Garafolo, L., & Gault, F. P. (1957). An exploration of abdominal potentials. *Journal of Comparative and Physiological Psychology, 50,* 519–523.

Davis, R. C., Garafolo, L., & Kveim, K. (1959). Conditions associated with gastrointestinal activity. *Journal of Comparative and Physiological Psychology, 52,* 466–475.

Diamanti, A., Bracci, F., Gambarara, M., Ciofetta, G. C., Sabbi, T., Ponticelli, A., Montecchi, F., Marinucci, S., Bianco, G., & Castro, M. (2003). Gastric electric activity assessed by electrogastrography and gas emptying scintigraphy in adolescents with eating disorders. *Journal Pediatr Gastroenterol Nutr, 37,* 35–41.

Dubois, A., & Mizrahi, M. (1994). Electrogastrography, gastric emptying, and gastric motility. In J. Z. Chen, & R. W. McCallum (Eds.), *Electrogastrography: Principles and applications* (pp. 247–256). New York: Raven Press.

Familoni, B. O., Bowes, K. L., Kingma, Y. J., & Cote, K. R. (1987). Can transcutaneous electrodes diagnose gastric electrical abnormalities? *Digestive Diseases and Sciences, 32,* 909.

Feldman, M., & Schiller, L. (1983). Disorders of gastrointestinal motility associated with diabetes mellitus. *Annals of Internal Medicine, 98,* 378–384.

Furness, J. B., & Costa, M. (1980). Types of nerves in the enteric nervous system. *Neuroscience, 5,* 1–20.

Geldof, H., van der Schee, E. J., van Blankenstein, M., & Grashuis, J. L. (1983). Gastric dysrhythmia; an electrogastrographic study. *Gastroenterology, 84,* 1163.

Geldof, H., van der Schee, E. J., & Grashuis, J. L. (1986). Accuracy and reliability of electrogastrography (EGG). *Gastroenterology, 90,* 1425.

Gianaros, P. J., Quigley, K. S., Mordkoff, J. T., Stern, R. M. (2001). Gastric myoelectrical and autonomic cardiac reactivity to laboratory stressors. *Psychophysiology, 38,* 642–652.

Ghoos, Y. F., Maes B. D., Geypens, B. J., Mys, G., Hiele, M. I., Rutgeerts, P. J., & Vantrappen, G. (1993). Measurement of gastric emptying rate of solids by means of a carbon-labeled octanoic acid breath test. *Gastroenterology, 104,* 1640–1647.

Hamilton, J. W., Bellahsene, B. E., Reichelderfer, M., Webster, J. H., & Bass, P. (1986). Human electrogastrograms. Comparison of surface and mucosal recordings. *Digestive Diseases and Sciences, 31,* 33–39.

Hinder, R. A., & Kelly, K. A. (1977). Human gastric pacesetter potentials: Site of origin and response to gastric transection and proximal vagotomy. *American Journal of Physiology, 133,* 29–33.

Hölzl, R., Loffler, K., & Muller, G. M. (1985). On conjoint gastrography or what the surface gastrograms show. In R. M. Stern, & K. L. Koch (Eds.), *Electrogastrography: Methodology, validation, and applications* (pp. 89–115). New York: Praeger.

Huisinga, J. D. (2001). Physiology and pathophysiology of the interstitial cells of Cajal: From bench to bedside, II: gastric motility: lessons from mutant mice on slow waves and innervation. *American Journal of Physiology, 281,* G1129–G1134.

Jednak, M. A., Shadigian, E. M., Kim, M. S., Woods, M. L., Hooper, F. G., Owyang, & Hasler, W. L. (1999). Protein meals reduce nausea and gastric slow wave dysrhythmic activity in first trimester pregnancy. *American Journal of Physiology, 277,* G855–G861.

Jones, K. R., & Jones, G. E. (1985). Pre- and postprandial EGG variation. In R. M. Stern, & K. L. Koch (Eds.), *Electrogastrography: Methodology, validation and applications* (pp. 168–181). New York: Praeger.

Kelly, K. A., Code, C. F., & Elveback, L. R. (1969). Patterns of canine gastric electrical activity. *American Journal of Physiology, 217,* 461–470.

Kim, T. W., Beckett, E. A. H., Hanna, R., et al. (2002) Regulation of pacemaker frequency in the murine gastric antrum. *Journal of Physiology* (Lond), *538,* 145–157.

Kingma, Y. J. (1989). The electrogastrogram and its analysis. *Critical Reviews in Biomedical Engineering, 17,* 105–124.

Koch, K. L. (2002). Electrogastrography. In M. M. Schuster, M. D. Crowell, & K. L. Koch (Eds.), *Schuster atlas of gastrointestinal motility, 2nd ed.* (pp. 185–202). Hamilton: Decker.

Koch, K. L., & Stern, R. M. (1985). The relationship between the cutaneously recorded electrogastrogram and antral contractions in man. In R. M. Stern, & K. L. Koch (Eds.), *Electrogastrography: Methodology, validation, and applications* (pp. 116–131). New York: Praeger.

Koch, K. L., Stewart, W. R., & Stern, R. M. (1987). Effects of barium meals on gastric electromechanical activity in man: A fluorscopic-electrogastrophic study. *Digestive Diseases and Sciences, 32,* 1217–1222.

Koch, K. L., Stern, R. M., Bingaman, S., & Eggli, D. (1991). Satiety, stomach volume and gastric myoelectrical activity during solid-phase gastric emptying: A study of healthy individuals. *Journal of Gastrointestinal Motility, 3,* 187.

Koch, & Stern (2004). *Handbook of electrogastrography.* New York: Oxford University Press.

Koch, K. L., & Stern, R. M. (1993). Electrogastrography. In D. Kumar, & D. Wingate (Eds.), *An illustrated guide to gastrointestinal motility* (pp. 290–307). London: Churchill Communications Europe.

Koch, K. L., Tran, T. N., Stern, R. M., Bingaman, S., & Sperry, N. (1993). Gastric myoelectrical activity in premature and term infants. *Journal of Gastrointestinal Motility, 5,* 41–47.

Koch, K. L., Hong, S.-P., & Xu, L. (2000). Reproducibility of gastric myoelectrical activity and the water load test in patients with dysmotility-like dyspepsia symptoms and in control subjects. *Journal of Clinical Gastroenterology, 12,* 125–129.

Kwong, N. K., Brown, B. H., Whittaker, G. E., & Duthie, H. L. (1970). Electrical activity of the gastric antrum in man. *British Journal of Surgery, 12,* 913–916.

Lacy, B. E., Koch, K. L., & Crowell, M. D. (2002). Manometry. In M. M. Schuster, M. D. Crowell, & K. L. Koch, *Schuster atlas of gastrointestinal motility, 2nd ed.* (135–150). Hamilton: Decker.

Lavigne, M. E., Wiley, Z. D., Meyer, J. H., Martin, P., & MacGregor, I. L. (1978). Gastric emptying rates of solid food in relation to body size. *Gastroenterology, 74,* 1258–1260.

Lee, K., Chey, W., Tai, H., & Yajima, H. (1978). Radioimmunoassay of motilin: Validation and studies on the relationship between plasma motilin and interdigestive myoelectric activity in the duodenum of dog. *Digestive Diseases and Sciences, 23,* 789–795.

Levine, M. E., Muth, E. R., Williamson, M. J., & Stern, R. M. (2004). Protein-predominant meals inhibit the development of gastric tachyarrhythmia, nausea and the symptoms of motion sickness. *Alimentary Pharmacology, & Therapeutics, 19,* 583–590.

Lin, H. C., & Hasler, W. L. (1995). Disorders of gastric emptying. In T. Yamada (Ed.), *Textbook of gastroenterology* (pp. 1318–1346). Philadelphia: Lippincott.

Lin, Z., & Chen, J. Z. (1994). Comparison of three running spectral analysis methods. In J. Z. Chen, & R. W. McCallum (Eds.), *Electrogastrography: Principles and applications* (pp. 75–98). New York: Raven Press.

McNearney, T., Lin, X., Shrestha, J., et al. (2002). Characterization of gastric myoelectrical rhythms in patients with systemic sclerosis using multichannel surface electrogastrography. *Digestive Diseases, & Sciences, 47,* 690–698.

Meyer, J. H. (1987). Motility of the stomach and gastroduodenal junction. In L. R. Johnson, J. Christensen, E. D., Jacobsen, & S. G. Schultz (Eds.), *Physiology of the gastrointestinal tract* (pp. 613–630). New York: Raven Press.

Meyer, J. H., Gu, Y. G., Dressman, J., & Amidon, G. (1986). Effect of viscosity and flow rate on gastric emptying of solids. *American Journal of Physiology, 250,* G161–G164.

Meyer, J. H., MacGregor, I. L., Gueller, R., Martin, P., & Cavalieri, R. (1976). 99Tc-tagged chicken liver as a marker of solid food in the human stomach. *American Journal of Digestive Diseases, 21,* 296–304.

Meyer, J. H., Ohashi, H., Jehn, D., & Thompson, J. B. (1981). Size of liver particles emptied from the human stomach. *Gastroenterology, 80,* 1489–1496.

Mintchev, M. P., Otto, S. J., & Bowes, K. L. (1997). Electrogastrography can recognize gastric electrical uncoupling in dogs. *Gastroenterology, 112,* 2006–2011.

Mirizzi, N., & Scafoglieri, V. (1983). Optimal direction of the electrogastrographic signal in man. *Medical and Biological Engineering and Computing, 2l,* 385–389.

Moraes, E. R., Toncon, L. E., Baffa, O., Oba-Kunyioshi, A. S., & Wakai, R. (2003). Adaptive, autoregressive spectral estimation for analysis of electrical signals of gastric origin. *Physiol. Meas., 24,* 91–106.

Morgan, K. G., Schmalz, P. F., & Szurszewski, J. H. (1978). The inhibitory effects of vasoactive intestinal polypeptide on the mechanical and electrical activity of canine antral smooth muscle. *Journal of Physiology, 282,* 437–450.

Muth, E. R., Koch, K. L, & Stern, R. M. (2000). Significance of autonomic nervous system activity in functional dyspepsia. *Digestive Diseases and Sciences, 45,* 854–863.

Muth, E. R., Koch, K. L., Stern, R. M., & Thayer, J. F. (1999). Effect of autonomic nervous system manipulations on gastric myoelectrical activity and emotional responses in healthy human subjects. *Psychosomatic Medicine, 61,* 297–303.

Muth, E. R., Stern, R.M., & Koch, K. L. (1996). Effects of vection-induced motion sickness on gastric myoelectric activity and oral-cecal transit time. *Digestive Diseases and Sciences, 41,* 330–334.

Muth, E. R., Thayer, J. F., Stern, R. M., Friedman, B. H., & Drake, C. (1998). The effect of autonomic nervous system activity on gastric myoelectrical activity: Does the spectral reserve hypothesis hold for the stomach? *Biological Psychology, 71,* 265–278.

Nelsen, T. S., & Kohatsu, S. (1968). Clinical electrogastrography and its relationship to gastric surgery. *American Journal of Surgery, 116,* 215–222.

Ogawa, A., Mizuta, I., Fukunaga, T., Takeuchi, N., Honaga, E., Sugita, Y., Mika, A., Inoue, Y., & Takeda, M. (2004). Electrogastrography abnormality in eating disorders. *Psychiatry Clinical Neuroscience, 58,* 300–310.

Read, N. W., An-Janabi, M. N., Bates, T. E., Holgate, A. M., Cann, P. A., Kinsman, R. I., McFarlane, A., & Brown, C. (1985). Interpretation of the breath hydrogen profile obtained after ingesting a solid meal containing unabsorbable carbohydrate. *Gut, 26,* 834–842.

Riezzo, G., Castellana, R. M., De Bellis, T., Laforgia, F., Indrio, F., & Chilorio, M. (2003). Gastric electrical activity in normal neonates during the first year of life: effect of feeding with breast milk and formula. *Journal of Gastroenterology, 38,* 836–843.

Riezzo, G., Porceli, P., Guerra, V., & Giorgio, I. (1996). Effects of different psychophysiological stressors on the cutaneous electrogastrogram in healthy subjects. *Archives of Physiology and Biochemistry, 104,* 282–286.

Roman, C., & Gonella, J. (1987). Extrinsic control of digestive tract motility. In L. R. Johnson, J. Christensen, E. D., Jacobsen, & S. G. Schultz (Eds.), *Physiology of the gastrointestinal tract* (pp. 507–553). New York: Raven Press.

Sarna, S. K. (2002). Myoelectrical and contractile activities of the gastrointestinal tract. In M. M. Schuster, M. D. Crowell, & K. L. Koch (Eds.), *Schuster atlas of gastrointestinal motility, 2nd ed.* (pp. 1–18). Hamilton: Decker

Schlegel, J. F., & Code, C. F. (1975). The gastric peristalsis of the interdigestive housekeeper. In G. Vantrappen (Ed.), *Proceedings from the Fifth International Symposium on Gastrointestinal Motility* (p. 321). Herentals, Belgium: Typoff Press.

Sciarretta, G., Furno, A., Mazzoni, M., Garagnani, B., & Malagut, P. (1994). Lactulose hydrogen breath test in orocecal transit assessment. Critical evaluation by means of scintigraphic method. *Digestive Diseases and Sciences, 39*, 1505–1510.

Smallwood, R. H. (1978). Analysis of gastric electrical signals from surface electrodes using phase-lock techniques. Part 2: System performance with gastric signals. *Medical and Biological Engineering and Computing, 16*, 513–518.

Smallwood, R. H., & Brown, B. H. (1983). Non-invasive assessment of gastric activity. In P. Rolfe (Ed.), *Non-invasive physiological measurements* (Vol. II). London: Academic Press.

Smout, A. J. P. M. (1980). *Myoelectric activity of the stomach: Gastroelectromyography and electrogastrography*. Thesis, Erasmus University, Rotterdam.

Smout, A. J. P. M., van der Schee, E. J., & Grashuis, J. L. (1980a). What is measured in electrogastrography? *Digestive Diseases and Sciences, 25*, 179–187.

Smout, A. J. P. M., van der Schee, E. J. , & Grashuis, J. L. (1980b). Postprandial and interdigestive gastric electrical activity in the dog recorded by means of cutaneous electrodes. In J. Christensen (Ed.), *Gastrointestinal motility* (pp. 187–194). New York: Raven Press.

Smout, A. J. P. M., Jebbink, H. J. A., & Samson, M. (1994). Acquisition and analysis of electrogastrographic data: The Dutch experience. In J. Z. Chen, & R. W. McCallum (Eds.), *Electrogastrography: Principles and applications* (pp. 3–30). New York: Raven Press.

Stemper, T. J., & Cooke, A. R. (1975). Gastric emptying and its relationship to antral contractile activity. *Gastroenterology, 69*, 649–653.

Stern, R. M., & Koch, K. L. (Eds.) (1985). *Electrogastrography: Methodology, validation, and applications*. New York: Praeger.

Stern, R. M., Koch, K. L., Leibowitz, H. W., Lindblad, I., Shupert, C., & Stewart, W. R. (1985). Tachygastria and motion sickness. *Aviation Space and Environmental Medicine, 56*, 1074–1077.

Stern, R. M., Koch, K. L., Stewart, W. R., & Lindblad, I. M. (1987). Spectral analysis of tachygastria recorded during motion sickness. *Gastroenterology, 92*, 92–97.

Stern, R. M., Crawford, H. E., Stewart, W. R., Vasey, M. W., & Koch, K. L. (1989). Sham feeding: Cephalic-vagal influences on gastric myoelectric activity. *Digestive Diseases and Sciences, 34*, 521–527.

Stern, R. M. Koch, K. L., & Vasey, M. W. (1990). The gastrointestinal system. In J. T. Cacioppo, & L. G. Tassinary (Eds.), *Principles of Psychophysiology, physical, social, and inforential elements* (pp. 294–314). Cambridge: Cambridge University Press.

Stern, R. M., Vasey, M. W., Hu, S., & Koch, K. L. (1991). Effects of cold stress on gastric myoelectic activity. *Journal of Gastrointestinal Motility, 3*, 225–228.

Stern, R. M., & Koch, K. L. (1994). Using the electrogastrogram to study motion sickness. In J. Z. Chen, & R. W. McCallum (Eds.), *Electrogastrography: Principles and applications* (pp. 199–218). New York: Raven Press.

Stern, R. M., & Koch, K. L. (1996). Motion sickness and differential susceptibility. *Current Directions in Psychological Science, 5*, 115–120.

Stern, R. M., & Stacher, G. (1982). Recording the electrogastrogram from parts of the body surface distant from the stomach. *Psychophysiology, 19*, 350.

Stern, R. M., & Koch, K. L., & Muth, E. R. (2000). Gastrointestinal system. In J. T. Cacioppo, L. G. Tassinary, & G. G. Berntson (Eds.), *Handbook of Psychophysiology*, 2nd ed. (pp. 294–314). Cambridge: Cambridge University Press.

Stern, R. M., Jokerst, M. D., Levine, M. E., & Koch, K. L. (2001). The stomach's response to unappetizing food: Cephalic-vagal effects on gastric myoelectric activity. *Neurogastroenterology and Motility, 13*, 151–154.

Stern, R. M., Vitellaro, K., Thomas, M., Higgins, S. C., & Koch, K. L. (2004). Electrogastrographic biofeedback: A technique for enhancing normal gastric activity. *Neurogastroenterology and Motility, 16*, 753–757.

Stoddard, C. J., Smallwood, R. H., & Duthie, H. L. (1981). Electrical arrhythmias in the human stomach. *Gut, 22*, 705–712.

Thompson, D. G., Richelson, E., & Malagelada, J. R. (1982). Perturbation of gastric emptying and duodenal motility through the central nervous system. *Gastroenterology, 83*, 1200–1206.

Thunberg, L. (1989). Interstitial cells of Cajal. In J. D. Wood (Ed.), *Handbook of physiology, The gastrointestinal system* (pp. 349–386), Section 6, Vol 1, Part 1. Bethesda, MD: American Physiological Society.

Uijtdehaage, S. H. J., Stern, R. M., & Koch, K. L. (1992). Effects of eating on vection-induced motion sickness, cardiac vagal tone and gastric myoelectric activity. *Psychophysiology, 29*, 193–201.

Van der Schee, E. J., Smout, A. J. P. M., & Grashuis, J. L. (1982). Applications of running spectrum analysis to electrogastrographic signals recorded from dog and man. In M. Wienbeck (Ed.), *Motility of the digestive tract* (pp. 241–250). New York: Raven Press.

Vantrappen, G., Hostein, J., Janssens, J., Vanderweerd, M., & De Wever, I. (1983). Do slow waves induce mechanical activity? *Gastroenterology, 84*, 1341.

Vantrappen, G., Janssens, J., Peeters, T. L., Bloom, S. R., Christofides, N. D., & Hellemans, J. (1979). Motility and the interdigestive migrating motor complex in man. *Digestive Diseases and Sciences, 24*, 497–500.

ver Hagen, M. A. M. T., Luijk, H. D., Samsom, M., and Smout, A. J. P. M. (1998). Effect of meal temperature on the frequency of gastric myoelectrical activity. *Neurogastroenterolog, & Motility, 10*, 175–181.

Wolf, S., & Wolff, H. G. (1943). *Human gastric function*. New York: Oxford.

Wolf, S. (1943). Relation of gastric function to nausea in man. *Journal of Clinical Investigations, 22*, 877–882.

Wood, J. D. (2002). Neural and humoral regulation of gastrointestinal motility. In M. M. Schuster, M. D. Crowell, & K. L. Koch (Eds.), *Atlas of gastrointestinal motility, 2nd ed*. (pp. 19–42) Hamilton: Decker.

You, C. H., & Chey, W. Y. (1984). Study of electromechanical activity of the stomach in humans and in dogs with particular attention to tachygastria. *Gastroenterology, 86*, 1460–1468.

Xu, G., & Zhou, Y. (1983). Modulated effect of acupuncture on gastroelectrical activity. *Acupuncture Research, 8*, 1–6.

10 The Respiratory System

TYLER S. LORIG

1. INTRODUCTION

Often overlooked in psychophysiology, the respiratory system is remarkably complicated and sensitive to a variety of psychological variables. Scientists have examined this system since the time of Galen and even before (Sternbach et al., 2001).

Over the intervening years some have argued for what has perhaps been an overly influential role for respiration. Feleky (1916) argued that the ratio between inspiration and expiration was intimately connected to psychological state and personality. Nielsen and Roth (1929) reviewed more than 20,000 spirometry records and identified ten breathing patterns that they argued were associated with the heritability of some traits. Sutherland, Wolf, and Kennedy (1938) stated the "respiratory curve is as constant and characteristic of an individual as his handwriting" and suggest that it is closely related to personality. Although few recent studies have sought to connect personality and respiration, it is clear that some individuals possess common respiratory patterns. This has led some to establish categories for these respiratory types or the *"personalite' ventalitoire"* (Shea & Guz, 1992).

More often than overestimating respiration's role in psychophysiology, this process is often ignored. In psychophysiology, respiration has been far overshadowed by research on the heart, brain, and electrodermal activity (Harver & Lorig, 2000). Wientjes and Grossman (1998) have effectively argued that it is respiration's susceptibility to voluntary influences that led early psychophysiologists to look elsewhere for physiological phenomena to study.

When respiration has been recorded, it is most often done to account for artifacts in other measures of more interest to the investigator (Grossman, 1983). Because of the coupling between breathing and cardiac output, heart rate changes as a function of the respiratory cycle. This phenomenon is called respiratory sinus arrhythmia (RSA) and for those interested in the cardiovascular system, it makes respiration an intervening variable. In fact, the degree of dissociation between heart rate and respiration has become of great interest in recent years since the "tight-ness" of this coupling can be viewed as an index of the vagal control of the heart (Berntson, Cacioppo, & Quigley, 1993). In addition to influencing cardiac activity, respiration can be a potent source of noise in electrodermal recordings as well (Rittweger, Lambertz, & Langhorst, 1997).

Part of the problem associated with measuring respiration in psychophysiology is that our needs are often so different from those of respiratory medicine. The past decade has provided tremendous advances in data and approaches related to respiratory health. Medical approaches to respiration are direct. They have been systematic and a number of standards exist for making lung function measurements (Evans & Scanlon, 2003). Almost all measurements of lung function in medical settings are made using spirometry. Even though this can be a very valuable technique in psychophysiology, many research questions limit the use of this approach. During a spirometric evaluation, the patient is usually nose clipped and breathes through a tube placed into the mouth. Though not invasive in the typically sense, it is psychologically invasive because it often centers the patient or subject's attention on the process of respiration (Han et al., 1997). In a medical setting, a technician making the recording encourages the patient to exhale even after the person feels their lungs fully exhausted. Certainly, this type of subject-experimenter interaction is foreign to most psychophysiological laboratories. Research questions seeking to relate cognition or emotional change to respiration must take a somewhat different approach and often use continuous measurements such as thoracic distention, pressure, or temperature as dependent variables while the tasks of interest are performed. These measurements provide less precise information about respiratory volume than spirometric approaches and don't often provide information about blood gasses. Even so, they may be preferred in some situations because they do not invade the psychological dimensions of the task. Carefully habituating subjects to spirographic evaluation can also be accomplished (Ritz, 2004) but requires great care and tasks that demand attention from subjects.

Few would argue that respiration's primary function is gas exchange. Oxygen is delivered to the blood stream

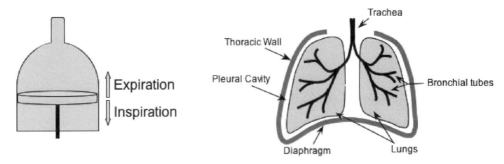

Figure 10.1. The left panel illustrates the principle by which the lungs operate. As the piston or diaphragm moves down, the pressure inside the vessel is reduced and air flows in to equalize the pressure. The right panel illustrates the placement of the lungs and diaphram in the thoracic cavity.

and carbon dioxide is removed by the actions of this system. Certainly the literature in medicine has emphasized this role and much research has been conducted to evaluate chemosensory receptors in the wall of blood vessels, absorption of oxygen into the blood, integrity of the lungs and alveoli, and many other portions of this system (Comroe, 1974). For psychophysiologists however, gas exchange is but one of several important functions. The respiratory system also acts to modulate the air necessary for speech, the pressure necessary to bring odors to the olfactory mucosa, and it anticipates the metabolic demands of cognitive and muscular activity (Collet et al., 1999). Furthermore, the interaction of this system with cardiac and other autonomic systems is a remarkable illustration of the functional complexity and cross-system integration of the nervous system.

Respiration is important in a number of illnesses of interest to psychologists such as asthma, which is widely studied for its psychological dimensions. From a respiratory perspective, it is associated with increased respiratory resistance or reduced airflow (Ritz, 2004). Persons experiencing an asthma attack must exert more effort to inhale because of narrowed air passages. This increased ventilatory effort is, in itself, a cue for breathing difficulty and may serve to provide positive feedback exacerbating respiratory difficulty (Harver & Mahler, 1998).

At its essence, the respiratory system is mechanical. Muscles control the filling of air sacks and these sacks are, in turn, connected to the outside world through air passages. Figure 10.1 illustrates the similarity of this system to a piston. The left panel of the figure shows a piston in a bottle. Movement of the piston is analogous to the contraction of the diaphragm. When the diaphragm contracts, the piston moves down, it creates an area of low pressure that causes air to flow into the bottle or lungs. The right panel of the figure illustrates the schematic nature of the mechanical system. Integrity of the air passages, sacks, and muscles all influence the system because it is controlled though multiple feedback loops. As an example, diminished air intake in one inhalation leads to subsequent increases in muscle activity producing increasing lung expansion and airflow. If resistance is increased in the system, volume will be decreased even though rate of flow

is high in just the same way that a nozzle on water hose increases the speed of the water but decreases the volume. The mechanical nature of this system belies its complexity. Because respiration is an essential component of life, it broadly influences activity in other systems. Similarly, it is mutually dependent on many other systems in the body for its regulation.

2. NEURAL CONTROL

The fact that breathing "is a truly strange phenomena of life caught midway between the conscious and unconscious" (Richards, 1953) is only suggestive of the system's diverse sources of regulation. Clearly, breathing is under voluntary control and just as clearly, it is not. Under ideal conditions, respiratory activity is a harmonious product of both sources of control. This harmony may breakdown in cases of pathology or under periods of stress to the system.

2.1. Autonomic control of respiration

Like most muscles systems, respiration depends upon feedback loops for its regulation. This feedback arises from a large number of receptor types including mechanoreceptors and chemoreceptors. In the case of the respiratory system, receptors in the walls of the airways (slowly adapting receptors – SARs) increase their activity in response to stretch associated with the volume of inhaled air (Hlastala & Berger, 1996). SARs provide negative feedback to the system via the vagus nerve. The action of these receptors is responsible for the Hering-Breuer reflex, a lengthening of the exhalatory phase of the cycle in response to distention of the airway wall.

In addition to SARs, Rapidly Adapting Receptors also influence the system by way of the vagus. These receptors are found on the epithelium of the airways and are responsive to both mechanical and chemosensory irritation. Activity in these receptors results in reflexive coughing (Hlastala & Berger, 1996). Particulates in the air and some chemicals such as chlorine activate these receptors which are more dense in the upper airways. This system is distinct from the trigeminally based irritation sensors in the nasal cavity and mouth.

Feedback to the respiratory system is also influenced by chemoreceptors in the arterial system. Theses receptors are found in a variety of arteries but those most influential to regulation of the respiratory system are the carotid bodies that are found in the carotid arteries. A second and slightly less influential set of chemoreceptors, the aortic bodies, is found in the wall of the aorta. Both the carotid and aortic bodies communicate with the central nervous system by way of the glossopharyngeal nerve. Receptors in both structures are sensitive to circulating levels of blood gases including oxygen and carbon dioxide and also blood pH (Hlastala & Berger, 1996). Because of the extreme vascularity of the carotid bodies in particular, even small reductions in oxygen lead to increased activity in the receptors. Similarly, activity in the nerve is also increased when CO_2 is abundant. These changes in blood gas increase activity in the nerve and subsequently the muscles of respiration. Through this mechanism, hypoxic events lead to increased ventilatory effort often including prolonged inhalation and gasping (Fung & St. John, 1995).

The arterial system is just one source for chemosensory regulation of breathing. There are also centrally located receptors sensitive to oxygen, CO_2, and pH in cerebrospinal fluid. Research by Harada et al. (1985) has demonstrated that perfusion of a rat brain in vitro leads to with increased levels of CO_2 or decreased O_2 leads to increased phrenic nerve output. This nerve is responsible for the contraction of the diaphragm. Hlastala and Berger (1996) review these data and propose two distinct areas or chemoreceptive zones. Both zones are on the ventral surface of the medulla with the larger zone at the level of the VIIIth nerve and the other is more caudal and closer to the midline.

Central mechanisms coordinate the input from these mechano and chemoreceptors and generate output to control the muscle groups associated with breathing. Several different areas of the brain contribute to the automatic regulation of the system and these areas differ from those used in voluntary control. As an example of this differential regulation, individuals afflicted with Ondine-Curse syndrome selectively lose the ability to automatically regulate breathing but are able to breathe by voluntary effort. This syndrome can arise in patients who have undergone surgery to transect the ventrolateral cervical spinal cord (bilaterally). This surgery is sometimes used for regulation of intractable pain and severs ascending pain projections. Descending pathways to the phrenic nerve are also disturbed however. Persons undergoing this procedure must be artificially ventilated during sleep because conscious regulation of breathing is necessary for their survival.

The descending fibers associated with automatic respiration arise in three different areas of the brain stem (Hlastala & Berger, 1996). These three groups of nuclei are located bilaterally in the pons, ventral and dorsal medulla. All of these respiratory groups have cells that increase their responding during inhalation and provide excitatory output to muscles as well as cells that inhibit spinal areas associated with output to respiratory muscles systems. Pathways between the respiratory groups and in the spinal cord provide internal feedback and regulation.

2.2. Voluntary regulation

Voluntary regulation of breathing ultimately uses the same muscles as automatic regulation but the pathways to those muscles differ. For instance, the spinal pathways that ultimately lead to the phrenic nerve and the nerves that control the intercostals travel through the corticospinal tract in the posterior-lateral portion of the cord. Output to those same nerves and muscles associated with automatic control travel in ventral pathways in the cord. Additionally, the nuclei that give rise to the fibers in these pathways are quite different. Because most automatic control can be associated with the brain stem (including the pons), voluntary control is much more complicated and involves cortical and diencephalic regions (Hlastala & Berger, 1996).

Much of the feedback for voluntary regulation comes from somatic receptors that relay information about the relative distention of thoracic muscles. This input comes to somatosensory areas of the thalamus and is relayed to diverse parts of the cortex and basal ganglia (Bramann, 1995). Cortical areas interact with basal ganglia and the medullary respiratory groups in coordinating output to the nerves and muscles associated with respiration. Instigation of the voluntary act of breathing, like the instigation of other voluntary acts, obviously involves multiple cortical systems but remains largely unknown. Curiously, because breathing can produce artifactual findings in fMRI research, there is great interest in the cortical components of respiration. Recent research on sniffing has indicated different mechanisms associated with voluntary sniffs versus odors arising in nonvoluntary inspirations (Sobel et al., 1998). Findings in this domain are bound to add tremendously to our knowledge of the cortical components of voluntary respiratory activity.

3. THE MECHANICAL SYSTEM

As mentioned previously, breathing is clearly a mechanical activity that is mutually dependent on vast feedback networks. This mechanical system consists of several interconnected parts that all function in unison but can have relatively independent regulation. Nasal congestion, as an example, may take place without altering patency of airways closer to the lungs (Eccles, 1996).

3.1. Functional anatomy

3.1.1. Lungs

The lungs are often characterized as air filled sacks. In fact, they are collections of much smaller sacks called alveoli that are connected to air passages. These sacks are plentiful (Comroe (1974) estimated 30 million), richly vascularized, and thin-walled. The massive surface area (approximately

140 m^2 (Johnson & Miller, 1968)) of these sacks and their thin walls make gas exchange fast and efficient. There are two types of cells that make up the wall of the alveoli. Type I cells form most of the volume of this wall and are the epithelial cells through which gases are exchanged. Type II cells are less plentiful but produce a surfactant-like phospholipid that reduces surface tension across the wall of the alveolar sack leading to more rapid gas exchange. The bronchial tubes that serve the lungs form three distinct regions in the right lung each with its collection of millions of alveoli. These lead to formation of three lung lobes: the lower, middle, and upper. The left lung, which is slightly smaller than the right, has only two lobes. Volume of the normal adult human lungs is approximately 5l (Hlastala & Berger, 1996).

3.1.2. Muscles

The primary muscle of external respiration (breathing) is the diaphragm. This is a large domed muscle (see Figure 10.1) that separates the thoracic cavity from the abdominal cavity. When contracted, the muscle flattens increasing the volume of the thoracic cavity. This creates an area of low pressure inside the cavity and airflows into the lungs to fill the volume. The lungs, which are highly elastic, are passive in this process. Diaphragmatic muscle spasms, also known as hiccups, are common and not necessarily indicative of other pathology.

In addition to the diaphragm, muscles of the ribs also contribute to breathing. The intercostal muscles are interconnected to the ribs. The external intercostals are the most superficial and their contraction leads to the lateral expansion of the rib cage. The contraction of these muscles and the diaphragm produce the majority of the muscular effort to inhale a bolus of air (DeTroyer, Gorman, & Gandevia, 2003). Exhalation is largely passive and is the result of gravity and the elasticity of the rib fascia and thoracic cavity. Rapid relaxation of the external intercostals and diaphragm leads to rapid exhalations. The role of the internal intercostals in this operation is controversial. A variety of reports suggest that these muscles act in opposition to the external intercostals and pull the ribs down thereby assisting in forced exhalation. In experiments with dogs, De Troyer and colleagues (1985) found that the internal intercostals function to further expand the ribs. Thus these two sets of intercostals muscles tend to both overlap in function and both act to expand the rib cage. At the margins of the ribs, the shallow insertion angle of the muscles leads to slight competition between these muscle groups for "opening" the ribs. This suggests that whereas both diaphragm and intercostals work to expand the volume of the thorax during inhalations, exhalation and even forced exhalation, are largely passive. More recent findings in humans (Wilson et al., 2001) have confirmed the effects the internal intercostals on exhalations. They found that these muscles, functioning on the lower ribs, do contract to increase expiration. Forced expirations may also involve abdominal muscles that, through their contraction, force the diaphragm further up into the thorax pushing out additional air.

3.1.3. Airways

The trachea is the most commonly described portion of the airways but the nasal and oral cavities, larynx, and bronchial tubes are also important features of the airway. At the upper end of the airway, the nose is a remarkable air sampling system. Air is pulled through the two external openings (nares) into the nasal cavity. This cavity has three boney protuberances called turbinates that increase the turbulent airflow allowing a relatively small volume of air to reach the olfactory mucosa while the majority of airflow is pulled into the trachea. Despite the enormous volume of air that flows through this system, it is capable of resisting drying under most conditions. Muscles of the nares contract during respiration and can be used to evaluate breathing.

Breathing may also take place through the mouth in some cases. Unlike the nose, this system dries easily and is not typically the preferred route for inspiration despite having half the ventilatory resistance of the nasal channel. Expired air, which tends to have increased humidity due to gas exchange, is less problematic. Inhaled air passes into the pharynx and past the epiglottis. The epiglottis folds up during inhalation opening the airway and down during swallowing to prevent liquids from entering (Hlastala & Berger, 1996).

The next portion of the airway is the larynx. In humans, this cartilaginous enlargement of the airway includes the vocal chords and is responsible for speech. The thyroid gland also occupies space in this area. Enlargement of the thyroid or pathology of the larynx may affect the air passage and increase airway resistance.

The trachea begins immediately below the larynx and divides into the left and right bronchial tubes. Like the lungs, the right bronchus is slightly larger in diameter than the left. These bronchi divide again and again. After some 24 divisions or generations, they connect to the alveoli (Ritz et al., 2002).

The trachea and bronchial tubes are sections of U-shaped cartilage bound by muscle tissue lined with an inner layer of epithelial and support cells. These cells contain cilia and other cells that secret mucous. Inflammation of these epithelial cells is commonly known as *bronchitis* and leads to excessive mucous production. As the cilia move this mucous (and foreign objects) back toward the mouth, reflexive contraction of the internal intercostals and abdominals (coughing) pushes short bursts of air and mucous out of the mouth. Additionally, the swelling of this tissue increases ventilatory effort causing the muscles of the system to expend more energy and thus requiring more ventilation to address the energy demands of that increased load in a positive feedback loop. Obviously, this problem is exacerbated by exertion and helps explain the "exhaustion" often reported by persons recovering from bronchitis or other pulmonary obstructive diseases.

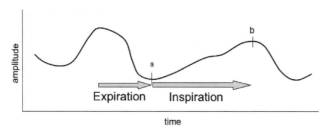

Figure 10.2. Typical output from piezoelectric belt transducer.

3.2. Measurement and quantification

Measurement and quantification of all types of pulmonary function have been aided immensely by the recent publication of guidelines for lung function measurements (Ritz et al., 2002). Readers should consult this report for specific details related to individual types of measurements. The descriptions of various techniques in this chapter are meant to help investigators make choices about which of the many respiratory parameters they may wish to evaluate.

Measurements of the mechanical aspects of respiration are straightforward and often quite simple. Most of these measurements depend upon changes in the volume of the thorax and abdomen and may be considered as a form of plethysmography. A variety of devices have been produced to make these measurements. Among the simplest is the respiratory belt (Grossman, 1967). This is a belt or tube that is affixed to the subject usually under the arms and around the chest and often a second belt is placed around the lower abdomen. The belt contains a sensor that is responsive to stretch. As the subject inhales, the volume of their upper thorax increases and stretches the device. In the past, these sensors have been, air filled bellows, strain gauges, mercury filled tubes, inductive coils and, most recently, fiber optic loops (Davis et al., 1999). The most commonly used belt method is currently a piezoelectric device. These are robust, don't leak air or mercury and provide reliable signals that can be incorporated into most electrophysiological recording systems. Pennock (1990) evaluated piezo-based respiratory belts and found that they were relatively linear compared to measurements made with a screen pneumotachometer. Figure 10.2 represents output typical of such a piezoelectric device.

The tracing in Figure 10.2 appears simple and is artifact free. Quantification of this signal is also straightforward but requires defining both the interests of the investigator and the parameters of the system. Peak exhalation is defined as the minima of the waveform between two cycles and is labeled as "a" on the graph. Peak inspiration is the maxima and is labeled as "b." It is an easy matter to evaluate the difference in these two points to find how much the chest changed during the inspiration. Counting the number of inspirations in a minute gives the rate of inspiration but the data contain far more information. Table 10.1 illustrates the variety of measurements that can be made from the simple waveform presented in Figure 10.2.

Only a few of these measurements are in common use but they serve to illustrate the complexity of the problem. Selection of the proper technique is related to the hypothesis, the way the data are acquired and the method used to reduce those data. Too often, an experimenter will seek to measure respiration then purchase the instrumentation to do so and find themselves at the end of the experiment left with still more questions about the respiration data. Perhaps worse, they will find themselves with a psychological variable that has no effect on *respiratory rate* and conclude that respiration was insensitive to their manipulation. In fact, many different parameters of respiration might have changed because *respiratory rate* is among the least sensitive (Wientjes & Grossman, 1998). This insensitivity is what led early researchers to adopt new metrics such as the inspiration/expiration ratio in the early twentieth century (Feleky, 1916).

In order to choose the proper technique, the investigator must consider, in depth, the mechanisms that lead physiological variables to change. If, for instance, one were concerned about cognitive problems related to subjects working at high altitude, the first mechanism to consider would be oxygen deprivation. Although such deprivation might lead to higher breathing rates, it will certainly lead to reduced blood levels of O_2 no matter the respiratory rate. In this example, the investigator should select a technique that, when mathematically reduced, will produce a direct measurement of the amount of oxygen in the blood over time so that it can be correlated with cognitive performance over time. It would be reasonable to add rate as a secondary measure but this would add relatively little to the findings. On the other hand, using respiratory rate exclusively would be highly problematic because rate is a very poor proxy for blood oxygen level. Respiratory patterns can be surprisingly complicated. A subject faced with a task may suspend breathing for several seconds. They may also immediately take a deep breath then suspend breathing. Breathing may become shallow or show a pattern of slow inhalations followed by brief periods of exhalations. Over minutes, one can expect that increases in metabolic demands will be equilibrated with both breathing and cardiovascular activity. Shorter epochs can be and often are much more variable and inconsistent with metabolic conditions. With respiration, just as with any psychophysiological dependent variable, the investigator must consider how the numbers that will ultimately be entered into their analysis will truly represent the psychological and physiological processes under investigation.

Although the respiratory belt has several advantages, it also suffers from several real problems. One problem is related to the transducer itself. Pulling the belt too tight leaves the transducer at the upper limit of its range and will produce "clipping" or a ceiling effect. Using a more loosely fitting belt can be equally problematic because only large inhalation may stretch the belt enough to produce a recording. Even with a properly fitting belt, individual differences in breathing lead some individuals to produce

Table 10.1. List of measurements that can be obtained from breathing transducers

Measurement	How obtained
Frequency/Rate	Mean number of peaks per minute
Inspiratory Volume (relative)	Base to peak or integration
Expiratory Volume (relative)	Base to peak or integration
Inspiration/Expiration Ratio	Computed
Inspiratory duration (absolute)	Base to peak duration
Expiratory duration (absolute)	Base to peak duration
Duration ratio	Computed
Complexity (frequency)	Spectral analysis combined with examination of the amplitudes of non-dominant frequencies

more abdominal distention making a belt placed under the arm pits insensitive to breathing. It is possible and often preferable to use a second belt placed over the abdomen (Grossman, 1967). Doing so, however, may increase subject discomfort. No mater how many belts are used, this method always provides external feedback because the belt must tighten during breathing resulting in greater constriction of the chest wall. Such feedback can make subjects far more aware of their breathing pattern and more likely to adopt response strategies that are different from less invasive procedures (Han et al., 1997). Finally, because the subject is often seated during testing, non-respiratory movements can stretch the transducer causing artifacts.

Similar to the respiratory belt is inductive plethys-mography, here the subject wears a broad band and more recently, a "shirt" that contains sensors responsive to abdominal stretch and distention. The LifeShirt® (Wilhelm, Roth, & Sackner, 2003) is a new and interesting technique that may prove very helpful in the field of respiratory measurement. This is a continuous ambulatory monitoring garment for cardiovascular and respiratory measures (VivoMetrics, Ventura, CA) that collects a variety of data available for telemetry or later download and analysis. Like impedance pneumography, investigators attracted to using this device to obtain continuous cardiovascular measures will also get respiratory signals from inductance plethysomography recording devices. This technique uses changes in magnetic flux of wires embedded in the shirt to estimate thoracic volume and respiratory activity. It provides data on rib and abdominal excursions that lead to the calculation of many respiratory parameters including tidal volume, respiratory timing, and inspiratory flow. The system can also contain noninvasive blood gas monitors in addition to a variety of sensors not associated with respiration. As several reviews point out, techniques such as this offer the opportunity to make detailed measurements of subject physiology in real-life settings and emergencies.

Another technique that makes use of the distention of the chest wall and abdomen is magnetometry. In this technique, as the subject's abdomen moves, magnet flux is sensed and the position can be plotted. This 3-D space can be differentiated into a change score that can be viewed like the output from a respiratory belt. Levine and colleagues (Levine et al., 1991) report good results using sources placed on the ventral and dorsal surfaces in predicting tidal volume. Recently, McCool, Wang, and Ebi (2002) have introduced a portable version of this device.

In some situations such as a driving simulator or cockpit, it is possible to use cramped space to the experimenter's advantage. Casali, Wierwille, and Cordes (1983) used a proximity indicator to estimate the location of the abdomen during breathing. Although certainly not applicable to all situations, this technique had the advantage of being less invasive although it may be more susceptible to movement artifacts.

Whole body plethysmography refers to using the fluctuating volume of a chamber containing the subject to determine respiratory activity (Ries, 1989). The air supply to the subject originates outside the chamber. As air is pulled into the lungs, the change in chest volume reduces the volume of the chamber. In the past, the chambers were water filled but more recent approaches use an air filled chamber and pressure transducers. This remains a widely used method in medicine and has particular advantages for measuring lung capacity in laboratory animals (Rozanski & Hoffman, 1999).

Another important measurement of thoracic volume is impedance pneumography. This technique measures the impedance of the thorax as it changes during respiration. This is a viable and interesting technique but is not often employed. Even though few investigators actively seek to measure respiration this way, it is often used to measure the heart via impedance cardiography. Recently, Ernst and colleagues (Ernst et al., 1999) have devised a way to extract impedance pneumography data from impedance cardiography recordings. This approach uses standard tetrapolar electrodes for impedance cardiography. The pneumographic signal can be derived from ΔZ (or ΔZd derived by integration of dZ/dt) by first using a digital filter to eliminate high frequency and cardiac activity and then demeaning or removing the signal offset. Ernst and colleagues (1999) compared this derived signal with both spirometry and strain gauge recordings of the chest and found high coherences for the derived measure and spirometry. In fact, the derived signal was a

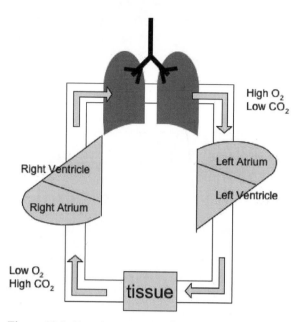

Figure 10.3. Function anatomy of gas distribution.

better predictor of the spirographic record than was the strain gauge. Because of the recent growth in impedance cardiography research, respiratory research may inadvertently gain new data and appreciation due to this analytic procedure.

Electromyography of the intercostals may also prove a useful technique under some conditions. If the investigator is measuring EKG from the chest wall in a position near the intercostals, these electrodes may also pick up activity from these respiratory muscles that, through filtering, can provide respiratory information (Pauly, 1957). Additionally, as mentioned previously, activity in the *nares dialator* can be monitored with electromyographic techniques (Sasaki & Mann, 1976).

4. THE GAS SYSTEM

The mechanical activity of the lungs, diaphragm and airways all serve the purpose of facilitating gas exchange with the blood. Oxygen in inhaled air passes through the wall of the alveoli and carbon dioxide diffuses from the blood into the alveoli and is expelled during exhalation.

4.1. Functional anatomy

Figure 10.3 shows a diagram of the functional anatomy of the gas distribution system. Air that is rich with oxygen and low in carbon dioxide fills the lungs and specifically, the alveoli. Here passive diffusion takes place across the cell membrane and pulmonary capillaries. Oxygen, in low concentration in the blood, flows into the capillaries and carbon dioxide that is in high concentration in the blood diffuses into the alveoli. This newly oxygenated blood flows into the left atrium and ventricle then provides the rest of

the body a supply of oxygen. As cellular metabolism takes place, the amount of oxygen in the blood is reduced and the supply of carbon dioxide increased. These products flow through the blood into the right side of the heart and are pumped into the lungs where gas exchange occurs with the air (Guyton & Hall, 2000).

4.2. Measurement and quantification

There are many different approaches to measuring the gasses associated with respiration. Among the most simple and reliable is pressure (Carroll et al., 1992). Because inspired air flows into the lungs through the nose and mouth, a cannula connected to a pressure transducer can readily measure the pressure changes during breathing. Like the mechanical measurements mentioned above, the output of such a device produces a record very much like the respiratory belt. Unlike the belt, this type of measurement is far less prone to movement artifacts. Any movement of the cannula itself, however, can produce far less effective recordings. A variety of respiratory pressure devices are available that were primarily designed to monitor sleep apnea. Most use a small soft nasal cannula that fits in the nose and over the ears and is often used to deliver oxygen in home medical applications.

Similar to pressure transduction, temperature transducers may also be used to measure breathing. Because air is warmed in the lungs before being exhaled, a temperature sensor can readily detect exhalations. Inhalations can also cool the transducer if sufficiently forceful. Like the pressure transducer, this device is very sensitive to positioning and requires some means to fix its position on the face. Some transducers have a nose or mouth clip to facilitate this process. One additional caveat about this type of sensor is its response speed or time constant. Thermocouples and thermisters used in these devices tend to be rather slow and sluggish in response to rapid changes in temperature. A few devices of this type respond rapidly and investigators interested in the shape of the breathing cycle should be certain that they use a device fast enough to record the responses of interest. Although normal respiratory activity has a cycle of approximately 0.3 Hz (approximately 18 inspirations per minute), the shape of the wave will change much faster and require capturing phenomena of 2.0 Hz and possibly higher. As an example, inhalation of a malodor causes rapid cessation of the inspiration (Frank, Dulay, & Gestland, 2003). In cases such as this, a temperature transducer would be a very poor choice because it tends to be less sensitive to the inspiratory phase of the cycle and slow to react to the change in breathing.

Sound may also be an effective means of determining breathing cycle. A small microphone placed at the nares will record clearly different sounds for inhalation and exhalation allowing the investigator to make a determination of respiratory cycle. Such devices are most often used for recording snoring but can be adapted to record normal breathing sounds by integrating the output of the microphone. As one might imagine, this technique is prone to artifacts from ambient noise. Such artifacts can easily overwhelm the small changes that are due to respiratory activity. Furthermore, should the subject speak, the output from the microphone has the potential to saturate the amplifiers and delay subsequent recordings. Que and colleagues (Que et al., 2002) recently reported on a more sophisticated approach to this problem. Using a tracheal microphone, in a technique they call phonospirometry, they analyzed sounds related to air flow in the lungs and were able to estimate a variety of respiratory parameters including tidal volume. They report that their measures corresponded well to more classic procedures and did not require subject to use mouthpiece or nose clip.

Spirometry is the most widely used technique for evaluating respiratory activity and can be accomplished with a variety of devices. The original spirometers required subjects to use a mouthpiece and nose clamp. Their exhalations were used to displace water under a bell. The volume of the displaced water was used to determine the volume of gas (under pressure) that was expired. More sophisticated devices added simple gas analysis to this operation. Modern approaches to spirometry seldom use water displacement and gas analysis is now far more specific.

Although subjects continue to use a mouthpiece and nose clip, the air they exhale now flows through a tube and fills a bellows or activates a small turbine or pressure transducer attached to a screen. In fact, portable devices now make it possible to collect data with a handheld computer and lightweight spirometry tube that produce data that are comparable to laboratory spirometers (Mortimer et al., 2003). Spirometry tends to concentrate on one phase of the breathing cycle at a time and provides the experimenter with a volume X time plot of the inhalation or, more commonly, the exhalation. Almost all specific respiratory measurements are conducted using spirometery (see Table 10.1). These will be detailed later in this chapter.

In addition to measuring the volume of air inspired or exhaled, it is also common to assess the efficiency of the gas exchange using a gas analysis system. In such a system, the analytic apparatus samples expired air. This apparatus may be a general-purpose analytic system such as a gas chromatograph or a system designed to specifically analyze a particular respiratory gas such as carbon dioxide. In fact, carbon dioxide monitoring is relatively common. Both oxygen and carbon dioxide monitoring equipment provide numeric readouts and most provide a linear analog voltage referred to that readout for connection to recording equipment producing a volume X time recording. Investigators interested in this type of analysis should be concerned about the timing of the analysis. Some devices respond relatively slowly and may not give breath-by-breath responses making the volume X time recording less valuable.

Although not specifically related to spirometery or other respiratory measurements *per se*, non-invasive measure-

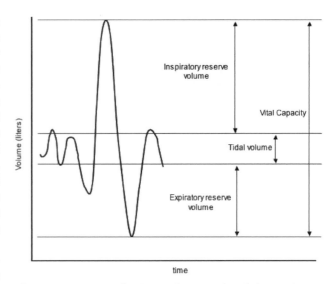

Figure 10.4. A typical spirographic record and the respiratory measurements that can be obtained from this method (adapted from Hlastala & Berger, 1996).

ment of blood gas may be an important part of understanding respiration and its psychophysiological components. Recently, pulse oximetry has become available to record parameters related to blood gases. This technique requires that a transducer, much like a photoplethysmograph be placed on the subject's skin. The pulse oximeter provides an estimate of the percentage of hemoglobin that is saturated with oxygen. This device works similarly to a photoplethysmograph except that it detects the ratio of absorbed light for two different light sources, one of which is specifically absorbed by oxygen bound hemoglobin. This technique provides a rapid readout but is very sensitive to the nature of the vascular bed over which the sensor is placed (Allen, 2004).

5. SPECIFIC RESPIRATORY MEASUREMENTS

Because of the importance of respiratory function to well-being and other physiological systems, it is extensively measured in medical settings. These measurements are standardized and can have a variety of uses for psychophysiologists interested in this system. Ritz and colleagues (2002), in their guidelines for psychophysiological research on respiration, provide a full list of such measurements. Furthermore, subjects undergoing this testing follow a prescribed protocol involving several forced breathing maneuvers. Typical values for many of these measurements are presented in Hlastala and Berger (1996) and some are discussed below. Figure 10.4 shows the relationship of several of these measures to a spirographic record. Some of the more commonly used measures are presented below.

Respiratory frequency (f) is the number of respiratory cycles occurring in one minute. This value ranges from about 12–15 respirations per minute under resting conditions.

Tidal volume (V_T) is the normal volume of air inhaled after an exhalation. It is highly variable but averages about 0.5l.

Vital capacity (V_C) is the volume of a full expiration. This metric depends upon size of the lungs, elasticity, integrity of the airways, and other parameters therefore it is highly variable between subjects. Values may range from 2l to 7l for adults.

Residual volume (V_R) is the volume that remains in the lungs following maximum exhalation. Like other measures that depend upon the size of the chest and lungs, this tends to be highly variable ranging from 1.4l to 1.9l in larger subjects.

Compliance (C) is a measure of the elasticity of the thoracic area. It may be applied to the lungs (C_L), chest wall (C_{CW}) or thorax (C_T). Conceptually it is the resistance to change in response to pressure. Highly compliant lungs, for instance, change in accord with external pressure changes. Thus, one may calculate compliance by determining the ratio of the change in volume (of the lungs or thorax) to changes in pressure. It should be noted that because this is an absolute measure, it is non-linear with respect to lung volume. Volume decreases disproportionately as lungs reach their maximal distention (Hlastala & Berger, 1996).

6. PSYCHOLOGICAL/FUNCTIONAL RELEVANCE

Because adequate ventilation is necessary for all physiological systems to function, it is little surprise that alteration of respiration leads to a cascade of changes throughout the body. Such changes affect the entire functioning of the organism including producing physiological and psychological effects. Some of these effects lead to artifacts in recording of the heart or functional imaging. But, as the preceding sections have shown, a diffuse network controls the respiratory system. The actions of this diffuse network lead many different psychological functions to alter respiration.

6.1. Respiratory effects as artifacts

6.1.1. Skin conductance

Skin conductance and other forms of electrodermal activity (EDA) are dramatically influenced by respiration. Asking subjects to make a deep breath is often used to validate the responsiveness and integrity of the recording system. Despite the sensitivity of EDA to respiratory changes, removal of artifacts due to respiration is difficult. EDA is multiply caused (Dawson, 2002) and rhythmic variations are not tightly coupled to respiratory cycle (Rittweger, Lambertz, & Langhorst, 1997). Recently, Schneider and colleagues (2003) have introduced a technique for identification of respiratory artifacts. It is too soon to know if this technique will enter widespread use for the correction of respiratory effects on EDA.

6.1.2. Heart

The effects of respiratory cycle on the heart are well known to psychophysiologists. The heart period, the time between successive beats, grows longer during exhalations leading to fewer beats per minute. During inhalation, heart period is shorter and consequently, heart rate appears to increase during this phase of respiration. This oscillatory interaction between the heart and respiratory system is know as respiratory sinus arrhythmia (RSA) and is the result of the influence of a variety of different physiological systems. Normally, evaluation of this interaction can produce an estimate of vagal tone in a subject. A full description of these interactions is beyond the scope of this chapter but the reader is referred to the chapter on cardiovascular psychophysiology in this volume for more extensive explanation of this phenomenon. Voluntary ventilation may introduce noise into this system and adversely influence estimates of vagal tone (Wilhelm, Grossman, & Coyle, 2004). Previous findings have indicated that even small changes such as missing an R spike can adversely affect such findings (Berntson & Stowell, 1998).

6.1.3. fMRI

Because functional magnetic resonance imaging (fMRI) is blood oxygenation level dependent (BOLD), it is reasonable to assume that the system that brings oxygen to the blood would be important in regulating the measured response. Consider this example. Subjects are asked to view a variety of pictures that are meant to evoke fear as well as a group of control pictures. Based on subjective ratings, the fear-producing pictures are effective in their emotional evocation and there are clear differences between the BOLD responses for the two picture types. One might conclude that the brain areas showing increased BOLD response during the fear pictures would be associated with the production of that emotion. In some ways they would, but not perhaps in the ways expected by the experimenters. Fear leads to increased ventilation rate and ventilatory effort (Boiten, Frijda, & Wientjes, 1994) due to airway constriction. Likewise, heart rate increases as does stroke volume (Sinha, Lovallo, & Parsons, 1992). Are the differences found in the brain's BOLD response the cause of these changes or their result? Furthermore, because of increases in stroke volume of the heart or the volume of the rib cage, the physical movement of the brain or volumetric disturbances in the magnetic field may impair the ability to accurately image the subjects during the fear evocation.

Correction of breathing and cardiac-related artifacts in fMRI is still controversial and a variety of papers have recently appeared suggesting several approaches. One of the most common is to gate or mask the responses during the different portions of the breathing cycle. Investigators might choose just the peak inspiratory phase of the cycle to make their measurements in BOLD responses or use a digital filter to isolate only BOLD changes in frequencies higher than respirations (Brosch, et al., 2002; Zhu et al., 2003).

6.2. Respiratory changes as a result of psychological influence

6.2.1. Emotion

Emotion has long been known to influence respiration. Descriptions of "breath taking" beauty and fear inducing an inability to "catch one's breath" have been a part of literature and folklore into the ancient past. As mentioned previously, Feleky (1916) recorded the ratio between inspiration and expiration and was able to identify a set of primary emotions. Others followed (Dudley, 1969), but relatively little research has been conducted related to emotion where respiration was the primary physiological variable of interest. Boiten, Fijda, and Wientjes (1994) review this literature and conclude that the major dimensions of emotion that alter respiratory activity are continua of calm-excited and active versus passive coping. They argue that it may be possible to make finer discriminations but the relative paucity of research and interest in this field has impaired our understanding of these phenomena. Subsequent research by Boiten (1998) has specifically addressed the effects of emotion on respiration using both chest and abdominal respiratory strain gauges. Subjects watched short video presentations designed to evoke a variety of emotions. Subjects altered their respiration patterns depending upon the content of the movies with more positive affect being associated with shorter inspiratory cycles. A scene that evoked disgust, led to respiratory pauses. Interestingly, without careful analysis, such pauses might be misinterpreted because long pauses would lead to lower respiratory rates. Such findings serve to illustrate the insufficiency of rate as a helpful measure of respiratory activity. Recently, Gomez, Stahel, and Danuser (2004) conducted a study evaluating respiratory responses to affective pictures confirming the importance of the continua proposed by Boiten and colleagues.

6.2.2. Asthma

Within psychophysiology, asthma is the most widely studied topic related to respiration. The National Institutes of Health report that, in the United States, approximately 15 million persons suffer from this chronic inflammatory disease of the airways. Asthma can be triggered by a reaction to environmental irritants but it is also often triggered by even the suggestion of irritants. Furthermore, it is clearly exacerbated by other stressors in sufferer's psychological environment. In their recent review of the psychological aspects of asthma, Lehrer et al. (2002) describe the nature of these stressors along with potential triggering mechanisms. They advocate the efficacy of symptom recognition and biofeedback for control of the cascade leading to airway constriction.

Ritz (2004) provides an excellent overview of this complicated and important area of research that is beyond the scope of this chapter. Just as the lungs are multiply controlled, so are the airways. The feedback, neural, and humoral regulation all interact and make delineating mechanisms of influence in this system difficult. Even so, the importance of this topic requires addressing the mechanisms at work.

6.2.3. Cognitive activity

Clearly, the reduction of the amount of oxygen in the blood stream can produce grave consequences related to brain function and cognitive ability. These hypoxic events may be related to extreme systems break down such as heart fibrillation, drowning, or suffocation but they may also be related to far less dramatic causes. Sleep apnea (Aloia et al., 2004), nocturnal asthma (Bender & Annett, 1999), and even scuba diving (Slosman et al., 2004) have some cognitive sequelae.

There is little evidence that breathing pattern, so long as it supplies sufficient oxygen, affects cognitive activity. The exception to this statement is a maneuver called "forced unilateral breathing." This exercise originated in yogic training and several studies have demonstrated that occlusion of the left or right nostril alters cognitive function. This is an interesting, varied and surprisingly large literature. Werntz, Bickford, and Shannahoff-Khalsa (1987) found that occlusion of the left or right nostril produces increased EEG amplitudes in the contralateral hemisphere. Contrary to most interpretations of increased EEG amplitude, this finding was interpreted as increased cortical activity and was used to account for behavioral differences associated with the "activated" hemisphere. A different study (Block, Arnott, Quigley, & Lynch, 1989), examined this breathing style on verbal test performance and spatial tasks finding effects for both gender, nostril and task. Males in this study performed spatial tasks better when breathing through the right nostril and the opposite response was found for women. A slightly more recent study by Jella and Shannahoff-Khalsa (1993) found that both men and women showed improved performance during left nostril breathing contradicting the earlier effect in males. Although inconsistent, the preponderance of the literature suggests that right nostril breathing is associated with better verbal performance and left nostril breathing is associated with better spatial performance. These findings have been interpreted as being the result of increased activation in the hemisphere contralateral to the nostril with airflow. Recently, this idea has been extended to research on emotional tones in a dichotic listening paradigm (Saucier et al., 2004).

Although a full review of this literature is inappropriate for this chapter, these studies rarely propose a mechanism by which uninostril breathing might alter hemispheric and/or cognitive activity. Nasal cycle, an alternating ultradian rhythm associated with increased patency of the left or right nostril, is poorly understood and often uncontrolled in these studies. Furthermore, the odor environment in which these studies are conducted is not described. Lorig et al. (1989) demonstrated that nasal versus mouth breathing had a profound influence on EEG and Lorig and coworkers (Lorig, 1999; Lorig, Malin, & Horwitz, 2005) later found that performance of verbal and other symbolic tasks can be impaired when the subject is challenged with an odor. Because the olfactory system projects ipsilaterally, left nostril breathing of odorized air could lead to poorer performance on verbal or symbolic tasks than right nostril breathing due to intrahemispheric competition. Because no air supply is truly odor-free, this simple and overlooked effect has the potential to account for much of the data in this literature. No study has, however, directly evaluated the connection of odor to the cognitive literature related to unilateral nostril breathing.

7. OTHER RESPIRATORY FUNCTIONS

Although breathing is normally associated with gas exchange, it is also an avenue for other functions related to the movement of air. As indicated in the preceding paragraph, odor acquisition is also a function of the respiratory system. Similarly, the muscles of respiration are also used for controlling the air for speech. Although such functions are certainly not the most important aspects of respiration, they are inextricably linked to the gas exchange system and will be briefly included here.

7.1. Odor acquisition

Humans show a remarkable ability to "tune out" odors (Zelano et al., 2005) despite the fact that they have excellent olfactory sensitivity (Lorig, 1999). Recent evidence from several different laboratories has demonstrated odor-related changes in brain activity despite an absence of awareness for the odor (Kirk-Smith et al., 1983; Lorig et al., 1990, 1991; Sobel et al., 1999; Kline et al., 2000; Jacob et al., 2001). With clear evidence of odor effects even when subjects don't notice their presence, it appears likely that each inhalation brings new olfactory information to the nervous system. Certainly, this phenomenon is true of other animals. Freeman and Schnieder (1982) and also Chaput (1986) found that the pattern of electrical activity on the olfactory bulb of rabbits was dependent on respiratory cycle. They suggested that the initiation of an inspiration triggered a "template" related to the odor to which the animal was conditioned. Buonviso et al. (2003) found that the primary component of rhythmic activity in the bulb of rats was dependent upon the respiratory cycle. Lorig and colleagues (Lorig et al., 1996), examined the effect of breathing pattern on chemosensory evoked potentials in humans and found that they differed as a function of whether stimuli were delivered in concert with inspiration or out of phase with this cycle further suggesting the production of such an odor template. In a related fMRI study, Sobel and coworkers (Sobel et al., 1998) found that sniffing produced activation patterns different than smelling,

further illustrating that respiratory activity serves to synchronize a variety of neural sub-systems related to odors and their anticipation.

In a recent study, Kay (2005) describes findings that illustrate how the olfactory-respiratory system is controlled. Based primarily on coherence data, it appears that as odor becomes available, activity in the bulb triggers hippocampal activity that forms a re-entrant loop with the bulb and also descends to influence control of the diaphragm. The odor signals an increase in respiratory effort resulting in sniffing. In a curious way, this process is similar to vision. Availability of visual input leads to movement of the eyes to focus the image on the fovea leading to better discrimination. In the case of olfactory stimuli, sniffing is the movement and this changes the dynamics of airflow in the nasal cavity leading to a change in the distribution of chemicals in the mucosa. Although we have not yet found the olfactory epithelium analog of the fovea, the behavior equivalent is clearly present because previous behavioral research has indicated that sniffing is the most efficient and information-rich way in which to evaluate odors (Laing, 1983).

Recently, it has been suggested that respiratory activity is reflexively truncated in response to a bad odor (Frank et al., 2003). For some time, it has been known that airborne malodors and irritants can affect breathing including reducing tidal volume (Warren et al., 1992) but only recently has a reflexive mechanism been proposed that might be related to odor hedonics. The argument for the reflexive nature is based on the rapidity of this inspiratory cessation. Inhalatory restriction starts at approximately 300 msec following odor availability. Reaction times to these odors tend to be more than 100 msec later (Overbosch et al., 1989) suggesting that the cessation takes place well before detection. Although this is hardly conclusive evidence of a reflexive connection, it does raise the strong possibility that some hedonic information is encoded prior to the action of central nervous system resources necessary for odor detection.

7.2. Speech

Another important aspect of breathing is providing a medium for speech sounds. Although often overlooked as a function of breathing, this is an important problem for subjects requiring artificial ventilation. Coordination of laryngeal movements with enforced lung movements and the availability of an air supply is often difficult to learn. Relatively few reports describe the pathways and mechanisms by which ventilatory movements are coordinated with speech production. It seems likely that such coordination is a product of feedback between cortical speech areas and the areas associated with voluntary breathing although a recent study with cats highlights the importance of the midbrain. Davis and colleagues (Davis et al., 1996) found that the periaqueductal gray area was associated to both respiratory and laryngeal output and their findings suggest that it integrates activity for these sets of muscles.

8. CONCLUSIONS

Like the actions of the heart, respiration is clearly a critical and life sustaining process. As might be expected of any process so important to survival, it is multiply controlled and affects many systems of the body. Likewise, it receives broad input for its regulation. Traditionally, psychophysiology has concentrated on other dependent variables. When respiration was measured it was often used as a covariate or control for the variables of primary interest. Clinical medicine, however, routinely examines the activity of this system and has developed many effective strategies for its assessment. It is within medicine that most of the advances in respiratory measurement have been made in the past few decades.

It is always difficult to imagine what the future holds in a research area. Technical and computational advances will certainly continue. There are already strong trends for more portable devices to measure respiration. Additionally, it is likely that the availability of high level mathematical programming languages designed to work with real data (e.g., MATLAB, LabView, etc.) will have a major impact on the ways that this seemingly simple waveform are viewed. It is also clear that advances such as ambulatory monitoring will lead to new and important insights about respiration in the real world. The fact that a system, ambulatory or not, provides simultaneous measures of so many interrelated dependent variables will beg for more sophisticated analyses than are currently being conducted. One might imagine a mathematical function indicating a parameter called metabolic respiratory demand. Such a function would be based on the long-term, nonlinear multiple regression between blood oxygen saturation, cardiac output and inspiratory volume. Knowing two of the variables should predict the third and the deviance between the predicted and actual values for inspiratory volume might be an indicator of "voluntary override." It would certainly be a curious twist of fate that the characteristic that turned early psychophysiologists away from studying this system (Wientjes & Grossman, 1998), would become an important area of study in the following century.

It is genuinely puzzling that a system with such broad effects on the brain and body is so relatively unstudied by psychophysiologists. There is far more to this system than it appears. Perhaps, as Wientjes and Grossman (1998) have suggested, we will find new insights into the areas of emotion and cognition in the loose coupling of respiration to the other systems of our bodies.

REFERENCES

Allen, K. (2004). Principles and limitations of pulse oximetry in patient monitoring. *Nursing Times, 100*, 34–37.

Aloia, M. S., Arnedt, J. T., Davis, J. D., Riggs, R. L., & Byrd, D. (2004). Neuropsychological sequelae of obstructive sleep apnea-hypopnea syndrome: a critical review. *Journal International Neuropsychological Society, 10*, 772–785.

Bender, B. G., & Annett, R. D. (1999). Neuropsychological outcomes of nocturnal asthma. *Chronobiology International, 16*, 695–710.

Berntson, G. G., Cacioppo, J. T., & Quigley, K. S. (1993). Respiratory sinus arrythmia: Autonomic origins, psychological mechanisms, and psychophysiological implications. *Psychophysiology, 30*, 183–196.

Berntson, G. G., & Stowell, J. R. (1998). ECG artifacts and heart period variability: don't miss a beat. *Psychophysiology, 35*, 127–132.

Block, R. A., Arnott, D. P., Quigley, B., & Lynch, W. C. (1989). Unilateral nostril breathing influences lateralized cognitive performance. *Brain and Cognition, 9*, 181–190.

Boiten, F. A,. Frijda, N. H., & Wientjes, C. J. (1994). Emotions and respiratory patterns: review and critical analysis. *International Journal of Psychophysiology, 17*, 103–128.

Bramann, S. S. (1995). The regulation of normal lung function. *Allergy Procedings. 16*, 223–226.

Brosch, J. R., Talavage, T. M., Ulmer, J. L., & Nyenhuis, J. A. (2002). Simulation of human respiration in fMRI with a mechanical model. *IEEE Transactions on Biomedical Engineering, 49*, 700–707.

Buonviso, N., Amat, C., Litaudon, P., Roux, S., Royet, J. P., Farget, V., & Sicard, G. (2003). Rhythm sequence through the olfactory bulb layers during the time window of a respiratory cycle. *European Journal of Neuroscience, 17*, 1811–1819.

Carroll, N., Clague, J. E., Pollard, M. N., Horan, M. A., Edwards, R. H., & Calverley, P. M. (1992). Portable maximum respiratory pressure measurement – a comparison with laboratory techniques. *Journal of Medical Engineering Technology, 16*, 82–86.

Casili, J. G., Wierwille, W. W., & Cordes, R. E. (1983). Respiratory measurement: Overview and new instrumentation. *Behavior Research Methods, Instruments, and Computers, 15*, 401–405.

Chaput, M. A. (1986). Respiratory-phase-related coding of olfactory information in the olfactory bulb of awake freely-breathing rabbits. *Physiology and Behavior, 36*, 319–324.

Collet, C., Deschaumes-Molinaro, C., Delhomme, G., Dittmar, A., & Vernet-Maury, E. (1999). Autonomic responses correlate to motor anticipation. *Behavioral Brain Research, 29*(63), 71–79.

Comroe, J. H. (1974). *The physiology of respiration, 2nd edition.* Chicago: Year Book Medical Publishers.

Davis, C., Mazzolini, A., Mills, J., & Dargaville, P. (1999). A new sensor for monitoring chest wall motion during high-frequency oscillatory ventilation. *Medical Engineering Physics, 21*, 619–623.

Davis, P. J., Zhang, S. P., Winkworth, A., & Bandler, R. (1996). Neural control of vocalization: respiratory and emotional influences. *Journal of Voice, 10*, 23–38.

De Troyer, A., Gorman, R. B., & Gandevia, S. C. (2003). Distribution of inspiratory drive to the external intercostals muscles in humans. *Journal of Physiology, 546*, 943–954.

De Troyer, A., Kelly, S., Macklem, P. T., Zin, W. A. (1985). Mechanics of intercostal space and actions of external and internal intercostal muscles. *Journal of Clinical Investigation, 75*, 850–7.

Dudley, D. L. (1969). *Psychophysiology of respiration in health and disease.* New York: Appelton-Century-Crofts.

Eccles, R. (1996). A role for the nasal cycle in respiratory defence. *European Respiration Journal, 9*, 371–379.

Ernst, J. M., Litvack, D. A., Lozano, D. L., Cacioppo, J. T., & Berntson, G. G. (1999). Impedance pneumography: Noise as signal in impedance cardiography. *Psychopysiology*, *36*, 333–338.

Evans, S. E., & Scanlon, P. D. (2003). Current practice in pulmonary function testing. *Mayo Clinic Procedings*, 78, 758–763.

Feleky, A. (1916). The influence of emotions on respiration. *Journal of Experimental Psychology*, *1*, 218–222.

Frank, R. A., Dulay, M. F., & Gestland, R. C. (2003). Assessement of the sniff magnitude test as a clinical test of olfactory function. *Physiology and Behavior*, *78*, 195–204.

Freeman, W. J., & Schneider, W. (1982). Changes in spatial patterns of rabbit olfactory EEG with conditioning to odors. *Psychophysiology*, *19*, 44–56.

Fung, M.-L., & St. John, W. M. (1995). Expiratory neural activities in gasping induced by pharyngeal stimulation and hypoxia. *Respiration Physiology*, *100*, 119–127.

Gomez, P., Stahel, W. A., Danuser, B. (2004). Respiratory responses during affective picture viewing. *Biological Psychology*, *67*, 359–373.

Grossman, P. (1983). Respiration, stress and cardiovascular function. *Psychophysiology*, *20*, 284–300.

Grossman, S. A. (1967). *A textbook of physiological psychology*. New York: Wiley.

Guyton, A. C., & Hall, J. E. (2000). *Textbook of Medical Physiology*, *10th ed*, New York: W. B. Saunders.

Han, J. N., Stegen, K., Cauberghs, M., & Vande Woestijne, K. P. (1997). Influence of awareness of the recording of breathing on respiratory pattern in healthy humans. *European Respiratory Journal*, 10, 161–166.

Harada, Y., Kuno, M., & Wang, Y. Z. (1995). Differential effects of carbon dioxide and pH on central chemoreceptors in the rat in vitro. *Journal of Physiology*, *368*, 679–693.

Harver, A., & Lorig, T. S. (2000). Respiration. In Cacioppo, et al. (eds.), *The Handbook of Psychophysiology*, *2nd ed.*, pp. 265–293.

Harver, A., & Mahler, D. A. (1998). Perception of increased resistance to breathing. In H. Kostes & A. Harver (eds.), *Self-management of asthma*. New York: Marcel Dekker, pp. 147–193.

Hlastala, M. P., & Berger, A. J. (1996). *Physiology of respiration*. New York: Oxford University Press.

Jella, S. A., & Shannahoff-Khalsa, D. S. (1993). The effects of unilateral forced nostril breathing on cognitive performance. *International Journal of Neuroscience*, *73*, 61–68.

Jacob, S., Kinnunen, L. H., Metz, J., Cooper, M., & McClintock, M. K. (2001). Sustained human chemosignal unconsciously alters brain function. *Neuroreport*, *8*, 2391–2394.

Johnson, R. L. Jr., & Miller, J. M. (1968). Distribution of ventilation, blood flow and gas transfer coefficient. *Journal of Applied Physiology*, *25*, 1–15.

Kay, L. M. (2005). Theta oscillations and sensorimotor performance. *Procedings of the National Academies of Science*, *102*, 3863–3868.

Kirk-Smith, M., Van Toller, C., & Dodd, G. (1983). Unconscious odour conditioning in human subjects. *Biological Psychology*, *17*, 221–231.

Kline, J. P., Schwartz, G. E., Dikman, Z. V., & Bell, I. R. (2000). Electroencephalographic registration of low concentrations of isoamyl acetate. *Consciousness and Cognition*, *9*, 50–65.

Laing, D. G. (1983). Natural sniffing gives optimum odour perception for humans. *Perception*, *12*, 99–117,

Lehrer, P., Feldman, J., Giardino, N., Song, H. S., & Schmaling, K. (2002). Psychological aspects of asthma. *Journal of Consulting and Clinical Psychology*, *70*, 691–711.

Levine, S., Silage, D., Henson, D., Wang, J. Y., Krieg, J., LaManca, J., & Levy, S. (1991). Use of a triaxial magnetometer for respiratory measurements. *Journal of Applied Physiology*, *70*, 2311–2321.

Lorig, T. S. (1999). On the similarity of odor and language processing. *Neuroscience and Biobehavioral Reviews*, *23*, 391–398.

Lorig, T. S., Herman, K. B., Schwartz, G. E., & Cain, W. S. (1990). EEG activity during administration of low concentration odors. *Bulletin of the Psychonomic Society*, *28*, 405–408.

Lorig, T. S., Huffman, E., DeMartino, A., & DeMarco, J. (1991). The effects of low concentration odors on EEG activity and behavior. *Journal of Psychophysiology*, *5*, 69–77.

Lorig, T. S., Malin, E. L., & Horwitz, J. E. (2005). Odor mixture alters neural resources during symbolic problem solving. *Biological Psychology*, *69*, 205–216.

Lorig, T. S., Matia, D. C., Peszka, J. J., & Bryant, D. N. (1996). The effects of active and passive stimulation on chemosensory event-related potentials. *International Journal of Psychophysiology*, *23*, 199–205.

Lorig, T. S., Schwartz, G. E., Herman, K. B., & Lane, R. (1988). Brain and Odor II: EEG activity during nose and mouth breathing. *Psychobiology*, *16*, 285–287.

McCool, D. F., Wang, J., & Ebi, K. L. (2002). Tidal volume and respiration timing derived from a portable ventilation monitor. *Chest*, *122*, 684–691.

Mortimer, K. M., Fallot, A., Balmes, J. R., & Tager, I. B. (2003). Evaluating the use of a portable spirometer in a study of pediatric asthma. *Chest*, *123*, 1899–1907.

Nielsen, J., & Roth, P. (1929). Clinical spirography. *Archive of Clinical Medicine*, *43*, 132–138.

Overbosch, P., de Wijk. R., de Jonge, T. J., & Koster, E. P. (1989). Temporal integration and reaction times in human smell. *Physiology and Behavior*, *45*, 615–626.

Pauly, J. E. (1957). Electromyographic studies of human respiration, *Chicago Medical School Quarterly*, *18*, 80–88.

Pennock, B. E. (1990). Rib and abdominal piezoelectric film belts to measure ventilatory airflow. *Journal of Clinical Monitoring*, *6*, 276–283.

Que, C. L., Kolmaga, C., Durand, L. G., Kelly, S. M., & Macklem, P. T. (2002). Phonospirometry for noninvasive measurement of ventilation: methodology and preliminary results. *Journal of Applied Physiology*, *93*, 1515–1526.

Richards, D. W., Jr. (1953). The nature of cardiac and pulmonary dsypnea. *Circulation*, *7*, 15–29.

Ries, A. L. (1989). Measurement of lung volumes. *Clinical Chest Medicine*, *10*, 177–186.

Rittweger, J., Lambertz, M., & Langhorst, P. (1997). Influences of mandatory breathing on rhythmical components of electrodermal activity. *Clinical Physiology*, *17*, 609–618.

Ritz, Thomas (2004). Probing the psychophysiology of the airways: Physical activity, experience emotion and facially expressed emotion. *Psychophysiology*, *41*, 809–821.

Ritz, T., Dahme, B., Dubois, A. B., Folgering, H., Fritz, G. K., Harver, A., Kotses, H., Lehrer, P. M., Ring, C., Steptoe, A., & Van de Woestijne, K. P. (2002). Guidelines for mechanical lung function measurements in psychophysiology. *Psychophysiology*, *39*, 546–67.

Rosanski, E. A., & Hoffman, A. M. (1999). Pulmonary function testing in small animals. *Clinical Technique in Small Animal Practice*, *14*, 237–41.

Saucier, D. M., Tessem, F. K., Sheerin, A. H., & Elias, L. (2004). Unilateral forced nostril breathing affects dichotic listening for emotional tones. *Brain and Cognition*, *55*, 403–405.

Sasaki, C. T., & Mann, D. G. (1976). Dilator naris function. *Archive of Otolaryngology, 102*, 365–367.

Schneider, R., Schmidt, S., Binder, M., Schafer, F., & Walach, H. (2003). Respiration-related artifacts in EDA recordings: introducing a standardized method to overcome multiple interpretations. *Psychological Reports, 93*, 907–920.

Sinha, R., Lovallo, W. R., & Parsons, O. A. (1992). Cardiovascular differentiation of emotions. *Psychosomatic Medicine, 54*, 422–435.

Slosman, D. O., De Ribaupierre, S., Chicherio, C., Ludwig, C., Montandon, M. L., Allaoua, M., Genton, L., Pichard, C., Grousset, A., Mayer, E., Annoni, J. M., & De Ribaupierre, A. (2004). Negative neurofunctional effects of frequency, depth and environment in recreational scuba diving: the Geneva "memory dive" study. *British Journal of Sports Medicine, 38*, 108–114.

Sobel, N., Prabhakaran, V., Desmond, J. E., Glover, G. H., Goode, R. L., Sullivan, E. V., & Gabrieli, J. D. (1998). Sniffing and smelling: Separate subsystems in human olfactory cortex. *Nature, 392*, 282–286.

Sobel, N., Prabhakaran, V., Hartley, C. A., Desmond, J. E., Glover, G. H., Sullivan, E. V., & Gabrieli, J. D. (1999). Blind smell: brain activation induced by an undetected air-borne chemical. *Brain, 122*, 209–217.

Sternbach, G. L., Varon, J., Fromm, R. E., Sicuro, M., & Basket, P. J. (2001). Galen and the origins of artificial ventilation, the arteries and the pulse. *Resuscitation, 49*, 119–122.

Sutherland, G. F., Wolf, A., & Kennedy, F. (1938). The respiratory fingerprint of the nervous system. *Medical Record, 148*, 101–103.

Shea, S. A., & Guz, A. (1992). *Personnalite ventilatoire* – An overview. *Respiration Physiology, 87*, 275–291.

Warren, D. W., Walker, J. C., Drake, A. F., & Lutz, R. W. (1992). Assessing the effects of odorants on nasal airway size and breathing. *Physiology and Behavior, 51*, 425–430.

Werntz, D. A., Bickford, R. G., & Shannahoff-Khalsa, D. (1987). Selective hemispheric stimulation by unilateral forced nostril breathing. *Human Neurobiology, 6*, 165–171.

Wientjes, C. J. F., & Grossman, P. (1998). Respiratory psychophysiology as a discipline: introduction to the special issue. *Biological Psychology, 49*, 1–8.

Wilhelm, F. H., Grossman, P., & Coyle, M. A. (2004). Improving estimation of cardiac vagal tone during spontaneous breathing using a paced breathing calibration. *Biomedical Science Instrumentation 40*, 317–24.

Wilhelm, F. H., Roth, W. T., & Sackner, M. A. (2003). The LifeShirt. An advanced system for ambulatory measurement of respiratory and cardiac function. *Behavior Modification, 23*, 671–679.

Wilson, T. A., Legrand, A., Gevenois, P. A., & De Troyer, A. (2001). Respiratory effects of the external and internal intercostal muscles in humans. *Journal of Physiology, 530*, 319–330.

Zelano, C. Bensafi, M., Porter, J., Mainland, J., Johnson, B., Bremner, E., Telles, C., Khan, R., & Sobel, N. (2005). Attentional modulation in human primary olfactory cortex. *Nature Neuroscience, 8*, 114–120.

Zhu, H., Goodyear, B. G., Lauzon, M. L., Brown, R. A., Mayer, G. S., Law, A. G., Mansinha, L., & Mitchell, J. R. (2003). *Medical Physics, 30*, 1134–1141.

11 The Sexual Response

ERICK JANSSEN, NICOLE PRAUSE, AND JAMES H. GEER

1. PROLOGUE

Although physiological responses during sexual activity have been explored as early as in the 1800s (e.g., Mendelsohn, 1896, who described "pulse curves" (EKGs) during sexual intercourse), the first systematic attempts to understand the psychophysiology of sexual response should probably be dated in the first part of the twentieth century, originating with writings on sexual physiology (e.g., Van de Velde, 1926; Dickinson, 1933). These works predated the research of Kinsey and colleagues (Kinsey, Pomeroy, Martin, & Gebhard, 1953), who provided an extensive description of the physiological changes that accompany sexual arousal, and Masters and Johnson (1966), who observed sexual responses in over 650 individuals and summarized their work in a model that has been the stimulus for much psychophysiological research. Initially, researchers relied on direct observation and the use of extragenital measures such as heart rate, respiration, and sweat gland activity to index sexual arousal. Zuckerman (1971), after reviewing the then available literature, concluded that extragenital measures were not specific to sexual arousal. Zuckerman's review of the literature, coupled with Masters and Johnson's (1966) report that myotonia and genital vasocongestion were the most reliable indicators of sexual arousal, accounts for the trend in the field toward the development and use of genital response measures.

2. PHYSICAL CONTEXT

2.1. Anatomical substrate

2.1.1. Men

The principal focus of genital response measurement in men is the penis. The key structures mediating erection are the corpora cavernosa and spongiosum. The two corpora cavernosa are surrounded by a thick fibrous sheath, the tunica albuginea, and share a perforated septum that allows them to function as a single unit. The corpora contain a meshwork of small, interconnected compartments (lacunar spaces), which are lined by vascular endothe-lium and separated by bonds of collagen and smooth muscle (trabeculae). The function of the corpora cavernosa is purely erectile. The corpus spongiosum, which expands to form the glans, also acts as a urinary conduit and an organ of ejaculation. On erection, the corpus spongiosum and the glans develop a modest turgidity.

With the exception of some minor branches from the scrotal and epigastric arteries, the blood supply to the penis is furnished by the two branches of the internal iliac artery, the internal pudendal arteries. After giving off the perineal arteries, they become the penile arteries, which branch off to become a complex of arteries that supplies the penis. Of particular interest are the paired dorsal and cavernous, or deep, arteries of the penis. The dorsal arteries give off circumflex branches and supply blood to the glans penis. The cavernosal arteries run along the middle of each corpus cavernosum, giving off helicine arteries, which open directly into the lacunar spaces (Kirby, 2004). Blood leaves the penis via a number of venous systems, including a network that lies between the smooth muscles and the tunica albuginea. The corpora cavernosa and spongiosum are surrounded by striated muscles. The most important ones, the bulbospongiosus and the ischeocavernosus, support the erect penis and also contract during ejaculation.

2.1.2. Women

The external female genital area is known as the vulva. This area is rich in nerve endings and heavily vascularized. The labia majora, also known as the outer lips, surround the labia minora, or inner lips, which enclose an area called the vestibule. The labia minora fuse to form the clitoral prepuce and fuse under the vaginal opening to form the frenulum. During sexual arousal, the clitoris and the labia minora become engorged, and the latter can increase in diameter by two to three times during sexual excitement (Masters & Johnson, 1966).

The clitoris is composed of the clitoral shaft or corpus, the crura, and the clitoral head or glans. The clitoral body is formed from two corpora cavernosa and a single corpus spongiosum. The bulbs of the clitoris (formerly vestibular bulbs) were only recently characterized (O'Connell, 1998) and are analogous to the corpus spongiosum in men. The clitoral shaft becomes engorged with blood during sexual arousal but women do not have a subalbugineal layer that would reduce venous outflow producing rigidity (Berman, Adhikari, and Goldstein, 2000).

The organ that has been the principal focus of psychophysiological measurement in women is the vagina. The vagina is an almost anaerobic collapsed canal (Levin, 2003) that is more a potential than a permanent space. The canal is formed by two layers. The innermost layer is a nonsecretory, squamous epithelium made of many transverse folds or 'rugae' (Krantz, 1950). Rugae are more prominent in the lower third of the vagina and are thought to provide accordion-like distensibility (Droegemueller, 1992). The epithelium is lined by a lamina propria, which is thick, vascularized connective tissue composed of elastic fibers and a network of blood vessels. Transudate from these blood vessels contributes to vaginal lubrication when forced, by increased pressure in the vessels, through the epithelium to coalesce from sweat-like droplets forming a smooth, lubricative film on the vaginal wall. Small amounts of lubrication are also supplied by the paired greater vestibule, or Bartholin's glands. The two layers are surrounded by the muscularis, or circular smooth muscle (Levin, 1992), which is covered by longitudinal smooth muscle and a fibrous sheath allowing expansion.

Vaginal blood supply originates with the uterine artery, internal iliac artery, and the vaginal artery. The vaginal artery consists of multiple arteries on each side of the pelvis and branches to the anterior and posterior surfaces of the vagina. Vascular responding of the erectile tissues of the introitus and extending to the clitoris is, as with the penis, controlled by the nerves that pass through the nervi erigentes from the sacral plexus. In comparison to men, much less is known about the vascular mechanisms involved in the female genital response.

2.2. Neural/humoral control

2.2.1. Neurophysiology of erection

Erection is essentially a hydrodynamic manifestation, weighing arterial inflow against venous outflow. Cavernous smooth muscles, which are in a tonically contracted state when the penis is flaccid, relax during penile erection (Andersson and Wagner, 1995). This lowers the corporal vascular resistance and results in increased blood flow to the penis. Venous return is diminished by means of a passive occlusion of the subtunical veins pressed against the tunica albuginea.

The spinal cord contains all the necessary components for the coordination and initiation of penile erection (McKenna, 2000). The tone of the penile vasculature and smooth muscles is controlled by both contractant and relaxant factors, which themselves are modulated by local and central processes (Andersson, 2001, 2003). Although the cholinergic, parasympathetic nervous system is the primary proerectile system, normal erection also requires participation of the sympathetic and somatic nervous systems. Parasympathetic nerve endings are sparse in the corpora cavernosa and play primarily a role in the initiation of vasodilatation (Saenz de Tejada et al., 2004). Sympathetic pathways mediate anti-erectile as well as erectile effects. Erection requires inhibition of sympathetically controlled vasoconstriction in the penis, but also activation of sympathetic pathways in the pelvis to assist blood flow to the penis (McKenna, 2000). In addition, full rigidity is dependent on the contraction of striated perineal muscles.

Nonadrenergic noncholinergic (NANC) transmitters, found in both adrenergic and cholinergic nerves (Andersson, 2001), play a central role in penile erection. At present, nitric oxide (NO) is considered to be the principle mediator of corporeal smooth muscle relaxation (Burnett, 1997). NO stimulates the production of cGMP, the second messenger molecule responsible for smooth muscle relaxation. cGMP levels are regulated by the enzyme phosphodiesterase (PDE), of which several subtypes exist. Drugs like sildenafil (Viagra), vardenafil (Levitra), and tadalafil (Cialis) exert their effect by blocking the degradation of cGMP through the inhibition of phosphodiesterase-5, which is relatively specific to the penis (it is found in lower concentrations elsewhere, including lungs and aorta). This thus facilitates erection by increasing bioavailable cGMP in the penis (Gonzalez-Cadavid, Ignarro, & Rajfer, 1999; Wagner & Mulhall, 2001).

Our understanding of the supraspinal control of erection lags behind that of the local neurophysiological and biochemical processes (Bancroft, 2000; McKenna, 1998, 2000, 2001). The presence of descending tonic inhibition has been demonstrated in studies in animals and in humans with spinal cord transections or injury, and is believed to be under control of the nucleus paragigantocellularis, or nPGi, and mediated by serotonin (Giuliano and Rampin, 2000). Serotonin, however, can also have facilitory effects, depending on receptor location and subtype, and this may be relevant to the sometimes conflicting findings on sexual effects of serotonin agonists and antagonists (Andersson, 2001). Other areas that are relevant to penile erection include the amygdala, hippocampus, locus coerulus, periaqueductal gray, and hypothalamus (Bancroft, 2000), of which the medial preoptic area (MPOA) is believed to have a function in the processing of sensory stimuli and the paraventricular nucleus (PVN) in the integration of genital and nongenital autonomic processes (McKenna, 2001).

2.2.2. Neurophysiology of vaginal arousal

Considerably less is known about the neurophysiology of genital response in women than is known about the mechanisms of penile erection. The vaginal epithelium, blood vessels, and smooth muscle are innervated by the sympathetic and parasympathetic divisions of the autonomous nervous system. The striated muscles that surround the vagina are innervated by the somatic nervous system (Levin, 1992). The clitoris, which contains nerve endings similar in number to those found in the male penis (Bancroft, 1989), is innervated by the pudendal nerve.

A number of peptides and neurotransmitters have been located in the female genital tissues. Among these are nitric oxide (NO) and vasoactive intestinal polypeptide (VIP; McKenna, 2002). Hoyle et al. (1996) failed to find NO synthase, the enzyme that manufactures nitric oxide, in approximately half of a group of pre- and postmenopausal women. According to Levin (1997), the available data point to VIP as the likely major neurotransmitter controlling vaginal blood flow and lubrication.

Central mechanisms of sexual arousal are becoming increasingly investigated in women, particularly as peripheral interventions appear relatively ineffective in improving women's self-reported sexual experiences (Basson, McInnes, Smith, Hodgson, & Koppiker, 2002; Laan et al., 2002). Research suggests that women, although reporting similar levels of arousal[1], display less amygdal activation to sexual stimuli than men (Hamann, Herman, Nolan, & Wallen, 2004). Although counterintuitive (if the amygdala are viewed primarily as an emotion center), the authors suggest that it may be more appropriate to view the amygdala as relevant to motivational processes. However, emotional responses to sexual stimuli appear more predictive of levels of sexual desire in men than in women (Prause, Janssen, & Hetrick, 2003). The use of stimuli that are equally effective in men and women is critical when exploring gender differences in neural activation to sexual stimuli, as otherwise findings may reflect simple differences in sexual arousal levels (cf. Janssen et al., 2003).

Recent research examining sexual functioning in women with spinal cord injuries has provided additional insight into the control of sexual response. Sipski et al. (2001) documented a relationship between sympathetic activation and level of genital vasocongestion in response to sexual stimulation, supporting the conclusion of studies in able-bodied women that sympathetic afferents are important in sexual arousal (Meston & Gorzalka, 1996; Meston & Heiman, 1998). Although Whipple and Komisurak (2002) have suggested that the vagus nerve may be the primary afferent, the mechanism by which genital stimulation uses sympathetic pathways to reach the brain is still debated.

2.2.3. Hormonal control

A number of studies have examined the effects of anti-androgens and exogenous androgens in men. There is also literature on the effects of sexual activity or erotic stimuli on hormone levels. However, the most relevant evidence on the role of sex hormones in men comes from studies in hypogonadal men. These studies have shown that within weeks after androgen withdrawal a decline in sexual desire occurs. When considering erectile func-

tion, a more complex picture emerges. Erections during sleep (nocturnal penile tumescence or NPT) are reduced by androgen depletion and restored with androgen replacement. On the other hand, erections to visual erotic stimuli have been found to continue in spite of androgen withdrawal, although the degree and duration of response may be decreased, (Bancroft, 1995). These findings have led to the distinction between androgen dependent and independent erectile responsiveness (Bancroft, 1989). Variations in androgen levels are, however, not believed to lead to variations in sexual behavior and responsiveness, unless variations are significant, as found in hypogonadal men or in adolescents around the time of puberty (Bancroft, 1989; Halpern, Udry, & Suchindran, 1998).

Most studies on the relationship between reproductive hormones and sexual responsiveness in women have assessed these variables across the menstrual cycle (Meuwisen and Over, 1992). Several studies have found that the level of subjective sexual arousal evoked by fantasy, erotic film, and audiotaped stories and genital physiological response to visual sexual stimuli remains stable across phases of the menstrual cycle (Hoon, Bruce, & Kinchloe, 1982; Meuwissen & Over, 1993; Morrell, Dixen, Carter, & Davidson, 1984; Slob, Koster, Radder, & Van der Werff ten Bosch, 1990), whereas some have found higher subjective sexual arousal during periovulatory than during follicular phases (e.g., Graham, Janssen, & Sanders, 2000) and others found vaginal pulse amplitude changes to be higher in premenstrual than in periovulatory phases (Meuwissen & Over, 1993; Schreiner-Engel, Schiavi, Smith, & White, 1981). Among the factors that may explain this lack of consistency in findings, are differences in the method used for determining cycle phase, variations in experimental design, and differences in subject characteristics (Hedricks, 1994).

Increasingly, researchers are exploring the role of other hormones, such as estrogens, oxytocin, and prolactin in sexual response in men and (pre- and postmenopausal) women. Estrogens are necessary for normal vaginal lubrication, and vaginal dryness associated with menopause can be decreased using hormone replacement therapy. Levels of circulating oxytocin increase during sexual arousal and peak during orgasm in both women and men (e.g., Gimpl and Fagrenholz, 2001). Also, a role for orgasmic-released prolactin as an "off switch" of sexual arousal has been proposed (see Kruger et al., 2005) although the evidence is still inconclusive and other mechanisms may be involved, especially in women (Levin, 2003).

Recently, researchers using evoked response potentials (ERP) have found that P300 amplitudes to sexually (or reproductivity) relevant stimuli increase during ovulation (Krug, Plihal, Fehm, & Born, 2000). Changes in ERP responses to nonsexual stimuli, however, have not been found consistently, and when ERP differences were attributed to menstrual cycle phase, did not appear to affect performance in cognitive tasks (Johnston &

---

[1] However, the questionnaire used in this study asked about physical arousal (i.e., did not explicitly ask about sexual arousal: Hanann, 2004, personal communication.

Oliver-Rodriguez, 1997; O'Reilly, Cunningham, Lawlor, Walsh, & Rowan, 2004; Walpurger, Pietrowsky, Kirschbaum, & Wolf, 2004). Thus, although menstrual cycle phase may not consistently affect overt responses or behavior, it does appear to have an effect on attention to sexual stimuli. For these reasons, although the impact of menstrual cycle effects on laboratory findings remains to be established, controls for menstrual phase are advised.

3. SOCIAL CONTEXT

3.1. Measurement milieu

The following discussion of the measurement context in sexual psychophysiological research will only touch upon a few relevant issues. For a more extensive discussion, see Janssen (2002), Prause and Janssen (2006), and Rowland (1999). For the discussion of the political context of sex research in general and sexual psychophysiology in particular, see Bancroft (2005).

3.1.1. Ethical issues

Guidelines for the ethical treatment of research participants (e.g., American Psychological Association, 1992) apply "in spades" to research on sexuality. Due to the personal nature of the inquiry, researchers must be sensitive to the concerns of research participants to ensure both the confidentiality of the data and the comfort and well-being of participants. Particularly important is the clear and understandable description of the details concerning genital response measurement, presentation of sexual stimuli, and of any collection of information concerning sexual practices or attitudes. Thus, participants in sex research are told a great deal about the nature of the studies they take part in, and the effects of this approach are not clear. Amoroso and Brown (1973), in a study on demand characteristics in sex research, found that participants attached to electrical recording devices rated stimuli as more erotic than participants rating the same stimuli outside the laboratory. In another study, Hicks (1970) found that experimenter moods and behaviors influenced both physiological records and subjective reports.

To prevent disease transmission, genital devices should be cleaned using disinfectants such as glutaraldehyde (e.g., Cidex Plus) or ortho-phthalaldehyde (e.g., Cidex OPA). These disinfectants function, depending on how long the devices are immersed, as low- or high-level disinfectants or sterilants. Genital measurement devices require a minimum of high-level disinfection, which destroys all pathogenic microorganisms (bacteria, fungi, and viruses) except for endospores. High-level disinfection has been found to kill Herpes Simplex-II (Morokoff, Myers, Hay, & Flora, 1988), but it is unclear whether it also kills Human Papillomavirus (HPV). Until evidence documents the effectiveness of such cleaning agents in destroying HPV, we recommend a prewash with sodium dodecyl sulfate (SDS). SDS is a common component in shampoo (where it is often listed as sodium lauryl sulfate) that has been shown to kill both HIV and HPV (Howett et al., 1999). Another goal of cleaning is to prevent tissue (e.g., vulvar) irritation. Tissue irritation can result from contact with disinfectants if they are not carefully rinsed off with sterile water.

3.1.2. Volunteer biases

A number of studies have explored differences between volunteers and nonvolunteers for sexuality studies. Differences have been found in sexual experience, frequencies of sexual activity, sex guilt, exposure to erotic materials, and sexual attitudes (e.g., Bogaert, 1996; Morokoff, 1986; Plaud et al., 1999; Strassberg & Lowe, 1995; Wiederman, 1999; Wolchik, Braver, & Jensen, 1985). Some of these studies found psychophysiological studies to be the most susceptible to volunteer biases. However, other studies have failed to find differences between volunteers and nonvolunteers for sex research on personality traits such as extraversion and neuroticism (Farkas et al., 1978), social desirability (Wolchik et al., 1983), and religiosity (Wiederman, 1999). Furthermore, in most cases, the differences that have been found are relatively small. Perhaps more important than differences in averages, however, is whether the *range* of relevant behaviors, attitudes, or experiences is represented in a volunteer sample. For example, Laan and Everaerd (1995), in a meta-analysis of psychophysiological studies involving approximately 300 women, found that 22% of participants had experienced some form of sexual abuse, a proportion similar to that found in the general population. Characteristics of volunteers may, even within a study, affect some variables but not others. Saunders et al. (1985), for example, found volunteer effects on negative affect in response to sexual films, but not on self-reported sexual arousal. Ultimately, the question is not whether differences exist between volunteers and nonvolunteers, but whether such differences influence the validity of our findings and conclusions. That is, the real question is whether the factors responsible for nonparticipation are related to the variables of interest (cf. Tourangeau, 2004).

3.2. Response agreement and within- vs. between-participant designs

A common finding in psychophysiological sex research is that correlations between subjective and genital responses are lower in women than in men (e.g., Laan & Everaerd, 1995). This has lead researchers to speculate about possible gender differences in the role of genital feedback in subjective sexual arousal (e.g., Laan and Janssen, in press). Although correlations tend to be higher in men than in women, discordant response *patterns* have been found as frequently in men. An increasing number of studies have shown that experimental manipulations may modify men's degree of erection although not affecting their subjective sexual arousal (Bach, Brown, and Barlow, 1999; Delizonna et al., 2001; Janssen & Everaerd, 1993; Lankveld and v. d. Hout, 2004). Such findings challenge the notion that subjective sexual arousal in men is strongly influenced by feedback from (changes in) their genitals. Thus, although researchers are largely focusing on the possible explanation of gender differences in correlations between response levels, discordant response *patterns* occur in both men and women, and are not well understood.

Most commonly, correlations between genital and subjective measures of sexual arousal are evaluated in a between-participant design. In this approach, the data used for the computation of correlations are collected across a set of subjects. The resultant statistic reflects the degree to which the two measures covary to a single stimulus presentation. It tells us nothing about individual differences in the relationship between genital and subjective feeling states. In addition, this approach is especially problematic with VPA, a signal that has a relative scale and cannot be calibrated at present, complicating the interpretation of between-subject correlations. Using standardized scores may be an improvement, but this approach forces a normal distribution upon the data and implies linearity of changes that may or may not exist. Although within-participant approaches give us more information about covariance between physiological and subjective responses, they suffer from the problem that response levels will vary from person to person, leading to differences in the range covered by the data. Korff and Geer (1983) applied a within-participant approach that is less sensitive to this problem. Instead of calculating within-participant correlations using the data collected during one sexual stimulus, they computed correlations between stimulus intensity (photos varying in erotic value) and genital change in women. They found, using that methodology, very high within-participant correlations. Within-participant designs also permit the use of the relationship as a dependent variable, allowing researchers to explore how the relationship itself may vary across conditions or individuals.

3.3. Range of applications

Psychophysiological methods are being employed in the exploration of an increasingly broad array of basic and applied questions. The topics include the relationship between subjective and physiological sexual arousal; the interaction between sexual arousal and other emotional states; the activation and inhibition of sexual response; the habituation and conditioning of sexual arousal; the psychophysiology of sexual motivation, desire, and orgasm; the effects of drugs, hormones, and aging on sexual responsivity; the association between sexual orientation and sexual arousal; and the effects of exposure to erotica or pornography on sexual attitudes and behavior. On a more applied level, sexual psychophysiology is used in studies focusing on the detection and diagnosis of sexual dysfunctions and problematic sexual preferences (e.g., pedophilia), and on the assessment of the effectiveness of pharmacological and psychological treatments. Rather

than attempt to review all research areas (for a collection of reviews, see Janssen, in press) we will briefly discuss two categories of clinical psychophysiological research.

3.3.1. Applications concerning arousal and response problems

One of the earliest applications of genital response measurement involves the diagnosis of erectile dysfunction. One of the central questions in the differential diagnosis of erectile dysfunction is to what degree the problem stems from peripheral (e.g., vascular, neurological) problems. Two types of psychophysiological paradigms have been used to evaluate men with erectile dysfunctions. The waking erectile assessment (WEA) approach involves the presentation of erotic stimuli and the determination of whether a normal penile response occurs. The other approach consists of recording erections during sleep to determine if normal nocturnal penile tumescence (NPT) occurs. Sakheim et al. (1985) reported 80% diagnostic accuracy in identifying functional versus organically impaired men using a waking assessment paradigm. Janssen et al. (1994a), found similarly high predictive values using a procedure in which patients were presented with combinations of visual, tactile, and cognitive stimuli.

Although early studies in men with premature ejaculation failed to find evidence for atypical response patterns, more recent studies have both confirmed and challenged some assumptions about the mechanisms involved in ejaculatory problems (see for review, Rowland, Tai, & Brummett, in press). For instance, rapid ejaculation in men with premature ejaculation occurs mainly in response to (vibro) tactile genital stimulation, not to erotic stimulation in general. Also, subjective sexual arousal levels are not higher in men with premature ejaculation than in sexually functional men, suggesting that the former are not "hyperaroused," although heart rate during sexual stimulation tends to accelerate in men with premature ejaculation, although it decelerates in sexually functional controls, suggesting that differences in autonomic control exist between men with and without premature ejaculation. Less is known about inhibited or retarded ejaculation.

Vaginal photoplethysmography (see section 4.1.2.3.) does not consistently differentiate women with and without sexual problems (Morokoff & Heiman, 1980), nor is it clear that it should because the measure is relative. However, some researchers have documented reduced VBV for women with arousal problems (Palace & Gorzalka, 1990; Wincze, Hoon, & Hoon, 1976), reported reduced VPA during penetration film clips for women with dyspareunia (Wouda et al., 1998), identified women with sildenafil-responsive arousal and orgasm problems (Basson & Brotto, 2003), predicted orgasm latency (Laan & van Lunsen, 2002), and identified radical hysterectomy patients with extensive vaginal deenervation (Maas et al., 2004).

Individual differences in the relationship between genital and subjective sexual responses may increasingly become a focus in the development and evaluation of interventions for sexual problems in women. Drugs like sildenafil have been found to increase genital blood flow, although not necessarily affecting subjective sexual arousal in women. New pharmacological interventions are being developed that target central mechanisms, including dopamine agonists to increase sexual desire (Bechara, Bertolino, Casabe, & Fredotovich, 2004; Beharry, Hale, Wilson, Heaton, & Adams, 2003; Caruso et al., 2004; Everaerd & Laan, 2000, see also Rosen et al., in press). However, some of the effects of these agents resemble those of addictive substances and this warrants caution. More importantly, considering the variable relationship between subjective and genital sexual responses in women, the development of any type of treatment, ideally, should involve the evaluation of both genital and subjective responses.

3.3.2. Applications concerning specific object preferences

The second type of clinical application involves sexual object preferences. Psychophysiological methods have been used to both diagnose and track the progress of treatment of individuals whose sexual preferences involve adolescent or preadolescent children (e.g., Seto, 2001, in press). Although adult men with no pedophilic preferences can show sexual arousal to pedophilic stimuli (e.g., Hall, Hirschman, and Oliver, 1995), the use of psychophysiological methods within clinical samples has been found to have high predictive validity. Recent meta-analyses found that genital response to depictions of children was the single best predictor of sexual offense recidivism, exceeding all other indicators of sexual deviancy and any developmental, personality, or demographic variable (Hanson and Bussiere, 1998; cf. Kuban et al., 1999; Seto, 2001).

Similarly, sexual aggressive men and rapists have been studied using psychophysiological methods. Barbaree et al. (1979) reported significant correlations between a statistic obtained by dividing the percent of erection to rape cues by the percent of erection to cues of consenting heterosexual activity and the frequency of previously reported rapes as well as with the tendency to commit violent rapes. Lohr, Adams, and Davis (1997) reported that whereas men with sexually coercive histories showed greater penile responding to coercive cues, males with no history also yielded some arousal to those same cues. Similarly, Janssen et al. (2002) found that male college students with no history of offending who scored low on a measure of sexual inhibition proneness, showed erectile responses to depictions of rape that were indistinguishable from their responses to consensual sexual films. These findings makes clear the fact that arousal to a particular stimulus category does not necessarily correspond with behavior. In women there are reports of rape victims responding with vaginal lubrication and even orgasm during a sexual assault (Levin and van Berlo, 2004). Laan et al. (1994) found that women responded equally with genital arousal to male- versus female-oriented erotica even though the women reported that they found the female-oriented erotica more arousing. Again, care must be taken before one accepts genital responding as the "golden rule" of sexual arousal, and thus sexual object preference. Sexual arousal, as is true for other emotional states, is a complex phenomenon that expresses itself in multiple response systems that are not always closely tied together.

4. INFERENTIAL CONTEXT

4.1. Mensuration and quantification

The following discussion will not cover all possible measures but will only include those that are most widely used.

4.1.1. Male genital measurement devices

The first to measure genital response in men was a simple electromechanical transducer (Ohlmeyer, Brilmayer, & Hullstrung, 1944) that provided a binary signal of the presence or absence of erection. Current research in male sexual arousal relies primarily on continuous measures of penile volume, circumference, and rigidity.

4.1.1.1. *Volume.* Freund (1963) developed an air volumetric plethysmograph. Less widely used variants of this technique have been described by Fisher et al. (1965), who used water instead of air, and McConaghy (1976). The plethysmograph is positioned on the participant by the experimenter, who places a sponge-rubber ring and plastic ring with an inflatable cuff over the penis. A glass cylinder with a funnel at the top is fitted over the other components, and the cuff is inflated with air. Changes in the size of the penis result in displacement of air, which can be detected by a pressure transducer.

Volumetric devices can be calibrated in terms of absolute penile volume and have the advantage of offering high sensitivity. A limitation of this technique, however, is that it does not allow for the determination of the source of change (e.g., circumference or length). In addition, the apparatus is relatively complex, cumbersome, and sensitive to temperature and movement artifacts.

4.1.1.2. *Circumference.* Originally described by Fisher and colleagues (1965), the first circumferential measure, the mercury-in-rubber strain gauge, was adapted from a similar transducer used by Shapiro and Cohen (1965). The device consists of a hollow rubber tube filled with mercury and sealed at the ends with platinum electrodes. The operation of the mercury-in-rubber strain gauge depends upon penile circumference changes that cause the rubber tube to stretch or shorten, thus altering the cross-sectional area of the column of mercury within the tube. The resistance of the mercury inside the tube varies directly with its cross-sectional area, which in turn is reflective of changes in the circumference of the penis. Variations of the mercury-in-rubber gauge have been described by Bancroft et al. (1966), Jovanovic (1967), and Karacan (1969).

Another type of penile strain gauge is the electromechanical strain gauge developed by Barlow and co-workers (1970). This device is made of two arcs of surgical spring material joined with two mechanical strain gauges. These gauges are flexed when the penis changes in circumference, producing changes in their resistance. The resistance changes are in turn coupled through a bridge circuit to a polygraph or computer. The electromechanical gauge does not fully enclose the penis. For this reason, it is more sensitive to movement artifacts and less suitable for studies on nocturnal penile tumescence (NPT) than the mercury-in-rubber gauge. However, mechanical strain gauges are quite sensitive and more rugged than their rubber counterparts. Both types of strain gauge are available from Behavioral Technology, Inc. (Salt Lake City, Utah) and the rubber strain gauge is also manufactured by Hokanson, Inc. (Bellevue, Washington).

4.1.1.3. *Comparison studies on volume and circumference measures.* Freund, Langevin, and Barlow (1974) compared the volumetric device with Barlow's electromechanical strain gauge. They presented a group of men slides of male and female nudes. Their results indicated that volumetric plethysmography is more sensitive to changes in penile tumescence. However, considering the type and number of stimuli used, and the absence of a check for habituation, their conclusion most likely pertains to relatively low response levels. McConaghy (1974) compared his adaptation of the volumetric device with a mercury strain gauge. He showed his subjects 10-second shots of male and female nudes that were inserted in a neutral film. In his paper he provides some example recordings, but no statistical analyses. In 1987, Wheeler and Rubin compared the mercury gauge and Freund's volumetric device, using erotic film excerpts, in 6 subjects. In contrast to Freund et al. (1974), they did not find any evidence for a higher sensitivity of the volumetric device. In addition, the authors reported that the volumetric device was more difficult to use and displayed more artifacts than the strain gauge (however, they did not use an inflatable cuff, Kuban et al., 1999). The absence of systematic differences in Wheeler and Rubin's (1987) study may due to the possibility that their film stimuli induced higher response levels than the slides used by Freund and colleagues.

More recently, Kuban et al. (1999) compared the mercury gauge and volumetric device in 42 heterosexual men who were presented with sexual slides and audiotaped narratives. They found that the two devices were comparable at 'high' response levels (>2.5 mm circumference change), where correlations exceeded .80. In contrast, correlations were nonsignificant at lower response levels, where only the volumetric device differentiated responses to images of adult and pubescent females from other (prepubescent) stimuli. Unfortunately, Kuban et al.'s (1999) conclusions were based on between-participant comparisons of low

and high responders, instead of on low and high (i.e., within-participant) response *levels*. Undetermined differences between the two groups (e.g., in attitudes or experience) may have contributed to the findings, rendering as premature the authors' suggestion that lower circumferential responses may be less valid.

Due to the ease of their use, penile strain gauges have remained relatively popular in laboratory use (e.g., Bach et al., 1999; Delizonna et al., 2001; Hoffmann et al., 2004). A number of in vitro studies have shown that both the mercury-in-rubber and the electromechanical strain gauge demonstrate linear outputs, high test-retest reliability, high stability over time, and minor sensitivity to temperature (e.g., Karacan, 1969; Farkas et al., 1979; Earls and Jackson, 1981; Richards et al., 1985; Richards et al., 1990; Janssen et al., 1997). Nowadays, the mercury-in-rubber strain gauge is also available in versions filled with an indium-gallium alloy, which is considered to be even less sensitive to temperature than mercury (Richards et al., 1985).

A potential concern with the use of circumferential measures is the suggestion that penile circumference may show a slight decrease at the onset of sexual arousal (McConaghy, 1974; Abel et al., 1975; Laws and Bow, 1976; see also Kuban et al., 1999). A brief decrease in circumference may represent a problem in that it may be incorrectly interpreted as a decrease in sexual response. Further, it has also been noted that strain gauges may be unreliable at the upper end of the tumescence curve (Earls et al., 1983). This may represent a limitation if the measures are to be used for determining the full range of erectile capacity.

Laws (1977), who was the first to compare the two strain gauges in vivo, found discrepancies in measurement with the two devices. Unfortunately, he obtained data from only one participant. Janssen et al. (1997) compared the two penile strain gauges, using indium-gallium instead of mercury for the rubber gauge, in a group of 25 sexually functional men. In addition, they compared two different calibration methods, using a circular and an oval shaped device. The electromechanical gauge calibrated on the circular device reported greater circumference changes. Circumference changes were not different when the oval calibration device was used. In addition, the findings suggested that the electromechanical gauge is more sensitive to changes in penile circumference during initial stages of erection than the rubber gauge, a conclusion that is consistent with earlier in vitro findings (Earls and Jackson, 1981; Richards et al. 1985), and that should be taken into consideration when comparing the advantages and disadvantages of volumetric and circumferential measures (cf. Kuban et al., 1999 and Wheeler and Rubin, 1987, who compared volumetry with the mercury-in-rubber gauge).

4.1.1.4. *Rigidity.* One of the first attempts to measure penile rigidity was made by Karacan et al. (1978), who reported the use of "buckling pressure" as a dependent variable in penile responding. This method uses a device that measures the axial force required for the bending

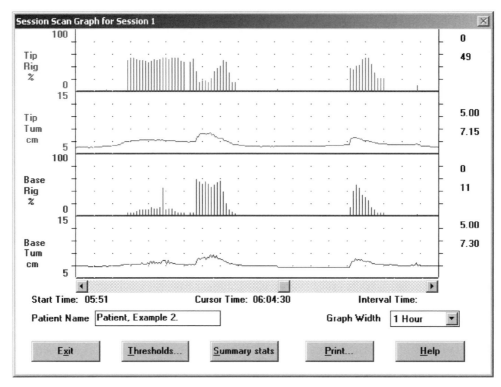

Figure 11.1. Example of output of the RigiScan. The vertical lines represent rigidity and the continuous ones penile circumference as measured at the base (bottom two signals) and the tip (top two signals) of the penis.

of the penis. Although it is mainly used in clinical studies (e.g., Goldstein et al., 2000), and has some predictive value, basic information on the validity and reliability of this method is still largely absent (Schiavi, 1992). Also, the rationale that is typically provided for preferring the measurement of axial over radial rigidity (i.e., intercourse involves mostly axial forces), though sensible, lacks an empirical basis. Other noncontinuous, discrete methods for indexing rigidity include stamp tests, the Snap Gauge, and the Erectiometer (Slob et al., 1998).

Bradley and Timm (1985) first described the RigiScan Plus monitor (Timm Medical Technologies, Eden Prairie, MN), an instrument designed to measure continuously both circumference and radial rigidity, and that can be used in real-time or ambulatory mode. The device consists of a recording unit, that can be strapped around the waist or thigh, and has two loops, one that can be placed around the base of the penis and the other just behind the corona. Each loop contains a cable that is tightened at discrete time intervals. Circumference is measured at 15-second intervals. The Rigiscan takes its first rigidity measure when a 20% increase in circumference is detected. This is repeated every 30 seconds (see Figure 11.1). To measure rigidity, the loops tighten a second time after circumference is measured, with a force of 2.8 Newton.

The Rigiscan represents the first practical measure of continuous rigidity, and has gained wide acceptance, particularly in clinical research. However, there are no published data on the test-retest reliability of the Rigiscan.

Information on the reliability of the device over longer periods of usage is pertinent because in contrast to strain gauges, where routine calibration allows for the test of linearity over time and where replacement is viable, a Rigiscan is typically used for a number of years. The importance of developing a calibration method for the Rigiscan is stressed by the finding of Munoz, Bancroft, and Marshall (1993) that different Rigiscan devices can record different degrees of rigidity. In their study, Munoz et al. (1993) developed a system that provided a relatively constant circumference with variable rigidity. Using this system they found that the Rigiscan underestimated circumference, in particular at lower levels of rigidity. This finding was confirmed by a comparison between the performance of the Rigiscan and a mercury-in-rubber strain gauge in the measurement of NPT (Munoz et al., 1993).

The measurement procedure used by the Rigiscan also raises questions about its potential reactivity. The extent to which the tightening of the loops may induce or modify sexual responses has not been assessed. Relevant to this, Munoz et al. (1993) found fewer NPT episodes in a group of men with erectile problems when a mercury-in-rubber strain gauge was used together with a Rigiscan as compared to nights during which only a strain gauge was used.

The two main arguments in support of the development and usage of rigidity measures have face validity: (1) Penile circumference is not a reliable predictor of rigidity, and (2) rigidity is the ultimate, behaviorally relevant measure of erectile capacity. Regarding the first assertion, two studies have been cited frequently. Wein and associates (1981) reported that significant changes in penile circumference occurred in 23% of normal control patients without sufficient increases in rigidity for vaginal penetration. Earls et al. (1988) reported finding discrepancies in circumference and participants' perception of erectile sufficiency for intromission. Wein et al. (1981), however, based their conclusions on the measurement of buckling force, which lacks proper validation (Schiavi, 1992). As for the second study, it is well established that the perception of erectile responses is biased in patient groups (Sakheim et al., 1987; Janssen and Everaerd, 1993). More importantly, however, with the availability of the Rigiscan, studies would be expected to test the relationship between circumference and rigidity. Remarkably, only one study to date has explored the relationship between the Rigiscan's base and tip circumference and rigidity measures (Levine and Carroll, 1994), and found correlations of $r = .87$ and $r = .88$, respectively.

Regarding the second issue, the key problem in erectile dysfunction is considered to involve a lack of rigidity (e.g., Giesbers et al., 1987). However, the question of what level of rigidity is sufficient has not yet been answered. Wabrek et al. (1986) and Wagner et al. (1986) gathered normative data on vaginal penetration pressure and found that it varied among positions (e.g., supine versus kneeling) and that it was lower during conditions of sexual stimulation. These studies indicate that, at present, any clinical criterion for deciding whether an erection is sufficiently rigid for penetration is a predictor, rather than an absolute measure, of erectile functionality in interactions with a partner.

4.1.1.5. *Other measures of genital response in men.* Less widely used measures involve the assessment of penile temperature, penile arterial pulse amplitude, and penile EMG. Thermistor devices have been designed to detect temperature changes that may accompany penile tumescence. Solnick and Berrin (1977) found a relatively high concordance between temperature changes and penile circumference. Webster and Hammer's results (1983) supported their findings.

Bancroft and Bell (1985) developed a reflectance photometer for the measurement of penile arterial pulse amplitude. The components of this device are similar to those used in the vaginal photometer, described later. It has been suggested that penile pulse amplitude may provide an index of arterial inflow related to generalizable penile tumescence (Rosen and Beck, 1988). However, the currently available data are insufficient to warrant a judgment on the usefulness of the penile photometer.

Wagner and Gerstenberg (1988) first described electrical activity in the cavernous tissues of the penis, using needle electrodes, and found that the perception of visual sexual stimuli resulted in decreased smooth muscle activity (Wagner & Gerstenberg, 1988; Gerstenberg et al., 1989; Wagner et al., 1989). Although one of the most sensitive measures of male genital response at present, the reliabil-

ity of the technique is still controversial. Various investigators have failed to reproduce the original findings. More problematic, however, is that the interpretation of the signal is hampered by the lack of information on its characteristic features and by the absence of standardized recording techniques. The recording of penile EMG is susceptible to sources of interference such as pelvic and penile muscle contractions, cross-talk due to cardiac action, and respiration (Jüneman et al., 1994). The non-invasive alternative, using surface electrodes, has been less well studied and also may be expected to be sensitive to interference. However, work on a consensus in measuring penile EMG is in progress and recommendations have been made for research that could increase our understanding of the electrophysiology of the corpora cavernosa (Sasso et al., 1997; Jiang et al., 2003).

4.1.2. Female measures

One of the first devices designed to measure female physiological sexual arousal recorded vaginal pH, as an indicator of lubrication (Shapiro et al., 1968). This method proved technically difficult and intrusive (Berman et al., 2001; Wagner & Levin, 1978) and researchers tended to document inconsistent and highly localized pH changes (Wagner & Levin, 1984). A second device, a mechanical strain gauge, was developed to measure clitoral enlargement in women with enlarged clitori from congenital adrenal hyperplasia (CAH), but the device has not been tested in nonclinical samples (Karacan, Rosenbloom, & Williams, 1970). A third, balloon-like device was developed to measure uterine contractions (Bardwick, 1967; Jovanovic, 1971), and another one for vaginal pressure (Berman et al., 2001), but the uterine device proved problematic because its placement could be painful and the device was occasionally extruded (Rosen and Beck, 1988). More recently, researchers are attempting to quantify clitoral blood flow and clitoral size changes using Doppler ultrasonography (Bechara et al., 2004; Khalifé & Binik, 2003; Munarriz, Maitland, Garcia, Talakoub, & Goldstein, 2003). Although the measurements appear to be reliable across analysts (Berman et al., 2001), currently the method requires a technician to hold the device in place during measurement (Khalife, Binik, Cohen, & Amsel, 2000). Finally, researchers are exploring the utility of electromyography, with concentric needle electrodes, in evaluating clitoral autonomic innervation and genital sensitivity (Yilmaz, 2002, 2004). However, further research is needed to further establish its validity and to determine the role of genital sensitivity in sexual arousal.

4.1.2.1. *Oxygenation and thermal clearance.* Levin and Wagner (1978) described a method in which a heated oxygen probe is used to detect changes in oxygen pressure (pO2) in the vaginal wall. The device consists of an oxygen electrode and a suction cup that is held on the vaginal wall by a partial vacuum generated in the cup. It is assumed that the more blood present in the tissues, the greater the amount of oxygen will be perfused across the vaginal epithelium. Using this device, it is possible to reliably determine the level of oxygen in the blood of the tissues located beneath the device. The actual dependent variable used is pO2, which is expressed in millimeters mercury.

The same device can also measure heat dissipation into the tissues under the transducer. This approach measures the amount of energy (e.g., milliwatts) that is required to keep the temperature of a heated thermistor constant. The heated oxygen probe has contributed to our understanding of the mechanisms underlying genital response in women (Levin, 1992) and the technique has been replicated (Sommer, 2001). An advantage of the device is that it is relatively free of movement artifacts. Disadvantages are the intrusiveness of the procedure and the need to limit duration of measurement sessions to protect the vaginal mucosa from damage from heat and suction needed to hold the device in place (Levin, 1992).

4.1.2.2. *Temperature.*
Fisher and Osofsky (1968) and Fisher (1973) used a thermistor to measure vaginal temperature and found that vaginal temperature reflects core temperature and is relatively insensitive to changes in sexual arousal. Fugl-Meyer, Sjogren, and Johansson (1984) described a radiotelemetric method for measuring vaginal temperature, using a battery-powered transducer mounted on a diaphragm ring. They reported decreases in vaginal temperature, measured during masturbation and intercourse, that were speculated to be the result of vaginal wall edema during sexual arousal (Wagner and Levin, 1978). Advantages of the device include its usability in natural settings. However, in view of the conflicting reports, replication is needed to establish the value of vaginal temperature as a measure of sexual arousal.

Henson et al. (1978) designed a transducer for measuring labial temperature. One thermistor monitors ambient room temperature, another monitors changes in skin temperature at an extragenital site, and a final thermistor is attached to the labia minora using a brass clip. Labial temperature of 9 of the 10 participants in Henson et al.'s study (1978) increased in response to an erotic film. Slob et al. (1990) and Slob et al. (1991) also found an increase in labial temperature in the majority of participants during the presentation of erotic stimuli. Slob et al. (1990) compared women with and without diabetes mellitus and found initial labial temperatures to be lower in the diabetic women. Differences between the two groups disappeared when participants were matched on initial labial temperature.

4.1.2.3. *Vaginal and labial pulse amplitude/blood volume.*
The most widely used method for monitoring genital responses in women is vaginal photoplethysmography. This technique uses a vaginal photometer, originally used by Palti and Bercovici (Palti & Bercovici, 1967) and refined by Sintchak and Geer (1975) and Hoon, Wincze, and Hoon (1976). The device, made by Behavioral Technology, Inc.

(Salt Lake City, Utah), is made of clear acrylic plastic and is shaped like a menstrual tampon. Embedded in the front end of the probe is a light source that illuminates the vaginal walls. Light is reflected and diffused through the tissues of the vaginal wall and reaches a photosensitive cell surface mounted within the body of the probe. Changes in the resistance of the cell correspond to changes in the amount of back-scattered light reaching the light-sensitive surface. It is assumed that a greater back-scattered signal reflects increased blood volume in the vaginal blood vessels (Levin, 1992). Hoon et al. (1976) introduced an improved model of the vaginal photometer that substituted an infrared LED (light-emitting diode) for the incandescent light source and a phototransistor for the photocell. These innovations reduced potential artifacts associated with blood oxygenation levels, problems of hysteresis, and light history effects. The vaginal photometer is designed so that it can be easily placed by the participant. A shield can be placed on the probe's cable so that depth of insertion and orientation of the photoreceptive surface is known and held constant (Geer, 1983; Laan, Everaerd, & Evers, 1995).

The photometer yields two analyzable signals. The first is the DC signal, which is thought to provide an index of the total amount of blood (Hatch, 1979), often abbreviated as VBV (vaginal blood volume). The second is the AC signal, often abbreviated as VPA (vaginal pulse amplitude), which is thought to reflect phasic changes in the vascular walls that result from pressure changes within the vessels (Jennings et al., 1980; see Figure 11.2). Although both signals have been found to reflect responses to erotic stimuli (e.g., Geer, Morokoff, & Greenwood, 1974; e.g., Hoon, Wincze, & Hoon, 1976), their exact nature and source is unknown. Heiman et al. (2004) compared, in 12 women, VPA and genital volume changes as measured using MRI, and found no significant correlations between the two. Heiman and Maravilla (in press) suggested it may be possible that at moderate levels of arousal the vaginal probe might detect changes to vaginal tissue that do not correspond with other genital blood volume changes. (Interestingly, however, the same study reported higher correlations with subjective sexual arousal for VPA than for MRI variables.) The interpretation of the relationship between the photometer's output and the underlying vascular mechanisms is hindered by the lack of a sound theoretical framework (Levin, 1992) and of a calibration method allowing transformation of its output in known physiological events. At present, most researchers describe their findings in relative measures, such as mm pen deflection or change in microVolts. Levin (1997) stated that one of the basic assumptions underlying use of the plethysmograph is that changes in VBV and VPA always reflect local vascular events. In his discussion of findings from studies on the effects of exercise and orgasm on VBV and VPA, however, he suggests that the signals are likely to reflect rather complex interactions between sympathetic and parasympathetic regulatory processes and between circulatory and vaginal blood pressure. However, Prause et al. (2005) found that, whereas VPA

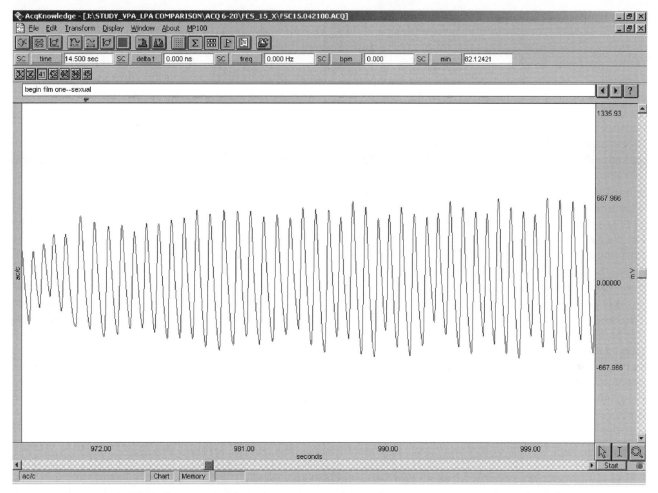

Figure 11.2. Example of a Vaginal Pulse Amplitude (VPA) signal obtained from the vaginal photo-plethysmograph.

discriminated between sexual, sexually threatening, and threatening film stimuli, blood pressure (while increased during all three conditions) did not.

The construct validity of VPA is better established than that of VBV. Researchers have reported high correlations between VPA and VBV, particularly with stronger sexual stimuli, but others have found low or no concordance between the two signals (Heiman, 1976; Meston and Gorzalka, 1995). VPA appears to be more sensitive to changes in stimulus intensity than VBV (Geer et al., 1974; Osborn & Pollack, 1977). VPA also corresponds more closely with subjective reports of sexual arousal than VBV (Heiman, 1977). Finally, VBV changes in response to increases in *general* arousal, indicating that VBV is less specific to sexual arousal than VPA (Laan, Everaerd, & Evers, 1995). Two studies have directly assessed the sensitivity and specificity of VPA (Laan et al., 1995; Prause, Cerny, & Janssen, 2005). Both studies measured responses of sexually functional women to sexual, anxiety inducing, sexually threatening, and neutral film excerpts, and found maximal increases in VPA to the sexual stimulus and moderate increases to the sexually threatening film. (Participants also reported intermediate levels of sexual arousal to the sexual-threat stimulus.) On both studies, VPA did not increase in response to anxiety-inducing stimuli. These results demonstrate response specificity of vaginal vasocongestion to sexual stimuli.

The study by Prause et al. (2005) included the comparison of VPA with a new measure of genital blood flow, the labial photoplethysmograph. Labial pulse amplitude (LPA), as measured by the labial photoplethysmograph, exhibited a degree of specificity to sexual stimuli that was similar to that found for VPA. Additionally, the labial photoplethysmograph demonstrated greater resistance to movement artifacts and a slightly higher correspondence with subjective measures of sexual arousal. Because it is worn externally, researchers can verify the placement of the device by visual inspection. The labial photoplethysmograph, though somewhat more difficult to place and less comfortable than its vaginal counterpart, warrants further development.

4.1.2.4. Comparison studies on temperature and pulse amplitude/blood volume. The literature comparing genital response measures in women is scant. Only one study has compared the measurement of vaginal temperature with vaginal blood flow (Gillan & Brindley, 1979).

However, that study used an atypical photometer (with more than one photocell). No studies have been published on the direct comparison of heat oxygenation and vaginal plethysmography. In contrast, various studies have been reported on the relationship between labial temperature and vaginal blood flow. Henson and Rubin (1978) and Henson, Rubin, and Henson (1982) compared changes in VBV and labial temperature in response to sexual films. Both measures were found to increase during stimulation, although there were large individual differences. Henson and Rubin (1978) found a low, nonsignificant correlation between VBV and labial temperature. Further, only correlations between labial temperature and subjective arousal were significant, leading to the suggestion that physiological changes in the labia might be more easily perceived than intravaginal changes. Although vaginal responses tended to decrease more quickly after stimulus presentations, neither instrument returned to pre-stimulus baseline levels.

In two other studies, C. Henson, Rubin, and Henson (1979) and D. Henson, Rubin, and Henson (1979) compared labial temperature with both the VPA and VBV signals of the vaginal plethysmograph. D. Henson et al. (1979) determined that, although there was considerable intrasubject consistency in response patterns and amplitudes across two recording sessions, labial temperature was the most consistent on both parameters. In the second study, C. Henson et al. (1979) found high correlations between subjective arousal and both VPA and labial temperature changes. VBV correlated less strongly with subjective arousal and returned to baseline more slowly than either VPA or labial temperature.

With respect to the advantages and disadvantages of each device. D. Henson et al. (1979) noted that ambient temperature control is a requirement for use with the labial clip but not with the vaginal transducer. In contrast, movement artifacts are more common with the vaginal probe, and reliable measurement with the thermistor is not precluded by the menses (there are, as yet, no published reports of vaginal photometer readings during menses). Levin (1997) asserted that the output of the vaginal measure, and in particular VBV, is readily invalidated because the photometer can slide over the lubricated epithelium, illuminating new areas of tissue.

Another important difference between the two devices is that the labial thermistor uses an absolute unit of measurement (°C), whereas changes in vaginal blood flow are relative. Further, it is not yet known to what extent factors related to individual variations in anatomy and to physiological characteristics, such as resting levels of vaginal muscular tone and vaginal moistness, may affect the amplitude of the vaginal blood flow signal. Finally, although sensitivity of the probe to temperature appears to be minimal, it is in fact the temperature of the light source that is most often a concern. It is not implausible that vaginal temperature itself can alter the probe's output, thus confounding the data (Beck, Sakheim, & Barlow, 1983).

Rogers et al. (1985), in a study on genital responses during sleep, used a measure of integrated VPA and muscle-contraction pressure, which enabled the detection of movement and muscle contractions. It may prove valuable to extend the current design of the vaginal plethysmograph with additional measures of muscle-contraction pressure and temperature.

4.1.3. Cross-sex measurement devices

The desire to directly compare sexual responses in men and women has been the impetus for the development of several measurement devices. Unfortunately, the challenge reaches beyond the mere development of a measure that can be used in similar locations, and is complicated by differences in the innervation and vascularization of the male and female genitalia.

4.1.3.1. *Anal blood flow and muscle activity.* Bohlen and Held (1979) described a device to monitor intra-anal pressure changes and pulse waves. The design of the probe was based on the observation that genital changes associated with the experience of sexual arousal are a result of increased blood volume and muscle tension throughout the pelvic area (Masters and Johnson, 1966). The device consists of a photometer and pressure transducer encased in a silicone rubber body. An adaptation of this design was used by Carmichael et al. (1994) to measure anal electromyographic activity and blood flow during orgasm. They found that although men and women did not differ in anal muscle tone during baseline testing, higher initial levels of blood flow were measured in women. During both sexual arousal and orgasm, men demonstrated higher levels of anal blood flow and muscle activity.

4.1.3.2. *Temperature.* Thermistors have been used to measure genital temperature in both sexes but the measurements are obtained from different structures. In contrast, thermography can be used in cross-sex comparisons (Seeley et al., 1980). The methodology is not widely used because it is costly and intrusive. Seeley et al. (1980) compared thermographic images of a male participant engaging in masturbation and a female participant engaging in masturbation. Their results suggested that thermography indeed reflected the presence of sexual arousal. However, the relationship of temperature to physiological events in the genitalia, regardless of the methodology used, is unclear, as studies have not been done to relate thermographic data to vascular responses.

4.1.3.3. *Brain and pelvic imaging.* Positron emission tomography (PET) and functional magnetic resonance imaging (fMRI) are fairly recent additions to the toolbox of psychophysiologists and have enabled the investigation of blood flow (including size and position) changes of relevant structures and areas in the pelvis and genitalia as well as in the brain during sexual response. In women, the use of pelvic fMRI has shown that the anterior vaginal wall is stretched and the uterus elevated during coitus, but that the uterus does not balloon as was previously thought (Faix, Lapray, Callede, Maubon, & Lanfrey, 2002; Weijmar-Schultz, van Andel, Sabelis, & Mooyaart, 1999). The finding that the anterior vaginal wall stretches is relevant because it is unknown how the signal of the vaginal photoplethysmograph may be affected by such changes. In men, it has been found that the penis during intercourse in "missionary position" obtains the shape of a boomerang, with approximately one third of its length consisting of the internal root (Weijmar-Shultz et al., 1999). In women, researchers have isolated the clitoris as a target organ, as it exhibits the most sizeable genital changes during sexual arousal (Suh et al., 2004) and clitoral measurements appear reliable (Maravilla et al., 2003). Investigators are still debating, however, whether MRI can document vaginal atrophy in post-menopausal women, and it also remains to be established exactly what physiological changes contribute to the output (Deliganis et al., 2002).

Brain-imaging studies make a unique contribution to the literature because they, in contrast to research in animal models and neurological patients, can be used to study brain mechanisms in nonclinical human populations. Studies using PET and fMRI have found activation during the processing of visual sexual stimuli of the occipototemporal cortex, orbitofrontal cortex, parietal lobules, putamen, amygdala, insula, claustrum, hypothalamus, as well as the deactivation of several areas of the lateral temporal cortex (Stoleru and Mouras, in press, Canli and Gabrieli, 2004).

Future research will, through the comparison of different populations and types of stimuli, undoubtedly refine our understanding of the role of specific brain areas and systems in sexual response and behavior. For example, imaging techniques can be applied to the study of gender differences in brain activation to different stimulus modes (e.g., visual, tactile, auditory, imaginary) as well as stimulus characteristics (e.g., heterosexual/homosexual, explicit/romantic, aggressive). Similarly, brain-imaging techniques can be used in research on sexual dysfunction (e.g., Stoleru et al., 2003) and its treatment (e.g., Montorsi et al., 2003). Stoleru and colleagues (2003) found that men with low sexual desire exhibited less activation of parietal regions (involved in emotional and motor imagery) and decreased *deactivaction* of the medial orbitofrontal cortex (involved in the inhibition of motivated behavior) as compared to a control sample. When it comes to treatment, Montorsi and colleagues (2003a, 2003b) evaluated, also using fMRI, the effects of the first officially approved centrally acting drug for the treatment of erectile dysfunction, apomorphine, in men with psychogenic problems. Apomorphine was associated with increased activation of parietal areas and, consistent with Stoleru and colleagues' (2003) findings, greater deactivation of the medial OFC.

These examples merely serve to illustrate the potential for brain-imaging methods to lead to new insights and hypotheses in the study of sexual response. Yet, researchers in this area face a number of challenges. For instance, the study of central processes using imaging techniques would benefit from the inclusion of measures of peripheral (genital and spinal) mechanisms. Unfortunately, the use of genital measures in MRI scanners is at present problematic (cf. Montorsi et al., 2003a). Also, it is unclear to what degree other autonomic (e.g., cardiovascular, respiratory) processes may be a confound, and thus threaten internal validity, in imaging studies of sexual arousal, which further emphasizes the need for including additional physiological measures. For example, Arnow and colleagues (2002) found correlations in the range of .3 and .5 between changes in respiration and changes in penile tumescence, introducing the possibility that the relationship between brain activation and sexual response in their study was mediated by (or reflected) changes in respiration. Another matter that requires attention involves the reliance on relatively large numbers of (often discrete) sexual stimuli. In contrast to traditional psychophysiological sex studies, imaging approaches have relatively specific requirements for the averaging of responses over time and across stimuli, making it more challenging to control for the effects of habituation, sensitization, or boredom. This may be especially problematic if differences in brain activation between groups of patients and controls or men and women really reflect differences in, for example, the speed of or propensity for habituation.

Although research in this area is increasingly guided by theoretical models (e.g., Redoute et al., 2000), most imaging studies still rely on "emotionally neutral" control stimuli. Progress in this area will depend on the use of designs and reference conditions that will allow the assessment of the specificity of changes (increases or decreases) to *sexual* systems by comparing sexual with other emotional stimuli. Although brain-imaging techniques represent a promising approach to the study of neural structures and processes, they are, like any other emergent technique, subject to methodological (e.g., the reliance on subtraction methods) and conceptual (e.g., the presence or absence of differential brain activation does not necessarily prove or rule out a role for a specific region) challenges, and researchers should be critical of the assumptions underlying the collection and interpretation of brain-imaging data (Cacioppo et al., 2003).

4.1.4. Measurement of subjective sexual arousal

The construct of sexual arousal, its necessary and sufficient conditions, its phenomenology, and its distinction from other components of sexual response (e.g., sexual desire), is receiving renewed and growing interest from researchers (e.g., Everaerd, Laan, & Both, 2003; Graham et al., 2004; Rowland, 1999). Although the physiological measurement of sexual arousal is a maturing science, the operationalization and assessment of subjective sexual arousal is still relatively undeveloped and poses challenges of its own. According to Mosher's (1980) involvement theory, subjective sexual arousal consists of awareness of physiological sexual arousal, sexual affects, and affect-cognition blends. Mosher, Barton-Henry, and Green (1988) developed a scale that measures these three dimensions but, while one of the few self-report measures with known psychometric properties (see Mosher, 1998), is rarely used in its original form. Most researchers use adaptations of this measure or comparable questions derived from the work of others (e.g., Heiman & Rowland, 1983; Henson et al., 1979).

Some researchers also use continuous measures of sexual arousal. Wincze, Hoon, and Hoon (1977) first reported on a lever capable of swinging through a 90° arc that participants could operate to indicate their degree of sexual arousal. Other researchers (e.g., Janssen et al., 1997; Laan et al., 1995) have employed a variant of this technique using horizontally placed sliders with lights providing subjects with feedback. Although rating scales and continuous measures have been found to yield roughly equivalent results (Steinman et al., 1981), both approaches have their disadvantages. One disadvantage of discrete measures of subjective sexual arousal is that they are retrospective in nature. The use of a continuous measure requires participants to monitor their response continuously, and thus may yield distractions or lead to "spectatoring" (Masters & Johnson, 1970). Thus, the reactivity of this measure may depend on participant characteristics (e.g., clinical versus nonclinical), a possibility that warrants more research. An obvious advantage of the continuous measure is that it allows for the evaluation of subjective responses throughout an entire stimulus episode. Peak levels of sexual arousal may be comparable with continuous and discrete measures, but *when* the peak occurs can be determined only with continuous measures. In addition, continuous measures allow for the calculation of within-participant correlations. With physiological measures where calibration of the signal is not possible (e.g., VPA), within-participant correlations are more reliable and informative than between-participant correlations.

4.2. Signal recording and processing

In contrast to many other areas of psychophysiological research, no guidelines exist for the measurement of sexual arousal, and the current lack of standardization of signal recording, processing, and analysis, complicates the evaluation and comparison of research findings[2]. Signal processing and data reduction appear to be the most significant sources of error variability. Although the more commonly used measurement systems (Contact Precision Instruments, Boston, MA; BIOPAC Systems, Inc., Goleta, CA) come with software containing basic signal processing tools, procedures for artifact detection and removal,

especially relevant in the analysis of VPA, are not standardized in these programs and often are not described in sufficient detail in publications. Automated algorithms exist in related fields for correcting artifacts similar to those seen in VPA (Kaiser & Findeis, 1999; Linden & Estrin, 1988) and could vastly decrease VPA processing time and increase standardization. Others have attempted to use Fourier analysis to select relevant VPA components (Polan, 2003; Wouda et al., 1998), but this approach is still confounded by movement artifacts that may cross into the desired frequency band (Prause & Janssen, 2004).

Another source of error in sexual response measurement is related to variations in device placement. Although measurement devices are usually put in place by participants, visual inspection of placement could increase measurement accuracy and reliability. However, with measures such as penile strain gauges, "improper" device selection or placement cannot always be prevented. For example, a gauge that fits well on a flaccid penis may prove too small for an erect penis. Placement of the vaginal plethysmograph can be standardized by using a shield (Geer, 1983; Laan et al. 1995) and this practice is recommended. A placement shield, however, will not prevent inaccurate readings due to (phasic or tonic) muscle contractions. As for the labial thermistor, little is known about the effects of placement and how changes in size or volume of the labia affect the output of the device. In view of this, we emphasize the importance of carefully checking all genital response data for outliers before performing statistical analyses.

Meuwissen and Over (1993) and Julien and Over (1981) examined whether the Law of Initial Values (LIV) applies to the measurement of genital responses and reported inconsistent findings. Not uncommonly, positive instead of negative correlations are found between baseline and response levels (e.g., Heiman et al., 2004, reported baseline-response level correlations of $r = 0.89$ for VPA and $r = 0.84$ for clitoral volume in women). Recent reconceptualizations of LIV (e.g., Jin, 1992) propose that within the middle range of initial states, higher initial values are expected to be related to greater (not smaller) reactivity. Only when an initial value reaches its upper limit, a tendency to reversed responses may occur. Although LIV may account for a portion of the variance, more research is needed to determine how it relates to constitutional (e.g., anatomical differences) and physiological factors in psychophysiological sex studies.

4.3. Models of sexual response

One of the first models of sexual response was introduced by Havelock Ellis in 1906. His two-stage model differentiates between a stage of "building up" (tumescence) and climactic release (detumescence). This model was extended by Moll (1908/1912) who described a *curve of voluptuousness* which consisted of four phases: the build-up of sexual excitement (the ascending limb), a high, stable level

---

[2] In 1998, SexLab, a listserve with companion website (www.indiana.edu/~sexlab) was established to facilitate standardization and stimulate discussion of methodological issues among sexual psychophysiologists.

of sexual excitement (the equable voluptuous sensation), orgasm (the acme), and the cessation of the sexual impulse (the decline).

4.3.1. The sexual response cycle

Although initially introduced as little more than a frame of reference, Masters and Johnson's (1966) four-stage model is probably the best-known model of sexual response to date. The model, reminiscent of Moll's curve of voluptuousness, describes the genital and extragenital responses that occur in humans during sexual behavior. The phases are (1) excitement phase, (2) plateau phase, (3) orgasmic phase, and (4) resolution phase. Although few would dispute the impact of Masters and Johnson's model on subsequent research and the development of sex therapy, it has been subjected to serious criticism. For example, the separation of sexual response into four discrete stages has been challenged (Robinson, 1976). The distinction between excitement and plateau phases is especially problematic, as there is no empirical support for an identifiable plateau phase. Similarly, the universality of the model has been questioned (Tiefer, 1991). Also, Masters and Johnson did not describe adequately their methods and their data were not quantified nor presented in a form that permits evaluation by others. Finally, the studies were restricted to the observation of physiological changes; psychological factors were not measured.

Kaplan (1977, 1979) presented a modification of Masters and Johnson's model in which she replaced their first stage by a "desire" phase. Her second and third phase, the excitement and orgasm phase, are similar to Masters and Johnson's first and third phases. Kaplan's model has been influential in the formulation of the American Psychiatric Association's diagnostic manuals since the *Diagnostic and Statistical Manual III* (APA, 1980).

4.3.2. Cognitive-affective models

Models of sexual response such as Masters and Johnson's suggest that some preprogrammed mechanism exists that is activated by adequate sexual stimulation (Janssen & Everaerd, 1993). They fail, however, to describe what exactly constitutes effective stimulation. In fact, Masters and Johnson's definition of the term is circular: Effective stimulation produces a response, and a response is evidence for effective stimulation. Another problem with models such as Masters and Johnson's is that they do not provide an explanation for the many regulatory processes related to sexual response, nor do they account for the many variations in subjective experience of sexual response and the complicated variation in stimulus and response parameters from such models.

Although a number of other sexual response models have been proposed over the years (e.g., Bancroft, 1989; Byrne, 1977), only a few originated from or are based on psychophysiological research. One such model was proposed by Barlow (1986). In a series of studies, he found support for a number of factors differentiating men

with erectile problems from men without sexual problems Together, these findings provided the basis for his model, which emphasizes the interaction between autonomic activation and cognitive processes. Sexual response patterns are conceptualized as forming either a positive or a negative feedback system, both starting with the perception of an explicit or implicit demand for sexual performance. This results in either positive or negative affective evaluations, both triggering autonomic arousal. The increase in autonomic arousal enhances attention for those features of the sexual situation that are most salient. Continued processing of erotic cues produces genital response, and ultimately leads to sexual approach behavior. Continued processing of nonerotic issues (e.g., consequences of not responding) interferes with sexual arousal and ultimately leads to avoidance behavior. By combining cognitive-affective and physiological features of sexual response, this type of conceptual approach holds genuine promise of yielding substantial theoretical progress.

Barlow's original model was based on studies of men. Palace (1995a) presented a similar model, based on studies in sexually functional and dysfunctional women, in which the summation of autonomic arousal and perceived and expected levels of genital response leads to an optimal sexual response. The model is based on studies showing that increased autonomic arousal and positive false feedback can enhance sexual responses in women (Palace, 1995b; Palace & Gorzalka, 1990). Thus, Palace emphasizes the relevance of expectations, as does Barlow (see also Wiegel et al., 2005), and both models emphasize the interaction between autonomic and cognitive processes and highlight the importance of feedback.

In constructing their models, Barlow and Palace both recognize the complexity of the interrelationships among response components, yet they essentially treat sexual arousal as a unified construct. Instances of discordance, however, suggest that genital and subjective sexual responses are, at least to a certain degree, under the control of different mechanisms (Bancroft, 1989). Janssen, Everaerd, Spiering, and Janssen (2000) presented a model that highlights the interaction between automatic (unconscious) and controlled (conscious) cognitive processes and proposes that different levels of processing can differentially affect subjective and physiological sexual arousal. The model states that unconscious processes are relevant to explaining the automaticity of the genital response, whereas subjective feelings of sexual arousal are believed to be under control of higher-level, conscious cognitive processing (see also Janssen and Everaerd, 1993; Laan and Everaerd, 1995; Laan and Janssen, in press). Support for the model is provided by studies exploring the role of unconscious processes in the activation of genital responses and sexual meaning (e.g., Janssen et al., 2000; Spiering et al., 2003; Spiering et al., 2004). A basic assumption of the model is that sexual stimuli may convey more than one meaning. Thus automatic and controlled cognitive processes may help explain differences in outcome in situations that convey sexual meaning while simultaneously activating negative meanings. Janssen et al. (2000) proposed that in these situations, automatic processing of sexual meaning initiates genital response, whereas controlled processing of negative meaning may result in decreased or nonsexual subjective experience.

5. EPILOGUE

Psychophysiology has matured into an important approach in studies on human sexuality. In addition to a growing number of studies on basic mechanisms of sexual response, an impressive body of practical information has accumulated, particularly related to the study of dysfunctions and to methods for the assessment of sex offenders. Progress in the laboratory study of human sexuality, however, is contingent upon methodological advancements. More than 15 years ago, Rosen and Beck (1988) noted that methods in sexual psychophysiology are based more on the availability and ease of use of particular transducers than upon a sound understanding of the underlying processes of sexual arousal. These concerns are still relevant today. For example, Rosen and Beck questioned the reliance on the vaginal photometer, pointing out that basic physiological studies (e.g., Wagner & Ottesen, 1980) "highlighted serious limitations in the vaginal photoplethysmograph as an adequate measure of genital engorgement" (p. 340). The development of new measures, especially of genital response in women, would indeed be a welcome contribution to the field of sexual psychophysiology.

Although the variable relationship between genital responses and subjective reports of sexual arousal in women has been documented extensively, and while experiential and laboratory differences have been found to influence this relationship (for review see Prause & Janssen 2006), the mechanisms involved are not well-understood. More generally, our understanding of the role of feedback from the genitals, and how it interacts with other processes that affect behavior, is still limited. Harking back to the early views of James-Lange, there is a continuing interest in peripheral feedback. Lang's (1994) discussion of the importance of that view and the more contemporary perspectives in emotion theory (e.g., Damasio, 1994) reemphasize the importance of the question of the role of feedback, and possible gender differences therein.

The role of individual differences has, as yet, not received much attention in sexual psychophysiology. Bancroft and Janssen (2000, 2001) proposed a model that postulates that sexual response depends on the balance between sexual excitation and inhibition, and that individual differences exist in the propensity for both. Just as future sexual response models should, at least ideally, attempt to incorporate predictions about the interrelationships between physiological and subjective responses, sexual psychophysiology could benefit from the development of conceptual approaches that contribute to our understanding of individual differences in sexual response and

behavior. This would be especially relevant in respect to questions about the development of problematic or unusual response (e.g., sexual dysfunction, paraphilic interests) and behavioral (e.g., sexual "compulsivity," sexual risk taking) patterns. Although such approaches could include the exploration of both general and more specific, sexuality-related (e.g., sexual inhibition proneness or erotophilia/phobia) aspects of personality, they also should include the consideration of interindividual variability in response patterning as reflected by, for example, individual differences in conditionability (Hoffmann, 2005).

Another unanswered question alluded to earlier is how to conceptualize and deal with the fact that sexuality is often surrounded with both positively and negatively valenced emotions. Some research suggests that sexual arousal may simply be a case of a highly arousing positive emotional state (Carretie, Hinojosa, & Mercado, 2003), whereas other studies have shown that sexual stimuli are processed differently from other emotional stimuli and are processed differently by the two genders (Geer & Manguno-Mire, 1997). Although it has been argued (Everaerd, 1988) that sexual arousal should be considered to be among the emotions, it is not clear whether its study would benefit most from a discrete or dimensional (e.g., circumplex) theoretical approach. What's more, some may contend that sexual arousal is not a prototypical emotion exactly *because* it often involves the co-activation of positive and negative affect, where other emotions are assumed to show stability in valence. However, findings of studies combining within- and between-subjects approaches increasingly challenge the notion that negative and positive emotions are mutually exclusive (e.g., Larsen, McGraw, & Cacioppo, 2001; Scollon, Diener, Oishi, & Biswas-Diener, 2005). Also, imaging studies (e.g., Canli, 2004; Cunningham, Raye, & Johnson, 2004) suggest "that positive and negative do not subtract from one another in our brains in the way that circumplex models tell us they should" (Zautra & Davis, 2004, p. 1099; cf. Cacioppo & Berntson, 1994). Either way, the advantage that the study of the sexual emotions holds is the specificity of the genital response. Although there is some independence of genital responding and subjective or cognitive events, there is also amazing specificity. Certainly there is no other domain in emotion and psychophysiology in which the physiological response system is as closely tied to the feeling state and stimuli under study.

Albertus Magnus noted, in the 1200s, that "pleasure is attached to intercourse so that it will be more desired, and thus generation will continue" (Book IX, Ch 3, Kitchell & Resnick, 1999). This is the premise that suggests that living animals are "prewired" to respond to relevant stimuli and engage in behaviors that will insure perpetuation of the species. Evolutionary psychology with its emphasis on natural selection is directly related to such a conceptualization. Three areas have been the principal focus in evolutionary approaches to sexuality: mate selection, jealousy, and attractiveness (Allgeier & Wiederman, 1994).

Psychophysiology provides a useful tool for the study and advancement of these research areas.

The future lies, we believe, in the amalgamation of interdisciplinary efforts. Specifically, the explosion of methodologies for assessing brain function will have a powerful impact. As methodologies become increasingly available to study the individual's brain functioning in naturalistic settings, our theories and conceptualizations may be altered dramatically. This does not mean that the measurement of peripheral processes and genital responses will become lost in the shuffle. It appears that peripheral feedback is important and information only from central events will not have the full picture available. In a similar vein, increasing attention to cognitive psychology and the neurosciences with the availability of sophisticated experimental paradigms will play an increasingly important role in the study of sexuality. The combination of studying brain function, cognitive and affective processes, and peripheral mechanisms can be expected to provide researchers with novel, powerful, multi-method approaches that will advance our understanding of the psychophysiology of sexual response and behavior.

REFERENCES

Abel, G. G., Blanchard, E. B., Barlow, D. H., & Mavissakalian, M. (1975). Identifying specific erotic cues in sexual deviations by audiotaped descriptions. *Journal of Applied Behavior Analysis*, 8, 247–260.

American Psychological Association (1992). Ethical principles of psychologists and code of conduct. *American Psychologist* 47, 1597–1161.

Amoroso, D. M., & Brown, M. (1973). Problems in studying the effects of erotic material. *Journal of Sex Research* 9, 187–195.

Andersson, K. E., & Wagner, G. (1995). Physiology of penile erection. *Physiological Review* 75, 191–236.

Arnow, B. A., Desmond, J. E., Banner, L. L., Glover, G. H., Solomon, A., Polan, M. L., et al. (2002). Brain activation and sexual arousal in healthy, heterosexual males. *Brain, 125*(Pt. 5), 1014–1023.

Bancroft, J. (1989). *Human sexuality and its problems*. Edinburgh: Churchill Livingstone.

Bancroft, J. (1995). Are the effects of androgens on male sexuality noradrenergically mediated? Some consideration of the human. *Neuroscience and Biobehavioral Reviews, 2*, 1–6.

Bancroft, J. (1999). Central inhibition of sexual response in the male: A theoretical perspective. *Neuroscience & Biobehavioral Reviews, 23*, 763–784.

Bancroft, J. (2004). *Annual Review of Sex Research*, 15, 1–39.

Bancroft, J., & Bell, C. (1985). Simultaneous recording of penile diameter and penile arterial pulse during laboratory-based erotic stimulation in normal subjects. *Journal of Psychosomatic Research*, 29, 303–313.

Bancroft, J. & Janssen, E. (2000). The dual control model of male sexual response: A theoretical approach to centrally mediated erectile dysfunction. *Neuroscience and Biobehavioral Review, 24*, 571–579.

Bancroft, J. & Janssen, E. (2001) Psychogenic erectile dysfunction in the era of pharmacotherapy: A theoretical approach. In Mulc-

ahy, J. (Ed.), Male sexual function: A guide to clinical management. Totowa, NJ: Humana Press, 79–89.

Bancroft, J., Jones, H. G., & Pullan, B. P. (1966). A simple transducer for measuring penile erection with comments on its use in the treatment of sexual disorder. *Behavior Research and Therapy* 4, 239–241.

Barbaree, H. E., Marshall, W. L., & Lanthier, R. (1979). Deviant sexual arousal in rapists. *Behavior Therapy and Research* 17, 215–222.

Barlow, D. H. (1986). Causes of sexual dysfunction: The role of anxiety and cognitive interference. *Journal of Consulting and Clinical Psychology* 54, 140–157.

Barlow, D. H., Becker, R., Leitenberg, H., & Agras W. (1970). A mechanical strain gauge for recording penile circumference change. *Journal of Applied Behavior Analysis*, 6, 355–367.

Basson, R., & Brotto, L. A. (2003). Sexual psychophysiology and effects of sildenafil citrate in oestrogenised women with acquired genital arousal disorder and impaired orgasm: A randomised controlled trial. *BJOG: an International Journal of Obstetrics & Gynaecology, 110*, 1014–1024.

Basson, R., McInnes, R., Smith, M. D., Hodgson, G., & Koppiker, N. (2002). Efficacy and safety of sildenafil citrate in women with sexual dysfunction associated with female sexual arousal disorder. *Journal of Women's Health & Gender-Based Medicine, 11*, 367–377.

Bechara, A., Bertolino, M. V., Casabe, A., & Fredotovich, N. (2004). A double-blind randomized placebo control study comparing the objective and subjective changes in female sexual response using sublingual apomorphine. *Journal of Sexual Medicine, 1*, 209–214.

Beck, J. G., Sakheim, D. K., & Barlow, D. H. (1983). Operating characteristics of the vaginal photoplethysmograph: some implications for its use. *Archives of Sexual Behavior* 12, 43–58.

Beharry, R. K., Hale, T. M., Wilson, E. A., Heaton, J. P., & Adams, M. A. (2003). Evidence for centrally initiated genital vasocongestive engorgement in the female rat: Findings from a new model of female sexual arousal response. *International Journal of Impotence Research, 15*, 122–128.

Berman, J. R., Berman, L. A., Lin, H., Flaherty, E., Lahey, N., Goldstein, I., et al. (2001). Effect of sildenafil on subjective and physiologic parameters of the female sexual response in women with sexual arousal disorder. *Journal of Sex & Marital Therapy, 27*, 411–420.

Bogaert, A. F. (1996). Volunteer bias in human sexuality research: Evidence for both sexuality and personality differences in males. *Archives of Sexual Behavior, 25*, 125–140.

Bohlen, J. G., & Held, J. P. (1979). An anal probe for monitoring vascular and muscular events during sexual response. *Psychophysiology*, 16, 318–323.

Bradley, W. E., Timm, G. W., Gallagher, J. M., & Johnson, B. K. (1985). New method for continuous measurement of nocturnal penile tumescence and rigidity. *Urology, 26*, 4–9.

Burnett, A. L. (1997). Nitric Oxide in Penis: Physiology and Pathology. *Journal of Urology* 157, 320–324.

Cacioppo, J. T., & Berntson, G. G. (1994). Relationship between attitudes and evaluative space: A critical review, with emphasis on the separability of positive and negative substrates. *Psychological Bulletin, 115*, 401–423.

Canli, T. (2004). Functional Brain Mapping of Extraversion and Neuroticism: Learning From Individual Differences in Emotion Processing. *Journal of Personality, 72*, 1105–1132.

Carmichael, M. S., Warburton, V. L., Dixen, J., & Davidson, J. M. (1994). Relationships among cardiovascular, muscular, and oxytocin responses during human sexual activity. *Archives of Sexual Behavior, 23,* 59–79.

Caruso, S., Agnello, C., Intelisano, G., Farina, M., DiMari, L., & Cianci, A. (2004). Efficacy and safety of daily intake of apomorphine. *Urology, 63,* 955–959.

Cranston-Cuebas, M. A. & Barlow, D. H. (1990). Cognitive and affective contributions to sexual functioning. *Annual Review of Sex Research* 1:119–161.

Cunningham, W. A., Raye, C. L., & Johnson, M. K. (2004). Implicit and explicit evaluation: fMRI correlates of valence, emotional intensity, and control in the processing of attitudes. *Journal of Cognitive Neuroscience, 16,* 1717–1729.

Damasio, A. (1994). *Descartes' Error.* New York: Putnam & Sons.

Deliganis, A. V., Maravilla, K. R., Heiman, J. R., Carter, W. O., Garland, P. A., Peterson, B. T., et al. (2002). Female genitalia: Dynamic mr imaging with use of ms-325 initial experiences evaluating female sexual response. *Radiology, 225,* 791–799.

Dickinson, R. L. (1933). *Human sex anatomy.* Baltimore: Williams and Wilkins.

Droegemueller, W. (1992). Anatomy. In *Comprehensive Gynecology,* A. L. Herbst, D. R. Mishell, M. A. Stenchever, & W. Droegemueller (Eds), pp. 43–78. St. Louis: Mosby Year Book.

Earls, C. M. & Jackson, D. R. (1981). The effects of temperature on the mercury-in-rubber strain gauge. *Journal of Applied Behavioural Analysis, 3,* 145–149.

Earls, C. M., Marshall, W. L., Marshall, P. G., Morales, A., & Surridge, D. H., 1983. Penile elongation: A method for the screening of impotence. *Journal of Urology,* 139: 90–92.

Earls, C. M., Morales, A., & Marshall, W. L. 1988. Penile sufficiency: An operational definitation. *Journal of Urology* 139:536–538.

Everaerd, W. 1988. Commentary on sex research: Sex as an emotion. *Journal of Psychology and Human Sexuality,* 2: 3–15.

Everaerd, W., & Laan, E. (2000). Drug treatments for women's sexual disorders. *Journal of Sex Research, 37,* 195–204.

Everaerd, E., Laan, E., & Both, S. (Eds.) (2003). *Sexual Appetite, Desire and Motivation Energetics of the Sexual System.* Amsterdam: Royal Dutch Academy of Sciences.

Farkas, G. M., Evans, I. M., Sine, L. F., Eifert, G., Wittlieb, E., & Vogelmann-Sine, S. (1979). Reliability and validity of the mercury-in-rubber strain gauge measure of penile circumference. *Behavior Therapy, 10,* 555–561.

Fisher, C., Gross, J., & Zuch, J. (1965). Cycle of penile erection synchronous with dreaming (REM) sleep. *Archives of General Psychiatry, 12,* 27–45.

Fisher, S. (1973). *The female orgasm.* New York: Basic Books.

Fisher, S., & Osofsky, H. (1967). Sexual Responsiveness in Women: Psychological Correlates. *Archives of General Psychiatry, 17,* 214–226.

Fleck, K., & Polich, J. (1988). P300 and the menstrual cycle. *Electroencephalography & Clinical Neurophysiology, 71,* 157–160.

Freund, K. (1963). A laboratory method for diagnosing predominance of hemo- or hetero-erotic interest in the male. *Behaviour Research and Therapy, 1,* 85–93.

Freund, K., Langevin, R., & Barlow, D. (1974). Comparison of two penile measures of erotic arousal. *Behaviour Research and Therapy, 12,* 355–359.

Fugl-Meyer, A. R., Sjogren, K., & Johansson, K. (1984). A vaginal temperature registration system. *Archives of Sexual Behavior, 13,* 247–260.

Geer, J. H. (1983). *Measurement and methodological considerations in vaginal photometry.* Paper presented at the meeting of the International Academy of Sex Research, Harriman, NY.

Geer, J. H. & Manguno, G. M. (1997). Gender differences in Cognitive Processes in Sexuality. *Annual Review of Sex Research, 9,* 90–124.

Geer, J. H., Morokoff, P., & Greenwood, P. (1974). Sexual arousal in women: The development of a measurement device for vaginal blood volume. *Archives of Sexual Behavior, 3,* 559–564.

Gerstenberg, T. C., Nordling, J., Hald, T., & Wagner, G. (1989). Standardized evaluation of erectile dysfunction in 95 consecutive patients. *Journal of Urology, 141,* 857–862.

Giesbers, A. A. G. M., Bruins, J. L., Kramer, A. E. J. L., & Jonas, U. (1987). New methods in the diagnosis of impotence: Rigiscan penile tumescence and rigidity monitoring and diagnostic papaverine hydrocloride injection. *World Journal of Urology, 5,* 173–176.

Gillian, P., & Brindley, G. S. (1979). Vaginal and pelvic floor responses to sexual stimulation. *Psychophysiology, 16,* 471–481.

Gimpl, G., & Fahrenholz, F. (2001). The oxytocin receptor system: Structure, function and regulation. *Physiological Reviews, 81,* 629–683.

Gonzalez-Cadavid, N. F., Ignarro, L. J., & Rajfer, J. (1999). Nitric oxide and the cyclic GMP system in the penis. *Molecular Urology, 3*(2), 51–59.

Graham, C. A., Sanders, S. A., Milhausen, R., & McBride, K. (2004). Turning on and turning off: A focus group study of the factors that affect women's sexual arousal. *Archives of Sexual Behavior, 33,* 527–538.

Hall, G. C. N., Hirschman, R., & Oliver, L. L. (1995). Sexual arousal and arousability to pedophilic stimuli in a community sample of normal men. *Behavior Therapy, 26,* 681–694.

Halpern, C. T, Udry, J. R, & Suchindran, C. (1998). Monthly measures of salivary testosterone predict sexual activity in adolescent males. *Archives of Sexual Behavior, 27,* 445–65.

Hamann, S., Herman, R. A., Nolan, C. L., & Wallen, K. (2004). Men and women differ in amygdala response to visual sexual stimuli. *Nature Neuroscience, 7,* 411–416.

Hatch, J. P. (1979). Vaginal photoplethysmography: Methodological considerations. *Archives of Sexual Behavior, 8,* 357–374.

Hedricks, C. A. (1994). Sexual Behavior across the menstrual cycle: A biopsychosocial approach. *Annual Review of Sex Research, 5,* 122–172.

Heiman, J. R. (1976). Issues in the use of psychophysiology to assess female sexual dysfunction. *Journal of Sex and Marital Therapy, 2,* 197–204.

Heiman, J. R. (1977). A psychophysiological exploration of sexual arousal patterns in females and males. *Psychophysiology, 14,* 266–274.

Henson, C., Rubin, H. B., & Henson, D. (1979). Women's sexual arousal concurrently assessed by three genital measures. *Archives of Sexual Behavior, 8,* 459–469.

Henson, D. E., & Rubin, H. B. (1978). A comparison of two objective measures of sexual arousal of women. *Behaviour Research and Therapy, 16,* 143–151.

Henson, D. E., Rubin, H. B., & Henson, C. (1979). Analysis of the consistency of objective measures of sexual arousal in women. *Journal of Applied Behavior Analysis, 12,* 701–711.

Henson, D. E., Rubin, H. B., & Henson, C. (1982). Labial and vaginal blood volume responses to visual and tactile stimuli. *Archives of Sexual Behavior, 11,* 23–31.

Hicks, R. G. (1970). Experimenter effects on the physiological experiment. *Psychophysiology, 7,* 10–17.

Hoffmann, H., Janssen, E., & Turner, S. L. (2004). Classical conditioning of sexual arousal in women and men: Effects of varying awareness and biological relevance of the conditioned stimulus. *Archives of Sexual Behavior, 33,* 1–11.

Hoon, P. W., Wincze, J. P., & Hoon, E. F. (1976). Physiological assessment of sexual arousal in women. *Psychophysiology, 13,* 196–204.

Hoon, P., Bruce, K., and Kinchelow, G. (1982). Does the menstrual cycle play a role in erotic arousal? *Psychophysiology, 19,* 21–26.

Howett, M. K., Neely, E. B., Christensen, N. D., Wigdahl, B., Krebs, F. C., Malamud, D., et al. (1999). A broad-spectrum microbicide with virucidal activity against sexually transmitted viruses. *Antimicrobial Agents & Chemotherapy, 43*(2), 314–321.

Hoyle, C. H., Stones, R. W., Robson, T., Whitley, K., and Burnstock, G. (1996). Innervation of vasculature and microvasculature of the human vagina by NOS and neuropeptide-containing nerves. *Journal of Anatomy, 188,* 633–644

Janssen, E. (2002). Psychophysiological measures of sexual response. In M. W. Wiederman & B. E. Whitley (Eds.), *Handbook for conducting research on human sexuality.* Mahwah, NJ: Erlbaum, 139–171.

Janssen, E. (Ed.) (in press). *The Psychophysiology of Sex.* Bloomington, IN: Indiana University Press, in press.

Janssen, E., Carpenter, D., & Graham, C. (2003). Selecting films for sex research: Gender differences in erotic film preference. *Archives of Sexual Behavior, 32,* 243–251.

Janssen, E., & Everaerd, W. (1993). Determinants of male sexual arousal. *Annual Review of Sex Research, 4,* 211–245.

Janssen, E., Everaerd, W., Spiering, M., & Janssen, J. (2000). Automatic processes and the appraisal of sexual Stimuli: Toward an information processing model of sexual arousal. *Journal of Sex Research, 37*(2), 8–23.

Janssen, E., Everaerd, W., van Lunsen, H., & Oerlemans, S. (1994a). Validation of a psychophysiological Waking Erectile Assessment (WEA) for the diagnosis of male erectile disorder. *Urology, 43,* 686–695.

Janssen, E., Everaerd, W., van Lunsen, H., & Oerlemans, S. (1994b). Visual stimulation facilitates penile responses to vibration. *Journal of Consulting and Clinical Psychology, 62,* 1222–1228.

Janssen, E., Vissenberg, M., Visser, S., & Everaerd, W. (1997). An in vivo comparison of two circumferential penile strain gauges: Introducing a new calibration method. *Psychophysiology, 34,* 717–720.

Janssen, E., Vorst, H., Finn, P., & Bancroft, J. (2002). The Sexual Inhibition (SIS) and Sexual Excitation (SES) Scales: II. Predicting psychophysiological response patterns. *Journal of Sex Research, 39,* 127–132.

Jennings, J. R., Tahmoush, A. J., & Redmont, D. P. (1980). Noninvasive measurement of peripheral vascular activity. In I. R. Martin & P. H. Venables (Eds.), *Techniques in psychophysiology.* New York: Wiley.

Jin, P. (1992). Toward a reconceptualization of the law of initial value. *Psychological Bulletin, 111,* 176–184.

Johnston, V. S., & Oliver-Rodriguez, J. C. (1997). Facial beauty and the late positive component of event-related potentials. *Journal of Sex Research, 3,* 188–198.

Jovanovic, U. J. (1967). Some characteristics of the beginning of dreams. *Psychologie Fortschung, 30,* 281–306.

Jovanovic, U. J. (1971). The recording of physiological evidence of genital arousal in human males and females. *Archives of Sexual Behavior, 1,* 309–320.

Julien, E. and Over, R. (1981). Male sexual arousal and the law of initial value. *Psychophysiology, 18,* 709–711.

Jünemann, K. P., Scheepe, J., Persson-Jünemann, C., Schmidt, P., Abel, K., Zwick, A., Tschada, R., & Alken, P. (1994). Basic experimental studies on corpus cavernosum electromyography and smooth-muscle electromyography of the urinary bladder. *World Journal of Urology, 12,* 266–273.

Kaiser, W., & Findeis, M. (1999). Artifact processing during exercise testing. *Journal of Electrocardiology, 32*(Suppl), 212–219.

Kaplan, H. S. (1977). Hypoactive sexual desire. *Journal of Sex and Marital Therapy, 3,* 3–9.

Kaplan, H. S. (1979). *Disorders of sexual desire.* New York: Brunner/Mazel.

Karacan, I. (1969). A simple and inexpensive transducer for quantitative measurements of penile erection during sleep. *Behavior Research Methods and Instrumentation, 1,* 251–252.

Karacan, I., Rosenbloom, A., and Williams, R. L. (1970). The clitoral erection cycle during sleep. *Psychophysiology, 7,* 338.

Karacan, I., Salis, P. J., Ware, J. C., Dervent, B., Williams, R. L., Scott, F. B., Attia, S. L., & Beutler, L. E. (1978). Nocturnal penile tumescence and diagnosis in diabetic impotence. *American Journal of Psychiatry, 135,* 191–197.

Karama, S., Lecours, A. R., Leroux, J.-M., Bourgouin, P., Beaudoin, G., Joubert, S., et al. (2002). Areas of brain activation in males and females during viewing of erotic film excerpts. *Human Brain Mapping, 16,* 1–13.

Kirby, R. (2004). *An Atlas of Erectile Dysfunction.* New York: Parthenon Publishing.

Kitchell, K., & Resnick, I. M. (1999). *Albertus Magnus De Animalibus: A Medieval Summa Zoologica.* Baltimore: Johns Hopkins Press.

Korff, J., & Geer, J. H. (1983). The relationship between sexual arousal experience and genital response. *Psychophysiology, 20,* 121–127.

Khalife, S., Binik, Y. M., Cohen, D. R., & Amsel, R. (2000). Evaluation of clitoral blood flow by color doppler ultrasonography. *Journal of Sex & Marital Therapy, 26,* 187–189.

Krug, R., Plihal, W., Fehm, H. L., & Born, J. (2000). Selective influence of the menstrual cycle on perception of stimuli with reproductive significance: An event-related potential study. *Psychophysiology, 37,* 111–122.

Kuban, M., Barbaree, H. E., & Blanchard, R. (1999). A comparison of volume and circumference phallometry: Response magnitude and method agreement. *Archives of Sexual Behavior, 28,* 345–359.

Laan, E., & Everaerd, W. (1995). Determinants of female sexual arousal: Psychophysiological theory and data. *Annual Review of Sex Research, 6,* 32–76.

Laan, E., Everaerd, W., Bellen, G. van, & Hanewald, G. (1994). Women's sexual and emotional responses to male- and female produced erotica. *Archives of sexual behavior, 23,* 153–170.

Laan, E., Everaerd, W., & Evers, A. (1995). Assessment of female sexual arousal: Response specificity and construct validity. *Psychophysiology, 32,* :476–485.

Laan, E. & Janssen, E. (in press). How do men and women feel? Determinants of subjective experience of sexual arousal. In E. Janssen (Ed.), *The Psychophysiology of Sex.* Bloomington, IN: Indiana University Press, in press.

Laan, E., & van Lunsen, R. H. W. (2002). *Orgasm latency, duration and quality in women: Validation of a laboratory sexual stimulation technique*. Paper presented at the International Academy of Sex Research (IASR), Hamburg, Germany.

Laan, E., van Lunsen, R. H., Everaerd, W., Riley, A., Scott, E., & Boolell, M. (2002). The enhancement of vaginal vasocongestion by sildenafil in healthy premenopausal women. *Journal of Women's Health & Gender-Based Medicine, 11*, 357–365.

Lang, P. J. (1994). The varieties of emotional experience: A meditation on James–Lange Theory. *Psychological Review, 101*, 211–221.

Lankveld, J. van, Hout, M. A. van den (2004). Increasing Neutral Distraction Inhibits Genital but not Subjective Sexual Arousal of Sexually Functional and Dysfunctional Men. *Archives of Sexual Behavior, 33*, 549–558.

Larsen, J. T., McGraw, P., & Cacioppo, J. T. (2001). Can people feel happy and sad at the same time? *Journal of Personality and Social Psychology, 81*, 684–696.

Laws, D. R. (1977). A comparison of the measurement characteristics of two circumferential penile transducers. *Archives of Sexual Behavior, 6*, 45–51.

Laws, D. R., & Bow, R. A. (1976). An improved mechanical strain gauge for recording penile circumference changes. *Psychophysiology, 13*, 596–599.

Laws, D. R., & Holmen, M. L. (1978). Sexual response faking by pedophiles. *Criminal Justice and Behavior, 5*, 343–356.

Levin, R. J. (1992). The mechanisms of human female sexual arousal. *Annual Review of Sex Research, 3*, 1–48.

Levin, R. J. (1997). Assessing human female sexual arousal by vaginal plethysmography: A critical examination. *Sexologies: European Journal of Medical Sexology, 6*, 25–31.

Levin, R. (2003). Is prolactin the biological 'off switch' for human sexual arousal? *Sexual and Relationship Therapy, 18*, 237–243.

Levin, R. J., & Wagner, G. (1978). Haemodynamic changes of the human vagina during sexual arousal assessed by a heated oxygen electrode. *Journal of Physiology, 275*, 23–24.

Levine, L. A., & Carroll, R. A. (1994). Nocturnal penile tumescence and rigidity in men without complaints of erectile dysfunction using a new quantitative analysis software. *Journal of Urology, 152*, 1103–1107.

Linden, W., & Estrin, R. (1988). Computerized cardiovascular monitoring: Method and data. *Psychophysiology, 25*, 227–234.

Lohr, B. A., Adams, H. E., & Dacis, J. M. (1997). Sexual arousal to erotic and aggressive stimuli in sexually coercive and noncoersive men. *Journal of Abnormal Psychology, 106*, 230–242.

Maas, C. P., ter Kuile, M. M., Laan, E., Tuijnman, C. C., Weijenborg, P. T., Trimbos, J. B., et al. (2004). Objective assessment of sexual arousal in women with a history of hysterectomy. *BJOG: an International Journal of Obstetrics & Gynaecology, 111*, 456–462.

Maravilla, K. R., Heiman, J. R., Garland, P. A., Cao, Y., Carter, W. O., Peterson, B. T., et al. (2003). Dynamic mr imaging of the sexual arousal response in women. *Journal of Sex & Marital Therapy, 29*, 71–77.

Masters, W. H., & Johnson, V. E. (1966). *Human sexual response*. New York: Little, Brown and Company.

Masters, W. H. , & Johnson, V. E. (1970). *Human sexual inadequacy*. New York: Little, Brown and Company.

McConaghy, N. (1974). Measurements of change in penile dimensions. *Archives of Sexual Behavior, 3*, 381–388.

Mendelsohn, M. (1896). Ist das Radfahren als eine gesundheidsgemässe uebung anzusehen und aus ärtzlichen gesichtspunkten zu empfehlen? *Deutsche Medicinische Wochenschrift, 22*, 383–384.

Meston, C. M., & Gorzalka, B. B. (1996). Differential effects of sympathetic activation on sexual arousal in sexually dysfunctional and functional women. *Journal of Abnormal Psychology, 105*, 582–591.

Meston, C. M., & Gorzalka, B. B. (1995). The effects of sympathetic activation on physiological and subjective sexual arousal in women. *Behaviour Research and Therapy, 3*, 651–664.

Meston, C. M., & Heiman, J. R. (1998). Ephedrine-activated physiological sexual arousal in women. *Archives of General Psychiatry, 55*, 652–656.

Meuwissen, I., & Over, R. (1992). Sexual arousal across phases of the human menstrual cycle. *Archives of Sexual Behavior, 21*, 101–119.

Meuwissen, I., & Over, R. (1993). Female sexual arousal and the law of initial value: Assessment at several phases of the menstrual cycle. *Archives of Sexual Behavior, 22*, 403–413.

Moll, A. (1912) *The sexual life of the child*. New York: Macmillan.

Montorsi, F., Perani, D., Anchisi, D., Salonia, A., Scifo, P., Rigiroli, P., et al. (2003). Apomorpine-induced brain modulation during sexual stimulation: A new look at central phenomena related to erectile dysfunction. *International Journal of Impotence Research, 15*(3), 203–209.

Morokoff, P. J., & Heiman, J. (1980). Effects of erotic stimuli on sexually functional and dysfunctional women. Multiple measures before and after sex therapy. *Behavior Research and Therapy, 18*, 127–137.

Morokoff, P. J., Myers, L. S., Hay, J., & Flora, M. N. (1988). Effectiveness of a procedure for disinfecting the vaginal photoplethysmograph contaminated with herpes simplex virus type 2. *Archives of Sexual Behavior, 17*(4), 363–369.

Morrell, M. J., Dixen, J. M., Carter, S., & Davidson, J. M. (1984). The influence of age and cycling status on sexual arousability in women. *American Journal of Obstetric Gynecology, 148*, 66–71.

Mosher, D. L. (1998). Multiple indicators of subjective sexual arousal. In C. M. Davis, W. L. Yarber, R. Bauserman, G. Schreer, & S. L. Davis, (Eds.), *Handbook of sexuality-related measures*. Thousand Oaks, CA: Sage.

Munoz, M. M., Bancroft, J., & Marshall, I. (1993). The performance of the Rigiscan in the measurement of penile tumescence and rigidity. *International Journal of Impotence Research, 5*, 69–76.

Ohlmeyer, P., Brilmayer, H., & Hullstrong, H. (1944). Periodische organge im schlaf II. Pfluengers. *Archiv fuer die Gesamta Physiologic, 249*, 50–55.

O'Reilly, M. A., Cunningham, C. J., Lawlor, B. A., Walsh, C. D., & Rowan, M. J. (2004). The effect of the menstrual cycle on electrophysiological and behavioral measures of memory and mood. *Psychophysiology, 41*, 592–603.

Osborn, C. A., & Pollack, R. H. (1977). The effects of two types of erotic literature on physiological and verbal measures of female sexual arousal. *Journal of Sex Research, 13*, 250–256.

Palace, E. M., & Gorzalka, B. B. (1990). The enhancing effects of anxiety on arousal in sexually dysfunctional and functional women. *Journal of Abnormal Psychology, 99*, 403–411.

Palace, E. M. (1995a). A cognitive-physiological process model of sexual arousal and response. *Clinical Psychology, Science and Practice, 2, 4*, 370–384.

Palace, E. M. (1995b). Modification of dysfunctional patterns of sexual response through autonomic arousal and false physiological feedback. *Journal of Consulting and Clinical Psychology, 63*, 604–615.

Palti, Y., & Bercovici, B. (1967). Photoplethysmographic study of the vaginal blood pulse. *American Journal of Obstetrics and Gynecology, 97*, 143–153.

Polan, M. L., Desmond, J. E., Banner, L. L., Pryor, M. R., McCallum, S. W., Atlas, S. W., et al. (2003). Female sexual arousal: A behavioral analysis. *Fertility & Sterility, 80*, 1480–1487.

Prause, N., Cerny, J., & Janssen, E. (2005). The labial photoplethysmograph: A new instrument for assessing genital hemodynamic changes in women. *Journal of Sexual Medicine, 2*, 58–65.

Prause, N., & Janssen, E. (2004). *Four approaches to the processing of vaginal pulse amplitude (VPA) signals.* Poster presented at the International Academy of Sex Research (IASR), Helsinki, Finland.

Prause, N., & Janssen, E. (2006). Vaginal photoplethysmography. In I. Goldstein, C. M. Meston, S. Davis, & A. Traish (Eds.), *Textbook of female sexual dysfunction.* New York: Taylor & Francis, 359–367.

Prause, N., Janssen, E., & Hetrick, W. P. (2003). The role of attention and affective response to sexual cues in the experience of sexual desire and sexual arousal. *Psychophysiology, 40* (Supp 1), S69.

Richards, J. C., Bridger, B. A., Wood, M. M., Kalucy, R. S., & Marshall, V. R. (1985). A controlled investigation into the measurement properties of two circumferential penile strain gauges. *Psychophysiology, 22*, 568–571.

Richards, J. C., Kalucy, R. S., Wood, M. M., & Marshall, V. R. (1990). Linearity of the electromechanical penile plethysmograph's output at large expansions. *Journal of Sex Research, 27*, 283–287.

Robinson, P. (1976). *The modernization of sex.* New York: Harper.

Rogers, G. S., Van de Castle, R. L., Evans, W. S., & Critelli, J. W. (1985). Vaginal pulse amplitude response patterns during erotic conditions and sleep. *Archives of Sexual Behavior, 14*, 327–342.

Rosen, R. C., & Beck, J. G. (1988). *Patterns of sexual arousal.* New York: Guilford Press.

Rosen, R. C., & Rosen, L. R. (1981). *Human Sexuality.* New York: Knopf.

Rosen et al. (in press). Sexual Dysfunction, Sexual Psychophysiology & Psychopharmacology: Laboratory studies in sexual psychopharmacology in men and women. In E. Janssen (Ed.), *The Psychophysiology of Sex.* Bloomington, IN: Indiana University Press, in press.

Rowland, D., Tai, W., & Brummett, K. (in press). Interactive Processes in Ejaculatory Disorders: Psychophysiological considerations. In E. Janssen (Ed.), *The Psychophysiology of Sex.* Bloomington, IN: Indiana University Press, in press.

Sakheim, D. K., Barlow, D. H., Abrahamson, D. J., & Beck, J. G. (1987). Distinguishing between organogenic and psychogenic erectile dysfunction. *Behaviour Research and Therapy, 25*, 379–390.

Sakheim, D. K., Barlow, D. H., & Beck, J. G. (1985). Diurnal penile tumescence: A pilot study of waking erectile potential in sexual functional and dysfunctional men. *Sexuality and Disability, 4*, 68–97.

Sasso, F., Stief, C. G., Gulino, G., Alcini, E. Jüneman, K. P., Gerstenberg, T., Merckx, L., & Wagner, G. (1997). Progress in corpus cavernosum electromyography (CC-EMG): Third international workshop on corpus cavernosum electromyography (CC-EMG). *International Journal of Impotence Research, 1*, 43–45.

Saunders, D. M., Fisher, W. A., Hewitt, E. C., & Clayton, J. P. (1985). A Method For Empirically Assessing Volunteer Selection Effects: Recruitment Procedures and Responses to Erotica. *Journal of Personality and Social Psychology, 49*,

Schiavi, R. C. (1992). Laboratory methods for evaluating erectile dysfunction. In R. C. Rosen, and S. R. Leiblum (Eds), *Erectile disorders: Assessment and treatment.* New York: Guilford Press, pp. 55–71.

Schreiner-Engel, P., Schiavi, R. C., Smith, H., & White, D. (1981). Sexual arousability and the menstrual cycle. *Psychosomatic Medicine, 43*, 199–214.

Scollon, C. N., Diener, E., Oishi, S., & Biswas-Diener, R. (2005). An experience sampling and cross-cultural investigation of the relation between pleasant and unpleasant emotion. *Cognition and Emotion, 19*, 27–52.

Seeley, F., Abramsen, P., Perry, L., Rothblatt, A., & Seeley, D. (1980). Thermogenic measures of sexual arousal: A methodological note. *Archives of Sexual Behavior, 9*, 77–85.

Seto, M. (in press). Psychophysiological Assessment of Paraphilic Sexual Interests. In E. Janssen (Ed.), *The Psychophysiology of Sex.* Bloomington, IN: Indiana University Press, in press.

Shapiro, A., & Cohen, H. (1965). The use of mercury capillary length gauges for the measurement of the volume of thoracic and diaphragmatic components of human respiration: A theoretical analysis and a practical method. *Transactions of the New York Academy of Sciences, 26*, 634–649.

Shapiro, A., Cohen, H., DiBianco, P., & Rosen, G. (1968). Vaginal blood flow changes during sleep and sexual arousal in women. *Psychophysiology, 4.* 349.

Sintchak, G., & Geer, J. H. (1975). A vaginal plethysmograph system. *Psychophysiology, 12*, 113–115.

Sipski, M. L., Alexander, C. J., & Rosen, R. (2001). Sexual arousal and orgasm in women: Effects of spinal cord injury. *Annals of Neurology, 49*, 35–44.

Slob, A. K., Ernste, M., & Werff-ten Bosch, J. van der (1991). Menstrual cycle phase and sexual arousability in women. *Archives of Sexual Behavior, 20*, 567–577.

Slob, A. K., Koster, J., Radder, J. K., & Werff-ten Bosch, J. van der (1990). Sexuality and psychophysiological functioning in women with diabetes mellitus. *Journal of Sex and Marital Therapy, 2*, 59–69.

Slob, A. K., Steyvers, C. L., Lottman, P. E., van der Werff ten Bosch, J. J., Hop, W. C. (1998). Routine psychophysiological screening of 384 men with erectile dysfunction. *Journal of Sex and Marital Therapy, 24*, 273–279.

Solnick, R., & Berrin, J. E. (1977). Age and male erectile responsiveness. *Archives of Sexual Behavior, 6*, 1–9.

Sommer, F., Caspers, H. P., Esders, K., Klotz, T., & Engelmann, U. (2001). Measurement of vaginal and minor labial oxygen tension for the evaluation of female sexual function. *Journal of Urology, 165*, 1181–1184.

Spiering, M., Everaerd, W., & Laan, E. (2004). Conscious Processing of Sexual Information: Mechanisms of Appraisal. *Archives of Sexual Behavior, 33*, 369–380.

Spiering, M., Everaerd, W., & Janssen, E (2003). Priming the sexual system: Implicit versus explicit activation. *Journal of Sex Research, 40*, 134–145.

Stoleru, S. & Mouras, H. (in press). Brain Functional Imaging Studies of Sexual Desire and Arousal in Human Males. In E. Janssen (Ed.), *The Psychophysiology of Sex.* Bloomington, IN: Indiana University Press, in press.

Stoleru, S., Redoute, J., Costes, N., Lavenne, F., Le Bars, D., Dechaud, H., et al. (2003). Brain processing of visual sexual stimuli in men with hypoactive sexual desire disorder. *Psychiatry Research: Neuroimaging, 124*(2), 67–86.

Strassberg, D. S., & Lowe, K. (1995). Volunteer bias in sexuality research. *Archives of Sexual Behavior, 24*, 369–382.

Suh, D. D., Yang, C. C., Cao, Y., Heiman, J. R., Garland, P. A., & Maravilla, K. R. (2004). Mri of female genital and pelvic organs during sexual arousal. *Journal of Psychosomatic Obstetrics & Gynecology, 25*, 153–163.

Tiefer, L. (1991). Historical, scientific, clinical, and feminist criticisms of "The Human Sexual Response Cycle" model. *Annual Review of Sex Research. 2*, 1–23.

Van de Velde, T. H. (1926). *Ideal marriage: Its physiology and technique*. New York: Random House.

Wabrek, A. J., Whitaker, K. F., McCahill, D., & Woronick, C. L. (1986). Vaginal penetration pressure: a pilot study. *World Congress of Sexology – Proceedings*, 55–61.

Wagner, G., & Gerstenberg, T. (1988). Human in vivo studies of electrical activity of corpus cavernosum (EACC). *Journal of Urology, 139*, 327A.

Wagner, G., Gerstenberg, T., & Levin, R. J. (1989). Electrical activity of corpus cavernosum during flaccidity and erection of the human penis: A new diagnostic method? *Journal of Urology, 142*, 723–725.

Wagner, G., & Levin, R. J. (1978). Vaginal fluid. In E. Hafez and T. Evans (Eds.), *The human vagina*. Amsterdam: Elsevier.

Wagner, G., & Levin, R. J. (1984). Human vaginal pH and sexual arousal. *Fertility and Sterility, 41*, 389–394.

Wagner, G., & Mulhall, J. (2001). Pathophysiology and diagnosis of male erectile dysfunction. *BJU International, 88*(Suppl. 3), 3–10.

Wagner, G., Wabrek, A. J., & Dalgaard, D. (1986). Vaginal penetration pressure: a parameter in impotence diagnosis? *World Journal of Urology, 4*, 250–251.

Walpurger, V., Pietrowsky, R., Kirschbaum, C., & Wolf, O. T. (2004). Effects of the menstrual cycle on auditory event-related potentials. *Hormones and Behavior, 46*, 600–606.

Webster, J. S., & Hammer, D. (1983). Thermistor measurement of male sexual arousal. *Psychophysiology, 20*, 115–115.

Wein, A. J., Fishkin, R., Carpiniello, V. L., & Malooy. T. R. (1981). Expension without significant rigidity during nocturnal penile tumescence testing: A potential source of misinterpretation. *Journal of Urology, 126*, 343–344.

Weijmar Schultz, W., van Andel, P., Sabelis, I., Mooyaart, E. (1999). Magnetic resonance imaging of male and female genitals during coitus and female sexual arousal. *British Medical Journal, 319*, 1596–1600.

Wheeler, D., & Rubin, H. B. (1987). A comparison of volumetric and circumferential measures of penile erection. *Archives of Sexual Behavior, 16*, 289–299.

Whipple, B., & Komisaruk, B. R. (2002). Brain (pet) responses to vaginal-cervical self-stimulation in women with complete spinal cord injury: Preliminary findings. *Journal of Sex & Marital Therapy, 28*, 79–87.

Wiederman, M. W. (1999). Volunteer bias in sexuality research using college student participants. *Journal of Sex Research, 36*, 59–66.

Wincze, J. P., Hoon, E. F., & Hoon. P. W. (1976). Physiological responsivity of normal and sexually dysfunctional women during erotic stimulus exposure. *Journal of Psychosomatic Research, 20*, 445–451.

Wolchik, S. A., Braver, S. L., & Jensen, K. (1985). Volunteer bias in erotica research: Effects of intrusiveness of measure and sexual background. *Archives of Sexual Behavior, 14*, 93–107.

Wouda, J. C., Hartmen, P. M., Bakker, R. M., Bakker, J. O., van de Weil, H. B. M., Schultz, W., et al. (1998). Vaginal plethysmography in women with dyspareunia. *Journal of Sex Research, 35*, 141–147.

Yilmaz, U., Kromm, B. G., & Yang, C. C. (2004). Evaluation of autonomic innervation of the clitoris and bulb. *Journal of Urology, 172*, 1930–1934.

Yilmaz, U., Soylu, A., Ozcan, C., & Caliskan, O. (2002). Clitoral electromyography. *Journal of Urology, 167*, 616–620.

Zuckerman, M. (1971). Physiological measures of sexual arousal in the human. *Psychological Bulletin, 75*, 297–329.

12

The Skeletomotor System: Surface Electromyography

LOUIS G. TASSINARY, JOHN T. CACIOPPO, AND ERIC J. VANMAN

The brain recalls just what the muscles grope for; no more, no less...(Faulkner, 1936, p. 143)

The principal function of the nervous system is the coordinated innervation of the musculature. Its fundamental anatomical plan and working principles are understandable only on these terms. (Sperry, 1952, p. 298)

INTRODUCTION

The sophistication of the skeletomuscular system enables the vast repertoire of adaptive reflexes and skilled actions characteristic of behavior. The electrophysiological signals associated with active muscles have been of interest for centuries due to the complexity of their organization and dynamics, their clinical applications, and their value as indices of and possible contributors to behavioral processes.

In this chapter, we provide an introduction specifically to psychophysiological research on the skeletomotor system.[1] We begin by reviewing the history of this research and by articulating some of the major issues, limitations, and advantages of surface electromyography (EMG) as a noninvasive measure of muscular activity. We then review briefly the physiological basis of EMG and summarize guidelines for surface EMG recording in humans. We continue with a discussion of the social context for EMG recording and of psychophysiological principles and common paradigms that have emerged from research on the skeletomotor system. For EMG signals to be of theoretical significance, one must consider conjointly the historical, physical, social, and inferential contexts in which these signals are acquired.

HISTORICAL CONTEXT

In this section we identify two distinct themes in the development of electromyography in psychophysiology.

---

[1] Additional information on electromyography generally can be found in Basmalian nand DeLuca (1985), Johnson and Pease (1997), Loeb and Gans (1986), or Ludin (1995).

The first is the history of the physiology of the muscles, which derives from the writings of the early Greek philosophers, and from the scientific renaissance in the seventeenth century. The second is the history of psychophysiological research, which began in earnest with the work of such figures as Duchenne (1990/1862), Spencer (1870), Darwin (1873/1872), and James (1890), all of whom emphasized relatively subtle patterns of muscular actions as a way of characterizing and understanding human behavior generally.

Muscle physiology

The history of muscle physiology can be traced back to the fourth century B.C.E., when Aristotle provided clear descriptions of coordinated motor acts (e.g., locomotion and the importance of the mechanism of flexion) in his books *De Motu Animalium* and *De Incessu Animalium*. The field of neurophysiology can be traced to Franceso Redi's deduction in 1666 that the shock of the electric ray fish (*Torpedo torpedo*) emanated from specialized muscle tissue (Wu, 1984). It was not until the early nineteenth century, however, that a sensitive instrument for measuring small electric currents was invented (i.e., the galvanometer). In 1833, Carlo Matteucci used such a device to demonstrate an electrical potential between an excised frog's nerve and its damaged muscle. Du-Bois Reymond, a student of the renowned physiologist Johannes Müller, built upon Matteucci's then recent publication, eventually publishing the results of an extensive series of investigations on the electrical basis of muscular contraction as well as providing the first *in vivo* evidence of electrical activity in human muscles during voluntary contraction (Basmajian & De Luca, 1985).

The study of the thermodynamics of muscle contraction owes a debt to another of Muller's students, Hermann Ludwig Ferdinand von Helmholtz. Fueled by the desire to abolish the notion of vital forces underlying muscular actions, von Helmholtz began an investigation into the chemical transformations occurring in frog muscle during contraction. Put simply, he reasoned that the heat of combustion combined with the transformation of food material should produce a quantity of heat measurable at the muscle surface during contraction. By stimulating an isolated muscle through its nerve and employing a sensitive thermocouple he was able to demonstrate a rise in temperature during contraction. This demonstration not only provided the experimental basis for his classic paper on the conservation of energy, but also proved instrumental in focusing subsequent investigations on the central problem of understanding the physiochemical processes involved in converting neural energy to mechanical work (Hill, 1959).

Based on experimental observations using electrical stimulation, muscle physiologists during the eighteenth and early nineteenth century attributed graded muscular responses to graded variations in the intensity of the stimulation. Until late in the nineteenth century, many erroneously inferred from the strong correlation between the intensity of exogenous electrical stimulation and the intensity of contraction that the actual size of the neural impulses was proportional to the stimulus intensity. Experimental work around the turn of the century (e.g., Lucas 1909), however, challenged this belief, strongly suggesting that graded muscular responses resulted from the firing of individual contractile units rather than from variation in the size of the nerve impulse. Direct evidence for the "all-or-none" character of the response of muscle fibers was finally obtained by Frederick Pratt and his colleagues in the early 1900s (Pratt, 1917; Pratt & Eisenberger, 1919). They applied graded electrical stimulation to individual muscle fibers while simultaneously photographing the spatial displacement of mercury droplets sprinkled previously over the muscle surface and observed that additional fibers contracted coincident with each quantal step in the displacement of a mercury droplet.[2] The foundations of modern electromyography were finally laid in the 1930s with publications of Adrian and Bronk (1929), Lindsley (1935), Jacobson (1927), and the introduction of the differential amplifier (Mathews, 1934).

Skeletomotor activation and patterning

Detecting myoelectric signals using surface electrodes remained difficult throughout the nineteenth and early twentieth centuries. Electrically stimulating a muscle cutaneously was considerably simpler, however. Perhaps best known for this work was Guillaume Duchenne de Boulogne, who used this technique in the mid-nineteenth century to investigate the dynamics and function of the human facial muscles in vivo (Duchenne, 1990/1862). Not surprisingly, Charles Darwin corresponded with Duchenne in an effort to evaluate his own observations about facial

expressions and emotion (Cuthbertson, 1990), as well as those observations of earlier writers with whom he was familiar (see Tassinary & Geen, 1990; Geen & Tassinary, 2002).

Darwin's interest in muscular action was based upon his belief that many behaviors were in part inherited. He focused his inquiry on the expression of emotions in man and animals to buttress this belief and presaged contemporary studies of the patterns of muscle contractions and facial actions that are undetectable to the naked eye with his conclusion that "... whenever the same state of mind is induced, however feebly, there is a tendency through the force of habit and association for the same movements to be performed, though they may not be of the least use" (Darwin, 1873/1872, p. 281).

The somatic elements of William James's (1884) theory of emotions and the various motor theories of thinking prevalent at the turn of the century (e.g., Washburn, 1916) further fueled interest in objective measures of subtle or fleeting muscle contractions. Among the more creative procedures used to magnify tiny muscular contractions were sensitive pneumatic systems used to record finger movements during conflict situations (Luria, 1932) as well as elaborate lever-based systems to record subtle tongue movements during thinking (Thorson, 1925). Sensitive and specific noninvasive recordings, however, awaited the development of metal surface electrodes, vacuum tube amplifiers, and the cathode-ray oscilloscope early in this century which enabled the pioneering work of Edmund Jacobson (1927; 1932) on electrical measurements of muscle activity during imagery. The results of these studies and others (e.g., Davis, 1938) demonstrated that EMG responses were evoked by psychologically relevant tasks (e.g., recall a poem), were minute and highly localized, and often occurred in the part of the body that one would use had the task called for an overt response. This work was subsequently criticized primarily for not definitively achieving mentally quiescent comparison periods (e.g., Humphrey, 1951; Max, 1937), but successful replications of this early work using different comparison tasks have been reported (McGuigan, 1966; 1978).

Enduring issues

Subsequent research using surface EMG has extended these early observations, documenting patterns of covert skeletomotor activity that differentiate both within and between emotional and cognitive processes (e.g., see reviews by Cacioppo, Klein, Berntson, & Hatfield, 1993; Fridlund & Izard, 1983; McGuigan, 1978; Tassinary & Cacioppo, 1992) as well as between normal and clinical populations (e.g., van Boxtel, Goudswaard, & Janssen, 1983; Gehricke & Shapiro, 2001; Hazlett, McLeod & Hoehn-Saric, 1994; Wolf et al., 2004). The enduring important issues in this research include the extent to which recorded EMG responses reflect specific or global

---

[2] Interested readers may wish to consult Fulton (1926), Huxley (1980), Keynes and Aidley (1991), or Needham (1971) for more in-depth coverage of the history of muscle physiology.

activation, as well as to what extent they reflect characteristics of the situation, the individual, or the processing task. Not surprisingly, it has proven advantageous to monitor multiple EMG responses across time using sophisticated designs with multiple control conditions and to employ time-locked recording procedures. For example, Cacioppo, Bush, and Tassinary (1992) examined simultaneously the effect of communicative intent and stimulus valence, using both social and asocial stimuli, on EMG activity at five discrete sites on the face. Their results suggest (1) that facial EMG activity continues to be modulated by both affective and communicative processes even when it is too subtle to produce a clearly perceptible expression and (2) that muscles in the brow and periocular regions are more responsive differentially to both processes than muscles in either the forehead, cheek, or perioral regions.

Two general features of the physical architecture of the skeletomotor system also present some enduring inferential challenges to surface EMG recording. First, is the sheer number of muscles. Most of the striated muscles are bilaterally symmetrical in pairs, with several hundred distinct muscles throughout the human body. Second is the alluring aggregate simplicity of the muscle as a functional unit. That is, from such a perspective, each striated muscle can be characterized as a linear actuator, with the potential states being limited to onset of contraction, offset of contraction, and relaxation (Tomovic & Bellman, 1970). The structural arrangements of the striated muscles as agonist-antagonist pairs, or through their interdigitation, however, expand dramatically the number of actions that can be achieved using these deceptively simple elements. The relatively small number of muscles in the head and face, for instance, have been estimated to enable the encoding of some 6,000 to 7,000 appearance changes (Izard, 1971; see Figure 12.1).

The challenges that derive from these architectural features are several. First, it is feasible to obtain measurements over only a small number of muscles in the human body in any given experiment. Yet because the action of the striated muscles is multiply determined, monitoring activity from a single site may only provide global or ambiguous information about the associated psychological or behavioral process. Ekman (1982) observed, for instance, that emotions, with the possible exception of happiness, cannot be identified by the activity of a single muscle, echoing an earlier call for the necessity of recording from more than one muscle group during emotional reactions (Lindsley, 1951).

Second, many movements can be achieved by the actions of different or differently activated striated muscles. Electromyographic responses may therefore appear unreliable if the focus is solely on the behavioral output rather than the mechanisms by which these movements were achieved (e.g., Gans & Gorniak, 1980; Kelso, Tuller, Vatikiotis-Bateson, & Fowler, 1984). Third, the imperfect selectivity of surface electrodes and the close proxim-

ity of the various striated muscles make it difficult to pinpoint exactly which muscles are contracting. Hence, when using surface electrodes, it is typically appropriate to refer to EMG signals as reflecting activity from sites or regions (e.g., *zygomaticus major* muscle region). Fourth, surface EMG recording, although noninvasive, can be obtrusive and potentially reactive. Electrodes attached to the surface of the skin with wires connected to preamplifiers, for instance, can restrict an individual's movement or make the individual tense or self-conscious, or sensitive to experimental demand characteristics. Finally, although acknowledged standards for the placement of surface electrodes to detect activity in particular muscles or muscle regions do exist (i.e., Fridlund & Cacioppo, 1986; Zipp, 1982), these have not been adopted universally (see Andreassi, 1995, p. 149; McGuigan, 1994, p. 225) and, consequently, comparisons across laboratories or across individuals and sessions within laboratories remain somewhat problematic.

Progress has been made in overcoming many of these limitations (e.g., De Luca & Knaflitz, 1992; Kumar & Mital, 1996; Fridlund & Cacioppo, 1986; Tassinary, Cacioppo, & Geen, 1989), and this progress is reviewed in the sections that follow. In addition, surface EMG recording offers several unique advantages that complement the study of overt behavior through traditional means. First, EMG responses, in contrast to measures such as response latencies or verbal reports, can be collected continuously without the individual's attention or labor. Second, the detection and quantification of EMG signals as a measure of muscle activation can be performed with the assistance of computers more sensitively, reliably, and quickly than can fine-grain analyses of overt behavior (Tuomisto, Johnson, & Schmidt, 1996; cf. Cohn, Zlochower, Lien, & Kanade, 1999; Himer, Schneider, Koest, & Heimann, 1991). Third, analyses of subtle somatic patterns and their time course may provide a means of differentiating underlying mechanisms of control over similar overt behaviors (Allain et al., 2004; Ghez & Krahauer, 2000; Hasbroucq et al., 2001).

Finally, many subtle psychological processes or events are not accompanied by visually perceptible actions or significant visceral changes (e.g., Graham, 1980; Rajecki, 1983). Darwin (1873/1872) recognized this limitation in the study of emotional expressions, stating that "the study of expression is difficult, owing to the movements being often extremely slight, and of a fleeting nature" (p. 12). It is now clear that fast or low-level changes in EMG activity can occur without leading to any visible movements. Facial expressions, for instance, result from displacements of skin and connective tissue due to the contraction of muscles that create folds, lines, and wrinkles in the facial skin and the movement of landmarks such as the brows and corners of the mouth (e.g., Rinn, 1991). Although muscle activation must occur if these facial distortions are to be achieved, it is possible for muscle activation to

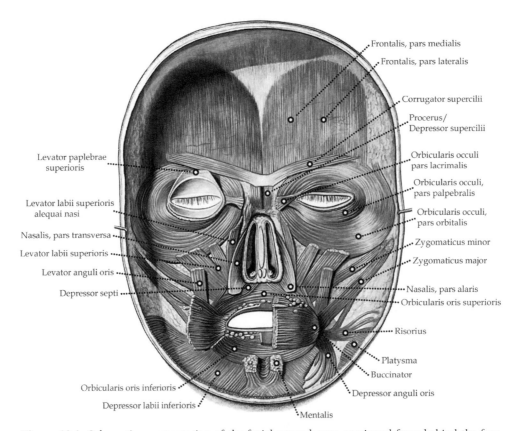

Levator paplebrae superioris

Levator labii superioris alequai nasi

Nasalis, pars transversa

Levator labii superioris

Levator anguli oris

Depressor septi

Frontalis, pars medialis

Frontalis, pars lateralis

Corrugator supercilii

Procerus/ Depressor supercilii

Orbicularis occuli pars lacrimalis

Orbicularis occuli, pars palpebralis

Orbicularis occuli, pars orbitalis

Zygomaticus minor

Zygomaticus major

Nasalis, pars alaris

Orbicularis oris superioris

Risorius

Platysma

Buccinator

Depressor anguli oris

Orbicularis oris inferioris

Depressor labii inferioris

Mentalis

Figure 12.1. Schematic representation of the facial musculature, as viewed from behind the face (modified from Figure 137 of Pernkopf, 1980). Overt facial expressions are based on contractions of the underlying musculature sufficiently intense to result in perceptible dislocations of the skin. More common perceptible effects of strong bilateral contractions of the depicted facial muscles include the following, divided into the major regions of the face. Muscles of the lower face: *depressor anguli oris*, pulls lip corners downward; *depressor labii inferioris*, depresses lower lip; *orbicularis oris* (*superioris* and *inferioris*), tightens, compresses, protrudes, and/or inverts lips; *mentalis*, elevates chin boss and protrudes lower lip; *platysma*, wrinkles skin of neck and may draw down both lower lip and lip corners. Muscles of the middle face: *buccinator*, compresses and tightens cheeks, forming dimples; *levator labii superioris alaequai nasi*, raises center of upper lip and flares nostrils; *nasalis pars alaris*, tightens or flares the ala of the nose; *nasalis pars transversa*, produces transverse wrinkles across the nose and may pull down the medial part of nose; *depressor septi*, pulls down septum and protrudes upper lip; *levator labii superioris*, raises upper lip and flares nostrils, exposing canine teeth; *zygomaticus major*, pulls lip corners up and back; *zygomaticus minor*, draws the upper lip backward, upward and outward; *risorius*, retracts lip corners. Muscles of the upper face: *corrugator supercilii*, draws brows together and downward, producing vertical furrows between brows; *procerus/depressor supercilii*, pulls medial part of the brows downward and may wrinkle skin over bridge of nose; *frontalis pars lateralis*, raises outer brows, producing horizontal furrows in lateral regions of forehead; *frontalis pars medialis*, raises inner brows, producing horizontal furrows in medial region of the forehead; *levator palpebrae superioris*, raises and pulls back upper eyelids; *orbicularis oculi pars orbitalis*, tightens skin surrounding eyes, causing "crow's feet" wrinkles; *orbicularis pars palpebrae*, tightens skin around eyes, causing lower eyelids to rise; *orbicularis oculi pars lacrimalis*, compresses the lachrymal sacs and facilitates effective tearing. Descriptions are consistent with those in Hislop and Montgomery (2002), Ekman and Friesen (1978), Gray (1918/2000), Izard (1971), Kendall and McCreary (1993), and Weaver (1977).

occur in the absence of any overt action if the activation is weak or transient or if the overt response is very rapid, suppressed or aborted (see Cacioppo et al., 1992). This holds for nonfacial striated muscles as well (see Coles, Gratton, Bashore, Eriksen, & Donchin, 1985; de Jong, Coles, Logan & Gratton, 1990; McGarry & Franks, 1997; Lutz, 2003).

In the face, the uncoupling of muscle activation and observable movement is due in part to the structure and elasticity of the facial skin, fascia, and adipose tissue, as well as due to the unique architecture of the facial musculature. The muscles of expression are attached to other muscles, bones, or a superficial musculoaponeurotic system (SMAS; Mitz, 1976; Kikkawa, Lemke, & Dortzvbach, 1996) that extends throughout the cervicofacial area; not unlike a loose chain, the facial muscles can be pulled a small distance (i.e., contracted slightly) before exerting a significant force on the points to which they are anchored. In addition, the elasticity of the SMAS, facial skin, and adipose tissue forms a complex low-pass mechanical filter,

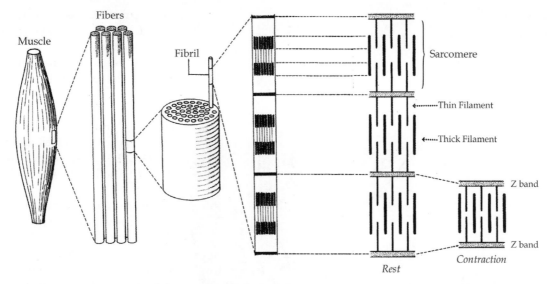

Figure 12.2. Diagram of the structure of the muscle with increasing magnification going from left to right. The bottom right corner of the figure illustrates the microgeometric changes that occur with contraction. (Modified from Figure 10.7 of Schmidt-Nielsen, 1997).

attenuating the visible effects of very brief or slight contractions yet allowing the displacement and bulging of the face due to sustained or moderate contractions (Partridge, 1966; Waters, 1992; Gousain, Amarante, Hyde, & Yousif, 1996)

In summary, measures of EMG and of observable muscular actions each have unique advantages and disadvantages. Neither is necessarily better or more capable of capturing completely the information provided by the other. A general congruence between the results based on EMG recordings and those obtained through fine-grain analyses of overt behavior is to be expected given the physiological basis of the surface EMG (see what follows), although EMG recordings and fine-grain behavioral observations do not coincide completely (Ekman, 1982; Girard et al., 1997). Therefore, the wealth of information that exists regarding nonverbal behavior during such processes as sleeping, thinking, communicating, dissimulating, and feeling (see Feldman & Rime, 1991; Russell & Fernández-Dols, 1997; Tyron, 1991) provides a rich theoretical resource for research on subtler, more fleeting responses or on underlying mechanisms.

PHYSICAL CONTEXT

An understanding of the physical system one is studying and the bioelectrical principles underlying its responses serve several important purposes. These include the development of operational definitions and procedures, the ability to discriminate signal from artifact, the maintenance of a safe environment for both experimenters and research participants (see Greene, Turetsky, & Kohler, 2000) and, ultimately, the guidance of inferences based on physiological data (see Cacioppo, Tassinary, & Berntson, this volume, Chapter 1). In this section, therefore, we review the physical basis of the surface EMG.

Anatomical and physiological basis of the surface electromyogram

Muscles perform many different functions (Smith & Kier, 1989). Their orchestrated activation maintains posture, causes reflexive movements, and produces both spontaneous and voluntary movements that occur across many different scales of space and time.[3]

Fundamentally, muscle is a tissue that both generates and transmits force. Striated muscle, in particular, is a hierarchical material made up of a very large number of parallel fibers whose diameters are orders of magnitude smaller than a millimeter and yet may be up to several centimeters in length (see Figure 12.2). The term "striated" comes from the fact these fibers are actually bundles of thinner structures, known as *fibrils*, which have repeating cross striations throughout their length known as Z-lines or Z-bands. Electron microscopy reveals that between these striations (an area know as the *sarcomere*) are a series of thick and thin filaments bound together by a system of molecular cross-linkages. The thick filaments are made up of the protein myosin and lie in the center of the sarcomere between the thin filaments. The thin filaments are composed of the proteins actin, tropomyosin, and troponin, are discontinuous and are attached either at one end or the other of the sarcomere. During contraction, conformational changes in the cross-linkages lead to only very slight changes in the length of the filaments but cause substantial changes in the distance between Z bands as the thick filaments slide in between the thin filaments (Schmidt-Nielsen, 1997).

[3] A detailed description of the central organization and control of the motor system, although important, is beyond the scope of the present chapter. Interested readers can consult Kandel, Schwartz, and Jessell (2000) for an overview and a recent review article by Morecraft et al. (2004) for more detailed information on the central organization and control of the facial motor system in particular. See also Solodkin, Hlustik, & Buccino, this volume, Chapter 22.

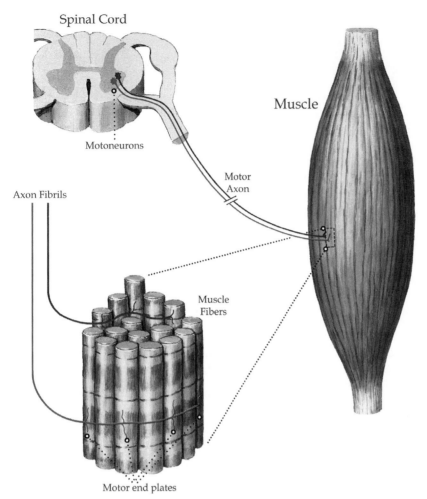

Figure 12.3. Diagram of two motor units. (Modified from slide 3705 of Netter, 1991).

Each striated muscle is innervated by a single motor nerve whose cell bodies are located primarily in the anterior horn of the spinal cord or, in the case of the muscles of the head, in the cranial nerves of the brain stem. All behavior – that is, all actions of the striated muscles regardless of the brain processes involved – result from neural signals traveling along these motor nerves. For this reason, the set of lower motor nerves has been designated the final common pathway (Sherrington, 1923/1906).

The motor nerve traveling to the muscle consists of axons of numerous individual motoneurons, which as a collective are referred to as a motoneuron pool. Each motoneuron axon divides into a number of small branches, termed axon fibrils, just before reaching the muscle; each axon fibril, in turn, forms a junction, called a motor end plate, on an individual muscle fiber. Each motoneuron innervates a number of interspersed muscle fibers within a muscle, and each muscle fiber is usually innervated by only one motoneuron. The spatial distribution of motor endplates on the muscle surface is not random but forms at most a few clusters (typically only one) and these are referred to as innervation zones. An important functional consequence of this structure is that muscle fibers do not contract individually but rather the entire set of muscle fibers innervated by a single

motoneuron contracts in consonance. Therefore, the most elementary functional unit within the final common pathway is the motoneuron cell body, its axon, its axon fibrils, and the individual muscle fibers innervated by these axon fibrils. This functional physiological entity is called the motor unit, a concept proposed by Liddell and Sherrington (1925) and subsequently quantified by Eccles and Sherrington (1930) (see Figure 12.3).

The axons of the motoneurons within a motoneuron pool vary in diameter and this structural feature also has important functional consequences. Generally, the smaller the diameter of a motoneuronal axon, the smaller the number of axon fibrils, the smaller the number of muscle fibers it innervates, and the smaller the size of its cell body. Hence, activation of muscle via small motoneurons produces smaller and more precise actions than activation of the same muscle by the depolarization of large motoneurons. In addition, the smaller the diameter of the motoneuron, the lower the critical firing threshold of its cell body and the more fatigue resistant (i.e., greater glycolytic capacity) are the muscle fibers it innervates. These relationships constitute the size principle (Henneman, 1980) and it contributes to our ability to control force in a smooth and graded fashion. More specifically, the initial force of contraction produced by a muscle is attributable to small motoneurons discharging intermittently and then discharging more frequently. Stronger muscle contractions are attributable to the depolarization of increasingly large motoneurons within the motoneuron pool concurrent with increases in the firing rates of the smaller motoneurons already active. As muscle contraction approaches maximal levels, further increases in force are attributable primarily to the entire pool of motoneurons firing more rapidly. This cascade of processes appears to be regulated by unidimensional increases in the aggregate neural input to the motoneuronal pool, a process referred to as "common drive" (De Luca & Erim, 1994; Brown, 2000).[4]

The number of muscle fibers innervated per motoneuron, known as the innervation ratio, varies even more dramatically across than within muscles. Consistent with the principles outlined in the preceding, muscles with low

[4] Although the size principle provides an elegant explanation for many phenomena related to the "voluntary" control of force there is some evidence that the principle may not hold when multi-degree of freedom muscles are involved, a phenomenon referred to as task-dependent muscle partitioning (see Desmedt & Godaux, 1981; Abbs, Gracco, & Blair, 1984).

innervation ratios are capable of producing actions more rapidly and with greater precision than are muscles with high innervation ratios. For example, the small extrinsic muscles of the eye, which are capable of very fast and fine movements, have innervation ratios around 10:1, whereas the relatively large and more slowly acting postural muscles, such as the gastrocnemius (i.e., superficial foot extensor muscle of the calf), have innervation ratios of around 2000:1 (Loeb & Ghez, 2000).

The depolarization of a motoneuron results in the quantal release of acetylcholine at the motor end plates. The activating neurotransmitter acetylcholine is quickly metabolized by the enzyme acetylcholinesterase so that continuous efferent discharges are required for continued propagation of muscle action potentials (MAPs) and fiber contraction. Nonetheless, the transient excitatory potential within a motor end plate can lead to a brief (e.g., 1 ms) depolarization of the resting membrane potential of the muscle cell and a MAP that is propagated bidirectionally across the muscle fiber with constant velocity and undiminished amplitude. The MAP travels rapidly along the surface of the fiber and flows into the muscle fiber itself via a system of T-tubules, thus ensuring that the contraction (known as a twitch) involves the entire fiber. The physiochemical mechanism responsible for the "twitch" involves a complex yet well-characterized self-regulating calcium-dependent interaction between the actin and myosin molecules.

A small portion of the changing electromagnetic field confederated with these processes passes through the extracellular fluids to the skin and it is these voltage fluctuations that constitute the major portion of the surface EMG signal. The voltage changes that are detected in surface EMG recording do not emanate from a single MAP but rather from MAPs traveling across many muscle fibers within a motor unit (i.e., motor unit action potential, or MUAP) and, more typically, from MAPs traveling across numerous motor fibers due to the activation of multiple motor units. Thus, the EMG does not provide a direct measure of tension, muscular contraction, or movement but rather the electrical activity associated with these events. More specifically, the surface EMG signal represents the ensemble electromagnetic field detectable at the surface of the skin at a given moment in time. Normally, both the details of the individual MAPs and the precise muscular origins of the signal are not recoverable (cf. Khan, Bloodworth, Woods, 1971). Reliable, valid, and sensitive information about the aggregate actions (or inactions) of motoneuron pools across time, however, can nonetheless be obtained by careful attention to the elements of surface EMG recording and analysis (e.g., see Cacioppo, Marshall-Goodell, & Dorfman, 1983; Lippold, 1967; De Luca & Knaflitz, 1992).

SIGNAL DETECTION

In this section we outline principles and technical issues involved in obtaining valid measures of EMG activity. As outlined above, the ensemble surface EMG signal emanating from the muscle is the result of the spatio-temporal summing of a quasi-random train of MUAPs. The aggregate signal is characterized by a frequency range of several hertz to over 500 Hz and by amplitudes ranging from fractions of a microvolt to over a thousand microvolts. These frequency and amplitude characteristics are broader than most bioelectrical signals of interest to psychophysiologists, and they overlap a variety of disparate bioelectrical signals (e.g., the electroencephalogram and the electrocardiogram) as well as the ubiquitous external 50/60 Hz signals emanating from most AC-powered equipment (see Marshall-Goodell, Tassinary, & Cacioppo, 1990). Consequently, the detection of EMG signals from a localized muscle region requires careful attention to noise reduction and grounding practices, electrode site preparation and placement, and appropriate differential preamplification and preliminary signal conditioning in order to eliminate extraneous electrical noise, minimize the detection of irrelevant bioelectrical signals, and enhance the signal-to-noise ratio.

Noise reduction and grounding

Noise has been defined by many authors as simply any unwanted signal. In the present context, it is important to note that EMG signals can be obscured by noise from many sources. These include but are not limited to external electrical sources, physiological responses whose frequency and amplitude characteristics overlap those for EMG recording, EMG signals emanating from task-irrelevant muscles (i.e., cross-talk), and EMG signals from target sites that result from "irrelevant" actions presumed to be minimized or eliminated by the design of the experiment (e.g., movement artifacts).

The most problematic exogenous electrical noise in the laboratory is narrowband noise because it arises from several common sources, radiates through walls and air, and overlaps in frequency with the EMG signal. For example, 50/60-Hz noise emanates from AC power lines, lights, relays, and transformers. Televisions, video monitors, and most computer terminals use cathode-ray tubes (CRTs), and these tend to generate high-frequency electrical noise (ranging from 15 kHz to several MHz). Although many EMG preamplifiers include filters to eliminate such noise, filters are neither completely selective nor entirely effective. Special-purpose notch filters, for example, attenuate frequencies to a varying degree on both sides of 50/60 Hz – a bandwidth that can represent a significant portion of the total power in an EMG signal – and strong signals in the high frequency range can appear under the "alias" of small signals in the EMG bandwidth. It is therefore important to minimize electrical noise prior to amplification. This can be done through appropriate placement and shielding of equipment and careful grounding of the research participant and laboratory equipment (Bramsley, Bruun, Buchthal, Guld, & Petersen, 1967; Fridlund & Cacioppo, 1986; McGuigan, 1979). Wideband noise (white noise) is usually attributable to the Brownian motion intrinsic to electronic devices. This noise is unavoidable but can be minimized by keeping electrode impedances low, amplifier filters set tightly to the proper bandwidth, and using calibrated high-grade equipment.

With respect to grounding, a research participant affixed with electrodes should be grounded at one and only one point on her or his body and any equipment touched by the participant should ideally be nonconductive. If multichannel recordings are to be made, the grounds for each channel should be strapped together and a single ground electrode attached. This procedure further minimizes 50/60 Hz noise in the recordings and enhances the safety of the participant by eliminating the possibility of ground loops (i.e., unintended current flow due to imperfect grounding).

Biological noise includes all endogenous signals that are not part of the bioelectrical signal of interest. In the sections that follow, we outline several procedures for minimizing biological noise. The careful and correct placement of a ground electrode, however, does not prevent artifacts from cross-talk, one of the primary sources of biological noise. Put simply, this is because the impedance into the ground electrode tends to exceed the access impedance of the volume-conductive tissues between the spurious current source and the recording electrode(s). Additional details and discussions are provided by Loeb and Gans (1986) and Basmajian and De Luca (1985).

Electrode selection and placement

Psychophysiologists, nearly without exception, use surface rather than needle or fine-wire electrodes for EMG recording. This is due primarily to the noninvasive nature of surface recording and to the fact that the research questions posed thus far by psychophysiologists involve muscles or sets of muscles rather than motor units within muscles. Surface EMG electrodes are less sensitive to exact anatomical placement because they detect the summated MAPs from an indeterminate cluster of motor units rather than a single unit.[5] This aggregate response develops in an orderly manner such that surface EMG recordings correlate well with the overall level of contraction of muscle groups underlying and near the electrodes, especially when limb movement is constrained and contractions are neither minimal nor maximal (Lawrence & DeLuca, 1983; Lippold, 1967).

Because most EMG amplifiers are AC coupled the electrical stability of the electrodes is not as important as, for instance, when recording skin conductance (see Dawson, Schell, & Filion, this volume). Nonpolarizing electrodes such as silver-silver chloride electrodes, however, can be used very effectively in nearly all recording situations. Tin, stainless steel, gold, or the platinum family of noble met-

als can be used effectively in many recording situations, although the lack of chemical equilibrium at the metal-electrolyte junction does make this class of electrode inherently more noisy and susceptible to artifact. In addition, stainless steel may be contraindicated when recording low-frequency, low-amplitude signals (Cooper, Osselton, & Shaw, 1980). As a result, the silver-silver chloride electrode is – in most research applications – the electrode of choice.

Surface electrodes can be constructed to be either active or passive. If passive, the electrode consists simply of a detection surface. If active, the input impedance of the electrode is made artificially high using proximal microelectronics.[6] Essentially, these microelectronics consist of a low-gain differential preamplifier with very high-input and very low-output impedances built into the electrode housing. Locating the first stage of high-impedance amplification as close as possible to the detection surfaces renders this class of electrodes relatively insensitive to the vagaries of the electrode-skin interface; and the low output impedance minimizes artifacts due to any movement of the cable connecting the electrode to the main amplifier. These advantages are obtained, however, at the cost of increased noise levels, higher expense, and typically much greater mass. Surface electrodes are also available in a variety of sizes. Electrodes with small detection surfaces and housings allow closer interelectrode spacing and consequently higher selectively. Such factors as the electrode size, electrode positioning and interelectrode distance over a particular site can affect the detected EMG signals and hence should be held constant across experimental conditions. For example, a smaller spacing shifts the bandwidth to higher frequencies and lowers the amplitude of the signal.

Fridlund and Cacioppo (1986) found that electrodes with 0.5-cm diameter detection surfaces and 1.5-cm diameter housings are used commonly for limb and trunk EMG recording, and miniature electrodes with 0.25-cm diameter detection surfaces and 0.5- or 1.0-cm diameter housings are used for facial EMG recording. They and others (Basmajian & De Luca, 1985) advocated, based on a variety of criteria, the use of a 1.0-cm interdetector surface spacing whenever possible. Given a circular detection surface, however, the inter detection-surface spacing is limited by the diameter of the electrodes. This is unfortunate because, *ceteris paribus*, the larger the size of the detection surfaces, the larger the amplitude of the signal that will be detected and the smaller the electrical noise that will be generated at the skin detection-surface interface. Some investigators have advocated the use of a rectangular rather than a circular detection surface based on the reasoning that a "bar" will, in general, intersect more fibers (De Luca, 1997). No empirical research, to our knowledge, has explicitly addressed the issue but simulation studies have been conducted (see Farina, Ceson, & Merletti, 2002).

[5] Placement with respect to the innervation zone of the muscle, however, is an important consideration because both the amplitude and frequency spectrum of the EMG signal vary as a function of this spatial relationship.

[6] Further discussion of these two different classes of surface electrodes can be found in Basmajian and De Luca (1985).

Regardless of the optimal detection surface geometry, however, only closely spaced electrodes and differential amplification can yield spatially selective surface EMG recordings. For example, using only these two basic procedures, a study of the human nasal musculature demonstrated a remarkable degree of specificity with passive surface EMG electrodes (Bruintjes, von Olphen, Hillen, & Weijs, 1996).

Specification of surface electrode placements over target muscle groups is important to ensure that findings are comparable across individuals, sessions, or laboratories. Several studies offer empirically and anatomically derived recommendations for EMG recording for facial, masticatory, and articulatory muscle activity using subdermal electrodes (e.g., Compton, 1973; Fridlund & Cacioppo, 1986; Isley & Basmajian, 1973; O'Dwyer, Quinn, Guitar, Andrews, & Neilson, 1981; Seiler, 1973; Vitti et al., 1975), and additional studies have examined the reliability of EMG measurements in relatively large, well-defined muscles (Gans & Gorniak, 1980; Komi & Buskirk, 1970; Martin, 1956), as well as offered suggestions for the placement of surface electrodes (see Cram, Kasman, & Holtz, 1998). This research supports a general principle of electrode orientation for spatially sensitive and specific differential recording over a given muscle region. Put directly, electrodes should be placed proximal and oriented parallel to voltage gradients of interest and, simultaneously, be placed distal and oriented perpendicular to voltage gradients of extraneous signal sources (e.g., other muscles). Successful implementation of this principle is limited by the underlying anatomy, the magnitude of interfering signals, the availability of reliable anatomical landmarks, and the presence of task-related complications (e.g., obstruction of vision).

For specific electrode placements on the face,[7] Tassinary et al. (1989) provided relevant data for the *corrugator supercilii*, *depressor supercilii*, and *zygomaticus major* muscle regions, regions that have proven informative in studies of emotion. Based on anatomical data regarding the location of these muscles (see Figure 12.1), several experiments were conducted to isolate the sites for surface EMG recording that met the general principle outlined in the preceding. Participants twice posed a series of facial actions and expressions while facial EMG activity was recorded. The activity of a specific muscle or set of muscles was verified using the Facial Action Coding System (FACS, Ekman & Friesen, 1978). The surface recording sites identified as providing both sensitive and relatively selective measures of activation of specific muscle regions are illustrated in the top panel of Figure 12.4.

Tassinary, Vanman, Geen, and Cacioppo (1987) provided relevant data for recording over the perioral muscle region and, in particular, for detecting silent language processing. Five sites in the perioral region were compared for their ability to differentiate facial actions due to the acti-

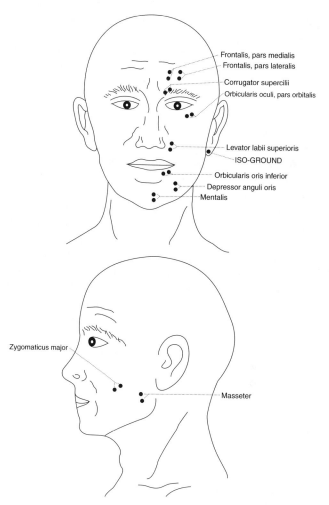

Figure 12.4. Suggested electrode placements for suface EMG recording of the facial muscles, based on Fridlund and Cacioppo (1986). (Modified and redrawn from Figure 6 of Cacioppo et al., 1990c).

vation of discrete facial muscles in the perioral region. In addition to four sites located over the *mentalis, orbicularis oris superior, orbicularis oris inferior*, and *depressor anguli inferioris* (see Figure 12.1), a standard electrode site (i.e., "chin"), recommended by Davis (1952) and routinely used in sleep research (Pivik, this volume, Chapter 27) to measure general perioral EMG activity, was included. Activation of specific muscles or sets of muscles was again achieved by poses and was verified using the FACS. Following their correct performance of the poses on two separate occasions, participants were asked to read affectively neutral passages silently, subvocally, and aloud. Only EMG responses recorded over the *mentalis, orbicularis oris inferior*, and "chin" muscle regions differentiated quiescent baseline activity from silent reading. Of these three sites, only the site over the *orbicularis oris inferior* muscle region demonstrated high discriminant validity when poses activating this versus proximal superficial muscles were contrasted.[8]

---

[7] To record muscle activity involved in movements of the limbs and neck, Zipp (1982) recommended placements first identified by Davis (1952).

[8] This is to be expected for the "chin" site because the distances between the electrodes are sufficiently large that recordings over this region should be sensitive but nonselective.

Site preparation

Surface EMG electrodes can be attached to the skin in a variety of ways, but the most common is via double-sided adhesive tape. A highly conductive medium (paste or gel) is used routinely between skin and the detection-surface. This medium serves to stabilize the interface between the skin and each detection surface through minimizing movement artifacts (by establishing an elastic connection between the detection surface and the skin), reducing inter-electrode impedances (by forming a conductive pathway across the keratinized layers of the skin), and stabilizing the hydration and conductivity of the skin surface.

Prior to the application of the conductive medium and electrodes, the designated site on the skin surface is usually cleaned to remove dirt and oil and typically abraded gently to lower interelectrode impedances to 5 or 10 kΩ. The electrodes are then commonly affixed in a bipolar configuration, as illustrated in Figure 12.4. The proximity of the ground electrode to the EMG sites being monitored is less important than the impedance of the skin-ground contact in helping to minimize extraneous electrical noise in EMG recording. Consequently, care and reflection can and should be used to ensure a stable and low-impedance connection to ground. Finally, to avoid obstructing movement due to the attachment of surface electrodes, thought should be given to the orientation of electrode collars and wires. Electrode wires, for instance, should be draped and secured to minimize distraction, annoyance, or obstruction of movement or vision.

Preamplification and signal conditioning

Electromyographic signals are "small" in two ways: They have low voltage and low current. An amplifier supplies both voltage gain (turning low into high voltages), which can he controlled by the investigator, and current gain, a function of the ratio of the input and output impedances of the amplifier. Electromyographic signals are amplified using differential amplifiers wherein the difference signal between two electrodes (with respect to a third, ground electrode) is amplified and carried through the signal processing chain. Any bioelectrical or extraneous electrical signal that is common to both electrodes (the "common-mode" signal) is therefore attenuated (see Marshall-Goodell et al., 1990).

An older and more traditional method of recording EMG signals is referred to as monopolar and involves the placement of one electrode over each target site (i.e., muscle or muscle group) of interest. The difference signal between the activity recorded at each target site and a common reference electrode (which, in theory, is in contact with an isoelectric site on the participant's body) is amplified and carried through the signal processing chain. However, the *bipolar* method is now the most commonly used method of recording EMG signals. Electrode pairs are aligned parallel to the course of the muscle fibers, and this alignment –

coupled with the high common-mode rejection capable of modern differential amplifiers – produces relatively sensitive and selective recording of the activity of the underlying muscle groups (Basmajian & De Luca, 1985; see also Cooper et al., 1980, Chapter 3).

Monopolar or "common reference" recording is characterized by (1) a much more general pickup region than bipolar recording and (2) an increased sensitivity to variations in the absolute level of electrical activity, assuming the ground electrode reflects an isoelectric state. Bipolar recording, in contrast, is more sensitive to variations in the gradient of electrical activity between the two active electrodes and is less susceptible to cross-talk. An elaboration of traditional bipolar recording, referred to as double-differential recording, promises to be even more spatially selective (De Luca & Merletti, 1988; Lowery, Stoykov, & Kuiken, 2003). In the simplest version of this technique, three rather than two detection surfaces are placed in a line over the muscle of interest. Detection surfaces d_1 and d_2 are fed into one differential amplifier, detection surfaces d_2 and d_3 are fed into a second differential amplifier, and the outputs of the two differential amplifiers are fed into yet a third differential amplifier. The argument is that synchronous activity detected in pairs d_1-d_2 and d_2-d_3 indicates a source of electrical activity that did not propagate along the contracting muscle (i.e., crosstalk) and that the addition of the second stage of differential amplification will remove such influences. This particular technique can be seen as a simple unidimensional linear spatial filter, and both theoretical and experimental research suggest that even greater spatial resolution in surface EMG recording is possible with more complex weighted electrode arrays (Disselhorst-Klug, Silny, & Rau, 1997; Lynn, Bettles, Hughes, & Johnson, 1978).

A schematized representation of a sequence of raw EMG signals is presented in the upper panel of Figure 12.5. As noted in the preceding, some filtering of the raw EMG signal is performed to increase the signal-to-noise ratio, decrease 50/60 Hz or ECG/EEG artifact, and reduce cross-talk. The primary energy in the bipolar recorded surface EMG signal lies between approximately 10 and 200 Hz (Hayes, 1960; van Boxtel, Goudswaard, & Shomaker, 1984). Between 10 and 30 Hz, this power is due primarily to the firing rates of motor units; beyond 30 Hz, it is due to the shapes of the aggregated motor unit action potentials (Basmajian & De Luca, 1985). Attenuating the high frequencies in the EMG signal (e.g., using 500-Hz low-pass filters) reduces amplifier noise but rounds peaks of the detected motor unit action potentials. Retaining sharp signal peaks may be important for waveform or spectral analysis but is less critical for obtaining overall estimates of muscle tension. Attenuating the low frequencies (e.g., using 90 Hz high-pass filters) reduces 50/60 Hz noise from AC power lines, EEG and EKG artifacts, and to some extent, cross-talk (due to the intervening tissue's preferential transmission of low frequencies) but also eliminates a significant and sizable portion of the target

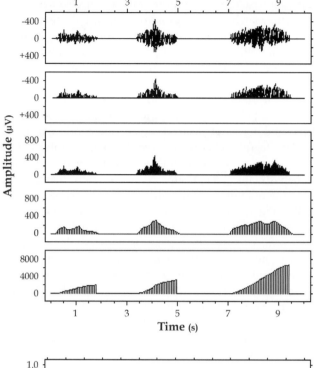

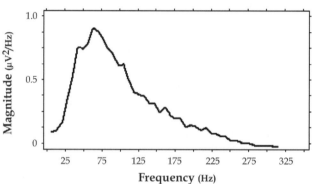

Figure 12.5. Common alternative representations of the surface EMG signal. The top five smaller panels depict three distinct non-fatigued responses. Going from top to bottom: the first represents "raw" (amplified and band-pass filtered only) waveforms; the second, half-wave rectified waveforms; the third, full-wave rectified waveforms; the fourth, "smoothed" waveforms; and the fifth, true integrated waveforms. The larger bottom panel depicts what one of these responses might look like if represented in the frequency domain. (Modified from Figure 7 of Cacioppo et al., 1990c).

EMG signal. Use of an overly restricted EMG signal passband may result in inaccurate appraisal of the level and form of EMG activity or a failure to detect small changes in the level of EMG activity. Hence, selection of an EMG detection passband must proceed based on susceptibility to artifact, presence of extraneous electrical noise at the source and high frequency noise internal to the amplifier, consideration of the amplitude of the EMG signals to be detected, need to minimize cross-talk, and variations across conditions in muscular fatigue. A passband from 10 to 500 Hz is satisfactory for most psychophysiological recording situations (van Boxtel, 2001); if low-frequency artifact and cross-talk are problematic, then a 20 or 30 Hz high-pass filter may be used (possibly in combination with

the double-differential recording technique) but the investigator should realize one consequence of this selection is that weak signals from the target muscle may also be attenuated.[9]

The two most common signal conditioning techniques are integration and smoothing, terms that are often confused. True *integration* is the temporal summation or accumulation of EMG activity, whereas *smoothing* typically refers to performing integration with a built-in signal decay and is accomplished either by low-pass filtering or some type of signal averaging. Because the total energy in the EMG signal in any epoch of time is roughly equivalent to the rectified and smoothed EMG response, considerable economy in terms of data acquisition and signal processing can be achieved by rectification and smoothing prior to digitization when frequency components of the raw signal are not of interest.

The most frequently used on-line "smoother" in psychophysiological research remains the *contour following* integrator, an electronic device consisting primarily of a precision rectifier connected to a simple first-order low-pass filter. Its output represents a running average of ongoing EMG activity by providing a varying voltage proportional to the envelope of the EMG signal. Short time constants provide sensitivity to momentary fluctuations in EMG signals and so are useful when measuring a rapidly changing EMG signal. A long time constant blurs rapid changes and hence the associated output can severely underestimate or overestimate EMG signal amplitude at any point in time as well as compromise precise measurements of response onset and offset. Conversely, if EMG signals that vary slowly are of primary interest, relatively short time constants may be too sensitive to momentary EMG fluctuations and the economic advantages of smoothing will he sacrificed. Despite the popularity of simple contour following integrators, a variety of more sophisticated quantitations that overcome many of these limitations have been available generally for two decades (Paynter filters, pulsed sampling integrators, etc.; see Loeb & Gans, 1986).

QUANTIFICATION AND ANALYSIS

Many investigators have performed frequency analyses on surface EMG recordings to determine whether there are shifts in the EMG spectra (i.e., changes in magnitude or power across frequency) as a function of some psychological or physiological variable. A particularly robust finding is that shifts in the central tendency of the EMG spectra (e.g., median frequency) are associated with muscle fatigue (e.g., Mulder & Hulstijn, 1984; Merletti, 1994; van

[9] One important implication is that a failure to find significant treatment differences in EMG activity could be due to the selection of an inappropriate recording bandpass rather than to an actual absence in EMG activity across treatments. It is often advisable, therefore, to use a wide bandpass during recording and subsequently apply filters to copies of the stored data.

Boxtel, Goudswaard, & Janssen, 1983). The persistent lack of attention to spectral analyses of the surface EMG in psychophysiology, however, continues to be attributable primarily to the fact that sophisticated spectral analyses have proven no more sensitive to psychological processes than relatively inexpensive amplitude and time-based analyses (Dollins & McGuigan, 1989; McGuigan, Dollins, Pierce, Lusebrink, & Corus, 1982).

Signal representation

Electromyographic activity unfolds over time and, like many other psychophysiological responses, the complexity of the raw signal enjoins data reduction. Whether represented in the time, amplitude, or frequency domains the first step involves the conversion of the digitized signal to a descriptive (e.g., physiological) unit of measurement. The numbers assigned to EMG signals of different amplitudes depend on: (1) the electrical unit chosen for description of the signal, (2) the accuracy of the calibration procedure and amplifier's gain setting, and (3) the type of integration method and length of time constant or reset criterion used. Here we focus on the first two factors; interested readers can consult Fridlund and Cacioppo (1986) and Basmajian and De Luca (1985) for additional details.

EMG activity as a voltage-time function.

EMG signals can be viewed as a voltage-time function, where the ordinate represents bounded signal amplitudes and the abscissa represents discrete intervals of time. The quantification of the amplitudes at each unit of time is determined by the direction and magnitude of the measured voltage and is expressed typically in units of microvolts (μV). The EMG voltage-time envelope, like the motor unit action potential, is bipolar and asymmetrical about electrical zero.

Most psychophysiological research using EMG has focused on some variation of EMG signal amplitude as the dependent variable. Simple averaging of the raw EMG amplitudes is uninformative, however, because the nature of the signal ensures that the average expected value is zero. Counting or averaging the peaks in the EMG signal, or tallying its directional changes or zero crossings, are relatively easy methods to implement and are useful for gauging differences in EMG activity provided a sufficiently high sampling rate is used (Loeb & Gans, 1986, Chapter 17). Lippold (1967) maintained that the total energy in an EMG signal at a given moment in time, or what he referred to as the integrated EMG signal, represents overall muscular contraction more accurately than the number or average amplitude of peaks in the EMG signal. Subsequent research has largely corroborated Lippold's assertion (Basmajian & De Luca, 1985; Goldstein, 1972). As discussed above, muscles consist of large numbers of homogeneous units, generating similarly sized action potentials all recruited at similar levels of effort. Consequently, increments in the level of effort are generally found to be more accurately reflected in an

integral-based measure rather than in a frequency-based measure, such as the zero-crossing or inflection count per unit time, which will tend to saturate (i.e., increasing firing rate will differentially affect the area under the amplitude-time envelope, rather than the number of zero-crossings or inflections). However, EMG signals consisting of low rates of widely varying spikes (e.g., those generated by small numbers of recruited motor units or closely spaced differential electrodes) generate poorly fused and noisy integrals, whereas the zero-crossing or simple inflection counts may reflect more accurately the level of effort (Loeb & Gans, 1986, Chapter 17). The irony, therefore, is that the ubiquitous parameter used routinely to quantify EMG activity (i.e., integration) works best, theoretically, when the movements are *forceful*, *overt* and *extended* in duration, whereas the typical psychophysiological laboratory environment results in movements that are *weak*, *covert*, and *epigrammatic*. Recent laboratory results consistent with this reasoning suggest that simple inflection counting is specifically sensitive to covert activation (e.g., less than 10 μVs). (Tassinary, 2005; see Figure 12.6). Such methods, though intriguing, remain highly experimental. We therefore focus the remainder of our review on the more commonly used integration methods.

The phrase "integrated EMG" has been used in this research to refer to the output of several different quantification techniques. Two of the most common parameters in contemporary research are the arithmetic average of the rectified and smoothed EMG signal and the root-mean-square (rms) of the raw EMG signal.[10] Both processing techniques transform the EMG voltage-time function into a waveform that is nonnegative and bounded in time and amplitude. The moment-by-moment amplitude of this function represents an estimate of the total energy of the signal across time; the mean amplitude of this voltage-time function represents the average level of electrical energy emanating from the underlying muscle region(s) during a given recording epoch; and the integral of this function (e.g., the sum of the amplitudes) represents the total electrical activity (i.e., the size of the response) emanating from the underlying muscle region(s) during the recording epoch.

One unfortunate consequence of the traditional focus on the amplitude domain of the EMG signal is that the form of the response across time has been largely ignored (see Cacioppo, Martzke, Petty, & Tassinary, 1988; Hess et al., 1989). A notable exception is Malmo's (1965) use of "EMG gradients" (Davis & Malmo, 1951), defined as an "[e]lectromyographic (EMG) voltage that rises continuously

---

[10] The rms of the EMG signal is calculated by summing the squares of each EMG amplitude within a recording bin, and performing the square root. The rms is superior to mean rectified amplitude as a measure of sinusoidal alternating current and Basmajian and DeLuca (1985) have extended this argument to motor unit action potentials as well. It is of interest to note that the measures of mean amplitude, rms amplitude, and total electrical energy are closely related mathematically, with each emphasizing a different aspect of the amplitude distribution of a waveform. Interested readers may wish to consult Dorfman and Cacioppo (1990).

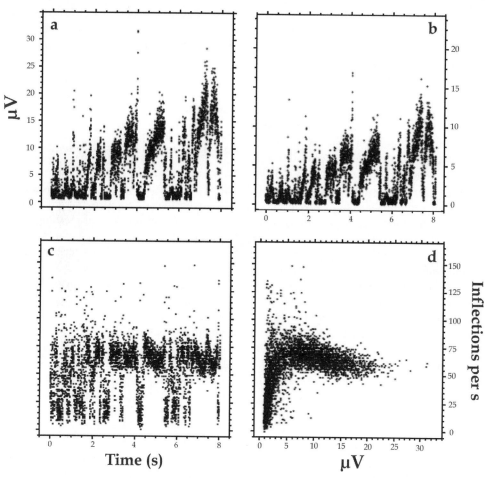

Figure 12.6. Four different plots of three different ways of representing the same eight minutes of EMG activity recorded over the left *zygomaticus major* muscle region of a single female subject while watching an amusing episode from the film *Much Ado About Nothing* (1993). The EMG signal was bandpass filtered (3–1000 Hz) and sampled at 6000 Hz. The data displayed represent discrete values computed over nonoverlapping intervals 100 ms in duration. Panel a: Root mean square values of the EMG activity expressed as a function of time. Panel b: Amplitude-weighted inflection counting of the EMG activity expressed as a function of time. Panel c: Simple inflection counting of the EMG activity expressed as a function of time. Panel d: Simple inflection counting expressed as a function of the root mean square. Data from Tassinary (2005). As is visually apparent in Panels a and b, there is very little difference between the root mean square and amplitude-weighted inflection counting representations, both of which are integral-based measures. In stark contrast, the simple inflection counting representation shown in Panel c, a frequency-based measure, appears unrelated to either of the prior representations. Panel d, however, reveals a very striking relationship between the root mean square and simple inflection counting representations; that is, the frequency of inflections increases rapidly from 0 to approximately 10 microvolts of EMG activity as indexed by the root mean square and then remains remarkably constant for further increases in EMG activity.

during motor performance or mental activity and falls precipitately at the end" (Malmo & Malmo, 2000, p. 145; see also Malmo, 1975). Electromyographic gradients are still used successfully to assess variations across time in tonic muscle tension; these gradients are depicted by plotting EMG amplitude for two or more consecutive recording epochs (e.g., Braathen & Svebak, 1994; Rimehaug & Sveback, 1987; Ritz et al., 1999).

Baselines

As in psychophysiology generally, it is often desirable to obtain response measures that are uncontaminated by the basal (prestimulus) level of activity. The notion of basal activity, however, can be ambiguous when applied to EMG signals. This is because the true physiological baseline for EMG activity is zero; hence, the lowest empirical baseline for EMG recording is actually the level of noise in the recording system.

In laboratory practice, muscles seldom show zero activity because the alert research participant is rarely completely relaxed. It is therefore important to consider the EMG activity that exists in the absence of experimental stimuli in order to assess individual differences and also to help achieve a measure of the experimental treatments free from prestimulus EMG activity. In assessing basal EMG activity, care is required to avoid any confounding of measurements with task-irrelevant activity (e.g., adaptation, fatigue, apprehension). The procedures commonly used include recording during prestimulus periods and recordings during pseudotrials (Johnson & Lubin, 1972; Jennings & Gianaros, this volume, Chapter 34). The use of pseudotrials has the advantage that assessments are obtained under conditions that – except for the lack of experimental stimuli – are identical to the experimental trials.

A closed-loop baseline procedure offers an alternative to the use of pseudotrials (McHugo & Lanzetta, 1983). Briefly, the presentation of experimental stimuli or treatments is programmed to be contingent on acceptably low levels of somatic activity across the recording sites. Task-specific EMG responses are thus quantified while minimizing the confounding effects of extraneous muscular activity or basal differences in somatic activity across treatments, a procedure that is reminiscent of Jacobson's (1932) use of progressive relaxation in studies of EMG and imagery. A closed-loop baseline procedure also has the advantage over simple change scores in that time series and waveform moment analyses (Dorfman & Cacioppo, 1990) can be performed with fewer restrictions. A potential liability of the closed-loop procedure, however, is that both the speed and accuracy with which acceptably low levels of EMG activity are achieved may be partially a function of experimental condition or idiosyncratic strategies, and designs employing this procedure may shape participants inadvertently in subtle ways that complicate interpretation. For this reason, most EMG-based psychological investigations have not employed this procedure, whereas some variant of this procedure is used routinely in investigations of physiological constructs such as muscle fatigue (Roy et al., 1997).

SOCIAL CONTEXT

Psychophysiological research was once thought to be exempt from the laboratory artifacts that have led others to consider the physical and social context in which the research was conducted (e.g., Rosenthal & Rosnow, 1969). The vulnerability of physiological responses to instructional sets (Sternbach, 1966), intentional distortions (e.g., Ekman, 1985; Honts, Devitt, Winbush, & Kircher, 1996), ethnicity (e.g., Rankin & Campbell, 1955; Vrana & Rollock, 1998), and social presence (e.g., Cacioppo, Rourke, Marshall-Goodell, Tassinary, & Baron, 1990; Geen & Bushman, 1989) vitiates this notion. Nowhere is this vulnerability more apparent in psychophysiology than in studies of the skeletomotor system (Cacioppo, Petty, & Tassinary, 1989). The evidence clearly suggests that vigilance with respect to these factors can contribute to the construction of more sensitive, artifact-free psychophysiological experimentation and, hence, to stronger inferences (Cacioppo, Marshall-Goodell, & Gormezano, 1983; Gale & Baker, 1981).

Social factors have been found also to moderate the influence of nonsocial factors on physiological responding.

This point, too, is perhaps clearest in studies of skeletomotor response. The expression of emotion, for instance, can be magnified, attenuated, or masked because of the presence of others and comprehensive psychophysiological theories must accommodate such moderating influences (see reviews by Cacioppo & Petty, 1986; Gardner, Gabriel, & Diekman, 2000).

Social factors as laboratory artifacts

Gale and Baker (1981) noted that experimenter-participant interactions are particularly important in psychophysiology because the procedures may involve touching, partial removal of clothing, skin abrasion, and the application and removal of sensors. This somewhat unique and extended interaction may result in participants becoming anxious, distracted, or aware of the experimenter's expectations and significant laboratory artifacts may be introduced.

Demand characteristics

To the extent that participants can discern the experimental hypotheses and manipulate their actions accordingly, EMG studies are vulnerable to experimental demand confounds (Orne, 1962). Fridlund and Izard (1983) argued that many facial EMG studies of emotion and emotional imagery could be interpreted in terms of demand characteristics. Specifically, they reasoned that placing multiple electrodes on a person's face can make the person acutely aware of her or his facial expressions. Participants who desired to please the experimenter or contribute to "science" might alter their expressions in accordance with what they believed were the experimental hypotheses. Particularly susceptible, they suggested, were studies in which the experimental hypothesis was obvious, such as the early studies of facial EMG activity during emotional imagery (e.g., Schwartz, 1975). Not all prior research using facial EMG to study emotion was susceptible to this interpretation (see Cacioppo & Petty, 1981a), and more recent studies whose designs minimized experimental demands have continued to find that subtle emotions can be discriminated using facial EMG (Cacioppo et al., 1992; McHugo, Lanzetta, & Bush, 1991; Hess, Banse, & Kappas, 1995; Greenwald, Cook, & Lang, 1989; Dimberg, 1997).

Although experimental demands do not appear to be necessary for facial EMG patterning to emerge during emotions, they nevertheless remain a potential source of bias. Procedures contrived to minimize such biases include: (1) providing participants with plausible alternative hypotheses; (2) employing cover stories that divert attention away from the physiological recording; (3) utilizing engaging experimental tasks; (4) placing multiple non-functional sensors over other areas of the body to reduce the salience of the functional sensors; and (5) designing the laboratory setting to be comfortable and free of unnecessary equipment. The level of experimental demand can also be assessed directly either through a funnel debriefing procedure that involves gradually revealing more and more of the hypothesis to participants while gauging their awareness of the hypothesis, or by including a "simulation" condition in which the EMG study is described explicitly to a naive group of participants who are then asked to predict how they would or should respond in such a situation.[11]

Evaluation apprehension

Naive participants may be apprehensive about participating in research involving the use of electrodes and electrical recording equipment. Such apprehension, although possibly of interest in its own right, may create a level of tension or hypervigilance in the participant that is unrepresentative and that can obscure the effects of the experimental treatments. This apprehension is in addition to the potential apprehension that participants may feel about being evaluated by experimenters who are presumably experts in human behavior. Rosenthal (1966) suggested that this "evaluation apprehension" may also lead participants to distort their actions in a socially desirable fashion. If an experimenter's behavior or experimental treatment makes participants especially anxious or aware that they are being evaluated, then the data may be significantly biased.

Procedures for minimizing evaluation apprehension, in addition to those outlined in the preceding section, include: (1) providing a tour of portions of the laboratory to prospective participants to brief them on the tasks and procedures involved in the study prior to seeking informed consent or scheduling them for participation; (2) substituting "sensor" or "biosensor" for "electrode" when communicating with participants; (3) allowing time before the beginning of the experimental procedures for participants to adapt to the laboratory; (4) using buffer trials or tasks to allow adaptation to the experimental procedure; (5) employing a closed-loop baseline to ensure participants are not unduly tense or aroused prior to initiating the next trial; and (6) minimizing the sense participants may have that they are being scrutinized by automating procedures, assuring them that their responses are anonymous, and using unobtrusive monitoring methods (e.g., hidden cameras; see Kappas, Hess, & Kleck, 1990) during the experiment.

Social factors as determinants

In the previous section, we saw that the nature of the interaction between the experimenter and participant is a source of both bias in psychophysiological research and a means for its solution. In this section, we briefly review illustrative research demonstrating how social factors can also moderate the influence of nonsocial factors on EMG responses.

Audience effects

The classic observations of Charles Darwin (1872/1873) suggested that facial expressions of emotion were universal. Most members of both the scientific community and the lay public, however, would undoubtedly agree that felt emotions are not always accompanied by perceptible expressions. According to an influential "neurocultural" model proposed by Paul Ekman (1972) to explain communalities and variations in facial expressions, a given emotion will not always be displayed in the same fashion due to the influence of personal habits, situational pressures, and cultural norms. In an early study on such "display rules," Japanese or American students were exposed to a disgusting film while being videotaped unobtrusively or with an authoritarian experimenter present (Friesen, 1972). Results revealed that both the Japanese and American students displayed revulsion while viewing the film in solitude, but the Japanese students masked their feelings of revulsion by smiling during the film when the experimenter was present. A study of racial bias suggested the opposite dissociation between expression and self-report may occur as well when examining covert responses (Vanman, Paul, Ito, & Miller, 1997). In the context of a cooperative task, White participants tended to report more liking for Black partners while simultaneously showing greater increases in the EMG activity recorded over the brow region, a result indicative of greater negative affect and interpreted by the authors as evidence of racial prejudice (see also Dambrun, Despres, & Guimond, 2004). In a subsequent study, racial bias indicated by EMG activity – but not self-reports – was related to White participants' preferences for a Black or White applicant for a fellowship (Vanman, Saltz, Nathan, & Warren, 2004). The ability of affective stimuli to evoke small but reliable changes in facial EMG activity even in the absence of awareness (e.g., Ravaja, Kallinen, Saari, & Keltikangas-Jarvinen, 2004; Tassinary, Orr, Wolford, Napps, & Lanzetta, 1984; Wexler, Warrenburg, Schwartz, & Janer, 1992) combined with the possibility that minute levels of activity may be imperceptible to both observers and producers (Max, 1932; Epstein, 1990) provides a plausible explanation for why such covert responses may be less susceptible to audience effects.

The influence of an observer on people's facial expressions of emotion emphasizes the multiple roles played by behavioral responses. Because the skeletomotor system is the only means individuals have of approaching, avoiding, or modifying elements in their physical environment, one might expect that overt somatic responses in part reflect or serve to gratify certain goals or desires. An individual who accidentally touches a hot platter is likely to exhibit a rapid

---

[11] For instance, Cacioppo, Petty, Losch, and Kim (1986) placed a small set electrodes on the head and neck as well as on the face and body of their participants who were told that this array of sensors was placed around their brain to help isolate and identify the involuntary neural processes involved in processing pictoral stimuli. To the extent that the electrodes on the body and the nonfunctional electrodes on the neck and head diverted attention from voluntary facial actions, which debriefng suggested they did, then this explanation was both accurate factually and successful at minimizing experimental demand.

withdrawal, just as an individual who smells a foul odor is likely to express disgust and rapidly either stop breathing or rapidly exhale (Tassinary, 1985).

The skeletomotor system is also an individual's primary means of communication and of effecting change in the social environment. It is not surprising, therefore, that overt somatic responses such as facial expressions can be affected strongly by the perceived presence of observers. Kraut and Johnson (1979), for instance, related the observed frequency of smiling to simultaneously occurring events in a wide range of naturalistic settings (e.g., bowling alleys, public walkways, hockey arenas). Their results indicated that people were most likely to smile while speaking with other people; they were significantly less likely to smile perceptibly to a presumable positive event (e.g., bowling a strike) when their faces were unobserved than observed. Related findings have been reported by Chovil (1991), Fridlund (1991), Gilbert, Fridlund, and Sabini (1987), Jäncke & Kaufman, 1994 and Jäncke (1996). Fridlund (1994) argued forcefully that such results provide strong evidence against the two-factor neurocultural model and strong evidence for a one-factor behavioral ecology model. A wide variety of results (e.g., Cacioppo et al., 1992; Geen, 1992; Hess, Banse & Kappas, 1995; Davis et al., 1995; Vanman et al., 1997; see also Russell, Bachorowski, & Fernández-Dols, 2003), however, suggest that a more rather than less inclusive and sophisticated model is necessary and this prevision is consistent with the multitude of neural systems contributing to the coordination and control of the facial musculature (Fanardjian & Manvelyan, 1987; Jenny & Saper, 1987; Petrides, Cadoret, & Maxkey, 2005).

Facial expressions of emotion are not the only somatic responses that are affected by the presence of observers. Chapman (1974), for instance, monitored EMG activity over the forehead region as participants listened to a story while unobserved, watched by a concealed observer, or watched by an unconcealed observer. Chapman found that EMG activity over the forehead region was higher during the story when the participant was observed than when unobserved and slightly though not significantly higher when the observer was present than when concealed. Groff, Baron, and Moore (1983) further demonstrated that the presence of observers led to more vigorous motor responses. These data fit well with observations made as far back as the late 1890s (Triplett, 1898), demonstrating that an individual's performance on a task can be altered dramatically simply by moving the task from a nonsocial to a social context. Zajonc (1965) organized much of this research with his proposal that the presence of conspecifics lowered the threshold for the single most likely response to a task (see reviews by Geen & Gange, 1977; Bond & Titus, 1983). The important point here is that not only performance but also physiological responses such as EMG activity have been found to vary as a function of the presence of observers (see Cacioppo & Petty, 1986, pp. 658–664).

Mimicry

Mimicry refers in this context to the elicitation of a localized motor response through witnessing the same response being performed by another. Evidence for motor mimicry includes such demonstrations as wincing at another's pain (Vaughan & Lanzetta, 1980), straining at another's effort (Markovsky & Berger, 1983), and spontaneously imitating another's evident emotion (Dimberg, 1982, 1990; Lundqvist & Dimberg, 1995). Motor mimicry in psychology has traditionally been conceptualized as primarily intrapersonal, representing either primitive empathy, a conditioned emotional response based on one's direct experience, or an expression of vicarious emotion (Allport, 1968), and as such is closely related to the concept of emotional contagion (Hatfield, Cacioppo, & Rapson, 1993; Hess, Philippot, & Blairy, 1999). Consistent with this framework, Dimberg (1982; 1990) reported that subtle decreases in EMG activity over the *corrugator supercilii* muscle region and increases in EMG activity over the *zygomaticus major* muscle region were observed when participants viewed pictures of smiling faces, whereas the opposite pattern of facial EMG activity was observed when participants viewed pictures of angry faces. Lanzetta and his colleagues (Englis, Vaughan, & Lanzetta, 1982; Lanzetta & Englis, 1989) provided evidence that counterempathic as well as empathic processes can result in subtle changes in facial EMG activity.

Studies by Bavelas and colleagues (Bavelas, Black, Lemery, & Mullett, 1986; Bavelas, Black, Chovil, Lemery, & Mullett, 1988) suggest the form and intensity of *visible* motor mimicry is influenced strongly by the communicative significance of the mimesis. For instance, in their earlier study, the victim of what appeared to be a painful injury was either increasingly or decreasingly visible to the observing participant. Results revealed that the pattern and timing of the observer's motor mimicry was affected significantly by the visibility of the victim. Subsequent research has found that differences in emotional empathy due to different attachment styles also affect motor mimicry (Sonnby-Borgström & Jönsson, 2003), but that neither mimicry nor imitation necessarily have cognitive sequelae (see Graziano et al., 1996). Thus, the research on mimicry is consistent with the preceding suggestion that social factors can influence somatic responding in the service of interpersonal (i.e., communicative) goals as well as personal feelings and emotions (cf. Gallese, 2003).

INFERENTIAL CONTEXT

One of the challenges in psychophysiological research involving surface EMG is to create paradigms that allow strong inferences (Platt, 1964) about psychological constructs based on somatic responses. Cacioppo et al. (1990) proposed that much of the variety and complexity in the experimental paradigms in this area can be characterized in terms of the function (Independent vs. Dependant variable) and the proximal origin (Endogenous vs.

Exogenous) of a somatic response, resulting in four generic paradigms referred to as Outcome, Conditional Probability, Reflex Probe, and Manipulated Response paradigms. Within these general paradigms, answers have been sought to questions regarding the psychological, behavioral, and health significance of somatic activity and the extent to which skeletomotor activity reflects specific or global activation; phasic, tonic, or modulated thresholds for activation; and characteristics of the stimulus situation or the individual's disposition.

Outcome paradigm

Outcome paradigms continue to be the most prevalent in psychophysiology. The essence of such paradigms is that a psychological or behavioral process is manipulated while one or more physiological (e.g., EMG) responses are monitored. Edmund Jacobson's (e.g., 1932) pioneering EMG studies mentioned at the beginning of this chapter are cases in point as are any studies based on subtractive or additive factors methodology (Sternberg, 1969; Cacioppo & Petty, 1986).

For over half a century, studies conducted within this general paradigm on phasic EMG responses have found that reliable and oftentimes minute patterns of EMG activity accompany thought, emotion, and imagery despite large variations within and between individuals (e.g., Bartholow, Fabiani, Gratton, & Bettencourt, 2001; Bakker, Boschker, & Chung, 1996; Cacioppo, Petty, Losch, & Kim, 1986; Lang, Greenwald, Bradley, & Hamm, 1993; Malcolm, Von, & Horney, 1989; Sloan, Bradley, Dimoulas, & Lang, 2002; Shaw, 1940). In an illustrative early study, Schwartz, Fair, Salt, Mandel, and Klerman (1976) reported that clinically depressed subjects displayed higher levels of EMG activity over the brow muscle region (*corrugator supercilii*) and lower levels of EMG activity over the cheek muscle region (*zygomaticus major*) when they imagined unpleasant experiences than when they imagined pleasant ones. Nondepressed subjects displayed patterns similar to those produced by the depressed subjects, but the pattern accompanying unpleasant imagery was attenuated in the nondepressed subjects. Numerous studies conducted since have expanded upon these basic findings and consistently demonstrated that affect-laden stimuli, whether imagined or perceived, result in similarly patterned changes in the facial musculature (e.g., Arndt, Allen, & Greenberg, 2001; Gehricke & Shapiro, 2001; Hu & Wan, 2003; Jänke, 1996). Much of this research has demonstrated that both EMG activity over the brow and cheek regions vary inversely as a function of the affective valence of the stimulus. However, in a recent study that used affective pictures, sounds, and words as stimuli, Larsen, Norris, and Cacioppo (2003) found that positive affect decreased and negative affect increased activity over the brow region, but only positive affect affected activity over the cheek region. Larsen et al. concluded that *zygomaticus major* may not be reciprocally activated by positive and negative affect, although

the extent of the generality of this specificity is not known yet. Additional recent studies have also begun to examine muscles hypothesized to be linked to specific emotional states (i.e., disgust) as opposed to generalized affect (Stark et al., 2005).

Although, as we have noted, most EMG research in psychophysiology has focused primarily on specific phasic changes in EMG activity, a parallel tradition of research has focused on general or tonic changes in tension, activation, or arousal (see reviews by Freeman, 1931; Duffy, 1962; Malmo & Malmo, 2000; van Boxtel & Jessurun, 1993). Germana (1974), for instance, suggested that although skilled or habitual actions are characterized by a well-orchestrated patterning of skeletomotor activity, response uncertainty leads to a general activation of the musculature. He speculated that general activation across functionally disparate muscle regions signifies extensive preparation for overt behavior, and proposed that both novel and partially conditioned stimuli are the most likely to produce response uncertainty. Interestingly, recent research provides partial support for Germana's suggestion that generalized somatic activation during response uncertainty reflects an equalization of response probabilities (e.g., see Fabiani, Gratton, & Federmeier, this volume, Chapter 4), and this suggestion has been incorporated into a heuristic model of emotion (Cacioppo, Berntson, & Klein, 1992) via the proposal that psychologically relevant somatic activity may range from completely undifferentiated tonic activation to emotion-specific patterns of phasic activation.

Research with respect to motivational states has tended to focus on the significance of EMG gradients in the task-irrelevant musculature (e.g., Rimehaug & Svebak, 1987). In an illustrative study, participants played one of two versions of a video game that required they stop a "ball" from passing across the screen by maneuvering a video "bat" to intercept the ball (Svebak, Dalen, & Storfjell, 1981). In the easy version, an unimpeded ball bounced across the screen in approximately 3 s, whereas in the difficult version the ball traveled at approximately twice this rate. Both versions required the subject to engage in continuous performance for 150 s, and EMG activity was recorded over the forearm flexor of the passive arm during baseline and task periods. Results revealed the EMG gradient associated with the difficult game to be significantly steeper than that associated with the easy game. Van Boxtel and Jessurun (1993) also reported strong EMG gradients recorded from the forehead, brow, and lip muscle regions during performance on difficult and extended tasks, and concluded that such activity provides a sensitive index of the degree of exerted mental effort.

In a similar vein but on a shorter time scale, Davis (1940) recorded EMG activity over several muscle regions (e.g., forearm extensors) as participants performed a choice reaction time task under unwarned, fixed foreperiod or variable foreperiod conditions. Davis observed that (a) EMG activity was higher in the foreperiod when the participant was warned as opposed to unwarned, (b) EMG activity began to rise approximately 200–400 ms following the warning signal and continued to rise until the overt response was completed, and (c) EMG activity was higher (and reaction time shorter) with a fixed than variable foreperiod. Davis concluded that the EMG responses during the foreperiod reflected preparation for the upcoming response. In a similar paradigm, van Boxtel, Damen, and Brunia (1996) recorded EMG activity over several pericranial muscle regions as participants performed a fixed foreperiod simple reaction time task involving either an auditory or visual reaction signal. The responses were performed with the hand or foot. Throughout the warning interval they observed that (a) neck muscle EMG activity remained relatively unchanged, (b) forehead, brow and lip EMG activity systematically increased, and (c) periocular, cheek, and temple EMG activity systematically decreased. Van Boxtel et al. interpreted this pattern of activation in the task-irrelevant pericranial musculature to be in the service of increasing perceptual sensitivity rather than facilitating response preparation.

There is thus no more consensus within the EMG field than within other fields of psychophysiology regarding which measure best reflects general motivation, tension, or activation. Meyer (1953) suggested eyeblink rate provided the best overall measure of generalized tension and Meyer, Bahrick, and Fitts (1953) reported that individuals who score high on anxiety inventories also have high blink rates. Rossi (1959) found a similar relationship, however, between manifest anxiety scores and EMG activity over the forearm extensors. Similarly, Davis, Malmo, and Shagass (1954) administered white-noise blasts at 1 minute intervals to both normals and individuals with anxiety disorders. Results revealed that although the noise blast evoked a slightly larger EMG response over the forearm extensor region in the anxious than normal individuals, the more significant difference occurred during recovery following the stressor. The elevation in EMG activity in normals was sharply delimited, returning to basal levels within seconds of the termination of the noise burst, whereas the elevation in EMG in the anxious subjects lingered.

Fridlund, Hatfield, Cottam, and Fowler (1986) replicated and extended these findings using EMG measures over the head, neck, and limbs. Participants first rested quietly for 15 minutes and then were exposed to 5 minutes of 105 dB binaural white-noise stimulation. High, in contrast to low, anxious participants exhibited higher levels of EMG activity primarily over the head and neck preceding the stimulus and more generally during the stimulus. An idiographic principal components analyses of EMG activity during these periods failed to reveal evidence for a general, intercorrelated tensional factor; instead, the EMG elevations in the highly anxious subjects consisted largely of uncorrelated response bursts. This pattern of EMG responses was interpreted to indicate a state of heightened activation or a lower threshold for activation. Consistent with this interpretation, Britt and Blumenthal (1992) reported that the latencies of auditory startle responses in participants low

in state anxiety were intensity dependent, whereas those high in state anxiety responded with equal latency regardless of stimulus intensity.

Woodworth and Schlosberg (1954, pp. 173–179) suggested that EMG activity, particularly in the neck region (e.g., splenius, upper trapezius), may be a somewhat unique indicator of the level of activation due to the possibility that a disproportionate share of proprioceptive impulses to the central nervous system originated in this muscle region. This suggestion is interesting in light of the sparse evidence for the notion of a coherent tensional factor (e.g., see Fridlund, Fowler, & Pritchard, 1980). In accord with this suggestion, Eason and White (1961) had subjects perform a variety of vigilance tasks (e.g., rotary tracking) while recording EMG activity over the splenius, upper trapezius, lower trapezius, and the deltoid and biceps of the right arm. The major finding in these studies was that the general level of EMG activity (most consistently that recorded over the neck muscles) varied as a function of the effort subjects expended on tasks. Waersted and Westgaard (1996) recorded surface EMG activity from 20 different sites while participants performed a complex 2-choice reaction time task designed to demand continuing attention yet require minimal activity. The major finding in this study was that attention-related activity was most clearly observed over the frontalis and upper trapezius muscle regions.

In summary, substantial increases in task difficulty, the subjective effort expended on tasks, or stress have been found to lead to elevated EMG activity during preparatory periods as well as during the performance of effortful engaging tasks. In addition, an inhibition of EMG activity over irrelevant musculature is sometimes observed during such tasks, particularly when the response to the task is well practiced (e.g., see Germana, 1974; Goldstein, 1972; Brunia & van Boxtel, 2000).

Double-dissociation design. Whether changes in EMG activity reflect particular actions or general somatic attitudes often has important theoretical implications. The double-dissociation design (Teuber, 1955) is considered to be one of the more powerful in this regard. This experimental design is so named because (a) one or more treatments that should evoke a specific response is contrasted with one or more treatments that should not evoke the expected response, and (b) one or more measures of the target response are included as well as one or more measures of a nontarget response. The former establishes discriminant validity of the treatments, whereas the latter demonstrates the discriminant validity of the responses.

To illustrate, there has long been a hypothesis that silent-language processing is associated with increased activation of the speech (e.g., perioral) musculature (see McGuigan, 1978). As McGuigan (1970) noted previously, there are a number of studies demonstrating that EMG activity over the perioral musculature increased from basal levels when individuals engaged in silent-language processing. These results alone are not particularly informative because such a psychophysiological outcome could be attributed to aspects of the task that had nothing to do with speech processing per se. A slight tensing of lips, for example, might be associated with orthographic or auditory processing or possibly to general increases in tension or arousal due to concerns about task performance. The inclusion of nonspeech as well as speech tasks addresses the first of these interpretational problems, and the measurement of EMG activity over nontarget as well as target sites addresses the second.

In most applications of the double-dissociation paradigm, different subjects or stimuli are used to achieve treatments that theoretically should and should not evoke a specific somatic action or pattern. In a particularly comprehensive series of studies, McGuigan and Bailey (1969) recorded EMG activity over the chin, tongue, and forearm muscle regions while subjects silently read, memorized prose, listened to prose, listened to music, and attentively listened to "nothing." Results revealed that EMG activity over the perioral musculature was uniquely associated with the performance of silent language tasks.

Double dissociation with constant stimuli. Although the outcome observed by McGuigan and Bailey (1969) is consistent with the hypothesis that silent-language processing leads to increased perioral EMG activity, Cacioppo and Petty (1979b; 1981b) noted that the grounds for such an inference would be strengthened further if the participants and the physical characteristics of the target stimuli were held constant within the double-dissociation paradigm. To achieve this refinement, EMG activity was monitored over the inferior *orbicularis oris* and the superficial forearm flexor muscle regions while participants evaluated a series of trait adjectives presented visually. The treatment conditions were altered by varying systematically the dimension of evaluation rather than by varying either participants or stimuli. Specifically, for half of the trait adjectives participants were asked to evaluate the stimulus semantically ("Is the following descriptive of you?"), and for the other half they were asked to evaluate the stimulus graphemically ("Is the following printed in uppercase letters?"). Results revealed EMG activity over the perioral region to be greater during the semantic task, whereas EMG activity over the nonpreferred forearm did not differ as a function of task. Because the type of stimulus presented or type of participant tested was held constant, the inference that silent-language semantic processing involving short-term memory leads to increased EMG activity over the perioral muscle region appears more secure.

It must be noted, however, that inferences derived from outcome paradigms are tentative at best when using even the most rigorous of designs. The data obtained from additive and subtractive factors designs in general, as well as double dissociation designs in particular, are indeterminate to the extent that continuous causal functions are dichotomized arbitrarily (Cook & Campbell, 1979, p. 12),

the underlying mechanisms are nonlinear (McClelland, 1979), or relevant factors are overlooked (Cacioppo, Petty, & Morris, 1985). The continuing controversy over the evidence for parallel brain systems for item memory and category knowledge (Knowlton & Squire, 1993; Nosofsky & Zaki, 1998; Smith & Minda, 2001) illustrates clearly the diagnostic limitations of interpretations based solely on the results from such designs.

Conditional probability paradigm

Most psychologists, like many psychophysiologists, have sought to use physiological data to infer psychological or behavioral constructs such as anxiety, emotion, deception, and depression. Typically, the target physiological events have been identified as those that have been shown to vary as a function of the theoretical construct of interest. Electromyographic activity over the forehead region has been of interest, for instance, because anxiety, tension, and mental effort are often accompanied by increased EMG activity over this site. However, knowing that the manipulation of a psychological or behavioral factor leads to this particular skeletomotor response does not logically imply that this response indexes the psychological or behavioral factor. Put succinctly, the probability of Event A given Event B cannot be assumed to equal the probability of Event B given Event A, and the former cannot even be derived unless both the latter and the probability of Event B given the absence of Event A are known. Put more concretely, the utility of a skeletomotor response to serve as an index of a theoretical construct is weakened by the occurrence of such responses in the absence of the construct of interest (see Cacioppo, Tassinary, & Bernston, this volume, Chapter 1).

Although one cannot logically identify all possible factors that might influence a target response or response pattern, its ability to index a theoretical construct can be defined as the extent to which the construct of interest is present given the presence of the target response or response pattern. That is, one can block on the presence or absence of a skeletomotor response (or on variations of this response) and analyze the extent to which the construct of interest is evident. In so doing, an endogenous skeletomotor response pattern functions as the independent rather than the dependent variable.

Cacioppo et al. (1988) utilized a conditional probability paradigm to examine the extent to which specific forms of EMG response over the brow region indexed particular emotions evoked during an interview. As noted above, previous research has demonstrated that mild negative imagery and unpleasant sensory stimuli tend to evoke greater EMG activity over the brow (*corrugator supercilli*) and less EMG activity over the cheek (*zygomaticus major*) and ocular (*orbicularis oculi*) muscle regions than mild positive imagery and pleasant sensory stimuli. This previous research did not address whether facial EMG responses provided a sensitive and specific index of particular emotions, however, because there are a multiplicity of events that can affect facial EMG activity. To address this question directly, Cacioppo et al. (1988) obtained both facial EMG and audiovisual recordings while individuals were interviewed about themselves. A while later individuals were asked to describe what they had been thinking during specific segments of the interview marked by distinctive EMG responses over the brow region in the context of ongoing but stable levels of activity elsewhere in the face. Consistent with the notion that the expressive components of emotion are "...sometimes brought unconsciously into momentary action by ludicrously slight causes." (Darwin, 1872/1873, p. 184), inconspicuous EMG responses over the *corrugator supercilii* muscle region were observed to covary with subtle variations in emotion during the interview even though the overt facial expressions evinced by subjects were rated similarly across conditions by observers. Furthermore, it was reasoned that certain forms of EMG activity in the context of an interview, such as brief jagged bursts rather than sustained smooth mounds, would be especially predictive of variations in emotion due primarily to theoretical differences in the probability of such responses in the absence of emotion. Smooth modulations in EMG activity over the brow region were thus hypothesized to reflect equally both paralinguistic signaling and emotional expression, whereas abrupt modulations in EMG activity over the same region were hypothesized to be much less likely to be associated with paralinguistic signaling. Support for this reasoning was also found. These results illustrate the power of the conditional probability paradigm and provide evidence that specific patterns of facial EMG response can actually index variations in emotion, at least within this limited context.

Shimizu and Inoue (1986) completed a study of sleep and dreams that bears on the utility of perioral EMG activity as a marker of silent-language processing. Electroencephalographic (EEG), electrooculographic (EOG), perioral EMG, and nonoral EMG activity were recorded during sleep. Participants were awakened during either rapid eye movement (REM) or Stage 2 sleep, as determined by inspection of the EEG and EOG recordings. When participants reported dreaming they were asked whether or not they had been speaking in their dreams. Dream recall during REM sleep occurred in approximately 80% of the awakenings, and it occurred during Stage 2 sleep in approximately 28% of the awakenings. Awakenings without dream recall were excluded from further analyses, as were awakenings preceded by phasic discharges in the perioral musculature that were accompanied by any whispering or vocalization. Results revealed that when phasic discharges over the perioral musculature were observed within the 30s preceding the awakening, subjects reported having been speaking in their dreams in 88% of the awakenings from REM sleep and 71% of the awakenings during State 2 sleep. Moreover, when phasic discharges over the perioral musculature were not observed within the 30s preceding the awakening, subjects reported having been

speaking in their dreams in only 19% of the awakenings from REM sleep and in none of the awakenings during Stage 2 sleep.

In summary, previous research has indicated (a) that situations in which participants report emotional reactions are accompanied by patterned EMG activity in the facial musculature, (b) that effortful tasks that require cognitive resources influence the EMG activity in task-irrelevant muscles, and (c) that silent language processing is accompanied by EMG activity in the perioral musculature. The research reviewed in this section further suggests that autochthonous EMG activity can be used to mark episodes of affect and silent-language processing in some limited contexts.

Reflex probe paradigms

Reflexes generally refer to any automatic reaction of the nervous system to stimuli impinging upon the body or arising within it (Merton, 1987).[12] Although there have been clear analytical attempts to define the concept of the reflex in precise logical and empirical terms from within both physiology (Sherrington, 1923/1906) and psychology (Skinner, 1931), the definition of the reflex and the functional significance of reflexes in the intact organism remain active topics of research (e.g., Berkinblit, Feldman, & Fulson, 1986).

From a physiological perspective, reflexes can be defined as a discrete type of behavior mediated by a reflex arc, thus providing both functional and structural constraints on the definition (Gallistel, 1980). Structurally, a reflex arc is an anatomical entity consisting of: (a) receptors tuned to transduce specifiable classes of environmental stimuli into neural signals; (b) sensory neurons that conduct the output signals from the receptors to the central nervous system (CNS); (c) mediators, either a single synapse or a small set of interneurons, that relay the sensory output to an appropriate subset of motoneurons or neurohumoral cells; (d) motoneurons or neurohumoral cells that conduct the signal from the CNS to particular effectors; and (e) the effectors themselves, which affect the environment as a function of neural and/or hormonal input.

Since the turn of the century, the scientific study of the reflex has proceeded in two directions. Disciplines concerned with the control of movement (e.g., neurophysiology) have generally followed the tradition of Sherrington (1923/1906) and examined reflexes as integral to the regulation of behavior. Predicated on this view of the reflex as a relatively invariant unit of behavior, the accompanying research and theory has focused on specifying the rules by which reflexes combine to generate coordinated, goal-directed movements.

In neurology and psychophysiology, however, the reflex is viewed in a manner more consistent with the behaviorist generalization of the concept articulated by Skinner (1931). In the field of neurology this conceptualization led

[12] The reader further interested in the history of the reflex is encouraged to consult the monographs by Fearing (1930), Liddell (1960), or Swazey (1969).

initially to widespread confusion, with the early part of the century referred to as an open season for the "hunting of the reflex" (Wartenberg, 1946). During this time, any stimulus-response correlation was "fair game" to be named and reified. An unfortunate result was that many reflexes were "discovered" by one author after another, each time renamed and claimed to be unique. However, it is now possible to use parameters of reflex responses as markers of CNS function because of increasingly detailed information about the neural circuits mediating specific reflexes (Davis, Walker, & Myers, 2003) and the publication of detailed guidelines for the EMG recording of reflexes (e.g., Blumenthal et al., 2005).

As a tool in the investigation of psychological processes, surface electromyography provides an ongoing record of muscular activity while minimally interfering with the behavior under study. The unique advantage of the reflex probe paradigm, however, is that it allows estimation of changes in the excitability of spinal and brainstem motor structures that may be manifest in neither overt behavior nor in peripheral EMG activity. The use of the reflex as a probe into ongoing psychological processes further exemplifies the examining of variations in reflex characteristics as a function of third variables. Although Skinner (1931) intended this experimental procedure to be used to quantify the influences of external variables on the reflex behavior of intact organisms, the logic of the situation allows one to use variations in reflex strength as an indicant of internal psychological processes as well. In the former case the focus is on the description of behavior, whereas in the latter case one infers the operation of either intervening variables or hypothetical constructs.

Early investigations of reflexes revealed that psychological factors (i.e., attention) affected aspects of reflex responsivity. Clinical neurologists looked upon these influences as nuisance variables, factors that could increase the likelihood of both false positives and false negatives in their diagnosis of CNS function. The enormous potential to use such procedures in psychophysiological investigations, however, was apparent from the turn of the century (Dodge, 1911; Golla & Antonovitch, 1929). Surprisingly, for reasons that remain somewhat unclear (see Ison & Hoffman, 1983), the use of this technique remained sporadic until the mid-1960s, when the power of the reflex probe paradigm for psychophysiological inference was first seen most clearly in the work on attention (Anthony, 1985), activation, and response preparation (Brunia & Boelhouwer, 1988). More recently, it has been conscripted to reveal the motivational substrate of affective processes (e.g., Bradley, Cuthbert, & Lang, 1999; see Bradley & Lang, this volume, Chapter 25).

Reviews of numerous experiments on the modulation of the blink reflex by manipulations affecting attention have concluded that the amplitude and/or latency of the blink can be used in specific situations to measure how attention is allocated to different sensory modalities (Anthony, 1985; Hackley, 1999). Specifically, in paradigms in which the subject is warned of an impending target stimulus, the amplitude of the blink is reliably enhanced or suppressed in the warning interval as a function of the match or mismatch, respectively, between the modalities of the two stimuli. In addition, reliable changes in the degree of facilitation or inhibition across the warning interval suggest that the selective allocation of attention may begin as early as the onset of the warning stimulus but that the rate of allocation speeds up dramatically approximately 2 s before the onset of the target stimulus.

Brunia and Boelhouwer (1988) reviewed a large and well-established body of experiments on the modulation of Achilles tendon, Hoffman, and blink reflex amplitude as a function of a wide range of tasks. They concluded that such changes in amplitude are a function of both aselective (i.e., activation) and selective (i.e., response preparation) processes and associate these hypothetical processes with major pathways in the central nervous system; aselective activation effects are hypothesized to be the result of activity in the reticulo-spinal and reticulo-bulbar pathways, and selective preparation effects are hypothesized to be the result of activity in the cortico-spinal and cortico-bulbar pathways. They also presented evidence to suggest that three distinct independent phases in the reflex amplitude function exist in the interval between the presentation of a warning stimulus and the execution of a movement, and argue that these empirically defined phases can be linked to the information processing operations of stimulus evaluation, motor preparation, and response execution. Finally, they (see also Davis, 1940; van Boxtel et al., 1996) presented evidence that there are situations in which changes in reflex amplitude (a) are redundant with nonprobed surface EMG activity (after the onset of the imperative stimulus), (b) stand in contraposition to surface EMG activity (during the foreperiod in an already activated muscle), and (c) occur in the absence of surface EMG activity (during the foreperiod in task-irrelevant muscles and, after practice, in the task relevant muscles as well).

Over the past two decades the reflex probe technique (specifically, the blink reflex) has been employed increasingly in psychophysiology to investigate basic affective processes, although these were preceded by much earlier investigations (Burtt & Tuttle, 1925). Bradley et al. (1999) reviewed the literature to date and evaluated the theoretical implications of this research. Although the exact time course of affective as well as attentional modulation of the blink reflex are sensory modality and task dependent (Neumann, Lipp, & Pretorius, 2004; Vanman, Boehmelt, Dawson, & Schell, 1996), sufficient consistency across studies exists to support the proposition that reflex modulation by affective valence occurs principally in the context of contemplative situations that both enthrall and induce. Viewed in this manner, augmented blink amplitudes observed during the perception of menacing events signalize the prefatory activation of defense or avoidance responses. Conversely, attenuated blink amplitudes observed during the perception of enticing events signalize the prefatory activation of consummatory or approach responses.

In summary, the reflex probe paradigm has been useful when simply recording surface EMG activity has proven to be either insensitive or polysemous. In these contexts, variations in reflex amplitudes have been used to track the allocation of attention, the recruitment of motivational systems, and the preparation for action. It is important to note, however, that this paradigm is inherently more intrusive, potentially less efficient, and only possibly more sensitive than either of the previous two paradigms. The decision regarding which paradigm to use in a given application depends heavily on the nature of the question asked as well as on the social context of the experiment.

Manipulated response paradigm

Questions about the contributions of skeletomotor actions to psychological states or processes have been addressed also by manipulating skeletomotor actions to achieve the desired configuration, verifying the configuration using some observational procedure such the FACS, and measuring the outcome variables of interest (e.g., subjective states, autonomic responses). Although skeletomotor actions have occasionally been manipulated through explicit operant conditioning procedures (e.g., Hefferline, Keenan, & Harford, 1959; Hutchinson, Pierce, Emley, Proni, & Sauer, 1977; Laurenti-Lions et al., 1985; Kleinke & Walton, 1982), the most common approaches have been to instruct subjects either to exaggerate or suppress general skeletomotor configurations (e.g., McCanne & Anderson, 1987; Cacioppo et al., 1992) or to achieve a particular pose by unobtrusively varying the actions of individual muscles (e.g., Strack, Martin, & Stepper, 1988; Larsen, Kasimatis, & Frey, 1992).

In an illustrative study utilizing the muscle-by-muscle induction variant of this general approach, Levenson, Ekman, and Friesen (1990) instructed participants to contract individual muscles until prototypes of the expressions of happiness, sadness, fear, anger, disgust, or surprise were constructed. The construction of each emotional expression was preceded by the construction of a nonemotional expression. Each expression was held for 10 s and was subsequently verified as having been achieved using the FACS. Averaged data during emotional faces minus that during nonemotional ones revealed that the (a) anger face was associated with elevated heart rate, skin conductance levels, and palmar skin temperature, (b) fear and sad faces were associated with elevated heart rate and skin conductance levels, (c) disgust face was associated with elevated skin conductance levels, and (d) the happy and surprise faces were associated with relatively unchanged levels of heart rate, finger temperature, and skin conductance.

Results obtained using the muscle-by-muscle induction paradigm have occasionally been inconsistent and are often open to alternative explanations (see Tourangeau & Ellsworth, 1979; Boiten, 1996). Methodological issues that may contribute to inconsistent results and flawed interpretations include (a) improper controls for somatic tension or effort, (b) floor and ceiling effects in emotional responding, and (c) the inherent difficulties associated with specifying and constructing appropriate expressions with naturalistic durations and trajectories while simultaneously controlling for the intensity and the inconspicuousness of the facial configurations. Relevant commentaries and reviews are provided by Cappella (1993), Hager and Ekman (1981), Laird (1984), Levenson (1992), and Neumann and Strack (2000).

Vaughan and Lanzetta (1981) employed the exaggeration-suppression variant of this paradigm to assess the possible influence of facial expressions on vicarious emotional arousal. Subjects were exposed to a videotaped model displaying pain, ostensibly from receiving electric shocks. One group of subjects was instructed to inhibit any facial expressions when the model was shocked, a second group was instructed to amplify their facial expressions when the model was shocked, and a third (control) group received no instructions about modulating their facial expressions. Results revealed that the amplify group exhibited larger skin conductance responses, heart rate increases, and facial EMG activity in response to the model's display of pain than the other two groups, which did not differ from one another.

Wells and Petty (1980) tested the hypothesis that affect-pertinent bodily movements might similarly influence attitudinal responses toward a persuasive appeal. Specifically, head movements (nodding in agreement or wagging in disagreement) were chosen for study because of their strong association with agreeing and disagreeing responses in a wide variety of cultures (Eibl-Eibesfeldt, 1972) and vertical head movements led to greater agreement with the message in both cases than did horizontal head movements. A conceptual replication and extension of this work by Cacioppo, Priester, and Berntson (1993) found similar compatibility effects for arm flexion and extension, a finding reminiscent of a related compatibility effect reported by Hugo Münsterberg over a century ago (as cited in Bebbe-Center, 1932, p. 339; cf. Foerster & Strack, 1997). This work has recently been extended further, demonstrating the ability of surreptitious feedback from particular facial muscles to ameliorate implicit racial bias (Ito, Chiao, Devine, Lorig, & Cacioppo, 2006).

APPLICATIONS

As described throughout this chapter, surface EMG has proven valuable in studying a wide variety of basic psychological and behavioral processes. This technique has also proven useful in applied contexts. In what follows we list a few general areas to illustrate the breadth of its application.

Detection of deception

The physiological detection of deception, both in research and forensic settings, routinely involves monitoring autonomic reactions to a series of test questions. Regardless of the test used (i.e., Control Question, Concealed Knowledge, or Relevant/Irrelevant), the validity of the test depends on the ability of a pattern of physiological responses to sensitively and specifically index deceit (see Iacono, this volume, Chapter 29). Not surprisingly, the possibility that countermeasures might be used to defeat or distort the polygraph exam has raised concerns about it usefulness (Lykken, 1998). By pressing their toes hard against the floor or biting their tongues, for example, examinees can generate autonomic responses that foil the polygraph exam (e.g., Honts, Hodes, & Raskin, 1985). In an attempt to prevent such physical countermeasures from undermining the validity of the exam, Honts, Raskin, and Kircher (1987) recorded surface EMG activity from the examinee's gastrocnemius and temporalis (i.e., jaw closing muscle of the temple) during a typical exam. Such measurement enabled the detection of 80 percent of the research participants who used either tongue biting or toe pressing to defeat the exam, thus auguring the addition of surface EMG to the list of physiological measures used in the routine detection of deception. Surprisingly, nearly two decades have passed since this seminal publication and surface EMG measurement in either research or forensic polygraphy remains the exception. We believe this is likely because surface EMG is perceived (incorrectly) to be a recondite technique only applicable to the use of physical countermeasures and some studies suggest that purely mental countermeasures might be equally effective in defeating either the control question or the concealed knowledge test (Honts, Raskin, & Kircher, 1994; Honts, Devitt, Winbush, & Kircher, 1996; cf. Olivers & Nieuwenhuis, 2005). As such, it finds occasional application as a manipulation check (Honts et al., 1994) but is not used routinely to improve the predictive validity of the lie detection test.

Polysomnography

For at least the past 40 years it has been known that sleep is not a unitary phenomenon but rather a multistage process. In general, the transition from wakefulness to sleep is accompanied by a decrease in alpha activity (8–13 Hz), a general slowing of EEG activity, a prominence of activity in the theta range (3–7 Hz), and the occurrence of vertex sharp waves. During the transition between wakefulness and Stage 1, slow horizontal eye movements occur, blink rate declines, and muscle tonus is generally reduced relative to waking levels (Perry & Goldwater, 1987). Stage 2 sleep is typically defined by the sporadic presence of two unique EEG waveforms (K-complexes and spindles) and the relative absence of delta activity (.5–2 Hz). Stages 3 and 4, also know as "slow-wave sleep," are typically differentiated from Stage 2 and from each other by the relative proportion of delta activity. Rapid eye movement (REM) sleep is defined by the occurrence of a relatively low-voltage, mixed frequency EEG, the absence of K complexes

and spindles, the presence of sporadically occurring eye movements, and markedly decreased tonus in the pericranial musculature (Ancoli-Israel, 1997; Pivik, this volume, Chapter 27).

The facial muscles are somewhat unique with respect to the rest of the musculature because they appear, paradoxically, to show both distinctly decreasing tonus as a function of sleep depth (Jacobsen et al., 1964; Jacobsen et al., 1965) as well as to be responsive precisely to the processing of both internal (Shimizu & Inoue, 1986) and external stimuli (Sumitsuji et al., 1980). This clear differentiation of tonic levels from phasic activity allowed a team of researchers (Leifting et al., 1994) to use chin EMG alone to differentiate between wakefulness and sleep (using tonic EMG levels) and between quiet (non-REM) and paradoxical (REM) sleep (using phasic EMG parameters) in young infants. In addition, an investigation of the influence of sleep on the muscles of the upper airway (Wheatley et al., 1993) revealed that a decided drop in the tonic level of activity in the alar nasalis muscle occurred coincident with the onset of stage 2 sleep. Surface EMG has also been used effectively to study (a) leg spasms in nocturnal myoclonus ("restless leg syndrome"), (b) abdominal actions in airway apneas (breathing difficulties due to paradoxical sleep-related epiglottal collapse), and (c) nocturnal bruxism, or tooth grinding (see Pressman & Orr, 1997).

Headache and stress reduction

A popular use of surface EMG is in clinical biofeedback for tension headache and stress reduction. This use stemmed from a clinical report by Budzynski and Stoyva (1969), who used EMG activity from a bilateral forehead site over the *frontalis*. In a typical clinical regimen, patients hear tones or clicks whose pitch or rate varies with the envelope of the smoothed, rectified electromyogram and they learn to lower the tone or click rate by relaxing their muscles. Such a procedure was promulgated as a treatment for muscle contraction ("tension") headache, but this procedure was soon extended to general stress management (e.g., Stoyva & Budzynski, 1974).

The rash of frontalis EMG biofeedback studies published in biofeedback's halcyon days consisted mostly of case reports and uncontrolled clinical trials (see Alexander & Smith, 1979, for review), and the claimed incremental efficacy over simple relaxation or meditation techniques remains controversial. The 1980s witnessed a devaluation of the role of muscle tension in "tension" headache (Chun, 1985), and an emphasis on vascular dysfunction, secondary ischemia, and nocigenic metabolites in the etiology (Pikoff, 1984). The past two decades, however, have seen a revival in the use of surface EMG in both the diagnosis and treatment of tension headaches. EMG levels in the neck and forehead of children prone to severe headache, for example, have been reported to be both higher and more variable than those of matched group of controls during the performance of cognitive tasks (Pritchard, 1995), with similar results reported for adults (Bansevicius & Sjaastad, 1996; Jensen, 1999). At least one study has also found trapezius or frontalis EMG biofeedback training to be significantly more effective in the treatment of tension headaches than simple progressive relaxation therapy (i.e., Arena et al., 1995).

Psychosomatic medicine researchers in the 1940s and 1950s were interested in painful, idiopathic muscular contractions occurring in stress or conflict (see Malmo, 1965, for a review), and these examples of "symptom specificity" have occasionally been treated with EMG biofeedback to relax the muscles. Somewhat surprisingly, the mean level of surface EMG activity has been found to be unrelated to the development of pain during stressful conditions (Bansevicius, Westgaard, & Jensen, 1997), while EMG activity recorded surreptitiously during rest periods, is particularly predictive of future muscle pain (Veiersted, 1994).

Physical medicine and rehabilitation

The use of EMG biofeedback in physical medicine was pioneered by John Basmajian in the early 1960s and soon led to the widespread use of surface EMG to enhance recovery of function in muscles that were rendered nonfunctional by stroke, illness, and accidents. In the rehabilitation setting, feedback derived from the surface EMG signal is used, depending upon the disorder, either to relax or tense spastic muscles or to activate atrophied or functionally denervated muscles (see Basmajian, 1989).

Electromyographic biofeedback in rehabilitation is now standard procedure. With respect to diagnosis, there are also promising results in the use of the surface EMG signal to classify muscle impairments in persons with lower back pain (Roy et al., 1997; Oddsson et al., 1997). These techniques are based on the phenomenon of the compression of the power spectral density spectrum of the EMG signal towards lower frequencies during sustained contractions and the fact that this change is associated with the metabolic concomitants of muscle fatigue. Using the different ways in which EMG median frequency parameters change as a function of contraction duration and muscle site, as well as the symmetry of activation during the early part of the contraction, these investigators have shown the surface EMG signal to perform significantly better than conventional clinical parameters at correctly classifying patients with and without lower back pain. EMG biofeedback in the treatment of asthma, however, has proven to be of limited effectiveness (Ritz et al., 2004).

Miscellaneous

Surface EMG is a noninvasive, precise way of measuring muscular contraction in an ongoing fashion in situations where observation is too imprecise, awkward, or costly. In addition to those uses we detailed above, surface EMG continues to used profitably to: (a) quantify muscle tension in ergonomics (see Kumar & Mital, 1996,

for a review), such as evaluating computer "mouse" use (Harvey & Peper, 1997), evaluating the comfort of automobile head rests (Lamotte et al., 1996), or evaluating stress and pain responses among supermarket cashiers (Lundberg et al., 1999; Rissen et al., 2000); (b) assess photophobia by quantifying "squinting" (Stringham et al., 2003); (c) measure precisely the onset, magnitude, and offset of responses in reaction time tasks, including incipient responses that precede the overt response (e.g., McGarry & Franks, 1997; Allain et al., 2004); (d) discern the specific muscles that maintain posture, coordinate gait, and participate in highly skilled acts (e.g., Trepman et al., 1994); (e) evaluate the effectiveness of television commercials (e.g., Hazlett & Hazlett, 1999; cf. Detenber et al., 2000); and (f) enable the continuous discrimination of adequate vs. inadequate anesthesia during surgery (see Paloheimo, 1990, for a review).

With the decreasing expense of the instrumentation required for sensitive and precise EMG measurement, the availability of guidelines and standards, and the emergence of conceptual frameworks and paradigms to aid in the interpretation of EMG responses, surface EMG promises to continue to find even wider application.

CONCLUSION

Theories proposed over a century ago attempted to explain many psychological processes entirely in terms of peripheral skeletomotor actions. This resulted in an exciting and active period for psychophysiology, but the disconfirmation of categorical predictions made by these motor theories was inevitable given the simplicity of the theories and the newness of the technology. Consequently, this premature peak of activity was followed by a downturn in interest in transient or weak skeletomotor actions during the middle of the past century. Nonetheless, many interesting results from this early period have been replicated and extended. Coupled with advances in signal acquisition and analysis, these data are ever increasingly being incorporated into sophisticated theoretical frameworks based on a more complete understanding of the integrated actions of the central and peripheral nervous systems. Major directions we foresee in the coming decade include (a) further refinement of the spatial and temporal patterning that characterizes specific organismic-environmental transactions, (b) continuing research on incipient actions of the skeletomotor system and their dynamic relation to ongoing mind/brain processes, (c) the continuing broadening of the inferential paradigms to include noninvasive brain imaging and brain stimulation methods (e.g., Iwase et al., 2002; Wrase et al., 2003; see Jahanshahi & Rothwell, 2000), (d) the continued development of an "emotional wardrobe" (see Picard, 1997; Stead et al., 2004) to enable "co-located" collaborative environments (see Mandryk & Inkpen, 2004; cf., Rani et al., 2004), and (e) the continued diagnostic and therapeutic use of EMG in psychopathology and rehabilitative medicine.

ACKNOWLEDGMENTS

The chapter represents a revision and update of a previous chapter by Tassinary and Cacioppo (2000).

REFERENCES

Abbs, J. H., Gracco, V. L. & Blair, C. (1984). Functional muscle partitioning during voluntary movement: Facial muscle activity for speech. *Experimental Neurology*, *85*, 469–479.

Adrian, E. D. & Bronk, D. W. (1929). The discharge of impulses in motor nerve fibers. Part II. The frequency of discharge in reflex and voluntary contractions. *Journal of Physiology*, *67*, 119–51.

Alexander, A. B., & Smith, D. D. (1979). Clinical applications of EMG biofeedback. In R. I Gatchel & K. P. Price (Eds.), *Clinical applications of biofeedback: Appraisal and status* (pp. 112–33). New York: Pergamon.

Allain, S., Carbonnell, L., Burle, B., Hasbroucq, T., & Vidal, F. (2004). On-line executive control: An electromyographic study. *Psychophysiology*, *41*, 113–16.

Allport, G. W. (1968). The historical background of modern social psychology. In G. Lindzey & E. Aronson (Eds.), *The handbook of social psychology* (2nd ed.). Menlo Park, CA: Addison-Wesley.

Ancoli-Israel, S. (1997). The polysomnogram. In M. R. Pressman & W. C. Orr (Eds.), *Understanding Sleep: The evaluation and treatment of sleep disorders* (pp. 177–91). Washington, DC: American Psychological Association.

Andreassi, J. L. (1995). *Psychophysiology: Human behavior and response* (3rd Ed.). Hillsdale, NJ: Lawrence Erlbaum Associates.

Anthony, B. I. (1985). In the blink of an eye: Implications of reflex modifcation for information processing. *Advances in Psychophysiology*, *1*, 167–218.

Arndt, J., Allen, J. J. B., & Greenberg. J. (2001). Traces of terror: Subliminal death primes and facial electromyographic indices of affect. *Motivation and Emotion*, *25*, 253–277.

Arena, J. G., Bruno, G. M., Hannah, S. L., & Meador, K. (1995). A comparison of frontal electromyographic biofeedback training, trapezius electromyographic biofeedback training, and progressive relaxation therapy in the treatment of tension headache. *Headache*, *35*, 411–419.

Bansevicius, D. & Sjaastad, O. (1996). Cervicogenic headache: The influence of mental load on pain level and EMG of the shoulder-neck and facial muscle. *Headache*, *36*, 372–78.

Bansevicius, D., Westgaard, R. H., & Jensen, C. (1997). Mental stress of long duration: EMG activity, perceived muscle tension, fatigue, and pain development in pain-free subjects. *Headache*, *37*, 499–510.

Bains, A. E. (1918). Studies in electro-physiology (animal and vegetable). London: G. Routledge & Sons.

Bakker, F. C., Boschker, M. S. J., & Chung, T. (1996). Changes in muscular activity while imagining weight lifting using stimulus or response propositions. *Journal of Sport and Exercise Psychology*, *18*, 313–24.

Bartholow, B. D., Fabiani, M., Gratton, G., & Bettencourt, B. A. (2001). A psychophysiological examination of cognitive processing of affective responses to social expectancy violations. *Psychological Science*, *12*(3), 197–204.

Basmajian, J. V. (1989). *Biofeedback: Principles and practice for clinicians* (3rd ed.). Baltimore: Williams & Wilkins.

Basmajian, J. V. & De Luca, C. J. (1985). *Muscles alive: Their functions revealed by electromyography* (5th ed.). Baltimore: Williams & Wilkins.

Baveles, J. B., Black, A., Chovil, N., Lemery, C. R., & Mullett, J. (1988). Form and function in motor mimicry: Topographic evidence that the primary function is communicative. *Human Communication Research*, *14*, 275–299.

Bavelas, J. B., Black, A., Lemery, C. R., & Mullett, J. (1986). "I show how you feel": Motor mimicry as a communicative act. *Journal of Personality and Social Psychology*, *50*, 322–329.

Beebe-Center, J. G. (1932). *The Psychology of Pleasantness and Unpleasantness*. New York: D. Van Nostrand Company, Inc.

Berkinblit, M. B., Feldman, A. G., & Fulson, O. I. (1986). Adaptability of innate motor patterns and motor control mechanisms. *Behavioral and Brain Sciences*, *9*, 585–638.

Blumenthal, T., Cuthbert, B. N., Filion, D. L., Hackley, S., Lipp, O. V., & van Boxtel, A. (2005). Committee report: Guidelines for human startle eyeblink electromyographic studies. *Psychophysiology*, *42*, 1–15.

Boiten, F. (1996). Autonomic response patterns during voluntary facial action. *Psychophysiology*, *33*, 123–131.

Bond, C. F. & Titus, L. J. (1983). Social facilitation: A meta-analysis of 241 studies. *Psychological Bulletin*, *94*, 265–92.

Braathen, E. T. & Sveback, S. (1994). EMG response patterns and motivational styles as predictors of performance and discontinuation in explosive and endurance sports among talented teenage athletes. *Personality and Individual Differences*, *17*, 545–56.

Bradley, M., Cuthbert, B. N., Lang, P. J. (1999). Affect and the startle reflex. In M. E. Dawson, A. Schell, A. Boehmelt (Eds.), *Startle modification: Implications for neuroscience, cognitive science, and clinical science* (pp. 157–83). Stanford, CA: Cambridge University Press.

Bramsley, G. R., Bruun, G. Buchthal, F., Guld, C. & Petersen, H. S. (1967). Reduction of electrical interference in measurements of bioelectrical potentials in a hospital. *Acta Polytechnica Scandanavia Electrical Engineering Series*, *15*, 1–37.

Britt, T. W. & Blumenthal, T. D. (1992). The effects of anxiety on motoric expression of the startle response. *Personality and Individual Differences*, *13*, 91–7.

Brown, P. (2000). Cortical drives to human muscles: The Piper and related rhythms. *Progress in Neurobiology*, *60*, 97–108.

Bruintjes, T. D., van Olphen, A. F., Hillen, B., & Weijs, W. A. (1996). Electromyography of the human nasal muscles. *European Archives of Otorhinolaryngology*, *253*, 464–69.

Brunia, C. H. M. & Boelhouwer, A. J. W. (1988). Reflexes as tools: A window in the central nervous system. *Advances in Psychophysiology*, *3*, 1–67.

Brunia, C. H. M. & van Boxtel, G. J. M. (2000). Motor preparation. In J. T. Cacioppo, L. G. Tassinary and G. Bernston (Eds.), *The Handbook of Psychophysiology*. New York: Cambridge University Press.

Budzynski, T. H., & Stoyva, I. M. (1969). An instrument for producing deep muscle relaxation by means of analog information feedback. *Journal of Applied Behavior Analysis*, *2*, 231–37.

Burtt, H. E. & Tuttle, W. W. (1925). The patellar tendon reflex and affective tone. *American Journal of Psychology*, *36*, 553–61.

Cacioppo, J. T., Berntson, G. & Klein, D. J. (1992). What is an emotion? The role of somatovisceral afference, with special emphasis on somatovisceral "illusions." *Review of Personality and Social Psychology*, *14*, 63–98.

Cacioppo, J. T., Bush, L. K., & Tassinary, L. G. (1992). Microexpressive facial actions as a function of affective stimuli: Replication and extension. *Personality and Social Psychology Bulletin, 18,* 515–26.

Cacioppo, J. T., Klein, D. J., Berntson, G., & Hatfield, E. (1993). The psychophysiology of emotion. In M. Lewis & J. M. Haviland (Eds.), *Handbook of emotions* (pp. 119–42). New York: Guilford.

Cacioppo, J. T., Marshall-Goodell, B. S. & Dorfman, D. D. (1983). Skeletal muscular patterning: Topographical analysis of the integrated electromyogram. *Psychophysiology, 20,* 269–83.

Cacioppo, J. T., Marshall-Goodell, B. S. & Gormezano, I. (1983). Social psychophysiology: Bioelectrical measurement, experimental control, and analog-to-digital data acquistion. In J. T. Cacioppo & R. E. Petty (Eds.), *Social psychophysiology: A sourcebook* (pp. 666–92). New York: Guilford Press.

Cacioppo, J. T., Martzke, J. S., Petty, R. E. & Tassinary, L. G. (1988). Specific forms of facial EMG response index emotions during an interview: From Darwin to the continuous flow hypothesis of affect-laden information processing. *Journal of Personality and Social Psychology, 54,* 592–604.

Cacioppo, J. T., & Petty, R. E. (1979a). Attitudes and cognitive response: An electrophysiological approach. *Journal of Personality and Social Psychology, 37,* 2181–199.

Cacioppo, J. T. & Petty, R. E. (1979b). Lip and nonpreferred forearm EMG activity as a function of orienting task. *Biological Psychology, 9,* 103–13.

Cacioppo, J. T. & Petty, R. E. (1981a). Electromyograms as measures of extent and affectivity of information processing. *American Psychologist, 36,* 441–56.

Cacioppo, J. T. & Petty, R. E. (1981b). Electromyographic specificity during covert information processing. *Psychophysiology, 18,* 518–23.

Cacioppo, J. T. & Petty, R. E. (1986). Social processes. In M. G. H. Coles, E. Donchin, & S. Porges (Eds.), *Psychophysiology: Systems, processes, and applications* (pp. 646–79). New York: Guilford Press.

Cacioppo, J. T., Petty, R. E., Losch, M. E. & Kim, H. S. (1986). Electromyographic activity over facial muscle regions can differentiate the valence and intensity of affective reactions. *Journal of Personality and Social Psychology, 50,* 260–268.

Cacioppo, J. T., Petty, R. E. & Morris, K. (1985). Semantic, evaluative, and self-referent processing: Memory, cognitive effort, and somatovisceral activity. *Psychophysiology, 22,* 371–84.

Cacioppo, J. T., Petty, R. E. & Tassinary, L. G. (1989). Social psychophysiology: A new look. *Advances in Experimental Social Psychology, 22,* 39–91.

Cacioppo, J. T., Priester, J. T., & Berntson, G. (1993). Rudimentary determinants of attitudes: II. Arm flexion and extension have differential effects on attitudes. *Journal of Personality and Social Psychology, 65,* 5–17.

Cacioppo, J. T., Rourke, P. A., Marshall-Goodell, B. S., Tassinary, L. G. & Baron, R. S. (1990). Rudimentary physiological effects of mere observation. *Psychophysiology, 27,* 177–86.

Cacioppo, J. T., & Tassinary, L. G. (1989). The concept of attitude: A psychophysiological analysis. In H. L. Wagner & A. S. R. Manstead (Eds.), *Handbook of psychophysiology: Emotion and social behaviour.* Chichester: Wiley.

Cacioppo, J. T. & Tassinary, L. G. (1990a). Inferring psychological significance from physiological signals. *American Psychologist, 45,* 16–28.

Cacioppo, J. T. & Tassinary, L. G. (1990b). Psychophysiology and psychophysiological inference. In J. T. Cacioppo & L. G. Tassinary (Eds.). *Principles of psychophysiology* (pp. 3–33). New York: Cambridge University Press.

Cacioppo, J. T. Tassinary, L. G., & Fridlund, A. (1990c). The skeletomotor system. In J. T. Cacioppo & L. G. Tassinary (Eds.), *Principles of psychophysiology* (pp. 325–84). New York: Cambridge University Press.

Cappella, J. N. (1993). The facial feedback hypothesis in human interaction: Review and speculation. *Journal of Language and Social Psychology, 12,* 13–29.

Chapman, A. J. (1974). An electromyographic study of social facilitation: A test of the "mere presence" hypothesis. *British Journal of Psychology, 65,* 123–28.

Chovil, N. (1991). Social determinants of facial displays. *Journal of Nonverbal Behavior, 15,* 141–54.

Chun, W. X. (1985). An approach to the nature of tension headache. *Headache, 25,* 188–89.

Cohn, J. F., Zlochower, A. J., Lien, J. & Kanade, T. (1999). Automated face analysis by feature point tracking has high concurrent validity with manual FACS coding. *Psychophysiology, 36,* 35–43.

Coles, M. G. H., Gratton, G., Bashore, T. R., Eriksen, C. W., & Donchin, E. (1985). A psychophysiological investigation of the continuous flow model of human information processing. *Journal of Experimental Psychology: Human Perception and Performance, 11* 529–53.

Compton, R. W. (1973). Morphological, physiological, and behavioral studies of the facial musculature of the Coati (Nasua). *Brain, Behavior, and Evolution, 7,* 85–126.

Cook, T. D. & Campbell, D. T. (1979). *Quasi-Experimentation: Design and analysis issues for field settings.* Boston: Houghton Mifflin

Cooper, R., Osselton, J. W., & Shaw, J. C. (1980). *EEG technology* (3rd ed.). London: Butterworth.

Cram, J. R., Kasman, G. & Holtz, J. (1998). *Introduction to surface EMG.* Boston: Jones & Bartlett Publishers.

Cuthbertson, R. A. (1990). The highly original Dr. Duchenne. In R. A. Cuthbertson (Ed. & Trans.), *The mechanism of human facial expression* (pp. 225–41). New York: Cambridge University Press.

Dambrun, M., Despres, G., & Guimond, S. (2004). On the multifaceted nature of prejudice: Psychophysiology responses to ingroup and outgroup ethnic stimuli. *Current Research in Social Psychology, 8,* 187–204.

Darwin, C. (1873). *The expression of the emotions in man and animals.* New York: Appleton. (Original work published 1872)

Davis, J. F. (1952). *Manual of surface electromyography.* Montreal: Laboratory for Psychological Studies, Allan Memorial Institute of Psychiatry.

Davis, J. F., & Malmo, R. B. (1951). Electromyographic recording during interview. *American Journal of Psychiatry, 107,* 908–16.

Davis, J. F., Malmo, R. B., & Shagass, C. (1954). Electromyographic reaction to strong auditory stimulation in psychiatric patients. *Canadian Journal of Psychology, 8,* 177–86.

Davis M., Walker D. L., Myers K. M. (2003). Role of the amygdala in fear extinction measured with potentiated startle. *Annals of the New York Academy of Science, 985,* 218–32.

Davis, R. C. (1938). The relation of muscle action potentials to difficulty and frustration. *Journal of Experimental Psychology, 23,* 141–58.

Davis, R. C. (1940). *Set and muscular tension.* Indiana University Publications, Science Series No. 10.

Davis, W. J., Rahman, M. A., Smith, L. J., Burns, A., Senecal, L., McArthur, D., Halpern, J. A., Perlmuter, A., Sickels, W., & Wagner, W. (1995). Properties of human affect induced by static color slides (IAPS): Dimensional, categorical and electromyographic analysis. *Biological Psychology, 41*, 229–53.

de Jong, R., Coles, M. G., Logan, G. D. & Gratton, G. (1990). In search of the point of no return: The contol of response processes. *Journal of Experimental Psychology: Human Perception and Performance, 16*, 164–82.

De Luca, C. J. & Erim, Z. (1994). Common drive of motor units in regulation of muscle force. *Trends in Neuroscience, 17*, 299–305.

De Luca, C. J. & Knaflitz, M. (1992). *Surface electromyography: What's new?* Torino, Italy: C.L.U.T Editrice.

De Luca, C. J. & Merletti, R. (1988). Surface myoelectric signal cross-talk among muscles of the leg. *Electroencephalography and Clinical Neurophysiology, 69*, 568–75.

De Luca, C. J. (1997). The use of surface electromyography in biomechanics. *Journal of Applied Biomechanics, 13*, 135–63.

Desmedt, J. E. & Godaux, E. (1981). Spinal motoneuron recruitment in man: Rank deordering with direction but not with speed of movement. *Science, 214*, 933–36.

Detenber, B. H., Simmons, R. F., & Reiss, J. E. (2000). The emotional significance of color in television presentations. *Media Psychology, 2*, 331–55.

Dimberg, U. (1982). Facial reactions to facial expressions. *Psychophysiology, 19*, 643–47.

Dimberg, U. (1990). Gender differences in facial reactions to facial expressions. *Biological Psychology, 30*, 151–59.

Dimberg, U. (1997). Social fear and expressive reactions to social stimuli. *Scandinavian Journal of Psychology, 38*, 171–74.

Disselhorst-Klug, C., Silny, J. & Rau, G. (1997). Improvement of spatial resolution in surface-EMG: A theoretical and experimental comparison of different spatial filters. *IEEE Transactions on Biomedical Engineering, 44*, 567–74.

Dodge, R. B. (1911). A systematic exploration of a normal knee jerk, its technique, the form of muscle contraction, its amplitude, its latent time and its theory. *Zeitschrift fur Allgemeine Physiologie, 12*, 1–58.

Dollins, A. B. & McGuigan, F. J. (1989). Frequency analysis of electromyographically measured covert speech behavior. *Pavlovian Journal of Biological Science, 24*, 27–30.

Dorfman, D. & Cacioppo, J. T. (1990). Waveform moment analysis: Topographical analysis of nonrhythmic waveforms. In J. T. Cacioppo and L. G. Tassinary (Eds.), *Principles of psychophysiology* (pp. 661–707). New York: Cambridge University Press.

Duchenne, G. B. (1990). *The mechanism of human facial expression* (R. A. Cuthbertson, Editor & Trans.). New York: Cambridge University Press. (Original work published 1862)

Duffy, E. (1962). *Activation and behavior*. New York: Wiley.

Eason, R. G., & White, C. T. (1961). Muscular tension, effort, and tracking difficulty: Studies of parameters which affect tension levels and performance efficiency. *Perceptual and Motor Skills, 12*, 331–72.

Eccles, J. C. & Sherrington, C. S. (1930). Number and contraction values of individual motor-units examined in some muscles of the limb. *Proceedings of the the Royal Society, 106B*, 326–57.

Eibl-Eibesfeldt, I. (1972). Similarities and differences between cultures in expressive movement. In R. A. Hinde (Ed.), *Nonverbal communication*. Cambridge: Cambridge University Press.

Ekman, P. (1972). Universal and cultural differences in facial expressions of emotion. In J. Cole (Ed.), *Nebraska symposium on motivation*, (Vol. 19, pp. 207–18). Lincoln: University of Nebraska Press.

Ekman, P. (1982). Methods for measuring facial action. In K. R. Scherer & P. Ekman (Eds.), *Handbook of methods in nonverbal behavior research* (pp. 45–90). Cambridge: Cambridge University Press.

Ekman, P. (1985). *Telling lies: Clues to deceit in the marketplace, politics, and marriage*. New York: Norton.

Ekman, P., & Friesen, W. V. (1978). *Facial action coding system (FACS): A technique for the measurement of facial actions*. Palo Alto, CA: Consulting Psychologists Press.

Englis, B. G., Vaughan, K. B., & Lanzetta, J. T. (1982). Conditioning of counter-empathic emotional responses. *Journal of Experimental Social Psychology, 18*, 375–391.

Epstein, L. H. (1990). Perception of activity in the *zygomaticus major* and *corrugator supercilii* muscle regions. *Psychophysiology, 27*, 68–72.

Fanardjian, V. V. & Manvelyan, L. R. (1987). Mechanisms regulating the activity of facial nucleus motoneurons-IV. Influences from brainstem structures. *Neuroscience, 20*, 845–53.

Farina, D., Cescon, C. & Merlietti, R. (2002). Influence of anatomical, physical, and detection-system parameters on surface EMG. *Biological Cybernetics, 86*(6), 445–56.

Faulkner, W. (1936). *Absalom, Absalom!* New York: Random House.

Fearing, F. (1930). *Reflex action: A study in the history of physiological psychology*. Baltimore: Williams & Wilkins.

Feldman, R. S. & Rime, B. (1991). *Fundamentals of nonverbal behavior*. New York: Cambridge University Press.

Foerster, J. & Strack, F. (1997). Motor action in retrieval of valenced information: A motor congruence effect. *Perceptual and Motor Skills, 85*, 1419–1427.

Freeman, G. L. (1931). Mental activity and the muscular processes. *Psychological Review, 38*, 428–47.

Fridlund, A. J. (1991). Sociality of solitary: Potentiation by an implicit audience. *Journal of Personality and Social Psychology, 60*, 229–240.

Fridlund, A. J. (1994). *Human facial expression: An evolutionary view*. San Diego, CA: Academic Press.

Fridlund, A. J., & Cacioppo, J. T. (1986). Guidelines for human electromyographic research. *Psychophysiology, 23*, 567–89.

Fridlund, A. J., Fowler, S. C., & Pritchard, D. A. (1980). Striate muscle tensional patterning in frontalis EMG biofeedback. *Psychophysiology, 17*, 47–55.

Fridlund, A. J., Hatfield, M. E., Cottam, G. L., & Fowler, S. C. (1986). Anxiety and striate-muscle activation: Evidence from electromyographic pattern analysis. *Journal of Abnormal Psychology, 95*, 228–36.

Fridlund, A. J., & Izard, C. E. (1983). Electromyographic studies of facial expressions of emohons and patterns of emotions. In J. T. Cacioppo & R. E. Petty (Eds.), *Social psychophysiology: A sourcebook* (pp. 243–86). New York Guilford Press.

Friesen, W. V. (1972). *Cultural differences in facial expression in a social situation: An experimental text of the concept of display rules*. Unpublished doctoral dissertation, University of California, San Francisco.

Fulton, J. F. (1926). *Muscular contraction and the reflex control of movement*. Baltimore: Williams & Wilkins.

Gale, A., & Baker, S. (1981). In vivo or in vitro? Some effects of laboratory environments, with particular reference to the psychophysiological experiment. In M. J. Christie & P. G.

Mellet (Eds.), *Foundations of psychosomatics*. Chichester: Wiley.

Gallistel, C. R. (1980). *The organization of action: The new synthesis*. Hillsdale, NJ: Erlbaum.

Gallese, V. (2003). The roots of empathy: The shared manifold hypothesis and the neural basis of intersubjectivity. *Psychopathology, 36*, 171–80.

Gans, C., & Gorniak, G. C. (1980). Electromyograms are repeatable: Precautions and limitations. *Science, 210*, 795–97.

Gardiner, W. L., Gabriel, S., & Diekman, A. B. (2000). Interpersonal Processes. In J. T. Cacioppo, L. G. Tassinary and G. Bernston (Eds.), *The Handbook of Psychophysiology*. New York: Cambridge University Press.

Graziano, W. G., Smith, S. M., Tassinary, L. G., Sun, Chien-Su., & Pilkington, C. (1996). Does imitation enhance memory for faces? Four converging studies. *Journal of Personality and Social Psychology, 71*(5), 874–87.

Geen, R. G. & Bushman, B. J. (1989). The arousing effects of social presence. In H. Wagner & A. Manstead (Eds.), *Handbook of Social Psychophysiology* (pp. 261–82). Chichester: Wiley.

Geen, R. G., & Gange, J. J. (1977). Drive theory of social facilitation: Twelve years of theory and research. *Psychological Bulletin, 84*, 1267–1288.

Geen, T. R. (1992). Facial expressions in socially isolated primates: Open and closed programs for expressive behavior. *Journal of Research in Personality, 26*, 273–80.

Geen, T. R. & Tassinary, L. G. (2002). The mechanization of expression in John Bulwar's Pathomyotonia. *American Journal of Psychology, 115*(2), 275–300.

Gehricke, J., & Shapiro, D. (2001). Facial and autonomic activity in depression: Social context differences during imagery. *International Journal of Psychophysiology, 41*, 53–64.

Germana, J. (1974). Electromyography: Human and general. In R. F. Thompson & M. M. Patterson (Eds.), *Bioelectric recording techniques: Part C: Receptor and effector processes* (pp. 155–63). New York: Academic Press.

Ghez, C. & Krahauer, J. (2000). The organization of movement. In E. R. Kandel, J. H. Schwartz, & T.M. Jessel, (Eds.), *Principles of neural science* (4th ed.), pp. 653–73. New York: Elsevier.

Gilbert, A. N., Fridlund, A. J. & Sabini, J. (1987). Hedonic and social determinants of facial displays to odors. *Chemical Senses, 12*, 355–363.

Girard, E., Tassinary, L. G., Kappas, A., Gosselin, P. & Bontempo, D. (1997). The covert-to-overt threshold for facial actions: An EMG study. *Psychophysiology, 34*, S38.

Goldstein, J. B. (1972). Electromyography: A measure of skeletal muscle response. In N. S. Greenheld & R. A. Sternbach (Eds.), *Handbook of psychophysiology* (pp. 329–66). New York: Holt, Rinehart & Winston.

Golla, F. & Antonovitch, S. (1929). The relaxation of muscular tonus and the patellar reflex to mental work. *Journal of Mental Science, 75*, 234–41.

Gousain, A. K., Amarante, M. T. J., Hydem J. S., & Yousif, N. J. (1996). A dynamic analysis of changes in the nasolabial fold using magnetic resonance imaging: Implications for facial rejuvination and facial animation surgery. *Plastic and Reconstructive Surgery, 98*, 622–36.

Graham J. L. (1980). A new system for measuring nonverbal responses to marketing appeals. *1980 AMA Educator's Conference Proceedings, 46*, 340–43.

Gray, H. (2000). *Anatomy of the Human Body* (20th Ed.). New York: Bartlby.Com. (Original work published 1918).

Greene, W. A., Turetsky, B., & Kohler, C. (2000). The skeletomotor system: Surface electromyography. In J. T. Cacioppo, L. G. Tassinary and G. Bernston (Eds.), *The Handbook of Psychophysiology*. New York: Cambridge University Press.

Greenwald, M. K., Cook, E. W. & Lang, P. J. (1989). Affective judgment and psychophysiological response: Dimensional covariation in the evaluation of pictorial stimuli. *Journal of Psychophysiology, 3*, 51–64.

Groff, B. D., Baron, R. S., & Moore, D. L. (1983). Distraction, attentional conflict, and drivelike behavior. *Journal of Experimental Social Psychology, 19*, 359–80.

Hackley, S. (1999). Implications of blink reflex research for theories of attention and consciousness. In M. E. Dawson, A. M. Schell, & A. H. Böhmelt (Eds.), *Startle modification: Implications for neuroscience, cognitive science, and clinical science* (pp. 137–56). New York: Cambridge University Press.

Hager, J. C., & Ekman, P. (1981). Methodological problems in Tourangeau and Ellsworth's study of facial expression and experience of emotion. *Journal of Personality and Social Psychology, 40*, 358–62.

Harvey, R. & Peper, E. (1997). Surface electromyography and mouse use. *Ergonomics, 40*, 781–789.

Hasbroucq, T., Burle, B., Akamatsu, M., Vidal, F., & Possamai, C. A. (2001). An electromyographic investigation of the effect of stimulus-response mapping on choice reaction time. *Psychophysiology, 38*(1), 157–62.

Hatfield, E., Cacioppo, J. T., & Rapson, R. L. (1993). *Emotional Contagion*. New York: Cambridge University Press.

Hayes, K. J. (1960). Wave analyses of tissue noise and muscle action potential. *Journal of Applied Physiology, 15*, 749–52.

Hazlett, R. L., McLeod, D. R., Hoehn-Saric, R. (1994). Muscle tension in generalized anxiety disorder: Elevated muscle tonus or agitated movement? *Psychophysiology, 31*, 189–95.

Hazlett, R. L. & Hazlett, S. Y. (1999). Emotional response to television commercials: Facial EMG vs. self-report. *Journal of Advertising Research, 39*, 7–23.

Hefferline, R. F., Keenan, B., & Harford, R. A. (1959). Escape and avoidance conditioning in human subjects without their observation of the response. *Science, 130*, 1338–39.

Henneman, E. (1980). Organization of the motoneuron pool: The size principle. In V. E. Mountcastle (Ed.), *Medical physiology: Vol. 1* (14th ed., pp. 718–41). St. Louis: Mosby.

Hess, U., Banse, R. & Kappas, A. (1995). The intensity of facial expression is determined by underlying affective state and social situation. *Journal of Personality and Social Psychology, 69*, 280–288.

Hess, U., Kappas, A., McHugo, G. J., & Kleck, R. E. (1989). An analysis of the encoding and decoding of spontaneous and posed smiles: The use of facial electromyography. *Journal of Nonverbal Behavior, 13*, 121–37.

Hess, U., Philipot, P. & Blairy, S. (1999). Mimicry: Facts and fiction. In P. Phillipot, R. Feldman, & E. Coats (Eds.), *The social context of nonverbal behavior: Studies in emotion and social interaction* (pp. 213–41). New York: Cambridge University Press.

Hill, A. V. (1959). The heat production of muscle and nerve, 1848–1914. *Annual Review of Physiology, 21*, 1–18.

Hislop, H. J. & Montgomery, J. (2002). *Daniels and Worthingham's Muscle Testing: Techniques of Manual Examination* (7th Ed.). Philadelphia: W.B. Saunders Company.

Himer, W., Schneider, F., Koest, G. & Heimann, H. (1991). Computer-based analysis of facial action: A new approach. *Journal of Psychophysiology, 5*, 189–95.

Hinsey, J. C. (1940). The hypothalamus and somatic responses. In J. F. Fulton, S. Walter & A. M. Frantz (Eds.), *Research publications of the Association for Research in Nervous and Mental Disease: Vol. 20* (pp. 657–685). Baltimore: Williams & Wilkins.

Honts, C. R., Devitt, M. K., Winbush, M., Kircher, J. C. (1996). Mental and physical countermeasures reduce the accuracy of the concealed knowledge test. *Psychophysiology, 33*, 84–92.

Honts, C. R., Hodes, R. L., & Raskin, D. C. (1985). Effects of physical countermeasures on the physiological detection of deception. *Journal of Applied Psychology, 79*, 177–87.

Honts, C. R., Raskin, D. C., & Kircher, J. C. (1987). Effects of physical countermeasures and their electromyographic detection during polygraph tests for deception. *Journal of Psychophysiology, 1*, 241–47.

Honts, C. R., Raskin, D. C., & Kircher, J. C. (1994). Mental and physical countermeasures reduce the accuracy of polygraph tests. *Journal of Applied Psychology, 79*, 252–59.

Hu, S., & Wan, H. (2003). Imagined events with specific emotional valence produce specific patterns of facial EMG activity. *Perceptual and Motor Skills, 97*, 1091–99.

Humphrey, G. (1951). *Thinking*. New York: Wiley.

Hutchinson, R. R., Pierce, G. E., Emley, G. S., Proni, T. J., & Sauer, R. A. (1977). The laboratory measurement of human anger. *Biobehavioral Reviews, 1*, 241–59.

Huxley, A. F. (1980). *Reflections on muscle*. Liverpool: Liverpool University Press.

Isley, C. L., & Basmajian, J. V. (1973). Electromyography of the human cheeks and lips. *Anatomical Record, 176*, 143–48.

Ison, J. R., & Hoffman, H. S. (1983). Reflex modification in the domain of startle: II. The anomalous history of a robust and ubiquitous phenomenon. *Psychological Bulletin, 94*, 3–17.

Iswase, M., Ouchi, Y., Okada, H., Yokoyama, C., Nobezawa, S., Tsukada, H., Takeda, M., Yamashita, K., Takeda, M., Yamaguti, K., Kuratsune, H., Shimizu, A., & Watanabe, Y. (2002). Neural substrates of human facial expression of pleasant emotion induced by comic films: A PET study. *Neuroimage, 17*(2), 758–68.

Ito, T. A., Chaio, K. W., Devine, P., Lorig, T., & Cacioppo, J. T. (2006). The influence of facial feedback on race bias. *Psychological Science, 17*(3), 256–61.

Izard, C. E. (1971). *The face of emotion*. New York: Appleton-Century-Crofts.

Jacobsen, A., Kales, A., Lehmann, D., and Hoedmaker, F. S. (1964). Muscle tonus in human subjects during sleep and dreaming. *Experimental Neurology, 10*, 418–24.

Jacobsen, A., Kales, A., Zweizig, J. R., and Kales, J. (1965). Special EEG and EMG techniques for sleep research. *American Journal of EEG Technology, 18*, 5–10.

Jacobson, E. (1927). Action currents from muscular contractions during conscious processes. *Science, 66*, 403.

Jacobson, E. (1932). Electrophysiology of mental activities. *American Journal of Psychology, 44*, 677–94.

Jahanshahi, M. & Rothwell, J. (2000). Transcranial magnetic stimulation studies of cognition: An emerging field. *Experimental Brain Research, 131*(1), 1–9.

James, W. (1884). What is an emotion? *Mind, 9*, 188–205.

James, W. (1890). *The principles of psychology*. New York: Holt.

Jäncke, K. & Kaufmann, N. (1994). Facial EMG responses to odors in solitude and with an audience. *Chemical Senses, 19*(2), 99–111.

Jäncke, L. (1996). Facial EMG in an anger-provoking situation: Individual differences in directly anger outwards or inwards. *International Journal of Psychophysiology, 23*, 207–14.

Jenny, A. B. & Saper, C. B. (1987). Organization of the facial nucleus and corticofacial projection in the monkey: A reconsideration of the upper motor neuron facial palsy. *Neurology, 37*, 930–39.

Jensen, R. (1999). Pathophysiological mechanisms of tension-type headache: a review of epidemiological and experimental studies. *Cephalagia, 19*(6), 602–21.

Johnson, E. W., & Pease, W. S. (1997). *Practical myography*, 3rd ed. Baltimore: Williams & Wilkins.

Johnson, L. C. & Lubin, A. (1972). On planning psychophysiological experiments: Design, measurement, and analysis. In N. S. Greenheld & R. A. Sternbach (Eds.), *Handbook of psychophysiology* (pp. 125–58). New York: Holt, Rinehart & Winston.

Kandel, E. R., Schwartz, J. H. & Jessel, T. M. (2000). *Principles of neural science*, 4th ed. New York: Elsevier.

Kappas, A., Hess, U., & Kleck, R. E. (1990). The periscope box: A nonobtrusive method of providing an eye-to-eye video perspective. *Behavior Research Methods, Instruments & Computers, 22*, 375–76.

Kelso, J. A. S., Tuller, B., Vatikiotis-Bateson, E., & Fowler, C. A. (1984). Functionally specific articulatory cooperation following jaw perturbations during speech: Evidence for coordinative structures. *Journal of Experimental Psychology: Human Perception and Performance, 10*, 812–32.

Kendall, F. & McCreary, E. K. (1993). *Muscles: Testing and Function*, 4th ed. Baltimore: Williams & Wilkins.

Khan, S. D., Bloodworth, D. S. & Woods, R. H. (1971). Comparative advantages of bipolar abraded skin surface electrodes over bipolar intramuscular electrodes for single motor unit recording in psychophysiological research. *Psychophysiology, 8*, 635–47.

Kikkawa, D. O., Lemke, B. N., & Dortzbach, R. K. (1996). Relations of the superficial musculoaponeurotic system to the orbit and characterization of the orbitomalar ligament. *Opthalmic Plastic and Reconstructive Surgery, 12*, 77–88.

Kleinke, C. L. & Walton, J. H. (1982). Influence of reinforced smiling on affective responses in an interview. *Journal of Personality and Social Psychology, 42*, 557–65.

Knowlton, B. J. & Squire, L. R. (1993). The learning of categories: Parallel brain systems for item memory and category knowledge. *Science, 262*, 1747–49.

Komi, P. V., & Buskirk, E. R. (1970). Reproducibility of electromyographic measurements with inserted wire electrodes and surface electrodes. *Electromyography, 10*, 357–67.

Kraut, R. E., & Johnson, R. E. (1979). Social and emotional messages of smiling: An ethological approach. *Journal of Personality and Social Psychology, 37*, 1539–53.

Kumar, S. & Mital, A. (1996) (Eds.). *Electromyography in ergonomics*. London: Taylor & Francis.

Laird, J. D. (1984). The real role of facial response in the experience of emotion: A reply to Tourangeau and Ellsworth, and others. *Journal of Personality and Social Psychology, 47*, 909–17.

Lamotte, T., Priez, A., Lepoivre, E., Duchene, J. et al. (1996). Surface electromyography as a tool to study head rest comfort in cars. *Ergonomics, 39*, 781–96.

Lang, P. J., Greenwald, M. K., Bradley, M. M., and Hamm, A. O. (1993). Looking at pictures: Affective, facial, visceral, and behavioral reactions. *Psychophysiology, 30*, 261–73.

Lanzetta, J. T. & Englis, B. G. (1989). Expectations of cooperation and competition and their effects on observers' vicarious emotional responses. *Journal of Personality and Social Psychology*, *56*, 543–54.

Larsen, J. T., Norris, C. J., & Cacioppo, J. T. (2003). Effects of positive and negative affect on electromyographic activity over *zygomaticus major* and *corrugator supercilii. Psychophysiology*, *40*, 776–85.

Larsen, R. J., Kasimatis, M. & Frey, K. (1992). Facilitating the furrowed brow: A unobtrusive test of the facial feedback hypothesis applied to unpleasant affect. *Cognition and Emotion*, *6*, 321–38.

Laurenti-Lions, L., Gallego, J., Chambille, B., Vardon, G. & Jacquemin, C. (1985). Control of myoelectrical responses through reinforcement. *Journal of the Experimental Analysis of Behavior*, *44*, 185–93.

Lawrence, J. H. & De Luca, C. J. (1983). Myoelectrical signal vs. force relationship in different muscles. *Journal of Applied Physiology*, *54*, 1653–59.

Leifting, B., Bes, F., Fagioli, I., and Salzarulo, P. (1994). Electromyographic activity and sleep states in infants. *Sleep*, *17*, 718–22.

Levenson, R. W. (1992). Autonomic nervous system differences among emotions. *Psychological Science*, *3*, 23–7.

Levenson, R. W., Ekman, P., & Friesen, W. (1990). Voluntary facial action generates emotion-specific autonomic nervous system activity. *Psychophysiology*, *27*, 363–84.

Liddell, E. G. T. & Sherrington, C. S. (1925). Recruitment and some other features of reflex inhibition. *Proceedings of the Royal Society of London (Biology)*, *97*, 488–518.

Liddell, E. G. T. (1960). *The discovery of the reflexes*. Oxford: Clarendon.

Lindsley, D. B. (1935). Electrical activity of human motor units during voluntary contraction. *American Journal of Physiology*, *114*, 90–9.

Lindsley, D. B. (1951). Emotion. In S. S. Stevens (Ed.), Handbook of Experimental Psychology (pp. 473–516). New York: Wiley.

Lippold, O. C. J. (1967). Electromyography. In P. H. Venables & I. Martin (Eds.), *Manual of psychophysiological methods* (pp. 245–298). New York: Wiley.

Loeb, G. E., & Gans, C. (1986). *Electromyography for experimentalists*. Chicago: University of Chicago Press.

Loeb, G. E. & Ghez, C. (2000). The motor unit and muscle action. In E. R. Kandel, J. H. Schwartz, & T.M. Jessel, (Eds.), *Principles of neural science* (4th ed.), pp. 674–93. New York: Elsevier.

Lowery, M. M., Stoykov, N. S. & Kuiken, T, A, (2003). Independence of myoelectic control signals examined using a surface EMG model. *IEEE Transactioin on Biomedical Engineering*, *50*(6), 789–93.

Lucas, K. (1909). The "all-or-none" contraction of amphibian skeletal muscle. *Journal of Physiology*, *38*, 113–33.

Lundberg, U., Dohns, I. E., Melin, B., Sandsjo, L., Palmerud, G., Kadefors, R., Ekstrom, M., & Parr, D. (1999). Psychophysiological stress responses, muscle tension, and neck and shoulder pain among supermarket cashiers. *Journal of Occupational Health Psychology*, *4*, 245–55.

Lundqvist, L. O. & Dimberg, U. (1995). Facial expressions are contagious. *Journal of Psychophysiology*, *9*, 203–211.

Luria, A. R. (1932). *The nature of human conflicts*. New York: Liveright.

Lutz, R. S. (2003). Covert muscle excitation is outflow from the central generation of motor imagery. *Behavioural Brain Research*, *140*(1–2), 149–63).

Lykken, D. (1998). *A tremor in the blood: Uses and abuses of the lie detector* (2nd Ed.). New York: Plenum.

Lynn, P. A., Bettles, N. D., Hughes, A. D. & Johnson, S. W. (1978). Influences of electrode geometry on bipolar recordings of the surface electromyogram. *Medical and Biological Engineering and Computing*, *16*, 651–60.

Malcolm, R., Von, J. M., & Horney, R. A. (1989). Correlations between facial electromyography and depression. *Psychiatric Forum*, *15*, 19–23.

Malmo, R. B. (1965). Physiological gradients and behavior. *Psychological Bulletin*, *64* 225–34.

Malmo, R. B. (1975). *On emotions, needs, and our archaic brain*. New York: Holt, Rinehart & Winston.

Malmo, R.B. & Malmo, H. P (2000). On electromyographic (EMG) gradients and movement-related brain activity: significance for motor control, cognitive functions, and certain psychopathologies. *International Journal of Psychophysiology*, *38*, 145–209.

Mandryk, R. L. & Inkpen, K. M. (2004). Physiological indicators for the evaluation of co-located collaborative play. *Proceedings of the 2004 ACM conference on Computer supported cooperative work*, Chicago, Il. (pp. 102–11).

Markovsky, B., & Berger, S. M. (1983). Crowd noise and mimicry. *Personality and Social Psychology Bulletin*, *9*, 90–6.

Martin, I. (1956). Levels of muscle activity in psychiatric patients. *Acta Psychologica*, *12*, 326–41.

Marshall-Goodell, B., Tassinary, L. G., & Cacioppo, J. T. (1990). Principles of bioelectrical measurement. In J. T. Cacioppo & L. G. Tassinary (Eds.), *Principles of psychophysiology* (pp. 113–48). New York: Cambridge University Press.

Mathews, B. H. C. (1934). A special purpose amplifier. *Journal of Physiology (London)*, *81*, 28.

Max, L. W. (1932). Myoesthesis and "imageless thought". *Science*, *76*, 235–36.

Max, L. W. (1937). An experimental study of the motor theory of consciousness: IV. Action-current responses in the deaf during awakening, kinaesthetic imagery and abstract thinking. *Journal of Comparative Psychology*, *24*, 301–44.

McCanne, T. R., & Anderson, J. A. (1987). Emotional responding following experimental manipulation of facial electromyographic activity. *Journal of Personality and Social Psychology*, *52*, 759–68.

McClelland, J. L. (1979). On the time relations of mental processes: An examination of systems in cascade. *Psychological Review*, *86*, 287–330.

McGarry, T. & Franks, I. (1997). A horse race between independent processes: Evidence for a phantom point of no return in the preparation of a speeded motor response. *Journal of Experimental Psychology: Human Perception and Performance*, *23*, 1533–42.

McGuigan, F. J. (1966). *Thinking: Studies of Covert Language Processes*. New York: Appleton-Century-Crofts.

McGuigan, F. J. (1970). Covert oral behavior during the silent performance of language. *Psychological Bulletin*, *74*, 309–26.

McGuigan, F. J. (1978). *Cognitive psychophysiology: Principles of covert behavior* Englewood Cliffs, NJ: Prenice–Hall.

McGuigan, F. J. (1979). *Psychophysiological measurement of covert behavior: A guide for the laboratory*. Hillsdale NJ: Erlbaum.

McGuigan, F. J. (1994). *Biological psychology: A cybernetic science*. Engelwood Cliffs, NJ: Prentice Hall.

McGuigan, F. J., & Bailey S. C. (1969). Logitudinal study of covert oral behavior during silent reading. *Perceptual and motor skills*, *28*, 170.

McGuigan, F. J., Dollins, A., Pierce, W., Lusebrink, V., & Corus, C. (1982). Fourier analysis of covert speech behavior. *Pavlovian Journal of Biological Science, 17*, 49–52.

McHugo, G., & Lanzetta, J. T. (1983). Methodological decisions in social psychophysiology. In J. T. Cacioppo & R. E. Petty (Eds.), *Social psychophysiology: A sourcebook* (pp. 630–65). New York: Guilford Press.

McHugo, G., Lanzetta, J. T. & Bush, L. (1991). The effect of attitudes on emotional reactions to expressive displays of political leaders. *Journal of Nonverbal Behavior, 15*, 19–41.

Merletti, R. (1994). Surface electromyography: Possibilities and limitations. *Journal of Rehabilitative Science, 7*, 24–34.

Merton, P. A. (1987). Reflexes. In R. L. Gregory (Ed.), *The Oxford companion to the mind*. New York: Oxford University Press.

Meyer, B. U., Werhahn, K., Rothwell, J. C., Roericht, S., & Fauth, C. (1994). Functional organization of corticonuclear pathways to motoneurones of lower facial muscles in man. *Experimental Brain Research, 101*, 465–72.

Meyer, D. R. (1953). On the interaction of simultaneous responses. *Psychological Bulletin, 20*, 204–20.

Meyer, D. R., Bahrick, H. P., & Fitts, P. M. (1953). Incentive, anxiety, and the human blink rate. *Journal of Expenmental Psychology, 45*, 183–287.

Mitz, V. (1976). The superfcal musculo-apneurotic system (SMAS) in the parotid and cheek area. *Plastic and Reconstructive Surgery, 58*, 80–88.

Morecraft, R. J. Stilwell-Morecraft, K. S., & Rossing, W. R. (2004). The motor cortex and facial expression: New insights from neuroscience. *The Neurologist, 10*(5), 235–49.

Morris, H. & Anson, B. J. (1966). *Human anatomy: A complete systematic treatise* (12th ed.). New York: McGraw-Hill.

Mulder, T. & Hulstijn, W. (1984). The effect of fatigue and repetition of the task on the surface electromyographic signal. *Psychophysiology, 21*, 528–34.

Needham, D. M. (1971). *Machina carnis: The biochemistry of muscular contraction in its historical development*. London: Cambridge University Press.

Neumann, D. L., Lipp, O. V., & Pretorius, N. R. (2004). The effects of lead stimulus and reflex stimulus modality on modulation of the blink reflex at very short, short, and long lead intervals. *Perception and Psychophysics, 66*, 141–51.

Neumann, R., & Strack, F. (2000). Experiential and nonexperiential routes of motor influence on affect and evaluation. In H. Bless & J. P. Forgas (Eds.), *The message within: The role of subjective experience in social cognition and behavior* (pp. 52–68). Philadelphia, PA: Psychology Press.

Nosofsky, R. M. & Zaki, S. R. (1998). Dissociations between categorization and recognition in amnesic and normal individuals: An exemplar-based interpretation. *Psychological Science, 9*, 247–55.

Oddsson, L. I. E., Giphart, J. E., Buijs, R. J. C., Roy, S. H., Taylor, H. P., & De Luca, C. J. (1997). Development of new protocols and analysis procedures for the assessment of LBP by surface EMG techniques. *Journal of Rehabilitation Research and Development, 34*, 415–26.

O'Dwyer, N. J., Quinn, P. T., Guitar, B. E., Andrews, G., & Neilson, P. D. (1981). Procedures for verification of electrode placement in EMG studies of orofacial and mandibular muscles. *Journal of Speech and Hearing Research, 241*, 273–88.

Olivers, C. N. L. & Nieuwenhuis, S (2005). The beneficial effect of concurrent task-irrelevant mental activity on temporal attention. *Psychological Science, 16*(4), 265–69.

Orne, M. T. (1962). On the social psychology of the psychological experiment: With particular reference to demand characteristics and their implications. *American Psychologist, 17*, 776–83.

Paloheimo, M. (1990). Quantitative surface electromyography (qEMG): Applications in anaesthesiology and critical care [Supplementum 93]. *Acta Anaesthesiologica Scandinavica, 34*, 1–83.

Partridge, L.D. (1966). Signal handling characteristics of load-moving muscle in man. *American Journal of Physiology, 210*, 1178–91.

Petrides, M., Cadoret, G., & Mackey, S. (2005). Orofacial somatomotor responses in the macaque mokey homologue of Broca's area. *Nature, 435*, 1235–38.

Perry, T. J. and Goldwater, B. C. (1987). A passive behavioral measure of sleep onset in high-alpha and low alpha subjects. *Psychophysiology, 24*, 657–65.

Picard, R. W. (1997). *Affective Computing*. Cambridge: MIT Press.

Pikoff, H. (1984). Is the muscular model of headache still viable? *Headache, 24*, 186–98.

Platt, J. R. (1964). Strong inference. *Science, 146*, 347–53.

Pratt, F. H. (1917). The all-or-none principle in graded response of skeletal muscle. *American Journal of Physiology, 44*, 517–42.

Pratt, F. H., & Eisenberger, J. P. (1919). The quantal phenomena in muscle: Methods with further evidence of the all-or-none principle in graded response for the skeletal fibre. *American Journal of Physiology, 49*, 1–54.

Pritchard, D. (1995). EMG levels in children who suffer from severe headache. *Headache, 35*, 554–56.

Pressman, M. R. & Orr, W. C. (Eds.) (1997). *Understanding sleep: The evaluation and treatment of sleep disorders*. Washington, DC: American Psychological Association.

Rajecki, D. W. (1983). Animal aggression: Implications for human aggression. In R. G. Geen & E. J. Donnerstein (Eds.), *Aggression: Theoretical and empirical reviews: Vol. 1* (pp. 189–211). New York: Academic Press.

Rani, P., Sarkar, N., Smith, C. A., & Kirby, L. D. (2004). Anxiety detecting robotic system – Towards implicit human-robot collaboration. *Robotica, 22*, 85–95.

Rankin, R. E. & Campbell, D. (1955). Galvanic skin response to negro and white experimenters. *Journal of Abnormal and Social Psychology, 51*, 30–3.

Ravaja, N., Kallinen, K., Saari, T., & Keltikangas-Jarvinen, L. (2004). Suboptimal exposure to facial expressions when viewing video messages from a small screen: Effects on emotion, attention, and memory. *Journal of Experimental Psychology: Applied, 10*, 120–131.

Rimehaug, T. & Sveback, S. (1987). Psychogenic muscle tension: The significance of motivation and negative affect in perceptual-cognitive task performance. *International Journal of Psychophysiology, 5*, 97–106.

Rinn, W. E. (1991). Neuropsychology of facial expression. In R. Feldman & B. Rimé (Eds.). *Fundamentals of Nonverbal Behavior*. New York: Cambridge University Press.

Rissen, D., Melin, B., Sandsjo, L., Dohns, I., & Lundberg, U. (2000). Surface EMG and psychophysiological stress reactions in women during repetitive work. *European Journal of Applied Physiology, 83*, 215–22.

Ritz, T., Dahme, B., & Claussen, C. (1999). Gradients of facial EMG and cardiac activity during emotional stimulation. *Journal of Psychophysiology, 13*(1), 3–17.

Ritz, T., Dahme, B. & Roth, W. T. (2004). Behavioral interventions in asthma: Biofeedback techniques. *Journal of Psychosomatic Research, 56*, 711–20.

Rosenthal, R. & Rosnow, R. (Eds.) (1969). *Artifact in behavioral research*. New York: Academic Press.

Rosenthal, R. (1966). *Experimenter effects in behavior research*. New York: Appleton-Century-Crofts.

Rossi, A. M. (1959). An evaluation of the manifest anxiety scale by the use of electromyography. *Journal of Experimental Psychology*, *58*, 64–9.

Roy, S. H., De Luca, C., Emley, M., Oddsson, L. I. E., Buijis, R. J. C., Levins, J., Newcombe, D. S., & Jabre, J. F. (1997). Classification of back muscle impairment based on the surface electromyographic signal. *Journal of Rehabilitation Research and Development*, *34*, 405–14.

Russell, J. A., Bachorowski, J. & Fernández-Dols, J. M. (2003). Facial and Vocal Expressions of Emotion. *Annual Review of Psychology*, *54*, 329–349.

Russell, J. A. & Fernández-Dols, J. M. (Eds.) (1997). *The psychology of facial expression*. New York: Cambridge University Press.

Schmidt-Nielsen, K. (1997). *Animal physiology: Adaptation and environment* (5th Ed.). New York: Cambridge University Press.

Schwartz, G. E. (1975). Biofeedback, self-regulation, and the patterning of physiological processes. *Amencan Scientist*, *63*, 314–24.

Schwartz, G. E., Fair, P. L., Salt, P., Mandel, M. R., & Klerman, G. L. (1976). Facial muscle patterning to affective imagery in depressed and nondepressed subjects. *Science*, *192*, 489–91.

Seiler, R. (1973). On the function of facial muscles in different behavioral situations: A study based on the muscle morphology and electromyography. *American Journal of Physical Anthropology*, *38*, 567–72.

Shaw, W. A. (1940). The relation of muscular action potentials to imaginal weight lifting. *Archives of Psychology*, No. 247.

Sherrington, C. S. (1923). *The integrative actions of the nervous system*. New Haven, CT: Yale University Press. (Original work published 1906.)

Shimizu, A, & Inoue, T. (1986). Dreamed speech and speech muscle activity. *Psychophysiology*, *23*, 210–15.

Skinner, B. F. (1931). The concept of the reflex in the description of behavior. *The Journal of General Psychology: Expenmental, Theoretical, Clinical, and Historical Psychology*, *5*, 427–57.

Sloan, D. M., Bradley, M. M., Dimoulas, E., & Lang, P. J. (2002). Looking at facial expressions: Dysphoria and facial EMG. *Biological Psychology*, *60*, 79–90.

Smith, R. R., Kier, W. M. (1989). Trunks, tongues, and tentacles: Moving with skeletons of muscle. *American Scientist*, *77*, 28–35.

Smith, J. D. & Minda, J. P. (2001). Journey to the center of the category: The dissociation in amnesia between categorization and recognition. *Journal of Experimental Psychology: Human Learning, Memory & Cognition*, *27*(4), 984–1002.

Sonnby-Borgström, M. & Jönsson, P. (2003). Models-of-self and models-of-others as related to facial muscle reactions at different levels of cognitive control. *Scandanavian Journal of Psychology*, *44*, 141–51.

Spencer, H. (1870). *Principles of Psychology* (2nd ed.). London: Williams & Norgate.

Sperry, R. (1952). Neurology and the mind-brain problem. *American Scientist*, *40*, 291–312.

Stark, R., Walter, B., Schienle, A. & Vaitl, D. (2005). Psychophysiological correlates of disgust and disgust sensitivity. *Journal of Psychophysiology*, *19*(1), 50–60.

Stead, L., Goulev, P., Evans, C., & Mamdani, E. (2004). The emotional wardrobe. *Personal and Ubiquitous Computing*, *8*, 282–90.

Sternbach, R. A. (1966). *Principles of psychophysiology*. New York: Academic.

Sternberg, S. (1969). The discovery of processing stages: Extensions of Donder's method. *Acta Psychologica*, *30*, 276–315.

Stoyva, J., & Budzynski, T. (1974). Cultivated low arousal: An anti-stress response? In L. V. DiCara (Ed.). *Recent advances in limbic and autonomic nervous system research* (pp. 370–94). New York: Plenum Press.

Strack, F., Martin, L. L., & Stepper, J. (1988). Inhibitory and facilitatory conditions of the human smile: A nonobtrusive test of the facial feedback hypothesis. *Journal of Personality and Social Psychology*, *54*, 768–77.

Stringham, J. M., Fuld, K., & Wenzel, A. J. (2003). Action spectrum for photophobia. *Journal of the Optical Society of America*, *20*(10), 1852–58.

Sumitsuji, N., Nan'no, H., Kuwata, Y., and Ohta, Y. (1980). The effects of the noise due to the jet airplane to the human facial expression (EMG study), EEG changes and their manual responses at the various sleeping stages of the subjects. *Electromyography and Clinical Neurophysiology*, *20*, 49–72.

Svebak, S., Dalen, K., & Storfjell, O. (1981). The psychological significance of task-induced tonic changes in somatic and autonomic activity. *Psychophysiology*, *18*, 403–09.

Tassinary, L. G. (1985). *Odor hedonics: Psychophysical, respiratory and facial measures*. Unpublished doctoral dissertation, Dartmouth College.

Tassinary, L. G. (2005). Improving the sensitivity and specificity of facial electromyography. *Psychophysiology*, *42*, S121.

Tassinary, L. G. & Cacioppo. J. T. (1992). Unobservable facial actions and emotion. *Psychological Science*, *3*, 28–33.

Tassinary, L. G. & Cacioppo, J. T. (2000). The skeletomotor system: Surface electromyography. In J. T. Cacioppo, L. G. Tassinary and G. Bernston (Eds.), *The Handbook of Psychophysiology*. New York: Cambridge University Press.

Tassinary, L. G. & Geen, T. R. (1990). James Parsons (1705–1770): A forgotten pioneer in the psychophysiology of emotion. *Psychophysiology*, *27*, S69.

Tassinary, L. G., Cacioppo, J. T., & Geen, T. R. (1989). A psychometric study of surface electrode placements for facial electromyographic recording: I. The brow and cheek muscle regions. *Psychophysiology*, *26*, 1–16.

Tassinary, L. G., Orr, S. P., Wolford, G., Napps, S. E., & Lanzetta, J. T. (1984). The role of awareness in affective information processing: An exploration of the Zajonc hypothesis. *Bulletin of the Psychonomic Society*, *22*, 489–92.

Tassinary, L. G., Vanman, E., Geen, T. R. & Cacioppo, J. T. (1987). Optimizing surface electrode placements for facial EMG recordings: Guidelines for recording from the perioral muscle region. *Psychophysiology*, *24*, 615–16.

Teuber, H. L. (1955). Physiological psychology. *Annual Review of Psychology*, *6*, 267–94.

Tobin, R. M., Graziano, W. G., Vanman, E. J. & Tassinary, L. G. (2000). Personality, emotional experience, and efforts to control emotions. *Journal of Personality and Social Psychology*, *79*(4), 656–69.

Thorson, A. M. (1925). The relation of tongue movements to internal speech. *Journal of Experimental Psychology*, *8*, 1.

Tomovic, R. & Bellman, R. (1970). A systems approach to muscle control. *Mathematical Biosciences*, *8*, 265–77.

Tourangeau, R., & Ellsworth, P. C. (1979). The role of facial response in the experience of emotion. *Journal of Personality and Social Psychology*, *37*, 1519–31.

Trepman, E., Gellman, R. E., Solomon, R., Murthy, K. R., Micheli, L. J. & De Luca, C. (1994). Electromyographic analysis of standing posture and demi-plié in ballet and modern dancers. *Medicine and Science in Sports and Exercise, 26*, 771–82.

Triplett, N. (1898). The dynamogenic factors in pacemaking and competition. *Amencan Journal of Psychology, 9*, 507–33.

Tuomitso, M. T., Johnston, D. W. & Schmidt, T. F. H. (1996). The ambulatory measurement of posture, thigh acceleration, and muscle tension and their relationship to heart rate. *Psychophysiology, 33*, 409–15.

Tyron, W. W. (1991). *Activity measurement in psychology and medicine*. New York: Plenum Press.

van Boxtel, A. (2001). Optimal signal bandwidth for the recording of surface EMG activity of facial, jaw, oral, and neck muscles. *Psychophysiology, 38*, 22–34.

van Boxtel, A., Goudswaard, P., & Janssen, K. (1983). Absolute and proportional resting EMG levels in muscle contrachon and migraine headache pahents. *Headache, 23*, 215–22.

van Boxtel, A., Goudswaard, P., & Janssen, K. (1983). Changes in EMG power spectra of facial and jaw-elevator muscles during fatigue. *Journal of Applied Physiology, 54*, 51–8.

van Boxtel, A., Goudswaard, P., & Shomaker, L. R. B. (1984). Amplitude and bandwidth of the frontalis surface EMG: Effects of electrode parameters. *Psychophysiology, 21*, 699–707.

van Boxtel, A. & Jessurun, M. (1993). Amplitude and bilateral coherency of facial and jaw-elevator EMG activity as an index of effort during a two-choice serial reaction task. *Psychophysiology, 30*, 589–604.

van Boxtel, A., Damen, E. J. P., and Brunia, C. H. M. (1996). Anticipatory EMG responses of the pericranial muscles in relation to heart rate during a warned simple reaction time task. *Psychophysiology, 33*, 576–83.

Vanman, E. J., Boehmelt, A. H., Dawson, M. E., & Schell, A. M. (1996). The varying time course of attentional and affective modulation of the startle eyeblink response. *Psychophysiology, 33*, 691–97.

Vanman, E. J., Paul, B. Y., Ito, T. A., & Miller, N. (1997). The modern face of prejudice and structural features that moderate the effect of cooperation on affect. *Journal of Personality and Social Psychology, 73*, 941–59.

Vanman, E. J., Saltz, J. L., Nathan, L. R., & Warren, J. A. (2004). Racial discrimination by low-prejudiced Whites: Facial movements as implicit measures of attitudes related to behavior. *Psychological Science, 15*, 711–14.

Vaughan, K. B., & Lanzetta, 1. T. (1981). The effects of modification of expressive displays on vicarious emotional arousal. *Journal of Experimental Social Psychology, 17*, 16–30.

Vaughan, K. B., & Lanzetta, J. T. (1980). Vicarious instigation and conditioning of facial expressive and autonomic responses to a model's expressive display of pain. *Journal of Personality and Social Psychology, 13*, 909–23.

Veiersted, K. B. (1994). Sustained muscle tension as a risk factor for trapezius myalgia. *International Journal of Industrial Ergonomics, 14*, 333–39.

Vitti, M., Basmajian, J. V., Ouelette, P. L., Mitchell, D. L., Eastman, W. P., & Seaborn, R.D. (1975). Electromyographic investigations of the tongue and circumoral muscular sling with fine-wire electrodes. *Journal of Dental Research, 54*, 844–49.

Vrana, S. R. & Rollock, D. (1998). Physiological response to a minimal social encounter: Effects of gender, ethnicity, and social context. *Psychophysiology, 35*, 462–69.

Waersted, M. & Westgaard, R. H. (1996). Attention-related muscle activity in different body regions during VDU work with minimal physical activity. *Ergonomics, 39*, 661–76.

Washburn, M. F. (1916). *Movement and imagery: Outlines of a motor theory of the complexer mental processes*. Boston: Houghton Mifflin.

Wartenberg, R. (1946). *The examination of reflexes: A simplification*. Chicago: Year Book Publishers.

Waters, K. (1992). A physical model of facial tissue and muscle articulation derived from computer tomography data. *Visualization in Biomedical Computing, 1808*, 574–83.

Weaver, C. V. (1977). Descriptive anatomical and quantitative variation in human facial musculature and the analysis of bilateral asymmetry. *Dissertation Abstracts International* (University Microfilms, No. 77-24, 305).

Wells, G. L., & Petty, R. E. (1980). The effects of overt head-movements on persuasion: Compatibility and incompatibility of responses. *Basic and Applied Social Psychology, 1*, 219–30.

Wexler, B. E., Warrenburg, S., Schwartz, G. E., & Jamner, L. D. (1992). EEG and EMG responses to emotion-evoking stimuli processed without conscious awareness. *Neuropsychologia, 30*, 1065–79.

Wolf, K., Mass, R., Kiefer, F., Eckert, K., Weinhold, N., Wiedemann, K., & Naber, D. (2004). The influence of olanzapine on facial expressions of emotions in schizophrenia – an improved facial EMG study. *German Journal of Psychiatry, 7*, 14–9.

Wheatley, J. R., Tangel, D. J., Mezzanotte, W. S., and White, D. P. (1993). Influence of sleep on the alae nasi EMG and nasal resistance in normal man. *Journal of Applied Physiology, 75*, 626–32.

Woodworth, R. S., & Schlosberg, H. (1954). *Experimental psychology* (Rev. Ed.) New York: Holt.

Wrase, J., Klein, S., Gruesser, S. M., Hermann, D., Flor, H., Mann, K., Braus, D. F., & Heinz, A. (2003). Gender differences in the processing of standardized emotional visual stimuli in humans: A functional magnetic resonance imaging study. *Neuroscience Letters, 348*(1), 41–5.

Wu, C. H. (1984). Electric fish and the discovery of animal electricity. *American Scientist, 72*, 598–607.

Zajonc, R. B. (1965). Social facilitation. *Science, 149*, 269–74.

Zipp, P. (1982). Recommendations for the standardization of lead positions in surface electromyography. *European Journal of Applied Physiology, 50*, 41–54.

Cellular and Humoral Systems

SECTION EDITOR: ESTHAR M. STERNBERG

13 The Neuroendocrinology of Stress

GREGORY A. KALTSAS AND GEORGE P. CHROUSOS

ABSTRACT

The *stress system* is among the most important and highly preserved systems in the organism. It is located and functions in both the central nervous system (CNS) and the periphery. Several external or internal stressful stimuli or *stressors* in association with higher cortical functions integrate and act at the level of the hypothalamus and the brain stem to activate the stress system. The latter maintains a basal circadian tone and responds to stressors in an appropriate attempt to maintain *homeostasis*. The CNS components of the stress system are the corticotrophin-releasing hormone (CRH)/arginine-vasopressin (AVP) and locus ceruleus-noradrenaline (LC-NA)/autonomic, mainly sympathetic, neurons of the hypothalamus and brain stem, respectively. The main effectors of the stress system include CRH, AVP, propiomelanocortin-derived peptides, glucocorticoids, and the catecholamines norepinephrine and epinephrine. Adequate responsiveness of the stress system to stressors is responsible for attaining homeostasis and achieving a sense of well-being. The *adaptive* or *stress response* depends not only on the intensity of the stressor but also on the inherent ability of the stress system to achieve and maintain an appropriate level and duration of activity. The stress response is influenced by both genetic and developmental factors. Nosologic disorders of homeostasis develop when there is an inappropriate level or duration response of the stress system to stressors. Inadequate or excessive and/or too brief or prolonged stress responses can be deleterious to the organism. The state of achieving survival at the expense of the psychologic and somatic well-being of an individual is called *chronic dyshomeostasis* or *allostasis*, or, even more to the point, *cacostasis*. Cacostasis accounts for major endocrine, metabolic, autoimmune, and psychiatric disorders.

INTRODUCTION

The neuroendocrine system plays a major role in the adaptation of the organism to stress and, hence, its survival as an individual and species (Chrousos and Gold, 1992; Habib et al., 2000). Under favorable conditions, functions that enhance growth, development, and reproduction, and thus survival of the self and species, are facilitated. Under threatening conditions, adaptations occur that help the individual survive the stressful environment, while searching for more favorable circumstances (Chrousos and Gold, 1992). Any potent enough *stressor*, that is, any real or perceived major threat to the stability of "*homeostasis*," or balances, places the organism in a *stress (threatened) state* and activates a "nonspecific, stereotypic," *adaptive response*, during which the brain interprets the stressor as threatening, thus responding in a progressively generalized and hence nonspecific way (Habib et al., 2000; Chrousos, 1998). Activation of the *stress system* leads to behavioral and peripheral changes that optimize the ability of the organism to adjust homeostasis and increases its chances of survival (Chrousos and Gold, 1992). The main central nervous system (CNS) components of this system are the corticotrophin-releasing hormone (CRH)/arginine-vasopressin (AVP) and locus ceruleus-noradrenaline (LC-NA)/autonomic (mainly sympathetic) neurons of the hypothalamus and brain stem (Chrousos, 1995). These respectively regulate the peripheral activities of the hypothalamic-pituitary-adrenal (HPA) axis and the systemic/adrenomedullary sympathetic nervous systems (SNS) (Chrousos and Gold, 1992). Activation of the HPA axis and LC-NA/autonomic system result in systemic elevations of glucocorticoids and catecholamines (Cas), which together with other products of the stress system, influence a variety of adaptive responses both at their baseline levels and/or at elevated levels which are encountered during the stress response (Elenkov et al., 1999).

During stress, cardiac output, and respiration are enhanced and blood flow is redirected to provide the highest perfusion to the brain and musculoskeletal system. The brain focuses on the perceived threat and stimulates behaviors that propel the organism to act accordingly (Habib et al., 2000). Endocrine programs of growth and reproduction are suppressed in order to save energy; catabolism is enhanced and fuel is used to supply the brain, heart, and muscles accompanied by increases in glucose levels, heart rate, and blood pressure (Chrousos and Gold, 1992). In addition, stress induces a state of immunomodulation particularly inhibiting innate and cellular immunity and favoring humoral immunity. In certain tissues, activation of the sympathetic system and the peripheral CRH-mast-cell-histamine axis, induces early proinflammatory activity, which has been referred to as *neurogenic inflammation* (Elenkov and Chrousos, 2002). This new understanding helps explain some well-known, but often contradictory, effects of stress on a variety of infectious, autoimmune/inflammatory, allergic, metabolic, adaptive, and neoplastic diseases. In this overview, the current understanding of the neuroendocrine components of the stress system and its interactions with other systems is presented and the physiologic and pathophysiologic implications of these interactions are briefly discussed.

ORGANIZATION OF THE STRESS SYSTEM

The brain circuits that initiate and maintain the stress response are illustrated in Figure 13.1. The HPA axis and the SNS are the afferent limbs of the stress system, whose main function is to maintain basal and stress-related homeostasis (Chrousos and Gold, 1992; Chrousos, 1995). The central components of this system are located in the hypothalamus and the brain stem. They include the parvocellular neurons of the paraventricular nuclei (PVN) of the hypothalamus that release CRH and AVP, the CRH neurons of the paragigantocellular and parabrachial nuclei of the brain stem, and the A1, A2, A3, and A6 (locus ceruleus, LC) mostly noradrenergic (NE) cell groups of the pons and medulla (the LC-NE system) (Chrousos and Gold, 1992). Paraventricular CRH neurons project to and innervate proopiomelanocortin (POMC)-containing neurons of the central stress system in the arcuate nucleus of the hypothalamus, as well as neurons of pain control areas of the hind brain and spinal cord (Figures 13.1 and 13.2). Activation of the stress system leads to CRH-induced secretion of POMC-derived and other opioid peptides, which enhance analgesia (Chrousos, 1995). These peptides also simultaneously inhibit the activity of the stress system by suppressing CRH and NE secretion (Chrousos and Gold, 1992).

CRH and AVP synergistically stimulate the secretion of corticotrophin (ACTH) hormone by the corticotroph cells of the anterior pituitary. This in turn stimulates adrenal steroidogenesis (mainly cortisol and androgens). CRH and AVP may act synergistically on other target tissues as well, both in the CNS and the periphery (Chrousos and Gold, 1992). Every hour, the parvocellular neurons secrete two or three mostly synchronous pulses of CRH and AVP into the hypophysial portal system. In early morning, the amplitudes of these pulses are highest, increasing the amplitude and apparent frequency of ACTH and cortisol secretory episodes (Chrousos and Gold, 1992; Chrousos, 1995). During acute stress, the amplitude of CRH and AVP pulses also increases, resulting in increases in the

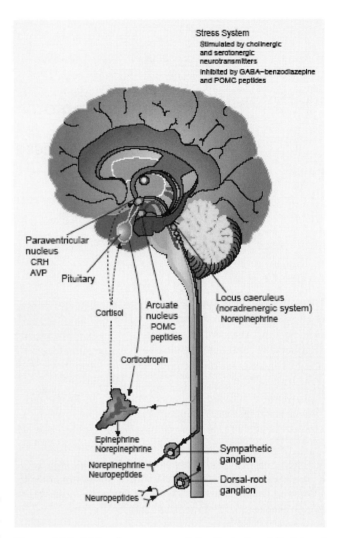

Figure 13.1. Major Components of the Central and Peripheral Stress System. The paraventricular nucleus and the locus ceruleus/noradrenergic system are shown along with their peripheral limbs, the pituitary-adrenal axis, and the adrenomedullary and systemic sympathetic systems. The hypothalamic corticotrophin-releasing hormone (CRH) and central noradrenergic neurons mutually innervate and activate each other, while they exert presynaptic autoinhibition through collateral fibers. Arginine vasopressin (AVP) from the paraventricular nucleus synergizes with CRH on stimulating corticotrophin (ACTH) secretion. The cholinergic and serotonergic neurotransmitter systems stimulate both components of the central stress system, while the gamma aminobutyric acid/benzodiazepine (GABA/BZD) and arcuate nucleus proopiomelanocortin (POMC) peptide systems inhibit it. The latter is directly activated by the stress system and is important in the enhancement of analgesia that takes place during stress (From Chrousos G. 1999. 1351–1362).

amplitude and apparent frequency of ACTH and cortisol pulses. In this case, the stress system recruits additional secretagogues of CRH, AVP, or ACTH, such as magnocellular AVP, and angiotensin II (Elenkov et al., 1999). Circulating ACTH of pituitary origin is the key regulator of glucocorticoid secretion from cells of the adrenal gland's *zona fasciculata*. Other hormones, including Cas, neuropeptide Y (NPY), and CRH are produced by the adrenal medulla and additional autonomic neural input to

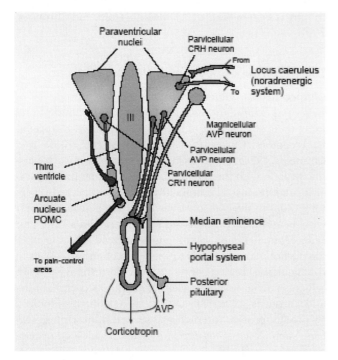

Figure 13.2. A Close-up View of the Paraventricular Nuclei of the Hypothalamus. Parvocellular CRH-and arginine vasopressin (AVP)-secreting neurons project to and secrete into the hypophysial portal system. Parvocellular CRH neurons also project to the brainstem to innervate neurons of the locus ceruleus/noradrenergic system. Magnocellular AVP-secreting neurons terminate at the posterior pituitary and secrete into the systemic circulation; they also have collateral terminals in the portal system, however. CRH is permissive for and stimulates pituitary corticotrophin (ACTH) secretion, while AVP has a major synergistic role with CRH in the secretion of ACTH. The arcuate proopiomelanocortin (POMC) nucleus is shown, along with the mutual innervations between CRH and POMC-peptide-secreting neurons (From Chrousos G., 1351–1362).

the adrenal cortex also influences glucocorticoid secretion (Elenkov et al., 1999).

The LC-NE system controls stress-induced stimulation of the arousal system as well as of the systemic sympathetic and sympathoadrenal nervous systems. The SNS, which originates in nuclei within the brain stem, gives rise to preganglionic efferent fibers that leave the CNS through the thoracic and lumbar spinal nerves ("thoracolumbar system"). Although this review will not address the parasympathetic nervous system (PSNS), it should be noted that it also participates in the stress response. Thus, Barrington's nucleus, the nucleus tractus solitarius, and the dorsal motor vagal nucleus, all components of the PSNS, control the differential activation of vagal and sacral parasympathetic efferent nerves that mediate gut responses to stress (Habib, Gold, and Chrousos, 2001). Furthermore the PSNS may facilitate or inhibit the effects of the SNS by respectively decreasing or increasing its activity.

The LC-NA system activates and is activated by the amygdala, which, acting in conjunction with the hippocampus and the anterior cingulate and prefrontal cortices, mediate focused attention of a perceived threat,

define the affective state of the individual and regulate fear-related behaviors (Brown et al., 1982). Most of the sympathetic preganglionic fibers terminate in ganglia located in the paravertebral chains that lie on either side of the spinal column; the remaining preganglionic sympathetic neurons terminate in prevertebral ganglia, which lie in front of the vertebrae (Chrousos and Gold, 1992). From these ganglia, postganglionic sympathetic fibers run to the tissues innervated by the SNS. Most postganglionic sympathetic fibers release NE. However, subpopulations of neurons also secrete other active substances including CRH, neuropeptide Y (NPY), somatostatin, and inflammatory mediators (Chrousos and Gold, 1992). In contrast to the SNS, the main neurotransmitter that mediates the action of the PSNS is acetylcholine (Habib, Gold, and Chrousos, 2001). The adrenal medulla contains chromaffin cells, embryologically and anatomically homologous to the sympathetic ganglia but unlike the postganglionic sympathetic nerve terminals, releases mainly epinephrine, and to a lesser extent NE in an approximate ratio of 4:1. Typical preganglionic sympathetic nerve terminals, whose main neurotransmitter is acetylcholine, innervate the chromaffin cells of the adrenal medulla (Chrousos, 1998).

NEUROENDOCRINE ALTERATIONS DURING THE STRESS RESPONSE

Role of stress system in maintaining basal and stress-related homeostasis

The stress system has a baseline, circadian activity, but also responds on demand to physical and emotional stressors through CRH, glucocorticoids, and Cas (Chrousos and Gold, 1992; Chrousos, 1998). These substances are major regulators of behavior, metabolism, cardiovascular function and thermogenesis, and adjust these functions according to the needs of the organism. The stress system integrates and responds to a great diversity of distinct circadian, neurosensory, blood-borne, and limbic signals. Functionally, the CRH/AVP and LC-NE systems seem to participate in a positive, reverberating feedback loop, so that activation of one system tends to activate the others as well (Chrousos and Gold, 1992; Chrousos, 1998). This includes projections of CRH- and AVP-secreting neurons from the lateral PVN to the central sympathetic regions in the brainstem, and conversely, projections of catecholaminergic fibers from the LC-NE system, via the ascending noradrenergic bundle, to the PVN in the hypothalamus. Thus, CRH and AVP stimulate norepinephrine secretion through their specific receptors, while norepinephrine stimulates CRH and AVP secretion through primarily α_1-noradrenergic receptors (Chrousos, 1995). Autoregulatory, ultrashort negative feedback loops are also present in these neurons, with CRH and norepinephrine collateral fibers acting in an inhibitory fashion on presynaptic CRH and α_2-noradrenergic receptors, respectively (Chrousos and Gold, 1992).

Table 13.1. Behavioral and physical adaptation during acute stress

Behavioral adaptation: adaptive redirection of behavior	Physical adaptation: adaptive redirection of energy
Increased arousal and alertness	Oxygen and nutrients directed to the CNS and stressed body sites
Increased cognition, vigilance and focused attention	Altered cardiovascular tone, increased blood pressure and heart rate
Euphoria or dysphoria	Increased respiratory rate
Heightened analgesia	Increased gluconeogenesis and lipolysis
Increased temperature	Detoxification from toxic products
Suppression of appetite and feeding behavior	Inhibition of growth and reproduction
Containment of the stress response	Containment of the inflammatory/immune response

The CRH, AVP, and noradrenergic neurons receive stimulatory input from the serotonergic, cholinergic, and histaminergic systems and inhibitory input from the gamma-aminobutyric acid (GABA)/benzodiazepine and opioid peptide neuronal systems of the brain (Chrousos and Gold, 1992; Chrousos, 1998). Centrally secreted substance P (SP) has inhibitory actions on hypothalamic CRH but not AVP neurons and stimulatory effects on the central noradrenergic system. Activation of the stress system leads to adaptive behavioral and physical changes (McEwen, 2002). Centrally, the behavioral changes include enhanced arousal and accelerated motor reflexes, improved attention span and cognitive function, reduced feeding, and sexual behavior, and increased ability to withstand pain (Table 13.1) (Chrousos and Gold, 1992). Peripherally, activation of the stress system results in increased sympathetic output, i.e., increased release of NE from sympathetic nerve terminals and epinephrine/NE from the adrenal medulla, as well as in increased secretion of glucocorticoids by the adrenal cortex (Chrousos, 1995). These changes result in physical adaptation that include changes in cardiovascular function, intermediary metabolism, and modulation of the immune and inflammatory reaction (Habib, Gold, and Chrousos, 2001). Thus, mobilization of stored energy with inhibition of subsequent energy storage and gluconeogenesis, sharpened focused attention on the perceived threat, increased cerebral perfusion rates, and cerebral glucose use, enhanced cardiovascular output and respiration, enhanced delivery of energy substrates to the skeletal muscles, inhibition of reproductive function and behavior, modulation of immune function, and decreased feeding and appetite, are all consequences of the activation of the stress system (Table 13.1) (Habib, Gold, and Chrousos, 2001).

The endocrine component of the stress system

Glucocorticoids. Glucocorticoids, the final products of HPA axis stimulation, are pleiotropic hormones and exert their effects via ubiquitously distributed intracellular receptors (Chrousos, 1995; Bamberger, Schulte, and Chrousos, 1996). The glucocorticoid receptor is a cytoplasmic protein with three major functional domains and several subdomains. The nonactivated glucocorticoid receptor resides in the cytosol in the form of a hetero-oligomer with heat shock proteins and immunophilins. The carboxyterminal region binds glucocorticoid and the middle portion domain binds to specific sequences of DNA in the regulatory regions of glucocorticoid-responsive genes (glucocorticoid-response elements) (Bamberger, Schulte, and Chrousos, 1996). The activated receptors also inhibit, by protein-protein interactions, several transcription factors, such as activator protein-1 (AP-1) which comprises c-jun/c-fos, and NF-kB, which are positive regulators of the transcription of several genes involved in the function and growth of nonimmune and immune cells (van der Saag, Caldenhoven, and van de, 1996). They also change the stability of mRNAs and, hence, the translation rates of several glucocorticoid-responsive genes and proteins (Table 13.2).

Glucocorticoids influence the traffic of circulating leukocytes and inhibit many functions of leukocytes and immune accessory cells. They suppress the immune activation of these cells, inhibit the production of cytokines and other mediators of inflammation, and cause proinflammatory cytokine resistance. Furthermore, glucocorticoids influence the secretion rates of specific proteins and alter the electrical potential of neuronal cells through mechanisms and remain to be elucidated (Gower, 1993). Glucocorticoids exert an inhibitory feedback on pituitary ACTH secretion, thus limiting the duration of the total tissue exposure to glucocorticoids and minimizing their basic catabolic, lipogenic, antireproductive, and immunosuppressive effect (Table 13.3) (Habib, Gold, and Chrousos, 2001). It seems that a dual receptor system for glucocorticoids exists in the CNS, including the glucocorticoid receptor type I, or mineralocorticoid receptor, that responds positively to low levels of glucocorticoids, and the glucocorticoid receptor type II, which responds to basal and stress levels (Habib, Gold, and Chrousos, 2001. Only the type II receptor appears to participate in the negative control feedback of the HPA axis (Habib, Gold, and Chrousos, 2001; Charmandari, Tsigos, and Chrousos, 2005). Several circadian immune functions cause disease-associated diurnal changes that correspond to plasma glucocorticoid levels (Chrousos and Gold, 1992).

Corticotrophin releasing hormone (CRH). CRH is one of the most potent factors that initiate and perpetuate the stress response affecting overall arousal and autonomic

Table 13.2. Genes that are regulated by glucocorticoids or glucocorticoid receptors

Site of action	Induced genes	Repressed genes
Immune System	IκB (NFκB inhibitor) Haptoglobin TCR z p21, p27 and p57 Lipocortin	Interleukins TNF-α IFN-γ E selectin ICAM-1 Cyclooxygenase 2 iNOS
Metabolic	PPAR-γ Tyrosine aminotransferase Glutamine synthase Glycogen-6-phosphatase PEPCK Leptin γ-Fibrinogen Cholesterol 7α hydroxylase C/EBP/β	Tryptophan hydroxylase Metalloprotease
Bone	Androgen receptor Calcitonin receptor Alkaline phosphatase IGF-BP-6	Osteocalcin Collagenase

Channels and transporters	Epithelium sodium channel (ENaC)
	  α, β, γ
	Serum and glucocorticoid –
	  induced kinase (SGK)
	Aquaporin	

Endocrine	βFGF VIP Endothelin RXR GHRH receptor Natriuretic peptide receptors	GR PRL POMC/CRH PTHP Vasopressin
Growth and development	Surfactant protein A, B, C	Fibronectin A-Fetoprotein NGF Erythropoetin G1 cyclins Cyclin-dependent kinases

bFGF, basic fibroblast growth factor; C/EBP/β CAAT-enchancer binding protein-beta; GR, glucocorticoid receptor, GHRH, growth hormone-releasing hormone, ICAM, intercellular adhesion molecule; IFN, interferon; IGF-BP, insulin growth factor-binding protein; IkB, inhibitory kappa B, iNOS, inducible nitric oxide synthase; NFkB, nuclear factor kB; NGF, nerve growth factor; PEPCK, phospho-enolpyruvate carboxykinase; POMC, propiomelanocortin; PPAR, peroxisome proliferator – activated receptor; PTHrP, parathyroid hormone – related protein; RXR, retinoid X receptor, SGK, serum and glucocorticoid-induced kinase; TCR, T-cell receptor; TNF-α, tumor necrosis factor-alpha, VIP, vasoactive intestinal peptide.

activation (Habib, Gold, and Chrousos, 2001). Administration of CRH antagonists is associated with suppression of many aspects of the stress response and CRH type 1 receptor (CRH-R1) knockout mice have a markedly deficient ability to mount an effective stress response (Smith et al., 1998). The presence of CRH neurons in the cerebral cortex is important for the behavioral effect of this peptide, particularly in the prefrontal areas which may be related with its effect on cognitive processing (Habib, Gold, and

Chrouros, 2001). In addition, the projection of CRH neurons to the brain stem and spinal cord is related with its actions on autonomic nervous system function, modulation of sensory input via ascending projections to the thalamus and reticular formation function (Chrouros, 1998).

CRH exerts its actions following binding to two distinct CRH receptors. CRH-R1 is the most abundant subtype found in the anterior pituitary as well as in the adrenal gland, skin, ovary and testis (Bale and Vale, 2004), whereas

Table 13.3. The principal action of glucocorticoids in humans highlighting some of the consequences of glucocorticoid excess

System/organ	Effect
Brain/CNS	Depression Psychosis
Eye	Glaucoma
Endocrine System	Reduction of LH, FSH release Reduction of TSH release Reduction of GH secretion Increase of appetite
Gastrointestinal tract	Increase in acid secretion (peptic ulceration)
Carbohydrate/lipid metabolism	Increased hepatic glycogen deposition Increased peripheral insulin secretion Increased gluconeogenesis Increased fatty acid production Overall diabetogenic effect Promotion of visceral obesity
Cardiovascular/Renal	Salt and water retention Hypertention
Skin/muscle/Renal	Protein catabolism/collagen breakdown Thinning of the skin Muscular atrophy
Bone	Reduction of bone formation Reduction of bone mass and development of osteoporosis
Growth and development	Reduction of linear growth
Immune system	Anti-inflammatory action Immunosuppression

CNS, central nervous system, GI, gastrointestinal; FSH, follicle-stimulating hormone; GH, growth hormone; LH, luteinizing hormone; TSH, thyroid stimulating hormone.

CRH-R2 is mainly expressed in the peripheral vasculature of the heart and subcortical structures of the brain (Habib, Gold, and Chouros, 2001). The diversity of CRH subtype and isoform expression is crucial in modifying the stress response through the actions of different ligands (CRH and CRH-related peptides) and intracellular signal systems (Bale and Vale, 2004). Central CRH administration produces a constellation behavioral effects including increased locomotor activity, increased sniffing, grooming and rearing in a familiar environment, assumption of a freeze posture, decreased feeding and sexual behavior and increased conflict behavior in an unfamiliar environment (Habib, Gold, and Chrousos, 2001). CRH is a also major anorexiogenic peptide, whose secretion is stimulated by NPY, a very potent orexiogenic peptide which

can also inhibit the LC-NA sympathetic system (Oellerich, Schwartz, and Malik, 1994). Changes in NPY levels may be of particular relevance to alterations in the activity of the stress system in conditions such as malnutrition, anorexia neurosa, and/or obesity (Oellerich, Schwartz, and Malik, 1994). The majority of these effects are blocked following the administration of specific CRH antagonists (Habib, et al., 2000).

CRH acts in the brain to activate the SNS (leading to subsequent increment in Ca release) with increased mean arterial pressure and heart rate inhibition of PSNS output (Kregel et al. 1990). In addition, the function of several interrelated neuronal pathways is increased, particularly those related to locus ceruleus, hippocampus, cerebral cortex, and lumbar spine (Habib, Gold, and Chrousos, 2001). Activation of the LC-NA system results in increased arousal and increased vigilance and its dysfunction may be related to the development of anxiety and depression (Habib, Gold, and Chrousos, 2001). In addition to CRH, several other CRH receptor ligands exist, with homology to CRH, including urocortin (Ucn I), Ucn II, and Ucn III (Bale and Vale, 2004). Although CRH seems to exert a mainly a stimulatory role in stress via the CRH R1 receptor, specific actions of UcnII and/or UcnIII on CRH R2 may be extremely important in altering stress sensitivity. In addition, UcnI exhibits a high affinity for both receptors and may also exert a regulatory action (Bale and Vale, 2004).

GABA agonists and benzodiazepines exert an inhibitory effect on CRH neurons, whereas cholinergic and serotonergic neurons stimulate CRH release (Habib, Gold, and Chrousos, 2001). Glucocorticoids exert a mainly inhibitory effect on the HPA axis, except on the CRH neurons in the amygdala and LC-NA, where their stimulatory effect is related in the perpetuation of the stress response (Spinedi, 1998).

CRH has also been localized in a variety of peripheral tissues including the adrenal medulla. Adrenomedullary CRH increases following autonomic nervous system stimulation and during stressful situation (Habib, Gold, and Chrousos, 2001). CRH can also be found in other tissues such as the testis, ovaries, pancreas, stomach, small intestine, uterus and placenta (Aguilera et al., 1987). Similarly, CRH immunoreactivity and mRNA have been detected in lymphocytes, where it plays a role in immune regulation (Elenkov and Chrousos, 2002). Systemic administration of specific CRH antiserum blocks the inflammatory exudate volume and cell number in carrageenin-induced inflammation, and inhibits stress-induced intracranial mast cell degranulation (Elenkov and Chrousos, 2002).

In addition, CRH administration to humans or nonhuman primates causes major peripheral vasodilation manifested as flushing and increased blood flow and hypotension. An intradermal CRH injection induces a marked increase in vascular permeability and mast cell degranulation, which is blocked by a CRH type 1 receptor antagonist (Theoharides et al., 1998). It appears that CRH activates mast cells via a CRH receptor type 1-dependent-mechanism, leading to release of histamine and other

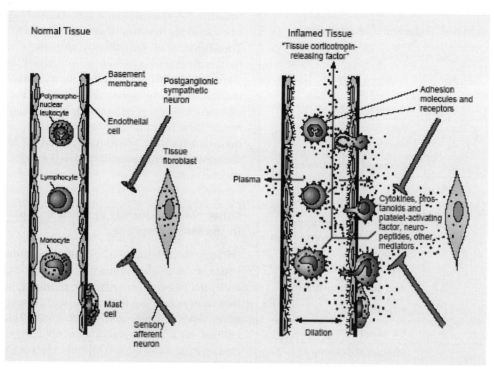

Figure 13.3. Major Components and Events of Inflammation. Quiescent circulating leukocytes, local immune accessory cells, and the terminals of peripheral postganglionic sympathetic and sensory afferent neurons are shown (left-hand panel). In inflamed tissue (right-hand panel), there is vasodilation, increased permeability of the vessel and exudation of plasma. Activated leukocytes and endothelial cells express adhesion molecules and adhesion-molecule receptors. Cells attach to the vessel wall and diapedesis takes place, with chemotaxis towards a chemokine gradient at the focus of inflammation. Activated circulating cells, migrant cells, local immune accessory cells, and peripheral nerves secrete cytokines, prostanoids, platelet activating factor, neuropeptides, and other mediators of inflammation. Some of these substances, such as interleukin-6, leukotrienes, complement component 5α, corticotrophin-releasing hormone, and transforming growth factor-β have chemokinetic activity. Some substances, such as the inflammatory cytokines tumor necrosis factor α, interleukin-1 and interleukin-6, escape in the systemic circulation, causing systemic symptoms and activating the hypothalamic-pituitary-adrenal axis. Because of such effects, these substances were historically referred to as "tissue corticotrophin releasing factor (CRF)" (From Chrousos G., 1351–1362).

contents of the mast cell granules that subsequently cause vasodilatation, increased vascular permeability and other manifestations of inflammation (Figure 13.3). Central, hypothalamic CRH influences the immune system indirectly, through activation of the end-products of the peripheral stress response, i.e., glucocorticoids and Cas. Peripherally secreted CRH at inflammatory sites (*peripheral* or *immune* CRH) influences the immune system directly, through local modulatory actions (Chrousos and Gold, 1992). Immune CRH has been shown in inflamed tissues of animals with experimentally induced aseptic inflammation, and in human tissues from patients with various autoimmune/inflammatory diseases, including rheumatoid arthritis, autoimmune thyroid disease, and ulcerative colitis. The identification of CRH-like immunoreactivity in the dorsal horn of the spinal cord, dorsal root ganglia and sympathetic ganglia support the hypothesis that the majority of immune CRH in early inflammation is of peripheral nerve rather than of immune cell origin (Habib, Gold, and Chrousos, 2001).

Argininine-vasopressin. AVP parvocellular neurons of the PVN of the hypothalamus have an important co-secretory role, and are activated together with CRH neurons during stress to achieve maximum secretion of ACTH (Koob et al., 1985). The subset of PVN neurons that co-secrete both of these peptides increases significantly during stress (Habib, Gold, and Chrousos, 2001), and during chronic or prolonged stress, there may be a shift in control of ACTH from CRH to AVP (Hauger and Aguilera, 1993). PVN CRH and AVP neurons also project to POMC neurons in the arcuate nucleus, which in turn inhibit LC-NA system neurons and pain control neurons of the hind brain and spinal cord (Habib, Gold, and Chrousos, 2001). AVP derived from magnocellular neurons has a major role in conserving body fluids and controlling plasma osmolality, and during hypovolemic stress, AVP becomes the principal ACTH secretagogue (Habib, Gold, and Chrousos, 2001). In addition to its endocrine and metabolic roles AVP has been implicated in some of the behavioral responses to stress (Habib, Gold, and Chrousos, 2001).

Table 13.4. Adrenergic responses of selected tissues

Organ or tissue	Receptor	Effect
Heart (myocardium)	β_1	Increased force of contraction Increased rate of contraction
Blood vessels	α β_2	Vasoconstriction Vasodilation
Kidney	β	Increased renin release
Gut	α, β	Decreased motility and increased sphincter tone
Pancreas	α β	Decreased insulin release Decreased glucagons release Increased insulin release Increased glucagon release
Liver	α, β	Increased glycogenolysis
Adipose tissue	β	Increased lipolysis
Most tissue	β	Increased calorigenesis
Skin	α	Increased sweating
Bronchioles	β_2	Dilation
Uterus	α β_2	Contraction Relaxation

The autonomic component of the stress response (LC-NA/Systemic Sympathetic and Adrenomedullary and Parasympathetic Systems)

The autonomic nervous system (ANS) (SNS and PSNS) responds rapidly to stressors and controls a wide range of systemic functions (Tsigos and Chrousos, 1994). The cardiovascular, respiratory, renal, endocrine and other systems, such as the gastrointestinal system, are regulated by either the SNS or PSNS, or both (Table 13.4) (Habib, Gold, and Chrousos, 2001). Reduction of parasympathetic nervous system activity results in removal of inhibition of the SNS, thus increasing sympathetic functions, while increased activity antagonizes the SNS (Charmandari, Tsigos, and Chrousos, 2005; Tsigos and Chrousos, 1994). Several immune functions are under the influence of SNS and catecholamines including lymphocyte traffic and circulation(Chrousos, 1995). Cas appear to have both inhibitory and stimulatory effects on macrophage activity. In addition to the "classic" neurotransmitters, acetylcholine and norepinephrine, both sympathetic and parasympathetic subdivisions of the autonomic nervous system include several subpopulations of target-selective and neurochemically coded neurons that express a variety of neuropeptides and, in some cases, adenosine triphosphate (ATP), nitric oxide, or lipid mediators of inflammation (Elenkov et al., 1999). Thus, CRH, NPY, somatostatin, and galanin are found in postganglionic noradrenergic vasoconstrictive neurons, while vasoactive intestinal peptide (IP), SP, and calcitonin gene-related peptide are found in cholinergic neurons (Habib, Gold, and Chrousos, 2001). Transmission in sympathetic ganglia is also modulated by neuropeptides released from preganglionic fibers and short interneurons, as well as by primary afferent nerve collaterals. These effects that underlie the characteristic phenomenology of behavioral, endocrine, visceral autonomic, and immune responses to stress are induced and maintained via the orchestrated interplay of several neurotransmitters systems in the brain (Figure 13.1) (Chrousos and Gold, 1992).

Other neuroendocrine systems that participate in the stress response

NPY, besides being a very potent stimulant of feeding behavior, exerts an important role in circadian rhythms and affects behavior, anterior pituitary hormone secretion, autonomic control, and other neurotransmitter systems (Habib, Gold, and Chrousos, 2001). Alteration of central NPY has been documented in stress and several mental disorders. Thus an inverse correlation has been shown between anxiety scores and NPY levels in depressed patients (Heilig and Widerlov, 1995). Several other systems, mainly including the dopaminergic system, also exert an effect on stress. Thus *mesocortical system* is involved in anticipatory phenomena and cognitive functions and is thought to exert a suppressive effect on the stress system (Chrousos and Gold, 1992). The *mesolimbic system* has a major role in motivation reinforcement and reward phenomena (Chrousos, 1998). Euphoria or dysphoria are also mediated through the mesocorticolimbic system and are affected by stress (Gold and Chrousos, 1999). Similarly, the *amygdala nuclei* are activated during stress mainly by catecholaminergic neurons and respond to emotional stressors that originate in cortical related areas. This is important for retrieval and emotional analysis of relevant information for any given stressor (Charmandari, Tsigos, and Chrousos, 2005).

Activation of the stress system also stimulates hypothalamic POMC-peptide secretion, such as α-MSH and β-endorphin. This reciprocally inhibits the activity of central components of the stress system and produces analgesia and, by stimulating the mesocorticolimbic system euphoria, may enhance dependence (Charmandari, Tsigos, and Chrousos, 2005). Activation of the stress system, either via the HPA-axis or the LC/NE system, elevates core temperature (Chrousos, 1998). In addition, CRH can mediate the pyrogenic effects of inflammatory cytokines, such as tumor necrosis factor α (TNF-α), interleukin-1, and -6 (IL-1 and IL-6) (Elenkov and Chrousos, 2002). Prolonged physical and psychological stress may also alter core temperature and suppress food intake (Habib, Gold, and Chrousos, 2001). This effect on appetite/satiety centers may be mediated via increased CRH or CRH-like peptides and/or decreased NPY levels and their actions on LC-NE/sympathetic system (Uehara et al., 1998). Furthermore, leptin, a satiety-stimulating polypeptide secreted by the white adipose tissue, is also involved reciprocally in these changes by directly suppressing NPY secretion or stimulating α-MSH secretion, the latter being a very potent anorexiogen (Charmandari, Tsigos, and Chrousos, 2005).

The last 20 years have provided evidence that certain cytokines, and particularly the pro-inflammatory ones, including tumor necrosis factor (TNF)-α, interleukin (IL)-1 and IL-6, activate both the HPA axis and the LC-NE/SNS system (Chrousos, 1995; Papanicolaou et al., 1996). Moreover, these cytokines induce anorexia/nausea, fatigue and/or depressive affect, hyperalgesia with or without headache, somnolence, sleep disturbances, temperature elevation or fever and increases of the basal metabolic rate, changes collectively referred to as *sickness behavior*. These cytokines also activate hepatic and other tissue synthesis of acute phase proteins, such as C-reactive protein, serum amyloid A, cell adhesion molecules, fibrinogen and plasminogen activator inhibitor 1, a phenomenon referred to as the *"acute phase reaction"*(Cutolo et al., 1998). Stress that is associated with an immune challenge has been called *immune* or *inflammatory stress*, which in fact is a combination of the sickness and classic stress syndromes, together with their effects on the pain/afferent neural systems and the acute phase reaction (Table 13.5) (Elenkov et al., 1999).

Emotions and psychological stress. Emotional responses are produced in the limbic system, which projects to several parts of the brain, including those involved in the initial activation and maintenance of the stress system thus explaining why emotional insults activate the stress system in humans (Chrousos and Gold, 1992). In humans the physiolological responses to social pressures, information overload, and rapid cultural change resemble those that are produced during physical stress and/or danger and outright threats to survival (Chrousos and Gold, 1992).

Genetics, development, environment, and the stress response

Vulnerability to stress effects may be the result of genetic, developmental, and environmental factors (Charmandari, Tsigos, and Chrousos, 2005). Many factors that determine individual stress responses are inherited. It is thought that approximately one half of reliable variance in personality traits is related to genetic influences but a significant amount of variance of the stress responses of individuals is also related to environmental factors, particularly at periods of increased brain plasticity during development (Chrousos, 1998). Depending on the genetic background of the individual, polymorphisms, such as those of CRH, AVP, and their receptors and/or regulators, and exposure to adverse stimuli in prenatal and/or postnatal life (developmental influences), there may be a failure to initiate and propagate appropriate stress responses to various stressors leading to various chronic states of either

Table 13.5. Inflammatory stress syndrome as a compound of two major biological programs of adaptation

Sickness syndrome	Classic stress syndrome
Anorexia/nausea	Anorexia/ Stimulation of Appetite*
Fatigue and/or Depressed Affect	Motivation/Stimulated Affect
Somnolence	Arousal
Hyperalgesia	Analgesia
Headache	
Elevated Temperature/ Fever	Antipyretic
Increased Metabolic Rate	Increased Metabolic Rate/ Return to Normal*
Acute Phase Reaction +++++	Acute Phase Reaction+
Molecular Effectors Inflammatory Cytokines/Mediators	CRH, AVP, Glucocorticoids, Catecholamines, Immune CRH

* Initially stimulation via CRH and catecholamines; then inhibition by glucocorticoids.

hyper- or hypoactivity of the stress system that can occur in any combination and degree of severity (Habib, Gold, and Chrousos, 2001). Excessive or sustained activation of the stress system during these critical periods may have profound effects on its function. These environmental triggers or stressors may have not a transient, but rather a permanent effect on the development of the HPA axis responses to stress, which may persist long after cessation of exposure to these hormones (Habib, Gold, and Chrousos, 2001; Charmandari, Tsigos, and Chrousos, 2005). In these early stages of development, exposure to psychological trauma sets into motion a cascade of mental changes that may result in long-term predisposition to anxiety, depression, or other stress related somatic illnesses (Maughan and McCarthy, 1997). Although no prospective studies exist, several observational studies have shown the presence of an association between the patterns of activity of the HPA-axis and the development of mood and/or anxiety disorders (Chrousos, 1998).

THE STRESS SYSTEM IN PHYSIOLOGY

Activation of the central CRH and LC-NE systems, and subsequent secretion of large amounts of glucocorticoids and Cas, affect virtually every cell of the body (Chrousos and Gold, 1992). This leads to extensive mobilization of energy stores in various systems. The heart's rate is accelerated and its force of contraction is grossly increased in an attempt to provide optimal blood supply to various tissues. Respiratory rate increases, and the bronchi dilate, providing maximum oxygen supply to the tissues to ensure adequate fuel consumption. Significant changes in blood flow result in redistribution of nutrients and oxygen (Chrousos and Gold, 1992). Endocrine adaptations also occur and preserve energy by ceasing function of various hormonal dependent behaviors. Thus the reproductive and growth axe and, to a lesser extent the thyrotrophin axis are temporarily shut off (Habib, Gold, and Chrousos, 2001). Activation of the HPA axis exerts profound modulatory effects on the immune system (Table 13.1). All these adaptations are protective and help to maintain homeostasis in the short run but can be damaging in the long run if the mediators are overproduced, underproduced, or dysregulated chronically (McEwen, 2002).

THE STRESS SYSTEM IN PATHOPHYSIOLOGY

In general, an appropriate stress response is of limited duration. The time-limited nature of this process renders its accompanying anti-growth, anti-reproductive, catabolic, and immunosuppressive effects temporarily beneficial and/or of no adverse consequences to the individual (Chrousos and Gold, 1992). In principle, there are four situations that can be related to either the intensity of the stressor an/or the response of the stress system that may be lead to dysregulation of the system (McEwen, 1998). This could be frequent exposure to stressful stimuli, lack of adaptation to repeated stressors, inability to shut off the stress response after the stressful stimulus is eliminated, and inadequate responses of the stress system to stressors (Figure 13.4) (McEwen, 1998). Chronic activation of the stress system may lead to a number of disorders, which are due to increased and/or prolonged secretion of stress mediators such as CRH, Cas, and/or glucocorticoids (Table 13.6).

SYSTEMIC EFFECTS DUE TO CHRONIC HYPERACTIVITY OF THE STRESS SYSTEM

Growth and development

During stress, the growth axis is inhibited at several levels. Prolonged activation of the HPA axis leads to suppression of GH secretion via CRH-induced increases in somatostatin secretion. Glucocorticoids also induce resistance in target tissues to the effects of both GH, insulin-like growth factor I (IGF-I) and other growth factors (Magiakou, Mastorakos, and Chrousos, 1994; Magiakou et al., 1994). The molecular mechanisms by which glucocorticoids suppress growth are complex, and involve both transcriptional and translational mechanisms that ultimately influence the GH receptor action (Bamberger, Schulte, and Chrousos, 1996). In several stress-related mood disorders accompanied by a hyperactive HPA axis, such as anxiety or melancholic depression, GH, and/or IGF-I concentrations

are significantly decreased, and the GH response to intravenously administered glucocorticoids is blunted. Children with anxiety disorders also may have short stature (Habib, Gold, and Chrousos, 2001). "Psychosocial short stature" is characterized by severely compromised height in children due to emotional deprivation. Such children display a significant decrease in GH secretion, which is fully restored within a few days following separation of the child from the adverse environment. Such children also exhibit a hyperactive HPA axis and amygdala (Skuse, 1996). Other consequences of hyperactive stress system include delayed growth and puberty; manifestations of the metabolic syndrome, such as premature adrenarche; visceral obesity, insulin resistance, and diabetes type II; hypertension; dyslipidemia; polycystic ovary syndrome (PCOS); sleep apnea; cardiovascular disease; and osteoporosis (Habib, Gold, and Chrousos, 2001).

Thyroid function

Thyroid function is also inhibited during stress. Activation of the HPA axis is associated with decreased production of thyroid-stimulating hormone (TSH), as well as inhibition of peripheral conversion of the relatively inactive thyroxine to the biologically active triiodothyronine (Benker et al., 1990). These alterations may be due to the increased concentrations of CRH-induced somatostatin and glucocorticoids. Somatostatin suppresses both TRH and TSH, while glucocorticoids inhibit the activity of the enzyme 5-deiodinase, which converts thyroxine to triiodothyronine. During inflammatory stress, inflammatory cytokines, such as TNF-a, IL-1, and IL-6, also activate CRH secretion and inhibit 5-deiodinase activity resulting in decreased T3 and increased rT3 levels (Chrousos and Gold, 1992; Tsigos and Chrousos, 2002).

Reproduction

The reproductive axis is inhibited at all levels by various components of the HPA axis. CRH suppresses the secretion of gonadotropin-releasing hormone (GnRH) either directly or indirectly, by stimulating arcuate POMC peptide-secreting neurons (Vamvakopoulos and Chrousos, 1994). Glucocorticoids also exert an inhibitory effect on GnRH neurons, pituitary gonadotrophs, and the gonads, and render target tissues of gonadal steroids resistant to these hormones (Tsigos and Chrousos, 2002; Chrousos, Torpy, and Gold, 1998). Suppression of gonadal function secondary to chronic activation of the HPA axis has been demonstrated in highly trained runners of both sexes and in ballet dancers (Habib, Gold, and Chrousos, 2001). The interaction between CRH and the hypothalamic-pituitary-gonadal axis is bi-directional, given that estrogen increases CRH gene expression via estrogen-response elements in the promoter region of the CRH gene (Vamvakopoulos and Chrousos, 1994). Therefore, the CRH gene is an important target of gonadal steroids and a potential mediator of

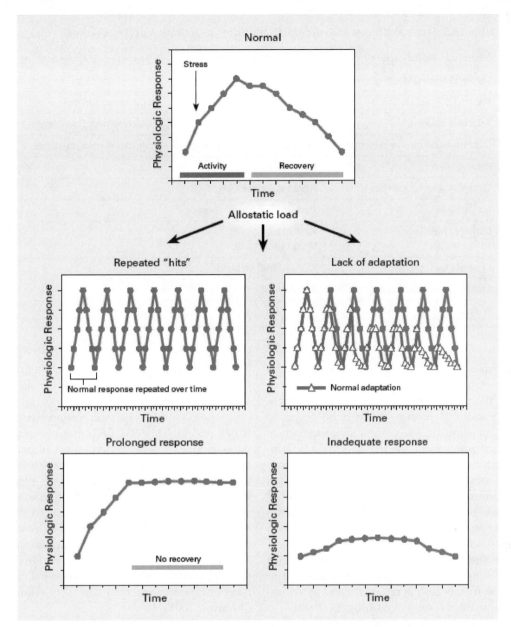

Figure 13.4. Types of allostatic (ability to handle stress) load. The top panel illustrates the normal allostatic response, in which a stressor initiates a response from the stress system and then is adequately turned off. The remaining panels illustrate four conditions that lead to allostatic load: repeated hits from multiple stressors, lack of adaptation, prolonged response due to delayed shutdown, and inadequate response that leads to compensatory hyperactivity of other\mediators (From Mc Ewen B., 171–179).

sex-related differences in the stress-response and the activity of the HPA axis.

Metabolism

In addition to their direct catabolic effects, glucocorticoids also antagonize the actions of GH and sex steroids on fat tissue catabolism (lipolysis) and muscle and bone anabolism (Charmandari, Tsigos, and Chrousos, 2005; Tsigos and Chrousos, 2002). Chronic activation of the stress system is associated with increased visceral adiposity, decreased lean body (bone and muscle) mass, and suppressed osteoblastic activity (a phenotype observed in patients with Cushing's syndrome). Some patients with melancholic depression, and patients with the metabolic syndrome (visceral obesity, insulin resistance, dyslipidemia, hypertension, hypercoagulation, atherosclerotic cardiovascular disease, sleep apnea), many of whom display increased HPA axis activity, exhibit similar clinical and biochemical manifestations (Gold and Chrousos, 1999; Tsigos and Chrousos, 2002; Pasquali et al., 1993). It has been shown that life-stress related hypersecretion of cortisol or tissue-limited hypersensitivity to glucocorticoids may deleteriously affect important physiologic

Table 13.6. States associated with hyperactivation or hypoactivation of the HPA axis

Increased HPA axis activity	Decreased HPA axis activity	Disrupted HPA axis activity
Severe chronic disease		
Melancholic depression	Atypical depression	Cushing syndrome
Anorexia neurosa	Seasonal depression	Glucocorticoid deficiency
Obsessive-compulsive disorders	Chronic fatigue syndrome	Glucocorticoid resistance
Panic disorders	Fibromyalgia	
Chronic excessive exercise	Adrenal suppression	
Malnutrition	Post glucocorticoid therapy	
Diabetes Mellitus	Post stress Drug withdrawal	
Central Obesity	Rheumatoid arthritis	
Childhood sexual abuse	Postpartum	
Pregnancy		

parameters, such as systemic blood pressure, lipid, and carbohydrate metabolism (Pasquali et al., 1993; Rosmond, Dallman, and Bjorntorp, 1998). Since increased gluconeogenesis is a cardinal feature of the stress response and glucocorticoids regulate insulin action and induce insulin resistance, activation of the HPA axis may also contribute to the poor control of diabetic patients with emotional stress or concurrent inflammatory or other diseases (Tsigos and Chrousos, 2002). Mild, chronic activation of the HPA axis has been shown in type I diabetic patients under moderate or poor glycemic control, and in type II diabetic patients who had developed diabetic neuropathy (Tsigos, Young, and White, 1993). Over time, progressive glucocorticoid-induced visceral adiposity and loss of lean body mass cause further insulin resistance and deterioration of glycemic control (Tsigos and Chrousos, 2002).

"Low turnover" osteoporosis is almost invariably seen in association with hypercortisolism and GH deficiency, and represents another example of the adverse effects of elevated cortisol concentrations and decreased GH/IGF-I concentrations on osteoblastic activity. Stress-induced hypogonadism and reduced concentrations of sex steroids may further contribute to the development of osteoporosis. Increased prevalence of osteoporosis has been demonstrated in young women with depression or a previous history of depression (Michelson et al., 1996).

Gastrointestinal function

PVN CRH induces inhibition of gastric acid secretion and emptying, while it stimulates colonic motor function (Tache et al., 1993). These effects are mediated by inhibition of the vagus nerve, which leads to selective inhibition of gastric motility, and by stimulation of the LC-NE-regulated sacral parasympathetic system, results

in selective stimulation of colonic motility. Therefore, CRH may be implicated in mediating the gastric stasis observed following surgery or during an inflammatory process, when central IL-1 concentrations are elevated (Suto, Kiraly, and Tache, 1994). CRH may also play a role in the stress-induced colonic hypermotility of patients with irritable bowel syndrome. Colonic contraction and pain in these patients may activate LC-NE-sympathetic neurons, forming a vicious cycle, which may account for the chronicity of the condition. Chronic activation of the HPA axis and/or the LC-NE-sympathetic system due to depletion of the opioid-peptide system, which mediates stress-induced analgesia, may also account for the lower pain threshold for visceral sensation reported in patients with functional gastrointestinal disorders (Habib, Gold, and Chrousos, 2001).

Psychiatric disorders

The syndrome of adult melancholic depression represents a typical example of dysregulation of the generalized stress response, leading to chronic dysphoric hyperarousal, activation of the HPA axis and the SNS, and relative immunosuppression (Elenkov et al., 1996; Elenkov and Chrousos, 1999). Patients suffering from the condition exhibit hypersecretion of CRH, elevated concentrations of norepinephrine in the CSF, which remain elevated even during sleep, and a marked increase in the number of PVN CRH neurons on autopsy (Gold and Chrousos, 1999). Some developmental environmental exposures may predispose to such syndromes. Childhood sexual abuse is associated with an increased incidence of adult psychopathology, as well as with abnormalities in HPA function. Sexually abused girls have a greater incidence of suicidal ideation, suicide attempts, and dysthymia compared to controls (De Bellis et al., 1994). In addition, they excrete significantly higher amounts of catecholamines and their metabolites, and display lower basal and CRH-stimulated ACTH concentrations compared to controls. However, the total and free basal and CRH-stimulated serum cortisol concentrations and 24h urinary free cortisol concentrations in these subjects are similar to those in controls. These findings reflect pituitary hyporesponsiveness to CRH, which may be corrected by the presence of intact glucocorticoid feedback regulatory mechanisms (De Bellis et al., 1994).

Other conditions may be associated with increased and prolonged activation of the HPA axis. These include anorexia nervosa (Ce Bellis et al., 1994), malnutrition, obsessive-compulsive disorder, panic anxiety, excessive exercise, chronic active alcoholism, alcohol and narcotic withdrawal, diabetes mellitus types I and II, visceral obesity, and perhaps, hyperthyroidism (Habib, Gold, and Chrousos, 2001). Both anorexia nervosa and malnutrition are characterized by a marked decrease in circulating leptin concentration and an increase in CSF NPY concentration, which could provide an explanation as to why the HPA axis in these subjects is activated in the presence of a profoundly hypoactive LC-NE-sympathetic system (Liu et al., 1994). Glucocorticoids, on the other hand, by stimulating NPY and by inhibiting the PVN CRH and the LC-NE-sympathetic systems may produce hyperphagia and obesity such as that observed in patients with Cushing's syndrome and many rodent models of obesity, including the Zucker rat (Charmandari, Tsigos, and Chrousos, 2005). Glucocorticoids have also been associated with leptin resistance, while Zucker rats are leptin receptor deficient with concurrent hypercorticosteronism and decreased LC-NE-sympathetic system activity (Habib, Gold, and Chrousos, 2001).

SYSTEMIC EFFECTS DUE TO CHRONIC HYPERACTIVITY OF THE STRESS SYSTEM

Hypoactivity of the stress system is characterized by chronically reduced secretion of CRH and norepinephrine and may be associated with hypoarousal states (Table 13.6). As a consequence, the activity of other systems increases as a result of lack of counterregulation, i.e., if cortisol secretion does not increase in response to stress, secretion of inflammatory cytokines (which are counterregulated by cortisol) increases (McEwen, 1998). Thus, patients with a typical or seasonal depression and chronic fatigue syndrome show chronic hypoactivity of the HPA axis in the depressive state and during the period of fatigue respectively (Habib, Gold, and Chrousos, 2001). Similarly, patients with fibromyalgia have been shown to have decreased 24-hour urinary free cortisol excretion when they develop fatigue (Ehlert, Gaab, and Heinrichs, 2001). In such cases a suboptimal HPA axis response to inflammatory stimuli would be expected to reproduce the glucocorticoid-deficient state and lead to relative resistance to infections and neoplastic diseases but

Table 13.7. States associated with hypercytokinemia

Trauma/ Burns
Infectious Illness
Autoimmune Inflammatory Disease
Allergic Inflammation
CNS Inflammation
Noninflammatory Stress
Obesity/Visceral Obesity
Ageing

increased susceptibility to autoimmune inflammatory disease (Elenkov et al., 1999). This has been shown in Fischer and Lewis rats, inbred strains characterized by their relative hyper- and hypo-HPA axis responsiveness and resistance or susceptibility, respectively, to inflammatory disease (Elenkov and Chrousos, 1999).

Patients with depression or anxiety have been shown to be more vulnerable to tuberculosis, both in terms of prevalence and severity of the disease (Sternberg et al., 1989; Sternberg et al., 1989). Similarly, stress has been associated with increased vulnerability to the common cold virus. A compromised innate and T helper-1 driven immunity may predispose an individual to these conditions. Furthermore, patients with rheumatoid arthritis, a T-helper-1 driven pattern of inflammatory disease, have a mild form of central hypocortisolism, as indicated by the normal 24-hour cortisol excretion despite the major inflammatory stress and diminished HPA axis responses to surgical stress (Elenkov and Chrousos, 2002). Therefore, dysregulation of the HPA axis may play a role in the development and/or perpetuation of T helper-1-type of autoimmune disease. The same theoretical concept may explain the high incidence of T helper-1 autoimmune diseases, such as rheumatoid arthritis and multiple sclerosis, observed following correction of hypercortisolism, in the postpartum period and in patients with adrenal insufficiency, who do not receive adequate replacement therapy (Chikanza et al., 1992; Magiakou et al., 1996).

STRESS, SYSTEMIC INFLAMMATION AND WELL-BEING

Like the stress response, the inflammatory reaction of an individual is crucial for survival of the self and species (Chrousos, 1998). Be it an inflammatory focus with spillover of inflammatory effector molecules into the systemic circulation or a truly generalized, systemic inflammatory reaction, the biological programs that are activated during inflammation have both synergistic and antagonistic actions (Table 13.7). For instance, inflammatory cytokines stimulate CRP production by the liver and this effect is potentiated by glucocorticoids, which, however, also inhibit the secretion of inflammatory cytokines (Chrousos and Gold, 1992). Most of the manifestations of sickness syndrome, including anorexia/nausea, fatigue and/or depressed affect, somnolence, hyperalgesia with or without headache, fever, and an increased metabolic rate, are all suppressed by glucocorticoids. Yet, peripheral neuronal CRH activated by stress or the inflammatory reaction, and substance P activated by the inflammatory reaction, both potentiate inflammation (Chrousos and Gold, 1992; Chrousos, 1995). Hypercytokinemia is not limited to conditions characterized by classic inflammatory stress, such as trauma and burns, infectious illnesses, autoimmune inflammatory diseases, and allergic inflammatory states (Table 13.4). Inflammatory phenomena in the CNS, such as Alzheimer's disease or schizophrenia, as well as noninflammatory stress, such as that of melancholic depression are associated with elevations of IL-6. Interestingly, obesity, especially the visceral type, is associated with chronic elevations of IL-6 in the circulation (see below).

The chronic pain and fatigue syndromes. Several chronic pain and fatigue syndromes, such as fibromyalgia and chronic fatigue syndrome, have been associated with chronic sickness syndrome manifestations, such as fatigue and hyperalgesia, and with hypoactivity of the stress system (Clauw and Chrousos, 1997) (Table 13.6). Interestingly, these clinical manifestations and the hypocortisolism of these patients are quite reminiscent of mild glucocorticoid deficiency (Addison's disease). Patients with glucocorticoid deficiency have elevated levels of proinflammatory cytokines such as IL-6 which may explain their typical sickness syndrome manifestations (Papanicolaou et al., 1996; Papanicolaou et al., 1998). It is tempting to speculate that patients with chronic pain and fatigue syndromes such as fibromyalgia and CFS suffer from an imbalance between the immune and inflammatory response and the stress response, which results in excessive sickness syndrome manifestations and diminished stress system counterregulation (Table 13.5).

Obesity as a chronic inflammatory state. Adipose tissue secretes large amounts of TNF-α and IL-6 in a neurally, hormonally and metabolically regulated fashion (Orban et al., 1999). The plasma levels of these cytokines are proportional to the body mass index (BMI) and are further elevated in patients with visceral obesity (Vgontzas et al., 1997). The secretion of inflammatory cytokines has a circadian pattern, with elevations in the evening and in the early morning hours (Vgontzas et al., 1999). This pattern is maintained in obese subjects, albeit at a higher level, is affected by the quality and quantity of sleep, and correlates with manifestations of the sickness syndrome. In obesity, hypercytokinemia is frequently associated with some manifestations of the sickness syndrome, such as fatigue and somnolence, and of the other biological programs that may be activated during the inflammatory reaction, especially

the acute phase reaction. Thus, obesity especially the visceral type, can be considered as a chronic inflammatory state, with many of the behavioral, immune, metabolic and cardiovascular sequel of such a state (Tables 13.6 and 13.7).

CONCLUSIONS

The stress system coordinates the adaptive response of the organism to stressors and plays an important role in maintenance of basal and stress-related homeostasis. Activation of the stress system leads to behavioral and physical changes that improve the ability of the organism to adapt and increase its chances for survival. However, an inadequate or excessive and prolonged response to stressors may impair growth and development, and may result in a variety of endocrine, metabolic, autoimmune, and psychiatric disorders. The development and severity of these conditions primarily depend on genetic, developmental and environmental factors. Medications that aim at antagonizing the central and peripheral activation of the stress system may be useful in states characterized by chronic hyperactivity of the stress system, whereas glucocorticoids may be useful in conditions characterized by chronic hypoactivity of the stress system.

REFERENCES

Aguilera, G., Millan, M. A., Hauger, R. L., & Catt, K. J. (1987). Corticotropin-releasing factor receptors: distribution and regulation in brain, pituitary, and peripheral tissues. *Ann N Y Acad Sci* 512, 48–66.

Bale, T. L., & Vale, W. W. (2004). CRF and CRF receptors: role in stress responsivity and other behaviors. *Annu Rev Pharmacol Toxicol* 44, 525–557.

Bamberger, C. M., Schulte, H. M., & Chrousos, G. P. (1996). Molecular determinants of glucocorticoid receptor function and tissue sensitivity to glucocorticoids. *Endocr Rev* 17(3), 245–261.

Benker, G., Raida, M., Olbricht, T., Wagner, R., Reinhardt, W., & Reinwein, D. (1990). TSH secretion in Cushing's syndrome: relation to glucocorticoid excess, diabetes, goitre, and the 'sick euthyroid syndrome'. *Clin Endocrinol* (Oxf) 33(6), 777–786.

Brown, M. R., Fisher, L. A., Spiess, J., Rivier, C., Rivier, J., & Vale, W. (1982). Corticotropin-releasing factor: actions on the sympathetic nervous system and metabolism. *Endocrinology* 111(3), 928–931.

Charmandari, E., Tsigos, C., & Chrousos, G. (2005). Endocrinology of the stress response. *Annu Rev Physiol* 67, 259–284.

Chikanza, I. C., Petrou, P., Kingsley, G., Chrousos, G., & Panayi, G. S. (1992). Defective hypothalamic response to immune and inflammatory stimuli in patients with rheumatoid arthritis. *Arthritis Rheum* 35(11), 1281–1288.

Chrousos, G. P. (1995). The hypothalamic-pituitary-adrenal axis and immune-mediated inflammation. *N Engl J Med* 332(20), 1351–1362.

Chrousos, G. P. (1998). Stressors, stress, and neuroendocrine integration of the adaptive response. The 1997 Hans Selye Memorial Lecture. *Ann N Y Acad Sci* 851, 311–335.

Chrousos, G. P., & Gold, P. W. (1992). The concepts of stress and stress system disorders. Overview of physical and behavioral homeostasis. *JAMA* 267(9), 1244–1252.

Chrousos, G. P., Torpy, D. J., & Gold, P. W. (1998). Interactions between the hypothalamic-pituitary-adrenal axis and the female reproductive system: clinical implications. *Ann Intern Med* 129(3), 229–240.

Clauw, D. J., & Chrousos, G. P. (1997). Chronic pain and fatigue syndromes: overlapping clinical and neuroendocrine features and potential pathogenic mechanisms. *Neuroimmunomodulation* 4(3), 134–153.

Cutolo, M., Sulli, A., Villaggio, B., Seriolo, B., & Accardo, S. (1998). Relations between steroid hormones and cytokines in rheumatoid arthritis and systemic lupus erythematosus. *Ann Rheum Dis* 57(10), 573–577.

De Bellis, M. D., Chrousos, G. P., Dorn, L. D., Burke, L., Helmers, K., Kling, M. A., Trickett, P.K., & Putnam, F.W. (1994). Hypothalamic-pituitary-adrenal axis dysregulation in sexually abused girls. *J Clin Endocrinol Metab* 78(2), 249–255.

De Bellis, M. D., Lefter, L., Trickett, P. K., & Putnam, F. W., Jr. (1994). Urinary catecholamine excretion in sexually abused girls. *J Am Acad Child Adolesc Psychiatry* 33(3), 320–327.

Ehlert, U., Gaab, J., & Heinrichs, M. (2001). Psychoneuroendocrinological contributions to the etiology of depression, posttraumatic stress disorder, and stress-related bodily disorders: the role of the hypothalamus-pituitary-adrenal axis. *Biol Psychol* 57(1–3), 141–152.

Elenkov, I. J., & Chrousos, G. P. (1999). Stress Hormones., Th1/Th2 patterns., Pro/Anti-inflammatory Cytokines and Susceptibility to Disease. *Trends Endocrinol Metab* 10(9), 359–368.

Elenkov, I. J., & Chrousos, G. P. (2002). Stress hormones, proinflammatory and antiinflammatory cytokines, and autoimmunity. *Ann N Y Acad Sci* 966, 290–303.

Elenkov, I. J., Papanicolaou, D. A., Wilder, R. L., & Chrousos, G. P. (1996). Modulatory effects of glucocorticoids and catecholamines on human interleukin-12 and interleukin-10 production: clinical implications. *Proc Assoc Am Physicians* 108(5), 374–381.

Elenkov, I. J., Webster, E. L., Torpy, D. J., & Chrousos, G. P. (1999). Stress, corticotropin-releasing hormone, glucocorticoids, and the immune/inflammatory response: acute and chronic effects. *Ann N Y Acad Sci* 876, 1–11.

Gold, P. W., & Chrousos, G. P. (1999). The endocrinology of melancholic and atypical depression: relation to neurocircuitry and somatic consequences. *Proc Assoc Am Physicians* 111(1), 22–34.

Gower, W. R., Jr. (1993). Mechanism of glucocorticoid action. *J Fla Med Assoc* 80(10), 697–700.

Habib, K. E., Gold, P. W., & Chrousos, G. P. (2001). Neuroendocrinology of stress. *Endocrinol Metab Clin North Am* 30(3), 695–728.

Habib, K. E., Weld, K. P., Rice, K. C., Pushkas, J., Champoux, M., Listwak, S., Webster, E. L., Atkinson, A. J., Schulkin, J., Contoreggi, C., Chrousos, G. P., McCann, S. M., Suomi, S. J., Higley, J. D., & Gold, P. W. (2000). Oral administration of a corticotropin-releasing hormone receptor antagonist significantly attenuates behavioral, neuroendocrine, and autonomic responses to stress in primates. *Proc Natl Acad Sci U S A* 97(11), 6079–6084.

Hauger, R. L., & Aguilera, G. (1993). Regulation of pituitary corticotropin releasing hormone (CRH) receptors by CRH: interaction with vasopressin. *Endocrinology* 133(4), 1708–1714.

Heilig, M., & Widerlov, E. (1995). Neurobiology and clinical aspects of neuropeptide. *Crit Rev Neurobiol* 9(2–3), 115–136.

Koob, G. F., Lebrun, C., Martinez, J. L., Jr., Dantzer R., Le Moal, M., & Bloom, F. E. (1985). Arginine vasopressin, stress, and memory. *Ann N Y Acad Sci* 444, 194–202.

Kregel, K. C., Overton, J. M., Seals, D. R., Tipton, C. M., & Fisher, L. A. (1990). Cardiovascular responses to exercise in the rat: role of corticotropin-releasing factor. *J Appl Physiol* 68(2), 561–567.

Liu, J. P., Clarke, I. J., Funder, J. W., & Engler, D. (1994). Studies of the secretion of corticotropin-releasing factor and arginine vasopressin into the hypophysial-portal circulation of the conscious sheep. II. The central noradrenergic and neuropeptide Y pathways cause immediate and prolonged hypothalamic-pituitary-adrenal activation. Potential involvement in the pseudo-Cushing's syndrome of endogenous depression and anorexia nervosa. *J Clin Invest* 93(4), 1439–1450.

Magiakou, M. A., Mastorakos, G., & Chrousos, G. P. (1994). Final stature in patients with endogenous Cushing's syndrome. *J Clin Endocrinol Metab* 79(4), 1082–1085.

Magiakou, M. A., Mastorakos, G., Oldfield, E. H., Gomez, M. T., Doppman, J. L., Cutler, G. B., Jr., Nieman, L. K., & Chrousos, G. P. (1994). Cushing's syndrome in children and adolescents. Presentation, diagnosis, and therapy. *N Engl J Med* 331(10), 629–636.

Magiakou, M. A., Mastorakos, G., Rabin, D., Dubbert, B., Gold, P. W., & Chrousos, G. P. (1996). Hypothalamic corticotropin-releasing hormone suppression during the postpartum period: implications for the increase in psychiatric manifestations at this time. *J Clin Endocrinol Metab* 81(5), 1912–1917.

Maughan, B., & McCarthy, G. (1997). Childhood adversities and psychosocial disorders. *Br Med Bull* 53(1), 156–169.

McEwen, B. S. (1998). Stress, adaptation, and disease. Allostasis and allostatic load. *Ann N Y Acad Sci* 840, 33–44.

McEwen, B. S. (2002). The neurobiology and neuroendocrinology of stress. Implications for post-traumatic stress disorder from a basic science perspective. *Psychiatr Clin North Am* 25(2), 469–94., ix.

Michelson, D., Stratakis, C., Hill, L., Reynolds, J., Galliven, E., Chrousos, G., & Gold, P. (1996). Bone mineral density in women with depression. *N Engl J Med* 335(16), 1176–1181.

Oellerich, W. F., Schwartz, D. D., Malik, K. U. (1994). Neuropeptide Y inhibits adrenergic transmitter release in cultured rat superior cervical ganglion cells by restricting the availability of calcium through a pertussis toxin-sensitive mechanism. *Neuroscience* 60(2), 495–502.

Orban, Z., Remaley, A. T., Sampson, M., Trajanoski, Z., & Chrousos, G. P. (1999). The differential effect of food intake and beta-adrenergic stimulation on adipose-derived hormones and cytokines in man. *J Clin Endocrinol Metab* 84(6), 2126–2133.

Papanicolaou, D. A., Petrides, J. S., Tsigos, C., Bina, S., Kalogeras, K. T., Wilder, R., Gold, P. W., Deuster, P. A., & Chrousos, G. P. (1996). Exercise stimulates interleukin-6 secretion: inhibition by glucocorticoids and correlation with catecholamines. *Am J Physiol* 271(3 Pt 1), E601–E605.

Papanicolaou, D. A., Wilder, R. L., Manolagas, S. C., & Chrousos, G. P. (1998). The pathophysiologic roles of interleukin-6 in human disease. *Ann Intern Med* 128(2), 127–137.

Pasquali, R., Cantobelli, S., Casimirri, F., Capelli, M., Bortoluzzi, L., Flamia, R., Labate, A. M., & Barbara, L. (1993). The hypothalamic-pituitary-adrenal axis in obese women with different patterns of body fat distribution. *J Clin Endocrinol Metab* 77(2), 341–346.

Rosmond, R., Dallman, M. F., & Bjorntorp, P. (1998). Stress-related cortisol secretion in men: relationships with abdominal obesity and endocrine., metabolic and hemodynamic abnormalities. *J Clin Endocrinol Metab* 83(6), 1853–1859.

Skuse, D., Albanese, A., Stanhope, R., Gilmour, J., & Voss, L. (1996). A new stress-related syndrome of growth failure and hyperphagia in children., associated with reversibility of growth-hormone insufficiency. *Lancet* 348(9024), 353–358.

Smith, G. W., Aubry, J. M., Dellu, F., Contarino, A., Bilezikjian, L. M., Gold, L. H., Chen, R., Marchuk, Y., Hauser, C., Bentley, C. A., Sawchenko, P. E., Koob, G. F., Vale, W., & Lee, K. F. (1998). Corticotropin releasing factor receptor 1-deficient mice display decreased anxiety, impaired stress response, and aberrant neuroendocrine development. *Neuron* 20(6), 1093–1102.

Spinedi, E., Johnston, C. A., Chisari, A., & Negro-Vilar, A. (1988). Role of central epinephrine on the regulation of corticotropin-releasing factor and adrenocorticotropin secretion. *Endocrinology* 122(5), 1977–1983.

Sternberg, E. M., Hill, J. M., Chrousos, G. P., Kamilaris, T., Listwak, S. J., Gold, P. W., & Wilder, R. L. (1989). Inflammatory mediator-induced hypothalamic-pituitary-adrenal axis activation is defective in streptococcal cell wall arthritis-susceptible Lewis rats. *Proc Natl Acad Sci U S A* 86(7), 2374–2378.

Sternberg, E. M., Young, W. S., III., Bernardini, R., Calogero, A. E., Chrousos, G. P., Gold, P. W., & Wilder, R. L. (1989). A central nervous system defect in biosynthesis of corticotropin-releasing hormone is associated with susceptibility to streptococcal cell wall-induced arthritis in Lewis rats 1. *Proc Natl Acad Sci U S A* 86(12), 4771–4775.

Suto, G., Kiraly, A., & Tache, Y. (1994). Interleukin 1 beta inhibits gastric emptying in rats: mediation through prostaglandin and corticotropin-releasing factor. *Gastroenterology* 106(6), 1568–1575.

Tache, Y., Monnikes, H., Bonaz, B., & Rivier, J. (1993). Role of CRF in stress-related alterations of gastric and colonic motor function. *Ann N Y Acad Sci* 697, 233–243.

Theoharides, T. C., Singh, L. K., Boucher, W., Pang, X., Letourneau, R., Webster, E., & Chrousos, G. (1998). Corticotropin-releasing hormone induces skin mast cell degranulation and increased vascular permeability, a possible explanation for its proinflammatory effects. *Endocrinology* 139(1), 403–413.

Tsigos, C., & Chrousos, G. P. (1994). Physiology of the hypothalamic-pituitary-adrenal axis in health and dysregulation in psychiatric and autoimmune disorders. *Endocrinol Metab Clin North Am* 23(3), 451–466.

Tsigos, C., & Chrousos, G. P. (2002). Hypothalamic-pituitary-adrenal axis., neuroendocrine factors and stress. *J Psychosom Res* 53(4), 865–871.

Tsigos, C., Young, R. J., & White, A. (1993). Diabetic neuropathy is associated with increased activity of the hypothalamic-pituitary-adrenal axis. *J Clin Endocrinol Metab* 76(3), 554–558.

Uehara, Y., Shimizu, H., Ohtani, K., Sato, N., & Mori, M. (1998). Hypothalamic corticotropin-releasing hormone is a mediator of the anorexigenic effect of leptin. *Diabetes* 47(6), 890–893.

Vamvakopoulos, N. C., & Chrousos, G. P. (1994). Hormonal regulation of human corticotropin-releasing hormone gene expression: implications for the stress response and immune/inflammatory reaction. *Endocr Rev* 15(4), 409–420.

van der Saag, P. T., Caldenhoven, E., & van de, S. A. (1996). Molecular mechanisms of steroid action: a novel type of cross-talk between glucocorticoids and NF-kappa B transcription factors. *Eur Respir J Suppl* 22, 146s–153s.

Vgontzas, A. N., Papanicolaou, D. A., Bixler, E. O., Kales, A., Tyson, K., & Chrousos, G. P. (1997). Elevation of plasma cytokines in disorders of excessive daytime sleepiness: role of sleep disturbance and obesity. *J Clin Endocrinol Metab* 82(5), 1313–1316.

Vgontzas, A. N., Papanicolaou, D. A., Bixler, E. O., Lotsikas, A., Zachman, K., Kales, A., Prolo, P., Wong, M. L., Licinio, J., Gold, P. W., Hermida, R. C., Mastorakos, G., & Chrousos, G. P. (1999). Circadian interleukin-6 secretion and quantity and depth of sleep. *J Clin Endocrinol Metab* 84(8), 2603–2607.

14 Reproductive Hormones

CHARLES T. SNOWDON AND TONI E. ZIEGLER

HISTORICAL BACKGROUND

Critical to understanding reproduction is an understanding of hormones. Hormones keep our bodies in balance. They are our chemical messengers. Hormones are secreted into the blood stream to maintain homeostasis. Endocrine and ductless glands, located throughout the body, release hormones into the blood stream affecting tissues in other parts of the body. Only within the latter half of the twentieth century have we understood the connection between the endocrine and nervous systems in their regulation of body function. The nervous system was considered the high-speed information track transmitting by electric stimuli whereas the endocrine system worked at a much slower pace but enacted long-term changes in the body. However, the nervous system not only carries information by electrical impulses from one cell to another but nerve endings also release chemical transmitters which, under some circumstances, circulate in the blood and, thus, can be considered endocrine gland products or hormones (Moore, 1978). To study hormones, it is essential to understand both neuroscience and endocrinology. This chapter examines the interaction of neural and endocrine systems on behavior, immunity, and reproductive function.

The concept of hormones and the endocrine glands was so complex that it took until the middle of the twentieth century to understand endocrinology. To recognize a gland or group of tissue as part of the endocrine system, one needed: (1) an anatomical recognition of glandular tissue, (2) a method to detect secretions from the gland, (3) glandular extracts to test that these secretions influenced other parts of the body, and (4) isolation of the pure hormone, determining its structure and synthesis (Doisy, 1936).

Much of early human behavior was based upon hormonal therapy. In prehistoric times, men ate the organs of their enemies after battle, drank their blood, or devoured extracts of their enemy's organs to obtain their bravery and, unknowingly, their hormones. The first deliberate use of hormone replacement occurred when French neurologist and physiologist, Charles Brown-Séquard (1817–1894), injected endocrine gland extracts from animals into humans to increase energy, or in the case of testicular injections, to rejuvenate "intellectual work and physical powers" (Brown-Séquard, 1889). These original experiments with animal testicular extracts were done by the physicians on themselves with reported increase in "strength, vigor and mental activity as well as increased contractility of the bladder" (Brown-Séquard, 1889). Within a few years, the procedure was called "organotherapy" and the techniques became an acceptable mode of therapeutics (Borell, 1976). Although interest in testicular extract injections faded, treatment with thyroid extracts was used to restore thyroid function in humans (Murray, 1891). Injections of adrenal extracts increased blood pressure (Abel & Crawford, 1897).

Infertility has long been a source of shame and worry. Anatomical description of the gonads and some understanding of their influence on the body were noted in antiquity. Many early societies had an understanding of the reproductive system (for review, see Medvei, 1982) and herbal and physical contraception was in use. Ovaries were described in Aristotle's time (384–322 B.C.) and his *History of Animals* described ovariectomy as a method to increase strength, endurance, and as a contraceptive device for animals. Ovariectomies may have been performed by the ancient Egyptians with the understanding that ovaries were necessary to conception. The importance of testicles was well known during antiquity. Early scholars debated the source of the genetic material, but many agreed with Aristotle that the testicles were the source of male genetic material and determined the sex of the child. Castration was practiced on a large scale, not only on slaves and defeated enemies, but also by the priesthood of various cults and on male attendants in harems. Castrated males, or eunuchs, were known to be sterile, and therefore, were sought after by women for love affairs because there was

Our research and the preparation of this chapter were supported by USPHS Grants MH 35215 and MH 58700. We thank Esther Sternberg for a detailed critique of the chapter.

no danger of pregnancy (Medvei, 1982). Hippocratic writings indicated that the menstrual cycle was known and that timing intercourse to the tenth day after the beginning of the period would increase one's chances for conception (Himes, 1936).

With the invention of microscopes in the seventeenth century, many advances in understanding the reproductive organs were made. The first descriptions of spermatozoa were made by van Leeuwenhoek and were referred to as "little animals of the sperm" or "animalcules"(Van Leeuwenhoek, 1678).

Isolation, purification and synthesis of hormones began in the early 1900s. Adrenaline (epinephrine) was the first hormone isolated (Aldrich, 1901) and synthesized. Estrogens, androgens, and corticosteroids were extracted, isolated, and synthesized in the 1920s and 1930s (Moore et al., 1929; Reichstein, 1936; Dodds et al., 1938). During this time, large quantities of estrogens were discovered in the urine of women, small amounts in the urine of men and tremendous amounts in the urine of pregnant mares. Extracts from pregnant mare urine have been the most popular hormone replacement for postmenopausal women (PREMARIN = PREgnant MARe urINe) until recently when long-term hormonal replacement has been considered risky.

In the 1950s, the neural connections to the endocrine system were beginning to be discovered. G. W. Harris suggested that the release of the pituitary hormones was controlled by humoral factors probably of hypothalamic origin (Harris, 1955). Extracts made from the hypothalamus were found to release some of the anterior pituitary hormones. After this, the race to isolate and identify the structure of the many releasing factors of the hypothalamus was begun by Schally and Guillemin, who worked independently of each other, to be the first to isolate and determine the structure of a releasing hormone. The structure of thyrotropin releasing hormone was first reported by Schally's lab. As reported in *Science*, "This race was monumental in that it lasted for 21 years, involved the creation of two rival teams of experts, and required investing time, money, and reputation in a venture seemed doomed to failure". The two scientists used techniques barely adequate for the job, faced skepticism from their colleagues, and were threatened with withdrawal of government funding if they didn't provide proof of a releasing hormone in a hurry (Wade, 1978). The two labs identified thyrotropin releasing hormone, gonadotropin releasing hormone, and somatostatin. For their perseverance, Schally and Guillemin shared the Nobel Prize in Physiology or Medicine in 1978.

The other large breakthrough was the development of methods to measure minute amounts of circulating and excreted hormones. The first methods were by bioassays. Bioassays measure the functional response of an organism, target organ, tissue, or group of cells to a hormone (Heist & Poland, 1992). For instance, the mouse Leydig cell bioassay for LH employs dispersed Leydig cells from

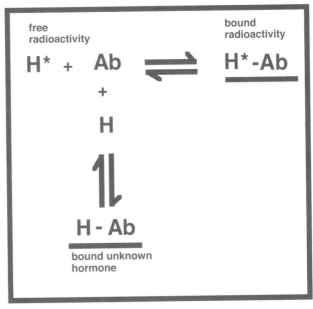

Figure 14.1. The principle of a competitive binding assay. Labeled hormone (H*), either radioactive or enzymatic, is combined with a specific antibody (Ab) made against the hormone (H) to produce labeled-antigen-antibody complexes. Unlabeled hormone also binds with specific antibody and produces antigen-antibody complexes. By separating the bound from the free, a ratio can be set up that will determine the percent bound. Standard amounts of the hormone can be used to create a standard curve and thereby interpret the concentration of the hormone of interest in the sample. Figure adapted from Yalow, 1992, p. 123, *Textbook of Endocrinology*, Wilson, Foster (Eds).

postpubertal male mice testes. The dispersed cells are target cells stimulated by the gonadotropin molecules (LH or CG) present in the sample (blood or urine) and produce a dose-response related increase in testosterone production (Ellingwood & Resko, 1980). Another bioassay uses the steroid-primed uterus of the rat to study oxytocin-induced contraction of the uterus. There are many types of bioassays for determining the biological activity of hormones.

In most cases, however, bioassays were replaced by radioimmunoassays (RIA) except when a difference between the biological response and the immune response was expected. The RIA has provided for both an increase in sensitivity and an increase in specificity. RIA was first developed by Rosalyn Yalow and Seymour Berson 1959 to measure insulin in humans (Yalow & Berson, 1959). Hormones exhibit antigenic properties when the molecular weight of the molecule is high enough. Where the molecular weight is low, such as with steroids, the molecule is conjugated to a higher molecular weight molecule. The underlying principles of RIA consist of combining a radiolabeled hormone with an antibody made specifically for the hormone of interest. The labeled hormone and the antibody produce an antigen-antibody complex where the molecules are bound tightly to each other (Figure 14.1). When an unlabelled hormone (found in blood or any bodily fluid) is added to the system, it competes with the labeled hormone for binding to the antibody

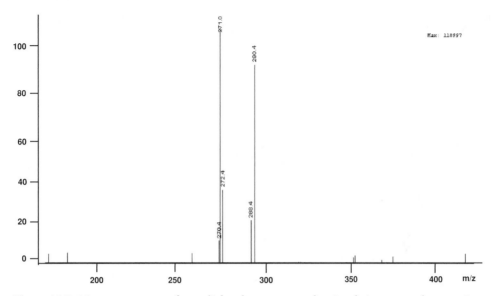

Figure 14.2. Mass spectrogram of estradiol and testosterone showing their mass-to-charge ratios.

and a displacement of radioactivity can be measured. Thus, a higher amount of radioactivity measured indicates less of the hormone of interest in the sample. RIAs have been used extensively since the 1960s to measure hormone concentration and can measure less than a picogram per milliliter of sample (10^{-12} gram per milliliter).

Recently, other methods of measuring hormones have been in use, which reduce the need to remove radioactive wastes. One of the more popular methods is an enzymeimmunoassay (EIA). EIAs have the same principle as RIAs except the hormone has an enzyme tag instead of a radioactive tag. The endpoint uses a color change measurable by spectrophotometry. EIAs have been shown to be as sensitive as RIAs, and in some cases, even more sensitive (Munro & Stabenfeldt, 1984). Other methods of measuring hormones make use of the chemical characteristics of the hormones. Chemical luminescence, fluorescence, chemical detection, and ultraviolet detection of High Pressure Liquid Chromatography (HPLC) separated hormones are all methods that are being used to identify or quantitate hormones.

Mass spectrometry via HPLC or Gas Chromatography encompasses techniques that have been available for many years but have only recently become a benchtop technique applicable to measurements of multiple hormones. These techniques, particularly LC/MS (liquid chromatography/mass spectrometry), can measure multiple hormones simultaneously at very low concentrations. Samples are separated by HPLC, usually using capillary columns that separate hormones to be measured in extremely low levels. The levels of steroid can be as low as subpicogram (femtogram) and can be measured in a volume as low as 1 microliter. Mass spectrometry measures the mass to charge ratio of an individual steroid. For instance, testosterone has a mass of 288 and depending upon the mobile phase (a mixture of buffers and solvents)

will take on electrons, such as hydrogen or sodium, and thereby will be identified at a mass of 289, 290, or 311. Once the mass and its charge are known, a steroid can be found readily and quantified by calibrating the steroid as a standard. All steroid or protein hormones can be measured this way as long as the chromatography method for separation of hormones is well developed. A mass spectral analysis of two steroids, estrone and testosterone, are shown as an on screen analyses in Figure 14.2. The two steroids have similar retention times using this particular method (estrone = 5.75, testosterone = 5.66 minutes) but different masses. Estrone, with a molecular weight of 270, is mainly ionized by hydrogen to yield a mass of 271. Testosterone, with a molecular weight of 288, is primarily ionized by two hydrogen ions to yield a mass of 290.4. These patterns of ionization provide the fingerprint of the individual steroids for identification. Through calibration, multiple steroids (or peptides) can be identified and quantified without the need for antibodies or concerns of cross-reactivities of RIAs or EIAs.

Hormones function by targeting specialized receptors that carry hormones into the cell nucleus where they bind to DNA and activate genes that transcribe proteins to activate enzymes that affect physiology and behavior. It has long been assumed that steroid receptors were activated only by binding with steroidal ligands, but recent work has demonstrated ligand- or steroid-independent activation of steroid receptors is possible and that nuclear receptors bind co-regulatory proteins that can determine whether a particular gene is transcribed or not. Proteins enhancing receptor activation are co-activators and those that suppress activation are co-repressors (Auger, 2004). Steroid receptor co-activators have been found in many tissues – reproductive tract, mammary gland, and brain (Molenda et al., 2003) and at least one of these co-activators (SRC-1) can influence the development of sex-specific

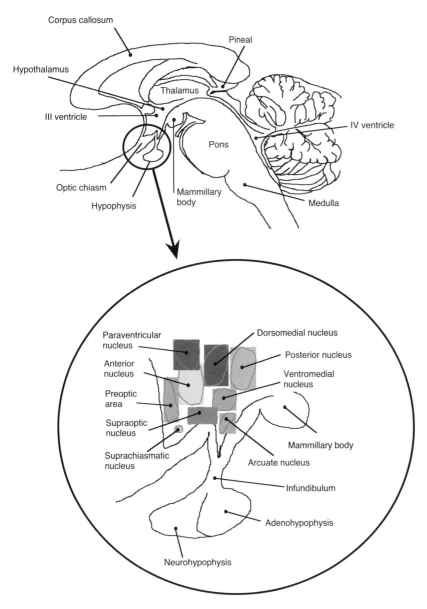

Figure 14.3. Drawing of the major parts of the brain. Circled part in the top diagram illustrates the position of the hypothalamus and pituitary. The hypothalamus and pituitary are shown in the enlarged circle. The hypothalamus is divided into nuclei named for their position. Nerve fibers extend from the hypothalamus into the infundibulum. Production and storage of LH, FSH, GH, TSH, ACTH, and prolactin occur in the adenohypophysis. Vasopressin and Oxytocin are produced in the hypothalamus and stored in the neurohypophysis.

brain morphology and behavior (Auger et al., 2000). Various neurotransmitters including dopamine, associated with motivational arousal and reward, can influence the expression of steroid receptors. What this means is that environmental events such as the behavior of a mate or various types of rewards may lead to expression of, for example, progestin receptors in females in the absence of progesterone. There are many implications of these findings for sexual differentiation and reproductive activation or inhibition (Auger, 2004).

PHYSICAL CONTEXT: ANATOMY AND PHYSIOLOGY OF THE NEUROENDOCRINE SYSTEM

Hypothalamus and pituitary

The brain influences the endocrine system through the hypothalamus (see Riskind & Martin, 1989). The hypotha-

lamus is an extension of the brain stem and is considered to be a phylogenetically ancient structure. The hypothalamus is below the thalamus and forms the walls and lower part of the third ventricle of the brain (Figure 14.3). The third ventricle is part of the fluid canal system that flows into the spinal cord. Links from other areas of the brain to the hypothalamus allow for social and behavioral, visceral, and autonomic controls. The hypothalamus is composed of areas referred to as the tuber cinereum, the infundibulum (also called the median eminence), and the mammillary bodies. Clusters of neurons are located here that secrete neurohormones for regulating the activity of the pituitary. The nerve clusters are named by position: supraoptic nucleus (SON), paraventricular nucleus (PVN), suprachiasmatic nucleus (SCN), ventromedial nucleus (VMN), dorsomedial nucleus (DMN), medial preoptic area (MPOA), arcuate nucleus (ARC), anterior nucleus, and the posterior nucleus. The clusters of neurons contain cell bodies whose axons extend into the infundibulum. Some axons extend into the neural, or anterior pituitary, whereas other neurons produce regulatory hormones that are transported from the median eminence to the anterior pituitary by the hypothalamic-pituitary portal circulation. A rich vascular supply allows transport of the hypothalamic regulatory hormones, neuropeptides, and neurotransmitters to the anterior pituitary.

The pituitary is divided into the anterior and posterior pituitary (also called the adenohypothesis and neurohypothesis). The anterior lobe is composed of three divisions: pars distalis, pars intermedia, and pars tuberalis. The hormone-producing cells are located in the pars distalis. The pars intermedia is very small and rudimentary in humans. The pars tuberalis is the upward extension of the anterior lobe and its attachment to the pituitary stalk. The posterior pituitary is an extension of the hypothalamus consisting of the infundibulum, the infundibular stem and the neural lobe. Two hormones, arginine vasopressin (AVP) and oxytocin (OT), are synthesized in the SON and PVN area of the hypothalamus, transported through elongated axons, and stored in the posterior lobe and from there released into the peripheral circulation. The anterior pituitary synthesizes adrenocorticotropin hormone (ACTH), growth hormone (GH), prolactin (PRL), thyroid stimulating hormone (TSH), luteinizing hormone (LH), follicle stimulating hormone (FSH), and in the pars intermedia, melanocyte-stimulating hormone (MSH) is produced in many mammals but not in adult humans. These hormones, in turn, regulate the hormones produced in the endocrine glands located throughout the body. Table 14.1 shows the relationship between the hypothalamus, pituitary, and target gland hormones.

Hypothalamic control of pituitary hormones can cause a positive release or an inhibitory release of hormones, as occurs with dopamine's inhibition of prolactin release. The anterior pituitary releases hormones in a pulsatile fashion into the blood where they travel to their target glands and exert effect. The hormones in the target glands feed back to both the hypothalamus and the pituitary. In this way the hormonal production of the endocrine glands is continuously monitored and regulated by the brain. The control of pituitary hormones is more complex than demonstrated in Table 14.1. For example, TRH also can stimulate the release of PRL from the pituitary whereas dopamine causes an inhibition of PRL release. OT stored in the posterior pituitary can stimulate the release of PRL (Mori et al., 1990). Although GnRH (gonadotropin releasing hormone) stimulates the release of both LH and FSH, the quantity of release of both these pituitary hormones changes during the ovarian cycle so that at ovulation LH is released as a large surge but during menses and the onset of follicular growth, FSH is released while LH is maintained at basal levels in the blood. More than 16 different neurotransmitters contribute to regulating LH and PRL (see Kordon et al., 1994 for an extensive review).

Table 14.1. Hypothalamic and pituitary hormones and their feedback control

Hypothalamic hormone	Pituitary hormone	Target gland	Feedback hormone
TRH	TSH	Thyroid	T_4 and T_3
GnRH	LH	Gonads	E_2 (women), T (men), P
	FSH	Gonads	Inhibin and (?) E_2 and T
SS	GH	Multiple	IGF 1
GHRH	GH	Multiple	IGF 1
DA, OT, TRH	Prl	Breast Gonads + brain	? E_2, T, P
CRH	ACTH	Adrenal	Cortisol
AVP	ACTH	Adrenal	Cortisol
DA, CRH, GABA	MSH	Skin, fetal adrenal	(?)

Key: ACTH, adrenalcorticotropin hormone; AVP, arginine vasopressin; CRH, corticotropin releasing hormone; DA, dopamine; E_2, estradiol; FSH, follicle stimulating hormone; GABA, gamma-amino-butyric acid; GH, growth hormone; GHRH, Growth hormone releasing hormone; GnRH, gonadotropin releasing hormone; IGF, insulin-like growth factor; LH, luteinizing hormone; MSH, melanocyte stimulating hormone; OT, oxytocin, P, progesterone; Prl, prolactin; SS, somatostatin; T, testosterone; TRH, thyrotropin releasing hormone; TSH, thyroid stimulating hormone.

Source: Adapted from Thorner et al. (1992).

Neurotransmitters control the secretion of releasing hormones and are secreted from neurons, which may be linked, to other neuronal inputs or to sensory neurons receptive to endogenous and exogenous cues. Neurotransmitters may have an inhibitory or a stimulatory effect. Small-molecule neurotransmitters mediate rapid reactions, whereas neuropeptides tend to modulate slower, ongoing brain functions. Small-molecule neurotransmitters consist of: acetylcholine, the amino acids such as glutamate, aspartate, GABA, glycine, the catecholamines such as dopamine, norepinephrine, epinephrine, serotonin, and histamine (Purves et al., 1997). Neuropeptides include enkephalins, endorphins, cholecystokinin (CCK), vasoactive intestinal peptide (VIP), neuropeptide-Y, AVP, OT, and angiotensin-II.

The main feedback control of anterior pituitary hormones comes from the release of steroids from the target endocrine glands. These include the adrenal gland, the thyroid gland, the gonads (ovaries and testes), the pancreas, the pineal and the placenta. Steroids secreted from these glands are released into the bloodstream to exert their effect on many tissues in the body. They also reach the pituitary and the hypothalamus to exert the negative feedback loop to control their own secretion.

Neurohypophysis hormones: oxytocin and arginine vasopressin

The nonapeptides, OT and AVP, are structurally closely related while serving distinct physiological roles. Both hormones consist of nine amino acids folded into a ring through a disulfide bridge with a terminal tripeptide side chain. The hormones differ by only two amino acids. Classically, OT is known for its control of milk release from the mammary gland and the contractions of the uterus during labor whereas AVP (also referred to as antidiuretic hormone) is involved with water balance. Actually both hormones serve many other functions within the body. They are involved in the processes of learning and memory, especially in a social context (Engelmann et al., 1996; Heinrichs et al., 2004). OT and AVP are released from the posterior pituitary into the bloodstream but they also serve a role in interneuronal communication. Both substances are released synaptically from axon terminals, dendrites and somata of hypothalamic neurons. Central actions include a variety of autonomic, endocrine and behavioral effects (Engelmann et al., 1996). Concentration of AVP and OT in the extracellular fluid of discrete brain areas is several orders of magnitude higher than peripheral levels in the blood.

The role of OT as a maternal hormone is without doubt. OT is not only responsible for milk letdown during nursing but is known for induction of contractions during labor. OT facilitates mother-infant interactions and has an inhibitory effect on aggressive behavior in rats (Giovenardi et al., 1997). Pairbond formation in monogamous prairie voles appears to be influenced by OT released centrally in the brain (Carter, 1998). OT may facilitate both social contact and attachment and the regulation of the parasympathetic functions (see below). OT inhibits CRH-mediated ACTH secretion in men. OT regulates receptor-mediated mechanisms within the amygdala involved in passive stress-coping strategies, which might be mediated via inhibitory influence on the local release of excitatory amino acids during stress (Ebner et al., 2004). OT has effects on female sexual receptivity (lordosis in rodents), penile erection, and male mounting behavior (Rao, 1995).

AVP, on the other hand, is associated with regulating defensive behaviors such as arousal, attention, or vigilance – increased aggressive behavior with an increase in sympathetic functions (Carter & Altemus, 1997). In monogamous male prairie voles, however, AVP induces pair bond formation and promotes parental behavior (Wang et al., 1994). AVP induces the contraction or relaxation of certain types of smooth muscle and it promotes the movement of water and sodium across responsive epithelial tissues, especially the kidney (Hadley, 1992).

Interestingly, these two peptides might be synergistic in promoting parenting behavior (Bales et al., 2004). OT and AVP have been shown to be anxiolytic (Uvnas-Moberg, 1997; Appenrodt et al., 1998; Dharmadhikari et al., 1997). Reducing the phobic responses to newborn infants is crit-ical to promoting parental behaviors ensuring the success of the offspring (Pryce, 1996).

The structure of the glands

The major glands secreting hormones are listed in Table 14.2, but many tissues in the body secrete chemical messengers. In the gastro-intestinal tract alone there are at least 10 hormones recognized. Other tissues that release chemical messengers are: skin, liver, kidney, heart, plasma, and various tissues releasing growth factors considered to be hormones. Here we briefly discuss the adrenal glands and then concentrate on the gonads with their communication to the brain and hypothalamus.

Adrenals

The adrenals are located directly above the kidneys and about one-tenth the size of kidneys. Each adrenal consists of two functionally distinct endocrine glands. The cortex is the steroid-secreting gland consisting of cells grouped into: the zona glomerulosa, zona fasciculata, and zona reticularis. The zona glomerulosa produces mineralocorticoids, such as aldosterone, which promotes sodium retention and potassium excretion, both regulating extracellular fluid volume (Bartter et al., 1956). The zona fasciculata and zona reticularis secrete glucocorticoids and androgens including dehydroepiandrosterone (DHEA) and androstenedione. The major human glucocorticoid is cortisol. The adrenal medulla is an endocrine gland derived from the neural crest. Epinephrine is the predominant catecholamine released from the medulla. The close anatomical coupling and functional interrelations between the adrenal cortex and medulla suggest that these two tissues may provide an integrated functional unit (Hadley, 1992).

Cortisol is well known for its role in the stress response and discussion of glucocorticoids can be found in other chapters. Both higher and lower amounts of cortisol than the physiological levels lead to disease states. Superphysiological levels can modulate mood, influence sleep patterns, cognition, and the reception of sensory input (McEwen, 1979). Cortisol has an inhibitory influence on the reproductive system. During prolonged stress, beta-endorphin, and CRH inhibit the release of GnRH. Stress causes the pituitary to be less sensitive to GnRH and glucocorticoids inhibit ovarian sensitivity to LH (Sapolsky, 1992), thus decreasing the likelihood of reproduction. Additionally, gonadal hormones influence the reactivity of the hypothalamic-pituitary-adrenal axis to stress. Estrogens enhance the HPA activity and androgens attenuate the response (Lund et al., 2004).

Epinephrine, synthesized and stored in the adrenal medulla is also released centrally from neurons, but is the primary catecholamine known to be released peripherally. The adrenal medulla is under the direct and exclusive control of the central nervous system. Functionally, catecholamines are neurochemical transducers that convert

Table 14.2. Endocrine glands in mammals and the major known hormones

Gland	Secreted hormone
Anterior pituitary	Growth Hormone
	Prolactin
	Melanophore stimulating hormone
	Adrenocorticotropin
	Luteinizing hormone
	Follicle stimulating hormone
	Thyroid stimulating hormone
Posterior pituitary	Arginine vasopressin
	Oxytocin
Thyroid gland	Thyroxin
	Calcitonin
Adrenal cortex	Glucocorticoids
	Corticosterone
	Cortisol
	Dihydroepiandosterone
	Mineralocorticoids
	Aldosterone
Adrenal medulla	Epinephrine
	Norepinephrine
	Enkephalins
	Endorphins
Kidney	Renin
	Angiotensin
Liver	Preangiotensin
Pancreas	Insulin
	Glucagon
Stomach and intestines	Gastrin
	Secretin
	Cholecystokinin
	Gastric inhibitory peptide
	Vasoactive inhibitory peptide
	Chymodium
	Motilin
	Neurotensin
	Substance P
	Gastrin releasing peptide
Pineal	Melatonin
Ovary	Estrogens
	Estradiol
	Estrone
	Progesterone
	Inhibin
Testes	Androgens
	Testosterone
	Dihydrotestosterone
	Androstenedione

electrical neural activity into physiological responses. Catecholamine effects are induced rapidly and dissipate quickly, unlike the slower, more prolonged effects of most hormones. The catecholamines maintain the constancy of the body's internal environment.

In summary, adrenal glands have both an endocrine and neural component. The main function of the adrenals is to maintain homeostasis. Through secretions of epinephrine by the adrenal medulla and glucocorticoids by the adrenal cortex, the body responds rapidly to a change in homeostasis with the release of neurally controlled epinephrine– or more slowly for a longer duration with release of the endocrine-controlled glucocorticoids.

Ovaries

The ovaries control reproduction in the female. Here ova are produced and the hormones that regulate the female sexual life are synthesized. Both the development of the ovum and the synthesis of steroid hormones are under the control of the hypothalamo-pituitary-ovarian axis. Figure 14.4 shows the reproductive organs of the human female. The ovaries lie laterally and posteriorly in the pelvic wall attached to the posterior surface of the broad ligament by a peritoneal fold termed the mesovarian. The ovary consists of three regions: the cortex containing the germinal epithelium and the follicles, the central medulla consisting of stroma and a hilum where the attachment of the ovary to the mesovarian ligament occurs (Carr, 1992). The primordial follicles lie near the periphery of the cortex and contain the primordial germ cells that give rise to the oocytes. The number of oocytes is fixed by birth in the female at about 1 million per ovary. The primordial follicles begin the process of meiosis within the embryo and became arrested in the prophase of mitosis by birth of the fetus. After puberty the endocrine system initiates the continued maturation of the follicles.

During each ovarian cycle six to 12 primary follicles develop into secondary follicles. The size of the oocyte and the number of layers of the granulosa cells that surround the ovum increase. A zona pellucida is formed and granulosa cells begin to develop. Usually only one or two follicles continue to develop beyond this stage and the others end in atresia. As a follicle develops, granulosa cells continue to mature and the interstitial tissue surrounding the follicle differentiates into two layers: theca externa and theca interna. As the follicle enlarges, a single large vesicle is formed. A mature follicle is called a Graafian follicle. The mechanisms controlling the rupture of the mature follicle involves the sequestering of leukocytes as part of the inflammatory process (Bonello et al., 2004) initiated by the release of LH from the pituitary. The LH causes rapid secretion of follicular steroid hormones and begins the conversion to secreting progesterone. At this time, the outside capsule of the follicle (theca externa) begins secreting proteolytic enzymes, weakening the capsular wall and increasing follicular swelling. New blood vessel growth occurs rapidly in the follicle wall and prostaglandins are secreted

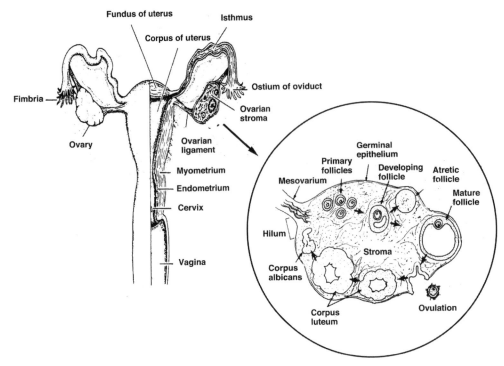

Figure 14.4. The reproductive organs of the human female. An enlargement of the ovary and the process of ovulation are shown in the circle. Parts of this figure were adapted from Niswender and Nett, 1988, p. 490, *The Physiology of Reproduction*, Knobil, Neill (Eds).

in the follicular tissues. The prostaglandins act as local hormones causing vasodilation of blood vessels (Guyton & Hall, 1996). Plasma flows into the follicle increasing the swelling, and the follicle ruptures. During ovulation, the fimbria of the uterine tubes (Fallopian tubes) spread over most of the medial surface of the ovary and provide wave-like movements to draw in the ovulated ova. The ovum moves down the Fallopian tubes where fertilization takes place. After fertilization the embryo moves into the fundus of the uterus where implantation and growth takes place. If fertilization does not take place, then prostagandins secreted by the endometrium of the uterus initiate lute-olysis of the corpus luteum. After the follicle ruptures, it fills with blood forming the corpus hemorrhagicum. Both granulosa cells and thecal cells begin increasing in number. The granulosa cells begin to accumulate large quantities of cholesterol in a process is termed luteinization. The corpus luteum is now formed and will remain large for about 14 days before regression.

Ovarian steroids are derived from the follicle and cor-pus luteum. There are three types: estrogens, androgens, and progestogens. During the follicular phase, estrogens are the major steroids secreted from the ovary whereas during the luteal phase and pregnancy, progesterone is the major steroid hormone secreted. Ovarian steroids, like all steroids including cortisol, are derived from choles-terol. Estradiol is biosynthesized from cholesterol via ste-riodogenic pathways shown in Figure 14.5. The thecal cells synthesize androgens, androstenedione, and testosterone, from cholesterol via pregnenolone, primarily through

dihydroepiandosterone. The androgens are transferred to the granulosa cells where they are aromatized to estro-gens. During follicular maturation the ability of granulosa cells to aromatize androgens into estradiol increases. Low levels of estradiol exert a negative feedback on pituitary LH. Peak levels of estradiol feed back to the hypothala-mus and pituitary to initiate the release of GnRH, which in turn releases LH and FSH. With the LH/FSH surge, progesterone biosynthesis begins in the granulosa cells. Progesterone acts on the hypothalamus to decrease LH and FSH secretion. As progesterone levels decline, pitu-itary gonadotropins begin secreting and initiate the next set of follicle growth. Other ovarian hormones help to reg-ulate the pituitary's influence on the ovary such as follicular activin, which exerts a positive release on FSH and follic-ular inhibin and follistatin that exert an inhibitory effect on FSH release.

At puberty, estrogens stimulate the continued develop-ment of the vagina, uterus, and oviducts. Secondary sexual characteristics developed at this time are due to estrogen secretion. However, ovarian androgens are also responsi-ble for some of the changes of puberty, such as pubic and axillary hair growth, acne, and sebaceous gland activity. Estrogen secretion also affects the distribution of fat and mammary growth and development typical to females.

Progesterone prepares and maintains the reproduc-tive tract for the embryo during pregnancy. Progesterone inhibits uterine contractions, increases the viscosity of the cervical mucus, promotes glandular development of the breast, and increases body temperature. The sequence of

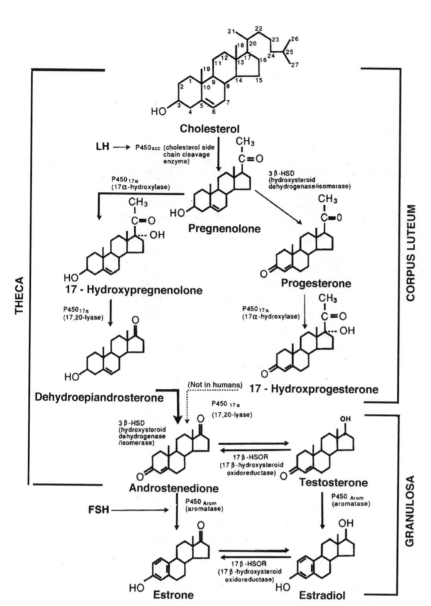

Figure 14.5. Steroidogenic pathway of ovarian steroids.

estrogen-primed tissue with increasing levels of progesterone has been implicated in triggering sexual behavior in many mammals.

Steroids and other hormones regulate specific target tissues by interacting with specific receptors. Hormone-specific receptors are located in plasma membranes, in the cell cytosol (cytoplasm) or in the nucleus. Estradiol receptors may bind with other substances that resemble estradiol. Many compounds, which bind to estrogen receptors, have estrogen-like effects on the body. Estrogen-like compounds, such as synthetic diethylstilbestrol or naturally occurring plant estrogens can mediate estrogen effects in the body producing physiological responses (Miksicek, 1993).

Ovulation occurs on average once every 28 days in the nonpregnant woman. However, many social and stressful events can influence cycle length or puberty onset. Olfactory cues from men can affect the length of ovarian cycles. The actual axillary secretions of men reduce the

variability in menstrual cycle lengths, whereas women's axillary secretions synchronize the onset of the menstrual cycle in recipient women (Preti et al., 1986; Cutler et al., 1986). Menstrual cycle synchrony has been demonstrated in women living in a college dormitory and among close friends (McClintock, 1971). Chemical signals from different times of a donor's cycle will either shorten (follicular cues) or lengthen (luteal cues) the recipient's cycle (Stern & McClintock, 1998). Factors of close bonding, or friendship, affect cycle synchrony (Goldman & Schneider, 1987; Weller & Weller, 1993, 1995). The presence of unrelated men in the home accelerate the timing of menarche in girls whereas the physical exposure of a related male may delay menarche (Surbey, 1990). (See subsequent sections for more details).

Testes

Testes produce both the sperm necessary for fertilization and the steroid hormones that regulate sperm production

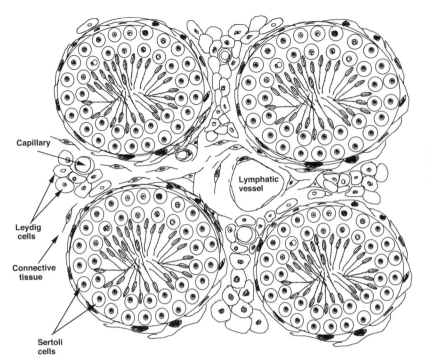

Capillary

Leydig
cells

Connective
tissue

Sertoli
cells

Lymphatic
vessel

Figure 14.6. Diagram of the testicular tissue in man showing the arrangement of the Sertoli cells with spermatocytes and the interstitial tissue containing the Leydig cells where testosterone is produced.

and male sexual life (Griffin & Wilson, 1992). The testes lie outside the abdominal cavity within the scrotal sac. Descent of the testes from the abdominal cavity where development takes place occurs during the latter two thirds of gestation. In the adult male, the testes have two components necessary for sexual function. Figure 14.6 shows the structures of the seminiferous tubules and the steroid producing Leydig cells. The tubules produce and transport the sperm to the excretory-ejaculatory ducts. Steroid-producing Leydig cells are located outside the seminiferous tubules. They contain lipid droplets of cholesterol that serve as a substrate for testosterone synthesis. Testosterone is metabolized from cholesterol by conversion to pregnenolone with subsequent 17-hydroxylation synthesis through dehydroepiandrosterone and androstenedione to testosterone as occurs in the ovary (Figure 14.5). Dehydroepiandrosterone and androstenedione are also end products of the Leydig cells but in small amounts and with low physiological potencies. Little testosterone is stored within the Leydig cells because the newly synthesized testosterone diffuses quickly into the blood from nearby capillary cells (Hadley, 1992).

The seminiferous tubules are filled with Sertoli cells that give rise to the spermatocytes. FSH interacts with receptors on the Sertoli cells to induce the synthesis of an androgen-binding protein (ABP). ABP is secreted into the lumen of the seminiferous tubules. The Leydig cells respond to LH stimulation and produce testosterone. Testosterone is also actively transported into the seminiferous tubules where it becomes bound to ABP within the Sertoli cells. The spermatocytes begin the process of maturation under the influence of testosterone. Mature sperm are stored in the epididymis where they develop the potential for fertilization and motility.

GnRH is released in an episodic manner into the hypophyseal portal system causing LH and FSH release in a pulsatile manner. The rate of secretion of LH, however, is controlled by the feedback action of gonadal steroids on the hypothalamus and the pituitary. Both testosterone and estradiol exert a negative feedback on LH. Testosterone can be converted to estradiol in the brain and pituitary. The ratio of testosterone to estradiol appears to influence the release of FSH (Sherins et al., 1982). FSH is also controlled by negative feedback from inhibin produced by the Sertoli cells under the influence of FSH.

Although testosterone is the main steroid secreted by the testes, it actually serves as a precursor for two types of active metabolites that have a higher biological activity than testosterone and provide the androgen effects on the body. Testosterone (T) can be reduced by 5-alpha-reductase to dihydrotestosterone (DHT). The conversion can take place in the prostate and seminal vesicles or in peripheral tissues. DHT mediates the growth promotion, differentiation, and functional aspects of male sexual development. The ratio of DHT to testosterone levels changes rapidly at the onset of puberty to favor the more potent DHT (Ginther et al., 2002). Alternatively, testosterone can be aromatized to estrogens in extraglandular tissues. Estrogens can act in concert with the androgens but more often estrogens have the opposite effect from androgens. Androgens can act directly on the brain to affect the male's behavior. Acting on other androgen-sensitive tissues, including accessory sex organs, androgens may affect behavior indirectly.

Sexual development into male or female proceeds from the establishment of genetic sex at the time of conception. Genetic sex governs the development of gonadal sex, which in turn, regulates the development of phenotypic sex, which is the differentiation of internal and external sex organs and the attainment of adult secondary sexual characteristics. In mammals the gonads and accessory glands develop toward the female unless influenced by the Y chromosome (Roberts, 1988). The Y chromosome triggers the genital ridges in the embryo to develop into testes rather than ovaries. The differentiation toward the male gonadal and body phenotype requires the inductive actions of gonadal androgens. Female ovarian and genital development may be considered an autonomous process requiring no hormonally active inductive substances. Removal of the gonads from indifferent embryos of either sex results in development of a female genotype (Bardin & Catterall, 1981). The timing of androgen exposure to the brain is important for physiological and behavioral processes. Deprivation of testosterone in the male animal during his species-specific critical time of brain differentiation will result in a female pattern of sexual dimorphic behavior (see below).

REPRODUCTIVE HORMONES AND IMMUNE DISEASES

Many autoimmune and rheumatic diseases occur at different rates in men and women suggesting a potential role for reproductive hormones in these disorders. For example, rheumatoid arthritis, Sjogren's (or dry-eye syndrome), systematic lupus erythematosis (lupus), scleroderma, and multiple sclerosis all occur much more often in women than in men and ankylosing spondylitis occurs much more often in men. Furthermore rheumatoid arthritis, lupus, and multiple sclerosis have typical onset during the peak reproductive years when estrogen and progestin levels are high whereas dry-eye syndrome appears to correlate with the onset of menopause (Butts & Sternberg, 2004). Despite the correlational evidence direct involvement of reproductive hormones is known for only a few of these diseases. Lupus can arise early in puberty and has decreased severity during menses, suggesting direct hormonal involvement. Oral contraceptives exacerbate symptoms, and women have high levels of estrogen and low levels of androgens. Experimental studies show that estradiol can block B-cell tolerance and induce a lupus-like syndrome in mice (Bynoe et al., 2000). High prolactin concentrations are associated with lupus and early death was induced with prolactin in an animal model of lupus (Walker et al., 1998).

Although the major steroid influences on rheumatoid arthritis are adrenal glucocorticoids, experimental animal studies suggest that long-term androgen treatment may protect cartilage from inflammatory breakdown. Estrogen may also be critical because symptoms are reduced during early pregnancy when estrogen levels are high (Cutolo, 1998). Dry-eye syndrome develops at the time of menopause suggesting that the reduction of gonadal steroids might influence the disease, but women with estrogen replacement therapy have a higher incidence of dry-eye syndrome and estradiol and progesterone treat-

ment of mice have significant effects on the expression of many genes regulating the lachrymal gland (Suzuki et al., 2002).

SOCIAL CONTEXT

Introduction

Many of the most interesting behavioral phenomena of life (behavioral sex differences, courtship, sex, parental care, aggression, cognition) are to some degree influenced by reproductive hormones, and psychophysiological research plays an important role in discovering the relative role of the hormones versus environmental and social factors influencing these phenomena.

We review seven broad areas here: What is the role of genes, hormones, and social environment on the development of sex differences? What is the interaction of hormones and social environment on puberty and reproductive maturation? How do hormones influence affiliative behavior, courtship, and pair bonding? Do hormones influence behavior across the ovarian cycle, and how do social interactions influence ovarian function? What is the relative role of hormones and social behavior on parental care? Are there sex differences in aggression and do these differences result from hormonal differences? Finally, how do reproductive hormones influence memory and cognition?

Development of behavioral sex differences

There is great diversity in how sex is determined biologically, and within mammals there are many places where sex determination can go awry. In mammals, the ovum always contains an X chromosome and sperm can be either X or Y, meaning that the father's sperm determines the sex of the offspring. In birds, however, males are homogametic (with two Z chromosomes) and ova contain either W or Z chromosomes, meaning that mothers determine the sex of their offspring (Breedlove, 1992). In some reptiles there are no sex chromosomes, and sex is determined by the temperature at which the eggs are incubated (Bull & Vogt, 1979). Some species of fish are sequentially hermaphroditic (female then male or male then female) – changing sex in response to the social structure of the group – or simultaneously hermaphroditic (trading sex roles and gametes during a sexual interaction (Demski, 1987). Postmaturational sex changes are influenced by social cues such as dominance interactions with larger individuals dominating. In some species sex is determined by relative size as a juvenile (Francis & Barlow, 1993).

In mammals, the Y chromosome contains a gene that stimulates fetal testes development, and secretions from the fetal testes lead to differentiation of male external genitalia and internal accessory organs. In the absence of testicular hormones or their receptors, female external genitalia and internal accessory organs develop. Thus, being female is the default value in mammalian fetal development (Eve had to precede Adam).

Research on rodents demonstrated that manipulation of fetal or perinatal hormone levels influenced the development of sex-typical behavior. Injections of testosterone to fetal females produced male-like behavior in adults. Subsequently, female rats injected with estrogen also displayed masculine behavior. How could this happen? Testosterone may be converted to estrogen by the aromatase enzyme found in the hypothalamus. In rodents, alpha-feto-protein binds plasma estrogen in female fetuses, preventing exposure of the female brain to maternal estrogen. Testosterone is not bound to alpha-feto-protein in the brain, where it is aromatized into estrogen and masculinizes neural structures (Breedlove, 1992). However, in spotted hyenas where females dominate males and have an extremely enlarged clitoris, infant females have very high levels of androgens although adult females do not exhibit high androgen levels (Van Jaarsveld & Skinner, 1991; Glickman et al., 1992).

Hormonal manipulations in nonhuman primates have used (a) injection of testosterone to females at various stages of fetal development and (b) administration of drugs to block testosterone secretion in males. Injections of testosterone to fetal females masculinized the expression of rough-and-tumble play and double-foot clasp mounts (Goy, 1970; Goy & Resko, 1972). Goy, Bercovitch, and McBrair (1988) used short-term doses of testosterone that did not masculinize genitalia and still reported increases in rough play and mounting behavior. Injections of diethylstilbestrol, a synthetic estrogen that often has masculinizing effects on human females, had little effect on male behavior but had a limited masculinizing effect on female macaques (Goy & Deputte, 1996). Wallen et al. (1995) injected fetal male monkeys with a gonadotropin releasing hormone antagonist to block testosterone secretion and found no effects on male behavior development.

Environment may influence sexual differentiation. Intrauterine position can affect sex-typical behavior and in hamsters females gestating between two male fetuses will give birth themselves to a higher proportion of male offspring than females gestated between two female fetuses (Clark & Galef, 1995). Postnatal social environments are also important. Goldfoot and associates (1984) reared rhesus macaques in isosexual groups and found aspects of behavior typical to each sex within the isosexual groups. In all-female groups, some showed male-like mounting and reduced female-like presenting; the opposite was found in all-male groups. Dimorphic behavior in rhesus macaques can be modulated by social experience and group composition.

In humans there are several hormonal disorders that provide analogs to the experiments with monkeys. Androgen-insensitive males have normal testes that secrete testosterone, but the receptor tissues are insensitive to testosterone. As a result, the internal accessory organs and external genitalia are female. Because the testes and adrenal glands secrete small amounts of estrogen, these androgen-insensitive males develop breasts and other female secondary sex characteristics at puberty. Generally, they discover they are genetic males only when they fail to menstruate. These genetic males identify themselves as female, suggesting the importance of sexual anatomy on sexual identification. (Breedlove, 1992).

A second disorder occurs when the enzyme needed to convert testosterone to dihydrotestosterone (5-alpha-reductase) is missing. Dihydrotestosterone is needed for the masculinization of external genitalia. A genetic male is born with testes inside the labia and an enlarged clitoris instead of a penis. In the Dominican Republic there is a population where this genetic disorder is relatively common. Children are typically reared as girls, but with the surge of testosterone at puberty leading to secondary sex characteristics, the children start taking on male roles and wearing men's clothes (Imperator-McGinley et al., 1979). The culture appears to support the social transition from girlhood to young manhood.

Fetal females can be exposed to exceptional levels of testosterone through congenital adrenal hyperplasia (CAH) where the adrenal gland lacks the enzyme needed to convert androstenedione to cortisol. Cortisol is not sufficient to stop production of ACTH, and thus the adrenal gland produces high levels of androgens. Some synthetic progestins and estrogens (e.g., diethylstilbestrol, used to sustain pregnancies in women with a history of hormonal insufficiency) also have androgenic effects.

The results are that genitals are often ambiguous at birth, with an enlarged clitoris that may resemble a penis and fused labia that resemble a scrotum. Ehrhardt and Money (1967) described the androgenized girls as becoming more tomboyish and athletic, preferring male playmates and male clothes and preferring career to marriage. But these tomboys of the 1960s sound like ideal feminist girls of the 2000s. More recent work (Berenbaum & Hines, 1992) also reports that girls with CAH prefer to play with male typical toys. Zucker and colleagues (1996) found that women with CAH recalled more cross-gender role behavior and expressed less comfort with their sense of "femininity" than unaffected cousins or sisters of similar age. Adult CAH women had lower rates of heterosexual fantasy and fewer heterosexual relationships. However, there were no differences between CAH women and controls in relationship status or sexual relations with women. Three women lived in a male gender role, two having been reared as boys and one having switched gender role during adolescence.

Meyer-Bahlburg and associates (1996) studied four CAH women who lived as men. Each had masculine childhood gender-role behavior, each was sexually attracted only to females, and each had changed gender gradually. A combination of gender-atypical behavioral image, a gender-atypical body image, and sexual attraction to women was involved in the gender change.

The work on ligand-independent activation and co-activation of nuclear steroid receptors by a variety of mechanisms including neurotransmitters described above (Auger, 2004) suggests that future research may discover many other mechanisms that influence sex-role determination and gender identity.

In summary, there is no simple role for reproductive hormones in sociosexual development. The social structure of rearing groups, the responses of parents to genital development, and individual difference appear to play important roles. The prenatal hormonal environment predisposes responses by caretakers toward infants and influences development. As Wallen concluded "Social context and biological predispositions are indispensable components in the development of behavioral sex differences" (1996, p. 377).

Influences on puberty and fertility

The social regulation of puberty has been well studied in rodents, where pheromonal control of reproductive maturation is clear (Vandenbergh, 1987). A female mouse exposed to the odor of an adult male reaches puberty sooner than expected, and a young female exposed to the odors of cycling females reaches puberty later than expected. In areas with high population density, female mice reach puberty at a much later age than do mice in low-density populations (Vandenbergh, 1987). Thus the social regulation of puberty has direct effects on regulating population density.

Social regulation of fertility is common in cooperatively breeding mammals, where only one or two females breed while the other females do not (canids, Moehlman & Hofer, 1997; voles, Carter et al., 1986; dwarf mongoose, Creel et al., 1992; naked mole rats, Faulkes & Abbott, 1997, Clarke & Faulkes, 1998; marmosets and tamarins, Snowdon, 1996; French, 1997). We followed the reproductive hormones of 31 postpubertal cotton-top tamarin females housed with mothers in intact families and found no evidence of ovulation (Snowdon, 1996), yet in golden lion tamarins French and Stribley (1987) demonstrated synchronous estrogen cycles between mothers and daughters. In both captive common marmosets (Saltzman et al., 1997) and pygmy marmosets (Carlson et al., 1997), some females ovulate within the natal family but do not become pregnant. Transfer of scents from the mother to a daughter newly paired with a novel male delayed the onset of ovulation compared with control females (Barrett et al., 1990; Savage et al., 1988). Stimulation by a novel male is also important (Widowski et al., 1990). Females removed from their mother and housed with a brother failed to ovulate, but the mere sight, sound, or smell of a novel male induced ovulation (Widowski et al., 1992). Clark and Galef (2001) report reproductive inhibition in female gerbils occurring between sisters but this is accentuated when an older, dominant female is present, so that reproduction is less likely with familiar males compared with novel males. Recent fathers had a higher latency of impregnating young females than other males.

There is little evidence of reproductive suppression in males in marmosets and tamarins (Ginther et al., 2001, 2002), but in spotted hyenas natal adult males had lower testosterone levels than immigrant males whose T levels directly correlated with social rank (Holekamp & Smale, 1998). The mechanism of reproductive inhibition in a cichlid fish is directly related to changes in size of gonadotropin-releasing hormone cells in the brain which become larger as males switch from subordinate to territorial and decrease as males switch from territorial to subordinate (Francis et al., 1993).

Puberty acceleration and delay in rodents, reproductive inhibition in cooperatively breeding mammals and dominance effects on fertility may seem to have little relevance to human reproduction, but social influences do affect human reproductive functioning.

Surbey (1990) found that girls experiencing the absence of father or of both parents prior to menarche reached puberty 4–5 months sooner than girls in biparental families. Family size, birth order, socioeconomic status, body weight, and height were similar between girls in biparental families and girls in father-absent families. Girls with stepfathers matured two months sooner than other girls, supporting the novel-male result with tamarins and gerbils. Mothers and daughters were highly correlated in age of menarche. Maternal age of menarche, years of contact with father, and stressful life events each affected the age of puberty in girls. Gerra et al. (1993) reported lower basal levels of luteinizing hormone in adolescent girls from divorced families compared with girls in intact families. Intense physical training or low body fat can lead to a delay in menarche or to anovulatory cycles in women already past menarche (Frisch, 2002). After exercise stress, girls from divorced families had lower responses of growth hormone and prolactin, suggesting other hormonal disorders in children of single-parent families.

Affiliation, bonding, and courtship

Although sexual behavior and parental care have been well studied, the precursors of courtship and pair bonding have been studied less (however, see Carter, 1998). In many species sexual contact is relatively brief, but in humans (and in many other socially monogamous or cooperatively breeding species) a long-term relationship involving nonconceptive sexual and affiliative behavior is established between mates. Such bonds can be evaluated by several methods: brief separations and reunions to see if affiliation is increased on reunions, intruder challenges when same-sex intruders are presented, and tests to choose between one's mate and another individual. These tests have been used to evaluate a mother-infant bond but less often to study the relationships between adults.

Recently, there has been increased interest in the hormonal correlates of pair bonding and affiliation. Female prairie voles, a monogamous species showing strong pair bonds, have increased oxytocin levels following the extensive vaginal cervical stimulation resulting from initial mating. After a prolonged mating bout, females form strong partner preferences. Intracerebral injections of oxytocin can facilitate pair-bond formation in female voles, and administration of oxytocin inhibitors can block pair formation (Carter, 1998).

In male voles, vasopressin administration influences partner choice and also leads to increased levels of territory defense and mate guarding. Increased levels of vasopressin may influence parental care in male prairie voles (Wang & Insel, 1996). The distribution of vasopressin receptor sites in the brain differs between monogamous and polygynous species of voles, and parallel differences as a function of breeding system are found in the distribution of oxytocin receptors in female voles (Wang & Insel, 1996). The vasopressin receptor, V1a, can be transferred from a male prairie vole (biparental) to a male meadow vole (promiscuous) inducing male meadow voles to mate for life. These genetically modified meadow voles have dopaminergic motivational circuits activated by vasopressin (Konner, 2004). Dopaminergic neural circuits are known to be active in the cravings expressed in addiction and substance abuse as well, suggesting that social attachment or pair bonds might be considered as a form of addictive disorder (Insel, 2003). However, oxytocin inhibits the development of tolerance to morphine and cocaine and attenuates symptoms of withdrawal (Kovacs et al., 1998). How can oxytocin related attachment be addictive if oxytocin blocks addictions?

Recent studies on both masturbatory and coital sex in men and women have reported an increase in prolactin at the time of orgasm (Exton et al., 2001, Krueger et al., 2003). Prolactin and dopamine have mutual inhibitory influences, and prolactin-releasing peptides can activate oxytocin cells (Zhu & Onaka, 2003). If we view the dopamine system as mediating arousal and the prolactin-oxytocin system as mediating arousal reduction or reward, then prolactin and oxytocin may have their major effects as "reward" hormones in positive social settings that can be conditioned to aspects of the mate (voice, appearance, odor) that serve to form and maintain a pair bond.

Adrenal steroids (corticosterone) are higher in monogamous voles than in polygynous voles (Carter, 1998), and oxytocin reduces levels of adrenal steroids in both rodents and humans (Carter & Altemus, 1997). Thus, one consequence of pair bonding may be reduction of stress hormones (Carter, 1998). Little is known about the hormonal basis of pair bonding in nonhuman and human primates. However, in the monogamous titi monkey, Mendoza and Mason (1997) found that (1) pairs spend much time in physical contact and (2) adrenal hormones rise to very high levels when mates are separated and return to normal levels at pair reunion. Wang et al. (1997) found fibers in the brains of common marmosets – monogamous primates – that had distributions of reactivity to vasopressin and oxytocin similar to those in monogamous voles. Future

research using minimally invasive methods is needed to evaluate the importance of oxytocin and vasopressin on pair bonding in primates.

Sexual behavior and changes over the menstrual cycle

Role of hormones in sexual behavior

Reproductive hormones appear to be important for copulatory behavior in many species. Removal of gonads prior to puberty may produce a failure to express sexual behavior, and removal of gonads after puberty can also reduce or eliminate sexual activity. Yet in primates (both human and nonhuman), sexual arousal and sexual behavior may continue for years after castration. Although testes size decreases and testosterone levels decline in men over 60, men over 80 can be sexually active. Correlations between testosterone and sexual activity are weak (Carter, 1992). Males who are hypogonadal due to Kallman's syndrome (a deficiency of gonadotropin-releasing hormone) have very low testosterone levels and do not experience puberty without hormonal supplementation. They also show low interest in sex, low sexual activity, and few nocturnal erections or emissions. When testosterone is administered, sexual interest does not appear within a year of injections. Although testosterone is not essential for sexual activity or interest, reduced testosterone levels generally correlate with lower sexual activity. Both surgical castration and administration of the antiandrogen-cyproterone acetate (CPA) can reduce sexually directed aggression in male sex offenders (Bradford, 1988) and low rates of recidivism occur after CPA administration. Bradford (1988) argued that consensual adult heterosexual relations are not affected by CPA.

Removal of ovaries or onset of menopause can reduce sexual activity, but the effects may be indirect because estrogen influences vaginal lubrication. In general, little is known about the effects of reproductive steroids on female sexuality (Carter, 1992).

Carter (1992) suggested that oxytocin be considered in studies of sexual behavior. Oxytocin is released during the contractions of the orgasmic response in humans of both sexes and during ejaculation in other species. Steroids, particularly estrogen and testosterone, can modulate oxytocin binding and release in the brain. Stimulation of breasts and other parts of the body during foreplay also releases oxytocin. Oxytocin may play a role in sexual satiation, in sperm transport into the uterus, and in promoting social bond formation in humans as it does in other species (Carter, 1998).

Prolactin may also be important. Prolactin levels increase at orgasm both coitus-induced and masturbation-induced in both men and women (Exton et al., 2001; Krueger et al., 2003). Prolactin is a dopamine antagonist and orgasm-released prolactin may provide a negative feedback loop to dopamine based sexual arousal (Krueger et al., 2002).

Changes in behavior over the ovarian cycle

Females of many species communicate ovulatory status by showing swellings of the genitals (chimpanzees, baboons) or marked changes in behavior (hamsters, rats, cats). However, in most pair-bonded species – including humans – physical or behavioral evidence of ovulation is not evident. This "concealed ovulation" has been described as adaptive for females to co-opt fathers for infant caretaking (Burley, 1979). Traditional theory holds that male mammals will have greatest reproductive success by mating with as many females as possible and deserting them before infants are born. Female mammals with greater parental certainty and the obligatory costs for gestation and lactation are obliged to provide infant care – so long as mothers can successfully rear infants alone (see Snowdon, 1997 for a summary and an alternative view). Biparental and cooperatively breeding species require helpers in addition to mothers to rear infants successfully, and concealed ovulation represents a method to "trick" males into staying long enough to engage in infant care. If the female is continuously receptive to copulation and conceals ovulation, males never know when a female becomes pregnant.

Several lines of evidence counter the idea of concealed ovulation. First, ovulation may be concealed from scientists but not from males of the species involved. In the cotton-top tamarin, Ziegler et al. (1993) transferred odors from ovulating females to recipient pairs each day. On the day of the donor female's ovulation, her scent induced higher rates of male erection and mounting of his own partner than did the donor female's scent from the remaining days of her cycle. Converse and colleagues (1995) showed elevated rates of male olfactory interest in females at the time of ovulation in pygmy marmosets. Ovulatory scents from a novel female common marmoset increased both sexual and investigative behaviors and testosterone levels in males in only 30 minutes (Ziegler et al., 2005). These same ovulatory odors induced activation of the anterior hypothalamus and medial preoptic areas as well as the hippocampus, temporal cortex, cerebellum, putamen, and anterior cingulate cortex using functional magnetic resonance imaging of awake conscious marmosets (Ferris et al., 2001, 2004). Cotton-top tamarin males exhibited increased levels of T and DHT during their mates' follicular phase suggesting some communication of female ovulatory state to prepare males for mating (Ziegler et al., 2004b).

In polygynous (Polygynous meaning one male mates with more than one female, not necessarily that female mates with more than one male which we would call polygamy) species copulations occur throughout the female cycle. However, successful mating depends on whether the female can control or pace sexual behavior. When captive monkeys and apes are paired within a small area, rates of copulation are higher than seen in the wild, and copulation occurs throughout the ovulatory cycle. When females are given control over whether to allow sexual access by males, copulation rates are much lower and more tightly linked to the time of ovulation (Graham & Nadler, 1990). Wallen (1990) reported lower levels of mating as well as mating more tightly linked to ovulation in large environments, where presumably the female has more control over mating. In rats, female-paced mating behavior differs from that where females cannot control mating (McClintock, 1984).

Female hormonal state is critical for sexual behavior and for social integration of rhesus monkey males into a group. Wallen and Tannenbaum (1997) found that females initiated proximity to males and groomed males only during the time of peak estradiol levels, times when ejaculations were most likely. They introduced ten adolescent males to a group of ovariectomized adult females and found, over a period of 2.5 years, no social interactions between males and females. Females were then injected with estradiol and within two days they were grooming and mating with the males. Affiliation with males remained high even after hormonal therapy was stopped. Tannenbaum and Wallen (1997) subsequently reported that novel males were more easily integrated into a female group during the breeding season (when female estrogen levels are high) than in the nonbreeding season. Elevated estrogen facilitates social interactions and social integration of males into macaque groups.

Wallen (1990) and Pfaus (1996) distinguished between desire and ability. The consummatory act of copulation must be carefully distinguished from the appetitive phase, and the appetitive phase must be clearly differentiated according to which partner initiates. Do humans have concealed ovulation and does sexual initiation or enjoyment change with the ovarian cycle? There are several problems have been identified in conducting such studies. Women who were told the purpose of a study – examining changes in sexual behavior over the cycle – reported high levels of arousal shortly before menstruation, whereas those uninformed about the goals of the study reported greater enjoyment close to ovulation (Englander-Golden et al., 1980).

A careful study of human sexual behavior over the ovulatory cycle must: (1) eliminate subjects using oral contraception, because oral contraceptives inhibit the cyclic fluctuations of ovarian hormones; (2) be aware that fear of pregnancy due to contraceptive failure may alter sexual patterns; and (3) distinguish clearly between which partner initiated sex and between initiation and acceptance of copulation. Furthermore, initiation (representing the appetitive or desire phase) must be clearly distinguished from enjoyment (the consummatory phase). Mateo and Rissman (1984) avoided some of these problems by studying lesbians. They found a significant increase in sexual initiations and orgasms by both partners at midcyle, although ovulation was not determined physiologically.

Testosterone may be important in female sexual responses. Morris and associates (1987) reported a midcycle increase in testosterone that correlated with the frequency of sexual initiation. Sherwin, Gelfand, and Brender (1985) studying premenopausal women with ovariectomies – found that administration of testosterone increased sexual desire, arousal, and frequency of sexual fantasies, whereas administration of estrogen and progesterone did not.

Many interesting questions remain concerning the role of reproductive hormones on sexual desire and responsiveness. Careful attention to the conceptual distinctions raised in the animal literature, coupled with use of hormonal assays to determine when ovulation really occurs (rather than simply inferring ovulation from menstruation), is critical for future research on human sexual behavior.

Menstrual synchrony

Menstrual cycle synchrony has been demonstrated in women who are close friends living in a college dormitory (McClintock, 1971). More recent studies have implicated the factors of close bonding or friendship, as well as time spent together, as affecting cycle synchrony (Goldman & Schneider, 1987; Weller & Weller, 1993, 1995).

Looking at menstrual synchrony under optimal conditions, Weller and Weller (1997) studied Bedouin women living in Israel. Bedouin women live together in close proximity and often share sleeping quarters. Society is sexually segregated, with little contact between sexes. Housing conditions are similar across all subjects with little use of oral contraceptives. Under these conditions, menstrual synchrony was found among all women in a family, among sisters who shared the same sleeping quarters, and among those who were close friends. However, no correlation existed between the degree of synchrony and either time spent together or degree of friendship.

McClintock (1971, 1984) suggested that olfactory cues provide the most plausible mechanisms for menstrual synchrony. Axillary secretions from men reduce the variability in menstrual cycle lengths in women. Stern and McClintock (1998) collected axillary secretions from women at different stages of ovulation and placed them above the lips of other women. Odors from women in the luteal phase (post-ovulation) decreased cycle length in recipients whereas odors from women in the follicular phase (pre-ovulatory) increased cycle length in recipients. These results support an olfactory mechanism, for menstrual synchrony.

The effects found even in an optimal study (like that of the Bedouin women) are small: a 20–25% shift toward synchrony from random expectations. Menstruation is easy to document, and it is used as a proxy for ovulation. But because ovulation has not been measured directly and because there is likely to be variation among women in when they ovulate relative to menstruation, the next generation of studies should measure ovulatory rather than menstrual synchrony. Functional explanations for synchrony are based on polygamous mating in species like rats, sheep, other ungulates, and polygynous primates where females can control mate choice through synchronous ovulation, but these explanations do not seem useful for explaining synchrony within families (Weller & Weller, 1997). Menstrual synchrony in humans remains an intriguing phenomenon in search of a function.

Ovarian hormones and stress

Ovarian hormones modulate physiological responses to stress. Postmenopausal middle-aged women showed heart rate increases during three stress tasks as well as increased systolic blood pressure in one of the tasks (Saab et al., 1989). Pregnant women had reduced diastolic blood pressure in response to serial subtraction, mirror image tracing and isotonic hand-grip tasks compared with their prepregnant responses and compared with a nonpregnant control group (Matthews & Rodin, 1992). The increased ovarian hormones of pregnancy and of pre-menopausal compared with postmenopausal women modulate the stress response. However, a study of performance in stress tests over the menstrual cycle found no effects of menstrual cycle on heart rate or blood pressure responses (Stoney et al., 1990).

Parental care

Maternal care

There is an extensive literature on the mechanisms of maternal care in a variety of species (Rosenblatt, 1992; Rosenblatt & Snowdon, 1996). Conceptually, it is important to distinguish between the onset and the maintenance of maternal care. The onset of maternal care appears to be influenced by the hormones of pregnancy and parturition. Thus, progesterone and estrogen are present at high levels through pregnancy and progesterone declines just before parturition, leading to increased levels of prolactin (to prepare the mammary tissue) and oxytocin, which stimulates uterine contractions and the milk letdown response from the nipple. Each of these hormones is involved in controlling the onset of maternal behavior, though the patterns and effects vary greatly across species.

Because estrogen and progesterone levels drop at parturition, maternal behavior must be maintained by stimuli from the infant rather than by any hormonal mechanism. Olfactory, auditory, and visual cues, nipple stimulation, and tactile contact with infants are all important stimuli for maintaining maternal care. Rabbits nurse infants only once a day, but even this brief nursing contact appears essential early in lactation to maintain maternal behavior. In sheep, where infants must follow mothers, oxytocin levels producing uterine contractions at parturition appear critical for forming a bond between mother and infant and facilitating maternal recognition of her infant based on its odors.

Surprisingly little evidence is available on the mechanisms influencing maternal behavior in primates. Pryce and colleagues (1988) showed in red-bellied tamarins that the quality of infant care shown by first-time mothers was dependent upon the levels of estrogen in late pregnancy. Females showing the normal pattern of elevated estrogen through the end of pregnancy displayed adequate maternal care, but first-time mothers with low levels of estrogen prior to birth had poor maternal care. Mothers with extensive infant care experience demonstrated no effect of estrogen levels in late pregnancy and maternal quality. Ziegler and colleagues (in preparation) found no relationship between maternal hormones late in gestation and infant survival in cotton-top tamarins, but found that estrogen levels predicted the sex ratio of the twins. Pryce, Doebeli, and Martin (1993) treated nulliparous common marmosets with the hormones of late pregnancy (progesterone and estrogen) and found increased motivation toward infant care. Marmosets and tamarins often require experience with caring for someone else's infants in order to be competent parents, but there is still a high level of poor parental care, especially with first-born infants (see Snowdon, 1996 for review).

Pryce (1996) developed a motivational model that integrates social learning, maternal experience, hormonal changes, and infant stimuli as factors in maternal care. Infant stimuli can elicit attraction, aversion, anxiety, and neophobia, with negative motivational states being high in females without prior infant experience. Preadult infant care experience changes the valence of infant stimuli toward more positive motivational states. Hormonal changes in late pregnancy (e.g., high levels of progesterone, estrogen, and prolactin) also lead to increased attraction to infant stimuli coupled with increased anxiety responses to infant crying. With the reinforcement that results from direct contact with infants and with learning which behaviors reduce crying, long-term memories are formed that make a mother less dependent on hormonal stimuli with successive infants.

This model, coupled with cognition about one's own infant, may apply to human mothers (Corter & Fleming, 1990). Pregnancy does not make women more interested in other people's babies, and first-time mothers report less responsiveness to their own fetus – especially early in pregnancy – compared with experienced mothers. Many first-time mothers showed the greatest responsiveness to infant stimuli and learned to discriminate their infant from others within a short period after parturition, suggesting that the hormones of late pregnancy play only an indirect role. Experienced mothers were more responsive to infant cries than first-time mothers, but only after the period of postpartum hormonal changes (Corter & Fleming, 1990). Fleming and associates (1997) found in both longitudinal and cross-sectional studies that feelings of nurturance grew during pregnancy and increased after parturition. The estrogen/progesterone ratio in late pregnancy predicted postpartum attachment. Women with low attachment had higher estrogen/progesterone ratios during weeks 20–35 of pregnancy than did women with high infant attachment, although there were no hormonal differences between these two groups at the end of pregnancy

or postpartum. Both estrogen and progesterone prime prolactin secretion. Fleming (1990) reported a significant positive correlation between cortisol levels and the amount of affectionate interactions with infants. She speculated that cortisol may arouse the mother, making her more attentive to cues from the infant, and that cortisol may lead mothers to recognize infant odors and vocalizations more readily, leading to stronger bonding.

One hormone that logically should be important in maternal behavior is prolactin, but there are few studies of prolactin levels and maternal care in human or nonhuman primates. Fleming (1990) reported that breast-feeding mothers (who should have higher prolactin levels) showed more affection toward infants, left the infants alone less often, and responded more contingently to infants than did mothers who bottle-fed infants. Warren and Shortle (1990) reported an increase in maternal responsiveness correlated with prolactin levels, and they found that prolactin levels in women increased with successive births. Tamarin mothers can control the time of their next ovulation through how they nurse. Mothers who tended to nurse both twins simultaneously ovulated significantly sooner after parturition than mothers who tended to nurse their twins sequentially (Ziegler et al., 1990).

Nonmaternal infant care

In many socially monogamous species, fathers and older siblings play important roles in infant care and often are necessary for the survival of infants (Savage et al., 1997; Snowdon, 1996). Biparental care or cooperative breeding is thought to result when maternal effort alone is not sufficient to rear infants successfully, especially during extreme variations in temperature or food availability. The structure of many human families is socially monogamous, so examination of the mechanisms leading to infant care by nonmaternal group members in socially monogamous birds and mammals has direct relevance to human parental care systems.

Ziegler (2000) reviewed studies on nonmaternal infant care in socially monogamous and cooperatively breeding birds, rodents, and primates, and found several common themes. Prolactin levels are elevated in caregivers, both biological parents and nonreproductive helpers, in cooperatively breeding birds and primates. In female mammals, maternal hormones and stimuli from the infant influence maternal care and prolactin levels, whereas in males stimuli from the pregnant female and from infants appear to be important.

Dixson and George (1982) reported that common marmoset males had elevated prolactin levels when caring for infants. Ziegler et al. (1996b) measured urinary prolactin before and after the birth of infants in male cotton-top tamarins. Fathers had significantly higher prolactin levels than nonfathers, and experienced fathers had higher prolactin levels than first-time fathers or sons who assist in infant care. The number of births a father had experienced and his prolactin levels were highly correlated.

Nursing mothers had postpartum prolactin levels similar to fathers, whereas mothers with miscarriages or infant deaths showed declining prolactin levels by the third week postpartum. Surprisingly, both first-time and experienced fathers had elevated prolactin levels in the weeks before their mates gave birth, suggesting that some communication between mates occurs during pregnancy to prepare males for infant care (Ziegler et al., 1996b; Ziegler, 2000).

Experienced cotton-top tamarin fathers had an elevated prolactin level in the last three months of pregnancy whereas less experienced fathers demonstrated an elevation of prolactin only in the last month before parturition (Ziegler & Snowdon, 2000). Subsequently, Ziegler et al. (2004a) found significant increases of androgens, estrogen, prolactin, and cortisol in the last two months before birth. Males displayed a significant increase in glucocorticoids exactly a week after the onset of glucocorticoid production by the adrenals of the fetus as seen in maternal urinary glucocorticoids, suggesting that fetus communicates to its father through the mother. This response was not consistent in less experienced parents, but less experienced pairs showed increased affiliative behavior in the last month of pregnancy.

In many species there is a reciprocal relationship between testosterone and prolactin (Ziegler, 2000). Males that care for infants have low testosterone levels while prolactin levels are elevated. In black tufted eared marmosets (Nunez et al., 2001) and Mongolian gerbils (Clark & Galef, 1999) testosterone levels are decreased during the time of infant care. However, other studies have found an important role for testosterone in parenting. In the biparental California mouse, Trainor and Marler (2001a) found that castrated males were actually more aggressive and less paternal than gonadally intact males. Trainor and Marler (2001b) found that paternal care was mediated by the reduction of testosterone to estrogen by the aromatase enzyme. When aromatase was blocked, males displayed poor parental care. Fathers had increased aromatase activity in the medial preoptic area, and there was a negative correlation between aromatase and progesterone (Trainor et al., 2003). Ziegler et al. (2000, 2004b) reported high levels of testosterone before and after birth in cotton-top tamarin fathers with an increase in both T and DHT in the five days prior to the mate's post-partum ovulation. In species where males must parent, defend a territory and mate with a female shortly after parturition, prolactin and testosterone are both present and may be equally important.

In human fathers those with lower testosterone and those with higher prolactin responded more to infant cries, but fathers hearing cries showed an increase in testosterone. Experienced fathers showed greater prolactin responsiveness to infant cries than first time fathers (Fleming et al., 2002). In a cross-sectional study fathers three weeks after infant birth had lower T levels than expectant fathers sampled 3 weeks before birth (Storey et al., 2000). In another study (Berg & Wynne-Edwards, 2001) fathers had lower T, lower cortisol and more samples with detectable estrogen than nonfathers. Much remains to be learned about the role of prolactin and testosterone in parental care in men and males of other species.

Aggression and dominance

Aggression and dominance behaviors are commonly thought to be more typical of males than females and thus under the influence of testosterone. However, the importance and role of testosterone in human aggression is controversial. Several typologies distinguish among different functional aspects of aggression, with the broadest distinction being between offensive aggression or dominance (thought to be under the control of testosterone) and defensive aggression (not linked with testosterone).

Albert, Walsh, and Jonik (1993) argued that testosterone is directly involved with offensive aggression in nonhumans, yet after reviewing several hundred studies they concluded that there are no consistent differences in testosterone levels between men who exhibit high versus low aggressiveness. Abnormal states such as hypogonadism or castration in men or hirsutism in females (where testosterone levels may be 200% above normal female levels) show neither increases of offensive aggression with increased testosterone nor decreased aggression with decreased testosterone. Albert et al. (1993) concluded that there are similarities between defensive aggression in humans and that displayed by nonhuman species, where mechanisms other than testosterone appear to be similar across species.

However, studies have rarely been long term. Recent studies covering longer time periods do show effects of hormone levels on aggression. Users of anabolic androgenic steroids showed higher levels of verbal aggression, indirect aggression, and impulsiveness than controls (Galligani et al., 1996). Although this study contradicts Albert et al. (1993), there were no data on these users prior to steroid use. Those likely to use steroids may already be more aggressive and impulsive.

Mazur and Booth (1998) reached the opposite conclusion. They argued that a single measure of testosterone could predict dominant or antisocial aggressive behaviors. The anticipation of competition leads to increases in testosterone, and after competition testosterone increases in winners and decreases in losers. Mazur and Booth (1998) developed a reciprocal model where testosterone levels vary as a function of the cumulative dominance interactions a man experiences along with his history of winning and losing, with testosterone being both a cause and a consequence of dominance interactions. This is an intriguing model that can only be evaluated by longitudinal studies with adequate sample sizes. One longitudinal study of more than 4,000 U. S. Air Force veterans found small, but statistically significant, negative correlations between testosterone and both education and income. Men with higher testosterone levels were more likely to be arrested for traffic violations and theft. Most interesting was an increase in testosterone just before and after a divorce and a decrease in testosterone with marriage (Mazur & Booth, 1998). Even though the correlations were significant, they were quite low and explained only a small amount of variance.

Stronger evidence comes from research on the "winner-effect" in animals. Hsu and Wolf (1999) tested a hermaphroditic fish where both the last and last but one experience in fighting affected the success in a subsequent contest. A winner effect lasted at least 48 hours. Trainor, Bird, and Marler (2004) injected castrated male California mice with testosterone (T) following an aggressive encounter. Males were more aggressive the following day than control males with the same fighting experience. Blocking the conversion of T to estradiol by injecting an aromatase inhibitor increased the aggression displayed. Oyegbile and Marler (2005) provided California mice with between zero and three winning experiences and found that three prior wins led to increased fighting success independent of intrinsic fighting ability and that winning at least two fights was associated with increased T levels. Thus, T increases the probability of winning and the experience of winning increases the levels of T.

Two sources of evidence question a simple model relating testosterone to offensive aggression. First, several studies of nonhuman species indicate that aggression is influenced by social, environmental, and cognitive variables. Second, there is increasing evidence (with human and nonhuman species) of dominance and offensive aggression by females that cannot easily be explained by testosterone.

Testing conditions often influence the outcome of contests. Castrated male wood rats fight as vigorously as intact males when tested in neutral arenas (Caldwell et al., 1984); castrated mice with no previous fighting experience do poorly, but males castrated after experiencing fights show normal levels of aggression (Scott & Fredericson, 1951). Wallen (1996) concluded that most aggressive behaviors (with the exception of rough-and-tumble play, which is under androgenic influence) are primarily influenced by social variables. Bester-Meredith and Marler (2001) cross fostered nonaggressive white-footed mice with territorially aggressive California mouse parents. Cross fostered pups displayed levels of territorial aggression similar to foster parents and also had high levels of arginine vasopressin in the bed nucleus of the stria terminalis, as did the California mouse foster parents. California mice are biparental and interestingly, the cross-fostering effects were observed only when fathers were present. Thus, even in nonhuman males, social and environmental variables are at least as important as hormones.

Recent data question the common assumptions about sex differences in offensive aggression. Because it has been assumed that there was little variance in female reproductive success but high variance in male success, offensive aggression was thought to benefit males more than females. In species of cooperatively breeding mammals only one or two females reproduce whereas the remaining females do not. In the golden lion tamarin, two independent studies have found high levels of sex-specific aggression. Male-male aggression was as common as female-female aggression, but the latter was often lethal whereas the former was not (Inglett et al., 1989; Kleiman, 1979). Field studies of a related species, the common marmoset have observed that when reproductive suppression fails and two females give birth at about the same time, one female attacks the offspring of the other often killing the infants (Lazaro-Perea et al., 2000). Because the two females are often related, this means that often a female is killing her nieces and nephews.

De Waal (1982) described sex differences in aggression among chimpanzees. Males frequently engaged in dominance interactions but were readily reconciled after fighting. Females engaged in aggressive interactions much less often, but when they did fight, females were less likely to reconcile and more likely to harm each other. Long-term field data show that dominant female chimpanzees have greater lifetime reproductive success – with more total offspring and with daughters reaching reproductive age earlier than daughters of subordinate females (Pusey et al., 1997). Thus, for marmoset and chimpanzee females, dominance contests are of critical importance. In other species, females are dominant to males (hamsters, Floody, 1983; spotted hyenas, Frank, 1986).

An epidemiological study of human couples found that women were more likely to initiate aggression than men. Magdol et al. (1997) studied all members of the 1972 birth cohort in a city in New Zealand at age 21. Of the women, 37% reported initiating aggression in the home compared with 22% of the men. Severe aggression was initiated by 18.6% of the women but by only 5.7% of the men. Men who committed severe aggression were more likely to be deviant on social and mental heath measures, whereas highly aggressive women were psychologically normal. This study contradicts popular beliefs about human aggression. It is unbiased – sampling an entire birth cohort in a population rather than using court or hospital records. The authors explained the results in terms of social norms. Men are reared to avoid being aggressive toward females and know they are more likely to be prosecuted if they do act aggressively. Women have fewer constraints on aggression and will be held less accountable by society. Although this study suggests that aggression is an "equal opportunity" behavior within the home that cannot be explained simply by testosterone, there is little evidence that women are as aggressive as men outside the family. In general, aggressive behavior is most likely the product of social, developmental, environmental, and cognitive variables interacting with hormones.

Hormonal effects on cognition

Much controversy concerns the degree to which there are gender differences in cognition, with meta-analyses of a large number of studies generally reporting small effect sizes for both verbal ability (Hyde & Linn, 1988) and mathematical ability (Hyde et al., 1990). Nonetheless, there are some specific sex differences where the effects, through small, appear to be consistent (Hampson & Kimura, 1992). Women tend to do better in tests of verbal abilities, perceptual speed and accuracy, and fine motor tasks, whereas males do better on spatial abilities, quantitative abilities, and tests of physical strength. Left-hemisphere brain damage has a more devastating effect on verbal IQ in men than in women, suggesting possible sex differences in lateralization (Hampson & Kimura, 1992). Women performed better on tests of spatial ability at menstruation, when estrogen and progesterone levels are low, compared with performance at the time of ovulation, when hormonal levels are high (Hampson & Kimura, 1992). Verbal tasks that involve reading lists, counting, or repeating syllables tend to show higher levels of performance at ovulation than at other times in the cycle. Hausmann et al. (2000) tested women at menstruation and in the luteal phase and reported significant differences on a mental rotation task but not on other spatial tasks. They measured steroid hormones and found a significant correlation between a woman's T levels and performance on the mental rotation task. McCormick and Teillon (2001) used a mental rotation task with women at different parts of the menstrual cycle and compared them with men. Men performed better than women at all stages of the cycle except at menstruation when there were no performance differences. Liben et al. (2002) experimentally manipulated steroid levels in adolescents being treated for delayed puberty and found sex differences in spatial performance but no relationship between administration of steroids or steroid levels and performance. The sex difference appeared to be independent of steroid levels.

What might account for these differences if steroid levels do not? Kimball (1989) noted that although boys perform better on standardized tests of math ability, girls receive better math grades in school. Either boys have greater experience with math, sex differences in learning styles are involved, or boys do better in novel testing situations than girls. Saucier et al. (2002) studied sex differences in navigational ability and found men did best using Euclidean information whereas women did best using landmark cues and the authors relate this to differences in experience. Finally, Lubinski et al. (2001) in a study of world-class math and science graduate students concluded that there were minimal sex differences and that the development of exceptional scientific expertise requires special educational experiences similar for both sexes.

Studies of variation over the menstrual cycle and in response to administration of steroids test the activational effects of hormones on performance but do not evaluate possible organizational effects. Hines and Sandberg (1996) studied women exposed to diethylstilbestrol during fetal development and found no differences between them and their untreated sisters on measures of verbal fluency, perceptual speed, or associative memory. Wegesin (1998) and Hall and Kimura (1995) assume that organizational effects underlie homosexuality. Wegesin (1998) reported that gay men performed like heterosexual women on both verbal and spatial tasks, whereas Hall and Kimura (1995) found gay men could not be easily categorized with either heterosexual men or women but that lesbians were more similar to heterosexual men than to any other group. The disparate results and the tenuous causal links between homosexuality and organizing effects suggest caution in interpreting such data.

Estrogen levels influence synaptic connections in the hippocampus, the brain area associated with formation of memory. Sherwin (see Wickelgren 1997) found that women treated with an estrogen blocker to suppress fibroid tumors decreased in verbal intelligence and also found improvement in women treated with estrogen compared with those taking a placebo. A few early trials with Alzheimer's patients showed improvements in verbal memory and attention with estrogen administration (Wickelgren, 1997). Studies of postmenopausal women with or without estrogen replacement therapy have shown that estrogen facilitates verbal memory but has no effect on visuospatial memory (Sherwin, 1997). Resnick and Maki (2001) compared a large sample of women receiving estrogen replacement therapy (ERT) compared with a sample matched for age and education. ERT women had higher visual retention scores, and increased skills in encoding, consolidation and recall on verbal learning tasks than untreated women. Furthermore, women starting ERT during the longitudinal study showed no cognitive decline over years compared with never-treated controls. fMRI measurements found women on ERT had greater blood flow to the hippocampus and mesial temporal lobe structures involved in memory. Together these studies that estrogen may facilitate visual and verbal memory and that ERT might be therapeutic in preventing or delaying the effects of cognitive aging.

INFERENTIAL CONTEXT

Many methods can be used to determine hormone concentrations. Likewise several types of samples can be collected from participants. Any bodily fluid will contain hormones, although not all hormones will be found in every body fluid. Hormones are released from the glands into the circulatory system where they can contact any tissue in the body. Hormones may be measured in blood, saliva, and ventricles of the brain, cerebral spinal fluid, scent secretions, ejaculates, urine, and feces. Selecting the type of body fluid to collect depends on the nature of the questions to be addressed, the amount of invasiveness that is permissible, the location of the individual (such as in primitive areas or in hospitals), and how frequently samples are needed (daily versus weekly). There are advantages and disadvantages to each type of body fluid used. For example, steroids are very small molecules and therefore can be found in most body fluids. Steroids can diffuse through cellular membranes and through tight junctions between cells provided they are unconjugated. Protein hormones, however, are much larger molecules that cannot diffuse between cells. Therefore, measurements of protein hormones are limited to blood and urine or in central nervous system fluids where they are released. The advantages and disadvantages of different sources will be described next.

Blood

Advantages. Measurement of hormone levels in the blood of animals and humans has been the most routine method used. Normative blood values for humans are known for most reproductive hormones. Samples can be collected throughout the day if there is a need to understand the changes in circulating hormones. Circulating hormones will show immediate changes in hormones in response to a stimulus, whereas measurements in other media may be delayed relative to timing in the blood. For instance, circulating cortisol will increase within minutes in response to an acute stressor.

Disadvantages. Measurement of circulating hormones requires venipuncture, which may cause pain and stress. Furthermore, blood samples provide information on the level of the hormone only at the time of sample collection, thus not accurately reflecting fluctuations in the blood levels due to pulsatile release or diurnal rhythms. For example, prolactin levels in the blood are known to change within minutes in response to factors such as sleep, exercise, stress and sexual stimulation. A more accurate measure of cortisol responses to social stressors, which influence cortisol changes over time, may best be seen in samples (e.g., urine or feces) that likewise accumulate the steroid over time. In small organisms repeated blood sampling depletes red blood cells, limiting the number of samples possible.

Saliva

Advantages. Saliva samples can be collected noninvasively from humans and from cooperating animals without restraint. Noninvasive sampling eliminates some ethical issues relating to studies directed at various age groups, such as infants and the elderly, and the physically and mentally handicapped. The concentrations of steroids in saliva correlate directly with the free levels of circulating steroids. Samples can be taken daily or more frequently without physical effects on the subject. Circulating steroids appear quickly in saliva.

Disadvantages. Protein hormones generally are not found in saliva, which limits measurement to steroid hormones. Most salivary steroid levels represent the free portion of circulating steroids and not total levels (a proportion of circulating steroids are bound to specific or nonspecific blood proteins and therefore are not available for binding to receptors). Enzymes within the saliva can metabolize steroids and therefore change their structure and the ability to measure them. Additionally, bacteria within the oral cavity can metabolize the steroids. False high values may occur if a small amount of blood enters the oral cavity due to lesions in the mouth. Conjugated steroids such as DHEAS cannot be measured in saliva because the conjugates will not filter into the saliva. Salivary steroid levels, like single venipuncture sampling, reflect the steroid level present in the blood only at that point in time. For chronic or longer term sampling, multiple salivary samples must be collected, or other bodily fluids must be used.

Urine

Advantages. Steroids, protein hormones, catecholamines, and neuropeptides can be found in the urine. These levels reflect an accumulation over time because hormones are filtered by the kidneys and stored in the bladder until urination. First morning void urine provides a concentrated sample that represents an overnight accumulation. Collection procedures can be performed daily. Indexing with creatinine (a metabolite that is excreted into the urine at a constant rate) can control for variability in urine concentration. Disease-related alterations in hormone metabolism can be monitored in the urine. Steroid hormones are usually found in very high amounts in urine due to the accumulation over time.

Disadvantages. Many hormones may be metabolized by the liver prior to excretion into the urine and therefore the specific metabolites that accurately reflect circulating hormones must be determined. Many steroid hormones are conjugated to glucuronides and sulfates prior to excretion Ziegler et al., 1989). In this form, the steroids cannot be measured by most antibodies and conjugated molecules must be liberated prior to analysis. Some protein hormones have a short half-life and therefore low levels may appear in the urine. For example prolactin, has a half-life of 12 minutes whereas LH has a half-life of 45 minutes (Yen and Jaffe, 1978). A lag may occur between peak blood levels of a hormone and appearance in urine. Thus, the LH peak found in the blood may be found the following day in the urine.

Feces

Advantages. Feces may be collected freely from free-ranging organisms where close contact is not possible. Steroid levels are found in large amounts in the feces. The fecal excretion of steroids reflects an accumulation over time and therefore adjusts for fluctuations in the hormones throughout the day.

Disadvantages. Most steroids are metabolized into many different steroid metabolites prior to excretion into the feces. The liver conjugates many steroids prior to release into the intestines. Some steroids, such as estradiol, are highly conjugated and may re-circulate before being fully excreted (Ziegler et al., 1996a). No protein hormones, neuropeptides, or catecholamines can be measured in the feces.

Metabolism of steroids

The measurement of steroids in blood has been thought to be fairly straightforward, and should represent the pure steroids released from the endocrine glands. However, some steroids, such as estradiol and estrone, can be conjugated quickly after release into the circulation and interconvert (Ruoff and Dziuk, 1994). A majority of estradiol can be converted to estrone and its conjugates within 5 minutes of its release (Ruoff and Dziuk, 1994). Therefore, the measurement of pure steroids in circulation may not always assess accurately the total amount of steroid unless one measures conjugated steroids as well. Human females and some primate species, such as common marmosets, have very high levels of estrone sulfate in circulation throughout the ovarian cycle (Nuñez et al., 1977; Harlow et al., 1984).

Steroid metabolites are a result of conversion of circulating steroids in the liver, although the stomach, intestines and some peripheral tissues also can metabolize steroids. The liver filters steroids from the blood and inactivates them by conjugation. Conjugation is the processes by which sulfate esters or glucuronates are attached to the steroid primarily by reduction of the A ring double bond and the 3-keto groups. The addition of sulfate or glucuronide acids makes the steroids water-soluble where they can then be removed from circulation by kidney filtration or released into the intestines by bile. Conjugation can be simple such as monoconjugates or complex such as di- or tri-conjugates consisting of both glucuronides and sulfates. When measuring steroids by an immune reaction as in RIA or EIA, the antibody does not always recognize the steroid in its conjugated form (Hodges and Eastman, 1984).

SUMMARY

Despite a fascination with reproductive processes that dates to antiquity, the modern study of reproductive hormones is barely five decades old. The development of assay methods to detect small amounts of hormones and the determination of hormonal structure and synthesis was needed to advance experimental research. We know that the regulation of hormones in the body is based on an intricate set of positive and negative feedback mechanisms involving multiple brain structures, the pituitary gland as well as peripheral glands. Current research on hormone receptor expression and the role of ligand-independent mechanisms of receptor expression promise an exciting future in understanding physical and behavioral sex differences. Reproductive hormones play an obvious role in sexual differentiation, in the control of puberty, in modulating behavior over the ovarian cycle and controlling courtship and sexual behavior. In a less obvious role

reproductive hormones are critical in preparing mothers for parental care and, in biparental species, including humans, preparing fathers as well. The hormones that function to maintain a parent-infant bond also appear to play an important role in pair bonding between adults. Reproductive hormones may also play an important role in dominance and aggressive behavior and may have some influence on spatial and verbal memory especially in aging. Reproductive hormones also play an important role in regulating immunological reactions and are increasingly being implicated in certain autoimmune disorders. At the same time, we have summarized in this review the important influences of early experience and social environment on hormonal function. Social relationships can affect the timing of menstrual cycles, the onset of puberty, the expression of competent parental behavior, the expression of dominance or aggressive behaviors and the maintenance of cognitive skills. It is the close interaction between social and physical environment and hormonal function that makes research on reproductive hormones exciting not just for endocrinologists, but also for psychophysiologists. Novel methods for noninvasive monitoring of hormonal function promise an exciting future for research with human participants.

REFERENCES

Abel, J. J., & Crawford, A. C. (1897). On the blood-pressure raising constituent of the suprarenal capsule. *Johns Hopkins Hosp. Bull.* 8, 151–7.

Albert, D. L., Walsh, M. L. & Jonik, R. H. (1993). Aggression in humans: What is its biological foundation? *Neurosci. Biobehav. Rev.* 17, 405–25.

Aldrich, T. B. (1901). A preliminary report on the active principle of the suprarenal gland. *Am. J. Physiol.* 5, 457–61.

Appenrodt E., Schnabel R., Schwarzberg H. (1998). Vasopressin administration modulates anxiety-related behavior in rats. *Physiol. Behav.* 64, 543–7.

Auger, A. P. (2004). Steroid receptor control of reproductive behavior. *Horm. Behav.* 45, 168–72.

Auger, A. P., Tetel, M. J. & McCarthy, M. M. (2000). Steroid receptor coactivator-1 (SRC-1) mediates the development of sex-specific brain morphology and behavior. *Proc. Nat. Acad. Sci. USA* 97, 7551–5.

Bales, K., Kim, A. J., Lewis-Reese, A. D. and Carter, C. S. (2004). Both oxytocin and vasopressin may influence alloparental behavior in male prairie voles. *Horm. Behav.* 45, 354–61.

Bardin, C. W., & Catterall, J. F. (1981). Testosterone: A major determinant of extragenital sexual dimorphism. *Science* 211, 1285–94.

Barrett, J., Abbott, D. H., & George, L. M. (1990). Extension of reproductive suppression by pheromonal cues in subordinate female marmoset monkeys (*Callithrix jacchus*). *J. Reprod. Fert.* 90, 411–18.

Bartter, F. C., Liddle, G. W., and Dunkin, L. E. Jr. (1956). The regulation of aldosterone secretion in man: The role of fluid volume. *J. Clin. Invest.* 35, 1306–15.

Berenbaum, S. A. & Hines, M. (1992). Early androgens are related to childhood sex-typed toy preferences. *Psych. Sci.* 3, 203–6.

Berg, S. J. & Wynne-Edwards, K. E. (2001). Changes in testosterone, cortisol and estradiol levels in men becoming fathers. *Mayo Clin. Proc*. 76, 582–92.

Bester-Meredith, J. K. & Marler, C. A. (2001). Vasopressin and aggression in cross-fostered California mice (*Peromyscus californicus*) and white-footed mice (*Peromyscus leucopus*). *Horm. Behav*. 40, 51–64.

Bonello, N., Jasper, M. J. and Norman R. J. (2004). Periovulatory expression of intercellular adhesion molecule-1 in the rat ovary. *Biol Reprod* 71, 1384–90.

Borell, M. (1976). Brown-Séquard's organotherapy and its appearance in America at the end of the nineteenth century. *Bull. Hist. Med*. 50, 309–20.

Bradford, J. M. W. (1988). Organic treatment for the male sex offender. *Ann. New York Acad. Sci*. 528, 193–202.

Breedlove, S. M. (1992). Sexual differentiation of brain and behavior. In J. B. Becker, S. M. Breedlove, & D. Crews (Eds.). *Behavioral Endocrinology* (pp. 39–68). Cambridge, MA: MIT Press.

Brown-Séquard, C. E. (1889). De quelques regles generales relatives a l'inhibition. *Arch. Physiol. Norm. Pathol. 5e, sér*.1:739–46.

Bull, J. J., & Vogt, R. C. (1979). Temperature dependent sex determination in turtles. *Science* 206, 1186–8.

Burley, N. (1979). The evolution of concealed ovulation. *Am. Nat*. 114, 835–58.

Butts, C. L. & Sternberg, E. M. (2004). Different approaches to understanding autoimmune rheumatic diseases: the neuroimmunoendocrine system. Best Practice and Research-Clinical Rheumatology. *Bailliere's Rhematol Rev*. 18, 125–39.

Bynoe, M. S., Grimaldi, C. M. & Diamond, B. (2000) Estrogen upregulates Bcl-2 and blocks tolerance induction of naïve B cells. *Proc. Nat. Acad. Sci*. USA 97, 2703–8.

Caldwell, G. S., Glickman, S. E., & Smith, E. R. (1984). Seasonal aggression independent of seasonal testosterone in woodrats. *Proc. Nat. Acad. Sci*. USA 81, 5255–7.

Carlson, A. A., Ziegler, T. E., & Snowdon, C. T. (1997). Ovulatory patterns of pygmy marmosets in intact and motherless families. *Am. J. Primatol*. 43, 347–55.

Carr, B. R. (1992). Disorders of the ovary and female reproductive tract. In J. D. Wilson and D. W. Foster (Eds.) *Textbook of Endocrinology*, 8th ed. (pp. 733–98). Philadelphia: Saunders Co.

Carter, C. S. (1992). Hormonal influences on human sexual behavior. In J. B. Becker, S. M. Breedlove, & D. Crews (Eds.), *Behavioral Endocrinology* (pp. 131–42). Cambridge, MA: MIT Press.

Carter, C. S. (1998). Neuroendocrine perspectives on social attachments and love. *Pyschoneuroendocrin*. 23, 779–818.

Carter, C. S., & Altemus, M. (1997). Integrative functions of lactational hormones in social behavior and stress management. *Ann. New York Acad. Sci*. 807, 164–74.

Carter, C. S., Getz, L. L. & Cohen-Parsons, M. (1986). Relationships between social organization and behavioral endocrinology in a monogamous mammal. *Adv. Stud. Behav*. 16, 109–45.

Clark, M. M. & Galef, B. G. Jr. (1995). A gerbil dam's fetal intrauterine position affects the sex ratios of litters she sires. *Physiol. Behav*. 57, 297–9.

Clark, M. M. & Galef, B. G., Jr. (1999). A testosterone-mediated trade-off between parental and sexual effort in male Mongolian gerbils (*Meriones unguiculatus*). *J. Comp. Psychol*. 113, 388–95.

Clark, M. M. & Galef, B. G. Jr. (2001). Socially induced infertility: familial effects on reproductive development of female Mongolian gerbils. *Anim. Behav*. 62, 897–903.

Clarke, F. M. & Faulkes, C. G. (1998). Hormonal and behavioural correlates of male dominance and reproductive status in captive colonies of the naked mole-rat, *Heterocephalus glaber*. *Proc Roy. Soc. Lond. B*. 265, 1391–9.

Converse, L. J., Carlson, A. A., Ziegler, T. E., & Snowdon, C. T. (1995). Communication of ovulatory state to mates by female pygmy marmosets, *Cebuella pygmaea*. *Anim. Behav*. 49: 615–21.

Corter, C. M., & Fleming, A. S. (1990). Maternal responsiveness in humans: Emotional, cognitive and biological factors. *Adv. Stud. Behav*. 19: 893–136.

Creel, S. R., Creel, N. M., Wildt, D. E., & Montfort, S. L. (1992). Behavioral and endocrine mechanisms of reproductive suppression in Serengeti dwarf mongooses. *Anim. Behav*. 43: 231–45.

Cutler W. B., Preti G., Krieger A., Huggins G. R., Garcia C. R., Lawley H. J. (1986). Human axillary secretions influence women's menstrual cycles: the role of donor extract from men. *Horm Behav*. 20, 463–73.

Cutolo, M. (1998). The roles of steroid hormones in arthritis. *Brit. J. Rheumatol*. 37, 597–601.

Demski, L. S. (1987). Diversity of reproductive patterns in teleost fishes. In D. Crews (Ed.) *Psychobiology of Reproductive Behavior: An Evolutionary Perspective* (pp. 1–27). Englewood Cliffs, NJ: Prentice-Hall.

De Waal, F. B. M. (1982). *Chimpanzee Politics: Power and Sex among the Apes*. New York: Harper & Row.

Dixson, A. F., & George, L. (1982). Prolactin and parental behavior in a male New World primate. *Nature* 229: 551–3.

Dharmadhikari, A., Lee, Y. S., Roberts, R. L., Carter, C. S. (1997). Exploratory behavior correlates with social organization and is responsive to peptide injections in prairie voles. *Ann N Y Acad Sci*. 807, 610–2.

Dodds, J. C., Goldberg, L., Lawson, W., & Robinson, R. (1938). Oestrogenic activity of certain synthetic compounds, *Nature* 141: 247–8.

Doisy, E. A. (1936). Sex hormones. Porter Lectures delivered at the University of Kansas School of Medicine (Lawrence).

Ebner K., Bosch O. J., Kromer S. A., Singewald N., Neumann I. D. (2005). Release of oxytocin in the rat central amygdala modulates stress-coping behavior and the release of excitatory amino acids. *Neuropsychopharm*. 30, 223–230.

Ehrhardt, A. A. & Money, J. (1967). Progestin-induced hermaphroditism: IQ and psychosocial identity in a study of ten girls. *J. Sex. Res*. 3, 83–100

Ellingwood W. E. & Resko, J. A. (1980). Sex differences in biologically active and immunoactive gonadotropins in the fetal circulation of rhesus monkeys. *Endocrinol*. 107: 902–7.

Engelmann, M., Wotjak, C. T., Neumann, I., Lidwig, M., & Landgraf, R. (1996). Behavioral consequences of intracerebral vasopressin and oxytocin: Focus on learning and memory. *Neurosci. Biobehav. Rev*. 20: 341–58.

Englander-Golden, P., Chung, H. S., Whitmore, M. R., & Dientsbier, R. A. (1980). Female sexual arousal and the menstrual cycle. *J. Human Stress* 6: 42–8.

Exton, M. S., Krueger, T. H. C., Koch, M., Paulsen, E., Knapp, W., Hartmann, U. & Schedlowski, M. (2001). Coitus-induced orgasm stimulates prolactin secretion in healthy subjects. *Psychoneurendo*. 26, 287–94.

Faulkes, C. G., & Abbott, D. H. (1997). The physiology of a reproductive dictatorship: Regulation of male and female reproduction by a single breeding female in colonies of naked mole rats. In N. G. Solomon & J. A. French (Eds.), *Cooperative Breeding in Mammals* (pp. 302–34). Cambridge University Press.

Ferris, C. F., Snowdon, C. T., King, J. A., Duong, T. Q., Ziegler, T. E., Ugurbil, K., Ludwig, R., Schultz-Darken, N. J., Wu, Z., Olson, D. P., Sullivan, J. M., Jr., Tannenbaum, P. L. & Vaughn, J. T. (2001). Functional imaging of brain activity in conscious monkeys responding to sexually arousing cues. *NeuroReport* 12, 2231–6.

Ferris, C. F., Snowdon, C. T., King, J. A., Sullivan, J. M. Jr., Ziegler, T. E., Ludwig, R., Schultz-Darken, N., Wu, Z., Olson, D. P., Tannenbaum, P. L., Einspanier, A., Vaughn, J. T., & Duong, T. Q. (2004). Imaging neural pathways associated with stimuli for sexual arousal in nonhuman primates. *J. Magnet. Res. Imag.* 19, 168–75.

Fleming, A. S. (1990). Hormonal and experiential correlates of maternal responsiveness in human mammalian mothers. In. N. A. Krasnegor & R. S. Bridges (Eds.), *Parenting: Biochemical, Neurobiological and Behavioral Determinants*, pp. 184–208. New York: Oxford University Press.

Fleming, A. S., Ruble, D., Krieger, H., & Wong, P. Y. (1997). Hormonal and experiential correlates of maternal responsiveness during pregnancy and the puerperium in human mothers. *Horm. Behav.* 31: 145–58.

Fleming, A. S., Corter, C., Stallings, J., & Steiner, M. (2002). Testosterone and prolactin are associated with emotional responses to infant cries in new fathers. *Horm. Behav.* 42, 399–413.

Floody, O. R. (1983). Hormones and aggression among female mammals. In B. B. Svare (Ed.), *Hormones and Aggression Behavior* (pp. 39–89). New York: Plenum.

Francis, R. C. & Barlow, G. W. (1993). Social control of primary sex differentiation in the Midas cichlid. *Proc. Nat. Acad. Sci. USA* 90, 10673–5.

Francis, R. C., Soma, K. & Fernald, R. D. (1993). Social regulation of the brain-pituitary-gonadal axis. *Proc. Nat. Acad. Sci. USA* 90, 7794–8.

Frank, L. G. (1986). Social organization of the spotted hyena, *Crocuta crocuta*. II. Dominance and reproduction. *Anim. Behav.* 34: 1510–27.

French, J. A. (1997). Proximate regulation of singular breeding in Callitrichid primates. In N. G. Solomon & J. A. French (Eds.), *Cooperative Breeding in Mammals*, pp. 34–75. New York: Cambridge University Press.

French, J. A., & Stribley, J. A. (1987). Ovarian cycles are synchronized between and within social groups of lion tamarins (*Leontopithecus rosalia*). *Am. J. Primatol.* 12: 469–78.

Frisch, R. E. (2002). *Female Fertility and the Body Fat Connection*. Chicago: University of Chicago Press.

Galligani, N., Renck, A., & Hansen, S. (1996). Personality profiles of men using anabolic steroids. *Horm. Behav.* 30: 170–5.

Gerra, G., Caccavari, R., Delsignore, R., Passeri, M., Fertonani Affini, G., Maestri, D., Monica, C., & Brambilla, F. (1993). Parental divorce and neuroendocrine changes in adolescents. *Acta. Psychiatr. Scand.* 87: 350–4.

Ginther, A. J., Ziegler, T. E. & Snowdon, C. T. (2001). Reproductive biology of captive male cotton-top tamarin monkeys as a function of social environment. *Anim. Behav.* 61, 65–78.

Ginther, A. J., Carlson, A. A., Ziegler, T. E. & Snowdon, C. T. (2002). Neonatal and pubertal development in males of a cooperatively breeding primate, the cotton-top tamarin (*Saguinus oedipus oedipus*). *Biol. Reprod.* 66, 282–90.

Giovenardi, M., Padoin, M. F., Cadore, L. P., & Lucion, A. B. (1997). Hypothalamic paraventricular nucleus, oxytocin, and maternal aggression in rats. *Ann. New York Acad. Sci.* 807: 606–9.

Glickman, S. E., Frank, L. G., Pavgi, S. & Licht, P. (1992). Hormonal correlates of masculinization in female spotted hyenas (*Crocuta crocuta*): 1. Infancy to sexual maturity. *J. Reprod. Fertil.* 95, 451–62.

Goldfoot, D. A., Wallen, K., Neff, D. A., McBrair, M. C., & Goy, R. E. (1984). Social influences on the display of sexually dimorphic behavior in rhesus monkeys: Isosexual rearing. *Arch. Sex Behav.* 13: 395–412.

Goldman, S. E., & Schneider, H. G. (1987). Menstrual synchrony: Social and personality factors. *J. Soc. Behav. Pers.* 2: 243–50.

Goy, R. W. (1970). Early hormonal influences on the development of sexual and sex-related behavior. In F. O. Schmitt (Ed.), *The Neurosciences: Second Study Program* (pp. 196–207). New York: Rockefeller University Press.

Goy, R. W., Bercovitch, F. B., & McBrair, M. C. (1988). Behavioral masculinization is independent of genital masculinization in prenatally androgenized female rhesus macaques. *Horm. Behav.* 22: 552–71.

Goy, R. W., & Deputte, B. L. (1996). The effects of diethylstilbestrol (DES) before birth on the development of masculine behavior in juvenile female rhesus monkeys. *Horm. Behav.* 30: 379–86.

Goy, R. W., & Resko, J. A. (1972). Gonadal hormones and behavior of normal and psuedohermaphroditic nonhuman female primates. *Rec. Prog. Horm. Res.* 28: 707–33.

Graham, C. E., & Nadler, R. D. (1990). Socioendocrine interactions in great ape reproduction. In T. E. Ziegler & F. B. Bercovitch (Eds.), *Socioendocrinology of Primate Reproduction* (pp. 33–58). New York: Wiley-Liss.

Griffin, J. E., & Wilson, J. D. (1992). Disorders of the testes and the male reproductive tract. In J. D. Wilson & D. W. Foster (Eds.), *Textbook of Endocrinology*, 8th ed. (pp. 799–852). Philadelphia: Saunders.

Guyton, A. C., & Hall, J. E. (1996). *Textbook of Medical Physiology*, 9th ed. Philadelphia: Saunders.

Hadley, M. E. (1992). Neurohypophysial hormones. In Endocrinology, pp.153–78. Englewood Cliffs, NJ: Prentice Hall.

Hall, J. A. Y., & Kimura, D. (1995). Sexual orientation and performance on sexually dimorphic motor tasks. *Arch. Sex. Behav.* 24, 395–407.

Hampson, E., & Kimura, D. (1992). Sex differences and hormonal influences on cognitive function in humans. In J. B. Becker, S. M. Breedlove, & D. Crews (Eds.), *Behavioral Endocrinology* (pp. 357–98). Cambridge, MA: MIT Press.

Harlow, C. R., Hearn, J. P., & Hodges, J. K. (1984). Ovulation in the marmoset monkey: Endocrinology, prediction and detection. *J. Endocrin.* 103: 17–24.

Harris, G. W. (1955). *Neural Control of the Pituitary Gland*. London: Arnold.

Hausmann, M., Slabbekoorn, D., van Goozen, S. H. M., Cohen-Kettenis, P. T., & Gunturkun, O. (2000). Sex hormones affect spatial abilities during the menstrual cycle. *Behav. Neurosci.* 114, 1245–50.

Heinrichs, M. Meinschmidt, G., Wippich, W., Ehlert, U. & Hellhammer, D. H. 2004. Selective amnesic effects of oxytocin on human memory. *Physiol Behav.* 83: 31–38.

Heist, E. K., & Poland, R. E. (1992). Bioassay methods. In C. B. Nemeroff (Ed.), *Neuroendocrinology* (pp. 21–38). Boca Raton, FL: CRC Press.

Himes, N. E. (1936). *Medical History of Contraception*. New York: Gamut.

Hines, M., & Sanberg, E. C. (1996). Sexual differentiation of cognitive abilities in women exposed to diethylstilbestrol (DES) prenatally. *Horm. Behav.* 30: 354–63.

Hodges, J. K., & Eastman, S. A. K. (1984). Monitoring ovarian function in marmosets and tamarins by the measurement of urinary estrogen metabolites. *Am. J. Primatol.* 6: 187–97.

Holekamp, K. E. & Smale, L. (1998) Dispersal status influences hormones and behavior in the male spotted hyena. *Horm. Behav.* 33: 205–16.

Hsu, Y. & Wolf, L. L. (1999). The winner and loser effect: Integrating multiple experiences. *Anim. Behav.* 57, 903–10.

Hyde, J. S., Fennema, E., & Lamon, S. J. (1990). Gender differences in mathematics performance: A meta-analysis. *Psych. Bull.* 107: 139–55.

Hyde, J. S., & Linn, M. C. (1988). Gender differences in verbal ability: A meta-analysis. *Psych. Bull.* 104: 53–69.

Imperator-McGinley, J., Peterson, R. E., Gautier, T., & Sturla, E. (1979). Androgens and the evolution of male sexual identity among male pseudohermaphrodites with 5 alpha reductase deficiency. *New England J. Med.* 300: 1233–7.

Inglett, B. J., French, J. A., Simmons, L. G., & Vires, K. W. (1989). Dynamics of intrafamily aggression and social reintegration in lion tamarins. *Zoo. Biol.* 8: 67–78.

Insel, T. R. (2003). Is social attachment an addictive disorder? *Physiol. Behav.* 79, 351–7.

Kleiman, D. G. (1979). Parent-offspring conflict and sibling competition in a monogamous primate. *Am. Nat.* 114: 753–60.

Kimball, M. M. (1989). A new perspective on women's math achievement. *Psych. Bull.* 105, 198–214.

Konner, M. (2004). The ties that bind, Attachment: the nature of the bonds between humans are becoming accessible to scientific investigation. *Science* 429: 705.

Kordon, C., Drouva, S. V., Escalera, G. M., & Weiner, R. I. (1994). Role of classic and peptide neuromediators in the neuroendocrine regulation of luteinizing hormone and prolactin. In E. Knobil & J. D. Neil (Eds.), *The Physiology of Reproduction*, 2nd ed. (pp. 1621–59). New York: Raven.

Kovacs, G. L., Sarnyai, Z, & Szabo, G. (1998). Oxytocin and addiction: A review. *Psychoneuroendo.* 23, 945–62.

Krueger, T. H. C., Haake, P., Hartmann, U., Schedlowski, M. & Exton, M. S. (2002). Orgasm-induced prolactin secretion: feedback control of sexual drive? *Neurosci Biobehav. Rev.* 26, 31–44.

Krueger, T. H. C., Haake, P., Chereath, D., Knapp, W., Janssen, O. E., Exton, M. S., Schedlowski, M., & Hartmann, U. (2003). Specificity of the neuroendocrine response to orgasm during sexual arousal in men. *J. Endocrin.* 177, 57–64.

Lazaro-Perea, C., Castro, C. S. S., Harrison, R., Araujo, A., Arruda, M. F. & Snowdon, C. T. (2000). Behavioral and demographic changes following the loss of the breeding female in cooperatively breeding marmosets. *Behav. Ecol. Sociobiol.* 48, 37–46.

Liben, L. S., Susman, E. J., Finkelstein, J. W., Chinchilli, V. M., Kunselman, S., Schwab, J., Dubas, J. S., Demers, L. M., Lookingbill, G., d'Archangelo, M. R., Krogh, H. R., & Kulin, H. E. (2002). The effects of sex steroids on spatial performance: A review and experimental clinical investigation. *Develop. Psych.* 38, 236–53.

Lubinski, D., Benbow, C. P., Shea, D. L., Eftekhari-Sanjani, H., & Halvorson, M. B. J., (2001) Men and women at promise for scientific excellence: Similarity not dissimilarity. *Psychol. Sci.* 12, 309–17.

Lund, T. D., Munson, D. J., Haldy, M. E. & Handa, R. J. 2004. Androgen inhibits, while oestrogen enhances, restraint-induced activation of neuropeptide neurons in the paraventricular nucleus of the hypothalamus. *J. Neuroendocrin.* 16:272–278.

Magdol, L., Moffitt, T. E., Caspi, A., Newman, D. L., Fagan, J., & Siva, P. A. (1997). Gender differences in partner violence in a birth cohort of 21 year olds: Bridging the gap between clinical and epidemiological approaches. *J. Clin. Consult. Psych.* 65: 68–78.

Mateo, S., & Rissman, E. F. (1984). Increased sexual activity during the mid-cycle portion of the human menstrual cycle. *Horm. Behav.* 18: 249–55.

Mathews, K. A., & Rodin, J. (1992). Pregnancy alters pressure responses to psychological and physical change. *Psychophys.* 29: 232–40.

Mazur, A., & Booth, A. (1998). Testosterone and dominance in men. *Behav. Brain Sci.* 21: 353–97.

McClintock, M. K. (1971). Menstrual synchrony and suppression. *Nature* 229: 244–5.

McClintock, M. K. (1984). Group mating in the domestic rat as a context for sexual selection: Consequences for the analysis of sexual behavior and neuroendocrine response. *Adv. Stud. Behav.* 14: 2–50.

McCormick, C. M. & Teillon, S. M. (2001). Menstrual cycle variation in spatial ability: relation to salivary cortisol. *Horm. Behav.* 39, 29–38.

McEwen, B. S. (1979). Influences of adrenocortical hormones on pituitary and brain function. In F. D. Baxter & G. G. Rousseau (Eds.), *Glucocorticoid Hormone Action* (pp. 467–92). New York: Springer-Verlag.

Medvei, V. C. (1982). *A History of Endocrinology*. Lancaster, U.K.: MTP Press.

Mendoza, S. P., & Mason, W. A. (1997). Attachment relationships in New World primates. *Ann. New York Acad. Sci.* 807: 203–9.

Meyer-Bahlburg, H. F. L., Gruen, R. S., New, M. I. Bell, J. J., Morishima, A., Shimshi, M. Bueno, Y., Vargas, Il, & Baker, S. W. (1996). Gender change from female to male in classical congenital adrenal hyperplasia. *Horm. Behav.* 30: 319–32.

Miksicek, R. J. (1993). Commonly occurring plant flavenoids have estrogenic activity. *Molec. Pharmacol.* 44: 37–43.

Moehlman, P. D., & Hofer, H. (1997). Cooperative breeding, reproductive suppression and body mass in canids. In N. G. Solomon & J. A. French (Eds.), *Cooperative Breeding in Mammals* (pp. 76–128). Cambridge University Press.

Molenda, H. A., Kilts, C. A., Allen, R. L. & Tetel, M. J. (2003). Nuclear receptor coactivator function in reproductive physiology and behavior. *Biol. Reprod.* 49, 1449–57.

Moore, C. R., Gallagher, T. F., & Koch, F. C. (1929). The effects of extracts of testis in correcting the castrated condition in the fowl and in the mammal. *Endocrinol.* 13: 367–74.

Moore, R. Y. (1978). Neuroendocrine regulation of reproduction. In S. S. C. Yen & R. B. Jaffe (Eds.), *Reproductive Endocrinology: Physiology, Pathophysiology and Clinical Management* (pp. 3–33). Philadelphia: Saunders.

Mori, M., Vigh, S., Miyata, A., Yoshihara, T., Oka, S., & Arimura, A. (1990). Oxytocin is the major prolactin releasing factor in the posterior pituitary. *Endocrinol.* 125: 1009–13.

Morris, N. M., Udry, J. R., Khan-Dawood, F., & Dawood, M. Y. (1987). Marital sex frequency and midcycle female testosterone. *Arch. Sex Behav.* 16: 27–37.

Munro, C., & Stabenfeldt, G. (1984). Development of a microtiter plate enzyme immunoassay for the determination of progesterone. *J. Endocrinol*. 101: 41–9.

Murray, G. R. (1891). Note on the treatment of myxedema by hypodermic injections of an extract of the thyroid gland of a sheep. *Br. Med. J*. 2: 796–7.

Niswender, G. D., & Nett, T. M. (1988). The corpus luteum and its control. In E. Knobil & J. D. Neill (Eds.), *The Physiology of Reproduction* (pp. 489–525). New York: Raven.

Nuñez, M., Aedo, A. R., Landgren, B. M., Cekan, S. Z., & Dicfalusy, E. (1977). Studies on the pattern of circulating steroids in the normal menstrual cycle. 6. Levels of oestrone sulphate and oestradiol sulphate. *Acta Endocrin*. 86: 621–33.

Nuñez, S., Fite, J. E., Patera, K. J., & French, J. A. (2001). Interactions among paternal behavior steroid hormones and parental experience in male marmosets (*Callithrix kuhlii*). *Horm. Behav*. 39, 70–82.

Oyegbile, T. O. & Marler, C. A. (2005) Winning fights elevates testosterone levels in California mice and enhances future ability to win fights. *Horm. Behav*. 48: 259–267.

Pfaus, J. G. (1996). Homologies of animal and human sexual behavior. *Horm. Behav*. 30: 187–200.

Preti, G., Cutler, W. B., Garcia, C. R., Huggins, G. R. & Lawley, H. J. (1986). Human axillary secretions influence women's menstrual cycles: The role of donor extract of females. *Horm. Behav*. 20, 474–82.

Pryce, C. R. (1996). Socialization, hormones and the regulation of maternal behavior in nonhuman simian primates. In J. S. Rosenblatt & C. T. Snowdon (Eds.), *Parental care: Evolution Mechanisms and Adaptive Strategies*, pp. 423–73. San Diego: Academic Press.

Pryce, C. R., Abbott, D. H., Hodges, J. K., & Martin, R. D. (1988). Maternal behavior is related to prepartum urinary estradiol levels in red-bellied tamarin monkeys. *Physiol. Behav*. 44: 717–26.

Pryce, C. R., Dobeli, M., & Martin, D. R. (1993). Effects of sex steroids on maternal motivation in the common marmoset (*Callithrix jacchus*): Development and application of an operant system with maternal reinforcement. *J. Comp. Psych*. 107: 99–115.

Purves, D., Augustine, G. J., Fitzpatrick, D., Katz, L. C., La Mantia, A. S., & McNamara, J. O. (Eds.) (1997). *Neuroscience*. Sunderland, MA: Sinauer Associates.

Pusey, A. I., Williams, J., & Goodall, J. (1997). The influence of dominance rank on the reproductive success of female chimpanzees. *Science* 277: 828–31.

Rao, G. M. (1995). Oxytocin induces intimate behaviors. *Ind. J. Med. Sci*. 49: 261–6.

Reichstein, T. (1936). Constituents of the adrenal cortex. *Helv. Chim. Acta*. 19: 402–12.

Resnick, S. M. & Maki, P. M. (2002). Effects of hormone replacement therapy on cognitive and brain aging. *Ann. N. Y. Acad. Sci*. 949: 203–14.

Riskind, P. N., & Martin, J. B. (1989). Functional anatomy of the hypothalamic-anterior pituitary complex. In L. J. Degroot (Ed.), *Endocrinology*, 2nd ed., vol. 1. (pp. 97–107). Philadelphia: Saunders.

Roberts, L. (1988). Zeroing in on the sex switch. *Science* 239: 21–3.

Rosenblatt, J. S. (1992). Hormone-behavior relations in the regulation of parental behavior. In J. B. Becker, S. M. Breedlove, & D. Crews (Eds.), *Behavioral Endocrinology*. (pp. 219–59). Cambridge, MA: MIT Press.

Rosenblatt, J. S., & Snowdon, C. T. (1996). *Parental Care: Evolution, Mechanisms and Adaptive Significance*. San Diego: Academic Press.

Ruoff, W. L., & Dziuk, P. J. (1994). Circulation of estrogens introduced into the rectum or duodenum in pigs. *Domes. Anim. Endocrin*. 11: 383–91.

Saab, P. G., Stoney, C. M., & McDonald, R. H. (1989). Premenopausal and postmenopausal women differ in their cardiovascular and neuroendocrine responses to behavioral stressors. *Psychophys*. 26: 270–80.

Saltzman, W., Severin, J. M., Schultz-Darken, N. J., & Abbott, D. H. (1997). Behavioral and social correlates of escape from suppression of ovulation in female common marmosets housed with the natal family. *Am. J. Primatol*. 41: 1–21.

Sapolsky, R. (1992). Neuroendocrinology of the stress response. In J. B. Becker, S. M. Breedlove, & D. Crews (Eds.), *Behavioral Endocrinology* (pp. 287–324). Cambridge, MA: MIT Press.

Saucier, D. M. Gren, S. M., Leason, J., MacFassen, A., Bell, S., & Elias, L. J. (2002). Are sex differences in navigation caused by sexually dimorphic strategies or by differences in the ability to use strategies? *Behav. Neurosci*. 116, 403–10.

Savage, A., Snowdon, C. T., Giraldo, H., & Soto, H. (1997). Parental care patterns and vigilance in wild cotton-top tamarins (*Saguinus oedipus*). In M. Norconk, A. Rosenberger, & P. A. Garber (Eds.), *Adaptive Radiations of Neotropical Primates* (pp. 187–99). New York: Plenum.

Savage, A., Ziegler, T. E., & Snowdon, C. T. (1988). Sociosexual development, pair-bond formation and maintenance, and mechanisms of fertility suppression in female cotton-top tamarins (*Saguinus oedipus*). *Amer. J. Primatol*. 14: 345–59.

Scott, J. P., & Fredericson, E. (1951). The causes of fighting in mice and rats. *Physiol. Zool*. 24, 273–309.

Sherins, R. J., Paterson, A. P., & Brightwell, D. (1982). Alteration in the plasma testosterone: estradiol ratio: An alternative to the inhibin hypothesis. *Ann. New York Acad. Sci*. 383: 295–306.

Sherwin, B. B. (1997). Estrogen and memory: Evidence from clinical studies. Paper presented at the society of Behavioral Neuroendocrinology (May, Baltimore).

Sherwin, B. B., Gelfand, M. M., & Brender, W. (1985). Androgen enhances sexual motivation in females: A prospective, cross-over study of sex steroid administration in the surgical menopause. *Psychosom. Med*. 4: 339–51.

Snowdon, C. T. (1996). Infant care in cooperatively breeding species. In J. S. Rosenblatt & C. T. Snowdon (Eds.), *Parental Care: Evolution, Mechanisms and Adaptive Strategies*. (pp. 643–89). San Diego: Academic Press.

Snowdon, C. T. (1997). The "nature" of sex differences: Myths of male and female. In P. A. Gowaty (Ed.), *Feminism and Evolutionary Biology*. (pp. 276–93). New York: Chapman & Hall.

Stern, K. & McClintock, M. K. (1998). Regulation of ovulation by human pheromones. *Nature* 392: 177–9.

Stoney, C. M., Owens, J. F., Matthews, K. A., Davis, M. C., & Caggiula, A. (1990). Influences of the normal menstrual cycle on physiologic functioning during behavioral stress. *Psychophys*. 27, 125–35.

Storey, A. E., Walsh, C. J., Quinton, R. & Wynne-Edwards, K. E. (2000). Hormonal correlates of paternal responsiveness in new and expectant fathers. *Evol. Hum. Behav*. 21, 79–95.

Surbey, M. K. (1990). Family composition and the timing of human menarche. In T. E. Ziegler & F. B. Bercovitch (Eds.), *Socioendocrinology of Primate Reproduction* (pp. 11–32). New York: Wiley-Liss.

Suzuki, T., Schaumberg, D. A., Sullivan, B. D., Liu, M., Richards, S. M., Sullivan, R. M., Dana, M. R., & Sullivan, D. A. (2002). Do estrogen and progesterone play a role in the dry eye or Sjogren's Syndrome? *Ann. N. Y. Acad. Sci.* 996: 223–5.

Tannenbaum, P. L., & Wallen, K. (1997). Sexually initiated affiliation facilitates rhesus monkey integration. *Ann. New York Acad. Sci.* 807: 578–82.

Thorner, M. O. Vance, M. L., Horvath, E., & Kovacs, K. (1992). The anterior pituitary. In J. D. Wilson & D. W. Foster (Eds.), *Textbook of Endocrinology*, 8th ed. (pp. 221–310). Philadelphia: Saunders.

Trainor, B. C. & Marler, C. A. (2001a). Testosterone, paternal behavior and aggression in the monogamous California mouse (*Peromyscus californicus*). *Horm. Behav.* 40, 32–42.

Trainor, B. C. & Marler, C. A. (2001b). Testosterone promotes paternal behavior in a monogamous mammal via conversion to oestrogen. *Proc. Roy Soc. Lond. B.* 269, 823–9.

Trainor, B. C., Bird, I. M., Alday, N. A., Schlinger, B. A. & Marler, C. A. (2003). Variation in aromatase activity in the medial preoptic area and plasma progesterone is associated with the onset of paternal behavior. *Neuroendocrin.* 78, 36–44.

Trainor, B. C., Bird, I. M., & Marler, C. A. (2004). Opposing hormonal mechanisms of aggression revealed through short-lived testosterone manipulations and multiple winning experiences. *Horm. Behav.* 45, 115–21.

Uvnas-Moberg, K. (1997). Physiological and endocrine effects of social contact. *Ann. New York Acad. Sci.* 807, 146–63.

Vandenbergh, J. G. (1987). Regulation of puberty and its consequences on population dynamics in mice. *Am. Zool.* 27: 891–8.

Van Jaarsveld, A. S. & Skinner, J. D. (1991). Plasma androgens in spotted hyenas (*Crocuta crocuta*); influence of social and reproductive development. *J. Reprod. Fertil.* 93, 195–201.

Van Leeuwenhoek, A. (1678). Observations de natis e semine genitali animalcules. *Philos. Trans. R. Soc.* 12: 1040.

Wade, N. (1978). Guillemin and Schally. *Science* 200: 279–82, 411–14, 510–13.

Walker, S. F., McMurray, R. W., Houri, J. M., Allen, S. H., Kiesler, D., Sharp, G. C. & Schlechte, J. A. (1998). Effects of prolactin in stimulating disease activity in systemic lupus erythematosus. *Ann. N. Y. Acad. Sci.* 840: 762–72.

Wallen, K. (1990). Desire and ability: Hormones and the regulation of female sexual behavior. *Neurosci. Biobehav. Rev.* 14: 233–41.

Wallen, K. (1996). Nature needs nurture: the interaction of hormonal and social influences on the development of behavioral sex differences in rhesus monkeys. *Horm. Behav.* 30: 364–78.

Wallen, K., Maestripieri, D., & Mann, D. R. (1995). Effects of neonatal testicular suppression with a GnRH antagonist on social behavior in group-living rhesus monkeys. *Horm. Behav.* 18: 431–50.

Wallen, K., & Tannenbaum, P. L. (1997). Hormonal modulation of sexual behavior and affiliation in rhesus monkeys. *Ann. New York Acad. Sci.* 807: 185–202.

Wang, Z., Ferris, C. F., & De Vries, G. J. (1994). Role of septal vasopressin innervation in paternal behavior in prairie voles (*Microtus ochrogaster*). *Proc. Nat. Acad. Sci. USA* 91: 400–4.

Wang Z., & Insel, T. (1996). Parental care in voles In: J. S. Rosenblatt & C. T. Snowdon (Eds) *Parental Care: Evolution Mechanisms and Adaptive Strategies.* (pp 361–384). San Diego: Academic Press.

Wang, Z., Moody, K., Newman, J. D., & Insel, T. (1997). Vasopressin and oxytocin immunoreactive neurons and fibers in the forebrain of male and female common marmosets (*Callithrix jacchus*). *Synapse* 27: 14–25.

Warren, M. P., & Shortle, B. (1990). Endocrine correlates of human parenting: A clinical perspective. In N. A. Krasnegor & R. S. Bridges (Eds.), *Mammalian Parenting: Biochemical, Neurobiological and Behavioral Determinants.* (pp. 209–26). New York: Oxford University Press.

Wegesin, D. J. (1998). A neuropsychological profile of homosexual and heterosexual men and women. *Arch. Sex. Behav.* 27, 91–108.

Weller, A., & Weller, L. (1993). Menstrual synchrony between mothers and daughters and between roommates. *Physiol. Behav.* 53: 943–9.

Weller, A., & Weller, L. (1995). The impact of social interaction factors on menstrual synchrony in the workplace. *Psychoneuroendocrin.* 20: 21–31.

Weller, A., & Weller, L. (1997). Menstrual synchrony under optimal conditions. Bedouin families. *J. Comp. Psych.* 111: 143–51.

Wickelgren, I. (1997). Estrogen stakes claim to cognition. *Science* 276: 675–8.

Widowski, T. M., Porter, T. A., Ziegler, T. E., & Snowdon, C. T. (1992). The role of males on the initiation, but not the maintenance, of ovarian cycling in cotton-top tamarins (*Saguinus oedipus*). *Am. J. Primatol.* 26: 97–108.

Widowski, T. M., Ziegler, T. E., Elowson, A. M., & Snowdon, C. T. (1990). The role of males in stimulation of reproductive function in female cotton-top tamarins. (*Saguinus oedipus*). *Anim. Behav.* 40: 731–41.

Yallow, R. S. (1992). Radioimmunoassay of hormones. In J. D. Wilson & D. W. Foster (Eds.), *Textbook of Endocrinology*, 8th ed. (pp. 1635–45). Philadelphia: Saunders.

Yallow, R. S., & Berson, S. A. (1959). Assay of plasma insulin in human subjects by immunological methods. *Nature* 184: 1648–9.

Yen, S. C., & Jaffe, R. B. (1978). *Reproductive Endocrinology: Physiology, Pathophysiology and Clinical Management*. Philadelphia: Saunders.

Zhu, L. L. & Onaka, T. (2003). Facilitative role of prolactin-releasing peptide neurons in oxytocin cell activation after conditioned fear stimuli. *Neurosci.* 118, 1045–53.

Ziegler, T. E. (2000). Hormones associated with non-maternal infant care: A review of mammalian and avian studies. *Folia Primatol.* 71: 6–21.

Ziegler, T. E., Sholl, S. A., Scheffler, G., Haggerty, M. A., & Lasley, B. L. (1989). Excretion of estrone, estradiol and progesterone in the urine and feces of the female cotton-top tamarin (*Saguinus oedipus oedipus*). *Am. J. Primat.* 17: 185–95.

Ziegler, T. E., Widowski, T. M., Larson, M. L., & Snowdon, C. T. (1990). Nursing does affect the duration of the post-partum to ovulation interval in the cotton-top tamarin (*Saguinus oedipus*). *J. Reprod. Fert.* 90: 563–70.

Ziegler, T. E., Epple, G., Snowdon, C. T., Porter, T. A., Belcher, A. M., & Kuderling, I. (1993). Detection of the chemical signals of ovulation in the cotton-top tamarin (*Saguinus oedipus*). *Anim. Behav.* 45: 313–22.

Ziegler, T. E., Scheffler, G., Wittwer, D. J., Schultz-Darken, N., J., Snowdon, C. T., & Abbott, D. H. (1996a). Metabolism of reproductive steroids during the ovarian cycle in two species of callitrichids, *Saguinus oedipus* and *Callithrix jacchus*, and estimation of the ovulatory period from fecal steroids. *Biol. Reprod.* 54, 91–9.

Ziegler, T. E., Wegner, F. H., & Snowdon, C. T. (1996b). Hormonal responses to parental and nonparental conditions in male cotton-top tamarin, *Saguinus oedipus*, a New World primate. *Horm. Behav.* 30: 287–97.

Ziegler, T. E., Wegner, F. H., Carlson, A. A., Lazaro-Perea, C. & Snowdon, C. T. (2000). Prolactin levels during the periparturitional period in the biparental cotton-top tamarin (*Saguinus oedipus*): interactions with gender, androgen levels and parenting. *Horm. Behav.* 38, 112–122.

Ziegler, T. E. & Snowdon, C. T. (2000). Preparental hormone levels and parenting experience in male cotton-top tamarins, *Saguinus oedipus*. *Horm. Behav.* 38, 159–167.

Ziegler, T. E., Washabaugh, K. F. & Snowdon, C. T. (2004a). Responsiveness of expectant male cotton-top tamarins, *Saguinus oedipus*, to mate's pregnancy. *Horm. Behav.* 45, 84–92.

Ziegler, T. E., Jacoris, S. & Snowdon, C. T. (2004b). Sexual communication between breeding male and female cotton-top tamarins (*Saguinus oedipus*) and its relationship to infant care. *Amer. J. Primatol.* 64, 57–69.

Ziegler, T. E., Schultz-Darken, N. J., Scott, J. J., Snowdon, C. T. & Ferris, C. F. (2005). Neuroendocrine response to female ovulatory odors depends upon social condition in male common marmosets, *Callithrix jacchus*. *Horm & Behav.* 47, 56–64.

Zucker, K. J., Bradley, S. J., Oliver, G., Blake, J., Fleming, S. & Hood, J. (1996). Psychosocial development of women with congenital adrenal hyperplasia, *Horm. Behav.* 30, 300–18.

15 Innate and Cell-Mediated Immunity: Basic Principles and Psychophysiological Influences

FIRDAUS S. DHABHAR

HISTORICAL CONTEXT

Throughout the history of medicine, physicians and philosophers have grappled with the question of whether and how different mental and emotional states affect health. Approximately 4,000 years ago, the Nei Ching, an ancient Chinese classic on internal medicine, laid out nine groups of disease-causing agents among which they listed "worry and imagination" (stress) as being able to upset the functioning of the spleen (immune system). Around the second century A.D., the Greek physician Galen observed that melancholic women were more susceptible to breast cancer than those who were sanguine. Closer to our times, there has been a tremendous interest from society and the scientific community in applying the principles and techniques of modern science towards understanding the age-old question of how states of mind might affect states of body and health. Solomon and Moos (1964) coined the term psychoimmunology to describe the field that examines interactions between psychological states and immune function (Solomon & Moos, 1964) and Ader and Cohen (1981) introduced the term psychoneuroimmunology that also represents the neuroendocrine connections between psychological states and immune function (Ader & Cohen, 1981). The history of the field is reviewed in Uchino, Kiecolt-Glaser, & Glaser, 2000. The past few decades have seen a tremendous increase in the number of scientific studies designed to examine how psychophysiology can influence immunology and vice versa (Steinman, 2004). Numerous different dimensions of immune function have been included in these investigations are discussed in excellent comprehensive reviews (e.g., Blalock, 1984; Dantzer & Kelley, 1989; Rabin et al., 1989; Bovbjerg, 1991; Dunn, 1995; Anisman et al., 1996a; Anisman et al., 1996b; Maier & Watkins, 1997; McEwen et al., 1997; Bucala, 1998;

Felten et al., 1998; Heijnen & Kavelaars, 1999; Vedhara, Fox, & Wang 1999; Pruett, 2001; Webster, Tonelli, & Sternberg, 2002; Irwin, 2002; Kiecolt-Glaser et al., 2002; Sanders & Straub, 2002; Straub & Besedovsky, 2003; Kelley, 2004) and books (e.g., Rabin, 1999; Schedlowski & Tewes, 1999; Sternberg, 2000; Ader, Felten, & Cohen, 2001) that have provided an updated integration of the field almost every year for the past two decades. Interestingly, the interactions between psychophysiological and immune factors are not unidirectional but are reciprocal in nature. It has also been shown that changes in immune function can have profound reciprocal psychological, behavioral, and physiological effects (for review see Black 1994; Miller 1998; Dunn 2000; Dantzer 2001; Capuron & Dantzer 2003; Harbuz 2003; Maier & Watkins 2003; Raison & Miller 2003; Straub 2004). Some scientifically based books that are written for a more general audience also make excellent and informative reading: (e.g., Sternberg, 2000; McEwen, 2002; Sapolsky, 2004). This chapter will focus on the mechanisms mediating innate and cell-mediated immunity and discuss relevant issues in the larger context of psychophysiological effects on immune function.

FACTORS MEDIATING INNATE & CELL-MEDIATED IMMUNITY

The major cellular and molecular components that make up innate and cell-mediated immune responses are discussed in the following sections. The reader is encouraged to keep in mind that each of the parameters discussed in the following sections can be measured and many of these parameters can be measured in peripheral blood, which is the most accessible and widely used compartment for studies involving human subjects. The interpretation of information obtained from such measurements depends on many factors such as the context, compartment, time point, and manner in which these measurements are made. These factors will be discussed later in this chapter.

Preparation of this chapter was supported by grants from the National Institutes of Health (AI48995) and The Dana Foundation Clinical Hypotheses Program in Mind Body Medicine.

INNATE IMMUNITY

Innate immunity is also known as native or natural immunity because components of the innate immune system are always present and ready to defend the organism (Abbas, Lichtman, & Pober, 2000; Roitt, Brostoff, & Male, 2001). Although innate immunity is sometimes considered primarily reactive against microbial pathogens, components of the innate immune system can also be involved in foreign antigen/body reactions and immunopathological reactions to self tissue. Innate immunity constitutes an effective mechanism for responding to and often eliminating pathogens early during an immune response. Therefore, components of innate immunity form the body's first line of defense and elements of the innate immune system can be activated within minutes of an immunological challenge. Components of the innate immune system include the following players:

Epithelial barriers. The only interfaces through which pathogens can enter the body are the skin, and the gastrointestinal, respiratory, and urinary genital tracts. Each of these interfaces has a specialized layer of continuous epithelial cells and associated mucosal tissues that form formidable innate defenses. In addition to acting as physical barriers, epithelial cells secrete and are covered by a host of anti-microbial peptides and enzymes that also confer protection. Each specialized epithelial barrier also has a host of other cellular components. For example, keratinocytes, mast cells and intra-epithelial or $\gamma\delta$-T cells are all present in skin and have important functions in host defense.

The complement system. The complement system is an important humoral component of innate immunity. It consists of critical circulating and membrane bound proteins that once triggered, participate in self-driven anti-microbial cascades. The complement cascade can be triggered by three major pathways: The classical pathway involves activation by antibodies bound on the microbial surface and as such is an example of the often-observed interplay between the innate and adaptive immune systems (discussed further in the following section). The alternative pathway is launched when specific complement proteins directly bind the microbial surface in the absence of counter-regulatory proteins (that are present to protect host cells). The lectin pathway is triggered when mannose-binding lectin (MBL, that is present in plasma) binds terminal mannose residues on microbial surface glycoproteins. Once activated, complemented-mediated microbe destruction involves punching osmotic holes into the microbial surface, opsonization of the microbe by complement factor C3b which facilitates removal by phagocytes that express C3b receptors, and chemoattraction, activation, and targeting of additional leukocytes to the site of microbial invasion.

Neutrophils & macrophages. Neutrophils and macrophages form the critical cellular phagocytic component of innate immunity. They arise from progenitor stem cells within the bone marrow that are of the myeloid lineage. The production of these leukocyte subpopulations is controlled by cytokines that are known as colony stimulating factors like IL-1, IL-3, IL7, and granulocyte macrophage colony stimulating factor (GMCSF) Circulating macrophages are known as monocytes. Monocytes mature into macrophages when they leave the circulation to enter tissues where they may undergo further activation and differentiation.

Neutrophils are among the first cells to enter tissue from the circulation following immune activation. They are critical for defense against bacterial and fungal infections and for the initial phases of wound healing. Although they are present in high proportions particularly in human blood, neutrophils have a short half-life and may die within hours after extravasating into tissues. Controlled neutrophil death occurs via the process of apoptosis although necrotic cell death is also observed during immunopathology. Neutrophils eliminate pathogens via phagocytosis followed by internal enzymatic destruction.

Macrophages closely follow neutrophils into sites of immune activation. They phagocytose and destroy antigens, pathogens, dead neutrophils, and damaged cells and tissues. In addition to phagocytosis, macrophages perform important functions like antigen presentation to T cells and therefore form a critical nexus between the innate and the adaptive immune systems. Macrophages are different from neutrophils in that they are capable of long-term survival after extravasation. In addition to macrophages that are recruited as monocytes from the blood, there are resident macrophages that are stationed in most tissues of the body. Macrophage differentiation can lead to the formation of specialized tissue specific forms like microglia in the CNS, Kupffer cells in liver, alveolar macrophages in lung, and osteoclasts in bone.

Neutrophils and macrophages have receptors that enable them to recognize microbes and specific microbial products. These receptors are thought to enable phagocytes to distinguish pathogens from self-antigens because they recognize molecules that are specific to microbes and generally not expressed by healthy self-tissue. Such receptors include mannose receptors that bind terminal mannose residues on microbial surface glycoproteins, N-formyl methionine peptide (FMLP) receptors, and receptors that specifically recognize acetylated low density lipoproteins specific for certain pathogens. In addition, macrophages bear toll-like receptors (TLRs) that are specific for certain fungi and gram negative and gram positive bacteria. These receptors are so named because they are homologous to the Toll protein which is critical for protecting Drosophilla from microbial pathogens. These cells may also express receptors for other microbe-specific products such as unmethylated bacterial DNA and double stranded viral RNA. In addition to an array of receptor mechanisms serving the innate immune functions performed by neutrophils and macrophages, these phagocytic cells also bear receptors that enable them to harness complement (complement receptors) and antibody (Fc receptors) mediated protective mechanisms.

The process of phagocytosis involves capturing extracellular pathogens into intracellular phagosomes. The phagocyte does this by extending a portion of its cell membrane all the way around the pathogen(s) until the membrane closes up and pinches off into the cytoplasm of the phagocyte. Phagosomes then combine with cytoplasmic lysosomes to form phagolysosomes. Pathogens are killed within phagolysosomes by several mechanisms which include the activation of anti-microbial systems consisting of lysosomal proteases, phagocyte oxidase which generates superoxide anions and free radicals, and inducible nitric oxide synthase, which generates NO, all of which have potent microbicidal effects.

Therefore, neutrophils and monocytes are extremely important cells of the innate immune system because they have the ability to recognize, phagocytose, and internally destroy an array of pathogens.

NK cells. NK cells are derived from lymphoid progenitor stem cells in the bone marrow, but do not express antigen-specific receptors that are seen on T and B cells. They form an important component of the innate immune system. They are not phagocytic cells, but kill cells that are infected by intracellular pathogens via lytic mechanisms which involve punching holes in the plasma membrane with the help of proteins like perforin followed by introducing other molecules into the target cell that activate enzymes that induce apoptosis of the infected cell. NK cells also secrete IFN-γ, that is a critical cytokine for macrophage activation. Interestingly, macrophages in turn produce cytokines like IL-12 which are potent activators of NK cells.

NK cells are thought to recognize infected cells through receptors for specific molecules that are only expressed on cells carrying intracellular pathogens. NK cells also express Fc receptors which enable them to play a role in antibody-dependent cytotoxicity. Another class of NK cell surface receptors is the family of killer inhibitory receptors which prevent NK cells from destroying self tissue. Killer inhibitory receptors recognize molecules like MHC I which is present on all healthy nucleated cells of the body. MHC I recognition prevents further NK activity. However, many microbes have evolved to induce cells to stop expressing MHC I after they are infected. This gives the pathogen a survival advantage by preventing recognition and elimination of the infected cell by cytolytic T cells (CTL). However, infected cells are now recognized by NK cells because they no longer express MHC I and thus fail to activate killer inhibitory receptors and this facilitates their elimination by NK cells.

Primary cytokines of innate immunity. Macrophages, NK cells, and other leukocytes of innate immunity secrete cytokines upon stimulation. These cytokines often act on the cells that produce them (autocrine effects) and on other target cells that may be adjacent (paracrine effects) or at a distance (endocrine effects). It is important to appreciate that many cytokines are secreted by different types of leukocytes and act on different target cells and therefore may be involved in mediating aspects of innate as well as adaptive immunity. TNF-α and IL-1 are perhaps the most important cytokine drivers of innate immunity. They recruit and activate neutrophils, macrophages and other leukocytes to the site of an innate immune reaction.

The principal cellular sources of TNF-α are macrophages and T cells. TNFα can exert a variety of effects on numerous different cells and tissues which include activation of endothelial cells and promotion of inflammatory and hemostatic cascades, neutrophil activation, fever production through central nervous system actions, stimulation of acute phase protein synthesis and secretion by the liver, breakdown of muscle and adipose tissue (cachexia), and stimulation of apoptosis of different cell types. Excess of TNF-α can also lead to clinically important and devastating effects. For example, TNF-α mediates toxic shock that occurs when macrophages produce systemically high levels of TNF-α, following activation of their lipopolyscharide (LPS) receptors by endotoxin (LPS) released from severe gram negative bacterial infections. Metabolic dysregulation, widespread intravascular coagulation and low blood pressure are hallmarks of toxic shock and are the result of high systemic levels of TNF-α.

The principal cellular sources of IL-1 are macrophages, keratinocytes, endothelial cells and some epithelial cells. IL-1 also activates endothelial cells, generates fever, and stimulates hepatic synthesis of acute phase proteins and can exert immuno-protective as well as immuno-pathological effects. In addition to these two cytokines, other components of the innate immune system like NK cells produce IFN-γ that is also produced by T cells and is a potent activator of macrophage function and also stimulates some classes of antibody responses. IFN-α and IFN-β that are critical for anti-viral immunity, are also produced by macrophages and other cells of the innate immune system. Other cytokines that are traditionally thought of as being mediators of adaptive immunity (e.g., IL-6, IL-10, IL-12, IL-15, and IL-18) are also secreted by macrophages in addition to T cells and act on various components of the innate immune system.

Acute phase proteins. Acute phase proteins are a family of proteins whose circulating levels increase sharply after infection. Plasma mannose-binding lectin (MBL) and C-reactive protein (CRP) are examples of acute phase proteins that also represent humoral components of innate immunity. MBL plays critical role by coating microbes through binding terminal mannose residues on microbial surface glycoproteins this enables microbial elimination via activating the complement system and by promoting phagocytosis. CRP similarly binds phosphorylcholine on the microbial surface and also promotes phagocytosis of coated microbes via binding the macrophage CRP receptor.

Innate immunity summary. The innate immune system is critical for rapid elimination of pathogens and are often the only line of available defense in case of primary encounters with pathogens to which the immune system has not been previously exposed. Specific responses to different types of microbial pathogens vary and are evolutionarily selected to best protect against these microbes. In general, extracellular pathogens are eliminated by the acute phase and complement systems and phagocytes. Intracellular pathogens are eliminated by NK cells and phagocytes. Components of the innate immune system are not only the body's first defenders, but also play the crucial role of activating the adaptive immune system (e.g., antigen presentation and activation of helper T cells by macrophages) and forming a crucial part of the effector mechanisms that are enlisted by an adaptive immune response (e.g., antibody-dependent cell-mediated cytotoxicity, Th1 cytokine stimulated activation of macrophage phagocytosis). Cytokines provide the critical links in communication between the cellular components of innate and adaptive immunity.

CELL-MEDIATED IMMUNITY (CMI)

CMI represents one arm of the adaptive immune system; the other arm being humoral immunity that is discussed in Chapter 16 (Humoral Immunity, V. Sanders). Traditionally, CMI reactions were defined as antigen-specific reactions that could be transferred from one organism to another only by the transfer of cells (later identified as T cells) and not by antibodies (Abbas et al., 2000; Roitt et al., 2001). Immune reactions orchestrated by helper T (Th) cells and effected by cytolytic T cells (CTLs), macrophages, and NK cells are known as CMI reactions. CMI reactions are critical for eliminating infections by intracellular pathogens because antibodies that mediate humoral immunity are ineffective for intracellular pathogens. Antigen specificity of these reactions is conferred by T cells whereas macrophages are among the most important effector cells either as directly activated phagocytes or as the cells that ultimately clear up CTL and NK cell-mediated destruction.

Antigen presenting cell and T cell interactions. Extracellular pathogens that are specifically phagocytosed by APCs and processed within vesicles are presented by MHC II molecules. Intracellular pathogens that are present in the cytoplasm are processed into peptides that are presented by MHC I molecules. APCs that present antigen in conjunction with MHC II molecules are also known as professional APCs. T cell activation occurs following specific cascades of interactions between the T cell and antigen presenting cell (APC) which involve antigen recognition in the context of MHC molecule presentation, cell-cell adhesion, and co-stimulation: (1) The T cell receptor complex interacts with MHC molecules on the APC to recognize antigen for which they are specific. (2) Integrins like LFA-1 on the T cell interact with ICAM-1 on the APC to stabilize cell-cell interactions that are crucial for T cell activation. (3) Co-stimulatory molecules like CD28 on T cells interact with B7–1 and B7–2 on APCs, and CD40L (CD154) on T cells interacts with CD40 on APCs to provide additional signals that are required for effective T cell activation.

Naïve, effector, & memory T cells. CMI involves antigen recognition by naïve and memory T cells at two largely distinct locations. Naïve T cells form within the thymus and are released into the circulation following positive and negative selection processes. Naïve T cells are activated when they encounter and recognize specific antigen in sentinel lymph nodes. Upon activation, naïve T cells proliferate and differentiate into effector and memory T cells. Effector T cells are responsible for elimination of pathogen whereas memory T cells are long-lived cells that are critical for mounting faster and more robust immune responses upon subsequent exposure to the same antigen. Once differentiated in sentinel lymph nodes, effector T cells can recognize the same antigen if detected anywhere in the body. These cells are again activated upon recognizing antigen under the appropriate antigen-presenting conditions. Activation of effector cells at sites of infection results in changes in phenotype that retain these cells at those sites. Cytokines, chemokines, and adhesion molecule cascades play a critical role in attracting, activating, and retaining antigen-specific effector T cells at sites of pathogen entry.

The adhesion molecule repertoire on the plasma membrane is particularly suited to maximize the probability that T cells in their different stages of differentiation will be exposed to antigen under the appropriate conditions. Therefore, naïve T cells express CD62L which enables them to attach to high endothelial venules within lymph nodes and increases the probability of their encountering APCs that may have trafficked to sentinel nodes following antigen entry. Activated effector and memory T cells on the other hand express ligands for E and P selectin which enable leukocyte rolling on activated endothelium and facilitate migration into tertiary immune tissues (skin, gut, etc.) that are often the sites of infection by intracellular pathogens. Effector and memory T cells also show increased expression of lymphocyte function-associated antigen-1 (LFA-1 a $\beta 2$ integrin) and very late activation antigen-4 (VLA-4, a $\beta 1$ integrin) which enable stronger adhesion to activated endothelium and transmigration into sites of infection. If an effector T cell encounters specific antigen, the cell is further activated at the tertiary site and retained at that site to stimulate or execute pathogen clearance. Effector cells that do not encounter specific antigen exit tissues through lymphatic vessels and re-enter the circulation. Memory T cells persist for long periods of time and constantly patrol tissues following surveillance trafficking patterns designed to maximize the probability of encounter with specific antigens for which they have memory.

Effector responses of CMI. Effector CMI responses can be divided into two broad categories: CD4+ Th cells activate phagocytes to destroy ingested pathogens that are contained within vesicles and CD8+ CTLs destroy all cells (phagocytic and nonphagocytic) that harbor cytoplasmic pathogens that are not contained within vesicles. This distinction is useful and important but not absolute as some CD4 T cells kill infected phagocytes and some CD8 T cells can activate phagocytes for destruction of pathogens within phagolysosomes.

Macrophage effector function. Upon recognition of antigens presented by macrophage MHC II molecules, effector CD4 T cells secrete Th1 cytokines like IFN-γ and stimulate CD40L-CD40 interactions that activate macrophages. Macrophage activation results in the production of transcription factors that in turn activate gene expression of nitric oxide synthase, proteases, and enzymes that generate reactive oxygen species all of which exert potent antimicrobial effects that were discussed earlier under "innate immunity." The requirement for activation by IFN-γ in addition to CD40L-CD40 interactions ensures that macrophages that are in close proximity to the Th cell (those that contain and are therefore able to present antigen) are mainly the ones that are activated. T cell stimulated macrophage effector function is especially important in cases where microbes have evolved to escape destruction in phagolysosomes and where additional T cell help enables macrophages to effectively eliminate such pathogens. In addition to eliminating pathogens, activated macrophages play several other important roles in CMI. They secrete cytokines like TNF-α and IL-1 and chemokines which activate endothelial cells and recruit additional leukocytes to the site of the CMI reaction. Macrophages are also critical for the clearance of apoptotic cells (e.g., neutrophils) and debris and hence pave the way for the resolution of inflammation.

CTL effector function. CD8+ cytolytic T cells (CTLs) are thus named because they kill infected cells and certain types of tumor cells by lysing as opposed to phagocytosing them. The classical method of CTL activation involves these cells recognizing antigen being presented in the context of MCH I molecules on the plasma membrane of an infected cell. CTLs can be activated by infected cells that present the antigen for which the CTL bears specificity. This specificity is expressed through the CTL T cell receptor. Adhesion molecules present on the CTL surface and interact with ligands (and vice versa) on the infected cell's plasma membrane and stabilize interactions between the

two cells. This enables the CTL to be activated and also enables the cell to go on to perform it's effector function with is to lyse the infected target cell.

A single CTL can successively kill many infected or target cells one after the other. Target cell lysis is accomplished by directed exocytosis of the CTLs granule contents at the site of closest approximation with its target cell. The products that are exocytosed consist of perforin which gets polymerized and embedded within the target cell plasma membrane to form pores through the membrane, and enzymes that induce DNA fragmentation and target cell apoptosis which travel into the target cell through perforin channels. CTL granule enzymes are called granzymes. Upon entry into the target cell, granzymes activate target cell caspases which then induce controlled cell death or apoptosis of the target cell. Fas ligand which is expressed by activated CTLs is thought to induce target cell apoptosis by activating target cell Fas (CD95) in some instances.

Importantly, phagocytes play an crucial role following CTL effector actions because it is these cells that ultimately clear up damaged and dead infected target cells that have been destroyed by CTL action. CTLs secrete IFN-γ at sites of activation. This further activates macrophages at sites of immune activation and enables them to more effectively process and destroy phagocytosed pathogens.

Cytokine regulators of cell-mediated immunity. Several different cytokines play important and specific roles in regulating different aspects of CMI. These functions are briefly described here. IL-12 is secreted by macrophages and professional APCs like dendritic cells. IL-12 is one of the most important initial drivers of CMI because it stimulates the differentiation of naïve Th cells to activated effector Th1 cells. It also stimulates both Th cells and CTLs to secrete IFN-γ, that as discussed earlier, is a potent macrophage activator and therefore a critical driver of the effector phase of CMI. IL-2 is produced by T cells. It promotes clonal expansion of antigen-activated T cells because it is a powerful autocrine T cell growth factor. TNF-α is secreted by macrophages and T cells at the site of antigen or pathogen detection. TNF-α is a potent initiator of the inflammatory cascade that launches the effector phase of CMI. It acts on endothelial cells to activate adhesion molecules which help recruit circulating leukocytes to the site of immune activation. TNF-α also helps activate leukocytes that are thus recruited to the site of immune activation. Thus, the prototypical Th1 cytokines, IL-12, IL-2, and IFN-γ play are crucial cytokine drives of CMI. In contrast, the Th2 cytokines, IL-4, IL-13, and IL-10 are important counter-regulatory factors that are thought to dampen CMI responses by inhibiting macrophage and Th1 cell activation and function. In contrast to Th1 cytokines that promote CMI, Th2 cytokines promote humoral immunity.

CMI reactions and the delayed type hypersensitivity (DTH) skin test. The CMI reactions described above can be modeled and measured by an in vivo immunological assay known as the DTH skin test. In this case, CMI reactions are elicited by injecting minute quantities of antigen into the skin of individuals to be tested. Healthy individuals who have been previously immunized or exposed to the antigen generally develop a positive immune response that is manifest as an increase in erythema and induration at the site of antigen injection. The name "Delayed Type Hypsersensitivity" comes from the fact that it takes 24 to 48 hours for circulating antigen-specific T cells to be recruited to the site of antigen administration, to be activated, and to subsequently activate effector cells that mediate the CMI reactions that result in detectable signs of a DTH response. The magnitude of erythema can be subjectively graded and the diameters of the area of induration recorded in millimeters. DTH is an example of Type IV hypersensitivity and involves a longer time course (24–48 h) for development of a detectable immune response compared to those seen with Type I (within minutes) or Types II and III (5–12 h) hypersensitivity reactions. DTH tests may be used clinically to gauge whether an individual has been previously exposed to an antigen or pathogen (e.g., the tuberculin skin test that tests for prior exposure to mycobacterium tuberculosis). DTH tests may also be used to examine whether an individual has developed effective immunity following vaccination. Such tests have been used to elucidate the extent of immunodeficiency (e.g., AIDS patients may progressively lose their ability to mount DTH reactions to commonly encountered antigens which may indicate a progressive loss of immunity to certain pathogens) (Birx et al., 1993).

Immune responses work in synchrony in vivo. It is helpful to categorize different aspects of the immune system into different categories such as innate versus adaptive, Th1 versus Th2 and so on. However, it is extremely important to bear in mind that most components of the immune system participate in most *in vivo* immune responses. Therefore, any given immune response will consist of cellular and molecular components of innate and adaptive immunity and Th1 as well as Th2 cellular and cytokine driver and regulatory systems. For example, some reactions, such as CMI reactions, are categorized as being an example of adaptive immunity. They consist more of CTL and macrophage driven responses that are predominantly stimulated by the Th1 family of cytokines. Other responses involve a greater contribution from B cell driven antibody or humoral responses and are stimulated by the Th2 family of cytokines. However, as discussed earlier, Th1 and Th2 cytokines play important counter-regulatory roles in most adaptive immune responses, and importantly, neutrophils, macrophages and NK cells, of the "innate" immune system often serve as critical effector cells for cellular and humoral immune responses.

Importance of leukocyte distribution & trafficking. The appropriate distribution of immune cells between organs in the body is crucial for the performance of the surveillance as well as effector functions of the immune system and is critical for supporting all types of immune responses. Rapid leukocyte trafficking into sites of immune activation is critical for effective immunoprotection (Sprent & Tough, 1994). Rapid and targeted leukocyte distribution also enables different components of the immune system to work together as discussed in the preceding section. The blood is an important conduit by which leukocytes travel from one body compartment to another and the blood is also perhaps the most important compartment that is sampled and studied especially for neuro-endocrine-immune studies involving human subjects. Therefore, it is important to understand the basic processes by which leukocytes traffic from body compartment to another.

Leukocytes travel from one area of the body to another by a combination of passive as well as active processes. Blood flow passively carries leukocytes throughout the circulatory system. Active processes triggered by cytokines and chemokines and mediated by changes in adhesion molecule expression or affinity, selectively retain specific leukocyte subpopulations at sites of immune activation. These active processes involve cascades of interactions between families of adhesion molecules and their ligands that may be present either on leukocytes or endothelial cells. The selectin family of adhesion molecules, consisting of L-selectin (CD62L), E-selectin (CD62E), and P-selectin (CD62P) and their respective ligands, are responsible for slowing leukocytes down by inducing leukocyte rolling on high endothelial venules within lymph node vasculature (CD62L) or on activated endothelial cells (CD62E and CD62P). Chemokines released by leukocytes, endothelial cells, and other cells at the site of immune activation are captured and presented by glycosaminoglycans on endothelial cells and they activate rolling leukocytes which begin to activate their cell surface integrins. Leukocyte surface integrins (e.g., CD18, CD11b) interact with endothelial ICAMs (e.g., CD54) to form stronger bonds that arrest leukocytes on the activated endothelium. Further activation cascades of integrins, ICAMS, and their respective ligands enable the activated leukocyte to transmigrate to leave the lumen of the blood vessel and enter extravascular tissue. Enzymes like matrix metalloproteases (MMPs) enable leukocytes to make their way through extracellular matrix to reach the site of immune activation.

PSYCHOPHYSIOLOGICAL INFLUENCES ON IMMUNE FUNCTION

Although it was traditionally thought that the immune system functioned largely autonomously from other physiological systems, a large body of evidence now shows that psychological and physiological factors can influence different immune parameters (For review see Ader et al., 2001). Solomon and Moos (1964) coined the term psychoimmunology to describe the field that examines interactions between psychological states and immune function (Solomon & Moos, 1964) and Ader and Cohen (1981) introduced the term psychoneuroimmunology that also represents the neuroendocrine connections between psychological states and immune function (Ader & Cohen, 1981).

Several key scientific findings have provided convincing and intriguing evidence for the number of molecular, cellular, and systems level pathways through which psychophysiology can influence the immune system. These findings and selected references and reviews describing them, are listed in the following section.

Immune cells and organs bear receptors for hormones and neurotransmitters and respond to ligands for these receptors. Such ligand-receptor effects (Weigent & Blalock, 1987) include those reported for catecholamines (Benschop et al., 1993; Madden & Felten, 1995; Heijnen and Kavelaars, 1999; Rouppe van der Voort, et al., 1999; Rouppe van der Voort et al., 2000; Sanders and Straub, 2002), glucocorticoids (Munck, Crabtree, & Smith, 1979; Miller et al., 1990; Munck & Naray-Fejes-Toth, 1992; Dhabhar et al., 1996; McEwen et al., 1997), opioid peptides (Faith et al., 1984; Weber & Pert, 1989; Adler et al., 1993; Carr et al., 1995; Carr, Rogers, & Weber, 1996; Jessop, 1998), growth hormone (Arkins, Dantzer, & Kelley, 1993; Malarkey et al., 2002), melatonin (Maestroni & Conti, 1996), leptin (La cava & Mataresse, 2004), calcitonin gene-related peptide (Asahina et al., 1995; Bulloch et al., 1995), neurotrophic factors (Torii et al., 1997), vasoactive intestinal peptide (Bellinger et al., 1996), neuropeptide Y (Jessop et al., 1992; Lambert & Granstein, 1998; Straub et al., 2000), prolactin (Arkins et al., 1993; Berczi, 1997; Clevenger, Freier, & Kline, 1998), oxytocin and vasopressin (Geenen et al., 1989), and androgens and estrogens (Draca, 1995; Da Silva, 1999; Ben-Eliyahu et al., 2000; Cutolo et al., 2004; Obendorf & Patchev, 2004).

Immune cells and organs have also been shown to synthesize various hormones and neurotransmitters that were traditionally thought to be the "property" of the nervous and endocrine systems (Jessop, 2002). Examples include proopiomelanocortin (POMC) peptides (Blalock, Harbour-McMenamin, & Smith, 1985; Jessop, Jukes, & Lightman, 1994; Blalock, 1999), adrenocortropic hormone (ACTH) (Jessop et al., 1995), endomorphins (Jessop et al., 2000), prolactin (Sabharwal et al., 1992), corticotrophin releasing factor (CRF) (Stephanou et al., 1990), corticosteroids (Vacchio, Papadopoulos, & Ashwell, 1994; Vacchio, Lee, & Ashwell 1999), and vasopressin (Jessop et al., 1995; Jessop, Murphy, & Larsen, 1995).

Elements of the nervous and endocrine systems have been shown to produce factors that were traditionally thought to belong exclusively to the immune system. For example, the pituitary has been shown to produce macrophage migration inhibition factor (MIF) that acts as an impor-

tant glucocorticoid counter-regulator (Bucala, 1998) and IL-18 has been shown to be produced by the adrenal cortex (Conti et al., 2000).

Different branches of the nervous system innervate specific immune organs. These innervations include those emanating from the sympathetic nervous system (Felten et al., 1987; Felten, 1993; Felten et al., 1993), the autonomic nervous system (Bulloch & Pomerantz, 1984; Tracey, 2002; Pavlov & Tracey, 2004), and from peptidergic nerves (Romano et al., 1991; Asahina et al., 1995; Kodali et al., 2004). Recently, the concept of the immunological reflex has been proposed that suggests that the nervous system, through cholinergic neurons may dampen immune responses as they occur (Tracey, 2002).

Immune responses can be behaviorally conditioned. A fundamental finding that in many ways launched modern field of psychoneuroimmunology came from seminal studies by Ader and Cohen (1975) that showed that immune responses can be behaviorally conditioned (Ader & Cohen, 1975; Bovbjerg, Ader, & Cohen, 1982; Ader & Cohen, 1991). In addition to showing the critical and intriguing link between the nervous and immune systems these conditioning studies have significant clinical implications for example for regulating the course of autoimmune diseases (Ader and Cohen, 1991). Importantly, conditioning studies have also been extended to human subjects which shows the significant clinical potential of behaviorally conditioning immune responses (Buske-Kirschbaum et al., 1992; Buske-Kirschbaum et al., 1994; Goebel et al., 2002).

Psychophysiological stressors affect immune function. The effects of stress on different parameters and aspects of immune function is perhaps the most widely studied connection between psychophysiological changes and immune function. Numerous groups of investigators have investigated this connection from different angles. The following reviews examine different aspects of the effects of stress on immune function (Zwilling, 1992; Herbert & Cohen, 1993; McEwen et al., 1997; Sheridan, 1998; Kiecolt-Glaser, 1999; Yang & Glaser, 2002; Cohen & Hamrick, 2003; Sephton & Spiegel, 2003; Hawkley & Cacioppo, 2004; Glaser, 2005). Specific examples include demonstrated relationships between stress reactivity and changes in immune parameters (Benschop et al., 1998; Cacioppo et al., 2002), chronic stress-induced suppression of wound healing (Kiecolt-Glaser et al., 2004), stress-induced suppression of recovery from surgery (Kiecolt-Glaser et al., 1998), chronic stress and susceptibility to infection (Glaser et al., 1987; Bonneau et al., 1991; Cohen, Tyrrell, & Smith, 1991; Sheridan et al., 1991; Bonneau, 1996; Cole & Kemeny, 1997; Sheridan et al., 1998; Sheridan et al., 2000; Buske-Kirschbaum et al., 2001), chronic stress-induced suppression of vaccine uptake (Kiecolt-Glaser et al., 1996; Glaser et al., 1998; Glaser et al., 2000), and the suggested relationships between stress and cancer susceptibility (Shavit et al., 1985; Brenner et al., 1990; Ben-Eliyahu et al., 1991; Bryla, 1996; Andersen et al., 1998; Kiecolt-Glaser, & Glaser 1999; Ben-Eliyahu, 2003; Lutgendorf et al., 2003; Pereira et al., 2003).

Exercise has also been shown to affect different immune parameters through physiological systems that are similar to those activated during stress (Pedersen & Hoffman-Goetz, 2000). In a recent paper, Epel et al. (2004) have shown that chronic perceived stress is correlated with accelerated telomere shortening in peripheral blood leukocytes (Epel et al., 2004). At first pass, a plausible explanation for such telomere shortening in immune cells was that the chronically stressed subjects may have experienced more infections. As a result, their immune cells may have been more activated by greater numbers of immune challenges, and may have gone through significantly higher numbers of cell divisions resulting in shorter telomeres. However, the relationship between stress and telomere shortening does not appear to be related to greater numbers of immune activating challenges experienced by high stress subjects. Thus, the high and low stress subjects did not show differences in proportions of naïve versus memory T cells, a ratio that reflects the "immunological experience" of an individual. Although much work remains to be done, this study is an important example of how clues obtained from different psychophysiological, immune, cellular, and molecular parameters can be pieced together to begin an understanding of an important phenomenon, namely accelerated cellular aging in the immune system that is related to psychological stress.

Although stress may be categorized in many ways, it is useful to classify stressors as being acute (lasting for minutes to hours) or chronic (lasting for weeks to months to years) (Dhabhar & McEwen, 1997; Dhabhar & McEwen, 2001). While working with these categories, it is also important to distinguish between single versus repeated stressors and recognize that repeated acute stressor may contribute significantly to chronic stress (Dhabhar, McEwen, & Spencer 1997). Dhabhar and McEwen have proposed a "stress spectrum model" that attempts to explain the bi-directional effects of acute versus chronic stress on immune function (Dhabhar & McEwen, 1997; Dhabhar & McEwen, 2001). The model also discusses the concept of resilience that biological organisms show in response to the transition from acute to chronic stress. It has been proposed that in healthy individuals acute stressors generally activate salubrious or health promoting aspects of psychophysiology whereas chronic stressors generally have maladaptive effects (Dhabhar, Miller, McEwen, & Spencer 1995; Dhabhar, 1998; Dhabhar and McEwen, 2001). The term "allostatic load" defines a useful concept for understanding the progressive "wear and tear" experienced by biological organisms as they attempt to maintain allostasis (homeostatic range of psychophysiological set points) in response to chronic stress exposure (McEwen, 1998; McEwen, 2002).

Decreased reactivity of the stress axes increases susceptibility to autoimmune disease. Interestingly, although most studies examining the effects of stress on immune function have shown stress to be immunosuppressive, an impressive body of work has clearly laid out the yin-yang relationships between physiological stress responses and regulation of immune function. These studies have shown that dysregulated stress reactivity can also have harmful consequences resulting in increased susceptibility to autoimmune and pro-inflammatory disorders (Mason, MacPhee, & Antoni 1990; Sternberg et al., 1992; Harbuz et al., 1997; Sternberg, 2001; Harbuz, Chover-Gonzalez, & Jessop 2003). In a series of seminal studies, Sternberg et al. (1989) showed that decreased HPA axis reactivity to inflammatory stimuli results in increased susceptibility to experimental arthritis (Sternberg et al., 1989; Sternberg et al., 1989; Sternberg et al., 1992). A similar role for HPA axis mediated endogenous immunoregulation has been shown for development of autoimmune thyroiditis, lupus erythematosus, and avian scleroderma in Obese strain (OS) chickens (Wick, Sgonc, & Lechner, 1998) and experimental autoimmune encephalomyelitis in rats (Whitacre, Dowdell, & Griffin, 1998). Complementing these pre-clinical studies, a series of elegantly conducted clinical studies (Buske-Kirschbaum & Hellhammer, 2003) have shown that patients with atopic dermatitis (Buske-Kirschbaum et al., 1997; Buske-Kirschbaum, Jobst, & Hellhammer, 1998; Buske-Kirschbaum, Geiben, & Hellhammer, 2001), and asthma (Buske-Kirschbaum et al., 2003) show decreased reactivity of their HPA axes. Studies of pediatric rheumatic diseases suggest a similar HPA axis deficiency coupled with other pro-inflammatory hormonal biases (Chikanza, Kuis, & Heijnen, 2000). Differences in NK cell stress reactivity and beta(2)-adrenoreceptor upregulation on PBMC have been observed in patients with systemic lupus erythematosus (Pawlak et al., 1999). A more complex role for sympathetic nervous system involvement in autoimmune disease has also been proposed (Kuis et al., 1996; Kavelaars et al., 1998).

Psychosocial interventions influence aspects of disease progression that may be mediated through immunological factors. (Kiecolt-Glaser & Glaser, 1992; Fawzy, 1995; van der Pompe et al., 1996; Blake-Mortimer et al., 1999; Miller & Cohen, 2001). Examples include psychosocial intervention involving weekly supportive group therapy and self-hypnosis for pain that increased survival of patients with metastatic breast cancer (Spiegel et al., 1989) and similar interventions that have been shown to decrease anxiety and stress and enhance immune function in women surgically treated for breast cancer (Andersen et al., 2004), cognitive behavioral stress management (CMSM) interventions for breast cancer (McGregor et al., 2004) and HIV+ patients (Antoni et al., 1990; Antoni et al., 2000; Antoni, 2003), exercise-related interventions for HIV+ patients (LaPerriere et al., 1994), and mindfulness-based stress reduction interventions for early stage breast and prostate cancer patients (Carlson et al., 2004). These studies suggest that psychosocial interventions may have clinically important benefits that affect stress status, immune function, and health or patients.

Other psychophysiological factors have been shown to affect immune parameters and health. Social support is an important factor that is positively correlated with immune function and health (Cohen, 1988; McGough, 1990; Lekander et al., 1996; Uchino, Cacioppo, & Kiecolt-Glaser 1996; Spiegel et al., 1998). The "physiology of marriage" has been suggested to exert both positive and negative effects immune function and health depending on the quality of the marriage (Robles & Kiecolt-Glaser, 2003). Anxiety was shown to affect anticipatory immune reactions in women receiving adjuvant chemotherapy for breast cancer (Fredrikson et al., 1993). Self-rated health is related to levels of circulating cytokines (Lekander et al., 2004). Prenatal stress (Coe et al., 2002) and early rearing conditions (Coe et al., 1992) have been shown to induce long-lasting effects on behavior (Roughton et al., 1998) and immune responses (Boccia et al., 1997) in adulthood in nonhuman primates (Coe, Lubach, & W. B. 1989; Gorman, Mathew, & Coplan 2002). Negative emotions (Kiecolt-Glaser et al., 2002) and behavior (Kiecolt-Glaser et al., 1993) have also been shown to affect endocrine and immune function. It has also been suggested that personality-related factors may affect immune responses (Segerstrom, 2000) and susceptibility to disease (Segerstrom, 2003). Studies have shown that psychological and mood disorders like depression (Herbert & Cohen, 1993; Maes, 1993; Maes, 1995; Irwin, 1999; Kiecolt-Glaser & Glaser, 2002), anxiety disorders (Koh & Lee, 1998), and post traumatic stress disorder (PTSD) (Watson et al., 1993; Ironson et al., 1997) have significant effects on endocrine and immune function. Recent studies have also shown that dysregulated circadian rhythms may have profound deleterious effects on immune function and health (Sephton, Sapolsky, Kraemer, & Spiegel, 2000; Sephton and Spiegel, 2003). The role of pain and the associated role of opioids in modulating immune function has been the subject of numerous studies (Page, Ben-Eliyahu, Yirmiya, & Liebeskind, 1993; Page & Ben-Eliyahu, 1997). Sleep dysregulation has been shown to have negative effects on immune function and health (Toth & Rehg, 1998; Van Cauter & Spiegel, 1999; Irwin, 2002; Irwin & Rinetti, 2004).

Changes within the immune system can affect the nervous and endocrine systems and have short- and long-term psychological effects. Interestingly, the interactions between psychophysiological and immune factors are not unidirectional but are reciprocal in nature. It has been suggested the immune system can act as a sensory organ for communicating information about changes in immune activation to the CNS (Blalock, 1984). Numerous studies have shown that changes in immune function can have profound reciprocal psychological, behavioral, and physiological effects (for review see: Besedovsky & Sorkin, 1977; Black, 1994; Miller, 1998; Dunn, 2000; Dantzer, 2001;

Capuron & Dantzer, 2003; Harbuz, 2003; Maier & Watkins, 2003; Raison & Miller, 2003; Straub, 2004). Examples of immune system effects on the nervous system include observed generation of sickness behavior by cytokines (Dantzer, 2001; Larson & Dunn, 2001), cytokine effects on sexual activity (Avitsur & Yirmiya, 1999), changes in circulating hormone levels, metabolic effects of immune activation (Besedovsky et al., 1975; Del Rey & Besedovsky, 1992; Besedovsky & del Rey, 2000), and immune activation induced depression in women with arthritis (Zautra et al., 2004). It is thought that the adaptive effects of this feedback from the immune system to the brain induce the individual to get more rest and stay out of harm's way to give the immune system the maximal chance for dealing with the wound, infection, or immune challenge at hand.

A body of literature related to sickness behavior (Opp & Imeri, 1999), now shows that changes in immune activation can have profound effects on sleep related parameters and sleep promotion (Krueger et al., 1994; Krueger & Majde, 2003; Opp & Toth, 2003; Toth & Hughes, 2004). Several pathways have been proposed to explain how immune messengers exert effects on the nervous and endocrine systems and on behavior (for review see Watkins, Maier, & Goehler, 1995; Goehler et al., 2000; Dantzer, 2001; Quan & Herkenham, 2002). These include direct CNS effects of cytokines entering the brain through circumventricular organs (Konsman, Kelley, & Dantzer, 1999), effects mediated through the vagus nerve (Laye et al., 1995; Watkins et al., 1995), effects mediated through actions on endothelial cells of the blood brain barrier (Quan, He, & Lai, 2003).

Importantly, it has been shown that aspects of mood disorders like depression may be mediated by CNS actions of cytokines (Miller, 1998; Yirmiya et al., 2000; Capuron et al., 2002; Raison and Miller, 2003) and that antidepressants may affect cytokine production (Kenis & Maes, 2002) and HPA axis function (Miller, Pariante, & Pearce 1999; Pariante & Miller, 2001). A series of landmark studies has elucidated the deleterious effects of cytokine induced depression during therapeutic interventions involving immunotherapy for diseases like hepatitis C (Raison et al., 2005), malignant melanoma (Capuron et al., 2002; Capuron et al., 2003) and other cancers (Capuron et al., 2001), and alleviated the risk of major depression and depression-induced noncompliance by pre-treatment of patients with anti-depressants (Musselman et al., 2001). These studies illustrate the clinical relevance of the profound reciprocal interactions that can take place between psychophysiological factors and the immune system.

MEASUREMENT OF INNATE AND CELL-MEDIATED IMMUNE PARAMETERS

Table 15.1 shows standard techniques for measuring some of the key immune parameters discussed earlier. (The reader is referred to *Current Protocols in Immunology* (2001) for more detailed descriptions of the protocols used

Table 15.1. Measurement of innate and cell-mediated immunity in human studies

Immune parameter	Analyte/site	Common assay technique
Innate immunity		
Neutrophil	Blood	Flow cytometry (FC)
	Tissue	Myeloperoxidase (MPO) assay
Monocyte	Blood	FC
NK cell	Blood	FC, CD16+CD56+
NK activity	Blood	In vitro lysis of target tumor cells
TNF-α, IL-1a, IL-1b	Plasma/serum	Immunoassay
	In vitro stimulated	Immunoassay
	Intracellular	FC
C-reactive protein	Plasma/serum	Immunoassay
Cell-mediated immunity		
T cell	Blood	FC, CD3+
T helper cell (Th)	Blood	FC, CD3+CD4+
Cytolytic T cell (CTL)	Blood	FC, CD3+CD8+
Naïve T cell	Blood	FC, CD3+CD45RA+CD45RB-
Activated/memory T cell	Blood	FC, CD3+CD45RA-CD45RB+
IFN-γ, IL-2, IL-12	Plasma/serum	Immunoassay
	In vitro stimulated	Immunoassay
	Intracellular	FC
DTH Test	Skin	Intradermal Ag injection
		Measurement of erythema & induration

to make the measurements shown in Table 15.1.) It is important to carefully evaluate how changes in any measured parameter might reflect the capacity of the subject to mount vivo immune responses in the context of the specific experiment or study at hand. In order to achieve this, one has to minimize potential confounding factors that come from the subject on whom the measurements are being made. Such factors, that are similar to potential confounding factors for most studies involving psychophysiology, include smoking, alcohol and caffeine intake, nutritional status, sleep patterns, physical activity (or lack thereof), use of medications, obesity, use of hormonal agents or contraceptives, and overall health status (for review see Kiecolt-Glaser & Glaser, 1988; Uchino et al., 2000) and can have significant effects on immune parameters (Pruett, Ensley, & Crittenden, 1993). The time of day of blood collection is also an important factor to keep constant because endocrine and cellular circadian rhythms can have significant effects on immune function.

Importance of the effects of stress on immune cell distribution. Immune cells or leukocytes circulate continuously from the blood, into various organs, and back into the blood. This circulation is essential for the maintenance of an effective immune defense network (Sprent and Tough,

1994). Because the blood is the most accessible and commonly used compartment for human studies, it is important to carefully evaluate how changes in blood immune parameters might reflect in vivo immune function in the context of the specific experiments or study at hand. Moreover, because most blood collection procedures involve a certain amount of stress, because all patients or subjects will have experienced stress in some manner, and because many studies of psychophysiological effects on immune function focus on stress, it is important to keep in mind the effects of stress on blood leukocyte distribution.

The numbers and proportions of leukocytes in the blood provide an important representation of the state of distribution of leukocytes in the body and of the state of activation of the immune system. Stress has been shown to induce a significant decrease in blood leukocyte numbers in fish (Pickford et al., 1971), mice (Jensen, 1969; Schwab et al., 2005), rats (Rinner et al., 1992; Dhabhar et al., 1994; Dhabhar et al., 1995), rabbits (Toft et al., 1993), horses (Snow, Ricketts, & Mason, 1983), nonhuman primates (Morrow-Tesch, McGlone, & Norman, 1993), and humans (Herbert & Cohen, 1993; Schedlowski et al., 1993). In fact, decreases in blood leukocyte numbers were used as an indirect measure for increases in plasma corticosterone before methods were available to directly assay the hormone (Hoagland, Elmadjian, & Pincus 1946). However, it is commonly assumed that in human studies, stress (especially acute stress) mainly induces an increase in blood leukocyte numbers. Many studies have indeed shown that stress can increase rather than decrease blood leukocyte numbers in humans (Naliboff et al., 1991; Schedlowski et al. 1993; Brosschot et al., 1994; Mills et al., 1995). In fact, stress-induced increases (rather than decreases) in blood leukocyte numbers are more commonly reported in human studies. This apparent contradiction is resolved when three important factors are taken into account. First, stress-induced increases in blood leukocyte numbers are observed following stress conditions that primarily result in the activation of the sympathetic nervous system. These stressors are often of a short duration (a few minutes) or are relatively mild (e.g., public speaking) (Naliboff et al., 1991; Schedlowski et al., 1993; Brosschot et al., 1994; Mills et al., 1995). Second, the increase in leukocyte numbers may be accounted for largely by stress- or catecholamine-induced increases in granulocytes, NK cells, and subpopulations of T cells (Naliboff et al., 1991; Schedlowski et al., 1993; Brosschot et al., 1994; Mills et al., 1995; Benschop, Rodriguez-Feuerhahn, & Schedlowski, 1996; Bosch et al., 2003). Because granulocytes form a large proportion of circulating leukocytes in humans (60–80% granulocytes) an increase in granulocyte numbers is reflected as an increase in total leukocyte numbers in contrast to rats and mice (10–20% granulocytes). Third, stress or pharmacologically-induced increases in glucocorticoid hormones induce a significant decrease in blood lymphocyte and monocyte numbers (Hoagland et al., 1946; Stein, Ronzoni, & Gildea, 1951; Schedlowski et al., 1993; Dhabhar et al., 1995; Dhabhar et al., 1996). Thus, stress conditions that result in a robust activation of the HPA axis will result in a decrease in blood leukocyte numbers. However, such conditions are more difficult to create with acute stressors that are generally used in human studies.

It has been proposed, that acute stress induces an initial increase followed by a decrease in blood leukocyte numbers according to the following pattern (Dhabhar and McEwen, 2001): Stress conditions which result in activation of the sympathetic nervous system, especially conditions which induce high levels of norepinephrine, may induce an increase in circulating leukocyte numbers. These conditions may occur during the very beginning of a stress response, very short duration stress (order of minutes), mild psychological stress, or during exercise. In contrast, stress conditions which result in the activation of the hypothalamic-pituitary-adrenal (HPA) axis induce a decrease in circulating leukocyte numbers. These conditions often occur during the later stages of a stress response, long duration acute stressors (order of hours), or during severe psychological, physical, or physiological stress. An elegant and interesting example in support of this hypothesis comes from Schedlowski et al. who measured changes in blood T cell and NK cell numbers as well as plasma catecholamine and corti-

sol levels in parachutists (Schedlowski et al., 1993). Measurements were made 2 hours before, immediately after, and 1 hour after the jump. Results showed a significant increase in T cell and NK cell numbers immediately (minutes) after the jump which was followed by a significant decrease 1 hour after the jump. An early increase in plasma catecholamines preceded early increases in lymphocyte numbers whereas the more delayed rise in plasma cortisol preceded the late decrease in lymphocyte numbers (Schedlowski et al., 1993). Importantly, changes in NK cell activity and antibody-dependent cell-mediated cytotoxicity (ADCC) closely paralleled changes in blood NK cell numbers, thus suggesting that changes in leukocyte numbers may be an important mediator of apparent changes in leukocyte "activity." Similarly, Rinner et al. have shown that a short stressor (1 min handling) induced an increase in mitogen-induced proliferation of T and B cells obtained from peripheral blood, whereas a longer stressor (2 h immobilization) induced a decrease in the same proliferative responses (Rinner et al., 1992). In another example, Manuck et al. showed that acute psychological stress induced a significant increase in blood CTL numbers only in those subjects who showed heightened catecholamine and cardiovascular reactions to stress (Manuck et al., 1991).

Therefore, it has been proposed that an acute stress response induces biphasic changes in blood leukocyte numbers (Dhabhar and McEwen, 2001). Soon after the beginning of stress (order of minutes) or during mild acute stress, or exercise, catecholamine hormones and neurotransmitters induce the body's "soldiers" (leukocytes) to exit their "barracks" (spleen, lung, marginated pool, and other organs) and enter the "boulevards" (blood vessels and lymphatics) (Dhabhar, 1998; Dhabhar et al., 2000; Dhabhar and McEwen, 2001). This results in an increase in blood leukocyte numbers, the effect being most prominent for NK cells and granulocytes. As the stress response continues, activation of the HPA axis results in the release of glucocorticoid hormones which induce leukocytes to exit the blood and take position at potential "battle stations" (skin, mucosal lining of gastro-intestinal and urinary-genital tracts, lung, liver, and lymph nodes) in preparation for immune challenges which may be imposed by the actions of the stressor (Dhabhar et al., 1995; Dhabhar & McEwen, 1996). Such a redistribution of leukocytes results in a decrease in blood leukocyte numbers, the effect being most prominent for T and B lymphocytes, NK cells, and monocytes. Thus, acute stress may result in a redistribution of leukocytes from the barracks, through the boulevards, and to potential battle stations within the body (Dhabhar & McEwen, 1999).

It is likely that stress-induced changes in leukocyte distribution are mediated by changes in either the expression, or affinity, of adhesion molecules on leukocytes and/or endothelial cells. It has been suggested that following stress or glucocorticoid-treatment, specific leukocyte subpopulations (being transported by blood and lymph through different body compartments) may be selectively retained in those compartments in which they encounter a stress- or glucocorticoid-induced "adhesion match" (Dhabhar, 1996; Dhabhar and McEwen, 1999). As a result of this selective retention, the proportion of some leukocyte subpopulations would decrease in the blood whereas it increases in the organ in which the leukocytes are retained (e.g., the skin) (Dhabhar and McEwen, 1996). We propose that adhesion molecules such as the selectins and their ligands, which mediate early adhesion events such as leukocyte rolling (McEver, 1994), are likely mediators of a stress-induced retention of blood leukocytes within the vasculature of target organs such as the skin and lymph nodes.

Support for the "selective retention" hypothesis comes from studies which show that prednisolone induces the retention of circulating lymphocytes within the bone marrow, spleen, and some lymph nodes thus resulting in a decrease in lymphocyte numbers in the thoracic duct and a concomitant decrease in peripheral blood (Spry, 1972; Cox & Ford, 1982). Moreover, glucocorticoid hormones also influence the production of cytokines (Danes & Araneo, 1989; Munck & Guyre, 1989), and lipocortins (Hirata, 1989) which in turn can affect the surface adhesion properties of leukocytes and endothelial cells (Issekutz, 1990). Further investigation of the effects of endogenous glucocorticoids (administered in physiologic doses, and examined under physiologic kinetic conditions) on changes in expression/activity of cell surface adhesion molecules and on leukocyte-endothelial cell adhesion is necessary.

In summary, when measuring immune responses, it is important to recognize the effects of acute and chronic stress on leukocyte distribution within the body. First, stress is an important focus for many studies examining the effects of psychophysiological factors on immune function. Second, even if stress is not the focus of the study per se, many clinical and experimental manipulations can be stressful and are likely to have unintended effects on immune parameters that need to controlled for and recognized. For example, an adrenergic surge experienced by some individuals upon seeing a physician or nurse approach with a blood collection syringe or even a blood pressure cuff (white coat effect) may stimulate the catecholamine stress response enough to induce a transient leukocytosis. Third, it is important to recognize the difference between transient changes in leukocyte numbers as seen during acute stress and more long-term changes that are likely to be observed during chronic stress. Fourth, because the blood is the most widely sampled compartment for experimental and diagnostic purposes, an understanding of the conditions of blood collection and how they may induce transient unintended changes in endocrine and immune parameters would be useful and beneficial.

Importance of intensity, concentration, and duration. It is also important to keep in mind the effects of intensity (e.g., experimental stressors involving public speaking (Kirschbaum, Pirke, & Hellhammer 1993) are much milder than those involving sky diving (Schedlowski et al., 1993) and concentration (e.g., amount of pharmacological agent administered) of the experimental manipulation under examination and the duration of manipulation or exposure (for review see Pruett, 2001). For studies that involve administering stress (Rinner et al., 1992; Wood et al., 1993) and pharmacological agents, it is not uncommon to observe bell-shaped or U-shaped relationships between the concentration of agent administered and the degree of changed observed in the measured immune parameter. For example, low physiological concentrations of endogenous glucocorticoid hormones have been shown to enhance skin cell mediated immunity whereas high pharmacological concentrations of endogenous glucocorticoids and low concentrations of their synthetic analogs like dexamethasone are potently immunosuppressive (Dhabhar and McEwen, 1999). One might expect to see similar relationships between other psychophysiological parameters and changes in immune function. Cases where such relationships are observed are important to clearly delineate and report just as cases where such relationships are not observed.

FUTURE DIRECTIONS

The past few decades have seen tremendous advances in our understanding of how psychophysiological factors can affect specific immune parameters or aspects of immune function. There is convincing evidence to show that there are connections between psychological and immunological responses that are mediated by physiological factors involving nerves, neurotransmitters, and hormones. Fortunately, each of these fields of research addressing these factors has also seen tremendous advances independently of the others. This presents a golden opportunity for integrational scientists such as those in the field of psychoneuroimmunology, to further the integration between psychophysiology and immune function. Tremendous advances have also been made in the technologies that allow integrational scientists to delve deeper and cast wider as they attempt to understand the biological mechanisms by which mind, physiology, and body work together. Technological advances that allow us to measure more, for longer and more accurately are an amazing asset while conducting multi-dimensional and interdisciplinary studies. For example, advances in flow cytometry allow the simultaneous analyses of multiple immune markers on a single cell and allow the gathering of information on these markers from thousands if representative cells. This greatly increases the amount of information and the accuracy of information that can be obtained about the cellular effects of psychophysiology on the number and relative proportions of immune cells as well as the capacity for adhesion, migration, activation, killing, antigen presentation, antigen specificity, or receptivity to a host of cytokines, hormones, and neurotransmitters. Similarly, advances in gene and protein arrays, that enable the simultaneous analysis of thousands of molecules from minute quantities of samples, have significantly increased our ability to examine the molecular effects of psychophysiological manipulations.

Future studies need to harness these and other technological advances with insightful collaboration between experts. It is extremely important to recognize that technology makes it relatively easy to perform multiple manipulations and make thousands of measurements but it is only using a well thought-out, carefully designed and collaborative approach involving experienced investigators from all relevant fields, that one is likely to be successful in identifying the most meaningful problems or questions and in obtaining relevant, useful and clinically applicable information.

In summary, the field of psychoneuroimmunology has made many advances in recent decades. Supported by the pioneering work of the founders of the field and studies that are currently combining state of the art techniques to tackle fundamental questions regarding the effects of psychophysiolgy on immune function, the field has made tremendous progress and been firmly established. Fortunately, there is also tremendous personal interest in this field – people the world over and from different walks of life are interested in understanding how their emotional health might affect their physical health. It behooves us not only to explain how psychophysiology affects immunology and health but to go one step further and understand and explain how an individual can harness their mind and body's natural defenses to maximize the salubrious effects of mind-body interactions. In the case of disease states, the field needs to better understand and explain how these interactions can be harnessed in a therapeutic setting to synergize with conventional medical approaches to rapidly and effectively bring relief to the patient with minimal side effects.

REFERENCES

Abbas, A. K., Lichtman, A. H. & Pober, J. S. (2000). *Cellular and molecular immunology*. Philadelphia: W. B. Saunders.

Ader, R. & Cohen, N. (1975). Behaviorally conditioned immunosuppression. *Psychosom Med* 37: 333–40.

Ader, R. & Cohen, N. (1981). *Psychoneuroimmunology*. New York: Academic Press.

Ader, R. & Cohen, N. (1991). Conditioning of the immune response. *Neth J Med* 39: 263–73.

Ader, R., Felten, D. L., & Cohen, N. (2001). *Psychoneuroimmunology*. San Diego: Academic Press.

Adler, M. W., Geller, E. B., Rogers, T. J., Henderson, E. E. & Eisenstein, T. K. (1993). Opioids, receptors, and immunity. *Adv Exp Med Biol* 335: 13–20.

Andersen, B. L., Farrar, W. B., Golden-Kreutz, D., Kutz, L. A., MacCallum, R., Courtney, M. E. & Glaser, R. (1998). Stress and immune responses after surgical treatment for regional breast cancer. *J Natl Cancer Inst* 90: 30–36.

Andersen, B. L., Farrar, W. B., Golden-Kreutz, D. M., Glaser, R., Emery, C. F., Crespin, T. R., Shapiro, C. L. & Carson, W. E., III (2004). Psychological, behavioral, and immune changes after a psychological intervention: a clinical trial. *J Clin Oncol* 22: 3570–80.

Anisman, H., Baines, M. G., Berczi, I., Bernstein, C. N., Blennerhassett, M. G., Gorczynski, R. M., Greenberg, A. H., Kisil, F. T., Mathison, R. D., Nagy, E., et al. (1996a). Neuroimmune mechanisms in health and disease: 1. Health. *Cmaj* 155: 867–74.

Anisman, H., Baines, M. G., Berczi, I., Bernstein, C. N., Blennerhassett, M. G., Gorczynski, R. M., Greenberg, A. H., Kisil, F. T., Mathison, R. D., Nagy, E., et al. (1996b). Neuroimmune mechanisms in health and disease: 2. Disease. *Cmaj* 155: 1075–82.

Antoni, M. H. (2003). Stress management effects on psychological, endocrinological, and immune functioning in men with HIV infection: empirical support for a psychoneuroimmunological model. *Stress* 6: 173–88.

Antoni, M. H., Cruess, S., Cruess, D. G., Kumar, M., Lutgendorf, S., Ironson, G., Dettmer, E., Williams, J., Klimas, N., Fletcher, M. A., et al. (2000). Cognitive-behavioral stress management reduces distress and 24-hour urinary free cortisol output among symptomatic HIV-infected gay men. *Ann Behav Med* 22: 29–37.

Antoni, M. H., Schneiderman, N., Fletcher, M. A., Goldstein, D. A., Ironson, G. & Laperriere, A. (1990). Psychoneuroimmunology and HIV-1. *J Consult Clin Psychol* 58: 38–49.

Arkins, S., Dantzer, R. & Kelley, K. W. (1993). Somatolactogens, somatomedins, and immunity. *J Dairy Sci* 76: 2437–50.

Asahina, A., Hosoi, J., Beissert, S., Stratigos, A., & Granstein, R. D. (1995). Inhibition of the induction of delayed-type and contact hypersensitivity by calcitonin gene-related peptide. *J Immunol* 154: 3056–61.

Asahina, A., Hosoi, J., Grabbe, S. & Granstein, R. D. (1995). Modulation of Langerhans cell function by epidermal nerves. *J Allergy Clin Immunol* 96: 1178–82.

Avitsur, R. & Yirmiya, R. (1999). The immunobiology of sexual behavior: gender differences in the suppression of sexual activity during illness. *Pharmacol Biochem Behav* 64: 787–96.

Bellinger, D. L., Lorton, D., Brouxhon, S., Felten, S. & Felten, D. L. (1996). The significance of vasoactive intestinal polypeptide (VIP) in immunomodulation. *Adv Neuroimmunol* 6: 5–27.

Ben-Eliyahu, S. (2003). The promotion of tumor metastasis by surgery and stress: immunological basis and implications for psychoneuroimmunology. *Brain behavior and immunity* 17 Suppl 1: S27–36.

Ben-Eliyahu, S., Shakhar, G., Shakhar, K. & Melamed, R. (2000). Timing within the oestrous cycle modulates adrenergic suppression of NK activity and resistance to metastasis: possible clinical implications. *Br J Cancer* 83: 1747–54.

Ben-Eliyahu, S., Yirmiya, R., Liebeskind, J. C., Taylor, A. N. & Gale, R. P. (1991). Stress increases metastatic spread of a mammary tumor in rats: evidence for mediation by the immune system. *Brain Behav Immun* 5: 193–205.

Benschop, R. J., Geenen, R., Mills, P. J., Naliboff, B. D., Kiecolt-Glaser, J. K., Herbert, T. B., van der Pompe, G., Miller, G. E., Matthews, K. A., Godaert, G. L., et al. (1998). Cardiovascular and immune responses to acute psychological stress in young and old women: a meta-analysis. *Psychosom Med* 60: 290–6.

Benschop, R. J., Oostveen, F. G., Heijnen, C. J. & Ballieux, R. E. (1993). Beta 2-adrenergic stimulation causes detachment of natural killer cells from cultured endothelium. *Eur J Immunol* 23: 3242–3247.

Benschop, R. J., Rodriguez-Feuerhahn, M. & Schedlowski, M. (1996). Catecholamine-induced leukocytosis: early observations, current research, and future directions. *Brain, Behavior, & Immunity* 10: 77–91.

Berczi, I. (1997). Pituitary hormones and immune function. *Acta Paediatr Suppl* 423: 70–5.

Besedovsky, H. & Sorkin, E. (1977). Network of immune-neuroendocrine interactions. *Clin Exp Immunol* 27: 1–12.

Besedovsky, H., Sorkin, E., Keller, M. & Muller, J. (1975). Changes in blood hormone levels during the immune response. *Proc Soc Exp Biol Med* 150: 466–70.

Besedovsky, H. O. & del Rey, A. (2000). The cytokine-HPA axis feed-back circuit. *Z Rheumatol* 59 Suppl 2: II/26–30.

Birx, D. L., Brundage, J., Larson, K., Engler, R., Smith, L., Squire, E., Carpenter, G., Sullivan, M., Rhoads, J. & Oster, C. (1993). The prognostic utility of delayed-type hypersensitivity skin testing in the evaluation of HIV-infected patients. Military Medical Consortium for Applied Retroviral Research. *J. Acquired Immune Deficiency Syndromes* 6: 1248–1257.

Black, P. H. (1994). Immune system-central nervous system interactions: effect and immunomodulatory consequences of immune system mediators on the brain. *Antimicrobial Agents & Chemotherapy* 38: 7–12.

Blake-Mortimer, J., Gore-Felton, C., Kimerling, R., Turner-Cobb, J. M. & Spiegel, D. (1999). Improving the quality and quantity of life among patients with cancer: a review of the effectiveness of group psychotherapy. *Eur J Cancer* 35: 1581–6.

Blalock, J. E. (1984). The immune system as a sensory organ. *J Immunol* 132: 1067–70.

Blalock, J. E. (1999). Proopiomelanocortin and the immune-neuroendocrine connection. *Ann N Y Acad Sci* 885: 161–72.

Blalock, J. E., Harbour-McMenamin, D. & Smith, E. M. (1985). Peptide hormones shared by the neuroendocrine and immunologic systems. *J Immunol* 135: 858s–861s.

Boccia, M. L., Scanlan, J. M., Laudenslager, M. L., Berger, C. L., Hijazi, A. S. & Reite, M. L. (1997). Juvenile friends, behavior, and immune responses to separation in bonnet macaque infants. *Physiol Behav* 61: 191–8.

Bonneau, R. H. (1996). Stress-induced effects on integral immune components invovled in herpes simplex virus (HSV)-specific memory cytotoxic T lymphocyte activation. *Brain, Behav, Immun* 10: 139–63.

Bonneau, R. H., Sheridan, J. F., Feng, N. & Glaser, R. (1991). Stress-induced effects on cell-mediated innate and adaptive memory components of the murine immune response to herpes simplex virus infection. *Brain, Behavior, Immun* 5: 274–95.

Bosch, J. A., Berntson, G. G., Cacioppo, J. T., Dhabhar, F. S. & Marucha, P. T. (2003). Acute stress evokes selective mobilization of T cells that differ in chemokine receptor expression: A potential pathway linking immunologic reactivity to cardiovascular disease. *Brain, Behavior, Immun* 17: 251–9.

Bovbjerg, D., Ader, R. & Cohen, N. (1982). Behaviorally conditioned suppression of a graft-versus-host response. *Proc Natl Acad Sci U S A* 79: 583–5.

Bovbjerg, D. H. (1991). Psychoneuroimmunology. Implications for oncology? *Cancer* 67: 828–32.

Brenner, G. J., Cohen, N., Ader, R. & Moynihan, J. A. (1990). Increased pulmonary metastases and natural killer cell activity in mice following handling. *Life Sciences* 47: 1813–19.

Brosschot, J. F., Benschop, R. J., Godaert, G. L., Olff, M., De Smet, M., Heijnen, C. J. & Ballieux, R. E. (1994). Influence of life stress on immunological reactivity to mild psychological stress. *Psychosom Medicine* 56: 216–24.

Bryla, C. M. (1996). The relationship between stress and the development of breast cancer: a literature review. *Oncol Nurs Forum* 23: 441–8.

Bucala, R. (1998). Neuroimmunomodulation by macrophage migration inhibitory factor (MIF). *Ann N Y Acad Sci* 840: 74–82.

Bulloch, K., McEwen, B. S., Diwa, A. & Baird, S. (1995). Relationship between dehydroepiandrosterone and calcitonin gene-related peptide in the mouse thymus. *Am J Physiol* 268: E168–73.

Bulloch, K. & Pomerantz, W. (1984). Autonomic nervous system innervation of thymic-related lymphoid tissue in wildtype and nude mice. *J Comp Neurol* 228: 57–68.

Buske-Kirschbaum, A., Geiben, A. & Hellhammer, D. (2001). Psychobiological aspects of atopic dermatitis: an overview. *Psychother Psychosom* 70: 6–16.

Buske-Kirschbaum, A., Geiben, A., Wermke, C., Pirke, K. M. & Hellhammer, D. (2001). Preliminary evidence for Herpes labialis recurrence following experimentally induced disgust. *Psychother Psychosom* 70: 86–91.

Buske-Kirschbaum, A. & Hellhammer, D. H. (2003). Endocrine and immune responses to stress in chronic inflammatory skin disorders. *Ann N Y Acad Sci* 992: 231–40.

Buske-Kirschbaum, A., Jobst, S. & Hellhammer, D. H. (1998). Altered reactivity of the hypothalamus-pituitary-adrenal axis in patients with atopic dermatitis: pathologic factor or symptom? *Ann N Y Acad Sci* 840: 747–54.

Buske-Kirschbaum, A., Jobst, S., Psych, D., Wustmans, A., Kirschbaum, C., Rauh, W. & Hellhammer, D. (1997). Attenuated free cortisol response to psychosocial stress in children with atopic dermatitis. *Psychosomatic Medicine* 59: 419–26.

Buske-Kirschbaum, A., Kirschbaum, C., Stierle, H., Jabaij, L. & Hellhammer, D. (1994). Conditioned manipulation of natural killer (NK) cells in humans using a discriminative learning protocol. *Biol Psychol* 38: 143–55.

Buske-Kirschbaum, A., Kirschbaum, C., Stierle, H., Lehnert, H. & Hellhammer, D. (1992). Conditioned increase of natural killer cell activity (NKCA) in humans. *Psychosom Med* 54: 123–32.

Buske-Kirschbaum, A., von Auer, K., Krieger, S., Weis, S., Rauh, W. & Hellhammer, D. (2003). Blunted cortisol responses to psychosocial stress in asthmatic children: a general feature of atopic disease? *Psychosom Med* 65: 806–10.

Cacioppo, J. T., Berntson, G. G., Malarkey, W. B., Kiecolt-Glaser, J. K., Sheridan, J. F., Poehlmann, K. M., Burleson, M. H., Ernst, J. M., Hawkley, L. C. & Glaser, R. (1998). Autonomic, neuroendocrine, and immune responses to psychological stress: the reactivity hypothesis. *Ann N Y Acad Sci* 840: 664–73.

Capuron, L. & Dantzer, R. (2003). Cytokines and depression: the need for a new paradigm. *Brain Behav Immun* 17 Suppl 1: S119–24.

Capuron, L., Gumnick, J. F., Musselman, D. L., Lawson, D. H., Reemsnyder, A., Nemeroff, C. B. & Miller, A. H. (2002). Neurobehavioral effects of interferon-alpha in cancer patients: phenomenology and paroxetine responsiveness of symptom dimensions. *Neuropsychopharmacology* 26: 643–52.

Capuron, L., Hauser, P., Hinze-Selch, D., Miller, A. H. & Neveu, P. J. (2002). Treatment of cytokine-induced depression. *Brain Behav Immun* 16: 575–80.

Capuron, L., Neurauter, G., Musselman, D. L., Lawson, D. H., Nemeroff, C. B., Fuchs, D. & Miller, A. H. (2003). Interferon-alpha-induced changes in tryptophan metabolism. relationship to depression and paroxetine treatment. *Biol Psychiatry* 54: 906–14.

Capuron, L., Ravaud, A., Gualde, N., Bosmans, E., Dantzer, R., Maes, M. & Neveu, P. J. (2001). Association between immune activation and early depressive symptoms in cancer patients treated with interleukin-2-based therapy. *Psychoneuroendocrinology* 26: 797–808.

Carlson, L. E., Speca, M., Patel, K. D. & Goodey, E. (2004). Mindfulness-based stress reduction in relation to quality of life, mood, symptoms of stress and levels of cortisol, dehydroepiandrosterone sulfate (DHEAS) and melatonin in breast and prostate cancer outpatients. *Psychoneuroendocrinology* 29: 448–74.

Carr, D. J., Carpenter, G. W., Garza, H. H. J., Bake, M. L. & Gebhardt, B. M. (1995). Cellular mechanisms involved in morphine-mediated suppression of CTL activity. *Adv Exp Med & Biol* 373: 131–139.

Carr, D. J., Rogers, T. J. & Weber, R. J. (1996). The relevance of opioids and opioid receptors on immunocompetence and immune homeostasis. *Proc Soc Exp Biol Med* 213: 248–57.

Chikanza, I. C., Kuis, W. & Heijnen, C. J. (2000). The influence of the hormonal system on pediatric rheumatic diseases. *Rheum Dis Clin North Am* 26: 911–25.

Clevenger, C. V., Freier, D. O. & Kline, J. B. (1998). Prolactin receptor signal transduction in cells of the immune system. *J Endocrinol* 157: 187–97.

Coe, C. L., Kramer, M., Kirschbaum, C., Netter, P. & Fuchs, E. (2002). Prenatal stress diminishes the cytokine response of leukocytes to endotoxin stimulation in juvenile rhesus monkeys. *J Clin Endocrinol Metab* 87: 675–81.

Coe, C. L., Lubach, G. & Ershler, W. B. (1989). Immunological consequences of maternal separation in infant primates. In Eds. M. Lewis and J. Worobey., *Infant stress and coping*. 45. New York: Jossey-Bass.

Coe, C. L., Lubach, G. R., Schneider, M. L., Dierschke, D. J. & Ershler, W. B. (1992). Early rearing conditions alter immune responses in the developing infant primate. *Pediatrics* 90: 505–9.

Cohen, S. (1988). Psychosocial models of the role of social support in the etiology of physical disease. *Health Psychol* 7: 269–97.

Cohen, S. & Hamrick, N. (2003). Stable individual differences in physiological response to stressors: implications for stress-elicited changes in immune related health. *Brain Behav Immun* 17: 407–14.

Cohen, S., Tyrrell, D. A. J. & Smith, A. P. (1991). Psychological stress and susceptibility to the common cold. *New Engl J. Med* 325: 606–12.

Cole, S. W. & Kemeny, M. E. (1997). Psychobiology of HIV infection. *Crit Rev Neurobiol* 11: 289–321.

Conti, B., Sugama, S., Kim, Y., Tinti, C., Kim, H. C., Baker, H., Volpe, B., Attardi, B. & Joh, T. (2000). Modulation of IL-18 production in the adrenal cortex following acute ACTH or chronic corticosterone treatment. *Neuroimmunomodulation* 8: 1–7.

Cox, J. H. & Ford, W. L. (1982). The migration of lymphocytes across specialized vascular endothelium. IV. Prednisolone acts at several points on the recirculation pathway of lymphocytes. *Cell. Immunol.* 66: 407–22.

Current Protocols In Immunology. New York: John Wiley.

Cutolo, M., Sulli, A., Capellino, S., Villaggio, B., Montagna, P., Seriolo, B. & Straub, R. H. (2004). Sex hormones influence on the immune system: basic and clinical aspects in autoimmunity. *Lupus* 13: 635–8.

Da Silva, J. A. (1999). Sex hormones and glucocorticoids: interactions with the immune system. *Ann N Y Acad Sci* 876: 102–17; discussion 117–8.

Danes, R. A. & Araneo, B. A. (1989). Contrasting effects of glucocorticoids on the capacity of T cells to produce the growth factors interleukin 2 and interleukin 4. *Eur J Immunol* 19: 2319–25.

Dantzer, R. (2001). Cytokine-induced sickness behavior: where do we stand? *Brain Behav Immun* 15: 7–24.

Dantzer, R. & Kelley, K. W. (1989). Stress and immunity: an integrated view of relationships between the brain and the immune system. *Life Sciences* 44: 1995–2008.

Del Rey, A. & Besedovsky, H. O. (1992). Metabolic and neuroendocrine effects of pro-inflammatory cytokines. *Eur J Clin Invest* 22, Suppl. 1: 10–15.

Dhabhar, F. S. (1998). Stress-induced enhancement of cell-mediated immunity. In Eds. S. M. McCann, J. M. Lipton, E. M. Sternberg et al., *Neuroimmunomodulation: Molecular, Integrative Systems, and Clinical Advances*. Ann NY Acad Sci 840: 359–372.

Dhabhar, F. S. & McEwen, B. S. (1996). Stress-induced enhancement of antigen-specific cell-mediated immunity. *J. Immunology* 156: 2608–15.

Dhabhar, F. S. & McEwen, B. S. (1997). Acute stress enhances while chronic stress suppresses immune function in vivo: A potential role for leukocyte trafficking. *Brain Behavior & Immunity* 11: 286–306.

Dhabhar, F. S. & McEwen, B. S. (1999). Enhancing versus suppressive effects of stress hormones on skin immune function. *PNAS, USA* 96: 1059–64.

Dhabhar, F. S. & McEwen, B. S. (2001). Bidirectional Effects Of Stress & Glucocorticoid Hormones On Immune Function: Possible Explanations For Paradoxical Observations. In Eds. R. Ader, D. L. Felten and N. Cohen., *Psychoneuroimmunology, 3rd ed*. San Diego: Academic Press.

Dhabhar, F. S., McEwen, B. S. & Spencer, R. L. (1997). Adaptation to prolonged or repeated stress – Comparison between rat strains showing intrinsic differences in reactivity to acute stress. *Neuroendocrinology* 65: 360–8.

Dhabhar, F. S., Miller, A. H., McEwen, B. S. & Spencer, R. L. (1996). Stress-induced changes in blood leukocyte distribution – role of adrenal steroid hormones. *J. Immunology* 157: 1638–44.

Dhabhar, F. S., Miller, A. H., McEwen, B. S. & Spencer, R. L. (1995). Effects of stress on immune cell distribution – dynamics and hormonal mechanisms. *J. Immunology* 154: 5511–27.

Dhabhar, F. S., Miller, A. H., McEwen, B. S. & Spencer, R. L. (1996). Stress-induced changes in blood leukocyte distribution – role of adrenal steroid hormones. *J Immunology* 157: 1638–44.

Dhabhar, F. S., Miller, A. H., Stein, M., McEwen, B. S. & Spencer, R. L. (1994). Diurnal and stress-induced changes in distribution of peripheral blood leukocyte subpopulations. *Brain Behav Immun* 8: 66–79.

Dhabhar, F. S., Satoskar, A. R., Bluethmann, H., David, J. R. & McEwen, B. S. (2000). Stress-Induced Enhancement of Skin Immune Function: A Role For IFNγ. *PNAS, USA* 97: 2846–51.

Draca, S. R. (1995). Endocrine-immunological homeostasis: the interrelationship between the immune system and sex steroids involves the hypothalamo-pituitary-gonadal axis. *Panminerva Med* 37: 71–6.

Dunn, A. J. (1995). Interactions between the nervous system and the immune system: Implications for psychopharmacology. In Eds. F. E. Bloom and D. J. Kupfer., *Psychopharmacology – The fourth generation of progress*. 719–31. New York: Raven.

Dunn, A. J. (2000). Cytokine activation of the HPA axis. *Ann N Y Acad Sci* 917: 608–17.

Epel, E., Blackburn, E. H., Lin, J., Dhabhar, F. S., Adler, N. E., Morrow, J. D. & Cawthon, R. M. (2004). Accelerated telomere shortening in response to life stress. *PNAS* 101: 17312–15.

Faith, R. E., Liang, H. J., Murgo, A. J. & Plotnikoff, N. P. (1984). Neuroimmunomodulation with enkephalins: enhancement of human natural killer (NK) cell activity in vitro. *Clin Immunol Immunopathol* 31: 412–8.

Fawzy, F. I. (1995). A short-term psychoeducational intervention for patients newly diagnosed with cancer. *Supportive Care in Cancer* 3: 235–8.

Felten, D. L. (1993). Direct innervation of lymphoid organs: substrate for neurotransmitter signaling of cells of the immune system. *Neuropsychobiol* 28: 110–12.

Felten, D. L., Felten, S. Y., Bellinger, D. L., Carlson, S. L., Ackerman, K. D., Madden, K. S., Olschowki, J. A. & Livnat, S. (1987). Noradrenergic sympathetic neural interactions with the immune system: structure and function. *Immunol Rev* 100: 225–60.

Felten, D. L., Felten, S. Y., Bellinger, D. L. & Madden, K. S. (1993). Fundamental aspects of neural-immune signaling. *Psychotherapy & Psychosomatics* 60: 46–56.

Felten, S. Y., Madden, K. S., Bellinger, D. L., Kruszewska, B., Moynihan, J. A. & Felten, D. L. (1998). The role of the sympathetic nervous system in the modulation of immune responses. *Adv Pharmacol* 42: 583–7.

Fredrikson, M., Furst, C. J., Lekander, M., Rotstein, S. & Blomgren, H. (1993). Trait anxiety and anticipatory immune reactions in women receiving adjuvant chemotherapy for breast cancer. *Brain Behav Immun* 7: 79–90.

Geenen, V., Robert, F., Defresne, M. P., Boniver, J., Legros, J. J. & Franchimont, P. (1989). Neuroendocrinology of the thymus. *Horm Res* 31: 81–4.

Glaser, R. (2005). Stress-associated immune dysregulation and its importance for human health: a personal history of psychoneuroimmunology. *Brain Behav Immun* 19: 3–11.

Glaser, R., Kiecolt-Glaser, J. K., Malarkey, W. B. & Sheridan, J. F. (1998). The influence of psychological stress on the immune response to vaccines. *Ann N Y Acad Sci* 840: 649–55.

Glaser, R., Rice, J., Sheridan, J., Fertel, R., Stout, J., Speicher, C., Pinsky, D., Kotur, M., Post, A., Beck, M., et al. (1987). Stress-related immune suppression: health implications. *Brain Behav Immun* 1: 7–20.

Glaser, R., Sheridan, J., Malarkey, W. B., MacCallum, R. C. & Kiecolt-Glaser, J. K. (2000). Chronic stress modulates the immune response to a pneumococcal pneumonia vaccine. *Psychosom Med* 62: 804–7.

Goebel, M. U., Trebst, A. E., Steiner, J., Xie, Y. F., Exton, M. S., Frede, S., Canbay, A. E., Michel, M. C., Heemann, U. & Schedlowski, M. (2002). Behavioral conditioning of immunosuppression is possible in humans. *Faseb J* 16: 1869–73.

Goehler, L. E., Gaykema, R. P., Hansen, M. K., Anderson, K., Maier, S. F. & Watkins, L. R. (2000). Vagal immune-to-brain communication: a visceral chemosensory pathway. *Auton Neurosci* 85: 49–59.

Gorman, J. M., Mathew, S. & Coplan, J. (2002). Neurobiology of early life stress: nonhuman primate models. *Semin Clin Neuropsychiatry* 7: 96–103.

Harbuz, M. (2003). Neuroendocrine-immune interactions. *Trends Endocrinol Metab* 14: 51–2.

Harbuz, M. S., Chover-Gonzalez, A. J. & Jessop, D. S. (2003). Hypothalamo-pituitary-adrenal axis and chronic immune activation. *Ann N Y Acad Sci* 992: 99–106.

Harbuz, M. S., Conde, G. L., Marti, O., Lightman, S. L. & Jessop, D. S. (1997). The hypothalamic-pituitary-adrenal axis in autoimmunity. *Ann N Y Acad Sci* 823: 214–24.

Hawkley, L. C. & Cacioppo, J. T. (2004). Stress and the aging immune system. *Brain Behav Immun* 18: 114–9.

Heijnen, C. J. & Kavelaars, A. (1999). The importance of being receptive. *J Neuroimmunol* 100: 197–202.

Herbert, T. B. & Cohen, S. (1993). Depression and immunity: A meta-analytic review. *Psychol. Bull.* 113: 472–86.

Herbert, T. B. & Cohen, S. (1993). Stress and immunity in humans: a meta-analytic review. *Psychosom Med* 55: 364–79.

Hirata, F. (1989). The role of lipocortins in cellular function as a second messenger of glucocorticoids. In Eds. R. P. Schleimer, H. N. Claman and A. Oronsky., *Anti-inflammatory steroid action – Basic and clinical aspects*. 67–95. San Diego: Academic Press.

Hoagland, H., Elmadjian, F. & Pincus, G. (1946). Stressful psychomotor performance and adrenal cortical function as indicated by the lymphocyte reponse. *J. Clin. Endocrinol.* 6: 301–11.

Ironson, G., Wynings, C., Schneiderman, N., Baum, A., Rodriguez, M., Greenwood, D., Benight, C., Antoni, M., LaPerriere, A., Huang, H. S., et al. (1997). Posttraumatic stress symptoms, intrusive thoughts, loss, and immune function after Hurricane Andrew. *Psychosom Med* 59: 128–41.

Irwin, M. (1999). Immune correlates of depression. *Adv Exp Med Biol* 461: 1–24.

Irwin, M. (2002). Effects of sleep and sleep loss on immunity and cytokines. *Brain Behav Immun* 16: 503–12.

Irwin, M. (2002). Psychoneuroimmunology of depression: clinical implications. *Brain Behav Immun* 16: 1–16.

Irwin, M. R. & Rinetti, G. (2004). Disordered sleep, nocturnal cytokines, and immunity: interactions between alcohol dependence and African-American ethnicity. *Alcohol* 32: 53–61.

Issekutz, T. B. (1990). Effects of six different cytokines on lymphocyte adherence to microvascular endothelium and in vivo lymphocyte migration in the rat. *J Immunol* 144: 2140–6.

Jensen, M. M. (1969). Changes in leukocyte counts associated with various stressors. *J. Reticuloendothelial Soc* 8: 457–65.

Jessop, D., Biswas, S., D'Souza, L., Chowdrey, H. & Lightman, S. (1992). Neuropeptide Y immunoreactivity in the spleen and thymus of normal rats and following adjuvant-induced arthritis. *Neuropeptides* 23: 203–7.

Jessop, D. S. (1998). Beta-endorphin in the immune system–mediator of pain and stress? *Lancet* 351: 1828–9.

Jessop, D. S. (2002). Neuropeptides: modulators of immune responses in health and disease. *Int Rev Neurobiol* 52: 67–91.

Jessop, D. S., Chowdrey, H. S., Lightman, S. L. & Larsen, P. J. (1995). Vasopressin is located within lymphocytes in the rat spleen. *J Neuroimmunol* 56: 219–23.

Jessop, D. S., Jukes, K. E. & Lightman, S. L. (1994). Release of alpha-melanocyte-stimulating hormone from rat splenocytes in vitro is dependent on protein synthesis. *Immunol Lett* 41: 191–4.

Jessop, D. S., Major, G. N., Coventry, T. L., Kaye, S. J., Fulford, A. J., Harbuz, M. S. & De Bree, F. M. (2000). Novel opioid peptides endomorphin-1 and endomorphin-2 are present in mammalian immune tissues. *J Neuroimmunol* 106: 53–9.

Jessop, D. S., Murphy, D. & Larsen, P. J. (1995). Thymic vasopressin (AVP) transgene expression in rats: a model for the study of thymic AVP hyper-expression in T cell differentiation. *J Neuroimmunol* 62: 85–90.

Jessop, D. S., Renshaw, D., Lightman, S. L. & Harbuz, M. S. (1995). Changes in ACTH and beta-endorphin immunoreactivity in immune tissues during a chronic inflammatory stress are not correlated with changes in corticotropin-releasing hormone and arginine vasopressin. *J Neuroimmunol* 60: 29–35.

Kavelaars, A., de Jong-de Vos van Steenwijk, T., Kuis, W. & Heijnen, C. J. (1998). The reactivity of the cardiovascular system and immunomodulation by catecholamines in juvenile chronic arthritis. *Ann N Y Acad Sci* 840: 698–704.

Kelley, K. W. (2004). From hormones to immunity: the physiology of immunology. *Brain Behav Immun* 18: 95–113.

Kenis, G. & Maes, M. (2002). Effects of antidepressants on the production of cytokines. *Int J Neuropsychopharmacol* 5: 401–12.

Kiecolt-Glaser, J. & Glaser, R. (2002). Depression and immune function: Central pathways to morbidity and mortality. *J Psychosom Res* 53: 873–9.

Kiecolt-Glaser, J. K. (1999). Norman Cousins Memorial Lecture 1998. Stress, personal relationships, and immune function: health implications. *Brain Behav Immun* 13: 61–72.

Kiecolt-Glaser, J. K. & Glaser, R. (1988). Methodological issues in behavioral immunology research with humans. *Brain Behav Immun* 2: 67–78.

Kiecolt-Glaser, J. K. & Glaser, R. (1992). Psychoneuroimmunology: can psychological interventions modulate immunity? *J Consult Clin Psychol* 60: 569–75.

Kiecolt-Glaser, J. K. & Glaser, R. (1999). Psychoneuroimmunology and cancer: fact or fiction? *Eur J Cancer* 35: 1603–7.

Kiecolt-Glaser, J. K., Glaser, R., Gravenstein, S., Malarkey, W. B. & Sheridan, J. (1996). Chronic stress alters the immune response to influenza virus vaccine in older adults. *PNAS USA* 93: 3043–7.

Kiecolt-Glaser, J. K., Malarkey, W. B., Chee, M., Newton, T., Cacioppo, J. T., Mao, H. Y. & Glaser, R. (1993). Negative behavior during marital conflict is associated with immunological down-regulation. *Psychosom Med* 55: 410–2.

Kiecolt-Glaser, J. K., Marucha, P. T., Malarkey, W. B., Mercado, A. M. & Glaser, R. (1995). Slowing of wound healing by psychological stress. *Lancet* 346: 1194–6.

Kiecolt-Glaser, J. K., McGuire, L., Robles, T. F. & Glaser, R. (2002). Emotions, morbidity, and mortality: new perspectives from psychoneuroimmunology. *Annu Rev Psychol* 53: 83–107.

Kiecolt-Glaser, J. K., McGuire, L., Robles, T. F. & Glaser, R. (2002). Psychoneuroimmunology and psychosomatic medicine: back to the future. *Psychosom Med* 64: 15–28.

Kiecolt-Glaser, J. K., Page, G. G., Marucha, P. T., MacCallum, R. C. & Glaser, R. (1998). Psychological influences on surgical recovery. Perspectives from psychoneuroimmunology. *Am Psychol* 53: 1209–18.

Kirschbaum, C., Pirke, K. M. & Hellhammer, D. H. (1993). The 'Trier Social Stress Test' – a tool for investigating psychobiological stress responses in a laboratory setting. *Neuropsychobiology* 28: 76–81.

Kodali, S., Ding, W., Huang, J., Seiffert, K., Wagner, J. A. & Granstein, R. D. (2004). Vasoactive intestinal peptide modulates Langerhans cell immune function. *J Immunol* 173: 6082–8.

Koh, K. B. & Lee, B. K. (1998). Reduced lymphocyte proliferation and interleukin-2 production in anxiety disorders. *Psychosom Med* 60: 479–83.

Konsman, J. P., Kelley, K. & Dantzer, R. (1999). Temporal and spatial relationships between lipopolysaccharide-induced expression of Fos, interleukin-1beta and inducible nitric oxide synthase in rat brain. *Neuroscience* 89: 535–48.

Krueger, J. M. & Majde, J. A. (2003). Humoral links between sleep and the immune system: research issues. *Ann N Y Acad Sci* 992: 9–20.

Krueger, J. M., Toth, L. A., Floyd, R., Fang, J., Kapas, L., Bredow, S. & Obal, F., Jr. (1994). Sleep, microbes and cytokines. *Neuroimmunomodulation* 1: 100–9.

Kuis, W., de Jong-de Vos van Steenwijk, C., Sinnema, G., Kavelaars, A., Prakken, B., Helders, P. J. & Heijnen, C. J. (1996). The autonomic nervous system and the immune system in juvenile rheumatoid arthritis. *Brain Behav Immun* 10: 387–98.

La cava, A. & Matarese, G. (2004). The weight of leptin in immunity. *Nature Reviews Immunology* 4: 371–9.

Lambert, R. W. & Granstein, R. D. (1998). Neuropeptides and Langerhans cells. *Exp Dermatol* 7: 73–80.

LaPerriere, A., Ironson, G., Antoni, M. H., Schneiderman, N., Klimas, N. & Fletcher, M. A. (1994). Exercise and psychoneuroimmunology. *Med Sci Sports Exerc* 26: 182–90.

Larson, S. J. & Dunn, A. J. (2001). Behavioral effects of cytokines. *Brain Behav Immun* 15: 371–87.

Laye, S., Bluthe, R. M., Kent, S., Combe, C., Medina, C., Parnet, P., Kelley, K. & Dantzer, R. (1995). Subdiaphragmatic vagotomy blocks induction of IL-1 beta mRNA in mice brain in response to peripheral LPS. *Am J Physiol* 268: R1327–31.

Lekander, M., Elofsson, S., Neve, I. M., Hansson, L. O. & Unden, A. L. (2004). Self-rated health is related to levels of circulating cytokines. *Psychosom Med* 66: 559–63.

Lekander, M., Furst, C. J., Rotstein, S., Blomgren, H. & Fredrikson, M. (1996). Social support and immune status during and after chemotherapy for breast cancer. *Acta Oncol* 35: 31–7.

Lutgendorf, S. K., Cole, S., Costanzo, E., Bradley, S., Coffin, J., Jabbari, S., Rainwater, K., Ritchie, J. M., Yang, M. & Sood, A. K. (2003). Stress-related mediators stimulate vascular endothelial growth factor secretion by two ovarian cancer cell lines. *Clin Cancer Res* 9: 4514–21.

Madden, K. S. & Felten, D. L. (1995). Experimental basis for neural-immune interactions. *Physiological Rev.* 75: 77–106.

Maes, M. (1993). A review on the acute phase response in major depression. *Rev Neurosci* 4: 407–16.

Maes, M. (1995). Evidence for an immune response in major depression: a review and hypothesis. *Prog Neuropsychopharmacol Biol Psychiatry* 19: 11–38.

Maestroni, G. J. & Conti, A. (1996). Melatonin and the immune-hematopoietic system therapeutic and adverse pharmacological correlates. *Neuroimmunomodulation* 3: 325–32.

Maier, S. F. & Watkins, L. R. (1997). Cytokines for psychologists: implications for bi-directional immune-to-brain communication for understanding behavior, mood, and cognition. *Psychol Rev* 105: 83–107.

Maier, S. F. & Watkins, L. R. (2003). Immune-to-central nervous system communication and its role in modulating pain and cognition: Implications for cancer and cancer treatment. *Brain Behav Immun* 17 Suppl 1: S125–31.

Malarkey, W. B., Wang, J., Cheney, C., Glaser, R. & Nagaraja, H. (2002). Human lymphocyte growth hormone stimulates interferon gamma production and is inhibited by cortisol and norepinephrine. *J Neuroimmunol* 123: 180–7.

Manuck, S. B., Cohen, S., Rabin, B. S., Muldoon, M. F. & Bachen, E. A. (1991). Individual differences in cellular immune response to stress. *Psychol Sci* 2: 111–5.

Marsland, A. L., Bachen, E. A., Cohen, S., Rabin, B. & Manuck, S. B. (2002). Stress, immune reactivity, and susceptibility to infectious disease. *Phsyiology & Behavior* 77: 711–6.

Mason, D., MacPhee, I. & Antoni, F. (1990). The role of the neuroendocrine system in determining genetic susceptibility to experimental allergic encephalomyelitis in the rat. *Immunology* 70: 1–5.

McEver, R. P. (1994). Selectins. *Curr. Opinion Immunol.* 6: 75–84.

McEwen, B. S. (1998). Protective and damaging effects of stress mediators: allostasis and allostatic load. *NEJM* 338: 171–9.

McEwen, B. S. (2002). The end of stress as we know it. Washington, DC: Dana Press.

McEwen, B. S., Biron, C. A., Brunson, K. W., Bulloch, K., Chambers, W. H., Dhabhar, F. S., Goldfarb, R. H., Kitson, R. P., Miller, A. H., Spencer, R. L., et al. (1997). Neural-endocrine-immune interactions: The role of adrenalcorticoids as modulators of immune function in health and disease. *Brain Res Rev* 23: 79–133.

McGough, K. N. (1990). Assessing social support of people with AIDS. *Oncol Nurs Forum* 17: 31–5.

McGregor, B. A., Antoni, M. H., Boyers, A., Alferi, S. M., Blomberg, B. B. & Carver, C. S. (2004). Cognitive-behavioral stress management increases benefit finding and immune function among women with early-stage breast cancer. *J Psychosom Res* 56: 1–8.

Miller, A. H. (1998). Neuroendocrine and immune system interactions in stress and depression. *Psychiatr Clin North Am* 21: 443–63.

Miller, A. H., Pariante, C. M. & Pearce, B. D. (1999). Effects of cytokines on glucocorticoid receptor expression and function. Glucocorticoid resistance and relevance to depression. *Adv Exp Med Biol* 461: 107–16.

Miller, A. H., Spencer, R. L., Stein, M. & McEwen, B. S. (1990). Adrenal steroid receptor binding in spleen and thymus after stress or dexamethasone. *American Journal of Physiology* 259: E405–E412.

Miller, G. E. & Cohen, S. (2001). Psychological interventions and the immune system: a meta-analytic review and critique. *Health Psychol* 20: 47–63.

Mills, P. J., Berry, C. C., Dimsdale, J. E., Ziegler, M. G., Nelesen, R. A. & Kennedy, B. P. (1995). Lymphocyte subset redistribution in response to acute experimental stress: effects of gender, ethnicity, hypertension, and the sympathetic nervous system. *Brain Behav Immun* 9: 61–69.

Morrow-Tesch, J. L., McGlone, J. J. & Norman, R. L. (1993). Consequences of restraint stress on natural killer cell activity, behavior, and hormone levels in Rhesus Macaques (*Macaca mulatta*). *Psychoneuroendocrinol.* 18: 383–95.

Munck, A., Crabtree, G. R. & Smith, K. A. (1979). Glucocorticoid receptors and actions in rat thymocytes and immunologically stimulated human peripheral lymphocytes. *Monogr. Endocrinol.* 12: 341–55.

Munck, A. & Guyre, P. M. (1989). Glucocorticoid physiology and homeostasis in relation to anti-inflammatory actions. In Eds. R. P. Schleimer, H. N. Claman and A. Oronsky, *Anti-inflammatory steroid action – basic and clinical aspects*. 30–47. San Diego: Academic Press.

Munck, A. & Naray-Fejes-Toth, A. (1992). The ups and downs of glucocorticoid physiology. Permissive and suppressive effects revisited. *Molec Cell Endocrinol* 90: C1–C4.

Musselman, D. L., Lawson, D. H., Gumnick, J. F., Manatunga, A. K., Penna, S., Goodkin, R. S., Greiner, K., Nemeroff, C. B. & Miller, A. H. (2001). Paroxetine for the prevention of depression induced by high-dose interferon alfa. *N Engl J Med* 344: 961–6.

Naliboff, B. D., Benton, D., Solomon, G. F., Morley, J. E., Fahey, J. L., Bloom, E. T., Makinodan, T. & Gilmore, S. L. (1991). Immunological changes in young and old adults during brief laboratory stress. *Psychosom Med* 53: 121–32.

Obendorf, M. & Patchev, V. K. (2004). Interactions of sex steroids with mechanisms of inflammation. *Curr Drug Targets Inflamm Allergy* 3: 425–33.

Opp, M. R. & Imeri, L. (1999). Sleep as a behavioral model of neuro-immune interactions. *Acta Neurobiol Exp (Wars)* 59: 45–53.

Opp, M. R. & Toth, L. A. (2003). Neural-immune interactions in the regulation of sleep. *Front Biosci* 8: d768–79.

Page, G. G. & Ben-Eliyahu, S. (1997). The immune-suppressive nature of pain. *Semin Oncol Nurs* 13: 10–5.

Page, G. G., Ben-Eliyahu, S., Yirmiya, R. & Liebeskind, J. C. (1993). Morphine attenuates surgery-induced enhancement of metastatic colonization in rats. *Pain* 54: 21–8.

Pariante, C. M. & Miller, A. H. (2001). Glucocorticoid receptors in major depression: relevance to pathophysiology and treatment. *Biol Psychiatry* 49: 391–404.

Pavlov, V. A. & Tracey, K. J. (2004). Neural regulators of innate immune responses and inflammation. *Cell Mol Life Sci* 61: 2322–31.

Pawlak, C. R., Jacobs, R., Mikeska, E., Ochsmann, S., Lombardi, M. S., Kavelaars, A., Heijnen, C. J., Schmidt, R. E. & Schedlowski, M. (1999). Patients with systemic lupus erythematosus differ from healthy controls in their immunological response to acute psychological stress. *Brain Behav Immun* 13: 287–302.

Pedersen, B. K. & Hoffman-Goetz, L. (2000). Exercise and the immune system: regulation, integration, and adaptation. *Physiol Rev* 80: 1055–81.

Pereira, D. B., Antoni, M. H., Danielson, A., Simon, T., Efantis-Potter, J., Carver, C. S., Duran, R. E., Ironson, G., Klimas, N. & O'Sullivan, M. J. (2003). Life stress and cervical squamous intraepithelial lesions in women with human papillomavirus and human immunodeficiency virus. *Psychosom Med* 65: 427–34.

Pickford, G. E., Srivastava, A. K., Slicher, A. M. & Pang, P. K. T. (1971). The stress response in the abundance of circulating leukocytes in the Killifish, Fundulus heteroclitus. I The cold-shock sequence and the effects of hypophysectomy. *J. Exp. Zool.* 177: 89–96.

Pruett, S. B. (2001). Quantitative aspects of stress-induced immunomodulation. *Int Immunopharmacol* 1: 507–20.

Pruett, S. B., Ensley, D. K. & Crittenden, P. L. (1993). The role of chemical-induced stress responses in immunosuppression: a review of quantitative associations and cause-effect relationships between chemical-induced stress responses and immunosuppression. *J Toxicol Environ Health* 39: 163–92.

Quan, N., He, L. & Lai, W. (2003). Endothelial activation is an intermediate step for peripheral lipopolysaccharide induced activation of paraventricular nucleus. *Brain Res Bull* 59: 447–52.

Quan, N. & Herkenham, M. (2002). Connecting cytokines and brain: a review of current issues. *Histol Histopathol* 17: 273–88.

Rabin, B. S. (1999). *Stress, Immune Function, and Health*. New York, Wiley-Liss.

Rabin, B. S., Cohen, S., Ganguli, R., Lysle, D. T. & Cunnick, J. E. (1989). Bidirectional interaction between the central nervous system and the immune system. *Crit Rev Immunol* 9: 279–312.

Raison, C. L., Broadwell, S. D., Borisov, A. S., Manatunga, A. K., Capuron, L., Woolwine, B. J., Jacobson, I. M., Nemeroff, C. B. &

Miller, A. H. (2005). Depressive symptoms and viral clearance in patients receiving interferon-alpha and ribavirin for hepatitis C. *Brain Behav Immun* 19: 23–7.

Raison, C. L. & Miller, A. H. (2003). Depression in cancer: new developments regarding diagnosis and treatment. *Biol Psychiatry* 54: 283–94.

Rinner, I., Schauenstein, K., Mangge, H., Porta, S. & Kvetnansky, R. (1992). Opposite effects of mild and severe stress on *in vitro* activation of rat peripheral blood lymphocytes. *Brain, Behav., Immun.* 6: 130–40.

Robles, T. F. & Kiecolt-Glaser, J. K. (2003). The physiology of marriage: pathways to health. *Physiol Behav* 79: 409–16.

Roitt, I. M., Brostoff, J. & Male, D. K. (2001). *Immunology*. London: Gower Medical Publishing.

Romano, T. A., Felten, S. Y., Felten, D. L. & Olschowka, J. A. (1991). Neuropeptide-Y innervation of the rat spleen: another potential immunomodulatory neuropeptide. *Brain Behav Immun* 5: 116–31.

Roughton, E. C., Schneider, M. L., Bromley, L. J. & Coe, C. L. (1998). Maternal endocrine activation during pregnancy alters neurobehavioral state in primate infants. *Am J Occup Ther* 52: 90–8.

Rouppe van der Voort, C., Kavelaars, A., van de Pol, M. & Heijnen, C. J. (1999). Neuroendocrine mediators up-regulate alpha1b- and alpha1d-adrenergic receptor subtypes in human monocytes. *J Neuroimmunol* 95: 165–73.

Rouppe van der Voort, C., Kavelaars, A., van de Pol, M. & Heijnen, C. J. (2000). Noradrenaline induces phosphorylation of ERK-2 in human peripheral blood mononuclear cells after induction of alpha(1)-adrenergic receptors. *J Neuroimmunol* 108: 82–91.

Sabharwal, P., Glaser, R., Lafuse, W., Varma, S., Liu, Q., Arkins, S., Kooijman, R., Kutz, L., Kelley, K. W. & Malarkey, W. B. (1992). Prolactin synthesized and secreted by human peripheral blood mononuclear cells: an autocrine growth factor for lymphoproliferation. *Proc Natl Acad Sci U S A* 89: 7713–6.

Sanders, V. M. & Straub, R. H. (2002). Norepinephrine, The Beta-Adrenergic Receptor, and Immunity. *Brain, Behavior, and Immunity* 16: 290–332.

Sapolsky, R. M. (2004). *Why Zebras Don't Get Ulcers*. New York: W. H. Freeman and Company.

Schedlowski, M., Falk, A., Rohne, A., Wagner, T. O. F., Jacobs, R., Tewes, U. & Schmidt, R. E. (1993). Catecholamines induce alterations of distribution and activity of human natural killer (NK) cells. *J Clin Immunol* 13: 344–51.

Schedlowski, M., Jacobs, R., Stratman, G., Richter, S., Hädike, A., Tewes, U., Wagner, T. O. F. & Schmidt, R. E. (1993). Changes of natural killer cells during acute psychological stress. *J Clin Immunol* 13: 119–26.

Schedlowski, M. & Tewes, U. (1999). *Psychoneuroimmunology*. Amsterdam, Kluwer Academic Publishers.

Schwab, C. L., Fan, R., Zheng, Q., Myers, L. P., Hebert, P. & Pruett, S. B. (2005). Modeling and predicting stress-induced immunosuppression in mice using blood parameters. *Toxicol Sci* 83: 101–13.

Segerstrom, S. C. (2000). Personality and the immune system: models, methods, and mechanisms. *Annals of behavioral medicine: a publication of the Society of Behavioral Medicine* 22: 180–90.

Segerstrom, S. C. (2003). Individual differences, immunity, and cancer: lessons from personality psychology. *Brain behavior and immunity* 17 Suppl 1: S92–7.

Sephton, S. & Spiegel, D. (2003). Circadian disruption in cancer: a neuroendocrine-immune pathway from stress to disease? *Brain Behav Immun* 17: 321–8.

Sephton, S. E., Sapolsky, R. M., Kraemer, H. C. & Spiegel, D. (2000). Early Mortaility in Metastatic Breast Cancer Patients with Absent or Abnormal Diurnal Cortisol Rhythms. *Journal of the National Cancer Institute* 92: 994–1000.

Shavit, Y., Terman, G. W., Martin, F. C., Lewis, J. W., Liebeskind, J. C. & Gale, R. P. (1985). Stress, opioid peptides, the immune system, and cancer. *J Immunol* 135: 834s–837s.

Sheridan, J. F. (1998). Stress-induced modulation of anti-viral immunity – Normal Cousins Memorial Lecture 1997. *Brain Behav Immun* 12: 1–6.

Sheridan, J. F., Dobbs, C., Jung, J., Chu, X., Konstantinos, A., Padgett, D. & Glaser, R. (1998). Stress-induced neuroendocrine modulation of viral pathogenesis and immunity. *Ann N Y Acad Sci* 840: 803–8.

Sheridan, J. F., Feng, N., Bonneau, R. H., Allen, C. M., Huneycutt, B. S. & Glaser, R. (1991). Restraint stress differentially affects anti-viral cellular and humoral immune responses in mice. *J Neuroimmunol* 31: 245–55.

Sheridan, J. F., Padgett, D. A., Avitsur, R. & Marucha, P. T. (2004). Experimental models of stress and wound healing. *World J Surg* 28: 327–30.

Sheridan, J. F., Stark, J. L., Avitsur, R. & Padgett, D. A. (2000). Social disruption, immunity, and susceptibility to viral infection. Role of glucocorticoid insensitivity and NGF. *Ann N Y Acad Sci* 917: 894–905.

Snow, D. H., Ricketts, S. W. & Mason, D. K. (1983). Hematological responses to racing and training exercise in Thoroughbred horses, with particular reference to the leukocyte response. *Equine Vet J* 15: 149–54.

Solomon, G. F. & Moos, R. H. (1964). Emotions, immunity and disease. *Arch Gen Psychiat* 11: 657–69.

Spiegel, D., Bloom, J. R., Kraemer, H. C. & Gottheil, E. (1989). Effect of psychosocial treatment on survival of patients with metastatic breast cacer. *Lancet* 2: 888–91.

Spiegel, D., Sephton, S. E., Terr, A. I. & Stites, D. P. (1998). Effects of psychosocial treatment in prolonging cancer survival may be mediated by neuroimmune pathways. *Ann N Y Acad Sci* 840: 674–83.

Sprent, J. & Tough, D. F. (1994). Lymphocyte life-span and memory. *Science* 265: 1395–1400.

Spry, C. J. F. (1972). Inhibition of lymphocyte recirculation by stress and corticotropin. *Cell Immunol* 4: 86–92.

Stein, M., Ronzoni, E. & Gildea, E. F. (1951). Physiological responses to heat stress and ACTH of normal and schizophrenic subjects. *Am J Psych* 6: 450–5.

Steinman, L. (2004). Elaborate interactions between the immune and nervous systems. *Nat Immunol* 5: 575–81.

Stephanou, A., Jessop, D. S., Knight, R. A. & Lightman, S. L. (1990). Corticotrophin-releasing factor-like immunoreactivity and mRNA in human leukocytes. *Brain Behav Immun* 4: 67–73.

Sternberg, E. M. (2000). *The Balance Within*. New York: W.H Freeman and Company.

Sternberg, E. M. (2001). Neuroendocrine regulation of autoimmune/inflammatory disease. *J Endocrinol* 169: 429–35.

Sternberg, E. M., Chrousos, G. P., Wilder, R. L. & Gold, P. W. (1992). The stress response and the regulation of inflammatory disease. *Ann Intern Med* 117: 854–66.

Sternberg, E. M., Glowa, J., Smith, M., Calogero, A. E., Listwak, S. J., Aksentijevich, S., Chrousos, G. P., Wilder, R. L. & Gold, P. W. (1992). Corticotropin releasing hormone related behavioural and neuroendocrine responses to stress in Lewis and Fischer rats. *Brain Research* 570: 54–60.

Sternberg, E. M., Hill, J. M., Chrousos, G. P., Kamilaris, T., Listwak, S. J., Gold, P. W. & Wilder, R. L. (1989). Inflammatory mediator-induced hypothalamic-pituitary-adrenal axis activation is defective in streptococcal cell wall arthritis-susceptible Lewis rats. *Proc Natl Acad Sci USA* 86: 2374–8.

Sternberg, E. M., Young, W. S., Bernadini, R., Calogero, A. E., Chrousos, G. P., Gold, P. W. & Wilder, R. L. (1989). A central nervous system defect in biosynthesis of corticotropin releasing hormone is associated with susceptibility to streptococcal cell wall-induced arthritis in Lewis rats. *Proc Natl Acad Sci USA* 86: 4771–5.

Straub, R. H. (2004). Complexity of the bi-directional neuroimmune junction in the spleen. *Trends Pharmacol Sci* 25: 640–6.

Straub, R. H. & Besedovsky, H. O. (2003). Integrated evolutionary, immunological, and neuroendocrine framework for the pathogenesis of chronic disabling inflammatory diseases. *Faseb J* 17: 2176–83.

Straub, R. H., Schaller, T., Miller, L. E., von Horsten, S., Jessop, D. S., Falk, W. & Scholmerich, J. (2000). Neuropeptide Y cotransmission with norepinephrine in the sympathetic nerve-macrophage interplay. *J Neurochem* 75: 2464–71.

Toft, P., Svendsen, P., Tonnesen, E., Rasmussen, J. W. & Christensen, N. J. (1993). Redistribution of lymphocytes after major surgical stress. *Acta Anesthesiol Scand* 37: 245–9.

Torii, H., Yan, Z., Hosoi, J. & Granstein, R. D. (1997). Expression of neurotrophic factors and neuropeptide receptors by Langerhans cells and the Langerhans cell-like cell line XS52: further support for a functional relationship between Langerhans cells and epidermal nerves. *J Invest Dermatol* 109: 586–91.

Toth, L. A. & Hughes, L. F. (2004). Macrophage participation in influenza-induced sleep enhancement in C57BL/6J mice. *Brain Behav Immun* 18: 375–89.

Toth, L. A. & Rehg, J. E. (1998). Effects of sleep deprivation and other stressors on the immune and inflammatory responses of influenza-infected mice. *Life Sci* 63: 701–9.

Tracey, K. J. (2002). The inflammatory reflex. *Nature* 420: 853–9.

Uchino, B. N., Cacioppo, J. T. & Kiecolt-Glaser, J. K. (1996). The relationship between social support and physiological processes: a review with emphasis on underlying mechanisms and implications for health. *Psychol Bull* 119: 488–531.

Uchino, B. N., Kiecolt-Glaser, J. K. & Glaser, R. (2000). Psychological Modulation of Cellular Immunity. In Eds. J. T. Cacioppo, L. G. Tassinary and G. G. Berntson., *Handbook of Psychophysiology*, pp. 1054. Cambridge: Cambridge Press.

Vacchio, M. S., Lee, J. Y. & Ashwell, J. D. (1999). Thymus-derived glucocorticoids set the thresholds for thymocyte selection by inhibiting TCR-mediated thymocyte activation. *J Immunol* 163: 1327–33.

Vacchio, M. S., Papadopoulos, V. & Ashwell, J. D. (1994). Steroid production in the Thymus: Implications for thymocyte selection. *J Exp Med* 179: 1835–1846.

Van Cauter, E. & Spiegel, K. (1999). Sleep as a mediator of the relationship between socioeconomic status and health: a hypothesis. *Ann N Y Acad Sci* 896: 254–61.

van der Pompe, G., Antoni, M., Visser, A. & Garssen, B. (1996). Adjustment to breast cancer: the psychobiological effects of psychosocial interventions. *Patient Educ Couns* 28: 209–19.

Vedhara, K., Fox, J. D. & Wang, E. C. (1999). The measurement of stress-related immune dysfunction in psychoneuroimmunology. *Neurosci Biobehav Rev* 23: 699–715.

Watkins, L. R., Goehler, L. E., Relton, J. K., Tartaglia, N., Silbert, L., Martin, D. & Maier, S. F. (1995). Blockade of interleukin-1 induced hyperthermia by subdiaphragmatic vagotomy: evidence for vagal mediation of immune-brain communication. *Neurosci Lett* 183: 27–31.

Watkins, L. R., Maier, S. F. & Goehler, L. E. (1995). Cytokine-to-brain communication: a review & analysis of alternative mechanisms. *Life Sci* 57: 1011–26.

Watson, I. P., Muller, H. K., Jones, I. H. & Bradley, A. J. (1993). Cell-mediated immunity in combat veterans with post-traumatic stress disorder. *Med J Aust* 159: 513–6.

Weber, R. J. & Pert, A. (1989). The periaqueductal gray matter mediates opiate-induced immunosuppression. *Science* 245: 188–90.

Webster, J. I., Tonelli, L. & Sternberg, E. M. (2002). Neuroendocrine regulation of immunity. *Annu Rev Immunol* 20: 125–63.

Weigent, D. A. & Blalock, J. E. (1987). Interactions between the neuroendocrine and immune systems: common hormones and receptors. *Immunol Rev* 100: 80–107.

Whitacre, C. C., Dowdell, K. & Griffin, A. C. (1998). Neuroendocrine influences on experimental autoimmune encephalomyelitis. *Ann N Y Acad Sci* 840: 705–16.

Wick, G., Sgonc, R. & Lechner, O. (1998). Neuroendocrine-immune disturbances in animal models with spontaneous autoimmune diseases. *Ann NY Acad Sci* 840: 591–8.

Wood, P. G., Karol, M. H., Kusnecov, A. W. & Rabin, B. S. (1993). Enhancement of antigen-specific humoral and cell-mediated immunity by electric footshock stress in rats. *Brain Behav Immun* 7: 121–34.

Yang, E. V. & Glaser, R. (2002). Stress-induced immunomodulation and the implications for health. *Int Immunopharmacol* 2: 315–24.

Yirmiya, R., Pollak, Y., Morag, M., Reichenberg, A., Barak, O., Avitsur, R., Shavit, Y., Ovadia, H., Weidenfeld, J., Morag, A., et al. (2000). Illness, cytokines, and depression. *Ann NY Acad Sci* 917: 478–87.

Zautra, A. J., Yocum, D. C., Villanueva, I., Smith, B., Davis, M. C., Attrep, J. & Irwin, M. (2004). Immune activation and depression in women with rheumatoid arthritis. *J Rheumatol* 31: 457–63.

Zwilling, B. (1992). Stress affects disease outcomes. Confronted with infectious disease agents, the nervous and immune systems interact in complex ways. *ASM News* 58: 23–5.

16 Psychosocial Effects on Humoral Immunity: Neural and Neuroendocrine Mechanisms

VIRGINIA M. SANDERS, NICHOLAS KIN, AND GEORG PONGRATZ

A major goal over the past 30 years has been to establish not only the mechanisms by which immunophysiology is affected by the host response to psychosocial factors, but also the mechanisms by which *Psychophysiology* is affected by the host response to antigen. In this chapter, we will discuss the evidence that indicates a role for psychosocial factors in modulating the level of humoral-mediated defense mechanisms in the body and vice versa, as well as technical approaches used in experimental designs to measure the status of humoral immunity.

1. HISTORICAL CONTEXT

Our ability to combat the many microorganisms that gain entry into our bodies depends on an intact immune system that functions to recognize and eliminate the invading microorganisms to maintain homeostasis. It was first discovered that the immune mechanisms for defense included those that were not specific for any particular microorganism and those that were exquisitely specific for one microorganism over another. The most well-recognized non-specific mechanism involves the process of phagocytosis by macrophages, which prevents the spread of microorganisms from their point of entry into the host. However, a number of deadly organisms such as encapsulated pneumococci do not adhere well to phagocytic cells. It is thought that humoral immune mechanisms evolved to provide a soluble antibody molecule that specifically recognizes and binds to a particular bacteria to help it adhere more readily to phagocytic cells for more efficient phagocytosis and destruction. Likewise, for intracellular microorganisms such as viruses and parasites, specific humoral immune mechanisms evolved to neutralize the activity of these microorganisms before they entered cells. These humoral immune mechanisms are mediated by T and B lymphocytes that are able to use cell surface receptors to recognize invading microorganisms specifically, and with high affinity. A B cell that receives cell contact and cytokine help from a T cell will produce an antibody to either neutralize or destroy a low number of invading pathogens.

One of the earliest studies to suggest that a relationship existed between the immune status and mental state of an individual was a study in 1919, which showed that psychosocial factors imposed upon a host with pulmonary tuberculosis decreased the phagocytic capacity of cells within the blood to eliminate the pathogen (Ishigami, 1919). The findings from this study suggested that the high rate of death from tuberculosis in the Japanese young might be related to the depression that ensued from "overtaxation of the mind" by a school system that dictated severe entrance examinations and had overcrowded learning conditions. Although the finding from this study was pioneering, it was ignored by the scientific community for a number of years, but is now considered by some to be the first documented venture into the area of psychoneuroimmunology.

Other studies soon followed that showed a similar relationship between an individual's mental state and immune status. The high incidence of industrial workers succumbing to the common cold and pneumonia in the 1920s was the impetus for the design of studies to determine if a relationship existed between a worker's perception of fatigue and their susceptibility to infection. This possibility was first tested with rabbits, in which a state of fatigue increased disease susceptibility to, and mortality from, *Streptococcus pneumoniae* (Bailey, 1925). What was most interesting about this study was that the rabbits were made less susceptible to infection if they were routinely exercised before inducing a state of fatigue, a topic that will be discussed later in this chapter.

In 1936, Selye (Selye, 1936; 1946) introduced the concepts of stress and stressor. Stress was defined as a biological response to a noxious stimulus, such as heat or cold, that induced activation of the hypothalamic-pituitary-adrenal axis (HPA). Stressor was defined as the noxious stimulus itself. Selye described a myriad of structural changes that occurred during the biological response to stress, including the appearance of lymphoid organ atrophy. This finding was the first to relate a stress-induced change in HPA activity to a change in immune system architecture. Today, the list of stressors has expanded

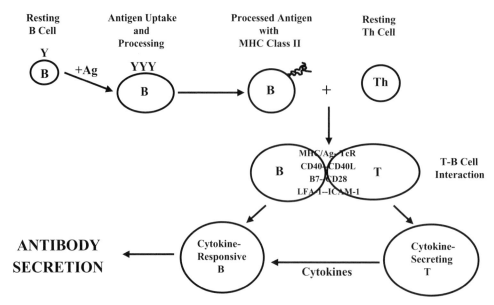

Figure 16.1. Diagram of the stages of T cell and B cell participation in the production of cytokines and antibodies. In this model the B cell binds, processes, and re-expresses antigen on the cell surface in association with MHC Class II molecules. The complex of MHC Class II and antigen is recognized by the T cell receptor associated with a resting Th cell. The presentation and recognition of MHC/antigen in conjunction with other T cell- and B cell-associated adhesion and costimulatory molecules allows a physical interaction to occur which is essential for the activation of both cells. The activation of these cells renders the Th cell capable of producing and secreting cytokines and the B cell capable of responding to the cytokines. As a result of cytokine stimulation of the activated B cell, the B cell is able to further differentiate into an antibody-secreting cell. In addition, the intracellular messengers generated as a consequence of cell activation are shown, as are the adhesion and costimulatory molecules that induce and strengthen the interaction between the T cell and B cell.

to include non-noxious stimuli, such as psychological stress.

By the 1960s, studies by Solomon and Moos showed that a relationship existed between psychological and immunological profiles of individuals afflicted with the immune-mediated disease rheumatoid arthritis (Solomon & Moos, 1964; Solomon & Moos, 1965). These studies introduced the concept that emotions could influence disease, introduced the area of psychoimmunology to the health science field, and, more importantly, emphasized the need for interdisciplinary approaches to (understanding the relationship between psychological factors and immunity). Some fifteen years later, a series of experiments were performed to show that humoral immune suppression could be conditioned (Ader & Cohen, 1975; Cohen et al., 1979). The latter studies are considered the cornerstone for the area of psychoneuroimmunology, providing the first experimental evidence to show that a link existed between a psychological process and immune system function.

The cellular, biochemical, and molecular mechanisms by which psychosocial factors affect humoral immune status is an area of active research. The endogenous molecules that most likely mediate effects on humoral immunity include neuroendocrine hormones, opioid peptides, neuropeptides, and sympathetic neurotransmitters. An understanding of the mechanisms by which these molecules modulate the level of humoral immunity and vice versa,

coupled with an increased availability of sensitive and reliable techniques to evaluate humoral immune status, will help us to define the relationship that exists between psychological and immunological states. Furthermore, any drug, disease, or psychosocial factor that either stimulates or inhibits hormone, neurotransmitter, or neuropeptide production and/or release might likewise be expected to alter the level of humoral immunity.

2. PHYSICAL CONTEXT

2.1. The T-helper cell-dependent antibody response

Figure 16.1 outlines the sequence of events leading to antibody production by a B cell, and these events are reviewed in detail elsewhere (Parker, 1993; Vitetta et al., 1989). This figure is presented not only to emphasize the complexity of the antibody response to antigen, but also to make clear that neuroendocrine hormones, opioid peptides, and neurotransmitters can regulate any cellular activity along this pathway, if the receptors for these modulators are expressed on the cells participating in the response. Initially, antigen is introduced into the immune system. The immunoglobulin (Ig) receptor expressed on the surface of the B cell, together with associated signaling molecules, is known as the B cell receptor (BCR). The Ig receptor binds antigen, whereas the BCR complex transmits signals to the B cell interior. The capping of the antigen/BCR complex also triggers receptor endocytosis into endosomal compartments where antigen dissociates from the Ig molecule. Further processing of the antigen occurs in the lysosomal compartment to form small peptide fragments. These peptide fragments encounter Major Histocompatibility Complex Class II (MHCII) molecules as vesicles containing the peptides fuse with vesicles containing newly synthesized MHCII. The peptide/MHCII complex is then expressed on the B cell surface for presentation of the peptide antigen to the CD4$^+$ T cell receptor (TCR), which is restricted to the recognition of that specific peptide in association with MHCII.

During the cell-cell interaction between the CD4+ T cell and B cell, the T cell not only activates the B cell, but also provides the cytokines necessary for B cell growth and differentiation into an antibody-secreting cell. Two CD4$^+$ T cell subsets have been identified and are characterized by the cytokines they secrete following cellular activation. These cells are collectively referred to as T-helper (Th) cells. Th1 cells secrete interferon (IFN)-gamma and IL-2, whereas Th2 cells secrete IL-4, IL-5, IL-6, IL-10, and transforming growth factor (TGF)-beta. The cytokines are involved in determining the antibody isotype produced by B cells, that is, IFN-gamma-producing Th1 cells induce mouse B cells to produce IgG$_{2a}$, IL-4-producing Th2 cells induce mouse B cells to produce IgG$_1$ and IgE, and TGF-beta-producing Th2 cells induce B cells to produce IgA.

In addition to the TCR interaction with peptide/MHCII, the binding of CD86 (also known as B7–2) on the B cell to CD28 on the T cell is also important. CD28 is constitutively expressed on the Th cell. In contrast, CD86 is expressed at low levels on splenic B cells, but is upregulated following B cell activation. In addition, the interaction between CD40L on the T cell and constitutively expressed CD40 on the B cell plays an important role in regulating the process of antibody production by the B cell. In summary, the initial interaction between the B cell and Th cell is a critical event that determines if the B cell will differentiate into an antibody-secreting cell. Therefore, any factor that alters antigen recognition, binding, processing, or presentation by a B cell to a T cell, cell surface molecule expression on a Th cell/B cell, or cytokine production by a Th cell, will consequently result in a change in the level of antibody produced by a B cell.

2.2. Neuroendocrine hormones and immunity

Activation of the HPA is induced by physical stressor, as first suggested by Selye (Selye, 1936; Selye, 1946), and by psychological stressors, such as academic stress (Malarkey et al., 1995). An understanding of the mechanisms by which the HPA axis is activated to release various biological mediators, and the mechanisms by which these mediators influence immune responsiveness, is an area under

much investigation. The reader is referred to the following reviews for a more detailed discussion of the role of the HPA in immunity (Harbuz, 2003; Harbuz et al., 2003; Jessop, 2002; Webster & Sternberg, 2004; Webster et al., 2002) and to recent articles suggesting a role for the HPA axis in mood disorders (Muller et al., 2004) and depression/anxiety (Strohle & Holsboer, 2003).

Interleukin-1 (IL-1) is a biological molecule that is released by an activated immune cell. Interleukin-1 also increases the production of corticotrophin releasing hormone (CRH) by neurons located in the paraventricular nucleus of the hypothalamus. These neurons project through the median eminence and terminate on the hypophyseal portal vessels that transport CRH to the anterior pituitary to act as a potent secretagogue for adrenocorticotropin (ACTH). The adrenal cortex, in turn, responds to the ACTH by increasing the rate of secretion of glucocorticoids that exert a suppressive effect on humoral immunity, except for IgE. In addition, because the hypothalamus is an area within the CNS that controls efferent sympathetic nerve activity, an IL-1β-induced increase in hypothalamic nerve activity and the level of CRH secretion from the hypothalamus (Akiyoshi et al., 1990; Chuluyan et al., 1992; Fleshner et al., 1995; Sapolsky et al., 1987) may also enhance the level of efferent sympathetic nerve activity and the rate of norepinephrine release in the periphery. For example, peripheral IL-1β administration induced c-fos expression in CRH-producing cells in the paraventricular nucleus of the hypothalamus, suggesting that IL-1β increased hypothalamic neuronal activity, which translated into an increase in efferent sympathetic nerve activity (Ericsson et al., 1994). The role played by the SNS in regulating humoral immunity will be discussed in the next section of this chapter.

Both T and B lymphocytes have been reported to release CRH protein and express CRH mRNA (Karalis et al., 1997). However, another finding suggested that the proposed CRH made by lymphocytes may actually be urocortin, which is a new member of the CRH family and which uses the same receptor as CRH to mediate an effect on cell activity (Bamberger et al., 1998). But in 2003, another group reported that immunoreactive CRH is produced within human T and B cells, and that this peptide was not urocortin (Baker et al., 2003), indicating that lymphocytes indeed produce CRH. Specific receptors for CRH are expressed on immune cells (Audhya et al., 1991; Smith et al., 1986; Webster et al., 1990). The effects of CRH on T cell function appear to be suppressive on cytokine production and cytokine receptor expression. (Singh, 1989; Singh & Leu, 1990). CRH exerts a suppressive effect on B cell proliferation (McGillis et al., 1989; Venihaki et al., 2003), and inhibits antibody production (Aebischer et al., 1994; Leu & Singh, 1993), possibly via an effect of CRH on accessory cells, as opposed to a direct effect on B cells themselves (Aebischer et al., 1994). When CRH is injected into the brain, IgG production in response to a T cell-dependent antigen is suppressed (Friedman & Irwin, 2001; Irwin, 1993), reportedly through a mechanism that involves activation of the sympathetic nervous system (SNS) and stimulation of the beta-adrenergic receptor on B cells, as opposed to a direct effect of CRH. If CRH is over-expressed in mice, chronic activation of the HPA occurs, accompanied by a loss of B cells, decreased IgG produc-tion, and impaired isotype switching (Murray et al., 2001). In addition, CRH transgenic mice fail to form germinal centers that are critical for B cell antibody production, via a mechanism that appears to involve an effect on follic-ular dendritic cell function (Murray et al., 2004). Thus, the actions of CRH within the brain or in the periphery appear to suppress peripheral T and B cell functions that are important for the ultimate production of antibody by a B cell, either via a direct effect or via activation of the SNS.

Glucocorticoids inhibit antigen-specific antibody pro-duction after a primary immunization, but not after a sec-ondary response (Wallgren et al., 1994). Also, various stres-sors, such as acute alcohol exposure (Han & Pruett, 1995) and inescapable shock (Fleshner et al., 1996) inhibit both cytokine and antibody production via a mechanism that partially involves an elevated level of glucocorticoids. How-ever, it is interesting to note that glucocorticoids are not associated exclusively with immune suppression. Gluco-corticoids appear to cause a shift to a Th2-slanted immune response, also as discussed in detail in recent reviews (Franchimont, 2004; Riccardi et al., 2002). This shift to a Th2 cytokine profile may be partially responsible for the enhancing effect of glucocorticoids on the level of IgE in individuals with asthma and atopy (Akdis et al., 1997; Kimata et al., 1995). For example, more Th2 cells mak-ing more IL-4 may induce more B cells to switch to the production of IgE. In addition, glucocorticoids may syn-ergize with Th2 cell-derived IL-4 to increase the level of B cell isotype switching to IgE by a B cell (Jabara et al., 1991; Jabara et al., 1993; Wu et al., 1991), via a mecha-nism that involves an upregulation of CD40L on the Th2 cell to deliver a more intense activation/switching signal to the B cell via CD40 (Jabara et al., 2001). These find-ings suggest that the concentration of glucocorticoids at the site of action may be important. For example, the level of stress, an activity that induces glucocorticoid release, is an important factor that determines the effect that stress will induce on immunocompetence, with moderate stress increasing the level of immune responsiveness and intense stress decreasing it (Dhabhar, 2002; Weiss et al., 1989). On the other hand, a low level of glucocorticoid signaling, because of a decreased level of either the hormone, level or sensitivity of the receptor, or both, may also be detri-mental during a stress-related circumstance, as has been discussed recently (Raison & Miller, 2003). Thus, any drug, disease, or psychosocial factor that either stimulates or inhibits CRH or glucocorticoid production/release might likewise be expected to alter the level of antibody-mediated immunity.

2.3. The sympathetic neurotransmitter norepinephrine and immunity

Over the years, four key discoveries documented that a link exists between the immune system and the SNS: (1) The discovery that the parenchyma of primary lymphoid organs, such as bone marrow and thymus (Bulloch & Pomerantz, 1984; Calvo, 1968; Felten et al., 1985; Williams & Felten, 1981) and secondary lymphoid organs, such as spleen, lymph nodes, gut-associated lymphoid tissue, and bronchiole-associated lymphoid tissue (Butter et al., 1988; Reilly et al., 1976; Riegele, 1929; Williams & Felten, 1981; Williams et al., 1981) was innervated. These findings indi-cate that the anatomy existed for the neurotransmitter to be released within close proximity to the immune cells that were primarily responsible for generating an immune response against antigens; (2) The discovery that the sym-pathetic neurotransmitter norepinephrine was released from the sympathetic nerve terminals in the spleen upon the administration of either antigen or cytokine (Del Rey et al., 1981; Felten et al., 1987; Fuchs et al., 1988; Lorton et al., 1990; Shimizu et al., 1994); (3) The discovery that lymphoid cells expressed the beta-2-adrenergic receptor (β_2AR) that could bind norepinephrine (Sanders et al., 2001), indicating that the machinery for transducing a norepinephrine signal directly to the immune cell was available; and 4) The discovery that norepinephrine reg-ulated the level of T and B lymphocyte activity via a cAMP- and PKA-mediated mechanism (Madden et al., 1995), indicating a mechanism by which the brain was able to communicate with peripheral immune cells. These findings suggest that a mechanism exists to explain the antibody changes that occur when an individual is exposed to a psychosocial stressor that affects some component of SNS activation and/or beta-2-adrenergic receptor (β_2AR) expression/function. This area of research has become quite exciting in recent years because of the data obtained using molecular tools to study cytokine and antibody immunobiology, techniques which will be discussed later in this chapter.

In vivo, norepinephrine depletion or administration of a non-selective βAR antagonist in adult animals either increases (Kruszewska et al., 1995) or decreases the T cell-dependent antibody response (Alaniz et al., 1999; Hall et al., 1982; Kasahara et al., 1977; Kohm & Sanders, 1999; Livnat et al., 1985), with the latter finding suggesting that norepinephrine enhances baseline immune cell activity and is necessary for maintaining an optimal level of anti-body production *in vivo*. Likewise, results obtained *in vitro* support the finding that norepinephrine induces an enhancing effect on the level of antibody normally pro-duced by a B cell *in vivo* (Burchiel & Melmon, 1979; Roper et al., 1990; Sanders & Munson, 1984a; Sanders & Munson, 1984b; Sanders & Powell-Oliver, 1992; Teh & Paetkau, 1976; Watson et al., 1973). To study this effect on a more mechanistic level *in vivo*, IgG$_1$ production and germinal center formation were found to decrease in *scid* mice depleted of norepinephrine prior to reconstitution with Ag-specific Th2 cells and B cells, an effect that was reversed by the administration of a β_2AR agonist (Kohm & Sanders, 1999).

In general, naive T cells and Th1 cells, but not Th2 cells, express the β_2AR as determined by radioligand binding, immunofluorescence, mRNA analysis, and cell function analysis (Ramer-Quinn et al., 1997; Sanders et al., 1997; Swanson et al., 2001). Resting B lymphocytes preferentially express the β_2AR, also {#3958; #1066; #1013; #8; #2649}. For a more detailed review of β_2AR expression by immune cell subsets, the reader is referred to the following comprehensive review article (Sanders et al., 2001). Classically, stimulation of the β_2AR initiates an intracellular signaling cascade leading to adenylyl cyclase activation, cAMP accumulation, and PKA activation. An increased level of intracellular cAMP decreased the level of IFN-γ production by an unfractionated population of CD4+ T cells (Betz & Fox, 1991; Borger et al., 1998; Paul-Eugene et al., 1992; Snijdewint et al., 1993; Van der Pouw-Kraan et al., 1992) and the β_2AR-selective agonist terbutaline decreased the level of IFN-γ by resting and activated Th1 cells (Ramer-Quinn et al., 1997; Sanders et al., 1997). In contrast, when naive CD4+ T cells were exposed to norepinephrine at the time of naïve T cell activation under conditions that promoted the development of Th1 cells, the progeny Th1 cells produced higher levels of IFN-γ upon restimulation with antigen in comparison to progeny Th1 cells generated in the absence of norepinephrine (Swanson et al., 2001). The β_2AR-selective agonist terbutaline failed to affect the level of IL-4 production by either unsorted CD4$^+$ T cells or Th2 cell clones, likely because Th2 cells do not express the β_2AR (Sanders et al., 1997). Therefore, norepinephrine may selectively influence naive and Th1 cell cytokine production, but not that by Th2 cells.

β_2AR stimulation on a CD40L/IL-4-activated B cell *in vitro* was found to increase the *rate* of mature IgG$_1$ transcription, without affecting class switch recombination to IgG$_1$ or mature IgG$_1$ transcript stability (Podojil & Sanders, 2003). This result was supported *in vivo* when norepinephrine depletion or administration of an antagonist decreased the serum level of Th2-dependent IgG$_1$, disrupted formation of germinal centers in the spleen, and decreased the level of antigen-induced CD86 expression on B cells (Kohm & Sanders, 1999). Because the Th2 cell does not appear to express the β_2AR (Sanders et al., 1997), the effect of norepinephrine on the level of IgG$_1$ produced by a B cell *in vivo* appears to be a direct one.

CD86 is a costimulatory molecule on the B cell, which appears to serve two functions. First, CD86-mediated stimulation of CD28 expressed on the surface of T cells exerts a critical regulatory influence on T cell cytokine production and surface molecule expression, thus indirectly influencing B cell function by modulating the level of "help" that the B cell receives from a T cell. Second, stimulation of CD86 sends a signal directly into the B cell to regulate the level of antibody production (Kasprowicz et al., 2000). β_2AR stimulation on a B cell was reported to increase the level of CD86 expressed on, and IgG$_1$ produced by, a B cell (Kasprowicz et al., 2000), and the β_2AR-induced upregulation of CD86 is dependent on the activation of NF-kB (Kohm et al., 2002). The mechanism by which this effect occurs appears to involve a CD86- and β_2AR-induced increase in B cell expression of the transcription factor Oct-2 and its coactivator OCA-B, respectively, as well as the binding of each protein to the 3'-IgH enhancer region (Podojil et al., 2004), a region of the genome that regulates the rate at which IgG1 is produced. Taken together, these findings suggest that an immune receptor-induced signaling pathway induced by CD86 may cooperate with a nervous system receptor-induced signaling pathway induced by the β_2AR to regulate the *rate* of mature IgG$_1$ transcription.

Taken together, psychological responses that involve activation of components of the CNS, such as the HPA, or the SNS, may affect immune cell activity via endogenous molecules released by these organ systems and, thus, induce the immune changes that are often associated with individuals experiencing various psychological responses to a variety of psychological factors.

3. SOCIAL CONTEXT

3.1. Psychological factors: Association with changes in parameters of humoral immunity

A number of studies have shown that a correlation exists between factors that alter psychophysiological states, such as mood alterations, depression, and acute/chronic stress with changes in the humoral arm of the immune system. It is important to note that most of these studies have measured the level of antibody produced against the endogenous latent herpesvirus, Epstein-Barr virus (EBV), or the exogenous influenza virus. Epstein-Barr virus is a latent virus that requires an intact cell-mediated immune response to maintain control over its expression, although, a rise in anti-herpesvirus antibody is often measured as an indicator that a cell-mediated immune response may be compromised in an infected individual. Nonetheless, for both EBV and influenza virus, the antibody response that develops is used to reflect the ability of B cells to produce antibody against the viruses, with the help of CD4$^+$ T cells. Thus, an assessment of humoral immune status can be used as an indicator of the status of both Th and B lymphocyte immunity at a given time point in time during the response to a stressor. Although some limitations exist with these studies, a review of their findings is necessary in order to formulate educated hypotheses about the impact that psychophysiological factors may have on immune interactions that must occur for the generation of a humoral immune response against antigen.

3.1.1. Stress

A number of excellent review articles have summarized the findings indicating that a connection exists between stress and immunity (Black, 2002; Marsland et al., 2002; Padgett & Glaser, 2003; Segerstrom & Miller, 2004; Yang & Glaser, 2002). A particularly enlightening meta-analytic study of 30 years of inquiry summarizes how the degree of stress – subacute, acute, and chronic – differentially affected different aspects of cellular and humoral immunity, and that age and disease played a role in modulating the effect induced (Segerstrom & Miller, 2004). The following summary focuses on the key findings with regard to the effect of stress on humoral immunity.

A number of studies indicated that psychological and physical stress increases the susceptibility of animals and humans to microbial and viral pathogens (Sanders, 2000). In animals, a number of stress paradigms were used to study the relationship between stress and humoral immunity. For example, the stress of crowding and heat (Beard & Mitchell, 1987; Edwards & Dean, 1977; Mashaly et al., 2004), restraint stress (Feng et al., 1991; Yorty & Bonneau, 2003; Yorty & Bonneau, 2004), forced exercise (Reyes & Lerner, 1976), and electric shock (Cao et al., 2004; Kusnecov et al., 1992) significantly delayed the development of antibody production. In contrast, a few studies using a stress and viral infection model system showed either no change or an increase in anti-viral antibody responses (Beard & Mitchell, 1987; Chang & Rasmussen, 1965; Yamada et al., 1964). However, as suggested by two other studies (Feng et al., 1991; McLean, 1982), stress may delay anti-viral antibody production and, hence, the effect of stress on humoral immune status could be misinterpreted if the antibody production is measured at only one point in time. Thus, although the cumulative antibody level generated against a pathogen may be unchanged in stressed individuals, the rate at which these antibodies are made may be the difference between an individual's ability to mount an early antibody response against a viral infection.

In humans, the majority of studies on the effects of stress on the humoral immune response have used natural stress paradigms, such as academic examinations stress, bereavement, stress associated with HIV-1 infection, and stress due to caring for a patient with progressive dementia. The majority of results obtained in these paradigms suggest that stress reduces humoral immunity; however, a few contradictory results have been obtained. The secretory immune system and, in particular secretory IgA (sIgA) that is present in mucosal membranes, provides the body with a first line of defense against invading pathogens. In a pioneering 1983 study, the effect of academic stress was examined in 64-first year dental students (Jemmott et al., 1983). The results showed that sIgA secretion rates were diminished from baseline during high-stress periods as compared to low-stress periods. In addition, the inter-individual responses revealed secretion of IgA was elevated at all time points in subjects who showed a great need to establish and maintain warm personal relationships. In contrast to all other subjects, in those students who exhibited an inhibited need for power, the IgA secretion did not return to baseline and continued to decline through the final low-stress period.

However, the type of academic stressor may have been the important factor that determined whether a change in salivary sIgA occurred during a given test period. Recent studies using a variety of acute academic stressors showed that significant increases (Ring et al., 2000; Willemsen et al., 1998; Willemsen et al., 2000) and decreases (Deinzer et al., 2000) occurred in the level of sIgA before and after a stressful academic activity. For example, one study showed that no significant change occurred in the sIgA levels of students before and after a *written* examination, but that a significant increase occurred after an *oral* presentation (Lowe et al., 2000). Another study recently confirmed that a written exam did not increase sIgA levels, and extended this finding to show that no change occurred in sIgA before the exam when perceived stress and cortisol levels were high (Ng et al., 2003). More recent results show that salivary samples from female students experiencing stress during exams had higher levels of EBV-specific IgG and IgA (Sarid et al., 2004) and that students with positive personality traits, with or without hypnosis, exhibited greater immune competence as indicated by T and B cell counts (Gruzelier et al., 2001). These findings suggest that the type of a specific academic stressor may induce changes in sIgA levels that are not necessarily reflected by the level of perceived stress or the stress-related changes in cortisol.

In addition to a change in salivary IgA levels, the effect of academic stress on the ability to mount an immune response to a hepatitis B vaccination was studied in 48 medical students (Glaser et al., 1992). In this study, students were administered a series of three hepatitis B vaccinations over an extended period of examinations. To assess the levels of perceived psychological stress, the students filled out a Profile of Mood States (POMS), Perceived Stress Scale (PSS), and an Interpersonal Support Evaluation List (ISEL). Results of this study revealed that although all of the students had seroconverted at the six-month interval, only 25% of the students had seroconverted at the one-month interval. Further analysis of the perceived psychological stress data revealed that the students who seroconverted at one month were significantly less anxious than those who seroconverted later. Thus, stress may delay the production of antibody in response to viral antigen challenge, suggesting that it may be important to monitor seroconversion in individuals who are experiencing stress, such as healthcare workers starting a new job, military personnel who are being transferred overseas, or elderly people who are moving to group care facilities, before exposing them to situations that increase their exposure to potential pathogens.

Consistent with the above study, a recombinant DNA hepatitis vaccine was utilized to assess the effects of perceived psychological stress on vaccination efficacy in medical students (Jabaaij et al., 1993). The effects of stress on both the initiation phase and the boost phase were examined. Results of this study also showed that stress reported at month 2 during the initiation phase of the immune response had a negative influence on antibody production. Another study indicated that the perception of mild, intermittent stress affected long-term maintenance of an antibody response against influenza virus in healthy adults (Burns et al., 2003). However, a more recent study showed that perceived stress either a few days before, or at the time of, influenza virus vaccination were not associated with a change in the antibody response, but that perceived stress 10 days after vaccination appeared to associate with a change in the antibody response, independently of other variables such as cortisol levels (Miller et al., 2004). Thus, perceived stress may play a role in the development and/or maintenance of an anti-viral antibody response.

Another recent study (Burns et al., 2002b) using undergraduate students who had received a series of EBV vaccinations showed that, in students performing an arithmetic task, salivary cortisol levels were higher in those students with high serum EBV antibody titers when compared to those with low titers. In contrast, using cardiac reactions as an indicator of SNS activation, reactions were greater in those students with low antibody titers. Taken together, this pattern of results suggested that both the HPA axis and the SNS are involved in regulating immune status following EBV vaccination, although the exact mechanism responsible for mediating the observed effects remain unclear. These findings lend some support to results from a subsequent study indicating that participants with above normal stress exposures were at a greater risk of having a low antibody titer against EBV (Burns et al., 2002a).

The effects of chronic stress associated with caregiving have also been studied. Caregivers of a relative with a progressive dementia experience high levels of distress and produce high levels of antibody against the endogenous latent herpesvirus (Kiecolt-Glaser et al., 1991; Kiecolt-Glaser et al., 1987). On the other hand, if exposed to an exogenous virus, such as influenza, the caregiver tends to produce less antibody than sex-, age-, and socioeconomically matched controls (Kiecolt-Glaser et al., 1996). Likewise, elderly caregivers of spouses with dementia showed an increase level of HPA activation, as indicated by salivary cortisol levels, and a decreased anti-HBV IgG response to influenza vaccine (Vedhara et al., 1999). However, when elderly caregivers received cognitive-behavioral stress management intervention, an increase in anti-influenza IgG was noted when compared to caregivers without intervention and non-caregivers (Vedhara et al., 2003). In contrast, young caregivers of spouses with multiple sclerosis showed no signs of immune suppression or enhancement, as measured by anti-influenza antibody titers and IFN-gamma/IL-4 levels (Vedhara et al., 2002). However, one study reported that no change occurred between young and elderly adults in their ability to develop increased levels of anti-influenza antibody (Brydak et al.,

2003). In response to a pneumococcal bacterial vaccine, the IgG antibody response in spousal caregivers is also decreased when compared to controls (Glaser et al., 2000). Thus, these findings suggest that differences may exist between caregivers due to age and/or the psychological burden associated with caring for spouses with different diseases.

In a study to examine the effects of stress on the ability to develop an immune response to a novel antigen (Snyder et al., 1990), women were immunized with the novel antigen keyhole limpet hemocyanin (KLH) and serum IgG was measured before immunization, 3 weeks following immunization, and at 8 weeks following immunization. Although the correlations were not significant, specific trends for antibody production were noted. First, more stressful events, either good or bad, were correlated with lower antigen-specific IgG at 3 weeks. Second, more good stressful events correlated with higher levels of IgG at 8 weeks. And third, women who reported more bad stressful events exhibited lower IgG at 8 weeks.

One commonly occurring stressful event is conjugal bereavement. Results of one study revealed that although there were no differences in T and B cell counts at one or two months after the spouse's death, cell proliferation in response to mitogens was significantly decreased (Schleifer et al., 1983). The results from this study suggested that suppression of mitogen-induced lymphocyte proliferation was a direct consequence of bereavement and not a consequence of major changes in diet, activity levels, alcohol, tobacco, drug use, or weight changes following death of a spouse. Although serum Ig levels were not reported in this study, the decreased proliferation to PWM, a mitogen that stimulates both B and T cells, suggests that the stress of bereavement may decrease both T and B cell function.

In a pilot study of 11 asymptomatic HIV-1 seropositive men, the effect of life stressors and coping style on CD4+ T cell numbers was assessed (Goodkin et al., 1992). Results of this study indicated that a significant correlation existed between the occurrence of a major life stressor over the previous year and total lymphocyte count. In addition, the low stress groups had higher CD4+ T cell counts than did high stress groups. Thus, the stress associated with HIV-1 infection may alter an individuals CD4+ Th cell population, which, in turn, could eventually lead to a decreased level of antibody production from the B cells that rely on CD4+ Th cells for "help." A more recent study showed that cognitive-behavioral stress management in HIV-infected men produced short-term increases in anti-herpesvirus IgG that were accompanied by a decrease in urinary cortisol and norepinephrine levels, as well as a reduction in the symptoms of depression (Antoni, 2003b). More details on this specific area of research can be found in the following comprehensive review (Antoni, 2003a).

In conclusion, the majority of studies presented above indicate that stress has a dampening effect on the humoral immune response in humans, but that the type of stress, the level of stress perception, age, and the inclusion of intervention therapy, may profoundly affect the response. At present, the mechanisms whereby stress leads to either a delay in the mounting of an antibody response or a decrease in the levels of antibody produced overall are unclear. This is where translational studies that are designed to relate basic science findings from mice and humans into one study will move the field forward, as suggested in one review on norepinephrine, beta-adrenergic receptors, and immunity (Sanders & Straub, 2002).

3.1.2. Mood

On a daily basis, humans are subjected to a variety of positive and negative experiences that have mood altering consequences, such as accomplishing a task, getting a promotion at work, losing keys, or having an argument with a loved one. A tight relationship between stress and the regulation of immune function has been documented in many studies (see previous section on stress) but less is known about the influence of the hedonic tone on immune function. Hedonic tone or mood states affect our daily lives and can be manipulated easily by conscious recall of emotional situations (Futterman et al., 1992). A within-subject analysis strategy was utilized to assess the effect that daily mood changes have on sIgA production to a novel antigen (Stone et al., 1987). Subjects in the study were orally administered a novel protein antigen and were asked to keep a daily diary. For a period of 8 weeks, sIgA that was specific for the novel antigen was measured 3 times a week from parotid saliva. The results of this study indicated that the level of sIgA directed against a novel antigen was lower on days in which daily diaries reported a high negative mood as compared to higher levels on days in which diaries reported a high positive mood. These studies were further confirmed in 1994 with a larger sample size (n = 96) over a 12-week sampling period (Stone et al., 1994). In 2004, a study reported that depressed and non-depressed female Japanese undergraduates, who were required to either write about unpleasant experiences or suppress their emotional response about them, showed differential regulation of sIgA levels in saliva (Takagi & Ohira, 2004). For example, writing about negative experiences was positively correlated to improved mood states in both depressed and non-depressed subjects. However, writing about negative emotions increased sIgA selectively in the depressed group only. Also, in a study undertaken with 105 students from Florida, who lived in neighborhoods more or less damaged by hurricane Andrew, the severity of disaster the subject has gone through was found to inversely correlate with sIgA levels (Rotton & Dubitsky, 2002).

A second strategy to assess the possibility that daily mood changes influence humoral immune status involved a process that "artificially" induces alterations in mood state in a laboratory setting. Results show that sIgA in saliva increases following the viewing of humorous videotape. In addition, female viewers who watched non-humorous videotape, and then wept openly, showed a significant decrease in sIgA when compared to subjects who did not weep openly (Labott et al., 1990). Another study was done to investigate weather negative or positive mood induction has a short-term influence on the rate of sIgA secretion (Hucklebridge et al., 2000). Surprisingly, both negative and positive mood states were correlated with an increase in sIgA concentration as well as sIgA secretion rate. In this study, the change in sIgA secretion rate and concentration were observed within minutes of mood manipulation, suggesting that the effect was on the transepithelial secretory process rather than an effect on B-cell function directly. Interpreting these data can be difficult as many parameters are able to influence sIgA levels. For example, the activation state of the autonomic nervous system has been shown to directly control transepithelial sIgA transport in the submandibular salivary gland of the rat (Carpenter et al., 1998) and sIgA concentration and rate of secretion parallels the diurnal pattern of cortisol with a declining phase in the morning (Hucklebridge et al., 1998; Zeier et al., 1996).

Interestingly, mood changes provoked by watching a humorous video (laughter) compared to watching a non-humorous video about weather information were found to differentially affect immunoglobulin isotype pattern generated in patients with atopic keratoconjunctivitis (Kimata, 2004). After watching the humorous video, cedar pollen-specific IgE, as well as IgG4, was decreased, whereas cedar pollen-specific IgA levels were increased in the tears. This group was also able to show that the decrease in allergen specific IgE measured whereas watching humorous films improved bronchial hyperresponsiveness in patients with allergic asthma. Pathophysiological relevance was demonstrated in a study investigating the role of emotional style on susceptibility to two strains of rhinoviruses that cause the common cold (Cohen et al., 2003). The data showed that an increased tendency to experience positive emotions was associated with a decreased susceptibility to both strains of virus, but not vice versa (Cohen et al., 2003). In addition to providing new information about a relationship between psychological factors and the level of humoral immunity, these types of studies may be very important therapeutically. For example, if creating a positive mood change with either a humorous video or through recall of positive events either enhances sIgA or decreases allergen-specific IgE production, then these types of mood altering strategies may be useful in obtaining an increased level of protection against viral and bacterial pathogens, as well as a decrease in the severity of allergic symptoms.

3.1.3. Depression

Results from previous studies designed to examine immune parameters in depression are somewhat conflicting (Stein et al., 1991). Much of this conflict may be due to an inadequate number of controls. Therefore, for ease of presentation, a series of well controlled studies will be presented, starting with those showing a correlation with immune suppression. A 1984 study examined eighteen patients hospitalized for major depressive disorder (Schleifer et al., 1984). Blood samples were taken from patients and controls and the absolute number of B and T cells, the percentage of B and T cells, and the ability of PBMC to proliferate in response to three mitogens was assessed. Results of this study showed that depressed patients exhibited decreases in all parameters measured. Thus, this early study indicated that the level of depression correlated with immune suppression.

When the Flinders sensitive line (FSL) rat, which is used as a genetic animal model of depression, was compared to the Flinders resistant line (FRL) rat used as controls depressive rats showed no change in the Th2 cell-dependent IgG1 response to KLH, but a decrease in the Th1 cell-dependent IgG2a (Friedman et al., 2002). In addition, IFN-gamma production was decreased in splenocytes obtained from immunized FLS rats compared to FRL rats after restimulation with KLH in vitro. In mice, chronic sequential exposure to a mild stressor can mimic symptoms of depression and was used to investigate the role of depression in T-cell independent versus T-cell dependent antibody responses (Silberman et al., 2004). After 6 weeks, stressor-exposed mice showed a significant decrease in T cell-dependent antibody production compared to non-exposed mice. Further, the authors were able to show that T cells obtained from stressor-treated animals were more sensitive to inhibitory signals delivered by corticosterone. Another study demonstrated that a direct link existed between major depression in humans and the level of cellular immunity against varicella-zoster-virus. The VZV-specific responder cell frequency in major depressed patients (n = 11) was significantly reduced compared to healthy controls (n = 11) of same age and sex implicating reduced VZV-specific cellular immunity in depressed individuals (Irwin et al., 1998). Thus, the majority of findings suggested that a state of immunosuppression exists in depressed individuals.

In contrast, another study showed that minor and major depressed patients have significantly higher serum antibody titers to the autoantigens phosphatidylserine and thromboplastin, as compared to non-depressed controls (Maes et al., 1993). To clearly address the possible correlation between depression and humoral immunity, further experimentation is necessary. To obtain a clearer picture, these experimental designs should include an analysis of complete antibody isotype profiles, a measurement of T cell cytokine profiles, and flow cytometric analysis of all CD4+ and B lymphocyte subsets. It is important that all of these parameters be measured in the same patient, and that repeated measures be taken over time to examine the possibility that the immune changes measured may be due to other psychological variables, such as daily mood changes. It will also be important to measure neuroendocrine parameters in parallel with measurements of immune parameters. Previous studies indicated that a number of neuroendocrine changes are present in some depressed patients, including alterations in CNS

neurotransmitter function, as measured by alterations in metabolites of both norepinephrine and serotonin in blood, CSF, and urine (Zis & Goodwin, 1982), abnormalities in the HPA axis, as measured by blunted ACTH responses to CRH (Gold et al., 1984; Gold et al., 1988; Sachar, 1982), and abnormalities in autonomic nervous system function, as measured by changes in plasma catecholamine levels (Potter, 1984; Rudorfer et al., 1985). In a recent study, the humoral response and the role of catecholamines and corticosterone were analyzed in a chronic mild stress model of depression in mice (Silberman et al., 2004). Although the T cell-dependent antibody response was decreased, the change did not appear to correlate with any changes induced in norepinephrine or glucocorticoids, but did appear to correlate with the sensitivity of receptors on T cells for the neurotransmitter and hormone. It is also important that age-matched controls be utilized in all analyses. As discussed earlier, some of the conflicts in the interpretation of the data collected thus far may be due to the different methods used to categorize depressed patients. Thus, a study that utilizes different depression categorization methods may provide useful information. Although many previous studies have not included patients with unipolar and bipolar depression because studies would provide a better understanding of the effects of depression on humoral immunity. Finally, depression and humoral immunity should be evaluated in patients involved in drug and behavior therapy programs to determine if treatments that decrease depressive symptoms concomitantly change neuroendocrine and humoral immune parameters.

Two scenarios emerge upon review of previous studies that were designed to examine if a correlation existed between depression and the level of humoral immunity. Studies revealed that the level of depression correlated with either immune suppression or enhancement. Although these two scenarios are somewhat opposite to each other, both scenarios indicate that changes occur in immune status when an individual becomes depressed. It is possible that some of the differences between the two scenarios are due to the methods utilized to classify depressed patients, especially because those who showed immunosuppression were categorized for depression based on Research Diagnostic Criteria (RDC), whereas the *Diagnostic and Statistical Manual of Mental Disorders* (DSM-III) rating system was used to categorize patients who showed immunoenhancement. In addition, the studies that suggest the level of depression correlated with immune enhancement utilized two-color flow cytometric analysis, a technique that may be more sensitive than the rosette formation technique utilized in the other studies that reported immune suppression.

3.2. Psychological intervention

Psychological factors, such as mood, depression, and stress, may have a negative impact on the humoral immune system. This suggests that psychological intervention may have beneficial effects on humoral immunity. A few intervention strategies that are commonly used in the area of psychotherapy include relaxation techniques, exercise, classical conditioning, and self-disclosure. In addition, the degree of social support and personal coping styles are often important factors in effective psychotherapy. Although the effects that these types of psychotherapies have on humoral immunity have not been examined mechanistically, the studies conducted thus far suggest that psychological intervention therapies may provide beneficial effects, particularly in individuals who have dampened humoral immune responses due to age or HIV-1 infection.

3.2.1. Relaxation

Two studies indicated that relaxation has a positive effect on the humoral immune system in humans. In the first study, salivary sIgA and serum antibody levels were examined in either control subjects or in subjects that practiced a daily relaxation technique (Green et al., 1988a). Results of this study indicated that following the first relaxation session, sIgA was significantly higher in the relaxation group than in controls. In addition to sIgA, serum IgA, IgG, and IgM levels also increased during the relaxation-training period in the relaxation subjects. In a second study, the effect of relaxation on changes in T helper cell percentages during examination stress was examined (Kiecolt-Glaser et al., 1986). Results of this study indicated that the percentage of T helper cells decreased during examination periods in both the relaxation group and controls. However, further analysis revealed that not all students practiced the relaxation technique with the same frequency (range 5 to 50 times). Thus, a regression analysis revealed that an increased frequency of relaxation practice was associated with a higher percentage of T helper cells in the blood during examinations. A more recent study showed that daily relaxation increased salivary IgA secretion rate after 20 min of relaxation, and was higher in individuals who practiced relaxation for a few weeks prior to saliva sampling (Green et al., 1988b). Serum IgA, IgG, and IgM also increased over the relaxation practice period. Likewise, in newspaper room workers supplied with soothing music during stressful periods, salivary IgA was increased as the level of stress decreased (Brennan & Charnetski, 2000). In addition, the effect of a 10-week cognitive-behavioral stress management intervention on the level of anti-HSV-2 IgG titers in a group of mildly symptomatic HIV-infected gay men showed that the level of cortisol and IgG were reduced in the stress management group, and that home relaxation practice in the stress management group reduced the cortisol and IgG titers even more (Cruess et al., 2000).

3.2.2. Exercise

Previous studies indicate that exercise has a beneficial effect on psychophysiological well-being (Callaghan, 2004; Guszkowska, 2004). Acute or moderate exercise is associated with a decrease in anxiety state and mood alterations.

Studies that examined the effects of long-term exercise programs showed positive effects of exercise in healthy people and in clinical populations, regardless of gender or age (Guszkowska, 2004). The beneficial effects of long-term exercise programs include a reduction in anxiety, depression, and negative mood, accompanied by improvements in self-esteem and cognitive functioning (Callaghan, 2004).

Findings from studies on psychoneuroimmune interactions suggested that stress, mood, anxiety, and depression altered the level of humoral immunity. For example, indicators of negative affective style, including differences in brain electrical measures of activation asymmetry and magnitude of emotion-modulated startle, were found to predict when a weak antibody response to influenza vaccination would occur (Rosenkranz et al., 2003), suggesting that a relationship existed between negative affective style and the ability to produce antibody in vivo. Thus, therapies such as exercise, which reduce the severity of these affective states, may also alter the level of humoral immunity. Other examples include studies showing that regular physical activity in older men was associated with a more robust primary immune response (Smith et al., 2004) and that a regular routine of moderate, physical activity may prevent detrimental stress-induced neuroendocrine and immunological effects (Fleshner, 2000).

One review of previous studies suggested that either brief graded-maximal or short-term submaximal exercise was associated with increases in serum antibody (Nieman, 1991). For example, two studies utilizing moderate exercise training showed that moderate exercise – walking for 45 minutes at 60% VO_2 max – was associated with increases in serum IgM, IgG, and IgA (Nehlsen-Cannarella et al., 1991a; Nehlsen-Cannarella et al., 1991b). In addition, one study reported that individuals who participated in a 10-week aerobic exercise training program exhibited an increase in the number of circulating $CD4^+$ T cells and B cells (LaPerriere et al., 1994a), whereas another study using physically active versus sedentary rats reported an increase in B-1 cells and natural IgM (Elphick et al., 2003a; Elphick et al., 2003b).

Although the exact mechanisms by which exercise alters humoral immunity are unknown. One possible mechanism may involve activation of the SNS and HPA, as well as the release of endogenous opiates. One study found that beta-adrenergic blockade suppressed the exercise-induced changes in antibody, IL-2, IFN-gamma, and mitogen-induced proliferation (Kohut et al., 2004). In addition, data showed that an increased clearance of tumor cells from the lung occurred in physically active rats versus sedentary controls (Jonsdottir & Hoffmann, 2000), suggesting that exercise may enhance lung immunity preferentially.

If it is true that psychological states suppress humoral immunity, then the possibility exists that exercise might be a good intervention therapy for individuals infected with HIV-1, who have both decreased immunity and increased depression/anxiety. A few studies have been conducted to examine this possibility (Dudgeon et al., 2004; LaPerriere et al., 1994b) and suggested that exercise has beneficial effects for HIV-1 infected individuals because it reduced anxiety, fatigue, anger, and depression (Florijin & Geiger, 1991; LaPerriere et al., 1991; Rigsby et al., 1992; Schlenzig et al., 1989), increased (LaPerriere et al., 1991; Rigsby et al., 1992; Schlenzig et al., 1989) or stabilized the CD4$^+$ T cell count (Dudgeon et al., 2004; Florijin & Geiger, 1991), and decreased viral load (Dudgeon et al., 2004).

The effect of exercise on the primary and secondary antibody response, especially the response after vaccination, is only beginning to be investigated. One study reported a positive relationship between habitual physical activity and baseline antibody concentration that remained elevated 12 months post-vaccination (Whitham & Blannin, 2003). In addition, another study reported that 2 weeks of physical activity was sufficient to increase the level of a secondary antibody response and, thus, may provide a useful strategy to enhance the antibody response to vaccination in humans (Kapasi et al., 2003).

3.2.3. Conditioning

One type of behavioral conditioning involves the illness-induced taste aversion paradigm. To condition a taste aversion response, a test animal is given a distinctly flavored solution, such as a dilute saccharin solution or chocolate milk, which serves as the conditioned-stimulus (CS). This exposure is followed by an intraperitoneal injection of a toxic agent that causes gastrointestinal distress, such as cyclophosphamide or lithium chloride, which serves as the unconditioned-stimulus (UCS). Since the mid 1970s, a number of studies have been conducted by Ader, Cohen, and others to investigate the effects of behavioral conditioning on both humoral and cell-mediated immune responsiveness (reviewed by Ader & Cohen, 1993; Cohen et al., 1994).

In an initial study (Ader & Cohen, 1975), the effects of taste aversion conditioning on humoral immune responsiveness was assessed by conditioning rats with saccharin solution (CS) and an intraperitoneal injection of cyclophosphamide (UCS), which induced nausea and, more importantly, immune suppression. Three days after conditioning, the rats were injected with sheep erythrocytes (SRBC), a T cell-dependent antigen, and were then allowed to drink the saccharin solution (CS) again. Six days later, serum antibody titers were measured. The results of this study showed that the conditioned rats receiving saccharin (CS) at the time of SRBC injection had lower antibody titers when compared to conditioned rats that had not received saccharin at the time of sRBC injection. Thus, a conditioned suppression of the antibody response had occurred. This experiment was repeated with similar findings by a second group (Rogers et al., 1976), with the exception that this group found it necessary to have two re-exposures to the CS in order to see a significant decrease in antibody titer. In addition, a 1988 study showed that the timing of re-exposure to the CS has a pro-

found effect on the ability of the CS to induce humoral immune suppression (Kusnecov et al., 1988).

Although the above studies showed that immunosuppression was linked to a conditioned stimulus, it was unclear as to whether B cells and/or T cells were affected. In an attempt to clarify which population of cells was altered, a conditioning protocol similar to the protocol described above was utilized in concert with either the T cell-dependent antigen SRBC or the T cell-independent antigen *Brucella abortus* (Wayner et al., 1978). The results of this study indicated that the T cell-independent antigen induced no change in antibody titers in the conditioned *versus* non-conditioned control rats, in contrast to the decrease measured when the T cell-dependent antigen was used. Thus, T cells may be the target cell of the conditioned taste aversion. However, in contrast to the results obtained in rats, a study conducted in mice reported that a conditioned antibody response could be induced with a T-independent antigen (Cohen et al., 1979), suggesting that B cells are the target cell of the conditioned taste aversion. Taken together, the data suggested that the cell populations responding to the conditioned response might differ depending on the species being studied.

The data obtained from animal conditioned immunosuppression studies suggested the possibility of using an alternative therapy for patients with autoimmune diseases, especially those who are currently treated with large doses of immunosuppressive agents that possess toxic side effects. Because the reported data implicate both B and T cells as targets of the conditioned response, conditioned immunosuppressive therapy may be particularly beneficial in diseases, such as Alzheimer's disease, multiple sclerosis, and systemic lupus erythematosus, all of which are diseases in which both B and T cells contribute to pathogenesis. However, it is clear from animal models that further experimentation is necessary with regard to the number of training sessions for conditioning necessary for beneficial effects, as well as the optimal time of exposure to the CS.

Although some studies have shown that an unconditioned stimulus, such as cyclophosphamide appears to condition immune suppression, other studies showed that when antigen was used as the unconditioned stimulus, immune enhancement could be conditioned. In 1993, a study was conducted in mice to determine if antigen could be used as the unconditioned stimulus (UCS) to enhance humoral responsiveness (Ader et al., 1993). In this study, intraperitoneal injections of the antigen keyhole limpet hemocyanin (KLH), the unconditioned stimulus, were paired with a chocolate milk drinking solution, the conditioned stimulus. Mice were given either three CS-UCS pairings at three week intervals, each consisting of intraperitoneal injection of a very low dose of KLH + the chocolate milk drink, or just the chocolate milk drink. Results of this study showed that there was an enhancement of the anti-KLH antibody response when conditioned mice were re-exposed to both the CS and a minimally immunogenic dose of KLH. Other studies showed that a single exposure to a conditioned stimulus, when associated with exposure to the unconditioned stimulus of antigen, could induce immune enhancement of the antigen-specific IgG response upon re-exposure to the conditioned stimulus (Madden et al., 2001; Ramirez-Amaya & Bermudez-Rattoni, 1999). In contrast, a more recent study challenges these findings to show that one-trial conditioned immune enhancement of an antibody response was found to not occur with all protein antigens tested as the unconditioned stimulus (Espinosa et al., 2004). The idea that conditioning may enhance antibody production to low doses of antigen suggests some exciting possibilities for future use in vaccination protocols in which the antigen used for vaccination is difficult to obtain because of limited quantities or limited financial resources. Thus, it appears that a humoral immune response can be conditioned for either suppression or enhancement.

3.2.4. Social support and coping styles

A 1992 study suggests that social support may play an important role in an individual's response to a vaccination (Glaser et al., 1992). In this study, which was designed to determine the effects of examination stress on the ability to generate an immune response to hepatitis B antigen, medical students were given a series of three hepatitis vaccinations on days when they had examinations. Results of this study showed that students who reported greater social support also produced higher antibody titers to hepatitis B surface antigen (HpBsAg) at the time of the third booster inoculation. A study was also designed to examine the relationship between stress, social support, coping, and immune function in elderly women, revealed that women experiencing high-stress exhibited lower CD4$^+$/CD8$^+$ T cell ratios than women experiencing low stress (McNaughton et al., 1990). The lower CD4$^+$/CD8$^+$ T cell ratios were partly due to increases in the number of CD8$^+$ T cells in women experiencing either high stress or less satisfaction with emotional social support. Thus, it appears that not only the quantity of social support, but also the quality of social support may be important. In addition, the results of this study showed that CD4$^+$ T cell number was significantly related to the endorsement of a greater percentage of problem-focused coping. Social support may also be beneficial for HIV-1-infected individuals. A previous study of 49 HIV-1-positive male hemophiliacs revealed that a low availability of attachment (AVAT) score was associated with a significant decline in CD4$^+$ T cell count over a five-year period (Theorell et al., 1995). Two previous studies have also indicated that coping styles may alter immunity in HIV-1-infected individuals (Goodkin et al., 1992; Mulder et al., 1995). A study of 11 asymptomatic HIV-1-positive males showed that passive coping style and high stress were associated with a decline in total lymphocyte number over a one-year period (Goodkin et al., 1992). In addition, in both low stress and high stress individuals who were active copers, there was a trend, although

not significant, toward an increased number of CD4$^+$ T cells, when compared to low and high stress individuals who utilized a passive coping style. A second study of 51 HIV-1-infected men, which included a one-year follow-up, showed that active coping strategy was also associated with a decrease in clinical progression (Mulder et al., 1995).

Depression has been associated with an increase in the level of IFN-gamma produced by T cells (Seidel et al., 1995; Seidel et al., 1996). For example, a decrease in IFN-gamma production was found to occur in individuals with multiple sclerosis who had a reduction in depression (Mohr et al., 2001). In contrast, IFN-gamma production appeared to be more readily reduced in patients with poor social support, as opposed to those with good support (Mohr & Genain, 2004). In another study, social support was found to buffer the effects of stress on the level of sIgA produced such that support lowered the amount secreted after the stressful task was completed (Ohira, 2004). Interestingly, it was reported that acute stress paradigms that had distinct effects on autonomic nervous system activity were coupled to distinct changes in the amount of salivary IgA secreted (Bosch et al., 2001), namely that a memory task increased IgA, whereas a surgical video decreased IgA, most notably IgA1.

In conclusion, although the mechanisms by which intervention strategies, such as relaxation, exercise, conditioning, coping, and self-disclosure, enhance humoral immunity are not fully understood, the studies presented above suggest that these intervention strategies have beneficial effects on the level of humoral immunity. Furthermore, although the benefits of these therapies may be minor for young, non-stressed, and healthy individuals, they seem to provide the most beneficial effects for individuals who are experiencing either increased levels of stress and/or who are somewhat immunocompromised, such as the elderly and HIV-1-infected individuals. Taken together, these studies suggest that the most beneficial strategies to ward off a pathogen need to include approaches that ensure both a healthy mind and a healthy body.

4. INFERENTIAL CONTEXT

4.1. Experimental design for PNI studies involving humoral immunity

Although the study of psychoneuroimmunology (PNI) has been ongoing for the past 100 years (Biondi & Zannino, 1997), many of the earliest studies in this field merely reported observations that immune function appeared to be modulated by physiological stressors. The general hypothesis was that stress leads to an increased incidence of disease by either prolonging disease symptoms, increasing susceptibility to infection, weakening protective immune mechanisms, or decreasing vaccination efficiency [reviewed by (Biondi & Zannino, 1997; Cohen & Herbert, 1996)].

4.1.1. Selection of study groups/controls

The initial phase of all scientific studies is to establish the study objectives and a hypothesis so that a proper study group can be generated. In regards to a PNI study, it is very important that the initial hypothesis encompass psychological/behavioral, neuroendocrine and immune parameters. For example, various psychosocial disorders and interventions have been, and are continuing to be, studied for psychoneuroimmunomodulation. One of the most important criteria for a well-designed PNI study is the selection of a proper or comparable control group. Without a well-designated control group, it is difficult to interpret data that are obtained. In addition, study subjects should be grouped based on one, several, or many of the following parameters, depending on the objectives of the study. These parameters include age, gender, disease history and drugs used, lifestyle, such as diet, alcohol and caffeine consumption, and smoking, sleep pattern, personality, and social status (Biondi & Zannino, 1997; Cohen & Herbert, 1996). The importance of each of these parameters must be defined before the study begins. In most cases, one parameter will be more important than another. For example, immunological status/competency – the ability to mount an immune response/antibody response – has been linked to exercise. With this information a study designed to determine the ability of an individual to mount an immune response during and/or following a specific stress response, has to be controlled for exercising subjects. For example if the control group contains individuals who frequently exercise, whereas the experimental group contains subjects who rarely exercise, then the results of an immunological analysis of these subjects may be skewed by factors not properly controlled for in this study. In any scientific study, especially those performed *in vivo*, it is important to remember that many systems in the body are connected and one system may be influencing other systems. To properly control for such events, it is important to set rigid criteria for test subject selection. It is difficult to draw clear conclusions from many previous studies in the PNI area due to the lack of proper age, gender, and lifestyle-matched controls.

4.1.2. Define background levels

Prior to the initiation of a PNI study, it is necessary to obtain a background profile for each of the test subjects (Kiecolt-Glaser & Glaser, 1992), in order to be able to conclude if changes occurred during the experimental testing period. Depending on the specific psychological, neurological, and immunological parameters that will be examined, a variety of tests must be performed to determine each individual's background resting levels. To rule out effects of diurnal variation, samples utilized to assess background levels should be collected at the same time of day as the test samples. In addition, for studies, which examine the effects of stress, it may be important to gather two separate background samples, one prior to the first day of study and one on the first day of the study, prior to the application of the stressor.

4.1.3. Sample collection and analysis

As reviewed in this chapter, the cellular and humoral immune systems and the CNS, HPA, and SNS are connected in many intricate ways with regulatory mechanisms occurring within the individual systems, as well as between the systems. Therefore, in order to link immunological changes to psychological and neurophysiological changes, it is important that PNI studies include simultaneous analysis of physical, psychological, immune, and neuroendocrine parameters. As discussed above, a few important physical characteristics, which should be recorded for the study group, include age, gender, weight, height, diet, drugs, lifestyle, and social status. Additional physical parameters that may be important to monitor include nutritional status, vaccine history, disease history, allergic status, number of subjects housed together, and the infectious state of subjects sharing the same house. In addition to physical factors, a number of psychological factors (reviewed above in section 3.0) can alter humoral and cellular immunity including mood changes, depression, stress, degree of social support, and personal motivation. Thus, it is particularly important that these psychological states be monitored with questionnaires either throughout the study, or on the days when samples are collected for analysis of immune and neuroendocrine parameters.

Previous PNI studies suggested that changes in psychological and neuroendocrine factors alter both the humoral and cellular immune systems. In addition, soluble factors produced during humoral and cellular immune responses may regulate each other. Thus, it is important for initial studies to include measurements of both humoral and cellular immune parameters. Initial analysis of immunity should include: (1) immunofluorescence staining of peripheral blood samples to determine the percentages of B cells, T cells (CD4$^+$ and CD8$^+$), NK cells, and macrophages; (2) measurement of both serum and salivary IgA levels by ELISA; (3) measurement of the capacity of peripheral blood T cells to secrete cytokines following anti- CD3 stimulation; (4) measurement of the ability of T and B cells to proliferate in response to mitogens; and (5) measurement of the ability of NK cells to lyse target cells. To obtain a better understanding of which neuroendocrine factor(s) may be altering the immune response, it is important to measure the levels of ACTH, cortisol, epinephrine, and norepinephrine that are present in the blood and saliva.

4.2. Analysis of humoral immunity

The earlier sections of this chapter discuss the process of antibody production in an immune response, as well as the other organ systems that influence this humoral immune response. Understanding the mechanism(s) by which antibody is produced and the non-immune factors that can enhance or inhibit antibody production are important. However, it is also necessary to understand the techniques that are used to measure the level of antibody produced and to determine specific features about the antibody produced, including antigenic specificity, antibody isotype or class, and affinity of the antibody for its antigen.

The following section focuses on techniques that are used to examine antibody production in animal and human systems. In some cases, such as the diagnosis of viral or bacterial infections, human serum can be tested directly for the presence of antibodies to these different antigens. However, if the goal is to define the mechanism by which a disease develops, it may be difficult to study a human model due to the limited reagents and limited sample material available for analysis. To circumvent these limitations, many scientists use mouse models because the mouse mimics many human diseases, and the assay reagents are easily accessible. Additional animal model systems utilized in psychoneuroimmunology research include rat, rabbit, and goat (Lingrel et al., 1985; Miyoshi et al., 1985; Peters & Theofilopoulos, 1977; Silagi & Schaefer, 1986; Talmadge, 1985).

4.2.1. Detection of antibody production in animals and humans

The techniques that will be described below are used to analyze the humoral (antibody) response in both the human and mouse systems. The limitations in human studies stem from the limited study material, usually only serum, versus multiple organs that can be examined in the mouse, such as the spleen and lymph nodes, in addition to serum. Over the past few decades, assay systems have been refined and are now able to detect nanogram to picogram quantities of antibody per milliliter of sample tested, as compared to sensitivity levels of microgram quantities detected in the earlier assay systems. Although a variety of techniques have been used to measure antibody levels and antibody parameters, the authors of this chapter recommend the techniques described below. To aid in the design of future PNI studies we have included the mechanism of detection, sensitivity of the assay, and the advantages and disadvantages for each technique.

4.2.2. Mechanism, sensitivity, advantages/disadvantages

Enzyme-linked immunosorbent assay (ELISA). The design and sensitivity of the ELISA are similar to the RIA (Engvall & Perlman, 1971; Macy et al., 1988). The ELISA can be used to test antiserum or purified antibody for its antigenic specificity, isotype, and quantity. A solid surface (96-well plate) is coated with an antigen or capture antibody. The antiserum sample is then added and allowed to bind to the coated plate. The plate is washed to remove unbound antibody and an enzyme-conjugated (alkaline phosphatase, horseradish peroxidase) detecting antibody is added. The

detecting antibody will bind to specific antibody that has bound to the capture antigen or antibody, and a soluble substrate is added to the plate. If the enzyme-conjugated detecting antibody is present, it will convert the substrate and result in a colorimetric reaction. The degree of substrate conversion can be measured using an ELISA reader, which determines the optical density of each well. To determine the antibody concentration in each sample well, the optical density readings of the sample wells are compared to the optical density readings of a standard curve. Both the capture antigen/antibody and detecting antibody can help to define the antigenic specificity and isotype of the bound antibody present in the antiserum. The sensitivity of the ELISA assay ranges from 0.0001–0.001 micrograms per milliliter (100 pg –1 ng/ml) of sample. The disadvantage of this system is that it requires purified antigens and antibodies for capturing and detecting antibody. The advantages include the ability to determine antigen concentration, isotype and specificity, its high sensitivity, good reproducibility, and the requirement for small amounts of sample antiserum (Adamkiewicz et al., 1984; Li, 1985).

ELISPOT. The ELISPOT assay is a modification of the ELISA that uses cells instead of cell supernatants or antiserum to assay for antibody production (Czerkinsky et al., 1983; Sedgwick & Holt, 1983). This system allows for the determination of the number of cells in a population that are producing antibody, as well as, the level of antibody produced by the cells in the sample population. As in the ELISA, wells are coated with a capture antigen or antibody. Instead of adding antiserum or cell supernatants to the wells, activated cells are added to the wells. The cells are allowed to secrete antibody for a limited period of time. Because the wells are coated with a capture antibody/antigen, antibody secreted by the cells that is specific for the capture antigen/antibody will bind to the plate and remain there when the cells are lysed and the plates are washed. After the plates are washed, an enzyme-linked detecting antibody is added. If antibody from the antiserum has bound to the wells, then the detecting antibody will bind to the captured antibody. An insoluble substrate is added to the wells that can be converted by the enzyme conjugated to the detecting antibody. In contrast to the ELISA assay, which employs a soluble substrate to determine antibody concentration using optical density readings, the ELISPOT assay uses an insoluble substrate that will generate "spots" where antibody has been secreted from cells. These spots can then be counted to determine the number of cells from the starting population that are secreting antibody. One disadvantage to this system is that there is no standard curve to quantify antibody levels. Therefore, samples must be compared to each other instead of a known standard. The ELISPOT is more practical than the Jerne plaque assay because sample wells can be stored before counting, and therefore do not require immediate analysis (Czerkinsky et al., 1983; Sedgwick & Holt, 1983).

Immunofluorescence. The surface or intracellular expression of certain proteins can increase or decrease following the activation of immune cells. Immunofluorescence analysis with fluorescently tagged antibodies or probes can help to identify whether the immune cell expresses the protein of interest. Although immunofluorescence is most commonly used in conjunction with flow cytometric analysis to examine protein expression on either the surface or inside of individual immune cells, when tissue samples are available, immunofluorescence can also be used in combination with histochemical techniques to localize protein expression within a particular tissue. It is now possible to sort specific populations of cells using a Fluorescence Activated Cell Sorter (FACS). The principle is the same as the flow cytometric analysis, however the labeled cells can be collected and placed into culture where functional readouts can be measured.

Quantitative real-time PCR. In the course of immune cell activation, the expression of a variety of genes is altered. Quantitative real-time PCR is a powerful tool to monitor the differential expression of genes on the mRNA level. The technique was first described by Higuchi (Higuchi et al., 1993) and the principle behind it has not changed since. In an ideal PCR reaction the amplified product doubles every cycle. The formation of those products can be detected by either unspecific intercalating dyes, such as SYBR Green I (Schmittgen & Zakrajsek, 2000; Schmittgen et al., 2000), specific probes against the PCR product, such as TaqMan probes (Gibson et al., 1996; Heid et al., 1996), or molecular beacons (Tyagi & Kramer, 1996). By using specific fluorescence-based detection systems, this technique allows the "real-time" monitoring of the accumulation of the PCR product, which is directly correlated to the intensity of the fluorescence signal. Ideally this signal follows an exponential curve (2^{cycle}) due to the *Nature* of the PCR reaction itself. Thereby, the Ct value of a specific sample is defined as that cycle (fractions of cycles are allowed) of the PCR reaction where the fluorescence signal of this specific sample can be detected, that is, is significantly higher than the background fluorescence and follows the exponential curve. Samples containing higher amounts of template will reach this detectable level of fluorescence (also called the threshold level) in an earlier cycle compared to samples with less template. By comparison of the Ct values of different samples, the relative expression of the template can be determined (Livak & Schmittgen, 2001; Meijerink et al., 2001; Pfaffl, 2001). For example, samples containing a high amount of mRNA will have a lower Ct value than one containing a lower amount.

Due to its very high sensitivity, real-time PCR is the method of choice to determine the relative expression of genes that are expressed at a very low level, such as cytokine genes (Overbergh et al., 1999), Ig heavy chain genes (Podojil & Sanders, 2003), or genes from samples containing limited numbers of cells, including flow sorted cells or laser capture microdissection samples (Glockner et al., 2000; Matsuzaki et al., 2004). Because of this high sensitivity it is important to control for differences in Ct values that may be due to sample processing by normalizing the results obtained for a particular gene of interest to the results for a gene that is constantly expressed in a cell – the so-called housekeeping gene, β-actin. The choice of the right housekeeping gene is a critical parameter and must follow certain procedures. Quantitative real-time PCR is the gold standard in evaluating and confirming results obtained from high-throughput technologies to study gene expression, such as microarray expression analysis (Rajeevan et al., 2001).

Microarray expression analysis. A first approach to determine if a given transcriptional alteration occurred in immune cells due to a certain treatment or stimulus is to use microarray expression analysis. The principle behind this technique involves the hybridization of fluorescently tagged cDNA to oligonucleotide- or cDNA-probes on a solid surface. To obtain the labeled cDNA, RNA is isolated from cell samples and is reverse transcribed in the presence of fluorescently labeled nucleotides. After the hybridization process, the fluorescence signal of each spot can be digitally processed and directly correlated with the amount of specific mRNA that is present in the cell sample. Relative expression patterns of up to >40,000 genes can be measured in one sample simultaneously and are calculated by sophisticated algorithms. By comparison of the expression patterns obtained from different samples, genes that are regulated differentially can be identified. The characteristic pattern of expression is then used as "sig*Nature*" of the cell to determine various cellular parameters, such as the state of cell activation or lineage commitment (Alizadeh & Staudt, 2000; Zan et al., 2001). The characteristic pattern of expression also suggests the involvement of certain intracellular signaling pathways, which can be confirmed subsequently by using standard protein identification techniques, such as western blot analysis. The vast amount of data that can be obtained from one single microarray analysis is certainly the advantage of this technique, but this vast amount of data also contributes to certain disadvantages, such as a high number of false positive results and relative low sensitivity when compared to real-time PCR (Hatfield et al., 2003). Thus, it is absolutely necessary to confirm results obtained with microarray analysis by another quantitative method, such as real-time PCR (Rajeevan et al., 2001). Successful application of the microarray technique is dependent on good coordination and planning of the physiological experiment, including selection of proper time points and positive controls, microarray technique, including use of custom arrays vs. commercial arrays, and bioinformatics, including type of data processing and presentation (McShane et al., 2003).

5. SUMMARY

This chapter describes the evidence that neuroendocrine hormones and the sympathetic neurotransmitter norepinephrine are involved in modulation of humoral immunity. It should be evident that a neuroendocrine-immune relationship indeed exists and that it influences the physiology and pathophysiology normally associated with each system individually. Data support the hypothesis that a disturbance in one component of the communication loop influences the functioning of another component and, thus, may contribute to both short- and long-term health consequences. By studying the mechanisms by which the multiple organ systems integrate with each other to function normally, we will gain better insight into how pathological processes develop from perturbation of the organism as a whole. Such insights will aid in the development of new therapeutic approaches and interventions that will contribute to the treatment and prevention of psycho- and immunopathology, as well as contribute to the enhancement of an individual's well being.

ACKNOWLEDGMENTS

The authors wish to thank the research funds provided to our laboratory by the National Institutes of Health AI37326, AI47420, T32 AI0055411, and the Deutsche Forschungsgemeinschaft (Po 801/1–1).

REFERENCES

Adamkiewicz, J., Nehls, P., & Rajewsky, M. F. (1984). Immunological methods for detection of carcinogen-DNA adducts. *IARC Scientif Publ 59*, 199–215.

Ader, R., & Cohen, N. (1975). Behaviorally conditioned immunosuppression. *Psychosom MedPsychosom Med 37*, 333–40.

Ader, R., & Cohen, N. (1993). Psychoneuroimmunology: conditioning and stress. *Annu Rev Psychol 44*, 53–85.

Ader, R., Kelly, K., Moynihan, J. A., Grota, L. J., & Cohen, N. (1993). Conditioned enhancement of antibody production using antigen as the unconditioned stimulus. *Brain Behav Immun 7*, 334–43.

Aebischer, I., Stampfli, M. R., Zurcher, A., Miescher, S., Urwyler, A., Frey, B., Luger, T., White, R. R., & Stadler, B. M. (1994). Neuropeptides are potent modulators of human in vitro immunoglobulin E synthesis. *J Immunol 24*, 1908–13.

Akdis, C. A., Blesken, T., Akdis, M., Alkan, S. S., Heusser, C. H., & Blaser, K. (1997). Glucocorticoids inhibit human antigen-specific and enhance total IgE and IgG4 production due to differential effects on T and B cells in vitro. *Eur J Immunol 27*, 2351–57.

Akiyoshi, M., Shimizu, Y., & Saito, M. (1990). Interleukin-1 increases norepinephrine turnover in the spleen and lung in rats. *Biochem Biophys Res Commun 173*, 1266–70.

Alaniz, R. C., Thomas, S. A., Perez-Melgosa, M., Mueller, K., Farr, A. G., Palmiter, R. D., & Wilson, C. B. (1999). Dopamine beta-hydroxylase deficiency impairs cellular immunity. *Proc Natl Acad Sci USA 96*, 2274–8.

Alizadeh, A. A., & Staudt, L. M. (2000). Genomic-scale gene expression profiling of normal and malignant immune cells. *Curr Opin Immunol 12*, 219–25.

Antoni, M. H. (2003a). Stress management and psychoneuroimmunology in HIV infection. *CNS Spectr 8*, 40–51.

Antoni, M. H. (2003b). Stress management effects on psychological, endocrinological, and immune functioning in men with HIV infection: empirical support for a psychoneuroimmunological model. *Stress 6*, 173–88.

Audhya, T., Jain, R., & Hollander, C. S. (1991). Receptor mediated immunomodulation by corticotropin-releasing factor. *Cell Immunol 134*, 77–84.

Bailey, G. H. (1925). The effect of fatigue upon the susceptibility of rabbits to intratracheal injections of type I pneumococcus. *Am J Hyg 5*, 175–85.

Baker, C., Richards, L. J., Dayan, C. M., & Jessop, D. S. (2003). Corticotropin-releasing hormone immunoreactivity in human T and B cells and macrophages: colocalization with arginine vasopressin. *J Neuroendocrinol 15*, 1070–4.

Bamberger, C. M., Wald, M., Bamberger, A. M., Ergun, S., Beil, F. U., & Schulte, H. M. (1998). Human lymphocytes produce urocortin, but not corticotropin-releasing hormone. *J Clin Endocrinol Metab 83*, 708–11.

Beard, C. W., & Mitchell, B. W. (1987). Effects of environmental temperatures on the serologic responses of broiler chickens to inactivated and viable Newcatle disease vaccines. *Avian Dis 31*, 321–6.

Betz, M., & Fox, B. S. (1991). Prostaglandin E2 inhibits production of Th1 lymphokines but not of Th2 lymphokines. *J Immunol 146*, 108–13.

Biondi, M., & Zannino, L.-G. (1997). Psychological stress, neuroimmunomodulation, and susceptibility to infectious diseases in animals and man: A review. *Psychother Psychosom 66*, 3–26.

Black, P. H. (2002). Stress and the inflammatory response: a review of neurogenic inflammation. *Brain Behav Immun 16*, 622–63.

Borger, P., Hoekstra, Y., Esselink, M. T., Postma, D. S., Zaagsma, J., Vellenga, E., & Kauffman, H. F. (1998). Beta-adrenoceptor-mediated inhibition of IFN-gamma, IL-3, and GM-CSF mRNA accumulation in activated human T lymphocytes is solely mediated by the beta2-adrenoceptor subtype. *Am J Respir Cell Mol Biol 19*, 400–7.

Bosch, J. A., de Geus, E. J., Kelder, A., Veerman, E. C., Hoogstraten, J., & Amerongen, A. V. (2001). Differential effects of active versus passive coping on secretory immunity. *Psychophysiology 38*, 836–46.

Brennan, F. X., & Charnetski, C. J. (2000). Stress and immune system function in a newspaper's newsroom. *Psychol Rep 87*, 218–22.

Brydak, L. B., Machala, M., Mysliwska, J., Mysliwski, A., & Trzonkowski, P. (2003). Immune response to influenza vaccination in an elderly population. *J Clin Immunol 23*, 214–22.

Bulloch, K., & Pomerantz, W. (1984). Autonomic nervous system innervation of thymic related lymphoid tissue in wild-type and nude mice. *J Comp Neurology 228*, 57–68.

Burchiel, S. W., & Melmon, K. L. (1979). Augmentation of the in vitro humoral immune response by pharmacologic agents. I: An explanation for the differential enhancement of humoral immunity via agents that elevate cAMP. *Immunopharmacology 1*, 137–50.

Burns, V. E., Carroll, D., Drayson, M., Whitham, M., & Ring, C. (2003). Life events, perceived stress and antibody response to influenza vaccination in young, healthy adults. *J Psychosom Res 55*, 569–72.

Burns, V. E., Carroll, D., Ring, C., Harrison, L. K., & Drayson, M. (2002a). Stress, coping, and hepatitis B antibody status. *Psychosom Med 64*, 287–93.

Burns, V. E., Ring, C., Drayson, M., & Carroll, D. (2002b). Cortisol and cardiovascular reactions to mental stress and antibody status following hepatitis B vaccination: a preliminary study. *Psychophysiology 39*, 361–8.

Butter, C., Healey, D. G., Agha, N., & Turk, J. L. (1988). An immunoelectron microscopical study of the expression of Class II MHC and a T lymphocyte marker during chronic relapsing experimental allergic encephalomyelitis. *J Neuroimmunol 20*, 45–51.

Callaghan, P. (2004). Exercise: a neglected intervention in mental health care? *J Psychiatr Ment Health Nurs 11*, 476–83.

Calvo, W. (1968). The innervation of the bone marrow in laboratory animals. *J Anat 123*, 315–28.

Cao, L., Martin, A., Polakos, N., & Moynihan, J. A. (2004). Stress causes a further decrease in immunity to herpes simplex virus-1 in immunocompromised hosts. *J Neuroimmunol 156*, 21–30.

Carpenter, G. H., Garrett, J. R., Hartley, R. H., & Proctor, G. B. (1998). The influence of nerves on the secretion of immunoglobulin A into submandibular saliva in rats. *J Physiol 512 (Pt 2)*, 567–73.

Chang, S. S., & Rasmussen, A. F. (1965). Stress induced suppression of interferon production in virus-infected mice. *Nature 205*, 623–4.

Chuluyan, H. E., Saphier, D., Rohn, W. M., & Dunn, A. J. (1992). Noradrenergic innervation of the hypothalamus participates in adrenocortical responses to interleukin-1. *Neuroendocrinology 56*, 106–11.

Cohen, N., Ader, R., Green, N., & Bovbjerg, D. (1979). Conditioned suppression of a thymus-independent antibody response. *Psychosom Med 41*, 487–91.

Cohen, N., Moynihan, J. A., & Ader, R. (1994). Pavlovian conditioning of the immune system. *Int Arch Allergy Immunol 105*, 101–6.

Cohen, S., Doyle, W. J., Turner, R. B., Alper, C. M., & Skoner, D. P. (2003). Emotional style and susceptibility to the common cold. *Psychosom Med 65*, 652–7.

Cohen, S., & Herbert, T. B. (1996). Health psychology: Psychological factors and physical disease from the perspective of human psychoneuroimmunology. *Annu Rev Psychol 47*, 113–42.

Cruess, S., Antoni, M., Cruess, D., Fletcher, M. A., Ironson, G., Kumar, M., Lutgendorf, S., Hayes, A., Klimas, N., & Schneiderman, N. (2000). Reductions in herpes simplex virus type 2 antibody titers after cognitive behavioral stress management and relationships with neuroendocrine function, relaxation skills, and social support in HIV-positive men. *Psychosom Med 62*, 828–37.

Czerkinsky, C. C., Nilsson, L.-A., Nygren, H., Ouchterlony, O., & Tarkowski, A. (1983). A solid-phase enzyme-linked immunospot (ELISPOT) assay for the enumeration of specific antibody-secreting cells. *J Immunol Methods 65*, 109–21.

Deinzer, R., Kleineidam, C., Stiller-Winkler, R., Idel, H., & Bachg, D. (2000). Prolonged reduction of salivary immunoglobulin A (sIgA) after a major academic exam. *Int J Psychophysiol 37*, 219–32.

Del Rey, A., Besedovsky, H. O., Sorkin, E., Da Prada, M., & Arrenbrecht, S. (1981). Immunoregulation mediated by the sympathetic nervous system II. *Cell Immunol 63*, 329–34.

Dhabhar, F. S. (2002). Stress-induced augmentation of immune function – the role of stress hormones, leukocyte trafficking, and cytokines. *Brain Behav Immun 16*, 785–98.

Dudgeon, W. D., Phillips, K. D., Bopp, C. M., & Hand, G. A. (2004). Physiological and psychological effects of exercise interventions in HIV disease. *AIDS Patient Care STDS 18*, 81–98.

Edwards, E. A., & Dean, L. M. (1977). Effects of crowding of mice on humoral antibody formation and protection to lethal antigenic challenge. *Psychosom Med 39*, 19–24.

Elphick, G. F., Greenwood, B. N., Campisi, J., & Fleshner, M. (2003a). Increased serum nIgM in voluntarily physically active rats: a potential role for B-1 cells. *J Appl Physiol 94*, 660–7.

Elphick, G. F., Wieseler-Frank, J., Greenwood, B. N., Campisi, J., & Fleshner, M. (2003b). B-1 cell (CD5+/CD11b+) numbers and nIgM levels are elevated in physically active vs. sedentary rats. *J Appl Physiol 95*, 199–206.

Engvall, E., & Perlman, P. (1971). Enzyme-linked immunosorbent assay (ELISA): Quantitative assay of immunoglobulin G. *Immunochem 8*, 871–9.

Ericsson, A., Kovacs, K. J., & Sawchenko, P. E. (1994). A functional anatomical analysis of central pathways subserving the effects of interleukin-1 on stress-related neuroendocrine neurons. *J Neurosci 14*, 897–913.

Espinosa, E., Calderas, T., Flores-Mucino, O., Perez-Garcia, G., Vazquez-Camacho, A. C., & Bermudez-Rattoni, F. (2004). Enhancement of antibody response by one-trial conditioning: contrasting results using different antigens. *Brain Behav ImmunBrain Behav Immun 18*, 76–80.

Felten, D. L., Felten, S. Y., Bellinger, D. L., Carlson, S. L., Ackerman, K. D., Madden, K. S., Olschowki, J. A., & Livnat, S. (1987). Noradrenergic sympathetic neural interactions with the immune system: Structure and function. *Immunol Rev 100*, 225–60.

Felten, D. L., Felten, S. Y., Carlson, S. L., Olschowka, J. A., & Livnat, S. (1985). Noradrenergic and peptidergic innervation of lymphoid tissue. *J Immunol 135(2)*, 755s–765s.

Feng, N., Pagniano, R., Tovar, C. A., Bonneau, R. H., Glaser, R., & Sheridan, J. F. (1991). The effect of restraint stress on the kinetics, magnitude, and isotype of the humoral immune response to influenza virus infection. *Brain Behav Immun 5*, 370–82.

Fleshner, M. (2000). Exercise and neuroendocrine regulation of antibody production: protective effect of physical activity on stress-induced suppression of the specific antibody response [In Process Citation]. *Int J Sports Med* 2000 May; 21 Suppl 1:S14–9 *21 Suppl 1*, S14–S19.

Fleshner, M., Brennan, F. X., Nguyen, K., Watkins, L. R., & Maier, S. F. (1996). RU-486 blocks differentially suppressive effect of stress on in vivo anti-KLH immunoglobulin response. *Am J Physiol 271*, R1344–R1352.

Fleshner, M., Goehler, L. E., Hermann, J., Relton, J. K., Maier, S. F., & Watkins, L. R. (1995). Interleukin-1 beta induced corticosterone elevation and hypothalamic NE depletion is vagally mediated. *Brain Res Bull 37*, 605–10.

Florijin, Y., & Geiger, A. (1991). Community based physical activity program for HIV-1 infected persons. Proceedings of the Biological Aspects of HIV Infection Conference.

Franchimont, D. (2004). Overview of the actions of glucocorticoids on the immune response: a good model to characterize new pathways of immunosuppression for new treatment strategies. *Ann N Y Acad Sci 1024*, 124–37.

Friedman, E. M., Becker, K. A., Overstreet, D. H., & Lawrence, D. A. (2002). Reduced primary antibody responses in a genetic animal model of depression. *Psychosom Med 64*, 267–73.

Friedman, E. M., & Irwin, M. (2001). Central CRH suppresses specific antibody responses: effects of beta-adrenoceptor antagonism and adrenalectomy. *Brain Behav Immun 15*, 65–77.

Fuchs, B. A., Albright, J. W., & Albright, J. F. (1988). Beta-adrenergic receptor on murine lymphocytes: Density varies with cell maturity and lymphocyte subtype and is decreased after antigen administration. *Cell Immunol 114*, 231–45.

Futterman, A. D., Kemeny, M. E., Shapiro, D., Polonsky, W., & Fahey, J. L. (1992). Immunological variability associated with experimentally-induced positive and negative affective states. *Psychol Med 22*, 231–8.

Gibson, U. E., Heid, C. A., & Williams, P. M. (1996). A novel method for real time quantitative RT-PCR. *Genome Res 6*, 995–1001.

Glaser, R., Kiecolt-Glaser, J. K., Bonneau, R. H., Malarkey, W., Kennedy, S., & Hughes, J. (1992). Stress-induced modulation of the immune response to recombinant hepatitis B vaccine. *Psychosom Med 54*, 22–9.

Glaser, R., Sheridan, J., Malarkey, W. B., MacCallum, R. C., & Kiecolt-Glaser, J. K. (2000). Chronic stress modulates the immune response to a pneumococcal pneumonia vaccine. *Psychosom Med 62*, 804–7.

Glockner, S., Lehmann, U., Wilke, N., Kleeberger, W., Langer, F., & Kreipe, H. (2000). Detection of gene amplification in intraductal and infiltrating breast cancer by laser-assisted microdissection and quantitative real-time PCR. *Pathobiology 68*, 173–9.

Gold, P. W., Chrousos, G., Kellner, C., Post, R., Roy, A., Augerinos, P., Schulte, H., & Oldfield, E. (1984). Psychiatric implications of basic and clinical studies with corticotropin-releasing factor. *Am J Psychiatry 141*, 619–27.

Gold, P. W., Goodwin, F. K., & Chrousos, G. P. (1988). Clinical and biochemical manifestations of depression: relation to the neurobiology of stress. *N Engl J Med 319*, 413–20.

Goodkin, K., Fuchs, I., Feaster, D., Leeka, J., & Dickson-Rishel, D. (1992). Life stressors and coping style are associated with immune measures in HIV-1 infection-a preliminary report. *Int J Psychiatry Med 22*, 155–72.

Green, M. L., Green, R. G., & Santoro, W. (1988a). Daily relaxation modifies serum and salivary immunoglobulins and psychophysiologic symptom severity. *Biofeedback Self Regul 13*, 187–99.

Green, M. L., Green, R. G., & Santoro, W. (1988b). Daily relaxation modifies serum and salivary immunoglobulins and psychophysiologic symptom severity. *Biofeedback Self Regul 13*, 187–99.

Gruzelier, J., Smith, F., Nagy, A., & Henderson, D. (2001). Cellular and humoral immunity, mood and exam stress: the influences of self-hypnosis and personality predictors. *Int J Psychophysiol 42*, 55–71.

Guszkowska, M. (2004). [The effects of exercise on anxiety, depression and mood states]. *Psychiatr Pol 38*, 611–20.

Hall, N. R., McClure, J. E., Hu, S. K., Tare, N. S., Seals, C. M., & Goldstein, A. L. (1982). Effects of 6-hydroxydopamine upon primary and secondary thymus dependent immune responses. *Immunopharmacology 5*, 39–48.

Han, Y. C., & Pruett, S. B. (1995). Mechanisms of ethanol-induced suppression of a primary antibody response in a mouse model for binge drinking. *J Pharmacol Exp Ther 275*, 950–7.

Harbuz, M. (2003). Neuroendocrine-immune interactions. *Trends Endocrinol Metab 14*, 51–2.

Harbuz, M. S., Chover-Gonzalez, A. J., & Jessop, D. S. (2003). Hypothalamo-pituitary-adrenal axis and chronic immune activation. *Ann N Y Acad Sci 992*, 99–106.

Hatfield, G. W., Hung, S. P., & Baldi, P. (2003). Differential analysis of DNA microarray gene expression data. *Mol Microbiol 47*, 871–7.

Heid, C. A., Stevens, J., Livak, K. J., & Williams, P. M. (1996). Real time quantitative PCR. *Genome Res 6*, 986–94.

Higuchi, R., Fockler, C., Dollinger, G., & Watson, R. (1993). Kinetic PCR analysis: real-time monitoring of DNA amplification reactions. *Biotechnology* (NY) *11*, 1026–30.

Hucklebridge, F., Clow, A., & Evans, P. (1998). The relationship between salivary secretory immunoglobulin A and cortisol: neuroendocrine response to awakening and the diurnal cycle. *Int J Psychophysiol 31*, 69–76.

Hucklebridge, F., Lambert, S., Clow, A., Warburton, D. M., Evans, P. D., & Sherwood, N. (2000). Modulation of secretory immunoglobulin A in saliva; response to manipulation of mood. *Biol Psychol 53*, 25–35.

Irwin, M. (1993). Brain corticotropin-releasing hormone- and interleukin-1-beta-induced suppression of specific antibody production. *Endocrinol 133*, 1352–60.

Irwin, M., Costlow, C., Williams, H., Artin, K. H., Chan, C. Y., Stinson, D. L., Levin, M. J., Hayward, A. R., & Oxman, M. N. (1998). Cellular immunity to varicella-zoster virus in patients with major depression. *J Infect Dis 178 Suppl 1*, S104–108.

Ishigami, T. (1919). The influence of psychic acts on the progress of pulmonary tuberculosis. *Am Rev Tuberc 2*, 470–84.

Jabaaij, L., Grosheide, P. M., Heijtink, R. A., Duivenvoorden, H. J., Ballieux, R. E., & Vingerhoets, A. J. J. M. (1993). Influence of perceived psychological stress and distress on antibody response to low dose rDNA hepatitis B vaccine. *J Psychosom Res 37*, 361–9.

Jabara, H. H., Ahern, D. J., Vercelli, D., & Geha, R. S. (1991). Hydrocortisone and IL-4 induce IgE isotype switching in human B cells. *J Immunol 147*, 1557–60.

Jabara, H. H., Brodeur, S. R., & Geha, R. S. (2001). Glucocorticoids upregulate CD40 ligand expression and induce CD40L-dependent immunoglobulin isotype switching. *J Clin Invest 107*, 371–8.

Jabara, H. H., Loh, R., Ramesh, N., Vercelli, D., & Geha, R. S. (1993). Sequential switching from mu to epsilon via gamma 4 in human B cells stimulated with IL-4 and hydrocortisone. *J Immunol 151*, 4528–33.

Jemmott, J. B., Borysenko, M., Chapman, R., Borysenko, J. Z., McClelland, D. C., Meyer, D., & Benson, H. (1983). Academic stress, power motivation, and decrease in secretion rate of salivary secretory immunoglobulin A. *Lancet 1*, 1400–2.

Jessop, D. S. (2002). Neuropeptides: modulators of immune responses in health and disease. *Int Rev Neurobiol 52*, 67–91.

Jonsdottir, I. H., & Hoffmann, P. (2000). The significance of intensity and duration of exercise on natural immunity in rats. *Med Sci Sports ExercMed Sci Sports Exerc 32*, 1908–12.

Kapasi, Z. F., Catlin, P. A., Adams, M. A., Glass, E. G., McDonald, B. W., & Nancarrow, A. C. (2003). Effect of duration of a moderate exercise program on primary and secondary immune responses in mice. *Phys Ther 83*, 638–47.

Karalis, K., Muglia, L. J., Bae, D., Hilderbrand, H., & Majzoub, J. A. (1997). CRH and the immune system. *J Neuroimmunol 72*, 131–6.

Kasahara, K., Tanaka, S., & Hamashima, Y. (1977). Suppressed immune response to T-cell dependent antigen in chemically sympathectomized mice. *Res Commun Chem Pathol Pharmacol 18*, 533–42.

Kasprowicz, D. J., Kohm, A. P., Berton, M. T., Chruscinski, A. J., Sharpe, A. H., & Sanders, V. M. (2000). Stimulation of the B cell receptor, CD86 (B7–2), and the beta-2-adrenergic receptor intrinsically modulates the level of IgG1 produced per B cell. *J Immunol 165*, 680–90.

Kiecolt-Glaser, J. K., Dura, J. R., Speicher, C. E., Trask, O. J., & Glaser, R. (1991). Spousal caregivers of dementia victims: Longitudinal changes in immunity and health. *Psychosom Med 53*, 345–62.

Kiecolt-Glaser, J. K., & Glaser, R. (1992). Psychoneuroimmunology: Can psychological interventions modulate immunity? *J Consult Clin Psychol 60*, 569–75.

Kiecolt-Glaser, J. K., Glaser, R., Gravenstein, S., Malarkey, W. B., & Sheridan, J. (1996). Chronic stress alters the immune response to influenza virus vaccine in older adults. *Proc Natl Acad Sci USA 93*, 3043–7.

Kiecolt-Glaser, J. K., Glaser, R., Shuttleworth, E. C., Dyer, C. S., Ogrocki, P., & Speicher, C. E. (1987). Chronic stress and immunity in family caregivers of Alzheimer's disease victims. *Psychosom Med 49*, 523–35.

Kiecolt-Glaser, J. K., Glaser, R., Strain, E., Stout, J., Tarr, K., Holliday, I., & Speicher, C. E. (1986). Modulation of cellular immunity in medical students. *Behav Med J Behav Med 9*, 5–21.

Kimata, H. (2004). Differential effects of laughter on allergen-specific immunoglobulin and neurotrophin levels in tears. *Percept Mot Skills 98*, 901–8.

Kimata, H., Lindley, I., & Furusho, K. (1995). Effect of hydrocortisone on spontaneous IgE and IgG4 production in atopic patients. *J Immunol 154*, 3557–66.

Kohm, A. P., Mozaffarian, A., & Sanders, V. M. (2002). B cell receptor- and beta-2-adrenergic receptor-induced regulation of B7–2 (CD86) expression in B cells. *J Immunol 168*, 6314–22.

Kohm, A. P., & Sanders, V. M. (1999). Suppression of antigen-specific Th2 cell-dependent IgM and IgG1 production following norepinephrine depletion in vivo. *J Immunol 162*, 5299–5308.

Kohut, M. L., Thompson, J. R., Lee, W., & Cunnick, J. E. (2004). Exercise training-induced adaptations of immune response are mediated by beta-adrenergic receptors in aged but not young mice. *J Appl Physiol 96*, 1312–22.

Kruszewska, B., Felten, S. Y., & Moynihan, J. A. (1995). Alterations in cytokine and antibody production following chemical sympathectomy in two strains of mice. *J Immunol 155*, 4613–20.

Kusnecov, A. V., Grota, L. J., Schmidt, S. G., Bonneau, R. H., Sheridan, J. F., Glaser, R., & Moynihan, J. A. (1992). Decreased herpes simplex viral immunity and enhanced pathogenesis following stressor administration in mice. *J Neuroimmunol 38*, 129–137.

Kusnecov, A. W., Husband, A. J., & King, M. G. (1988). Behaviorally conditioned suppression of mitogen-induced proliferation and immunoglobulin production: effect of time span between conditioning and reexposure to the conditioning stimulus. *Brain Behav Immun 2*, 198–211.

Labott, S. M., Ahleman, S., Wolever, M. E., & Martin, R. B. (1990). The physiological and psychological effects of the expression and inhibition of emotion. *Behav Med 16*, 182–9.

LaPerriere, A., Antoni, M. H., Ironson, G., Perry, A., McCabe, P., Klimas, N., Helder, L., Schneiderman, N., & Fletcher, M. A. (1994a). Effects of aerobic exercise training on lymphocyte subpopulations. *Int J Sports Med 15*, s127–s130.

LaPerriere, A., Fletcher, M. A., Antoni, M. H., Klimas, N. G., Ironson, G., & Schneiderman, N. (1991). Aerobic exercise training in an AIDS risk group. *Int J Sports Med 12*, s53–s57.

LaPerriere, A., Ironson, G., Antoni, M. H., Schneiderman, N., Klimas, N., & Fletcher, M. A. (1994b). Exercise and psychoneuroimmunology. *Med Sci Sports Exerc 26*, 182–190.

Leu, S. J., & Singh, V. K. (1993). Suppression of in vitro antibody production by corticotropin-releasing factor neurohormone. *J Neuroimmunol 45*, 23–29.

Li, C. K. (1985). ELISA-based determination of immunological binding constants. *Molec Immunol 22*, 321–7.

Lingrel, J. B., Townes, T. M., Shapiro, S. G., Wernke, S. M., Liberator, P., & Menon, A. G. (1985). Structural organization of the alpha and beta globin loci of the goat. *Progress in Clinical and Biological Research 191*, 67–79.

Livak, K. J., & Schmittgen, T. D. (2001). Analysis of relative gene expression data using real-time quantitative PCR and the 2(-Delta Delta C(T)) Method. *Methods 25*, 402–8.

Livnat, S., Felten, S. Y., Carlson, S. L., Bellinger, D. L., & Felten, D. L. (1985). Involvement of peripheral and central catecholamine systems in neural-immune interactions. *J Neuroimmunol 10*, 5–30.

Lorton, D., Hewitt, D., Bellinger, D. L., Felten, S. Y., & Felten, D. L. (1990). Noradrenergic reinnervation of the rat spleen following chemical sympathectomy with 6-hydroxydopamine: Pattern and time course of reinnervation. *Brain Behav Immun 4*, 198–222.

Lowe, G., Urquhart, J., & Greenman, J. (2000). Academic stress and secretory immunoglobulin A. *Psychol Rep 87*, 721–2.

Macy, E., Kemeny, M., & Saxon, A. (1988). Enhanced ELISA: How to measure less than 10 picograms of a specific protein (immunogobulin) in less than 8 hours. *FASEB J 2*, 3003–09.

Madden, K. S., Boehm, G. W., Lee, S. C., Grota, L. J., Cohen, N., & Ader, R. (2001). One-trial conditioning of the antibody response to hen egg lysozyme in rats. *J Neuroimmunol 113*, 236–9.

Madden, K. S., Sanders, V. M., & Felten, D. L. (1995). Catecholamine influences and sympathetic neural modulation of immune responsiveness. *Ann Rev Pharmacol Toxicol 35*, 417–48.

Maes, M., Meltzer, H., Jacobs, J., Suy, E., Calabrese, J., Minner, B., & Raus, J. (1993). Autoimmunity in depression: increased antiphospholipid autoantibodies. *Acta Psychiatr Scand 87*, 160–6.

Malarkey, W. B., Pearl, D. K., Demers, L. M., Kiecolt-Glaser, J. K., & Glaser, R. (1995). Influence of academic stress and season on 24-hour mean concentrations of ACTH, cortisol, and beta-endorphin. *Psycho Neuroendocrinology 20*, 499–508.

Marsland, A. L., Bachen, E. A., Cohen, S., Rabin, B., & Manuck, S. B. (2002). Stress, immune reactivity and susceptibility to infectious disease. *Physiol Behav 77*, 711–16.

Mashaly, M. M., Hendricks, G. L., 3rd, Kalama, M. A., Gehad, A. E., Abbas, A. O., & Patterson, P. H. (2004). Effect of heat stress on production parameters and immune responses of commercial laying hens. *Poult Sci 83*, 889–94.

Matsuzaki, S., Canis, M., Vaurs-Barriere, C., Pouly, J. L., Boespflug-Tanguy, O., Penault-Llorca, F., Dechelotte, P., Dastugue, B., Okamura, K., & Mage, G. (2004). DNA microarray analysis of gene expression profiles in deep endometriosis using laser capture microdissection. *Mol Hum Reprod 10*, 719–28.

McGillis, J. P., Park, A., Rubin-Fletter, P., Turck, C., Dallman, M. F., & Payan, D. G. (1989). Stimulation of rat B-lymphocyte proliferation by corticotropin-releasing factor. *J Neurosci Res 23*, 346–52.

McLean, R. G. (1982). Potentiation of Keystone virus infection in cotton rats by glucocorticoid-induced stress. *J Wildl Dis 18*, 141–8.

McNaughton, M. E., Smith, L. W., Patterson, T. L., & Grant, I. (1990). Stress, social support, coping resources, and immune status in elderly women. *J Nerv Ment Dis 178*, 460–1.

McShane, L. M., Shih, J. H., & Michalowska, A. M. (2003). Statistical issues in the design and analysis of gene expression microarray studies of animal models. *J Mammary Gland Biol Neoplasia 8*, 359–74.

Meijerink, J., Mandigers, C., van de Locht, L., Tonnissen, E., Goodsaid, F., & Raemaekers, J. (2001). A novel method to compensate for different amplification efficiencies between patient DNA samples in quantitative real-time PCR. *J Mol Diagn 3*, 55–61.

Miller, G. E., Cohen, S., Pressman, S., Barkin, A., Rabin, B. S., & Treanor, J. J. (2004). Psychological stress and antibody response to influenza vaccination: when is the critical period for stress, and how does it get inside the body? *Psychosom Med 66*, 215–23.

Miyoshi, I., Yoshimoto, S., Kubonishi, I., Fujishita, M., Ohtsuki, Y., Yamashita, M., Yamato, K., Hirose, S., Taguchi, H., Niiya, K., & et al. (1985). Infectious transmission of human T-cell leukemia virus to rabbits. *Int J Cancer 35*, 81–5.

Mohr, D. C., & Genain, C. (2004). Social support as a buffer in the relationship between treatment for depression and T-cell production of interferon gamma in patients with multiple sclerosis. *J Psychosom Res 57*, 155–8.

Mohr, D. C., Goodkin, D. E., Islar, J., Hauser, S. L., & Genain, C. P. (2001). Treatment of depression is associated with suppression of nonspecific and antigen-specific T(H)1 responses in multiple sclerosis. *Arch Neurol 58*, 1081–6.

Mulder, C. L., Antoni, M. H., Duivenvoorden, H. J., Kauffmann, R. H., & Goodkin, K. (1995). Active confrontational coping predicts decreased clinical progression over a one-year period in HIV-infected homosexual men. *J Psychosom Res 39*, 957–65.

Muller, M. B., Uhr, M., Holsboer, F., & Keck, M. E. (2004). Hypothalamic-pituitary-adrenocortical system and mood disorders: highlights from mutant mice. *Neuroendocrinology 79*, 1–12.

Murray, S. E., Lallman, H. R., Heard, A. D., Rittenberg, M. B., & Stenzel-Poore, M. P. (2001). A genetic model of stress displays decreased lymphocytes and impaired antibody responses without altered susceptibility to Streptococcus pneumoniae. *J Immunol 167*, 691–8.

Murray, S. E., Rosenzweig, H. L., Johnson, M., Huising, M. O., Sawicki, K., & Stenzel-Poore, M. P. (2004). Overproduction of corticotropin-releasing hormone blocks germinal center formation: role of corticosterone and impaired follicular dendritic cell networks. *J Neuroimmunol 156*, 31–41.

Nehlsen-Cannarella, S. L., Nieman, D. C., Balk-Lamberton, A. J., Markoff, P. A., Chritton, D. B., Gusewitch, G., & Lee, J. W. (1991a). The effects of moderate exercise training on immune response. *Med Sci Sports Exerc 23*, 64–70.

Nehlsen-Cannarella, S. L., Nieman, D. C., Jessen, J., Chang, L., Gusewitch, G., Blix, G. G., & Ashley, E. (1991b). The effects of acute moderate exercise on lymphocyte function and serum immunoglobulin levels. *Int J Sports Med 12*, 391–8.

Ng, V., Koh, D., Mok, B. Y., Chia, S. E., & Lim, L. P. (2003). Salivary biomarkers associated with academic assessment stress among dental undergraduates. *J Dent Educ 67*, 1091–4.

Nieman, D. C. (1991). The effects of acute and chronic exercise on immunoglobulins. *Sports Med 11*, 183–201.

Ohira, H. (2004). Social support and salivary secretory immunoglobulin A response in women to stress of making a public speech. *Percept Mot Skills 98*, 1241–50.

Overbergh, L., Valckx, D., Waer, M., & Mathieu, C. (1999). Quantification of murine cytokine mRNAs using real time quantitative reverse transcriptase PCR. *Cytokine 11*, 305–312.

Padgett, D. A., & Glaser, R. (2003). How stress influences the immune response. *Trends Immunol 24*, 444–8.

Parker, D. C. (1993). T cell-dependent B cell activation. *Ann Rev Immunol 11*, 331–60.

Paul-Eugene, N., Kolb, J. P., Calenda, A., Gordon, J., Kikutani, H., Kishimoto, T., Mencia-Huerta, J. M., Braquet, P., & Dugas, B. (1992). Functional interaction between beta-2-adrenoceptor agonists and Interleukin-4 in the regulation of CD23 expression and release and IgE production in human. *Molec Immunol 30*, 157–64.

Peters, C. J., & Theofilopoulos, A. N. (1977). Antibody-dependent cellular cytotoxicity against murine leukemia viral antigens: studies with human lymphoblastoid cell lines and human peripheral lymphocytes as effector cells comparing rabbit, goat, and mouse antisera. *J Immunol 119*, 1089–96.

Pfaffl, M. W. (2001). A new mathematical model for relative quantification in real-time RT-PCR. *Nucleic Acids Res 29*, e45.

Podojil, J. R., Kin, N. W., & Sanders, V. M. (2004). CD86 and beta2-adrenergic receptor signaling pathways, respectively, increase Oct-2 and OCA-B Expression and binding to the 3'-IgH enhancer in B cells. *J Biol Chem 279*, 23394–404.

Podojil, J. R., & Sanders, V. M. (2003). Selective regulation of mature IgG1 transcription by CD86 and beta2-adrenergic receptor stimulation. *J Immunol 170*, 5143–51.

Potter, W. Z. (1984). Psychotherapeutic drugs and biogenic amines: current concepts and therapeutic implications. *Drugs 28*, 127–43.

Raison, C. L., & Miller, A. H. (2003). When not enough is too much: the role of insufficient glucocorticoid signaling in the pathophysiology of stress-related disorders. *Am J Psychiatry 160*, 1554–65.

Rajeevan, M. S., Ranamukhaarachchi, D. G., Vernon, S. D., & Unger, E. R. (2001). Use of real-time quantitative PCR to validate the results of cDNA array and differential display PCR technologies. *Methods 25*, 443–51.

Ramer-Quinn, D. S., Baker, R. A., & Sanders, V. M. (1997). Activated Th1 and Th2 cells differentially express the beta-2-adrenergic receptor: A mechanism for selective modulation of Th1 cell cytokine production. *J Immunol 159*, 4857–67.

Ramirez-Amaya, V., & Bermudez-Rattoni, F. (1999). Conditioned enhancement of antibody production is disrupted by insular cortex and amygdala but not hippocampal lesions. *Brain Behav Immun 13*, 46–60.

Reilly, F. D., McCuskey, P. A., & Meineke, H. A. (1976). Studies of the hematopoietic microenvironment. VIII. Adrenergic and cholinergic innervation of the murine spleen. *Anat Rec 185*, 109–118.

Reyes, M. P., & Lerner, A. M. (1976). Interferon and neutralizing antibody in sera of exercised mice with coxsackievirus B-3 myocarditis. *Proc Soc Exp Biol Med 151*, 333–8.

Riccardi, C., Bruscoli, S., & Migliorati, G. (2002). Molecular mechanisms of immunomodulatory activity of glucocorticoids. *Pharmacol Res 45*, 361–68.

Riegele, L. (1929). Uber die mikroscopische Innervation der Milz. *Z Zellforschmikrosk Anat 9*, 511–33.

Rigsby, L., Dishman, R. K., Jackson, A. W., Maclean, G. S., & Raven, P. B. (1992). Effects of exercise training on men seropositive for the human immunodeficiency virus-1. *Med Sci Sports Exerc 24*, 6–12.

Ring, C., Harrison, L. K., Winzer, A., Carroll, D., Drayson, M., & Kendall, M. (2000). Secretory immunoglobulin A and cardiovascular reactions to mental arithmetic, cold pressor, and exercise: effects of alpha-adrenergic blockade. *Psychophysiology 37*, 634–43.

Rogers, M. P., Reich, P., Strom, T. B., & Carpenter, C. B. (1976). Behaviorally conditioned immunosuppression: replication of a recent study. *Psychosom Med 38*, 447–51.

Roper, R. L., Conrad, D. H., Brown, D. M., Warner, G. L., & Phipps, R. P. (1990). Prostaglandin E2 promotes IL-4-induced IgE and IgG1 synthesis. *J Immunol 145*, 2644–51.

Rosenkranz, M. A., Jackson, D. C., Dalton, K. M., Dolski, I., Ryff, C. D., Singer, B. H., Muller, D., Kalin, N. H., & Davidson, R. J. (2003). Affective style and in vivo immune response: neurobehavioral mechanisms. *Proc Natl Acad Sci USA 100*, 11148–52.

Rotton, J., & Dubitsky, S. S. (2002). Immune function and affective states following a natural disaster. *Psychol Rep 90*, 521–4.

Rudorfer, M. V., Ross, R. J., Linnoila, M., Sherer, M. A., & Potter, W. Z. (1985). Exaggerated orthostatic responsivity of plasma norepinephrine in depression. *Arch/GenPsychiatry 42*, 1186–92.

Sachar, E. J. (1982). Endocrine abnormalities in depression. In, E. S. Paykel, ed. New York: Guilford, pp. 191–201.

Sanders, V. M., Baker, R. A., Ramer-Quinn, D. S., Kasprowicz, D. J., Fuchs, B. A., & Street, N. E. (1997). Differential expression of the beta-2-adrenergic receptor by Th1 and Th2 clones: Implications for cytokine production and B cell help. *J Immunol 158*, 4200–10.

Sanders, V. M., Iciek, L., and Kasprowicz, D. (2000). Psychological Factors and Humoral Immunity. In Handbook of Psychphysiology, L. T. J. Cacioppo, and G. Berntson, ed. New York: Cambridge University Press, pp. 425–55.

Sanders, V. M., Kasprowicz, D. J., Kohm, A. P., & Swanson, M. A. (2001). Neurotransmitter receptors on lymphocytes and other lymphoid cells. In Psychoneuroimmunology (3rd ed.), R. Ader, D. Felten, & N. Cohen, eds. San Diego: Academic Press, pp. 161–96.

Sanders, V. M., & Munson, A. E. (1984a). Beta-adrenoceptor mediation of the enhancing effect of norepinephrine on the murine primary antibody response in vitro. *J Pharmacol Exp Ther 230(1)*, 183–92.

Sanders, V. M., & Munson, A. E. (1984b). Kinetics of the enhancing effect produced by norepinephrine and terbutaline on the murine primary antibody response in vitro. *J Pharmacol Exp Ther 231(3)*, 527–31.

Sanders, V. M., & Powell-Oliver, F. E. (1992). Beta-2-adrenoceptor stimulation increases the number of antigen-specific precursor B lymphocytes that differentiate into IgM-secreting cells without affecting burst size. *J Immunol 148*, 1822–8.

Sanders, V. M., & Straub, R. H. (2002). Norepinephrine, the beta-adrenergic receptor, and immunity. *Brain Behav Immun 16*, 290–332.

Sapolsky, R., Rivier, C., Yamamoto, G., Plotsky, P., & Vale, W. (1987). Interleukin-1 stimulates the secretion of hypothalamic corticotropin-releasing factor. *Science 238*, 522–4.

Sarid, O., Anson, O., Yaari, A., & Margalith, M. (2004). Academic stress, immunological reaction, and academic performance among students of nursing and physiotherapy. *Res Nurs Health 27*, 370–7.

Schleifer, S. J., Keller, S. E., Camerino, M., Thornton, J. C., & Stein, M. (1983). Suppression of lymphocyte stimulation following bereavement. *JAMA 250*, 374–7.

Schleifer, S. J., Keller, S. E., Meyerson, A. T., Raskin, M. J., Davis, K. L., & Stein, M. (1984). Lymphocyte function in major depressive disorder. *Arch/GenPsychiatry 41*, 484–6.

Schlenzig, C., Jager, H., & Rieder, H. (1989). Supervised physical exercise leads to psychological and immunological improvement in pre-AIDS patients. Proceedings of the 5th International AIDS Conference, 337–330.

Schmittgen, T. D., & Zakrajsek, B. A. (2000). Effect of experimental treatment on housekeeping gene expression: validation by real-time, quantitative RT-PCR. *J Biochem Biophys Methods 46*, 69–81.

Schmittgen, T. D., Zakrajsek, B. A., Mills, A. G., Gorn, V., Singer, M. J., & Reed, M. W. (2000). Quantitative reverse transcription-polymerase chain reaction to study mRNA decay: comparison of endpoint and real-time methods. *Anal Biochem 285*, 194–204.

Sedgwick, J. D., & Holt, P. G. (1983). A solid-phase immunoenzymatic technique for the enumeration of specific antibody-secreting cells. *J Immunol Methods 57*, 301–9.

Segerstrom, S. C., & Miller, G. E. (2004). Psychological stress and the human immune system: a meta-analytic study of 30 years of inquiry. *Psychol Bull 130*, 601–30.

Seidel, A., Arolt, V., Hunstiger, M., Rink, L., Behnisch, A., & Kirchner, H. (1995). Cytokine production and serum proteins in depression. *Scand J Immunol 41*, 534–8.

Seidel, A., Arolt, V., Hunstiger, M., Rink, L., Behnisch, A., & Kirchner, H. (1996). Increased CD56+ natural killer cells and related cytokines in major depression. *Clin Immunol Immunopathol 78*, 83–5.

Selye, H. (1936). A syndrome produced by diverse noxious agents. *Nature 138*, 132–130.

Selye, H. (1946). The general adaptor syndrome and the diseases of adaptation. *J Clin Endocrinol 6*, 117–230.

Shimizu, N., Hori, T., & Nakane, H. (1994). An interleukin-1-beta-induced noradrenaline release in the spleen is mediated by brain corticotropin-releasing factor: an in vivo microdialysis study in conscious rats. *Brain Behav Immun 7*, 14–23.

Silagi, S., & Schaefer, A. E. (1986). Successful immunotherapy of mouse melanoma and sarcoma with recombinant interleukin-2 and cyclophosphamide. *J Bioll Resp Modif 5*, 411–22.

Silberman, D. M., Ayelli-Edgar, V., Zorrilla-Zubilete, M., Zieher, L. M., & Genaro, A. M. (2004). Impaired T-cell dependent humoral response and its relationship with T lymphocyte sensitivity to stress hormones in a chronic mild stress model of depression. *Brain Behav Immun 18*, 81–90.

Singh, V. K. (1989). Stimulatory effect of corticotropin-releasing factor neurohormone on human lymphocyte proliferation and interleukin-2 receptor expression. *J Neuroimmunol 23*, 257–62.

Singh, V. K., & Leu, S.-J. C. (1990). Enhancing effect of corticotropin-releasing neurohormone on the production of interleukin-1 and interleukin-2. *Neuroscience Letters 120*, 151–4.

Smith, E. M., Morrill, A. C., Meyer III, W. J., & Blalock, J. E. (1986). Corticotropin releasing factor induction of leukocyte-derived immunoreactive ACTH and endorphins. *Nature 321*, 881–882.

Smith, T. P., Kennedy, S. L., & Fleshner, M. (2004). Influence of age and physical activity on the primary in vivo antibody and T cell-mediated responses in men. *J Appl Physiol 97*, 491–8.

Snijdewint, F. G., Kalinski, P., Wierenga, E. A., Bos, J. D., & Kapsenberg, M. L. (1993). Prostaglandin E2 differentially modulates cytokine secretion profiles of human T helper lymphocytes. *J Immunol 150*, 5321–9.

Snyder, B. K., Roghmann, K. J., & Sigal, L. H. (1990). Effect of stress and other biopsychosocial factors on primary antibody response. *J Adolesc Health Care 11*, 472–9.

Solomon, G. F., & Moos, R. H. (1964). Emotions, immunity, and disease: A speculative theoretical integration. *Arch/Gen Psychiatry 11*, 657–74.

Solomon, G. F., & Moos, R. H. (1965). The relationship of personality to the presence of rheumatoid factor in asymptomatic relatives of patients with rheumatoid arthritis. *Psych Med 27*, 350–60.

Stein, M., Miller, A. H., & Trestman, R. L. (1991). Depression, the immune system, and health and illness. *Arch/GenPsychiatry 48*, 171–7.

Stone, A. A., Cox, D. S., Valdimarsdottir, H., Jandorf, L., & Neale, J. M. (1987). Evidence that secretory IgA antibody is associated with daily mood. *J Personality Soc Psychol 52*, 988–93.

Stone, A. A., Neale, J. M., Cox, D. S., Napoli, A., Valdimarsdottir, H., & Kennedy-Moore, E. (1994). Daily events are associated with a secretory immune response to an oral antigen in men. *Hlth Psychol 13*, 440–6.

Strohle, A., & Holsboer, F. (2003). Stress responsive neurohormones in depression and anxiety. *Pharmacopsychiatry 36 Suppl 3*, S207–214.

Swanson, M. A., Lee, W. T., & Sanders, V. M. (2001). IFN-gamma Production by Th1 Cells Generated from Naive CD4(+) T Cells Exposed to Norepinephrine. *J Immunol 166*, 232–40.

Takagi, S., & Ohira, H. (2004). Effects of expression and inhibition of negative emotions on health, mood states, and salivary secretory immunoglobulin A in Japanese mildly depressed undergraduates. *Percept Mot Skills 98*, 1187–98.

Talmadge, J. E. (1985). Immunoregulation and immunostimulation of murine lymphocytes by recombinant human interleukin-2. *J Biol Resp Modif 4*, 18–34.

Teh, H. S., & Paetkau, V. (1976). Regulation of immune responses. II. The cellular basis of cyclic AMP effects on humoral immunity. *Cell Immunol 24*, 220–9.

Theorell, T., Blomkvist, V., Jonsson, H., Schulman, S., Berntorp, E., & Stigendal, L. (1995). Social support and the development of immune function in human immunodeficiency virus infection. *Psychosom Med 57*, 32–6.

Tyagi, S., & Kramer, F. R. (1996). Molecular beacons: probes that fluoresce upon hybridization. *Nat Biotechnol 14*, 303–8.

Van der Pouw-Kraan, T., Van Kooten, C., Rensink, I., & Aarden, L. (1992). Interleukin (IL)-4 production by human T cells: differential regulation of IL-4 vs. IL-2 production. *J ImmunolEur J Immunol 22*, 1237–41.

Vedhara, K., Bennett, P. D., Clark, S., Lightman, S. L., Shaw, S., Perks, P., Hunt, M. A., Philip, J. M., Tallon, D., Murphy, P. J., et al. (2003). Enhancement of antibody responses to influenza vaccination in the elderly following a cognitive-behavioural stress management intervention. *Psychother Psychosom 72*, 245–52.

Vedhara, K., Cox, N. K., Wilcock, G. K., Perks, P., Hunt, M., Anderson, S., Lightman, S. L., & Shanks, N. M. (1999). Chronic stress in elderly carers of dementia patients and antibody response to influenza vaccination. *Lancet 353*, 627–31.

Vedhara, K., McDermott, M. P., Evans, T. G., Treanor, J. J., Plummer, S., Tallon, D., Cruttenden, K. A., & Schifitto, G. (2002). Chronic stress in nonelderly caregivers: psychological, endocrine and immune implications. *J Psychosom Res 53*, 1153–61.

Venihaki, M., Zhao, J., & Karalis, K. P. (2003). Corticotropin-releasing hormone deficiency results in impaired splenocyte response to lipopolysaccharide. *J Neuroimmunol 141*, 3–9.

Vitetta, E. S., Fernandez-Botran, R., Myers, C. D., & Sanders, V. M. (1989). Cellular interactions in the humoral immune response. *Adv Immunol 45*, 1–105.

Wallgren, P., Wilen, I. L., & Fossum, C. (1994). Influence of experimentally induced endogenous production of cortisol on the immune capacity in swine. *Veterinary Immunol Immunopathol 42*, 301–16.

Watson, J., Epstein, R., & Cohn, M. (1973). Cyclic nucleotides as intracellular mediators of the expression of antigen-sensitive cells. *Nature 246*, 405–9.

Wayner, E. A., Flannery, G. R., & Singer, G. (1978). Effects of taste aversion conditioning on the primary antibody response to sheep red blood cells and *Brucella abortus* in the albino rat. *Physiol Behav 21*, 995–1000.

Webster, E. L., Tracey, D. E., Jutila, M. A., Wolfe, S. A. J., & DeSouza, E. B. (1990). Corticotropin-releasing factor receptors in mouse spleen: Identification of receptor-bearing cells as resident macrophages. *Endocrinol 127*, 440–52.

Webster, J. I., & Sternberg, E. M. (2004). Role of the hypothalamic-pituitary-adrenal axis, glucocorticoids and glucocorticoid receptors in toxic sequelae of exposure to bacterial and viral products. *J Endocrinol 181*, 207–21.

Webster, J. I., Tonelli, L., & Sternberg, E. M. (2002). Neuroendocrine regulation of immunity. *Annu Rev Immunol 20*, 125–63.

Weiss, J. M., Sundar, S. K., Becker, K. J., & Cierpial, M. A. (1989). Behavioral and neural influences on cellular immune responses: effects of stress and interleukin-1. *J Clin Psychiatry 50*, 43–53.

Whitham, M., & Blannin, A. K. (2003). The effect of exercise training on the kinetics of the antibody response to influenza vaccination. *J Sports Sci 21*, 991–1000.

Willemsen, G., Ring, C., Carroll, D., Evans, P., Clow, A., & Hucklebridge, F. (1998). Secretory immunoglobulin A and cardiovascular reactions to mental arithmetic and cold pressor. *Psychophysiology 35*, 252–9.

Willemsen, G., Ring, C., McKeever, S., & Carroll, D. (2000). Secretory immunoglobulin A and cardiovascular activity during mental arithmetic: effects of task difficulty and task order. *Biol Psychol 52*, 127–41.

Williams, J. M., & Felten, D. L. (1981). Sympathetic innervation of murine thymus and spleen: A comparative histofluorescence study. *AnatRec 199*, 531–42.

Williams, J. M., Peterson, R. G., Shea, P. A., Schmedtje, J. F., Bauer, D. C., & Felten, D. L. (1981). Sympathetic innervation of murine thymus and spleen: Evidence for a functional link between the nervous and immune systems. *Brain Res Bull 6(1)*, 83–94.

Wu, C. Y., Sarfati, M., Heusser, C., Fournier, S., Rubio-Trujillo, M., Peleman, R., & Delespesse, G. (1991). Glucocorticoids increase the synthesis of immunoglobulin E by interleukin 4-stimulated human lymphocytes. *J Clin Invest 87*, 870–7.

Yamada, A., Jensen, M. M., & Rasmussen, A. F. (1964). Stress and susceptibility to viral infections. III. Antibody response and viral retention during avoidance learning stress. *Proc Soc Exp Biol Med 116*, 677–80.

Yang, E. V., & Glaser, R. (2002). Stress-induced immunomodulation and the implications for health. *Int Immunopharmacol 2*, 315–24.

Yorty, J. L., & Bonneau, R. H. (2003). Transplacental transfer and subsequent neonate utilization of herpes simplex virus-specific immunity are resilient to acute maternal stress. *J Virol 77*, 6613–9.

Yorty, J. L., & Bonneau, R. H. (2004). Impact of maternal stress on the transmammary transfer and protective capacity of her-pes simplex virus-specific immunity. *Am J Physiol Regul Integr Comp Physiol 287*, R1316–R1324.

Zan, H., Komori, A., Li, Z., Cerutti, A., Schaffer, A., Flajnik, M. F., Diaz, M., & Casali, P. (2001). The translesion DNA polymerase zeta plays a major role in Ig and bcl-6 somatic hypermutation. *Immunity 14*, 643–53.

Zeier, H., Brauchli, P., & Joller-Jemelka, H. I. (1996). Effects of work demands on immunoglobulin A and cortisol in air traffic controllers. *Biol Psychol 42*, 413–23.

Zis, A. P., & Goodwin, F. K. (1982). *The amine hypothesis*. In, E. S. Paykel, ed. New York: Guilford, pp. 175–90.

Thematic
Psychophysiology

SECTION EDITOR: JOHN T. CACIOPPO

17 Behavioral Genetics

A. COURTNEY DeVRIES AND RANDY J. NELSON

INTRODUCTION

Behavioral genetics is the study of the relationship between genes and behavior. There are four main issues addressed by this scientific discipline: (1) understanding the extent to which individual behavioral differences are evoked by the effects of genes, (2) identifying genes that affect individual differences in behavior, (3) determining how the interaction between genes and the environment affect the development of behavior, and (4) discovering what genetic changes are involved in the evolution of a behavior (Maxson, 2002). The vast majority of behavioral genetics studies have been conducted in nematodes (*Caenorhabditis elegans*), fruit flies (*Drosophilia melanogaster*), honey bees (*Apis mellifera*), mice (*Mus musculus*), or humans (*Homo sapiens*). This bias reflects complete, or nearly complete, genomic sequences in these species, and in the case of the nonhuman animals, the ease with which genetic mutants can be generated and maintained.

An appreciation of behavioral genetics is important in understanding psychophysiology. At its core, psychophysiology aims to illuminate the interrelationships among physiology, psychology, brain, and behavior (Cacioppo et al., 2006). Genes are inherited, but they are also responsive to the environment from conception and guide the development of structure-function relationships. The genes that produce physiological or behavioral phenotypes that fail to promote survival and reproductive success are omitted from the genome by natural selection, whereas genes underlying successful survival and reproductive output are retained. Differential expression of genes accounts for the plasticity, variability, and adaptability that forms the foundation of the psychophysiological approach (Cacioppo et al., 2006).

The field of behavioral genetics emerged far in advance of its name. The two general approaches in the field (i.e., genealogical and evolutionary) are traditionally considered to have arisen from the writings of two cousins in the nineteenth century: Charles Darwin and Sir Francis Galton. Indeed, the term genetics was coined in 1909,

just two years before Galton's death. Galton's work provoked modern studies of the causes of individual variation among human behaviors, especially cognition, personality, psychopathology, and addictions (Galton & Galton, 1997). He studied extensive family records to discern the inherited tendency of complex traits, often making comparisons between parents and their children and between monozygotic (identical) and dizygotic (fraternal) twins. This approach is especially relevant to psychophysiology and behavioral neuroscience. Darwin's writings stimulated modern research on the genetics of so-called adaptive behaviors in humans and nonhuman animals. The approach of studying the adaptive context of a behavior is more common in behavioral ecology than psychophysiology, but we believe that this approach is important for revealing relationships about genes and behavior that could also have translational value for humans. Indeed, evolutionary psychology has informed several traditional subdisciplines in Psychology including social, personality, developmental, and cognitive psychology (Buss, 1999; Durrant and Ellis, 2003).

It has been more than a half-century since Watson and Crick described the structure of deoxyribose nucleic acid (DNA), and concluded their report with perhaps the most profound understatement in the history of science, *viz.*, "It has not escaped our notice that the specific pairing we have postulated immediately suggests a possible copying mechanism for the genetic material" (Watson & Crick, 1953a). Identification of the helical structure of DNA offered insights into how genes are copied, how genes undergo mutation, and how they function (Watson & Crick, 1953b). Within five years after Watson and Crick described the structure and function of DNA, the importance of genes for understanding behavior was emphasized (Ginsburg, 1958). Ginsburg argued that genetics was a critical tool for understanding behavior because of the following reasons: (1) genetics can be used to dissect behavior into its fundamental units, (2) genes can be used to study the neural, endocrine, and other mechanisms underlying behavior, (3) genetics can be used as a tool to study the effects of the environment on behavior, and (4) understanding genetics is critical to understand the evolution of behavior. Since the initial discovery of DNA, the biological sciences have made enormous progress in understanding the genetic, molecular, and cellular processes underlying normal function, as well as how aberrations in these processes lead to disease. Importantly, the field of molecular genetics appears to be on the threshold of even greater insights into biological mechanisms, linking genotype to phenotype. Because behavior represents an important phenotype, the number of behavioral genetics studies has grown exponentially in recent years. It would seem that the time is ripe for developing a major link between psychophysiology and behavioral genetics.

Methods in behavioral genetics

Screening animals to link a phenotype and genotype can proceed in either of two directions (Figure 17.1): (1) forward genetic screens begin with a phenotype and involve screening the genome to identify the gene or genes responsible for the phenotype, or (2) reverse genetic screens begin with animals possessing a mutated gene and involve extensive behavioral testing to describe the phenotype. Prior to recent advances in mutagenic and transgenic technologies, most behavioral genetics studies began with a phenotype then worked toward identifying candidate genes. Traditionally, in behavioral genetics, there have been two global approaches to reveal genetic contributions to nonhuman behavior: (1) crossing experiments and (2) selection experiments. To be successful, each type of study must be conducted in a constant environment. In both crossing and selection experiments, the most difficult problem is to choose suitable "units of behavior" for genetic analyses.

This problem of the appropriate phenotypic character is not unique for behaviorists. Gregor Mendel's good fortune and genius was to choose characteristics in his pea plants that were clear-cut and could be quantified easily. In Mendel's case, each "unit" (i.e., height of the plant, seed color, seed texture, etc.) essentially corresponded to a single gene. Mendel's laws of inheritance can be applied successfully to predict inheritance of several monogenic disorders (such as Duchenne muscular dystrophy), however, there is little chance that a single gene will directly control a complex human behavioral, cognitive, or personality trait. Intelligence is a classic example; it is a hypothetical construct that defies precise definition, but is commonly assessed through the use of IQ tests. Overall, studies reveal a moderate to strong heritability for IQ in childhood and adulthood, respectively (Bouchard and McGue, 2003). However, despite a clear genetic influence on IQ, there has been no definitive identification of a gene or group of genes that influence performance on IQ tests or other measures of intelligence in humans. Interestingly, the popular press announced the discovery of the "intelligence

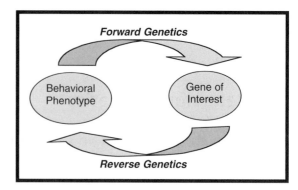

Figure 17.1. A *forward genetic screen* involves beginning with a behavioral trait then screening the genome to identify which gene or group of genes is responsible for the phenotype. Techniques utilized in forward genetics include QTL mapping and selective breeding. A reverse genetic screen involves mutating a gene, then performing behavioral tests to determine the phenotype. Techniques utilized in reverse genetics include targeted mutations, use of antisense, and viral gene transfection.

gene" during the late summer of 1999. The study in question had reported that overexpression of the gene for the NMDA receptor 2B (NR2B) in the forebrains of transgenic mice was associated with enhanced activation of NMDA receptors, which improved performance in various learning and memory tasks (Tang et al., 1999). The authors concluded that their "...results suggest that genetic enhancement of mental and cognitive attributes such as intelligence and memory in mammals is feasible" (Tang et al., 1999). Although not much evidence exists in humans for a role of the NMDA 2B receptor in intelligence, it has been implicated in susceptibility to obsessive compulsive disorder (Arnold et al., 2004) and schizophrenia (Di Maria et al., 2004). Again, it is unlikely that intelligence or any other complex behavior is regulated by a single gene.

Selection studies. Walter Rothenbuhler's work with honeybees (*Apis mellifera*) represents one of the best, early examples of choosing a simple behavior when attempting to study the influences of genes on behavior. Rothenbuhler proposed a two-gene model to explain the phenotypic variance observed in the removal of dead brood from honey bee colonies (Rothenbuhler, 1964a, b). Rothenbuhler's model proposed that a single locus controls the uncapping of brood cells containing dead pupae, whereas a second locus controls the removal of the corpses from the cells. He referred to strains of bees that uncap cells and remove dead larva as "hygienic" bees. In contrast, worker bees of the so-called "unhygienic" strains essentially ignore cells containing dead larvae. The progeny obtained by crossing the two strains are unhygienic, which suggests that the unhygienic trait is dominant. Rothenbuhler (1964b) back-crossed the hybrids from 29 colonies to the recessive, hygienic strain with the following results: (1) approximately 31% uncapped cells containing dead larvae, but did not remove the corpses (these were designated uuRr), (2) approximately 21% did not uncap cells, but would remove dead larvae placed in the colony by an experimenter (Uurr), (3) approximately 27% exhibited the unhygienic phenotype and failed to uncap cells or remove corpses (UuRr), (4) approximately 21% exhibited the hygienic phenotype and both uncapped cells and removed corpses (uurr). Thus, the proportion of the four phenotypic classes did not differ significantly from equality (25% per group) and supported the hypothesis that this behavior was influenced by two pairs of alleles, one of which controlled the expression of the uncapping pattern and the other that controlled the removal of dead larvae. However, these Mendelian results do not imply that a single locus controls the development and activation of the physiological machinery required for uncapping cells or removing dead larvae. Indeed, if unhygienic worker bees are provided with sufficient stimuli, they will begin to engage in hygienic behaviors, albeit at much lower levels than the hygienic strain. Thus, it was concluded that the U and u alleles actually serve as "behavioral switches" that determine the threshold at which the uncapping pattern is initiated (Roethenbuhler, 1964a). Indeed, modern molecular genetic techniques and quantitative trait loci (QTL) linkage mapping (described below) have revealed that the genetic basis of hygienic behavior may be more complex than originally proposed by Roethenbuhler (1964a), and that many genes are likely to contribute to this behavior (Lapidge et al., 2002). Seven suggestive QTLs were associated with hygienic behavior and each controlled only between 9–15% of the observed phenotypic variance in the characteristic.

Crossing studies. There are many other examples of complex behaviors that inherit completely or not at all. For example, duck courtship displays consist of a series of behavioral patterns that are well conserved throughout the duck family. Konrad Lorenz (1966) referred to one such behavioral pattern as the "down-up" display in which a drake dips his bill into the water and then by rapidly lifting his head, generates a plume of water. This courtship pattern is not observed, however, in the pintail (*Dafila acuta*) or in the yellow-billed teal (*Nettion flaviroster*). If individuals from these two species are bred, then the down-up display reappears in its typical form in the F_1 hybrids, which suggests that the absence of the down-up behavior in pintail and teals is mediated by different, recessive, species-specific blocking mechanisms (Lorenz, 1966). Presumably, the recombination of genes in the F_1 hybrids removes the constraints on the down-up behavior such that it is again performed in response to the appropriate social stimuli. However, the best test of this hypothesis would involve back-crossing the hybrids to the parental species, but as is common among such hybrids, they are infertile (Manning, 1967).

Although these so-called breeding experiments have become considered out-dated by many behavioral geneticists, there have been recent calls for their reinstatement (Phillips et al., 2002). Crossing and selection experiments can provide an important approach to understanding complex genetic and environmental interactions associated with both typical and aberrant behavioral processes. The use of controlled breeding experiments in genetic mapping is described in the following section in more detail.

Quantitative trait loci (QTL) linkage mapping. Some traits such as eye color are controlled by a single gene and fall within a few distinct phenotypic classes. In the case of such traits, if the genotype is known, then the phenotype can be predicted, and if phenotype is known, then the genotype can be predicted. For example, if a baby has blue eyes, then we know its genotype; if this individual grows up and fathers a child with a brown-eyed woman whose mother had blue eyes and father had brown eyes, then we can confidently predict the genotype of the offspring based on eye color. Such discrete phenotypes are called discontinuous traits.

Other traits such as intelligence, anxiety, learning abilities, or height, however, do not fall into discrete phenotypic classes. Rather, when a population is analyzed for these traits, a continuous distribution, often bell-shaped, is found. Indeed, most behavioral traits appear to follow a *polygenic* pattern of inheritance which leads to a continuum of phenotypes (Fisher, 1918; Wright, 1921). Continuous traits are often assigned a quantitative value and are referred to as quantitative traits. In keeping with the terminology, the loci controlling these traits are called quantitative trait loci or QTL.

Thus, the QTL contain the allelic variants (polymorphisms) that underlie individual variation in behavior. QTL tend to have only a small effect on phenotype as compared to Mendelian mutations (Flint, 2003). Overall, the proportion of the phenotypic variance that is attributed to QTL tends to be quite small, (i.e., less than 10% in most mouse studies) (Flint, 2003), and because there are a large number of genes with relatively small individual contributions to the phenotype, quantitative traits are a much greater challenge to map than Mendelian traits. Small sequence differences that may slightly alter behavior, for example contributing less than 5% to phenotypic variance, can easily be missed. Mapping of QTL involves identifying chromosomal regions that contain the genes that influence quantitative traits. Typically, quantitative traits are regulated by several genes and also may be responsive to environmental factors.

The first primitive version of QTL was used to map patterns of pigmentation in bean seeds (Sax, 1923). However, a dearth of easily identifiable, segregating genetic markers (DNA used as "landmarks" on the chromosome) limited the applicability of QTL analyses for nearly 60 years. It was not until polymerase chain reaction (PCR) became commonly available in the 1980s that polymorphisms of a single nucleotide became readily detectable and molecular markers were easily detected and plentiful. In mice, detecting QTL often involves crossbreeding two behaviorally distinct inbred strains to produce the F_1 generation, then inter-mating the F_1 generation or backcrossing the F_1 generation to either of the parental strains to produce the F_2 generation (Flint, 2004). Analysis of molecular markers (i.e., polymorphisms) then signals which chromosomal segments segregated with the trait of interest. A goal in mapping these markers is to eventually identify the actual protein coding genes which affect the variation of a trait. The markers that are used for gene mapping to a region of a chromosome are usually DNA variants, including restriction fragment length polymorphisms (RFLPs), simple sequence length polymorphisms (SSLPs), and single nucleotide polymorphisms (SNPs) (Plomin et al., 2000; Plomin and Crabbe, 2000). These markers are used in mapping because: (1) many of them are closely spaced on the linkage map of each chromosome, and (2) they do not affect the measured traits. However, the mapping is fairly imprecise, and even with as many as 1000 animals, if the contribution of the QTL to the behavioral trait is less than 10%, the 95% confidence interval of the QTL will still include approximately 10 centimorgans (see Figure 17.2) and could include hundreds to thousands of genes (Flint, 2004). Mapping resolution can be improved further by repeating the loci mapping in heterogeneous stock, which reduces the QTL confidence interval to a few centimorgans (Mott et al., 2000).

Mapping QTL can be expensive, labor intensive, and tedious, but it provides a useful tool for exploring the genetic bases of complex psychological traits. For example, to identify a genetic basis for emotionality, behavioral and quantitative trait analyses were performed on approximately 900 mice from an F_2 intercross (Flint et al., 1995). The progenitors belonged to inbred mouse strains that were selected for either high or low open field activity (DeFries et al., 1978). The authors of the QTL study chose to use co-variation between exploratory behavior (a locomotor response) and defecation (an autonomic response) as an index of emotionality because there is no known physiological mechanism that can explain the covariation between these two measures. Yet, selection studies in both mice and rats suggest that these behaviors are genetically correlated; rodents bred to exhibit high locomotor responses in novel environments tend to excrete fewer fecal boli whereas rodents bred for high novelty-induced defecation tend to become immobile in novel environments (Flint et al., 1995). Indeed, QTL mapping identified three loci on mouse chromosomes 1, 12, and 15 that influenced four measures of emotionality (open field activity, Y-maze activity, defecation in novel environments, and open arm exploration in the elevated plus maze). Although the mouse study does not have sufficiently high mapping resolution to identify the specific genes regulating emotionality, it does suggest that variation at only three loci

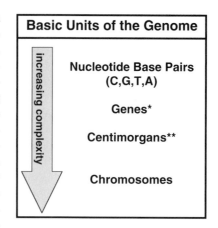

Figure 17.2. The basic units of the genome. The *sequence of nucleotides that is translated into RNA are the genes. The average genetic distance is approximately one million base pairs (i.e., 1 centimorgan**). Within this interval, there is a 1% chance of recombination. Chromosomes are species-specific collections of pieces of DNA. Mice have a chromosomal complement that includes 19 autosomes (non sex chromosomes) and the X and Y sex chromosomes. Humans have 22 autosomes and the X and Y sex chromosomes.

account for a large proportion of the observed individual differences in emotionality among the mice.

A similar study mapped QTL in an F_2 intercross of Roman high avoidance and Roman low avoidance strain of rats selectively bred to exhibit differential fear responses (Fernandez-Teruel et al., 2002). Roman high and low avoidance rats have well characterized behavioral profiles and have been extensively studied in anxiety paradigms. Several QTL with test-specific effects on measures of anxiety were identified, but only one QTL, which was located on rat chromosome 5, influenced behavior in several behavioral tests of anxiety (active avoidance, conditioned fear, elevated plus maze, and open field; Fernandez-Teruel et al., 2002). Whether allelic variation in homologous genes in other species affects emotionality and anxiety remains to be determined, but there is some evidence that rat chromosome 5 (which contains the anxiety QTL) is partially syntenic with human chromosome 1p, which contains a QTL that influences neuroticism (see the following section; Flint 2004). Unfortunately, the mapping resolution in both species was too low to definitively conclude that the same gene affects the trait in humans and rats.

QTLs underlying individual differences in behavior have been mapped in several species including nemotodes (Segalat, 1999), fruit flies (Sokalowski, 1999), honey bees (Ruppell et al., 2004a; b), and humans (reviewed in Plomin and Crabbe, 2000; Ferreira, 2004). Studies involving non-human animals can exploit selective breeding to produce extreme phenotypes for the behavior of interest prior to attempting to map the genetic basis of the behavior. The most challenging aspects of conducting behavioral QTL studies in humans are (1) detecting the QTL, (2) obtaining high resolution mapping, and (3) enrolling a large enough cohort to be able to detect loci that may be contributing only 5–10% of the total phenotypic variance (Flint, 2004). Indeed, few QTL studies attempting to map human personality traits have sufficient sample size or power to detect small genetic effects.

In studies of humans, two primary approaches are used to identify genes relevant to a specific trait or behavior: (1) Linkage analysis and (2) allelic association (also called linkage disequilibrium). In linkage analysis, several DNA sequence polymorphisms that are near (or within) a gene of interest are used to track the inheritance of a disease-causing mutation in that gene. Linkage analysis has been successful at identifying the causal agents for single gene (monogenic) disorders such as Huntington Disease or Duchenne muscular dystrophy, but this method is not particularly informative about genetic effects for polygenic traits of most interest to psychophysiologists or other behavioral neuroscientists.

Allellic association is also called linkage disequilibrium. It is the non-random association of alleles at two or more loci on a chromosome. It describes a situation in which co-occurrence of a specific DNA marker and a disorder is at a higher frequency than would be predicted by random chance. For example, allellic association has been used to find an allele for the phospholipase A2 (PLA2) gene that is associated with depression among unipolar patients with at least 3 depressive episodes (Papadimitriou et al., 2003). This followed the observation of co-segregation in one family pedigree of bipolar affective disorder with Darier's disease. The gene of interest is on chromosome 12q23–q24.1; linkage and association studies revealed that PLA2, which is located nearby, may be involved in affective disorders. Eight alleles were examined, but only one was found to correlate with depression. Molecular studies can now investigate structural changes in this gene that may contribute to depressed affect (Papadimitriou et al., 2003).

Two QTLs for neuroticism have been identified though comparison of sibling genotypes and responses on depression and anxiety questionnaires (Nash et al., 2004). Interestingly, location of the QTLs was different for male sibling pairs (chromosome 6p) and female sibling pairs (chromosome 1p), which suggests that the genetic mechanism underlying neuroticism in humans may be sexually dimorphic (also see Fullerton et al., 2003; Abkevich et al., 2003). Putative QTLs for several disorders and traits related to neuroticism, including susceptibility for anxiety (Fullerton et al., 2003) and major depression (Nurnberger et al., 2001), also have been mapped to chromosome 1. The nature of genetic contribution to complex psychological traits and psychiatric disorders is not well understood (Flint et al., 1995). There has been only limited success in mapping psychiatric disorders in humans, which suggests that many genes contribute to the phenotype, each with a very small effect. Furthermore, because human populations are outbred and there is great individual variation in diet, medication, stress exposure, SES, and other environmental factors, statistical power tends to be low for most studies (Farrall, 2004).

No single genetic approach is likely to provide a comprehensive understanding of complex behaviors, and understanding behavioral traits with multiple genetic and environmental determinants represents one of the greatest challenges for genetic analysis (Phillips et al., 2002). Despite the use of QTL, once a trait is mapped, it is common to change the experimental focus to identifying individual genes (Phillips et al., 2002; Farrall, 2004). As the number of QTL mapping studies increase, and resolution of genetic mapping improves, the number of genes known to influence any given behavior will increase substantially. Yet, it will be difficult to isolate the effects of any single gene amid the contributions of other genetic and environmental influences (Phillips et al., 2002; Plomin & Crabbe, 2000). Furthermore, once the key genes underlying a behavior have been identified, determining the mechanisms through which the genetic variants affect behavior will be a major undertaking. The following sections discuss the process of identifying candidate genes.

Transgenic and knockout models. The development of gene targeting strategies in mice has revolutionized biological sciences (Sung et al., 2004). In order to inactivate, or "knockout," a gene, molecular biologists rearrange the nucleotide sequence that encodes for the gene of interest. This has been accomplished for an astounding number of murine genes during the past fifteen years. Although now fairly routine, the creation of a mouse with targeted disruption (i.e., knockout) of a specific gene is a labor intensive process that combines several low probability events. The majority of mutant mice to date have been generated through pronuclei injection or homologous recombination in embryonic stem (ES) cells (Muller, 1999). Transgenic mice are generated via a procedure that involves injecting DNA consisting of the sequence of interest and an enhancer or promoter into the pronucleus of a one-cell mouse embryo (Bockamp et al., 2002). The DNA integrates into the genome, becomes functional and is passed on to subsequent generations. One potential shortcoming of the technique is that the transgene integrates into the genome at a random site and as a result may affect the function of surrounding genes. In contrast, homologous recombination in ES cells precisely determines the integration site of the mutated gene when producing a "knockout" or "knockin" mouse.

To begin, mouse embryonic stem cells are harvested from a mouse blastocyst (embryo) and cultured. A targeting vector is engineered to contain two homologous regions that flank a positive selection marker, such as the neomycin phosphotransferase gene (Sung et al., 2004). The vector is then introduced into the cultured ES cells either by microinjection or electroporation transfection. Homologous recombination will then incorporate a very small number of the altered genes into the DNA of the ES cells. PCR can be used to detect the cells in which homologous recombination has occurred. The mutated ES cells are inserted into otherwise normal mouse blastocysts, then implanted into surrogate (pseudopregnant) mothers (Sung, 2004). Within developing mice, all of the descendant cells from the cloned stem cells will have the altered gene; the descendant cells of the original blastocyst cells will have wild-type (i.e., unaltered) genes. The resultant mouse, possessing copies of both mutant and wild-type (WT) cells is called a chimera. If the mutated stem cells are incorporated into the germ lines (the cells destined to become the sperm or ova), then some of the gametes will contain the mutant gene (Sung et al., 2004). Chimeric mice are then bred with wild-type mice; some of the offspring produced will be heterozygous for the mutation, that is, possess one copy of the mutant gene. If the heterozygous mice are interbred, then according to Mendelian segregation approximately one fourth of their offspring will be homozygous for the mutation, one fourth will be homozygous WT and half will be heterozygous for the mutant gene. These homozygous mice can be interbred to produce pure-lines of mice with the gene in question knocked-out (Sung et al., 2004). The product for which the gene typically encodes will be missing from all of the progeny. Behavioral performance is typically compared among WT ($^{+/+}$), heterozygous ($^{+/-}$), and homozygous ($^{-/-}$) mice in which the gene product is produced normally, usually produced at reduced levels (i.e., knockdowns), or completely missing, respectively, though this assumption must be confirmed by directly assaying the gene product.

One limitation to the interpretation of behavioral data from knockout mice is that the targeted gene is missing throughout ontogeny (Nelson, 1997). Thus, any functional deficits may be due to the missing gene product at the time of behavioral testing and/or due to the absence of the gene product during key developmental processes throughout ontogeny. Furthermore, mutations of genes that are essential for normal development can induce embryonic lethality or produce profound deficits that limit or preclude behavioral testing. It also is possible that compensatory or redundant mechanisms might be activated when a gene is disrupted. For example, in mice lacking the gene for the neuronal isoform of nitric oxide synthase (nNOS$^{-/-}$), there is a 20% increase in the expression of the endothelial isoform of nitric oxide synthase (Burnett et al., 1996). A compensatory mechanism may spare behavioral function, and cloud interpretation of the normal contribution of the gene to behavior.

The availability of "inducible" or "conditional" knockouts, in which a specific gene can be inactivated at any point during development, or only inactivated in tissue-specific cells, will provide an important tool to circumvent the problem of ontogenetic interactions (Nelson & Young, 1998). Region- or cell-specific promoters are combined with genes that can be activated at any time by specific events induced by the investigators (e.g., exposure to tetracycline, ecdysone, or interferon; reviewed in Lewandoski, 2001). These substances bind to a special promoter transgenically attached to the gene of interest and terminate expression of a gene. In principal, restricted gene inactivation also can be accomplished in any tissue, at any developmental stage with Cre-loxP mediated gene targeting (Gu et al., 1994). This transgenic strategy is based on the Cre-loxP recombination system of bacteriophage P1 and can mediate loxP recombination in both ES cells or mice (Gu et al., 1994). This bacteriophage site-directed recombination method requires two mouse strains be developed and mated; one containing the *cre* transgene in a cell-type or developmental stage-specific manner and a second strain that has the gene of interest flanked by two loxP sites. In the resulting offspring, Cre-loxP site specific recombination will occur, thereby deleting the target gene only in the cells where *cre* is expressed while tissues not expressing *cre* will not be affected (Gu et al., 1994). Ecdysone, an insect hormone, also can be used to inactivate a gene during any point of pregnancy because it easily crosses the placenta-blood barrier and has no noticeable nonspecific effects in rodents (No et al., 1996). The widespread availability of inducible knockout and transgenic mice should prove extremely useful in behavioral studies because they will provide a method of studying genetic influences on behavior in the absence of ontogeny issues that often obscure interpretation of knockout mouse behavior. Furthermore, by testing conditional knockouts prior to and after gene deactivation, the potential confound of differential genetic background effects can be eliminated (Lee et al., 1998). Although thousands of genetic knockouts have been created, only a small proportion of these knockouts have been thoroughly phenotyped. Importantly, many knockouts have been examined in behavioral tests, but display no significant behavioral impairments (e.g., Nelson & Young, 2000). In contrast, some knockouts have exhibited phenotypes that appear to be highly influenced by the background strain, laboratory environment, or an interaction between these two factors (Wahlsten et al., 2003).

Random mutagenesis. Random mutagenesis involves exposing male mice of an inbred strain to a chemical mutagen. In behavioral neuroscience, the most commonly used chemical mutagen is N-ethy-N-nitrosourea (ENU). It typically induces point mutations by modifying A-T base pairs. The mutations can lead to allelic alterations that begin a cascade of physiological changes and ultimately affect behavior. ENU mutagenesis is a major forward genetics screening strategy with the goal of finding genes that can cause variation in a behavioral trait (Maxson, 2002). Dominant mutants are detected in the first generation of progeny, whereas recessive mutants are detected in subsequent generations. Because the ENU-induced mutations occur at random, it is advantageous to be able to house large numbers of animals and to employ "high throughput" behavioral testing. Once an intriguing behavioral phenotype has been identified, the chromosomal location and the DNA sequence of each mutant gene is determined. Unfortunately, sometimes identifying the gene responsible for the altered phenotype is difficult. For example, fitness-1 (fit-1) mice were initially described in 1990, but it was not until 13 years later that the gene mutation responsible for inducing hematopoietic metabolic abnormalities was identified (Klebig et al., 2003; reviewed in Sung et al., 2004). Large-scale mouse behavioral mutagenesis projects are currently ongoing at the Jackson Laboratory, Northwestern University, Oak Ridge Laboratories, the University of Tennessee, and elsewhere.

The mutagenesis approach also has been applied successfully to *C. elegans* (reviewed in Jorgensen & Mango, 2002) and *Drosophila melanogaster* (St. Johnston, 2002) using ethyl methane sulphonate, X-ray irradiation and insertion of P-transposable elements. The invertebrate models have several advantages over the vertebrate models including: (1) it is inexpensive to maintain large colonies, (2) the generation time is short (10 days for flies and 3 days for roundworms [*C. elegans*]), (3) they generate large numbers of offspring, and (4) they have many fewer chromosomes (4 for flies and 6 for roundworms) and genes (approximately 15,000 for flies and 20,000 for roundworms). Importantly, the completion of the human and fly genome projects has revealed that 178 out of 287 known human disease genes have known homologues in flies (Rubin et al., 2000; Fortini et al., 2000). The disadvantages of using flies and roundworms in behavioral genetics studies are (1) a fairly limited behavioral repertoire and (2) a relatively uncomplicated CNS, although most of the major vertebrate neurotransmitters systems have been confirmed in roundworms and flies (Wolf & Heberlein, 2003). Indeed, flies are an intriguing model for studying drug effects and addiction. For example, to screen for gene mutations that influence ethanol-induced behavior, large numbers of flies are rotated through an apparatus that releases ethanol vapor then quantifies the behavioral changes that follow (Park et al., 2000). Following exposure to ethanol vapor, flies exhibit behavioral changes that are similar to those observed among intoxicated humans, including increased locomotor activity at low concentrations versus decreased locomotor activity and loss of postural control at high concentrations. However, if a mutation is induced in the pka-RII (a protein kinase A regulatory subunit) gene, the flies exhibit improved coordination in a climbing task following ethanol exposure (Park et al., 2000). Similarly, PKA-RIIβ mutant mice voluntarily consume more ethanol, and are less sensitive to the sedative effects, than WT mice (Thiele et al., 2000). Thus, flies have been invaluable for elucidating signal transduction pathways, and it appears that they also may be a valuable tool in studying genetic influences on behavior.

Genetic screens in lower invertebrates have been used repeatedly to identify modifiers of preexisting genetic defects (i.e., modifier screens). Generally, animals with a genetic defect that produces a distinctive phenotype are exposed to random mutagenesis techniques and screened for mutations that reverse the phenotype. Recently, the first such screen was successfully used in mice to identify mutations capable of ameliorating congenital thrombocytopenia (reduced platelet count; Carpinelli et al., 2004).

Modifier screens provide a more sensitive background in which to detect changes in phenotype (Curtis, 2004). Usefulness of this technique in behavioral genetics of a complex behavior is limited by the absence of high throughput behavioral protocols for complex behaviors; an exception is circadian locomotor behavior which involves automated measurement of locomotor activity.

Viral vectors to transfer genes. Viruses have evolved to transfer genes into infected cells. This ability has been exploited to deliver experimental or therapeutic gene treatment to individuals. Among the various types of viruses used to transfer genes (retroviruses, adenovirus, adeno-associated virus, herpesvirus, and poxvirus) the use of retroviruses has become most prevalent because they provide high gene transfer efficiency and relatively high therapeutic gene expression in the recipient cells (Walther & Stein, 2000). The methodology of viral gene transfer is beyond the scope of this chapter but has been thoroughly reviewed in the literature (Walther & Stein, 2000; Lowenstein & Castro, 2001). Recent advances in the use of viral vectors to transfer genes include improvement of infectivity and the duration of novel gene expression, which is critical to improve the safety and efficacy of RNA- and DNA-viral vectors (see Walther & Stein, 2000 for a review). However, viral vectors have inherent risks such as toxicity, activation of the recipients' immune system, and viral recombination and further improvements are necessary before this method of gene therapy is clinically dependable. (Walther & Stein, 2000). However, the use of viral vectors to transfer genes to understand the genetic contribution to behavior is becoming an important tool (Lowenstein & Castro, 2001).

The behavioral effects of gene manipulations have been studied using primarily inbred rodent strains. However, one the goals of behavioral genetics should be to understand how naturally occurring genetic changes may have shaped evolution of a complex social behavior. An interesting example of such a phenomenon has been investigated in monogamous rodents using viral vectors. Most mammals are polygynous, which means that the males and females associate only during mating, and as a result females provide a large proportion, if not all, of the resources necessary to raise the progeny. Fewer than 3% of mammalian species are reported to exhibit a monogamous social system in which long-term pair bonds are formed between males and females and the fathers contribute to the raising of the young (Carter et al., 1995). How and why some mammals evolved to exhibit monogamy are intriguing questions. The explanation at an ultimate level of analysis involves whether maximal male reproductive fitness can be achieved by abandoning the female after fertilization and searching out additional mates versus remaining to assist in raising the progeny (Krebs & Davies, 1993). The proximate explanation may involve differential expression of a single gene, the vasopressin V1a receptor (V1aR). Much of the work related to understanding the proximate regulation of monogamy has been conducted in vole species because there are several closely related species that vary in social structure from monogamous to polygynous. For example, prairie voles and pine voles are monogamous; males and females form social bonds and provide biparental care. In contrast, montane voles and meadow voles are polygynous; males and females do not form social bonds and only females provide parental care. Although the V1aR gene sequence is highly conserved among vole species, there is an alteration in the repetitive microsatellite DNA in the 5′ regulatory region of the gene that is associated with social system (Young et al., 1999). Thus, the pattern of V1aR expression in vole brains is substantially different between monogamous and polygynous species (Lim et al., 2004; Young et al., 1999). A similar pattern of increased V1aR also has been reported in monogamous versus polygynous *Peromyscus* species (Bester-Meredith et al., 1999). Furthermore, transgenic mice that carry the prairie vole V1aR coding sequence and flanking regions, exhibit patterns of V1aR expression that are more similar to prairie voles than WT mice (Young et al., 1999). The transgenic mice with the altered V1aR expression also are more social than WT mice. Furthermore, increasing V1aR expression in ventral pallidum of polygynous meadow voles through viral vector-mediated gene transfer results in a shift in behavior that more closely resembles monogamy than polygyny (Lim et al., 2004). The genetically manipulated meadow voles exhibited a clear social preference for their partner versus a stranger, and spend four times as much time in physical contact with the stimulus animals as the unmanipulated meadow voles (Lim et al., 2004).

Taken together, these data suggest that differential gene regulation, rather than a mutation in the coding region, accounts for species differences in propensity to exhibit social behavior among prairie voles. These data suggest that a single gene polymorphism alters receptor expression and vastly influences behavior. Presumably, not all regions that express V1aR are involved in pair bonding, but the pattern in the ventral pallidum (high in monogamous voles low in polygynous voles) provided strong inference (Insel et al., 1994). Indeed, injecting V1aR antagonist directly into the ventral pallidum prevents the formation of partner preferences (Lim et al., 2004). Thus, converging evidence from several molecular, genetic, and pharmacological techniques provides evidence that altering expression of a single gene (that of course may have pleiotropic or epistatic effects) can influence the formation of partner preference, the establishment of pair bonds and potentially the expression of a monogamous versus polygynous social system.

Antisense and gene function. Gene expression in adult animals can be modified through the use of "antisense technology." The DNA in the nucleus of each cell contains specific coding instructions for peptides. This "message" is carried by messenger ribonucleic acid (mRNA) from the nucleus to the cytosol where protein production occurs. The mRNA sequence that codes for the protein is referred to as the "sense" strand because it provides the message with the instructions for making the protein. Once the mRNA sequence for a certain protein is known, a piece of DNA can be generated that consists of 10–30 complementary bases to the sense mRNA. This piece of DNA (oligodeoxynucleotide) is referred to as "antisense" because it consists of a sequence of bases that is the mirror image of the "sense" message (Galderisi et al., 1999). After entering a cell, the antisense binds to the mRNA and prevents the production of the protein that is normally coded by the mRNA.

One early use of antisense in behavioral neuroscience research examined sexual behavior in female rats (Mani et al., 1994). Typically, high estrogen concentrations provoke the expression of progesterone receptors in the ventromedial nuclei of the hypothalamus and elsewhere. Activation of these hypothalamic progesterone receptors promotes reproductive behavior in female rats. However, when sexually receptive females were treated with progesterone receptor (PR) antisense they did not display appropriate sexual behaviors. Follow-up assays confirmed low gene expression of PR in the hypothalamus. In contrast, females treated with the sense oligonucleotides, which do not bind the mRNA nor disrupt translation, displayed normal sexual behaviors (Mani et al., 1994).

Use of antisense is warranted when pharmaceutical techniques are not available, are nonspecific, or have undesirable side effects. For example both experimental and clinical data have implicated brain α2-adrenoceptors in the regulation of many psychophysiological measures, including sexual behaviors, anxiety, and stress-coping behaviors (Tanaka et al., 2000), but the results of pharmacological interventions are often inconsistent (Shishkina et al., 2001). Lack of specific ligands for selectively blocking activation of any of the three unique α2-adrenoceptor subtypes (α2A, α2B, and α2C) may be partially responsible for the conflicting reports. Thus, antisense technology is superior to current pharmacological methods in elucidating the role of α2-adrenoceptors in behavior because the antisense strands can discriminate among the mRNA encoding for the three isoforms. Indeed, administration of antisense oligodeoxynucleotides to inhibit α2A-adrenoceptor expression in the locus coeruleus decreases anxiety-like behaviors in the elevated plus maze (Shishkina et al., 2001).

Gene expression assays. Another relatively new technology that has become extremely useful in both behavioral genetics and behavioral neuroscience is the DNA gene array (although RNA arrays are also used). The gene array technology represents a fusion between genomics and computer microprocessor manufacturing to provide high throughput monitoring of gene expression. The underlying principal of gene arrays is hybridization of complementary strands of nucleic acid (i.e., A-T and G-C for DNA; A-U and G-C for RNA; Nisenbaum, 2002). Essentially, the gene of interest is represented by a miniscule spot containing probes (usually cDNA or oligonucleotide) that are affixed to a glass slide (or occasionally nylon matrix) in a precise location (Phimister, 1999). Purified RNA is obtained from the samples, then reverse transcribed, labeled with a fluorescent dyes and placed on the gene-chip to allow hybridization. Once the microarray has been processed, the relative levels of gene expression for several thousand genes can be deduced based on the fluorescent signal associated with each probe spot. This is obviously a dramatic increase in throughput as compared to the older molecular biology methods where only one or two genes could be assessed. However, due to the staggering volumes of data that can be derived from a single gene chip, it is necessary to use software to help with data mining and extracting the biologically important, as compared to unimportant, gene expression levels. Also, because the gene array only provides relative information about gene expression, an additional method, such as quantitative real-time PCR must be conducted on individual samples. In behavioral neuroscience, gene arrays might be used to determine relative gene expression during the onset of a behavior, or a change in developmental state, or among individuals that vary in the frequency of a given behavior or behavioral state. Honey bees (*Apis mellifera*) provide an exquisite example of how pheromones can mediate social influences on gene expression and age-related shifts in behavior. Honey bees have a complex social system in which pheromones are an important means of communication. For the first two weeks of their life, honey bees typically perform tasks within the hive, such as brood care (Grozinger et al., 2003). As they age, their physiology and behavior changes, they become better adapted to foraging for nectar and pollen outside of the hive, such that the last several weeks of their lives are spent foraging (Grozinger et al., 2003). In fact, microarray analysis revealed that the profiles of gene expression in the brains of bees are substantially different in bees that are foraging versus providing brood care (Grozinger et al., 2003; Whitfield et al., 2003) and it appears that a pheromone secreted by the queen (queen mandibular pheromone or QMP) regulates the genetic and behavioral changes that accompany the shift from brood care to foraging. Indeed, repeated exposure to a swipe of queen mandibular pheromone consistently activates several genes that are correlated with brood care and suppresses genes that correlate with foraging behavior. Thus, the queen may regulate the shift from hive work to foraging, essentially controlling the division of labor within the colony, through secretion of QMP (Grozinger et al., 2003). These data suggest great genomic plasticity in adult honey bee brains.

The heritability of behavior

The major goal of behavioral genetics is to understand what accounts for individual variation in traits. The methods of quantitative genetics (e.g., Falconer & Mackay, 1996; Flint, 2003; Phillips et al., 2002) are used to assess the relative roles of genes and environment in individual differences in behavior. As noted, selection and crossing are used in nonhuman animals. In humans and nonhuman animals, the similarities among relatives and non-relatives can be compared. Essentially, these methods allow the individual phenotypic variance to be partitioned into two components: (1) genetic (V_g) and (2) environmental (V_e). This variance is usually expressed as the ratio of genotypic to total variance (i.e., $h^2 = V_g/V_T$, where h^2 = heritability, V_g = variability attributable to genetic variation, and V_T = total phenotypic variability observed in the population); this ratio is known as the heritability of the trait (Griffiths et al., 1999). If either V_g or V_e are known, the other can be obtained by subtraction; i.e., $V_g = V_T - V_e$ and $V_e = V_T - V_g$. This ratio can vary from zero to one. Importantly, there are no traits that have heritability values of zero or of one. Therefore, *all* behaviors have both genetic and environmental contributions. A heritability quotient of .6 means that 60% of the observed population variability is due to genetic variability and this would be a high genetic influence. A heritability quotient of .3 is considered a moderate genetic influence, whereas a heritability quotient of .1 is considered a small genetic influence.

Although central to many facets of behavioral genetics, there are problems with the concept of the heritability quotient. First, total variation is comprised of variability attributable to genetic variation plus variability attributable to environmental variation plus any variation attributable to the interaction between genetic and environmental factors (i.e., $V_g + V_e + V_{e \times g}, = V_T$) (Griffiths et al., 1999). Usually, $V_{e \times g}$ is assumed to be negligible and is typically not considered; thus, as noted above, the formula for determining total variance is usually reduced to $V_g + V_e = V_T$. It is not always apparent that this assumption is warranted because in many cases the effects of genes and environment are not additive, but rather truly interactive (multiplicative and probably non-linear) (Rice & Borecki, 2001). $V_{e \times g}$ suggests that some individuals are genetically more sensitive to environmental influences than others (Silventoinen, 2003).

The explanatory power of heritability ratios is limited, however, to the specific population studied and only in the environment in which the study was conducted (Rice & Borecki, 2001). If the population or the environment changes, then the heritability estimate also will change (Nicholson, 1990). For example, human body height is influenced by genetics, environment, and an interaction between genetics and environment. Although reports regarding the heritability of body height vary greatly, it appears that body height has a heritability of approximately .8 (Silventoinen, 2003). Although this is a very high heritability, this value does not have any predictive value about other populations and does not suggest low environmental influences. For example, some of the variability in reported heritability ratios of height may reflect socioeconomic differences between study populations. For example, heritability of height is reduced when environmental conditions are poor (Silventoinen et al., 2000). Furthermore, parent-offspring correlations for body height can vary by nation (Mueller, 1976). Indeed, average height has consistently increased over the last several generations among inhabitants of industrialized nations, an effect that is more likely to be explained by increased standards of living than genetics alone (Silventoinen, 2003). Thus, heritability statements provide no basis for predictions about the expression of the trait in question for any specific individual and it is not a measure of genetic control over a phenotype.

Finally, even if the assumptions of additivity between genetic and environmental variances are accepted, heritability only measures the *relative* variability of genetic and environmental contributions, and not the degree to which a trait is inherited, as often claimed. For example, suppose the environment is held constant during a study to determine the contribution of genetic factors to impulsivity, then $V_e = 0$, $V_g = V_T$, and heritability = 1. In contrast, if genetically identical mice are used to examine impulsivity, then $V_g = 0$ and heritability is essentially zero. The extent to which the trait is genetically encoded or inherited is not likely different in the two studies. Therefore, heritability is not an estimate of the degree to which a trait is transmitted genetically. Despite this caution, many people have erroneously used heritability estimates to argue the extent to which a trait is innate (e.g., Jensen, 1973; Herrnstein & Murray, 1994). However, when heritability is high, phenotypic selection is more likely to be successful than when heritability is low. For example, treadmill running endurance in rats was assessed and within each of three generations, the two highest performing pairs and two lowest performing pairs were bred (Koch et al., 1998). The average distance traveled in the founder group was approximately 400 m; after three generations of selective breeding the average distance traveled among low endurance rats had not changed substantially, however, the average distance traveled by the high endurance rats had increased to approximately 650 m. The heritability was determined to be approximately 0.40, that is, 40% of variability in running endurance between high and low endurance rats was due to heritable factors (Koch et al., 1998).

It is now well accepted and documented that in all cases examined including in humans, individual differences in behavioral traits is a function of both genetic and environmental variability. In other words, heritability is neither 0 nor 1 in any studied outbred population. The interesting issues that extend beyond the so-called nature-nurture controversy and will become more central to behavioral genetics include: (1) identifying the genes that affect variance in a trait, (2) understanding how genes interact with each other and with the environment to affect phenotype, and (3) discovering the genetic mechanisms underlying population and species diversity in behavioral phenotypes. Molecular biology and genetics are critical approaches to

addressing these issues. The first step is well underway, *viz.*, identifying all of the genes through the various genome projects. Once these genes are identified, the function of those genes must be ascertained. Studies that identify genes that contribute to behavior and studies that determine the environmental contribution to gene expression are well underway. As genetic tools become more available and inexpensive, these tools will become a large part of psychophysiology research (Plomin & Crabbe, 2000). Completion of the primary genome projects will aid in that goal.

The genome projects

The genome of any individual consists of the DNA strands that comprise the chromosomes in the nucleus of its diploid cells. Each chromosome is comprised of one molecule of DNA. Human have 23 pairs of chromosomes: 22 autosomes and 2 sex chromosomes, termed X and Y. The immediate goal of the genome projects is to determine the sequence of the nucleotide bases (i.e., adenine [A], cytosine [C], guanine [G], or thymine [T]) of the nuclear genome of a single representative (or in some cases, several representatives) of a species. This goal in final and draft forms has been realized for *E. coli*, which has a genome size of 47 Mb (megabases), *C. elegans* which has a with a genome size of 100 Mb, *D. melanogaster* with a genome size of 165 Mb, and *Homo sapiens* with a genome size of ~2900 Mb, (Lander et al., 2001; Morton, 1991); identification of the genome is nearing completion for *Mus musculus*, an important model in mammalian genetics and a useful model in behavioral and biomedical sciences, which has a genome size of approximately 2500 Mb (International Human Genome Sequencing Consortium, 2001; Mouse Genome Sequencing Consortium, 2002).

It is important to note that most of the genome does not reflect coding genes. Indeed, it has been estimated that only 3–5% of the human genome encodes for genes (Lander et al., 2001). For mice and humans (and other mammals for which a draft of the genome is available), it is estimated that there is about one gene per 100,000 bases (International Human Genome Sequencing Consortium, 2001; Mouse Genome Sequencing Consortium, 2002; Rat Genome Sequencing Project Consortium, 2004). The function of non-coding DNA remains to be specified (Gardiner, 1995). The parts of DNA that specify the amino acid sequence of the protein that the gene encodes are called exons; the DNA areas that are interspersed between exons, which are trimmed from the RNA transcript prior to translation into protein, are called introns. Genes are also associated with regulatory regions that interact with other genes and binding proteins to regulate transcription of the gene.

Genomes contain a large quantity of repetitive sequences, which far exceeds the number of sequences necessary for protein-coding genes. For example, >50% of the human genome reveals repeat sequences (Lander et al., 2001).

The sequence variation defining a polymorphism involves either alteration of a single DNA base pair (i.e., single nucleotide polymorphism, or SNP) or tandem lengths of DNA that occur repetitively, with various numbers of repeat elements present in different individuals.

Several different types of repeats have been described including transposon-derived repeats (~45% in human), simple sequence repeats (SSR), and segmental duplications. Of these, SSRs, which are also termed satellite DNA, have been most useful in behavioral genetics. Generally, satellite DNAs show enormous variability among individuals, especially in the number of tandem repeats at a given locus. Units of repetition may be very short (e.g., di- and trinucleotide repeats [also termed microsatellites]) or contain longer DNA sequences known as Variable Number of Tandem Repeats (VNTRs). This variability has been important as a marker for individual variation in several behavioral traits (see the following section).

The number of protein coding genes can be estimated in the genome once the entire sequence is known for a given species. The number of genes in humans has been estimated to be between 35,000–45,000 genes. Also, the amino acid sequence in each protein can be deduced from the coding nucleotide triplets in the gene's structural region as the genome is finely identified.

The mitochondria in each cell also contain DNA; this DNA codes for some of the proteins involved in cellular energy metabolism. This DNA has been sequenced for many organisms including humans. Neurological effects of variants of these mitochondrial genes have been reported, which are important in typical and impaired behavior (Wallace, 1999, 2001).

Gene-environment interactions and behavior

Although genes and environment are often considered separate factors influencing physiology and behavior, genetic factors also can influence the impact of some environmental factors on the development of a particular trait. For example, a person may have a genetic variant that is known to increase his or her risk for developing emphysema from tobacco smoking, an environmental factor. If that person never smokes, then emphysema will not likely develop. Two more subtle examples of an interaction between genes and environment are provided in the following section.

Maternal care in rats. As with human mothers, maternal care varies greatly among rat mothers. Stable individual differences in time spent licking, grooming, and archback nursing (LG-ABN) emerge during the first week postpartum (Champagne et al., 2003). Such naturally occurring variations in the expression of maternal behavior are associated with differences in estrogen-inducible oxytocin receptors in the MPOA (Champagne et al., 2001). Offspring of mothers that exhibit high levels of LG-ABN display life-long attenuation of stress responses, decreased fearfulness, and enhanced cognitive ability (Liu et al.,

1997, 2000; Caldji et al., 1998; Francis et al., 1999). These individual differences in maternal care are transmitted across generations; LG-ABN mothers produce daughters that become high LG-ABN mothers, whereas low LG-ABN mothers produce daughters that become low LG-ABN mothers (Francis et al., 1999). Cross-fostering studies confirm that these behavioral and physiological traits are transmitted across generations via a non-genomic mechanism. In rats, a functional link has been established between central oxytocin receptor levels and behavioral differences in maternal care (Champagne et al., 2001; Francis et al., 1999; Insel & Shapiro, 1992), and oxytocin receptor binding in the MPOA of the hypothalamus is greater in high LG-ABN females as compared with low LG-ABN mothers (Champagne et al., 2001; Francis et al., 1999). Estrogen regulation of oxytocin receptors in the MPOA is dependent on the alpha but not beta estrogen receptor subtype (Young et al., 1998; Champagne et al., 2003).

In addition to altering oxytocin receptor binding, exposure to high LG-ABN produces an increase in glucocorticoid receptor gene expression in the hippocampus, which presumably contributes to efficient regulation of the hypothalamic-pituitary-adrenal (HPA) axis throughout life (McCormick et al., 2000). These effects on GR gene transcription in high LG-ABN offspring are achieved through decreased DNA methylation, and increased histone acetylation and nerve growth factor-induced gene A (NGFI-A, a transcription factor) binding to the GR promoter (Weaver et al., 2004). DNA methylation affects the promoter region of a gene and provides long-term gene silencing (Egger et al., 2004). Thus, the demethylation that occurs soon after birth as a result of exposure to high LG-ABN, presumably results in a significant increase in GR gene expression (Weaver et al., 2004). Furthermore, acetylation of the histones promotes transcription factor binding to the promoter sites. These differences in DNA methylation and histone acetylation exist between high and low LG-ABN offspring by postnatal day 6 and persisted into adulthood. The effects were reversed by cross-fostering high LG-ABN offspring to low LG-ABN mothers on the first day of life (Weaver et al., 2004). Thus, these maternally induced epigenetic influences (i.e., factors that influence phenotype without altering the genotype) persist into adulthood and can be passed on to subsequent generations. The extent to which such organizational effects of glucocorticoids, induced by relative subtle alteration in neonatal environment, apply to humans remains unspecified.

Monoamine oxidase A and human violence. Over a decade ago, a genetic study of a large Dutch kindred with a family history of impulsive violence (including attempted sexual assault, arson, and battery) was undertaken. Urine samples from the aggression study participants revealed disturbed monoamine metabolism; further genetic analysis identified a point mutation in the monoamine oxidase A (MAOA) gene (Brunner et al., 1993). The mutation produces an early stop codon, which renders the affected males of this family completely devoid of MAOA activity (Brunner et al., 1993). The gene for MAOA is located on the X chromosome, so men have only one copy of the gene and if mutated exhibit impulsive behavior. In contrast, female obligate carriers of the mutated gene exhibit normal intelligence and behavior, presumably because the women have two X chromosomes, and therefore two copies of the MAOA gene. Subsequent work confirmed that male transgenic mice in which the gene for MAOA was deleted, also displayed elevated aggressive behavior (Cases et al., 1995; Shih, 2004; Holschneider et al., 2001). The correspondence between the rodent and human data suggests that the influence of MAOA on aggressive behavior is well conserved across species. However, the mutation described in the Dutch family is relatively rare, produces an extreme change in MAOA activity, and is not likely to account for a large proportion of variation in human aggression and violence. There is wide variability in MAOA activity in the normal population. For example, a repeat length polymorphism (VNTR) located upstream of exon 1 in the MAO A regulatory region contains four common alleles that have between three and five repeats of a 30-base pair (bp) sequence (Sabol et al., 1998). In vitro experiments indicate that these allelic differences in humans could result in two to ten-fold differences in transcriptional activity in the MAOA gene (Sabol et al., 1998). In all of the cell lines, the constructs that contained human alleles 2 and 3 (which have 3.5 or 4 copies of the 30 bp repeat, respectively) were expressed at significantly higher levels than the constructs containing alleles 1 and 4 (which have 3 or 5 copies of the 30 bp repeat, respectively; Sabol et al., 1998). When polymorphic variation in this 30 bp VNTR in the promoter region of the MAOA gene was assessed in a community sample of men, those with alleles 2 or 3 (the high transcription variants) exhibited reduced serotonergic responsivity and scored higher on a composite measure of aggressiveness and impulsivity than men with either of the other two alleles (Manuck et al., 2000). Furthermore, the high activity MAOA allele 3 also was more common among boys who were identified by parents and teachers as being persistently aggressive (Beitchman et al., 2004). Thus, both complete absence of MAOA activity (humans and mice) and increased MAOA activity within the physiological range (humans) are associated with increased aggressive behavior.

How important are environmental influences on a complex behavior such as aggression? In a recent path breaking study (Caspi et al., 2002), young men in New Zealand who were part of a long-term developmental study were examined for a link between anti-social behavior and high versus low activity MAO A. The cohort of 1037 people (52% male) was assessed every two to three years between the ages of 3 and 26 years. Remarkably, nearly 97% of the original birth cohort remained in the study at age 26. Between the ages of 3 and 11 years, 8% of the study children experienced "severe" maltreatment, 28% experienced "probable"

maltreatment, and 64% experienced no maltreatment (Caspi et al., 2002). The maltreated groups did not differ in MAO A activity from the group that was not mistreated, thereby implying that genotype did not influence exposure to maltreatment. However, among the maltreated groups, individuals with low MAOA gene expression had a higher likelihood to develop adult antisocial and aggressive behaviors than maltreated children with a genotype conferring high levels of MAO A expression (Caspi et al., 2002). These results may partially explain why not all victims of maltreatment develop into abusers themselves. Genes can moderate an individual's responsiveness to environmental perturbations. Allelic variation in MAOA activity also interacts with early environment in rhesus monkeys to influence the expression of aggressive behavior (Newman et al., 2005). Studies on gene–environment interactions promise to be highly informative in behavioral genetic studies of psychophysiology.

Twin studies provide insight into genotype x environment interaction. The comparison of physical and psychological measures in monozygotic (MZ) and dizygotic (DZ) twins provides an important tool for studying the interaction between genotype and environment (Boomsma et al., 2002; Legrand et al., 2005). MZ twins are genetically identical (or in rare cases, nearly identical), while DZ twins share 50% of their segregating genes on average. Thus, any heritable disorder will be more concordant in MZ than DZ twins. Twin studies also offer the added advantages of (1) removing the potential confound of age differences between siblings, (2) increasing similarities in prenatal and post-natal influences and environment experienced by the siblings, and (3) increasing certainty of shared paternity (Boomsma et al., 2002; see Figure 17.3). Using MZ and DZ twins from six European Union countries, it was determined that the heritabilities for resting blood pressure range from 44–66% for diastolic blood pressure and 52–66% for systolic blood pressure, and that 50% of the variance in blood pressure is due to genetic factors (Evans et al., 2003). Only in Finish twins did there appear to be an effect of shared environmental factors on resting blood pressure. The MZ-DZ design also has been used to confirm genetic and environmental influences on blood lipid concentrations (Knoblauch et al., 2000). QTL linkage analysis was then performed on the DZ subset (MZ twins are not useful in linkage studies because they are genetically identical) and strong evidence was provided for linkage at a chromosome 13q locus with HDL, LDL, total cholesterol, and body weight. Thus, the study led to the identification of a new gene that decreases blood lipid concentrations in apparently healthy humans (Knoblauch et al., 2000).

Twin studies also have been used to estimate heritable versus environmental influences on complex behavioral disorders, including vulnerability toward conduct disorder, adult antisocial behavior, drug dependence, and alcohol dependence (Hicks et al., 2004). General vulnerability toward these externalizing disorders among 17 year old twins was highly heritable ($h^2 = .8$); disorder-specific

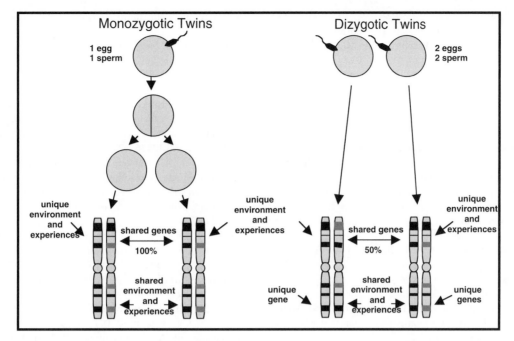

Figure 17.3. Twins are an effective way to assess genetic and environmental contributions to behavior in humans. Monozygotic (identical) twins develop from a single fertilized egg and share 100% of their segregating genes and some environmental influences and life experiences. Dizygotic (fraternal) twins develop from two separate fertilized eggs and share, on average, 50% of their segregating genes and some environmental influences and life experiences. Thus, any physiological or behavioral characteristic with a genetic influence is revealed through higher concordance among monozygotic than dizygotic twins.

vulnerabilities also were detected for each of these externalizing disorders except adult antisocial behavior (Hicks et al., 2004). Of course, exhibiting an "externalizing disposition" does not preordain an individual to behavioral disorders, there are many socially acceptable/beneficial ways in which externalizing tendencies could be expressed (i.e., engaging in high-risk occupations or hobbies).

What are the implications of behavioral genetics?

Researchers in the field of behavioral genetics have asserted that many behaviors, including aggression, impulsivity, homosexuality, parenting, learning, and nurturing have a genetic basis. A growing scientific and popular focus on genes and behavior has contributed to a resurgence of behavioral genetic determinism – the belief that genetics is the major factor in determining behavior. This contradicts the dominant *zeitgeist* in North American psychology during most of the twentieth century in which behaviorism prevailed. Fueled by John B. Watson's impressive writings early in the twentieth century that only *overt* behavior could be considered the rightful topic of scientific studies on behavior, introspection was shed as a method of data collection. Paired with the distaste of North Americans for the misuse of genetics in the form of eugenics, the pendulum of the nature-nurture controversy stayed far in the range of "nurture" for most of the century. Watson's famous assertion ruled out a significant role for genes: "Give me a dozen healthy infants, well formed, and my own specified world to bring them up in and I'll guarantee

to take any one at random and train him to become any type of specialist I might select – doctor, lawyer, artist, merchant, chief, and yes, even beggar-man and thief, regardless of his talents, penchants, tendencies, abilities, vocations, and race of his ancestors. There is no such thing as an inheritance of capacity, talent, temperament, mental constitution, and behavioral characteristics" (Watson, 1925). During the first decade of the twenty-first century, the pendulum may be swinging too far into genetic regulation of behavior (Plomin & Crabbe, 2000). Variation in behavior is a result of both environmental and genetic factors.

It would be useful to move beyond the nature-nurture controversy. The issue of considering whether behaviors are inbred, written indelibly in our genes as immutable biological imperatives, or whether environment is more important in shaping cognition and behavior, remains a false dichotomy. Behaviors only exist in the context of environmental influence. Regardless, the debate ignites again every few years, in response to genetic analyses of traits such as criminality, intelligence, or homosexuality, traits that bear significant social, legal, and political characteristics that are weighted with social, political, and legal meaning. Ethicists, politicians, and members of society will have to wrestle with the social consequences of finding genes tightly associated with behavioral traits.

REFERENCES

Abkevich, V., Camp, N. J., Hensel, C. H., Neff, C. D., Russell, D. L., Hughes, D. C., Plenk, A. M., Lowry, M. R., Richards, R. L.,

Carter, C., Frech, G. C., Stone, S., Rowe, K., Chau, C. A., Cortado, K., Hunt, A., Luce, K., O'Neil, G., Poarch, J., Potter, J., Poulsen, G. H., Saxton, H., Bernat-Sestak, M., Thompson, V., Gutin, A., Skolnick, M., Shattuck, D., and Cannon-Albright, L. 2003. Predisposition locus for major depression at chromosome 12q22–12q23.2. *American Journal of Human Genetics*, 73:1271–81.

Arnold, P. D., Zai, G., and Richter, M. A. 2004. Genetics of anxiety disorders. *Current Psychiatry Reports*, 6:243–254.

Beitchman, J. H., Mik, H. M., Ehtesham, S., Douglas, L., and Kennedy, J. L. 2004. MAOA and persistent, pervasive childhood aggression. *Molecular Psychiatry, 9*:546–547.

Bester-Meredith, J. K., Young, L. J., and Marler, C. A. 1999. Species differences in paternal behavior and aggression in *Peromyscus* and their associations with vasopressin immunoreactivity and receptors. *Hormones and Behavior*, 36:25–38.

Blonigen, D. M. and Krueger, R. F. 2005. Human quantitative genetics of aggression. In *Biology of Aggression*. Edited by R. J. Nelson. New York: Oxford University Press.

Bockamp, E., Maringer, M., Spangenberg, C., Fees, S., Fraser, S., Eshkind, L., Oesch, F., and Zabel, B. 2002. Of mice and m odels: improved animal models for biomedical research. *Physiological Genomics*, 11:115–32.

Buss, D. M. 1999. *Evolutionary Psychology: The New Science of the Mind*. Boston: Allyn and Bacon.

Boomsma, D., Busjahn, A., and Peltonen, L. 2002. Classical twin studies and beyond. *Nature Review*, 3:872–882.

Bouchard, J. T. and McGue M. 2003. Genetic and environmental influences on human psychological differences. *Journal of Neurobiology 54*:4–45.

Burnett, A. L., Nelson, R. J., Calvin, D., Demas, G. E., Klein, S. L., Kriegsfeld, Dawson, T. M., & Snyder, S. H. 1996. Nitric oxide-dependent penile erection in mice lacking neural nitric oxide synthase. *Molecular Medicine*, 2:288–296.

Brunner, H. G., Nelen, M., Breakefield, X. O., Ropers, H. H., and van Oost, B. A. 1993. Abnormal behavior associated with a point mutation in the structural gene for monoamine oxidase A. *Science*, 262:578–580.

Cacioppo, J. T., Tassinary, L. G., and Berntson, G. G. 2006. Psychophysiological science. In *Handbook of Psychophysiology* (3rd ed.). Cacioppo, J. T., Tassinary, L. G., and Berntson, G. G. (Eds). Cambridge University Press: New York.

Caldji, C., Tannenbaum, B., Sharma, S., Francis, D., Plotsky, P., and Meaney, M. J. 1998. Maternal care during infancy regulates the development of neural systems mediating the expression of fearfulness in the rat. *Proceedings of the National Academy of Sciences (USA)*, 95:5335–5340.

Carpinelli, M. R., Hilton, D. J., Metcalf, D., Antonchuk, J. L., Hyland, C. D., Mifsud, S. L., Di Rago, L., Hilton, A. A., Willson, T. A., Roberts, A. W., Ramsay, R. G., Nicola, N. A., and Alexander, W. S. 2004. Suppressor screen in Mpl−/−mice: c-Myb mutation causes supraphysiological production of platelets in the absence of thrombopoietin signaling. *Proceedings of the National Academy of Sciences of the United States of America*, 101:6553–8.

Carter, C S, DeVries, A. C., and Getz, L L. 1995. Physiological substrates of mammalian monogamy: the prairie vole model. *Neuroscience and Biobehavioral Reviews*, 19:303–314.

Cases, O., Seif, I., Grimsby, J., Gaspar, P., Chen, K., Pournin, S., Muller, U., Aguet, M., Babinet, C., Shih, J. C., et al. 1995. Aggressive behavior and altered amounts of brain serotonin and norepinephrine in mice lacking MAOA. *Science*, 268:1763–1766.

Caspi A, McClay J, Moffitt T E, Mill J, Martin J, Craig I W, Taylor A, and Poulton R. 2002. Role of genotype in the cycle of violence in maltreated children. *Science*, 297:851–854.

Champagne, F., Diorio, J., Sharma, S., and Meaney, M. J. 2001. Naturally occurring variations in maternal behavior in the rat are associated with differences in estrogen-inducible central oxytocin receptors. *Proceedings of the National Academy of Sciences (USA)*, 98:12736–12741.

Champagne, F. A., Weaver, I. C., Diorio, J., Sharma, S., and Meaney, M. J. 2003. Natural variations in maternal care are associated with estrogen receptor alpha expression and estrogen sensitivity in the medial preoptic area. *Endocrinology*.144:4720–4724.

Curtis, D. J. 2004. Modifier screens in the mouse: Time to move forward with reverse genetics. *Science*, 101: 7209–7210.

DeFries, J. C., Gervais, M. C., and Thomas, E. A. 1978. Response to 30 generations of selection for open-field activity in laboratory mice. *Behavior Genetics*, 8:3–13.

Di Maria, E., Gulli, R., Begni, S., De Luca, A., Bignotti, S., Pasini, A., Bellone, E., Pizzuti, A., Dallapiccola, B., Novelli, G., Ajmar, F., Gennarelli, M., and Mandich, P. 2004. Variations in the NMDA receptor subunit 2B gene (GRIN2B) and schizophrenia: a case-control study. *American Journal of Medical Genetics. B. Neuropsychiatriatric Genetics*, 128B:27–29.

Durrant, R. and Ellis, B. 2003. Evolutionary psychology. In: *Handbook of Psychology, Vol. 3: Biological Psychology*. Edited by M. Gallagher and R. J. Nelson. New York: Wiley & Sons.

Egger, G., Liang, G., Aparicio, A., and Jones, P. A. 2004. Epigenetics in human disease and prospects for epigenetic therapy. *Nature*, 429:457–463.

Evans, A., Van Baal, C. M., McCarron, P., delange, M., Soerensen, T. I. A., deGeus, E. J. C., Kyvik, K., Pedersen, N. L., Spector, T. D., Andrew, T., Patterson, C., Whitfield, J. B., Zhu, G., Martin, N. G., Kaprio, J., Boomsma, D. I. 2003. The genetics of coronary heart disease: the contribution of twin studies. *Twin Research*, 6:432–441.

Falconer, D. S. & McKay, T. F. C. 1996. *Introduction to quantitative genetics. 4th ed.* Harlow UK: Longman.

Farrall, M. 2004. Quantitative genetic variation: a post-modern view. *Human Molecular Genetics*, 3:R1–7.

Fernandez-Teruel, A., Escorihuela, R. M., Gray, J. A., Aguilar, R., Gil, L., Gimenez-Llort, L., Tobena, A., Bhomra, A., Nicod, A., Mott, R., Driscoll, P., Dawson, G. R., and Flint, J. 2002. A quantitative trait locus influencing anxiety in the laboratory rat. *Genome Research*, 12: 618–26.

Ferreira, M. A. 2004. Linkage analysis: principles and methods for the analysis of human quantitative traits. *Twin Research*, 7:513–530.

Fisher, R. A. 1918. The correlation between relatives on the supposition of Mendelian inheritance. *Transactions of the Royal Society of Edinburgh*, 52: 399–433.

Flint J. 2003. Analysis of quantitative trait loci that influence animal behavior. *Journal of Neurobiology*, 54:46–77.

Flint, J., Corley, R., DeFries, J. C., Fulker, D. W., Gray, J. A., Miller, S. Collins, A. C. 1995. A simple genetic basis for a complex psychological trait in laboratory mice. *Science*, 269:1432–5.

Fortini, M. E., Skupski, M. P., Boguski, M. S., and Hariharan, I. K. 2000. A survey of human disease gene counterparts in the *Drosophila* genome. *The Journal of Cell Biology, 150*:F23–30.

Francis, D. D., Diorio, J., Liu, D., and Meaney, M. J. 1999, Non-genomic transmission across generations of maternal behavior and stress responses in the rat. *Science*, 286:1155–1158.

Fullerton, J., Cubin, M., Tiwari, H., Wang, C., Bomhra, A., Davidson, S., Miller, Fairburn, C., Goodwin, G., Neale, M. C., Fiddy, S., Mott, R., Allison, D. B., and Flint, J. 2003. Linkage analysis of extremely discordant and concordant sibling pairs identifies quantitative-trait loci that influence variation in the human personality trait neuroticism. *American Journal of Human Genetics*, 72:879–90.

Galderisi, U., Cascino, A., and Giordano, A. 1999. Antisense oligonucleotides as therapeutic agents. *Journal of Cellular Physiology*, 181:251–257.

Galton, D. J. and Galton C. J. 1997. Francis Galton: his approach to polygenic disease. *Journal of the Royal College of Physicians of London*, 31:570–3.

Gardiner, K. 1995. Human genome organization. *Current Opinion in Genetics and Development*, 5:315–322.

Ginsburg, B. E. 1958. Genetics as a tool in the study of behavior. *Perspectives in Biology and Medicine*, 1:397–424.

Griffiths, A. J. F., Gelbart, W. M., Miller, J. H. and Lewontin, R. C. 1999. *Modern Genetic Analysis*. 7th Edition. W. H. Freeman & Sons, New York.

Grozinger, C. M., Sharabash, N. M., Whitfield, C. W., and Robinson, G. E. 2003. Pheromone-mediated gene expression in the honey bee brain. *Proceedings of the National Academy of Sciences (USA)*, 100:14519–14525.

Gu, H., Marth, J. D., Orban, P. C., Mossmann, H., and Rajewsky, K. 1994. Deletion of a DNA polymerase beta gene segment in T cells using cell type-specific gene targeting. *Science*, 265:103–106.

Herrnstein, R. J. and Murray, C. 1994. *The Bell Curve: Intelligence and Class Structure in American Life*. New York: Free Press.

Hicks BM, Krueger RF, Iacono WG, McGue M, and Patrick CJ. 2004. Family transmission and heritability of externalizing disorders: a twin-family study. *Archives of General Psychiatry*, 61:922–928.

Holschneider, D. P., Chen, K., Seif, I., and Shih, J. C. 2001. Biochemical, behavioral, physiologic, and neurodevelopmental changes in mice deficient in monoamine oxidase A or B. *Brain Research Bulletin*, 56:453–462.

Insel, T. R. and Shapiro, L. E. 1992. Oxytocin receptors and maternal behavior. *Annals of the New York Academy of Science*, 652:122–141.

Insel, T. R., Wang, Z. X., and Ferris, C. F. 1994. Patterns of brain vasopressin receptor distribution associated with social organization in microtine rodents. *Journal of Neuroscience*, 14:5381–5392.

International Human Genome Sequencing Consortium. 2001. Initial sequencing and analysis of the human genome. *Nature*, 409: 860–921.

Jensen, A. R. 1973. Personality and scholastic achievement in three ethnic groups. *British Journal of Educational Psychology*, 43:115–125.

Jorgensen, E. M. and Mango, S. E. 2002. The art and design of genetic screens: *Caenorhabditis elegans*. *Nature Reviews. Genetics*, 3:356–69.

Klebig, M. L., Wall, M. D., Potter, M. D., Rowe, E. L., Carpenter, D. A., and Rinchik, E. M. 2003. Mutations in the clathrin-assembly gene Picalm are responsible for the hematopoietic and iron metabolism abnormalities in fit1 mice. *Proceedings of the National Academy of Sciences of the United States of America*, 100:8360–5.

Koch, L. G., Meredith, T. A., Fraker, T. D., Metting, P. J., and Britton SL. 1998. Heritability of treadmill running endurance in rats. *American Journal of Physiology*, 275:R1455–R1460.

Knoblauch, H., Müller-Myhsok, B., Busjahn, A., Ben Avi, L., Bähring, S., Baron, H., Heath S. C., Uhlmann, R., Faulhaber, H-D., Shpitzen, S., Aydin, A., Reshef, A., Rosenthal, M., Eliav, O., Mühl, A., Lowe, A., Schurr, D., Harats, D., Jeschke, E., Friedlander, Y., Schuster, H., Luft, F. C., Leitersdorf, E. 2000. A cholesterol-lowering gene maps to chromosome 13q. *Am. J. Hum. Genet.*, 66:157–166.

Krebs, J. R. and Davies, N. B. 1993. *An Introduction to Behavioural Ecology*. Blackwell Scientific, Oxford.

Lander ES, Linton LM, Birren B, Nusbaum C, Zody MC, Baldwin J, Devon K, Dewar K, Doyle M, FitzHugh W, Funke R, et al. 2001. Initial sequencing and analysis of the human genome. *Nature*, 409:860–921.

Lapidge, K. L., Oldroyd, B. P., and Spivak, M. 2002. Seven suggestive quantitative trait loci influence hygienic behavior of honey bees. *Naturwissenschaften*, 89:565–868.

Lee, P., Morley, G., Huang, Q., Fischer, A., Seiler, S., Horner, J. W., Factor, S., Vaidya, D., Jalife, J., and Fishman, G. I. 1998. Conditional lineage ablation to model human diseases. *Proceedings of the National Academy of Sciences of the United States of America*, 95:11371–6.

Legrand, L. N., Iacono, W. G. and McGue, M. 2005. Predicting addiction. *American Scientist*, 93:140–147.

Lewandoski, M. 2001. Conditional control of gene expression in the mouse. *Nature Reviews Genetics*, 2:743–755.

Lim, M. M., Wang, Z., Olazabal, D. E., Ren, X., Terwilliger, E. F., and Young, L. J. 2004. Enhanced partner preference in a promiscuous species by manipulating the expression of a single gene. *Nature*, 429:754–757.

Lin, S. H., Kiyohara, T., and Sun, B. 2003. Maternal behavior: activation of the central oxytocin receptor system in parturient rats? *Neuroreport*, 14:1439–1444.

Liu, D., Diorio, J., Tannenbaum, B., Caldji, C., Francis, D., Freedman, A., Sharma, S., Pearson, D., Plotsky, P. M., and Meaney, M. J. 1997. Maternal care, hippocampal glucocorticoid receptors, and hypothalamic-pituitary-adrenal responses to stress. *Science*, 277:1659–1662.

Liu, D., Diorio, J., Day, J. C., Francis, D. D., and Meaney, M. J. 2000. Maternal care, hippocampal synaptogenesis and cognitive development in rats. *Nature* 3:799–806.

Lorenz, K. Z. 1966. *Evolution and the Modification of Behaviour*. Methuen, London.

Lowenstein, P. R. and Castro, M. G. 2001. Genetic engineering within the adult brain: Implications for molecular approaches to behavioral neuroscience. *Physiology and Behavior*, 73:833–839.

Mani, S. K., Blaustein, J. D., Allen, J. M., Law, S. W., O'Malley, B. W., and Clark, J. H. 1994. Inhibition of rat sexual behavior by antisense oligonucleotides to the progesterone receptor. *Endocrinology*, 135:1409–1414.

Manning, A. 1967. *Introduction to Animal Behavior*. Addison-Wesley, Reading, MA.

Manuck, S. B., Flory, J. D., Ferrell, R. E., Mann, J. J., and Muldoon, M. F. 2000. A regulatory polymorphism of the monoamine oxidase-A gene may be associated with variability in aggression, impulsivity, and central nervous system serotonergic responsivity. *Psychiatry Research, 95*:9–23.

Maxson, S. 2002. Behavioral genetics. In: *Handbook of Psychology: Biological Psychology*. Vol. 3. Edited by M. Gallagher and R. J. Nelson. New York Wiley & Sons.

McCormick, J. A., Lyons, V., Jacobson, M. D., Noble, J., Diorio, J., Nyirenda, M., Weaver, S., Ester, W., Yau, J. L., Meaney, M. J., Seckl, J. R., and Chapman, K. E. 2000. 5′-heterogeneity of glucocorticoid receptor messenger RNA is tissue specific: differential regulation of variant transcripts by early-life events. *Molecular Endocrinology, 14*:506–517.

Morton, N. E. 1991. Parameters of the human genome. *Proceedings of the National Academy of Science (USA)*, 88:7474–7476.

Mott, R., Talbot, C. J., Turri, M. G., Collins, A. C., and Flint, A. J. 2000. Method for fine mapping quantitative trait loci in outbred animal stocks. *Proceedings of the National Academy of Sciences of the United States of America*, 97:12649–54.

Mouse Genome Sequencing Consortium. 2002. Initial sequencing and comparative analysis of the mouse genome. *Nature*. 420: 520–562.

Mueller, W. H. 1976. Parent-child correlations for stature and weight among school aged children: A review of 24 studies. *Human Biology*, 48: 379–397.

Muller, U. 1999. Ten years of gene targeting: targeted mouse mutants, from vector design to phenotype analysis. *Mechanisms of Development*, 82:3–21.

Nash, M. W., Huezo-Diaz, P., Williamson, R. J., Sterne, A., Purcell, S., Hoda, F., Cherny, S. S., Abecasis, G. R., Prince, M., Gray, J. A., Ball, D., Asherson, P., Mann, A., Goldberg, D., McGuffin, P., Farmer, A., Plomin, R., Craig, I. W. and Pak, C. 2004. Genomewide linkage analysis of a composite index of neuroticism and mood-related scales in extreme selected sibships. *Human Molecular Genetics*, 13:2173–82.

Nelson, R. J. 1997. The use of genetic "knock-out" mice in behavioral endocrinology research. *Hormones and Behavior*, 31:188–196.

Nelson, R. J. and Young, K. A. 1998. Behavioral effects of targeted disruption of specific genes. *Neuroscience & Biobehavioral Reviews*, 22:453–462.

Nisenbaum, L. K. 2002. The ultimate chip shot: can microarray technology deliver for neuroscience? *Genes, Brain and Behavior*, 1:27–34.

Newman TK, Syagailo YV, Barr CS, Wendland JR, Champoux M, Graessle M, Suomi SJ, Higley JD, Lesch KP. 2005. Monoamine oxidase: A gene promoter variation and rearing experience influences aggressive behavior in rhesus monkeys *Biological Psychiatry*, 57:167–172.

Nicholson, I. R. 1990. Are heritability estimates generalizable? Lack of evidence from cross-sample correlations. *Social Biology* 37:147–61.

No, D., Yao, T.-P. and Evans, R. M. 1996. Ecdysone-inducible gene expression in mammalian cells and transgenic mice. *Proceedings of the National Academy of Sciences. (USA)*, 93:3346–3351.

Nurnberger, J. I. Jr., Foroud, T., Flury, L., Su, J., Meyer, E. T., Hu, K., Crowe, R., Edenberg, H., Goate, A., Bierut, L., Reich, T., Schuckit, M., and Reich, W. 2001. Evidence for a locus on chromosome 1 that influences vulnerability to alcoholism and affective disorder. *The American Journal of Psychiatry*, 158:718–24.

Papadimitriou, G N., Dikeos, D. G., Souery, D., Del-Favero, J., Massat, I., Avramopoulos, D., Blairy, S., Cichon, S., Ivezic, S., Kaneva, R., Karadima, G., Lilli, R., Milanova, V., Nothen, M.,

Oruc, L., Rietschel, M., Serretti, A., Van Broeckhoven, C., Stefanis, C., and Mendlewicz, J. 2003. Association between the phospholipase A2 gene and unipolar affective disorder: A multicentre case-control study. *Psychiatric Genetics*, 13:211–220.

Park, S. K., Sedore, S. A., Cronmiller, C., and Hirsh, J. 2000. Type II cAMP-dependent protein kinase-deficient *Drosophila* are viable but show developmental, circadian, and drug response phenotypes. *Journal of Biological Chemistry*, 275:20588–20596.

Phillips, T. J., Belknap, J. K., Hitzemann, R. J., Buck, K. J., Cunningham, C. L., and Crabbe, J. C. 2002. Harnessing the mouse to unravel the genetics of human disease. *Genes, Brain, and Behavior*, 1:14–26.

Phimister, B. 1999. Going global. *Nature Genetics*, 21: 1–1.

Plomin, R. and Crabbe, J. 2000. DNA. *Psychological Bulletin*, 126:806–828.

Plomin, R., DeFries, J. C., McClearn, G. E., and McGuffin, P. 2000. *Behavioral Genetics. Fourth edition*. New York: Worth.

Rat Genome Sequencing Project Consortium. 2004. Genome sequence of the brown norway rat yields insights into mammalian evolution. *Nature*. 428: 493–521.

Rice, T. K. and Borecki, I. B. 2001. Familial resemblance and heritability. *Advances in Genetics*, 42:35–44.

Rothenbuhler, W. C. 1964a. Behavior genetics of nest cleaning of honey-bees. I. Responses of four inbred lines to disease killed broods. *Animal Behaviour*, 12:578–583.

Rothenbuhler, W. C. 1964b. Behavior genetics of nest cleaning of honey-bees. IV. Responses of F_1 and backcross generations to disease-killed brood. *American Zoologist*, 4:111–123.

Rubin, G. M., Hong, L., Brokstein, P., Evans-Holm, M., Frise, E., Stapleton, M., and Harvey, D. A. 2000. *A Drosophila* complementary DNA resource. *Science*, 287:2222–4.

Ruppell, O., Pankiw, T., and Page, R. E. 2004a. Pleiotropy, epistasis and new QTL: the genetic architecture of honey bee foraging behavior. *Journal of Heredity*, 95:481–491.

Rueppell, O., Pankiw, T., Nielsen, D. I., Fondrk, M. K., Beye, M., and Page, R. E. 2004b. The genetic architecture of the behavioral ontogeny of foraging in honeybee workers. *Genetics*, 167:1767–1779.

Sabol, S. Z., Hu, S., and Hamer, D. 1998. A functional polymorphism in the monoamine oxidase A gene promoter. *Human Genetics*, 103:273–279.

Sax, K., 1923. The association of size difference with seed-coat pattern and pigmentation in *Phaseolus vulgaris*. *Genetics*, 8:552–560.

Segalat, L. 1999. Genetic analysis of behavior in the nematode, *Caenorhabditis elegans*. In: B. C. Jones & P. Mormede (Eds.) *Neurobehavioral genetics: Methods and applications*. (pp. 373–381) Boca Raton: CRC.

Shih, J. C. 2004. Cloning, after cloning, knock-out mice, and physiological functions of MAO A and B. *Neurotoxicology*, 25:21–30.

Shishkina, G. T., Kalinina, T. S., Sournina, N. Y., and Dygalo, N. N. 2001. Effects of antisense to the α2A-adrenoceptors administered into the region of the locus ceruleus on behaviors in plusmaze and sexual behavior tests in sham operated and castrated male rats. *Journal of Neuroscience*, 21:726–731.

Silventoinen, K. 2003. Determinants of variation in adult body height. *Journal of Biosocial Sciences*, 35: 263–285.

Silventoinen K, Kaprio J, Lahelma E, Koskenvuo M. 2000. Relative effect of genetic and environmental factors on body height: differences across birth cohorts among Finnish men and women. *American Journal of Public Health*, 90:627–630.

Sokalowski, M. B. 1999. Genetic analysis of food search behavior in the fruit fly, *Drosphilia melanogaster*. In: B. C. Jones & P. Mormede (Eds.) *Neurobehavioral genetics: Methods and applications*. (pp. 357–364) Boca Raton: CRC.

St Johnston, D. 2002. The art and design of genetic screens: *Drosophila melanogaster*. *Nature Reviews. Genetics* 3:176–88.

Sung, Y. H., Song, J., and Lee, H-W. 2004. Functional genomics approach using mice. *Journal of Biochemistry and Molecular Biology*, 37:122–32.

Tanaka, M., Yoshida, M., Emoto, H., and Ishii, H. 2000. Noradrenaline systems in the hypothalamus, amygdala and locus coeruleus are involved in the provocation of anxiety: basic studies. *European Journal of Pharmacology*, 405:397–406.

Tang, Y.-P., Shimizu, E., Dube, G. R., Rampon, C., Kerchner, G. A., Zhuo, M., Liu, G., and Tsien, J. Z. 1999. Genetic enhancement of learning and memory in mice *Nature*, 401, 63–69.

Thiele, T. E., Willis, B., Stadler, J., Reynolds, J. G., and Bernstein, I. L., McKnight, G. S. 2000. High ethanol consumption and low sensitivity to ethanol-induced sedation in protein kinase A-mutant mice. *The Journal of Neuroscience*, *20*:RC75:1–6.

Thoday, J. M., 1960. Location of polygenes. *Nature*, 191: 368–370.

Wallace, D. C. 1999. Mitochondrial diseases in man and mouse. *Science*, 283:1482–1488.

Wallace, D. C. 2001. Mitochondrial defects in neurodegenerative disease. *Mental Retardation and Developmental Disabilities Research Review*, 7:158–166.

Wahlsten, D., Metten, P., Phillips, T. J., Boehm, S. L. 2nd., Burkhart-Kasch, S., Dorow, J., Doerksen, S., Downing, C., Fogarty, J., Rodd-Henricks, K., Hen, R., McKinnon, C. S., Merrill, C. M., Nolte, C., Schalomon, M., Schlumbohm, J. P., Sibert, J. R., Wenger, C. D., Dudek, B. C., and Crabbe, J. C. 2003. Different data from different labs: lessons from studies of gene-environment interaction. *Journal of Neurobiology*, 54:283–311.

Walther, W. and Stein, U. 2000. Viral vectors for gene transfer: a review of their use in the treatment of human diseases. *Drugs*, 60: 249–271.

Watson, J. B. 1925. *Behaviorism*. Norton, New York.

Watson, J. D. and Crick, F. H. C. 1953a. Molecular structure of nucleic acids: a structure for deoxyribose nucleic acid. *Nature*, 171: 737–738.

Watson, J. D. and Crick, F. H. C. 1953b. Genetical implications of the structure of deoxyribosenucleic acid. *Nature*, 171, 964–967.

Weaver, I. C. G., Cervoni, N., Champagne, F. A., D'Alessio, A. C., Sharma, S., Seckl, J. R., Dymov, S., Szyf, M., Meaney, M. J. 2004. Epigenetic programming by maternal behavior. *Nature Neuroscience*, 7, 847–854.

Whitfield, C. W., Cziko, A. M., and Robinson, G. E. 2003. Gene expression profiles in the brain predict behavior in individual honey bees. *Science*, 302:296–299.

Wolf, F. W. and Heberlein, U. 2003. Invertebrate models of drug abuse. *Journal of Neurobiology*, 54:161–78.

Wright, S. 1921. Systems of mating. *Genetics*, 6:111–178.

Young, L. J., Nilsen, R., Waymire, K. G., MacGregor, G. R., and Insel, T. R. 1999. Increased affiliative response to vasopressin in mice expressing the V1a receptor from a monogamous vole. *Nature*, 400: 766–768.

Young, L. J., Wang, Z., Donaldson, R., and Rissman, E. F. 1998. Estrogen receptor alpha is essential for induction of oxytocin receptor by estrogen. *Neuroreport*, 9:933–936.

18 Probing the Mechanisms of Attention

MICHAEL I. POSNER, M. ROSARIO RUEDA, AND PHILIPP KANSKE

ABSTRACT

This chapter emphasizes the many methods currently being employed to study brain networks related to attention. We seek to set current studies into a historical background of efforts to understand how the brain selects among stimuli and resolves competing responses. We examine attention as an organ system with networks of neural areas related to several major functions such as maintaining the alert state, orienting to sensory events and resolving conflict between responses. We consider the anatomy and circuitry of these networks and examine the role of genes and experience in their normal development and of various pathologies. Finally we examine how our current knowledge of the psychophysiology of attention illuminates traditional issues in cognition about how attention operates.

The field of attention is one of the oldest in psychology. At the turn of the twentieth century Titchener (1909) called attention "the heart of the psychological enterprise." Attention is relatively easy to define subjectively as in the classical definition of William James who said: "Everyone knows what attention is. It is the taking possession of the mind in clear and vivid form of one our of what seem several simultaneous objects or trains of thought." (James, 1890, p. 403). However, this subjective definition does not provide hints that might lead to an understanding of mechanisms of attention that can illuminate its physical basis in terms of underlying physiological process nor clarify its normal development and pathologies. For these goals it is useful to think about attention as an organ system with its own anatomy and circuitry that develops in early life under the control of genes and experience. This will be the focus of our chapter.

The modern history of attention as an organ can be started with the important studies of Maruzzi and Magoun (1949) on the reticular activating system. About the same time, Hebb (1949) called attention to the importance of networks of neural areas (cell assemblies and phase sequences) in building conscious representation of stimulus input (see Posner & Rothbart, 2004 for a review of Hebb's contribution). In the last fifty years there has been steady progress in the development of methods that allow us to probe the mechanisms of attention at a physiological level. It is the development of these methods and their use to probe attentional networks that seems most relevant to the current handbook.

In this chapter we first trace history of the development of methods that allow study of attentional separately from other cognitive functions. We examine the methods used to link attention to underlying brain mechanisms including studies of lesioned patients, recording of electrical activity noninvasively in humans or by use of implanted electrodes and efforts to understand the genes related to attention. These include the use of microelectrodes in alert animals beginning in the 1970s and early studies of neuroimaging using hemodynamic methods starting in the 1980s. After our historical review, we examine current studies within cognitive psychology to get an idea of the functions of networks in vigilance, visual search, and cognitive control tasks. We then examine the anatomical networks that underlie these functions using whenever possible the combined methods that have developed over the last half century to explore neural networks. We then consider evidence of how genes and experience shape the development of attentional networks. At the end we return to some of the major questions in cognition that concern attention and review their current state.

MODERN HISTORY

1950s

D. O. Hebb (1949) argued that all stimuli had two effects. One of these, following the studies of Maruzzi and Magoun, involved the reticular activating system and worked to keep the cortex tuned in the waking state, whereas the other used the great sensory pathways and

The authors would like to thank Prof. Mary K. Rothbart for her participation in this research and colleagues at the University of Oregon and the Sackler Institute at Weill Medical College of Cornell University.

provided information about the nature of the stimulating event.

In the early 1950s, Colin Cherry (Cherry, 1953) initiated an epic series of experiments designed to examine how subjects selected stimuli that were presented simultaneously to each ear. A major result was that rapid presentation of pairs of digits one to each ear, led people to recall of all digits presented to the right ear first, followed by all presented to the left. Broadbent (1958) summarized these and other results by suggesting that a peripheral short-term memory system buffers sensory input prior to a filter, which selects a channel of entry (in this case an ear) and sends information to a limited capacity perceptual system.

A second line of attention research that emerged from studies conducted in the Second World War involved the study of sustained attention during vigilance tasks (Mackworth & Mackworth, 1956). During continuous tasks subjects tended to miss more signals as the task continued. Changes in the EEG suggested that there was an increase in a sleep-like state.

1960s

One of the big developments of the 1960s involved the ability to average electrical signals from the scalp to develop the event-related potential, as a series of electrical events time locked to the stimulus. The technique was applied to the study of attention. In 1965 Sutton (Sutton et al., 1965) reported that surprising or unexpected cognitive events, of the type that might be closely inspected produced a strong positive wave in the scalp potential called the P 300. This component has and continues to play an important role in attention research (Donchin & Cohen, 1967; Rugg & Coles, 1995).

At about the same time Gray Walter reported that the brain produced a marked DC shift during the period following a warning and prior to a target, this was called the contingent negative variation and was viewed as a sign that alerting was taking place (Walter et al., 1964). Reaction time improved markedly over the first 500 milliseconds following the warning and often, errors increased with warning interval, producing a tradeoff between speed and accuracy. This finding suggested that warning effects did not improve the accrual of information but instead made it faster to attend to the input and thus sped the response (Posner, 1978).

1970s

The work of Hubel and Wiesel (1968) using microelectrodes to probe the structure of the visual system began in the early 1960s. However, before this method could be applied to attention it was necessary to adapt the microelectrode technique to alert animals. This was accomplished in the early 1970s by Evarts (1968) and applied by Mountcastle (1978) and Wurtz, Goldberg, and Robinson (1980) to examine mechanisms of visual attention in the superior colliculus and parietal lobe. Their findings suggested the importance of both of these areas to a shift of visual attention. It had been known for many years that patients with lesions of the right parietal lobe could suffer from a profound neglect of space opposite the lesion. The findings of "attention related cells" in the posterior parietal lobe of alert monkeys suggested that these cells might be responsible for the clinical syndrome.

An impressive result from the microelectrode work, was that the time course of parietal cell activity seemed to follow a visual stimulus by 80–100 milliseconds. Beginning in the 1970s, Hillyard (van Voorhis & Hillyard, 1978) and other investigators explored the use of scalp electrode to examine time differences between attended and unattended visual locations. They found that the N1 and P2 components of the visual event related potential showed changes due to attention starting at about 100 milliseconds after input. These finding showed likely convergence of the latency of psychological processes as measured by ERPs in human subjects and cellular processes measured in alert monkeys. This finding was a very important development for mental chronometry because it suggested that scalp recordings could accurately reflect the underlying temporal structure of brain activity.

1980s

Posner (1980) studied the use of a cue in an otherwise empty visual field as a way of moving attention to a target. Electrodes near the eyes were used to insure there were no eye movements and because only one response was required there was no way to prepare the response differently depending upon the cue, making it clear that whatever changes were induced by the cue were covert and not due to motor adjustment of the eyes or hand.

It was found that covert shifts could enhance the speed of responding to the target even in a nearly empty field. Within half a second, one could shift attention to a visual event and, when it indicated a likely target at another location, move attention to enhance processing at the new location. It was shown (Shulman, Remington, & McClean, 1979) that response times to probes at intermediate locations were enhanced at intermediate times as though attention actually moved through the space and that it was possible to prepare to move the eyes to one location while moving attention covertly in the opposite direction (Posner, 1980). Whether attention moves through the intermediate space and how free covert attention is from the eye movement systems are still disputed matters (LaBerge, 1995; Rizzolatti et al., 1987), suggesting the limitation of purely behavioral studies.

At the time, it was also hard to understand how a movement of attention could possibly be executed by neurons. Subsequently it was shown that the population vector of a set of neurons in the motor system of a monkey could carry out what would appear behaviorally, as a mental rotation (Georgopoulos et al., 1989). After that finding, a covert shift of attention did not seem too far-fetched.

It had been reported that patients with lesions of the parietal lobe could make same-different judgments concerning objects that they were unable to report consciously (Volpe, LeDoux, & Gazzaniga, 1979). It was possible to follow this result in more analytic cognitive studies. What did a right parietal lesion do that made access to material on the left side difficult or impossible for consciousness and yet still left the information available for other judgments?

This puzzle was partially answered by the systematic study of patients with different lesion locations in the parietal lobe, the pulvinar and the colliculus. These lesions all tended to show neglect of the side of space opposite the lesion. But in a detailed cognitive analysis it was clear that they differed in showing deficits in specific mental operations involved in shifting attention (Posner, 1988). These studies supported a limited form of brain localization. The hypothesis was that different brain areas executed individual mental operations or computations such as disengaging from the current focus of attention (parietal lobe), moving or changing the index of attention (colliculus), and engaging the subsequent target (pulvinar). If this hypothesis were correct it might explain why Lashley thought the whole brain was involved in mental tasks. Perhaps it's not the whole brain, but a widely dispersed network of quite localized neural areas.

1990s to Date

In the late 1980s, the Washington University School of Medicine was developing a PET center led by Marc Raichle. These studies helped establish neuroimaging as a means of exploring brain activity during cognitive functions in general and the study of attention in particular. (Posner & Raichle, 1994, 1998). In general, these studies have shown that most cognitive tasks, including those that are designed to separate mechanisms of attention, have activated a small number of widely scattered neural areas. Some people have argued that these areas are specific for domains of function like language, face perception, or episodic memory (Kanwisher & Duncan, 2004). In the area of attention it has been more frequent to consider the mental operations or computations carried out by a particular area (Corbetta & Shulman, 2002; Posner, 2004). These two ideas are not mutually exclusive. It is certainly possible to talk about the set of areas that are involved in language and at the same time maintain that the areas carry out different computations within that domain.

The findings from neuroimaging that cognitive tasks involve a number of different anatomical areas has led to an emphasis on tracing the time dynamics of these areas during tasks involving attention. Because shifts of attention can be so rapid it is difficult to follow them with hemodynamic imaging. To fill this role, algorithms have been developed (Scherg & Berg, 1993) to relate the scalp distribution recorded from high density electrical or magnetic sensors on or near the skull to brain areas active during hemodynamic imaging (see Dale et al., 2000, for a review). In some areas of attention there has been extensive validation of these algorithms (Heinze et al., 1994) and they allow precise data on the sequence of activations during the selection of visual stimuli (see Hillyard, Di Russo, & Martinez, 2004 for a review). The combination of spatial localization with hemodynamic imaging and temporal precisions from electrical recording has provided an approach to the networks underlying attention.

At the turn of the century the overall sequence of the human genome had been accomplished (Venter et al., 2001). Although humans have a common genome there are differences among individuals, in many genes (polymorphisms). These differences make it possible to examine particular genes related to individual differences in behavior and in brain activity (Goldberg & Weinberger, 2004; Mattay & Goldberg, 2004).

COGNITIVE STUDIES

The cognitive approach to attention provides a variety of models and conceptual frameworks for brain studies. Perhaps the most general issue is whether to think of attention as one thing or as a number of somewhat separate issues. A classic distinction in the field is to divide attention by considering separately the intensive and selective aspects (Kahneman, 1973). Attentional states vary. They include slow wave sleep, coma, rapid eye movement sleep, and degrees of wakefulness that may vary over the course of the day (dirurnal rhythm), time on task or following warnings. These states can be contrasted with selective attention that involves the mechanisms in committing resources to some particular event.

In this chapter we follow a division of attention into three distinct networks: one of these involves a change of state and is called alerting. The other two are closely involved with the selection and are called orienting and executive control (Posner & Petersen, 1990). Alerting deals with the intensive aspect of attention related to how the organism achieves and maintains the alert state. Orienting deals with selective mechanisms operating on sensory input. The idea that new sensory stimuli lead to an orienting reflex goes back to the classic studies of Sokolov (1963) on peripheral changes underlying the orienting reflex, but much new has been learned about the brain systems involved. The executive network deals with conflict among competing responses and related to issues such as the development of self-regulation not only of thoughts but also of feelings and behavior (Rueda, Posner, & Rothbart, 2004). Although in much of our behavior all of these networks are involved simultaneously, the distinction allows us to review somewhat different literatures.

ALERTING

The state of wakefulness and arousal is influenced by internal and external signals (Hackley & Valle-Inclan, 1998). Intrinsic or tonic alertness clearly changes over the course of the day from sleep to waking and within the waking state from sluggish to highly alert. Originally these effects were thought to involve a single mechanism, the reticular activating system, but current research considers the interplay of a number of midbrain neural modulators such as norepinephrine and dopamine to be involved. In all tasks involving long periods of processing the role of changes of state may be important. Thus vigilance or sustained attention effects probably rest at least in part on changes in tonic alerting system.

The presentation of an external stimulus can also increase alertness. The clearest case can be observed as a reduction in reaction times in tasks in which a warning signal is presented prior to a target. This effect is partly automatic as it can occur with an auditory accessory event, which does not predict a target. It is partly due to voluntary actions based on the information about the time of the upcoming target. These effects can be observed as a general DC shift in electrical activity of the EEG called the contingent negative variation (Walter et al., 1964). However, more specific negative shifts may also be seen in particular structures depending upon the target or activity required in the task (Rosler, Heil, & Roder, 1997).

Alertness reflects the state of the organism for processing information and is an important condition in all tasks. It is also possible distinguish effects of alertness on sensory input from its effect on motor systems (Sanders, 1998).

ORIENTING

When examining a visual scene there is the general feeling that all information about it is available. However, careful experimental studies (Rensink, O'Regan & Clark, 1997; Rock & Guttman, 1981) have shown that this is not the case. Important semantic changes can occur in the scene without any report of the observer provided they take place away from the focus of attention and cues that are normally effective in producing a shift of attention such as luminance changes or movement are suppressed. These findings, called change blindness, underlie the importance of attention shifts for normal conscious perception.

The study of visual orienting has often involved the use of visual search tasks in which a particular object is defined as a target (Treisman & Gelade, 1980). Visual search has been used to study limits to the amount of information contained in a scene that is passed on to higher processing (Broadbent, 1958; Treisman & Gelade, 1980). A widely used metaphor for this capacity limit (Cavanagh, 2004) views attention orienting as a spotlight that enables examination of details within the spotlight while reducing what can be reported outside the spotlight.

When the target differs in a single element from all the background reaction times generally are similar irrespective of the number of elements as though they pop out from the background. However, when the target and background have attributes in common reaction times generally increase linearly with the number of background elements, conjunction search (Treisman & Galade, 1980). The idea of conjunction search suggests a single focus of attention that is moved at all over the visual display. Indeed when the array is large, eye movements are a major vehicle for moving the focus of attention from one location to another. However, similar results can be obtained even when the eyes are fixed and this underlies the idea that attention can be viewed as a covert spotlight.

Several recent studies suggest the existence of multiple spotlights (Yantis, 1992; Kramer & Hahn, 1995). Awh and Pashler (2000) were able to demonstrate that just an extension in size of the spotlight is not sufficient to explain all of the extant data. However, it seems that the size of the selection region can vary extensively in correspondence to what is demanded by the task (Klein & McCormick, 1989). The minimal selection region within a fixation can be described as a covert acuity limit (Intriligator & Cavanagh, 2001). Cavanagh (2004) argues for another limitation he calls coding singularity. Within the selection region it is not possible to further scrutinize details, instead a single label is passed on for the entire region (Nakayama, 1990). Of course coding singularity is the basis for the acuity limit but the acuity limit determines the minimum selection region.

Visual orienting is an important model because of the close coordination between overt motor activity and internal covert selection. Overt and covert shifts of attention often go together. Shifts in gaze seem to be preceded by covert orienting of attention. This tight linkage between covert and overt orienting is supported by neuroimaging data showing extensive overlap in the corresponding brain regions. The behavioral and imaging data support the oculomotor readiness hypothesis (Klein, 1980; see also "pre-motor theory," Rizzolatti et al., 1987) stating that endogenous covert orienting is the preparation of an eye movement. However, the two predictions arising from this hypothesis, faster eye movements to attended locations and facilitated detection of events at locations to which an eye movement is being prepared, have not been completely supported (Klein, 2004; Hunt & Kingstone, 2003). It is possible that endogenous covert and overt orienting are isolable systems. Klein (2004) formulates three conclusions: "There is a tight linkage between saccade execution and covert visual orienting ... overt and covert orienting are exogenously activated by similar stimulus conditions (and) endogenous covert orienting of attention is not mediated by endogenously generated saccadic programming."

Although head or eye movements can achieve overt orienting, most research on overt orienting has concentrated on one type of eye movement, namely saccades. If subjects are required to perform a saccade to a peripheral target, the saccadic reaction time is shortened when a fixation or another peripheral signal is turned off shortly, about 100–200 ms, before the target appears (gap effect) (Schiller, Sandell, & Maunsell, 1987). Klein and colleagues (Klein & Kingstone, 1993; Taylor, Kingstone, & Klein, 1998) proposed a three-component-model explaining this pattern: An offset of any stimulus in the environment can increase alertness by functioning as a warning signal. As depicted above, reaction times decrease with increasing alertness. Also, because of the disappearance of a signal the oculomotor system will be exogenously disengaged and there has to be an endogenous disengagement of the oculomotor system as in the natural environment objects of fixation rarely disappears.

A task that is widely used to study endogenous control of overt orienting is the anti-saccade task in which a saccade away from a target is to be performed. However, Klein (2004) points out that this procedure is "messy" as it includes more than one endogenous orienting computation. The endogenous attentional computation as well as the endogenous execution of the saccade has to be performed. Additionally, an exogenously controlled saccade to the target has to be inhibited. The oculomotor capture paradigm (Theeuwes et al., 1998) explicitly enables exploration of the interaction between exogenous and endogenous orienting. Results of this research and the evidence provided above suggest a competition of endogenous and exogenous signals for control of the oculomotor system (Klein, 2004).

Another important characteristic of the orienting network is an inhibitory function. Inhibition in general in cognitive tasks is inferred from an increase in reaction time or an increased error rate. In orienting tasks when a peripheral cue is presented more than 300 ms before a target, inhibition takes place at the location of the cue and reaction time at that location increases. This effect called inhibition of return (IOR) (Posner & Cohen, 1984) suggested that the initial exogenous shift of attention to the cued location has been terminated and a return to that location is now inhibited. IOR can also be observed in tasks in which not only one peripheral cue is presented as described above (single-cue procedure) but also when a center cue is presented between the presentation of the peripheral cue and the target (double-cue procedure). Fuentes and colleagues (Fuentes, Vivas, & Humphreys, 1999) demonstrate that when more complex stimuli are presented at the cued location, and thus inhibited, they were less likely to elicit semantic priming compared to primes presented at an uncued location. These authors also applied Erikson's flanker paradigm (Erikson & Hoffman, 1972, 1973), which consists of the presentation of a central stimulus (e.g., an arrow) accompanied by either congruous (arrows pointing in the same direction) or incongruous (arrows pointing in the opposite direction) stimuli. When the flankers are presented at the cued location, contrary to the usual results, congruous flankers produced longer RTs compared to incongruous flankers. Fuentes (2004) called this effect inhibitory tagging, a mechanism temporally inhibiting "the links between the activated representations of inhibited stimuli and their appropriate response." Data from parietal and schizophrenic patients show that IOR and inhibitory tagging, although both affecting stimuli at already explored regions are separate inhibitory mechanisms (Vivas, Humphreys, & Fuentes, 2003; Fuentes et al., 2000). IOR fulfills an important function as it prevents re-examination of locations that have already been explored

(Klein, 2000). As alertness is increased with changing environmental conditions, it seems as if orienting and alerting bias the organism for novelty and change.

EXECUTIVE ATTENTION

An important vehicle for studying executive attention is to induce conflict between response tendencies particularly where the person is to execute the subdominant response while suppressing the dominant tendency (Botvinick et al., 2001). For example, in the Stroop task, a dominant because well-learned response (reading a color word) has to be oppressed in favor of a less dominant response (naming the color a word is printed in). The flanker task would be another example in which a target stimulus is surrounded either by congruent or incongruent flankers for a conflicting response situation. Executive attention is also required in error commission, in working memory tasks (Baddeley, 1993) or in problem solving.

Executive attention has been examined by developing neural network models. A theoretical model dealing with executive, controlling functions of attention has been presented by Cohen, Aston-Jones, and Gilzenrat (2004) by modifying an earlier model of the Stroop task (Cohen, Dunbar, & McClelland, 1990). The model is made up of units, which are organized in two pathways, a color naming pathway and a word pathway. Each pathway contains stimulus units projecting to associative units, which project to verbal response units. If the connections are stronger in the word pathway the model will be biased towards reading the word and not naming the color, similar to human behavior. To be able to also explain the human capability of overriding this prepotent response tendency – to name the color and not read the word – the model was modified. Task demand units were included each of which matches to a certain task (read a word or name the color). As these task demand units are connected to the associative units in the corresponding pathway, activation of a task demand unit will modulate the activity of these associative units and bias the system. It is now possible for the model to not read a word in favor of naming its color and thus to show executive control.

Similar models have been proposed to account for other functions of the executive attention network. Botvinick and colleagues (2004) demonstrated that adding a conflict monitoring unit to models of different tasks could account for behavioral and neuroscientific results, that occur with making an error.

Another approach to executive attention is to examine similarities between orienting to information in long-term memory and orienting to sensory information. A mechanism similar to inhibition of return in the orienting network has been described by Fuentes (2004). With sufficiently long intervals between the presentation of a semantically related prime and target (Neely, 1977) or the presentation of a semantically unrelated cue between prime and target (similar to the double cue procedure), negative priming was observed. Taken together with the results

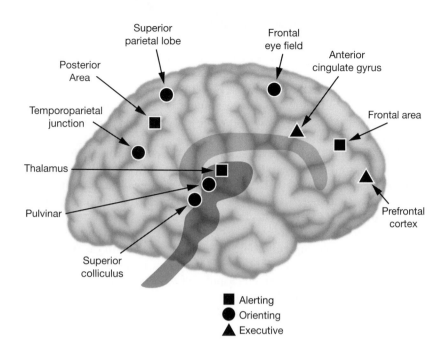

Figure 18.1. This figure illustrates brain areas involved in three attention networks. The alerting network (squares) includes thalamic and cortical sites related to the brain's norepinepherine system. The orienting network (circles) is centered on parietal sites (discussed in the following section) and the executive network (Triangles) includes the anterior cingulate and other frontal areas.

from studies (described above) examining how orienting and executive attention co-act when primes or flankers are presented at locations subject to IOR the bias for novelty seems to be "a pervasive property of the attention system" (Fuentes, 2004).

As indicated above cognitive theories of attention continue to be essential in understanding attentional phenomena, in the era of new methods such as neuroimaging.

ANATOMICAL NETWORKS

In this section we outline studies using all of the methods cited in our historical introduction to indicate the common anatomy and circuitry of attentional networks involved in alerting, orienting, and executive control. These are illustrated in cartoon form in Figure 18.1.

ORIENTING TO SENSORY EVENTS

The vast majority of studies of the physical basis of attention have involved orienting to sensory events, particularly visual events. The findings of these studies provide the basis for our limited understanding of how to approach brain mechanisms of attention. In this field a basic distinction is between those brain areas that are influenced by acts of orienting (sites) and those that are parts of the orienting network itself and thus the sources of the orienting influence. Although our discussion focuses mainly on vision, it is limited to the sources of the attention effect that appear to be similar in other modalities (Macaluso, Frith & Driver, 2000; Driver, Eimer, & Macaluso, 2004).

Sites and sources. Normally all sensory events act both to contribute to a state of alertness and to orient attention (Hebb, 1949). In order to distinguish the brain areas that are involved in orienting (See Figure 18.1) from the sites at

which they operate it is useful to separate the presentation of a cue indicating where a target will occur from the presentation of the target requiring a response (Posner, 1980; Corbetta & Shulman, 2002). This methodology has been used for behavioral studies with normal people (Posner, 1980); patients (Posner, 1988) and monkeys (Marrocco & Davidson, 1998); and in studies using scalp electrical recording (Hillyard, DiRusso, & Martinez, 2004) and event related neuroimaging (Corbetta & Shulman 2002).

Studies using event related fMRI have shown that following the presentation of the cue and before the target is presented a network of brain areas become active (Corbetta & Shulman, 2002; Kastner et al., 1999; Hillyard, DiRusso, & Martinez, 2004). These include the superior parietal lobe, temporal parietal junction and frontal eye fields shown in Figure 18.1. There is widespread agreement about the identity of these areas (see Orienting areas in Figure 18.1) but there remains a considerable amount of work to do in order to understand the function of each area.

When a target is presented at the cued location it is processed more efficiently than if no cue had been presented. The brain areas influenced by orienting will be those which that would normally be those used to process the target. For example, in the visual system orienting can influence sites of processing in the primary visual cortex, or, or in a variety of extra striate visual areas where the computations related to the target are performed. Orienting to target motion influences area MT (V5) while orienting to target color will influence area V4 (Corbetta et al., 1991). This principle of activation of brain areas also extends to higher-level visual input as well, for example, attention to faces modifies activity in the face sensitive area of the fusiform gyrus (Wojciulik, Kanwisher, & Driver, 1998). The finding that attention can modify activity in primary visual areas (Posner & Gilbert, 1999) has been of particularly important because the microcircuitry of this brain area has been more extensively studied than another other.

When multiple targets are presented they tend suppress the normal level of activity they would have produced if presented in isolation (Kastner et al., 1999). This finding has become the cornerstone of one of the most popular views of attention in which emphasis is placed on competition between potential targets within each relevant brain area (Desimone & Duncan, 1995). This view places less stress upon top-down control or at least emphasizes that top-down control emerges from bottom-up competition.

Functional anatomy. Work with stroke patients showed that lesions of many brain areas result in difficulty shifting attention to locations or objects that were conveyed directly to the damaged hemisphere (Rafal, 1998). In neurology these patients would be said to be suffering from extinction in that when simultaneous stimuli are presented to both hemispheres only the one going to the undamaged hemisphere is consciously perceived. Experimental studies suggested that we could define different forms of extinction due to lesions of the parietal lobe, the midbrain or the thalamus (Posner, 1988). Data in the 1980s suggested that operations of disengage (parietal lobe), move (superior colliculus), and engage (pulvinar) were computed in different brain areas that formed a vertical network that together performed the task of orienting.

More recent studies involving both patients and imaging seem to support this general approach to localization, but suggest somewhat different separation of the operations involved. A paradox of the lesions studies of the early 1980s was that the superior parietal lobe seemed to be the area most related to producing a difficulty in disengaging from a current focus of attention. Yet most clinical data seemed to support the idea that clinical extinction arose from more from lesions of the temporal-parietal junction. Event related imaging studies have served to reconcile this difference (Corbetta & Shulman, 2002). There seem to be two separate regions both of which can both produce difficulty in shifting attention in contralesional space, but for quite different reasons. Lesions of the temporal-parietal junction are important when a novel or unexpected stimulus occurs (Corbetta & Shulman, 2002; Friedrich et al., 1998; Karnath, Ferber, & Himmelbach, 2001). When functioning normally, this area allows disengaging from a current focus of attention to shift to the new event. This area is most critical in producing the core elements of the syndrome of neglect or extinction in both humans and monkeys although the exact location of the most critical area may differ between the two species. In addition, there is much clinical evidence that in the human there is lateralization in the right temporal parietal junction that may be more important to the deficit than the left (Mesulam, 1981; Perry & Zeki, 2000).

A different region, the superior parietal lobe, seems to be critical for voluntary shifts of attention following the cue. In one event-related fMRI study (Corbetta et al., 2000) this region was active following a cue informing the person to shift attention covertly to the target. The region is part of a larger network that includes frontal eye fields and the superior colliculus that appears to orchestrate both covert shift of attention and eye movements toward targets (Corbetta, 1998). When people voluntarily move their attention from location to location while searching for a visual target this brain area is also active.

There is evidence from other patient groups indicating brain areas involved in shifting attention. For example, patients with Alzheimer's disease involving degeneration in the superior parietal lobe (Parasurman et al., 1992) have difficulty in dealing with central cues that inform them to shift their attention. There is also evidence that lesions of the superior colliculus may be involved in the preference for novel locations rather than locations to which one has already oriented (Sapir et al., 1999). Patients with lesions of the thalamus (most likely the pulvinar) also show subtle deficits in visual-orienting tasks that may be related to the access to the ventral information-processing stream. It seems that a vertical network of brain areas related to voluntary eye movements and to processing novel input are critical elements of orienting, but a precise model including a role for all of these areas is still lacking.

It is also necessary to reexamine the role of alerting in the cueing effects. There has been a great deal of evidence that damage to the right frontal lobe and to the right parietal lobe can produce difficulty in maintaining the alert state (for a summary see Posner & Petersen, 1990). However, recent work with fMRI has indicated that using a cue to warn a subject that a target will occur shortly activates a left hemisphere network (Coull et al., 1996; Coull, Nobre, & Frith, 2001; Nobre, 2004). Thus there are apparently roles for both the right a left hemisphere in the alerting process. It appears that right hemisphere centers are most important for tonic alertness, but the left hemisphere areas may play a more important role in phasic alerting produced by warning signals.

Circuitry. Cellular studies have shown that attention toward the location of an impending target can alter the baseline of cellular activity (Desimone & Duncan, 1995). This finding suggests that cuing attention to a location can induce changes in the visual system that altar the processing of a target. Evidence from high-density electrical activity suggests that cuing attention influences prestriate activity occurring 100–150 milliseconds after input. This information may in some circumstances then be fed back to influence activity within the primary visual cortex and perhaps also the thalamic relays of the visual information (O'Connor et al., 2002). These studies suggest a circuitry by which parietal activity can influence the visual analysis of a visual target, but direct evidence linking the more dorsal attention system with the more ventral object analysis system is still lacking.

The study of visual orienting has provided strong evidence that scalp recording can give an accurate time course for the operation of generators found active in fMRI studies. Hillyard and associates (Hillyard, DiRusso, & Martinez, 2004) have exploited the fact that early visual areas are retinotopically organized. They have identified an early ERP component (C1) with the primary visual cortex operation at 50 or so milliseconds after input, they have shown that posterior P1 and N1 arise in prestriate areas. This work has led to the interesting finding that a cue to location does not influence the initial V1 activity but is fed back to influence later striate cortex component (Martinez et al., 2001).

It is likely that we still do not have the final answer as to the exact operations that occur at each location even in a relatively simple act like shifting attention to a novel event. Nonetheless, the data provide considerable convergence between clinical, neurophysiological, imaging and cognitive methods. The results of attentional studies as with many other areas of cognition support the general idea of localization of component operations.

Transmitters. It is very important to be able to link the neurosystem results, that suggest brain areas related to attention, with cellular and synaptic studies that provide more details as to the local computations. One strategy for doing so is to study the pharmacology of each of the attention networks (Marrocco & Davidson, 1998). To carry out these tests it is important to be able to study monkeys who are able to use cues to direct attention to targets. Fortunately cueing studies can be run successfully in monkeys.

A series of pharmacological studies with alert monkeys have related each of the attentional networks we have discussed with specific chemical neuromodulators (Davidson & Marrocco, 2000; Marrocco & Davidson, 1998). The component of alerting related to the influence of warning signal appears to involve the cortical distribution of the brain's norepinephrine (NE) system arising in the locus coeruleus of the midbrain. Drugs like clonidine and guanfacine that act to block NE, reduce or eliminate the normal effect of warning signals on reaction time, but have no influence on orienting to the target location (Marrocco & Davidson, 1998).

Cholinergic systems arising in the basal forebrain play a critical and important role in orienting. Lesions of the basal forebrain in monkeys interfere with orienting attention (Voytko et al., 1994). However, it does not appear that the site of this effect is in the basal forebrain. Instead it appears to involve the superior parietal lobe. Injections of scopolamine directly into the lateral interparietal area of monkeys, a brain area containing cells, which are influenced by cues about spatial location, have been shown to have a large effect on the ability to shift attention to a target. Systemic injections of scopolamine have a smaller effect on effect on covert orienting of attention than do local injections in the parietal area (Davidson & Marrocco, 2000). Cholinergic drugs do not affect the ability of a warning signal to improve performance and thus there appears to be double dissociation that relates NE to the alerting

network and Ach (actylcholine) to the orienting network. These observations in the monkey have also been confirmed by similar studies in the rat (Everitt & Robbins, 1997) and by studies of nicotine in humans. Of special significance in the rat, studies comparisons of the cholinergic and dopaminergic mechanisms have shown that only the former influence the orienting response.

The evidence relating Ach to the orienting network and NE to the alerting network provides strong evidence of dissociation between the different attentional networks. In the next section we show that the frontal executive network is closely related to dopamine as a neural modulator.

EXECUTIVE ATTENTION NETWORK

Executive control is most needed in situations which situations, which involve planning or decision-making, error detection, novel responses, and in overcoming habitual actions (Shallice, 1988). Although these concepts are somewhat vague, a more explicit version of the idea of executive attention stresses the role of attention in monitoring conflict between computations occurring in different brain areas (Botvinick et al., 2001). Although this view may not be adequate to explain all of the existing data, it provides a useful model for summarizing much of what is known.

Functional anatomy. A very large number of functional imaging studies have examined tasks that involve executive attention. These "thinking" tasks often activate a wide range of frontal areas. For example, (Duncan et al., 2000) examined verbal, spatial and object tasks selected from intelligence tests that all had in common a strong loading on the factor of general intelligence (g). These items were contrasted with perceptually similar control items that did not require the kind of attention and thought involved in problem solving. This subtraction led to differential activity in two major areas. One was the anterior cingulate and the second was lateral prefrontal cortex.

Moreover, manipulations of the content of material have often shown that the same areas may be active irrespective of whether the stimuli are spatial, verbal, or visual objects. This has led some to conclude that the frontal lobes may be an exception to the specific identification of brain areas with mental operations that we have discussed for orienting (Duncan & Owen, 2000).

A specific comparison of three conflict tasks within one study (Stroop, spatial conflict, and flanker) showed two areas of common activation by the three tasks (Fan et al., 2003). These were the anterior cingulate and a left lateralized area of the prefrontal cortex (area 10). A summary of many imaging studies using the Stroop task or variants of it that involved conflict among elements (Bush, Luu, & Posner, 2000) showed consistent action in the dorsal anterior cingulate.

An event-related functional MRI study of the Stroop effect used cues to separate presentation of the task instruction from reaction to the target (McDonald et al., 2000). Lateral prefrontal areas were responsive to cues indicating whether the task involved naming the word or dealing with the ink color. The cue did not activate the cingulate. When the task involved naming the ink color the cingulate was more active on incongruent than congruent trials. This result reflects the general finding that lateral areas are involved in representing specific information over time (working memory), whereas medial areas are more related to the detection of conflict.

Another cue to the functional activity in these areas comes from studies of generating the use of a word. In a typical version of this task, subjects are shown a series of forty simple nouns (e.g., hammer) (Raichle et al., 1994). In the experimental condition they indicate the use of each noun (for example, hammer -> pound). In the control condition, they simply read the word aloud. The difference in activation between the two tasks illustrates what happens in the brain when subjects are required to develop a very simple thought, in this case how to use a hammer. Practice that is sufficient to automatize the responses results in eliminating the activation of the anterior cingulate and lateral areas, but increases activity in the anterior insula which is active during word reading, but reduced during generating a new use. These results illustrate that the anatomy of this high-level cognitive activity is similar enough among individuals to produce focal average activations that are both statistically significant and reproducible.

Circuitry. To examine the time course of these activations it is possible to use a large number of scalp electrodes to obtain scalp signatures of the generators found active in imaging studies. (Abdullaev & Posner, 1998). When subjects obtain the use of a noun, there is an area of positive electrical activity over frontal electrodes starting about 150 milliseconds after the word appears. This early electrical activity is generated by the large area of activation in the anterior cingulate.

A left prefrontal area (anterior to the classical Broca's area) begins to show activity about 200 milliseconds after the word occurs. This area appears to be activated when the task involves a semantic content, but the early time course of the activation and its close relation to the cingulate seem to make it more related to attention to semantic content. The left posterior brain area found to be more active during the processing of the meaning of visual words did not appear until a much later time (500 milliseconds). This activity is near the classical Wernicke's area; lesions of which are known to produce a loss of understanding of meaningful speech. An examination of correlations among distant electrodes showed evidence of the transfer of information from left frontal electrodes to the posterior area at about 450 milliseconds into the task (Nikolaev et al., 2002).Because the response time for this task was about 1,100 milliseconds this would leave time for the generation of related associations needed to solve the task.

These studies provide a start in understanding the functional roles of different brain areas in carrying out executive control. The medial frontal area appears most related to the executive attention network and is active when there is conflict among stimuli and responses. It may be serving as a monitor of conflict, but it is possible that it plays other roles as well. The lateral prefrontal area seems to be important in holding in mind the information relevant to the task. Even when a single item is presented, it may still be necessary to hold it in some temporary area while other [whereas is not correct while means at the same time as] brain areas retrieve information relevant to the response. Together these two areas are needed to solve nearly any problem, that depends upon attention to the retrieval of stored information. Both of these areas could be said to be related to attention, or one might identify only the medial area with attention and the lateral one with working memory. In either case they begin to give us a handle on how the brain parses high tasks into individual operations that are carried out in separate parts of the network.

Lesion studies. Classical studies of strokes of the frontal midline including the anterior cingulate showed a pervasive deficit of voluntary behavior (Damasio, 1994; Kennard, 1955). Patients with akinetic mutism can orient to external stimuli and follow people with their eyes, but they do not initiate voluntary activity. Recent studies of patients with small lesions of the anterior cingulate (Ochsner et al., 2001; Turken & Swick, 1999) show deficits in conflict related tasks, but these patients frequently recover from their deficits suggesting that other areas may also be involved. In some cases lesions of the mid frontal area in children and adults may produce permanent loss of future planning and appropriate social behavior (Damasio, 1994). Early-childhood damage in this area can produce permanent deficits in decision-making tasks that require responses based on future planning (Anderson et al., 2000).

Cellular mechanisms. The anterior cingulate and lateral frontal cortex are target areas of the ventral tegmental dopamine system. All of the dopamine receptors are expressed in layer five of the cingulate, which in turn is connected to many other important cortical areas (Goldman-Rakic, 1988).

The association of the anterior cingulate with high-level attentional control may seem rather odd because this is clearly a phylogenetically old area of the brain. Although the anterior cingulate is an ancient structure, there is evidence that it has evolved significantly in primates. Humans and great apes appear to have a unique cell type found mainly in layer V of the anterior cingulate and insula, a cell type not present in other primates (Nimchinsky et al., 1999). These cells also undergo a rather late development in line with the findings that executive control systems develop strongly during later childhood (Allman, 2001) (see also next section). Although the precise function of this cell is not known, high correlations between its volume and encephalization suggest a likely role in higher cortical functioning. The proximity of these cells to vocalization areas in primates led Nimchinksy and colleagues to speculate that these cells may link emotional and motor areas, ultimately resulting in vocalizations that convey emotional meaning. There is as yet no direct evidence linking the cellular architecture of the anterior cingulate to activity detected during neuroimaging studies.

Several replicated human genetic studies demonstrate an association of one of the dopamine receptor genes D4 (DRD4) located on chromosome 11p15.5 and an attentional disorder common in childhood (attention deficit/hyperactivity disorder or ADHD) (Swanson et al., 2000). About 50% of the ADHD cases have a 7-repeat allele whereas only about 20% ethnically matched control subjects have a 7-repeat allele. However, a direct comparison of children with ADHD who either have or do not have the 7 repeat allele suggest that attentional abnormalities are more common in those children without the 7 repeat (Swanson et al., 2000). The authors suggest that there are different routes to ADHD only some of which involve a specific reduction in cognitive ability.

INDIVIDUAL DIFFERENCES

Although there is strong evidence of common networks underlying cognitive processes, there are also individual differences in details that influence the efficiency of these networks. Individual differences are likely to reflect both genes and experience. The rapid development of fMRI methods has begun to provide a basis for understanding differences among individual brains both anatomically and in terms of functional activations. These differences are to be expected because people are not identical in their thoughts, feelings, or behaviors. Several studies have shown that individual differences in functional activation can be reliably assessed (Miller et al., 2002; Reiss, Backus, & Heeger, 2000).

To study these individual differences an attention networks test (ANT) has been used to examine the efficiency of the three brain networks we have described in the previous section (Fan et al., 2002). As illustrated in Figure 18.2 the test provides three scores that represent the skill of each individual in the alerting, orienting, and executive networks. In a sample of 40 normal persons each of these scores were reliable over repeated presentations.

The ability to measure differences in attention among adults raises the question of the degree to which attention is heritable. In order to deal with this issue, the attention network test was used to study 26 pairs of monozygotic and 26 pairs of dyzygotic same sex twins (Fan, Fossella, & Posner, 2001). Strong correlations between the monozygotic twins for the executive network, led to an estimate of heritability of the executive network of .89. Because of the small sample, the estimate of 95% confidence interval for heritability is between .3 and .9. In fact a more recent study

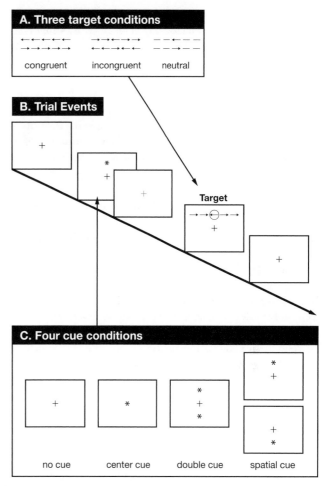

Figure 18.2. A schematic of the Attention Network Test. The task requires a left key press when the central arrow points left and a right key press when it points right. The arrow is surrounded by flankers is pointing in the same (congruent) or opposite direction (incongruent). Before the target cues inform the person of when and where a target will appear. At the bottom of the figure are three subtractions that yield information on the efficiency of three attentional networks. (Adapted from Fan et al., 2002).

using a somewhat different task has failed to show heritability among children with the flanker task (Stins et al., 2004), although they did find substantial heritability with another executive attention task, the Stroop task. Possibly this discrepancy related to the importance of errors in the child data. Nonetheless, these data overall support a role for genes in executive attention.

The Attention Network Test (ANT see Figure 18.1) has been used to examine candidate genes related to chemical neuromodulators of attentional networks. Alleles of two cholinergic genes have been found to influence a visual search task related to the orienting network (Parasuraman, Greenwood, Kumar, & Fossella, 2004), whereas alleles of several dopamine genes influence performance in the flanker task and when compared produced a significant difference in activation in the anterior cingulate (Fossella et al., 2002; Fan et al., 2003). Alleles of additional gene (COMT) have been found to relate to a different conflict related phenotype (Diamond et al., 2004).

Studies have also examined the role of genetic differences in the strength of activation of networks involved in attention and memory in fMRI studies (Mattay & Goldberg, 2004). These studies demonstrate that at least part of the variability in strength of activation is due to having different versions (alleles) of genes related to the network.

Genetic differences observed to date account for only a small part of the variance found in behavior and imaging. However, a major contribution of these differences is that they serve as clues to the genes involved in network development. These genes can be examined in comparative animal studies to address questions like how genes related to hippocampal development may have affected behavior in species even before there was a hippocampus. These genes can also be examined in species for which the hippocampus plays a role in forms of memory that may be precursors of the explicit recollection found to be its role in humans. In the case of the DRD4 gene, which in humans is related to attention deficit disorder (Swanson et al., 2000) and to the normal monitoring of conflict in the mouse, seems to be related to exploration of the environment (Grandy & Kruzich, 2004; Han, Touathaigh, & Koch, 2004). These studies have the potential of improving our understanding of the role of genes in shaping the networks common to all humans.

Gene by environment interactions. One reason for the relatively modest effect of genetic alleles in accounting for behavioral differences may be that they interact with experience during development of the network. The existence of gene by environment interaction is not controversial, and it is well known that gene expression can be influenced by the microenvironment in the brain area where it is expressed. Moreover, there is ample evidence that in primates, gene expression can be influenced by events, which, like maternal separation, can be a part of human development (Soumi, 2003). These findings make more important the examination of how attentional networks actually develop during infancy and childhood, a topic to which we turn in the next section.

DEVELOPING NETWORKS OF ATTENTION

A study using the child version of the attention network test (Rueda et al., 2004), examined the development of the attentional networks in a cross-sectional study involving 6– and 10-year-old children and adults. Results indicated no changes in the orienting scores in the age range studied, whereas alertness showed evidence of change up to and beyond age 10. Executive attention measured by conflict resolution scores appeared stable after age 7 up to adulthood. These findings are placed in context below.

Orienting

Studies of orienting summarized in Ruff and Rothbart (1996) have suggested that only voluntary movement speed and the accuracy of termination continue to improve in late childhood. The ANT involves a very simple sense of orienting to visual locations that uses the ability of a peripheral cue to redirect attention to one of two places above and below fixation and therefore, would appear to be a task whose requirements would suggest an early developmental course. Most of the work in this area, including developmental studies summarized by Trick and Enns (1998) compares valid and invalid cue conditions (cost plus benefit) and thus provide stronger evidence of the time to disengage and reorient from an attended location. Studies made under conditions where orienting involved an invalid cue and thus required a voluntary shift of attention have shown that the time to disengage from a cued location is reduced with age, but the movement of attention toward a peripheral cue shows no change between six year olds and adults (Akhtar & Enns, 1989). They also found that children show a strong tendency for an interaction between orienting and conflict that is reduced between 5-year-olds and adults.

Alerting

During the first year of life, children show a remarkable development of their ability to achieve and maintain alert states. However, there are still considerable differences between children and adults in both speed of preparation from alerting cues and maintenance of that preparation (Morrison, 1982). Both preparation and vigilance might be playing a role in the differences found in alertness among children and adults in the child ANT study. These phasic and tonic aspects of alertness may influence RT when alertness is measured by comparing trials with and without warning cues. Age differences in preparation certainly affect RT to cued trials, whereas differences in vigilance might affect non-cued trials.

A study by Berger, et al. (2000) showed that 5-year-old children reduce their reaction time to stimuli that are preceded by an alert cue although, unlike the adults, children showed reduced RT benefits with cue-target intervals greater than 500 ms, suggesting increased difficulty for children to maintain preparation produced by the alerting cue. Moreover, young children have increased difficulty compared to older children and adults when dealing with situations that require more complex strategies to prepare, as when the interval between the alert cue and the target varies across trials.

On the other hand, Lin, Hsiao, and Chen (1999) examined sustained attention abilities in 6–15 year-olds using the Continuous Performance Test (CPT). They found progressive improvement in performance (measured by hits and false alarms) with age, reaching asymptotic levels around age 13. The percentage of children that complete the CPT at preschool ages is informative of their ability to sustain attention. Levy (1980) found that less than 50% of the children between 3 and 4 years of age were able to complete the test, whereas the percentage increased to 70% for children between 4 and $4\frac{1}{2}$ years old and was close to 100% after that age.

The influence of phasic and tonic components on the efficiency of alertness has been compared between 6 and 10 year-olds and adults (Rueda et al., in process). In this experiment, participants performed 4 blocks of trials of a Go/No-Go task with a low percentage (25%) of Go trials. To examine differences in phasic alertness the presence (75% of the trials) or absence (25% of the trials) and the time interval (simultaneous, short, and long) between the warning cue and the target were all manipulated. Compared to trials with no warning cue, children and adults showed reduced RT to targets preceded by a cue, but only adults showed reduced RT when cue and target were presented simultaneously. In this experiment, both 6- and 10-year-old children showed a continuous increase in RT across blocks, whereas adults had equivalent RTs in all blocks. In addition, 6-year-old children showed greater percentage of omissions than 10 year-olds and adults. Interestingly, this difference was significant only when no warning cue was presented or when cue and target were presented simultaneously, whereas no age differences were found when the warning cue preceded the target, especially at long cue-target intervals. Taken together, these results suggest that children seem to have greater difficulty than adults sustaining attention during extended task performance. This difference appears to be more remarkable for young children, although their reduced vigilance can be overcome by presenting warning cues with some time in advance. The influence of warning signals on performance may vary with age because of the greater difficulty children have in retaining the set toward task instructions.

Executive attention

The finding of little or no development in the executive network after age 7 in the child ANT study may not extend to more difficult executive tasks as those involving strategic decisions or other functions like rule-holding, planning, set switching, and so on. However, developmental studies of executive attention have shown the greater development of conflict resolution to happen between 2 and 6 years of age (Rueda, Posner, & Rothbart, submitted).

Infant studies have stressed the relative lack of executive control during the first year of life (Ruff & Rothbart, 1996). However, a sign of the control of cognitive conflict is found at the end of the first year of life. Infants younger than 12 months fail to search for an object hidden in a location when previously trained to reach for the object in a different location. After the first year, children develop the ability to inhibit the prepotent response toward the trained location, and successfully reach for the object in the new location (Diamond, 1991).

From two years of age and older, children are able to perform simple conflict tasks in which their reaction time can be measured. The Spatial Conflict Task (SCT; Gerardi-Caulton, 2000) induces conflict between the identity and the location of an object. Between 2 and 4 years of age, children progressed from an almost complete inability to carry out the task to relatively good performance.

Although 2-year-old children tended to perseverate on a single response, 3 year-olds performed at high accuracy levels, although, like adults, they responded more slowly and with reduced accuracy to incompatible trials (Gerardi-Caulton, 2000; Rothbart et al., 2003). The detection and correction of errors is another form of action monitoring. While performing the SCT, 2 1/2 and 3-year-old children showed longer RT following erroneous trials than following correct ones, indicating that children were noticing their errors and using them to guide performance in the next trial. However, no evidence of slowing following an error was found at 2 years of age (Rothbart et al., 2003). A similar result with a different time frame was found when using a version of the Simple Simon game. In this task, children are asked to execute a response when a command is given by one stuffed animal, while inhibiting responses commanded by a second animal (Jones, Rothbart, & Posner, 2003). Children of 36–38 months were unable to inhibit their response and showed no slowing following an error, but at 39–41 months, children showed both an ability to inhibit and a slowing of reaction time following an error. These results suggest that between 30 and 39 months children greatly develop their ability to detect and correct erroneous responses and that this ability may relate to the development of inhibitory control.

The importance of being able to study the emergence of executive attention is enhanced because cognitive measures of conflict resolution in these laboratory tasks have been linked to aspects of children's temperament. Signs of the development of executive attention by cognitive tasks relate to a temperamental measure obtained from caregiver reports called effortful control (Gerardi-Caulton, 2000; Rothbart, Ellis, & Posner, 2004). Children relatively less affected by conflict received higher parental ratings of temperamental effortful control and higher scores on laboratory measures of inhibitory control (Gerardi-Caulton, 2000). We regard effortful control as reflecting the efficiency with which the executive attention network operates in naturalistic settings.

Empathy is strongly related to effortful control, with children high in effortful control showing greater empathy (Rothbart, Ahadi, & Hershey, 1994). To display empathy towards others requires that we interpret their signals of distress or pleasure. Imaging work in normals shows that sad faces activate the amygdala. As sadness increases, this activation is accompanied by activity in the anterior cingulate as part of the attention network (Blair et al., 1999). It seems likely that the cingulate activity represents the basis for our attention to the distress of others.

Developmental studies have identified different routes to the successful development of conscience. The internalization of moral principles appears to be facilitated in fearful preschool-aged children, especially when their mothers use gentle discipline (Kochanska, 1995). A strongly reactive amygdala would provide the signals of distress that would easily allow empathic feelings toward others and improve socialization abilities. In the absence of this form of control development of the cingulate would allow appropriate attention to the signals provided by amygdala activity. Consistent with its influence on empathy, effortful control also appears to play a role in the development of conscience. In addition, internalized control is facilitated in children high in effortful control (Kochanska et al., 1996). Thus, two separable control systems, one reactive (fear) and one self-regulative (effortful control) appear to regulate the development of conscience.

Some developmental studies have been carried out using ERPs and conflict tasks aimed at understanding the brain mechanisms that underlie the development of executive attention. In one of these studies, a flanker task was used to compare conflict resolution in three groups of children aged 5 to 6, 7 to 9, and 10 to 12, and a group of adults (Ridderinkhof & van der Molen, 1995). In this study, developmental differences were examined in two ERP components, one related to response preparation (LRP) and another one related to stimulus evaluation (P3). The authors found differences between children and adults in the latency of the LRP, but not in the latency of the P3 peak, suggesting that developmental differences in the ability to resist interference are mainly related to response competition and inhibition, but not to stimulus evaluation.

In adult studies, the N2 has been related to situations that require executive control (Kopp, Rist, & Mattler, 1996) and has been directly associated to activation coming from the anterior cingulate cortex (van Veen & Carter, 2002). We have recently conducted an ERP study in which we used the child-friendly version of the flanker task used in the child ANT study with 4-year-old children and adults (Rueda et al., 2004). Adults showed larger N2 for incongruent trials over the mid frontal leads. Four-year-old children also showed a larger negative deflection for the incongruent condition at the mid frontal electrodes that, compared to adults, had a larger size, greater amplitude, and were extended over a longer period of time. Whereas the frontal effect was evident for adults at around 300 ms post-target, children did not show any effect until approximately 550 ms after the target. In addition, the effect was sustained over a period of 500 ms before the children's responses, in contrast with only 50 ms in the case of adults. The difference observed between children and adults over the frontal channels differed from other components observed at mid parietal channels. For both children and adults, we found a greater positivity for incongruent trials over mid parietal leads. For adults, this effect was observed at approximately 400 ms post-target, in the time window of the P3, whereas it was more delayed in the case of children (between 800 and 1100 ms post-target). This parietal effect could reflect developmental differences in the difficulty of evaluating the display depending on the congruence of surrounding flankers, while the frontal effect could reveal differences in the time course of conflict resolution.

Another important difference between 4-year-old children and adults was the distribution of effects over the scalp. In adults, the frontal effects appear to be focalized on the mid-line, whereas in children the effects were observed mostly at pre-frontal sites and in a broader number of channels, including the mid-line and lateral areas. In addition, the effect on the P3 appears to be left lateralized in the adult data but lateralized to the right side in the children. The focalization of signals in adults as compared to children is consistent with neuroimaging studies conducted with older children, where children appear to activate the same network of areas as adults when performing similar tasks, but the average volume of activation appears to be remarkably greater in children compared to adults (Casey et al., 1997; Durston et al., 2002; Casey et al., 2002). Altogether, these data suggest that the brain circuitry underlying executive functions becomes more focal and refined as it gains in efficiency. This maturational process involves not only greater anatomical specialization but also reducing the time these systems need to resolve each of the processes implicated in the task.

ATTENTIONAL PATHOLOGIES

Attention is a very frequent symptom of many forms of psychopathology. However, without a real understanding of the neural substrates of attention, this has been a somewhat empty classification. This situation has been changed with the systematic application of our understanding of attentional networks to pathological issues. Viewing attention in terms of underlying neural networks provides a means of classifying disorders that differs from the usual DSM IV symptom related criteria. A number of abnormalities involving attention, including Alzheimer's dementia, anxiety, attention deficit hyperactivity disorder (ADHD), autism, borderline personality disorder, depression, and schizophrenia have been studied either with the attention network task (Fan et al., 2002), that measures the efficiency of all three networks (see Figure 18.2) or with parts of the task that measure one or two of the networks. These studies have shown that different disorders are associated with problems in different networks, although there is not a one to one relation between diagnosis and disorder. Below we review a number of common disorders in relation to abnormalities in attentional networks.

ALERTING

Patients with anterior and posterior right hemisphere damage have problems when tasks are given without warning (Posner et al., 1987; Robertson et al., 1998). This arises because patients, like young children, have very long RTs in the absence of warning. Robertson has argued that the inability to maintain the alert state absent a warning signal is a major contributor to the reduced attention to the side of space opposite the lesion found more strongly in patients with right than with left posterior lesions.

A study using the ANT has shown that normal elderly persons also show dramatically larger alerting effects than young adults, resembling what is found with children

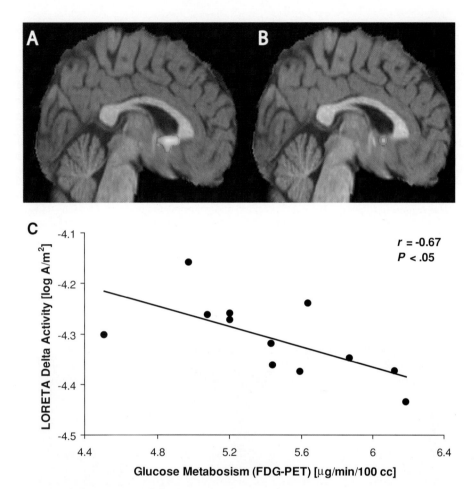

Plate 1. Reciprocal relation between delta activity and glucose metabolism. In a recent study integrating concurrently recorded electric (28-channel scalp EEG) and metabolic ([^{18}F]-2-fluoro-2-deoxy-D-glucose positron emission tomography, FDG-PET) measures of brain activity, melancholic depression was characterized by (A) significantly increased delta current density (see yellow-red colors), as assessed with LORETA (see Section 8.2.3.); and (B) significantly decreased glucose metabolism (see blue colors). Statistical maps are thresholded at P < .05 (corrected) and displayed on a representative structural MRI. In psychiatrically healthy subjects, a significant negative correlation between delta current density and glucose metabolism in the subgenual prefrontal cortex emerged (C). Adapted from Pizzagalli et al. (2004) with permission.

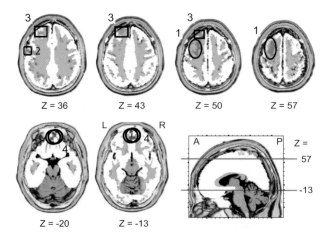

Plate 2. Example of LORETA findings highlighting relations between resting intracerebral EEG sources and approach-related behavior. Whole-brain analyses showing voxel-by-voxel correlations between resting alpha2 (10.5–12 Hz) current density and response bias toward reward-related cues for 18 healthy subjects. Six axial brain slices (head seen from above, nose up, L = left, R = right; A = anterior, P = posterior) are shown. Alpha2 current density within both dorsolateral prefrontal regions (clusters #1–3; see green colors) and ventromedial prefrontal regions (cluster #4; see blue colors) was negatively correlated with reward bias, indicating that higher resting activity within these regions was associated with stronger reward bias. Adapted from Pizzagalli et al. (2005).

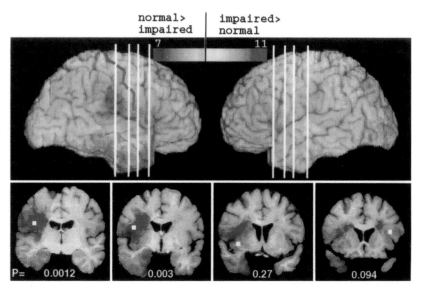

Plate 3. Lesion overlap map created with Map-3. In this study 108 subjects performed emotion recognition task. Color (*scale* at *top*) encodes the difference in the density of lesions between the subjects with the lowest and those with the highest scores. Thus, *red regions* correspond to locations at which lesions resulted in impairment more often than not, and *blue regions* correspond to locations at which lesions resulted in normal performance more often than not. *p* values indicating statistical significance are shown in *white* for voxels in four regions (*white squares*) on coronal cuts (*bottom*) that correspond to the *white vertical lines* in the 3-D reconstructions (*top*). (From Adolphs et al., 2000, used with permission.)

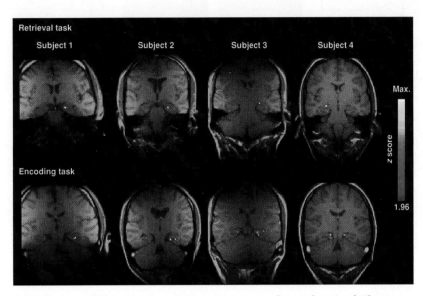

Plate 4. Mesial temporal lobe activations during memory encoding and retrieval. The top row shows activations in the subiculum of the hippocampus during the retrieval memory task that were greater for words corresponding to previously seen than unseen line drawings (Subjects 1, 2, and 3) or greater for line drawings corresponding to previously seen than unseen words (Subject 4). The bottom row shows activations in the parahippocampal cortex during the encoding memory task that were greater for novel than for repeated color scenes (Subjects 1, 2, and 3) or greater for novel than for repeated line drawings (Subject 4). (From Gabrieli et al., 1997, used with permission.)

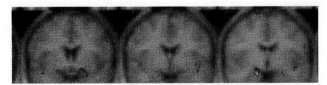

Plate 5. Bilateral activation of amygdala in response to subliminal presentation of fearful faces compared to happy faces (From Whalen et al., 1998, used with permission).

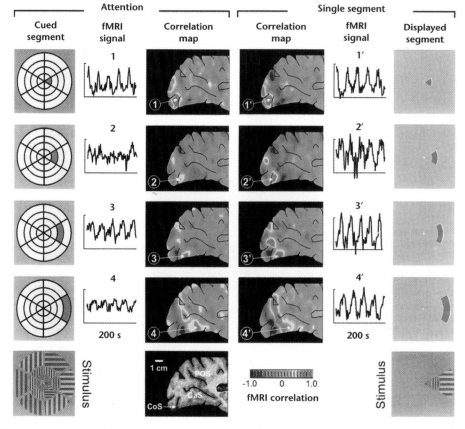

Plate 6. Retinotopic attentional modulation compared to activation evoked by cued targets alone. Cued segment (left column) shows schematic sequence of target segments cued for attentional scrutiny. Stimulus (bottom left) is actual target array. FMRI signal (left) shows signal modulation of individual voxels at sites indicated on adjacent correlation maps. Temporal phase shift of the signal at each site identifies the corresponding locus of attention. Correlation maps show sites where timing of modulation was positively correlated (red) or anti-correlated (blue) with the timing of attentional shifts. Displayed segment (right column) shows schematic sequence of single segments presented during otherwise identical control experiment. Composite of single segments shown in stimulus bottom right. FMRI Signal and correlation map on right show results of control experiment. Structural MRI (bottom) is a parasagittal section (13.6 mm left of midline) through occipital lobe in same plane as correlation maps. Sulcal landmarks; CaS, calcarine sulcus; CoS, collateral sulcus; POS; parieto-occipital sulcus. (From Brefczynski and DeYoe, 1999, used with permission)

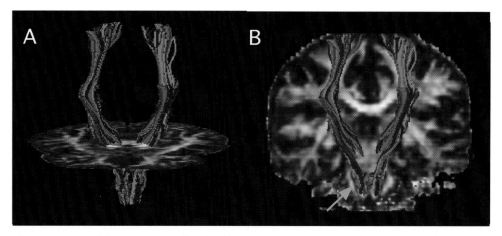

Plate 7. Image of the cortico-spinal path of humans using DTI. These figures show in blue, corticospinal fibers going from cortical motor and sensory areas, in their way to brain-stem and spinal cord. **a.** Descending fibers shown in three dimensions, crossing through an axial structural MRI. **b.** Same fibers superimposed to a coronal MRI slice. Note how the right and left parts of the pathway get close together at the level of the medulla where they will cross over to the contralateral side. *Courtesy of K. Arfanakis. Department of Biomedical Engineering. Illinois Institute of Technology (IIT).*

(Fernandez-Duque & Black, in press). The study also found that the normally developing adults and Alzheimer's patients showed the same elevated alerting scores, but only the Alzheimer's patients showed increased difficulty in resolving conflict (see executive attention section).

ADHD. Studies of ADHD have linked the disorder to aspects of both attention and sensation seeking (Swanson et al., 2001). Many theories of ADHD have suggested a deficit in executive functions (Barkley, 1997). However, in early work using a spatial orienting task, the most compelling deficit appeared to be a difficulty in maintaining the alert state in the absence of a warning signal (Swanson et al., 1991). This difficulty might arise from right hemisphere damage, which has also been reported to be a feature in many studies of ADHD.

More recent studies using the ANT have also shown problems with alerting, again mostly due to the inability to hold the alert state when no warning signal was used. In one study (Booth, Carlson, & Tucker, 2002), the ANT was used to attempt to discriminate the inattentive subtype from normals and the combined subtype. The alerting network best distinguished the different forms of ADHD, with inattentive children showing less ability to maintain the alert state in the absence of warning signals.

Neuroimaging studies of ADHD children have generally shown right frontal, cingulate and basal ganglia deficits (Casey et al., 1997). Because right frontal areas have been related both to problems with the alert state and with inhibitory control there could be links between the ANT results and these imaging studies, but this research has not yet been conducted.

Casey, Durston, and Fossella (2001) used three different tasks that rely upon different processes (stimulus selection, response selection, and response execution) to analyze executive functions in different types of developmental disorders (Schizophrenia, Sydenham's Chorea, Tourette's Syndrome, and ADHD). They suggest that each of the cognitive operations is implemented in a particular basal ganglia-thalamo-cortical circuit. Stimulus processing seems to be related to connections between basal ganglia, thalamus and the dorso-lateral prefrontal cortex, whereas response processing is associated with connections of sub-cortical structures to the lateral orbital frontal cortex. Schizophrenic patients exhibited deficits in stimulus election, Sydenham's chorea in response selection, Tourette's syndrome children in response execution, and ADHD children in both stimulus selection and response execution, suggesting that specific cognitive operations related to executive attention can be independently damaged.

For a number of years it has been thought that ADHD related to problems with dopamine and other catecholamine (Wender, 1971). In molecular genetics research, the dopamine theory found support in replicated findings that one allele (7 repeat) of the dopamine 4 receptor gene is over-represented in children with ADHD and also is associated with a temperament featuring high sensation seeking

(see Swanson et al., 2001 for a recent summary). Sensation seeking is a lower order construct of extraversion. This finding has been well replicated for the syndrome of ADHD, but has not been found to produce a cognitive deficit in executive function (Swanson et al., 2000). One study of children with and without the 7 repeat allele confirmed it is associated with ADHD, but showed that it was not associated with the cognitive deficit that usually accompanies ADHD (Swanson et al., 2000). This finding led to the suggestion that there may be two routes to ADHD. One route would involve a temperamental extreme of sensation seeking (or extraversion), the frequency of which might be increased by the presence of the repeat version of the Dopamine 4 receptor gene. This route need not involve a cognitive deficit. A second route to ADHD would involve cognitive deficits that might either be genetic, or due to early brain injury or other experiential factors.

ORIENTING

Anxiety and depression. There is much new information explicating the role of attention in anxiety, depression, and mood disorders. In a series of studies, sub-clinical college students with high scores on trait anxiety were cued to attend to a location by a positive, negative, or neutral face. Trials on which the cue to the location was negative and invalid produced longer reaction times for the trait anxiety subjects (Fox, Ricardo, & Dutton, 2002; Fox et al., 2001). These results replicate and extend previous studies by Derryberry and Reed (1994), and together they suggest that trait anxiety influences the ability to disengage particularly from threat stimuli. Derryberry and Reed suggest that this finding may be dependent upon relatively low levels of effortful control. Those subjects high in effortful control but suffering from depression did not have difficulty disengaging from negative affect.

A symptom of depression is the tendency to dwell on negative ideation (Beck, 1976). Vasey and Macleod (2001) have reviewed recent studies on trait anxious children, finding evidence for the children making threatening interpretations of ambiguous stimulus material, overestimating the likelihood of future negative events, and showing a negative bias toward threatening information. Negative bias has also been noted in children's speeding of detection of dot probes in the vicinity of threatening words (Bijttebier, 1998; Schippel et al., 2003). In temperament research, the ability to control attention was found to be negatively related to negative affect (Derryberry & Rothbart, 1988; Rothbart, Ahadi, & Evans, 2000), congruent with the interpretation that good attentional mechanisms may serve to protect against negative ideation. Children who have had a history of abuse have also been found to be hypersensitive to the recognition of angry faces, misclassifying objectively neutral faces as actually angry (Pollak & Kistler, 2002). Together these findings suggest that both temperament and experience can influence aspects of attention toward threat stimuli, perhaps by both enhancing the boundary of classification and increasing the time to dwell on these stimuli. Because orienting to cues and targets can be studied in children from birth onward (Pollak & Kistler, 2002) it would be possible to use these findings to obtain more information on the effect of anxiety on normal development and to determine the degree to which it predicts later problems, given stressful experience.

The brain systems related to unipolar depression have been explored in a number of imaging studies (Drevets & Raichle, 1998; Liotti et al., 2003). These studies have generally shown the importance of midline frontal areas including the anterior cingulate and orbital prefrontal cortex. In normal persons these areas are related to the experience and control of emotion (Bush, Luu, & Posner, 2000), behavior and cognition (Drevets, 2000), and self-image (Gusnard et al., 2003). The areas appear to function abnormally in depressed persons exposed to material producing a sad mood, whether or not they were currently depressed. The overlap between brain activities in currently depressed people with those who have suffered from depression in the past may explain the frequent occurrence of multiple depressive bouts.

Autism. Autism is a disorder that has been linked to the orienting system (Akshoomoff, Pierce, & Courchesne, 2002; Landry & Bryson, in press). It is well known that autistic persons do not normally orient to faces. However, Landry and Bryson report their difficulty in orienting in tasks that involve non-social stimuli similar to those used in the ANT. Similar deficits in the ability to disengage and move attention have been reported in autism in relation to abnormal development of the cerebellum (Akshoomoff, Pierce, & Courchesne, 2002). We do not know if this abnormality is due only to cerebellar deficits because many of the patients also show parietal abnormalities as well. Rodier (2002) has some evidence that the abnormalities found in autism might relate to a gene associated with migration of cells in early development.

EXECUTIVE FUNCTION

Borderline. Borderline personality disorder is characterized by very great lability of affect and problems in interpersonal relations. In some cases, patients are suicidal carry out self-mutilation. Because this diagnosis has been studied largely by psychoanalysts and has a very complex definition, it might at first be thought of as a poor candidate for a specific pathophysiology involving attentional networks. However, we focused on the temperamentally based core symptoms emotionality and difficulty in self-regulation. We found that patients were very high in negative affect and relatively low in effortful control (Rothbart, Ahadi, & Evans, 2000), and defined a temperamentally matched control group of normal persons without personality disorder who were equivalent in these two dimensions. Our study with the ANT found a deficit specific in the executive attention network in borderline patients (Posner et al., 2002). Preliminary imaging results suggested over-

generalization of responding in the amygdala and reduced responding in the anterior cingulate and related midline frontal areas (Posner et al., 2002). Patients with higher effortful control and lower conflict scores on the ANT were also the most likely to show the effects of therapy. This methodology shows the utility of focusing on the core deficits of patients, defining appropriate control groups based on matched temperament, and using specific attentional tests to help determine how to conduct imaging studies.

Schizophrenia. A number of years ago, never medicated schizophrenic patients were tested both by imaging and with a cued detection task similar to the orienting part of the ANT. At rest, these subjects had shown a focal decrease in cerebral blood flow in the left globus palidus (Early et al., 1989) a part of the basal ganglia with close ties to the anterior cingulate. The subjects showed a deficit in orienting similar to what we had shown for left parietal patients (Early et al., 1989). When their visual attention was engaged, they had difficulty in shifting attention to the right visual field. However, they also showed deficits in conflict tasks, particularly when they had to rely on a language cue. It was concluded that the overall pattern of their behavior was most consistent with a deficit in the anterior cingulate and basal ganglia, parts of a frontally based executive attention system. This deficit in orienting rightward has been replicated in first break schizophrenics, but does not seem to be true later in the disorder (Maruff et al., 1995), nor does this pattern appear to be part of the genetic predisposition for schizophrenia (Pardo et al., 2000). First break schizophrenic subjects often have been shown to leave hemisphere deficits and there have been many reports of anterior cingulate and basal ganglia deficits in patients with schizophrenia (Benes, 1999). It appears that the anterior cingulate may be part of a much larger network of frontal and temporal structures that operate abnormally in schizophrenia (Benes, 1999).

A recent study using the ANT cast some light on these results (Wang et al., 2005) in this case the schizophrenic patient were chronic and they were compared with a similarly aged control group. The schizophrenic patients had a much greater difficulty resolving conflict than did the normal controls. The deficit with these patients was also much larger than that found for borderline personality patients, however, there was still a great deal of overlap between the patients and normal indicating that the deficit is not suitable for making a differential diagnosis. The data showed a much smaller orienting deficit of the type that had been reported previously. These findings suggest that there is a strong executive deficit in chronic schizophrenia, as would be anticipated by the Benes theory. It remains to be determined whether this deficit is prior to the initial symptoms or whether it develops with the disorder.

Chromosome 22q11.2 deletion syndrome. This syndrome is a complex one that involved a number of abnormalities including facial and heart but also a mental retardation that is due to deletion of a number of genes. It is known that the children are at a high risk for the development of schizophrenia. Among the genes that are deleted in this syndrome is the COMT gene, which has been associated with a conflict task (Diamond et al., 2004) and with schizophrenia (Egan et al., 2001). In light of these findings it was to be expected that the disorder would produce a large executive deficit (Simon et al., 2005; Sobin et al., 2004). Sobin has suggested in a further paper that the deficit in resolving conflict is associated the ability to inhibit a blink following a cue that a loud noise would be presented shortly (pre-pulse inhibition). The authors suggest that the association of the high-level attention and pre-pulse inhibition deficit suggests a pathway that includes both the basal ganglia and the anterior cingulate.

Many neurological and psychiatric disorders produce a difficulty in attention. Data to date suggest that disorders have specific influences on attentional networks. However, a number of disorders influence the same network (e.g., schizophrenia, borderline and Alzheimer's dementia affect executive attention) and the same disorder can influence more than one network (e.g., schizophrenia may affect both the executive and orienting network although perhaps at different stages of the disorder). These findings reduce the utility of attention as a means of classifying disorders, but they may be useful in suggesting methods of treatment at least of the attentional symptoms.

RESOLVING ENDURING ISSUES IN ATTENTION

Modularity

There has been a great deal of discussion in the cognitive psychology literature of the concept of modularity. These discussions have often defined modularity in a way which required a system to be unaffected by top down (attentional) influences in order to be modular. According to this view only a very few vertical sensory and motor systems could be modular (Fodor, 1983). However, the evidence that even primary sensory systems can be modulated by attention makes it unlikely that any higher-level brain systems will meet the criterion of modularity so defined.

Imaging data provides a rather different perspective on modularity. The material reviewed in this chapter suggests that even brain networks that reflect voluntary activity such as executive attention may be modular in the sense that very specific brain areas perform computations reflecting their component operations. This form of modularity does not suggest that these mechanisms will operate in the same way irrespective of strategy or context. However, they do provide a starting place for linking cellular and genetic mechanisms to brain areas and then to cognitive operations and behavior.

Early and late selection

One of the oldest issues in the field of attention is how early in processing can attention influence input. This issue arose before there was much discussion of specific brain mechanisms of attention. Many empirical studies were done to determine if attentional changes showed up as alterations in the beta (decision) parameter of a signal detection analysis or whether instead they involved changes in the dí (sensory) parameter.

Although many elegant studies were conducted attempting to clarify this issue, there has been no final resolution (although it seems likely that both parameters can be varied by some experimental conditions).

The early versus late question can be resolved into three somewhat interdependent issues. (1) How early in the nervous system can attention influence stimulus input? The results suggest that it can be as early as V1 (Posner & Gilbert, 1999) under some conditions, but more often attention influence is in extrastriate visual areas (Kastner et al., 1999). (2) How quickly after input can attention influence information processing? Again the cellular and physiological data indicate that it can be about as early as clear evidence of cortical processing can be obtained, although in many situations the influence is not present until 80–100 milliseconds after stimulus onset (Martinez et al., 2001). The timing issue is of particular importance because activation of a particular brain area may be either along the input pathway, or could be due to feedback from higher areas. (3) What does early selection mean for the processing of information both selected and unselected? Here the answer is more complex. It seems to mean that certain aspects of complex scenes may be available for conscious report whereas other aspects will only be available if they succeed in producing reorienting. Unattended objects, however, may still be processed to fairly high levels and the processing itself may summon attention. The depth of cognitive processing of unattended objects and the possibility of attention to higher level codes suggests that early selection does not have the cognitive consequence originally implied. Selecting one stimulus over others does not mean that unselected items will not produce a reorienting of attention or still influence behavior.

Priming

Priming refers to the influence of one event on the processing of subsequent events. Behavioral studies suggested that reaction time could be improved to a target by the presentation of a stimulus (prime) that shares a part of the same pathway. Priming can occur in either of two ways. In one way a stimulus activates a pathway automatically and a second stimulus that shares the same pathway is improved in performance (Posner, 1978). These effects can occur even when the prime is presented and masked so that subjects are not able to report its identity. Although there has been a great deal of dispute about how to measure conscious processing, it appears clear that priming can occur when subjects are unable to report even when stopped in the middle of the trial the nature of the prime (Cheesman & Merikle, 1984). Most unconscious priming has been of sensory or semantic codes, but under some conditions

(Dehaene et al., 2003) even responses can be primed without explicit knowledge of the nature of the prime.

A second way that priming can occur is if a person attends to some feature that will be shared by the target. For example, if people are taught that the word "animal" should be interpreted as a body part, the target finger will be primed. The priming is from the subject's attention to body part not from automatic activation of finger by the prime animal.

Data from imaging studies of priming by input and by attention support this distinction by showing very different effects on neural activity in the primed area. If priming occurs automatically by input the target shows reduced activation of the primed cells. On the other hand, attending to an area will enhance neural activity and increase the effect of the target (Corbetta et al., 1991).

The newer imaging data shows the reality of the distinction between automatic priming and priming by attention. However, it is not at all clear how the brain brings about similar changes in performance sometimes by reducing and sometimes by increasing the activity of the target. This puzzle remains to be explained by future studies.

Relation to neuropsychology

The ability to image the human brain has also provided new perspectives for neuropsychologists in their efforts to understand, diagnose and treat insults to the human brain that might occur as the result of stroke, tumor, traumatic injury, degenerative disease, or errors in development (Fernandez-Duque & Posner, 2001).

As we have argued, attention networks have anatomical and functional independence, but that they also interact in many practical situations. Damage to a node of these networks, irrespective of the source, produces distinctive neuropsychological deficits. This principle has been best established with respect to damage to the parietal lobe. Studies have shown that damage to parietal neurons that occur in stroke, due to degeneration in Alzheimer's disease, blocking of cholinergic input, due to lesions of nucleus bassalis, temporary damage from transcranial magnetic stimulation, direct injections of scopolamine, or closed head injury all lead to difficulties in using cues to process targets in the visual field opposite the major insult. Recently, normal persons who have one or two copies of the (4 allele of the apolipoprotein E APOE4) gene which increases the risk of Alzheimer's disease, have also been shown to have increased difficulty in orienting attention and in adjusting the spatial scale of attention, however, they had no difficulty with maintaining the alert state (Greenwood et al., 2000).

In one sense the convergence between imaging, lesions and pharmacology in terms of cognitive effect is obvious. If computations of parietal neurons lead to shifts of visual attention damage to these neurons should produce difficulties. Yet there has been the notion in neuropsychology that localization is not as important as the cause of the lesion. Moreover, there has also been the argument that imaging does not provide a good account of the computations that can predict the effect of damage (Uttal, 2001). Here we see that the imaging results provide clear evidence of the importance of areas of the parietal lobe in shifts of attention and damage to these areas regardless of cause or organism interferes with orienting.

In addition, to efforts to better understand the nature of the brain disorder there have been efforts to adopt these ideas related to the physical basis of attention to for rehabilitation. Some recent studies have tried to rehabilitate specific attentional networks (Sohlberg et al., 2000; Sturm et al., 1997). These studies suggest that rehabilitation procedures should focus on the particular attentional operations of the lesioned area, while at the same time considering the contribution of those deficits to other attentional functions.

In one study (Sturm et al., 1997), a computerized rehabilitation program was designed to try to enhance specific attentional networks. The authors concluded from these findings that vigilance and alertness are the most fundamental functions in the hierarchy, and that selective attention and divided attention recruit these functions for their normal operation. Another study that utilized a practice-oriented therapy (attention process therapy) with brain-injured patients showed an overall improvement in performance (Sohlberg et al., 2000). In some tasks the group that had relatively high vigilance scores showed better effects of the therapy in agreement with the Sturm idea.

A third rehabilitation study tested the possible interaction between vigilance and orienting by training patients to increase their self-alertness, and exploring whether the rehabilitation of self-alertness had an impact on patients' neglect (i.e., orienting deficit) (Robertson et al., 1995). Exogenous alertness was used as a basis for training patients to self-alert. External warning signals were presented, and patients were instructed to generate a self-alertness signal in response to it. Exogenous alertness, as produced by a loud noise, depends on a thalamo-mesencephalic path and is relatively unimpaired in right parietal patients. After the training procedure was explained, the patient started the task and at variable intervals the experimenter knocked on the table while at the same time saying "Attend!" in a loud voice. At the next stage in the training, it was the patient who shouted "Attend!" each time the experimenter knocked on the table. Later, the patient would do both the knocking and the vocal command, first loudly, then subvocally, and finally mentally. Patients were encouraged to try this self-alertness method in their everyday life. This rehabilitation training not only improved patient's self-alertness, but also reduced the extent of their spatial neglect.

Taken together, these findings reveal benefits of systematically analyzing interactions and dissociations of the attentional networks, instead of treating attention as a monolithic concept. They also demonstrate that behavioral therapy can be successful in improving vigilance skills. The availability of imaging as a means of examining brain networks prior to and following rehabilitation have provided opportunities for fine-tune both behavioral and pharmacological interventions. For example, both cognitive behavioral and pharmaceutical therapies have been reported to be about equally effective in the treatment of severe depression. Mayberg (2003) found that the two worked on entirely different parts of the impaired network. Although the cognitive behavioral theory improved cortical parts of the network involved with attention, the pharmaceutical therapy tended to improve subcortical parts of the network. This study shows the importance of taking a network approach to intervention, the additional of genetic information may further improve an understanding of who might benefit from particular forms of therapy.

REFERENCES

Abdullaev, Y. G. & Posner, M. I. (1998). Event-related brain potential imaging of semantic encoding during processing single words. *Neuroimage*, 7: 1–13.

Akhtar, N. & Enns, J. T. (1989). Relations between covert orienting and filtering in the development of visual attention. *Journal of Experimental Child Psychology*, 48: 315–344.

Akshoomoff, N., Pierce, K., & Courchesne, E. (2002). The neurobiological basis of autism from a developmental perspective. *Developmental Psychopathology*, 14(3): 613–34.

Allman, J. (2001). The anterior cingulate cortex: The evolution of an interface between emotion and cognition. In A. Damasio, et al (eds.), *Unity of Knowledge. Annals of New York Academy of Science*, 935: 107–117.

Anderson, S. W., Damasio, H., Tranel, D. & Damasio, A. R. (2000). Long-term sequelae of prefrontal cortex damage acquired in early childhood. *Developmental Neuropsychology*, 18(3): 281–296.

Awh, E. & Pashler, H. (2000). Evidence for split attentional foci. *Journal of Experimental Psychology: Human Perception and Performance*, 26: 834–46.

Baddeley, A. D. (1993). Working memory or working attention? In A. D. Baddeley & L. Weiskrantz (Eds.), *Attention: Selection, Awareness, & Control.* (pp. 152–170). Oxford: Clarendon Press.

Barkley, R. A. (1997). Behavioral inhibition, sustained attention, and executive functions: Constructing a unifying theory of ADHD. *Psychological Bulletin*, 121: 65–94.

Beauregard, M., Levesque, J. & Bourgouin, P. (2001). Neural correlates of conscious self- regulation of emotion. *Journal of Neuroscience*, 21: RC165: 1.

Benes, F. (1999). Model generation and testing to probe neural circuitry in the cingulate cortex of postmortem schizophrenic brains. *Schizophrenia Bulletin*, 24: 219–229.

Berger, A., Jones, L, Rothbart, M. K. & Posner, M. I. (2000). Computerized games to study the development of attention in childhood. *Behavioral Research Methods and Instrumentation*, 32: 290–303.

Bijttebier, P. (1998). Monitoring and blunting coping styles in children. Unpublished doctoral thesis. Catholic University of Leuven, Belgium.

Bisley, J. W. & Goldberg, M. E. (2003). Neuronal activity in the lateral intraparietal area and spatial attention. *Science*, 299: 81–86.

Blair, R. J. R., Morris, J. S., Frith, C. D., Perrett, D. I. & Dolan, R. J. (1999). Dissociable neural responses to facila expression of sadness and anger. *Brain*, 1222: 883–893.

Booth, J., Carlson, C. L. & Tucker, D. (2001). Cognitive inattention in the ADHD subtypes. Paper presented at the 10th meeting of the *International Society for Research in Child and Adolescent Psychopathology*, Vancouver, Canada.

Botvinick, M. M., Braver, T. S., Barch, D. M., Carter, C. S. & Cohen, J. D. (2001). Conflict monitoring and cognitive control. *Psychological Review*, 108: 624–652.

Botvinick, M., Braver, T. S., Yeung, N., Ullsperger, M., Carter, C. S., Cohen, J. D. (2004). Conflict monitoring: Computational and empirical studies. In M. I. Posner (Ed.), *Cognitive Neuroscience of Attention*. New York: Guildford 91–104.

Broadbent, D. E. (1958). *Perception and Communication*. New York: Pergamon.

Bronson, M. B. (2000). *Self-Regulation in Early Childhood*. New York: Guilford Press.

Bush, G., Luu, P. & Posner, M. I. (2000). Cognitive and emotional influences in the anterior cingulate cortex. *Trends in Cognitive Science*, 4/6: 215–222.

Casey, B. J., Durston, S. & Fossella, J. A. (2001). Evidence for a mechanistic model of cognitive control. *Clinical Neuroscience Research*, 1: 267–282.

Casey, B. J., Thomas, K. M., Davidson, M. C., Kunz, K., Franzen, P. L. (2002). Dissociating striatal and hippocampal function developmentally with a stimulus-response compatibility task. *Journal of Neuroscience*, 22: 8647–8652.

Casey, B. J., Trainor, R. J., Orendi, J. L., Schubert, A. B., Nystrom, L. E., Giedd, J. N., Castellanos, F. X., Haxby, J. V., Noll, D. C., Cohen, J. D., Forman, S. D., Dahl, R. E. & Rapoport, J. L. (1997). A developmental functional MRI study of prefrontal activation during performance of a go-no-go task. *Journal of Cognitive Neuroscience*, 9: 835–847.

Cavanagh, P. (2004). Attention routines and the architecture of selection. In M. I. Posner (Ed.), *Cognitive Neuroscience of Attention*. (pp. 29–44). New York: Guilford Press.

Cherry, E. C. Some experiments on the recognition of speech with one and two ears. *Journal of the Acoustical Society*, 25: 975–979.

Cheesman, J. & Merikle, P. M. (1984). Priming with and without awareness. *Perception and Psychophysiology*, 36: 387–395.

Cohen, J. D., Dunbar, K. & McClelland, J. L. (1990). On the control of automatic processes: A parallel distributed processing model of the Stroop effect. *Psychological Review*, 97(3): 332–361.

Cohen, J. D., Aston-Jones, G. & Gilzenrat, M. S. (2004). A systems level theory on attention and cognitive control. In M. I. Posner (Ed.), *Cognitive Neuroscience of Attention*. (pp. 29–44). New York: Guilford Press.

Corbetta, M. (1998). Frontoparietal cortical networks for directing attention and the eye to visual locations: Identical, independent, or overlapping neural systems? *Proceedings of the National Academy of Science*, 95: 831–838.

Corbetta, M., Kincade, J. M., Ollinger, J. M., McAvoy, M. P. & Shulman, G. (2000). Voluntary orienting is dissociated from target detection in human posterior parietal cortex. *Nature Neuroscience*, 3: 292–297.

Corbetta, M., Miezin, F. M., Dobmeyer, S., Shulman, G. L. & Petersen, S. E. (1991). Selective and divided attention during visual discriminations of shape, color, and speed: Functional anatomy by positron emission tomography. *Journal of Neuroscience*, 11: 2383–2402.

Corbetta, M. & Shulman, G. L. (2002). Control of goal-directed and stimulus-driven attention in the brain. *Nature Neuroscience Reviews*, 3: 201–215.

Coull, J. T., Frith, C. D., Frackowiak, R. S. & Grasby, P. M. (1996). A fronto-parietal network for rapid visual information processing: A PET study of sustained attention and working memory. *Neuropsychologia*, 34(11): 1085–1095.

Coull, J. T., Nobre, A. C. & Frith, C. D. (2001). The noradrenergic alpha2 agonist clonidine modulates behavioural and neuroanatomical correlates of human attentional orienting and alerting. *Cerebral Cortex*, 11(1): 73–84.

Dale, A. M., Liu, A. K., Fischi, B. R., Buckner, R., Beliveau, J. W., Lewine, J. D. & Halgren, E. (2000), Dynamic statistical parameter mapping: Combining fMRI and MEG for high resolution cortical activity. *Neuron*, 26: 55–67.

Damasio, A. (1994). *Descartes Error: Emotion, Reason and the Brain*. New York: G. P. Putnam.

Davidson, M. C. & Marrocco, R. T. (2000). Local infusion of scopoplamine into intraparietal cortex slows cover orienting in rhesus monkeys. *Journal of Neurophysiology*, 83: 1536–49.

Davidson, R. J., Putnam, K. M. & Larson, C. L. (2000). Dysfunction in the neural circuitry of emotion regulation: A possible prelude to violence. *Science*, 289: 591–594.

Dehaene, S., Artiges, E., Naccache, L., Martelli, C., Viard, A., Schurhoff, F., Recasens, C., Martinot, M. L. P., Leboyer, M. & Martinot, J. L., (2003). Conscious and subliminal conflicts in normal subjects and patients with schizophrenia: The role of the anterior cingulate. *Proceedings of the National Academy of Sciences of the USA*, 100(23): 13722–13727.

Derryberry, D. & Reed, M. A. (1994). Temperament and the self-organization of personality. *Development and Psychopathology*, 6: 653–676.

Derryberry, D. & Rothbart, M. K. (1988). Arousal, affect, and attention as components of temperament. *Journal of Personality and Social Psychology*, 55: 958–966.

Desimone, R., Duncan, J. (1995). Neural mechanisms of selective visual attention. *Annual Review of Neuroscience*, 18: 193–222.

Diamond, A., Briand, L., Fossella, J. & Gehlbach, L. (2004). Genetic and neurochemical modulation of prefrontal cognitive functions in children. *American Journal of Psychiatry*, 161: 125–135.

Diamond, A. (1991). Neuropsychological insights into the meaning of object concept development. In S. Carey, & R. Gelman (Eds.), *The Epigenesis of Mind: Essays on Biology and Cognition* (pp. 67–110). Hillsdale, NJ: Lawrence Erlbaum Associates.

Donchin, E. & Cohen, L. (1967). Average evoked potentials and intermodal selective attention. *EEG and Clinical Neurophysiology*, 22: 537–546.

Drevets, W. C. (2000). Neuroimaging studies of mood disorders. *Biological Psychiatry*, 18: 813–829.

Drevets, W. C. & Raichle, M. E. (1998). Reciprocal suppression of regional cerebral blood flow during emotional versus higher cognitive processes: Implications for interactions between emotion and cognition. *Cognition and Emotion*, 12: 353–385.

Driver, J., Eimer, M. & Macaluso, E. (2004). Neurobiology of human spatial attention: Modulation, generation, and integration. In N. Kanwisher & J. Duncan, (Eds.), *Attention and Performance XX: Functional Brain Imaging of Visual Cognition*, 267–300.

Duncan, J. & Owen, A. M. (2000). Common regions of the human frontal lobe recruited by diverse cognitive demands. *Trends in Neurosciences*, 23: 475–483.

Duncan, J., Seitz, R. J., Kolodny, J., Bor, D., Herzog, H. Ahmed, A., Newell, F. N. & Emslie, H. (2000). Aneural basis for general intelligence. *Science*, 289: 457–460.

Durston, S., Thomas, K. M., Yang, Y., Ulug, A. M., Zimmerman, R. D. & Casey, B. J. (2002). A neural basis for the development of inhibitory control. *Developmental Science*, 5: F9–F16.

Early, T. S., Posner, M. I., Reiman, E. M. & Raichle, M. E. (1989). Hyperactivity of the left stiato-pallidal projection, Part I: Lower level theory. *Psychiatric Developments*, 2: 85–108.

Egan, M. F., Goldberg, T. E., Kolachana, B. S., Callicott, J. H., Mazzanti, C. M., Straub, R. E., Goldman, D. & Weinberger, D. R. (2001). Effect of COMT Val108/158 Met genotype on frontal lobe function and risk for schizophrenia. *Proceedings of the National Academy of Sciences of the USA*, 98: 6917–22.

Eriksen, C. W. & Hoffman, J. E. (1972). Temporal and spatial characteristics of selective encoding from visual displays. *Perception & Psychophysics*, 12: 201–204.

Eriksen, C. W. & Hoffman, J. E. (1973). The extent of processing noise elements during selective encoding from visual displays. *Perception and Psychophysics*, 14: 155–160.

Evarts, E. V. (1968). Relation of the pyramidal tract activity to force exerted during voluntary movement. *Journal of Neurophysiology*, 31: 14–27.

Everitt, B. J. & Robbins, T. W. (1997). Central cholinergic systems and cognition. *Annual Review of Psychology*, 48: 649–684.

Fan, J., Flombaum, J. I., McCandliss, B. D., Thomas, K. M., & Posner, M. I. (2003). Cognitive and brain mechanisms of conflict. *Neuroimage*, 18: 42–57.

Fan, J., Fossella, J. A., Summer T. & Posner, M. I. (2003). Mapping the genetic variation of executive attention onto brain activity. *Proceedings of the National Academy of Sciences of the USA*, 100: 7406–11.

Fan, J., McCandliss, B. D., Sommer, T., Raz, M. & Posner, M. I. (2002). Testing the efficiency and independence of attentional networks. *Journal of Cognitive Neuroscience*, 3(14): 340–347.

Fan, J., Wu, Y., Fossella, J., & Posner, M. I. (2001). Assessing the heritability of attentional networks. *BioMed Central Neuroscience*, 2: 14.

Fernandez-Duque, D. & Black, S. (2006). Attentional networks in normal aging and Alzheimer's disease. *Neuropsychology*. 20, 133–143.

Fernandez-Duque, D. & Posner, M. I. (2001). Brain imaging of attentional networks in normal and pathological states. *Journal of Clinical and Experimental Neuropsychology*, 23: 74–93.

Fodor, (1983). *Modularity of Mind*. Cambridge, MA: MIT Press.

Fossella, J., Sommer, T., Fan, J., Wu, Y., Swanson, J. M., Pfaff, D. W. & Posner, M. I. (2002). Assessing the molecular genetics of attention networks. *BMC Neuroscience*, 3: 14.

Fox, E., Ricardo, R., & Dutton, K. (2002). Attentional bias for threat: Evidence for delayed disengagement from emotional faces. *Cognition and Emotion*, 16: 355–379.

Fox, E., Russo, R., Bowles, R. J. & Dutton, K. (2001). Do threatening stimuli draw or hold attention in subclinical anxiety? *Journal of Experimental Psychology – General*, 130: 681–700.

Friedrich, F. J., Egly R., Rafal, R. D. & Beck, D. (1998). Spatial attention deficits in humans: A comparison of superior parietal and temporal-parietal junction lesions. *Neuropsychology*, 12(2): 193–207.

Fuentes, L. J. (2004). Inhibitory processing in the attentional networks. In M. I. Posner (Ed.), *Cognitive Neuroscience of Attention*. (pp. 29–44). New York: Guilford Press.

Fuentes, L. J., Boucart, M., Vivas, A. B., Álvarez, R. & Zimmerman, M. A. (2000). Inhibitory tagging in inhibition of return is affected in schizophrenia: Evidence from the Stroop task. *Neuropsychology*, 14: 134–140.

Fuentes, L. J., Vivas, A. B. & Humphreys, G. W. (1999). Inhibitory tagging of stimulus properties in inhibition of return: Effects on semantic priming and flanker interference. *Quarterly Journal of Experimental Psychology: Human Experimental Psychology*, 52: 149–164.

Gall, S., Kerschreiter, R. & Mojzisch, A. (2002). *Handbuch Biopsychologie und Neurowissenschaften*. Bern, Switzerland: Verlag Hans Huber.

Georgopoulos, A. P., Lurito, J. T., Petrides, M., Schwartz, A. B. & Massey, J. T. (1989). Mental rotation of the neuronal population vector. *Science*, 243: 234–236.

Gerardi-Caulton, G. (2000). Sensitivity to spatial conflict and the development of self-regulation in children 24–36 months of age. *Developmental Science*, 3/4: 397–404.

Goldberg, T. E. & Weinberger, D. R. (2004). Genes and the parsing of cognitive processes. *Trends in Cognitive Science*, 8: 325–335.

Goldman-Rakic, P. S. (1988). Topography of cognition. Parallel distributed networks in primate association cortex. *Annual Review of Neuroscience*, 11: 137–156.

Grandy, D. K. & Kruzich, P. J. (2004). A molecular genetic approach to the neurobiology of attention utilizing dopamine receptor-deficient mice. In M. I. Posner (Ed.), *Cognitive Neuroscience of Attention*. New York: Guilford, pp. 260–268.

Greenwood, P. M., Sunderland, T., Friz, J. L. & Parasuraman, R. (2000). Genetics and visual attention: Selective deficits in healthy adult carriers of the epsilon 4 allele of the apolipoprotein E gene. *Proceedings of National Academy of Sciences, USA*, 97: 11661–11666.

Gusnard, D. A., Ollinger, J. M., Shulman, G. L., Cloninger, C. R., Price, J. L., Van Essen, D. C. & Raichle, M. E. (2003). Persistence and brain circuitry. *Proceedings of the National Academy of Sciences of the United States*, 100: 3479–3484.

Hackley, S. A. & Valle-Inclan, F. (1998). Automatic alerting does not speed late motoric processes in a reaction-time task. *Nature*, 391: 786–788.

Han, C. J., O'Tuathaigh, C. M. & Koch, C. (2004). A practical assay for attention in mice. In M. I. Posner (Ed.), *Cognitive Neuroscience of Attention*. New York: Guilford, pp. 294–312.

Hebb, D. O. (1949). *Organization of Behavior*. New York: John Wiley & Sons.

Heinze, H. J., Mangun, G. R., Burchert, W., Hinrichs, H., Scholtz, M., Muntel, T. F., Gosel, A., Scherg, M., Johannes, S., Hundeshagen, H., Gazzaniga, M. S. & Hillyard, S. A. (1994). Combined spatial and temporal imaging of brain activity during visual selective attention in humans. *Nature*, 372: 543–546.

Hillyard, S. A., Di Russo, F. & Martinez, A. (2004). The imaging of visual attention. In N. Kanwisher & J. Duncan (Eds.), *Functional Neuroimaging of Visual Cognition Attention and Performance XX* (pp. 381–390).

Holroyd, C. B. & Coles, M. G. H. (2002). The neural basis of human error processing: Reinforcement learning, dopamine and the error related negativity. *Psychological Review*, 109: 679–709.

Hubel, D. & Wiesel, T. N. (1968). Receptive field and functional architecture of the monkey striate cortex. *Journal of Physiology* (London), 195: 215–243.

Hunt, A & Kingstone, A. (2003). Covert and overt voluntary attention: Linked or independent. *Cognitive Brain Research*, 18: 102–105.

Intriligator, J. & Cavanagh, P. (2001). The spatial resolution of visual attention. *Cognitive Psychology*, 43: 171–216.

James, W. (1890). *Principles of Psychology*. New York: Holt.

Jones, L. B., Rothbart, M. K. & Posner, M. I. (2003). Development of executive attention in preschool children. *Developmental Science*, 6: 498–504.

Jonides, J. (1981). Voluntary versus automatic control over the mind's eye's movement. In J. B. Long & A. D. Baddeley (Eds.), *Attention and Performance IX* (pp. 187–203). Hillsdale, NJ: Erlbaum.

Kahneman, D. (1973). *Attention and Effort*. Englewood Cliffs, NJ: Prentice Hall.

Kanwisher, N. & Duncan, J. (Eds.). (2004). Functional neuroimaging of visual cognition. *Attention and Performance XX*. Oxford U.K.: Oxford University Press.

Karnath, H-O., Ferber, S. & Himmelbach, M. (2001). Spatial awareness is a function of the temporal not the posterior parietal lobe. *Nature*, 411: 95–953.

Kastner, S., Pinsk, M. A., De Weerd, P., Desimone, R. & Ungerleider, L. G. (1999). Increased activity in human visual cortex during directed attention in the absence of visual stimulation. *Neuron*, 22: 751–761.

Kennard. M. A. (1955). The cingulate gyrus in relation to consciousness. *Journal of Nervous Mental Disorders*, 121(1): 34–9.

Klein, R. M. (1980). Does oculomotor readiness mediate cognitive control of visual attention? In R. Nickerson (Ed.), *Attention and Performance*, 259–276. New York: Academic Press.

Klein, R. M. (2000). Inhibition of return. *Trends in Cognitive Sciences*, 4: 138–147.

Klein, R. M. (2004). On the control of visual orienting. In M. I. Posner (Ed.), *Cognitive Neuroscience of Attention*. (pp. 29–44). New York: Guilford Press.

Klein, R. M. & Kingstone, R. M. (1993). Why do visual offsets reduce saccadic latencies? *Behavioral and Brain Sciences*, 16: 583–4.

Klein, R. M. & McCormick, P. (1989). Covert visual orienting: Hemifield-activation can be mimicked by zoom lens and mid-location placement strategies. *Acta Psychologica*, 70: 235–250.

Kochanska, G. (1995). Children's temperament, mothers' discipline, and security of attachment: Multiple pathways to emerging internalization. *Child Development*, 66: 597–615.

Kochanska, G., Murray, K., Jacques, T. Y., Koenig, A. L. & Vandegeest, K. A. (1996). Inhibitory control in young children and its role in emerging internationalization. *Child Development*, 67: 490–507.

Kramer, A. F. & Hahn, S. (1995). Splitting the beam: Distribution of attention over noncontiguous regions of the visual field. *Psychological Science*, 6: 381–386.

LaBerge, D. (1995). *Attentional Processing*. Cambridge, MA: Harvard University Press.

Landry, R. & Bryson, S. E. (2004). Impaired disengagement of attention in young children with autism. *Journal of Child and Adolescent Psychiatry*. 45, 1115–1122.

Levy, F. (1980). The development of sustained attention (vigilance) and inhibition in children: Some normative data. *Journal of Child Psychology*, 27: 77–84.

Lin, C. C. H., Hsiao, C. K. & Chen, W. J. (1999). Development of sustained attention assessed using the continuous performance test among children 6–15 years of age. *Journal of Abnormal Child Psychology*, 27(5): 403–412.

Liotti, M., Mayberg, H. S., McGinnis, S., Brannan, S. L. & Jerabeck, P. (2003). Unmasking disease-specific cerebral flow abnormalities: Mood challenge in patients with remitted unipolar depression. *American Journal of Psychiatry*, 159: 183–186.

Macaluso, E., Frith, C. D. & Driver, J. (2000). Modulatilon of human visual cortex by cross-modal spatial attention. *Science*, 289: 1204–1208.

Mackworth, J. F. & Mackworth, N. H. (1956). The overlapping of signals for decisions. *American Journal of Psychology*, 69: 26–47.

Marrocco, R. T. & Davidson, M. C. (1998). Neurochemistry of attention. In R. Parasuraman (Ed.), *The Attentive Brain*. Cambridge, MA: MIT Press, 35–50.

Martinzez, A., DiRusso, F., Anllo-Vento, L. Sereno, M., Buxton, R., Hillyard, S. (2001). Putting spatial attention on the map: Timing and localization of stimulus selection processing striate and extrastriate visual areas. *Vision Reseach*, 41: 1437–1457.

Maruff, P., Currie, J., Hay, D., McArthur-Jackson, C. & Malone, V. (1995). Asymmetries in the covert orienting of visual spatial attention in schizophrenia. *Neuropsychologia*, 31: 1205–1223.

MacDonald, A. W., Cohen, J. D., Stenger, V. A. & Carter, C. S. (2000). Dissociating the role of the dorsolateral prefrontal and anterior cingulate cortex in cognitive control. *Science*, 288: 1835–1838.

Mattay, V. S. & Goldberg, T. E. (2004). Imaging genetic influences in human brain function. *Current Opinion in Neurobiology*, 14 (2): 239–247.

Mayberg, H. S. (2003). Modulating dysfunctional limbic-cortical circuits in depression: Towards development of brain-based algorithms for diagnosis and optimized treatment. *British Medical Bulletin*, 65: 193–207.

Mesulam, M.-M. (1981). A cortical network for directed attention and unilateral neglect. *Annals of Neurology*, 10: 309–325.

Miller, M. B., Van Horn, J. D., Wolford, G. L., Handy T. C., Valsangkr-Smyth, M., Inati, S., Grafton, S., and Gazzaniga, M. S. (2002). Extensive individual differences in brain activations associated with episodic retrieval are reliable over time. *Journal of Cognitive Neuroscience*, 14: 1200–1214.

Morrison, F. J. (1982). The development of alertness. *Journal of Experimental Child Psychology*, 34: 187–199.

Mountcastle, V. M. (1978). The world around us: Neural command functions for selective attention. *Neuroscience Research Progress Bulletin*, 14(Suppl): 1–47.

Moruzzi, G. & Magoun, H. W. (1949). Brainstem reticular formation and activation of the EEG. *EEG and Clinical Neurophysiology*, 1: 455–473.

Nakayama, K. (1990). The iconic bottleneck and the tenuous link between early processing and perception. In Colin Blakemore (Ed.), *Vision: Coding and Efficiency* (pp. 411–422). Cambridge: Cambridge University Press.

Neely, J. H. (1977). Semantic priming and retrieval from lexical memory: Roles of inhibitionless spreading activation and limited-capacity attention. *Journal of Experimental Psychology: General*, 106: 226–254.

Nikolaev, A. R., Ivanitsky, G. A., Ivanitsky, A. M., Abdullaev, Y. G. & Posner, M. I. (2001). Short-term correlation between frontal and Wernicke's areas in word association. *Neuroscience Letters*, 298: 107–110.

Nimchinsky, E. A., Gilissen, E., Allman, J. M., Perl, D. P., Erwin, J. M. & Hof, P. R. (1999). A neuronal morphologic type unique to humans and great apes. *Proceedings of the National Academy of Science*, 96: 5268–5273.

Nobre, A. C. (2004). Probing the flexibility of attentional orienting in the human brain. In M. I. Posner (Ed.), *Cognitive Neuroscience of Attention*. New York: Guilford, pp. 157–179.

O'Connor, D. H., Fukui, M. M., Pinsk, M. A., Kasnter, S. (2002). Attention modulates responses in the human lateral geniculate nucleus. *Nature Neuroscience*, 5(11): 1203–1209.

Ochsner, K. N., Bunge, S. A., Gross, J. J. & Gabrieli, J. D. E. (2002). Rethinking feelings: An fMRI study of the cognitive regulation of emotion. *Journal of Cognitive Neuroscience*, 14: 1215–1229.

Ochsner, K. N., Kossyln, S. M., Cosgrove, G. R., Cassem, E. H., Price, B. H., Nierenberg, A. A. & Rauch, S. L. (2001). Deficits in visual cognition and attention following bilateral anterior cingulotomy. *Neuropsychologia*, 39: 219–230.

Parasuraman, R., Greenwood, P. M., Haxby, J. B. & Grady, C. L. (1992). Visuospatial attention in dementia of the Alzheimer type. *Brain*, 115: 711–733.

Parasuraman, R., Greenwood, P. M., Kumar, R. & Fossella, J. et.al. (2005). Beyond heritability: Neurotransmitter genes differentially modulate visuospatial attention and working memory. *Psychological Science*.16, 200–207.

Pardo, P. J., Knesevich, M. A., Vogler, G.P, Pardo J. V., Towne, B., Clonninger, C. R. & Posner, M. I. (2000). Genetic and state variables of neurocognitive dysfunction in schizophrenia: A twin study. *Schizophrenia Bulletin*, 26: 459–477.

Perry, R. J. & Zeki, S. (2000). The neurology of saccades and covert shifts of spatial attention. *Brain*, 123: 2273–2293.

Pollak, S. D. & Kistler, D. J. (2002). Early experience is associated with the development of categorical representations for facial expressions of emotion. *Proceedings of the National Academy of Sciences of the United States*, 99: 9072–9076.

Posner, M. I. (1978). *Chronometric Explorations of Mind*. Hillsdale, NJ: Lawrence Erlbaum Associates.

Posner, M. I. (1980). Orienting of attention. The 7th Sir F. C. Bartlett Lecture. *Quarterly Journal of Experimental Psychology*, 32: 3–25.

Posner, M. I. (1988). Structures and functions of selective attention. In T. Boll and B. Bryant (Eds.), *Master Lectures in Clinical Neuropsychology and Brain Function: Research, Measurement, and Practice, American Psychological Association* (pp. 171–202).

Posner M. I. (Ed.) (2004). *Cognitive Neuroscience of Attention*. New York: Guilford.

Posner, M. I. (2004). The achievements of brain imaging: Past and present. To appear in N. Kanwisher & J. Duncan (Eds.), *Attention and Performance XX*, Oxford University Press (pp. 505–528).

Posner, M. I. & Cohen, Y. A. (1984). Components of visual orienting. In H. Bouma & D. G. Bouwhuis (Eds.), *Attention and Performance X*, (pp. 513–556), Hillsdale, NJ: LEA.

Posner, M. I. & Gilbert, C. D. (1999). Attention and primary visual cortex: *Proceedings of the National Academy of Science of U.S.A.*, 96/6: 2585–2587.

Posner, M. I., Inhoff, A., Friedrich, F. J. & Cohen, A. (1987). Isolating attentional systems: A cognitive-anatomical analysis. *Psychobiology*, 15: 107–121.

Posner, M. I. & Petersen, S. E. (1990). The attention system of the human brain. *Annual Review of Neuroscience*, 13: 25–42.

Posner, M. I. & Raichle, M. E. (1994). *Images of Mind*. Scientific American Books.

Posner, M. I. & Raichle, M. E. (Eds.) (1998). Neuroimaging of cognitive procsses. *Proceedings of the National Academy of Sciences of the U.S.*, 95: 763–764.

Posner, M. I. & Rothbart, M. K. (1998). Attention, self-regulation and consciousness. *Philosophical Transactions of the Royal Society of London B*: 353: 1915–1927.

Posner, M. I. & Rothbart, M. K. (2000). Developing mechanisms of self-regulation. *Development and Psychopathology*, 12: 427–441.

Posner, M. I. & Rothbart, M. K. (2004). Hebb's Neural networks support the integration of psychological science. *Canadian Psychologist*, 45: 265–278.

Posner, M. I., Rothbart, M. K., Vizueta, N., Thomas, K. M., Levy, K., Fossella, J., Silbersweig, D. A., Stern, E., Clarkin, J. & Kernberg, O. (2003). An approach to the psychobiology of personality disorders. *Development and Psychopathology*, 15(4): 1093–1096.

Rafal, R. (1998). Neglect. In R. Parasuraman (Ed.), *The Attentive Brain*. Cambridge, MA: MIT Press (pp. 711–733).

Raichle, M. E., Fiez, J. A., Videen, T. O., McCleod, A. M. K., Pardo, J. V., Fox, P. T. & Petersen, S. E. (1994). Practice-related changes in the human brain: Functional anatomy during nonmotor learning. *Cerebral Cortex*, 4: 8–26.

Rainville, P., Duncan, G. H., Price, D. D., Carrier, B. & Bushnell, M. C. (1997). Pain affect encoded in human anterior cingulated but not somatosensory cortex. *Science*, 277: 968–970.

Reiss, D., Backus, B. T. & Heeger, D. J. (2000). Activity in primary visual cortex predicts performance in a visual detection task. *Nature Neuroscience*, 3: 940–945.

Rensink, R. A., O'Regan, J. K., & Clark, J. J. (1997). To see or not to see: The need for attention to perceive changes in scenes. *Psychological Science*, 8(5): 368–373.

Ridderinkhof, K. R. & van der Molen, M. W. (1995). A psychophysiologicl analysis of developmental differences in the ability to resist interference. *Child Development*, 66: 1040–1056.

Rizzolatti, G., Riggio, L., Dascola, I. & Umilta, C. (1987). Reorienting attention across the horizontal and vertical meridians: Evidence in favor of the premotor theory of attention. *Neuropsychologia*, 25: 31–40.

Robertson, I. H., Mattingley, J. B., Rorden, C. & Driver, J. (1998). Phasic alerting of neglect patients overcomes their spatial deficit in visual awareness. *Nature*, 395: 169–172.

Robertson, I. H., Tegnér, R., Tham, K., Lo, A. & Nimmo-Smith, I. (1995). Sustained attention training for unilateral neglect: Theoretical and rehabilitation implications. *Journal of Clinical and Experimental Neuropsychology*, 17(3): 416–430.

Rock, I. & Gutman, D. (1981). The effects of inattention on form perception. *Journal of Experimental Psychology: Human Perception and Performance*, 7: 502–534.

Rodier, P. M. (2002). Converging evidence for brain stem injury during autism. *Development and Psychopathology*, 14: 537–559.

Rosler, F., Heil, M. & Roder, B. (1997). Slow negative brain potentials as reflections of specific modular resources of cognition. *Biological Psychology*, 21: 109–141.

Rothbart, M. K., Ahadi, S. A. & Evans, D. E. (2000). Temperament and personality: Origins and outcomes. *Journal of Personality and Social Psychology*, 78: 122–135.

Rothbart, M. K., Ahadi, S. A. & Hershey, K. (1994). Temperament and social behavior in children. *Merrill-Palmer Quarterly*, 40: 21–39.

Rothbart, M. K., Ellis, L. K. & Posner, M. I. (2004). Temperament and self-regulation. In R. F. Baumeister & K. D. Vohs (Eds.), *Handbook of Self-Regulation: Research, Theory, and Applications*, New York: Guilford Press, 18: 357–370.

Rothbart, M. K., Ellis, L. K., Rueda, M. R. & Posner, M. I. (2003). Developing mechanisms of conflict resolution. *Journal of Personality*, 71(6): 1113–1143.

Rueda, M. R., Fan, J., McCandliss, B., Halparin, J. D., Gruber, D. B., Pappert, L. & Posner, M. I. (2004). Development of attentional networks in childhood. *Neuropsychologia*, 42: 1029–1040.

Rueda, M. R., Holtz, F., Posner, M. I. & Fuentes, L. (in process). Factors influencing the development of alertness. Manuscript in preparation.

Rueda, M. R., Posner, M. I. & Rothbart, M. K. (2005). Development of executive attention: Contributions to the emergence of self-regulation. *Developmental Neuropsychology 28*, 573–599.

Rueda, M. R., Posner, M. I., Rothbart, M. K. & Davis-Stober, C. P. (2004). Development of the time course for processing conflict: An event-related potentials study with 4 year olds and adults. *BMC Neuroscience*, 5: 39.

Ruff, H. A. & Rothbart, M. K. (1996). *Attention in early development: Themes and variations*. New York: Oxford University Press.

Rugg, M. D. & Coles, M. G. H. (1995). *Electrophsyiology of Mind*. Oxford: Oxford University Press.

Sanders, A. (1998). *Elements of Human Performance*. Mahwah N. J.: LEA.

Sapir, A., Soroker, N., Berger, A. & Henik, A. (1999). Inhibition of return in spatial attention: Direct evidence for collicular generation. *Nature Neuroscience*, 2(12): 1053–1054.

Scherg, M. & Berg, P. (1993). *Brain Electrical Source Anlaysis*. Version 2.0 NeuroScan, Herndon, VA.

Schiller, P. H., Sandell, J. H. & Maunsell, H. R. (1987). The effect of frontal eye field and superior colliculus lesions on saccadic latencies in the Rhesus monkey. *Journal of Neurophysiology*, 57(4): 1033–1049.

Schippel, P., Vasey, M. W., Cravens-Brown, L. M. & Bretveld, R. A. (2003). Suppressed attention to rejection, ridicule, and failure cues: A unique correlate of reactive but not proactive aggression in youth. *Journal of Clinical Child & Adolescent Psychology*, 32: 40–55.

Shallice, T. (1988). *From Neuropsychology to Mental Structure*. New York: Cambridge University Press.

Shulman, G. L. Remington, R. W. & McClean, J. P. (1979). Moving attention through space. *Journal of Experimental Psychology: Human Perception and Performance*, 5: 522–526.

Simon, T. J., Bish, J. P., Bearden, C. E., Ding, L., Ferrante, S., Nguyen, V., Gee, J., McDonald-McGinn, D., Zackai, E. H. & Emanuel, B. S. (2005). A multi-level analysis of cognitive dysfunction and psychopathology associated with chromosome 22q11.2 deletion syndrome in children 17: 753–784.

Sobin, C., Kiley-Brabeck, K., Daniels, S., Blundell, M., Anyane-Yeboa, K. & Karayiorgou, M. (2004). Networks of attention in children with the 22q11 deletion syndrome. *Developmental Neuropsychology*, 26: 611–626.

Sohlberg, M. M., McLaughlin, K. A., Pavese, A., Heidrich, A. & Posner, M. I. (2000). Evaluation of attention process therapy training in persons with acquired brain injury. *Journal of Clinical and Experimental Neuropsychology*, 22: 656–676.

Sokolov, E. N. (1963). Higher nervous functions: The orienting reflex. *Annual Review of Physiology*, 25: 545–580.

Soumi, S. J. (2003). Gene-environment interactions and the neurobiology of social conflict. *Annals of New York Academy of Science*, 1008: 132–139.

Stroop, J. R. (1935). Studies of interference in serial verbal reactions. *Journal of Experimental Psychology*, 18: 643–662.

Stins, J. F., van Baal, CGM, A. Tinca, Polderman, J. C., Verhulst, F. C. & Boomsma, D. I. (2004). Heritability of Stroop and flanker performance in 12-year-old children. *BMC Neuroscience*, 5: 49.

Sturm, W., Willmes, K., Orgass, B. & Hartje, W. (1997). Do specific attention effects need specific training. *Neurological Rehabilitation*, 7: 81–103.

Sutton, S., Nraren, M., Zubin, J., & John, E. R. (1965). Evoked potential correlates of stimulus uncertainty. *Science*, 150: 1187–1188.

Swanson, J., Deutsch, C., Cantwell, D., Posner, M., Kenndy, J., Barr, C., Moyzis, R., Schuck, S., Flodman, P., & Spence, A. (2001). Genes and attention-deficit hyperactivity disorder. *Clinical Neuroscience Research*, 1(3): 207–216.

Swanson, J. M., Kraemer, H. C., Hinshaw, S. P., Arnold, L. E., Conners, C. K., Abikoff, H. B., Clevenger, W., Davies, M., Elliott, G. R., Greenhill, L. L., Hechtman, L., Hoza, B., Jensen, P. S., March, J. S., Newcorn, J. H., Owens, E. B., Pelham, W. E., Schiller, E., Severe, J. B., Simpson, S., Vitiello, B., Wells, K., Wigal, T. & Wu, M. (2001). Clinical relevance of the primary findings of the MTA: Success rates based on severity of ADHD and ODD symptoms at the end of treatment. *Journal of the American Academy of Child & Adolescent Psychiatry*, 40(2): 168–179.

Swanson, J., Oosterlaan, J., Murias, M., Moyzis, R., Schuck, S., Mann, M., Feldman, P., Spence, M. A., Sergeant, J., Smith, M., Kennedy J. & Posner, M. I. (2000). ADHD children with 7-repeat allele of the DRD4 gene have extreme behavior but normal performance on critical neuropsychological tests of attention *Proceedings of the National Academy of Sciences, USA*, 97: 4754–4759.

Swanson, J. M., Posner, M. I., Potkin, S., Bonforte, S., Youpa, D., Cantwell, D. & Crinella, F. (1991). Activating tasks for the study of visual-spatial attention in ADHD children: A cognitive anatomical approach. *Journal of Child Neurology*, 6: S119–S127.

Taylor, T., Kingstone, A. F. & Klein, R. M. (1998). Visual offsets and oculomotor disinhibition: Endogenous and exogenous contributions to the gap effect. *Canadian Journal of Experimental Psychology*, 52: 192–200.

Theeuwes, J., Kramer, A. F., Han, S. & Irwin, D. E. (1998). Our eyes do not always go where want them to go: Capture of the eyes by new objects. *Psychological Science*, 9: 379–385.

Titchener, E. B. (1909). *Experimental Psychology of the Thought Processes*. New York: Macmillan.

Treisman, A. M. & Gelade, G. (1980). A feature-integration theory of attention. *Cognitive Psychology*, 12: 97–136.

Trick, L. M. & Enns, J. T. (1998). Lifespan changes in attention: the visual search task. *Cognitive Development*, 13: 369–386.

Turken, A. U. & Swick, D. (1999). Response selection in the human anterior cingulate cortex. *Nature Neurosceince*, 2(10): 920–924.

Uttal, W. R. (2001). *The New Phrenology: The Limits of Localizing Cognitive Processes in the Brain*. Cambridge MA: MIT Press.

Vasey, M. W. & Macleod, C. (2001). Information-processing factors in childhood-anxiety: A review and developmental perspective. In M. E. Vasey & M. R. Dadds (Eds.), *The Developmental Psychopathology of Anxiety*, (pp. 253–277). New York: Oxford University Press.

van Veen V, Carter CS: (2002). The timing of action-monitoring processes in the anterior cingulate cortex. *Journal of Cognitive Neuroscience*, 14: 593–602.

Van Voorhis, S. T. & Hilyard, S. A. (1977). Visual evoked potential and selective attention to points in space. *Perception and Psychophysiology*, 1: 54–62.

Venter, J. C., Adams, M. D., Myers, E. W., Li, P. W., Mural, R. J., Sutton et al., (2001). The sequence of the human genome. *Science*, 291: 1304–1335.

Vivas, A. B., Humphreys, G. W. & Fuentes, L. J. (2003). Inhibitory processing following damage to the parietal lobe. *Neuropsychologia*, 41: 1531–1540.

Volpe, B. T., LeDoux, J. E. & Gazzaniga, M. S. (1979). Information processing of visual stimuli in an extinguished visual field. *Nature*, 282: 1947–52.

Voytko, M. L., Olton, D. S., Richardson, R. T., Gorman, L. K., Tobin, J. R. & Price, D. L. (1994). Basal forebrain lesions in monkeys disrupt attention but not learning and memory. *Journal of Neuroscience*, 14(1): 167–186.

Walter, W. G., Cooper, R., Aldridge, V. J., McCallum, W. C. & Winter, A. L. (1964). Contingent negative variation: an electrical sigh of sensorimotor association and expectancy in the human brain. *Nature*, 203: 380–384.

Wang, K. J., Fan, J., Dong, Y., Wang C., Lee, T. M. C. & Posner, M. I. (2005). Selective impairment of attentional networks of orienting and executive control in schizophrenia. *Schiz. Res.* 78, 235–241.

Wender, P. (1971). *Minimal Brain Dysfunction in Children*. New York: Wiley-Liss.

Wojciulik, E., Kanwisher, N. & Driver, J. (1998). Covert visual attention modulates face-specific activity in the human fusiform gyrus: fMRI study. *Journal of Neurophysiology*, 79(3): 1574–1578.

Wurtz, R. H., Goldberg, E. & Robinson, D. L. (1980). Behavioral modulation of visual responses in monkey: Stimulus selection for attention and movement. *Progress in Psychobiology and Physiological Psychology*, 9: 43–83.

Yantis, S. (1992). Multi-element visual tracking: Attention and perceptual organization. *Cognitive Psychology*, 3: 295–340.

19 Integrative Physiology: Homeostasis, Allostasis, and the Orchestration of Systemic Physiology

GARY G. BERNTSON AND JOHN T. CACIOPPO

1. INTRODUCTION

Since the seminal work of Walter Cannon, the concept of homeostasis has been a major force in the historical development of views of autonomic regulation and control. The homeostatic construct also importantly shaped many twentieth century psychological concepts and theories, including models of reinforcement, motivation, perception, personality, and psychosomatic disorders. This construct has been particularly salient in psychophysiology and behavioral medicine, because of the putative role of homeostatic processes in the regulation of autonomic and neuroendocrine systems. The present chapter will explore the current status of the homeostatic model, and the emergence of modern concepts of allostasis and allodynamic regulation.

A second aim of the chapter is to consider the underlying neural systems and mechanisms that give rise to autonomic regulation and psychophysiological relationships. A complication in drawing clear psychophysiological relations is the fact that these associations cut across systems and processes represented at distinct levels of conceptualization and analysis. One goal of multi-level integrative analyses is to bring the concepts, processes and terms of the two levels of analysis into registration, to permit a more accurate appreciation of the underlying links and organizations (Cacioppo et al., 2000). The construct of fear, for example, has a long tradition in psychology and brain systems mediating this state are beginning to be elucidated. What is less clear is how brain *processes*, not just areas and structures, give rise to fear – that is, how the physiological and psychological domains map onto one another. Rapprochement between psychological and physiological constructs and theories will likely require refinements in conceptualization and quantification within both the physiological and psychological domains. Integrative analysis across psychological and physiological levels is still very much a work in progress and psychophysiology resides at a critical intersection to pursue this integration. In considering the psychophysiology of the autonomic nervous system, the present chapter will identify some aspects of a broad framework that may contribute to the emergence of a true *neuropsychophysiology*.

1.1. Homeostasis and homeodynamic regulation

1.1.1. Origins of the homeostatic concept

The notion of natural balancing or equilibrium-seeking tendencies may be traced back as early as Hippocrates (Cofer & Appley, 1964). The term homeostasis, and the contemporary negative feedback model of homeostatic regulation has a more recent history. Claude Bernard (1878/1974) reflected on the relative constancy of the internal environment (*mileau intérieur*) of living creatures. This constancy was seen to reflect an organism's ability to stabilize the cellular environment, despite powerful entropic forces that threaten to disrupt the biological order essential for life. Mechanisms underlying this constancy permit warm-blooded creatures to live what Bernard termed a "free and independent life" (Bernard, 1878/1974, p 89). Cannon (1929,1939) extended this perspective, coining the term *homeostasis* to refer to the processes by which the *constancy of the fluid matrix* is maintained. The concept of homeostasis was so central to Cannon's view that he virtually equated homeostatic adjustments with adaptive responses.

Cannon's concepts significantly shaped contemporary views of autonomic regulation and control. Legacies from the Cannon era include the concepts that (1) the autonomic nervous system is reflexively regulated for homeostasis, (2) the sympathetic and parasympathetic branches generally exert opposing effects on end organs, and (3) the sympathetic and parasympathetic branches are subject to reciprocal central control. From a homeostatic perspective, the concept of reciprocal control is natural. A reciprocal pattern of autonomic control would maximize autonomic resources in the maintenance of a homeostatic set point as the two branches would act synergistically in this process. The concepts of homeostasis and reciprocal control were echoed in Fulton's (1949) influential *Textbook of Physiology*: "The autonomic nerves . . . . are the regulators concerned with emergency mechanisms, with repair, and with preservation of the constancy of the internal environment" (Fulton, 1949, p. 222); and "In the reflex regulation of the heart rate, the sympathetic and parasympathetic nervous systems are reciprocally linked in their central representations" (Fulton, 1949, p. 668). Homeostasis remains the dominant organizing concept of autonomic function in the contemporary physiological literature, and the notion of reciprocal control of the autonomic branches continues to be advanced. Malliani (1999), for example, asserts: "In most physiological conditions, sympathetic and vagal activities modulating heart period undergo a reciprocal regulation" (p. 111).

The concept of homeostasis has also had a powerful impact on psychophysiological theory. Homeostatic compensatory adjustments were viewed by Lacey (1956) as an important secondary, reflexive contributor to observed patterns of psychophysiological response, while Obrist (1981) considered homeostatic processes to contribute more directly to the primary response. In his construct of cardiac-somatic coupling, for example, Obrist viewed heart rate responses in behavioral contexts to reflect, at least in part, homeostatic adjustments associated with increased metabolic demands.

The concept of reciprocal control of the autonomic branches also has had a continuing influence on psychophysiological constructs. Examples include Wenger's classic index ($\bar{A}$) of *autonomic balance* along a continuum extending from sympathetic to parasympathetic dominance (Wenger, 1941). A more recent example is the application of the ratio of low to high frequency heart rate variability (LF/HF ratio) as an index of *sympathovagal balance* (e.g., Malliani, 1999).

1.1.2. Some mechanisms of homeostasis

A number of factors contribute to the relative constancy of internal states. These include peripheral processes such as buffering systems of the blood that maintain plasma pH, and the inherent elasticity of the vasculature that tends to minimize pressor variations due to changes in blood volume. These mechanisms are included in the general class of peripheral *autoregulatory* processes that contribute to stability in physiological dimensions (see Dworkin, 1993).

In contrast to peripheral autoregulatory processes, central reflex mechanisms have generally been of greater interest in psychophysiology. An important aspect of the homeostatic model is that reflexive networks achieve sensitivity to the functional state of some regulated dimension (e.g., blood pressure), by means of visceral feedback (e.g., via baroreceptors), and generate compensatory responses to restore detected imbalances. Like the thermostatic control of room temperature, homeostatic reflexes may operate as feedback controlled servomechanisms, continually adjusting autonomic outflow to compensate for perturbations in the target dimension. This is the classic feedback-controlled model of homeostasis.

A. Schematic Baroreflex Circuit

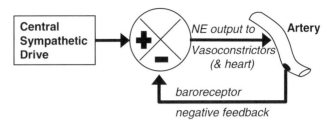

B. Human Baroreceptor Cardiac Reflex

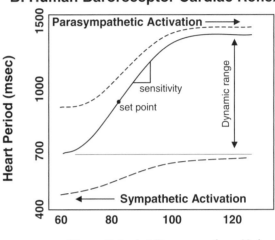

Figure 19.1. A. A basic servocontrolled homeostatic system with negative feedback **B.** Baroreceptor-cardiac reflex function in humans. The solid line illustrates changes in heart period with variations in mean arterial pressure. The solid dot depicts the resting blood pressure set point, the slope of the line represents the sensitivity of the reflex, and the distance from the minima to the maxima is the dynamic range. Note that increases in blood pressure yield an increase in parasympathetic activation and a reciprocal decrease in sympathetic activity. The dashed lines illustrate the separate sympathetic and parasympathetic contributions during selective blockades of the other branch. (Data are derived from Robinson et al., 1966; see Berntson, Cacioppo, & Quigley, 1993).

1.1.3. A prototypic homeostatic mechanism: The baroreceptor-heart rate reflex

As illustrated in Figure 19.1, a typical feedback-controlled homeostatic system is characterized by a set-point that represents the regulatory level or the central tendency of the regulatory system (see Table 19.1). Deviations from this regulated level contribute to the critical feedback control signal that triggers a compensatory response. These homeostatic features are instantiated in the baroreceptor-cardiac reflex depicted in Figure 19.2. As illustrated in this figure, an increase in blood pressure triggers (via baroreceptor afferents) a reflexive withdrawal of cardiac sympathetic tone and a reciprocal increase in vagal outflow to the heart. The coordinated changes in the two autonomic branches synergistically lead to a decrease in heart rate and ventricular contractility, which contribute to a reduction in cardiac output. These responses and the associated

Table 19.1. Regulatory parameters

1. *Set point*:
   The set point is the functional status that is actively regulated, and physiologically defended, by compensatory responses to perturbations. In the absence of over-riding perturbations, it can be indexed by the central tendency of the regulated dimension.

2. *Operating Characteristics*:
   (a) *Dynamic range*. The dynamic range characterizes the limits of a compensatory process. It represents the regulatory capacity of the system, and is generally expressed as the difference between the maximal and minimal asymptotes of the response (e.g. the maximal and minimal heart rates seen to perturbations of blood pressure associated with the baroreceptor-heart rate reflex).

   (b) *Sensitivity (threshold and "gain")*. Sensitivity represents the threshold of perturbation in the regulated dimension that is just capable of initiating compensatory responses, and gain is the magnitude or compensatory capacity of the initiated response. This is often represented as the slope of the response function (e.g., the compensatory change in heart rate to a unit change in blood pressure).

   (c) *Linearity*. This refers to the shape of the activation (response) function across the dynamic range of control. Deviations from linearity represent variations in gain along the response function for a given increment in the relevant stimulus (deviation from regulatory level). In physiological systems, response functions are often sigmoidal, but in many cases, may be approximated by a linear function within the typical operating ranges.

   (d) *Temporal dynamics*. Temporal (dynamic) aspects of the control system, including dimensions such as latency, time course, recovery time, frequency response, and phase lag.

   (e) *Stability*. Stability of a process is its reliability or reproducibility, for a given set of conditions. Variations may be random (noise), or systematic (e.g., hysteresis resulting from baroreceptor adaptation, so that the heart rate for an given blood pressure may differ for an increasing pressor ramp than for a decreasing ramp).

withdrawal of sympathetic tone to the vasculature tend to oppose the pressor perturbation.

1.2. Beyond homeostasis: Homeodynamic regulation

Based on the work of Pavlov, Cannon recognized that learned autonomic adjustments could be made in anticipation of a visceral perturbation (Cannon, 1928). Such anticipatory responses can not be viewed as mere reflexive adjustments to a physiological perturbation. More recently, Dworkin has re-emphasized the potential importance of higher learning processes in homeostatic regulation (Dworkin, 1993; Dworkin & Dworkin, this volume). Dworkin proposes that by appropriately calibrated

conditioned responses, learned autonomic adjustments may minimize or preclude homeostatic disturbances from otherwise perturbing stimuli. Dworkin outlines a sophisticated control-theory framework for homeostatic regulation, incorporating anticipatory *feed-forward* components. This model offers an important advance over traditional feedback-controlled models of homeostatic regulation. Although not incompatible with the homeostatic concept, the existence of anticipatory controls highlights an important limitation of the simple feedback model of homeostatic regulation illustrated in Figure 19.1.

In addition to these basic lower-level reflexes, autonomic regulation is also impacted by higher central processes. When blood pressure goes up, baroreceptor reflexes tend to compensate by driving heart rate (and hence cardiac

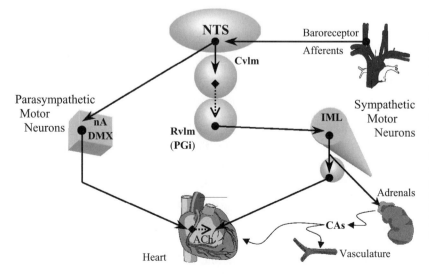

Figure 19.2. Summary of brainstem systems underlying baroreceptor cardiac reflex. Baroreceptor afferents project to nucleus tractus solitarius (NTS), which in turn leads to activation of parasympathetic motor neurons in the nucleus ambiguus (nA) and dorsal motor nucleus of the vagus (DMX). The NTS also activates the caudal ventrolateral medulla (Cvlm) which in turn inhibits the rostral ventrolateral medulla (Rvlm), leading to a withdrawal of excitatory drive on the sympathetic motor neurons in the intermediolateral cell column of the cord (IML). Abbreviations: ACh, acetylcholine; CAs, catecholamines; NE, norepinephrine; PGi, paragigantocullar nucleus (partially coextensive with Rvlm).

output) down. Consequently, blood pressure and heart rate often show a negative covariation. During stress, however, both blood pressure and heart rate may increase in apparent violation of the baroreflex pattern, and the increase in heart rate can further contribute to the pressor response in a distinctly non-homeostatic fashion. Although not homeostatic, this may be highly adaptive in providing the metabolic resources for effective response (fight or flight). It is now clear that a range of stressors, including moderate cognitive stressors, can reduce the gain or set-point of the baroreceptor-heart rate reflex (Lucini et al., 2002; Steptoe & Sawada, 1989; Van Roon et al., 2004). By suppressing baroreceptor reflexes, together with more direct descending controls over autonomic source nuclei, higher neural systems can by-pass or override homeostatic reflexes. This allows for a more flexible allostatic (other level) pattern of autonomic control, in which organ systems can be regulated at alternative (allostatic) levels in the face of changing circumstances.

Summary. The considerations above suggest that the simple feedback-control, set-point model may not adequately represent the complexity of visceral regulation. Moreover, the emphasis on static levels and the fixedness implied by the term *homeostasis* does not capture the variability and dynamic features of visceral control systems. A more appropriate construct may be that of *homeodynamic regulation*, which recognizes the fact that regulatory mechanisms are multiple and complex, including both feedback and feedforward components, as well as multiple levels of control extending from lower reflexes to descending regulation from higher neurobehavioral substrates. The concept of homeodynamic regulation does imply a single regulatory level, but recognizes that variations around this level may be rather broad, reflecting the operations of multiple dynamic influences. This represents an important conceptual advance over the rigidity implied by the term homeostasis.

1.3. Heterostasis, allostasis, and allodynamic regulation

1.3.1. Heterostasis
Although variations in gain, dynamic range or other operating characteristics can alter the efficiency, capacity, and time course of regulatory processes, as long as the regulatory set-point remains constant these processes could be subsumed under the construct of homeodynamic regulation. Selye (1973), however, argued that regulatory levels are not rigidly fixed, but may be actively altered in the face of exogenous challenges or pathogens. For Selye, homeostatic processes may continue to operate at the basic regulatory level, being sensitive to *internal* physiological stimuli that signal deviations from a regulated set point. According to Selye, however, *exogenous* stimuli may reset regulatory levels, either directly or via a humoral route, to facilitate resistance or adaptation to the exogenous stressor. Such readjustments of set-point deviate from homeo-

static or homeodynamic processes, as they represent active alterations of the regulatory level. In contrast to homeostasis, Selye applied the term *heterostasis* to this class of regulatory adjustment (from the Greek *heteros* meaning "other" or "different" and *stasis* meaning "fixity" or "lack of movement").

An example of heterostatic regulation is a fever, which differs from hyperthermia arising from a thermoregulatory failure (e.g., due to extreme heat or exercise). Instead, illness-induced fever reflects the adoption of a higher set-point, which is actively regulated and defended. An artificial reduction in body temperature during a fever is met with active compensatory thermogenic processes (e.g., shivering, metabolic thermogenesis, behavioral thermoregulation; Romanovsky, 2004; Werner, 1988). The elevation in temperature associated with a fever may be of benefit in mobilizing energy resources to combat infections or other adaptive challenges. Because a fever reflects the adoption of a *new* regulatory set point, it is more appropriately considered a heterostatic rather than a homeostatic or homeodynamic process. Selye (1973) emphasized the role of hormones and the chemical environment in heterostatic regulation. As will be considered below, however, modulation of regulatory mechanisms can also arise from central process and these processes may mediate or interact with changes in the hormonal and chemical environment of the body.

1.3.2. Allostasis
More recently, Sterling and Eyer (1988) introduced the term *allostasis*, (from the Greek *allos*, meaning "other") to capture the complexities of visceral regulation. Sterling and Eyer recognized that regulatory levels are not fixed, but may be flexibly adjusted to meet changing demands. Although allostasis also entails the concept of changing regulatory set-points, the construct is conceptualized more broadly than Selye's heterostasis. The allostatic concept of Sterling and Eyer incorporates the view that many visceral dimensions are regulated by multiple interacting mechanisms that are subject to a wide range of modulatory influences. Blood pressure, for example, is not constant throughout the day, but shows systematic fluctuations associated with circadian cycles of sleep and waking and with varying diurnal patterns of activity throughout the day. These alterations in set-point are not consonant with simple homeostatic or homeodynamic models. Nor do they necessarily involve the exogenous agents or pathological conditions of Selye's model. Rather, they are seen as reflecting the natural adaptive readjustment of regulatory levels in view of changing physiological demands.

An additional feature of Sterling and Eyer's concept of allostatic regulation is that it reflects the operations of higher neural systems that control and integrate a broad range of more basic "homeostatic" reflexes. Consequently, allostatic control is not constrained to a single functional dimension or even to a large set of parallel regulatory processes. Rather, allostatic control may achieve greater flexibility in maintaining integrative regulation across visceral functions. In the regulation of a functional end-point such as maintenance of circulation, for example, higher neural systems can modulate a wide range of functional dimensions that influence this end-point. These include heart rate, cardiac contractility, vascular tone, blood pressure, and renal function; each of which can alter cardiovascular dynamics and can be in turn adjusted by a combination of autonomic and neuroendocrine influences. An implication of this integrative model is that the end-point of regulation may not be adequately characterized by a single dimension of visceral function, such as sympathetic outflow, heart rate, vascular tone, or blood pressure. In view of the multiplicity and integrative nature of allostatic control, central abnormalities that contribute to hypertension, for example, may not be effectively normalized by clinical treatment of a single visceral parameter (e.g., diuretics or beta-blockers). This is because allostatic regulatory processes are speculated to control many response parameters in the regulation of the target visceral dimension. Treatment of one dimension may merely lead to a compensatory alteration in another, which may maintain the abnormal regulated state of blood pressure. This concept has substantive implications for behavioral medicine, an issue to which we will return below (see Inferential Context).

Summary. The term heterostasis was proposed by Selye to reflect the alterations in regulatory levels that may be triggered by exogenous stimuli. The concept of allostasis was subsequently introduced by Sterling and Eyer to represent a wider set of central integrative controls over visceral regulation, related to both endogenous and exogenous conditions. The construct of allostasis subsumes and broadens Selye's concept of heterostasis, and is particularly significant for psychophysiology because rostral brain systems that underlie behavioral processes can exert complex patterns of regulation over neuroendocrine and autonomic function. Consequently, the optimal approach to understanding and alleviation of stress-related disorders is not merely the identification and palliation of a peripheral pathology. Rather, the origins of the dysregulation must be sought in central-visceral interactions (Thayer & Lane, 2000). Similarly, consideration of the central integrative processes that give rise to physiological responses may help to clarify psychophysiological relations, a subject to which we will return below.

1.3.3. Allodynamic regulation

The constructs of homeostasis and homeodynamic regulation both entail a relatively fixed regulatory set-point, although the homeodynamic concept explicitly recognizes the dynamic features of regulatory systems. The notion of heterostasis and the broader concept of allostasis similarly assume a regulatory set-point, although both emphasize the fact that regulatory levels may be variable, rather than fixed. It remains unclear, however, whether deviations from a fixed functional level universally represent

an allostatic-like adoption of a new set-point. We will consider below (see Physical Context) the possibility that at least some physiological changes associated with behavioral states may reflect the active inhibition of set-point regulation, rather than the adoption of an altered regulatory level. This is an issue of fundamental importance for conceptions of the nature of visceral control and for its health implications.

In view of these considerations, we introduce as a heuristic starting point the construct of *allodynamic regulation* (see Table 19.1). This construct is intended to broadly subsume the wide range of regulatory processes represented by the concepts of homeostasis, homeodynamic regulation, heterostasis, and allostasis. In addition, the allodynamic concept recognizes the potential limitations of regulatory processes, and the possibility that visceral reactions may not always be regulated about a set-point level.

2. PHYSICAL CONTEXT

2.1. Classical baroreceptor reflex and homeostatic regulation

Figure 19.2 presents a schematic depiction of the basic baroreceptor reflex circuit (Dampney et al., 2003; Spyer, 1990). Baroreceptor afferents increase their rate of firing in response to an increase in blood pressure and this afferent activity is conveyed to the nucleus of the tractus solitarius (NTS) in the medulla, which is the primary visceral receiving area in the brainstem. The NTS issues direct and indirect excitatory projections to vagal motor neurons in the nucleus ambiguus and the dorsal motor nucleus, leading to a reflexive increase in parasympathetic outflow. The NTS also projects to a "depressor area" in the caudal ventrolateral medulla (CVLM), which in turn inhibits sympathoexcitatory neurons of a "pressor area" in the rostral ventrolateral medulla (RVLM). This leads to a decrease in activity of the sympathetic motor neurons in the intermediolateral cell column of the cord. Through this circuitry, baroreceptors achieve reciprocal reflexive control over sympathetic and parasympathetic outflows and contribute to the homeostatic feedback-regulation of blood pressure.

2.2. Complexities in autonomic control

This homeostatic feedback-controlled model is elegant in its simplicity and, together with the construct of a set-point or regulatory level, could contribute to the relative stability of blood pressure over time. This simple model, however, belies the complexity of cardiovascular control (for a more comprehensive model, see Van Roon et al., 2004). Although baroreceptor reflexes importantly serve to oppose transient blood pressure perturbations, they may not wholly account for the long-term stability of blood pressure. Like other interoceptors, baroreceptors are subject to adaptation and it has been argued that they cannot reliably report steady-state levels (Dworkin, 1993). Although more recent studies raise the possibility that this adaptation may

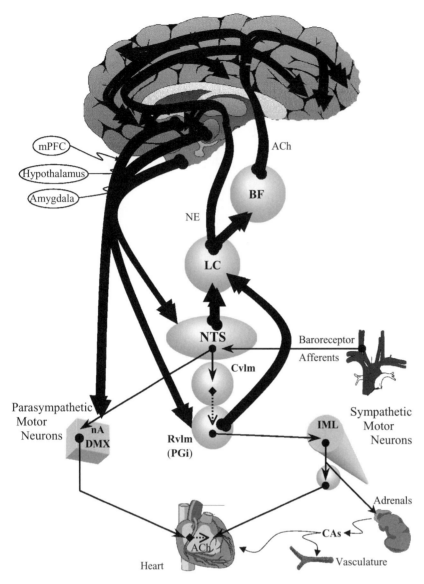

Figure 19.3. Expansion of the baroreflex circuit of Figure 19.2, to illustrate the ascending and descending pathways to and from rostral neural areas such as the medial prefrontal cortex (mPFC), hypothalamus (Hypo), and amygdala. Ascending systems include routes from the rostral ventrolateral medulla (Rvlm) and the nucleus of the tractus solitarius (NTS) to the locus coeruleus (LC) noradrenergic system, and indirectly to the basal forebrain (BF) cortical cholinergic system. Abbreviations: ACh, acetylcholine; CAs, catecholamines; NE, norepinephrine; PGi, paragigantocullar nucleus (partially coextensive with Rvlm).

brainstem are closely regulated by chemoreceptive feedback from blood gases, but can be modulated or overridden by higher-level systems associated with vocalization, anticipation of exercise, affective modulation of respiration, or volitional breath-holding (Harper, 1996). These latter influences appear to be mediated by descending pathways from the hypothalamus, amygdala, and the cerebral cortex. As illustrated in Figure 19.3, these structures project to autonomic regulatory substrates in the brainstem, including the NTS and the ventrolateral medulla, as well as to lower central autonomic motor neurons (Chen & Toney, 2003; Neafsey, 1990; Sequeira et al., 2000; Shih, Chan, & Chan, 1995; Wallace, Magnuson & Gray, 1992). Of particular relevance for psychophysiology is the fact that the rostral sources of these descending projections include limbic and forebrain areas that have been implicated in behavioral processes. Stimulation or lesions of these rostral structures have been shown to be capable of facilitating, inhibiting, or even bypassing basic brainstem autonomic reflexes to modulate autonomic outflow in a direct fashion (Inui et al., 1995; Koizumi & Kollai, 1981; Neafsey, 1990; Oppenheimer & Cechetto, 1990; Sequeira et al., 2000; Sevoz-Couche et al., 2003; Spyer, 1990). Stimulation of the central nucleus of the amygdale or the hypothalamus, for example, can inhibit barosensitive neurons in the rostral ventrolateral medulla (Gelsema et al., 1989) as well as the baroreflex response (Sevoz-Couche et al., 2003). It is likely that descending influences such as these serve as the conduit by which psychological stressors can inhibit the baroreflex and yield a concurrent increase in blood pressure and heart rate in direct opposition to this reflex (see also Van Roon et al., 2004).

Although baroreceptor reflexes may exert a classical pattern of reciprocal control over the autonomic branches, rostral systems appear to be much more flexible. The traditional concept of reciprocal central control of the autonomic branches has undergone considerable qualification in the light of contemporary findings, and it is now apparent that the two autonomic branches can vary reciprocally, coactively, or independently (Table 19.2; Berntson, Cacioppo, & Quigley, 1991, 1993; Berntson et al., 1994; Koizumi & Kollai, 1992; see Van Roon et al., 2004). Descending influences from higher neural systems are

not be complete, steady-state levels of blood pressure are also regulated by a variety of factors, including peripheral (autoregulatory) processes, hormonal influences, and brainstem generators of autonomic tone that are at least in part independent of baroreceptor activity. Adding to this complexity are the contributions of rostral neural systems and anticipatory modulations of lower autonomic mechanisms.

2.3. Rostral influences

Rostral neural structures exert potent controls over brainstem regulatory systems. Respiratory mechanisms of the

Table 19.2. Conceptual models of autonomic regulation

Set point	Operating characteristics	
	Fixed	Variable
Fixed	Homeostatic	Homeodynamic
Variable	Allostatic	Allodynamic

capable of modulating the operating characteristics of brainstem homeostatic mechanisms, and can generate highly flexible patterns of autonomic outflow. Hypothalamic stimulation, for example, can evoke each of the basic modes of reciprocal, coactive, or independent changes in the activity of the autonomic branches (Koizumi & Kollai, 1981; Shih, Chan, & Chan, 1995). These descending integrative influences likely serve as important substrates for allodynamic regulation of the viscera.

Clearly, autonomic state cannot be viewed as lying along a single reciprocal autonomic continuum extending from sympathetic dominance at one end to parasympathetic dominance at the other. Although reflex systems may tend toward reciprocal patterns of control, higher neurobehavioral networks exert a much broader and more flexible range of controls over the autonomic branches. When considering rostral influences, sympathetic and parasympathetic activities are more properly conceptualized by a bivariate autonomic plane (Figure 19.4). This parallels the somatic motor system, where extensor and flexor muscles are subject to reciprocal innervation by spinal reflexes. Reflexes that excite motor neurons for a given muscle (e.g., flexion and limb withdrawal from a pain stimulus) also inhibit the opponent (extensor) motor neurons. Despite this reciprocal innervation at the spinal cord level, we can volitionally contract both flexor and extensor muscles concurrently, as in a stiff-arm.

2.4. Afferent links and ascending influences

Of particular relevance for emerging neurobehavioral models of the links between psychological processes and autonomic control is the fact that interactions between rostral and caudal neural systems are bidirectional (see Figure 19.3). The potential role of visceral afference in higher level processes has long been of interest to psychologists, but has proven very difficult to characterize and quantify. Although the role of visceral afference in emotion and cognition remains speculative (see Cacioppo, Berntson, & Klein, 1992; Damasio, 1994), empirical findings document potent influences of visceral afferent information in central nervous system functions. Baroreceptor afferents to the brainstem represent the afferent limb of reflexes which subserve basic homeostatic functions. Visceral afferents, however, play a much broader and far more flexible role in behavioral processes. Baroreceptor activation, for example, has been shown to modulate afferent pain transmission and reduce pain perception (Dworkin

et al., 1994; Edwards et al., 2002). Visceral afferents may also impact more directly on activity in higher brain systems. Ascending projections from brainstem autonomic substrates project directly to forebrain areas that have been implicated in neurobehavioral processes, including the amygdala, cerebral cortex and basal forebrain cholinergic system (Aston-Jones et al., 1996; Berntson, Sarter, & Cacioppo, 2003; Zardetto-Smith & Gray, 1995).

As depicted in Figure 19.3, baroreceptor afferents terminate in the nucleus of the tractus solitarius (NTS). In addition to participating in local reflex circuits, baroreceptor afferent activity is relayed via the NTS to the nucleus paragigantocellularis (PGi), which provides a tonic drive on sympathetic motor neurons (Figure 19.3; for review see Berntson, Sarter, & Cacioppo, 2003). Consequently, the PGi (which is coextensive with the rostral ventrolateral

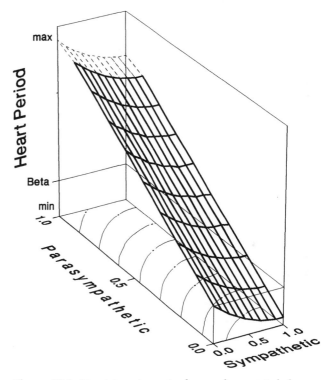

Figure 19.4. Bivariate autonomic plane and associated chronotropic effector surface. The plane bounded by the parasympathetic and sympathetic axes represents all possible combinations of sympathetic and parasympathetic activities (on a relative scale from 0 to 1). The effector surface overlying the autonomic plane represents the chronotropic state of the target organ, expressed in heart period, for all loci within autonomic space (see Berntson et al., 1993 for details on derivation). Parasympathetic activation exerts relatively linear effects on heart period, whereas sympathetic activation yields somewhat nonlinear effects. The dotted surface at maximal levels of parasympathetic activation represents the ambiguity in effects at this extreme. For illustrative purposes, the relative lengths of the axes are scaled in proportion to relative dynamic ranges of control of the autonomic branches, and Beta represents the "intrinsic" heart period in the absence of autonomic input. The curved lines on the autonomic plane represent isoeffector contours projected from the effector surface onto the autonomic plane. These contour lines illustrate loci on the autonomic plane that yield equivalent chronotropic effects.

medullary pressor area) would be expected to be highly sensitive to the state of activity in the sympathetic branch. The PGi also projects to the locus coeruleus, a structure that has been implicated in arousal and anxiety (Aston-Jones et al., 1996; Berntson et al., 1998, 2003), and the LC in turn issues an ascending noradrenergic projection to the limbic system and cerebral cortex. The activity of this ascending noradrenergic pathway would thus be expected to be modulated by the level of sympathetic tone.

In addition to its direct projections to limbic areas, the locus coeruleus also projects to the basal forebrain, which is the primary source of cholinergic innervation of the cortex (for review see, Sarter & Bruno, 1997). This cholinergic projection appears to enhance cortical processing, and has been implicated in cognitive and attentional processes (Sarter & Bruno, 1997). Degeneration of the basal forebrain-cortical cholinergic system is considered one of the major neuropathological conditions leading to the attentional and cognitive decline in Alzheimer's disease. In contrast, increased activity in this cholinergic system has been suggested to underlie cognitive aspects of anxiety, by virtue of the enhanced processing of anxiogenic stimuli (Berntson et al., 1998, 2003). The prototypic anxiolytic agents, the benzodiazepine receptor agonists such as chlordiazepoxide (*Librium*) and diazepam (*Valium*), appear to exert their anti-anxiety actions, at least in part, by attenuating activity in the basal forebrain cholinergic system. These ascending pathways likely mediate the affective and cognitive effects of visceral afference.

Over a century ago, William James (1884) proposed that the perception of visceral afferent information may constitute an important component of emotional experience (see Cacioppo, Berntson, & Klein, 1992). Research on human subjects with high spinal transections (quadriplegia or tetraplegia) has not yielded strong support for the necessary involvement of visceral activity and associated visceral afference in emotion (Chwalisz, Diencer, & Gallagher, 1988). This, however, does not rule out an important modulatory role of visceral afference in emotion (see Cacioppo, Berntson, & Klein, 1992). High spinal cord transections do disrupt descending control of sympathetic outflow, but eliminate neither parasympathetic responses nor vagally conveyed visceral afference. Further, given the modulatory role of norepinephrine and acetylcholine on cortical activation and reactivity, the ascending pathways of Figure 19.3 would be expected to enhance cortical/limbic processing generally. Hence, ascending visceral afference may be more likely to prime or bias, rather than strictly determine, affective states. Affective and autonomic reactivity may be driven by a cognitively related top-down activation (e.g., in affective imagery) of the descending system depicted in Figure 19.3, and the resulting autonomic reactivity may further bias rostral systems toward the processing of affective stimuli via ascending pathways. Alternatively, visceral afference may yield a bottom-up priming of cognitive/affective processing even in the absence of an affective context via the pathways in Figure 19.3.

The early study of Schachter and Singer (1962) on emotional priming by epinephrine was consistent with this model, although serious questions have been raised over the generality of these results (Cacioppo, Berntson, & Klein, 1992; Reisenzein, 1983). More recent work offers substantial support to the view that visceral afference can modulate higher cognitive/emotional processing. Vagal stimulation or systemic administration of epinephrine has been reported to enhance cortical processing and to potentiate memories in rats and humans, and these effects can be blocked or attenuated by vagotomy, inactivation of the NTS, or by direct infusions of adrenergic blockers into the basal forebrain or the amygdala (Berntson et al., 2003; Cahill & Alkire, 2003; Clark et al., 1999; Hassert, Miyashita, & Williams, 2004; Williams & Clayton, 2001). Visceral afference also appears to play an important role in the allodynamic regulation of body temperature, as the fever associated with behavioral stress or exogenous mitogens appears to be mediated at least in part by a vagal afferent message (Hansen et al., 2001). Further work is clearly needed in this area, but the existing data are in accord with the bidirectional interaction among rostral and caudal neural substrates in the control of affective and autonomic reactivity.

Summary. Both ascending and descending neural systems appear to participate in affective states and autonomic control. Although the contributions of descending pathways have been more fully studied, ascending visceral information may prove to be equally important in biasing psychological processes and mediating psychophysiological relations. Findings at a neurobiological level focus attention on the complex interactions between central systems, autonomic regulation, and peripheral afferent signals. The convergence of visceral afference on common rostral neural systems, together with the hierarchical, integrative control these systems exert on lower autonomic substrates, likely contributes to the broader integration of behavioral and autonomic processes implied by the concept of *allodynamic regulation*. Homeostatic mechanisms can be highly adaptive, but there are many conditions in which it may not be optimal to maintain a fixed steady-state. In view of the limitless adaptive challenges an organism can encounter, it is hardly surprising that evolutionary pressures led to the development of sophisticated learning mechanisms that support behavioral flexibility and adaptability in overcoming these challenges. It would be most surprising if these same evolutionary pressures ignored the control of autonomic and neuroendocrine functions that provide the visceral support for adaptive response.

3. PSYCHOLOGICAL CONTEXT

3.1. The cardiac-somatic hypothesis: Psychophysiology and metabolic demands

The relationships between somatic effort, metabolic demand, and autonomic regulation have led to the suggestion that cardiovascular reactions in psychological contexts can be attributable to metabolic factors. Based on the apparent correspondence between the direction and magnitude of cardiac change and variations in somatic response, Obrist proposed that "the metabolically relevant relationship or linkage between cardiac and somatic events is also relevant to behavioral events" (Obrist et al., 1970, p. 570). Obrist recognized, however, that many psychological tasks are metabolically trivial and that the cardiac response in psychological contexts often exceeds that expected on the basis of metabolic demands (Obrist, 1981; Turner, 1994). This is clearly apparent in the autonomic responses that can be invoked, in absence of somatic response, in curarized animals (Dworkin & Dworkin, 1990) and paralyzed human subjects (Berntson & Boysen, 1990).

Obrist later revised the concept of cardiac-somatic coupling, arguing that the fundamental linkage between cardiac and somatic events is attributable to a central coupling rather than peripheral metabolic feedback (Obrist, 1970, 1981). According to this view, it is not the somatomotor response, per se, that triggers cardiovascular responses but rather the central command for motor action. A strong test of the revised cardiac-somatic hypothesis would require measures of central somatic motor outflows in paralyzed subjects. Data relevant to this issue was provided by a study of Dworkin and Dworkin (1990) in which cardiovascular variables and somatic nerve activities were concurrently recorded in a paralyzed rat preparation during the course of discriminative Pavlovian conditioning. Even under complete paralysis, animals evidenced consistent discriminative conditioning (to footshock), as evidenced by EEG desynchronization, somatic (tibial) nerve activity, and cardiovascular responses. Both the conditioned (CR) and unconditioned (UR) central somatic responses entailed an increase in tibial nerve activity. From the standpoint of the cardiac-somatic hypothesis, this was consistent with the tachycardia observed as a UR to shock, but was at variance with the overall bradycardia to the CR despite the associated increase in somatic nerve activity.

Summary. Metabolic effects associated with somatic effort are known to trigger potent reciprocal autonomic adjustments, and this potential contribution needs to be considered in psychophysiological studies. Metabolic effects in many behavioral contexts, however, are insufficient in magnitude or in the wrong direction to account for observed cardiac responses to changing psychological states. There is little doubt that rostral central systems orchestrate coordinated somatic and autonomic responses, and do so in a fashion which transcends simple reflexive adjustments.

3.2. The neuropsychophysiological perspective

The allodynamic model and the rostral neuroanatomical systems depicted in Figure 19.3 suggest a considerable richness in the neurobiological substrates underlying psychophysiological relations. The *neuropsychophysiological* perspective affords the basis for a powerful multilevel analysis of the links between psychological processes and visceral functions. The value of this perspective lies in the fact that psychophysiology can both inform and be informed by neurobiological data, constructs, and theories. The parallels between the central organization and evolution of the somatic and autonomic systems (Folkow, 2000) have not always been fully appreciated and this has sometimes led to unrealistic expectations of simple isomorphic relations between psychological processes and autonomic states.

Illustrative is the pessimism expressed by Obrist (1981) over the use of heart rate in the psychophysiological study of behavioral processes. Commenting on the fact that attention to environmental events is often associated with a decrease in heart rate (HR) whereas increased HR is typically observed in active avoidance, Obrist remarks "... both types of conditions have an obvious attentional component. If we assume for the moment that a decrease in HR is indicative of the attentional factor, then it must be overridden by some other aspect of the task during shock avoidance. It is anything but a parsimonious situation and leads to interpretive difficulties." (Obrist, 1981, p. 198). But since attentional responses frequently entail a decrease in behavioral activity, it may be instructive to substitute the term "behavior" for "HR" in the above comment. Given our understanding of the multiple determinants of behavior, the mere occurrence of a decrease in behavior can not be taken to imply attention nor can an increase in behavior be interpreted as a lack of attention (see Cacioppo & Tassinary, 1990). This is insufficient reason to be disillusioned over the study of behavior, or for that matter, of heart rate. In both cases, a more productive strategy would be to define and disentangle the multiple determinants and processes operative in a given context, and to clarify the underlying relationships and mechanisms.

3.2.1. Rostral descending influences and the modes of autonomic control

Rostral neurobehavioral systems can exert relatively direct and selective influences on central autonomic outflows and their actions may not adhere to simple principles of homeostasis and reciprocal control (Recordati, 2002). Rather, descending systems are capable of evoking a wide range of autonomic modes of control. The autonomic origins of the cardiac responses of humans subjects to orthostatic stress (assumption of an upright posture) and to typical psychological stressors (mental arithmetic, reaction time, and a speech stress task) were evaluated by pharmacological blockades that yielded quantitative estimates of the sympathetic and parasympathetic contributions to cardiac response (Berntson et al., 1994a; Berntson et al., 1994b; Cacioppo et al., 1994). At the group level, the orthostatic and psychological stressors yielded an essentially equivalent pattern of heart rate increase, characterized by sympathetic activation and parasympathetic withdrawal. For

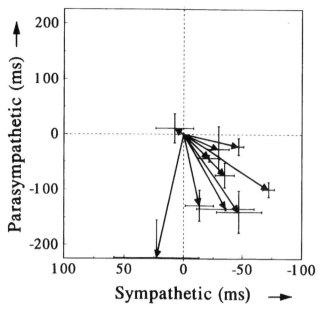

Figure 19.5. Individual patterns of response to stress depicted on the autonomic plane. The intersection of the dotted lines in the center of the graph represents the basal resting state, and the arrows depict the individual response vectors along the sympathetic and parasympathetic axes, with the peak response at the arrowheads. Vectors were derived from independent estimates of the contributions of the autonomic branches under selective pharmacological blockades. Note that some subjects responded primarily with parasympathetic withdrawal, some primarily with sympathetic activation, and some with reciprocal sympathetic activation and parasympathetic withdrawal. These individual response vectors were stable. Three stressors were used (mental arithmetic, a reaction time task, and a speech stressor), and the error bars at the tip of each response vector illustrate the standard errors of the response across the three tasks. Units on the axes are in milliseconds of heart period. (Figure is adapted from Berntson, Cacioppo, Binkley et al., 1994).

the orthostatic stressor, the cardiac response reflected a relatively tight reciprocal central control of the autonomic branches, as evidenced by the significant negative correlation between the responses of the autonomic branches across subjects ($r = -0.71$). Although the group response to psychological stressors was similar, there were considerable individual differences in the pattern of response, and there was no significant correlation between responses of the autonomic branches. The individual patterns of autonomic response were highly reliable across different psychological stressors, but subjects differed considerably in their mode of response. As illustrated in Figure 19.5, some subjects showed primarily sympathetic activation, some reciprocal sympathetic activation and parasympathetic withdrawal, and others primarily parasympathetic withdrawal.

Individual differences in the pattern of autonomic response may have special relevance to psychophysiological relations and psychosomatic disorders. Cardiovascular reactivity to acute laboratory stressors can predict endocrine and immune responses to stress, with high heart rate reactors showing greater changes in cortisol, natural-killer cell activity, and T cell activation (Bachen et al., 1995;

Bosch et al., 2003; Cacioppo, 1994; Cacioppo et al., 1995; Sgoutas-Emch et al., 1994). As illustrated in Figure 19.5, however, there can be sizeable individual differences in the autonomic origins of heart rate responses to stress, and these distinct autonomic modes of control may have differential implications for neuroendocrine and immune responses. It is the sympathetic component of the heart rate response, rather than the parasympathetic component or the heart rate response *per se*, that is most predictive of neuroendocrine and immune reactions to stress (Bosch et al., 2003; Cacioppo, 1994; Cacioppo et al., 1995). This is in keeping with the finding that some immune responses to laboratory stressors can be prevented by selective sympathetic blockade (Bachen et al., 1995; Benschop et al., 1994).

Summary. Descending projections of rostral neurobehavioral systems confer a high degree of flexibility over patterns of autonomic outflow, and can lead to reciprocal, coactive, or independent changes in the activities of the autonomic branches. The allodynamic model incorporates the central integrative nature of behavioral, neuroendocrine, and visceral control, and affords a more comprehensive framework for psychophysiology than does the more limited construct of homeostasis. The allodynamic model also fosters a neuropsychophysiological perspective that recognizes that psychophysiology can both inform and be informed by neurobiological analyses.

4. INFERENTIAL CONTEXT

The homeostatic model emerged from the early physiological literature, and continues as an important organizing construct in both physiology and psychophysiology. There is considerable appeal to the elegant simplicity of the homeostatic construct and the associated reciprocal model of autonomic control. These models, however, do not provide a comprehensive conceptualization of autonomic control in behavioral contexts. Deviations from the reciprocal homeostatic model were recognized in the early physiological literature, but it has been psychophysiological findings that have offered the strongest evidence against these restrictive constructs. The allodynamic model subsumes homeostatic processes, but offers a more comprehensive framework for psychophysiology.

The neuropsychophysiological perspective is particularly relevant within the allodynamic framework, as allodynamic systems quintessentially entail higher central integrative processes. Psychophysiology entails a multi-level approach to the study of the mind-body problem and the relations between psychological and physiological processes. Historically the discipline was often forced to bridge the wide chasm between cognitive and psychological operations on the one hand and rather peripheral physiological dimensions on the other. This was attributable largely to the accessibility of peripheral measures and the relative lack of knowledge of brain systems underlying cognitive and behavioral processes. Although early electroencephalographic studies did obtain more direct measures of brain function, they did not offer much anatomical precision and they focused largely on global states of sleep and arousal. Within the past several decades, however, emerging understandings of neurobiological systems and explosive developments within behavioral and cognitive neuroscience now permit much more direct and specific studies of the central mediators of psychophysiological relations, which is the essence of neuropsychophysiology. Psychophysiological data provide the ultimate subject matter for neurobehavioral studies and the means for validating neurobiological models. At the same time, knowledge of underlying neural mechanisms can inform and constrain psychophysiological theories and facilitate interpretation of psychophysiological data.

4.1. Neuropsychophysiology: Peripheral mappings, measurement, and quantification

The fact that the autonomic branches can be independently controlled has substantial implications for psychophysiological theory and measurement. The autonomic space model (Figure 19.4) suggests that meaningful psychophysiological measures of dually innervated organs require attention to the specific autonomic origins of the end organ state (Berntson et al., 1991). That is, a change in heart rate associated with sympathetic activation may have considerably different psychological and physiological significance than an equivalent change due to parasympathetic withdrawal. Although heart rate measures may continue to have utility in psychophysiology, there is an inherent source of variance that is not adequately parsed by measures of heart rate alone. This variance is relegated to error, and tends to obscure lawful psychophysiological relationships.

The importance of neurophysiologically meaningful measurement of psychophysiological signals is not limited to the heart. Other dually innervated organs, such as the iris of the eye are subject to the similar considerations. Pupillary diameter is a joint function of parasympathetically innervated sphincter (pupillary constrictor) muscle and sympathetically innervated radial (dilator) muscle (see Cohen, this volume). Although there is a degree of reciprocity among the autonomic controls of the iris, changes in pupillary diameter can arise from distinct central systems and can be differentially influenced by the autonomic branches (Loewy, 1990). Parasympathetic control is predominant in accommodation and light reflexes, whereas variation in sympathetic activity is the primary determinant of pupillary responses in behavioral and stress contexts. Again, similar end organ responses arising from different modes of autonomic control may have distinct psychophysiological implications.

Careful elucidation of peripheral autonomic end-organ mappings is important from the perspective of measurement. Equally important are the implications of peripheral mappings for conceptual models and psychophysiological theories. The autonomic space concept of Figure 19.4 is not a mere measurement model, but has substantial implications for psychophysiological concepts. In an early influential theory, Eppinger and Hess (1915) proposed a classification of people as vagally dominant (vagotonic) or sympathetically dominant (sympathicotonic). This view entailed not only a bipolar concept of autonomic control, but a dichotomous individual differences model of autonomic balance. The subsequent studies of Wenger (1941) suggested that "autonomic balance," at best, is continuous rather than dichotomous. More recent studies outlined above (Psychological Context) reveal that the pattern of autonomic response cannot be characterized even along a single continuum, but requires a bivariate model of autonomic control. These findings mandate a more comprehensive conceptualization of the relations between psychological processes, the modes of autonomic control, and potential dispositional biases in psychophysiological disorders.

4.2. Neuropsychophysiology: Central mappings and the relation between psychological processes and brain systems

Evidence outlined above indicates that rostral neural systems can modulate autonomic control in a fashion that is not easily reconciled with a simple homeostatic model. As illustrated in Figure 19.3, there are multiple descending neurobehavioral systems that serve to orchestrate and integrate behavioral, autonomic, and neuroendocrine responses. A greater appreciation of the functional contributions of these systems (i.e., a clarification of the mappings between psychological and neural processes) is likely to contribute to the understanding of complex psychophysiological relations. As neurobehavioral mechanisms are increasingly elucidated, joint studies of psychological and neural functions can be mutually informative.

The literature on arousal offers an example of the mutual benefits of an integrative approach across levels of analysis (behavioral and physiological) and provides an illustration of the increasing complexity of autonomic control at higher levels of the neuraxis. Arousal has been an important concept in physiology, psychology, and psychophysiology over the past five decades. Much of the impetus for arousal theories and for concepts of the role of general arousal in behavior came from work in the 1940s and 1950s on the brainstem reticular formation (for review see Magoun, 1963). Historically, the reticular formation was viewed as a relatively undifferentiated, highly interconnected set of neurons that exerted relatively nonspecific activational effects on rostral neural systems. Results of early stimulation, lesion and recording studies led to the construct of an Ascending Reticular Activating System (ARAS), which was believed to regulate the state of arousal of cortical and neurobehavioral systems (Magoun, 1963). The ARAS model resonated with psychologists because it was recognized that, apart from associative or structural determinants of behavior, there were important motivational or activational (arousal) contributions (Hebb, 1955; Duffy, 1957). The construct of general arousal is appealing in its inherent simplicity and parsimony, which is likely one reason it has been so resilient in the face of contradictory evidence. Even early studies revealed that the effects of arousal were not truly generalized and that behavioral and cortical arousal could be dissociated (Bradley & Elkes, 1953; Feldman & Waller, 1962). Moreover, psychophysiological measures commonly purported to be indices of arousal (e.g., heart rate, EDR) often do not covary highly with each other or with behavioral performance (e.g., see Lacey, 1959, 1967). Autonomic control, at least that arising from higher-level neurobehavioral substrates, does not lie along a single arousal continuum and does not reflect a simple homeostatic process. Paralleling the emerging recognition of the limitations of the construct of general arousal in psychology and psychophysiology were developments in neuroscience. These included a growing appreciation that the reticular formation was not as nonspecific as originally conceived. More refined neuroanatomical methods and neurochemical markers revealed a great deal of differentiation within what was classically considered an undifferentiated system (Sarter, Bruno, & Berntson, 2003). It is now apparent that there are multiple ascending activating systems, each having differential patterns of afferent input, dissimilar projection fields, and distinct neurochemical mediators (Krout, Belzer, & Loewy, 2002; Robbins et al., 1998). These include ascending noradrenergic, dopaminergic, cholinergic and serotonergic systems. The precise roles of these ascending systems in behavior and autonomic control remain to be fully elucidated, but their functions are clearly differentiated. The mesolimbic dopaminergic system has been implicated in reward, incentive, and behavioral activation (Robbins et al., 1998; Gray & McNaughton, 1996); the locus coeruleus noradrenergic system in cortical and motivational arousal (Aston-Jones et al., 1996); the cholinergic system in cortical/cognitive processing (Robbins & Everitt, 1995; Sarter & Bruno, 1997), and the serotonergic system in attention and behavioral inhibition (Robbins & Everitt, 1995; Gray & McNaughton, 1996). Each of these neurobehavioral systems have distinct anatomical projections, differentiated roles in behavioral processes, and distinct links to autonomic control systems. In contrast to the early work on the ARAS and on autonomic control, psychological, psychophysiological, and neurobiological data concur that neither arousal nor autonomic control can be viewed as a unitary process along a single continuum.

Research on arousal systems illustrates the mutual benefit of multilevel analyses. Psychological, psychophysiological, and physiological perspectives were each essential for ultimate progress in this area. Although psychological concepts of generalized arousal antedated the emergence of the ARAS construct, it required neurophysiological studies on the reticular formation to crystallized this construct and embody it within a neuroanatomical substrate. In the light of current understandings, the ARAS model may seem primitive, but it represented an important conceptual advance at the time. The ARAS, for example, offered the first viable psychobiological account for why an organism did not simply lie inert in the absence of evocative environmental stimuli (Hebb, 1955). Psychological and psychophysiological data provided the early support for the ARAS construct, but it was those same disciplines that ultimately posed the strongest challenges to the concept of generalized arousal. Moreover, it was findings and perspectives from those same disciplines that ultimately spearheaded efforts to refine both the ARAS construct and the homeostatic model of autonomic control.

4.3. Neuropsychophysiology of stress-related disorders

Psychophysiological disorders have often been viewed as homeostatic dysfunctions (e.g., Cannon, 1932; Holmes & Ripley, 1955; Selye, 1956), and stress has been defined by some researchers as a state of threatened homeostasis (Johnson et al., 1992). The homeostatic construct, however, has been applied so broadly, across such a diverse range of phenomena, that its status as an explanatory construct warrants re-examination and refinement.

Although homeostatic processes and disturbances may impact health, more recent attention has shifted to the potential health implications of allostatic or allodynamic regulation. It is important to recognize that the mere labeling of a condition as a homeostatic or allodynamic dysfunction contributes little to scientific understanding. For meaningful progress, the origins, mechanisms and implications of dysfunctions ultimately must be clarified. The significance of the constructs of homeostasis, allostasis, or allodynamic regulation lies more in the strategic guidance they offer for research efforts, and in the directions and potential mechanisms that they focus attention on.

4.3.1. Psychophysiological disorders as specific homeostatic dysfunctions

Some researchers have considered psychophysiological disorders as manifestations of constitutional dispositions toward specific patterns of autonomic response to stress. An historical example is the Eppinger and Hess (1915) constitutional model, as considered above. According to this view, exaggerated activity in one of the autonomic branches can bias toward specific disorders such as asthma (parasympathetic) or Raynaud's disease (sympathetic). Further consistent with this notion of a dispositional bias were the reports of Moos and Engel (1962) and Malmo (1975) of exaggerated psychophysiological reactivity appearing specifically in organ systems that evidenced psychosomatic dysfunctions. Hypertensive patients, for example, were reported to respond to stress with exaggerated cardiovascular responses, whereas arthritic patients were more likely to show EMG abnormalities around affected joints. Although these patterns of psychophysiological response could represent consequences of the specific disorders rather than markers of inherent dispositions, some prospective studies are consistent with the dispositional model. The normotensive offspring of hypertensive parents are at risk for the subsequent development of hypertension, and several studies have reported exaggerated basal or reactive cardiovascular activity in these individuals even prior to the development of hypertension (Fredrickson & Matthews, 1990; Maver, Strucl, & Accetto, 2004; Turner, 1994).

Additional support for constitutional contributions to hypertension comes from animal models. The spontaneously hypertensive rat (SHR) and the borderline hypertensive rat (BHR) represent potentially important genetic models of hypertension. SHR and BHR animals may also display exaggerated cardiovascular reactions to challenge stimuli (Kirby et al., 1989) and a regimen of behavioral stress can transform normotensive BHR animals to permanently hypertensive (Sanders & Lawler, 1992). Exaggerated sympathetic activity appears to contribute importantly to the conditions leading to hypertension in these animals (Korner, 1995a) and to cardiovascular disorders in humans (Grassi, 2004). These findings are consistent with a dispositional bias interacting with a stress context. SHR rats, and some hypertensive humans, show a lowered sensitivity of baroreceptor reflexes that could be interpreted to reflect an underlying homeostatic deficit (Head, 1995; Korner, 1995c; Maver et al., 2004; Watkins et al., 1996). This is intriguing in view of the fact that behavioral stress, which is known to suppress baroreflexes and increase sympathetic outflow, is able to exacerbate the hypertensive condition in the BHR rat. Although this model of homeostatic dysfunction has appeal, it is at best oversimplified. Baroreflexes can buffer short-term changes in blood pressure but do not appreciably contribute to long-term blood pressor regulation. Baroreceptor damage in humans or sino-aortic denervation in animals manifests primarily in acute blood pressure lability rather than chronic hypertension and basal hypotension may even be apparent (Franchini & Krieger, 1992; Robertson et al., 1993). These findings do not rule out the possibility that homeostatic deficits contribute to hypertension, but they do suggest that hypertension is not simply a baroreflex anomaly. The complexity and interactions of the determinants of hypertension may be more in keeping with a model of allodynamic regulation.

4.3.2. Generalized features of stress: Allostatic load

In addition to the multitude of specific regulatory deficits that may underlie stress-related disorders, more generalized features of stress have been recognized. For Cannon (1932) these were related to the generalized activation of the sympathetic nervous system. Selye (1956) further developed the generalized model of stress response, but shifted the focus from the autonomic nervous system to the pituitary adrenocortical system. In addition to potential specific reactions to stressors, Selye (1956) argued that the stressors typically elevate adrenocorticosteroid hormones, a component of what he termed the General Adaptation Syndrome (GAS). In Selye's view, autonomic activation contributes primarily to the initial reaction to stress (the alarm stage) whereas the adrenocorticosteroid response was considered to represent the generalized and persistent effect of stress (the resistance stage). Adrenocorticosteroids have widespread effects on insulin release and metabolic processes, muscle contractile strength, psychological states, and immune functions. The corticosteroid response was viewed by Selye as an adaptive mobilization to counter stress challenges, through syntoxic actions such as anti-inflammatory effects that minimize tissue damage, and catatoxic actions that enhance bodily defenses. In the GAS model, if the stress is not adequately resolved, defensive resources are ultimately depleted and the individual becomes increasingly susceptible to disease (exhaustion phase).

The generalized consequences of stressors continue to attract attention. Although the negative effects of stress are often the focus of psychophysiological studies, it is important to recognize that stress reactions can confer positive benefit in dealing with adaptive challenges and can protect and restore vital functions. The adaptive utility of stress reactions were inherent in Selye's (1973) syntoxic and catatoxic features of the stress response, and it is increasingly recognized that acute stress may enhance immune reactions (Bosch et al., 2005; Dhabhar, 2003). Moreover, moderate early stress has been shown to enhance development and improve vigor of organisms, and mild infant stress may reduce subsequent stress effects in adulthood (Gandelman, 1992; Meaney et al., 1996).

Severe or prolonged stress, however, may have negative consequences (McEwen & Wingfield, 2003; Seckl & Meaney, 2004). McEwen and Steller (1993) argue that specific patterns of stress response may vary considerably across individuals and contexts, but that they also show common allostatic features. In contrast to simple homeostatic systems that are focused around a set point on a single dimension (e.g., blood pressure), allostatic systems entail multiple dimensions that are integrated and orchestrated by central, autonomic, and endocrine processes. Within allostatic systems, functional set points are subject to change, and disturbances in one dimension may lead to compensatory fluctuations in another. McEwen and Stellar (1993) propose that repeated or prolonged allostatic fluctuations extract a physiological cost, a sort of "wear and tear" that they term *allostatic load*. This allostatic load is seen to be cumulative, and to dispose toward a broad range of stress pathologies, such as atherosclerosis and hypertension (McEwen & Stellar, 1993). A wide variety of psychosocial stressors, for example, have been suggested to confer an aggregate risk for acute myocardial infarction as revealed in one of the larger cohorts studied (INTERHEART study; Rosengren et al., 2004). This risk was independent of physical and demographic variables and was comparable to that of hypertension and obesity. An aggregate score putatively reflecting global allostatic load has been reported to predict not only physical health outcomes but the cognitive and functional decline associated with aging (Karlamangla et al., 2002; Seeman et al., 2001).

Glucocorticoids assume special importance in allostatic load and the consequences of stress because they modulate a wide range of functions. Adrenal steroid secretion is under the control of pituitary ACTH, which in turn is regulated by hypothalamic corticotropin releasing hormone (CRH). In addition to its role in adrenocortical control, CRH has been implicated as a trigger of the central stress response (de Kloet, 2003; Gray & Bingaman, 1996). This circuit is regulated by an inhibitory glucocorticoid feedback signal which modulates CRH release. One of the consequences of stress is the allostatic alteration of the operating level of this system, yielding higher basal levels of CRH and glucocorticoids (see Schulkin et al., 1994; McEwen & Wingfield, 2003 for reviews). The hippocampus is an important target site of the glucocorticoids, where binding serves to dampen or shut off stress related CRH release from the hypothalamus. But repeated stress can trigger atrophy of pyramidal dendrites in the hippocampus (via conjoint actions of glucocorticoids and excitatory amino acids), and severe and prolonged stress may even lead to loss of hippocampal neurons (McEwen & Wingfield, 2003; Sapolsky, 2003; Uno et al., 1989). This could lead to higher than normal levels of glucocorticoids during stress and impose a further allostatic load due to impaired feedback regulation, which may further contribute to stress pathology.

In addition, social but not physical stressors have been reported to foster a specific allostatic adjustment entailing glucocorticoid resistance associated with alterations in glucocorticoid receptor processes. Despite normal levels of immunomodulatory glucocorticoids, animals with glucocorticoid insensitivity display exaggerated immune reactions, which under some conditions may in fact be potentially life-threatening (Quan et al., 2003). Other neural, neuroendocrine, metabolic, and immune pathways also likely contribute to the health consequences of stress and allostatic load, and in the aggregate may underlie the generalized relations between allostatic load and health.

Summary. Stress reactions may entail both specific and generalized features, arising from homeostatic and allodynamic processes. Consequently, stress related pathology may not be conceptualized adequately within a restricted homeostatic framework. Stress disorders arising from allodynamic disturbances may have multiple origins in complex interacting systems, where disturbances in one domain may manifest in another, and compensatory responses can be orchestrated across several functional domains. Consequently, treatment strategies directed to a single perturbed target dimension (e.g., blood pressure) may not be optimal, as they may simply result in compensatory changes in another dimension that could perpetuate the disturbance. An important issue for future research is the extent to which allostatic "load" represents a truly generalized consequence of stress or to what extent it may manifest differentially based on the individual and the stress context.

4.3.3. Specific consequences of stress

Although broad indices of allostatic load focus on the generalized consequences of stress, more organ- or function-specific effects may also be apparent with allostatic or allodynamic disturbances. Allostatic load has been conceptualized as an aggregate state of allostatic processes, but may be comprised of a number of more specific conditions or relations. The *metabolic syndrome* is a diagnostic classification based on a cluster of risk factors including hypertension, insulin resistance, and central adiposity, which forebodes an increased risk for cardiovascular morbidity and mortality and type II diabetes (Reaven, 2005). Measures of allostatic load include many markers of the metabolic syndrome, as well as additional parameters that expand the boundaries of the concept of allostatic load (e.g., see Seeman et al., 2001). That is, the concept of allostatic load is considerably broader than that of the metabolic syndrome, which raises an important question as to whether this represents a conceptual advantage or disadvantage. The generalized predictive abilities of the allostatic load construct may be due to a critical *interaction* among the systems, dimensions, and parameters which serve to measure and define it. Alternatively, allostatic load may provide a global predictor of health outcome because of the aggregate predictive relations among components with relatively independent risk factors. If the former is true, parsing allostatic load into component predictors may degrade the predictive power, whereas if the latter is the case, such a parsing may lead to more system- or function-specific predictors. This is an important distinction, because the two options have different implications for research strategies. If risk factors are independent, then they can be studied in relative isolation, although an aggregate measure may still have some utility in predicting health outcomes. If the risk factors interact, however, then the overall risk status cannot be adequately determined by isolated studies of individual risk factors, regardless of how many are included.

In this regard, Reaven (2005) has recently questioned the predictive utility of the concept of metabolic syndrome over its individual dimensions. If the metabolic syndrome is merely an aggregate of independent predictors, then the selective focus on specific relations between individual factors and allodynamic systems and health would be appropriate. That is, the appearance of insulin resistance alone, in the absence of other components of the metabolic syndrome, may be a sufficient indication for treatment and for the specific treatment strategy to resolve the insulin resistance (Raeven, 2005). The ongoing development of cardiovascular risk factor profiles is increasingly making an important contribution to risk stratification for cardiovascular disorders (Rosengren et al., 2004; Wood, 2001). If this merely reflects the identification of a set of orthogonal dimensions that allow an aggregate risk assessment, then the individual dimensions can be studies independently, and a disturbance in a single dimension might suggest a treatment strategy focused on that specific anomaly. In contrast, if the risk factors are interacting, then isolated studies of the individual dimensions will never capture the full health implications of a group of risk factors. Moreover, if studies were limited to independent assessments, interactions between factors may never be known. Reality probably lies somewhere between these extremes. It will be important for future research to elucidate the manifestations of homeostatic or allostatic disorders that relate to specific physiological dimensions as well as those that entail more complex multi-system interactions. It is important that the latter not be disregarded, however, as a comprehensive understanding of an organism and its adaptation can only be achieved by the interactions of its parts and its transactions within the physical and social worlds (Cacioppo et al., 2000).

4.3.4. Allodynamic processes: protective and restorative functions

Although the discussion above has focused on physiological disturbances and negative health outcomes, homeostatic, allostatic, and allodynamic adjustments likely evolved because of their adaptive value and their positive benefit to health and survival. Autonomic, neuroendocrine and immune systems are orchestrated in part to buffer the organism against effects of internal and external changes by regulatory and restorative devices. Alterations from a constant homeostatic state may have highly beneficial effects in the short run, despite potential negative effects over longer periods of time (see Cacioppo & Berntson, 2006; McEwen & Seeman, 1999). Stress-related allostatic adjustments can improve wound healing and moderate stress may even enhance long-term immunological function and protective processes (Dhabhar, 2003; Dhabhar & Viswanathan, 2005). Alternative levels of regulation in allostasis, which may themselves be subject to change over time and circumstance, can be adaptive or maladaptive depending in part on the physical and social environment and the status of the organism. The focus of the above discussion of allostatic load has been on biological substrates and physical systems, but these systems are influenced powerfully by psychological states and the social world.

Although stress pathology is increasingly being elucidated, the neurobehavioral processes and transduction mechanisms that link stress to health outcomes are less well understood. What constitutes a stress and how the system reacts may differ from individual to individual. Individuals who approach active coping tasks with the belief that they can meet the task demands ("challenge appraisals") show primarily cardiac activation to the task, whereas those harboring a belief that they cannot meet task demands ("threat appraisals") show primarily vascular activation (Tomaka et al., 1997). These different reactions may have distinct health outcomes, and stressors may have positive as well as negative effects. For example, early stress can promote stress "immunization," entailing a genetic reprogramming that can lead to lower stress reactivity throughout life (Levine, Haltmeyer, & Karas, 1967; Meaney, 2001). Autonomic, endocrine and immune reactions serve important regulatory and restorative functions that buffer adaptive challenges. This may be accomplished through homeostatic-like processes that defend the steady state or through allostatic adjustments that defy homeostasis. Generally adaptive, these processes in some circumstances may have negative outcomes. The design for a brain and stress physiology that worked well through early evolution may have maladaptive aspects, especially as longevity has increased well beyond the reproductive years. Even those reactions with negative dimensions often have positive effects on other dimensions, and the focus on positive, buffering, and restorative functions is an important emphasis in the recent literature (see Cacioppo & Berntson, 2006).

4.4. The allodynamic perspective

Homeostatic processes contribute importantly to adaptive function, but the simple feedback-controlled homeostatic model with its fixed operating set point does not adequately represent the complexity of psychophysiological regulation. Organ systems are complexly controlled and allodynamically regulated by integrative neural, autonomic and endocrine systems. Regulatory levels and other operating characteristics are not rigidly fixed, but can be adaptively varied to face existing or anticipated demands. The allodynamic model affords a more comprehensive framework for psychophysiology than does the homeostatic construct. As considered above, the allodynamic model has substantive implications for psychophysiological measurement, constructs of physiological response, theories of psychophysiological relationships, and strategies for clinical intervention.

The neuropsychophysiological perspective is particularly important in studies of allodynamic regulation and dysregulation, as the links between psychological processes and physiological outcomes may be highly complex and dependant on central integrative systems. Studies of these intervening systems can both inform and be informed by psychophysiological relations. Because mappings between terms and concepts among closely related levels of analysis are likely to be simpler than those between more remote levels, the neuropsychophysiological perspective offers a viable bridging strategy for clarifying psychophysiological relations. This perspective does not challenge the importance of contributions from research limited to the psychological, psychophysiological, or neural levels of analysis. Rigorous independent research at each of these levels is crucial. The ultimate development of psychophysiology, however, will be substantially enhanced by meaningful interdisciplinary multilevel analyses.

REFERENCES

Aston-Jones, G., Rajkowski, J., Kubiak, P., Valentino, R. J. and Shipley, M. T. (1996). Role of the locus coeruleus in emotional activation, *Progress in Brain Research, 107*, 379–402.

Bachen, E. A., Manuck, S. B., Cohen, S., Muldoon, M. F., Raibel, R., Herbert, T. B., & Rabin, B. S. (1995). Adrenergic blockade ameliorates cellular immune responses to mental stress in humans. *Psychosomatic Medicine, 57*, 366–372.

Bard, P. (1960). Anatomical organization of the central nervous system in relation to control of the heart and blood vessels. *Physiological Review, 40 (Suppl 4)*, 3–21.

Benschop, R. J., Nieuwenhuis, E. E. S., Tromp, E. A. M., Godart, G. L. R., Ballieux, R. E. and van Doornen, L. P. J. (1994). Effects of β-adrenergic blockade on immunologic and cardiovascular changes induced by mental stress, *Circulation, 89*, 762–769.

Bernard, C. (1878). Leçons sur les phénomènes de la vie communes aux animaux et aux végétaux. Paris: B. Baillière et Fils. (Lectures on the phenomena of life common to animals and plants, 1974, translated by H. E. Hoff, R Guillemin, and L. Guillemin. Springfiled, Ill: Thomas.)

Bernard, C. (1879). Leçons sur les phénomènes de la vie communes aux animaux et aux végétaux. Paris: B. Baillière et Fils.

Berntson, G. G. & Boysen, S. T. (1990). Cardiac indices of cognition in infants, children and chimpanzees. In C. Rovee-Collier & L. Lipsitt (Eds.), *Advances in infancy research*. Vol 6. (pp. 187–220). New York: Ablex.

Berntson, G. G., Cacioppo, J. T., Binkley, P. F., Uchino, B. N., Quigley, K. S. & Fieldstone, A. (1994a). Autonomic cardiac control: III. Psychological stress and cardiac response in autonomic space as revealed by pharmacological blockades. *Psychophysiology, 31*, 599–608.

Berntson, G. G., Cacioppo, J. T., & Quigley, K. S. (1991). Autonomic Determinism: The modes of autonomic control, the doctrine of autonomic space, and the laws of autonomic constraint. *Psychological Review, 98*, 459–487.

Berntson, G. G., Cacioppo, J. T., & Quigley, K. S. (1993). Cardiac psychophysiology and autonomic space in humans: Empirical perspectives and conceptual implications. *Psychological Bulletin, 114*, 296–322.

Berntson, G. G., Cacioppo, J. T. & Quigley, K. S. (1994b). Autonomic cardiac control. I. Estimation and validation from pharmacological blockades. *Psychophysiology, 31*, 572–585.

Berntson, G. G., Cacioppo, J. T., Quigley, K. S., & Fabro, V. J. (1994c). Autonomic space and psychophysiological response. *Psychophysiology, 31*, 44–61.

Berntson, G. G., Cacioppo, J. T., & Quigley, K. S. (1995). The metrics of cardiac chronotropism: Biometric perspectives. *Psychophysiology, 32*, 162–171.

Berntson, G. G., Sarter, M., & Cacioppo, J. T. (1998). Anxiety and cardiovascular reactivity: The basal forebrain cholinergic link. *Behavioural Brain Research, 94*, 225–248.

Berntson, G. G., Sarter, M. & Cacioppo, J. T. (2003). Ascending visceral regulation of cortical affective information processing. *European Journal of Neuroscience, 18*, 2103–2109.

Blessing, W. W. (1997). *The lower brainstem and bodily homeostasis*. New York: Oxford.

Bosch, J. A., Berntson, G. G., Cacioppo, J. T., Dhabhar, F. S., & Marucha, P. T. (2003). Acute stress evokes a selective mobiliza-

tion of T cells that differ in chemokine receptor expression: A potential pathway linking immunologic reactivity to cardiovascular disease. *Brain, Behavior & Immunity, 17*, 251–259.

Bosch, J. A., Berntson, G. G., Cacioppo, J. T., & Marucha, P. T. (2005). Differential mobilization of functionally distinct Natural Killer subsets during acute psychological stress. *Psychosomatic Medicine, 67*, 366–375.

Bradley, P. B., & Elkes, J. (1953). The effect of atropine, hyoscyamine, physostigmine, and neostigmine on the electrical activity of the brain of the conscious cat. *Journal of Physiology (London), 120*, 14P–15P.

Cacioppo, J. T. (1994). Social neuroscience: Autonomic, neuroendocrine, and immune responses to stress. *Psychophysiology, 31*, 113–128.

Cacioppo J. T. & Berntson, G. G. (2006) The brain, homeostasis and health: balancing demands of the internal and external milieu. In Friedman, H. S. & Cohen Silver, R. (Eds.) *The Oxford Handbook of Health Psychology*. New York: Oxford University Press.

Cacioppo, J. T., Berntson, G. G., Binkley, P. F., Quigley, K. S., Uchino, B. N., & Fieldstone, A. (1994). Autonomic cardiac control. II. Basal response, noninvasive indices, and autonomic space as revealed by autonomic blockades. *Psychophysiology, 31*, 586–598.

Cacioppo, J. T., Berntson, G. G., & Klein, D. J. (1992). What is an emotion? The role of somatovisceral afference, with special emphasis on somatovisceral "illusions". *Review of Personality and Social Psychology, 14*, 63–98.

Cacioppo, J. T., Berntson, G. G., Sheridan, J. F., & McClintock, M. K. (2000). Multi-level integrative analyses of human behavior: The complementing nature of social and biological approaches. *Psychological Bulletin, 126*, 829–843.

Cacioppo, J. T., Crites, S. L., & Garnder, W. L. (1996). Attitudes to the right: Evaluative processing is associated with lateralized late positive event-related brain potentials. *Personality and Social Psychology Bulletin, 22*, 1205–1219.

Cacioppo, J. T., Klein, D. J., Berntson, G. G., & Hatfield, E. (1993). The psychophysiology of emotion. In R. Lewis & J. M. Haviland (Eds.), *The handbook of emotions* (pp 119–142). New York: Guilford Press.

Cacioppo, J. T., Malarkey, W. B., Kiecolt-Glaser, J. K., Uchino, B. N., Sgoutas-Emch, S. A., Sheridan, J. F., Berntson, G. G., & Glaser, R. (1995). Heterogeneity in neuroendocrine and immune responses to brief psychological stressors as a function of autonomic cardiac activation. *Psychosomatic Medicine, 57*, 154–164.

Cacioppo, J. C. & Tassinary, L. G. (1990). Inferring psychological significance from physiological signals. *American Psychologist, 45*, 16–28.

Cacioppo, J. T., Uchino, B. N., Crites, S. L., Snydersmith, M. A., Smith, G., Berntson, G. G. & Lang, P. J. (1992). The relationship between facial expressiveness and sympathetic activation in emotion: A critical review, with emphasis on modeling underlying mechanisms and individual differences. *Journal of Personality and Social Psychology, 62*, 110–128.

Cahill, L. & Alkire, M. T. (2003) Epinephrine enhancement of human memory consolidation: Interaction with arousal at encoding. *Neurobiology of Learning and Memory, 79*, 194–198.

Cannon, W. B. (1928). The mechanism of emotional disturbance of bodily functions. *New England Journal of Medicine, 198*, 877–884.

Cannon, W. B. (1929). Organization for physiological homeostasis. *Physiological Reviews, 9*, 399–431.

Cannon, W. B. (1932). *The wisdom of the body*. New York: Norton.

Cannon, W. B. (1939). *The wisdom of the body*. (2nd Ed.). London: Kegan Paul, Trench, Trubner & Co.

Cechetto, D. F. and Saper, C. B. (1990). Role of the cerebral cortex in autonomic function. In A. D. Loewy and K. M. Spyer (Eds.), *Central regulation of autonomic function* (pp. 208–233) New York: Oxford.

Chen, Q. H., & Toney, G. M. (2003). Identification and characterization of two functionally distinct groups of spinal cord-projecting paraventricular nucleus neurons with sympathetic-related activity. *Neuroscience, 118*, 797–807.

Chwalisz, K., Diener, E., & Gallagher, D. (1988). Autonomic arousal feedback and emotional experience: Evidence from the spinal cord injured. *Journal of Personality and Social Psychology, 54*, 820–828.

Clark, K. B., Naritoku, D. K., Smith, D. C., Browing, R. A. & Jensen, R. A. (1999). Enhanced recognition memory following vagus nerve stimulation in human subjects. *Nature Neuroscience, 2*, 94–98.

Cofer, C. N., & Appley, M. H. (1964). *Motivation: Theory and research*. New York: John Wiley.

Damasio, A. R. (1994). *Descartes Error*. New York: Grosset/Putnam.

Dampney, R. A., Polson, J. W., Potts, P. D., Hirooka, Y., & Horiuchi, J. (2003). Functional organization of brain pathways subserving the baroreceptor reflex: studies in conscious animals using immediate early gene expression. *Cellular and Molecular Neurobiology, 23*, 597–616.

Danielsen, E. H., Magnuson, D. J., & Gray, T. S. (1989). The central amygdaloid nucleus innervation of the dorsal vagal complex in rat: a Phaseolus vulgaris leucoagglutinin lectin anterograde tracing study. *Brain Research Bulletin, 22*, 705–715.

de Kloet, E. R. (2003). Hormones, brain and stress. *Endocrine Regulation, 37*, 51–68.

Dhabhar, F. S. (2003). Stress, leukocyte trafficking, and the augmentation of skin immune function. *Annals of the New York Academy of Sciences, 992*, 205–217.

Dhabhar, F. S., & Viswanathan, K. (2005). Short-term stress experienced at the time of immunization induces a long-lasting increase in immunological memory. *American Journal of Physiology: Regulatory, Integrative and Comparative Physiology, 289*, R738–R744.

Ditto, B., & France, C. (1990). Carotid baroreflex sensitivity at rest and during psychological stress in offspring of hypertensives and non-twin sibling pairs, *Psychosomatic Medicine, 52*, 610–620.

Duffy, E. (1957). The psychological significance of the concept of "arousal" or "activation". *Psychological Review, 64*, 265–275.

Dunn, A. J., & Berridge, C. S. (1990). Physiological and behavioral responses to corticotropin-releasing factor administration: Is CRF a mediator of anxiety or stress responses. *Brain Research Reviews, 15*, 71–100.

Dworkin, B. R. (1993). *Learning and physiological regulation*. Chicago: Univ. Chicago Press.

Dworkin, B. R., & Dworkin, S. (1990). Learning of physiological responses: I. Habituation, sensitization, and classical conditioning. *Behavioral Neuroscience, 104*, 298–319.

Dworkin, B. R., & Dworkin, S. (1999). Heterotopic and homotopic classical conditioning of the baroreflex. *Integrative Physiology and Behavioral Science, 34*, 158–176.

Dworkin, B. R., Elbert, T., Rau, H., Birbaumer, N., Pauli, P., Droste, C. & Brunia, C. H. (1994). Central effects of baroreceptor activation in humans: attenuation of skeletal reflexes and pain perceptions. *Proceedings of the National Academy of Sciences, 91*, 6329–6333.

Edwards, L., McIntyre, D., Carroll, D., Ring, C. & Martin, U. (2002). The human nociceptive flexion reflex threshold is higher during systole than diastole. *Psychophysiology, 39*, 678–681.

Elam, M., Svensson, T. H., & Thoren, P. (1974). Differentiated cardiovascular afferent regulation of locus coeruleus neurons and sympathetic nerves. *Brain Research, 358*, 77–84.

Elridge, F. L. (1994). Central integration of mechanisms in exercise hyperpnea. *Medical Sciences in Sports and Exercise, 26*, 319–327.

Eppinger, H., & Hess, L. (1915). *Vagotonia: A clinical study in vegetative neurology* (trans. W. M. Kraus & S. E. Jelliffe). New York: The Nervous and Mental Disease Publishing Co.

Feldman, S. M., & Waller, H. J. (1962). Dissociation of electrocortical activation and behavioral arousal. *Nature, 196*, 1320–1322.

Folkow, B. (2000). Perspecties on the integrative functions of the 'sympatho-adrenomedullary system'. *Autonomic Neuroscience, 83*, 101–115.

Franchini, K. G., & Krieger, E. M. (1992). Carotid chemoreceptors influence arterial pressure in intact and aortic-denervated rats. *American Journal of Physiology, 262*, R677–683.

Fredrickson, M., & Matthews, K. A. (1990). Cardiovascular responses to behavioral stress and hypertension: A meta-analytic review. *Annals of Behavioral Medicine, 12*, 30–39.

Fulton, J. F. (1949). *Textbook of Physiology* (16th ed.). Philadelphia: Saunders.

Gairard, A., Pernot, F., Bergmann, C., & van Overloop, B. (1994). Ions, parathyroids, and genetic hypertension. *American Journal of Medical Science, 307* (Suppl 1), S126–129.

Gandelman, R. (1992). *The psychobiology of behavioral development*. New York: Oxford.

Gebber, G. L. (1990). Central determinants of sympathetic nerve discharge. In A. D. Loewy and K. M. Spyer (Eds.), *Central regulation of autonomic function*. (pp. 126–144). New York: Oxford.

Gelsema, A. J., Agarwal, S. K., & Calaresu, F. R. (1989). Cardiovascular responses and changes in neural activity in the rostral ventrolateral medulla elicited by electrical stimulation of the amygdala of the rat. *Journal of the Autonomic Nervous System, 27*, 91–100.

Grassi, G. (2004). Sympathetic and baroreflex function in hypertension: implications for current and new drugs. *Current Pharmaceutical Design, 10*, 3579–3589.

Gray, J. A., & McNaughton, N. (1996). The neuropsychology of anxiety: Reprise. *Nebraska Symposium on Motivation, 43*, 61–134.

Gray, T. S. (1993). Amygdaloid CRF pathways. Role in autonomic, neuroendocrine, and behavioral responses to stress. *Annals of the New York Academy of Sciences, 697*, 53–60.

Gray, T. S., & Bingaman, E. W. (1996). The amygdala: corticotropin-releasing factor, steroids, and stress. *Critical Reviews in Neurobiology, 10*, 155–168.

Guyenet, P. G. (1990). Role of the ventral medulla oblongata in blood pressure regulation. In A. D. Loewy and K. M. Spyer (Eds.), *Central regulation of autonomic function*. (pp. 134–167). New York: Oxford.

Hansen, M. K, O'Connor, K. A., Goehler, L. E., Watkins, L. R., & Maier, S. F. (2001). The contribution of the vagus nerve in interleukin-1beta-induced fever is dependent on dose. *American*

Journal of Physiology: Regulatory, Integrative & Comparative Physiology, 280, R929–934.

Harper, R. M. (1996). The cerebral regulation of cardiovascular and respiratory functions. *Seminars in Pediatric Neurology, 3*, 13–22.

Hassert, D. L., Miyashita, T., & Williams, C. L. (2004). The effects of peripheral vagal nerve stimulation at a memory-modulating intensity on norepinephrine output in the basolateral amygdala. *Behavioral Neuroscience, 118*, 79–88.

Head, G. A. (1995). Baroreflexes and cardiovascular regulation in hypertension. *Journal of Cardiovascular Pharmacology, 26*, S7–16.

Hebb, D. O. (1955). Drives and the CNS (Conceptual nervous system). *Psychological Review, 62*, 243–254.

Hillyard, S. A., Mangun, G. R., Woldorff, M. G., & Luck, S. J. (1995). Neural systems mediating selective attention. In M. S. Gazzaniga (Ed.), *The cognitive neurosciences*. (pp. 665–681). Cambridge: MIT Press.

Holmes, T. H., & Ripley, H. S. (1955). Experimental studies on anxiety reactions. *American Journal of Psychiatry, 111*, 921–929.

Hurley, K. M., Herbert, H., Moga, M. M., & Saper, C. B. (1991). Efferent projections of the infralimbic cortex of the rat. *Journal of Comparative Neurology, 308*, 249–276.

Inui, K., Murase, S., & Nosaka, S. (1994). Facilitation of the arterial baroreflex by the ventrolateral part of the midbrain periaqueductal grey matter in rats. *Journal of Physiology, 477*, 89–101.

Inui, K., Nomura, J., Murase, S., & Nosaka, S. (1995). Facilitation of the arterial baroreflex by the preoptic area in anaesthetized rats. *Journal of Physiology, 488*, 521–531.

Ito, T. A., Thompson, E., & Cacioppo, J. T. (2004). Tracking the timecourse of social perception: the effects of racial cues on event-related brain potentials. *Personality and Social Psychology Bulletin, 30*, 1267–1280.

Iwata, J., & LeDoux, J. E. (1988). Dissociation of associative and nonassociative concomitants of classical fear conditioning in the freely behaving rat. *Behavioral Neuroscience, 102*, 66–76.

James, W. (1884). What is an emotion? *Mind, 9*, 188–205.

Janssen, B. J., Tyssen, C. M., Struijker Boudier, H. A., & Hutchins, P. M. (1992). 24-hour homeodynamic states of arterial blood pressure and pulse interval in conscious rats. *Journal of Applied Physiology, 73*, 754–761.

Johnson, E. O., Kamilaris, T. C., Chrousos, G. P., & Gold, P. W. (1992). Mechanisms of stress: A dynamic overview of hormonal and behavioral homeostasis. *Neuroscience and Biobehavioral Reviews, 16*, 115–130.

Karlamangla, A. S., Singer, B. H., McEwen, B. S., Rowe, J. W., & Seeman, T. E. (2002). Allostatic load as a predictor of functional decline. MacArthur studies of successful aging. *Journal of Clinical Epidemiology, 55*, 696–710.

Kirby, R. F., Callahan, M. F., McCarty, R., & Johnson, A. K. (1989). Cardiovascular and sympathetic nervous system responses to an acute stressor in borderline hypertensive rats (BHR). *Physiology & Behavior, 46*, 309–313.

Koizumi, K., & Kollai, M. (1981). Control of reciprocal and non-reciprocal action of vagal and sympathetic efferents: Study of centrally induced reactions. *Journal of the Autonomic Nervous System, 3*, 483–501.

Koizumi, K. & Kollai, M. (1992). Multiple modes of operation of cardiac autonomic control: development of the ideas from Cannon and Brooks to the present, *Journal of the Autonomic Nervous System, 41*, 19–30.

Korner, P. I. (1995a). Cardiovascular hypertrophy and hypertension: causes and consequences. *Blood Pressure (Suppl), 2*, 6–16.

Korner, P. I. (1995c). Cardiac baroreflex in hypertension: role of the heart and angiotensin II. *Clinical & Experimental Hypertension, 17*, 425–439.

Korner, P. I., & Angus, J. J. (1992). Structural determinants of vascular resistance properties in hypertension. Haemodynamic and model analysis. *Journal of Vascular Research, 29*, 293–312.

Krout, K. E., Belzer, R. E., Loewy, A. D. (2002). Brainstem projections to midline and intralaminar thalamic nuclei of the rat. *Journal of Comparative Neurology, 448*, 53–101.

Lacey, J. I. (1956). The evaluation of autonomic responses: Toward a general solution. *Annals of the New York Academy of Sciences, 67*, 123–164.

Lacey, J. I. (1959). Psychophysiological approaches to the evaluation of psychotherapeutic process and outcome. In E. A. Rubinstein & M. B. Parloff (Eds.), *Research in psychotherapy* (pp. 160–208). Washington: APA.

Lacey, J. I. (1967). Somatic response patterning and stress: Some revisions of activation theory. In M. H. Appley & R. Trumbull (Eds.), *Psychological stress: Issues in research* (pp. 4–44). New York: Appleton-Century-Crofts.

Lewis, S. J., Verberne, A. J. M., Robinson, T. G., Jarrott, B., Louis, W. J., & Beart, P. M. (1989). Excitotoxin-induced lesions of the central but not basolateral nucleus of the amygdala modulate the baroreceptor heart rate reflex in conscious rats. *Brain Research, 494*, 232–240.

Levine, S., Haltmeyer, G. C., & Karas, G. G. (1967). Physiological and behavioral effects of infantile stimulation. *Physiology & Behavior, 2*, 55–59.

Loewy, A. D. (1990). Autonomic control of the eye. In A. D. Loewy and K. M. Spyer (Eds.), *Central regulation of autonomic function* (pp. 268–285). New York: Oxford.

Lidberg, L., & Wallin, B. G. (1981). Sympathetic skin nerve discharges in relation to amplitude of skin resistance responses. *Psychophysiology, 18*, 268–271.

Lucini, D., Norbiato, G., Clerici, M., Pagani, M. (2002). Hemodynamic and autonomic adjustments to real life stress conditions in humans. *Hypertension, 39*, 184–188.

Luiten, P. G., ter Horst, G. J., Karst, H., & Steffens, A. B. (1985). The course of paraventricular hypothalamic efferents to autonomic structures in medulla and spinal cord. *Brain Research, 329*, 374–378.

Lundin, S., Ricksten, S.-E., & Thoren, P. (1984). Interaction between "mental stress" and baroreceptor reflexes concerning effects on heart rate, mean arterial pressure and renal sympathetic activity in conscious spontaneously hypertensive rats. *Acta Physiologica Scandinavica, 120*, 273–281.

Magoun, H. W. (1963). *The waking brain*. Springfield: Charles C. Thomas.

Malliani, A. (1999). The pattern of sympathovagal balance explored in the frequency domain. *News in Physiological Science, 14*, 111–117.

Malmo, R. T. (1975). *On emotions, needs, and our archaic brain*. New York: Holt, Rinehart & Winston.

Maver, J., Strucl, M., & Accetto, R. (2004). Autonomic nervous system activity in normotensive subjects with a family history of hypertension. *Clinical Autonomic Research, 14*, 369–375.

McEwen, B. S., Chattarji, S. (2004). Molecular mechanisms of neuroplasticity and pharmacological implications: the example of tianeptine. *European Journal of Neuropsychopharmacology, 14 (Suppl 5),* S497–502.

McEwen, B. S., & Seeman, T. (1999). Protective and damaging effects of mediators of stress. Elaborating and testing the concepts of allostasis and allostatic load. *Annals of the New York Academy of Science, 896,* 30–47.

McEwen, B. S., & Stellar, E. (1993). Stress and the individual: Mechanisms leading to disease. *Archives of Internal Medicine, 153,* 2093–2101.

McEwen, B. S., & Wingfield, J. C. (2003). The concept of allostasis in biology and biomedicine. *Hormones and Behavior, 43,* 2–15.

Meaney, M. J. (2001). Maternal care, gene expression, and the transmission of individual differences in stress reactivity across generations. *Annual Review of Neuroscience, 24,* 1161–1192.

Meaney, M. J., Diorio, J., Francis, D., Widdowson, J., LaPlante, P, Caldji, C., Sharma, S., Seckl, J. R., & Plotsky, P. M. (1996). Early environmental regulation of forebrain glucocorticoid receptor gene expression: implications for adrenocortical responses to stress. *Developmental Neuroscience, 18,* 49–72.

Montagu, J. D., & Coles, E. M. (1966). Mechanisms and measurement of the galvanic skin response. *Psychological Bulletin, 65,* 261–279.

Moos, R. H., & Engle, B. T. (1962). Psychophysiological reactions in hypertensive and arthritic patients. *Journal of Psychosomatic Medicine, 6,* 227–242.

Neafsey, E. J. (1990). Prefrontal cortical control of the autonomic nervous system: anatomical and physiological observations. *Progress in Brain Research, 85,* 147–166.

Ness, T. J., Fillingim, R. B., Randich, A., Backensto, E. M., & Faught, E. (2000). Low intensity vagal nerve stimulation lowers human thermal pain thresholds. *Pain, 86,* 81–85.

Nosaka, S., Nakase, N., & Murata, K. (1989). Somatosensory and hypothalamic inhibitions of baroreflex vagal bradycardia in rats. *Pflugers Archives, 413,* 656–666.

Obrist, P. A., (1981). *Cardiovascular psychophysiology: A perspective.* Plenum, New York.

Obrist, P. A., Webb, R. A., Sutterer, J. R., & Howard, J. L. (1970). The cardiac-somatic relationship: Some reformulations. *Psychophysiology, 6,* 569–587.

Oppenheimer, S. M., & Cechetto, D. F. (1990). Cardiac chronotropic organization of the rat insular cortex. *Brain Research, 533,* 66–72.

Pascoe, J. P., Bradley, D. J., & Spyer, K. M. (1989). Interactive responses to stimulation of the amygdaloid central nucleus and baroreceptor afferent activation in the rabbit. *Journal of the Autonomic Nervous System, 26,* 157–167.

Powell, D. A., Goldberg, S. R., Dauth, G. W., Schneiderman, E., & Schneiderman, N. (1972). Adrenergic and cholinergic blockade of cardiovascular responses to subcortical electrical stimulation in unanesthetized rabbits. *Physiology & Behavior, 8,* 927–936.

Quan, N., Avitsur, R., Stark, J. L., He, L., Lai, W., Dhabhar, F., & Sheridan, J. F. (2003). Molecular mechanisms of glucocorticoid resistance in splenocytes of socially stressed male mice. *Journal of Neuroimmunology, 137,* 51–58.

Reaven, G. M. (2005). The metabolic syndrome: requiescat in pace. *Clinical Chemistry, 51,* 931–938.

Recordati, G. (1984). The functional role of the visceral nervous system. A critical evaluation of Cannon's "homeostatic" and "emergency" theories. *Archives Italienes de Biologie, 122,* 248–267.

Recordati, G. (2002). The visceral nervous system and its environments. *Journal of Theoretical Biology, 214,* 293–304.

Reisenzein, R. (1983). The Schachter theory of emotion: Two decades later. *Psychological Bulletin, 94,* 239–264.

Robbins, T. W., & Everitt, B. J. (1995). Arousal systems and attention. In M. S. Gazzaniga (Ed.), *The cognitive neurosciences.* (pp. 703–729). Cambridge: MIT Press.

Robbins, T. W., Granon, S., Muir, J. L., Durantou, F., Harrison, A., Everitt, B. J. (1998). Neural systems underlying arousal and attention. Implications for drug abuse. *Annals of the New York Academy of Science, 846,* 222–237.

Robertson, D., Hollister, A. S., Biaggioni, I., Netterville, J. L., Mosqueda-Garcia, R., & Robertson, R. M. (1993). The diagnosis and treatment of baroreflex failure. *New England Journal of Medicine, 329,* 1449–1455.

Robinson, B. F., Epstein, S. E., Beiser, G. D. & Braunwald, E. (1966). Control of heart rate by the autonomic nervous system. *Circulation Research, 14,* 400–411.

Romanovsky, A. A. (2004). Do fever and anapyrexia exist? Analysis of set point-based definitions. *American Journal of Physiology: Regulatory and Integrative Comparative Physiology, 287,* R992–995.

Rosengren, A., Hawken, S., Ounpuu, S., Sliwa, K., Zubaid, M., Almahmeed, W. A., Blackett, K. N., Sitthi-amorn, C., Sato, H., & Yusuf, S. (2004). Association of psychosocial risk factors with risk of acute myocardial infarction in 11119 cases and 13648 controls from 52 countries (the INTERHEART study): case-control study. *Lancet, 364,* 953–62.

Rowell, L. B. (1986). *Human circulation regulation during physical stress.* New York: Oxford.

Sanders, B. J., & Lawler, J. E. (1992). The borderline hypertensive rat (BHR) as a model for environmentally-induced hypertension: a review and update. *Neuroscience and Biobehavioral Reviews, 16,* 207–217.

Sapolsky, R. M. (2003). Stress and plasticity in the limbic system. *Neurochemical Research, 28,* 1735–1742.

Sarter, M. (1994). Neuronal mechanisms of the attentional dysfunctions in senile dementia and schizophrenia: two sides of the same coin? *Psychopharmacology, 114,* 539–550.

Sarter, M., & Bruno, J. P. (1997). Cognitive functions of cortical acetylcholine: toward a unifying hypothesis. *Brain Research Reviews, 23,* 28–46.

Sarter, M., Bruno, J. P., & Berntson, G. G. (2003). Reticular activating system. In Nadel, L. (Ed.), *Encyclopedia of Cognitive Science.* Vol. 3 (pp 963–967). London: Nature Publishing Group.

Schachter, S., & Singer, J. E. (1962). Cognitive, social, and physiological determinants of emotional state. *Psychological Review, 69,* 379–399.

Schulkin, J., McEwen, B. S., & Gold, P. W. (1994). Allostasis, amygdala, and anticipatory angst. *Neuroscience and Biobehavioral Reviews, 18,* 385–396.

Schwaber, J. S., Kapp, B. S., Higgins, G. A., & Rapp, P. R. (1982). Amygdaloid and basal forebrain direct connections with the nucleus of the solitary tract and the dorsal motor nucleus. *Journal of Neuroscience, 10,* 1424–1438.

Seckl, J. R., & Meaney, M. J. (2004). Glucocorticoid programming. *Annals of the New York Academy of Sciences, 1032,* 63–84.

Selye, H. (1973). Homeostasis and heterostasis. *Perspectives in Biology and Medicine, 16,* 441–445.

Selye, H. (1956). *The stress of life.* New York: McGraw Hill.

Seeman, T. E., McEwen, B. S., Rowe, J. W., & Singer, B. H. (2001). Allostatic load as a marker of cumulative biological risk: MacArthur studies of successful aging. *Proceedings of the National Academy of Sciences, 98,* 4770–4775.

Sequeira, H., Viltart, O., Ba-M'Hamed, S., & Poulain, P. (2000). Cortical control of somato-cardiovascular integration: neuroanatomical studies. *Brain Research Bulletin, 53*, 87–93.

Sevoz-Couche C, Comet MA, Hamon M, Laguzzi R. (2003). Role of nucleus tractus solitarius 5-HT3 receptors in the defense reaction-induced inhibition of the aortic baroreflex in rats. *Journal of Neurophysiology. 90*, 2521–2530.

Sgoutas-Emch, S. A., Cacioppo, J. T., Uchino, B. N., Malarkey, W., Pearl, D., Kiecolt-Glaser, J. K., & Glaser, R. (1994). The effects of an acute psychological stressor on cardiovascular, endocrine, and cellular immune response: A perspective study of individuals high and low in heart rate reactivity. *Psychophysiology, 31*, 264–271.

Shih, C. D., Chan, S. H., & Chan, J. Y. (1995). Participation of hypothalamic paraventricular nucleus in the locus coeruleus-induced baroreflex suppression in rats. *American Journal of Physiology, 269*, H46–52.

Sokolov, E. N. (1963). *Perception and the conditioned reflex.* New York: MacMillan.

Spyer, K. M. (1989). Neural mechanisms involved in cardiovascular control during affective behavior. *Trends in Neuroscience, 12*, 506–513.

Spyer, K. M. (1990). The central nervous organization of reflex circulatory control. In A. D. Loewy and K. M. Spyer (Eds.), *Central regulation of autonomic function.* (pp. 1168–1188). New York: Oxford University Press.

Steptoe, A., & Sawada, Y. (1989). Assessment of baroreceptor reflex function during mental stress and relaxation. *Psychophysiology, 26*, 140–147.

Sterling, P, & Eyer, J. (1988). Allostasis: A new paradigm to explain arousal pathology. In S. Fisher & J. Reason (Eds.). *Handbook of Life Stress, Cognition and Health.* (pp. 629–649). New York: John Wiley & Sons.

Stitt, J. T. (1979). Fever versus hyperthermia. *Federation Proceedings, 38*, 39–43.

Thayer, J. F., & Lane, R. D. (2000). A model of neurovisceral integration in emotion regulation and dysregulation. *Journal of Affective Disorders, 61*, 201–216.

Tomaka, J., Blascovich, J., Kibler, J., & Ernst, J. M. (1997). Cognitive and physiological antecedents of threat and challenge appraisal. *Journal of Personality and Social Psychology, 73*, 63–72.

Turner, J. R. (1994). *Cardiovascular reactivity and stress.* New York: Plenum

Uno, H., Tarara, R., Else, J. G., Suleman, M. A., & Sapolsky, R. M. (1989). Hippocampal damage associated with prolonged and fatal stress in primates. *Journal of Neuroscience, 9*, 1705–1711.

Van Roon, A. M., Mulder, L. J., Althaus, M., & Mulder G. (2004). Introducing a baroreflex model for studying cardiovascular effects of mental workload. *Psychophysiology, 41*, 961–981.

Venables, P. H., & Christie, M. J. (1980). Electrodermal activity. In I. Martin & P. H. Venables (Eds.). *Techniques in psychophysiology* (pp. 3–67). Chichester: Wiley & Sons.

Wallace, D. M., Magnuson, D. J. & Gray, T. S. (1992). Organization of amygdaloid projections to brainstem dopaminergic, noradrenergic, and adrenergic cell groups in the rat. *Brain Research Bulletin, 28*, 447–454.

Watkins, L., Grossman, P., & Sherwood, A. (1996). Noninvasive assessment of baroreflex control in borderline hypertension: comparison with the phenylephrine method. *Hypertension, 28*, 238–243.

Wenger, M. A. (1941). The measurement of individual differences in autonomic balance. *Psychosomatic Medicine, 3*, 427–434.

Werner, J. (1988). Functional mechanisms of temperature regulation, adaptation and fever: complementary system theoretical and experimental evidence. *Pharmacology & Therapeutics, 37*, 1–23.

Williams, C. L., & Clayton, E. C. (2001). Contributions of brainstem structures in modulation memory storage processes. In Gold, P. E. & Greenough, W. T. (Eds.). *Memory consolidation: Essays in honor of James L. McGaugh.* (pp. 141–163). Washington, D.C.: American Psychological Association.

Wood, D. (2001). Established and emerging cardiovascular risk factors. *American Heart Journal, 141*, 49–57.

Zardetto-Smith, A. M., & Gray, T. S. (1995). Catecholamine and NPY efferents from the ventrolateral medulla to the amygdala in the rat. *Brain Research Bulletin, 38*, 253–260.

20 Developmental Psychophysiology: Conceptual and Methodological Issues

NATHAN A. FOX, LOUIS A. SCHMIDT, HEATHER A. HENDERSON, AND PETER J. MARSHALL

HISTORICAL PRECEDENT

Developmental psychophysiology is the study of behavior – physiology relations in infants and young children. Issues that are commonly studied by psychophysiologists with adult populations such as cognitive processing, cognition-emotion interactions, or responses to stress, may be examined in populations of young children as well. For example, utilizing age appropriate paradigms, interested researchers have investigated infant visual attention through the measurement of cardiac orienting (Field, 1979; Sameroff, Cashmore, & Dykes, 1973); others have examined infant discrimination of human faces by recording event-related potentials (de Haan & Nelson, 1997; Nelson & Collins, 1991, 1992; Parker et al., 2005). Such research has been quite valuable in revealing the links between physiological responses and behavior in infants and children of different ages. When multiple ages are utilized, such studies have also revealed age-related differences in physiology-behavior linkages (Richards, 1985, 1989).

Developmental psychophysiology, however, may offer the greater promise of revealing the processes by which both physiology and behavior change together over time. Such an approach necessitates a three-tier investigation. First, there must be a description of age-related changes in behavioral performance and physiological response. Second, there must be an attempt to describe how the physiological system itself is developing and changing over time, often as a function of the stimuli that are being studied. Third, there should be some attempt at integration of physiology and behavior. An example of this approach may be seen in the study of infant memory for faces. Such research has utilized event-related potentials (ERPs), examining multiple age groups (Nelson & Collins, 1991, 1992). These studies find decreasing latency and increasing amplitude of particular components of the ERP with age (see Nelson, 1994; Nelson & Monk, 2001 for reviews). In several other areas of developmental study, decreasing latency and increasing amplitude of specific ERPs have further been linked to improved cognitive

performance including memory performance (Howard & Polich, 1985) and response monitoring (Segalowitz et al., 2004; Santesso, Segalowitz, & Schmidt, 2006a) across childhood. Together, these studies demonstrate the links between developmental changes in the characteristics of physiological measures and the underlying cognitive processes. While these findings are an important first step, the developmental psychophysiologist should ask the next set of questions. Specifically, it seems critical when one studies a system that changes over time to understand what parameters of that system contribute to the response being measured. In the case of the increasing amplitude and decreasing latency of the ERP, we need to know what physical and physiological changes have occurred over developmental time, which may contribute to these changes in the ERP. For example, it is possible that changes in myelination of brain areas thought to be putatively involved in the behavior may affect the latency of the response. There may be changes in skull thickness or cortico-cortical connections that affect the pattern of the response. As well, there are clearly certain cognitive processes involved in the development of face recognition and discrimination, for example, which contribute to the behavioral response. Finally, while direct comparisons between adult and child behaviors may not be appropriate (i.e., each group may solve a particular problem with different strategies and perhaps with different underlying neural mechanisms), similarities in performance between age groups or deficits in one group may be useful for raising hypotheses about the underlying bases of the behavior. In a recent paper, Schacter, Kagan, and Leichtman (1995) reviewed studies of adult clinical populations who showed patterns of amnesia for episodic memory or confabulatory behaviors. Many of these adult subjects had injury to areas of the prefrontal region. Indeed, the clinical data on brain damaged adults seem to indicate that injury to certain areas of the prefrontal cortex may be associated with source memory deficits. Schacter, Kagan, and Leichtman (1995) drew a comparison between the responses of adult brain damaged patients to the behaviors that young children exhibit when tested for episodic or source memory. While they did not suggest that the processes responsible for adult or child errors were similar, they do raise interesting hypotheses regarding the role of the prefrontal region in episodic memory.

Thus, developmental psychophysiology has the opportunity to study not only changes in response systems over age, but also the processes underlying this change. Not only must change in the response system be measured but it must be understood as a function of the physical and psychological maturation of the organism under study. These added elements of developmental change create a new level of complexity (Emde & Walker, 1976; Richards, 1989; Snidman et al., 1995) in contrast to the psychophysiological study of adult populations.

MODELS OF DEVELOPMENT

Developmental change has been modeled in many different ways and the model one adopts as well as the processes one examines will determine the questions that are asked. There are a number of different models of development, each of which emphasizes differentially the role of environment and biology in influencing behavior. Application of one of these models to a particular study will influence the manner in which questions are asked and variables are measured.

Biologically determined models of development. These models postulate that development is a function of the unfolding of predetermined biological processes. The underlying structures of the brain develop and connect with one another via predetermined processes, which have a great deal to do with the action and expression of certain genes (Edelman, 1987). Thus, neurons within the neuroblast migrate and generate particular layers of cortical and sub-cortical structures during embryonic development similarly for all individuals in the absence of toxic environments (e.g., in utero exposure to drugs, alcohol, or radiation) (Huttenlocher, 1979; Sidman & Rakic, 1973). Similarly, the formation of the nuclei responsible for cardio-respiratory control and vagal innervation of the heart occur in a standard developmental timetable except in the presence of toxic environmental effects. Of course, even in instances of well-programmed neural development, there are individual differences in the outcome of such growth, which may be the result of differences in intrauterine environments and the timing of particular stressors or intrauterine conditions upon development (Huttenlocher, 1979). Such differences reflect a critical variable, which must be taken into account in any developmental model. The timing with which certain environmental events impact upon pre-programmed biological growth is a critical area of study. Ultimately though, in biological models of development, the timing of neural development is thought to be pre-programmed and to occur in an orderly fashion in the absence of negative environmental events.

Critical period models of development. A second model of development is one that takes into account environmental input and emphasizes the criticality of the timing at which this input is presented. This model is best thought of as reflecting the concept of a critical period. The idea of a critical period is that there is a window of opportunity through which particular environmental input will have a major influence on the organization of behavior (Hubel & Wiesel, 1970). For example, there is some evidence that exposure to language during the early years of life is critical for the adequate formation of appropriate language ability (Lenneberg, 1967; Petitto, 1993). There are, in addition, other sensory modalities (e.g., audition, vision) that are thought to develop in human infants and children via critical period models (see Maurer, 2005 for a recent Special Issue on the topic). Such a notion implies that exposure prior to, or after, this window of opportunity will not have the same effect upon the neural organization underlying this behavior (however, see Mills, Coffey-Corina, & Neville, 1994). In addition, this model implies that appropriate exposure during the critical period will lead to the organization of structures in such a way that they will henceforth underlie the more mature behavioral pattern. The critical period model of development is akin to an "innoculation" model in that appropriate development necessitates input at a particular time. Neural reorganization occurs as a function of this input, which then underlies subsequent behavior. This reorganization of behavior is a second process, which plays an important role in our understanding of behavioral change. Once the infant has received the appropriate environmental input he/she is protected ("innoculated") from other competing environmental inputs.

Stage models of development. A third model of development is one in which development is explained as a series of different periods of reorganization of both physiology and behavior (Case, 1992; Fischer, 1983, 1987; Thatcher, 1991, 1994). Such a model is a derivative of Piaget's view of development. Piaget viewed development as comprising a continuous process of the organism accommodating and assimilating environmental information. At particular points in development, an individual's interpretation of the information changes qualitatively as he/she moves, for example, from a sensorimotor view to a more concrete operational one. For example, at a certain age, Piaget observed that young children were more influenced by the perceptual properties of objects than by rules of conservation. Once a child understands that the quantity of a liquid does not change if poured from a tall, thin to a low, round beaker they have mastered a new stage of understanding. At these transition moments, there are both behavioral and accompanying physiological reorganizations, which reflect changes in the manner in which the child operates on the world. There is interesting, though indirect physiological evidence to support this view. Thatcher, Walker, and Giudice (1987) examined changes in intra- and inter-hemispheric coherence of the EEG across multiple age points. Thatcher et al. found what they described as lawful patterns of reorganization of coherence both within and between the left and right hemispheres. The ages at which these changes occurred seemed to correspond to periods of cognitive reorganization proposed by Piaget. A number of "stage" or re-organization models describe the transformation of existing behavioral/cognitive structures at particular periods of time into more sophisticated structures for the purpose of assimilating new and more complex information (Case, 1992; Fischer, 1980). Further, behavioral/cognitive re-organization is supposedly mimicked at the neural level (Fischer 1987; Fischer & Rose, 1994). For example, in a re-analysis of longitudinal EEG data collected by Matousek and Petersén (1973) John (1977) described distinct periods of reorganization of power in anterior to posterior scalp locations, which coincided with age periods thought to represent times of cognitive change. In a more discrete study of brain-behavior relations, Bell and Fox (1992) reported on changes in EEG power recorded from the frontal scalp leads in infants who had and had not mastered an object permanence task (A not B). This task is thought to involve the activity of the dorsolateral frontal cortex (Diamond & Goldman-Rakic, 1983, 1986, 1989). The timing of changes in behavior and EEG for successful infants was tightly locked so that reorganization of behavior and EEG (reflected not only in power but also coherence) was similar in scope.

Interactionist models of development. A fourth approach to the study of development is one that views the process as involving a continuous interaction between the genetic and biological disposition of the individual and environmental factors which impinge upon that individual (Gottlieb, 1976; Segalowitz & Schmidt, 2003). The goal of research is to understand the processes involved in gene-environment interactions. Accordingly, one must assess not only the biological/physiological status of the organism but also the manner in which various types of environmental contexts affect that status. Such an approach involves the study of individual differences and the role of the environment in affecting these differences. The study of individual differences is in fact a major topic in psychophysiology. Researchers have for some time recognized that individuals differ in their initial or baseline pattern of physiology and have attempted to take these differences into account when understanding subject response to stimulation (see Zahn, 1986, for a review). Indeed, a number of workers have given specific emphasis to the psychological meaning of these individual differences in physiology. For example, Davidson and colleagues have argued that resting patterns of asymmetrical frontal EEG activation reflects individual differences in the relative strength of approach versus withdrawal motivation tendencies (Davidson, 1984a, 1984b, 1995, 2000). Adults with greater relative right frontal EEG activation are more likely to respond to signs of impending danger or punish-

ment with a negative hedonic valence compared to adults exhibiting left frontal activation. Within the domain of autonomic activity, Porges has argued that individual levels of heart rate variability or vagal tone will affect the subject's reaction and subsequent recovery to a mild stressor (Porges, 1992). Individuals with low vagal tone are less likely to display significant cardiac orienting as compared to those with higher levels of vagal tone. Porges' work is unique in that he has extended these findings from adult to infant and child populations. Fox and colleagues have extended Davidson's model to examine temperamental differences among infants and young children. In a series of studies, Fox and his colleagues have shown that infants with resting right frontal EEG asymmetry are more likely to display distress and negative affect to unfamiliar stimuli as compared to infants with left frontal asymmetry (Calkins, Fox, & Marshall, 1996; Fox, Bell, & Jones, 1992). They have also shown that children displaying this pattern of right frontal asymmetry are more likely to show social withdrawal and reticence in a social situation with unfamiliar peers (Fox et al., 1995; Fox et al., 2001). Frontal EEG asymmetry has also been related to patterns of continuity and change in behavioral inhibition over time, with the best predictor of the tendency to be socially reticent with unfamiliar peers in the preschool years being the combination of temperamental negative affect and right frontal EEG asymmetry as assessed in infancy (Henderson, Fox, & Rubin, 2001).

While most developmental psychologists subscribe to the interactionist model to describe developmental processes, few studies actually capture the interactional component of the model (with some notable recent exceptions, see e.g., Fox et al., 2005). Most studies and researchers of individual differences are able to characterize the individual, and often the environment, but are less likely to describe the manner in which these factors mutually influence one another. Any understanding of development, however, must ultimately take into account such interaction. Such a model necessitates the integration of timing and reorganization of physiology as a function of experience and must take into account when exposure to certain events occurs and how this affects the organization of physiology and behavior.

Summary

Each of the four models described above provides important insight into developmental processes. There are clearly some changes that are primarily under "genetic" control (e.g., migration of nerve cells in the embryological development of the brain), other changes that necessitate environmental input at a particular point in time (e.g., the need for visual stimulation in the organization of the visual system), and still other changes that show transformations over time as a function of interaction with the environment (e.g., means-end ability). As such, the choice of a model will be a direct function of the processes under study. At a macro-level, there must be some integration of these frameworks for understanding the complex manner in which development occurs in the central nervous system. In the next section, we review two major psychophysiological systems (electrocortical and cardiovascular) and describe, where appropriate, how these systems have been examined in relation to the four models of development. We describe the historical precedent regarding each of these systems and review studies focusing on developmental issues.

PHYSICAL CONTEXT: SYSTEMS IN DEVELOPMENTAL PSYCHOPHYSIOLOGY

The electrocortical system: EEG and ERP measures

Overview. Like any system undergoing change, there are dramatic differences in activity of the EEG during the first two years of life. Changes in power and frequency of the EEG during this time period may be a function of certain developmental changes in specific brain parameters. For example, it is possible that changes in myelination of axons, changes in dendritic branching, and the sculpting of neuronal patterns (both in terms of cell proliferation and cell death) each affect the pattern of electrical energy recorded off the scalp. We know, however, precious little about the development of any of these physical parameters. The data on myelination of brain areas come from studies such as those conducted by Benes, Turtle, Khan, and Farol (1994) and Gilles, Shankle, and Dooling (1983). The data on dendritic changes and sculpting come from studies by Huttenlocher and colleagues (e.g., Huttenlocher, 1984; Huttenlocher & de Courten, 1987; Huttenlocher et al., 1982). None of these studies have directly linked anatomical changes to behavior.

The paucity of information regarding growth and development of the systems under study obviously makes interpretation of the pattern of responses being measured from these systems somewhat problematic. For example, adult alpha, recorded over the occipital cortex is defined as comprising the frequency band of 8 to 13 Hz. This frequency band seems to respond reliably to changes in visual attention (eyes-open versus eyes-closed produces alpha suppression). There is, however, little power in the 8 Hz to 13 Hz frequency band through late childhood. On the other hand, there is a reliable rhythm recorded over the occipital cortex, which is responsive in similar ways to visual input in the first year of life. The change in this frequency band may be of significance for understanding basic neural development as well as the relation between EEG and behavioral changes. That is, the increase in frequency of the "alpha rhythm" may tell us something about the development of the underlying neural generators in the thalamus, which are purportedly responsible for the generation of adult alpha rhythm (Nunez, 1981).

Developmental changes in psychophysiological measures may also reflect functional changes in the way the brain processes information. It is possible that certain brain structures are present early on but do not come "on line" until later in development. Changes in psychophysiological responses may thus be the result of the appearance of new functional operations rather than the physical maturation of any structures. For example, some patterns of electrical activity are less a result of anatomical variations and more a reflection of functional changes. One example is the pattern of frontal EEG asymmetry reported in infant and adult studies. Individuals may show a predominant asymmetry pattern at rest (either left or right frontal EEG asymmetry). But there are also clear shifts in these same individuals as a function of affective state or cognitive activity. For example, individuals with a pattern of resting left frontal EEG asymmetry may display right frontal EEG asymmetry in response to an aversive film clip (Jones & Fox, 1992; Tomarken, Davidson, & Henriques, 1990). These shifts seem to suggest that the pattern of changes in EEG asymmetry reflect functional changes in brain activation rather than anatomical differences. There may be, of course, developmental changes in the degree to which these functional differences emerge and are utilized. Nevertheless, individual differences in psychophysiological measures such as EEG asymmetry may reflect important functional rather than structural differences.

Historical background. Berger (1929, 1932a, 1932b) was the first to use the electroencephalogram (EEG) to assess human brain development. Berger found little brain electrical activity before one month of age, after which time EEG frequency and amplitude increased in the occipital region. Following Berger's important work, a number of longitudinal studies on EEG development were conducted with full-term and premature infants, with a focus on distinguishing between sleep and wake states. Overall, the early studies found that EEG frequency and amplitude increased during the first year of life in the full-term infant, while brain electrical activity of the premature infant was similar to the *in utero* infant (Dreyfus-Brisac & Monod, 1975). More recent studies have also noted reduced EEG amplitude in pre-term compared with fullterm infants (Duffy, Als, & McAnulty, 1990).

The early EEG studies were, however, limited on several fronts (Berger, 1932a, 1932b; Smith, 1938a, b, c, 1939). First, most of the studies were largely descriptive. They attempted to detail the development of various components of the EEG in the absence of any information regarding the physical development of the nervous system. Second, attempts at quantification of EEG frequency and amplitude were done by hand with a ruler, possibly limiting the precision of calculations; many of the early studies predated the use of computers and frequency analyzers. Third, adult parameters of state such as sleep staging were used to index EEG development in the infant. Fourth, the number of sites from which EEG was recorded were limited. A majority of studies only recorded from one or two scalp sites, possibly precluding the contribution of brain maturation in other regions relative to the sites collected.

Both clinicians and basic researchers have used the EEG as an instrument to understand complex brain-behavior relations. Traditionally, the EEG has been used in clinical settings to diagnose neuropathology. In this setting, the neurologist primarily uses qualitative interpretation of the EEG signal to understand brain anomalies such as seizures or tumor. More recently, quantitative EEG (qEEG) has been used in basic research settings by investigators interested in understanding issues related to normal as well as atypical brain development. For example, some researchers have examined changes in EEG frequency (Hagne, 1968, 1972) and coherence (Thatcher, Krause, & Hrybyk, 1986) in relation to brain maturation. Still others have related regional EEG activation to the emergence of particular functions in the developing brain. For example, patterns of frontal EEG activation have been examined in relation to emotional (Dawson et al., 1992; see also Fox, 1991, 1994; Fox et al., 1992) and cognitive development (Bell & Fox, 1994) during infancy as well as the development of maladaptive patterns of social and emotional responding in early childhood (Fox et al., 1996; Fox et al., 2001; Shankman et al., in press).

With the advent of new computer technologies, the collecting of ongoing high density EEG at a high rate of speed is now a reality. Such advances allow for reliable temporal resolution of underlying neurophysiology processes. Furthermore, unlike the more intrusive brain imaging procedures such as positron emission tomography (PET) and functional magnetic resonance imaging (fMRI), the EEG is a relatively noninvasive procedure, making it more tractable with pediatric populations. These methodological improvements and considerations, in combination with recent theoretical advances in the neurosciences, provide an exciting atmosphere for researchers interested in using the EEG to understand the developing human brain (Lewis & Stieben, 2004).

The use of EEG in understanding human brain development has been limited, however, largely because there have been relatively few longitudinal studies in which quantitative EEG has been used to assess brain maturation. In addition, the EEG suffers from poor spatial resolution. Neuroimaging techniques such as PET and fMRI have superior spatial resolution.

Studies relating EEG to early brain development. A number of longitudinal studies have been directed towards examining EEG frequency development during the first two years of life. Most of these studies examined posterior EEG frequency development and noted that a dominant EEG frequency emerged between 3 Hz to 5 Hz during the first 6 months of life and between 6 Hz to 8 Hz by the end of the first year. Smith (1938a, 1938b, 1938c, 1939) was one of the first researchers to examine EEG frequency development in the developing brain. Smith (1938b) noted that by age 3 to 4 months, a characteristic "alpha-like" rhythm

appeared in the occipital region in the human infant. The occipital rhythm increased to 6 Hz to 7 Hz by age 12 months (Smith 1938b, 1939, 1941). Smith (1938b) suggested that the onset of occipital activity at 3–4 months was linked to maturation of visual systems. Smith (1939, 1941) also noted a 7 Hz alpha-like frequency at age 3–4 months in the central region, which increased in frequency after 10 months. Smith (1941) speculated that this shift in pattern was linked to the emergence of reaching behavior in the infant. Lindsley (1939) also noted the development of an alpha-like rhythm between 3 Hz to 5 Hz in the occipital region at age 3–4 months, which increased to 6 Hz by age 12 months. Lindsley (1939) postulated that the development of this rhythm was related to the ontogeny of visual perception. Henry (1944) also reported a 3 Hz to 4 Hz rhythm in the occipital region at 3–4 months that increased to 7 Hz by age 12 months.

Following this early work, longitudinal studies of EEG frequency development waned for nearly three decades until the work of Hagne and her colleagues (Hagne, 1968, 1972; Hagne et al., 1973). Hagne's work is of particular importance for at least three reasons. First, unlike earlier studies, which calculated frequency data by hand, she performed frequency analyses using a fast Fourier transform. Second, Hagne recorded from multiple sites representing anterior and posterior regions of the brain. Third, Hagne was interested in relative power and peak frequency. Hagne (1968, 1972) reported that a delta (1.5 Hz to 3.5 Hz) to theta (3.5 Hz to 7.5 Hz) frequency ratio changed from 8 to 12 months, with increases in theta and decreases in delta. This pattern of change was a function of electrode location. Theta activity decreased in P3 and O1 between 8 and 10 months and increased between 10 and 12 months, while theta activity in C3 and Cz increased between 8 and 12 months. Still others (Mizuno et al., 1970) have examined relative power in the right occipital area using an alpha (7.17 Hz to 10.3 Hz)/delta (2.4 Hz to 3.46 Hz) quotient. Mizuno et al. (1970) found that this quotient increased from 1 to 12 months of age: There were increases in alpha activity and corresponding decreases in the delta band. Relative increases and decreases in band power have also been used as an index of EEG maturation, which in turn has been related to aspects of behavioral development. A relatively high level of low-frequency power (e.g., delta, theta) and a relative lack of higher-frequency power (e.g., alpha, beta) in the EEG has been associated with cognitive delays and attentional problems over a range of ages and contexts, including environmental adversity (Barry, Clarke, & Johnstone, 2003; Harmony et al., 1988; Marshall, Fox, & the BEIP Core Group, 2004; Satterfield, Cantwell, & Satterfield, 1974). There is some debate as to whether these deficits represent a maturational lag, or whether the EEG profile represents tonic hypoactivation (Barry, Clarke, & Johnstone, 2003).

We recently carried out an analysis of changes in EEG band power in a longitudinal sample from 5 months to 4 years of age (Marshall, Bar-Haim, & Fox, 2002). This study replicated many of the above findings from previous researchers, and established guidelines for the use of a 6 to 9 Hz band to represent alpha power from late in the first year of life and into early childhood. Other researchers have employed similar bands to study alpha-range rhythms: For example, Orekhova, Stroganova, and Posikera (2001) used a frequency band of 6.4 Hz to 10.0 Hz in a sample of infants aged 7–12 months to represent both posterior alpha rhythms as well as sensorimotor rhythms such as the mu rhythm. The classical mu rhythm occurs in the 7 Hz to 13 Hz range in adults, and is maximal over central sensorimotor areas. The amplitude of the mu rhythm is attenuated by voluntary movement and somatosensory stimulation (Gastaut, Dongier, & Courtois, 1954), but is minimally affected by changes in visual stimulation and is considered to be a somatosensory alpha rhythm that is sensitive to somatic afferent input and is distinct from the alpha range rhythms in more posterior regions (Kuhlman, 1978). Very few studies have addressed the development of the mu rhythm, although we have noted the appearance in infancy of a rhythm in the 6 Hz to 9 Hz band in the EEG power spectra over the central region (Marshall, Bar-Haim, & Fox, 2002). In terms of its relative contribution to the overall power spectrum, this rhythm is particularly prominent in the second year of life. Other researchers who have documented this rhythm have suggested a functional relation between the oscillation observed at central sites in infancy and early childhood and the mu rhythm in adults (Galkina & Boravova, 1996; Stroganova, Orekhova, & Posikera, 1999). The salience of the central sensorimotor rhythm in the EEG power spectra may not be coincidental, given that the second year after birth is a time of such intense development of locomotor ability. An additional, intriguing possibility is related to the observation that the amplitude of the mu rhythm in adults is not only related to movement *per se*, but is also sensitive to subtle variations in observed movements (Muthukumaraswamy & Johnson, 2004). Given the importance of imitative learning in social contexts in the second year of life, it is also possible that the salience of the mu rhythm is related to this capacity, as well as to the developing locomotor capacities of the infant.

EEG coherence has also been used as a measure in the study of brain development. EEG coherence is a measure of the phase relation of two processes at a specific frequency band. Coherence values range from 0 (there is no phase relation) to 1 (the two signals are either completely in or out of phase with each other). A number of researchers have speculated on the interpretation of changes in EEG coherence. Nunez (1981) has suggested that coherence between two EEG electrode locations may reflect the activity of axonal connections between two regions. Others have postulated that coherence values may be related to the activity of short- and long-fiber networks of the axons (Thatcher, Krause, & Hrybyk, 1986; Thatcher, Walker, & Giudice, 1987). Thatcher postulated that development in the cortex involves processes of increasing communication between regionally distinct locations as well

as increased differentiation of regions across the cortex. Thatcher utilized a ratio score of long to short distance coherence to demonstrate this model. By examining the coherence of long-distance sites (and assuming increases to reflect increased long distance communication) and examining the coherence between short-distance sites (and assuming decreases to reflect regional specialization) Thatcher, Walker, and Giudice (1987) were able to model the growth of the cerebral hemispheres across the first ten years of life. Thatcher, Walker, and Giudice (1987) reported that periods of major change in short- and long-distance coherence coincided with what appear to be major stage transitions in cognitive growth. This, he argued, is an indirect confirmation of his model of neural change as reflected in the EEG measure of coherence. More recently, Barry and colleagues have focused on changes in EEG coherence over middle childhood and have argued for particular methodological modifications in the interpretation of coherence, such as correcting for inter-electrode distances (Barry et al., 2005; Barry et al., 2004).

If, in fact, coherence reflects the connectivity between different regions, then it may change as a function of the degree to which that connectivity increases or decreases. Studies of both human (Huttenlocher, 1979; Huttenlocher et al., 1982) and non-human primate cortical development (Greenough & Volkmar, 1973) report that during early development there is an over-population of neurons in the cortex which, also during early development seem to be selectively pruned. Bell and Fox (1996) wondered whether these processes may be reflected in measures of EEG coherence and took as their model the timing of self-produced locomotion during the first year of life. They recorded EEG from four groups of 8-month-old infants who varied in the degree of experience they had with self-produced locomotion (one group was not yet crawling; a second group crawled for one to two weeks; a third group from three to six weeks and a fourth group had been crawling for more than 7 weeks). Bell and Fox argued that coherence measures should differ as a function of the degree of experience that infants had with crawling. This model of experience dependent changes in neural patterning was first proposed by Greenough (Greenough & Black, 1992; Greenough, Black, & Wallace, 1987) who predicted an inverted U-shaped function in the number of connections (with an increase at the onset of particular expected experiences and a decrease as pruning occurred once a particular competency had been mastered). Bell and Fox (1996) found this same inverted U-shape function for intra-hemispheric coherence in the EEG among the four groups. Infants with no experience in crawling showed less coherence than those with only a short period of crawling experience. By seven weeks of experience the level of coherence had again dropped.

Studies relating ERP morphology to early brain development. Developmentalists who subscribe to early critical periods are interested in how environmental input can affect brain development and the emergence of particular competencies during development. One such example is the acquisition of language. There seem to be critical periods around which particular components of language emerge. During the first half of the first year of post-natal life, all infants are capable of discriminating the sounds of any language across lexical boundaries. Thus, infants raised in an English-speaking environment in the United States are capable of discriminating across certain boundaries of Chinese or Japanese (Best, 1993). After six to eight months, this ability to discriminate any boundary seems to disappear and the child is only able to make these discriminations for their native language, the language to which they have been exposed. These changes clearly suggest the reorganization of neural centers as a function of language input and the critical period during which this reorganization is said to occur. ERP techniques have also been used to provide additional evidence of the neural changes underlying this reorganization (Cheour et al., 1998; Rivera-Gaxiola, Silva-Pereyra, & Kuhl, 2005). However, not all neural reorganization for language necessitates the input of oral communication. In a series of studies, Helen Neville and her colleagues have shown that congenitally deaf subjects differ from hearing subjects in the pattern of their ERP responses to language (Neville, Kutas, & Schmidt, 1982a, 1982b). Whereas hearing subjects displayed a prototypical left hemisphere distribution of the ERP in response to language stimuli, deaf subjects showed an opposite pattern (one of right hemisphere distribution). Neville reported that this pattern of right hemisphere activity in the ERP of deaf subjects might be a function of the type of language input that they receive. While hearing subjects receive oral auditory input, deaf subjects were more likely to receive visual-spatial input as communication. The type of language communication therefore reorganized the pattern of hemispheric dominance. These patterns of reorganization were reflected in the asymmetry of the ERP.

As with the EEG, particular characteristics of the ERP in early development have been related to certain aspects of brain maturation. For instance, the polarity of the mismatch negativity (MMN) in the auditory ERP has been found to related to global maturational status in newborns (Leppanen et al., 2004). Characteristics of the auditory and visual ERP responses have also been used to document deviations from the typical maturational sequence in at-risk clinical populations of newborns and infants who suffered particular insults or deprivations in fetal development (Black et al., 2004; Siddappa et al., 2004). In older infants and young children living in institutions in Bucharest, Romania, the ERP responses recorded to facial expressions of emotion were significantly smaller in amplitude compared with a group of never-institutionalized infants and young children (Parker, Nelson, & the BEIP Core Group, 2005) In addition, the early negative components such as the Nc and N170 did not show age-related changes in the institutionalized children, whereas particular changes were seen in terms of latency and amplitude changes with age in the never-institutionalized children.

Still other more recent ERP studies have attempted to link particular ERP components to individual differences in personality in older children. For example, we have recently examined the error-related negativity (ERN) in children and adults. The ERN is an ERP waveform that occurs approximately 100 ms following an error response of the realization of having erred. The source of the ERN is thought to be the anterior cingulate cortex (ACC). The ACC is known to play an important role in error detection and response monitoring. We have found in a sample of nonclinical 10-year-olds attenuated ERN responses in children classified as undersocialized (Santesso, Segalowitz, & Schmidt, 2005) and exaggerated ERN responses in children classified as high on obsessive compulsive behaviors (Santesso, Segalowitz, & Schmidt, 2006c).

While developmental ERP studies have long attempted to link certain ERP components to behavioral and psychological phenomena, there is increasing interest in the use of new techniques to localize these components in the brain. While localization of scalp-recorded brain potentials requires particular assumptions in order to overcome the "inverse problem" that is a fundamental constraint on such endeavors, recent advances have been made that allow researchers more accuracy in speculating about the possible origins of brain potentials in infants and children. Reynolds and Richards (in press) focused on the negative component known as the Nc, which is commonly observed in studies of visual recognition memory in infants (Nelson & Collins, 1992). Using spatial independent components analysis, the cortical source of the Nc was localized to specific areas of prefrontal cortex, including the medial and inferior parts of the frontal gyrus, as well as the anterior cingulate cortex. The study by Reynolds and Richards (in press) represents a particularly interesting application of combining novel statistical methods with new methods for recording EEG from high-density scalp arrays in infancy. The use of such techniques may prove very important in addressing some of the critical questions in the literature concerning the nature of early cortical development (de Haan, Johnson, & Halit, 2003; Gauthier & Nelson, 2001).

The cardiovascular system: Heart period and heart rate variability

Overview. The cardiovascular system is relatively well developed at birth and recording of the ECG is relatively easy even during the newborn period, thus providing researchers and clinicians with a useful and noninvasive means for assessing the developmental status of infants. Measures of heart period (the time interval between successive heart cycles, or the inter-beat interval) and heart rate variability (a general term used to refer to beat-to-beat changes in heart rate or heart period) serve as indices of autonomic nervous system regulatory activities and have been related to individual differences in attention, cognition, and emotion in both child and adult populations. The interpretation of the autonomic origins of cardiovascular response patterns, whether in the context of intra-individual responses to discrete stimuli or inter-individual differences in "baseline" cardiovascular patterns, is complicated by the fact that the parasympathetic and sympathetic branches of the ANS dually innervate the heart. Methodological advances, such as the incorporation of spectral analytic techniques into the analysis of heart rate variability data, however, allow for the isolation and quantification of particular sources of heart rate variability (Mezzacappa et al., 1994).

The ability to empirically link basic cardiovascular measures such as heart period to higher order cognitive processes such as attention and information processing has been particularly useful in the field of child development where researchers are faced with the difficulty of gathering information from infants who have yet to acquire language or complex motor behaviors. Thus, cardiovascular measures have become a useful tool for the study and assessment of sensory, perceptual, and cognitive development in infants. Conversely, infant development provides a useful means for studying the development of autonomic functioning and its role in psychological processes.

Beyond infancy, cardiovascular functioning has been related to the development of emotional and behavioral disorders in childhood and adolescence. Theoretically, the cardiovascular system has been related to problem behaviors based on the assumption that cardiovascular functioning is related to higher order cognitive processes such as information processing. In older children and adults, information processing expands beyond simply attending to stimuli in the environment to allocating attention between internal (i.e., self-focused) and external (i.e., other-focused) events.

Historical background. There are excellent reviews of the historical development of the use of cardiovascular measures with adult populations in psychological research (e.g., Hassett & Danforth, 1982). Cardiovascular measures were originally used as an index of general arousal or emotion. Darrow (1929) first documented adults' physiologically distinct responses to classes of stimuli differing in the extent to which they were psychologically arousing. Specifically, when adults were presented with disturbing or arousing words, Darrow recorded a rise in blood pressure along with increases in heart rate. In contrast, there were little or very slight drops in blood pressure in response to benign sensory stimuli. In addition, Darrow found that heart rate and respiration were more tightly coupled or associated during the psychologically arousing conditions compared to the more benign conditions. Together, Darrow's findings demonstrated that stimuli with distinct characteristics and psychological meanings evoked physiologically unique responses. In addition, increased respiratory-cardiac coupling under psychologically arousing conditions was attributed to increased autonomic arousal.

Ax (1953) extended Darrow's findings by demonstrating that specific emotions were associated with distinct physiological reaction patterns. During anger provocation in the laboratory, Ax found that adults responded with increased diastolic blood pressure and decreased heart rate. In contrast, there were fewer consistent reaction patterns during the induction of fear. Further, Ax noted that there was a greater coupling or association between physiological measures during anger induction. Ax interpreted these differences in the concordance of physiological measures as reflecting greater integration or organization during anger versus fear induction. From an evolutionary perspective, Ax related the increased physiological integration during anger reactions to a complete mobilization of resources, in contrast to a relative lack of integration or paralysis of bodily functions during fear reactions.

Lacey (1967) provided compelling ideas as well as empirical evidence to argue against general activation theories of emotion. Lacey argued that physiological activation could not simply be conceptualized as a uni-dimensional continuum in which the degree of physiological activation directly maps onto the intensity of emotion or behavior. Rather, Lacey proposed that activation is multidimensional and that physiological reaction patterns reflect not only the intensity but also the intended goal or aim of an emotion or behavior. In a series of experiments, Lacey reported that the direction of cardiovascular response was telling of a subject's intention (e.g., approach versus avoid/withdrawal) towards external stimuli. Through directional reactions, the cardiovascular system serves to meet the varying metabolic demands of the body. Cardiac decelerations in response to arousing stimuli were thought to reflect stimulus detection and active intake from the environment, while cardiac accelerations were thought to reflect active mental work, an internal focus, and the active filtering of irrelevant external stimuli.

The application of spectral analytic techniques to the study of both intra- and inter-individual differences in heart rate variability has allowed for more precise interpretations regarding the autonomic origins of these differences. Using power spectral analysis, heart rate signals are decomposed into a series of component frequencies, with each component contributing to the total variance in the signal. The distribution of the total variance across the frequency range studied is associated with particular sources of the heart rate variability and the related parasympathetic and sympathetic nervous system mediators (Akselrod et al., 1981, 1985). In adults, the majority of heart rate variability is contained within the frequency range of 0.0 Hz to 0.5 Hz, with the components ranging from 0.15 Hz to 0.5 Hz being referred to as high frequency (HF) and the components ranging from 0.04 Hz to 0.15 Hz being referred to as low frequency (LF). The HF band marks the component of heart rate variability associated with respiration or RSA (Hirsch & Bishop, 1981).

However, developmental changes in respiratory rate will affect the boundaries of this band. The influences of respiration on heart rate variability are mediated primarily by changes in parasympathetic control over the heart via the vagus nerve (Katona & Jih, 1975). Porges (1986) developed an algorithm to index cardiac vagal tone – a measure of heart rate variability due to respiration. Porges work was based on early theoretical work of Eppinger and Hess (1915) on vagotonia and how the balance in sympathetic and parasympathetic tone was related to clinical phenomena and the empirical work of Katona and Jih (1975) some six decades later providing anatomical and functional evidence to this end in animals. The cardiac vagal tone metric is derived from spectral power in the HF band as a measure of the magnitude of Respiratory Sinus Arrhythiniac, which in turn has been used as an index of vagal control over the heart. However, the predictive relations between RSA and cardiac vagal control are reduced by nonrespiratory parasympathetic contributions to heart rate variability and within-subject changes in respiratory parameters, making RSA an imperfect estimate of vagal cardiac control (see Bernston et al., 1997, for a review). Despite these limitations, RSA remains among the most selective noninvasive indices of parasympathetic cardiac control (Berntson, Cacioppo, & Quigley, 1993).

The neural origins of LF variability are more diffuse, being mediated by both the parasympathetic and sympathetic branches of the autonomic nervous system. Low frequency power varies with sympathetic control, but only under limited and very specific conditions (see Berntson et al., 1997 for a review). Measures of the LF/HF ratio have been used to index the balance between sympathetic and vagal cardiac control (e.g., Malliani et al., 1994). However, for several reasons including the fact that the PNS and SNS are not always reciprocally controlled, this method of estimating sympathovagal balance remains controversial (Berntson et al., 1997). Further, measurement of LF power requires HP data to be collected over a period of several minutes, with minimal motor movement and regular respiration (Snidman et al., 1995). These constraints are particularly challenging to overcome in work with infants and young children.

Sympathetic cardiac control has also been evaluated by measuring the duration of pre-ejection period (PEP); (Cacioppo et al., 1994). PEP is the period over which the left ventricle generates force, or the interval from the onset of ventricular depolarization to the beginning of ejection, and is inversely related to sympathetic inotropy (Binkley & Boudoulas, 1986). Systolic time intervals such as PEP can be derived from information provided by impedance cardiography, or from a combination of concurrent electrocardiographic, phonocardiographic, and pulse measurements. Although clearly more challenging to assess in children, PEP measures have recently been incorporated into studies of individual differences in young children (e.g., Buss et al., 2004).

In summary, advances in measurement techniques provide researchers with a means for empirically evaluating the specific relations between parasympathetic and sympathetic influences and a variety of cognitive, emotional, and behavioral measures (e.g., Mezzacappa et al., 1997). Due to the relative ease of isolating the parasympathetic influences on cardiac control, there have been more empirical studies relating psychological indices to vagal influences over the heart. Methods for non-invasively estimating sympathetic influences over the heart continue to be refined, however, as of yet there is no agreed upon measure (Berntson et al., 1997). Further, pragmatic constraints limit the extent to which methods for assessing sympathetic cardiac control can be applied to studies of infants and young children.

Cardiovascular psychophysiology is based, in part, on the premise that both the direction and magnitude of cardiovascular responses, are sensitive to stimulus characteristics and reflect not only the intensity of one's reaction but the intention as well. Cardiovascular measures can also serve as markers of individual differences in these reaction tendencies. The demonstration and articulation of these properties of the cardiovascular response system has triggered growing interest by developmental psychologists in cardiovascular development and in the development of ANS/CNS integration. As well, developmental psychologists have used cardiovascular measures and psychophysiological paradigms to index perceptual and cognitive processing abilities and risk status in preverbal infants. Finally, a good deal of developmental work has been completed on cardiovascular markers of individual differences in response tendencies in both cognitive and social domains.

SOCIAL, COGNITIVE, AND PSYCHOLOGICAL CONTEXTS

EEG and cognitive development: The case of the frontal lobes

There is a good deal of interest in the study of relations between maturation of specific brain areas and the development of cognitive processes (Bell & Fox, 1994; Diamond & Goldman-Rakic, 1989; Fox & Bell, 1990; Thatcher, 1994). One brain area that has held interest for both those interested in individual differences and those interested in cognitive-brain relations is the frontal region. The dorsolateral area of the frontal region is known to play a critical role in processes associated with working memory. Goldman-Rakic (Goldman-Rakic, 1987a, 1987b; Goldman-Rakic et al., 1983) and Diamond (Diamond & Goldman-Rakic, 1983, 1986, 1989; Diamond, Zola-Morgan, & Squire, 1989) have demonstrated how maturation of this area is critical in the performance of certain cognitive tasks which develop in the first and second years of life in the human infant. Diamond and colleagues (Diamond et al., 1997) have shown how variations in infant diet could affect infants with PKU and ultimately compromise their frontal functioning. There is, in addition, a good deal of speculation on the role that the frontal lobes might play in inhibition, planning, and executive function behaviors (Chelune et al., 1986; Dennis, 1991; Welsh, Pennington, & Groisser, 1991). The frontal cortex is also directly involved in multiple behavioral components associated with emotion such as the motor facilitation of emotion expression, the organization and integration of cognitive processes underlying emotion, and the ability to regulate emotions (Dawson, 1994; Fox, 1994).

Although a large corpus of evidence exists on EEG frequency development in posterior regions as noted earlier, there has been little research directed towards frontal EEG development. Much of the hesitation in examining frontal EEG involved the belief that the frontal lobes did not develop until later childhood. Neuro-imaging studies, however, suggest otherwise. Chugani and Phelps (1986) found an increase in glucose metabolism in the frontal cortex in human infants between 8 and 12 months, providing evidence for changes in frontal activity during the first year of life.

Developmental research with non-clinical populations utilizing measures of brain electrical activity (whether via EEG or ERP) has examined changes in frontal lobe activity over the first years of life (c.f. Bell & Fox, 1994, 1996). There are also studies that have utilized measures of EEG or ERP as dependent variables examining frontal response as a function of cognitive challenge (Nelson, 1994). As well, there are studies that have attempted to link these measures to known developmental changes in specific brain structures and the behaviors which purportedly are subsumed by those structures.

An example of this work may be found in the intersection of the work of Diamond and Goldman-Rakic (1989) and Bell and Fox (1992, 1994). Diamond and Goldman-Rakic utilized infant non-human primates and were able to show by ablation of specific regions of frontal cortex that performance on paradigms such as the delayed response task or Piaget's A not B task both involved maturation and integrity of the dorsolateral frontal cortex. Bell and Fox (1992) followed up to this work, recording EEG monthly from infants aged 6 to 12 months. At each session, infants were assessed on the A not B task. Bell and Fox (1992) found a correlation between EEG recorded over the frontal region and performance on the A not B task in human infants. Bell and Fox suggested that the EEG recordings reflected activity generated from the dorsolateral frontal cortex. Such studies are suggestive of the manner in which EEG may inform knowledge of cognitive development.

Fox and his colleagues (Fox & Bell, 1990; Fox et al., 1992) explored frontal lobe maturation during the latter half of the first year of post-natal life using frontal EEG frequency measures. EEG was recorded from left and right frontal, parietal, and occipital scalp locations monthly in a group of 13 healthy full-term infants from 7 until 12 months of age. A measure of relative power for each region using 6 Hz to 9 Hz/1 Hz to −4 Hz at each age was computed. The data revealed an increase in 6 Hz to 9 Hz power in the frontal region over age suggesting an increase in EEG power for the frontal region in the second half of the first year of life. These EEG data, in combination with the neuro-imaging findings mentioned earlier, suggest that the frontal lobes are active and developing during the latter half of the first year of postnatal life. Changes in EEG power in the frontal region during the latter half of the first year of postnatal life might reflect frontal lobe maturation.

Bell and Fox (1994) also examined EEG coherence values between anterior and posterior electrode locations in the same sample reported above. They found stronger coherence between the frontal and occipital sites across age compared with the frontal and parietal sites (see Bell & Fox, 1994). This pattern of long versus short distance coherence suggests the maturation of anterior and posterior connections over the second half of the first year of postnatal life which are necessary for the sequencing of complex behavior (Pribram, 1973).

Frontal EEG activation and the development of emotions

Based upon a series of studies completed with adults that indicated that the frontal region was involved in certain aspects of emotional behavior (Davidson, 1984a, 1984b), Fox and Davidson completed a series of papers in which they examined the relation between EEG asymmetry and the expression of emotion in human infants. Their first study (Davidson & Fox, 1982) investigated EEG in ten-month-old infants who viewed a videotape of an actress while the actress was smiling or crying. Davidson and Fox (1982) found, in two independent studies, that infants exhibited greater relative left frontal EEG activity when viewing the smiling face compared to when they viewed the crying face. Fox and Davidson (1984) interpreted these results as suggesting that the frontal region was specialized for the control of the expression of behaviors involved in approach and withdrawal. Emotions were one class of behaviors and that could be parsed into those associated with approach (such as joy or interest) or withdrawal (disgust, fear, distress) (see Fox, 1991).

In a subsequent test of this model, Fox and Davidson presented one- and two-day-old infants with different liquid tastes (sugar water, citric acid, and plain water) (Fox & Davidson, 1986a). They recorded EEG in response to the presentation of the tastes and found differences in asymmetry along the approach-withdrawal dimension. Further studies with ten-month-old infants who were responding to the approach of an unfamiliar adult (Fox & Davidson, 1987) or maternal separation (Fox & Davidson, 1988) confirmed the role of behaviors associated with either approach or withdrawal as being associated with left or right frontal EEG asymmetry. More recent studies on the issue of frontal EEG activity and the development of emotion have used other sensory modalities to induce emotion and examine corresponding changes in physiology. The auditory modality is one such example to which we now turn.

Studies of musical/auditory emotions.

Santesso, Schmidt, and Trainor (2006b) recently examined infants' psychophysiological responses to emotional infant direct (ID) speech and music. Although behavioral studies suggest that ID speech elicits appropriate emotional responses in infants (Fernald, 1993; Santesso, et al., 2006b) were interested in whether infants could differentiate the emotional content of ID speech using regional continuous EEG measures.

Nine-month-old infants were presented with pre-recorded samples of mothers saying, "Hey honey, come over here," that varied in both emotional intensity (e.g., intense versus calm) and valence (e.g., pleasant versus unpleasant). For example, comforting (low intensity, positive valence), surprised (high intensity, positive valence), and fearful (high intensity, negative valence) voices were used and presented while infants' regional EEG and heart rate measures were continuously recorded. Santesso et al. (2006b) found that the emotional intensity of the ID speech was directly related to the overall frontal EEG power, such that greater power was related to greater emotional intensity. The fearful ID speech elicited the greatest absolute frontal EEG power, followed by the surprised and finally the comforting ID speech. These authors speculated that infants were responding to the *cognitive* aspects of ID speech, as increased EEG power during the first year of postnatal life is related to the cognitive/attentional properties of the stimuli (see Bell, 2002, for a review). Increasing the intensity of the ID speech (e.g., surprise/fearful ID speech) amplifies its emotional and attentional properties, thereby increasing the infants' external attention and interest. This corresponds to an increase in overall frontal EEG power (e.g., decreased activation). The comforting ID speech may encourage a decrease in EEG power (e.g., greater activation) and, therefore, more synchronous electrocortical activity, promoting emotional regulation. This interpretation was corroborated by the autonomic responses to the ID speech. Significant decelerations in heart rate were seen in response to both the positively and negatively valenced ID speech, which may signify either the infants' interest or their attentional engagement with speech stimuli. Thus, both central and autonomic measures suggest that infants are responding primarily to cognitive or attentional properties of ID speech, rather than emotional properties.

Similar to ID speech, ID music is a form of emotional communication between parents and infants. These musical registers facilitate both the creation of an emotional bond between parent and child, and the regulation of infants' emotional states (Rock, Trainor, & Addison, 1999; Trainor, 1996). As with ID speech, caregivers tend to make universal modifications to their singing directed toward infants (Rock, Trainor, & Addison, 1999; Trehub & Trainor, 1998; Trainor et al., 1997) that distinguish it from

adult-directed (AD) music (Trainor, 1996; Trehub, Unyk, & Trainor, 1993). Furthermore, infants are responsive to music, with innate (Masataka, 1999) preferences for ID to AD music (Trainor, 1996), and distinctive behavioral responses to the emotional content of the ID music (Rock, Trainor, & Addison, 1999). Although older children are able to extract emotional meaning and make emotional judgments about music (Scherer & Zentner, 2001; Trainor & Trehub, 1992), little is known about the basis for infants' reactions to musical emotions. Are infants' reactions based on the emotional quality of the songs, or are they rooted primarily in the attentional properties of the children's music, as appears to be the case with ID speech?

We (Hodgson-Minnie et al., 2006) next presented 9-month-old infants with 60-second excerpts of children's music varying in emotional valence and intensity while continuously recording their regional EEG and heart rate responses. The musical stimuli resembled either songs that infants would typically be exposed to in their natural environment (e.g., play-songs and lullabies) or unfamiliar, fearful music to which most infants of this age would not have been exposed. Infants, then, listened to three types of children's songs: familiar, joyful, play-song-like music (intense, pleasant emotion); fearful, unfamiliar style of children's music (intense, unpleasant emotion); and familiar, soothing, lullaby-like music (calm, pleasant emotion). It appears that the processing of children's musical emotions may tap into right frontal processes, rather than recruiting the differential left and right hemispheric activities noted with other stimulus modalities at this age and with older children and adults (e.g., Davidson, 1984, 1992, 2000; Fox, 1991, 1994). Greater relative right frontal EEG activity (e.g., less frontal EEG power) resulted from the presentation of both positively- and negatively-valenced children's musical emotions. Although this finding coincides with the idea that the right hemisphere dominates the processing of emotion (e.g., Heller, 1993; Gainotti, Caltagirone, & Zoccolotti, 1993), it is also important to note that the emotional prosody contained in the children's music is a salient feature for infants, and its detection has been linked to increased right hemispheric activity (Buchanan et al., 2000; Pihan, Altenmuller, & Ackermann, 1997). Perhaps infants of this age are focusing exclusively on the prosodic features of the children's music, resulting in a right hemispheric bias. In contrast to earlier findings with ID speech (Santesso et al., 2006b), overall frontal EEG power was linearly related to the affective *valence* of the children's music, such that greater relative EEG power corresponded to increases in the *positive* valence of the music. Again, the pattern of overall EEG power may reflect the cognitive aspects of emotion (Bell, 2002). For example, infants tend to respond behaviorally to play-songs with increased external awareness and attention, whereas they respond to lullabies with a greater internal focus (Rock, Trainor, & Addison 1999). Similar to the surprised ID speech, joyful children's songs may result in greater EEG power (e.g., decreased activation) due to the attentional properties of the music that promote greater social interactions. In contrast, the soothing, lullaby-like children's songs (resembling comforting ID speech) may promote emotional regulation through a decrease in overall frontal EEG power. One might expect the fearful children's music to encourage increased external attention and therefore greater frontal EEG power, as was seen with the fearful ID speech; however, in this case, this unfamiliar stimulus corresponded to the least relative frontal EEG power. Perhaps the fearful music activates more primitive, subconscious brain structures due to its negative quality. Conversely, perhaps the infants are unable to process the emotional quality of this unfamiliar, fearful music on a cognitive level due to their inexperience with this emotion in a musical context. Fear is one of the hardest emotions to express by music (Terwogt & van Grinsven, 1991) and is rarely included in children's songs. On the autonomic level, infants responded with heart rate decelerations to increasing attentional demands associated with the emotional stimuli. Infants' heart rate was inversely related to the intensity of the musical emotions, with more intense children's musical emotions (joyful, play-song-like and fearful music) eliciting heart rate decelerations, relative to the less intense stimuli (soothing, lullaby-like music). Infants exhibited a low heart rate in response to the intense, fearful stimulus, corresponding to external attention and interest (Berntson & Boysen, 1990), which would be required to assess any potential threats or dangers. Moreover, there was an association between the cognitive and autonomic attentional processes during the processing of the joyful and soothing children's music. Specifically, the joyful, play-song-like children's music promoted greater EEG power and heart rate decelerations, both of which are associated with external attention and emotional engagement. In contrast, soothing, lullaby-like music may promote self-regulation through the combination of heart rate accelerations associated with an internal attentional focus (Berntson & Boysen, 1990) and attenuated overall frontal EEG power. It appears that infants respond to the cognitive or attentional properties of the musical, auditory stimuli. However, both ID speech and ID music have relatively simplistic structural properties. It is unclear if this apparently attentional response would continue if the complexity of the music is increased to include orchestral, rather than ID, pieces.

Schmidt, Trainor, and Santesso (2003) addressed this question in a series of cross-sectional studies that examined infants' psychophysiological responses to orchestral music at 3, 6, 9, and 12 months of age. Infants were presented with a series of three 30-second orchestra excerpts varying in emotional valence and intensity (fear, sadness, and happy) while their regional EEG and heart rate responses were continuously recorded. With these increasingly complex pieces, infants were neither able to differentiate the valence nor the intensity of the emotional music on a psychophysiological level. However, clear developmental changes were observed in response to the emotion-laden orchestral music. First, while each excerpt served to increase overall brain activity in 3-month-old infants,

by 12 months of age, each of the affective pieces attenuated overall brain activity, perhaps exerting a "calming" influence and reflecting infants' interest and attention to the musical stimuli. Specifically, both frontal and parietal regions shifted from exhibiting a decrease in EEG power to an increase in EEG power in response to the orchestral pieces (collapsed across condition) with increasing age. The distribution of EEG activity also changed with age. The musical emotions exerted a more global influence during early development, resulting in equivalent measured EEG activation in frontal and parietal scalp regions at 3 and 6 months of age, and later shifted to a more localized effect on the frontal scalp region by 12 months of age. This change likely reflects the maturation of frontal lobe functioning. Finally, infants failed to show differential hemispheric responses to the music (collapsed across condition) until 12 months, at which time they displayed increased left hemispheric EEG activity (greater relative right hemispheric EEG power) in response to both the orchestral stimuli and baseline conditions. The authors believe that this pattern of hemispheric EEG asymmetry may reflect the development of emotional regulatory processes, involving the maturation of frontal lobe functioning between 9 and 12 months and the relative attenuation of frontal activity by 12 months. On an autonomic level, heart rate was attenuated in response to the music (collapsed across condition) early in development (e.g., at 3 and 6 months), perhaps reflecting interest in the novel musical stimuli. By 9 months, infants' heart rate accelerated in response to the music, suggesting an internal focus (Berntson & Boysen, 1990) and possibly the emergence of self-regulatory processes. By 12 months, however, there were no significant differences between resting and music conditions on heart rate, opening the possibility that either infants were able to self-regulate their emotional responses and arousal or that the orchestral music was too complex for them to extract any emotional significance. Unlike its structurally simpler musical counterparts, then, orchestral music was seemingly too complex for infants to process its emotional valence or intensity. It did, however, promote developmentally distinct psychophysiological reactions in infants across the first year of post-natal life, possibly reflecting the development of emotion regulatory processes crucial for successful social and emotional development.

FRONTAL EEG ACTIVATION AND THE DEVELOPMENT OF INDIVIDUAL DIFFERENCES IN TEMPERAMENT AND AFFECTIVE STYLE

Recent studies have shown that the pattern of resting frontal EEG alpha asymmetry reflects a predisposition to experience positive and negative emotion and is predictive of individual differences in affective style in healthy adults (see Davidson, 1993, 2000; Coan & Allen, 2004, for reviews) and children (Fox, 1991, 1994; Fox et al., 2001). Individuals who exhibit stable right frontal EEG asymmetry at rest are easily distressed, fearful, and shy, whereas those who exhibit stable left frontal EEG asymmetry at rest are socially outgoing and extraverted.

Individual differences in approach/withdrawal.

Both Davidson (1995; Wheeler, Davidson, & Tomarken, 1993) and Fox (1991) found that the pattern of resting or baseline frontal EEG asymmetry was itself a marker for the disposition of the subject to express affects associated with either approach or withdrawal. For example, Davidson and Fox (1989) reported that differences in tonic frontal EEG arousal predicted infants' emotional responses. Infants who displayed a pattern of greater relative right frontal EEG activation exhibited a shorter latency to cry to maternal separation at age 10 months compared with infants who display left frontal asymmetry. Together, these studies suggest that stable individual differences in frontal EEG (e.g., Fox et al., 1992) may reflect individual differences in temperamental characteristics of the individual. Additional work from Fox's laboratory with behaviorally inhibited toddlers and preschool children would seem to confirm this notion (Fox et al., 1995; Fox et al., 2001).

Studies of behaviorally inhibited and socially withdrawn children.

Behavioral inhibition reflects a tendency to display fear and wariness in response to novel stimuli (Kagan, Reznick, & Snidman, 1987). Behaviorally inhibited children display long latencies to approach novel stimuli, exhibit a high frequency of negative affect, and remain in close proximity to their mothers in response to the presentation of novel stimuli. Children who display this pattern of behavior towards novel social stimuli have been characterized as shy and timid. In addition, children who remain inhibited during the first few years of life are at risk for anxiety disorders in later childhood (Hirshfeld et al., 1992).

Calkins et al. (1996) examined frontal lobe development in a group of infants selected at 4 months of age for temperamental constellations thought to predict behavioral inhibition and shyness in early childhood. Eighty-one healthy infants were selected at 4 months of age from a larger sample of 207 using procedures similar to those reported by Kagan and Snidman (1991). Infants were observed in their homes at 4 months of age and videotaped as they responded to novel auditory and visual stimuli. The 81 infants were selected based upon their frequency of motor activity, and degree of positive and negative affect displayed in response to these novel stimuli. Three groups were formed on the basis of the infant's behavior at 4 months of age. The Negative group comprised infants who responded to the stimuli with high motor activity, high negative affect, and low positive affect. Kagan and Snidman (1991) found that this temperamental group of infants was behaviorally inhibited at 14 months of age. The Positive group comprised infants who responded with both high amounts of motor activity and positive affect, but low amounts of negative affect. A third group of infants, referred to as the Low responders, were characterized by their low levels activity, including motor activity and both positive and negative affect.

The infants were seen again in the laboratory at 9, 14, and 24 months, at which time EEG was recorded. At 14 months, each infant was observed interacting during a freeplay situation, and with a series of unfamiliar stimuli designed to elicit his or her response to novelty. The data revealed that infants who were easily distressed to novelty at 4 months of age exhibited greater relative right frontal EEG activation at 9 months as well as at 24 months compared with infants in the other two groups. These same infants displayed a greater number of behaviors reflecting inhibition at both 14 and 24 months of age compared to infants in either of the two other groups. It is also important to note that infants who displayed a pattern of stable right frontal EEG activity across the first two years of postnatal life tended to be more inhibited at both 14 and 24 months compared with infants who exhibited a pattern of stable left frontal EEG during this time (Fox, Calkins, & Bell, 1994).

These data suggest that greater activity in the right versus left frontal region may serve as a marker for infants' temperamental wariness in response to novelty. Infants who display a pattern of greater relative right frontal EEG activation appear less able to successfully regulate the arousal of negative affect, perhaps serving as a marker of subsequent behavioral inhibition in toddlers.

This pattern of frontal EEG asymmetry and inhibition is critical for understanding the development of social withdrawal in the school years. The preschool years coincide with the development of social skills and peer interactions, both of which are determinants of the child's subsequent social development. Children who are shy and socially reticent often fail to develop such skills, and as a result are at risk for social withdrawal, social anxiety, and internalizing problems during the early school years (Rubin, Stewart, & Coplan, 1995). Conversely, children who are aggressive and intrusive with other children often fail to develop social skills and peer relationships. This group of children may be at risk for externalizing problems during the early school years. The origins of both forms of maladaptive social behavior may be linked to emotion regulatory problems and frontal dysfunction.

In an attempt to examine this very issue, Fox et al. (1995) observed 48 4-year-old children during play in groups of four. These groups were comprised of children who were unfamiliar to one another, but of the same age and same sex. The play session consisted of five parts: (1) unstructured freeplay, (2) clean-up, (3) birthday speeches, (4) cooperation task, and (5) unstructured freeplay. The children were unobtrusively observed during this time and their social behaviors were subsequently coded for measures of social participation.

A composite measure of social reticence was computed from behaviors displayed during the play session. This composite included the following standardized measures: (1) proportion of anxious behavior, latency to first spontaneous utterance, proportion of reticent behavior (unoccupied and onlooking behavior) during freeplay, (2) proportion of unoccupied behavior during cleanup and cooperation task, (3) the inverse of duration of speech episode, and the inverse of total time talking during the speech episode.

Each child was seen individually some two weeks after the group visit at which time EEG was recorded for 3 minutes while the child was seated and attending to a visual stimulus. The data revealed that children who displayed a high proportion of anxious behavior and wariness in response to their peers during the play session exhibited greater relative right frontal EEG activation that was a function of less power (more activation) in the right frontal site relative to the left frontal site compared with their more sociable and less anxious peers.

Measures of frontal EEG activation have also been used in conjunction with behavioral measures to help elucidate the underlying motivations for different social behaviors in young children. We recently examined patterns of frontal EEG activation in relation to different forms of nonsocial behavior in preschoolers during a play session with unfamiliar peers: social reticence and solitary-passive behavior (Henderson et al., 2004). In contrast to solitary-passive children who occupy themselves with exploratory and constructive activities such as drawing and working on puzzles while in the company of unfamiliar peers, reticent children remain visually focused and oriented toward other children, yet do not join them in their activities. Both reticent and solitary-passive children showed a pattern of resting right frontal EEG asymmetry, which suggests that these different forms of solitude may share a common withdrawal motivation. However, reticent children also showed a pattern of increased generalized EEG activation (or decreased alpha power) across the scalp. This pattern of activation in consistent with animal studies demonstrating that generalized cortical activation can reflect activity in the central nucleus of the amygdala (e.g., Kapp, Supple, & Whalen 1994).

Measures of frontal EEG activation have also been used to examine the regulation of children's social behaviors. Fox et al. (1996) examined the interactions between resting frontal EEG asymmetry and social behavior during peer play in the prediction of behavior problems in preschoolers. Highly sociable children who were right frontally activated at rest were more likely to exhibit externalizing problems compared with sociable children who were left frontal. In addition, shy children who displayed greater relative right frontal EEG activity were more likely to exhibit internalizing problems compared with shy children who displayed greater relative left frontal EEG activity at rest. These findings suggest that individual differences in frontal EEG activation may play an important role in the development of maladaptive social behavior during the preschool years. Children who display greater relative right frontal EEG activation may not have the competencies such as verbal mediation skills and analytic abilities –

thought to be subserved by the left frontal region – which are necessary to successfully regulate affective arousal. Children who display a pattern of right frontal EEG activation and extreme social reticence or sociability may be at risk for subsequent affective and behavioral problems. Indeed, frontal dysregulation has been implicated in conduct disorders by others (Moffit & Henry, 1989).

Theall-Honey and Schmidt (2006) recently reported that the frontal EEG asymmetry measure was related to the processing of emotion in shy preschoolers. Shy preschoolers who exhibited greater relatively right frontal EEG activity had problems regulating emotion, particularly negative emotion compared with their non-shy counterparts. When presented with affective video-clips that induced fear and sadness or when asked to give a speech about an embarrassing moment, shy children who exhibited greater relative right frontal EEG activity displayed more nonverbal signs of anxiety during the presentation of these stimuli compared with nonshy children or those exhibiting greater relative left frontal EEG activity.

Similarly, in older children, Schmidt et al. (1999) found that frontal EEG measures were related to the processing of social stress in older children who were shy. Seven-year-olds who were shy exhibited significantly greater increases in right, but not left, frontal EEG activity in anticipation of giving a speech about an embarrassing moment. The findings from these latter two studies demonstrate that the frontal EEG measures may be used to index, in addition to trait-like measures, state or phasic changes related to the processing and regulation of emotion in shy children.

Studies of shy and socially anxious adults. Individual differences in frontal EEG were also shown to predict affective style and personality in young adults. Adults who displayed a pattern of greater relative right frontal EEG activation are likely score high on psychometric measures indexing behavioral inhibition (Sutton & Davidson, 1997) and to rate film clips more negatively (Tomarken et al., 1990) than those individuals display greater relative left frontal EEG activation. As well, young adults who are shy (Schmidt, 1999) and unsocial in a dyadic social interaction (Schmidt & Fox, 1994) are more likely to exhibit greater relative right frontal EEG activity compared with sociable adults.

EEG and the development of behavior problems in older children and adults

Psychophysiologists have long been interested in psychopathology. There is a long and rich history of research investigating the CNS responses via EEG and ERPs of clinical populations including patients diagnosed with schizophrenia, depression, and psychosis (Lahmeyer, Reynolds, Kupfer, & King, 1989; Miller & Lesser, 1988; Niznikiewicz et al., 1997; Pollock & Schneider, 1990; Pritchard, 1986). There have been also a number of studies of CNS responding with children who have been diagnosed with specific psychiatric disorders such as hyperactivity, attention deficit disorder, and conduct disorder (e.g., Chelune et al., 1986; Raine & Venables, 1987; Raine, Venables, & Williams, 1990a). These studies have, by and large, attempted to outline the physiological mechanisms that are associated with the cognitive or affective deficits seen in these child clinical populations.

The use of resting frontal EEG measures and individual differences in the patterning of resting frontal EEG asymmetry can shed light on some behavioral problems in older children. For example, we (Santesso et al., 2006a) have most recently found a pattern of greater relative resting right frontal EEG activity at rest in a group of nonclinical 10-year-olds who were reported to have more CBCL aggression than those displaying greater relative left frontal EEG activity at rest.

Over the past ten years, there has been an increased interest in processes associated with the development of psychopathology in children, along with a re-thinking of the manner in which these issues ought to be approached. In particular, the questions arise as to the origins and factors which predispose some children to certain conditions, or the environmental factors which contribute to these conditions, and ultimately, to the nature of the interaction between dispositions and environments which may be the ultimate cause of certain types of psychopathology in children (Cicchetti, 1993). Researchers have recognized that certain forms of child psychopathology (particularly internalizing or externalizing disorders) do not arise de novo but rather are the end product of multiple factors including infant or child temperament, parenting style, and certain environmental correlates (e.g., Cicchetti & Richters, 1993). Such an approach is analogous to the interactionist model detailed above and necessitates for the psychophysiologist an analysis at the level of individual differences in child or infant disposition and the effects of environments (or parenting) on these initial dispositions.

Studies of infants and children of depressed mothers.

An example of this approach would be the work currently being completed on the effects of maternal depression on infant physiology and ultimately on child behavioral outcome. Recent studies have begun to examine the effects of maternal depression on infant physiology (Dawson et al., 1992; Field et al., 1995). It is widely known that adults who are depressed display less positive affect and more anxiousness compared to their nondepressed counterparts. Depressed adults are also known to exhibit reduced left frontal EEG activation (Henriques & Davidson, 1991) and greater right frontal EEG activation (Schaffer, Davidson, & Saron, 1983; Henriques & Davidson, 1990) than nondepressed adults. Women who are depressed are known to display less positive affect and reduced levels of stimulation when interacting with their infants (Cohn & Tronick, 1989; Cohn et al., 1986; Field, 1986; Field et al., 1988). Infants of depressed mothers display less positive affect and increased irritability (Cohn et al., 1986; Field, 1986,

Field et al., 1985) and greater frontal EEG activation than infants of nonsymptomatic mothers (Dawson et al., 1992). The findings reported by Dawson and her colleagues were with infants who ranged in age from 11–17 months. A similar pattern of frontal EEG asymmetry has recently been documented in infants as early as the first six months of life (Field et al., 1995).

Field et al. (1995) recorded baseline EEG in infants of depressed and nondepressed adolescent mothers. Infants ranged in age from 3 to 6 months. EEG was recorded during an alert state of attention. Infants of depressed mothers exhibited greater right frontal activation compared to infants of nondepressed mothers. Collectively, these studies suggest that maternal depression may affect infant physiology in the first two years of life. The fact that maternal depression affects brain electrical activity is consistent with an interactionist approach to development. It is also possible that the pattern of frontal EEG asymmetry in infants of depressed mothers may reflect a heritable component of the mothers' depression. There have been relatively few studies in which the genetic basis of EEG patterns has been examined. Further, it remains unknown whether these patterns of EEG asymmetry as observed in infancy remain stable over time (given certain types of parenting and environments) or whether they change, and whether children who as infants displayed these EEG patterns present with behavioral difficulties as they get older. The answers to these questions, however, will require longitudinal study, which operationalize and assess the interactive processes involved in development.

Studies of adults with depression, anxiety, and psychosis.

A number of other studies have shown that the pattern of resting frontal EEG alpha (8 to 13 Hz) asymmetry is predictive of individual differences in affective style in some clinically depressed and anxious populations even when their symptoms are in remission. Individuals who exhibit stable patterns of greater relative right frontal EEG activity at rest are known to be at risk for depression (Henriques & Davidson, 1990, 1991) and anxiety-related disorders. Recent studies have also shown that adolescent females at familial risk for major depressive disorder (Miller et al., 2002) exhibit greater relative right frontal EEG activity at rest.

Still other studies have examined the relation between frontal EEG activity and affective style in populations characterized by clinical phenomena other than mood and anxiety disorders. For example, we (Jetha, Schmidt, & Goldberg, 2005) recently examined the pattern of resting frontal EEG alpha activity in relation to personality in a group of adults with major psychosis. Using recent frontal EEG activation/affective style models as a theoretical platform, we attempted to extend these findings to adults with schizophrenia. The relations among the pattern of resting (eyes open, eyes closed) regional EEG alpha activity and trait shyness and sociability were examined in 20 adults with schizophrenia (outpatients who attend a community-based treatment and rehabilitation center and who were classified as having low positive and negative symptoms). Interestingly, we found the predicted relation between high trait shyness and greater relative resting right frontal EEG activity, and high trait sociability and greater relative resting left frontal EEG activity only in adults with schizophrenia whose positive symptoms of the disorder were reduced. In other words, once the symptoms of the disorder were controlled, then and only then, did the predicted relations emerge. This provides further evidence for the notion that the pattern of frontal EEG activity may reflect a basic property of personality even in the disordered brain.

Other issues: Psychometric considerations of the frontal EEG asymmetry metric

Inherent in the definition that the frontal EEG asymmetry metric is trait-like is the notion that it is stable across time and context. There is growing support for this idea in both adults and children. For example, Davidson and his group (Tomarken et al., 1992) have found modest to good stability across 3 months on frontal EEG asymmetry measures. We have recently noted modest to good stability of frontal EEG alpha activity in another context, across different stages of sleep in non-clinical young adults (Schmidt et al., 2003). We have also examined short-term stability (i.e., second-by-second stability) on frontal EEG asymmetry measures in 9 month-infants (Schmidt, 2006) and 7-year-old children (Schmidt, 1996) and found that stable patterns of greater relative right frontal EEG activity were related to individual differences in temperament. Taken together, the frontal EEG asymmetry metric is stable across time, situation, and development.

Cardiovascular measures and the study of cognitive development

Berg and Berg (1979) emphasized the utility of cardiovascular and other autonomic measures in the study of developmental psychology due to the fact that these systems are relatively well-developed at birth and during infancy relative to the limited behavioral repertoire of same-aged infants. For example, the heart begins to beat by the fourth week post-conception and with the development of central control mechanisms, the heart becomes responsive to state changes (e.g., Groome et al., 1997). By 30 weeks post-conception heart rate changes are reliably associated with changes in internal states, such as changes in sleep cycles.

As with adults, infants demonstrate directional cardiac responses to external stimuli. The direction of change is directly related to the development of neural control over the heart. In both humans and rats, Porges reports monotonic increases in the extent of vagal control over the heart across gestational age (e.g., Porges, McCabe, & Yongue, 1982; Porges, 1983). At birth, infants show reliable heart rate accelerations in response to stimulation (airstreams), however, by 2.5 months of age infants show consistent heart rate decelerations in response to the same stimulus (Berg & Berg, 1979). Others have noted significant shifts in baseline levels of heart rate variability around 2 to 4 months of age (e.g., Attuel et al., 1986; Lewis et al., 1970). These shifts in baseline and reactive cardiac patterns may reflect a general physiological reorganization of the CNS reflecting increasing cortical control. By 3 to 4 months of age, infants show consistent heart rate decelerations in response to stimulation regardless of modality (i.e., visual, acoustic, and tactile stimuli). These decelerative responses are interpreted as reflecting infants' active processing of sensory events.

Infants do not simply respond indiscriminately to the environment, rather their orienting responses are sensitive to stimulus parameters. Even newborns show visual preferences for horizontal versus vertical gratings, curved versus straight contours, and novel versus repeated stimuli (Slater & Morison, 1991). These visual preferences are accompanied by larger and longer decelerative heart rate responses (e.g., Lewis et al., 1966; McCall & Kagan, 1967). The fact that infants can discriminate among such stimuli and that these discriminations are reflected in different patterns of heart rate change gave rise to important developments in experimental paradigms for work with infants. For example, the habituation/dishabituation paradigm (Graham & Clifton, 1966) provides a means for indexing fundamental cognitive processes such as attention, memory, and responsiveness to novelty, and continues to be used as an index of basic sensory capacities. Specifically, with repeated exposure to the same stimulus, behaviors (i.e., visual attention) and physiological responses (i.e., heart rate decelerations) become habituated, or less pronounced, reflecting an infant's waning attention. During dishabituation trials, a novel stimulus is presented and stimulus detection is marked by an increase in responding such as renewed visual attention or cardiac decelerations.

Differences in tonic and reactive cardiac responses can also serve as markers of individual differences in physical and/or cognitive status. For example, differences in parasympathetic tone have been related to levels of infant attentiveness and reactivity (Richards, 1987). Perinatal events (e.g., physical stress and recovery from maternal medication) have been reported to temporarily block the decelerative response (Adkinson & Berg, 1976) and more enduring conditions such as malnourishment have longer-term effects on cardiac reactivity (Lester, 1975). Thus, cardiovascular responses can serve as a means or apparatus for the study of development within particular domains of psychology including cognitive, sensory, and perceptual development, and in addition, as a means of assessing individual differences in the neurally mediated capacity to respond within these domains.

In order to serve as a marker of enduring individual differences, as opposed to simply differences in state, cardiac measures must show stability over time and over shifts in development and maturation (Porges, Doussard-Roosevelt, Portales, & Suess, 1994). Individual differences in cardiovascular measures including heart period and heart rate variability show little stability from birth until at least 3 months of age (Fracasso et al., 1994; Snidman et al., 1995; Stifter & Fox, 1990). For example Stifter and Fox (1990) found little stability from birth to 5 months of age on measures of heart period, heart rate variance and vagal tone, but moderate stability from 5 to 14 months of age. Similarly, Fracasso et al. (1994) assessed vagal tone and mean heart period during baseline and following the presentation of emotion-eliciting stimuli at four time points between 5 and 13 months of age. These measures were significantly related at all ages, with the magnitude of the correlations increasing with age. With older children, Fox and Field (1989) reported moderate stability in vagal tone and heart rate variability across a six-month period in a sample of preschool-aged children. Longer-term stabilities, from infancy into early childhood, were reported for both heart period and vagal tone by Porges et al. (1994). From 9 months until 3 years of age, heart period and vagal tone increased across the entire group, but children maintained their rankings relative to the group across the same time interval. Porges et al. (1994) further reported that the stability of heart period and vagal tone was similar in magnitude to the stability of maternal reports of temperament over the same time period. Baseline measures of RSA also show a good deal of stability in later childhood. For example, El-Sheikh (2005) recently reported a moderate level of temporal stability in baseline RSA over a two year period in children between the ages of 9 and 11 years.

Cardiovascular measures as indices of risk status

Premature neonates demonstrate different patterns of both tonic and reactive cardiovascular activity compared to full-term newborns. For example, premature infants, both those who are healthy and those who are at greater risk due to various medical complications, tend to have higher heart rates (e.g., Krafchuk, Tronick, & Clifton, 1983) and greater heart rate variability compared to full-term infants. Premature infants also demonstrate markedly different patterns of cardiovascular responding to environmental stimuli compared to full-term infants. Rose, Schmidt, and Bridger (1976) reported that sleeping preterm infants exhibited depressed cardiac responses to various tactile stimuli in comparison to full-term infants. Further, Krafchuk Tronick and Clifton (1983) found that in comparison to full-term infants, high-risk premature infants showed slower and smaller magnitude cardiac changes in response to auditory stimuli and in response to a dishabituation trial in which the head end of the infant's basinet was raised 2–3 inches and then released. Once the high risk group reacted to the stimuli, particularly the dishabituation stimulus, however, they took longer to habituate their cardiac response. This mix of hypo- and hyper-responsiveness was interpreted as reflecting the relative immaturity of the CNS. This pattern of reacting provides an infant with less control and flexibility with which to regulate his/her responses to the environment.

Global cardiac measures (i.e., heart period, heart period variability) have been used as a means for detecting gross dysfunction (i.e., severe brain damage versus all other infants) among neonates with a variety of clinical pathologies (e.g., Porges, 1983). Porges (1983) used vagal tone, thought to provide a more sensitive index of CNS functioning, to classify the same group of neonates along a continuum reflecting the severity of neuropathology. Higher vagal tone was associated with lower risk status. Higher vagal tone has also been associated with better cognitive outcomes by the end of the first year of life. For example, infants with higher vagal tone at birth had higher Bayley MDI scores at both 8 and 12 months compared to infants with lower vagal tone (Fox & Porges, 1985). Although children in the extremes of the distribution of vagal tone had consistent outcomes, there was not a perfect linear relationship. That is, not all children with low vagal tone performed poorly on the Bayley MDI. These findings raise the more general issue of how different patterns of early reactivity, as reflected in cardiovascular measures, affect, and are affected by, the nature of interactions with their surrounding environment, in particular, interactions with caregivers to promote development.

Cardiovascular measures and emotional development

In general, greater heart rate variability during the first year of life is associated with greater reactivity, both cardiovascular and behavioral, to environmental stimulation. These differences apply not only to sensory stimuli but to social stimuli which for young infants consists primarily of interactions with caregivers. Work by Fox (1989) suggests that these differences in global reactivity are associated with differences in self-regulation and the development of particular social behaviors.

In infants, differences in heart period variability have been associated with differences in facial expressivity. Specifically, 3-month-old infants with greater heart rate variability displayed longer duration interest expressions during face-to-face interactions with their mothers (Fox & Gelles, 1984). Stifter and Fox (1990) found that at five months of age, infants with greater heart rate variability displayed more negative expressions in response to an arm-restraint procedure used to elicit distress or anger in the laboratory. Stifter, Fox, and Porges (1989) further reported that 5 month olds with higher levels of heart rate variability expressed a greater number of positive emotional expressions especially in response to an approaching stranger. Thus, heart rate variability appears to be related to global reactivity or responsivity (both positive and negative) in early infancy.

Heart rate variability is also associated with infants' capacities to flexibly regulate their own reactions. Infants with greater heart rate variability at birth displayed more self-regulatory behaviors in response to an arm-restraint procedure at 5 months of age (Fox, 1989). Behaviors such as looks to mother, looks at self in the mirror, arm and leg thrusts, and vocalizations were coded as self-regulatory. Heart rate variability is likely related to self-regulatory behaviors via the common relations with infants' capacities to flexibly implement strategies for managing interactions with the environment. By the second year of life, differences in reactivity and regulation are apparent in children's behaviors in social contexts. At 14 months of age, children with high vagal tone approached an adult stranger more readily and spent less time in close proximity to mother during a laboratory visit. Vagal tone measured at 14 months of age related to the same infants' reactions and use of self-regulatory behaviors during their 5-month visit. Specifically, children with high vagal tone at 14 months of age expressed more negative affect during the 5 month visit and were more likely to have cried during the arm restraint procedure at 5 months, in comparison to children with low vagal tone.

Cardiovascular measures, as assessed during infancy, have concurrent relations to temperament and also predictive relations to temperament at later ages. For example, Porges, Doussard-Roosevelt, Portales, and Suess (1994) found that high vagal tone was related to maternal reports of difficult temperament at 9 months of age. Interestingly, while there were no concurrent relations between vagal tone and temperament ratings at the 3-year assessment, higher vagal tone as assessed at 9 months of age was predictive of maternal reports of less difficult temperament when the same children were 3 years old. Nine month vagal tone predicted 3-year temperament reports over-and-above, or independent of, the relations between 9-month and 3-year temperament reports. This apparent switch in the direction of relation between vagal tone and temperament is probably best explained by considering the influences of early temperament on infants' interactions with their environment and particularly their interactions with caregivers. High vagal tone during early infancy appears to be associated with greater global reactivity, which is likely interpreted by caregivers as "difficult." Vagal tone, however, is also related to infants' abilities to self-regulate their reactions. Thus, the capacity to self-regulate at 3 years of age is likely interpreted by caregivers as reflecting a relatively easy temperament. It may be that infants who are reactive to their environments from birth, in a sense, create more opportunities for learning how to flexibly regulate their own arousal. Reactivity likely leads to more contact with caregivers, leading to more socialization experiences surrounding issues of regulating reactivity. In contrast, less reactive infants may have fewer learning experiences surrounding issues of self-regulation. However, hypotheses regarding the ways in which reactivity, regulation, and socialization experiences interact to promote development have yet to be empirically examined.

Cardiovascular measures and the development of behavior problems in older children and adolescents

Individual differences in the tonic level of activation and in the degree of reactivity of the ANS have been related to the development of specific behavior problems. There have been mixed results relating tonic levels of autonomic activity to behavior problems. For example, in a prospective study of criminal behavior, Raine, Venables, and Williams (1990a) found that lower resting heart rate and fewer nonspecific skin conductance responses as assessed in a sample of 15-year-old boys were associated with an increased likelihood of criminal behavior at 24 years of age. These findings suggest that ANS underarousal may be associated with, and perhaps even causally, criminal behavior. This global pattern of underarousal may lead individuals to seek out stimulation, for example, by engaging in antisocial or criminal behaviors. In the studies by Raine and his colleagues, ANS underarousal has been hypothesized to be attributable to both reduced sympathetic modulation (Raine et al., 1990a, 1990b) and enhanced vagal modulation (Raine & Jones, 1987; Raine & Venables, 1984). In contrast, however, Zahn and Kruesi (1993) concluded that there were no consistent differences in tonic levels of arousal or generalized ANS activity between boys with behavior disorders and their same-aged peers. Indeed, in a recent review of studies Raine (1993) reported on the inconsistencies of the findings relating global underarousal to antisocial behaviors.

Using spectral analytic techniques, Mezzacappa et al. (1997) more directly examined the relations between adolescent boys' self-reports of antisocial behavior and autonomic regulatory influences over the heart. Mezzacappa et al. (1997) analyzed the transfer of respiratory variability to heart rate variability. This transfer can essentially be thought of as the heart rate response to quantified changes in respiration, with individual differences in the transfer dynamics implying differences in the central processing of cardiorespiratory interactions. Using this logic, the findings indicated that the central processing of respiratory-heart rate relations was disrupted in antisocial individuals, which would support the literature relating parasympathetic control to the integrity of regulatory processes (Porges, Doussard-Roosevelt, & Maiti, 1994).

In addition to tonic levels of autonomic arousal, antisocial behaviors have been related to unique patterns of autonomic reactions to various environmental stimuli. Autonomic reactivity has been related to the development of behavior problems through their common relations to orienting responses and orienting deficits. Cardiovascular reactivity can serve as an index of the orienting reflex which assesses the extent to which a subject attends to and processes an eliciting stimulus. Raine et al. (1990b) found that criminal behavior at 24 years of age was predicted by hyporeactive heart rate responses to auditory stimuli as assessed at 15 years of age. This pattern of hyporesponsivity was predictive of criminal behavior over-and-above the predictive effects of tonic heart rate, suggesting that the response deficit was not simply a function of lower overall physiological arousal, and that the deficit may be a risk factor for later criminal behavior.

Raine and his colleagues have recently expanded their work to explore patterns of psychophysiological responding which may serve to protect antisocial adolescents from continuing on to commit crimes in early adulthood. Specifically, they hypothesized that adolescents who engage in antisocial behaviors but who do not go on to commit crimes in adulthood, may have distinctly "hyper-reactive" patterns of physiological responding in comparison to both normals and those antisocial adolescents who go on to commit crimes in early adulthood (Raine, Venables, & Williams, 1995). Such a model goes against previous theories in which "adolescent-limited" antisocial individuals are seen as falling between their more resistant antisocial peers and their normal peers on a continuum of antisocial behavior. Indeed, Raine, Venables, and Williams (1995) reported that adolescent-limited antisocial individuals had higher resting heart rates and greater electrodermal orienting responses compared to their resistant antisocial peers. Raine, Venables, and Williams (1995) further reported that the adolescent-limited antisocial individuals had higher heart rates and greater electrodermal orienting responses compared to a sample of normal adolescents, however, these differences did not reach statistical significance. It is, therefore, difficult to deduce whether this pattern of greater autonomic arousal indeed reflects a unique protective mechanism against committing crime, or whether the adolescent-limited antisocial individuals simply respond autonomically like their non-antisocial peers. Regardless, the work of Raine and his colleagues, highlight the relation between both tonic and reactive patterns of autonomic responding and antisocial behaviors.

The direction of heart rate change in response to environmental stimuli has further been interpreted in the context of social information processing. Cardiac decelerations, as in work with infants, are interpreted as reflecting the active intake of information from the environment. This style of responding may serve as a marker of other-oriented-focused attention such as the experiences of empathy and sympathy. In contrast, cardiac accelerations are interpreted as reflecting the rejection of environmental inputs and may serve as a marker of a person's attempt to actively cope with personal distress or anxiety (e.g., Zahn-Waxler et al., 1995). For example, preschoolers who responded with cardiac decelerations to a videotape designed to induce sadness, were observed displaying more prosocial behavior and greater empathic concern in response to others' distress compared to children who responded with little or no cardiac deceleration. In contrast, children with lower tonic heart rates while viewing the sadness induction tape were observed demon-

strating more avoidance and joy reactions during others' distress.

In contrast to the findings linking cardiac hypo-activation to conduct problems, cardiac hyper-activation, may be related to behavior problems of an internalizing nature. Children who expressed few emotions while viewing a mood induction tape were found to have higher, more stable heart rates, lower vagal tone and to display less change in heart rate from baseline to the mood induction tape (Cole et al., 1996). This pattern of cardiovascular responding was interpreted as reflecting a resistance to external input and an increased focus on internal state. This pattern of high, stable heart rate is similar to that reported by Kagan and his colleagues relating cardiovascular measures to behavioral inhibition in children (e.g., Kagan, Reznick, & Snidman, 1987, 1988). In an examination of the changes in the frequency components of heart rate variability during cognitive challenge, Kagan, Reznick, and Snidman (1987, 1988) found that behaviorally inhibited children displayed greater shifts in the distribution of heart rate variability towards the LF band of the distribution. Kagan and colleagues interpreted this shift as reflecting an increase in sympathetic influences over the heart during the cognitive challenge. In a more direct examination of the associations between anxiety and sympathetic cardiac influences, Mezzacappa et al. (1997) used the change in LF heart rate variability with postural manipulations (supine to standing) as an indicator of sympathetic cardiac influences on heart rate. Sympathetic influences were positively correlated with adolescent boys' self-reports of anxiety.

INFERENTIAL CONTEXT: METHODOLOGICAL ISSUES IN THE PSYCHOPHYSIOLOGICAL STUDY OF INFANTS AND CHILDREN

There are obvious methodological issues involved in the recording of EEG, ERPs, or ECG in adult populations. These have been discussed in detail elsewhere, and there are published recommendations regarding standards of methods for each measure (Berntson et al., 1997; Pivik et al., 1993; Task Force, 1996). Additionally, there are unique methodological problems when using these measures with infants and young children. These include movement and muscle artifact, placement of electrodes, state changes of the infant or young child, definition of a "baseline" and the need to link physiology to behavioral response. It should be noted that these methodological issues are not specific to either EEG, ERPs, or ECG response acquisition but are common to the recording of all psychophysiological responses.

Movement and muscle artifact. Obviously, one cannot instruct infants or young children to sit still so as to record resting levels of physiology. As well, when presenting either auditory or visual stimuli it is not possible with infants or young children to issue instructions to pay attention to the stimulus or not to move. Therefore, recording of either autonomic or brain electrical activity is fraught with the possibility of confounding with unwarranted movement artifact. Researchers have attempted to design studies, which capture the young subject's attention for long enough periods of time so as to provide data for analysis. Further, developmental psychophysiologists have usually designed systems, which allow them the ability and flexibility to edit their physiological records for period of artifact. Nevertheless, the problem is a critical one for investigators wishing to study these populations. Studies, which do not report how they edited or artifact scored data or which do not report the ratio of artifact rejected to "good" data may be including points which are unwarranted.

Electrode placement. Prior to the advent of neuroimaging techniques such as MRI, the placement of electrodes was accomplished by the examination of brain geometry and topography via autopsy, and these findings were generalized to create a set of standard placement sites (Jasper, 1958). Jasper mapped what became accepted as an international set of placements of 20 electrodes over the scalp reflecting the major cortical divisions as well as the various sulci of the cortex. Unique sets of problems arise in the application of the 10–20 system for use with infants and young children. In the Jasper system, the placement of electrodes relies on a ratio of distances between anterior and posterior sites. It is unclear whether this same ratio exists across development or whether different regions of the brain mature, physically, at different rates, leading to differences in the relation between anterior to posterior growth. A number of researchers (e.g., Myslobodsky et al., 1990) have examined this problem, primarily again through autopsy, and have found that the 10–20 system does an adequate job in defining placement of electrodes across key cortical regions. With the advent of MRI, a number of studies have begun to examine the accuracy of electrode placement with respect to actual physical landmarks of cortical topography (Lagerlund et al., 1993). Overall, these studies have found that by and large the 10–20 system does a good job in defining the location of electrodes over significant cortical landmarks in adult populations. Less is known, however, about the adequacy of this system for use with infants and children. The issue of electrode placement is becoming less of a problem with the recent advent of dense arrays of EEG electrodes on some caps that include 128 and 256 sites.

State change. A third methodological issue involves the need to attend to the state of the subject, particularly when subjects are infants or young children. Again, it is not possible to issue instructions regarding level of attention to a task to these populations, nor is it always possible to time laboratory visits so that they are optimal for the level of attention that is necessary for the task. These issues are particularly salient for infants whose ability to main-

tain a particular state of attention may be fragile. Often researchers working with infants will time their assessments with the sleep wake and eating cycle of the child. Subjects are often seen prior to a feeding when they are awake and alert – or after a feeding and a sleep cycle. Aside from concern regarding the timing of the assessment, it is incumbent upon the researcher to monitor behavioral state so as to insure that the physiological responses that are recorded across subjects are done so consistently from the identical state.

Definition of a baseline. Very often psychophysiologists are interested in the change in response of a measure from a "resting baseline" to some other state, which has been elicited as a function of cognitive or affective challenge. Or, researchers are interested in individual differences in the level of resting state of a group of individuals (for measures of EEG, blood pressure, or heart rate). In all instances, the assumption underlying measurement of a resting baseline or a pre-challenge condition is that subjects are all in the same affective and cognitive state. While it is not always clear that this assumption is being met with adult populations, it is ever more difficult with infant and child populations. It is sometimes impossible to instruct subjects to remain in a particular state for a period of time. As well, state variability is great for very young infants. Researchers have met this challenge by presenting infants with certain types of stimuli which have a general appeal and create conditions of quiet attention across large groups of subjects. So, for example, Fox and colleagues present infants with a rotating bingo wheel which contains multi-colored bingo balls. This display captivates most infants' attention and EEG can be collected during these times as it remains relatively artifact free from movement. This event and the state it elicits from infants is one of focused attention, however, and is obviously different from the "resting baseline" collected in some adult studies. State control and equivalence of baseline are thus critical issues as you go up the developmental ladder.

Linking physiological responses to behavior. Monitoring behavior during the experiment leads to an additional critical methodological issue for studies with infant and young child populations. In the absence of self-report, it is necessary that infant or young child psychophysiological responses be anchored to behavior. If the researcher does not have this anchor, it will be difficult to interpret the physiological response that is being recorded. For example, in studies of infant face discrimination Nelson and his colleagues (e.g., Nelson & Collins, 1992) routinely test infants in behavioral paradigms to insure that they are able to make the types of discriminations that are being presented in the ERP study. The coordination of behavioral testing and ERP testing lends support to any interpretation these workers may have about neural processing of face discrimination. Fox (Fox, 1994; Fox & Davidson, 1986b) has argued that inference about physiological correlates of emotion response should only be made in the presence of observable behavioral measures such as facial or vocal expressions. In his work, there is a link between report of EEG activity during the expression of certain emotions and behavioral signs of these emotions. Obviously, as children develop and are able to provide self-report measures or appropriate motor responses these should be utilized in linking physiology to behavior. In general, however, physiological reactivity should be reported in infants or young children only in the presence of observable behavioral response.

Signal localization. Aside from these unique methodological issues, recording EEG and ERPs from infants and young children poses additional issues to researchers interested in the localization of these signals. These issues are, in some sense, above the very real concerns about localization that researchers have for the signals as recorded in adults. The morphological changes, which occur over development during the first years of postnatal life may influence the localization of the electrical activity emanating from the brain. These changes include myelination of certain brain areas as well as dendritic arborization (Greenough et al., 1987; Greenough & Volkmar, 1973). The little we know about neural development compounds the problem of accurate localization of source activity in the young infant. In addition, the fontenelle does not close in most infants until the second half of the first year of postnatal life. The fontenelle may in fact create an electrical "sink hole" around which there would be current flow. This might change the nature of the signals that are being transduced off the scalp. The use of today's systems and EEG caps with more dense array of electrodes to record brain electrical activity now permit current source density mapping to localize signals.

THOUGHTS ON THE STUDY OF DEVELOPMENTAL PSYCHOPHYSIOLOGY

Psychophysiology has lagged behind other branches of psychology in integrating knowledge of developmental processes into its approach to research. A survey of papers or posters presented over the past ten years at Psychophysiology conferences finds only a handful of presentations in which children are studied and fewer yet in which developmental questions are asked. Too often, when infants or children are studied, their responses are treated similarly to adult data. These populations have often been approached as if they are "little adults" and the measurements and interpretations of their responses are viewed against the background of group differences (infant, child, adult) attributed to "age." To some extent the lack of interest in developmental processes is changing within the Psychophysiological community. There is increased interest within cognitive neuroscience in the development of processes, such as memory or attention, which have been studied intensively within Psychophysiology. This renewed interest is coupled at a time with improved technology, which makes the psychophysiological study of developmental populations more accessible.

Through the integration of research in the areas of developmental psychology and psychophysiology, advances have been made in understanding the structural and functional developments of the autonomic and central nervous systems in infancy and childhood. Substantial progress has been made towards unraveling the intricate processes underlying development in these systems, and the relations these developments have to changes in cognition and behavior during childhood. The fact that children and adults differ in the organization of physiological systems, highlights the need to investigate the development of these systems in detail. As these systems become better understood, as they exist and develop in children, they contribute both conceptually and methodologically to our understanding of the development of basic psychological processes including cognition, perception, and emotion. Further, stable individual differences in the activity and reactivity of these systems provide insight into the basic processes involved in the development of both normal and problem behaviors.

REFERENCES

Adkinson, C. D., & Berg, W. K. (1976). Cardiac deceleration in newborns: Habituation, dishabituation, and offset responses. *Journal of Experimental Child Psychology, 21,* 46–60.

Akselrod, S., Gordon, D., Madwed, J. B., Snidman, N. C., Shannon, D. C., & Cohen, R. J. (1985). Hemodynamic regulation: Investigation by spectral analysis. *American Journal of Physiology, 249,* H867–H875.

Akselrod, S., Gordon, D., Ubel, R. A., Shannon, D. C., Barger, A. C., & Cohen, R. J. (1981). Power spectrum analysis of heart rate fluctuation: A quantitative probe of beat-to-beat cardiovascular control. *Science, 213,* 220–222.

Attuel, P., Leporho, M. A., Ruta, J., Lucet, V., Steinberg, C., Azancot, A., & Coumel, P. (1986). The evolution of the sinus heart rate and variability as a function of age from birth to 16 years. In E. F. Doyle (Ed.), *Pediatric cardiology: Proceedings of the second world congress 1985.* New York: Springer-Verlag.

Ax, A. F. (1953). The physiological differentiation between fear and anger in humans. *Psychosomatic Medicine, 15,* 433–442.

Barry, R. J., Clarke, A. R., & Johnstone, S. J. (2003). A review of electrophysiology in attention-deficit/hyperactivity disorder: I. Qualitative and quantitative electroencephalography. *Clinical Neurophysiology, 114,* 171–183.

Barry, R. J., Clarke, A. R., McCarthy, R., Selikowitz, M., Johnstone, S. J., & Rushby, J. A. (2004). Age and gender effects in EEG coherence: I. Developmental trends in normal children. *Clinical Neurophysiology, 115,* 2252–2258.

Barry, R. J., Clarke, A. R., McCarthy, R., & Selikowitz, M. (2005). Adjusting EEG coherence for inter-electrode distance effects: An exploration in normal children. *International Journal of Psychophysiology, 55,* 313–321.

Bell, M. A. (2002). Power changes in infant EEG frequency bands during a spatial working memory task. *Psychophysiology, 39,* 450–458.

Bell, M. A., & Fox, N. A. (1992). The relations between frontal brain electrical activity and cognitive development during infancy. *Child Development, 63*, 1142–1163.

Bell, M. A., & Fox, N. A. (1994). Brain development over the first year of life. Relations between electroencephalographic frequency and coherence and cognitive and affective behaviors. In G. Dawson & K. W. Fischer (Eds.), *Human behavior and the developing brain* (pp. 314–345). New York: Guilford Press.

Bell, M. A., & Fox, N. A. (1996). Crawling experience is related to changes in cortical organization during infancy: Evidence from EEG coherence. *Developmental Psychobiology, 29*, 551–561.

Benes, F. M., Turtle, M., Khan, Y., & Farol, P. (1994). Myelination of a key relay zone in the hippocampal formation occurs in human brain during childhood, adolescence and adulthood. *Archives of General Psychiatry, 51*, 477–484.

Berg, W. K., & Berg, K. M. (1979). Psychophysiological development in infancy: State, sensory function and attention. In J. D. Osofsky (Ed.), *Handbook of infant development* (pp. 283–343). New York: Wiley.

Berger, H. (1929). Uber das Elektrenkephalogramm des Menschen: I. *Archiv fur Psychiatri und Nervenkrankheiten, 87*, 527–570.

Berger, H. (1932a). Uber das Elektrenkephalogramm des Menschen: IV. *Archiv fur Psychiatri und Nervenkrankheiten, 97*, 6–26.

Berger, H. (1932b). Uber das Elektrenkephalogramm des Menschen: V. *Archiv fur Psychiatri und Nervenkrankheiten, 98*, 231–254.

Berntson, G. G., Bigger, J. T., Eckberg, D. L., Grossman, P., Kaufman, P. G., Malik, M., Nagaraja, H. N., Porges, S. W., Saul, J. P., Stone, P. H., & van der Molen, M. W. (1997). Heart rate variability: Origins, methods, and interpretive caveats. *Psychophysiology, 34*, 623–648.

Berntson, G. G., & Boysen, S. T. (1990). Cardiac indices of cognition in infants, children and chimpanzees. In C. Rovee-Collier & L. P. Lipsitt (Eds.), *Advances in Infancy Research* (pp. 187–220). Norwood, NJ: Albex.

Berntson, G. G., Cacioppo, J. T., & Quigley, K. S. (1993). Respiratory sinus arrhythmia: Autonomic origins, physiological mechanisms, and psychophysiological implications. *Psychophysiology, 30*, 183–196.

Best, C. T. (1993). Emergence of language-specific constraints in perception of non-native speech: A window on early phonological development. In B. de Boysson-Bardies, S. de Schonen, P. Jusczyk, P. MacNeilage, & J. Morton (Eds), *Developmental Neurocognition: Speech and face processing in the first year of life* (pp. 289–304). Boston: Kluwer Academic Publishers.

Binkley, P. F., & Boudoulas, H. (1986). Measurement of myocardial inotropy. In C. V. Leier (Ed.), *Cardiotonic drugs: A clinical survey* (pp. 5–48). New York: Marcel Dekker.

Black, L. S., deRegnier, R. A., Long, J., Georgieff, M. K., & Nelson, C. A. (2004). Electrographic imaging of recognition memory in 34–38 week gestation intrauterine growth restricted newborns. *Experimental Neurology, 190 Suppl 1*, S72–83.

Buchanan, T. W., Lutz, K., & Mirzazade, S. (2000). Recognition of emotional prosody and verbal components of spoken language: An fMRI study. *Cognitive Brain Research, 9*, 227–238.

Buss, K. A., Davidson, R. J., Kalin, N. H., & Goldsmith, H. H. (2004). Context-specific freezing and associated physiological reactivity as a dysregulated fear response. *Developmental Psychology, 40*, 583–594.

Cacioppo, J. T., Berntson, G. G., Binkley, P. F., Quigley, K. S., Uchino, B. N., & Fieldstone, A. (1994). Autonomic cardiac control. II. Basal response, noninvasive indices, and autonomic space as revealed by autonomic blockades. *Psychophysiology, 31*, 586–598.

Calkins, S. D., Fox, N. A., & Marshall, T. R. (1996). Behavioral and physiological antecedents of inhibited and uninhibited behavior. *Child Development, 67*, 523–540.

Case, R. (1992). The role of the frontal lobes in the regulation of cognitive development. Special Issue: The role of frontal lobe maturation in cognitive and social development. *Brain and Cognition, 20*, 51–73.

Chelune, G. J., Ferguson, W., Koon, R., & Dickey, T. O. (1986). Frontal lobe disinhibition in attention deficit disorder. *Child Psychiatry and Human Development, 16*, 221–234.

Cheour, M., Ceponiene, R., Lehtokoski, A., Luuk, A., Allik, J., Alho, K., et al. (1998). Development of language-specific phoneme representations in the infant brain. *Nature Neuroscience, 1*, 351–353.

Chugani, H. T., & Phelps, M. E. (1986). Maturational changes in cerebral function in infants determined by 18FDG positron emission tomography. *Science, 231*, 840–843.

Cicchetti, D. (1993). Developmental psychopathology: Reactions, reflections, projections. Special Issue: Setting a path for the coming decade: Some goals and challenges. *Developmental Review, 14*, 471–502.

Cicchetti, D., & Richters, J. E. (1993). Developmental considerations in the investigation of conduct disorder. Special Issue: Toward a developmental perspective on conduct disorder. *Development and Psychopathology, 5*, 331–344.

Coan, J. A., & Allen, J. J. (2004). Frontal EEG asymmetry as a moderator and mediator of emotion. *Biological Psychology, 67*, 7–49.

Cohn, J. F., Matias, R., Tronick, E. Z., Connell, D., & Lyons-Ruth, D. (1986). Face-to-face interactions of depressed mothers and their infants. In E. Z. Tronick & T. Field (Eds.), *Maternal depression and infant disturbance* (pp. 31–45). San Francisco: Jossey Bass.

Cohn, J. F., & Tronick, E. Z. (1989). Specificity of infants' response to mothers' affective behavior. *Journal of the American Academy of Child and Adolescent Psychiatry, 28*, 242–248.

Cole, P. M., Zahn-Waxler, C., Fox, N. A., Usher, B. A., & Welsh, J. D. (1996). Individual differences in emotion regulation and behavior problems in preschool children. *Journal of Abnormal Psychology, 105*, 518–529.

Darrow, C. W. (1929). Electrical and circulatory responses to brief sensory and ideational stimuli. *Journal of Experimental Psychology, 12*, 267–300.

Davidson, R. J. (1984a). Affect, cognition and hemispheric specialization. In C. E. Izard, J. Kagan, & R. B. Zajonc (Eds.), *Emotions, cognition and behavior* (pp. 320–365). New York: Cambridge University Press.

Davidson, R. J. (1984b). Hemispheric asymmetry and emotion. In K. R. Scherer & P. Ekman (Eds.), *Approaches to emotion* (pp. 39–57). Hillsdale, NJ: Erlbaum.

Davidson, R. J. (1992). Anterior cerebral asymmetry and the nature of emotion. *Brain and Cognition, 30*, 125–151.

Davidson, R. J. (1993). The neuropsychology of emotion and affective style. In M. Lewis & J. M. Haviland (Eds.), *Handbook of emotion* (pp. 143–154). New York: Guilford.

Davidson, R. J. (1995). Cerebral asymmetry, emotion, and affective style. In R. J. Davidson & K. Hugdahl (Eds.), *Brain asymmetry*. Cambridge, MA: MIT Press.

Davidson, R. J. (2000). Affective style, psychopathology, and resilience: Brain mechanisms and plasticity. *American Psychologist, 55*, 1196–1214.

Davidson, R. J., & Fox, N. A. (1982). Asymmetrical brain activity discriminates between positive versus negative stimuli in human infants. *Science, 218*, 1235–1237.

Davidson, R. J., & Fox, N. A. (1989). The relation between tonic EEG asymmetry and ten month old emotional response to separation. *Journal of Abnormal Psychology, 98*, 127–131.

Dawson, G. (1994). Development of emotional expression and emotion regulation in infancy: Contributions of the frontal lobe. In G. Dawson & K. W. Fischer (Eds.), *Human behavior and the developing brain* (pp. 346–379). New York, NY: The Guilford Press.

Dawson, G., Grofer Klinger, L., Panagiotides, H., Hill, D., & Spieker, S. (1992). Frontal lobe activity and affective behavior in infants of mothers with depressive symptoms. *Child Development, 63*, 725–737.

Dawson, G., Panagiotides, H., Grofer Klinger, L., & Hill, D. (1992). The role of frontal lobe functioning in the development of self-regulatory behavior in infancy. *Brain and Cognition, 20*, 152–175.

de Haan, M., & Nelson, C. A. (1997). Recognition of the mother's face by six-month-old infants: A neurobehavioral study. *Child Development, 68*, 187–210.

de Haan, M., Johnson, M. H., & Halit, H. (2003). Development of face-sensitive event-related potentials during infancy: A review. *International Journal of Psychophysiology, 51*, 45–58.

Dennis, M. (1991). Frontal lobe function in childhood and adolescence: A heuristic for assessing attention regulation, executive control, and the intentional states important for social discourse. *Developmental Neuropsychology, 7*, 327–358.

Diamond, A., & Goldman-Rakic, P. S. (1983). Comparison of performance on a Piagetian object permanence task in human infants and rhesus monkeys: Evidence for involvement of prefrontal cortex. *Society for Neuroscience Abstracts, 9*, 641.

Diamond, A., & Goldman-Rakic, P. S. (1986). Comparative development in human infants and infant rhesus monkeys of cognitive functions that depend on prefrontal cortex. *Society for Neuroscience Abstracts, 12*, 742.

Diamond, A., & Goldman-Rakic, P. S. (1989). Comparison of human infants and rhesus monkeys on Piaget's AB task: Evidence for dependence on dorsolateral prefrontal cortex. *Experimental Brain Research, 74*, 24–40.

Diamond, A., Prevor, M. B., Callender, G., & Druin, D. P. (1997). Prefrontal cortex cognitive deficits in children treated early and continuously for PKU. *Monographs of the Society for Research in Child Development, 62* (4, Serial No. 252).

Diamond, A., Zola-Morgan, S., & Squire, L. R. (1989). Successful performance by monkeys with lesions of the hippocampal formation on A-not-B and object retrieval, two tasks that mark developmental changes in human infants. *Behavioral Neuroscience, 103*, 526–537.

Dreyfus-Brisac, C., & Monod, N. (1975). The electroencephalogram of full term newborns and premature infants. In G. C. Lairy (Ed.), *Handbook of electroencephalography and clinical neurophysiology: Volume 6. The normal EEG throughout life* (pp. 6B-6–6B-30). Amsterdam. Elsevier.

Duffy, F. H., Als, H., & McAnulty, G. B. (1990). Behavioral and electrophysiological evidence for gestational age effects in healthy preterm and fullterm infants studied two weeks after expected due date. *Child Development, 61*, 1271–1286.

Edelman, G. M. (1987). *Neural Darwinism: The theory of neuronal group selection*. New York: Basic Books.

El-Sheikh, M. (2005). Stability of respiratory sinus arrhythmia in children and young adolescents: A longitudinal examination. *Developmental Psychobiology, 46*, 66–74.

Emde, R. N., & Walker, S. (1976). Longitudinal study of infant sleep: Results of 14 subjects studied at monthly intervals. *Psychophysiology, 13*, 456–461.

Eppinger, H. & Hess, L. (1915). *Vagotonia: a clinical study in vegetative neurology* [translated by Karua, W. M. and Jellife, S. E.]. New York: The Nervous and Mental Disease Publishing Company.

Fernald, A. (1993). Approval and disapproval: Infant responsiveness to vocal affect in familiar and unfamiliar languages. *Child Development, 64*, 674.

Field, T. (1986). Models for reactive and chronic depression in infancy. In E. Z. Tronick & T. Field (Eds.), *Maternal depression and infant disturbance* (pp. 47–60). San Francisco: Jossey-Bass.

Field, T. M. (1979). Visual and cardiac responses to animate and inanimate faces by young term and preterm infants. *Child Development, 50*, 188–194.

Field, T., Fox, N. A., Pickens, J., & Nawrocki, T. (1995). Relative right frontal EEG activation in 3- to 6-month-old infants of "depressed" mothers. *Developmental Psychology, 31*, 358–363.

Field, T., Healy, B., Goldstein, S., Perry, S., Bendall, D., Schanberg, S., Zimmerman, E., & Kuhn, C. (1988). Infants of depressed mothers show "depressed" behavior even with nondepressed adults. *Child Development, 59*, 1569–1579.

Field, T., Sandberg, D., Garcia, R., Vega-Lahr, N., Goldstein, S., & Guy, L. (1985). Prenatal problems, postpartum depression, and early mother-infant interaction, *Developmental Psychology, 12*, 1152–1156.

Fischer, K. W. (1980). A theory of cognitive development: The control and construction of hierarchies of skills. *Psychological Review, 87*, 477–531.

Fischer, K. W. (1983). Developmental levels as periods of discontinuity. *New Directions for Child Development, 21*, 5–20.

Fischer, K. W. (1987). Relations between brain and cognitive development. *Child Development, 58*, 623–632.

Fischer, K. W., & Rose, S. P. (1994). Dynamic development of coordination of components in brain and behavior: A framework for theory and research. In G. Dawson & K. W. Fischer (Eds.), *Human behavior and the developing brain* (pp. 3–66). New York: The Guilford Press.

Fox, N. A. (1989). Heart-rate variability and behavioral reactivity: Individual differences in autonomic patterning and their relation to infant and child temperament. In J. S. Reznick (Ed.), *Perspectives on behavioral inhibition*. Chicago: University of Chicago Press.

Fox, N. A. (1991). If it's not left, it's right: Electroencephalogram asymmetry and the development of emotion. *American Psychologist, 46*, 863–872.

Fox, N. A. (1994). Dynamic cerebral processes underlying emotion regulation. In N. A. Fox (Ed.), The development of emotion regulation: Behavioral and biological considerations. *Monographs of the Society for Research in Child Development* (pp. 152–166), *59* (2–3, Serial No. 240).

Fox, N. A., & Bell, M. A. (1990). Electrophysiological indices of frontal lobe development: Relations to cognitive and affective behavior in human infants over the first year of life. In A. Diamond (Ed.), The development and neural bases of higher cognitive functions. *Annals of the New York Academy of Sciences, 608*, 677–698.

Fox, N. A., & Davidson, R. J. (1984). Hemispheric substrates of affect: A developmental model. In N. A. Fox & R. J. Davidson (Eds.), *The Psychobiology of Affective Development* (pp. 353–382). Hillside, N.J: Erlbaum Press.

Fox, N. A., & Davidson, R. J. (1986a). Taste-elicited changes in facial signs of emotion and the asymmetry of brain electrical activity in human newborns. *Neuropsychologia, 24*, 417–422.

Fox, N. A., & Davidson, R. J. (1986b). Psychophysiological measures of emotion: New directions in developmental research. In C. E. Izard & P. Read (Eds.), *Measuring emotions in infants and children* Vol. II (pp. 13–47). New York: Cambridge University Press.

Fox, N. A., & Davidson, R. J. (1988). Patterns of brain electrical activity during the expression of discrete emotions in ten month old infants. *Developmental Psychology, 24*, 230–236.

Fox, N. A., & Field, T. (1989). Young children's responses to entry into preschool: Psychophysiological and behavioral findings. *Journal of Applied Developmental Psychology, 10*, 527–540.

Fox, N. A., & Gelles, M. (1984). Face-to-face interaction in term and preterm infants. *Infant Mental Health Journal, 5*, 192–205.

Fox, N. A., Bell, M. A., & Jones, N. A. (1992). Individual differences in response to stress and cerebral asymmetry. *Developmental Neuropsychology, 8*, 161–184.

Fox, N. A., Calkins, S. D., & Bell, M. A. (1994). Neural plasticity and development in the first two years of life: Evidence from cognitive and socioemotional domains of research. *Development and Psychopathology, 6*, 677–696.

Fox, N. A., & Davidson, R. J. (1987). EEG asymmetry in ten month old infants in response to approach of a stranger and maternal separation. *Developmental Psychology, 23*, 233–240.

Fox, N. A., Henderson, H. A., Rubin, K. H., Calkins, S. D., & Schmidt, L. A. (2001). Continuity and discontinuity of behavioral inhibition and exuberance: Psychophysiological and behavioral influences across the first four years of life. *Child Development, 72*, 1–21.

Fox, N. A., Nichols, K. E., Henderson, H. A., Rubin, K. H., Schmidt, L. A., Hamer, D. H., Ernst, M., & Pine, D. S. (2005). Evidence for a gene environment interaction in predicting behavioral inhibition in middle childhood. *Psychological Science, 16*, 921–926

Fox, N. A., & Porges, S. W. (1985). The relation between neonatal heart period patterns and developmental outcome. *Child Development, 56*, 28–37.

Fox, N. A., Rubin, K. H., Calkins, S. D., Marshall, T. R., Coplan, R. J., Porges, S. W., Long, J. M., & Stewart, S. (1995). Frontal activation asymmetry and social competence at four years of age. *Child Development, 66*, 1770–1784.

Fox, N. A., Schmidt, L. A., Calkins, S. D., Rubin, K. H., Coplan, R. J. (1996). The role of frontal activation in the regulation and dysregulation of social behavior during the preschool years. *Development and Psychopathology, 8*, 89–102.

Fracasso, M. P., Porges, S. W., Lamb, M. E., & Rosenberg, A. A. (1994). Cardiac activity in infancy: Reliability and stability of individual differences. *Infant Behavior and Development, 17*, 277–284.

Gainotti, G., Caltagirone, C., & Zoccolotti, P. (1993). Left/right and cortical/subcortical dichotomies in the neuropsychological study of human emotions. *Cognition and Emotion, 7*, 71–93.

Galkina, N. S., & Boravova, A. I. (1996). Formation of electroencephalographic mu- and alpha-rhythms in children during the second to third years of life. *Human Physiology, 22*, 540–545.

Gastaut, H., Dongier, M., & Courtois, G. (1954). On the significance of "wicket rhythms" in psychosomatic medicine. *Electroencephalography and Clinical Neurophysiology, 6*, 687.

Gauthier, I., & Nelson, C. A. (2001). The development of face expertise. *Current Opinion in Neurobiology, 11*, 219–224.

Gilles, F. H., Shankle, W., & Dooling, E. C. (1983). Myelinated tracts: Growth patterns. In F. H. Gilles, A. Leviton, & E. C. Dooling (Eds.), *The developing human brain: Growth and epidemiologic neuropathology* (pp. 117–183). Boston: John Wright-PSG.

Goldman-Rakic, P. S. (1987a). Development of cortical circuitry and cognitive function. *Child Development, 58*, 601–622.

Goldman-Rakic, P. S. (1987b). Circuitry of the prefrontal cortex and the regulation of behavior by representational knowledge. In F. Plum & V. Mountcastle (Eds.), *Handbook of physiology, Volume 5* (pp. 373–417). Bethesda, MD: American Physiological Society.

Goldman-Rakic, P. S., Isseroff, A., Schwartz, M., & Bugbee, N. (1983). The neurobiology of cognitive development. In M. M. Haith & J. J. Campos (Eds.), *Handbook of child psychology: Vol. II. Infancy and developmental Psychobiology* (pp. 281–344). New York: Wiley.

Gottlieb, G. (1976). The role of experience in the development of behavior and the nervous system. In G. Gottlieb (Ed.), *Neural and behavioral specificity, studies on the development of behavior and the nervous system Vol. 3.* New York: Academic Press.

Graham, F. K., & Clifton, R. K. (1966). Heart-rate changes as a component of the orienting response. *Psychological Bulletin, 65*, 305–320.

Greenough, W. T., & Black, J. E. (1992). Induction of brain structure by experience: Substrates for cognitive development. In M. R. Gunnar & C. A. Nelson (Eds.), *Minnesota Symposia on Child Psychology: Vol. 24. Developmental behavioral neuroscience* (pp. 155–200). Hillsdale, NJ: Erlbaum.

Greenough, W. T., Black, J., & Wallace, C. (1987). Effects of experience on brain development. *Child Development, 58*, 540–559.

Greenough, W. T., & Volkmar, F. R. (1973). Pattern of dendritic branching in the occipital cortex of rats reared in complex environments. *Experimental Neurology, 40*, 491–504.

Groome, L. J., Swiber, M. J., Atterbury, J. L., Bentz, L. S., & Holland, S. B. (1997). Similarities and differences in behavioral state organization during sleep periods in the perinatal infant before and after birth. *Child Development, 68*, 1–11.

Hagne, I. (1968). Development of the waking EEG in normal infants during the first year of life. In P. Kellaway & I. Petersén (Eds.), *Clinical electroencephalography of children* (pp. 97–118). New York: Grune & Stratton.

Hagne, I. (1972). Development of the EEG in normal infants during the first year of life. *Acta Pediatrica Scandinavica, (Suppl. 232)*, 25–32.

Hagne, I., Persson, J., Magnusson, R., & Petersen, I. (1973). Spectral analysis via fast Fourier transform of waking EEG in normal infants. In P. Kellaway & I. Petersén (Eds.), *Automation of clinical EEG* (pp. 103–143). New York: Raven Press.

Harmony, T., Alvarez, A., Pascual, R., Ramos, A., Marosi, E., Diaz de Leon, A. E., et al. (1988). EEG maturation on children with different economic and psychosocial characteristics. *International Journal of Neuroscience, 41*, 103–113.

Hassett, J., & Danforth, D. (1982). An introduction to the cardiovascular system. In J. T. Cacioppo & R. E. Petty (Eds.), *Perspectives in cardiovascular psychophysiology*. New York:Guilford.

Heller, W. (1993). Neuropsychological mechanisms of individual differences in emotion, personality, and arousal. *Neuropsychology, 7*, 476–489.

Henderson, H. A. (2004). *The interaction of reactivity and regulation in predicting monitoring: Effects of temperament*. Unpublished Doctoral dissertation, University of Maryland, College Park.

Henderson, H. A., Fox, N. A. & Rubin, K. H. (2001). Temperamental contributions to social behavior: The moderating roles of frontal EEG asymmetry and gender. *Journal of the American Academy of Child and Adolescent Psychiatry, 40*, 68–74.

Henderson, H. A., Marshall, P. J., Fox, N. A., & Rubin, K. H. (2004). Psychophysiological and behavioral evidence for varying forms and functions of nonsocial behavior in preschoolers. *Child Development, 75*, 251–263.

Henriques, J. B., & Davidson, R. J. (1990). Regional brain electrical asymmetries discriminate between previously depressed subjects and healthy controls. *Journal of Abnormal Psychology, 99*, 22–31.

Henriques, J. B., & Davidson, R. J. (1991). Left frontal hypoactivation in depression. *Journal of Abnormal Psychology, 100*, 535–545.

Henry, J. R. (1944). Electroencephalograms of normal children. *Monographs of the Society for Research in Child Development, 9* (3, Serial No. 39).

Hirsch, J. A., & Bishop, B. (1981). Respiratory sinus arrhythmia in humans: How breathing pattern modulates heart rate. *American Journal of Physiology, 241*, H620–H629.

Hirshfeld, D. R., Rosenbaum, J. F., Biederman, J., Bolduc, E. A., Faraone, S. V., Snidman, N., Reznick, J. S., & Kagan, J. (1992). Stable behavioral inhibition and its association with anxiety disorder. *Journal of the American Academy of Child and Adolescent Psychiatry, 31*, 103–111.

Hodgson-Minnie, L. D., Schmidt, L. A., Trainor, L. J., Santesso, D. L., & Sonnadara, R. (2006). *Frontal brain electrical activity (EEG) and heart rate responses to children's musical emotions in 9-month-old infants*. Manuscript in preparation.

Howard, L., & Polich, J. (1985). P300 latency and memory span development. *Developmental Psychology, 21*, 283–289.

Hubel, D. H., & Wiesel, T. N. (1970). The period of susceptibility to the physiological effects of unilateral eye closure in kittens. *Journal of Physiology (London), 206*, 419–436.

Huttenlocher, P. R. (1979). Synaptic density in human frontal cortex: Developmental changes and effects of aging. *Brain Research, 163*, 195–205.

Huttenlocher, P. R. (1984). Synapse elimination and plasticity in developing human cerebral cortex. *American Journal of Mental Deficiency, 88*, 488–496.

Huttenlocher, P. R., & de Courten, C. (1987). The development of synapses in striate cortex of man. *Human Neurobiology, 6*, 1–9.

Huttenlocher, P. R., de Courten, C., Garey, L. J., & Van der Loos, H. (1982). Synaptogenesis in human visual cortex: Evidence for synapse elimination during normal development. *Neuroscience Letters, 33*, 247–252.

Jasper, H. H. (1958). The ten-twenty electrode system of the International Federation. *Electroencephalography and Clinical Neurophysiology, 10*, 371–375.

Jetha, M. K., Schmidt, L. A., & Goldberg, J. O. (2005). Resting frontal brain activation asymmetry and shyness and sociability in schizophrenia [Abstract]. *Schizophrenia Bulletin, 31*(2), 455.

John, E. R. (1977). *Functional neuroscience: vol. 2. Neurometrics*. Hillsdale, NJ: Erlbaum.

Jones, N. A., & Fox, N. A. (1992). Electroencephalogram asymmetry during emotionally evocative films and its relation to positive and negative affectivity. *Brain and Cognition, 20*, 280–299.

Kagan, J., Reznick, J. S., & Snidman, N. (1987). The physiology and psychology of behavioral inhibition. *Child Development, 58*, 1459–1473.

Kagan, J., Reznick, J. S., & Snidman, N. (1988). Biological bases of childhood shyness. *Science, 240*, 167–171.

Kagan, J., & Snidman, N. (1991). Infant predictors of inhibited and uninhibited profiles. *Psychological Science, 2*, 40–44.

Kapp, B. S., Supple, W. F., & Whalen, P. J. (1994). Stimulation of the amygdaloid central nucleus produces EEG arousal. *Behavioral Neuroscience, 108*, 81–93.

Katona, P. G., & Jih, F. (1975). Respiratory sinus arrhythmia: A noninvasive measure of parasympathetic cardiac control. *Journal of Applied Physiology, 39*, 801–805.

Krafchuk, E. E., Tronick, E. Z., & Clifton, R. K. (1983). Behavioral and cardiac responses to sound in preterm neonates varying in risk status: A hypothesis of their paradoxical reactivity. In T. M. Field & A. Sostek (Eds.), *Infants born at risk: Physiological and perceptual processes* (pp. 99–128). New York: Grune & Stratton.

Kuhlman, W. N. (1978). Functional topography of the human mu rhythm. *Electroencephalography and Clinical Neurophysiology, 44*, 83–93.

Lacey, J. I. (1967). Somatic response patterning and stress: Some revisions of activation theory. In M. H. Apley & R. Trumbull (Eds.), *Psychological stress*. New York: Appleton-Century-Crofts.

Lagerlund, T. D., Sharbrough, F. W., Rack, C. R., Erickson, B., Strelow, D. C., Cicora, K. M., & Busacker, N. E. (1993). Determination of 10–20 system electrode locations using magnetic resonance image scanning with markers. *Electroencephalography and Clinical Neurophysiology, 86*, 7–14.

Lahmeyer, H. W., Reynolds, C. F., Kupfer, D. J., King, R. (1989). Biologic markers in borderline personality disorder: A review. *Journal of Clinical Psychiatry, 50*, 217–225.

Lenneberg, E. (1967). *Biological foundations of language*. New York: Wiley.

Leppanen, P. H., Guttorm, T. K., Pihko, E., Takkinen, S., Eklund, K. M., & Lyytinen, H. (2004). Maturational effects on newborn ERPs measured in the mismatch negativity paradigm. *Experimental Neurology, 190 Suppl 1*, S91–101.

Lester, B. M. (1975). Cardiac habituation of the orienting response to an auditory signal in infants of varying nutritional status. *Developmental Psychology, 11*, 432–442.

Lewis, M., Kagan, J., Campbell, H., & Kalafat, J. (1966). The cardiac response as a correlate of attention in infants. *Child Development, 37*, 63–71.

Lewis, M., & Stieben, J. (2004). Emotion regulation in the brain: Conceptual issues and directions for developmental research. *Child Development, 75*, 371–376.

Lewis, M., Wilson, C. D., Ban, P., & Baumel, M. H. (1970). An exploratory study of resting cardiac rate and variability from the trimester of prenatal life through the first year of postnatal life. *Child Development, 41*, 799–812.

Lindsley, D. B. (1939). A longitudinal study of the occipital alpha rhythm in normal children: Frequency and amplitude standards. *Journal of Genetic Psychology, 55*, 197–213.

Malliani, A., Pagani, M., & Lombardi, F. (1994). Physiology and clinical implications of variability of cardiovascular parameters with focus on heart rate and blood pressure. *American Journal of Cardiology, 73*, 3C–9C.

Marshall, P. J., Bar-Haim, Y., & Fox, N. A. (2002). Development of the EEG from 5 months to 4 years of age. *Clinical Neurophysiology, 113*, 1199–1208.

Marshall, P. J., Fox, N. A., & the BEIP Core Group (2004). A comparison of the electroencephalogram (EEG) between institutionalized and community children in Romania. *Journal of Cognitive Neuroscience, 16*, 1327–1338.

Masataka, N. (1999). Preference for infant-directed singing in 2-day-old hearing infants of deaf parents. *Developmental Psychology, 35*, 1001–1005.

Matousek, M., & Petersén, I. (1973). Frequency analysis of the EEG in normal children and adolescents. In P. Kellaway & I. Petersén (Eds.), *Automation of clinical electroencephalography* (pp. 75–102). New York: Raven Press.

Maurer, D. (2005). Introduction to the Special Issue on Critical Periods Rexamined: Evidence from human sensory development. *Developmental Psychobiology, 46*, 155–292.

McCall, R. B., & Kagan, J. (1967). Attention in the infant: Effects of complexity, contour, perimeter, and familiarity. *Child Development, 38*, 939–952.

Mezzacappa, E., Kindlon, D., Earls, F., & Saul, J. P. (1994). The utility of spectral analytic techniques in the study of the autonomic regulation of beat-to-beat heart rate variability. *International Journal of Methods in Psychiatric Research, 4*, 29–44.

Mezzacappa, E., Tremblay, R. E., Kindlon, D., Saul, J. P., Arseneault, L., Seguin, J., Pihl, R. O., & Earls, F. (1997). Anxiety, antisocial behavior, and heart rate regulation in adolescent males. *Journal of Child Psychology and Psychiatry, 38*, 457–469.

Miller, A., Fox, N. A., Cohn, J. F., Forbes, E. E., Sherrill, J. T., & Kovacs, M. (2002). Regional patterns of brain activity in adults with a history of childhood-onset depression: Gender differences and clinical variability. *American Journal of Psychiatry, 159*, 934–940.

Miller, B. L., & Lesser, I. M. (1988). Late-life psychosis and modern neuroimaging. *Psychiatric Clinics of North America, 11*, 33–46.

Mills, D. L., Coffey-Corina, S. A., & Neville, H. J. (1994). Variability in cerebral organization during primary language acquisition. In G. Dawson & K. Fischer (Eds.), *Human behavior and the developing brain* (pp. 427–455). New York: The Guilford Press.

Mizuno, T., Yamauchi, N., Watanabe, A., Komatsushiro, M., Takagi, T., Iinuma, K., & Arakawa, T. (1970). Maturation of patterns of EEG: Basic waves of healthy infants under 12 months of age. *Tahoka Journal of Experimental Matachewan*, 91–98.

Moffit, T. E., & Henry, B. (1989). Neuropsychological assessment of executive functions in self-reported delinquents. *Development and Psychopathology, 1*, 105–118.

Muthukumaraswamy, S. D., & Johnson, B. W. (2004). Changes in rolandic mu rhythm during observation of a precision grip. *Psychophysiology, 41*, 152–156.

Myslobodsky, M. S., Coppola, R., Bar-Ziv, J., & Weinberger, D. R. (1990). Adequacy of the international 10–20 electrode system for computed neurophysiologic topography. *Journal of Clinical Neurophysiology, 7*, 507–518.

Nelson, C. A. (1994). Neural correlates of recognition memory in the first postnatal year. In G. Dawson and K. W. Fischer (Eds.), *Human behavior and the developing brain* (pp. 269–313). New York: The Guilford Press.

Nelson, C. A., & Collins, P. F. (1991). Event-related potential and looking time analysis of infants' responses to familiar and novel events: Implications for visual recognition memory. *Developmental Psychology, 27*, 50–58.

Nelson, C. A., & Collins, P. F. (1992). Neural and behavioral correlates of visual recognition memory in 3- and 8-month-old infants. *Brain and Cognition, 19*, 105–121.

Nelson, C. A., & Collins, P. F. (1992). Neural and behavioral correlates of visual recognition memory in 4- and 8-month-old infants. *Brain and Cognition, 19*, 105–121.

Nelson, C. A., & Monk, C. (2001). The use of event-related potentials in the study of cognitive development. In C. A. Nelson & M. Luciana (Eds.), *Handbook of Developmental Cognitive Neuroscience* (pp. 125–136). Cambridge, MA: MIT Press.

Neville, H. J., Kutas, M., & Schmidt, A. (1982a). Event-related potential studies of cerebral specialization during reading: II. Studies of congenitally deaf adults. *Brain and Cognition, 16*, 316–337.

Neville, H. J., Kutas, M., & Schmidt, A. (1982b). Event-related potential studies of cerebral specialization during reading: I. Studies of normal adults. *Brain and Cognition, 16*, 300–315.

Niznikiewicz, M. A., O'Donnell, B. F., Nestor, P. G., Smith, L., Law, S., Karapelou, M., Shenton, M. E., & McCarley, R. W. (1997). ERP assessment of visual and auditory language processing in schizophrenia. *Journal of Abnormal Psychology, 106*, 85–94.

Nunez, P. (1981). *Electric fields of the brain*. New York: Oxford University Press.

Orekhova, E. V., Stroganova, T. A., & Posikera, I. N. (2001). Alpha activity as an index of cortical inhibition during sustained internally controlled attention in infants. *Clinical Neurophysiology, 112*, 740–749.

Parker, S. W., Nelson, C. A., & the BEIP Core Group (2005). The impact of early institutional rearing on the ability to discriminate facial expressions of emotion: An event-related potential study. *Child Development, 76*, 54–72.

Petitto, L. A. (1993). On the ontogenetic requirements for early language acquisition. In: de Boysson-Bardies, S. Schonen, P. Jusczyk, P. F. MacNeilage, & J. Morton (Eds.), *Developmental neurocognition: Speech and face processing in the first year of life*. NATO ASI series D: Behavioral and social sciences, Vol. 69 (pp. 365–383). Dordrecht, Netherlands: Kluwer Academic Publishers.

Pihan, H., Altenmuller, E., & Ackermann, H. (1997). The cortical processing of perceived emotion: A DC-potential study on affective speech prosody. *Neuroreport: An Internaltional Journal for the Rapid Communication of Research in Neuroscience, 8*, 623–627.

Pivik, R. T., Broughton, R. J., Coppola, R., Davidson, R. J., Fox, N., & Nuwer, M. R. (1993). Guidelines for the recording and quantitative analysis of electroencephalographic activity in research contexts. *Psychophysiology, 30*, 547–558.

Pollock, V. E., & Schneider, L. S. (1990). Quantitative, waking EEG research on depression. *Biological Psychiatry, 27*, 757–780.

Porges, S. W. (1992). Vagal tone: A physiologic marker of stress vulnerability. *Pediatrics, 90*, 498–504.

Porges, S. W. (1983). Heart rate patterns in neonates: A potential diagnostic window to the brain. In T. Field & A. Sostek

(Eds.), *Infants born at risk: Physiological and perceptual processes* (pp. 3–22). New York: Grune & Stratton.

Porges, S. W. (1986). Respiratory sinus arrythmia: Physiological basis, quantitative methods, and clinical implications. In P. Grossman, K. Jansen, & D. Vail (Eds.), *Cardiac respiratory and somatic psychophysiology* (pp. 223–264). New York: Guilford.

Porges, S. W., Doussard-Roosevelt, J. A., & Maiti, A. K. (1994). Vagal tone and the physiological regulation of emotion. In N. A. Fox (Ed.), *The development of emotion regulation: Biological and behavioral considerations* (pp. 167–188). *Monographs of the Society for Research in Child Development, 59* (2–3, Serial No. 240).

Porges, S. W., Doussard-Roosevelt, J. A., Portales, A. L., & Suess, P. E. (1994). Cardiac vagal tone: Stability and relation to difficulties in infants and 3-year-olds. *Developmental Psychobiology, 27,* 289–300.

Porges, S. W., McCabe, P. M., & Yongue, B. G. (1982). Respiratory-heart rate interactions: Physiological implications for pathophysiology and behavior. In J. Cacioppo & R. Petty (Eds.), *Perspectives in cardiovascular psychophysiology* (pp. 223–264). New York: Guilford.

Pribram, K. H. (1973). The primate frontal cortex: Executive of the brain. In K. H. Pribram, & A. R. Luria (Eds.), *Psychophysiology of the frontal lobes.*

Pritchard, W. S. (1986). Cognitive event-related potential correlates of schizophrenia. *Psychological Bulletin, 100,* 43–66.

Raine, A. (1993). *The psychopathology of crime: Criminal behavior as a clinical disorder.* San Diego, Academic Press.

Raine, A., & Jones, F. (1987). Attention, autonomic arousal, and personality in behaviorally disordered children. *Journal of Abnormal Child Psychology, 15,* 583–599.

Raine, A., & Venables, P. H. (1984). Tonic heart rate level, social class, and antisocial behavior in adolescents. *Biological Psychology, 18,* 123–132.

Raine, A., & Venables, P. H. (1987). Contingent negative variation, P3 evoked potentials, and antisocial behavior. *Psychophysiology, 24,* 191–199.

Raine, A., Venables, P. H., & Williams, M. (1990a). Relationships between central and autonomic measures of arousal at age 15 years and criminality at age 24 years. *Archives of General Psychiatry, 47,* 1003–1007.

Raine, A., & Venables, P. H., & Williams, M. (1990b). Autonomic orienting responses in 15-year-old male subjects and criminal behavior at age 24. *American Journal of Psychiatry, 147,* 933–937.

Raine, A., Venables, P. H., & Williams, M. (1995). High autonomic arousal and electrodermal orienting at age 15 years as protective factors against criminal behavior at age 29 years. *American Journal of Psychiatry, 152,* 1595–1600.

Reynolds, G. D., & Richards, J. E. (in press). Familiarization, attention, and recognition memory in infancy: an ERP and cortical source localization study. *Developmental Psychology.*

Richards, J. E. (1985). The development of sustained visual attention in infants from 14 to 26 weeks of age. *Psychophysiology, 22,* 409–416.

Richards, J. E. (1987). Infant visual sustained attention and respiratory sinus arrhythmia. *Child Development, 58,* 488–496.

Richards, J. E. (1989). Development and stability in visual sustained attention in 14, 20, and 26 week old infants. *Psychophysiology, 26,* 422–430.

Rivera-Gaxiola, M., Silva-Pereyra, J., & Kuhl, P. K. (2005). Brain potentials to native and non-native speech contrasts in 7- and 11-month-old American infants. *Developmental Science, 8,* 162–172.

Rock, A. M. L., Trainor, L. J., & Addison, T. L. (1999). Distinctive messages in infant-directed lullabies and play songs. *Developmental Psychology, 35,* 527–534.

Rose, S., Schmidt, K., & Bridger, W. H. (1976). Cardiac and behavioral responsivity to tactile stimulation in premature and full-term infants. *Developmental Psychology, 12,* 311–320.

Rubin, K. H., Stewart, S. L., & Coplan, R. J. (1995). Social withdrawal in childhood: Conceptual and empirical perspectives. In T. Ollendick & R. Prinz (Eds.), *Advances in Clinical Child Psychology* (Vol. 17, pp. 157–196). New York: Plenum Press.

Sameroff, A. J., Cashmore, T. F., & Dykes, A. C. (1973). Heart tare decelerations during visual fixation in human newborns. *Developmental Psychology, 8,* 117–199.

Santesso, D. L., Reker, D. L., Schmidt, L. A., & Segalowitz, S. J. (2006a). Frontal electroencephalogram activation asymmetry, emotional intelligence, and externalizing behaviors in 10-year-old children. *Child Psychiatry and Human Development, 36,* 311–328.

Santesso, D. L., Schmidt, L. A., & Trainor, L. J. (2006b). *Frontal brain electrical activity (EEG) and heart rate responses to affective infant-directed (ID) speech in 9-month-old infants.* Manuscript in preparation.

Santesso, D. L., Segalowitz, S. J., & Schmidt, L. A. (2005). ERP correlates of error monitoring in 10-year-old children are related to socialization. *Biological Psychology, 70,* 79–87.

Santesso, D. L., Segalowitz, S. J., & Schmidt, L. A. (2006c). Error-related electrocortical responses are enhanced in children with obsessive-compulsive behaviors. *Developmental Neuropsychology, 29,* 431–445.

Santesso, D. L., Segalowitz, S. J., & Schmidt, L. A. (2006d) Error-related electrocortical responses in 10-year-old children and young adults. *Developmental Science.*

Satterfield, J. H., Cantwell, D. P., & Satterfield, B. T. (1974). Pathophysiology of the hyperactive child syndrome. *Archives of General Psychiatry, 31,* 839–844.

Schacter, D. L., Kagan, J., & Leichtman, M. (1995). True and false memories in children and adults: A cognitive neuroscience perspective. *Psychology, Public Policy and Law, 2,* 411–428.

Schaffer, C. E., Davidson, R. J., & Saron, C. (1983). Frontal and parietal electroencephalogram asymmetry in depressed and nondepressed subjects. *Biological Psychiatry, 18,* 753–762.

Scherer, K. R., & Zentner, M. R. (2001). Emotional effects of music: Production rules. In P. N. Juslin & J. A. Sloboda (Eds.), *Music and Emotion: Theory and Research* (pp. 361–392). New York: Oxford University Press.

Schmidt, L. A.(1996). *The psychophysiology of self-presentation anxiety in seven-year-old children: A multiple measure approach.* Unpublished Doctoral Dissertation, University of Maryland, College Park, MD.

Schmidt, L. A. (1999). Frontal brain electrical activity in shyness and sociability. *Psychological Science, 10,* 316–320.

Schmidt, L. A. (2006). *Psychometric properties of resting frontal brain electrical activity (EEG) and their relation to temperament in 9-month-old human infants.* Manuscript in preparation.

Schmidt, L. A., Cote, K. A., Santesso, D. L., & Milner, C. E. (2003). Frontal electroencephalogram (EEG) alpha asymmetry during sleep: Stability and its relation to affective style. *Emotion, 3,* 401–407.

Schmidt, L. A., & Fox, N. A. (1994). Patterns of cortical electrophysiology and autonomic activity in adults' shyness and sociability. *Biological Psychology, 38*, 183–198.

Schmidt, L. A., Fox, N. A., Schulkin, J., & Gold, P. W. (1999). Behavioral and psychophysiological correlates of self-presentation in temperamentally shy children. *Developmental Psychobiology, 35*, 119–135.

Schmidt, L. A., Polak, C. P., & Spooner, A. L. (2005). Biological and environmental contributions to childhood shyness: A diathesis-stress model. In W. R. Crozier & L. E. Alden (Eds.), *The Essential Handbook of Social Anxiety for Clinicians* (pp. 33–55). United Kingdom: John Wiley & Sons.

Schmidt, L. A., Trainor, L. J., & Santesso, D. L. (2003). Development of frontal electroencephalogram (EEG) and heart rate (ECG) responses to affective musical stimuli during the first 12 months of post-natal life. [Special Issue on Affective Neuroscience], *Brain and Cognition, 52*, 27–32.

Segalowitz, S. J., Davies, P. L., Santesso, D., Gavin, W. J., & Schmidt, L. A. (2004). The development of the error negativity in children and adolescents. In M. Ullsperger & M. Falkenstein (Eds.), *Errors, Conflicts, and the Brain: Current Opinions on Performance Monitoring* (pp. 177–184). Leipzig: Max Planck Institute for Cognition and Neurosciences.

Segalowitz, S. J., & Schmidt, L. A. (2003). Developmental psychology and the neurosciences. In J. Valsiner & K. Connolly (Eds.), *Handbook of Developmental Psychology* (pp. 48–71). London: Sage Publishers.

Shankman, S. A., Tenke, C. E., Bruder, G. E., Durbin, C. E., Hayden, E. P., & Klein, D. N. (1995). Low positive emotionality in young children: Associations with EEG asymmetry. *Development and Psychopathology 17*, 85–98.

Siddappa, A. M., Georgieff, M. K., Wewerka, S., Worwa, C., Nelson, C. A., & Deregnier, R. A. (2004). Iron Deficiency Alters Auditory Recognition Memory in Newborn Infants of Diabetic Mothers. *Pediatric Research, 55*, 1034–1041.

Sidman, R. L., & Rakic, P. (1973). Neuronal migration with special reference to developing human brain: A review. *Brain Research, 62*, 1–35.

Slater, A., & Morison, V. (1991). Visual attention and memory at birth. In M. J. Weiss, & P. R. Zelazo (Eds.), *Newborn attention: Biological constraints and the influence of experience* (pp. 256–277). Norwood, NJ: Ablex.

Smith, J. R. (1938a). The electroencephalogram during normal infancy and childhood: I. Rhythmic activities present in the neonate and their subsequent development. *Journal of Genetic Psychology, 53*, 431–453.

Smith, J. R. (1938b). The electroencephalogram during normal infancy and childhood: II. The nature and growth of alpha waves. *Journal of Genetic Psychology, 53*, 455–469.

Smith, J. R. (1938c). The electroencephalogram during normal infancy and childhood: III. Preliminary observations on the pattern sequence during sleep. *Journal of Genetic III Psychology, 53*, 471–482.

Smith, J. R. (1939a). The "occipital" and "pre-central" alpha rhythms during the first two years. *Journal of Psychology, 7*, 223–226.

Smith, J. R. (1941). The frequency and growth of the human alpha rhythms during infancy and childhood. *Journal of Psychology, 11*, 177–198.

Snidman, N., Kagan, J., Riordan, L., & Shannon, D. C. (1995). Cardiac function and behavioral reactivity during infancy. *Psychophysiology, 32*, 199–207.

Stifter, C. A., & Fox, N. A. (1990). Infant reactivity and regulation: Physiological correlates of newborn and five-month temperament. *Developmental Psychology, 26*, 582–588.

Stifter, C. A., Fox, N. A., & Porges, S. W. (1989). Facial expressivity and heart rate variability in five- and ten-month-old infants. *Infant Behavior and Development, 12*, 127–137.

Stroganova, T. A., Orekhova, E. V., & Posikera, I. N. (1999). EEG alpha rhythm in infants. *Clinical Neurophysiology, 110*, 997–1012.

Sutton, S. K., & Davidson, R. J. (1997). Prefrontal brain asymmetry: A biological substrate of the behavioral approach and inhibition systems. *Psychological Science, 8*, 204–210.

Task Force of the European Society of Cardiology and the North American Society of Pacing and Electrophysiology. (1996). Heart rate variability: Standards of measurement, physiological interpretation, and clinical use. *Circulation, 93*, 1043–1065.

Terwogt, M. M., & van Grinsven, F. (1991). Musical expression of moodstates. *Psychology of Music, 19*, 99–109.

Thatcher, R. W. (1991). Maturation of the human frontal lobes: Physiological evidence for staging. Special Issue: Developmental consequences of early frontal lobe damage. *Developmental Neuropsychology, 7*, 397–419.

Thatcher, R. W. (1994). Psychopathology of early frontal lobe damage: Dependence on cycles of development. Special Issue: Neural plasticity, sensitive periods, and psychopathology. *Development and Psychopathology, 6*, 565–596.

Thatcher, R. W., Krause, P., & Hrybyk, M. (1986). Corticocortical association fibers and EEG coherence: A two compartmental model. *Electroencephalography and Clinical Neurophysiology, 64*, 123–143.

Thatcher, R. W., Walker, R. A., Giudice, S. (1987). Human cerebral hemispheres develop at different rates and ages. *Science, 236*, 1110–1112.

Theall-Honey, L. A., & Schmidt, L. A. (2006). Do temperamentally shy children process emotion differently than non-shy children? Behavioral, psychophysiological, and gender differences in reticent preschoolers. *Developmental Psychobiology, 48*, 187–196,

Tomarken, A. J., Davidson, R. J., & Henriques, J. B. (1990). Resting frontal brain asymmetry predicts affective responses to films. *Journal of Personality and Social Psychology, 59*, 791–801.

Tomarken, A. J., Davidson, R. J., Wheeler, R. E., & Kinney, L. (1992). Psychometric properties of resting anterior EEG asymmetry: Temporal stability and internal consistency. *Psychophysiology, 29*, 576–592.

Trainor, L. J. (1996). Infant preferences for infant-directed versus noninfant-directed playsongs and lullabies. *Infant Behavior and Development, 19*, 83–92.

Trainor, L. J., Clark, E. D., Huntley, A., & Adams, B. A. (1997). The acoustic basis of preferences for infant-directed singing. *Infant Behavior and Development, 20*, 383–396.

Trainor, L. J., & Trehub, S. E. (1992). The development of referential meaning in music. *Music Perception, 9*, 455–470.

Trehub, S. E., & Trainor, L. J. (1998). Singing to infants: Lullabies and play songs. In C. Rovee-Collier, L. P. Lipsilt, & H. Hayne (Eds.), *Advances in Infancy Research* (pp. 43–77). Stamford, Connecticut: Ablex Publishing Corporation.

Trehub, S. E., Unyk, A. M., & Trainor, L. J. (1993). Adults identify infant-directed music across cultures. *Infant Behavior and Development, 16*, 193–211.

Welsh, M. C., Pennington, B. F., & Groisser, D. B. (1991). A normative-developmental study of executive function: A window on prefrontal function in children. *Developmental Neuropsychology, 7*, 131–149.

Wheeler, R. E., Davidson, R. J., & Tomarken, A. J. (1993). Frontal brain asymmetry and emotional reactivity: A biological substrate of affective style. *Psychophysiology, 30*, 82–89.

Zahn, T. P. (1986). Psychophysiological approaches to psychophysiology. In M. G. H. Coles, E. Donchin, & S. W. Porges (Eds.), *Psychophysiology: Systems, processes, and applications* (pp. 508–610). New York: Guilford.

Zahn, T. P., & Kruesi, M. J. P. (1993). Autonomic activity in boys with disruptive behavior disorders. *Psychophysiology, 30*, 605–614.

Zahn-Waxler, C., Cole, P. M., Darby Welsh, J., & Fox, N. A. (1995). Psychophysiological correlates of empathy and prosocial behaviors in preschool children with behavior problems. *Development and Psychopathology, 7*, 27–48.

21 Interoception

BARRY R. DWORKIN

The focus of this chapter is the basic physiological properties of those sensory receptors that monitor the internal state of the body, and on the methods that are used to study them. Its content is intended to provide an appreciation of the range of biological phenomena that involve interoceptors, to explain the goals and procedures of interoception research, and to offer to researchers some practical suggestions and theoretical guidelines for interoception experiments.[1] The scope of the chapter is well characterized in the following quotation from an 1894 lecture by Pavlov.

… in the life of a complex organism the reflex is the most essential and frequent neural phenomenon. With its help a constant, correct, and precise correlation becomes established among the parts of an organism, and among the relationships between the organism as a whole and the surrounding conditions. And the starting point of the reflex is the irritation of the peripheral endings of centripetal nerves. These endings pervade all organs and all tissues. These endings must be visualized as extremely diverse, specific ones, each individually adapted, like the nerve endings of sense organs, to its own specific irritant of mechanical, physical, or chemical nature. Their effectiveness determines at each given moment the magnitude of, and fluctuations in, the activity of the organism. (Pavlov, 1940, p. 142)

SENSORY RECEPTORS

There are three generally recognized classes of sensory transducers:

(1) Exteroceptors, such as the photoreceptors of the eye, the hair cells of the cochlea, or the mechanoreceptors of the skin. These are located at or near the body surface, and are the basis of exteroception, the perception of mechanical and electromagnetic energy fields in surrounding space.

(2) Proprioceptors, such as skeletal muscle spindles, Golgi tendon organs, and joint strain receptors. These sense the velocity, orientation, and mechanical tension of the skeleton. They are the basis of proprioception: the control of skeletal reflexes, complex movement, and the perception of the orientation and action of the body in space.

(3) Interoceptors, such as mechano, thermo, and chemoreceptors, of the gut; stretch receptors of the atria, carotid arteries, and aorta; chemoreceptors of the carotid sinus, lipid receptors in the portal circulation, and metaboreceptors in the skeletal muscles. These are situated within the body cavities, and are the basis of visceral reflexes; and of interoception, the central neural representation of the blood vessels and visceral organs. They are the sensory radix of the vegetative infrastructure of higher animals.

Among the receptors, the first two classes are most readily accessible to stimulation and electrophysiological recording. As a consequence, their microanatomy and biophysical transduction mechanisms are well described, and to a large extent, modal selectivity, dynamic response characteristics and central connections have been analyzed. In contrast, the receptive field, generator structure, and pseudo-dendrite of a typical interoceptor are deep within a body cavity, and comparatively inaccessible.

It is much more difficult to stimulate the, comparatively inaccessible, receptive field of an interoceptor, and simultaneously record from its small, often unmyelinated, fiber. Consequently, the detailed properties and functions of interoceptors are less known than those of exteroceptors and proprioceptors. Nonetheless, anatomically, nearly ninety percent of the fibers of the vagus and more than fifty percent of the fibers of all autonomic nerves are afferent (Norgren, 1985, p. 145), and these fibers convey extensive information from interoceptors to the brain.

---

[1] Thus, the emphasis is on the physiological implications of visceral sensory mechanisms, not the psychological implications of visceral perception. Excluded are certain subjects dealing with specialized perceptions, for example, the awareness of heart beat (see next note) and a detailed discussion hunger and satiety. For a recent review of the role of the perception of visceral sensation in the control of food intake see (McHugh & Moran, 1985; Schwartz & Moran, 1996). Nociception is discussed in relation to interoceptor properties, but visceral pain and its mechanism is an extensive and separate subject.

INTEROCEPTOR TAXONOMY

The term "interoceptors" includes visceral receptors, but, is broader: "Visceral" is from "viscus," meaning an internal organ of the body; especially: one (as the heart, liver, or intestine) located in the great cavities of the trunk. For example, the entire small intestine or bladder is considered visceral; whereas, the skeletal muscles are not. Thus defined, the stretch receptors of the gut are all interoceptors; whereas, the nearly homologous, spindles, which regulate the mechanical function of the skeletal muscles, are not. The spindles and other skeletal mechanoreceptors are instead called proprioceptors. This distinction is logically consistent and reasonably clear, but adjacent to proprioceptors, the skeletal muscles also have other receptors, which respond to the metabolic state of the muscle tissue itself. These metaboreceptors fire with elevated lactic acid and diprotonated phosphate (H_2PO_4-) concentrations in the surrounding tissue; their activation augments muscle sympathetic nerve activity and partially opposes the local vasodilatory effects of metabolic products; they, thus, regulate the circulation, and ensure that each muscle receives the cardiac output fraction that fits its activity (Batman et al., 1994; Sinoway & Prophet, 1990). Metaboreceptors are neither proprioceptors or exteroceptors; they have many properties in common with interoceptors, but are not part of the "viscera" by the usual definition.

The metaboreceptor example points up that, in addition to its anatomy, the function of a receptor also must be accounted into the taxonomy: In general, within an organ or tissue there are (1) those sensory elements that serve a special host organ function, such as photoreceptors of the eye, the hair cells of the cochlea, the spindles of the skeletal muscles, or the stretch and mucosal chemoreceptors of the intestine; and (2) those that subserve more general tissue maintenance functions, such as do, the various metaboreceptors. Hence, a distinction can be appropriately drawn between receptors serving vegetative and those serving special organ functions.

Thus, to be complete, interoceptors should include all sensory receptors in visceral organs, plus other receptors, wherever located, that subserve local tissue metabolic functions. In addition, it is necessary to consider separately certain other cases where the anatomical position of a sensory ending and its effective receptive field do not obviously coincide. For example, some stretch receptors in the mesentery are activated with strong contraction of the muscular layers of adjacent intestine. Although, these are indisputably interoceptors, and their function seems obvious, there are other more subtle or ambiguous cases: For example, at least in part, the conscious perception of the heart beat, particularly in arrhythmia, depends on receptors situated in the chest wall and/or overlying skin.[2] Because their receptive field includes visceral structures,

should these striate muscle and/or cutaneous receptors appropriately be considered to be interoceptors? The general answer probably is no; but in a specific case, it may depend on the implications that are to be drawn from the observed effects. (And suppose, for argument, that the receptors in question were located on the pleural membrane instead of the chest wall, Would their classification be the same?)

Finally, certain authors have objected to the tacit identification of sensory receptors with one or the other branches of the autonomic nervous system (Jänig & Häbler, 1995). This concern is appropriate, and it should be yet further noted that the peripheral nervous pathway of a receptor cell's afferent process is not always a reliable basis for characterizing a receptor or receptor population: For example, the vagus is mostly composed of visceral afferents, but the vagus is, in fact, not a pure visceral nerve. Fibers from the larynx, via the recurrent laryngeal nerve, enter the vagus at the aortic arch; thence, course the full extent of the cervical vagus. Some of these fibers are afferent, and project to striate muscle spindles. In addition to these somatic proprioceptive afferents, the vagus also contains a population of general cutaneous sensory fibers, which are derived from its auricular ramus (Brodal, 1969). Thus, electrical stimulation of the cervical vagus can not be assumed to emulate a pure visceral afferent effect, and electrical activity that is recorded from the vagus may be partially somatic.

In biology, we *classify* things so that we can make observations on a few members of a class, and then use the result to make useful inferences to the other members of the same class. Definitions constrain conclusions: If a question concerns, for example, specific hemodynamic effects of low pressure atrial baroreceptors, the receptor population for study can be readily defined in terms of physiological and anatomical criteria, and the conclusions confidently applied back to the appropriate population. However, when more general questions are addressed, such as, "Is there conscious perception of moderate intestinal dilation?", the criteria are less pat.

More important than post hoc justification of inferences, definitions guide the design of a convincing experiment. For example, an intestinal perception hypothesis could be tested by applying a signal detection procedure to a balloon in the lumen. But, in parts of the intestine, in addition to the stretch receptors of the gut wall, balloon inflation might also distend the overlying abdominal skin. Suppose, in such an experiment, detection is found to be reliable, but that activation of the skin receptors has not been ruled out as a source of the sensory input, Is it reasonable to infer that, in general, intestinal dilation can be perceived? Probably not, But why? The ready answer is: Because the sensation is obviously from the skin, not the intestine! But, why are skin receptors not considered to be a legitimate source of visceral sensory input?

---

[2] See for example (Brenner & Jones, 1974; Paintal, 1972). For an excellent and extensive review of heart beat perception see (Jones, 1994); for a discussion of probable sources of mediation op. cit. pp. 156–160.

To overcome the limitation (on the target inference class) the intestinal perception experiment would need to incorporate appropriate controls. These could be achieved in two ways: (1) With a differential experiment in which the skin artifact is deliberately included in both the control and experimental stimulations, or (2) by refining the intraluminal stimulation technique to entirely exclude any skin artifact. In an animal study, inflation of an intraluminal balloon could be compared to "control" inflation of an adjacent extralumenal balloon. The control inflation would stimulate the skin, but not the luminal stretch receptors; the intraluminal inflation would stimulate both, and the difference would specifically measure the luminal stretch contribution. This design is satisfactory but requires surgical placement of the control balloon in the abdominal cavity; something which is obviously not appropriate in humans.

It is difficult to dilate an intestinal segment without some effect on overlying skin, but sometimes a more stringent experiment can be used to show that an observation also holds in a less stringent sense. For example, a relatively non-invasive procedure can be used to study differential detection in two adjacent intestinal segments: A catheter with two separately inflatable balloons spaced several centimeters apart (a Barthelheimer tube) can be passed per os into the intestine, with the subject is instructed to attempt to respond to one and only one of the two balloons as the signal, and the balloons inflated in a controlled quasi-random pattern. If the experiment shows that the separate inflations can be discriminated, the result would go beyond, but would definitely include, solid evidence of simple detection by intestinal distension. In fact, procedure of this kind has been successfully used (Adam, 1967, pp. 127–128) to study the sensory capability of the human duodenum.

It should be noted, here, that a hazard of using discrimination as the criterion of simple detection is the increased chance of the Type II error (the null hypothesis is inappropriately accepted). In general, experiments should be designed so as to minimize systematic error, but a draconian standard of evidence can obscure an important phenomenon; hence, in stating the conclusions of a highly differential experiment, negative outcomes should be interpreted with the same degree of caution as a positive ones.

Ultimately, any acceptable definition depends on the question that it serves, and the question devolves to the relationship between the experimental preparation and the target inference class. Every scientist appreciates that randomization is the crux of statistical inference; a valid proband always must be drawn at random from the applicable universe; in fact, a similar, but more general "sampling" principle governs any inference. It demands that an experimental preparation be, as nearly as possible, a *generic* example drawn from the target class: in other words, the properties of the preparation – at least, those properties that, arguably, are relevant to the putative effect – must be the same for all members of the inference class. For example, consider again the enteric perception experiment, if all intestinal segments were situated such that the overlying skin was stimulated by balloon dilation, the result would be convincingly applicable to all intestinal segments, and generally valid; however, because this is almost certainly not true, the inference only applies to those segments where the condition holds. Furthermore, general properties of the physiology and anatomy of the gut dictate that skin stimulation would not likely be a reliable sensory pathway for intestinal distention; thus, in experiments of this kind, an effect that depends on sensation in the overlying skin is appropriately considered an experimental artifact.

THE GENERAL BIOPHYSICAL PROPERTIES OF INTEROCEPTORS

Stimuli have the qualities of anatomical location, physical mode, intensity and its derivatives of time; but, although a particular receptor may be more efficiently activated by certain combinations of these qualities, most interoceptors are anatomically diffuse, polymodal, and simultaneously affected by both the level and rate of change of the stimulus.

Selectivity: For any sensory system, stimulus discriminability ultimately is determined by the properties of individual receptors. Studies of skin sensations of awake humans indicate that individual receptors can code a range of stimulus qualities. Intraneural micro-stimulation of individual afferent units can evoke sensations of intermittent tapping, vibration or tickle, or a perception of distinctly localized pressure: Quantitatively, depending on the unit stimulated, afferent impulse frequency may determine the magnitude of perceived pressure, or the frequency of perceived vibration (Ochoa & Torebjork, 1983).

In addition to unit properties, modern sensory physiology, kindled by the work of Adrian, Hartline, and Hubel and Weisel, has confirmed that comparatively simple assemblages of appropriately connected receptors can encode many additional stimulus properties; thus, in the central visual areas, there are cells that fire differentially to edges moving in a particular direction, even though, the retina itself, has no actual edge detecting cells. Due to the comparative inaccessibility of the visceral receptive fields, and visceral afferent nerve tracts, there are no direct observations of the sensory capabilities of functional interoceptor arrays, but most likely the organization is similar: We know for example, that the anal canal has "shearing" sensitive regions (Jänig & Häbler, 1995), and that probably similar shear sensitivity occurs in the upper gastrointestinal tract; and that these perceptions probably derive from spatially organized receptive fields composed of simple stretch (pressure) receptors. The regulatory implications of temporal convergence of activity from different receptors is not addressed by conventional systems analyses: the electrical activity from a visceral nerve is typically treated as a scalar quantity, represented by the rectified and integrated neurogram. Consider by analogy, trying to explain pattern detection or color vision from fluctuations in the averaged activity of the optic nerve.

For almost all receptors certain key steps in transduction are common: in particular, although some visual and auditory receptors hyperpolarize to certain stimuli, an adequate stimulus usually displaces the membrane potential toward zero. Because maintenance of the resting membrane potential depends on metabolically sensitive active processes, ionic selectivity of the plasma membrane, and the composition of the extracellular environment, depolarization is also a consequence of any cellular damage or extra-cellular change that is sufficient to disrupt either metabolism or structure, or affect the Nernst potential of a key ion. Hence, large parametric excursions, or moderate non-specific injury of the surrounding tissue will cause most receptors to begin firing, often rapidly, and to continue to fire, until the cell is actually devastated. For similar common biophysical reasons, all receptors are sensitive to ambient electrical currents, and most will also fire with application of mechanical pressure sufficient to produce significant membrane distortion. Beyond these ubiquitous membrane processes, transduction processes initiated by trans-membrane receptor molecules, may be multi-modal or non-specific. For example, chemoreceptors respond to both CO_2 and pH, and many gustatory receptors respond to several of the basic stimuli, and some vagal afferent fibers respond to both cholecystokinin and distention. In addition, the broad and overlapping sensitivity of many "pharmacological" receptor molecules is well documented.

Temporal properties: Receptors can be broadly characterized by their firing rate as a function of a step change of the stimulus in time. In a qualitative sense there are two separable aspects of this "step response": the accuracy or speed with which the receptor follows the rising edge of the step, and the stability of the asymptotic firing rate to the steady level of the plateau. In the somatomotor, the visual, and the auditory systems, receptor response speed is important, because it is often the limiting factor in system performance, but for the regulation of visceral function this is rarely the case: For most autonomic reflexes the sensory receptor mechanism is relatively fast, compared to the cumulative lag of the proximal stimulus dynamics, central processing and efferent mechanisms (Dworkin et al., 2000); thus, *interoceptor response speed is ordinarily not the limiting factor in determining autonomic control properties*.

However, in contrast to somatosensory, visual and auditory processes, which mostly engage phasic reflexes acting within seconds, many interoceptors are involved the feedback controlled steady state regulation of the basal value of physiological variables. Consequently, for interoceptors, the stability of the asymptotic firing rate to a constant stimulus is an extremely important issue. In fact, the steady state response properties of interoceptors, which are described and analyzed below, are difficult to reconcile with their putative function within a conventional negative feedback regulatory framework, and exactly how the sys-

tem actually works remains an open question (Dworkin, 1993).

Adaptation is the gradual decline in receptor firing to constant stimulation. Adaptation can be a striking and obvious effect: In the 1950s there were experiments in humans that employed stabilized retinal images, produced by special optical projectors (Race & Rosenbaum, 1966; Riggs et al., 1953). These experiments showed that "... with an essentially motionless retinal image prolonged fixation results in disappearance of objects from the field of view." (Riggs et al., 1953). Complete fading of the image can occur within several seconds. The stabilized image is a particularly graphic example, but receptor adaptation is ubiquitous: In every neural system, at every level of the animal kingdom, whenever receptor temporal properties have been accurately measured, adaptation has been found.

Mechanisms of adaptation: Various biochemical and physical factors account for receptor adaptation. For example, in Pacinian corpuscles, as in certain interoceptors, mechanical high pass filtering by the surrounding tissue is an important component of the adaptation mechanism (Lowenstein & Mendelson, 1965); however, even with removal of the mechanical filtration of the viscous lamellae or capsule, the generator potential of a naked receptor has a duration of less than 100 msec. (Lowenstein & Skalak, 1966). The range of the time scale of adaptation is such that receptors considered notable for being *slow* to adapt, such as muscle spindle, bee hair-plate, or slow crustacean stretch receptors, actually sustain generator potentials for only seconds or minutes.

Whether or not adaptation holds for every membrane bound receptor, neural or not, is unknown, but in most systems with the presence of persistent ligand levels, there is "down regulation" or reduced receptor sensitivity of both a fast and slow kind. There are various neurochemical mechanisms of adaptation; however, recovery of sensitivity after long-term ligand exposure probably requires protein synthesis (Axelrod, 1984; Browning, Brostrom, & Groppi, 1976; Deguchi & Axelrod, 1973; Gavin et al., 1974; Mallorga et al., 1980; Strulovici et al., 1984; Terasaki et al., 1978).

Interoceptor adaptation: When exposed to a static stimulus all known interoceptors eventually cease to fire; thus, the sensory manifestation of adaptation for visceral receptors, parallels that of the stabilized image for the retina. The central nervous system representation of any completely constant stimulus gradually fades, and is eventually obliterated; moreover, the constant component of a variable stimulus also disappears. So, for example, although the pulse variation of the blood pressure continues to be indefinitely reflected in corresponding fluctuations in the firing rate of the baroreceptor nerves, the mean arterial pressure (MAP), the central value around which the pulse pressure varies, gradually disappears from the afferent signal. Table 21.1 is taken from Chernigovskiy's (Chernigovskiy, 1967) extensive monograph.[3] It lists the

---

[3] For additional general references on interoceptor properties see (Mountcastle, 1980).

Table 21.1. This is abstracted from Chernigovskiy's (Chernigovskiy, 1967, pp. 228–29) extensive monograph. It lists the approximate time of adaptation for a number of carefully studied interoceptors. Note the actual time to adaptation given for the "very slow" adaptation receptors

Receptors	Adaptation speed	Adaptation class
Mechanoreceptors of the carotid sinus (cat)	25% of the initial impulse frequency within 6 sec of stimulation; the initial rapid phase of adaptation is practically absent.	Very slow
Mechanoreceptors of the aortic arch (rabbit)	Complete adaptation within 5–10 min.	Very slow
Mechanoreceptors of the atrium (cat)		Very slow
Mechanoreceptors of the urinary bladder (dog)	1. Complete adaptation within several fraction of a second (only 10–30 impulses). 2. Incomplete adaptation within 15–25 min.	Very slow
Mechanoreceptors of the urinary bladder (cat)	Complete adaptation within fractions of a second.	Very rapid
Various types of stretch receptors of the lungs (cat)	Not more than 5% of the initial impulse frequency within 10 sec. 1. Decrease in impulse frequency by 10–55% during the 2nd sec of stimulation. 2. Complete or almost complete adaptation by the end of the first sec of stimulation. These receptors are distinguished by a high threshold.	 Slow Very rapid

approximate time of adaptation (to a constant stimulus) for a number of carefully studied interoceptors: again especially note, what are actually rather rapid adaptation times of those receptors that Chernigovskiy saw fit to classify as being "very slow" to adapt. Figure 21.1 shows the response of a typical "slowly adapting" cardiovascular receptor to a constant stimulus at its receptive surface (Mifflin & Kunze, 1982).

INTEROCEPTORS AND STEADY-STATE PHYSIOLOGICAL REGULATION

Interoceptor adaptation poses some intractable and perplexing problems for conventional theories of physiological regulation, and because of this, its ubiquity has not been accepted without controversy. Many authors either have ignored evidence of receptor adaptation, or attempted to dismiss it as a technical artifact of the isolation and measurement procedure.[4] The analysis of the carotid baroreceptors by Landgren (Landgren, 1952) is typical. For carotid sinus pressures below 100 mmHg he found the usual rapid adaptation; however, above 100 mmHg, the time until "complete" adaptation was much longer. On the basis of this, he surmised that there was a term in the step response that represented a time invari-

ant pressure dependent firing rate, wrote the equation for the receptor as $Frequency = A(p) + Bt^{-.65}$, and explicitly characterized the baroreceptor response to pressures above 100 mmHg as "steady discharge." By including $A(p)$,

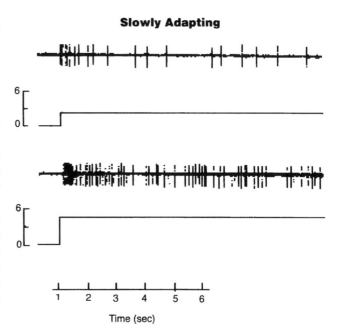

Slowly Adapting

Time (sec)

Figure 21.1. Slowly adapting low-pressure vagal receptor of the rat. The spike record shows the fall-off in firing in rate following application and maintenance of a stimulus step. Adaptation occurs with both high-and low-strength stimuli, but complete adaptation is usually more rapid with weaker stimulation. The classification as "slowly adapting" is made relative to other kinds of interoceptors, studied under similar conditions (see text).

[4] This idea has been prevalent in autonomic nervous system neurophysiology for many years. When, in 1969, as a student, I asked the influential autonomic nervous system neurophysiologist, Detlev Bronk, about the apparent ubiquity of receptor adaptation, and its implications for physiological regulation, he insisted that it was not a real phenomenon, but an artifact of damage inflicted by the dissection required to isolate the receptor.

a purely pressure dependent term, Landgren implicitly asserted that at higher pressures the baroreceptors did not fully adapt, and thus that they indefinitely continued to transmit steady-state pressure information. This result challenged the assertion that adaptation was ubiquitous; however, Langren observed receptors at constant pressure for no more than 10 minutes.[5] The firing rate, at that point in time, appeared stable and, because of this, he concluded, "The curve approaches a constant asymptotic value."

Given the putative role of the baroreceptors in blood pressure regulation, "steady discharge" to a constant pressure was an important finding. Langren's result was readily accepted as evidence that the baroreceptors indeed had sufficient long-term stability to regulate basal blood pressure. However, by the mid 1950s, baroreceptor "resetting"(McCubbin, Green, & Page, 1956) was experimentally demonstrated, and with it, serious doubts arose about whether the baroreceptors were involved in tonic blood pressure control.

The controversy about the baroreceptors points up a general problem in interpreting interoceptor adaptation data. In all cases, the temporal response establishes the regulatory limitations of the receptor; for example, if a receptor, which adapts to 50% of maximum firing rate in 20 seconds, is the afferent element of a phasic reflex that requires only a few seconds of firing to initiate, that receptor is "slowly adapting." For a baroreceptor, an orthostatic response to postural change fits that case well. On the other hand, if the same baroreceptor is assumed to sense mean blood pressure, it needs to maintain its firing rate for very much longer – in certain (quite conventional) conceptions of the regulatory process – possibly even for years. Thus, compared to the time scale of steady state blood pressure regulation (and this was the important physiological issue), observation of a receptors response for 10 minutes was too brief to make a useful inference.[6]

In sum, all interoceptors appear to adapt within seconds or minutes. Interoceptor adaptation has profound implications for control system models of long-term or steady state regulation: If the key assumption of the conventional regulatory paradigm – that some receptors continue to faithfully transduce the absolute level of physiological variables for many months, and can provide the sensory substrate of long-term central regulation – is valid, there should be many studies convincingly documenting hours or more of stable transduction by various interoceptors; in fact, there appear to be none whatsoever.

ACCOMMODATION

Accommodation is when stimulus change is sufficiently gradual that, because of adaptation, it fails to fully activate a receptor. As such, accommodation is simply another facet of adaptation. It is, however, an especially interesting facet, because it illustrates the regulatory implications of adaptation.

If a receptor adapts, given an appropriate stimulus rate of change (driving) function, it can be made to fire at a constant frequency. If the driving function is sufficiently gradual, the constant firing frequency can remain close to zero (Gray & Malcolm, 1951; Gray & Matthews, 1951). In other words, because of accommodation, a stimulus can increase from zero to the physiological maximum without ever changing the receptor's firing rate. A more precise and quantitative way of defining accommodation is in terms of the receptor transfer function: If a time domain step function response has a Laplace transform, $F(s)$, its transfer function, $T(s)$, is $F(s)$ divided by $1/s$, the transform of a zero time aligned step. The transform of the output function that describes a particular constant firing frequency R, is R/s. And, it follows that,

$$H(s) \cdot T(s) = \frac{R}{s};$$
$$H(s) = \frac{R}{sT(s)}$$

where $H(s)$ is the Laplace transform of the stimulus or driving function that will cause the receptor to fire continuously at constant frequency R. This relationship can be applied to the step function data for an interoceptor, and used to derive a cumulative stimulus drift function that will produce a constant, arbitrarily low, firing rate. For example, for feline right atrial mechanoreceptors Chapman and Pankhurst (Chapman & Pankhurst, 1976) found no evidence of time invariant firing in the atrial volume receptors, that is, the receptors adapted to a zero firing rate. At above the threshold volume, the firing rate was characterized by $Frequency = \frac{12Hz}{ml}(\frac{t}{1sec})^{-.24}$; thus, the transfer function for this receptor is, $T(s) = \frac{12Hz}{ml \cdot sec^{-.24}}\Gamma(.76)s^{.24}$, and the inverse of $H(s)$ for $R = 1$, a firing rate of one impulse per second, is $h(t) = \frac{ml}{12\Gamma(.76)\Gamma(1.24)}(\frac{t}{1sec})^{.24}$, which describes a volume drift curve that will evoke a constant rate of firing over the linear range of the receptor (from threshold to saturation). Solving this shows that as much as 0.5 ml of additional atrial volume can accumulate, within an hour,

---

[5] Because the empirically observed firing rates always include some random variability, appropriate statistics must be used to convincingly show that the firing rate actually approaches a final, non-zero, constant level. The assertion that a curve has reached "asymptotic level" means that the regression line fit to data on the terminus of the linear plot has a slope of zero to within an acceptable error. It is important to appreciate that Langren did not use an appropriate statistical criteria to evaluate the slope of the terminal firing rate, even within the specified 10-minute observation period.

[6] Langren's was an early and pioneering study, but similar criteria also characterize more recent interoceptor studies. For example, Mifflin and Kunze (Mifflin & Kunze, 1982) studied slowly and rapidly adapting low pressure receptors in the left superior vena cava of the rat (see Figure 21.1). For the slow receptors they observed substantial (60%) increases in threshold following 15-min exposures to pressures of 5 mmHg, which agreed with other results (Kappagoda & Padsha, 1980), and these, they explicitly claimed, did show time invariant firing. However, when their published data was reanalyzed with standard regression techniques and conservative criteria (Dworkin, 1993, p. 139), the firing rate had actually continued to decline substantially during the last 10 minutes of observation.

without perturbing the firing rate. Thus, under appropriate circumstances, even an "extremely slowly adapting" interoceptor can fully accommodate to a rate of volume change that would soon accrue to a substantial physiological error.

Is adaptation an experimental artifact?: A possible way to dismiss the physiological implications of interoceptor adaptation is to argue that adaptation is an artifact that results from damage inflicted in preparation for recording, on a receptor or its nerve. Because, direct quantitative measurement of interoceptor adaptation in situ is impractical (For one thing, accurately controlling the stimulation level in an intact animal is difficult), this assertion is extremely hard either to prove or refute.

The Russian visceral physiologists had an explicit theoretical commitment to brain mediated interoceptive regulation of the physiological state. They, thus, found the relentlessness of receptor adaptation particularly vexing, and were especially motivated to seek an alternative explanation that would mitigate the adaptation data. Their predicament had two aspects: first, if the primary interoceptor adapts, it is impossible for the brain to continuously acquire information from it, and, second, in addition to primary adaptation, observed ex situ, there was undeniable evidence for adaptation, resetting or habituation of many different in situ visceral reflexes.[7] Given these facts, and especially if the second phenomenon is actually a manifestation of the first, they asked, How can the brain have an important role in long-term regulation? Their putative explanations were: (1) primary receptor adaptation, observed *ex situ*, is an experimental artifact; and (2) adaptation of intact reflexes is due to an active inhibitory process that occurs in the brain, not at the interoceptor. To test these hypotheses, the leading Soviet sensory physiologist N. Chernigovskiy did an experiment that attempted to directly challenge the notion that the universally observed adaptation of visceral reflexes is a direct consequence of interoceptor adaptation (Chernigovskiy, 1967, pp. 230–34).

The experiment used a loop of intestine and its mesenteric nerves. Distending the segment stimulated mechanoreceptors in the wall, which through afferent nerves to the brain, caused a reflexive increase of blood pressure and respiratory rate. The investigators found that, following its increase, the blood pressure gradually returned toward normal as the wall tension was maintained constant for several minutes. This was exactly as expected, and the conventional explanation of this result is that the interoceptors of the gut wall eventually adapt to the constant stretch. However, in Chernigovskiy's experiment, once adaptation developed and the reflex magnitude diminished, the mesenteric nerve was subjected to transmission block by cooling it to 5°C. As would be expected,

the cold block, at that point in the protocol, was without effect on either the blood pressure or respiration. Again, the usual and obvious explanation is that there was no activity on the nerve to be blocked. But, a less readily explained result occurred when the temperature was returned to 37°C and afferent nerve conduction was reestablished: Blood pressure and respiration again rose, and the change was as large, or even larger, than to the original distention. Chernigovskiy argued that this proved that the receptor had continued to fire undiminished throughout the protocol; that the observed adaptation of the reflex was due only to a process somewhere central to the block, and, most important for the central regulatory theory, that information from the receptor had, in fact, continued to reach the brain. He said, "Thus, on the basis of these experiments it can be concluded that the apparent cessation of the reflex response takes place not in the least as a result of receptors' adaptation but is due to changes in the excitability of the vasomotor center which develops in the course of the reflex response itself."

These were interesting observations (c.f. Thomas E. Lohmeier, et al., 2004), but Chernigovskiy was almost certainly wrong in his conclusions. Besides the immediate effects of rewarming on the activity of the afferent nerve, which Chernigovskiy claimed (but did not explain how) he adequately controlled, his experiment had other probable pitfalls. In particular, along with stretch afferents, the mixed nerve of the pedicle contains motor, secretory, and vascular fibers, and cooling to 5°C would have blocked these efferent fibers and also probably lowered the temperature of the arterial blood supply and, thence, the tissue of the loop itself. Consequently, the vascular, and possibly thermal and motor, disturbance produced by the cold block would almost certainly have newly activated many different kinds of interoceptors, and the effects of this stimulation would not have become apparent until the afferent nerve was rewarmed.

Chernigovskiy's experiment is, nonetheless, informative for two reasons, first it illustrates some of the possible ways that interoception experiments can become confounded by failure to isolate pure afferent effects; second and more generally, it underlines that a well recognized authority on the physiology of interoceptors saw a serious inconsistency between the established ex situ adaptation characteristics of visceral sensory receptors and the participation of the central nervous system in long-term regulation of the physiological state. Clearly, he was troubled sufficiently by this disparity that he attempted a difficult experiment to reconcile interoceptor function with the conventional feedback regulation concepts of the prevalent regulatory theory.

In sum, adaptation is an established feature of all interoceptors which have been adequately studied. The erroneous conclusion that an interoceptor can have time independent functional activity derives from prematurely curtailing observations, or inaccurately measuring the terminal changes in firing rates. In all published cases, observation for periods even remotely comparable to the

---

[7] Chernogovskiy (1967) gives a many examples for intestinal reflexes, but the best documented example in the Western literature is the resetting blood pressure baroreflexes. See (Kezdi, 1962; Koushanpour & Kelso, 1972; Koushanpour & Kenfield, 1981; Kreiger, 1970; McCubbin et al., 1956).

time scale of steady-state physiological regulation have disclosed evidence of continued monotonically declining firing rates. The direct physiological implications are that, in all cases, information about the absolute stimulus magnitude is gradually distorted by an interoceptor, and after sufficient time, the visceral stimulus (similar to a stabilized visual image) probably fails to register altogether. Similarly, for accommodation, a sufficiently gradual rate of stimulus drift will not change the firing rate of the receptor, and the drift will elude detection and correction by regulatory mechanisms that depend at some link on sensory neural transduction.

EXPERIMENTAL METHODS IN INTEROCEPTOR RESEARCH

The experimental analysis of interoceptor function requires selective activation of the pathway(s) of interest. In general, researchers strive to confine and focus stimulation, so they know exactly what is being stimulated. There are a number of methods for accomplishing this; some of these can be used in humans, but others, because of their invasive and injurious nature can only be applied in animal studies. At present no interoceptive stimulation method for animals or humans that can be applied without the addition of specific control procedures to verify its effectiveness and/or specificity. The following describes some typical methods, their potential pitfalls, and usual controls.

Direct Nerve Stimulation: In principle, the most precise way to activate a particular fiber or circumscribed group of fibers is to surgically isolate and electrically stimulate them; however in practice, most sensory fibers are accessible to stimulation only after they have entered mixed nerves; thus, a satisfactory stimulation method depends on detailed knowledge of the relevant anatomy and physiology. For example, in humans the innervation of the tooth pulp is almost exclusively by nociceptive c-fibers, and it is possible to induce a relatively pure pain sensation by applying a dental probe electrode to the surface of a tooth (this is the principle of the "pulp tester" which has been used by dentists for many decades); however, with the conventional technique, current leakage to the gingiva reduces the accuracy of the stimulation, because the stray current activates mucosal receptors, producing additional non-pain sensations. Together, these factors degrade the accuracy and specificity of the tooth pain psychophysical function, which is obtained with this method (Zamir & Shuber, 1980). However, precise repeatable (within subject) stimulation of the pulp with a constant stimulation area (and current density) can be achieved with a tooth that has a vital pulp and a stable metal filling. The method involves imbedding the electrical contact in an individually molded, tightly fitted, rubber cap that completely insulates the electrode from the mucosa (Lee et al., 1985). It yields far better data than a simple hand held probe, but involves extensive preparations and is far more time consuming. Whether the effort is worthwhile again depends upon the question being asked: for example, does the hypothesis make highly quantitative predictions about pain as distinct from other oral sensations?

In another approach, when diverse pathways are unavoidably activated by an electrical stimulus, selective lesions often can be used to verify those component paths that are needed to produce the observed effect. For example, the general sensory effects of stimulation of the baroafferent pathways has been of increasing interest in recent years (Ghione, 1996). The rat vagus includes baroafferent fibers, and to study antinociceptive effects, Randich (Randich, Ren, & Gebhart, 1990) has used electrical stimulation of the whole central vagus as a technically simple means of activating these fibers. He controlled non-baroafferent effects by making selective ibotinic acid lesions in appropriate areas of the brain stem, and found that lesions placed in regions known to be involved in blood pressure control substantially blunted the antinociceptive effects of vagus stimulation, whereas other located lesions had less or no effect. This method is subject to all of the usual caveats for lesion procedures, but, in knowledgeable hands, can effectively help to verify the locus of mixed nerve stimulation effects. Specific lesions or nerve sections also can be used to limit the extent of non-electrical stimulation methods discussed below.

An additional issue about direct electrical stimulation of an afferent pathway is that, in general, the quantitative equivalence between electrical nerve stimulation and natural stimulus parameters is indeterminate: Higher stimulus current cannot be tacitly assumed to mimic stronger natural stimulation (although, as described above for cutaneous receptors, at a constant supra-threshold current, for certain kinds of individual fibers, the impulse rate of stimulation can have a useful physiological relationship to the properties of a distal stimulus). The general problem with using current strength as a stimulation variable is that, in a whole nerve, increasing current strength is more likely to recruit additional, smaller, fibers, than to more strongly activate those that are already recruited. In particular, when a nerve is composed of a mixture of myelinated and non-myelinated fibers, the myelinated fibers will be recruited at considerably lower current than the non-myelinated ones. Thus, it is often possible to selectively activate myelinated fibers, but not vise versa; furthermore, because "current" is determined by the local voltage gradient across the active neural membrane, the geometrical relationship between the stimulating electrode and nerve can strongly affect which fibers are actually stimulated at a particular current. On the whole the problem of electrically stimulating a mixed nerve is sufficiently complicated that another approach should be employed when the exact identity of the fibers stimulated is crucial; for example, when, to separate specific sensation from pain, large sensory fibers, but not c-fibers, need to be stimulated.

In the few cases of anatomically distinct nerves that are known to be physiologically homogeneous, electrical stimulation can be a clean and precise technique. Often the stringent requirements are met in only certain species. For example, the baroreceptors of the aortic arch reach the CNS through nerves that travel through the neck along the vagus and sympathetic trunk. These "aortic depressor nerves" (ADN) are very readily identified and isolated in the dog, rabbit, and rat; however, whereas the ADN of both the dog and rabbit also include many fibers from chemoreceptors in the arch, the rat ADN is composed entirely of pressure afferents. When the rat ADN is successfully isolated, it is a pure baroreceptor input.

The conclusion that a nerve is "pure" depends on several kinds of evidence. In some instances, it is possible to dissect the nerve over the entire course to the actual receptive field; then the effects of various stimuli at the receptors can be directly observed. This has been done for the rat ADN (Numao et al., 1985; Sapru, Gonzalez, & Krieger, 1981). Another important, and often more easily achieved criteria, is consistency of the response properties (or sensations) over a range of stimulus strength and rate parameters: Responses should monotonically relate to stimulation strength from threshold to saturation. This has also been done for the rat ADN (Dworkin & Dworkin, 1995; Dworkin, Dworkin, & Tang, 2000). Monotonicity is potentially a convincing criterion; however, for it to be so, the subject must be capable of expressing a wide range of responses, and all putative extraneous responses must be recorded. For example, the rat ADN enters the superior laryngeal nerve (SLN) near the carotid bifurcation, and the SLN is very much easier to identify and isolate than the much smaller ADN; it is thus technically easier to stimulate baroafferents within the SLN; however, the SLN contains numerous laryngeal afferents. Notwithstanding, for several typical baroreflex responses (including blood flow), Faber and Brody showed convincingly monotonic relationships between SLN stimulation parameters and depressor effects (Faber & Brody, 1983); however, because they used anesthetized rats, the effects of the laryngeal afferents were probably blunted or entirely eliminated. When the SLN is stimulated in conscious rats, the mixed effects of stimulation are depressor responses for low levels, often nothing at all for moderate levels, and clear pressor effects for stronger stimulation.

In sum, direct electrical stimulation of afferent nerve tracts can be a useful well controlled method for interoceptive stimulation,[8] but when modal specificity is important, controls are needed to verify that extraneous pathways are not being inadvertently activated.

Surgically isolated receptive fields: The usual goal of surgical isolation of a receptive field is to create a sensory surface to which stimuli may be applied with greater accuracy, convenience, and specificity than is possible in situ.

There are many examples of this method. Two illustrative ones are the isolated carotid sinus, and the isolated intestinal segment. A further advantage to using a surgically isolated receptive field is that the stimulus environment can be explicitly controlled, and the local sensory apparatus is less likely affected by endogenous physiological processes. An isolated intestinal loop is not inadvertently stimulated by the uncontrolled passage of chyme, and the arterial cul de sac can be stimulated, at an arbitrary pressure, independently of the systemic pressure.

The original carotid sinus cul de sac technique is attributed to Moissejeff (Heymans & Neil, 1958). It involves ligature of the internal and external carotid arteries (the former being tied cephalic to the sinus, carefully avoiding the carotid sinus nerve) and, cannulation of the central stump of the common carotid. Using this method, it is possible, by generating specific pulsatile or static pressures in the cannula, to accurately stimulate the carotid sinus baroreceptors. With a similar preparation, by irrigating the isolated sinus at constant pressure, the carotid chemoreceptors also can be independently stimulated. Although, in larger animals, such as the dog, it is possible to create a chronic isolated sinus preparation by anastomosing the common and internal carotid arteries, usually for chronic stimulation, a balloon is inserted into the carotid sinus via an incision in the common carotid artery, with a competent Circle of Willis, net brain blood flow is minimally affected. Balloons have been used to study the effects of carotid stimuli in intact conscious dogs and rats (Adam, 1967; Dworkin et al., 2000; Koch, 1932), and provided some of the earliest evidence that the carotid pressure receptors had general sensory effects.

The gut is an especially surgically tractable and plastic structure, and many ingenious methods have been invented for experimentally modifying its architecture and isolating its various regions. Everyone is familiar with Pavlov's innervated stomach pouches, which he used for collecting specimens of pure gastric juice in studies of the cephalic phase of digestion. Similar pouches and diverticuli can be constructed along the extent of the gastrointestinal tract, including completely isolated loops, which enter and exit at the external skin surface, preserve the nervous and vascular supply, and which if properly maintained, can be patent and functional for many years.[9] Various stimuli are easily applied to these cul de sacs and/or loops, which are readily distended by balloons or obturators, or irrigated with solutions of experimental compounds, such as acids, fats, or neurotransmitters. The more involved intestinal surgeries are more easily accomplished in the

---

[8] Direct nerve stimulation can rarely be used in normal humans; however, there are occasional opportunities to study patients. For example, stimulation of the carotid sinus nerve is sometimes used to control severe hypertension; some such patients have implanted pacemakers that can be externally controlled.

[9] Typical are Thiry-Vella loops, which are completely isolated sections of intestine. They are removed with the circulation and nerve supply intact, the ends are brought through and sutured to outside of the abdominal wall to form two papillae, and the remainder of the intestine reconnected with an end to end anastomosis. The resultant loop is easily accessible in a unanesthetized animal, and with reasonable care, various pressure, and thermal and chemical stimuli can be applied surreptitiously.

dog or monkey, because of the strength of their tissues and size of the structures, but it is also possible to make sophisticated surgical rearrangements of the gut in smaller animals, such as rabbits, or even rats (Bàrdos, Nagy, & Àdàm, 1980; Schwartz & Moran, 1996).

Observations of intestinal perception in humans are usually carried out with cannulas introduced per os or per anus; but, also at times, researchers have recruited, as research subjects, patients who have had medically prescribed ileostomy or colostomy procedures. Using stimuli produced by balloon inflation, Àdàm has done an extensive series of carefully controlled perceptual experiments with such subjects. These are discussed in more detail on pages 503 however we note here that using a surgically isolated receptive field does not automatically obviate the need for control procedures to exclude the effects of inadvertent stimulation of adjacent sensory structures: for example, distention of a carotid cul de sac or an isolated intestinal loop can inadvertently stretch overlying skin.

Non-invasive or minimally invasive methods for humans: These are techniques which are considered to involve only minimal risk for participating human subjects; however, "invasive" has a range of definitions, depending on who the subjects are, whom the procedure is performed by, and the extent to which the principal of intention of the procedure is therapeutic (versus purely scientific study). To a cardiologist, placing a catheter into the brachial artery of a heart patient may be considered minimally invasive; whereas, in most psychological research, a venous catheter is thought invasive, and even oral administration of approved drugs may be classified as invasive. Intent is possibly also as important as the actual manipulation. Almost everyone considers mild electric shock that is intended to produce even slight pain to be highly invasive; yet, the same or stronger electric current applied through the same electrodes, with the intention of producing muscle contraction or sweat secretion, might well be considered innocuous or "minimally invasive." In practice, what is "invasive" is determined by local (community) standards, and the arbiter is the legally constituted institutional review board (IRB) to which the investigator is professionally responsible. All human research must be approved by an IRB, and investigators are strongly advised to consult with the executives of the IRB at the earliest possible stage of research planning in order to obtain an estimate of the probable acceptability of what they plan to do. Often this can save much frustration and wasted time.

Minimally invasive procedures avoid penetration of the skin, and since the locus of stimulation in interoception studies is beneath the skin, and the skin is richly endowed with sensory receptors, the design problem often devolves to stimulating a structure under the skin without stimulating the skin itself. The proximal parts of the gastrointestinal tract are exceptions; where per os or per anus, access to the lumen can be achieved with minimal discomfort or risk; however, here also, if the stimulus involves distention of the lumen, distortion of the overlying skin is a potential source of extraneous sensation, for which appropriate controls must be devised and incorporated.

A novel stimulation technique can sometimes provide the key to an experiment that would otherwise appear to be impossible. Non-invasive stimulation of specific cardiovascular receptors presents an especially difficult problem: In addition to actual access, because the vascular system is both anatomically distributed and tightly coupled, the effects of locally applied stimuli propagate to, and influence, distant structures.

Pharmacological activation of the baroreceptors: Bolus injections of vasoactive drugs are technically the most straightforward methods for stimulating the baroreceptors. The injections are to an extent invasive in that they require venous access, and the drugs used are not without some inherent risk – a too rapid rise in blood pressure can be very dangerous; nonetheless, the procedures are considered a standard part of medical practice, and the drugs, which are readily available, have been extensively tested in humans.

Vasoactive drugs were first used to experimentally stimulate baroreceptors and study baroreflex gain in the late 1960s. The drug employed is phenylephrine, which has vasoconstrictor actions similar to the naturally occurring adrenergic neurotransmitter, norepinephrine, but is more stable than norepinephrine and, thus, more convenient to prepare and administer. The baroreflex gain measurement technique is known as the Oxford method (Smythe, Pascoe, & Storlien, 1989).[10]

Vasoconstrictors cause blood pressure to rise by increasing the peripheral resistance; the rise in blood pressure stimulates the high pressure baroreceptors, and the (cardiac inhibitory) baroreflex gain can be assessed by observing the fall in heart rate as a function of the rise in blood pressure or by changes in sympathetic nerve traffic. Phenylephrine, and similar drugs also have been used in behavioral studies of baroreceptor stimulation in humans (Rockstroh et al., 1988). Vasoactive drugs have the advantage that, if administered through an indwelling venous catheter, the actual administration is indistinguishable (to the subject) from that of a vehicle control. For behavioral studies, however, there are two substantial disadvantages to using vasoactive agents to stimulate the baroreceptors, first, most have direct excitatory effects on the CNS (Dworkin et al., 1979), and second, because vasoactive agents act by raising systemic blood pressure, the net blood pressure effects, which are key indices of barostimulation, are not directly observable.

Lower body negative pressure (LBNP): LBNP is a mechanically cumbersome, but physiologically straightforward technique for increasing the proportion of the circulating volume that is sequestered in the large veins,

---

[10] Angiotensin II has also been used for baroreceptor stimulation; however, it has few advantages when compared to norepinephrine analogs, and has the disadvantage of affecting the R-R interval independently of baroreflex mechanisms (Ismay, Lumbers, & Stevens, 1979).

primarily those in the legs. The removal of a volume aliquot from the central circulation, decreases the net venous return to the heart, reduces cardiac filling, and unloads low pressure receptors in the thoracic vascular bed. The LBNP apparatus consists of a large rigid cylindrical tank with a pneumatic seal at the waist. The tank encloses the entire lower body, and in the tank pressure is reduced with a pump, such as a domestic vacuum cleaner, usually by 10–40 mmHg, but sometimes by as much as 70 mmHg. (Larger negative pressures almost always produce syncope, but even pressures as low as −10 mmHg can produce periods of asystole in healthy individuals). It is probable that low levels of LBNP (<20 mmHg) selectively activate volume receptors, and that higher levels also engage the high pressure arterial receptors.

LBNP has been used in both physiological research to analyze reflex interactions in humans (Eckberg & Sleight, 1992), and to an extent, in psychophysiological research to study baroreceptor effects on sensory perception. For perceptual studies the method has the obvious disadvantage that the suction also activates receptors of the skin and pelvic organs, and convincing controls for these extraneous stimuli are difficult to implement. It should also be noted that, although apparently "non-invasive"; there are several reports of extended periods of asystole being induced in healthy volunteers by LBNP (Eckberg & Sleight, 1992, pp. 196–197).

Neck Suction: Distention of a surgically isolated carotid sinus cul de sac is the most widely accepted experimental barostimulation method, and a related, but non-invasive, external pressure stimulation method has been used in humans: The method depends upon the fact that the baroreceptors are actually stretch receptors in the arterial wall, and that although pressure inside the artery normally *pushes* the wall outward, the wall also can be artificially *pulled* outward by extravascular suction applied through an pneumatically sealed collar that encircles the neck. In the usual arrangement a constant or *static negative* pressure in the "neck chamber," sums with the natural pulsatile intracarotid *positive* pressure, and increases the average stretch of the sinus; thus, simulating an elevated mean arterial pressure (MAP). The neck chamber has been used extensively to study the peripheral physiology of the human baroreflex, but, as with LBNP, the "static pressure" neck chamber has a drawback for psychological studies: the neck suction activates receptors in the skin and deeper neck structures, and potentially has additional perceptual/behavioral effects that are unrelated to barostimulation. The static chamber is an effective, but non-specific, barostimulation method.

The usual "first line" strategy for dealing with stimulus non-specificity is to compare the experimental stimulus to an appropriate control stimulus, for example, suction applied to the skin a distance away from the target receptive field; however, for neck suction, a satisfactory way to do this has not been found. Some investigators have used positive neck pressure as the control procedure, but for

several reasons this is not very convincing (Elbert et al., 1988; Rockstroh et al., 1988). The solution to this problem provides an informative case study in designing a stimulation technique. In general, for any interoceptive stimulation method there are always several issues, which need to be considered; these are:

1. What is the effective natural stimulus for the target receptors?

2. Where are the target receptors located?

3. What non-target receptors could be affected?

4. What differences in modal sensitivity exist between the target and non-target receptors?

For the neck chamber, the first three were discussed above. As regards the fourth, an essential fact is that baroreceptors are at least as sensitive to changes in pulse pressure as to the mean pressure. Thus, instead of static or constant suction, it is possible to use sequences of brief cardiac cycle coordinated pressure changes to stimulate or inhibit baroreceptor activity. Eckberg had already shown that brief suction pulses applied randomly during various parts of the cardiac cycle differentially affected subsequent P-P intervals (Eckberg, 1976). However, because suction pulses were random, the barostimulation or inhibition effects that they produced were not controlled, and were transitory (lasting for only a single cycle). This was fully satisfactory for Eckberg's purposes, but limited the utility of the method for psychophysiological studies. To stimulate or inhibit the carotid receptors continuously for as long as several minutes, Eckberg's method was augmented by replacing the randomly produced suction pulses with computer generated cardiac-cycle-synchronized trains of repeatedly alternating pressure and suction pulses that were phase-locked to an R-wave trigger (Dworkin, 1988). Alternating suction during systole with positive pressure during diastole augmented the endogenous carotid sinus pulse pressure (CSPP), whereas reversing the phase relationship (via the valve operating computer program) created a control condition, in which the endogenous CSPP was actually decreased. This Phase Locked Neck Suction (PLNS) method produced heart rates 5–10% lower during stimulation compared to the control condition. Although the pulse pressure effects of the barostimulation condition (cardiac phase synchronized suction), and control condition (cardiac phase inverted suction) have very different cardiovascular effects, they are indistinguishable to the subject (Furedy, Rau, & Roberts, 1992).[11]

Comparison of PLNS and the original static neck chamber technique points up both the advantages and some of the "hidden" costs of specificity: Each method stimulates the baroreceptors; the static technique is a far simpler and, in fact, somewhat more effective in producing baroreflex

---

[11] For better pressure symmetry between conditions, a variable length atmospheric pressure pulse can separate the suction and positive pressure pulses (Rau, Elbert, Geiger, & Lutzenberger, 1992) methods have never been shown to be functionally different.

activation; on the other hand, the PLNS method is considerably more specific: the stimulation and control conditions differ only in baroreceptor activation. In general, it is not unusual for specificity to be obtained at the price of some loss in efficacy. No procedure is completely specific, and a control procedure, if it is efficient, will to some degree stimulate the target receptors. A similar example is found in studies of intestinal pressure sensitivity discussed below.

THE REGULATORY FUNCTIONS OF INTEROCEPTORS

The best studied and most generally accepted role of interoceptors is as afferent components in control loops that regulate the viscera. In fact, interoceptors are the first element of the feedback path of all reflex mechanisms of physiological regulation. In closed loop control systems, usually within broad parametric limits, the characteristics of the feedback path dictate the dynamics, and final level of the regulated variable (Dworkin et al., 2000). Because they occupy a crucial position, interoceptors are directly implicated in many medical conditions, and their properties, as simple transducers, are pivotal to important areas of basic psychophysiologic research.

For example, all of the following processes involve closed-loop control mechanisms that depend upon information derived from visceral sensory receptors: neural regulation of the circulation; the central control of food and fluid intake, energy balance, and electrolyte metabolism; the sensory substrate of behavioral reward, the afferent mechanisms of conditioned aversions, emotion and pain; the mechanisms of addiction and the treatment of substance abuse, non-compliance with medical regimens resulting from the aversiveness of treatment associated side effects, and the pathophysiology of certain psychosomatic conditions.

Specific interoceptors with well defined reflexogenic effects were not directly observed until the second half of the nineteenth century. In 1866, Cyon and Ludwig found that, in the rabbit, heart rate and blood pressure were reduced upon stimulation of the central end of a small nerve that runs along the common carotid artery, adjacent to but separate from the vago-sympathetic trunk.[12] They recognized that the "depressor nerve" conveyed sensation, and, further, proposed that its receptors were in the heart, and were part of a regulator of the heart rate and blood pressure. Eighty years later Bronk and Stella (Bronk & Stella, 1935) used the single fiber method of Adrian (Adrian, 1926) to systematically investigate the properties of the high pressure baroreceptors. Since then, the baroreceptors have been the most thoroughly studied interoceptors, and it is now well established that the "aortic depressor nerves," convey barosensory impulses from receptors

in the aortic arch and distal portion the carotid artery, and that these receptors, along with those in the sinus of the carotid bifurcation (those studied by Stella and Bronk), are the afferent limb of the blood pressure regulating buffer reflexes. The structural and quantitative dynamic aspects of the baroreflexes, and their relationship to the physiological state have been among the most extensively studied interoceptor mechanisms (Dworkin & Dworkin, 2004; Dworkin et al., 2000; Dworkin, Dworkin, & Tang, 2000, 2000; Sagawa, 1983).

Adrian's technique, which has been a key method in interoceptor research involves recording from a small bundle containing a few distinct fibers that have been carefully dissected from a whole nerve. Using this method, Bronk and Stella showed that for a given fiber over a moderate range of pressures there was an approximately linear relationship between intra-sinus pressure and firing rate, and, further, that specific fibers were above threshold and below saturation in only over a limited part of the physiological pressure range. Together, their observations established the important principle of parallel systems of within and between fiber (dynamic and channel) coding that appears to characterize all interoceptors.

As discussed above, most receptors require seconds or minutes to adapt, sufficient time for phasic reflexes, such as orthostasis or salivary secretion, to act. A key property of the negative feedback scheme is that the corrective efferent action of the reflex effectively removes the initiating stimulus from the receptor, and the receptor returns to its basal state, ready for subsequent reactivation. If the corrective action is not achieved within the time constraint of adaptation, of the reflex becomes ineffective and, other mechanisms, which are functionally different from conventional negative feedback, are recruited to restore the basal physiological state. These mechanisms are either non-neural and non-adapting, or neural and adapting. The former are well documented and exemplified by the pressure diuresis effects in the kidney, the latter, which probably involve homotopic conditioning, are presently not well understood, but are likely implicated in long-term regulation of key variables, such as, blood pressure (Dworkin, 1993, see Chapters 7 & 8).

Interoceptive conditioned reflexes: Although the concept of association among stimuli dates to before the British empiricists, the first systematic observations of conditioning in defined reflex systems were by Pavlov in 1897. Pavlovian or classically conditioned responses develop when a sensory conditioned stimulus (CS), which has a weak or no physiological effect, is repeatedly followed by a strong distinct physiological perturbation or unconditioned response (UCR). The UCR is itself produced by application of a second more potent unconditioned stimulus (UCS) that acts at the receptive field of a reflex. With each pairing or trial the physiological effect of the CS increases, and eventually the CS begins to elicit a conditioned response (CR) that mimics the unconditioned physiological reaction.

---

[12] Two years later in 1868, Hering and Breuer identified receptors in the lung which initiated respiratory reflexes. For a detailed history of the discovery of the baroreceptors see Heymans and Neil (Heymans & Neil, 1958, pp. 18–25).

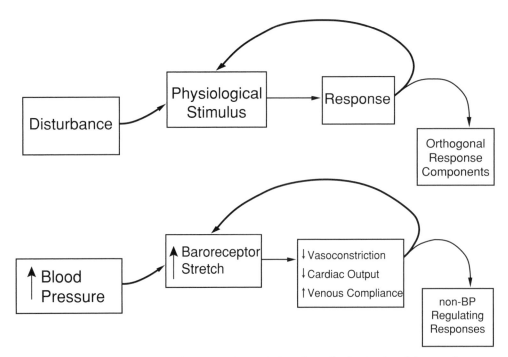

Figure 21.2. The general scheme of an unconditioned physiological reflex (top) and the specific example of the baroreflex (bottom). The leftmost box represents the initiating events of the DISTURBANCE. These events along with the non-orthogonal components of the RESPONSE determine the PHYSIOLOGICAL STIMULUS. The events of the DISTURBANCE form a sequence in time and, thus, the physiological component of the DISTURBANCE is, itself, a function of time. In the baroreflex example a rise in blood pressure distends the blood vessels, and thus stretches endings in the vessel walls. This causes depolarization and firing, which is propagated via afferent fibers in the aortic depressor nerve (ADN), the superior laryngeal nerve (SLN), the vagus and the glossopharyngeal nerve to synapses in nucleus of the solitary tract (NTS). Fibers from the NTS distribute to the cardioinhibitory and vascular depressor centers of the brain stem where efferent activity to the heart and blood vessels is modulated. With increased blood pressure, the modulation is achieved by (somatoinhibitory) reduction of arterial resistance, relaxation of the veins, reduction of the pressure and volume ejected in each cardiac cycle; and (parasympathetic excitatory) slowing of the heart. The net result of this action is a decrease in blood pressure toward the pre-rise baseline, which restores the stretch on the baroceptive endings to the original level, and thus terminates the reflex activity.

It has been thoroughly accepted for nearly 100 years that conditioning can directly modify visceral function. Pavlov's first conditioned reflexes, secretion of gastric juice and saliva, were both glandular responses, and since Pavlov, psychologists and physiologists have established a large literature on classical conditioning of autonomic reflexes, including salivary, sudomotor, cardiac, vascular, pupillary, and gastrointestinal.

Kinds of conditioned reflexes: The common CSs of the conditioning paradigm are sounds, lights, tastes and odors, but, pertinent to the topic of this chapter, various interoceptive stimuli, are also effective conditioned stimuli. In fact, on the basis of the sensory mode of the conditioned and unconditioned stimulus, there is a logical fourfold classification of conditioned reflexes:

(1) Extero-exteroceptive conditioned reflexes associate a weak exteroceptive stimulus such as, a sound, light or vibration, with a stronger, reflex eliciting, somatosensory stimulus such as electric shock.

Elaboration of extero-exteroceptive conditioned reflexes is usually technically straightforward and reliable;

and, typically, they are both rapidly acquired and stable. Extero-exteroceptive conditioned reflexes are most commonly used in research where the focus on is on such things as neurophysiological mechanisms of association; the effects of general variables such as stress, diet, or aging on the discrimination, acquisition, retention, or extinction; or in other studies where the need arises for a convenient generic fragment of learned behavior to be used as a dependent variable.

(2) Extero-interoceptive conditioned reflexes associate a weak exteroceptive stimulus such as a sound, light, or vibration with a stronger, reflex eliciting, visceral stimulus such as food induced gastric secretion, irritant induced salivation, or electrical baroreceptor activation.

Extero-interoceptive conditioned reflexes are usually more circumscribed in effect, and both the creation of the unconditioned stimulus and the measurement of the response are, technically, more involved than for extero-exteroceptive reflexes. Pavlov studied extero-interoceptive reflexes as components of the "cephalic" phase of digestion; however, he also extensively used conditioned salivation, as a "generic" learned response,

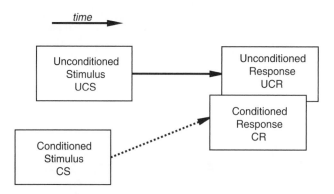

Figure 21.3. The traditional conception of the relationship among stimuli and responses in the classical conditioning paradigm

to study general aspects of association. In recent years, visceral conditioned reflexes have been only rarely used as general indices of behavior; however, there are many recent extero-interoceptive conditioning studies. These have concerned the role of context conditioned compensatory responses in the development of tolerance to drugs (Siegel, 1983; Siegel, Krank, & Hinson, 1987), and in adaptation to specific physiological stresses, such as induced shifts in blood pressure (Dworkin & Dworkin, 1995), blood glucose (Siegel, 1972) or temperature (Siegel, Krank, & Hinson, 1987).

(3) Intero-exteroceptive conditioned reflexes associate an interoceptive stimulus, such as distention of the small intestine, carotid sinus, or renal pelvis with an externally produced skeletal motor reflex, such as shock induced paw withdrawal. The usual goal is to estimate the detectability and discriminability of particular interoceptive stimuli. The conditioned response is a substitute for verbal behavior in infrahuman species, and, in certain special cases, with humans. Examples of this paradigm are discussed below with respect to visceral perception. In a variant of this paradigm the response is an operant, such as bar pressing, which is brought under control of an interoceptive stimulus, such as intra-intestinal pressure (Slucki, Adam, & Porter, 1965).

(4) Intero-interoceptive conditioned reflexes associate an interoceptive stimulus, such as distention of the small intestine, carotid sinus, or renal pelvis, or thermal stimulation of the stomach, or osmotic stimulation of the liver, with a visceral reflex, such as food induced gastric secretion or fluid load induced renal secretion, or the activation of baroreflex. More than 30 years ago Àdàm wrote:

It seems likely that temporary connections initiated by visceral receptors and affecting both vegetative and somatic functions are being continuously established and extinguished, while never becoming conscious. On the basis of our experimental data we suppose that the unconscious interoceptive sphere, too, has a 'memory', i.e., an ability to retain experience, which helps adaptation to changes in the environment. (Adam, 1967, pp. 139–40)

Outside of Eastern Europe intero-interoceptive conditioned reflexes have been little studied; technically, they are comparatively quite demanding: Elaborating a clearly defined intero-interoceptive reflex typically involves performing several separate chronic surgical procedures to prepare access for application of the conditioned and the unconditioned stimuli, and for measurement of the response. Nonetheless, the intero-interoceptive reflex is probably of great importance in physiological regulation. In the quotation from Pavlov which began this chapter the phrase "a constant, correct, and precise correlation becomes established among the parts of an organism" almost certainly refers to intero-interoceptive conditioning.

In fact, normal anatomical juxtaposition of receptors creates many arrangements in which the temporal requirements of conditioning are automatically satisfied. For example, the essence of coordinated GI function is that partially processed chyme leaves one segment and enters the next. In principle, intero-interoceptive conditioning could coordinate action among different parts of the gut. For example, distention in a proximal gut segment could trigger conditioned reflex secretion or motility in a more distal segment. If an oral segment had the necessary receptors, entering chyme could activate these and produce a conditioned stimulus; then, as the chyme entered the next segment, it could produce an unconditioned secretory or motor stimulus that completed the paradigm; thus, with sufficient repetition (conditioning trials), the distention of the oral segment would trigger digestive activity in the aboral segment, which would effectively anticipate arrival of the chyme, and improve its digestion. This intero-interoceptive paradigm parallels the extero-interoceptive

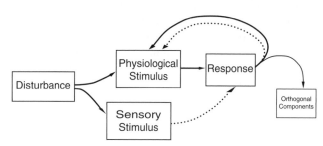

Figure 21.4. A modified conception of the classical conditioning paradigm for visceral reflexes that emphasizes the interaction between conditioned (dotted path) and unconditioned (solid path) reflexes. This revised scheme and terminology puts the conditioning process into a more biologically consistent framework: The Disturbance is an initiating event that changes the physiological and sensory state. It gives rise to a Sensory Stimulus and a Physiological Stimulus. The Sensory Stimulus is clearly the same as the conditioned stimulus, but there is ambiguity in the literature concerning the proper physiological identity of the unconditioned stimulus and unconditioned response. The unconditioned and conditioned responses are together equivalent to the Response; thus, the Response is the total regulatory reaction of the nervous system to the Disturbance (the "Orthogonal components" are other non-regulatory response components) (Dworkin, 1993, see Chapter 3).

paradigm, which Pavlov called the "cephalic phase" of digestion, wherein the sight or aroma of food is the conditioned stimulus that triggers anticipatory salivary or gastric secretion. The Russian physiologists took this general schema quite seriously. Their ideas remain provocative, but their experimental studies (see below) (Bykov, [1942] 1957, pp. 231–279; Bykov & Kurtsin, [1949] 1966, pp. 21–78) need to be replicated with better controls and appropriate statistical analyses.

When common drugs, such as morphine, or ethanol are repeatedly administered certain of their effects weaken, that is, the subject becomes tolerant to the drug. It is now accepted that conditioning of reflex compensatory responses elicited by the drug effects, is an important part of tolerance. The key studies establishing the role of conditioning in drug tolerance have effectively exploited the differential extero-interoceptive paradigm: specific environmental cues (tones, lights, odors, etc.) that could be manipulated were the CS, and the physiological effect of the drug was the UCS. Although the cumulative evidence from these studies showing that conditioning has a role in tolerance is convincing, there have been some contradictory reports. A plausible explanation of these exceptions is that "interoceptive" stimuli produced by the drug, during initial absorption, called "drug onset cues" (DOCs), can function as a potent CS, and "overshadow" explicitly manipulated, but less relevant, environmental stimuli. Because, these DOCs are inextricable from the drug administration, it is difficult to directly manipulate them; recently however, Siegel and his colleagues have described a series of trenchant experiments that convincingly distinguish the effects of the DOCs from the exteroceptive environmental cues (Kim, Siegel, & Patenall, 1999; Sokolowska, Siegel, & Kim, 2002). On the basis of their observations there appears to be little doubt that the DOCs have an important role in drug tolerance. However, whether the DOCs are, in fact, interoceptive stimuli, requires systematic exclusion of possible effects of the initial drug levels on the receptive fields of non-visceral receptors; for example, effects on visual or cutaneous receptors.

Heterotopic or homotopic conditioning: Within cases (1) and (4) above, it is possible to make the additional logical and biologically important distinction of whether the conditioned and unconditioned stimulus are applied in separate or the same sensory modes. For conventional or *heterotopic* conditioning, the CS and UCS are in *different sensory modes*; for example, the CS can be an auditory tone, followed by a UCS of an electric shock to a finger tip. After repeating this stimulus combination many times or "trials," a withdrawal reaction develops to the sound, and the emergence of this new response is evidence of conditioning. For *homotopic* conditioning, both the CS and UCS are applied in the *same sensory mode*. In a roughly parallel example, the CS would be a mild electric current applied on a finger tip, followed by a UCS of a *stronger* current on the same finger tip: With repetition, the withdrawal reaction to the milder CS current will gradually strengthen

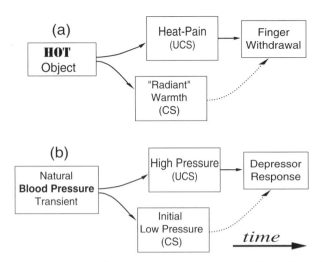

Figure 21.5. For the simple example of avoiding being burned by a sometimes hot object (**a**), homotopic conditioning effectively calibrates the sensory threshold of the defensive withdrawal reflex. By similarly calibrating visceral reflexes, such as the example of the baroreflex in (**b**), interoceptive homotopic conditioning could have an important role in autonomic regulation.

from what it was at the start. The *quantitative change* in the withdrawal response to the weaker current is the measure of conditioning.

There are many commonplace natural adaptations that fit the extero-exteroceptive *homotopic* paradigm. A simple case is the conditioned response that helps in avoiding burns from objects that are sometimes hot: the CS is the radiated warmth that is first sensed as the fingers approach the object, and the UCS is the heat-pain in the fingers on contact: The heat-pain activates a reflex withdrawal, and gradually with "experience," that is, with the accumulation of conditioning trails, the sensation of warmth, that is the CS by itself, triggers the protective withdrawal (see Figure 21.5). If the sensory effects of drug onset cues are, in fact, visceral, then drug tolerance probably involves intero-interoceptive homotopic conditioning. In addition to the morphine tolerance studies cited above, conditioned hyperthermia has been produced using a low dose of ethanol a CS, and a higher dose, which produces a clear hypothermia, as a UCS (Greeley et al., 1984). In ethanol thermic conditioning, the UCS is hypothermia, which is due to vasodilatation and consequent heat loss to the environment; the hypothermia activates compensatory metabolic reflexes, which become conditioned to the CS (Dworkin, 1993, for an analysis of the mechanism see pp. 109–115).

In fact, in a neurophysiological sense, the general properties and cellular anatomy of homotopic conditioning probably closely parallel those of heterotopic conditioning. This is because for most sensory systems, over a wide stimulus range, coding of stimulus magnitude is not confined to increased firing rate, but also involves successive recruitment of higher threshold receptor populations. For example, there are two classes of heat sensing receptors in the fingers: "warmth" receptors, which respond with

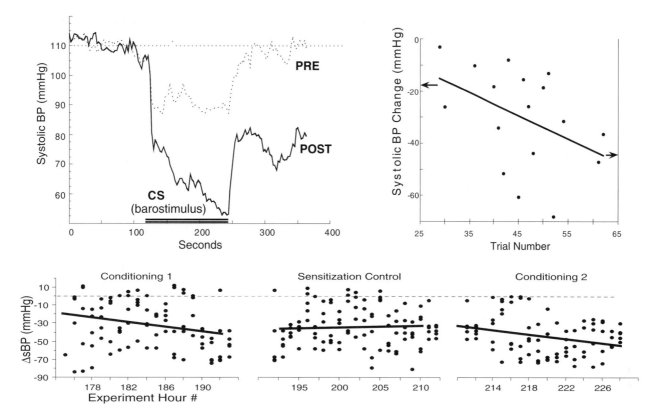

Figure 21.6. Homotopic conditioning of the baroreflex: A rat experiment in which the CS was A-fiber (25 μA, 100 μs, 100 ips) and the US, A + C-fiber stimulation (125 μA, 200 μs, 5 ips). Each sequence was 18 h (90 trials). The top left panel shows the response of a 5 Hz electrical stimulus (the CS) applied to the aortic depressor nerve of a rat, before (pre) and after (post) the CS had been paired with a 25 Hz UCS to the same nerve in a classical conditioning procedure. The top right panel shows the magnitude of the blood pressure response to the 5 Hz (CS) stimulus as a function of the number of conditioning trials (N.B. that the conditioned response is a blood pressure decrease). The effects are in the direction predicted for homotopic conditioning and statistically reliable. The bottom panel shows another homotopic conditioning experiment in which the CS was A-fiber (25 μA, 100 μs, 100 ips) and the US, A + C-fiber stimulation (125 μA, 200 μs, 5 ips). Each sequence was 18 h (90 trials). All of the effects are in the direction predicted for homotopic conditioning and statistically reliable.

increasing discharge rate to temperatures between 32 and 45°C, and heat-pain receptors that begin to fire at only >45°C. As discussed above, the baroreceptors also have this kind of intensity–channel coding arrangement: In their study of the carotid receptors, Bronk and Stella observed that: "...wide variation in threshold for different receptors" (Bronk & Stella, 1932; Bronk & Stella, 1935). Thus, just as do the separate modalities of heterotopic conditioning, the neural representations of the *different strength* homotopic CS and UCS probably enter the CNS over separate axons and project to different synapses.

In the laboratory, homotopic conditioning has been studied much less than heterotopic, in fact, hardly at all; but, there is nothing in conditioning theory that prefers that the CS and UCS be from different sensory modalities; to the contrary, among learning theorists, the usual notion is that the more similar or related are the CS and UCS, the more easily conditioning can occur. In fact, the paucity of research on homotopic conditioning is more likely due to certain practical difficulties in doing the experiments. Although, the homotopic CS is a

relatively weak stimulus, when applied at the receptive field of the unconditioned reflex, before any conditioning has taken place, it measurably activates the reflex. Thus, studying homotopic conditioning requires, at least, the ability to make a reliable *quantitative measurement* of the change of the conditioned response strength from the beginning and to the end of conditioning. For the comparison to be meaningful, the state of the subject must be stable, the response measurements accurate, and the proximal stimuli constant (see Figure 21.6). Because conditioning takes time, these stringent criteria must be met throughout the many hours, or even several days, of an experiment, and the difficulty in accomplishing all of this is probably why intero-interoceptive homotopic conditioning has not been more extensively investigated by psychophysiologists and regulatory physiologists.

Early work on interoceptive conditioning: Probably the first explicit description of an interoceptive conditioned reflex was in 1928 by Bykov and Ivanova (Bykov, [1942] 1957, pp. 246–7). They performed a urinary secretion conditioning experiment in which an unconditioned

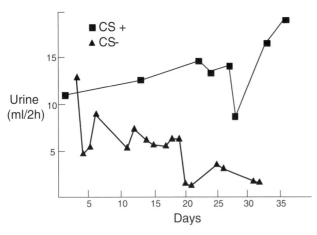

Figure 21.7. This Soviet era experiment used two distinctive stimuli. The "active" stimulus was the a distinctive room where the UCS was administered; the "differential" stimulus was a second dissimilar room, also equipped for measuring urine output. In the "active" room water was administered per rectum and urine collected; in the "differential" room, urine was collected, but no water was administered. The plot shows the daily urine output in the two rooms measured before any water was administered. Initially, the urine output in the differential room was nearly the same as it had been in the active room; this is a typical generalization effect in classical conditioning. As the trials progressed the rate of urine output in the differential room fell; at the same time the urine output in the reinforced room continued rising; thus, a discrimination formed. Bykov described several similar experiments with other dogs, one in which the water load was given by mouth, and another discrimination experiment that used two distinctive bell sounds as conditioned stimuli.

stimulus of 200 ml saline, was infused into a dog's stomach directly through a chronic trans-abdominal fistula. After giving approximately 25 infusions they began to observe that the dog secreted urine as soon as the gastric mucosa was wetted, before a physiologically significant amount of saline was introduced. Eventually they found that if saline was briefly introduced and removed, before it could be absorbed, urine flow developed that was of smaller magnitude, but of similar time course, to that caused by the full load. They designated this an intero-interoceptive conditioned reflex, because both the conditioned stimulus and unconditioned stimulus were interoceptive stimuli. Figure 21.7 describes a similar "discriminative" version of this experiment.

In other Russian experiments, designated "intero-exteroceptive," the conditioned stimulus was interoceptive, but the unconditioned stimulus was exteroceptive. For example, the conditioned stimulus of wetting the gastric mucosa was repeatedly paired with an electric shock to the paw, resulting in conditioned paw withdrawal. Airapetyantz, (Bykov, [1942] 1957, pp. 249–51) another of Bykov's coworkers demonstrated the formation of a discrimination between 26°C and 36°C intragastric water. After 150 trials in which a salivary unconditioned stimulus followed a 36° but not (otherwise identical) 26° water infusions, only the 36° stimulus produced a reliable flow of saliva. Airapetyantz and his associates also did a number of similar experiments with other intestinal interoceptors

as conditioned stimuli, for example, they formed discriminated salivary responses to pH and temperature stimuli in isolated intestinal segments.

The general conclusions of the Eastern European scientists were that interoceptive conditioned reflexes, when compared to their exteroceptive counterparts, required a larger and more variable numbers of trials to become stable; however, that once formed, interoceptive reflexes had the essential characteristics typical of exteroceptive reflexes, including inhibition of delay and susceptibility to disruption by novel stimuli (external inhibition).

IS DRIVE NECESSARY FOR FORMATION AND CONSOLIDATION OF A CONDITIONED RESPONSE?

The standard conception of the classical conditioning paradigm is shown in Figure 21.3; Figure 21.4 extends the paradigm for visceral reflexes to include the feedback mechanisms of regulation, and emphasizes that, for visceral reflexes, the conditioned response also can have important regulatory consequences. Nonetheless, both figures presume a similar, relatively uncomplicated, and traditional neurophysiological conception of classical conditioning: Beginning with Pavlov, and for the 50 years following him, the central dogma was that the temporal contiguity of a neutral stimulus and a reflex formed an association; however, McGaugh's work in the 1960s suggested that learning, especially consolidation, in distinction to formation of an association, might be affected by pharmacological manipulation of relatively non-specific central adrenergic and cholinergic mechanisms (McGaugh, 1966); also, that certain kinds of natural stimuli also might influence consolidation (McGaugh, 1989). There is evidence that aversive stimuli, such as shock, can enhance the retention; that shock also activates central adrenergic mechanisms, and that the amygdala and its major pathway, the striate terminalis, are involved in both the pharmacological and shock effects. If these findings prove valid for interoceptive reflexes, such "motivational" influences on conditioning could have implications for the plasticity of regulatory mechanisms.

In the preface to the 1957 English edition of *The Cerebral Cortex and the Internal Organs*, Bykov wrote, "The higher regulating apparatus determines and preserves the unity and integrity of all the complex executive organs and tissues, receiving information through the extero- and interoceptors. The cortex is *at every moment* determining the fate of every reaction of the organism." Reading Bykov's book leaves little doubt that he meant that there was a continuous formation and extinction of conditioned reflexes, with each successive association slightly changing the visceral regulatory network.

This view of an ongoing calculus, *continuously* reorganizing and adjusting the network to optimum (Dworkin, 1993, see Chapters 3 and 4) is possibly entirely correct; however, interoceptive conditioning also could be *saltatorial*: that is, new synaptic connections might form, or connection strengths be modified only infrequently and under special circumstances, for example, when the extant central visceral network does not adequately constrain the physiological state within limits that are compatible with the adjustment capacity of non-neural peripheral mechanisms (Dworkin, 1993, see Ch. 6 pp. 118–122). Thus, for central connections to be modified, in addition to stimulus association, a net homeostatic imbalance also might need to be present. By activating visceral receptors, the imbalance would, in a manner similar to shock or direct neurochemical manipulations, activate central adrenergic mechanisms (Gold, 1984), possibly via the amygdala (McGaugh, Cahill, & Roozendaal, 1996), and enable consolidation.

Traditional conceptions of learning distinguish between the classical and operant conditioning paradigms, and the suggestion of a dependence of synaptic modification on "homeostatic imbalance," inevitably brings to mind the operant model's distinctive features of motivation or drive; and reinforcement or drive reduction (Dworkin, 1993, see Chapters 7 and 8). However, there is a substantial difference: in the operant model, the strengthening of a particular response requires, specifically, that the response bring about (or at lest be well correlated with) a reduction of the homeostatic imbalance; whereas, in this "drive dependent" view of classical conditioning, the postulated neurochemical effects of the imbalance only must be present during and/or following the association of the CS and UCS.[13]

PERCEPTION OF THE VISCERA AND VISCERAL INFLUENCES ON BEHAVIOR

Historically "interoception" has had a number of different meanings. In addition to the well documented regulatory functions already discussed, interoceptors have been attributed more general perceptual functions that parallel those of the receptors of exteroception and proprioception. It is through exteroceptors that we develop a detailed functional model – a conscious perception – of the environment, and similarly through proprioceptors, that we apprehend the position and motion of the parts of our skeleton in space. The conscious perception of visceral states, and the control of autonomic and skeletal behaviors, including verbal reports of visceral stimuli are also potentially important. But unlike exteroception and proprioception, which are clearly phenomenologically valid,

robust, and functionally important, there remains some reasonable doubt about whether conscious perception of the viscera is other than a comparatively fragile laboratory curiosity. There is no doubt that, for most visceral organs, sufficiently strong stimulation produces a conscious perception of pain; however, although there has been extensive and excellent work on visceral perception, it is not entirely established whether, under normal circumstances, except for some special cases, such as gastric "hunger"[14] contractions, there is general awareness of sensations from sub-noxious stimuli in the *deep* internal organs. Furthermore, if substantial non-pain conscious awareness of the deep viscera does exist, its function, if any, is unknown.

Typical dictionary definitions distinguish "sensation" as the immediate result of a "sensory input" from "perception," which involves a combination of sensations, as well as memory of past sensations. Psychologists often further distinguish perception from discrimination, which is the ability to distinguish stimulus levels and/or stimulus qualities. This distinction is important; however, it is necessary to also recognize that without there being direct perception or discrimination of the stimulus, a visceral stimulus can have substantial effects on perception and sensation.

For example, baroreceptor activation reduces the arousal level; and attenuates both spinal level reflexes, and the reported painfulness of noxious stimuli (Dworkin et al., 1994). But, most naive human subjects can not reliably distinguish baroreceptor activation conditions from control conditions (Furedy et al., 1992); thus, baroreceptor activation, itself, is probably not directly perceived or discriminated. This is an example of where, without being directly perceived, a visceral stimulus can measurably affect behavior and the perception of other stimuli. Parallel phenomena have been described for the abdominal organs: For example, Kukorelli and Juhàsz showed that EEG synchronization and sleep could be induced by levels of sub-noxious stimulation of the intestine and abdominal nerves (Kukorelli & Juhàsz, 1976, 1977), which probably would not be directly perceived.

The control of ingestion is the most extensively studied and analyzed example of interoception. The first modern observations of intestinal perception were made by Walter B. Cannon with his student Washburn. Using simultaneous kymographic recording of intragastric pressure and behavioral responses, they observed a temporal relationship between gastric contractions and "hunger pangs"(Cannon & Washburn, 1912). These observations (in which Wasburn was the subject) are illustrated and described in Figure 21.8, and the accompanying legend. Largely on the basis of these and other "correlational" studies using kymographic or radiographic measures of intestinal movement, Cannon concluded that the experience of hunger derived from the perception of gastric

[13] The distinction between the classical, and operant or instrumental, paradigms is actually less definite: Although B. F. Skinner conceived of the operant response as a strictly random event (Skinner, 1981), in Neal Miller's reformulation of instrumental learning (Miller, 1959) response probabilities (which determine the order of the "response hierarchy") became a deterministic function of the motivational (drive) state, which, itself, is subject to classical conditioning. Especially for physiological regulatory responses, Miller's idea of a response-determining drive (interoceptive stimulus) state fittingly brings together instrumental, and drive dependent classical, conditioning.

[14] In fact, Cannon described hunger as, "a very disagreeable ache or pang or sense of gnawing or pressure which is referred to the epigastrium" (Cannon, 1939, p. 70); thus that hunger is a "non-noxious" interoception is at least arguable.

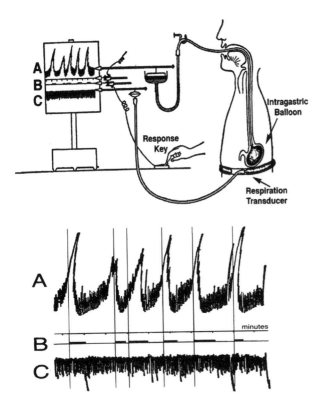

Figure 21.8. (top) Cannon's student, Washburn, learned to swallow a balloon, which registered the contractions of his stomach. Another transducer was placed around his abdomen to register the movement of his abdominal muscles. When Washburn perceived a "hunger pang" he pressed the response key. The entire set of events was recorded on a kymograph, a primitive polygraph device, as a function of time. (bottom) The record shows the relationship between the gastric contractions and the "pangs." Cannon concluded two thing from this record: first, that the perception was related to stomach contractions, not to movements of the abdominal wall, and second, that the contractions preceded the perception in time. Cannons original figure did not include the vertical cursors, which have been inserted in this version: he said that the "hunger pang was not recorded until the contraction had nearly reached its peak"; yet the cursors show that the "pang" marker always begins quite early in the contraction, and that the relationship is, in fact, more variable than might be expected from a simple coupling.

contractions.[15] However, by the mid-century a substantial body of data accumulated in conflict with Cannon's simple "gastric perception" model of hunger: For example, in humans, most of the stomach can be excised or the vagus nerve severed, without loss of either hunger motivation or the experience of hunger.

Nonetheless, in contrast to the clinical evidence that peripheral signals are not essential to the experience of *hunger*, sophisticated laboratory studies have clearly implicated gastrointestinal stimuli in the interoceptive control of *ingestion* (McHugh & Moran, 1985). Hunt showed that the osmotic pressure of the chyme influenced both gastric motility and the rate of gastric emptying; and that energy content and volume were also important control stimuli (Hunt, 1961; Hunt & Stubbs, 1975), and Mei found specific glucoreceptors in the small intestine (Mei, 1978). Additional studies of the control of motility, gastric emptying, and satiety, have focused on the role of gastric load, mechanical and chemical properties of intestinal contents, and various hormonal receptors, particularly those sensitive to, the octapeptide, cholecystokinin.

The work of McHugh, Moran, and Schwartz is especially notable in emphasizing the integration of various stimuli by individual interoceptors. For example, Schwartz and Moran (1996) have described the additive effect of cholecystokinin on the firing rate of intraluminal volume sensitive vagal afferents. Using a sophisticated rat preparation (see Figure 21.9, left), they showed that isolated single vagal afferents had polymodal sensitivity, "responding to both mechanical stimulation . . . and to exogenous administration of a peptide that is released by the duodenum presence of nutrients." Pre-treatment with cholecystokinin caused the vagal gastric mechano-sensitive afferents to fire at a higher rate for the same load. At concentrations of cholecystokinin, or at intragastric volumes, that individually were too low to activate the afferents, prior application of cholecystokinin produced rapid firing to the volume stimulus (see Figure 21.9, right); thus, operating within a classical regulatory mechanism, cholecystokinin and mechanoreceptor effects apparently summate and enhance the activity of the efferent limb of appropriate digestive reflexes. Because effects of the compound stimulus were effective at levels that individually were ineffective, at low stimulus levels, the effects have features of a multiplicative interaction. If the subthreshold levels used in the analysis are in the normal physiological range, then an interaction would have regulatory implications beyond simple summation; however, given the apparent linearity of the combined suprathreshold effects (see Figure 21.9) it is more probable that the afferents are polymodal and that the cholecystokinin and mechanical receptors, are distinct structures that independently produce additive effects. This means that either cholecystokinin *or* gastric load would have similar functional consequences in the CNS; in other words, that for reflex activation, neither depends upon the other.

In a conceptualization, somewhat reminiscent of the Russian School, Moran and Schwartz (Schwartz & Moran, 1996, p. 49) have emphasized the general perceptual nature of the complex stimulus patterns that arise in the gut: "Furthermore, we view the constellation of meal-related stimuli arising from several gastrointestinal compartments as comprising a context representative of the internal milieu during a meal. . . . Thus, it is critical to establish responses to individual properties

---

[15] Cannon also had a similar conception of thirst. William James anteceded Cannon at Harvard, and in Cannons time James's ideas about emotion were still influential. Although Cannon expressed doubt about the physiological basis of the peripheral emotion theory of James and Carl Lange, in fact, his conception of motivation unquestionably paralleled it.

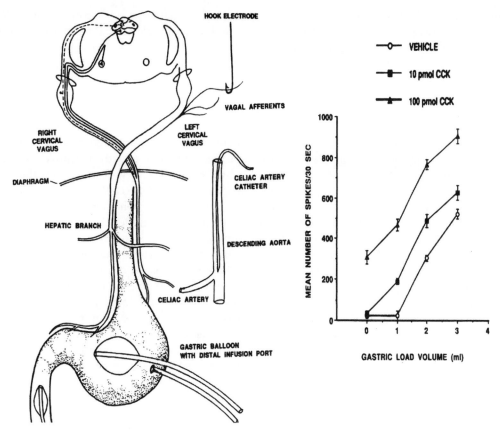

Figure 21.9. The preparation used by Schwartz and Moran for analysis of the interaction of the effects of cholecystokinin and mechanical (volume) distention on single vagal afferent fibers with receptors in the stomach. The left panel shows the experimental preparation, which enables simultaneous stimulation of gastric mechanoreceptors, infusion of CCK into the celiac artery and recording of afferent activity in single vagal fibers. The right panel shows the effect of various doses of CCK on the response of vagal afferents. Note that at higher doses the effect is additive.

and then elucidate the integrative capacities of sensory afferents responding to combinations of properties likely to occur in the context of a meal in the gastrointestinal tract." It remains to be determined whether, in understanding complex integrative processes, this quasi-cognitive formulation has advantages over explicit algebraic control-theoretic, or statistically based "autonomic space" (Berntson, Cacioppo, & Quigley, 1991) formulations of the same effects.

Innate and learned conscious perception: In that stimulation that does not normally reach consciousness can have detectable behavioral effects, it is arguable that given the possibility of learning, a non-conscious stimulus could eventually become conscious. For example, if a non-conscious *conditioning* stimulus affects general arousal or modifies the conscious perception of other stimuli, with appropriate discrimination training, a subject should be able to acquire the capability to estimate and report, at least indirectly, the presence and/or intensity of the *conditioning* stimulus itself. Discrimination training is known to be helpful in reestablishing bowel continence in adults (Whitehead & Schuster, 1983); it is also likely an important factor in the normal development of the perception

of bladder and rectal distention, and is almost certainly involved in the primary establishment of fecal and urinary continence. Experimental results, discussed below, indicate that the perception threshold for bowel distention can, in fact, be lowered with training.

Whether normal consciousness of interoceptive stimuli, any more so than consciousness of exteroceptive or proprioceptive stimuli, requires discrimination practice is not known. A more biological way of putting this same question is to ask, Does the neuroanatomy of interoception provide access to the neurophysiological substrates of consciousness, equivalent to that of exteroception or proprioception? Without doubt, various forms of this question tacitly motivate much of interoception research; however, at present, our understanding of what consciousness is (and isn't) neurophysiologically, and conceptually remains sufficiently immature that it is difficult to know where to start seeking an answer. Notwithstanding, it is clear that neither interoception or consciousness are homogeneous classes of phenomena, and that both interact with, are affected by, and effect changes in behavior; thus, without getting into the nature of consciousness, some useful distinctions can be drawn.

Visceral sensations have obvious and direct effects on behavior, but the selectivity and sensitivity of different tissues varies enormously. For conscious perception, and other effects on behavior, the strength of a stimulus and its anatomical site of application interact.

Strong visceral stimuli can function in two ways: First, because various unconditioned defensive reflexes confer a survival advantage, they were selected and well conserved during the evolutionary history of the species. Strong visceral stimuli can promptly activate these simple defensive reflexes that directly and efficiently ameliorate the visceral irritation. Second, in addition to specific reflexes, general mechanisms of behavioral reinforcement and learning were also established durnig evolution. Acting through these mechanisms, pain or discomfort of visceral origin mobilizes more complex and flexible sequences of behavior. In contrast to the specific reflexes, motivated sequences are not focused, and do not immediately ameliorate the initiating stimulus; however, because the reduction of pain or discomfort is a powerful behavioral reinforcer, *for a given individual*, those behavioral sequences, which reliably antecede pain reduction, have a high probability of being selected and strengthened by learning mechanisms.[16]

Distention of the urinary bladder is a straightforward example of both kinds of interoceptor effects: The muscle of the bladder wall, the detrusor, contains mechanoreceptors; extreme distention strongly activates these receptors and triggers an organized reflex that incites prompt "involuntary" enuresis; whereas, moderate bladder distention *motivates* a more elaborate and variable pattern of behavior that potentially leads to better controlled and more convenient micturition. This sequence is then reinforced by relief of the aversive sensations from the bladder. Another example of both mechanisms is mechanical or chemical stimulation of the nasal mucosa: Strong stimulation by an irritant produces greatly increased serous and mucous secretion, and sneezing, which together comprise a protective defensive reflex that can immediately clear the irritant from the upper respiratory tract; whereas, weaker stimulation *motivates* a more flexible and variable behavior pattern leading to more controlled expulsion of the irritant – for example, by blowing the nose into a handkerchief. Again, the successful sequence is reinforced by relief from the irritation.

In normal individuals both moderate and strong sensations from the mechanoreceptors of the detrusor are readily perceived, and the presence of a nasal irritant is also easily recognized. However, recognition of the irritant is not ipso facto required to activate simple reflexes, and awareness also may not be prerequisite for the irritant to have a motivational effect (Hefferline & Perera, 1963). Instead, the crucial factor is whether the neural activity, generated by the receptor, reaches the integrative centers where an appropriate effect is initiated.

It could be asserted that bladder distention and nasal irritation are special cases because, although the receptors involved are not actually on the body surface, they are just barely within it. In fact, this assertion has some merit, and in general, the distinction between exteroception and interoception is often not definite. A brief tour through the gastrointestinal tract illustrates this: From the top down, most everyone would agree that sensations of the lips are not interoception; most would also concur that sensations from the oral mucosa, and maybe even the pharynx should not be considered interoceptive. But, at the esophagus, the consensus would likely weaken. There are certainly reflexes, which are activated when things go wrong in the esophagus, there is pain (heartburn) and more moderate sensations as well. We perceive "burning" from too hot a beverage, and often even can sense the passage of a hot bolus down the tube; this is also true for very cold liquids or ice cream. We also are aware when something too large or dry has been swallowed and is having a difficult passage. On the whole, most sensations from the esophagus are unpleasant, but not necessarily "painful." Esophageal sensations are not as well defined as those from more oral loci: spatial discrimination is less precise, and stimulus qualities are not as distinct. Aside from the special case of sensations associated with hunger, there little if any evidence of any entirely non-painful sensation from receptors in the stomach.

Beginning at the bottom and proceeding orally the sequence is similar: The anus has clear and detailed sensation; the rectum certainly has pain, distention, and probably some amount of temperature sensitivity. Activation of receptors in both regions can trigger both direct reflexes and motivate more complex behaviors: for example, toilet use. However, above the sigmoid flexure perception is again more equivocal. There are some laboratory data which show that, below the pain threshold, the colon has sensitivity to distention, and that stimuli in the descending colon, which are only several centimeters apart, can, after special training, be discriminated. But there is no evidence that different qualities, such as temperature and pressure can be discriminated.

---

[16] Motivation might also be derived from positive sensations. Students of learning have long debated about the differences between the function of positive and negative sensations in eliciting reflexes and motivating behavior (Miller, 1959, 1966; Stellar & Stellar, 1985). For example, Pavlov used both weak acid and meat powder to elicit salivation (Pavlov, [1897] 1910). Acid is an obvious irritant, and the bicarbonate secretion of the salivary reflex neutralizes the acid, but is it reasonable to consider meat powder, in a parallel sense, also as an irritant? Probably not: The effects of the meat are more complicated, and this becomes evident when the acid or meat are used as behavioral reinforcers, to modify more general behavior, rather than as simple unconditioned stimuli. The reinforcing effects of the two on antecedent behavior are, in fact, opposite. Along related lines, the sensory effects of the intestinal hormone cholecystokinin have been the subject of vigorous debate. CCK produces satiety, i.e. simulating the sensory effects of a satisfactory meal (Smith & Gibbs, 1994), but at higher doses its effects more closely resemble nausea. Although nausea and satiety may have similar unconditioned effects on eating, the potential motivational consequences are likely quite different.

The small intestine has an extensive array of sensory receptors: Distention or surface irritation activates local peristaltic and other reflexes, which are mediated both by the intrinsic myenteric plexus, and extra-intestinal inter-segmental pathways. For example, stimulating the duo-denum or proximal jejunum by distention, acid or lipid, promptly inhibits gastric motility, and relaxes the stom-ach. Nonetheless, evidence of specific sub-pain level per-ception in either half of the small intestine is equivocal. Àdàm originally showed that sub-noxious balloon disten-tion of the duodenal wall causes desynchronization of the EEG (Àdàm et al., 1965). He eventually extended this fun-damental finding to a differential (two point) paradigm, which was mentioned above. The details of these stud-ies were described in his monograph on interoception and behavior (Àdàm, 1967). More recently, to explore the sensibility of distal intestinal segments, Àdàm stud-ied enterostomy patients. He found that some of these subjects could successfully discriminate moderate degrees of balloon distention of the small intestine; however, the subsequent inclusion of carefully designed control proce-dures in these studies showed that the apparent intero-ception was likely, at least in part, due to stretching of the overlying abdominal wall or the skin surrounding the papilla.

To do these enterostomy studies, Àdàm constructed a special intraintestinal catheter with an attached annular skin stimulation balloon. Using a similar but modified instrument, for colon stimulation in normal subjects, Hölzl extended Àdàm's findings, and developed a sophisticated signal detection analysis of the interaction of the skin and intraintestinal stimuli. In irritable bowel patients, Hölzl found that, depending on the temporal and spatial rela-tionship among the stimuli, skin stimulation can either summate with, or mask, intestinal stimulation (Holzl et al., 1996). Hölzl has also analyzed these effects in terms of intra or intersegmental convergence of the sensory fields. His results in normal subjects and patients indicate that detection of stimuli is possible without the subjects aware-ness, but that "localization" requires stimuli sufficiently strong to produce "conscious subjective sensation"(Hölzl, Erasmus, & Möltner, 1996).

Concerning the conscious perception of visceral stimuli, in 1967 Görgy Àdàm said,

In summarizing, we tend to believe that in man the majority of interoceptive impulses influence behaviour without, how-ever, causing any subjective sensation. . . . The question might now arise as to whether . . . visceral impulses entering con-sciousness actually occurs in conditions of normal life. It can be assumed that the interoceptive components of functions important for the individual (hunger, thirst) and socially (mic-turition, defecation) become conditioned in early childhood with exteroceptive stimuli, and the reinforcement of impulses other than these would constitute too great a stress for the higher nervous centers; in other words, to bring into con-sciousness such internal processes would be pathological.

– (Adam, 1967)

Although there remains little support for the notion that consciousness perception of the viscera can be "patholog-ical," research in the intervening 35 years has not substan-tially contradicted Àdàm's basic conclusion.

SUMMARY

(1) Almost all visceral structures have an extensive array of primary sensors, or interoceptors that are the sensory radix of the afferent limb of the dynamic visceral reflexes that stabilize the internal milieu. It is well accepted that many different unconditioned interoceptive reflexes have important physiological functions.

(2) Interoceptive stimuli can function as conditioned stimuli for visceral and somatic conditioned reflexes, and these intero-exteroceptive, or intero-interoceptive reflexes may coordinate of various visceral-visceral and visceral-somatic relationships. Interoceptive condition-ing is fruitful subject for further study with important implications for drug tolerance and autonomic regula-tion.

(3) The special case of the homotopic conditioned reflex, particularly the intero-interoceptive form, could have a central role in drug tolerance and in calibration of the sensitivity and dynamic characteristics of visceral regulators, such as the baroreflex.

(4) There is conscious perception of non-noxious stimuli from certain visceral organs; however as empha-sized throughout this chapter, the validity of this con-clusion depends on the definitions of "perception" and "visceral." For the most part, it can probably be said that normal perception of non-noxious stimuli is limited to special functions, such as hunger, or to special struc-tures, such as the bladder or rectum. There is a strong possibility that conscious perception in special struc-tures, especially those which communicate with the external environment, is not direct, and that perception exists, at least to a large degree, because of learned asso-ciations with more perspicuous proprioceptive and exte-roceptive stimuli during ontogeny. Aside from certain well recognized special cases, it is not clear that con-scious perception of visceral stimuli is important to nor-mal physiological function.

(5) Separate from conscious perception, there are well established effects of non-noxious interoceptive stim-uli on higher CNS function and on behavior. Appropri-ate interoceptive stimulation can affect satiety, modify reflex activity or pain perception and produce EEG syn-chronization and sleep. In addition to their direct con-sequences, these "non-conscious" CNS effects may be substrates of associative processes involved in the devel-opment of conscious visceral perception.

(6) All visceral sensory receptors adapt, and therefore do not to provide the continuous negative feed-back signals required steady state regulation through conventional control mechanisms. If interoceptors do participate in long-term regulation, the mechanism, by which they do, remains to be demonstrated. This is also an important area for future investigations.

REFERENCES

Adam, G. (1967). *Interoception and Behavior: An experimental study*. (R. Chatel & R. Slucki, Trans.). Budapest: Akademiai Kiado.

Àdàm, G., Preisich, P., Kukorelli, T., & Kelemen, V. (1965). Changes in human cerebral electrical activity in response to mechanical stimulation of the duodenum. *Electroencephalography and Clinical Neurophysiology, 18*, 409–415.

Adrian, E. D. (1926). The impulses produced by sensory nerve endings. Part 1. *Journal of Physiology, 61*, 49–72.

Axelrod, J. (1984). Stress hormones: Their interaction and regulation. *Science, 224*, 452–459.

Bàrdos, G., Nagy, J., & Àdàm, G. (1980). Thresholds of behavioral reactions evoked by intestinal and skin stimulation in rats. *Physiology and Behavior, 24*, 661–665.

Batman, B. A., Hardy, J. C., Leuenberger, U. A., Smith, M. B., Yang, Q. X., & Sinoway, L. I. (1994). Sympathetic nerve activity during prolonged rhythmic forearm exercise. *J Appl Physiol, 76*(3), 1077–1081.

Berntson, G. G., Cacioppo, J. T., & Quigley, K. S. (1991). Autonomic determainism: The modes of autonomic control, the doctrine of autonomic space, and the laws of autonomic constraint. *Psychological Review, 98*, 459–487.

Brenner, J., & Jones, J. M. (1974). Interoceptive discrimination in intact humans: Detection of cardiac activity. *Physiology and Behavior, 13*, 763–767.

Brodal, A. (1969). *Neurological Anatomy* (2nd ed.). New York: Oxford.

Bronk, D. W., & Stella, G. (1932). Afferent impulses in the carotid sinus nerve. *Journal of Cell and Comparative Physiology, 1*, 113–130.

Bronk, D. W., & Stella, G. (1935). The response to steady pressures of single end organs in the isolated carotid sinus. *The American Journal of Physiology, 110*, 708–714.

Browning, E. T., Brostrom, C. O., & Groppi, V. E., Jr. (1976). Altered adenosine cyclic 3',5'-monophosphaste synthesis and degradation by C-6 astrocytoma cells following prolonged exposure to norepinephrine. *Molecular Pharmacololgy, 12*, 32–40.

Bykov, K. M. ([1942] 1957). *The cerebral cortex and the internal organs*. (T. f. t. R. a. e. b. W. H. Gantt, Trans.). New York: Chemical Publishing Co.

Bykov, K. M., & Kurtsin, I. T. ([1949]1966). *The corticovisceral theory of the pathogenesis of peptic ulcer* (T. f. t. R. a. e. b. S. A. Corson, Trans.). Oxford: Pergamon Press.

Cannon, W. B. (1939). *The wisdom of the body*. (2nd ed.). New York: W. W. Norton and Company.

Cannon, W. B., & Washburn, A. L. (1912). An explanation of Hunger. *American Journal of Physiology, 29*, 441–455.

Chapman, K. M., & Pankhurst, J. H. (1976). Strain sensitivity and directionality in cat atrial mechanoreceptors in vitro. *Journal of Physiology, 259*, 405–426.

Chernigovskiy, V. N. (1967). *Interoceptors* (a. e. b. D. B. L. Translated from the Russian by G. Onischenko, Trans.). Washington: American Psychological Association.

Deguchi, T., & Axelrod, J. (1973). Supersensitivity and subsensitivity of the β-adrenergic receptor in pineal gland regulated by catecholamine transmitter. *Proceedings of the National Academy of Sciences, 70*, 24411–24414.

Dworkin, B. (1988). Hypertension as a learned response: The baroreceptor reinforcement hypothesis. In T. Elbert, W. Langosch, A. Steptoe & D. Vaitl (Eds.), *Behavioral medicine in cardiovascular disorders* (pp. 17–47). Chichester: John Wiley & So.

Dworkin, B. R. (1993). *Learning and Physiological Regulation*. Chicago: University of Chicago Press.

Dworkin, B. R., & Dworkin, S. (1995). Learning of physiological responses: II. Classical conditioning of the baroreflex. *Behavioral Neuroscience, 109*, 1119–1136.

Dworkin, B. R., & Dworkin, S. (2004). Baroreflexes of the rat. III. Open-loop gain and electroencephalographic arousal. *Am J Physiol Regul Integr Comp Physiol, 286*(3), R597–605.

Dworkin, B. R., Dworkin, S., & Tang, X. (2000). Carotid and aortic baroreflexes of the rat I: open-loop steady-state properties and blood pressure variability. *Am. J. Physiol. Regulatory integrative Comp. Physiol., 279*, R1910-R1921.

Dworkin, B. R., Elbert, T., Rau, H., Birbaumer, N., Pauli, P., Droste, C., et al. (1994). Central effects of baroreceptor activation in humans: Attenuation of skeletal reflexes and pain perception. *Proceedings of the National Academy of Sciences USA, 91*, 6329–6333.

Dworkin, B. R., Filewich, R. J., Miller, N. E., Craigmyle, N., & Pickering, T. G. (1979). Baroreceptor activation reduces reactivity to noxious stimulation: Implications for hypertension. *Science, 205*, 1299–1301.

Dworkin, B. R., Tang, X., Snyder, A., & Dworkin, S. (2000). Carotid and aortic baroreflexes of the rat II: open-loop frequency response and the blood pressure spectrum. *Am. J. Physiol. Regulatory integrative Comp. Physiol., 279*, R1922–R1933.

Eckberg, D. L. (1976). Temporal response patterns of the human sinus node to brief carotid baroreceptor stimuli. *Journal of Physiology, 258*, 769–782.

Eckberg, D. L., & Sleight, P. (1992). *Human Baroreflexes in health and Disease* (Vol. 43). Oxford: Clarendon Press.

Elbert, T., Lutzenberger, W., Rockstroh, B., Kessler, M., Pietrowsky, R., & Birbaumer, N. (1988). Baroreceptor stimulation increases pain threshold in borderline hypertensives. *Psychophysiology, 25*, 25–29.

Faber, J. E., & Brody, M. J. (1983). Reflex hemodynamic response to superior laryngeal nerve stimulation in the rat. *Journal of the Autonomic Nervous System, 9*, 607–622.

Furedy, J., Rau, H., & Roberts, L. (1992). Physiological and psychological differentiation of bidirectional baroreceptor carotid manipulation in humans. *Physiology and Behavior, 52*, 953–958.

Gavin, J. R., Rothe, J., Neville, J., D. M., De Meyts, P., & Buell, D. N. (1974). Insulin-dependent regulation of insulin receptor concentrations: A direct demonstration in cell culture. *Proceedings of the National Academy of Sciences, 71* (84–88).

Ghione, S. (1996). Hypertension-Associated Hypalgesia. *Hypertension, 28*, 494–504.

Gold, P. E. (1984). Memory Modulation: Roles of Peripheral Catecholamines. In L. R. Squire & N. Butters (Eds.), *Neuropsychology pf Memory* (pp. 566–578). New York: The Guilford Press.

Gray, J. A. B., & Malcolm, J. L. (1951). The excitation of touch receptors in a frog's skin. *Journal of Physiology, 115*, 1–15.

Gray, J. A. B., & Matthews, P. B. C. (1951). A comparison of the adaptation of the pacinian corpuscle with the accommodation of its own axon. *Journal of Physiology, 114*, 454–464.

Greeley, J., Le, D. A., Poulos, C. X., & Cappell, H. (1984). Alcohol is an effective cue in the conditional control of tolerance to alcohol. *Psychopharmacology, 83*, 159–162.

Hefferline, R. F., & Perera, T. B. (1963). Propioceptive discriminatin of a covert operant without its observation by the subject. *Science, 13*, 834–835.

Heymans, C., & Neil, E. (1958). *Reflexogenic areas of the cardiovascular system*. Boston: Little, Brown and Company.

Hölzl, R., Erasmus, L., Kröger, C., Whitehead, W. e., & Ottenjann, R. *Analysis of Visceral Hyperalgesia in Symptomatic Subgroups of the "Irritable Bowel Syndrome"* (Forschungberichte No. 29). Mannheim: Otto-Seltz-Institut (University of Mannheim).

Hölzl, R., Erasmus, L., & Möltner, A. (1996). Detection, discrimination and sensation of visceral stimuli. *Biological Psychology, 42*, 199–214.

Hunt, J. N. (1961). Osmotic control of gastric emptying. *Gastroenterology, 41*, 49–51.

Hunt, J. N., & Stubbs, D. F. (1975). The volume and energy content of meals as determinants of gastric emptying. *Journal of Physiology (London), 245*, 209–225.

Ismay, M. J. A., Lumbers, E. R., & Stevens, A. D. (1979). The action of angiotensin II on the baroreflex response of the conscious ewe and the conscious fetus. *The Journal of Physiology, 288*, 467–479.

Jänig, W., & Häbler, H.-J. (1995). Visceral-autonomic integration. In G. F. Gebhart (Ed.), *Visceral pain. Progress in pain research and management*. (Vol. 4, pp. 311–348). Seattle: IASP Press.

Jones, G. E. (1994). Perception of visceral sensations: A review of recent findings, methodologies, and future directions. *Advances in Psychophysiology, 5*, 55–192.

Kappagoda, C. T., & Padsha, M. (1980). Transducer properties of atrial receptors in the dog avter 60 min of increased atrial pressure. *Canadian Journal of Physiological Pharmacology, 59*, 837–842.

Kezdi, P. (1962). Mechanism of the carotid sinus in experimental hypertension. *Circulation Research, 11*, 145–152.

Kim, J. A., Siegel, S., & Patenall, V. R. (1999). Drug-onset cues as signals: intraadministration associations and tolerance. *J Exp Psychol Anim Behav Process, 25*(4), 491–504.

Koch, E. B. (1932). Die Irradiation der pressorezeptorischen Kreislaufreflexe. *Klinische Wochenschrift, 2*, 225–227.

Koushanpour, E., & Kelso, D. M. ed: (1972). Partition of the carotid sinus baroreceptor response in dogs between the mechanical properties of the wall and the receptor elements. *Circulation Research, 31*, 831–845.

Koushanpour, E., & Kenfield, K. J. (1981). Partition of carotid sinus baroreceptor response in dogs with chronic renal hypertension. *Circulation Research, 48*, 267–273.

Kreiger, E. M. (1970). Time course of baroreceptor resetting in acute hypertension. *American Journal of Physiology, 218*, 486–490.

Kukorelli, T., & Juhàsz, G. (1976). Electroencephalographic Synchronization induced by stimulation of the small intestine and splanchnic nerve in cats. *Electroencephalography and Clinical Neurology, 41*, 491–500.

Kukorelli, T., & Juhàsz, G. (1977). Sleep induced by intestinal stimulation in cats. *Physiology & Behavior, 19*, 355–358.

Landgren, S. (1952). On the excitation mechanism of the carotid barociceptors. *Acta Physiologica Scandinavia, 26*, 1–34.

Lee, M. H. M., Zaretsky, H. H., Ernst, M., Dworkin, B. R., & Jonas, R. (1985). The analgesic effects of aspirin and placebo on experimentally induced tooth pulp pain. *Journal of Medicine, 16*, 417–428.

Lowenstein, W. R., & Mendelson, M. (1965). Components of receptor adaptation in a Pacinian corpuscle. *Journal of Physiology, 177*, 377–397.

Lowenstein, W. R., & Skalak, R. (1966). Mechanical transmission in a Pacinian corpuscle: An analysis and a theory. *Journal of Physiology, 182*, 346–378.

Mallorga, P., Tallman, J. F., Henneberry, R. C., Hirata, F., Strittmatter, W. T., & Axelrod, J. (1980). Mepacrine blocks β-adrenergic agonist-induced desensitization in astrocytoma cells. *Proceedings of the National Academy of Sciences, 77*, 1341–1345.

McCubbin, J. W., Green, J. H., & Page, I. H. (1956). Baroreceptor function in chronic renal hypertension. *Circulation Research, 4*, 205–210.

McGaugh, J. L. (1966). Time-dependence processes in memory storage. *Science, 153*, 1351–1358.

McGaugh, J. L. (1989). Involvement of Hormonal and Neuromodulatory Systems in the Regulation of Memory Storage. *Annual Review of Neuroscience, 12*, 255–287.

McGaugh, J. L., Cahill, L., & Roozendaal, B. (1996). Involvement of the Amygdala in Memory Storage: Interaction with other brain systems. *Proc. Natl. Acad. Sci. USA, 93*, 13508–13514.

McHugh, P. R., & Moran, T. H. (1985). The Stomach: A conception of Its Dynamic Role in Satiety. *Progress in Psychobiology and Physiological Psychology, 2*, 197–232.

Mei, N. (1978). Vagal glucoreceptors in the small intestine of the cat. *Journal of Physiology (London), 282*, 485–506.

Mifflin, S. W., & Kunze, D. L. (1982). Rapid resetting of low pressure vagal receptors in the superior vena cava of the rat. *Circulation Research, 51*, 241–249.

Miller, N. E. (1959). Liberalization of basic S-R concepts; extensions to conflict behavior, motivation and social learning. In K. S. (Ed.), *Psychology: A study of a science* (Vol. 2, study 1, pp. 196–292). New York: McGraw-Hill.

Miller, N. E. (1966). Experiments relevant to learning theory and psychopathology. In W. S. Sahakian (Ed.), *Psychopathology today: Experimentation, theory, and research* (pp. 148–166). Itasca, IL: Peacock.

Mountcastle, V. (1980). *Medical physiology* (14th ed.). St. Louis: Mosby.

Norgren, R. (1985). Taste and the autonomic nervous system. *Chemical Senses, 10*, 143–161.

Numao, Y., Siato, M., Terui, N., & Momoru, K. (1985). The aortic nerve-sympathetic reflex in the rat. *Journal of the Autonomic Nervous System, 13*, 65–79.

Ochoa, J., & Torebjork, E. (1983). Sensations evoked by intraneural microstimulation of single mechanoreceptor units innervating the human hand. *Journal of Physiology, 342*, 633–654.

Paintal, A. S. (1972). Cardiovascular receptors. In E. Neil (Ed.), *Handbook of Sensory Physiology* (Vol. III/1). New York: Springer.

Pavlov, I. P. (1940). *Complete collected works* (Vol. 1). Moscow: Academy of Sciences of the USSR.

Pavlov, I. P. ([1897] 1910). *The work of the digestive glands* (T. f. t. R. b. W. H. Thompson, Trans. 2nd English ed.). London: Charles Griffin and Company.

Race, D., & Rosenbaum, M. (1966). Non-respiratory oscillations in systemic arterial pressure of dogs. *Circulation Research, 18*, 525–533.

Randich, A., Ren, K., & Gebhart, G. F. (1990). Electrical stimulation of cervical vagal afferents. II. Central relays for behavioral antinociception and arterial blood pressure decreases. *Journal of Neurophysiology, 64*(4), 1115–1124.

Rau, H., Elbert, T., Geiger, B., & Lutzenberger, W. (1992). PRES: The controlled noninvasive stimulation of the carotid baroreceptors in humans. *Psychophysiology, 29*(2), 165–172.

Riggs, L. A., Ratliff, F., Cornsweet, J. C., & Cornsweet, T. N. (1953). The Disappearance of Steadily Fixated Visual Test Objects. *J. Optical. Soc. of America, 43*(6), 495–501.

Rockstroh, B., Dworkin, B. R., Lutzenberger, W., Ernst, M., Elbert, T., & Birbaumer, N. (1988). The influence of baroreceptor activation on pain perception. In T. Elbert, W. Langosch, A. Steptoe & D. Vaitl (Eds.), *Behavioral Medicine in Cardiovascular Disorders* (pp. 49–60). Chichester: John Wiley & Sons.

Sagawa, K. (1983). Baroreflex conrol of systemic arterial pressure and vascular bed. In J. T. Shepherd & F. M. Abboud (Eds.), *Handbook of physiology: The cardiovascular system* (Vol. 3, pp. 453–496). Bethesda Md: American Physiological Society.

Sapru, H. N., Gonzalez, E., & Krieger, A. J. (1981). Aortic nerve stimulation in the rat: Cardiovascular and respiratory responses. *Brain Research Bulletin, 6*, 393–398.

Schwartz, G. J., & Moran, T. H. (1996). Sub-diaphragmatic Vagal Afferent Integration of Meal-Related Gastrointestinal Signals. *Neuroscience and Biobehavioral Reviews, 20*(1), 47–56.

Siegel, S. (1972). Conditioning of insulin-induced glycemia. *Journal of Comparative and Physiological Psychology, 89*, 233–241.

Siegel, S. (1983). Classical conditioning, drug tolerance, and drug dependence. In Y. Israel, F. B. Glaser, H. Kalant, R. E. Popham, W. Schmidt & R. G. Smart (Eds.), *Research advances in alcohol and drug problems* (Vol. 7, pp. 207–243). New York: Plenum Press.

Siegel, S., Krank, M. D., & Hinson, R. E. (1987). Anticipation of pharmacological and nonpharmacological events: Classical conditioning and addictive behavior. *Journal of Drug Issues, XX*, 83–109.

Sinoway, L., & Prophet, S. (1990). Skeletal muscle metaboreceptor stimulation opposes peak metabolic vasodilation in humans. *Circ Res*,66(6), 1576–1584.

Skinner, B. F. (1981). Selection by consequences. *Science, 213*, 501–504.

Slucki, H., Adam, G., & Porter, R. W. (1965). Operant discrimination of an interoceptive stimulus in rhesus monkeys. *Journal of the Experimental Analysis of Behavior, 8*, 405–414.

Smith, G. P., & Gibbs, J. (1994). Satiating effects of cholecystokinin. *Annals of the New York academy of Sciences, 713*, 236–241.

Smythe, G. A., Pascoe, W. S., & Storlien, L. H. (1989). Hypothalamic noradrenergic and sympathoadrenal control of glycemia after stress. *American Journal of Physiology, 256*, E231–E235.

Sokolowska, M., Siegel, S., & Kim, J. A. (2002). Intraadministration associations: conditional hyperalgesia elicited by morphine onset cues. *J Exp Psychol Anim Behav Process, 28*(3), 309–320.

Stellar, J. R., & Stellar, E. (1985). *The neurobiology of motivation and reward.* New York: Springer-Verlag.

Strulovici, B., Cerione, R. A., Kilpatrick, B. F., Caron, M. G., & Lefkowitz, R. J. (1984). Direct demonstration of impaired functionality of a purified desensitized beta-adrenergic receptor in a reconstituted system. *Science., 225*, 837–840.

Terasaki, W. L., Brooker, G., de Vellis, J., Inglish, D., Hsu, C., & Moylan, R. D. (1978). Involvement of cyclic AMP and protein synthesis in catecholamine refractoriness. In W. J. George & L. J. Ignarro (Eds.), *Advances in cyclic nucleotide research* (Vol. 9, pp. 33–52). New York: Raven Press.

Thomas E. Lohmeier, Eric D. Irwin, Martin A. Rossing, David J. Serdar, & Robert S. Kieval, Prolonged Activation of the Baroreflex Produces Sustained Hypotension Hypertension. 2004;43[part 2]:306–311).

Whitehead, W. E., & Schuster, M. M. (1983). Techniques for the assessment of the anorectal mechanism. In R. Hölzl & W. E. Whitehead (Eds.), *Psychophysiology of the Gastrointestinal Tract* (pp. 311–329). New York and London: Plenum Press.

Zamir, N., & Shuber, E. (1980). Altered pain perception in hypertensive humans. *Brain Research, 201*, 471–474.

22 The Anatomy and Physiology of the Motor System in Humans

ANA SOLODKIN, PETR HLUSTIK, AND GIOVANNI BUCCINO

INTRODUCTION

Sensation and volition, so far as they are connected with corporeal motions, are functions of the brain alone... The will operating in the brain only, by a motion begun there and propagated along the nerves, produces the contraction of the muscles.

– William Cullen (1710–1790)

The behavioral *repertoire* of humans is broad, extending from simple behaviors such as sensory perception to more complex cognitive behaviors like language or creativity. Interestingly, no matter how simple or complex are these behaviors, they share without exception the common feature that their expression is a motor act. For the motor system to implement this large variety of cognitive behaviors, there must be an evolutionary bias toward a highly sophisticated and expanded organization of the system. Indeed, according to some (Freund, 1983), association cortical motor regions are among the cortical areas that have changed the most from non-human to human primates. They further manifest a parallel increase in complexity of their connectivity patterns (Zilles et al., 1995). This means that while subcortical motor regions (from spinal cord to cerebellum and basal ganglia) might not be that dissimilar among mammals, cortical motor regions have changed significantly, reflecting a link between motor output and cognitive processing.

This chapter on motor physiology intends to provide an overview on how the nervous system has implemented the ability to produce complex motor behaviors in the human. Although the following sections will place special emphasis on "skilled" movements, some comments on rhythmic movements will also be included.

Coordination of movements between the upper limbs is a function highly distributed across the animal kingdom, from tetrapod taxa to primates (Iwaniuk & Whishaw, 1999). Although this coordination can be considered to be homologous across species, and although the movements *per se* are not very different between animal species and humans, there are two aspects of this homology to highlight: First is that there are at least two types of limb synchronization, one involving simpler, generally rhythmic, movements and another incorporating more complex movements. The simplest movements are generally associated with posture and locomotion and are, at least in part, controlled subcortically (Poppele & Bosco, 2003), generated in specialized circuits originally described as "motor pattern generators" (Grillner & Wallen, 1985; Pearson, 1995). By contrast, more complex movements, sometimes called "skilled" movements, have evolved to the highest levels in humans. In terms of evolutionary biology, motor skill refers to the "ability to solve a motor problem correctly, quickly, rationally and resourcefully" (Bernstein, 1996, cited in Wiesendanger, 1999). According to Wiesendanger (1999), the high degree of development of hand dexterity in hominids is reflected by the fact that they not only have the ability to use tools but are also able to fabricate them. In this context, the concept of hand dexterity implies goal-directed action that has been previously learned and practiced. Throughout evolution, the increase in hand skill, tool making and vertical locomotion (that freed the hands), has been accompanied by a parallel increase in the size of cortical motor association areas. Anatomically, this increase is specifically related to an increased volume of neuropil, reflecting an increase in the complexity of connectivity (Zilles et al., 1995).

Albeit somewhat artificial, an anatomical division of regions involved in the production of movement can be instructive in understanding the physiology of the human motor system (Figure 22.1). The brain stem and spinal cord can be viewed as the regions of the central nervous system that contain the interneuronal-motoneuronal networks responsible for the production of reflexive and rhythmic motor behaviors. These networks can be regulated by descending modulation from the cerebral cortex (to produce voluntary movements) or from sensory afferents from the peripheral nerves to produce reflexes. Sherrington (1906) called this the *final common pathway* to denote the fact that this is the final output from the whole system to the muscles. The Basal Ganglia and the Cerebellum are important regions of the Central Nervous System that play a crucial role in the coordination of

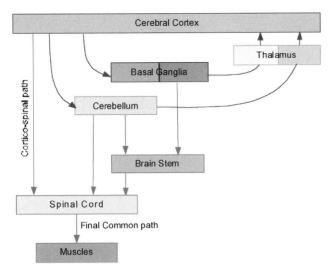

Figure 22.1. Diagram of the general organization of the Motor System in Humans. This figure depicts a simplified organization of the motor system in humans. Note the variety of descending pathways originating from the cerebral cortex that will finally convey into the final common pathway on its way to the effector muscles. The cerebellum (CRB) and the basal ganglia (BG) are important components of this system since they not only have descending inputs into the brain-stem, but also, they are part of closed loops from and to the cerebral cortex. Note that even when both loops pass through the thalamus towards the cerebral cortex, each one of them has a private line in different thalamic regions. *Modified from: Heimer L (1994). The human brain and spinal cord: functional neuroanatomy and dissection guide. 2nd. Ed. Springer Verlag.*

movement by exerting a modulatory influence on most of the cerebral cortex. These complex regions form two important re-entrant systems to the cerebral cortex (as seen in Figure 22.1), where they can produce widespread effects. Finally, the motor cortical regions are interesting to study particularly in the context of cognitive functions. Some of these cortical motor regions are among the regions that have suffered a large change through evolution, as commented previously (Freund, 1983), but others included in modern maps of motor anatomy (Rizzolatti, Luppino, & Matelli, 1998) are located mainly in the parietal lobule, and have not traditionally been considered integral areas for motor control. Because of the inherent importance of skilled movements in the evolution of species, including humans, this chapter will provide some specific examples (motor imagery, motor imitation, and motor learning) to illustrate potential interactions between movement production and higher cognitive functions.

METHODS FOR THE STUDY OF HUMAN MOTOR PHYSIOLOGY: HISTORICAL PERSPECTIVE

Neuroanatomical substrate of motor functions

To know the brain . . . is equivalent to ascertaining the material course of thought and will, to discovering the intimate history of life in its perpetual duel with external forces.
                    – Santiago Ramón y Cajal (1852–1934)

The concept and study of human motor function (along with all other brain functions) progressed greatly with advances in science and anatomy starting in the late 18th century, when sophisticated techniques of brain tissue fixation and sectioning provided a new window on the three-dimensional anatomy of the brain. Since Schwann proposed the cell theory in 1939, the field of histology and microscopic anatomy developed rapidly. In 1906, the Nobel Prize in Physiology or Medicine was awarded to Camillo Golgi and Santiago Ramón y Cajal in recognition

of their studies on the structure of the nervous system. In fact, their approach provided for the first time the notion of the neuron as the basic unit of the nervous system.

Regionally specific features of the central brain region were described by Betz (1874), making one of the first steps toward the microstructural, cytoarchitectonic parcellation of the entire human cerebral cortex, a task later pioneered by Campbell (1905), Elliot Smith (1907), and, most prominently, Brodmann (1909) (Figure 22.2). Cortical fields associated with motor function were further differentiated by the Vogts (Vogt & Vogt, 1919), who, among other advances, divided the premotor regions (BA 6) into two subregions, a division later justified by physiological differences in human and non-human primates.

Contemporary anatomical methods of the motor system are based on the visualization of specific groups of brain cells (both neurons and glia) using immunological methods. These cells are detected using specific antibodies against proteins present in cell organelles or in chemical elements contained in them (e.g., neurotransmitters). This method has uncovered specific groups of cells (e.g., pyramidal cells or glial and endothelial cells) as well as cells that contain specific neurotransmitters (e.g., GABA, glutamate, amines, NO) or specific proteins, some of which are present only in certain states (e.g., apoptosis, the process of programmed cell death). Since these techniques are performed *post-mortem*, they have facilitated construction of chemo-architectonic maps of the brain in humans as well as animals, thus permitting direct comparison among species. As an example of these neurochemical techniques, Figure 22.3 shows the giant Betz cells located in the primary motor cortex (M1) in humans detected with an antibody against a non-phosphorylated neurofilament protein called SMI-32. Note the great detail that can be achieved with this type of method. For an interesting example of these techniques, we refer the reader to the chemoarchitectonic maps based on the distribution of transmitter and neuromodulator receptors in the human brain (Zilles et al., 2002).

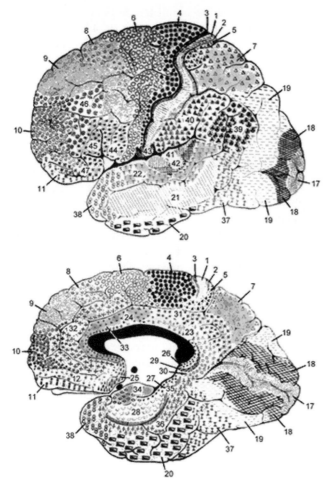

Figure 22.2. Brodmann's cytoarchitectonic map of the human cerebral cortex. These numbers are still commonly used to refer to different brain regions. The reason for its universal use is perhaps the fact that by describing anatomical differences among cortical areas, implicitly he provided a map for functional differences as well.

Relating brain lesions to motor deficits

Effects of brain lesions on human behavior have been observed for centuries. The Edwin Smith papyrus provided the first written record about a case of hemiplegia after (closed) head injury, as well as cases of motor and sensory deficits after spinal cord injury. In 1760, Arne-Charles Lorry demonstrated that damage to the cerebellum affects motor coordination (Finger, 1994).

Nineteenth-century physicians studied patients with lesions to understand the cortical localization of function, including language (Broca, 1861) and motor function. Hughlings Jackson and Charcot (Charcot, 1877; Jackson, 1863; Jackson, 1873), studied both irritative (seizure-generating) lesions and stroke, and summarized their observations of motor abnormalities. They proposed, along with other motor features, an orderly gross somatotopic arrangement of motor control. In the precentral gyrus (i.e., M1), the head subdivision was localized most ventrally and laterally near the lateral sulcus, hand and

arm dorsal to the head, and trunk and leg most superiorly and extending onto the medial surface of the hemisphere.

Subsequent lesion studies (Foerster, 1909; Freund, 1987) generally replicated earlier findings, rather than providing novel information on finer aspects of motor control. The reason for this is that cortical lesions are typically large (Bogousslavsky & Caplan, 1995) and affect several motor cortical areas and/or a substantial portion of each. On the other hand, deficits resulting from a cortical lesion and limited to certain fingers or certain arm movements were reported early in the twentieth century (Foerster, 1909; Foerster, 1936a). With the availability of non-invasive brain imaging (X-ray computed tomography, CT, or magnetic resonance imaging, MRI), small brain lesions can now be detected *in vivo*, allowing clinical-pathological correlations in patients with small and/or transient motor deficits. Taking advantage of these methodological advances, several recent clinical studies described either focal finger pareses or pareses with radial/ulnar predominance with small lacunes of the precentral gyrus revealed on MRI (e.g., Lee, Han, & Heo,

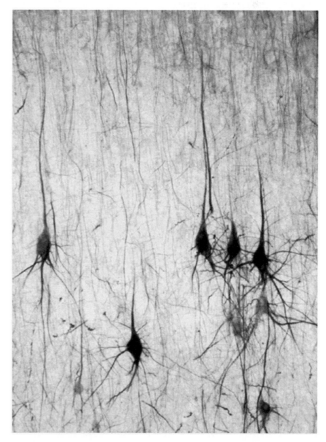

Figure 22.3. Microphotograph of human Betz cells in the human. These motor neurons were stained with an antibody against a non-phosphorylated neurofilament protein found only in pyramidal cells. The microphotograph from neurons located in layer V of the human primary motor cortex, give rise to some (not all) of the descending fibers of the corticospinal pathway that will terminate in the spinal cord.

1998). Although such cases have been known to clinicians, they were dismissed as uninformative exceptions in previous discussions of human motor cortical organization.

Nineteen-century pioneers of the lesion method, Broca and Wernicke, also made an important distinction between lesions located in the gray and the white matter, thus differentiating cortical syndromes from "conduction" syndromes. The concept of white matter or "conduction" syndromes was further developed by Dejerine and Liepmann and reached maximal expression with Norman Geschwind (1965), who described specific syndromes in both animals and men in terms of disconnections among cortical brain regions.

Geschwind's approach to understanding neurological deficits was important not only because he highlighted the connections among brain regions as being the recipients of function, but also because he included in his analysis the actual connectivity patterns of the brain. In fact, among his speculations was the suggestion that the increase in association cortical areas in man would provide new connectivity patterns (not present in animals) to explain the presence of novel interrelationships among areas producing new functions (like language). The limitation of this early perspective, however, is that neurological syndromes were still described as specific lesions in specific white matter pathways, perpetuating in some sense, the localizationist approach to behavior.

The connectionist approach however, has been constantly evolving, and as we will see in the last part of this section, new methodological approaches for the study of the physiology of the CNS in humans, like brain imaging, are making feasible a more comprehensive study of the relationship between brain and behavior.

Electrical stimulation and ablation studies

Proceeding from these observations on the effect of natural lesions, pioneering physiologists conducted animal vivisection experiments and electrical stimulation and ablation studies on animals, including monkeys and apes.

Flourens (1824) conducted ablation and stimulation experiments examining motor functions of the cerebellum (where his conclusions regarding its role in coordination of voluntary movements remain valid) and cerebral hemispheres (where his method was inappropriate and therefore his conclusions, incorrect). German physiologists Fritsch and Hitzig (1870) carried out electrical stimulation studies in a canine model. Their findings overthrew three theories that had stood since Flourens: they established cortical excitability, a role for the primary motor cortex in the mechanism of movements, and cerebral localization.

Building on the efforts of Jackson and of Fritsch and Hitzig, Ferrier published detailed studies (1873; 1875) of cortical localization in non-human primates. He thus established stimulation mapping as a reliable experimental method. Ferrier also proposed that motor centers, besides leading the "accomplishment of acts of volition", form the organic centers for the memory of "accomplished acts", that is, allow storage of learned movements. These early studies culminated in the work of Charles Scott Sherrington (1906), whose work "The Integrative Action of the Nervous System" formed the basic framework for the rest of the twentieth century. Similar information was also collected in the human, almost exclusively in patients planned for brain surgery (most often for epilepsy), rather than in healthy brains (but see: Bartholow, 1874).

Electrical stimulation of exposed cortical surface in patients scheduled for brain surgery (e.g., Cushing, 1909) confirmed the presence of somatotopic representations along the precentral and postcentral gyri (M1 and S1 respectively). Furthermore, an orderly arrangement was also found within the hand, where thumb was found most laterally and little finger most medially (Foerster, 1936b; Foerster & Penfield, 1930; Penfield & Boldrey, 1937). Most of these pioneering authors also commented on the complexity of the observed arrangement and the early researchers also reported on many complex features of primary motor cortex organization, such as overlapping functional codes of different movements and dynamic changes of function performed by a particular cortical location. For example, Jackson (1873) noted that although a single part of the body is represented "preponderating" (sic) in one area of the human precentral gyrus, it is also represented in other parts of the gyrus, though to a different degree and in different combinations with other body parts. Like Sherrington (on the instability of cortical point), Foerster observed that from a single precentral locus, repeated surface stimulation evokes a series of different movements of individual fingers, from which he concluded that each stimulation point on the motor cortex contains neurons representing different body parts (Foerster, 1936a). Finally, Penfield and Boldrey (1937) showed overlap of the motor cortical sites at which stimulation evoked movements of different fingers. They expressly warned against an oversimplified interpretation of their famous homunculus cartoon (See Figure 22.4).

Single-neuron recording in the cerebral cortex of awake, behaving primates (and, rarely, humans). Until the late 1970s, most human mental processes, including complex motor control, were not amenable to direct experimental analysis. Since that time, however, several different approaches have been developed to characterize the neural substrates of information processing.

Ed Evarts, studying the neural correlates of movement and, subsequently, Vernon Mountcastle and his colleagues, focusing on somatic sensation, helped establish the study of internal representations of specified behaviors by studying the activity of single neurons in the cerebral cortex in intact, awake, behaving primates that are trained to do particular motor or perceptual tasks. Human studies with cortical single-neuron recordings are rare. Goldring and Ratcheson (1972), for example, confirmed active and

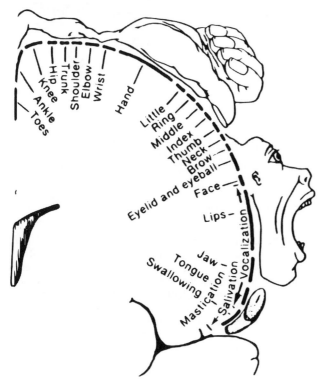

Figure 22.4. Somatotopic Organization of the primary motor cortex in Humans. Schematic representation of the location of different body parts within the primary motor cortex. Note that the areas that have the larger representations are the fingers, face and mouth. Even though when Penfield suggested a careful interpretation of the diagram since the divisions for each body part are overlapped, this diagram has been used extensively and sometimes over interpreted.

passive movement-related neuronal activity in human M1, while auditory and tactile stimuli produced no effect. For further examples see Engel et al. (2005).

These important studies (seldom done in humans) highlight the importance of the intrinsic features of the individual neuron with respect to function. However, they neglected the effects of ensembles of neurons in the generation of such behaviors. Additional methodological approaches, discussed in the following sections, provide a systems approach by determining the effects of activation at the population level on the production of motor behavior.

Electrophysiology methods

Electroencephalogram (EEG) – motor-related potentials. A noninvasive window on dynamic nervous system functioning was opened by the development of techniques to study nerve conduction and electroencephalography (EEG) by Sir Richard Caton in animals and Hans Berger in humans (1929). This methodological approach refers to the scalp recording of electrical field potentials generated on the surface of the cortical mantle. The analysis of this continuous EEG recording is based on the frequency of the signals and on the morphology of the waves.

In contrast, "evoked potentials" or "event-related potentials" (ERP) refer to changes in the patterns of activation produced by specific stimuli. The earliest experimental evoked potentials were described by Waldo in 1933, and the first EEG related to a human motor act was reported by Bates (1951), who described a negative potential after movement onset, originally interpreted as a re-afferent sensory evoked potential. Different instrumental settings were required to detect the very slow changes or DC shifts reflecting preparatory movement-related components of the EEG signal: contingent negative variation (CNV) (Walter et al., 1964) and the *Bereitschaftspotential* or readiness potential (BP/RP), (Kornhuber & Deecke, 1965), which are markers of motor preparation for externally cued or internally initiated movements, respectively. The RP initially localizes to the midline but its amplitude becomes greater over the hemisphere contralateral to the responding hand (for a review, see: Coles, 1989). Another motor-associated phenomenon is EEG (event-related) desynchronization (ERD), observed contralaterally to the moving hand. All of these electrophysiological phenomena – RP, CNV, and ERD – have been related to different aspects of motor programming and have also been investigated and found pathological in patients with motor dysfunction, such as dystonia (Kaòovskπ, 2002).

Magnetoencephalography (MEG). One of the great limitations of the classical electrophysiological techniques (EEG and ERP) is their inability to record and/or localize electrical field potentials from brain regions that do not originate on the brain surface or close to the scalp. This limitation does not apply to the relatively new technique of magnetoencephalography (MEG) that detects the magnetic field generated by the neuronal electrical activity (Hari & Kaukoranta, 1985). MEG technology has grown from a single-channel to multi-channel techniques, and currently achieves spatial localization of dipole sources down to a few millimeters. MEG has been used to map movement-related magnetic fields, (e.g., Antervo et al., 1983), and has contributed to study of motor control timing (because of its excellent temporal resolution) and complex motor control, such as the study of motor correlates of long-term skilled motor practice (Elbert et al., 1995).

Transcranial electrical and magnetic stimulation (TMS)

Although direct electrical stimulation of the human brain has been possible only with the use of invasive techniques during neurosurgical procedures (see, for instance, Penfield & Rasmussen, 1950), the knowledge gained with this method in animal experiments is impressive. Thus, it is not difficult to understand the tremendous value in developing a technique to stimulate motor regions in a non-invasive manner in neurologically intact humans. Such a technique should not have direct contact with the motor regions (i.e., performed outside of the skull), and at the same time, it should be painless. Electrical activation from the scalp (Levy, York, McCaffrey, & Tanzer, 1984) fulfills the first requirement but not the second. Hence, the alternative has been to induce electrical currents within the brain with time-varying magnetic fields (Faraday's law).

The history of magnetic stimulation is relatively recent (for review see Kobayashi & Pascual-Leone, 2003). The first report of a time-variable magnetic field producing physiological changes in the brain was written by d'Arsonval in 1896. In his study, a volunteer reported phosphenes and vertigo when his head was stimulated by a coil at 42 Hz (not surprising he got those effects since that is a high frequency by today's standards).

Several subsequent studies were performed, many by stimulation of peripheral nerves rather than cortex, but these studies led to methodological refinements regarding the quality of the magnetic pulse needed to produce a response with minimal risk to the subjects. In the study of Barker et al. (1985), brief transcranial magnetic stimulation pulses over the motor cortex excited the corticospinal pathway (from M1 to spinal cord) and generated electromyographic signals (motor evoked potentials, MEPs), with or without brief contractions in the peripheral muscles. TMS has been widely used since that time to study the motor system in humans, both healthy and diseased. TMS helps to assess the excitability of the primary motor cortex and the corticospinal pathway, which can be enhanced during spontaneous mild voluntary contraction (Mills, Murray, & Hess, 1987), motor preparation (Barker, Jalinous, & Freeston, 1985) or motor imagery (Rossini et al., 1999), as well as after successful motor recovery from hemiparetic stroke (Liepert et al., 1998). For this, it has become a clinical tool as well. More sophisticated physiological studies have shown that the facilitation of responses in hand muscles produced by voluntary contraction is also present when contralateral muscles are used, but not when a leg muscle is contracted. These results demonstrate a close functional influence of one cortical hemisphere on the other, probably involving neural activity at both spinal and cortical levels.

Motor evoked potentials can also be obtained by stimulation of the spinal cord (Figure 22.5) or the cerebellum. Not surprisingly in these cases, the latency of the MEPs is shorter and the conduction velocity is faster when compared to the stimulation in the primary motor cortex. These latter examples highlight further the value of TMS in assessing motor physiology.

Brain imaging

Following the development of quantitative methods for measuring whole brain blood flow and metabolism in animals by Kety and his colleagues (Landau et al., 1955), David Ingvar, Neils Lassen, and their Scandinavian colleagues introduced methods applicable to humans that permitted regional blood flow measurements by using scintillation detectors arrayed like a helmet over the head

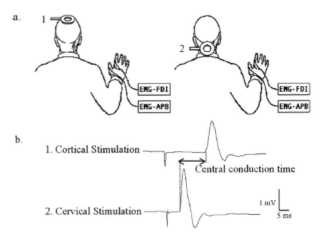

Figure 22.5. Principle of transcranial magnetic stimulation. **a.** Representation of the placement of the stimulating coil (on the scalp overlying the primary motor cortex and over the cervical spinal cord targeting the dorsal roots). These cartoons show also the recording sites on hand muscles (either the first dorsal *interosseus* (FDI) or the abductor *pollicis brevis* (APB)) where the motor evoked potentials are recorded. **b.** Panels showing the actual muscle response (MEPs) as a result of the stimulation at the level of the cortex (1) and in the spinal cord (2). Note the difference in latency for each response. The central conduction time is calculated by the difference between them. *From: Maeda and Pascual-Leone (2003). Transcranial magnetic stimulation: studying motor neurophysiology of psychiatric disorders. Psychopharmac. 168:359–376. With permission of Dr. Pascual-Leone.*

(Lassen et al., 1963). They subsequently demonstrated that blood flow changed regionally during changes in brain functional activity in humans (Ingvar & Risberg, 1965). This approach was not initially embraced by many neuroscientists or psychologists, an interesting indifference that was to disappear almost completely in the 1980s.

Applying image reconstruction techniques introduced in X-ray computed tomography, researchers envisioned another type of tomography, positron emission tomography (PET), which created *in vivo* autoradiograms of blood flow and glucose metabolism reflecting brain function (Ter-Pogossian et al., 1975). As expressed by Marcus Raichle (Raichle et al., 1983), "a new era of functional brain mapping began."

One of the advantages of PET is the possibility to simultaneously investigate different physiological processes. For example, studying regional cerebral blood flow (CBF) and cerebral metabolic rate of oxygen ($CMRO_2$) (Fox, Mintun, & Raichle, 1986) uncovered their uncoupling during cortical activation, which has provided a physiological mechanism to explain the functioning of subsequently developed functional MRI (see below).

Functional brain imaging with PET targeted many issues in the organization of the human motor system, (see, for example Passingham, 1998).

Magnetic resonance imaging (MRI) and spectroscopy (MRS). MRI has pushed non-invasive brain imaging yet another step further towards our understanding of the

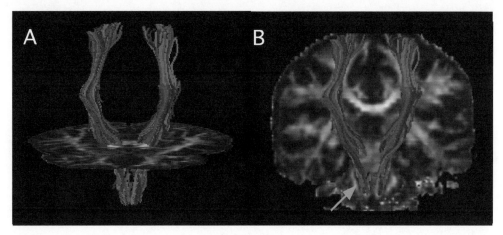

Figure 22.6. Image of the cortico-spinal path of humans using DTI. These figures show in blue, corticospinal fibers going from cortical motor and sensory areas, in their way to brain-stem and spinal cord. **a**. Descending fibers shown in three dimensions, crossing through an axial structural MRI. **b**. Same fibers superimposed to a coronal MRI slice. Note how the right and left parts of the pathway get close together at the level of the medulla where they will cross over to the contralateral side. *Courtesy of K. Arfanakis. Department of Biomedical Engineering. Illinois Institute of Technology (IIT).* (See color plate).

mind-brain relationship. MRI provides significantly higher sensitivity than other structural imaging techniques like CT in the detection of abnormal or malconfigured brain tissue, as well as providing higher resolution in the anatomical features of normal brains. The benefit of morphological MRI in detecting small brain lesions and thus allowing fine-grained lesion studies has been already mentioned. However, the main new feature of this methodology is that the MR scanner may be "tuned" to detect other properties of brain tissue (beyond anatomy), providing information on brain metabolism, function or connectivity. Magnetic resonance spectroscopy, functional MRI (fMRI) and diffusion tensor imaging (DTI) represent three such applications, and the acquired data from each MR modality can be easily integrated within the same studied brain.

Functional MRI takes advantage of similar tissue processes as other previous functional imaging methods, e.g., single photon emission computed tomography (SPECT) and PET, namely the rise in local metabolism and local cerebral blood flow with increased synaptic activity. The most frequently used blood oxygenation level-dependent (BOLD) fMRI technique (Ogawa et al., 1990) exploits the uncoupling of oxygen consumption and blood flow: changes in blood flow are accompanied by much smaller changes in oxygen consumption. Thus, the venous blood leaving active cerebral tissue contains relatively more oxygenated hemoglobin. Since hemoglobin oxygenation changes its magnetic properties, this change in blood oxygen content at the site of brain activation can be detected with MRI.

Free from the radiation load of emission-computed tomographic methods and faster in acquiring functional brain mapping data, fMRI has allowed an explosion of functional brain experiments to investigate brain responses to myriad tasks and stimuli, not in the least from

the motor domain. High spatial resolution has enabled the study of cortical organization on a millimeter scale for example, to study somatotopy within the hand area of the motor cortex (Hlustik et al., 2001). The reader is referred to review articles (e.g., Jezzard, Matthews, & Smith, 2001; Picard & Strick, 2001, and fMRI textbooks) and fMRI textbooks (Jezzard, Matthews, & Smith, 2001; Moonen & Bandettini, 1999) for examples of applications to the study of the motor system. It should be mentioned that fMRI (as well as other functional brain mapping techniques) is most useful when combined with (or preceded by) well-conceived behavioral experiments, as in the work of cognitive scientists (for review, see Posner & Raichle, 1994).

DTI can probe, *in vivo*, the intrinsic diffusion properties of water in deep tissues (Basser, Mattiello, & LeBihan, 1994). One of the most interesting aspects of DTI is that it describes not only the magnitude of the diffusion of water but also, the degree of "anisotropic diffusion" (diffusion in a preferential direction) and its primary direction. When DTI is applied to the central nervous system, it has revealed that the diffusion of water in the white matter is "anisotropic." The suggested reason for this anisotropy is the ordered structure of axons and myelin sheaths, which imposes a heavy constraint on the diffusion of water in directions perpendicular to the axons but not parallel to them. In this way, information about diffusion acquired with DTI can be translated into the detection and assessment of pathways in the brain as well as to changes in the pathways related to pathology. Diffusion tensor imaging is a promising technique that potentially can allow us to trace and measure, for the first time, pathways in the human brain *in vivo*. Figure 22.6 shows the path tracing of the corticospinal pathway in a human without neurological disease. The traced path has been superimposed on an anatomical MRI section in the axial and the coronal

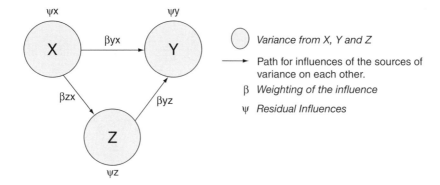

$$STRUCTURAL\ EQUATIONS: \quad X = \psi_x$$
$$Z = \beta_{zx}x + \psi_z$$
$$Y = \beta_{yx}x + \beta_{yz}Z + \psi_y$$

Figure 22.7. Theoretical Principle for the determination of the Structural equation models. This diagram shows a simple algorithm describing the effects of regions X, Y and Z onto each other (effective connectivity: element "β" plus an error variable Ψ representing unknown influences). An important aspect of the model, differentiating it from some other multivariate methods is that it explicitly represents directionality of effects since it assumes a causal relationship of one area over others with which it is anatomically connected. *Modified from: McIntosh and Gonzalez-Lima (1994). Structural Equation Modelling and its Application to Network Analysis in Functional Brain Imaging. Human Brain Mapping. 2: 2–22.*

planes. Note the origin of this pathway (in the cerebral cortex) descending through the brain stem to cross over at the level of the medulla. Refer to a recent review (Mesulam, 2005) for additional information.

Computer modeling

Computer science also has made a distinctive contribution to systems neuroscience. Learning and memory have been modeled by associative neural networks of Hopfield and others, and the back-propagation learning algorithm of Rumelhart and Hinton. They have shown that complex behaviors could arise from the intrinsic properties of neural nets. Computer models simulate some aspects of the activity of large populations of neurons, thus providing an environment for testing possible neural implementations of particular behaviors in the brain. Neuronal network properties go well beyond the properties of individual neurons and provide for the emergent properties that are commonly referred to as higher brain functions. Computational approaches along these lines, and especially when combined with psychophysics, as in the work of Terry Sejnowski, Steven Lisberger, Richard Andersen, Emilio Bizzi, and Tony Movshon, have been informative in suggesting explanations for functional properties and capabilities of specific neural systems. In the motor domain, for example, modeling suggested a possible mechanism of aligning cortical motor and somatosensory maps (Chen & Reggia, 1996).

An additional approach to computer modeling has been the construction of networks of activation based on PET

and fMRI imaging data. Several tactics have been proposed for using network analysis based on brain imaging data. Notable examples are principal and independent components analysis, and structural equation modeling (SEM). The description of brain imaging data using structural equation modeling as depicted in Figure 22.7 (Buchel & Friston, 1997; Gonzalez-Lima & McIntosh, 1994; Horwitz, Friston, & Taylor, 2000) has produced a conceptual change in the way we interpret such data. In particular, by characterizing networks of activation, SEM describes the functional influence of a specific anatomical brain region on other areas with which it is anatomically connected. The emphasis thereby changes from the individual brain regions active in each condition to the relationships among them. This functional influence of one region over others is called "effective connectivity." In the past, McIntosh and his collaborators (1999, 2000) have referred to the modulation of effective connectivity over time or over different conditions as "neural context" to denote the fact that a single anatomical region can play different roles depending on its interactions with regions with whom it is related. This means that behavior will be generated depending on the dynamics of the temporo-spatial relationships among brain regions. An example of SEM applied to the study of motor physiology can be found in this chapter in the section dedicated to motor imagery.

Combined methodology

Added power can be gained by combining different complementary research techniques within the same subject and study. For example, combination of fMRI and EEG/MEG yields data with both high structural resolution (benefit of fMRI) and high temporal resolution (EEG/EMG). In a different way, DTI allows more advanced network analysis of fMRI data by providing direct within-subject estimates of brain connections among the active regions.

Another approach combines functional mapping of active brain areas during specific behavioral conditions with subsequent studies of single neuronal activity in the corresponding areas in the brains of conscious monkeys carrying out essentially the same behavioral task. This combined approach in monkeys and humans promises to be a powerful tool for analyzing those complex higher-brain functions that have correlates in non-human primates.

THE ANATOMICAL ORGANIZATION OF THE MOTOR SYSTEM: A MODERN VIEW

In the previous section of this chapter, we highlighted the methods used for the study of motor physiology and anatomy in humans. However, even when not explicitly stated, the section also suggested the importance of neural networks for understanding motor control mechanisms. This section on anatomy of the motor system will emphasize pathways of the brain associated with motor control.

Concretely, we can consider the motor pathways as belonging to one of three distinct categories: Descending pathways that produce the actual movement; re-entrant circuits that modulate the ongoing activation of other motor circuits; and cortico-cortical pathways determining interactions among motor cortical regions. Because of the prominent role of the cortex in the generation of motor cognitive functions, our emphasis will be biased towards the latter connections.

Descending pathways

The role of the descending pathways includes not only the regulation of skeletal muscles (i.e., from reflexes to skilled voluntary movements), but also the regulation of smooth muscle for autonomic control. Descending pathways (e.g., cortico-spinal path) that originate in the cerebral cortex terminate in the brain stem for the control of head and face movements and in the spinal cord for the control of the rest of the body. These however, are not the only descending pathways. Additional paths originate in brain stem nuclei (red *nucleus*, vestibular *nuclei*, superior *colliculus*), also terminating in the spinal cord. Because of its prominent role in the control of voluntary movements in humans, we will limit our description to the descending pathways originating in the cortical regions, i.e., the corticospinal path. A depiction of this pathway in a human *in vivo* as seen with diffusion tensor imaging can be appreciated in Figure 22.6.

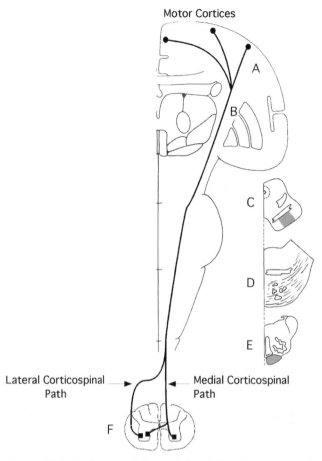

Figure 22.8. Trajectory of the medial and lateral corticospinal path. **a**: Corona radiata; **b**: Internal capsule; **c**: Midbrain; **d**: Pons; **e**: Medulla; **f**: Spinal cord. Note the somatotopic termination in the spinal cord, of the medial and lateral components of the pathway carrying information for proximal and distal movements respectively. *Modified from: Haines D. E. (1987) Neuroanatomy. An Atlas of Structures, Sections and Systems. Second Ed. Urban & Schwarzenberg, Germany.*

Corticospinal pathway. The neurons of origin of this pathway are located in several cortical regions (all displaying somatotopic organization). Among them, the primary motor (Brodmann's area 4; M1) and sensory (especially BA3; S1) cortices, the premotor regions (BA 6 medial and lateral or supplementary motor area: SMA and lateral premotor cortices: LPMC respectively), and the anterior cingulate motor area: CMA (BA 24). This descending pathway has two different components: one is a pathway that descends laterally in the spinal cord and controls the movements of the distal muscles (hands); the other is a medially descending pathway that controls the movements of the proximal muscles (trunk). Whereas the entire lateral corticospinal path crosses over to the contralateral side at the level of the medulla (resulting in a contralateral motor control of hands), the medial path does not cross. As a consequence, injury to the right primary motor cortex produces a deficit in the left hand and vice versa.

Figure 22.8 shows the trajectory of both components of the corticospinal path through the different levels of the brain (from cerebral cortex to spinal cord).

The corticospinal path originates in deep layers of several motor and sensory regions in the cerebral cortex. The axons of these neurons descend through the *corona radiata* and form a tight bundle descending in the internal capsule. The pathway continues on its way down forming the middle portion of the cerebral peduncles in the midbrain. After that, the compact bundle passes through the pons on its way to the medulla, where in its lower levels, all the fibers forming the lateral cortico-spinal path cross but the fibers forming the medial path do not. The final destination of the bundle is in the spinal cord, where these long axons synapse either in the motoneuronal pool, in the interneurons located in the middle portion of the central grey, or in the sensory neurons located in the posterior horn. As seen in Figure 22.8 the spinal cord also has a somatotopic organization: whereas the lateral corticospinal path terminates in the motorneuronal pool located in the lateral regions of the anterior horn, the medial path terminates bilaterally in the medial motoneuronal pool. In turn, the axons of the spinal motoneurons travel in the peripheral nerves to reach and synapse in the appropriate muscles.

The organization of the motor path that controls muscles in face and head have a very similar organization, except that the termination of the cortical neurons is not at the level of the spinal cord but at the level of the brain-stem (cortico-bulbar path), where they synapse with the cranial nerve nuclei in *lieu* of the spinal cord.

Re-entrant circuits

There are two important subcortical motor regions intimately related to the cortex: the basal ganglia and the cerebellum. These structures are sometimes referred to as forming an "extrapyramidal" system to distinguish them from the "pyramidal" corticospinal system. These structures modulate motor activation through two re-entrant circuits to the cortex via the thalamus.

Cerebellum. The cerebellum plays an important role in the coordination of fine movements and in the control of posture. This structure consists of a number of central nuclei surrounded by hemispheres whose intrinsic anatomy resembles the layered organization of the cerebral cortex. The cerebellum receives a variety of afferent inputs from subcortical regions in spinal cord and brainstem (reticular formation, inferior olive, vestibular system, raphe nuclei), conveying information for the control of reflexes involved in posture and eye position during head movements (Heimer, 1983). In addition, the cerebellum receives inputs from motor and sensory cortical regions, instantiating its role in the modulation of voluntary movements. Output from cerebellum terminates mostly in the red nucleus in the midbrain and the ventral lateral nucleus (VL) of the thalamus. This thalamic nucleus projects to several cortical motor regions, closing a loop between cerebellum and cortex. For a review of the cortical regions receiv-

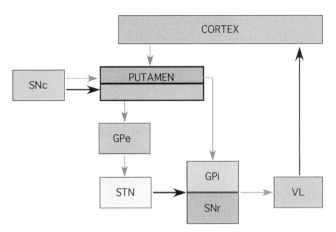

Figure 22.9. Direct and indirect motor paths between basal ganglia and cerebral cortex. Schematic representation of the two re-entrant motor circuits between the basal ganglia and the cerebral cortex. Excitatory projections are represented by the dark arrows and the inhibitory projections by the light grey. **SNc**: Substantia Nigra pars compacta; **SNr**: Substantia nigra pars reticulata; **GPe**: external portion of Globus pallidus; **GPi**: internal portion of Globus pallidus; **STN**: sub-thalamic nuclei; **VL**: ventral-lateral nucleus of thalamus.

ing indirect inputs from cerebellum see the work by Peter Strick (Middleton & Strick, 1997).

Basal ganglia. A primary function of the basal ganglia is motor control. The basal ganglia consist of two large structures, the caudate and lentiform *nuclei*. The lentiform *nucleus* is composed of the putamen and the *globus pallidus*. Due to similarities between the putamen and the caudate, some authors group them together under the term *striatum*.

Figure 22.9 shows the main inputs and outputs from the basal ganglia involved in motor control. By far, the cerebral cortex provides the main input to the basal ganglia through the putamen, with all cortical areas sending afferents to it. In addition, the putamen receives well-known dopaminergic input from the *sustantia nigra pars compacta*. Two paths loop back from the putamen to the cortex, one direct and the other indirect. The direct path goes to the internal *globus pallidus*, which in turn projects to thalamus, specifically the ventro-anterior and ventral lateral *nuclei*, (independent of the cerebellar input to these nuclei). The final part of the pathway originates in thalamus and projects to cortical motor regions. The indirect path goes from putamen to external *globus pallidus*, and from there, to the subthalamic nuclei. The path then projects to the internal *globus pallidus* and the *sustantia nigra pars reticulata* regions that project to VL thalamus and then to motor cortices. An interesting aspect of these two pathways is the large number of inhibitory connections (represented in Figure 22.9 with grey arrows producing double inhibitory effects). A number of researchers have attempted, with limited success, to apply this network to understanding the motor deficits of Parkinson's disease. What it is clear is that the basal ganglia are not only involved in the modulation of motor functions, but also play a role in cognitive functions (Middleton & Strick, 1994).

Cortico-cortical connections

Neurophysiological, cytoarchitectonic, and histochemical studies have radically altered our view on the cortical motor system over the last two decades. Until then, the prevailing notion was that the cortical motor system consisted of three main sectors: the primary motor cortex (M1), lying in the precentral gyrus, the premotor cortex (LPMC) located in the precentral gyrus in front of the primary motor cortex, and the supplementary motor area (SMA) on the mesial surface of the hemisphere. The primary motor cortex was thought to be involved in the actual execution of movements, while the premotor and the supplementary motor areas were thought to be more involved in motor planning. Numerous cytoarchitectonic and histochemical studies have challenged this view. Figure 22.10 shows a modern subdivision of the cortical motor areas originally proposed by Massimo Matelli and coworkers (1985). Figure 22.10 clearly illustrates that the organization of the motor system is more complex than previously thought. In fact, this system consists of numerous areas, each indicated in the monkey with the letter F (frontal) followed by a number. F1 corresponds to the classically defined primary motor cortex (area 4 of Brodmann); the premotor cortex (BA 6l) is further divided into a ventral premotor cortex (LPMCv) and a dorsal premotor cortex (LPMCd). The ventral premotor cortex consists of two distinct areas: area F5 (BA 44 in humans), rostrally located, and area F4 (LPMCv in humans), caudally located. The dorsal premotor cortex is also composed of two areas: area F2, rostrally located (rostral LPMCd in humans) and area F7 (caudal LPMCd in humans), caudally located. On the mesial surface of the hemisphere, the premotor cortex includes a caudal area (area F3, which corresponds to the classically defined SMA in humans) and a rostral area (area F6, also called pre-SMA in humans). An additional area shown in both species is the cingulate motor region (CMA or BA 24c and 23c).

Each of these cortical areas is not only anatomically distinct, but also functionally distinct, since they display specific motor representations of actions somototopically represented (e.g., hand or mouth). At the same time, motor acts involving a specific body part may be represented in several areas. This multiple motor representation of actions is due to the fact that each area codes for a different aspect of the action. For example, among other features, grasping an apple implies knowing *where* the apple is and *how* big it is. In order to grasp an object properly, one needs to localize it in space, code its pragmatic features, and determine the position of the body in relation to the object. Different areas of the motor system play a specific role in this coding.

All areas in the motor system are connected to additional regions of the cerebral cortex. Some of them (F1-

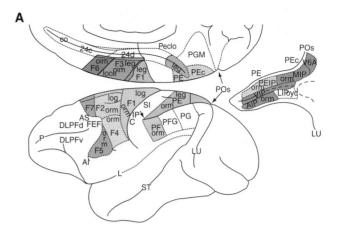

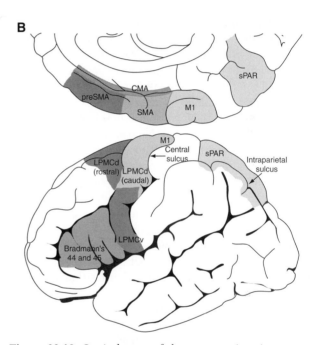

Figure 22.10. Cortical maps of the motor regions in macaque and humans. **A**: Cortical regions in the parietal and frontal lobes in the macaque. **B**: Cortical motor regions in humans. Similar colors between species suggest homology. *Modified from Rizolatti, Luppino and Matelli (1998). The organization of the cortical motor system: New concepts. Electr. Clin. Neurophysiol. 106: 283–296.*

F5, i.e., M1, posterior LPMCd, SMA, LPMCv, and Broca's area) are connected to specific areas located in the posterior parietal lobe, whereas some others (area F6 and area F7, i.e., preSMA and rostral LPMCd) are connected to the prefrontal cortex. Interestingly, while motor areas heavily connected to parietal regions project to spinal cord, motor areas heavily connected pre-frontal regions do not. Furthermore, areas functionally connected to the parietal lobule form a fronto-parietal circuit, devoted to a sensory-motor transformation necessary to act properly on an object and to perform actions accurately. In addition, whereas the prefrontal regions are more devoted to motor planning, cingulate motor regions are involved in motor control related to emotional expression.

It is beyond the scope of the present chapter to describe in detail all of the motor cortical circuits and their functional roles. We will consider three such circuits as examples of the organization of skilled movements. Although most data come from anatomical and physiological studies carried out in the monkey, there is increasing evidence that the same organization is also present in the human brain. When available, data will be reported to show a parallel functional organization in both species.

AIP-F5 circuit for grasping. Area F5 (BA 44 in humans) lies in the rostral part of F4 (LPMCv). Electrophysiological studies have shown that this area contains motor representations for both mouth and hand object-directed actions. Neurons found in this region discharge when one executes specific goal-directed actions like grasping a piece of food with the hand or the mouth, holding it, tearing and manipulating it. There are even neurons that discharge with specific types of grasping. Notable examples of this include precision grip (a prehension obtained opposing the index finger and the thumb, e.g. grasping a piece of food); finger prehension (obtained by opposing the thumb and the other fingers, e.g., grasping a pen); whole hand prehension (obtained by closing the whole hand around an object, e.g., grasping a little ball). Since their discovery, it has been proposed that these neurons build up a "vocabulary" of hand/mouth actions that, like words in a language, can be used in different contexts, whenever appropriate.

Besides motor properties, neurons in area F5 also encode visual features. Based on their visual properties, F5 neurons are divided into a) mirror neurons and b) canonical neurons. Mirror neurons (that will be described in a latter section in this chapter) are neurons that discharge not only when the monkey performs a specific object-directed action with the hand or the mouth, but also when it observes another individual (monkey or human) doing the same or a similar action. They are called "mirror" because the observed action seems to be reflected like in a mirror in the motor representation coded by the neuron. Canonical neurons are not different from mirror neurons as far as their motor properties are concerned, but their visual response is triggered by the observation of an object congruent to the type of action coded by the neuron. For example, if a canonical neuron codes precision grip, it may respond to the observation of a piece of food (which is an object normally grasped with a precision grip). It has been proposed that canonical neurons are able to "describe" the observed object in motor terms and therefore "translate" the pragmatic features integrating them into the appropriate action. Area F5 is intimately connected with the intraparietal area (AIP), an area located inside the intraparietal sulcus. Electrophysiological studies in neurons of area AIP show that they share common features with those of area F5. Most of these neurons discharge during the execution of hand and finger actions (like grasping), activation that in some of them can be modified by visual stimuli. During the act of grasping, for example, area AIP can extract relevant physical features of the object, whereas area F5 selects the most appropriate type of prehension among those present in the motor "vocabulary" of the area.

Although data coming from monkey studies are not easily comparable to those obtained in humans, there is increasing evidence from brain imaging studies that a fronto-parietal circuit like monkey AIP-F5 is also present. During an fMRI experiment in which participants were required to grasp and manipulate different objects, the main active areas were the LPMCv (including Broca's region) and an area inside the intraparietal sulcus in the parietal lobe, which could be considered the human homologue of area AIP (Binkofski et al., 1999). Furthermore, patients with lesions within the intraparietal sulcus, are not able to grasp and manipulate objects reinforcing the role of this area similar to that in non-human primates.

VIP-F4 circuit for space coding. Area F4 lies in the caudal part of the ventral premotor cortex in the monkey. In humans, it is the most ventral portion of the pre-central gyrus (LPMCv). Electrophysiological studies have shown that this area contains a motor representation of proximal arm and mouth actions, the data showing that neurons discharge during the execution of reaching movements directed towards or away from the body. F4 neurons also respond to visual and tactile stimuli. Hence, depending on their responses to sensory stimuli (visual and somatosensory), they can be uni- or bimodal. For instance, bimodal neurons respond not only to tactile, but also to visual stimuli presented in the space adjacent to the tactile receptive fields (personal space), thus forming a single responsive region that includes the skin and the space adjacent to it. Most interesting is the fact that the coordinate system in which visual receptive fields are coded is in somato-centered coordinates (i.e., their location is independent of eye position). Area F4 is connected with the ventral intraparietal area (VIP). Again, neurons of area VIP share common features with those of area F4 since they can be uni- or bimodal. What is the role of the VIP-F4 circuit? It has been proposed that this circuit plays a role in coding personal space by transforming the location of objects in space in order to execute appropriate movements to reach them.

Area F2-V6A-MIP circuit for online up-dating of grasping actions. Area F2 lies in the caudal part of the dorsal premotor cortex in the monkey and in the dorsal portion of the pre-central gyrus in humans (LPMCd). Electrophysiological studies have shown that this area has a rough somatotopic organization, with hindlimb movements located medial to the superior precentral dimple and forelimb movements located in the cortex lateral to it. A recent study (Fogassi et al., 2001) showed that this region displays (a) purely motor neurons, which discharge during grasping conditions; (b) visually modulated neurons, that are active during grasping accompanied with visual perception of an object; and (c) visuomotor neurons, that discharge during the perception of objects in the absence of any overt movement. Taken together, these data indicate that area F2, like area F5, plays an important role in the control of goal-directed hand actions. Area F2 receives its major visual inputs from area MIP, in the superior parietal lobule, and from area V6A in the occipital lobule. Although visual properties of area MIP are not very well-known, recent findings suggest that this area responds to the presentation of 3-dimensional objects. As for area V6A, it has been reported that neurons in this area are sensitive to the hand-target interactions, thus supporting its role in the visual monitoring of hand position in space. One can conclude that during grasping, the circuit F2–MIP/V6A could be updating on-line the configuration and the orientation of the hand when it reaches for objects.

MOTOR PHYSIOLOGY

Subcortical motor control: Reflexes and central pattern generators

The spinal cord and brain stem play an important role in the generation of movement because a large number of specialized motor circuits are located there. As an example, consider the generation of voluntary movements. Once voluntary movements are initiated, their production requires the activation of specialized circuits located in the spinal cord that in turn activates the corresponding muscles. Furthermore, since different segments of the spinal cord control different body parts, it is easy to understand that the production of complex movements requires the sequential activation of various levels of the spinal cord. In this section we will review two examples of such circuits: reflexes and central pattern generators.

Reflexes

Reflexes are stereotyped movements triggered by somatosensory stimulation. Spinal reflexes can be initiated by stimulation of receptors in the joints, muscles and the skin, with the resulting motor response controlled entirely within circuits located in the spinal cord and brain stem.

Is there a role for reflexive activity? Reflexes are ecologically important because they produce adaptive movements when integrated with centrally generated motor commands. Thus reflexes are an essential part of complex movements. For instance, multiple sensory stimulation is produced during coordinated movements (information coming from joints, muscles, and skin), providing feedback to the system to help with production of coordinated and smooth movements. When perturbations in the environment occur, sensory feedback information produces a reflexive response, making possible small adjustments in the ongoing movement. These adjustments are especially important in the control of tone in proximal musculature related to the maintenance of posture.

In early studies, reflexes were considered stereotyped unchangeable movements. Most recent observations, however, have shown that reflexes have a degree of flexibility and can adjust to changes in the external or internal environment. In other words, reflexes show plasticity. This feature makes them more interesting, since it implies a possible role in motor learning or recovery of motor function after neurological damage.

The stretch reflex. The stretch reflex is one of the better known reflexes since it is used in clinical practice, but it is also one of the simplest spinal reflexes, employing a neural circuit of few elements. This reflex is illustrated in Figure 22.11.

The stimulus that produces the quadriceps stretch reflex is typically a tap on the patellar tendon in the knee, although any action that stretches this muscle has the equivalent effect. When the muscle is stretched, sensory receptors (muscle spindles) located in the muscle fire in response. This produces electrical firing of the spindle afferents (called Ia afferents) that make direct synaptic contact with spinal motoneurons innervating the *quadriceps*. In other words, this network forms a loop, since it returns to the same muscle where the stimulated spindles are located. In addition, this type of circuit is called "monosynaptic" because it has a single synapse (between the Ia afferents and the motoneurons) in the spinal cord.

Since the synaptic contact between the Ia afferents and the motoneurons that innervate the *quadriceps* are excitatory, their activation triggers the motoneuron to fire, and in turn produces a contraction of this muscle.

While this is occurring, a concomitant pathway is involved in the reflex. The Ia afferent fiber activated by the stretch of the quadriceps muscle also makes a synaptic contact with inhibitory interneurons located in the spinal cord.

These interneurons inhibit the motoneurons innervating a knee flexor muscle (in this case the *semitendinosus*), an antagonist of the *quadriceps* (i.e., when it contracts, it produces the opposite movement), producing flexion of the knee in contrast to the extension produced by the *quadriceps*. The inhibition of the antagonist allows the *quadriceps* to contract easier since the *semitendinosus* relaxes. The end result of this balance is the well-known movement of leg (lift) when the patellar tendon is stimulated.

Because the inhibitory circuit includes more than one synapse (one between the Ia afferent and the interneurons and a second one between the interneurons and the motoneurons), the pathway is considered to be "polysynaptic."

The balance of excitation and inhibition between agonist and antagonist muscles is called "reciprocal inhibition" and the spinal circuit associated with it is called "reciprocal innervation." This important concept was described by one of the greatest physiologists ever to live who was already mentioned in the history section, Sherrington (1906), and refers to the fact that when a group of muscles is excited, the antagonist muscles to that first group of muscles are inhibited. The balance between excitation and inhibition

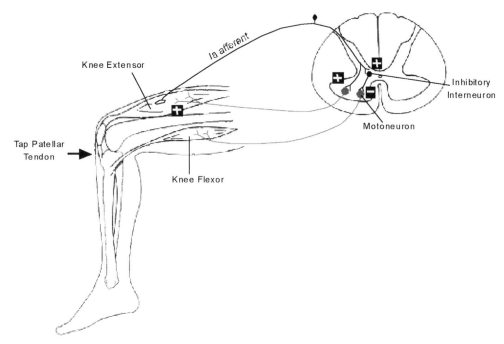

Figure 22.11. Circuit associated with the production of the flexor reflex in humans. Schematic representation of the two circuits associated with the generation of the knee jerk reflex. The monosynaptic circuit (marked with positive signs) is excited producing the contraction of the *quadriceps* muscle. At the same time, a polysynaptic circuit is involved with the difference that it involves inhibitory interneurons in the spinal cord (marked by the minus sign), that will produce a relaxation of the antagonist muscle. *Modified from Boron WF and Boulpaep EL. (2003) Medical Physiology. Saunders. Elsevier Science (USA).*

of reciprocal musculature is critical to the coordinated movement of the joints.

These examples of spinal reflexes illustrate a limited portion of what occurs constantly throughout the body to maintain posture. Sensory information is constantly delivered from the body. Control of posture (static or changing) requires incoming sensory information not only from muscles, tendons and skin but also from vestibular and visual receptors. These inputs originate in brain-stem, cerebellum and different levels of the spinal cord, and are integrated rapidly in the spinal cord through the activation of proprio-spinal paths whose function is the interconnection of different levels of the spinal cord and brain stem. The point of this example is to illustrate not only the apparent complexity of keeping posture (through activation of reflex activity) and the importance of reflexes in this control, but also, to illustrate the fact that all these adjustments are done automatically, without conscious control. This points out another feature of the motor system: Although we are aware of the initiation of some (voluntary) movements, not all movements are in the conscious realm. This fact becomes critical in situations where recovery of motor function is desired (after injury for instance) or for motor learning.

Central pattern generators (CPGs)

For years, the importance of network activation in the generation of motor behaviors by the CNS has been widely recognized. In this context, the motor system has often

been described as having a "hierarchical organization" (Wiesendanger & Wise, 1992) to define a situation where this complex system is composed of a number of relatively automatic subsystems capable of performing a specific task but also influenced by "general commands" initiated in higher levels or through sensory feedback (Arshavsky, 2003). This means that higher centers do not control individual elements within the lower circuits but rather, provide commands by which these latter networks can perform their tasks. The result of this organization is a highly efficient system.

Remarkable examples of these "autonomous centers" are what have been called: "Central Pattern Generators or CPGs." The CPGs have been associated with the control of automatic, basic motor patterns such as locomotion, respiration, swallowing, chewing, swimming, scratching, and defensive behaviors, among others.

Formally the CPGs are defined as the neuronal networks that produce a basic motor output in the absence of sensory feedback. More precisely, Marsden has defined the CPG as: "a set of muscle commands (or motor program) which are structured before movement begins and which can be sent to the muscle with the correct timing so that the entire sequence is carried out in the absence of peripheral feedback." What this means is that the direct electrical stimulation of specific circuits will produce rhythmic activation associated with complex motor acts as stepping or galloping, swimming, swallowing or breathing. Since stimulation in these studies is not "natural," the resulting

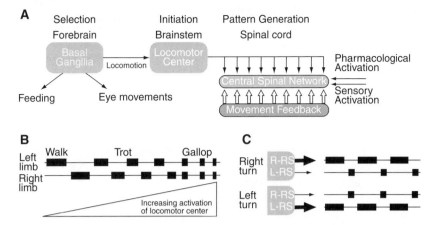

Figure 22.12. General organization of CPGs in vertebrates. Schematic representation of locomotion in vertebrates, that shows also the general organization of the CPGs. **a**: Forebrain structures initialize the spinal CPG activation. The resulting rhythmic activation is then modulated by sensory and pharmacological inputs. **b**: Representation of the interlimb coordination in quadrupeds. Note the alternation of the rhythm between both sides of the cord. **c**: Reticular activation leads to an asymmetrical pattern that will result in the animal turning to one side. *From: Grillner et al. (2000). The intrinsic function of a motor system-from ion channels to networks and behavior. Brain Res. 886: 224–236. With permission of S. Grillner.*

motor behavior is called "fictive behavior" (for instance "fictive locomotion" etc.) to denote their distance from the ecological movements. Such fictive movements tend to be more stereotyped than true ecological movements.

Although it has been suggested that the structure of CPGs are genetically determined and their physiology does not depend on experience, they in fact can be modulated by sensory feedback and descending inputs. Because this influence from descending inputs and sensory feedback changes their functioning, the preferred approach to studying CPGs has been by isolating them from these influences. The easiest way to do this has been to use invertebrates (Arshavsky, 2003; Grillner et al., 2000; Marder, 2000; Marder & Bucher, 2001). This approach has provided a large amount of information on the physiology and anatomy of CPGs. In vertebrates, the methods of choice have been the use of isolation methods such as spinalization (Jankowska et al., 1967; McCrea, 1998) where the spinal cord is isolated anatomically from higher regions of the central nervous system or by the administration of pharmacological agents such as *curare* that eliminates the proprioceptive sensory input to the cord (Kiehn & Kjaerulff, 1998).

In general, these studies have focused on CPGs that generate rhythmic activity present extensively throughout the phylogenetic scale, from invertebrates (like mollusks and crustacea) to vertebrates (including mammals). In the latter, CPGs are typically located at the level of the spinal cord (for locomotion and scratching) and at the level of the brainstem for other motor behaviors such as respiration, swallowing and chewing.

The general organization of CPGs in mammals is depicted in Figure 22.12 (Grillner et al., 2000) where the influence of descending systems and sensory information is shown to highlight the fact that these circuits are highly regulated. In order to understand better the physiology of these circuits, it is important to mention that all CPGs share several features:

(a) The intrinsic properties of the neurons within the CPGs are important in the generation of the rhythmic motor behaviors. For instance, some neurons of the circuit are driven by pacemaker neurons. So the rhythmic activity is generated by the synaptic contact between the pacemakers (or core oscillators) and other neurons that do not have a rhythmic activity on themselves.

(b) Even though it was previously thought that the generation of motor rhythmic behavior was solely through a chain of reflexes, the current view is that a central circuit generates the rhythmic patterns of activity including some reflexive activation (Marder & Bucher, 2001) and some other elements not part of the reflexive circuits.

(c) CPGs are regulated by neuromodulators. Depending on the function of the CPG, they receive inputs from descending, sensory or hormonal origins. The function of these inputs is to initiate the movement (descending control), whereas in other cases (hormonal, sensory), these inputs either terminate or regulate the rhythmic activity.

(d) Some complex motor behaviors might be produced by the coordination of one or more CPGs. A classic example is swimming (studied extensively in lampreys and frogs). Swimming behavior implies the simultaneous coordination of several body segments (up and down or right and left) and in consequence the coordination of several spinal segments is essential. In these animals, each spinal segment produces motor patterns that organize the local swimming movements (Marder & Bucher, 2001). It has been suggested that coordinated movements of the whole body result from the coupling of the individual CPGs along the cord. This coupling implies the simultaneous coordination of several CPGs and the regulation of independent movements by each one in the same fashion as the control of posture was described in a previous section.

(e) Rhythmic movements associated with CPGs tend to be stereotyped (especially fictive movements) and some studies suggest, might be genetically determined (Marder & Bucher, 2001).

Locomotion. Traditionally, the spinal cord has been associated with the generation of non-flexible, automatic, simple motor behaviors. However, the types of motor behaviors that can be generated through spinal circuits can be much more complex than previously thought. This section will discuss one such circuit that generates locomotion.

The generation of locomotion within the spinal cord is particularly interesting because it is present in humans and is quite complex in that it involves long motor sequences and can be modified. Unfortunately, locomotion in humans with reference to the presence of CPGs has been difficult to assess due to obvious experimental limitations. Nonetheless, lesions to the spinal cord provide some data on this topic, and this will be presented at the end of this section.

Locomotion in mammals. The study of CPGs and locomotion in mammals has employed several experimental approaches: (a) spinalization of the animals where the spinal cord is isolated from higher centers; (b) administration of pharmacological agents such as *curare* that prevents sensory proprioceptive information from reaching the spinal cord; and (c) isolation of spinal neurons forming the CPGs (as in invertebrates) in neonatal rats (but not mature animals).

The study of locomotion in mammals has a long history, beginning with the pioneering work of Sherrington (1910), who determined that the spinal cord of cats has enough reflexive-related circuitry to produce by itself the rhythmic flexor-extensor pattern during locomotion. Almost simultaneously, Brown (1911) performed more descriptive studies in spinalized plus deafferented (i.e., no sensory inputs) cats where he confirmed the ability of these animals to perform stepping behavior in the absence of afferent input. He suggested that the spinal cord contains intrinsic circuits able to produce locomotion. Today, several studies in deafferented and spinalized animals have shown that the spinal cord can produce what has been called "fictive locomotion", i.e., rhythmic patterns of activity in circuits that would drive rhythmic muscle movement (Marder, 2001). Furthermore, the most current theories (Jankowska et al., 1967) describing the CPGs for locomotion in mammals are a combination of reflex activation plus additional elements forming a complex circuit.

The existence of CPGs for locomotion have been demonstrated in several species with the interesting fact that the general organization seems quite similar in all species studied, even thought the locomotion patterns seem at some level very different (from swimming to walking to trotting or running).

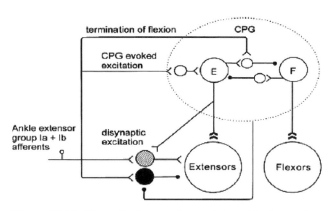

Figure 22.13. Theoretical network associated with the production of fictive locomotion in mammals. Schematic representation of the actual spinal generator. Inhibitory connections are represented by filled circles and excitatory connections by open forks. This model highlights the importance of reflexive activity between flexors and extensors. *From: McCrea (1998). Neuronal basis of afferent-evoked enhancement of locomotor activity. Ann. NY Acad. Sci. 860: 216–225. With permission of D.A. McCrea.*

Figure 22.13 depicts the hypothetical anatomical arrangement of a spinal CPG of the cat's spinal cord (McCrea, 1998). According to McCrea (2001) there are several relevant features of CPGs for locomotion in four paw mammals:

1. Since the rhythmic motor behavior during locomotion is stereotyped, the role of segmental reflexes circuits is to compensate for changes in the environment.

2. Fictive locomotion in decerebrate animals can be triggered by electrical stimulation of the midbrain or by the administration of adrenergic agents.

3. Afferent inputs can modulate the rhythmicity of locomotion. Even when it is clear that the rhythmic activation of neurons within the spinal cord during fictive locomotion is quite close to the activation during real movement, it is nevertheless not identical. More and more studies have shown the great relevance of sensory input as a determinant aspect of CPGs physiology especially for its role in adapting the CPGs activation to constant changes in the environment. The roles associated with sensory input are: Reinforcement of CPG activity related to load-bearing muscles; regulation of timing depending on the actual task performed and the facilitation of phase transitions (MacKay-Lyons, 2002).

4. Rhythmic activity is generated by the reciprocal inhibition of two sets of interneurons located on each side of the spinal cord – an extensor circuit and a flexor circuit – each exciting their corresponding motoneurons.

5. Supraspinal centers can regulate the activation of spinal CPGs for locomotion. Even though it is clear that CPGs can be activated in the absence of supraspinal centers, these regions play an important role in several aspects of locomotion, since they are crucial to the initiation of CPG activity and in controlling the intensity of their activity, maintaining equilibrium during locomotion, adapting limb movement to changes in external conditions and coordinating locomotion with other motor acts. Among the supraspinal regions that have been associated with this control are the primary motor and sensory cortical regions, the cerebellum, and the basal ganglia.

Locomotion in humans. Based on the large number of studies on locomotion in animal species, an obvious question is to what extent human walking can be understood using similar principles.

Intuitively, human walking has obvious differences with other types of mammalian locomotion. First, humans walk erect on two legs; at the moment of the contact with the ground, the leg is almost completely extended and the body part that touches the ground first is the heel. One of the consequences of this is that simultaneous activation of flexors and extensors is present at heel contact (rather than in phase like other animals) (Capaday, 2002). Furthermore, when people suffer complete transactions of the spinal cord, that is, the spinal cord is completely isolated from the rest of the supra-spinal regions, one would expect recovery of locomotion with direct electrical stimulation of the spinal cord. Unfortunately, as we know, this is not the case.

In contrast to these differences with other mammals, locomotion in humans shares some features with both mammals and with other classes. Among these parallels:

1. Some spinal control of locomotion in humans is performed through the regulation of reflexes, especially the stretch reflex, which is thought to make a high contribution to walking in humans.

2. Sensory input is critical to the control and modulation of walking in humans. One suggestion has been that the stance-to-swing transition is promoted when the hip is extended, and the load in ankle extensors is decreased (these changes captured by sensory receptors) (Capaday, 2002).

3. The corticospinal pathway is involved in the initiation of walking (Capaday et al., 1999).

4. Lastly is the question of the existence (or not) of locomotion CPGs proper in the human spinal cord. The presence of CPGs for human walking would have tremendous implications for recovery of spinal cord lesions, with the option of activating them (as in other species) through sensory inputs, neuromodulators (like dopamine or adrenaline), or with direct electrical stimulation. As mentioned, the answer is not clear and at first glance, seems implausible. However, favoring the notion that human walking is performed with the participation of CPGs, it is possible to elicit rhythmic activity within the spinal cord of humans with intact sensory inputs, suggesting the existence of specialized circuits. Human spinal CPGs are undoubtedly weaker than those of other mammals, because after complete spinal cord injury, pharmacological interventions do not produce walking in humans as they do in rats and cats. More promising results, however, have been seen after partial transection of the spinal cord, where a combination of pharmacological activation plus treadmill training has produced some improvement in locomotion of these patients.

MOTOR BEHAVIOR AND COGNITION

In the following sections, we will describe three examples of motor behavior closely related to complex cognitive functions. The idea is to provide a sense of the complexity of motor physiology in the context of cognitive processes. It is important, however, to understand that each of these examples (motor imagery, motor imitation, and motor learning) is intimately interrelated, even when presented as independent phenomena.

Motor imagery

Some cognitive psychologists (Annett, 1996) have suggested a distinction between two types of knowledge: explicit and implicit (or "knowing what" and "knowing how"). One of the features is that whereas explicit knowledge can easily be described verbally, implicit or procedural knowledge cannot. Motor acts tend to fall into the category of implicit knowledge, and as such, motor imagery can be considered the internal representation of the motor act.

Motor acts are triggered either by external sensory stimuli or by internal commands, implying that the central nervous system needs constantly to merge or transform sensory (or internal) codes into motor commands. As suggested by Passingham, Toni, and Rushworth (2000), this could be achieved through the use of what he calls "high-level representations" (or "cross-domain mappings" Wise, di Pellegrino, & Boussaoud, 1996) where stimuli and actions must be represented (see also the cortico-cortical connections section in this chapter). In other words, motor imagery could be considered the internal representation of previously learned movements.

In the most general sense, motor imagery refers to the "mental rehearsal of simple or complex motor acts that is not accompanied by overt body movements" (Jeannerod, 1995; Porro et al., 1996).

Although the definition appears simple, people asked to perform motor imagery do not make an unambiguous interpretation unless instructed more specifically. In particular, people generally perform this mental rehearsal of movements according to one of two strategies: (1) they produce a visual representation of their moving limb; or (2) they mentally simulate the movements associated with a kinesthetic feeling of the movement. In the first case, the person is a spectator of the movements (external imagery). We will refer to this behavior as visual imagery (VI). In the second case, the person is a performer (internal imagery). We will refer to this behavior as kinetic imagery (KI).

In fact, each of these strategies of motor imagery has different properties: For example, while KI is difficult to verbalize, VI is not. Whereas KI follows Fitt's law (i.e., the imagined movement associated with KI shows the same limitations as movements during execution), VI does not. This means that during KI, a person cannot perform movements at a higher rate than during overt execution, and this still holds after brain injury, when both execution and KI are diminished correspondingly. In contrast, during VI, a person can imagine movements that far exceed the physiological limitations of the execution (for review see Jeannerod, 1995). Moreover, certain physiological changes associated with KI mimic those occurring during execution, whereas during VI, they do not. For example, whereas electromyographic (EMG) activity during KI shows an increase in voltage in the muscles corresponding to movement execution, there are no such changes during VI (Fadiga et al., 1999). Furthermore, the excitability of the cortico-spinal pathway measured with transcranial magnetic stimulation is increased during KI but not VI (Abbruzzese et al., 1999; Fadiga et al., 1999; Rossini et al., 1999). In addition, if these imagery tasks involve strenuous movements, KI (but not VI) will show concomitant changes in autonomic function similar to those present during execution, including increases in heart and respiratory rates as well as in end-tidal PCO_2 (Decety et al., 1991; Oishi, Kasai, & Maeshima, 2000).

Since KI shares more physiological characteristics with the movement execution than does VI, it has been associated more closely with motor functions *per se* such as motor preparation, imitation and anticipation, restraining and the refining of motor abilities (Deiber et al., 1998; Jeannerod, 1995; Lotze et al., 1999; Stephan & Frackowiak, 1996). However, even when this correlation between motor execution and KI has been made, it is still not clear if KI and VI are sensory representations associated with the motor act or if they are in fact, true storage motor representations. This outstanding issue has been elucidated using a number of different techniques although the most revealing results have been obtained with functional brain imaging techniques. In the next section, we describe some conclusions that we have reached regarding motor imagery using modern techniques.

The physiology of motor imagery

With respect to imaging studies, several accounts of areas activated during KI or VI have been reported using PET or fMRI. Even though some of the studies do not differentiate between KI and VI, there are several features common to most of them (Jeannerod, 2001; Kim et al., 1995; Roland et al., 1980; Sanes, 1994; Stephan & Frackowiak, 1996). In general, studies have shown that several areas are activated during motor imagery tasks. Included in these active regions are the following: SMA, superior and inferior parietal lobule, LPMCd and LPMCv, pre-frontal areas, inferior frontal gyrus (BA44), superior temporal gyrus, M1, S1, secondary sensory area, insular cortex, anterior cingulate cortex, superior temporal gyrus, basal ganglia, and cerebellum. This extensive activation pattern suggests a complex distributed circuit. In studies that compared execution to motor imagery, it was found that even though the active areas tend to be similar between the two conditions, in general, volumes of activation are larger during execution than during motor imagery (Gerardin et al., 2000; Jeannerod, 2001; Stephan & Frackowiak, 1996). A controversial point in some of these studies is the role of M1 during imagery, since its activation is not seen consistently in all studies and if seen, it is always less active than during execution (Beisteiner et al., 1995; Fadiga et al., 1999; Hashimoto & Rothwell, 1999). The lack of M1 involvement during motor imagery has been explained as the way the system avoids overt movements during imagery.

In summary, these studies suggest that the volume of brain activation differs between execution and motor imagery and that with few exceptions the distribution of activation tends to be similar in the two conditions.

So we have here an interesting riddle: on the one hand it seems that executing a movement and having KI of the same movement produce similar patterns of activation in the brain. However, moving is not the same as imagining that one is moving. What is the difference? In the following section, we demonstrate how brain imaging data provided a novel perspective on human motor neurophysiology.

There is no doubt that studies in systems neuroscience have benefited tremendously from the development of techniques such as functional Magnetic Resonance Imaging (fMRI). However, image analysis in fMRI has generally focused on enumerating areas of activation under different behavioral conditions, rather than characterizing the networks involved in the generation of those behaviors. Thus, with respect to localizational assumptions, these studies are analogous to lesion analysis studies, and incorporate some of the same advantages and limitations.

An alternative approach has been the efforts by some to assess networks of activation through the evaluation of effective connectivity among areas activated during different behavioral conditions (Buchel & Friston, 1997; Gonzalez-Lima & McIntosh, 1994; Horwitz et al., 2000). These models provide an interesting new perspective on experimental design and data analysis since they give an analytical approach to understanding integrated systems.

Network analysis in motor imagery

What does it mean to understand networks of activity? One of the most interesting features of the physiology of the CNS is the influence of regions on each other by means of established anatomical connections. Interestingly, not only have these connectivity patterns increased through the evolution of the cerebral cortex (Zilles et al., 1995) but in addition, the patterns of connections are not random: not all regions connect with all regions but rather, form specific patterns of connections. In terms of physiology, it means that changes in one region produce concomitant changes in regions anatomically connected to it. Although brain imaging has provided maps of regional activation, thereby giving an initial understanding to the neural basis of cognition, so far, we have not been able to establish the effect that one particular region is exerting upon the

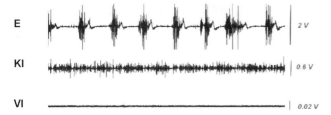

Figure 22.14. Electromyographic recordings during E, KI and VI. The upper trace shows EMG activation in the FDI during finger opposition movements. The second trace during KI and the third trace during VI. Muscle tone increased during KI but not during VI that did not differ from rest.

regions connected to it. Connectivity modeling is allowing us for the first time to quantify the effect of one region (node) over others. The directional effect of one region upon another as mentioned in the historical section, is called "effective connectivity."

Following this idea of connectivity analysis, the present section will describe effective connectivity in networks associated with three different conditions: execution of hand movements (E), and kinetic and visual imagery of these same movements (KI and VI). These networks can help to inform about a possible role of "motor imagery" in the improvement of motor skill in normal subjects and in recovery after neurological damage. In normal subjects, for instance, motor imagery is used by athletes and professional musicians, where it is called "mental rehearsal," to improve performance. By the same token, motor imagery is used therapeutically after stroke to stimulate recovery of motor abilities (Yaguez et al., 1999).

In a recent study, we aimed to understand the networks underlying hand motor imagery as compared to actual execution. This study was performed using fMRI (Solodkin et al., 2004). The first step in the study was to assess the subjects' ability to perform kinetic imagery: One of the issues during motor imagery is the difficulty detecting if people are actually performing the task correctly. In general, most people will tend to perform visual imagery rather than kinetic imagery. For this, and before the subjects were

scanned for the fMRI session, outside the scanner, they were asked to perform either a finger opposition movement and both kinetic and visual imagery of the same movement. During the task practice, EMG was recorded in the first dorsal *interosseus*, one of the muscles controlling the opposition of the thumb and the index fingers. The results of this part of the study are illustrated in Figure 22.14. During execution, the EMG showed the typical muscle spindles associated with the contraction of muscles. As expected, these spindles were not present during either type of imagery, since during these tasks, there was no overt movement of the fingers. However, the EMG recordings during kinetic and visual imagery were not identical; kinetic imagery produced an increase in muscle tone (seen by the amplitude of the recorded band) whereas the muscle tone during visual imagery was identical to rest. This observation not only demonstrated that the participants were performing kinetic imagery correctly, but also illustrates the fact that kinetic imagery is associated with motor preparation that involves a change in the voltage of the involved muscles, shifting them closer to the contraction threshold (they are facilitated).

Second, an fMRI study was performed: The task during the fMRI session was as follow: The fingers of the dominant hand were numbered from 1 to 4 (1 = index, 2 = middle, 3 = ring, 4 = pinky). Numbers from 1 to 4 appeared randomly on a screen, and for each one, subjects performed the corresponding finger-thumb opposition. The task was externally paced at a rate of 2 Hz. The motor task paradigm included the execution of those movements alternated with either one of the two imagery conditions (KI or VI).

Figure 22.15 shows the fMRI activation patterns for each condition (the arrows are pointing to the central sulcus for guidance).

Note that the volumes of activation in the primary motor cortex during execution are larger than that seen during kinetic imagery (Jeannerod, 1995; Kim et al., 1995), general trend for all areas during the imagery tasks.

Third, we determined the networks of activation: By determining networks of activation, Structural equation

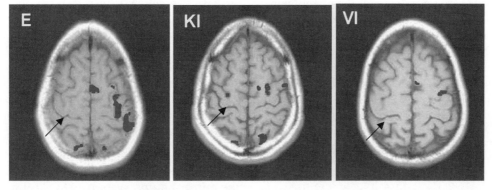

Figure 22.15. Single subject fMRI during E, KI and VI. Brain activation was seen in several sensory and motor areas during execution (E), kinetic imagery (KI) and visual imagery (VI). These axial slices depict regions at the level of the hand motor area of M1. For orientation purposes, the arrows are pointing to the central sulcus. Note that volumes of activation were much larger during E than during KI or VI. Since these are radiological images, the left side of the figure represents the right hemisphere.

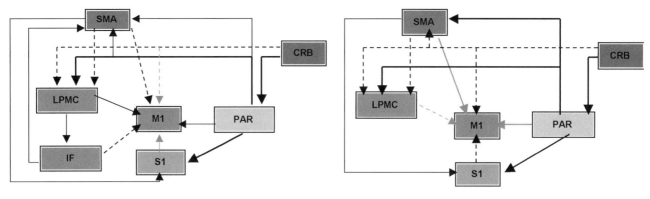

Execution of finger opposition

Kinetic imagery of finger opposition

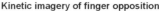

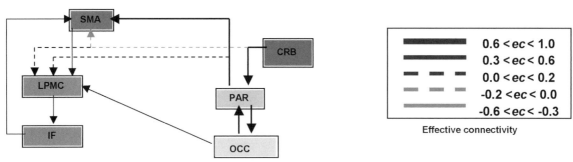

Visual imagery of finger opposition

Effective connectivity

Figure 22.16. Final networks for E, KI, and VI. This figure depicts the values of effective connections during the three experimental conditions. Note the close parallels between E and KI except in the connections between association motor areas and superior parietal lobule with M1. In contrast, the patterns of connectivity in the VI conditions were biased towards visual areas.

modeling (SEM) describes the functional influences among anatomical brain regions. The emphasis thereby changes from the individual brain regions active in each condition to the relationships among them. The results of the present study demonstrated that independent of the volumes of activation *per se*, there are clear differences (and similarities) in the networks for E, KI, and VI. The following figure shows the networks associated with each condition.

As shown in Figure 22.16, E and KI are closely related tasks, since they share several, identical parts of the network. The VI condition differs the most. These results show that resulting networks can differentiate among conditions that activate the same regions by means of effective connectivity values, but also they denote if they are facilitatory (positive) or not (negative). These parallels suggest that influences among areas involved in sensory-motor integration are kept constant during E and KI. Thus during KI and E, not only are similar areas active, but the relative influence of these areas on each other also remains constant. This notion reinforces further the idea of KI as a true motor behavior, a postulate also supported by behavioral data, since KI has been associated with motor preparation, imitation and anticipation, motor restraint, motor execution, and motor learning (Deiber et al., 1998; Jeannerod, 1995).

In contrast, there are some differences between E and KI. The most notable differences were found in the inputs

to M1. During KI, many of the inputs from association areas (PAR and SMA) to M1 are strong and negative compared to their effect during execution. These negative values could be interpreted as a suppression effect (McIntosh & Gonzalez-Lima, 1998) of SMA and PAR on M1, since during KI there are no overt movements. The fact that these connectivity values change from weak and positive to strong and negative during a task with no overt movements (KI) provides a new perspective on how the motor system might be encoding information. In other words, we have two closely related tasks (E and KI), involving activation in similar areas, and with several similar interrelationships. Yet even when the volumes of activation in M1 during KI are not that different, the influence exerted by SMA and PAR is opposite their influence during E. This exemplifies how network analysis can provide a new perspective on the neurophysiology of the motor system by describing how changes in the interrelationships among areas can generate different motor behaviors.

Understanding actions done by others: the mirror neuron system

The mirror neuron system in monkeys

Many of the original studies done in the mirror system used non-human primates as experimental subjects. Because of this, we will refer first to this data followed by studies in

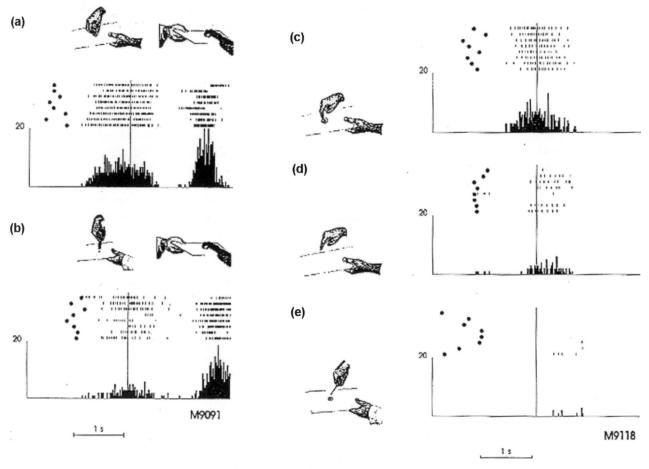

Figure 22.17. Mirror system in macaques. Firing patterns of neurons located in F5 from the observation and the execution of grasping movements. The discharge patterns of mirror neurons during action observation, are similar to execution (**(a)** left panel) or **(c)** but not during action observation when a tool is involved (**(b)** left panel) and **(e)** nor when the object is missing **(d)**. *Modified from: Rizzolatti et al. (1996). Premotor cortex and the recognition of motor actions. Cogn. Brain Res. 3: 131–141.*

humans. As previously stated, electrophysiological studies have shown that area F5 contains a motor representation of mouth and hand goal-directed actions (Rizzolatti et al., 1988). Some of the neurons in this area (mirror neurons) discharge during the execution of both hand and mouth goal-directed actions, and also respond when the monkey observes another monkey or a human performing the same or a similar action (Gallese et al., 1996; Rizzolatti et al., 1996). The visual properties of mirror neurons resemble those of neurons found in the superior temporal sulcus (STS) region. These neurons, like mirror neurons, respond to the visual presentation of goal-directed hand actions, of walking, turning the head, moving the hand and bending the torso (for a review see Carey, 1996). However, differently from mirror neurons described in area F5, neurons described in the STS region do not discharge during the execution of any of the actions that may trigger them visually. The congruence between the action motorly coded by the neuron and that triggering the same neuron visually may be very strict: in this case only the observation of an action which is identical to that coded by the neuron can activate it. More often, this congruence is broader; in this case, the observed and the executed action coded

by the neuron match the goal of the action rather than the movements necessary to execute it. Some important features of mirror neurons should be highlighted: during action observation they discharge only when a biological effector (a hand, for example) interacts with an object; if the action is performed with a tool the neuron does not discharge. Mirror neurons are not active either when the observed action is simply mimicked, that is, executed in the absence of the object. Finally, mirror neurons do not discharge during the mere visual presentation of an object (Figure 22.17). Up to now only mirror neurons related to hand actions were described. More recently it has been demonstrated that in area F5 there are also mirror neurons which discharge during the execution and observation of mouth actions. Not surprisingly, most of the mouth mirror neurons become active during the execution and observation of mouth feeding behaviors such as grasping, sucking or breaking food. However, some of these neurons respond during the execution and observation of oral communicative actions such as lip-smacking (Ferrari et al., 2003).

Since their discovery, the preferred hypothesis has been that mirror neurons might play an important role both in action recognition and action understanding (Jeannerod et al., 1995). If mirror neurons are responsible for action recognition, then these neurons should discharge also when the monkey cannot see the whole sequence of an action, provided that the goal of the observed action can be clearly inferred. A recent electrophysiological study (Umilta et al., 2001) supports the claim that mirror neurons may infer the goal of an action. In this experiment, two conditions were presented: in the first one (vision condition) the animal could see the whole sequence of a hand goal-directed action, in the second one (hidden condition) the final part of the action was hidden from the sight of the monkey by means of a screen. In this last condition, however, the animal was shown that an object, for example a piece of food, was placed behind the screen preventing the observation of the final part of the performed action. The results showed that mirror neurons discharge not only during the observation of action, but also when the final part of it is hidden. As a control, a mimicked action was presented in the same conditions. As expected, in this case, the neuron did not discharge either in the full vision condition or in the hidden condition.

Actions may be recognized also from their typical sound, when presented acoustically. For example, we can recognize that an individual is manipulating some keys simply from the typical sound this action produces, even when we cannot see the individual performing it. Besides visual properties, a recent monkey experiment has demonstrated that about 15% of mirror neurons also respond to the presentation of the sound typical for a specific action. These neurons are called audio-visual mirror neurons (Kohler et al., 2002). Audio-visual mirror neurons could be used to recognize actions done by other individuals, when presented acoustically. It has been argued that these neurons code the action content, which may be triggered either visually or acoustically, thus representing a possible step for the acquisition of language. It is worth noting that for anatomical and physiological reasons area F5 is considered the monkey homologue of human Broca's region (Binkofski & Buccino, 2004; Petrides & Pandya, 1984; Rizzolatti & Arbib, 1998).

The mirror neuron system in humans

There is increasing evidence that a mirror neuron system also exists in humans. Converging data supporting this notion come from experiments carried out with neurophysiological, behavioral, and brain imaging techniques.

Neurophysiological studies. The first evidence of the existence of a mirror neuron system in humans was provided by Fadiga et al. (1995). During this experiment, a single pulse with transcranial magnetic stimulation (TMS) was delivered while subjects were observing an experimenter performing various hand actions in front of them. As control condition, single pulse TMS was delivered during object observation, dimming detection and observation of arm movements. Motor evoked potentials (MEPs) were recorded from extrinsic and intrinsic hand muscles.

Results showed that during hand action observation, but not in the other conditions, there was an increase in the amplitude of the motor evoked potentials recorded from the hand muscles, normally recruited when the observed action is actually performed by the observer. These results were recently confirmed by Strafella and Paus (2000). Furthermore, using the same technique, Gangitano et al. (2001) found that during the observation of hand actions not only there is an increase of MEPs amplitude in the muscles involved in the actual execution of the observed action, but MEPs are modulated in a fashion strictly resembling the time-course of the observed action. Taken together, the TMS data support the notion of a mirror neuron system coupling action execution and action observation in terms of both the muscles involved and the temporal sequence of the action.

Similar to these results are those obtained by Cochin et al. (1999) using quantified electroencephalography (qEEG). In this study "mu" activity was blocked during both the observation and execution of various hand actions, when compared to rest. It is worth recalling that similar results were observed by Gastaut and Bert (1954), who noted the suppression of "mu" activity in humans during the movie presentation of various actions, results also obtained by Hari and co-workers using magnetoencephalography (MEG) (Makela et al., 1993). In this study it was found a suppression of 15–25 Hz activity originated in the precentral motor cortex, during the execution and, to a less extent, during the observation of object manipulation. All of these studies provide further evidence that observation and execution of action share common neural substrates.

Behavioral studies. Evidence in favor of the existence of a mirror neuron system also derives from neuropsychological studies using behavioral paradigms. Brass (2000) investigated how movement observation could affect movement execution in a stimulus-response compatibility paradigm. Using a reaction time paradigm, they contrasted the role of symbolic cues during the observation of finger movements and during the execution of the same finger movements. Subjects were faster to respond when the finger movement was the relevant stimulus. Moreover the degree of similarity between the observed and executed movement led to a further advantage in the execution of the observed movement. These results provide a strong evidence for an influence of the observed movement on the execution of that movement. Similar results were obtained by Craighero et al. (2002) in a study where subjects were required to prepare to grasp as fast as possible a bar oriented either clockwise or counter-clockwise, after presentation of a picture showing the right hand. Two experiments were carried out: in the first experiment the picture represented the final required position of the hand to grasp the bar, as seen through a mirror. In a second experiment, in addition to stimuli used in experiment one, other two pictures were presented, obtained rotating of 90° the hand shown in the pictures used in Experiment 1. In both experiments, responses of the subjects were faster when the hand orientation of the picture corresponded to that achieved by the hand at the end of action, when actually executed. Moreover the responses were globally faster when the stimuli were not rotated.

Brain imaging studies. All the cited studies provide little, if any, insight on the localization of the mirror neuron system in humans. This issue has been addressed by a number of brain imaging studies.

In an early positron emission tomography (PET) experiment aimed at identifying the brain areas active during action observation, Rizzolatti et al. (1996), comparing hand action observation with the observation of an object, found activation of Broca's region, the middle temporal gyrus and the superior temporal sulcus region. Broca's region is classically considered an area devoted to speech production. Recently, however, it has been demonstrated that in this area, a motor representation of hand actions is also present (Binkofski & Buccino, 2004; Binkofski et al., 1999; Ehrsson et al., 2000). Given the homology between Broca's area and area F5 in the monkey, (where mirror neurons were originally discovered), this study provided the first evidence on the anatomical localization of the mirror neuron system for hand actions in humans.

A recent fMRI study showed that in humans, the mirror neuron system is complex and related to different body actions performed not only with the hand, but also with the foot and the mouth. Buccino et al. (2001) asked subjects to observe video-sequences presenting different actions performed with the mouth, the hand and the foot, respectively. The actions shown were either transitive (the mouth/hand/foot acted on an object) or intransitive (the mouth/hand/foot action was performed without an object). The following actions were presented: biting an apple, grasping a cup, grasping a ball, kicking a ball, and pushing a brake. As a control, subjects were asked to observe a static image of each action.

The observation of both transitive and intransitive actions, compared to the observation of a static image of the same action, led to the activation of different regions in the premotor cortex and Broca's area, depending on the body part involved in the observed action. The different regions largely overlapped those where classical studies (Penfield & Rasmussen, 1950) had shown a somatotopically organized motor representation of the different effectors (Figure 22.18). Moreover, during the observation of transitive actions, distinct sectors in the inferior parietal lobule were active, including areas inside and around the intraparietal sulcus, with localization depending on the body part involved in the observed action. All activations found in this study are shown in Figure 22.18.

On the whole, this study strongly supports the claim that, as in the actual execution of actions, during action observation different, somatotopically organized fronto-parietal circuits are recruited (Jeannerod et al., 1995; Rizzolatti &

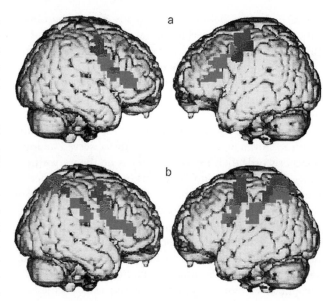

Figure 22.18. Mirror system in humans. Somatotopic fMRI activation in parietal and premotor regions during observation of intransitive (**a**) and transitive (**b**) actions in humans. Light: mouth related movements; Dark: hand related movements; Medium: foot related movements.

Fadiga, 1998). In this context, it is worth noting that mirror neurons, similar to those described in area F5, have recently been reported by Gallese et al. (2002) in the inferior parietal lobule of the monkey (area PF).

Contrast between the mirror system in humans and monkeys

As previously stated, in the monkey the mirror neuron system can be activated when the animal observes an experimenter, a member belonging to other species (nonconspecific), while performing a similar action motorly-coded by the neuron. A recent fMRI study (Buccino et al., 2004) addressed whether we recognize action performed by non-conspecifics using the same neural structures involved in the recognition of action performed by con-specifics (same species). In this study, normal subjects were asked to carefully observe different mouth actions performed by a man, a monkey, and a dog, respectively. Two kinds of mouth actions were visually presented: biting a piece of food and oral communicative actions (human silent speech, monkey lip-smacking, and silent dog barking). The results showed that during the observation of biting, there is a clear activation of the *pars opercularis* of the inferior frontal gyrus and of the inferior parietal lobule, regardless of the species performing the action. Interestingly, during the observation of oral communicative mouth actions, a different pattern of activation was observed, this time depending on the species performing them. During the observation of silent speech (human), there was a clear activation of Broca's area in both hemispheres, with a leftward asymmetry; during the observation of lip smacking (monkey) there was only a small bilateral activation in the *pars opercularis* of Broca's area, with no clear asymmetry between the two hemispheres. Finally during the observation of silent dog barking no activation was found in Broca's area, but activation was present only in the right superior temporal sulcus region. The results of the experiment strongly suggest that action performed by other individuals, including non-conspecifics, may be recognized in two different ways: for actions like biting or silent speech reading, there is a motor resonance of the cortical circuits involved in the actual execution of the observed actions. In other words their recognition relies on the mirror neuron system. For actions like barking, this resonance is missing. In the first case there is a "personal" knowledge of the action observed, in the sense that it is mapped on the observer's motor repertoire and therefore the observer has a direct, personal experience of its execution (e.g., I recognize it because I am able to do the same action I am looking at). In the second case, although the viewed actions are still recognized as biological motion (as suggested by the activation of the STS region), personal knowledge about these actions is lacking because the observer has no direct experience of the observed action in motor terms (e.g., I can approximately imitate a dog barking, but, as a matter of fact, I am not able to do it).

Finally, it is well known that we can recognize actions even when we look at point lights attached to the joints of an actor in motion. Early brain imaging studies on this issue demonstrated that observation of point-light biological motion leads to activation of superior temporal cortical areas. These early studies failed to show any activation in the motor system. The results of a very recent fMRI study, however, showed that areas responding selectively to point-light biological motion are found not only in the lateral and inferior temporal cortex but also in the premotor cortex. This result suggests that, although there is no direct matching between the observed action and the motor repertoire of the observer, in the case of point light biological motion the motor system is involved in filling in the simplified motor pattern obtained with point-lights and in "humanizing" the observed action.

MOTOR LEARNING AND MOTOR CORTICAL PLASTICITY

The areas of procedural learning, motor memory, and motor skill acquisition have been traditionally studied independently by different scientific disciplines. Psychology has a long tradition of studying human procedural memory and behavioral changes during skill acquisition without the possibility of observing the underlying cerebral processes. For the past 20+ years, neuroscience has emphasized the study of adult brain plasticity, including motor cortical plasticity, resulting from biological as well as environmental and behavioral changes. Finally, neurology and rehabilitation have studied deficits of motor behavior after stroke and re-gaining of motor skill during recovery and rehabilitation. Recently, noninvasive human imaging methods have provided a unique opportunity to combine the research methods across disciplines to allow a more complete picture of the issues involved. Understanding the mechanisms and the subsequent optimization of the motor learning process are desirable for different fields of human activity: developing and improving manual skills for a job, training in sports, and neurological rehabilitation.

Motor learning and motor memory

Motor learning has been studied within several disciplines, although the acquired knowledge has not been fully integrated across disciplines. Psychology has studied both acquisition of complex motor behavior (skill) (i.e., motor learning) and the storage and representation of this acquired knowledge (i.e., motor memory). It is generally accepted that knowledge of skills or procedural ("how") memory is distinct from knowledge of facts or declarative ("what") memory (Cohen & Squire, 1980; Squire, 1987b). Procedural memory is acquired incrementally, is modality-specific, does not allow for storage of individual events, and is usually associated with motor skill learning (Squire, 1987a). Most commonly, psychological theories view learning and memory in abstract terms, without any consideration of possible neuronal correlates of their proposed components. This is in contrast to similar endeavors from the neuroscience community (Fuster, 1995). Recently, the integrative field of cognitive neuroscience has been trying to focus simultaneous attention on both behavioral issues and neurobiological substrates and constraints imposed by the nervous system (e.g., Clegg, DiGirolamo, & Keele, 1998).

The term "motor learning" may be used in a broad sense in the psychological and neuroscience literature to encompass many processes, including the following (Strangman, 1998):

Adaptation: This is the simplest process during which existing behavior is modified or rescaled in response to environment. Examples of adaptation are habituation, sensitization, and vestibulo-ocular reflex (Raymond, Lisberger, & Mauk, 1996; Squire, 1987b).

Conditional motor association: This involves learning to associate an available motor response with a given stimulus (Halsband & Freund, 1990; Petrides, 1985, 1997). Most monkey learning studies belong into this category.

Finally, motor learning in the narrow sense is a process that leads to the acquisition of a novel response pattern that involves little or no functional trade-off for other movements. While adaptation and conditional motor association modify an existing behavior or connect it with a particular stimulus, motor learning enriches the individual's motor repertoire.

Motor learning may vary according to the type of motor control necessary for successful task performance

(Strangman, 1998). Tasks that do not rely on somatosensory feedback are called open-loop (e.g., dart throwing, penalty kick in soccer). The movements are usually so rapid (under 500 ms) that there is not enough time to process proprioceptive feedback. The second class of tasks is closed-loop, and such actions are mediated and error-corrected in real time by somatosensory feedback (e.g., gymnastics, figure skating). This dichotomy is somewhat artificial, as the amount of somatosensory feedback and subsequent self-correction can vary continuously. Still, considering the importance of proprioceptive input for cortical motor processing, it is likely that the amount of this internal feedback modulates the learning process in a significant way.

One of the issues addressed by research in motor learning is the transfer of training, that is, transfer of behavioral improvement on one task to a different task, a movement effector (e.g., from one hand to the other), or the environment (Adams, 1987). Performance benefit from practice on specific motor skills often does not correlate with, or transfer to, similar but non-identical tasks. Performance on these "transfer tasks" is usually substantially poorer for subjects that practiced the original but not the transfer task (Adams, 1987).

Practicing under highly structured conditions (different skills practiced in blocks) leads to faster learning but poorer transfer of skills than training by randomly mixing different skills. There seems to be a trade-off between practice variability and learning time on one hand, and between practice variability and behavior generalization on the other (Strangman, 1998).

There is not a clear understanding in the behavioral literature on the kind of practice that is the most beneficial. It is understood, though, that (a) subjects should distribute practice over time rather than participate in one massed practice session, (b) subjects should get feedback on how they are performing, and (c) the task should be easy enough to make at least occasional success possible (Strangman, 1998).

Neuroscience: Motor learning and memory in the brain

Neuroscience arrived at the topic of motor learning and memory from a different direction than the behavioral sciences. The speculative connection between the structure of the nervous system and acquisition of skilled behavior was made at least a hundred years ago. Ramón y Cajal mentions in his autobiography (1923) at a conference presentation in 1893 when he suggested the encoding of skill through modulation of neuronal connections. In this presentation, he offered an

explanation of the adaptation and professional skills (physical education, language operations, writing, playing the piano, mastering fencing, etc.) by the progressive strengthening of nervous pathways...excited by the pass of a wave, as well as by the creation of new cellular appendages (den-

dritic growth and elongation or branching of nervous collaterals, non-congenital), capable of improving the adjustment and extension of the contacts, and of organizing completely new relationships between neurons that were originally not connected.

– Translation Dr. Ana Solodkin

More recently, the discovery of plastic changes in the adult mammalian brain have provided new evidence to explain mechanisms of motor learning and memory. Most of the research has focused on primary motor and sensory cortices, since the anatomical and functional organization of these areas had been well described, thus simplifying the investigation of plastic changes. The following section will review the research on plasticity of the primary motor cortex, the area most relevant to motor learning.

Plasticity in animal and human M1

Several animal studies have demonstrated that the representations of muscles or movements in adult primary motor cortex can undergo plastic changes in response to peripheral or central lesions or altered experience. Motor maps have been shown to change in response to peripheral motor nerve lesions in the rat (Donoghue, Suner, & Sanes, 1990), repetitive cortical stimulation in the monkey (Nudo, Jenkins, & Merzenich, 1990), pharmacological modulation of intracortical inhibition in the rat (Jacobs & Donoghue, 1991), change of rat limb configuration (Sanes, Wang, & Donoghue, 1992), motor practice (Nudo, Wise, SiFuentes, & Milliken, 1996), or cortical lesions in the monkey (Nudo & Milliken, 1996; Nudo, Milliken, Jenkins, & Merzenich, 1996) found expansion of the motor cortical representations of muscles/movements that were used during a several week long session when monkeys learned to retrieve food pellets from small wells. In another primate study with long-term movement practice, M1 neurons that have been initially silent begin firing (Kennedy & Bakay, 1997). The extent of newly emerged cortical finger representation was correlated with recovery after stroke destroying the original finger representation (Nudo et al., 1996).

Several cellular mechanisms have been implicated to explain the observed plasticity, including unmasking or potentiation of existing but normally ineffective neural connections, axonal sprouting with new synapse formation, or a combination of these. Changes in motor maps after the application of bicuculline, an antagonist of the inhibitory neurotransmitter GABA (Jacobs & Donoghue, 1991), have been taken as evidence that a part of the wide network of available neural connections is functionally suppressed through intracortical inhibition. Long-term potentiation of cortico-cortical synapses has been observed in cat motor cortex (Keller, Arissian, & Asanuma, 1990), as has the appearance of new synapses after damage to deep cerebellar nuclei (Keller, Iriki, & Asanuma, 1990) or long-term thalamic stimulation (Keller, Arissian, & Asanuma, 1992). Increased synaptogenesis and early immediate gene c-fos expression have been associated with motor acrobatic learning in rat motor cortex (Kleim et al., 1996). Furthermore, the strength of intrinsic connections in M1 is dynamically modifiable through long-term potentiation (Aroniadou & Keller, 1995; Hess & Donoghue, 1994). Finally, the extent of horizontal connections has been shown to correlate well with the extent of plastic changes in motor cortical representations after transsection of efferent connections in the rat (Huntley, 1997).

Human motor plasticity

Changes of primary motor cortical organization have also been observed in adult humans. Expansion and shifts in motor maps occur after central or peripheral neurological lesion such as stroke (Weiller et al., 1993), amyotrophic lateral sclerosis (Kew et al., 1994), arm amputation (Kew et al., 1994; Pascual-Leone et al., 1996) and facial paralysis (Rijntjes et al., 1997). Remapping within M1 was suggested as one possible mechanism of motor function recovery after stroke (Weiller et al., 1993). One type of map change observed within M1 as a result of brain injury or disease was a shift of hand area laterally and ventrally, into the presumed face area, over a distance of up to 10 mm (Kew et al., 1994; Rijntjes et al., 1997; Weiller et al., 1993).

Similar changes have been described in the absence of motor system injury. Practice of Braille reading and motor learning caused expansion of scalp area from which movement could be evoked by transcranial stimulation (Pascual-Leone et al., 1993; Pascual-Leone, Grafman, & Hallett, 1994). Prolonged leg immobilization, on the other hand, caused shrinking of the scalp area for excitation of a leg muscle (Liepert, Tegenthoff, & Malin, 1995). Several studies of human motor learning have observed changes within M1 (Karni et al., 1995; Kawashima, Roland, & O'Sullivan, 1994; Pascual-Leone et al., 1995), even though M1 is only one of the multiple cerebral areas supposedly involved in motor learning (Halsband & Freund, 1993b). A newly acquired motor skill may take advantage of movement segments that are formed by combining neural units of M1 (segmental learning) and retrieved during the execution of the acquired skill (Asanuma & Keller, 1991). The possible anatomical substrate for the co-activation of an ensemble of neurons during skilled movement is the network of horizontal corticocortical connections observed within monkey M1 (Huntley & Jones, 1991).

Cortical activation size and learning

If one accepts the assumption that increasing skill and automaticity for a specific movement originates from changes of cortical motor function, the next question regards the character and direction of such changes. There is an intuitive concept that skill reflects efficiency at the cortical level and that such skill would translate into less cortical activation during functional imaging, implying either that neural units are firing less, fewer neural units are firing action potentials, or both. On the other hand, there is both nonhuman primate (see above) and human evidence that practice increases, rather than decreases the area of cortex associated with the practiced movement (at least in the time frame of several weeks).

Human motor learning studies have commonly reported that movement practice leads to recruitment of additional motor cortex, with the appearance of new active cortical fields (Kawashima et al., 1994), and expansion of the cortical territory corresponding to the practiced muscles/movements of several millimeters up to several centimeters (Karni et al., 1995; Pascual-Leone et al., 1995). Subjects who practiced a five-finger piano exercise for 2 hours a day for 5 days showed an enlarging motor cortical area targeting the long finger flexors and extensors, followed by a decreased threshold for activation as they learned the skill (Pascual-Leone et al., 1993).

Karni et al. (1995), compared fMRI activation caused by two sequential finger movements involving the same fingers. The sequences had five components and each involved fingers 2–5 touching the thumb in a particular order. One of the sequences was repeatedly practiced over several weeks. While the extent of cortex activated with either sequence was similar at the beginning of the study, after training the primary cortical activation by the practiced finger sequence was significantly larger than activation caused by the non-practiced sequence. The area of evoked response in M1 for the trained sequence did not extend beyond the hand representation, which was mapped in a subset of the subjects by independent finger movements. However, the amount of change in the rest of the motor map was not addressed to establish whether the learning was competing for cortical output neurons or instead whether it enhanced sharing of neurons. The relationship between the observed expansion and the localization of other hand movements was also not described. Finally, the study was limited to M1, although there is evidence that other motor and somatosensory regions participate in learning of new motor skills (see below).

In addition to investigating the effect of short- and medium-term experimental motor training on the motor cortex, correlation has also been sought between very long-term practice of skilled movements and the motor system. Although right-hand dominance for skilled movements is typical for humans, hand preference has also been observed in monkeys (Nudo et al., 1992). The monkey motor cortex controlling the preferred hand has been found to contain a larger and more complex hand area when studied with intracortical microstimulation (Nudo et al., 1992). Studies of human M1 structural asymmetry related to handedness have found asymmetry in the depth of the central sulcus, with the left hemisphere bigger than the right in right-handers, and a less prominent opposite asymmetry in left-handers (Amunts et al., 1996; White & Hardy, 1995). Microstructural asymmetry has been found in post-mortem brains, with a larger neuropil compartment (containing dendrites, axons, and synapses) in the left (dominant) motor cortex (Amunts et al., 1996). The authors suggest that this finding reflects a greater density of intracortical horizontal connections in the cortex serving the dominant hand (Amunts et al., 1996). Callosal connections from the opposite motor cortex comprise another possible source of increased connectivity, but callosal connection density is very low in the monkey motor hand areas and seems to be inversely related to the development of independent fine movements (Zant & Strick, 1978). Callosal connections have also been suggested to be a potential hindrance for independent movements of one hand (Gould et al., 1986). Another anatomical study did not find any asymmetry in the size of the precentral motor cortex in post-mortem human brains (White et al., 1997).

The effect of long-term bimanual practice (i.e., playing a musical keyboard instrument) on brain structure was studied by Amunts et al. (1997). The asymmetry of central sulcus depth observed in control subjects was diminished in musicians and this effect was proportional to the age of inception of music training. Similarly, finger-tapping performance of musicians was more symmetrical, due to significantly better performance of the nondominant left hand. A right-larger-than-left difference was found in the strength of cortical magnetic fields evoked by moving left versus right fingers in the primary motor cortex of string players (Elbert et al., 1995). All this evidence seems to further support the notion that long-term practice changes the motor cortex on both microscopic and macroscopic levels.

Contribution of other motor and somatosensory areas to motor learning

Regions other than M1 have also been implicated in motor learning and motor plasticity. Changes in the supplementary motor area (SMA), premotor cortex (LPMC), cingulate motor area (CMA), and areas of the parietal lobe have all been associated with motor skill acquisition (Halsband & Freund, 1993a).

Primate SMA neurons participate in preparatory rather than movement-related activity (Aizawa & Tanji, 1994; Wiesendanger, 1986) and their activity is modulated by learning. After a motor task (keypress movement in response to a visual trigger) had been extensively overtrained (12 months) in monkeys, very few, if any, SMA neurons remained active before movement onset (Aizawa et al., 1991). The authors suggest that SMA neuronal activity during a simple task is redundant and therefore eliminated over time to increase efficiency through division of labor. It might be inferred that even during a complex motor task, non-primary motor activation can be gradually eliminated at the same time-scale as the movement is increasingly encoded in M1. However, after M1 damage, SMA activity reappears (Aizawa et al., 1991). Similarly, in a human study of motor learning, SMA was active early during motor skill acquisition (Grafton, Hazeltine, & Ivry, 1998) but not later during transfer of skill from hand to arm. In contrast to these results and the theoret-

ical model they suggest, Jenkins et al. (1994) found SMA activation in a human study of motor sequence learning to be stronger during performance of a pre-learned sequence than during new learning. It is thus possible that some type of movement sequences becomes represented in the SMA rather than M1 over the course of learning. Human imaging studies using PET has also shown prominent activation of LPMC and parietal association cortex in early stages of motor learning (Jenkins et al., 1994).

Participation of primary somatosensory cortex in motor cortical plasticity

Primary somatosensory cortex is also thought to play a role in the plasticity of M1. While ablation of somatosensory cortex does not markedly worsen motor performance in the monkey (Asanuma & Arissian, 1984), it prevents learning of new motor skills (Pavlides, Miyashita, & Asanuma, 1993). The importance of S1 for motor learning is most likely due to processing of proprioceptive feedback, the absence of which degrades skilled movements (Bossom, 1974) and slows or blocks the acquisition of new motor skills (Rothwell et al., 1982). Changes in forelimb configuration have caused expansion of the M1 forelimb motor area into the representation of face in the rat (Sanes, Wang, & Donoghue, 1992).

As mentioned above, proprioceptive afferent information mainly reaches area 3a (Jones, 1983) and, to a lesser degree, area 3b (Heath, Hore, & Phillips, 1976), with further processing in area 2. It has been suggested that each of these areas has a separate somatotopic map in the monkey (Kaas et al., 1979) and these maps have been found to show plastic changes in response to manipulation of the periphery or cortex (Courtemanche, Sun, & Lamarre, 1997; Kaas, Florence, & Neeraj, 1997; Merzenich et al., 1984). Changes in the 3a map have been studied with training of fine touch on the skin (Recanzone, Merzenich, & Dinse, 1992) and after experimental cortical stroke in area 3b (Xerri et al., 1998). Acquisition of a motor skill dependent on fine touch caused reorganization in area 3b (Xerri et al., 1999), but it is not known whether area 3a also reorganizes during motor skill acquisition and whether it thus possibly contributes to the reorganization in M1.

REFERENCES

Abbruzzese, G., Assini, A., Buccolieri, A., Marchese, R., & Trompetto, C. (1999). Changes of intracortical inhibition during motor imagery in human subjects. *Neurosci Lett*, *263*(2–3), 113–116.

Adams, J. A. (1987). Historical review and appraisal of research on the learning, retention, and transfer of human motor skills [Review]. *Psychological Bulletin*, *101*(1), 41–74.

Aizawa, H., Inase, M., Mushiake, H., Shima, K., & Tanji, J. (1991). Reorganization of activity in the supplementary motor area associated with motor learning and functional recovery. *Experimental Brain Research*, *84*(3), 668–671.

Aizawa, H., & Tanji, J. (1994). Corticocortical and thalamocortical responses of neurons in the monkey primary motor cortex and their relation to a trained motor task. *Journal of Neurophysiology*, 71(2), 550–560.

Amunts, K., Schlaug, G., Jancke, L., Steinmetz, H., Schleicher, A., Dabringhaus, A., et al. (1997). Motor cortex and hand motor skills: Structural compliance in the human brain. *Human Brain Mapping*, 5(4), 206–215.

Amunts, K., Schlaug, G., Schleicher, A., Steinmetz, H., Dabringhaus, A., Roland, P. E., et al. (1996). Asymmetry in the human motor cortex and handedness. *Neuroimage*, 4(3 Pt 1), 216–222.

Annett, J. (1996). On knowing how to do things: a theory of motor imagery. *Brain Res Cogn Brain Res*, 3(2), 65–69.

Antervo, A., Hari, R., Katila, T., Poutanen, T., Seppanen, M., & Tuomisto, T. (1983). Cerebral magnetic fields preceding self-paced plantar flexions of the foot. *Acta Neurologica Scandinavica*, 68(4), 213–217.

Aroniadou, V. A., & Keller, A. (1995). Mechanisms of LTP induction in rat motor cortex in vitro. *Cerebral Cortex*, 5(4), 353–362.

Arshavsky, Y. I. (2003). Cellular and network properties in the functioning of the nervous system: from central pattern generators to cognition. *Brain Res Brain Res Rev*, 41(2–3), 229–267.

Asanuma, H., & Arissian, K. (1984). Experiments on functional role of peripheral input to motor cortex during voluntary movements in the monkey. *Journal of Neurophysiology*, 52(2), 212–227.

Asanuma, H., & Keller, A. (1991). Neuronal mechanisms of motor learning in mammals. [Review]. *Neuroreport*, 2(5), 217–224.

Barker, A. T., Jalinous, R., & Freeston, I. L. (1985). Non-invasive magnetic stimulation of the human motor cortex. *Lancet*, 1, 1106–1107.

Bartholow, R. (1874). Experimental investigations into the functions of the human brain. *American Journal of Medical Sciences (New Series)*, 67, 305–313.

Basser, P. J., Mattiello, J., & LeBihan, D. (1994). MR diffusion tensor spectroscopy and imaging. *Biophys J*, 66(1), 259–267.

Bates, J. (1951). Electrical activity of the cortex accompanying movements. *Journal of Physiology (London)*, 113, 240.

Beisteiner, R., Hollinger, P., Lindinger, G., Lang, W., & Berthoz, A. (1995). Mental representations of movements: Brain potentials associated with imagination of hand movements. *Electroencephalogr Clin Neurophysiol*, 96(2), 183–193.

Berger, H. (1929). Über des Elektrenkephalogramm des Menschen. *Archiv für Psychiatrie und Nervenkrankheiten*, 87, 527–570.

Betz, W. (1874). Anatomischer Nachweis zweier Gehirncentra. *Centralblatt für die medizinische Wissenschaften*, 12, 578–580, 595–599.

Binkofski, F., & Buccino, G. (2004). Motor functions of the Broca's region. *Brain Lang*, 89(2), 362–369.

Binkofski, F., Buccino, G., Stephan, K. M., Rizzolatti, G., Seitz, R. J., & Freund, H. J. (1999). A parieto-premotor network for object manipulation: Evidence from neuroimaging. *Exp Brain Res*, 128(1–2), 210–213.

Bogousslavsky, J., & Caplan, L. (Eds.), (1995). *Stroke syndromes*. Cambridge, England: Cambridge University Press.

Bossom, J. (1974). Movement without proprioception. *Brain Research*, 71(2–3), 285–296.

Brass, M., Bekkering, H., Wohlschlaeger, A., & Prinz, W. (2000). Compatibility between observed and executed finger movements: comparing symbolic, spatial and imitative cues. *Brain and Cognition*, 44, 124–143.

Broca, P. (1861). Remarques sur le siege de la faculte du language articule, suivives d'une observation d'aphemie (perte de la parole). *Bulletines de la Societe Anatomique*, 36, 330–357.

Brodmann, K. (1909). *Vergleichende Lokalisationslehre der Grosshirnrinde in ihren Prinzipien dargestellt auf Grund des Zellenbaues*. Leipzig: Barth.

Brown, T. G. (1911). The intrinsic factors in the act of progression in the mammal. *Proc Royal Soc*, B84, 308–319.

Buccino, G., Binkofski, F., Fink, G. R., Fadiga, L., Fogassi, L., Gallese, V., et al. (2001). Action observation activates premotor and parietal areas in a somatotopic manner: an fMRI study. *Eur J Neurosci*, 13(2), 400–404.

Buccino, G., Lui, F., Canessa, N., Patteri, I., Lagravinese, G., Benuzzi, F., et al. (2004). Neural circuits involved in the recognition of actions performed by nonconspecifics: an FMRI study. *J Cogn Neurosci*, 16(1), 114–126.

Buchel, C., & Friston, K. J. (1997). Modulation of connectivity in visual pathways by attention: cortical interactions evaluated with structural equation modelling and fMRI. *Cereb Cortex*, 7(8), 768–778.

Capaday, C. (2002). The special nature of human walking and its neural control. *Trends Neurosci*, 25(7), 370–376.

Capaday, C., Lavoie, B. A., Barbeau, H., Schneider, C., & Bonnard, M. (1999). Studies on the corticospinal control of human walking. I. Responses to focal transcranial magnetic stimulation of the motor cortex. *J Neurophysiol*, 81(1), 129–139.

Carey, D. P. (1996). 'Monkey see, monkey do' cells. Neurophysiology. *Curr Biol*, 6(9), 1087–1088.

Charcot, J. M. (1877). Contribution a l'étude des localisations dans l'écorce des hémispheres du cerveau. Observations relatives aux paralysies et aux convulsions d'origine corticale. *Revue Mensuelle de Médecine et de Chirurgie*, 1, 1–18, 113–123, 180–195, 357–376, 437–457.

Chen, Y., & Reggia, J. A. (1996). Alignment of coexisting cortical maps in a motor control model. *Neural Computation*, 8(4), 731–755.

Clegg, B. A., DiGirolamo, G. J., & Keele, S. W. (1998). Sequence learning. *Trends in Cognitive Sciences*, 2(8), 275–281.

Cochin, S., Barthelemy, C., Roux, S., & Martineau, J. (1999). Observation and execution of movement: similarities demonstrated by quantified electroencephalography. *Eur J Neurosci*, 11(5), 1839–1842.

Cohen, N. J., & Squire, L. R. (1980). Preserved learning and retention of pattern-analyzing skill in amnesia: dissociation of knowing how and knowing that. *Science*, 210(4466), 207–210.

Coles, M. G. (1989). Modern mind-brain reading: psychophysiology, physiology, and cognition. *Psychophysiology*, 26(3), 251–269.

Courtemanche, R., Sun, G. D., & Lamarre, Y. (1997). Movement-related modulation across the receptive field of neurons in the primary somatosensory cortex of the monkey. *Brain Research*, 777(1–2), 170–178.

Craighero, L., Bello, A., Fadiga, L., & Rizzolatti, G. (2002). Hand action preparation influences the responses to hand pictures. *Neuropsychologia*, 40(5), 492–502.

Cushing, H. (1909). A note upon the faradic stimulation of the postcentral gyrus in conscious patients. *Brain*, 32, 44–53.

Decety, J., Jeannerod, M., Germain, M., & Pastene, J. (1991). Vegetative response during imagined movement is proportional to mental effort. *Behav Brain Res*, 42(1), 1–5.

Deiber, M. P., Ibanez, V., Honda, M., Sadato, N., Raman, R., & Hallett, M. (1998). Cerebral processes related to visuomotor imagery and generation of simple finger movements studied with positron emission tomography. *Neuroimage*, 7(2), 73–85.

Donoghue, J. P., Suner, S., & Sanes, J. N. (1990). Dynamic organization of primary motor cortex output to target muscles in adult rats. II. Rapid reorganization following motor nerve lesions. *Experimental Brain Research*, 79(3), 492–503.

Ehrsson, H. H., Naito, E., Geyer, S., Amunts, K., Zilles, K., Forssberg, H., et al. (2000). Simultaneous movements of upper and lower limbs are coordinated by motor representations that are shared by both limbs: a PET study. *Eur J Neurosci*, 12(9), 3385–3398.

Elbert, T., Pantev, C., Wienbruch, C., Rockstroh, B., & Taub, E. (1995). Increased cortical representation of the fingers of the left hand in string players. *Science*, 270(5234), 305–307.

Engel, A. K., Moll, C. K., Fried, I., & Ojemann, G. A. (2005). Invasive recordings from the human brain: clinical insights and beyond. *Nature Reviews Neuroscience*, 6(1), 35–47.

Fadiga, L., Buccino, G., Craighero, L., Fogassi, L., Gallese, V., & Pavesi, G. (1999). Corticospinal excitability is specifically modulated by motor imagery: a magnetic stimulation study. *Neuropsychologia*, 37(2), 147–158.

Fadiga, L., Fogassi, L., Pavesi, G., & Rizzolatti, G. (1995). Motor facilitation during action observation: a magnetic stimulation study. *J Neurophysiol*, 73(6), 2608–2611.

Ferrari, P. F., Gallese, V., Rizzolatti, G., & Fogassi, L. (2003). Mirror neurons responding to the observation of ingestive and communicative mouth actions in the monkey ventral premotor cortex. *Eur J Neurosci*, 17(8), 1703–1714.

Ferrier, D. (1873). Experimental researches in cerebral physiology and pathology. *West Riding Lunatic Asylum Reports*, 3, 1–50.

Ferrier, D. (1875). Experiments in the brain of monkeys. *Proceedings of the Royal Society of London. Series B: Biological Sciences*, 23, 409–430.

Finger, S. (1994). *Origins of Neuroscience. A History of Explorations into Brain Function*. New York: Oxford University Press.

Flourens, M. J. P. (1824). *Recherches expérimentales sur les propriétés et les fonctions du systeme nerveux dans les animaux vertébrés*. Paris: Crevot.

Foerster, O. (1909). Über den Lähmungstypus bei corticalen Hirnherden. *Deutsche Zeitschrift für Nervenheilkunde*, 37, 349–414.

Foerster, O. (1936a). Motorische Felder und Bahnen. In H. Bumke & O. Foerster (Eds.), *Handbuch der Neurologie* (Vol. 6, pp. 1–357). Berlin: Springer-Verlag.

Foerster, O. (1936b). Symptomatologie der Erkrankungen des Grosshirns. Motorische Felder und Bahnen. In O. Bumke & O. Foerster (Eds.), *Handbuch der Neurologie* (Vol. 6, pp. 1–357). Berlin: Springer-Verlag.

Foerster, O., & Penfield, W. (1930). The structural basis of traumatic epilepsy and results of radical operation. *Brain*, 53, 99–120.

Fogassi, L., Gallese, V., Buccino, G., Craighero, L., Fadiga, L., & Rizzolatti, G. (2001). Cortical mechanism for the visual guidance of hand grasping movements in the monkey: A reversible inactivation study. *Brain*, 124(Pt 3), 571–586.

Fox, P. T., Mintun, M. A., & Raichle, M. E. (1986). Mapping Human Visual Cortex with Positron Emission Tomography. *Nature*, 323, 806–809.

Freund, H. J. (1983). Motor unit and muscle activity in voluntary motor control. *Physiol Rev*, 63(2), 387–436.

Freund, H. J. (1987). Motor deficits after cortical lesions in man. *Electroencephalogr Clin Neurophysiol Suppl*, 39, 81–82.

Fritsch, G., & Hitzig, E. (1870). Ueber die Elektrische Erregbarkeit des Grosshirns. *Arch. Anat. Physiol. Wiss. Med.*, 37, 300–332.

Fuster, J. M. (1995). *Memory in the Cerebral Cortex: An Empirical Approach to Neural Networks in the Human and Nonhuman Primate*. Cambridge, MA: MIT Press.

Gallese, V., Fadiga, L., Fogassi, L., & Rizzolatti, G. (1996). Action recognition in the premotor cortex. *Brain*, 119 (Pt 2), 593–609.

Gallese, V., Fogassi, L., Fadiga, L., & Rizzolatti, G. (2002). Action representation and the inferior parietal lobule. In W. Prinz & B. Hommel (Eds.), *Attention and performance XIX: Common mechanisms in perception and action* (pp. 334–355). Oxford, UK: Oxford University Press.

Gangitano, M., Mottaghy, F. M., & Pascual-Leone, A. (2001). Phase-specific modulation of cortical motor output during movement observation. *Neuroreport*, 12(7), 1489–1492.

Gastaut, H. J., & Bert, J. (1954). EEG changes during cinematographic presentation; moving picture activation of the EEG. *Electroencephalogr Clin Neurophysiol Suppl*, 6(3), 433–444.

Gerardin, E., Sirigu, A., Lehericy, S., Poline, J. B., Gaymard, B., Marsault, C., et al. (2000). Partially overlapping neural networks for real and imagined hand movements. *Cereb Cortex*, 10(11), 1093–1104.

Geschwind, N. (1965). Disconnection Syndromes in Animals and Man. *Brain*, 88, 237–294, 585–644.

Goldring, S., & Ratcheson, R. (1972). Human motor cortex: sensory input data from single neuron recordings. *Science*, 175(29), 1493–1495.

Gonzalez-Lima, F., & McIntosh, A. R. (1994). Neural Network Interactions Related to Auditory Learning Analyzed with Structural Equation Modelling. *Hum Brain Mapp*, 2, 23–44.

Gould, H., Cusick, C., Pons, T., & Kaas, J. (1986). The relationship of corpus callosum connections to electrical stimulation maps of motor, supplementary motor, and the frontal eye fields in owl monkeys. *Journal of Comparative Neurology*, 247, 287–325.

Grafton, S., Hazeltine, E., & Ivry, R. (1998). Abstract and effector-specific representations of motor sequences identified with PET. *Journal of Neuroscience*, 18, 9420–9428.

Grillner, S., Cangiano, L., Hu, G., Thompson, R., Hill, R., & Wallen, P. (2000). The intrinsic function of a motor system – from ion channels to networks and behavior. *Brain Res*, 886(1–2), 224–236.

Grillner, S., & Wallen, P. (1985). Central pattern generators for locomotion, with special reference to vertebrates. *Annu Rev Neurosci*, 8, 233–261.

Halsband, U., & Freund, H. J. (1990). Premotor cortex and conditional motor learning in man. *Brain*, 113(Pt 1), 207–222.

Halsband, U., & Freund, H. J. (1993a). Motor learning. *Curr Opin Neurobiol*, 3(6), 940–949.

Halsband, U., & Freund, H. J. (1993b). Motor learning. [Review]. *Current Opinion in Neurobiology*, 3(6), 940–949.

Hari, R., & Kaukoranta, E. (1985). Neuromagnetic studies of somatosensory system: principles and examples. *Prog Neurobiol*, 24(3), 233–256.

Hashimoto, R., & Rothwell, J. C. (1999). Dynamic changes in corticospinal excitability during motor imagery. *Exp Brain Res*, 125(1), 75–81.

Heath, C. J., Hore, J., & Phillips, C. G. (1976). Inputs from low threshold muscle and cutaneous afferents of hand and forearm to areas 3a and 3b of baboon's cerebral cortex. *Journal of Physiology (London), 257*(1), 199–227.

Heimer, L. (1983). *The Human Brain and Spinal Cord. Functional Neuroanatomy and Dissection guide.* (2nd ed.). New York: Springer-Verlag.

Hess, G., & Donoghue, J. P. (1994). Long-term potentiation of horizontal connections provides a mechanism to reorganize cortical motor maps. *Journal of Neurophysiology,71*(6), 2543–2547.

Hlustik, P., Solodkin, A., Gullapalli, R. P., Noll, D. C., & Small, S. L. (2001). Somatotopy in human primary motor and somatosensory hand representations revisited. *Cereb Cortex, 11*(4), 312–321.

Horwitz, B., Friston, K. J., & Taylor, J. G. (2000). Neural modeling and functional brain imaging: an overview. *Neural Netw, 13*(8–9), 829–846.

Huntley, G. W. (1997). Correlation between Patterns of Horizontal Connectivity and the Extent of Short-Term Representational Plasticity in Rat Motor Cortex. *Cerebral Cortex, 7*, 143–156.

Huntley, G. W., & Jones, E. G. (1991). Relationship of intrinsic connections to forelimb movement representations in monkey motor cortex: a correlative anatomic and physiological study. *Journal of Neurophysiology,66*(2), 390–413.

Ingvar, D. H., & Risberg, J. (1965). Influence of mental activity upon regional cerebral blood flow in man. A preliminary study. *Acta Neurol Scand Suppl, 14*, 183–186.

Iwaniuk, A. N., & Whishaw, I. Q. (1999). How skilled are the skilled limb movements of the raccoon (Procyon lotor)? *Behav Brain Res, 99*(1), 35–44.

Jackson, J. H. (1863). Convulsive spasms of the right hand and arm preceding epileptic seizures. *Medical Times and Gazette, 1*, 589.

Jackson, J. H. (1873). Observations on the localisation of movements in the cerebral hemispheres, as revealed by cases of convulsions, chorea and "aphasia". *West Riding Asylum Medical Reports, 3*, 175–195.

Jacobs, K. M., & Donoghue, J. P. (1991). Reshaping the Cortical Motor Map by Unmasking Latent Intracortical Connections. *Science, 251*, 944–947.

Jankowska, E., Jukes, M. G., Lund, S., & Lundberg, A. (1967). The effect of DOPA on the spinal cord. 6. Half-centre organization of interneurones transmitting effects from the flexor reflex afferents. *Acta Physiol Scand, 70*(3), 389–402.

Jeannerod, M. (1995). Mental imagery in the motor context. *Neuropsychologia, 33*(11), 1419–1432.

Jeannerod, M. (2001). Neural simulation of action: a unifying mechanism for motor cognition. *Neuroimage, 14*(1 Pt 2), S103–109.

Jeannerod, M., Arbib, M. A., Rizzolatti, G., & Sakata, H. (1995). Grasping objects: the cortical mechanisms of visuomotor transformation. *Trends Neurosci, 18*(7), 314–320.

Jenkins, I. H., Brooks, D. J., Nixon, P. D., Frackowiak, R. S., & Passingham, R. E. (1994). Motor sequence learning: a study with positron emission tomography. *Journal of Neuroscience, 14*(6), 3775–3790.

Jezzard, P., Matthews, P. M., & Smith, S. M. (2001). *Functional MRI: an introduction to methods*. Oxford: Oxford University Press.

Jones, E. G. (1983). The nature of the afferent pathways conveying short-latency inputs to primate motor cortex. In J. Desmedt (Ed.), *Motor Control Mechanisms in Health and Disease* (pp. 263–285). New York: Raven Press.

Kaas, J. H., Florence, S. L., & Neeraj, J. (1997). Reorganization of sensory systems of primates after injury [Review]. *Neuroscientist, 3*(2), 123–130.

Kaas, J. H., Nelson, R. J., Sur, M., Lin, C. S., & Merzenich, M. M. (1979). Multiple representations of the body within the primary somatosensory cortex of primates. *Science, 204*(4392), 521–523.

Kaðovskπ, P. (2002). Dystonia: a disorder of motor programming or motor execution? *Movement Disorders, 17*(6), 1143–1147.

Karni, A., Meyer, G., Jezzard, P., Adams, M. M., Turner, R., & Ungerleider, L. G. (1995). Functional MRI Evidence for Adult Motor Cortex Plasticityt during Motor Skill Learning. *Nature, 377*, 155–158.

Kawashima, R., Roland, P. E., & O'Sullivan, B. T. (1994). Fields in human motor areas involved in preparation for reaching, actual reaching, and visuomotor learning: a positron emission tomography study. *Journal of Neuroscience, 14*(6), 3462–3474.

Keller, A., Arissian, K., & Asanuma, H. (1990). Formation of new synapses in the cat motor cortex following lesions of the deep cerebellar nuclei. *Experimental Brain Research, 80*(1), 23–33.

Keller, A., Arissian, K., & Asanuma, H. (1992). Synaptic Proliferation in the Motor Cortex of Adult Cats after Long-Term Thalamic Stimulation. *Journal of Neurophysiology, 68*(1), 295–308.

Keller, A., Iriki, A., & Asanuma, H. (1990). Identification of neurons producing long-term potentiation in the cat motor cortex: intracellular recordings and labeling. *Journal of Comparative Neurology, 300*(1), 47–60.

Kennedy, P. R., & Bakay, R. A. (1997). Activity of single action potentials in monkey motor cortex during long-term task learning. *Brain Research, 760*(1–2), 251–254.

Kew, J. J., Ridding, M. C., Rothwell, J. C., Passingham, R. E., Leigh, P. N., Sooriakumaran, S., et al. (1994). Reorganization of cortical blood flow and transcranial magnetic stimulation maps in human subjects after upper limb amputation. *Journal of Neurophysiology, 72*(5), 2517–2524.

Kiehn, O., & Kjaerulff, O. (1998). Distribution of central pattern generators for rhythmic motor outputs in the spinal cord of limbed vertebrates. *Ann N Y Acad Sci, 860*, 110–129.

Kim, S. G., Jennings, J. E., Strupp, J. P., Andersen, P., & Ugurbil, K. (1995). Functional MRI of Human Motor Cortices during Overt and Imagined Finger Movements. *International Journal of Imaging Systems and Technology, 6*, 271–279.

Kleim, J. A., Lussnig, E., Schwarz, E. R., Comery, T. A., & Greenough, W. T. (1996). Synaptogenesis and Fos expression in the motor cortex of the adult rat after motor skill learning. *Journal of Neuroscience, 16*(14), 4529–4535.

Kobayashi, M., & Pascual-Leone, A. (2003). Transcranial magnetic stimulation in neurology. *Lancet Neurol, 2*(3), 145–156.

Kohler, E., Keysers, C., Umilta, M. A., Fogassi, L., Gallese, V., & Rizzolatti, G. (2002). Hearing sounds, understanding actions: action representation in mirror neurons. *Science, 297*(5582), 846–848.

Kornhuber, H. H., & Deecke, L. (1965). Hirnpotentialänderungen bei Willkürbewegungen und passiven Bewegungen des Menschen: Bereitschaftspotential und reafferente Potentiale. *Pflügers Arch Gesamte Physiol Menschen Tiere, 284*, 1–17.

Landau, W. M., Freygang, W. H., Jr., Roland, L. P., Sokoloff, L., & Kety, S. (1955). The local circulation of the living brain; values in the unanesthetized and anesthetized cat. *Transactions of the American Neurological Association, 80*, 125–129.

Lassen, N. A., Hoedt-Rasmussen, K., Sorensen, S. C., Skinhoj, E., Cronquist, S., Bodforss, B., et al. (1963). Regional Cerebral Blood Flow in Man Determined by Krypton. *Neurology*, *13*, 719–727.

Lee, P. H., Han, S. W., & Heo, J. H. (1998). Isolated weakness of the fingers in cortical infarction. *Neurology*, *50*(3), 823–824.

Levy, W. J., York, D. H., McCaffrey, M., & Tanzer, F. (1984). Motor evoked potentials from transcranial stimulation of the motor cortex in humans. *Neurosurgery*, *15*(3), 287–302.

Liepert, J., Miltner, W. H., Bauder, H., Sommer, M., Dettmers, C., Taub, E., et al. (1998). Motor cortex plasticity during constraint-induced movement therapy in stroke patients. *Neurosci Lett*, *250*(1), 5–8.

Liepert, J., Tegenthoff, M., & Malin, J. P. (1995). Changes of cortical motor area size during immobilization. *Electroencephalography & Clinical Neurophysiology*, *97*(6), 382–386.

Lotze, M., Montoya, P., Erb, M., Hulsmann, E., Flor, H., Klose, U., et al. (1999). Activation of cortical and cerebellar motor areas during executed and imagined hand movements: an fMRI study. *J Cogn Neurosci*, *11*(5), 491–501.

MacKay-Lyons, M. (2002). Central Pattern Generation of Locomotion: A review of the evidence. *Phys Ther*, *82*, 69–83.

Makela, J. P., Hari, P., Karhu, J., Salmelin, R., & Teravainen, H. (1993). Suppression of magnetic mu rhythm during parkinsonian tremor. *Brain Res*, *617*(2), 189–193.

Marder, E. (2000). Motor pattern generation. *Curr Opin Neurobiol*, *10*(6), 691–698.

Marder, E., & Bucher, D. (2001). Central pattern generators and the control of rhythmic movements. *Curr Biol*, *11*(23), R986–R996.

Matelli, M., Luppino, G., & Rizzolatti, G. (1985). Patterns of cytochrome oxidase activity in the frontal agranular cortex of the macaque monkey. *Behav Brain Res*, *18*(2), 125–136.

McCrea, D. A. (1998). Neuronal basis of afferent-evoked enhancement of locomotor activity. *Ann N Y Acad Sci*, *860*, 216–225.

McCrea, D. A. (2001). Spinal circuitry of sensorimotor control of locomotion. *J Physiol*, *533*(Pt 1), 41–50.

McIntosh, A. R. (1999). Mapping cognition to the brain through neural interactions. *Memory*, *7*(5–6), 523–548.

McIntosh, A. R. (2000). Towards a network theory of cognition. *Neural Netw*, *13*(8–9), 861–870.

McIntosh, A. R., & Gonzalez-Lima, F. (1998). Large-scale functional connectivity in associative learning: interrelations of the rat auditory, visual, and limbic systems. *J Neurophysiol*, *80*(6), 3148–3162.

Merzenich, M. M., Nelson, R. J., Stryker, M. P., Cynader, M. S., Schoppmann, A., & Zook, J. M. (1984). Somatosensory Cortical Map Changes Following Digit Amputation in Adult Monkeys. *Journal of Comparative Anatomy*, *224*, 591–605.

Mesulam, M. (2005). Imaging connectivity in the human cerebral cortex: the next frontier? *Annals of Neurology*, *57*(1), 5–7.

Middleton, F. A., & Strick, P. L. (1994). Anatomical evidence for cerebellar and basal ganglia involvement in higher cognitive function. *Science*, *266*(5184), 458–461.

Middleton, F. A., & Strick, P. L. (1997). Cerebellar output channels. *Int. Rev. Neurobiol.*, *41*, 61–82.

Mills, K. R., Murray, N. M., & Hess, C. W. (1987). Magnetic and electrical transcranial brain stimulation: physiological mechanisms and clinical applications. *Neurosurgery*, *20*(1), 164–168.

Moonen, C. T. W., & Bandettini, P. A. (Eds.). (1999). *Functional MRI*. Heidelberg: Springer Verlag.

Nudo, R. J., Jenkins, W. M., & Merzenich, M. M. (1990). Repetitive Microstimulation Alters the Cortical Representation of Movements in Adult Rats. *Somatosensory and Motor Research*, *7*, 463–483.

Nudo, R. J., Jenkins, W. M., Merzenich, M. M., Prejean, T., & Grenda, R. (1992). Neurophysiological correlates of hand preference in primary motor cortex of adult squirrel monkeys. *Journal of Neuroscience*, *12*(8), 2918–2947.

Nudo, R. J., & Milliken, G. W. (1996). Reorganization of movement representations in primary motor cortex following focal ischemic infarcts in adult squirrel monkeys. *J Neurophysiol*, *75*(5), 2144–2149.

Nudo, R. J., Milliken, G. W., Jenkins, W. M., & Merzenich, M. M. (1996). Use-dependent alterations of movement representations in primary motor cortex of adult squirrel monkeys. *J Neurosci*, *16*(2), 785–807.

Nudo, R. J., Wise, B. M., SiFuentes, F., & Milliken, G. W. (1996). Neural Substrates for the Effects of Rehabilitative Training on Motor Recovery after Ischemic Infarct. *Science*, *272*(5269), 1791–1794.

Ogawa, S., Lee, T. M., Nayak, A. S., & Glynn, P. (1990). Oxygenation-Sensitive Contrast in Magnetic Resonance Image of Rodent Brain at High Magnetic Fields. *Magnetic Resonance in Medicine*, *14*, 68–78.

Oishi, K., Kasai, T., & Maeshima, T. (2000). Autonomic response specificity during motor imagery. *J Physiol Anthropol Appl Human Sci*, *19*(6), 255–261.

Pascual-Leone, A., Cammarota, A., Wassermann, E. M., Brasil-Neto, J. P., Cohen, L. G., & Hallett, M. (1993). Modulation of motor cortical outputs to the reading hand of braille readers. *Annals of Neurology*, *34*(1), 33–37.

Pascual-Leone, A., Grafman, J., & Hallett, M. (1994). Modulation of cortical motor output maps during development of implicit and explicit knowledge. *Science*, *263*(5151), 1287–1289.

Pascual-Leone, A., Nguyet, D., Cohen, L. G., Brasil-Neto, J. P., Cammarota, A., & Hallett, M. (1995). Modulation of muscle responses evoked by transcranial magnetic stimulation during the acquisition of new fine motor skills. *Journal of Neurophysiology*, *74*(3), 1037–1045.

Pascual-Leone, A., Peris, M., Tormos, J. M., Pascual, A. P., & Catala, M. D. (1996). Reorganization of human cortical motor output maps following traumatic forearm amputation. *Neuroreport*, *7*(13), 2068–2070.

Passingham, R. (1998). Functional organisation of the motor system. In R. S. J. Frackowiak, K. J. Friston, R. D. Dolan & J. C. Mazziotta (Eds.), *Human Brain Function* (pp. 243–274). San Diego: Academic Press.

Passingham, R. E., Toni, I., & Rushworth, M. F. (2000). Specialisation within the prefrontal cortex: the ventral prefrontal cortex and associative learning. *Exp Brain Res*, *133*(1), 103–113.

Pavlides, C., Miyashita, E., & Asanuma, H. (1993). Projection from the sensory to the motor cortex is important in learning motor skills in the monkey. *Journal of Neurophysiology*, *70*(2), 733–741.

Pearson, K. G. (1995). Proprioceptive regulation of locomotion. *Curr Opin Neurobiol*, *5*, 786–791.

Penfield, W., & Boldrey, E. (1937). Somatic motor and sensory representation in the cerebral cortex of man as studied by electrical stimulation. *Brain*, *60*, 389–443.

Penfield, W., & Rasmussen, T. (1950). *The Cerebral Cortex of Man*. New York: Macmillan.

Penfield, W., & Rasmussen, T. (1950). *The cerebral cortex of man. A clinical study of localization of function*. New York: Macmillan.

Petrides, M. (1985). Deficits in non-spatial conditional associative learning after periarcuate lesions in the monkey. *Behavioral and Brain Research*, 16(2–3), 95–101.

Petrides, M. (1997). Visuo-motor conditional associative learning after frontal and temporal lesions in the human brain. *Neuropsychologia*, 35(7), 989–997.

Petrides, M., & Pandya, D. N. (1984). Projections to the frontal cortex from the posterior parietal region in the rhesus monkey. *J Comp Neurol*, 228(1), 105–116.

Picard, N., & Strick, P. L. (2001). Imaging the premotor areas. *Current Opinion in Neurobiology*, 11(6), 663–672.

Poppele, R., & Bosco, G. (2003). Sophisticated spinal contributions to motor control. *Trends Neurosci*, 26(5), 269–276.

Porro, C. A., Francescato, M. P., Cettolo, V., Diamond, M. E., Baraldi, P., Zuiani, C., et al. (1996). Primary motor and sensory cortex activation during motor performance and motor imagery: a functional magnetic resonance imaging study. *J Neurosci*, 16(23), 7688–7698.

Posner, M. I., & Raichle, M. E. (1994). *Images of mind*. New York: W. H. Freeman & Company.

Raichle, M. E., Martin, W. R. W., & Herscovitch, P. (1983). Brain Blood Flow Measured with Intravenous H$_2$^{15}O II: Implementation and Validation. *Journal of Nuclear Medicine, 24*, 790–798.

Ramon y Cajal, S. (1923). *Recuerdos de mi vida*. Madrid: J. Pueyo.

Raymond, J. L., Lisberger, S. G., & Mauk, M. D. (1996). The cerebellum: a neuronal learning machine? [Review]. *Science*, 272(5265), 1126–1131.

Recanzone, G. H., Merzenich, M. M., & Dinse, H. R. (1992). Expansion of the cortical representation of a specific skin field in primary somatosensory cortex by intracortical microstimulation. *Cerebral Cortex*, 2(3), 181–196.

Rijntjes, M., Tegenthoff, M., Liepert, J., Leonhardt, G., Kotterba, S., Muller, S., et al. (1997). Cortical reorganization in patients with facial palsy. *Ann Neurol*, 41(5), 621–630.

Rizzolatti, G., & Arbib, M. A. (1998). Language within our grasp. *Trends Neurosci*, 21(5), 188–194.

Rizzolatti, G., Camarda, R., Fogassi, L., Gentilucci, M., Luppino, G., & Matelli, M. (1988). Functional organization of inferior area 6 in the macaque monkey. II. Area F5 and the control of distal movements. *Exp Brain Res*, 71(3), 491–507.

Rizzolatti, G., & Fadiga, L. (1998). Grasping objects and grasping action meanings: the dual role of monkey rostroventral premotor cortex (area F5). *Novartis Found Symp*, 218, 81–95; discussion 95–103.

Rizzolatti, G., Fadiga, L., Gallese, V., & Fogassi, L. (1996). Premotor cortex and the recognition of motor actions. *Brain Res Cogn Brain Res*, 3(2), 131–141.

Rizzolatti, G., Luppino, G., & Matelli, M. (1998). The organization of the cortical motor system: new concepts. *Electroencephalogr Clin Neurophysiol*, 106(4), 283–296.

Roland, P. E., Skinhoj, E., Lassen, N. A., & Larsen, B. (1980). Different cortical areas in man in organization of voluntary movements in extrapersonal space. *J Neurophysiol*, 43(1), 137–150.

Rossini, P. M., Rossi, S., Pasqualetti, P., & Tecchio, F. (1999). Corticospinal excitability modulation to hand muscles during movement imagery. *Cereb Cortex*, 9(2), 161–167.

Rothwell, J. C., Traub, M. M., Day, B. L., Obeso, J. A., Thomas, P. K., & Marsden, C. D. (1982). Manual motor performance in a deafferented man. *Brain*, 105(Pt 3), 515–542.

Sanes, J. N. (1994). Neurophysiology of preparation, movement and imagery. *Behav Brain Sci*, 17, 221–223.

Sanes, J. N., Wang, J., & Donoghue, J. P. (1992). Immediate and delayed changes of rat motor cortical output representation with new forelimb configurations. *Cerebral Cortex*, 2(2), 141–152.

Sherrington, C. S. (1906). *The integrative action of the nervous system*. New York, N. Y.: C Scriber's Sons.

Sherrington, C. S. (1910). Flexion reflex of the limb, crossed extension reflex, and reflex stepping and standing. *J Physiol*, 40, 28–121.

Solodkin, A., Hlustik, P., Chen, E. E., & Small, S. L. (2004). Fine modulation in network activation during motor execution and motor imagery. *Cereb Cortex*, 14(11), 1246–1255.

Squire, L. R. (1987a). Divisions of long-term memory. In *Memory and Brain* (pp. 151–179). New York: Oxford University Press.

Squire, L. R. (1987b). *Memory and brain*. New York: Oxford University Press.

Stephan, K. M., & Frackowiak, R. S. (1996). Motor imagery – anatomical representation and electrophysiological characteristics. *Neurochem Res*, 21(9), 1105–1116.

Strafella, A. P., & Paus, T. (2000). Modulation of cortical excitability during action observation: a transcranial magnetic stimulation study. *Neuroreport*, 11(10), 2289–2292.

Strangman, G. E. (1998). *Modes of motor learning*. Unpublished Ph.D. dissertation, Brown University, Providence, Rhode Island.

Ter-Pogossian, M. M., Phelps, M. E., Hoffman, E. J., & Mullani, N. A. (1975). A positron-emission transaxial tomograph for nuclear imaging (PETT). *Radiology*, 114(1), 89–98.

Umilta, M. A., Kohler, E., Gallese, V., Fogassi, L., Fadiga, L., Keysers, C., et al. (2001). I know what you are doing: a neurophysiological study. *Neuron*, 31(1), 155–165.

Vogt, C., & Vogt, O. (1919). Allgemeine Ergebnisse unserer Hirnforschung. *Journal für Psychologie und Neurologie, 25*, 279–461.

Walter, W. G., Cooper, R., Aldridge, V. J., McCallum, W. C., & Winter, A. L. (1964). Contingent Negative Variation: An Electric Sign of Sensorimotor Association and Expectancy in the Human Brain. *Nature*, 203, 380–384.

Weiller, C., Ramsay, S. C., Wise, R. J., Friston, K. J., & Frackowiak, R. S. (1993). Individual patterns of functional reorganization in the human cerebral cortex after capsular infarction. *Ann Neurol*, 33(2), 181–189.

White, A., & Hardy, L. (1995). Use of different imagery perspectives on the learning and performance of different motor skills. *Br J Psychol*, 86(Pt 2), 169–180.

White, L. E., Andrews, T. J., Hulette, C., Richards, A., Groelle, M., Paydarfar, J., et al. (1997). Structure of the human sensorimotor system. II: Lateral symmetry. *Cereb Cortex*, 7(1), 31–47.

Wiesendanger, M. (1986). Recent developments in studies of the supplementary motor area of primates. *Rev Physiol Biochem Pharmacol*, 103, 1–59.

Wiesendanger, M. (1999). Manual dexterity and the making of tools – an introduction from an evolutionary perspective. *Exp Brain Res*, 128(1–2), 1–5.

Wiesendanger, M., & Wise, S. P. (1992). Current issues concerning the functional organization of motor cortical areas in nonhuman primates. *Adv Neurol*, 57, 117–134.

Wise, S. P., di Pellegrino, G., & Boussaoud, D. (1996). The premotor cortex and nonstandard sensorimotor mapping. *Can J Physiol Pharmacol*, 74(4), 469–482.

Xerri, C., Merzenich, M. M., Jenkins, W., & Santucci, S. (1999). Representational plasticity in cortical area 3b paralleling tactual-motor skill acquisition in adult monkeys. *Cerebral Cortex, 9*(3), 264–276.

Xerri, C., Merzenich, M. M., Peterson, B. E., & Jenkins, W. (1998). Plasticity of primary somatosensory cortex paralleling sensorimotor skill recovery from stroke in adult monkeys. *J Neurophysiol, 79*(4), 2119–2148.

Yaguez, L., Canavan, A. G., Lange, H. W., & Homberg, V. (1999). Motor learning by imagery is differentially affected in Parkinson's and Huntington's diseases. *Behav Brain Res, 102*(1–2), 115–127.

Zant, J., & Strick, P. (1978). The cells of origin of interhemispheric connections in the primate motor cortex. *Society for Neuroscience Abstracts, 4*, 308.

Zilles, K., Palomero-Gallagher, N., Grefkes, C., Scheperjans, F., Boy, C., Amunts, K., et al. (2002). Architectonics of the human cerebral cortex and transmitter receptor fingerprints: reconciling functional neuroanatomy and neurochemistry. *Eur Neuropsychopharmacol, 12*(6), 587–599.

Zilles, K., Schlaug, G., Matelli, M., Luppino, G., Schleicher, A., Qu, M., et al. (1995). Mapping of human and macaque sensorimotor areas by integrating architectonic, transmitter receptor, MRI and PET data. *J Anat, 187*(Pt 3), 515–537.

23 The Neural Basis of Affective and Social Behavior

RALPH ADOLPHS AND MICHAEL L. SPEZIO

INTRODUCTION

The processing of affectively and socially relevant information, long the purview of social psychology and psychiatry, has recently become a primary focus for cognitive neuroscience. The reasons for this are twofold: (1) the maturation of theoretical frameworks for understanding such information processing provided specific hypotheses that made neuroanatomical predictions; and (2) the advent of modern neuroscience methods, in particular functional neuroimaging, provided ways of testing those predictions. Of course, the predictions were not all formulated first and then simply tested, but as the data from neuroscience began to trickle in, major revisions in the theoretical framework and the hypotheses were undertaken at the same time. This has resulted in one of the most dynamic and interesting fields of scientific research, really a paradigm study in the philosophy of science, in which hypotheses and data continuously update one another.

Two historical texts, one by Charles Darwin (Darwin, 1872/1965) and the other by William James (James, 1884), have provided the impetus for many of the questions modern affective neuroscience has thought it has had to address. Darwin's book, *The Expression of the Emotions in Man and Animals*, provided three famous principles for understanding emotion and its relation to social communication: the idea that emotional expressions had evolutionarily antecedent bodily reactions whose primary adaptive nature had been co-opted for social purposes; the idea that emotions have an internal structure (specifically, his principle of antithesis); and, last but not least, the idea that emotions are a direct result of the nervous system, which mediates interactions between the brain and bodily affect in the expression of emotions (cf., Bernard, 1866).

James departed from Darwin's third principle – which emphasized the interaction between brain and bodily affect – to answer the question "What is an emotion?" in an eponymously entitled paper (James 1884). His answer was counterintuitive, and reactions to it have influenced the theoretical positions on emotion to this day. James proposed that bodily changes, or affects, directly follow the perception of some emotionally evocative stimulus ("exciting fact"), and that the perceptions of these bodily changes are simply identified as the emotion or feeling. James thought that the emotion/feeling only happened *after* the bodily changes had occurred, arguing against the idea that neural activity in preparation for the bodily changes could itself be perceived and give rise to emotion/feeling prior to or at the same time as the bodily changes.

Cognitive neuroscience has used the interactionist perspective Darwin proposed in investigating the mechanisms by which the brain processes both environmental stimuli in the generation of emotions and the concomitant physiological responses as they influence not only further emotional processing, but also higher order cognitive functions. The goal of incorporating emotional processing into a rigorous mechanistic understanding of cognition (Simon, 1979) is being actively pursued in cognitive neuroscience. Recent reviews on the relationship of emotion to memory (LaBar, 2003; Richter-Levin, 2004; Kensinger, 2004; McGaugh, 2004), to attention (Pessoa, Kastner, & Ungerleider, 2002; Pessoa & Ungerleider, 2004), and to decision making (Bechara, 2004; Bechara, Damasio, & Damasio 2003) illustrate the wide reach of emotional processing research within cognitive neuroscience. Some of the most surprising results in relating emotion to complex cognition, however, have come from the cognitive neuroscience of social behavior. Here, not only has emotional processing within localized brain networks been shown to strongly modulate social behavior, but there is evidence that emotional processing is in fact constitutive of and required for normal social behavior (Adolphs, Tranel, & Damasio, 2003; Adolphs, 2003, 2003; Anderson et al., 2000). That is, damage to key brain areas important for emotional processing impairs a range of social abilities, from judging emotion from faces or voices or bodily motion to profound social dysfunction.

Indeed, most structures that have been shown to be important in processing emotions have turned out to be important also for social behavior. These include (a) higher-order sensory cortices; (b) amygdala, ventral striatum, and orbitofrontal cortex; and (c) additional cortical regions such as the left prefrontal, right parietal, and anterior as well as posterior cingulate cortices. One can relate these three sets of regions, respectively, as implementing different sets of processes: (a) a perceptual representation of the stimuli and their constituent features, (b) an association of this perceptual representation with emotional response, cognitive processing, and behavioral motivation, and (c) the construction of an internal model of the social environment, involving representation of other people, their social relationships with oneself, and the value of one's actions in the context of a social group. To some extent these three sets of processes build on one another, although their interactions are complex.

SENSORY PROCESSING

Faces: visual cortex and the amygdala. A large literature has shown that humans pay attention to, make eye movements to, discriminate, categorize and recognize faces differently than other visual stimuli (Adolphs, 2002). These differences in processing at multiple levels are driven by the computational demands that faces present: they constitute a large class of stimuli that are all visually very similar, yet require rapid and accurate subordinate-level categorization and recognition. Their social significance and ubiquity also makes everyone an expert at such processing, at least for large classes of faces. While debate continues regarding the extent to which face processing is domain-specific (Kanwisher, 2000; Tarr & Gauthier 2000), it is clear that it differs from processing of other visual stimuli, whether in kind or degree, and that it consequently correlates with disproportionate engagement of certain neural structures.

In addition to processing the identity, age, and gender of faces, one socially very important aspect of face processing is emotional expression (Darwin, 1872/1965) including direction of eye gaze (Emery, 2000). Although it remains a rich topic in psychology and philosophy how to conceptualize the terms "emotion" and "expression" (Russell, Bachorowski, & Fernandez-Dols, 2003), and there is continuing debate regarding how best to classify the different emotional facial expressions, most investigators within cognitive neuroscience have followed the scheme pioneered by Paul Ekman. He and others identified happiness, fear, anger, disgust, and sadness, with possibly also surprise and contempt, as so-called "basic" emotions that could be reliably signaled by the face (Ekman, 1972, 1973; Tomkins 1962), and his stimuli remain the most widely used set (Ekman & Friesen, 1976).

More contentious has been a second argument of Ekman's: that these basic emotions are cultural universals. Based on cross-cultural studies, some investigators argued that the set of basic emotions can be recognized as such across all cultures, and furthermore that this is evidence for their innate basis (Ekman, 1972; Izard, 1971). More recent studies and meta-analyses have provided clear evidence that both culturally universal and specific factors contribute to recognition of emotional facial expressions: viewers from all cultures perform above chance levels in their ability to classify facial displays into emotion categories, but there is a further advantage if the race of the face shown in the stimulus matches that of the viewer (Russell & Fernandez-Dols, 1997; Elfenbein & Ambady 2002, 2002). There appears to be cultural learning (Sporer, 2001), such that increasing familiarity with the ethnicity of the faces shown as stimuli results in a graded increase in the accuracy with which they are recognized (Elfenbein, & Ambady, 2003).

Gender differences in the recognition of emotional facial expressions have also been reported, in line with the large literature on gender differences in processing emotional information more generally. Across studies, there is a consensus that females are more accurate than males, that such differences develop early (McClure, 2000), and that they depend also on the gender of the face shown in the stimulus (Erwin et al., 1992). There is even preliminary evidence that developmental gender differences in facial emotion processing are reflected in differences in the activation of certain brain structures, such as the amygdala (Killgore, Oki, & Yurgelun-Todd, 2001).

A large literature from functional imaging studies exists on face processing in extrastriate visual cortices; such work has shown, for example, that there are regions specialized to process different kinds of information from faces, such as information about identity and emotional expression (Hoffman & Haxby, 2000); that such processing draws on a distributed set of brain regions even though there is also specialization (Haxby et al., 2001); that facial expression and direction of gaze interact (Adams et al., 2003), and that such processing operates at several temporal scales (Adolphs, 2002). The amygdala is arguably the brain structure whose specific role in processing facial emotion has been investigated most intensely. Functional imaging studies have provided evidence that viewing facial expressions, especially fear, automatically engages the amygdala in normal individuals (Vuilleumier et al., 2001), and that abnormal amygdala activation can be seen in certain psychiatric populations with disorders of emotion (Rauch et al., 2000; Sheline et al., 2001; Davidson, 2002; Drevets, 2001). A large number of studies have reported disproportionate amygdala activation when viewing expressions of fear (Morris et al., 1996; Breiter et al., 1996; Phillips et al., 1998; Whalen et al., 2001). However, as in the case of the lesion studies (cf. below), other investigations have found evidence for amygdala processing of expressions other than fear, including either activations (Breiter et al., 1996) or deactivations (Morris et al., 1996) to happy faces, as well as activations to sad faces (Blair et al., 1999). At least some of these discrepancies in the literature may have arisen due to the interaction of facial emotion with other factors, such as context or direction of eye gaze, a topic that has been explored very recently.

The direction of eye gaze is an important source of information about individuals intention, and likely future behavior. Eye gaze is a key social signal in many species (Emery, 2000), especially apes and humans, whose white sclera makes the pupil more easily visible and permits better discrimination of gaze. Human viewers make preferential fixations onto the eye region of others' faces (Janik et al., 1978), a behavior that appears early in development and may contribute to the socioemotional impairments seen in developmental disorders like autism (Baron-Cohen, 1995). Eyes signal important information about emotional states, and there is evidence from functional imaging studies that at least some of this processing recruits the amygdala (Baron-Cohen et al., 1999; Kawashima et al., 1999; Wicker, Perrett et al., 2003). The interaction between facial emotion and direction of eye gaze has been explored only very recently. It was found that direct gaze facilitated processing of approach-oriented emotions such as anger, whereas averted gaze facilitated the processing of avoidance-oriented emotions such as fear (Adams & Kleck, 2003), and that this processing facilitation correlated with increased activation of the amygdala in a functional imaging study (Adams et al., 2003).

Some of the amygdala's contribution to the processing of facial emotion may rely on an initial, rapid evaluation of the stimulus, possibly in part via subcortical inputs (Morris, Ohman, & Dolan, 1999; Morris et al., 2001), followed by feedback modulation of visual cortex. The amygdala is known to receive input from visual cortex and to project back to temporal and occipital visual cortices, including striate cortex, in primates (Amaral & Price, 1984; Amaral, Behniea, & Kelly, 2003; Stefanacci & Amaral, 2000) probably including humans (Catani et al., 2003). A possible functional role for this anatomical connectivity is suggested by electrophysiological data: intracranial recordings from the human brain show that field potentials in both the amygdala (Krolak-Salmon et al., 2004; Oya et al., 2002) and in temporal visual cortex (Puce, Allison, and McCarthy, 1999) are modulated by emotional and/or social information. The time course of this field potential modulation – amygdala first, visual cortex next – is consistent with amygdala input giving rise to emotional modulation seen in the visual cortex. Dependence upon the amygdala for emotional discrimination in the temporal visual cortex is also suggested by recordings from single neurons in monkey temporal cortex (Sugase et al., 1999). In monkey temporal visual cortex, neurons encode discriminations between superordinate categories (e.g., face vs. non-face objects) earlier than they encode discrimination between facial emotions.

Some of the most convincing evidence for the amygdala's role in the emotional modulation of visual cortex comes from studying people who have amygdala lesions. Amygdala lesions eliminate the ability of fear faces to modulate activation in visual cortex, including the fusiform gyrus and occipital cortex (Vuilleumier et al., 2004). People without lesions to the amygdala and people who have lesions of the hippocampus alone continue to show modulation of brain activation in visual cortex by fear faces, compared to neutral faces. Thus, the amygdala appears to be required for robust modulation of visual cortex activation by facial emotions.

The requirement of the amygdala for face processing in normal social behavior is confirmed by lesion studies, many of which were actually carried out first and provided the impetus for the functional imaging studies. Several recent lesion studies reported rare patients with bilateral damage to the amygdala. Most of the impairments found were not seen in the more common unilateral cases, typically patients with neurosurgical temporal lobectomy for the treatment of epilepsy. The bilateral amygdala patients fell into three classes: most common (albeit still rare) were those who had complete bilateral amygdala damage as well as damage to surrounding structures from encephalitis. Yet more rare were those with bilateral but incomplete damage relatively restricted to the amygdala.

Following earlier indications that bilateral amygdala damage might impair aspects of face processing (Jacobson, 1986), the first study to demonstrate a selective impairment in recognition of emotion from faces also found this impairment to be relatively restricted to certain highly arousing emotions, especially fear (Adolphs et al., 1994). Some subsequent studies found a disproportionately severe impairment in recognizing fear (Adolphs, Tranel et al., 1995; Broks et al., 1998; Calder et al., 1996; Anderson & Phelps, 2000; Sprengelmeyer et al., 1999), whereas others found evidence for a broader or more variable impairment in recognizing multiple emotions of negative valence in the face, including fear, anger, disgust, and sadness (Adolphs et al., 1999; Adolphs, 1999; Schmolck & Squire, 2001) (Siebert, Markowitsch, & Bartel, 2003). Impairments in processing the direction of eye gaze have also been reported (Young et al., 1995).

Across the majority of studies, impairments in recognition of emotion have been found despite an often normal ability to discriminate perceptually among the same stimuli. Many patients with bilateral amygdala damage perform in the normal range on the Benton Face Matching Task (Benton et al., 1983), in which subjects are asked to match different views of the same, unfamiliar person's face, and they also perform normally in discriminating subtle changes in facial expression, even for facial expressions that they are nonetheless unable to recognize (Adolphs, Tranel, & Damasio, 1998; Adolphs & Tranel, 2000). A final piece of evidence for normal face perception is that some of the subjects with amygdala lesions are able to recognize a person's identity (Adolphs et al., 1994), as well as gender and age (Anderson & Phelps, 2000) from the face, even though they fail to recognize aspects of its emotional expression.

A single case to date, subject SM, has complete bilateral damage that is restricted to the amygdala (Adolphs et al., 1994). This subject has been especially informative because of the specificity of both her lesion and her impairment (Tranel & Hyman, 1990; Adolphs & Tranel, 2000). SM is a 40-year-old woman who has complete bilateral amygdala damage resulting from a rare disease (Urbach-Wiethe disease (Hofer, 1973)) On a series of tasks, she shows a relatively disproportionate impairment in recognizing the intensity of fear from faces alone, and a lesser impairment also in recognizing the intensity of related emotions such as surprise and anger (Adolphs et al., 1994). Her impairment is restricted to this class of emotions when asked to rate the intensity of basic emotions; however she also has a broader impairment in rating the degree of arousal of all negatively valenced emotions (Adolphs, Russell, & Tranel, 1999), as well as in making social judgments concerning the trustworthiness and approachability of people from their faces (Adolphs, Tranel, & Damasio, 1998), displaying a strong bias to issue judgments of trustworthiness independent of facial characteristics. SM also shows a distinct failure to make use of the eyes when judging emotion from faces, and an impairment in overt attention to fear faces (Adolphs et al., 2005). These results are consistent with the notion that the amygdala is required for effective processing of salient information signaling emotion in a face, and support theories implicating the amygdala in visual processing of emotion from the eyes.

Several different theories have been offered to explain the data thus far. We have suggested that the amygdala is involved principally in processing stimuli related to threat and danger (Adolphs & Tranel, 2000; Adolphs et al., 1999). Others have suggested that it instead triggers cognitive resources to help resolve ambiguity in the environment – under this explanation, both facial expressions of fear and of anger signal threat/danger, but fear differs from anger in that the source of the threat is ambiguous. It would then be the imperative to resolve this ambiguity that engages the amygdala (Whalen, 1999). This latter explanation would fit also with the substantial evidence for the amygdala's modulation of attentional processes in both animals (Holland & Gallagher, 1999) and humans (Holland & Gallagher, 1999; Anderson and Phelps, 2001), including a possible role for modulating spatial attention to facial expressions (Vuilleumier & Schwartz, 2001). It also fits with some reports (Whalen et al., 2001) that the amygdala is more important for recognizing fear from facial expressions than it is for recognizing anger, and with recent findings that the amygdala activation by fear and anger faces depends on the direction of gaze (Adams et al., 2003). Another explanation is that the amygdala is involved in processing a class of emotions that are of negative valence and high arousal (Adolphs, Russell, & Tranel, 1999), which may carve out an ecologically salient emotion category of which threat/danger is a subset. Yet a further possibility is that the emotions whose recognition depends most on the amygdala are related to behavioral withdrawal (Anderson, Spencer et al., 2000), where again threat/danger or fear are a subset of this class. Given these multiple interpretations, it seems plausible that the amygdala may instead participate primarily in a set of more basic processes that can all come into play in emotion recognition, but that do not translate neatly into any particular categories of emotion. One such more basic process, the one investigated in the present application's proposed studies, is that the amygdala is relatively specialized to process information from a particular feature, or set of features in the face – features that are particularly important for detecting threat, resolving ambiguity, and eliciting behavioral withdrawal when recognized. The expression and direction of gaze of the eyes would be one such candidate feature.

Unilateral damage to the amygdala results in a smaller magnitude of impaired recognition of emotion than does bilateral damage (Adolphs, Tranel et al., 1995). However, when larger samples of subjects are tested, impairments are also found: an impaired ability to learn new emotional facial expressions correlated with the extent of unilateral amygdala damage (Boucsein et al., 2001), and both (Adolphs et al. (2001) (sample N = 26) and (Anderson et al. (2000) (sample N = 23)) found evidence that subjects with unilateral damage due to temporal lobectomy were impaired, as a group, in their recognition of some negative emotions from facial expressions, despite intact basic visual perception (Mendola et al., 1999). The impairment was especially striking for fear (Adolphs, Tranel, & Damasio, 2001) but may extend to emotions related to withdrawal in general (Anderson, Spencer et al., 2000).

The studies of other patients with bilateral amygdala damage, as well as further considerations of data just from patient SM, raised important additional questions. One puzzling finding was that some patients who had complete, non-selective bilateral amygdala damage nonetheless appeared to perform normally on the same tasks that SM failed. This was puzzling because the lesions of these other patients included the entirety of the lesion present in SM, plus additional tissue. Several explanations could be entertained: first, it is important to note that SM's lesion was likely acquired developmentally, quite early in life, whereas the lesions of the other subjects were acquired in adulthood. Second, it is certainly possible to construct a model whereby additional brain damage actually improves performance due to a primary lesion (Kapur, 1996). Third, the patients were very rare and all different in many respects, so that performance differences might be due to other neuropsychological or demographic differences. In the end, while any of these possibilities might still be important, it turned out that (a) subjects perform variably from trial to trial, and (b) when data were reanalyzed, general impairments in emotion recognition were found to be present in all the subjects, although they did not appear to show up in exactly the same way (Schmolck & Squire, 2001). The picture that emerged should not have been unexpected, since it is the standard picture for thinking about how risk factors contribute to pathology: lesions of the amygdala interfere with certain basic emotional processes, and hence compromise recognition of fear from faces. But this effect interacts with damage to any other parts of the brain, age of acquisition of the lesion, background neuropsychology and personality of the subject, and indeed the particular context and task used to assess emotion recognition.

We can summarize the basic impairment that follows lesions of the human amygdala. Since subjects with amygdala lesions do not have basic discriminatory visuoperceptual impairments, it cannot be that they simply cannot discriminate certain visual features. Since they also don't have general conceptual/semantic impairments about emotions, it cannot be that they simply don't know what certain emotions mean. What patients with amygdala damage lack is the ability to link these two: the mechanism for using visual changes in a particular facial feature to obtain information about a particular emotion.

Voices: cortical and subcortical substrates. As in Darwin's work on human emotional expression (Darwin, 1872/1965), the quantity of cognitive neuroscience research into emotional processing in the facial/visual domain dwarfs that on processing emotion from the vocal/auditory domain. Yet there is an extensive literature on emotional cues in and processing of vocalizations in social contexts, and like the work on emotional processing from faces, the work on vocalizations utilizes an evolutionarily informed approach (cf., Scherer, 1988; Marler, 1984).

Study of emotional processing in the vocal/auditory domain focuses primarily on prosody in the voice. Prosody is defined as vocal information that cannot be ascertained from lexical information, and includes measures of pitch, duration, and amplitude (Monrad-Kohn, 1947). Acoustic measurements of prosodic components can be used in combinatorial algorithms to categorize basic emotions from voices alone with an accuracy of 60–70% (Scherer et al., 1991; van Bezooijen, Otto, & Heenan, 1983; van Bezooijen, 1984; Yildirim et al., 2004; Scherer, 1995), where chance performance is in the 10–20% range. Yet the categorization accuracy of human judges is higher than this, and it is of interest to determine the mechanism used by the brain to yield such effective emotional judgment from the voice.

Although the amygdala was seen to be required for effective processing of emotion from faces, the evidence for the amygdala's involvement in judgment of vocal emotion is less clear. While there is evidence for the activation of the amygdala by emotional prosody (Morris, Scott, & Dolan, 1999), and for the impairment of vocal emotion judgment after bilateral amygdala lesion (Scott et al., 1997), there is also evidence that bilateral lesions of the amygdala have no effect on such judgment (Adolphs & Tranel 1999).

However, an extensive study of patients with cortical lesions revealed several cortical areas that are important for such judgment (Adolphs, Tranel, & Damasio, 2002). The cortical areas whose lesions most affected emotional judgment from the voice include the frontal pole, the frontal operculum (including Broca's area), and the right frontal and anterior parietal cortex, including right somatosensory cortex. Impairments were worst for the emotions of fear, anger, and surprise, compared to happiness and sadness. In an important study of a single patient, a lesion to the right ventromedial prefrontal cortex eliminated the ability to judge vocal emotion while preserving propositional speech and syntactic prosody (Heilman, Leon, & Rosenbek, 2004).

Results from neuroimaging experiments are largely consistent with results from lesioned patients. Activations to vocal emotion are primarily right lateralized and have been seen in right frontoparietal areas (Buchanan et al., 2000), including the right frontal gyrus, the right inferior parietal lobule, the right middle temporal gyrus (Mitchell et al., 2003), the right ventromedial prefrontal cortex (Wildgruber et al., 2005), and both the left (Mitchell et al., 2003) and right (Wildgruber et al., 2005) superior temporal gyri. Superior temporal regions have also been implicated in discriminating angry vs. neutral prosody, absent semantic content of speech (Grandjean et al., 2005). As yet the mechanism for how emotional information from the voice is processed within these areas, and the temporal order by which these areas are brought online for judgment of vocal emotion, remains obscure. Nevertheless, the work thus far focuses increasing attention on the right hemisphere of the brain, particularly in the frontal and frontoparietal regions. The implication of superior temporal regions is somewhat more recent, and it will be important for future cognitive neuroscientific work on the judgment of vocal emotion to delineate what the specific function is of this area in emotional processing of voices.

Several of the areas implicated by lesion analysis and neuroimaging for judging vocal emotion (e.g., ventromedial prefrontal cortex, right somatosensory cortex) are known to be critical for normal social behavior (see below). In fact, psychopaths who show severely abnormal social behavior also exhibit impairments in judging emotion in the voice, and they are especially impaired at judging vocal fear (Blair et al., 2002). This observation is consistent with the notion that brain centers required for emotional processing, in this case of vocal emotion, are also required for normal social behavior.

SOCIAL JUDGMENT AND DECISION-MAKING

Orbitofrontal cortex. We now consider explicitly the importance for social judgment and decision making of brain areas that are strongly implicated in emotional processing. Probably the best example here is the orbitofrontal cortex, a region of the brain located on the ventral surface of the frontal lobes. The studies of orbitofrontal cortex began with a famous historical case, that of Phineas Gage (Damasio, 1994). Gage, a foreman working on the railway in Vermont, sustained a traumatic brain injury due to a tamping iron that exploded through his head. It was amazing that he survived the accident at all, but no less amazing were the specific cognitive changes that ensued. His basic intellect appeared unchanged, but long-term behaviors and dispositions relating to emotional responses to his environment and to other people had been dramatically altered. Whereas before the accident he was a respected, well liked, courteous, and amiable person, after the accident he became uncaring, rude, profane, and exhibited a gross disregard both for his own personal future and for other people. What had changed were emotional processes that contribute substantially to our concept of a personality.

Gage's case was notably resurrected in recent times by a further analysis of his likely brain lesion (Damasio et al., 1994), and by supplementation with data from modern patients who had sustained similar damage – not because of the passage of an iron rod through their head, but typically because of tumor resections of the frontal lobe or aneurysms of the anterior communicating artery (Damasio, 1994). These modern case studies permitted more controlled experimental investigations of the impairment, and eventually accrued to comprise a group of subjects that shared damage to ventral and medial sectors of the prefrontal cortex, all of whom exhibited a remarkably similar constellation of findings. They failed to elicit emotional psychophysiological responses to stimuli (Damasio, Tranel, and Damasio, 1990), they failed to elicit such responses in anticipation of future punishment (Bechara et al., 1996), and they failed to guide their behavior so as to avoid future punishment (or seek future reward) (Bechara et al., 1994). Their behavior was driven by what was immediately present, and did not take into account planning for the future. One of the major current theories of the function of this region of prefrontal cortex, Antonio Damasio's somatic marker hypothesis, draws on these findings and proposes that they are causally related (Damasio, 1994). In real life, all these patients fail to maintain lasting social relationships or jobs, a reflection of their dysfunction in this particular mechanism.

As the investigations of orbitofrontal cortex have accrued a sufficient number of cases, they have permitted some further specification of the neuroanatomy and the processes. For instance, dissociations have been found between damage in dorsolateral and ventromedial prefrontal cortex in relation to working memory and decision-making, respectively (Bechara et al., 1998). Damage to the right prefrontal cortex has been shown to result in more severe impairments in emotion processing than damage to left (Tranel, Bechara, & Denburg, 2002). And the impairments following damage to ventromedial prefrontal cortex have been shown to be distinct from any impairment in IQ, language function, or perception.

The above summarized findings are consistent with what is known about the connectivity of this region of the brain. Medial and ventral sectors of prefrontal cortex have been shown to constitute a densely interconnected network that obtains polysensory information, taste and smell information, and visceral information, and projects to autonomic control structures, such as the hypothalamus and periaqueductal grey area (Öngür & Price, 2000). They are consistent also with other data from functional imaging studies in humans, as well as from lesion and electrophysiological studies in animals.

The orbitofrontal cortex has also been implicated in social reasoning. Damage to this region impairs the ability to figure out that other people are being deceptive (Stuss, Gallup, & Alexander, 2001), and results in impaired performance in reasoning about social exchange using the Wason selection task (Stone et al., 2002; Adolphs, Bechara et al., 1995). These findings may reflect the above mentioned role for the orbitofrontal cortex in guiding social cognition by the elicitation of emotional states that serve to bias cognition, a role further supported by investigations of moral reasoning.

The role of specific brain structures in moral behavior has been investigated using social and moral dilemmas – choice options structured so that they conflict (Greene & Haidt, 2002). Such conflict may arise from short-term versus long-term goals, or from goals advantageous to oneself versus those advantageous for others or society as a whole. It is thus closely related to altruistic behavior, social cooperativity, and the cognitive processes that guide behavior in markets and that are described by economics. A subset of moral dilemmas involve one's own agency and trigger strong emotions in their consideration; these have been found to engage structures involved in emotion processing, such as the superior temporal sulcus, cingulate, and medial prefrontal cortices (Greene et al., 2001). Social cooperation in the prisoner's dilemma engages a similar set of structures, including orbitofrontal and anterior cingulate cortices as well as ventral striatum (Rilling et al., 2002). All of the above data on medial and orbital prefrontal cortex are consistent with a role for this region in guiding the strategic adoption of someone else's point of view – perhaps by triggering emotional states, by engaging simulation routines, or by more cognitive strategies.

The amygdala, take two. We encountered the amygdala earlier, when we discussed the recognition of emotions from faces. But the amygdala also plays a complex and more ubiquitous role in emotional aspects of social behavior (Aggleton, 2000). The mechanisms that underlie this role are best understood in animals, especially rodents, where they have been shown to draw on the amygdala's ability to modulate a large variety of response components and cognitive processes based on the emotional significance of the stimulus. Thus, the amygdala modulates attention, memory, and decision making, as well as many components of an emotional response (including behavioral, autonomic, and endocrine components), and all of these are highly relevant to regulating social behavior. It is still an open question to what extent the amygdala might actually be specialized to subserve social behavior as such, or whether it is simply involved in domain-general emotional processing that happens also to be important to social behavior.

The amygdala's functional complexity is mirrored in its vast array of connections with other brain structures: high-level sensory neocortices provide information about the stimulus, primarily to the lateral nucleus, and the amygdala projects back to much of neocortex, as well as to basal forebrain, hippocampus, and basal ganglia to modulate cognition, and to hypothalamic and brainstem nuclei to modulate emotional response (Amaral et al., 1992). It is precisely because of the complexity of the various processes in which the amygdala participates that it can effect a concerted change in cognition and behavior that plays out as an organized emotional reaction.

Beyond its role in recognition of basic emotions, the amygdala shows differential habituation of activation to faces of people of another race (Hart et al., 2000), and amygdala activation has been found to correlate with race stereotypes of which the viewer may be unaware (Phelps et al., 2000). However, the amygdala's role in processing information about race is still unclear: other brain regions, in extrastriate visual cortex, are also activated differentially as a function of race (Golby et al., 2001), and lesions of the amygdala do not appear to impair race judgments (Phelps, Cannistraci, & Cunningham, 2003).

Other kinds of social judgments also appear to involve the amygdala. In one study, patients with bilateral amygdala damage were found to be impaired in judging how much to trust another person from viewing their face: they all judged other people to look more trustworthy and more approachable than do normal viewers (Adolphs, Tranel, & Damasio, 1998), a pattern of impairment that is also consistent with the often indiscriminately friendly behavior of such patients in real life. The amygdala's role in processing stimuli related to potential threat or danger thus extends to the complex judgments on the basis of which we come to approach or trust other people.

Lesion studies of the amygdala's role in judging trustworthiness have been complemented by functional imaging studies. When normal subjects view faces of people judged to appear untrustworthy, activation is found in superior temporal sulcus, amygdala, orbitofrontal cortex as well as insular cortex (Winston et al., 2002), perhaps outlining a sequence of processes encompassing perception, judgment, and aspects of emotional response. Interestingly, some of the amygdala activation by untrustworthy looking faces is independent of factors such as gender, eye gaze, race, or emotional expression of the face (Winston et al., 2002). Given that much of the variance in the physical dimensions along which faces vary can be eliminated, yet still drive amygdala activation, one is led to assume that the amygdala activation reflects the judgments and inferences that subjects make about the face, rather than its perceptual properties. It will be important to test this idea directly by systematically manipulating the attributions that viewers make to a fixed set of social stimuli. An important future direction will be to examine the variance in viewers' personality traits in these social judgments, as has been done in two recent studies correlating amygdala activation to emotional expressions with viewers' extraversion (Canli et al., 2002) or anxious temperament due to polymorphism in the serotonin transporter promoter (Hariri et al., 2002). To the extent that amygdala activation covaries with differences in the personality of the viewer, rather than the physical composition of the stimulus, we may conclude that we are tapping processes more distal to perception and closer to judgment, decision making, and the interpersonal behaviors based on them.

Another class of social judgment made from faces is attractiveness, which can be manipulated by specific properties of faces. For instance, faces are perceived to look more attractive the more average or symmetrical they are, or with greater exaggeration of robusticity and neoteny features, all of which have been proposed to signal differential fitness. Moreover, such preferences by women can vary across the menstrual cycle (Penton-Voak et al., 1999), as do other aspects of their categorization of men (Macrae et al., 2002), possibly providing a link between mate preference and probability of conception. Judgments of attractiveness can reflect both aesthetic judgments (e.g., males can judge faces of both males and females to look beautiful) as well as motivational aspects (e.g., males prefer to look at beautiful female rather than beautiful male faces), two aspects that have been dissociated in functional imaging studies (Aharon et al., 2001). The motivational aspects of facial attractiveness appear to activate the ventral striatum (Kampe et al., 2001; Aharon et al. 2001) as well as orbitofrontal cortex (O'Doherty et al., 2003). These structures likely play a broad role in processing the motivational properties of stimuli: for instance, they are activated also when males find pictures of sportscars more rewarding than pictures of limousines or small cars (Erk et al., 2002). Ventral striatum and orbitofrontal cortex are reciprocally connected with the amygdala; all three structures can be thought of as components of a neural system that links sensory representations of stimuli with the social judgments we make about them on the basis of their motivational value. Given that the same structures that mediate social judgments also mediate more basic reward processing, one is led to wonder whether the former might be reducible to the latter, an issue taken up in the concluding section of this review.

SIMULATION AND SOCIAL COGNITION

"Simulation theory" advances the notion that processing involved in the perception of one's own bodily states is required for the accurate judgment of others' emotional states, via a partial simulation of those states within the person doing the judging (Goldman, 1992; Goldman & Sripada, 2005). Simulation theory has gained support from the discovery of "mirror neurons" in Rhesus monkeys and putative homologous neural functions in humans (Iacoboni et al., 2005; Rizzolatti & Craighero,

2004; Gallese, Keysers, & Rizzolatti, 2004). Mirror neurons were originally reported from recordings from single neurons in monkey motor area F5, and the unifying principle in their identification was that they showed nearly identical neuronal firing both when a monkey performed an action and when the monkey observed the same or a similar action performed by a human experimenter or another monkey (Gallese et al., 1996). They constitute approximately 20% of neurons in F5 (Gallese et al., 1996). Mirror neurons are classified as "strictly congruent" and "broadly congruent" based on the similarity between performed and observed action in generating neuronal firing, and approximately 1/3 of all mirror neurons in F5 were strictly congruent, with the remainder being broadly congruent. This class of neurons is not only observed in F5, but also in area 7b in the monkey parietal cortex (probably Von Economo's area PF, see Von Economo, 1929; Seltzer & Pandya, 1980; Seltzer & Pandya, 1994), which sends projections to area F5. Approximately 30% of area 7b neurons are active during performance and observations of similar actions (Rizzolatti & Craighero, 2004).

While there is only limited evidence of mirror neurons in the human brain (Hutchison et al., 1999), there is evidence of broadly overlapping neural tissue involved in both the sensation and in the judgment of emotion. This evidence comes from studies of the effects of lesions, from neuroimaging studies, and from studies examining the interference with emotional judgment due to transcranial magnetic stimulation. In all of these studies, it is not possible to speak strictly of mirror neurons, for although the studies identify large-scale similarity of brain areas involved in emotional sensation and judgment, in all cases the degree of overlap is partial only. This observation may be important in elucidating a mechanism of emotional judgment that prevents confusion between one's own emotional states and the inferred emotional states of others, something that strict mirroring in all areas could not allow. It is useful to keep in mind that simulation theory does not require nor postulate identity, but only a degree of overlap, between the neural processing involved in sensing and judging emotion.

The clearest evidence in support of the simulation theory of emotional judgment comes from studies involving the somatosensory cortex and insula. An intensive study of the cortical areas involved in the judgment of emotions from faces involved 108 subjects with focal brain lesions (Adolphs et al., 2000). All 108 lesions were mapped onto a single normal reference brain, so that their lesions could be directly compared and lesion density overlap images could be constructed. When one examined the subjects who had the lowest performance scores on each emotion, regardless of absolute performance, a consistent pattern emerged for all emotions: lesions in right ventral parietal cortex and right frontal cortex were systematically and significantly associated with impaired recognition of emotion. The sites within which lesions systematically resulted in impaired emotion recognition focused on ventral S-I and S-II (i.e., somatosensory cortex), with involvement in insula and anterior supramarginal gyrus, as well.

The requirement of somatosensory cortex for emotional judgment from faces alone has been confirmed by transcranial magnetic stimulation (TMS) (Pourtois et al., 2004). Judgments of fearful faces took longer when single pulse TMS was applied over right somatosensory cortex. The application of the TMS pulse occurred between 100 msec and 200 msec following onset of the facial image, suggesting that the processing of facial emotion in somatosensory cortex occurs very early on, perhaps in parallel with processing in the amygdala (see above).

The most straightforward interpretation of these findings is one that invokes simulation theory: we construct central images of the body state that would be associated with the visually observed emotion; that is, we imagine how the other person would feel by simulating some of the neural network activation involved in the feeling that way. Just as the brain recruits visual cortex both during visual perception and during visual imagery (Kosslyn, Ganis, & Thompson, 2003; Klein et al., 2004; Ganis, Thompson, & Kosslyn, 2004; Slotnick, Thompson, & Kosslyn, 2005), it recruits somatosensory cortex both during perception of one's own body state as well as during imagining how someone else feels.

The extensive study of lesioned patients described above also identified the right insula as important for emotional judgment from faces. The insula is also known to be strongly involved in sensations of disgust (Fitzgerald et al., 2004) and it strongly responds to images depicting bodily mutilation and contamination (Wright et al., 2004). A focused study of one patient, B., with extensive bilateral lesions including the anterior insula showed that the insula is required for the accurate judgment of disgust from faces. B. was not only impaired in the ability to judge disgust from gustatory stimuli (e.g., high salinity solution) or visual stimuli (e.g., images of food covered with cockroaches), he was unable to judge disgust from dynamic facial stimuli and he could not infer another person's disgust from events in a descriptive narrative (Adolphs, Tranel, & Damasio, 2003). These results are consistent with neuroimaging studies that robustly and repeatedly show insula activation when viewing facial expressions of disgust (Phillips et al., 1997; Wicker, Keysers et al., 2003). In the case of Wicker et al. (2003), the same participants were imaged either during olfaction with disgusting odors or during viewing of movies of facial disgust. An approximate 40% overlap in active brain voxels in the left insula and inferior frontal gyrus was seen in comparing the two conditions (olfaction vs. viewing), again providing support for the simulation of emotional states in the judgment of the emotional states of others.

The primary conclusion from the findings reviewed here is that there is a great deal of evidence for a simulation theory of judging others' emotions, although there is also debate regarding the scope of simulation in cognition (Saxe, 2005). The findings discussed here also fall under the theme already seen for the involvement of the amygdala and orbitofrontal cortex in social behavior. That is, brain areas important for emotional processing are also crucial for social cognition and therefore for normal social behavior. Simulation theory can also be extended to areas of social cognition that incorporate but go beyond emotional judgment, such as imitation, empathy, and theory of mind. We turn next to a consideration of these important topics in the cognitive neuroscience of social behavior.

IMITATION, EMPATHY, AND THEORY OF MIND

Within cognitive neuroscience, it is now possible to see a clear relationship between areas for emotional processing and key aspects of social behavior, such as imitation, empathy and theory of mind. Imitative behavior in humans is known to occur early in development and is thought to be critical for the normal development of social referencing, empathy, and theory of mind (Meltzoff & Moore, 1977; Meltzoff & Decety, 2003). Indeed, the mental imitation, or simulation, of another's actions and/or states is sometimes taken to be necessary for a full understanding of the other (Lipps, 1907; Lipps, 1903; Barresi & Moore, 1996). Imitation has been linked with emotional processing using two lines of evidence. The first is the observation that people with social behavior dysfunction that includes difficulty in judging another's emotion also show impairments in imitative behavior. One of the most striking examples of this association occurs in autism (Meltzoff & Decety, 2003; Sigman et al., 2004; Rogers et al., 1996; Rogers et al., 2003; Roeyers, Van Oost, & Bothuyne, 1998; Williams et al., 2001; Williams, Whiten, & Singh, 2004). Indeed, deficits in imitation are among the most robust and replicable social deficits observed in autism, from very early in development to late adulthood, along with deficits in understanding the emotional states of other people. The fact that autism leads to deficits in emotional understanding and in imitative behavior led theorists to propose that there is a relationship between the neural circuitry underlying both of these aspects of social behavior.

The second line of evidence associating emotion with imitation in social behavior comes from studies of empathic processing. Chartrand and Bargh (1999) showed that people who exhibit a greater ability to take the perspective of another person show a greater propensity for nonconscious imitative behavior (i.e., the "Chameleon Effect") and also that imitative behavior led to higher positive ratings of social behavior. It is important to distinguish the nonconscious imitation typically thought to be involved in emotional understanding and empathy from overt imitation without emotional overtones, since the latter may actually reduce activity in emotional processing (Leslie, Johnson-Frey, & Grafton, 2004). Both Carr et al. (2003) and Leslie, Johnson-Frey, and Grafton (2004) observed activation in the right inferior frontal cortex, and Carr et al. (2003) observed activation in the insula, during passive viewing of static and dynamic facial expressions

of emotion, respectively. Importantly, they saw increases of activation in these areas during imitation, compared to simply passive viewing. Since we have already seen these areas involved in emotional judgment, this evidence is consistent with the notion that imitative social behavior recruits areas necessary for the processing of emotion in social behavior.

A direct assessment of emotional processing within empathy is possible by studying people during the passive viewing of another person's pain. In one such study, women were imaged using fMRI both while they watched their significant others receive painful stimulation to the right hand and while they themselves received the same painful stimulation (Singer et al., 2004). A comparison of the observation vs. stimulation conditions revealed that observation alone activated those brain areas strongly associated with the emotional response to painful stimuli as opposed to somatosensory areas associated only with the perception of the stimulus itself. This result was extended by a recent study that examined brain activation during the viewing and assessment of pictures of hands and feet in painful positions (Jackson, Meltzoff, & Decety, 2005). Here, the network of brain areas active during the viewing of painful bodily positions was very similar to that identified by viewing a significant other undergoing painful stimulation. Areas included the anterior insular cortex and posterior part of the anterior cingulate, both known to associate with the affective response to pain. A strong correlation was observed between subjective ratings of pain in the images and activation of the posterior part of the anterior cingulate ($r = 0.83$).

Constructing an affective theory of mind about another person is necessary for social adaptive behavior. The work on the cognitive neuroscience of social behavior reviewed thus far provides strong evidence that neural networks for emotional processing are strongly involved in, and in several cases are required for, normal operation of an affective theory of mind. Normal emotional processing contributes to the accurate perception of emotions and emotional states relating to particular conditions, such as being in pain. The way in which this occurs appears to be via nonconscious imitative processes long postulated by simulation theories of the theory of mind. Moreover, it is possible that these imitative/simulational processes engage motivational systems for the deployment of resources for seeking out and processing of social information, and thus normal emotional processing could be implicated in mechanisms responsible for the strong social orientation in humans.

THE ROLE OF PSYCHOPHYSIOLOGY IN COGNITION

In this last section, we return to the question raised by William James in the Introduction and to his novel answer to it. It is notable that several of the structures discussed above play dual roles in social cognition and in triggering psychophysiological concomitants of emotional response in the body. For instance, we discussed the role of the amygdala in recognition of emotion from viewing other people's facial expressions, and its role in social judgments such as trustworthiness. But there is also a large literature documenting its role (specifically, that of the central nucleus of the amygdala) in autonomic responses, including changes in skin conductance, heart rate, blood pressure, and endocrine regulation. Similarly, in the case of orbitofrontal cortex, we pointed out that this structure plays roles in decision making as well as psychophysiological responses, and that in fact the latter have been postulated to play a direct causal role in the former. These observations raise a deep and unresolved issue that brings us right back to the question of James we had mentioned at the beginning of this chapter. Are psychophysiological responses involved in cognition as such, or are they merely epiphenomenal with respect to it? There is no question that thinking, remembering, deciding are often, perhaps even typically, associated with physiological changes in our bodies – but are the latter merely a consequence of the former, or, as Darwin suggested and William James emphasized, might the latter be antecedent to some components of the former?

The issue is very difficult to resolve empirically, but that has not stopped hypotheses. Foremost among these is the somatic marker hypothesis we discussed above. In its most general form, that hypothesis argues that subjective utility (value) is ultimately to be identified with actual or represented changes in the homeostatic parameters of an organism's body. So far, there is evidence in favor as well as against this idea, but none of it is at all decisive at this stage. Our own view is that the somatic marker hypothesis, in its general form, is extremely likely to be correct, even though some of its more specific interpretations (which in some cases are actually not the interpretations of its author) are very likely to be false.

Rather than debate the details of the somatic marker hypothesis here, which has been done substantially in several recent publications, we would like to add to it in providing perhaps an even more general conception of the role of the body in cognition. That conception is a fairly straightforward extension of the somatic marker hypothesis as originally stated: parameters of body states are computational. That is, just as parameters specifying electrical and neurotransmitter-related changes within the brain can be said to process information, so can parameters specifying changes in autonomic, endocrine, and musculoskeletal states of the body. The body, as well as the brain, performs computations and information processing.

In making sense of this speculation, two observations are important. First, the body does not process information in isolation, but as an adjunct to the information processing that occurs in the brain. Seen this way, the body might provide the brain with computational resources in the same way that the external environment might – just as we use pencil and paper to calculate math problems by relying on structured processes outside ourselves, so our brains might make use of changes in bodily parameters as

a kind of "somatic scratchpad." One might imagine that the brain triggers autonomic changes in the body, but that those triggers themselves do not yet make explicit the information required, just like the visual array at the level of the retina is sufficient to trigger visual representations, but not yet sufficiently explicit to constitute them. Once those psychophysiological changes have been triggered, they play out within the body, subject to the causal role and constraints of various organs and their interaction. That is a form of computation, provided it can be read out again and made use of by the brain.

Which brings us to the second important observation. The kind of computations in which the body might engage do differ, if not qualitatively then at least quantitatively, from those in which the brain typically engaged: they are analog rather than digital. Some (perhaps more than we usually acknowledge) neural computations are also analog, so this difference may not be as dramatic as we are at first inclined to think. Nonetheless, it is clear that at least a good portion of the information processing within the brain relies on the digital nature of action potentials, whereas essentially all of the information processing within the body relies on the analog interactions of joints, muscles, and hormones.

We take it that all of this sounds reasonable enough, except for one key point on which many readers are likely to get stuck in doubt. What kind of information, pray tell, is the body processing? Certainly, one would think, not visual information, or auditory information, or representations of abstract concepts (however those might be instantiated). Well, of course it processes somatic information, but that sounds like we are claiming the body processes somatic information in the same sense that the lens of the eye processes visual information; and that is not our claim here. The claim, rather, is that the body's somatic information processing is used by the brain to compute value. That is, somatic representations can be used to point to the value that events and situations in the environment provide, an idea that finds resonance in some recent philosophical theories (e.g., Prinz, 2004). That value, in turn, comes into play in guiding social behavior, and in decision making of all kinds.

REFERENCES

Adams, R. B, Gordon, H. L, Baird, A. A, Ambady, N. and Kleck, R. E. (2003). Effects of gaze on amygdala sensitivity to anger and fear faces. *Science, 300,* 1536.

Adams, R. B, and Kleck, R. E. (2003.) Perceived gaze direction and the processing of facial displays of emotion. *Psychological Science, 14,* 644–647.

Adolphs, R. (1999). The human amygdala and emotion. *The Neuroscientist, 5,* 125–137.

Adolphs, R. (2002). Recognizing emotion from facial expressions: psychological and neurological mechanisms. *Behavioral and Cognitive Neuroscience Reviews, 1,* 21–61.

Adolphs, R. (2003). Cognitive Neuroscience of Human Social Behavior. *Nature Reviews Neuroscience, 4,* 165–178.

Adolphs, R. (2003). Investigating the cognitive neuroscience of social behavior. *Neuropsychologia, 41*, 119–126.

Adolphs, R., Bechara, A., Tranel, Damasio, H., and Damasio, A. (1995). Neuropsychological approaches to reasoning and decision-making. In Y. Christen, A. Damasio, and H. Damasio (Ed.), *Neurobiology of Decision Making*, New York: Springer.

Adolphs, R., Damasio, H., Tranel, D., Cooper, G., and Damasio, A. R. (2000). A role for somatosensory cortices in the visual recognition of emotions as revealed by three-dimensional lesion mapping. *The Journal of Neuroscience, 20*, 2683–2690.

Adolphs, R., Gosselin, F., Buchanan, T. W., Tranel, T. W., Schyns, P. G., and Damasio, A. (2005). A mechanism for impaired fear recognition after amygdala damage. *Nature, 433*, 68–72.

Adolphs, R., J., Russell, A., and Tranel, D. (1999). A role for the human amygdala in recognizing emotional arousal from unpleasant stimuli. *Psychological Science, 10*, 167–171.

Adolphs, R., and Tranel, D. (1999). Intact recognition of emotional prosody following amygdala damage. *Neuropsychologia*, 37, 1285–1292.

Adolphs, R., and Tranel, D. (2000). Emotion recognition and the human amygdala. In J. P. Aggleton (Ed.), *The Amygdala. A Functional Analysis*, New York: Oxford University Press.

Adolphs, R., Tranel, D., and Damasio, A. (2003). Dissociable neural systems for recognizing emotions. *Brain and Cognition*, in press.

Adolphs, R., Tranel, D., and Damasio, A. R. (1998). The Human Amygdala in Social Judgment. *Nature, 393*, 470–474.

Adolphs, R., Tranel, D., and Damasio, H. (2001). Emotion recognition from faces and prosody following temporal lobectomy. *Neuropsychology, 15*, 396–404.

Adolphs, R., Tranel, D., and Damasio, H. (2002). Neural systems for recognizing emotion from prosody. *Emotion, 2*, 23–51.

Adolphs, R., Tranel, D., Damasio, H., and Damasio, A. (1994). Impaired recognition of emotion in facial expressions following bilateral damage to the human amygdala. *Nature, 372*, 669–672.

Adolphs, R., Tranel, D., Damasio, H., and Damasio, A. (1995). Fear and the human amygdala. *The Journal of Neuroscience, 15*, 5879–5892.

Adolphs, R., Tranel, D., Hamann, S., Young, A., Calder, A., Anderson, A., Phelps, E., Lee, G. P., and Damasio, A. R. (1999). Recognition of facial emotion in nine subjects with bilateral amygdala damage. *Neuropsychologia, 37*, 1111–1117.

Adolphs, R., Tranel, D., and Damasio, A. R. (2003). Dissociable neural systems for recognizing emotions. *Brain Cogn, 52*(1) 61–69.

Aggleton, J. (Ed.). (2000). *The Amygdala: A functional analysis*. New York: Oxford University Press.

Aharon, I., Etcoff, N. L., Ariely, D., Chabris, C. F., O'Connor, E., and Breiter, H. C. (2001). Beautiful faces have variable reward value: fMRI and behavioral evidence. *Neuron, 32*, 537–551.

Amaral, D. G., Behniea, H., and Kelly, J. L. (2003). Topographic organization of projections from the amygdala to the visual cortex in the macaque monkey. *Neuroscience, 118*(4), 1099–120.

Amaral, D. G., and Price, J. L. (1984). Amygdalo-cortical connections in the monkey (Macaca fascicularis). *J. Comp. Neurol, 230*, 465–496.

Amaral, D. G., Price, J. L., Pitkanen, A., and Carmichael, S. T. (1992). Anatomical organization of the primate amygdaloid complex. In J. P. Aggleton (Ed.), *The Amygdala: Neurobiological Aspects of Emotion, Memory, and Mental Dysfunction*. New York: Wiley-Liss.

Anderson, A. K., and Phelps, E. A. (2000). Expression without recognition: contributions of the human amygdala to emotional communication. *Psychological Science 11*, 106–111.

Anderson, A. K., and Phelps, E. A. (2001). Lesions of the human amygdala impair enhanced perception of emotionally salient events. *Nature, 411*, 305–309.

Anderson, A. K., Spencer, D. D., Fulbright, R. K., and Phelps, E. A. (2000). Contribution of the anteromedial temporal lobes to the evaluation of facial emotion. *Neuropsychology, 14*, 526–536.

Anderson, S. W., Damasio, H., Tranel, D., and Damasio, A. R. (2000). Long-term sequelae of prefrontal cortex damage acquired in early childhood. *Dev Neuropsychol, 18*(3), 281–96.

Baron-Cohen, S. (1995). *Mindblindness: an essay on autism and theory of mind*. Cambridge, MA: MIT Press.

Baron-Cohen, S., Ring, H. A., Wheelwright, S., Bullmore, E. T., Brammer, M. J., Simmons, A., and Williams, S. C. R. (1999). Social intelligence in the normal and autistic brain: an fMRI study. *European Journal of Neuroscience 11*, 1891–1898.

Barresi, J., and Moore, C. (1996). Intentional relations and social understanding. *Behavioral and Brain Sciences, 19*, 107–154.

Bechara, A., Damasio, A. R., Damasio, H., and Anderson, S. W. (1994). Insensitivity to future consequences following damage to human prefrontal cortex. *Cognition, 50*, 7–15.

Bechara, A., Damasio, H., Tranel, D., and Anderson, S. W. (1998). Dissociation of working memory from decision making within the human prefrontal cortex. *The Journal of Neuroscience*, 18, 428–437.

Bechara, A., Tranel, D., Damasio, H., and Damasio, A. R. (1996). Failure to respond autonomically to anticipated future outcomes following damage to prefrontal cortex. *Cerebral Cortex*, 6, 215–225.

Bechara, A. (2004). The role of emotion in decision-making: evidence from neurological patients with orbitofrontal damage. *Brain Cogn, 55*(1), 30–40.

Bechara, A., Damasio, H., and Damasio, A. R. (2003). Role of the amygdala in decision-making. *Ann N Y Acad Sci, 985*, 356–69.

Benton, A. L., Hamsher, K., Varney, N. R., and Spreen, O. (1983). *Contributions to Neuropsychological Assessment*. New York: Oxford University Press.

Bernard, Claude. (1866). *Leçons sur les propriétés des tissus vivants*. Paris: G. Ballière.

Blair, R. J., Mitchell, D. G., Richell, R. A., Kelly, S., Leonard, A., Newman, C., and Scott, S. K. (2002). Turning a deaf ear to fear: impaired recognition of vocal affect in psychopathic individuals. *J Abnorm Psychol 111*(4), 682–6.

Blair, R. J. R., Morris, J. S., Frith, C. D., Perrett, D. I., and Dolan, R. J. (1999). Dissociable neural responses to facial expressions of sadness and anger. *Brain, 122*, 883–893.

Boucsein, K., Weniger, G., Mursch, K., Steinhoff, B. J., and Irle, E. (2001). Amygdala lesion in temporal lobe epilepsy subjects impairs associative learning of emotional facial expressions. *Neuropsychologia, 39*, 231–236.

Breiter, H. C., Etcoff, N. L., Whalen, P. J., Kennedy, W. A., Rauch, S. L., Buckner, R. L., Strauss, M. M., Hyman, S. E., and Rosen, B. R. (1996). Response and habituation of the human amygdala during visual processing of facial expression. *Neuron, 17*, 875–887.

Broks, P., Young, A. W., Maratos, E. J., Coffey, P. J., Calder, A. J., Isaac, C., Mayes, A. R., Hodges, J. R., Montaldi, D., Cezayirli, E., Roberts, N., and Hadley, D. (1998). Face processing impairments after encephalitis: amygdala damage and recognition of fear. *Neuropsychologia, 36*, 59–70.

Buchanan, T. W., Lutz, K., Mirzazade, S., Specht, K., Shah, N. J., Zilles, K., and Jancke, L. (2000). Recognition of emotional prosody and verbal components of spoken language: an fMRI study. *Cognitive Brain Research*, 9, 227–238.

Calder, A. J., Young, A. W., Rowland, D., Perrett, D. I., Hodges, J. R., and Etcoff, N. L. (1996). Facial emotion recognition after bilateral amygdala damage: differentially severe impairment of fear. *Cognitive Neuropsychology*, 13, 699–745.

Canli, T., Sivers, H., Whitfield, S. L., Gotlib, I. H., and Gabrieli, J. D. E. (2002). Amygdala reposes to happy faces as a function of extraversion. *Science, 296*, 2191.

Carr, L., Iacoboni, M., Dubeau, M. C., Mazziotta, J. C., and Lenzi, G. L. 2003. Neural mechanisms of empathy in humans: a relay from neural systems for imitation to limbic areas. *Proc Natl Acad Sci USA*, 100(9), 5497–502.

Catani, M., Jones, G. L., Donato, R., and Hffytche, D. (2003). Occipito-temporal connections in the human brain. *Brain, 126*, 2093–2107.

Chartrand, T. L., and Bargh, J. A. (1999). The chameleon effect: the perception-behavior link and social interaction. *Journal of Personality and Social Psychology*, 76(6) 893–910.

Damasio, A. R. (1994). *Descartes' Error: Emotion, Reason, and the Human Brain*. New York: Grosset/Putnam.

Damasio, A. R., Tranel, D., and Damasio, H. (1990). Individuals with sociopathic behavior caused by frontal damage fail to respond autonomically to social stimuli. *Behav. Brain Res, 41*, 81–94.

Damasio, H., Grabowski, T., Frank, R., Galaburda, A. M., and Damasio, A. R. (1994). The return of Phineas Gage: Clues about the brain from the skull of a famous patient. *Science, 264*, 1102–1104.

Darwin, C. (1872/1965). *The Expression of the Emotions in Man and Animals*. Chicago: University of Chicago Press.

Davidson, R. J. (2002). Anxiety and affective style: role of prefrontal cortex and amygdala. *Biological Psychiatry. 51*, 68–80.

Drevets, W. C. (2001). Neuroimaging and neuropathological studies of depression: implications for the cognitive-emotional features of mood disorders. *Current Opinion in Neurobiology, 11*, 240–249.

Ekman, P. (1972). Universals and cultural differences in facial expressions of emotion. In J. Cole (Ed.), *Nebraska Symposium on Motivatio, 1971*, Lincoln, NE: University of Nebraska Press.

Ekman, P. (Ed.). (1973). *Darwin and facial expression: A century of research in review*. New York: Academic Press.

Ekman, P., and Friesen, W. (1976). *Pictures of facial affect*. Palo Alto, CA: Consulting Psychologists Press.

Elfenbein, H. A., and Ambady, N. (2002). Is there an in-group advantage in emotion? *Psychological Bulletin, 128*, 243–249.

Elfenbein, H. A., and Ambady, N. (2002). On the universality and cultural specificity of emotion recognition: A meta-analysis. *Psychological Bulletin*, 128, 203–235.

Elfenbein, H. A., and Ambady, N. (2003). When familiarity breeds accuracy: cultural exposure and facial emotion recognition. *Journal of Personality and Social Psychology*, 85, 276–290.

Emery, N. J. (2000). The eyes have it: the neuroethology, function and evolution of social gaze. *Neuroscience and Biobehavioral Reviews*, 24, 581–604.

Erk, S., Spitzer, M., Wunderlich, A. P., Galley, L., and Walter, H. (2002). Cultural objects modulate reward circuitry. *NeuroReport*, 13, 2499–2503.

Erwin, R. J., Gur, R. C., Gur, R. E., Skolnick, B., Mawhinney-Hee, M., and Smailis, J. (1992). Facial emotion discrimination: I. Task construction and behavioral findings in normal subjects. *Psychiatry Research, 42*, 231–240.

Fitzgerald, D. A., Posse, S., Moore, G. J., Tancer, M. E., Nathan, P. J., and Phan, K. L. (2004). Neural correlates of internally-generated disgust via autobiographical recall: a functional magnetic resonance imaging investigation. *Neurosci Lett*, 370(2–3), 91–6.

Gallese, V., Fadiga, L., Fogassi, L., and Rizzolatti, G. (1996). Action recognition in the premotor cortex. *Brain, 119*, 593–609.

Gallese, V., Keysers, C., and Rizzolatti, G. (2004). A unifying view of the basis of social cognition. *Trends Cogn Sci, 8*(9), 396–403.

Ganis, G., Thompson, W. L., and Kosslyn, S. M. (2004). Brain areas underlying visual mental imagery and visual perception: an fMRI study. *Brain Res Cogn Brain Res*, 20(2), 226–41.

Golby, A. J., Gabrieli, J. D. E., Chiao, J. Y., and Eberhardt, J. L. (2001). Differential responses in the fusiform region to same-race and other-race faces. *Nature Neuroscience*, 4, 845–850.

Goldman, A. (1992). In defense of the simulation theory. *Mind and Language*, 7, 104–119.

Goldman, A. I., and Sripada, C. S. (2005). Simulationist models of face-based emotion recognition. *Cognition*, 94(3), 193–213.

Grandjean, D., Sander, D., Pourtois, G., Schwartz, S., Seghier, M. L., Scherer, K. R., and Vuilleumier, P. (2005). The voices of wrath: brain responses to angry prosody in meaningless speech. *Nat Neurosci*, 8(2), 145–6.

Greene, J. D., and Haidt, J. (2002). How (and where) does moral judgment work? *Trends in Cognitive Science, 6*, 517–523.

Greene, J. D., Sommerville, R. B, Nystrom, L. E., Darley, J. M., and Cohen, J. D. (2001). An fMRI investigation of emotional engagement in moral judgment. *Science 293*, 2105–2107.

Hariri, A. R., Mattay, V. S., Tessitore, A., Kolachana, B., Fera, F., Goldman, D., Egan, M. F., and Weinberger, D. R. (2002). Serotonin transporter genetic variation and the response of the human amygdala. *Science, 297*, 400–403.

Hart, A. J., Whalen, P. J., Shin, L. M., McInerney, S. C., Fischer, H., and Rauch, S. L. (2000). Differential response in the human amygdala to racial outgroup vs ingroup face stimuli. *NeuroReport, 11*, 2351–2355.

Haxby, J. V., Gobbini, M. I., Furey, M. L., Ishai, M. L., Schouten, J. L., and Pietrini, P. (2001). Distributed and overlapping representation of faces and objects in ventral temporal cortex. *Science, 293*, 2425–2429.

Heilman, K. M., Leon, S. A., and Rosenbek, J. C. (2004). Affective aprosodia from a medial frontal stroke. *Brain Lang*, 89(3), 411–6.

Hofer, P. A. (1973). Urbach-Wiethe disease: a review. *Acta Derm. Venerol, 53*, 5–52.

Hoffman, E.A, and Haxby, J. V. (2000). Distinct representations of eye gaze and identity in the distributed human neural system for face perception. *Nature Neuroscience*, 3, 80–84.

Holland, P. C., and Gallagher, M. (1999). Amygdala circuitry in attentional and representational processes. *TICS*, 3, 65–73.

Hutchison, W. D., Davis, K. D., Lozano, A. M., Tasker, R. R., and Dostrovsky, J. O. (1999). Pain-related neurons in the human cingulate cortex. *Nature Neuroscience, 2*, 403–405.

Iacoboni, M., Molnar-Szakacs, I., Gallese, V., Buccino, G., Mazziotta, J. C., and Rizzolatti, G.. (2005). Grasping the intentions of others with one's own mirror neuron system. *PLoS Biol*, 3(3), e79.

Izard, C. (1971). *The face of emotion*. New York: Appleton-Century-Crofts.

Jackson, P. L., Meltzoff, A. N., and Decety, J. (2005). How do we perceive the pain of others? A window into the neural processes involved in empathy. *Neuroimage*, 24(3), 771–9.

Jacobson, R. (1986). Disorders of facial recognition, social behavior and affect after combined bilateral amygdalotomy and subcaudate tractotomy – a clinical and experimental study. *Psychological Medicine*, 16, 439–450.

James, W. (1884). What is an emotion? *Mind*, 9, 188–205.

Janik, S. W., Wellens, A. R., Goldberg, M. L., and Dell'Osso, L. F. (1978). Eyes as the center of focus in the visual examination of human faces. *Perceptual and Motor Skills*, 47, 857–858.

Kampe, K. K. W., Frith, C. D., Dolan, R. J., and Frith, U. (2001). Reward value of attractiveness and gaze. *Nature*, 413, 589.

Kanwisher, N. (2000). Domain specificity in face perception. *Nature Neuroscience*, 3, 759–763.

Kapur, N. (1996). Paradoxical functional facilitation in brain-behavior research. *Brain*, 119, 1775–1790.

Kawashima, R., Sugiura, M., Kato, T., Nakamura, A., Natano, K., Ito, K., Fukuda, H., Kojima, S., and Nakamura, K. (1999). The human amygdala plays an important role in gaze monitoring. *Brain*, 122, 779–783.

Kensinger, E. A. (2004). Remembering emotional experiences: the contribution of valence and arousal. *Rev Neurosci*, 15(4), 241–51.

Killgore, W. D., Oki, M., and Yurgelun-Todd, D. A. (2001). Sex-specific developmental changes in amygdala responses to affective faces. *NeuroReport*, 12, 427–433.

Klein, I., Dubois, J., Mangin, J. F., Kherif, F., Flandin, G., Poline, J. B., Denis, M., Kosslyn, S. M., and Le Bihan, D. (2004). Retinotopic organization of visual mental images as revealed by functional magnetic resonance imaging. *Brain Res Cogn Brain Res*, 22(1) 26–31.

Kosslyn, S. M., Ganis, G., and Thompson, W. L. (2003). Mental imagery: against the nihilistic hypothesis. *Trends Cogn Sci*, 7(3), 109–111.

Krolak-Salmon, P., Henaff, M. A., Vighetto, A., Bertrand, O., and Mauguiere, F. (2004). Early amygdala reaction to fear spreading in occipital, temporal, and frontal cortex: a depth electrode ERP study in human. *Neuron*, 42(4) 665–76.

LaBar, K. S. (2003). Emotional memory functions of the human amygdala. *Curr Neurol Neurosci Rep*, 3(5), 363–4.

Leslie, K. R., Johnson-Frey, S. H., and Grafton, S. T. (2004). Functional imaging of face and hand imitation: towards a motor theory of empathy. *Neuroimage* 21(2), 601–7.

Lipps, T. (1907). *Psychologische Untersuchungen*. Leipzig: Engelman.

Lipps, T. (1903). Einfühlung, innere Nachahmung und Organempfindug. *Arch. Gesamte Psychol*, 1, 465–519.

Macrae, C. N., Alnwick, K. A., Milne, A. B., and Schloerscheidt, A. M. (2002). Person perception across the menstrual cycle: hormonal influences on social-cognitive functioning. *Psychological Science*, 13, 532–537.

Marler, P. (1984). Animal communication: affect or cognition? In K. R. Scherer and P. Ekman. (Eds.). *Approaches to emotion*, Hillsdale, NJ: Earlbaum.

McClure, E. B. (2000). A meta-analytic review of sex differences in facial expression processing and their development in infants, children, and adolescents. *Psychological Bulletin*, 126, 424–253.

McGaugh, J. L. (2004). The amygdala modulates the consolidation of memories of emotionally arousing experiences. *Annual Review of Neuroscience*, 27, 1–28.

Meltzoff, A.N., and Decety, J. (2003). What imitation tells us about social cognition: a rapprochement between developmental psychology and cognitive neuroscience. *Philosophical Transactions of the Royal Society (London), Series B*, 358, 491–500.

Meltzoff, A.N., and Moore, M. K. (1977). Imitation of facial and manual gestures by human neonates. *Science*, 198, 74–78.

Mendola, J. D., Rizzo, J. F., Cosgrove, G. R., Cole, A. J., Black, P., and Corkin, S. (1999). Visual discrimination after anterior temporal lobectomy in humans. *Neurology*, 52, 1028–1037.

Mitchell, R. L., Elliott, R., Barry, M., Cruttenden, A., and Woodruff, P. W. (2003). The neural response to emotional prosody, as revealed by functional magnetic resonance imaging. *Neuropsychologia*, 41(10), 1410–21.

Monrad-Kohn, G. H. (1947). The prosodic quality of speech and its disorders: a brief survey from a neurologist's point of view. *Acta Psychiatrica Neurological Scandinavica*, 22, 255–269.

Morris, J.S, deGelder, B., Weiskrantz, L., and Dolan, R. J. (2001). Differential extrageniculostriate and amygdala responses to presentation of emotional faces in a cortically blind field. *Brain*, 124, 1241–1252.

Morris, J. S., Frith, C. D., Perrett, D. I., Rowland, D., Young, A. W., Calder, A. J., and Dolan, R. J. (1996). A differential neural response in the human amygdala to fearful and happy facial expressions. *Nature*, 383, 812–815.

Morris, J. S., Ohman, A., and Dolan, R. J. (1999). A subcortical pathway to the right amygdala mediating "unseen" fear. *PNAS*, 96, 1680–1685.

Morris, J. S., Scott, S. K., and Dolan, R. J. (1999). Saying it with feeling: neural responses to emotional vocalizations. *Neuropsychologia*, 37, 1155–1163.

O'Doherty, J., Winston, J. S., Critchley, H. D., Perrett, D. I., Burt, D. M., and Dolan, R. J. (2003). Beauty in a smile: the role of medial orbitofrontal cortex in facial attractiveness. *Neuropsychologia*, 41, 147–155.

Öngür, D., and Price, J. L. (2000). The organization of networks within the orbital and medial prefrontal cortex of rats, monkeys, and humans. *Cerebral Cortex*, 10, 206–219.

Oya, H., Kawasaki, H., Howard, M. A., and Adolphs, R. (2002). Electrophysiological responses in the human amygdala discriminate emotion categories of complex visual stimuli. *The Journal of Neuroscience*, 22, 9502–9512.

Penton-Voak, I. S., Perrett, D. I., Castles, D. L., Kobayashi, T., Burt, T. M., Murray, L. K., and Minamisawa, R. (1999). Menstrual cycle alters face preference. *Nature*, 399, 741–742.

Pessoa, L., Kastner, S., and Ungerleider, L. G. (2002). Attentional control of the processing of neural and emotional stimuli. *Brain Res Cogn Brain Res*, 15(1) 31–45.

Pessoa, L., and Ungerleider, L. G. (2004). Neuroimaging studies of attention and the processing of emotion-laden stimuli. *Prog Brain Res*, 144, 171–82.

Phelps, E. A., Cannistraci, C. J., and Cunningham, W. A. (2003). Intact performance on an indirect measure of race bias following amygdala damage. *Neuropsychologia*, 41, 203–209.

Phelps, E. A., O'Connor, K. J., Cunningham, W. A., Funayama, E. S., Gatenby, J. C., Gore, J. C., and Banaji, M. (2000). Performance on indirect measures of race evaluation predicts amygdala activation. *Journal of Cognitive Neuroscience*, 12, 729–738.

Phillips, M. L., Young, A. W., Scott, S. K., Calder, A. J., Andrew, C., Giampietro, V., Williams, S. C. R., Bullmore, E. T., Brammer, M., and Gray, J. A. (1998). Neural responses to facial and vocal expressions of fear and disgust. *Proc. R. Soc. London Series B*, 265, 1809–1817.

Phillips, M. L., Young, A. W., Senior, C., Brammer, M., Andrew, A., Calder, A. J., Bullmore, E. T., Perrett, D. I., Rowland, D., Williams, S. C. R., Gray, J. A., and David, A. S. (1997). A specific neural substrate for perceiving facial expressions of disgust. *Nature*, *389*, 495–498.

Pourtois, G., Sander, D., Andres, M., Grandjean, D., Reveret, L., Olivier, E., and Vuilleumier, P. (2004). Dissociable roles of the human somatosensory and superior temporal cortices for processing social face signals. *Eur J Neurosci* 20(12), 3507–15.

Prinz, J. (2004). *Gut Reactions*. New York: Oxford University Press.

Puce, A., Allison, T., and McCarthy, G. (1999). Electrophysiological studies of human face perception. III: Effects of top-down processing on face-specific potentials. *Cerebral Cortex, 9*, 445–458.

Rauch, S. L., Whalen, P. J., Shin, L. M., McInerney, S. C., Macklin, M. L., Lasko, N. B., Orr, S. P., and Pitman, R. K. (2000). Exaggerated amygdala response to masked facial stimuli in posttraumatic stress disorder: a functional MRI study. *Biological Psychiatry, 47*, 769–776.

Richter-Levin, G. (2004). The amygdala, the hippocampus, and emotional modulation of memory. *Neuroscientist*, 10(1), 31–39.

Rilling, J. K., Gutman, D. A., Zeh, T. R., Pagnoni, G., Berns, G. S., and Kilts, C. D. (2002). A neural basis for social cooperation. *Neuron, 35*, 395–405.

Rizzolatti, G., and Craighero, L. (2004). The mirror-neuron system. *Annu Rev Neurosci, 27*, 169–192.

Roeyers, H., Van Oost, P., and Bothuyne, S. (1998). Immediate imitation and joint attention in young children with autism. *Dev Psychopathol*, 10(3), 441–450.

Rogers, S. J., Bennetto, L., McEvoy, R., and Pennington, B. F. (1996). Imitation and pantomime in high-functioning adolescents with autism spectrum disorders. *Child Dev*, 67(5), 2060–73.

Rogers, S. J., Hepburn, S. L., Stackhouse, T., and Wehner, E. (2003). Imitation performance in toddlers with autism and those with other developmental disorders. *J Child Psychol Psychiatry*, 44(5), 763–81.

Russell, J. A., Bachorowski, J. A., and Fernandez-Dols, J. M. (2003). Facial and vocal expressions of emotion. *Annual Review of Psychology, 54*, 329–49.

Russell, J. A., and Fernandez-Dols, J. M., (Eds.). (1997). *The Psychology of Facial Expression*. Cambridge, MA: Cambridge University Press.

Saxe, R. (2005). Against simulation: the argument from error. *TICS*.

Scherer, K. R. (1995). Expression of emotion in voice and music. *Journal of Voice, 9*, 235–248.

Scherer, K. R., Banse, R., Wallbot, H. G., and Goldbeck, T. (1991). Vocal cues in emotion encoding and decoding. *Motivation and Emotion, 15*, 123–148.

Scherer, K. R. (1988). On the symbolic functions of vocal affect expression. *Journal of Language and Social Psychology, 7*, 79–100.

Schmolck, H., and Squire, L. R. (2001). Impaired perception of facial emotions following bilateral damage to the anterior temporal lobe. *Neuropsychology, 15*, 30–38.

Scott, S. K., Young, A. W., Calder, A. J., Hellawell, D. J., Aggleton, J. P., and Johnson, M. (1997). Impaired auditory recognition of fear and anger following bilateral amygdala lesions. *Nature, 385*, 254–257.

Seltzer, B., and Pandya, D. N. (1994). Parietal, temporal, and occipital projections to cortex of the superior temporal sulcus in the rhesus monkey: a retrograde tracer study. *Journal of Comparative Neurology, 343*, 445–463.

Seltzer, B., and Pandya, D. N. (1980). Converging visual and somatic sensory cortical input to the intraparietal sulcus of the rhesus monkey. *Brain Res*, 192(2), 339–51.

Sheline, Y. I., Barch, D. M., Donnelly, J. M., Ollinger, J. M., Snyder, A. Z., and Mintun, M. A. (2001). Increased amygdala response to masked emotional faces in depressed subjects resolves with antidepressant treatment: an fMRI study. *Biological Psychiatry, 50*, 651–658.

Siebert, M., Markowitsch, H. J., and Bartel, P. (2003). Amygdala, affect and cognition: evidence from 10 patients with Urbach-Wiethe disease. *Brain, 126*, 2627–2637.

Sigman, M., Dijamco, A., Gratier, M., and Rozga, A. (2004). Early detection of core deficits in autism. *Ment Retard Dev Disabil Res Rev*, 10(4), 221–33.

Simon, H. A. (1979). Information processing models of cognition. *Annual Review of Psychology, 30*, 365–396.

Singer, T., Seymour, B., O'Doherty, J., Kaube, H., Dolan, R. J., and Frith, C. D. (2004). Empathy for pain involves the affective but not sensory components of pain. *Science, 303*, 1157–1162.

Slotnick, S. D., Thompson, W. L., and Kosslyn, S. M. (2005). Visual Mental Imagery Induces Retinotopically Organized Activation of Early Visual Areas. *Cereb Cortex*.

Sporer, S. L. (2001). Recognizing faces of other ethnic groups: an integration of theories. *Psychology, Public Policy, and Law, 7*, 36–97.

Sprengelmeyer, R., Young, A. W., Schroeder, U., Grossenbacher, P. G., Federlein, J., Buttner, T., and Przuntek, H. (1999). Knowing no fear. *Proc. R. Soc. London Series B, 266*, 2451–6.

Stefanacci, L., and Amaral, D. G. (2000). Topographic organization of cortical inputs to the lateral nucleus of the macaque monkey amygdala: a retrograde tracing study. *J Comp Neuro,l* 421(1), 52–79.

Stone, V. E., Cosmides, L., Tooby, J., Kroll, N., and Knight, R. T. (2002). Selective impairment of reasoning about social exchange in a patient with bilateral libic system damage. *PNAS, 99*, 11531–11536.

Stuss, D. T., Gallup, G. G., and Alexander, M. P. (2001). The frontal lobes are necessary for 'theory of mind'. *Brain, 124*, 279–286.

Sugase, Y., Yamane, S., Ueno, S., and Kawano, K. (1999). Global and fine information coded by single neurons in the temporal visual cortex. *Nature, 400*, 869–872.

Tarr, M. J., and Gauthier, I. (2000). FFA: a flexible fusiform area for subordinate-level visual processing automatized by expertise. *Nature Neuroscience, 3*, 764–769.

Tomkins, S. S. (1962). *Affect, imagery, consciousness*. Vol. 1, 2. New York: Springer Verlag.

Tranel, D., and Hyman, B. T. (1990). Neuropsychological correlates of bilateral amygdala damage. *Archives of Neurology, 47*, 349–355.

Tranel, D., Bechara, A., and Denburg, N. L. (2002). Asymmetric functional roles of right and left ventromedial prefrontal cortices in social conduct, decision-making, and emotional processing. *Cortex*, 38(4), 589–612.

van Bezooijen, R. (1984). *The Characteristics and Recognizability of Vocal Expression of Emotions*. Dordrecht: Foris.

van Bezooijen, R., Otto, S. A., and Heenan, T. A. (1983). Recognition of vocal expressions of emotion. *Journal of Cross-Cultural Psychology*, 14, 387–406.

Von Economo, C. (1929). *The Cytoarchitectonics of the Human Cerebral Cortex*. London: Oxford University Press.

Vuilleumier, P., Armony, J. L., Driver, J., and Dolan, R. J. (2001). Effects of attention and emotion on face processing in the human brain. An event-related fMRI study. *Neuron, 30*, 829.

Vuilleumier, P., Richardson, M. P., Armony, J. L., Driver, J., and Dolan, R. J. (2004). Distant influences of amygdala lesion on visual cortical activation during emotional face processing. *Nature Neuroscience, 7*, 1271–1278.

Vuilleumier, P., and Schwartz, S. (2001). Emotional facial expressions capture attention. *Neurology, 56*, 153–158.

Whalen, P. J. (1999). Fear, vigilance, and ambiguity: initial neuroimaging studies of the human amygdala. *Current Directions in Psychological Science, 7*, 177–187.

Whalen, P. J., Shin, L. M., McInerney, S. C., Fischer, H., Wright, C. I., and Rauch, S. L. (2001). A functional MRI study of human amygdala responses to facial expressions of fear versus anger. *Emotion, 1*, 70–83.

Wicker, B., Perrett, D. I., Baron-Cohen, S., and Decety, J. (2003). Being the target of another's emotion: a PET study. *Neuropsychologia, 41*, 139–146.

Wicker, B., Keysers, C., Plailly, J., Royet, J. P., Gallese, V., and Rizzolatti, G. (2003). Both of us disgusted in my insula: the common neural basis of seeing and feeling disgust. *Neuron*, 40(3), 655–664.

Wildgruber, D., Riecker, A., Hertrich, I., Erb, M., Grodd, W., Ethofer, T., and Ackermann, H. (2005). Identification of emotional intonation evaluated by fMRI. *Neuroimage*, 24(4), 1233–1241.

Williams, J. H., Whiten, A., and Singh, T. (2004). A systematic review of action imitation in autistic spectrum disorder. *J Autism Dev Disord*, 34(3), 285–299.

Williams, J. H., Whiten, A., Suddendorf, T., and Perrett, D. I. (2001). Imitation, mirror neurons and autism. *Neurosci Biobehav Rev*, 25(4), 287–295.

Winston, J. S., Strange, B. A., O'Doherty, J., and Dolan, R. J. (2002). Automatic and intentional brain responses during evaluation of trustworthiness of faces. *Nature Neuroscience, 5*, 277–283.

Wright, P., He, G., Shapira, N. A., Goodman, W. K., and Liu, Y. (2004). Disgust and the insula: fMRI responses to pictures of mutilation and contamination. *Neuroreport* 15(15), 2347–2351.

Yildirim, S., Bulut, M., Lee, C. M., Kazemzaeh, A., Lee, S., Neumann, U., and Narayanan, S. (2004). *An acoustic study of emotions expressed in speech. Paper read at 8th International Conference on Spoken Language Processing, at Jeju Island*, Korea.

Young, A. W., Aggleton, J. P., Hellawell, D. J., Johnson, M., Broks, P., and Hanley, J. R. (1995). Face processing impairments after amygdalotomy. *Brain, 118*, 15–24.

24 Language

MARTA KUTAS, KARA D. FEDERMEIER, JENNY STAAB, AND ROBERT KLUENDER

The Brain – is wider than the sky –
For – put them side by side –
The one the other will contain –
With ease and you beside

The Brain is deeper than the sea –
For – hold them – Blue to Blue –
The one the other will absorb –
As Sponges – Buckets – do

The Brain is just the weight of God –
For – Heft them – Pound for Pound –
And they will differ – if they do –
As Syllable from Sound
        – Emily Dickinson, 1896

1. HISTORICAL CONTEXT

As Dickinson notes, the brain has a remarkable capacity that differentiates it from other sorts of material substances: the ability to intentionally represent, to impose its own internal order on perceptions of the outside world supplied to it via the senses. Although we often take this capacity for granted, it is no small feat that we are able to access, decipher, and interpret the thoughts of a woman who died well over a century ago. While many consider Dickinson to be an exceptionally gifted poet, her ability to exploit the representational capacity afforded by the brain through language is shared by all humans. This capacity allows us to analyze our own internal thought processes, to communicate with one another across distances of time and space, and to alter our environment by influencing one another's behavior.

It is this ability that intrigues language researchers and inspires them to plumb the depths of the language system in hopes of unmasking its intrinsic principles and underlying mechanisms. With the onset roughly half a century ago of the cognitive revolution, language quickly came into focus as one of the main puzzles of human cognition. The most fundamental reason for this puzzlement is that, at least *prima facie*, language is a behavioral phenomenon not found in any species other than our own. Moreover, language mediates virtually every aspect of human social and cultural interaction. Human beings are the only species in which language plays a role not just in the formation of mental representations, but in the interrelationships of such representations with each other and with the external environment as well. By understanding language, we thus not only gain a privileged window into the internal workings of the human mind, but also a way to comprehend how it relates to the outside world.

At this point in history, we already know something of the intrinsic principles and mechanisms of language. For example, we know that language is a multi-layered system, with principles that apply at different levels of organization, namely those of sound (phonetics and phonology), the word (morphology), the phrase and the sentence (syntax), the entire text, be it written or spoken (discourse and information structure), and meaning (semantics and pragmatics) – cf. section 3. We further know that because language is a serialized signal that unfolds sequentially in time and space, it must rely on the support of other cognitive systems, including attention and memory, both working and long-term.

Long-term memory provides a useful illustration of the difference between principles and mechanisms of language and between the often complementary interests of linguists and psycholinguists. Long-term memory plays an important role in the pairing of sound patterns with associated meanings at the level of individual lexical items, which must be accessed and retrieved during on-line processing. This process of "lexical access" is a major focus of investigation with respect to both psychological and neural mechanisms (see section 4). However, it is largely absent from purely linguistic discussions because, among the linguist's inventory of ontological primitives, the word is the most poorly defined. Even though linguists know a great deal about the principles governing word formation (morphology), they merely assume that words are taken from the lexicon when inserted into syntactic structures, as the mechanism(s) of lexical insertion remains largely unspecified.

More generally, the ontological status of linguistic principles, levels of organization, and mechanisms lies at the heart of three related but logically independent debates within linguistics and psycholinguistics, commonly referred to as competence versus performance, modularity, and psychological reality. With regard to the first, Chomsky (1965) has taken great pains to distinguish a language user's inherent knowledge of his or her native language (competence) from its implementation in real time and space (performance). The former is an abstract, idealized, almost Platonic set of mental representations distributed across a speech or sign community, whereas the latter is an imperfect individual reflection of this, subject to human cognitive limitations on attention and memory, etc. The prevailing view within linguistics for the past half century has been that competence rather than performance is the proper subject of the language researcher's investigation. This is because competence remains relatively stable over time – though subject to changes across generations as innovations make their way into the system – whereas performance is subject to the moment-to-moment vagaries of on-line processing. This is another reason why linguists have traditionally paid little attention to the mechanics of processes like lexical access: everyone is familiar with the effects of impaired memory on lexical access in the individual brain, but this has no impact whatsoever on the collective repository of lexical items in any given language.

However, while many linguists still adhere to a strict dichotomy between competence and performance, others have begun to challenge it: in recent years, performance-based accounts of a number of core linguistic facts usually attributed to competence – such as basic word order (Hawkins, 1994), and dependencies between discontinuous sentence elements, so-called "unbounded dependencies" (Hawkins, 1999; Kluender, 1998, 2005) – have emerged. During this same time period, a number of event-related brain potential (ERP), positron emission tomography (PET), and functional magnetic resonance imaging (fMRI) studies have investigated the precise role of working memory in the processing of unbounded dependencies (see section 4.3.2.1). The aim of these studies has been to determine whether syntactic mechanisms play a role over and above that of working memory in the processing of such structures, or whether the two are largely co-extensive.

The second debate centers around Fodor's (1983) claim that cognition is the result of a large number of autonomously functioning, highly specialized input modules feeding into a more general-purpose central processor. The role of input modules is to transform specific inputs from the sensory periphery into representations that can be handled by this central processor. Since an input system is dedicated to processing only one type of input, it is said to be "informationally encapsulated," i.e., insensitive to any source of information that falls outside its particular domain of specialization. It is also argued that the central processor has access only to the outputs of such modules and not to any intermediate representations that they may compute for their own internal purposes. Perhaps most importantly for present purposes, each input module is said to be associated with a fixed neural architecture.

This series of claims has had two major consequences for the study of language. First, language itself is taken to be a sort of macro-module, independent of other cognitive systems like attention and memory; this is essentially a reification of the competence/performance distinction. Second, levels of organization within the language system are often taken to be sub-modules that are informationally encapsulated from each other. This claim has been made most frequently with respect to lexical and syntactic levels of processing, which are argued to be impervious, during lexical access and initial syntactic parsing operations, to semantic and pragmatic factors, in turn argued to engage higher-level processes of interpretation solely under the purview of the central processor. On this view, contextual meaning should not initially influence how a word is identified by the lexical access module or how a string is parsed by the syntactic module. Lexical access and syntactic parsing operations are thus expected to be subserved by brain regions different from those that figure in semantic or pragmatic interpretation.

Psychophysiologically, this expectation has been investigated most thoroughly with respect to comparisons and interactions of syntactic and semantic processing (see section 4.3.2.2.2), although it is not always obvious how to isolate syntactic processing from the influence of other levels of organization. For example, a common experimental manipulation compares active and passive versions of the same sentence, the general assumption being that the two versions differ in syntactic structure alone. However, passivization affects not only the alignment of semantic (or "thematic"; cf. section 3) roles with syntactic positions (either agent or undergoer (patient) as subject of the sentence in active vs. passive sentences, respectively), but also the underlying information structure of the sentence. To illustrate, the "team of authors" is not only the subject, but also the topic of the active sentence *A team of authors wrote the chapter*, while "the chapter" forms part of the informational focus, or new information about the topic. These information structural statuses are reversed in the passive sentence *The chapter was written by a team of authors*, in which "the chapter" is the topic and the "team of authors" is part of the new informational focus. Linguists are not sure whether to assimilate information structure to syntactic or semantic levels of representation or to consider it a completely independent level of representation on its own, although it is recognized to play a role in sentence structure over and above purely syntactic considerations.

Information structure is not the only level of linguistic organization for which it is difficult to entertain claims of modularity. As mentioned above, processes of word formation are quite well understood by linguists, but the notion that morphology should constitute an independent, autonomous, informationally encapsulated level of organization (and/or processing) within the language system is almost certainly wrong. Morphological processes of word formation are known to interact extensively both with "lower" level phonological processes, as well as with "higher" level syntactic processes; for this reason, linguists refer to – and distinguish between – "morphophonological" and "morphosyntactic" processes. Phonological processes similarly play a role in both morphology and syntax; aside from the subdiscipline of morphophonology just mentioned, a very popular topic in psycholinguistics at the time of writing is the role that prosody plays in word segmentation and in syntactic parsing. It is even difficult to see how morphology could be entirely dissociated from semantics, as affixes typically involve a concomitant change in word meaning: *lion* vs. *lioness*, *child* vs. *children*, *rational* vs. *irrational*, *write* vs. *rewrite*.

Nevertheless, there is a long-standing controversy within morphology itself that does bear on issues of modularity: the difference between regular (rule-based) and irregular (more or less idiosyncratic) processes of word formation. Note that here the claim for modularity is based on a sub-sub-module of the language system. The controversy centers around whether regular and irregular processes of word formation constitute separate subsystems, each with unique principles and mechanisms (the "dual route" model), or whether these two processes share the same resources (the "single route" model). There is an extensive behavioral and computational literature devoted to this topic, and there have been a number of psychophysiological studies as well (section 4.2.1).

The third debate in linguistics is referred to as psychological reality: is there any evidence to be found for the levels of organization posited by linguists, and the principles claimed to apply to them, in the on-line processing of language, or are they merely explanatorily convenient, abstract constructs? First raised by Sapir (1933), nowadays this issue is generally cast more in terms of finding behavioral evidence for linguistic constructs, and thus has been rejected by some as irrelevant to issues of competence (Chomsky, 1980). Nonetheless, the current prevalent trend in linguistic departments in the United States is to add positions in psycho- and neurolinguistics, pointing to at least tacit recognition of the fact that linguistic theory construction in the 21st century requires a broader empirical base that also addresses questions of psychological reality.

To this end, research on the psychophysiology of language processing – using techniques such as ERPs, PET, and fMRI – has attempted to monitor how the brain reacts to experimental manipulations at various levels of linguistic organization. As noted above, the assumption is that language subprocesses are subserved by different anatomical and physiological substrates that generate distinct patterns of biological activity – and this assumption is neutral with respect to issues of competence vs. performance, modularity, and psychological reality. These patterns of biological activity can then be picked up by methods sensitive to fluctuations in electromagnetic and hemodynamic activity.

Psychophysiological studies of language processing are well-suited to examine issues of both representation and processing. Techniques with high spatial resolution, such as PET and fMRI, can help pinpoint brain areas important for language processing. Techniques with high temporal resolution, such as ERPs and eye-tracking, can help reveal how language processing unfolds over time; they can be used to track the availability of different sorts of linguistic information and the temporal course of their interactions. Additionally, studies of brain-damaged patients, in conjunction with the use of psychophysiological measures, can provide important insights about which brain areas are necessary and/or sufficient for certain types of linguistic processes, and about the relationship between language processing and other cognitive abilities. In this chapter, then, we consider the role of the brain in understanding and producing natural language utterances. We review how psychophysiologists have addressed this issue in the past and consider how these methods might best be employed in the future.

2. PHYSICAL CONTEXT

The physical context for language is the human brain – the only known physical system capable of language. And, although some parts of the brain have been more closely tied to language than others, nearly the whole brain seems to be involved to some extent. Language comprehension, for example, depends on subcortical and cortical neural systems that transduce, process, and identify the sensory information that constitutes language input. Language production, in turn, ultimately makes use of the motor cortical, basal ganglia, and cerebellar systems that enervate the muscles and coordinate the movements of the diaphragm, intercostal muscles, vocal folds, jaw, tongue, and lips (and/or arms, hands, and face). Both comprehension and production require that information be attended, held in working memory, and accessed from long-term memory, thereby involving hippocampal, medial temporal, frontal and parietal areas. These brain areas show varying degrees of specialization for various linguistic processes, and many appear to perform general functions – like sequencing or mapping between inputs/outputs and knowledge – that are necessary for language without being unique to it.

Of course, some parts of the brain are considered by most neuroscientists to be particularly concerned with the processing of language. One of these is an area of left frontal cortex (Brodmann's area, or BA 44 and 45) known as Broca's area, damage to which (often including underlying subcortical tissue and white matter) causes an aphasia characterized by halting, "telegraphic" speech (lacking in function words) but with reasonably good comprehension. Despite its obvious import in language production and the control of articulation, there has been some controversy over whether the apraxia of speech is due to malfunction of Broca's area (Hillis et al., 2004) or the underlying insula (Dronkers, 1996; Ackermann & Riecker, 2004). Whatever its precise role, there is ample evidence not only for its involvement in language processing but for functional subdivisions of this area (see Bookheimer, 2002).

For example, imaging studies have found activation in posterior aspects of the left frontal operculum (especially BA 44) associated with phonological encoding in production (see meta-analysis by Indefrey & Levelt, 2004) as well as with phoneme discrimination (Zatorre et al., 1996) and sequencing (Demonet et al., 1994) during comprehension. Some have suggested that the primary role of this area is to subserve articulatory-based working memory processes (Hickok & Poeppel, 2004). Similar arguments have been made for the role of the more medial portion of Broca's area in syntax. Lesions to Broca's area cause problems with the production (Friedman & Grodzinsky, 1997) and interpretation (Grodzinsky, 2000) of syntactically complex sentences, and this area has shown activation in many imaging studies comparing relatively simple to more complex syntactic structures (see 4.3.2.1). While some have taken this to mean that syntactic processing is mediated by Broca's area (e.g., Grodzinsky, 2000), others have suggested that it subserves general or syntax-specific aspects of working memory (Caplan & Waters, 1999; Caplan & Waters, 1999; Fiebach, Schlesewsky, & Friederici, 2001; Kaan and Swaab, 2002; Friederici, 2002).

Finally, anterior portions of Broca's area (BA 47, and the inferior part of BA 45) have been linked to semantic processing (reviewed in Bookheimer, 2002; Gabrieli, Poldrack, & Desmond, 1998). Thompson-Schill and colleagues have argued that this area is not specific to semantics but rather is involved in selection more generally, showing increased activation when competing, irrelevant information engenders high selection demands (1999; Kan & Thompson-Schill, 2004) and deficits in selection when damaged (Thompson-Schill et al., 1998). Others, however, have suggested that it is a more superior and posterior area that mediates selection (Martin & Chao, 2001; Wagner et al., 2001), linking the anterior portion of Broca's area with controlled semantic retrieval.

The functionally specific sub-areas that seem to make up the original "Broca's area" have thus been linked to language at the sound, structure, and meaning levels, especially for production but, to some extent, also for comprehension. What remains more controversial is whether the computations this brain area performs are language-specific or more general. Both lesion and imaging work suggest that Broca's area is especially critical for language functions, yet activity in this area has also been observed during non-linguistic tasks such as tone discrimination (Müller & Basho, 2004), motor imagery (Binkofski et al., 2000; Hanakawa et al., 2003), and imitation (Iacoboni et al., 1999; Leslie, Johnson-Frey, & Grafton, 2004), consistent with its being part of more general brain systems concerned with segmentation, planning, working memory, and/or selection processes, among others.

Another brain area closely linked to language is Wernicke's area (BA 22) in the left temporal/parietal cortex. Damage to this area produces a "fluent" aphasia and impaired comprehension; patients' speech has normal rate and rhythm together with many paraphasias (incorrect word substitutions) that render it nearly incomprehensible. Wernicke's area has traditionally been associated with language comprehension and semantics, though it too has been subdivided into functionally specific subareas.

The traditional "Wernicke's area," the posterior superior temporal gyrus (STG), has become closely linked to phonological decoding. Lesions to this area cause word deafness (especially, or even perhaps only, when bilateral: Poeppel, 2001; Buchman et al., 1986), and bilateral STG activation is consistently observed in speech comprehension tasks (Hickok & Poeppel, 2000, 2004). This area is also sensitive to the acoustic properties of speech (Binder et al., 2000; Scott et al., 2000), although left and right STG may mediate somewhat different aspects of acoustic processing (Ivry & Robertson, 1998). The left posterior STG seems to play a more crucial role for language *production*, as damage to this area causes a conduction aphasia marked by phonemic production difficulties at all levels (Anderson et al., 1999; Boatman, 2004). The anterior portion of the STG is also important for the analysis of speech (Scott & Wise, 2004), but it seems to play an additional role in the processing of language structure. Lesions to this portion of the STG are associated with syntactic processing deficits (Friederici, 2002; Dronkers et al., 2004), and imaging studies find increased activation in this area for sentences versus word lists (Stowe et al., 1999), for ungrammatical versus grammatical sentences (Meyer et al., 2002), as well as activation changes linked to syntactic priming (Noppeney & Price, 2004).

More inferior parts of the temporal lobe have come to be associated with processing at the interface between sound and meaning. Damage to the posterior portion of the middle temporal gyrus (MTG) has been associated with severe word comprehension and naming deficits (Dronkers et al., 2004). Activations in this area have been observed during word comprehension (Binder et al., 1997) and the processing of environmental sounds (Lewis et al., 2004), as well as in a meta-analysis of production imaging studies, where it has been linked to "conceptually driven lexical retrieval" (Levelt & Indefrey, 2004). Still more inferior areas, in the inferior temporal gyrus (ITG) and fusiform gyrus, seem to play a role in reading, naming, and concept retrieval. Stimulation of this "basal temporal language area" (in epileptic patients undergoing surgery) results in language deficits ranging from anomia to global expressive and receptive aphasias (Lüders et al., 1991). The fact that only transient aphasia results from damage to the basal temporal language area suggests that its functions are or can be duplicated by other brain areas (or, perhaps, that stimulation of this area disrupts language primarily through its connections with other language areas). Nevertheless, imaging studies suggest that activity in this area accompanies normal semantic-linguistic processing (Thompson-Schill et al., 1999; Chao, Haxby, & Martin, 1999). The "visual word form area" in the posterior fusiform is consistently activated in reading tasks (review in Cohen et al., 2002) and is sensitive to abstract orthographic properties (Polk & Farah, 2002). It has been hypothesized to be involved in the prelexical processing of letter strings, though it also becomes active in a variety of other (even non-visual) tasks (Price & Devlin, 2003).

The aforementioned brain areas classically associated with aphasia, and thus with language – Broca's area and Wernicke's area – are in the left cerebral hemisphere, leading to the now widely accepted view that the left hemisphere is the "verbal" hemisphere and the right is the "nonverbal hemisphere." However, it now seems that left-lateralization may be strong only for language production, with the right hemisphere playing a more important role in the integrative and pragmatic aspects of comprehension (for reviews see Joanette, Goulet, & Hannequin, 1990; Beeman & Chiarello, 1998). Right hemisphere damage has been associated with difficulties producing and comprehending both affective and linguistic prosody (Wymer, Lindman, & Booksh, 2002; Baum & Dwivedi, 2003) as well as with impairment in processing a variety of types of non-literal language, including indirect requests, sarcasm and speech acts (Kaplan et al., 1990; Champagne et al., 2003), connotations, jokes and humor. Right hemisphere damage has also been associated with more general problems drawing inferences and processing language at a discourse level. Correspondingly, imaging studies often observe bilateral – or even in some cases right-lateralized – activity in a variety of language tasks. For example, activity in right hemisphere homologues of left hemisphere language areas (inferior frontal gyrus, posterior superior temporal sulcus) has been seen in tasks requiring judgments of metaphorical meaning (Bottini et al., 1994), use of higher-level linguistic context (Kircher et al., 2001; St. George et al., 1999; Robertson et al., 2000), use of metalinguistic knowledge (Meyer, Friederici, & von Cramon, 2000), and monitoring of emotional prosody (Buchanan et al., 2000).

Overall, recent neuropsychological and imaging data suggest that a complex network of brain areas, including frontal, temporal, and parietal cortical areas in both hemispheres, along with associated subcortical structures, subserve normal language processing. A small set of these areas subserves functions that are so particular and so critical for language that damaging them causes severe and sometimes permanent language deficits. However, a larger set of areas also seems to make important contributions to language, albeit contributions whose loss can more readily be compensated for. As a result, the precise network involved in any given situation will depend heavily on the choice of experimental and control tasks and the methods used to process and analyze the data. When drawing conclusions from neuroimaging data, as from all types of psychophysiological data, it is thus important to recognize the inferential leaps required by and the inferential limitations inherent in mappings from physiology to psychology (see Chapter 1 and Sarter et al., 1996).

3. SOCIAL/COGNITIVE CONTEXT

For at least 100,000 years our species has used language to describe – and construct – the world around us. First, and perhaps most obviously, language provides a medium for the communication of thoughts via a structured stream of sound, or, in signed language, manual and facial gesture. Upon hearing or seeing language, comprehenders are somehow able to formulate a mental representation of the conceptual content of the spoken, written, or signed message, which can alter the comprehenders' mental state and affect subsequent behavior. Language thus provides the primary means of social interaction, enables the coordination of group action, and plays an organizing role in social relationships. Second, language enables us to transmit cultural knowledge such as customs and values.

The cognitive basis of this complex human skill involves representations and processes at a number of different levels, the regularities of which are investigated by subdisciplines within linguistics. Moving from sound to meaning, these disciplines include phonology, the study of linguistic sound patterns; morphology, the study of word formation; syntax, the study of hierarchical structure in individual utterances; information structure, the study of structure in spoken and written discourse; semantics, the study of context-invariant aspects of meaning; and pragmatics, the study of meaning in use. Although it is still unclear how traditional linguistic categories map onto brain structures and functions, it is important to consider the work of linguists as a relevant starting point for exploration of these issues.

Although our intuition may suggest that the fundamental unit of language is the word, linguistic research has shown that words are composed of more fundamental units known as phonemes and morphemes. Phonemes are categories of sounds considered equivalent to each other in a language and that distinguish one word from another: in *The cat sat on the mat*, the phonemes /k/, /s/, and /m/ recombine with the phonemes /æ/ and /t/ to form three different English words. Morphemes are the smallest units of meaning in a language: *cat* consists of three phonemes but only one morpheme, while *anti-dis-establish-ment-ari-an-ism* consists of seven morphemes, each contributing to the meaning of the word as a whole. This idea of building up meanings by combining representations at different levels is a recurrent one in linguistics because it helps explain the fact that we can express an infinite number of different meanings with a limited repertoire of speech sounds. Thus, phonemes are combined into morphemes, morphemes into lexemes (words), words into phrases, phrases into sentences, and sentences into discourses.

Just as words are built up out of individual sounds, sentences are built up from individual words. The relationship between words and sentences is complex and involves structure at a number of different levels. "Parsing" is the process of analyzing the input into a series of lexical units and mapping higher order structures onto those units in a consistent and eventually meaningful way.

Words are divided into "grammatical categories" (traditional parts of speech: noun, verb, etc.), and syntax is the study of the relations among them – grammatical, phrase structural, subcategorization, and thematic. "Grammatical relations" include the traditional parts of a sentence: subject, object, etc. Words combine to form phrases in hierarchical configurations ("phrase/tree structures") that encode grammatical relations. For example, the direct object of a verb is the noun phrase (NP) sister node of a verb (V); together, they form a verb phrase (VP). VP–>V NP is a "phrase structure rule." The entry of a word in the lexicon also specifies syntactic information. For example, not all verbs take direct objects: those that do are called transitive verbs, those that don't are intransitive. This distinction is captured in a verb's "subcategorization frame." Within the grammatical category of verbs, subcategories of verbs take different syntactic complementation options: the lexical entry of a transitive verb specifies that it takes an NP complement, while that of an intransitive verb specifies that it takes no complement at all. "Thematic relations" are also lexically specified, and they determine the types of semantic roles that a verb co-occurs with. Thus a transitive verb like *make* takes both an agent and a patient/undergoer, while an intransitive verb takes either an agent (as in *run*) or a patient/undergoer (as in *die*), but not both.

Psychophysiological techniques have been used to study language representations and processes at nearly all levels of analysis; the relevant methods, measures, and inferences will be reviewed briefly in the remainder of this chapter.

4. INFERENTIAL CONTEXT

4.1. What's the word?

From the brain's perspective, language is a mapping between physical inputs/outputs, in the form of written, spoken, or signed signals, and experiences, memories, and knowledge stored in long-term memory. One of the critical units for such mapping is the word. Psychophysiological methods have been aimed at better specifying the features of a word, the organization of different kinds of information associated with a word, and the various influences on word processing. One proposal is that information about words is represented in a mental "lexicon" containing both lower-level phonological and orthographic information, as well as higher-level information about a word's meaning and its various syntactic properties (when applicable), such as grammatical gender and subcategorization (though see Elman, 2004). On the standard model, recognizing a word activates this information in the lexicon, in a process known as "lexical access." This information, in turn, is used to combine the meanings of words

into phrases and the meanings of phrases into sentences and discourses.

In this section we consider how, where, and when the brain is able to distinguish between sensory input that is treated as language and other sorts of perceptual information, ERP effects of local and global frequency, and the sensitivity of ERPs to lexical word class and word meaning.

4.1.1. Lexical versus perceptual processing of word forms

Initially, a linguistic stimulus is just another sensory signal – a pattern of light hitting the retina or a constellation of sound pressure waves reaching the cochlea. It is not surprising, therefore, that the earliest brain responses to language are indistinguishable from those to other types of visual and auditory inputs. Eventually, however, the brain begins to categorize (and thus respond differentially to) the input, for example, as a visual string rather than a single object, as a familiar event rather than a novel one, as belonging to the class of stimuli that may be associated with meaning, and so forth. When and how these classifications unfold are critical questions that have been partially answered by psychophysiological studies.

Schendan, Ganis, and Kutas (1998) examined the time course of visual classification by comparing the ERP responses to object-like, word-like, and intermediate stimuli. Regardless of task, around 95 ms a negativity over midline occipital sites distinguished the response to single object-like stimuli from those to strings, followed 10 ms later by a further distinction between strings composed of real letters and non-letters. Thus in the scalp-recorded ERP the first sign of specialized processing of "linguistic" stimuli appears around 105 ms. Results from intracranial recording and fMRI studies suggest that such differentiations may be occurring in the posterior fusiform gyrus (Allison et al., 1994) and the occipitotemporal and inferior occipital sulci (Puce et al., 1996). Finally, random letter strings are differentiated from pronounceable letter strings and words beginning approximately 200 ms post-stimulus-onset in the ERP. Spatial imaging studies have revealed activations that differentiate words and pronounceable pseudowords from non-words and false fonts in left medial extrastriate regions (Petersen & Fiez, 1993). Magnetoencephalographic responses likewise point to an important role for occipito-temporal cortex in reading within 200 ms, delineating a systematic sequence of activations from basic visual feature processing to object-level analysis (Tarkiainen, Cornelissen, & Salmelin, 2002; Cornelissen et al., 2003). Overall, these results intimate a hierarchy in which visual responses become increasingly selective for classes of visual stimuli over time.

A similar time-course of categorizations seems to hold for auditory inputs as well, with the first distinction between meaningful and nonsense words in the ERP around 200 ms (Novick, Lovrich, & Vaughan, 1985). PET findings suggest that activity early in primary auditory cortex and posterior temporal areas is unlikely to be language specific. In contrast, responses in and around Wernicke's area seem to be more specific for words, as well as for tasks exacting phonological processing such as judging whether two words rhyme (Liotti, Gay, & Fox, 1994). Across modalities and methods, therefore, observations support the idea that the processing of words diverges from that of other types of stimuli within about 200 milliseconds, and that this differentiation occurs in secondary perceptual processing areas of the brain.

4.1.2. Repetition, frequency, and neighborhood effects

Once words have been categorized as such by the perceptual system, other factors – such as a word's frequency in the language as well as within an experimental setting (repetition) – begin to affect their neural analysis (see Van Petten et al., 1991). The brain is sensitive to event repetition at many levels, reflecting its recent experience with a particular physical form as well as its recent activation of a particular feature, concept or meaning. For proper names, Pickering and Schweinberger (2003) observed font-sensitive repetition effects between 180–220 ms, font-insensitive repetition effects between 220–300 ms, and later same "person" repetition effects, whether accessed via the name or the face. Repetition reliably decreases N400 amplitude (a negativity between 300–500 ms) to words both within and between modalities, as well as to orthographically legal, pronounceable pseudowords, whether these are derived from (and thus closely resemble) real words or not. Thus, although the N400 is often associated with semantic processing (section 4.2.2), its amplitude can be modulated even when there is no specific meaning to be retrieved (Deacon et al., 2004). N400 repetition effects are largest for immediate repetitions and can be seen even in amnestic patients (Olichney et al., 2000). Finally, the N400 is often followed by a late positivity (LPC) that is also sensitive to repetition (Rugg, 1990).

The first reported effects of word frequency – that is, of the system's global experience with a particular linguistic stimulus – manifest around the time (~150 ms or so) that letter strings begin to be differentiated from words and pronounceable pseudowords. This stage of visual processing seems to be sensitive to orthographic regularity (larger P150 to words and pseudowords than to letter strings) and, more generally, to the amount of experience accrued for a given perceptual form (larger P150 to high than to low frequency words; Proverbio, Vecchi, & Zani, 2004). Then, between 200 and 400 ms, the latency of a left anterior negativity ("frequency sensitive negativity" or FSN), subsuming the N280, is sensitive to the eliciting word's frequency of occurrence in the language (King & Kutas, 1998; Osterhout, Bersick, & McKinnon, 1997; Münte et al., 2001). For words in list format, N400 amplitude is also an inverse function of a word's eliciting frequency with all other factors held constant (see Figure 24.1).

The processing of a particular word or word-like stimulus not only depends on how recently and how often it was experienced, but also on the system's experience with

other, sufficiently similar, stimuli. "Lexical neighborhood density," which refers to the number of known words that differ from a given target by only a single letter (N-metric; Coltheart et al., 1977), also modulates N400 amplitudes: words and pseudowords with many lexical neighbors elicit larger amplitude N400s than those with fewer neighbors (Holcomb, Grainger, & O'Rourke, 2002).

4.1.3. Other lexical variables

During the 200–400 ms time range in which the ERP becomes sensitive to word frequency, effects of lexical class also appear – open class or content words, such as nouns, verbs, adjectives, and adverbs with significant semantic content, versus closed class or function words, such as articles, determiners, prepositions, and conjunctions with more relational content. FSN latency is sensitive to word frequency, irrespective of word class, though other negative components in this latency seem to be sensitive to lexical class *per se* (Brown, Hagoort, & ter Keurs, 1999; Münte et al., 2001). Content words elicit much larger N400s than function words, except when the latter is less expected than usual (King & Kutas, 1995); among function words, those with richer lexical semantic content elicit larger N400s than those with less (Kluender & Kutas, 1993a; McKinnon & Osterhout, 1996).

The ERP is also sensitive to further lexical subdivisions, such as that between nouns and verbs, showing both early and late differences in laterality, distribution, and sensitivity to potential and actual functional roles (Koenig & Lehmann, 1996; Khader et al., 2003; Federmeier et al., 2000). Within the category of nouns, those depicting a tangible, often pictureable, entity (concrete nouns) elicit larger N400s over frontal sites than do abstract nouns (Kounios & Holcomb, 1994), although less so within a supportive sentence context (Holcomb et al., 1999). The specific brain areas activated and reflected at the scalp seem to be influenced by the semantic content of words as well, differing for action versus perception related words, and within action verbs as a function of the body part involved (Pulvermüller, 2001).

4.2. Two of a kind: processing of word pairs

As previously noted, much language research has been aimed at determining the internal organization of the mental lexicon. To this end, a large number of studies have contrasted the responses to pairs of words (or other meaningful stimuli) that systematically vary along some dimension (orthography, phonology, morphology, semantics) as people make some decision about them. The pattern of sensitivity to types and degrees of similarity between the two stimuli – as well as interactions with task – have been used to address questions such as (among others): (1) what features constitute a lexical entry, (2) what resources and/or stages of processing are involved in the access and manipulation of various kinds of linguistic information, and (3) whether or not it makes sense to talk about an "amodal" representation of a concept that can be accessed via written, spoken, and signed words as well as via non-linguistic stimuli.

4.2.1. Orthographic, phonological and morphological relationships

As interfaces between the perceptual form of a word and its lexical and semantic properties, orthographic and phonological information are important components of most models of the lexicon. Several ERP studies have shown that the influences of these cues can be observed in the N400 time window and beyond. For example, in rhyme-judgment tasks, rhyming word pairs elicit a smaller negativity between 250–550 ms than do non-rhyming word pairs (Sanquist et al., 1980). When the rhyming pairs are orthographically dissimilar (moose-juice), reduced N400 amplitudes can be attributed to the phonemic similarity. However, when phonemic and orthographic similarity are crossed, Polich and colleagues (1983) found that both influence the amplitude of the N400, consistent with behavioral reports that orthography cannot be ignored during rhyme judgment. Rugg and Barrett (1987) further demonstrated that orthographic, and not just visual, similarity modulates N400 amplitude. However, the nature of the task seems to affect the expression of these effects: whereas semantic similarity effects obtain even under passive viewing conditions (more below), Perrin and Garcia-Larrea (2003) found that phonological similarity affected the N400 only when participants were making active judgments about the stimuli (though phonological effects on the N400 can be observed when the judgment itself is not about phonology; Liu, Perfetti, & Hart, 2003).

Morphological influences on word processing also have been observed in the ERP by around 250 ms. Morphological processing involves both the derivation of new words ("derivational morphology") and the marking of case, number, tense, and other word features ("inflectional morphology"). Several studies suggest that language users rapidly decompose words into their morphological constituents. McKinnon, Mark, & Osterhout (2003) observed larger N400s for pseudowords without morphemes (flermuf) compared to both real words and pseudowords with morphemes, suggesting that word-like stimuli are morphologically decomposed (even, in this case, for only partially productive morpheme stems, e.g., inceive). Dominguez, de Vega, and Barber (2004) compared morphological priming between pairs of Spanish words with a shared stem (hijo/hija [son/daughter]) to words that were not morphologically or semantically related, but shared a superficially similar stem (foco/foca [floodlight/seal]), and to those that were merely orthographically similar (rasa/rana [flat/frog]). They found that the brain rapidly distinguished between the morphologically- and superficially-related pairs; both elicited an initial amplitude reduction in the N400 time window, but this effect was sustained only for the morphologically (and thus semantically) similar pairs.

For many subsystems of inflectional morphology, regular patterns (e.g., in English past tense: stretch/stretched; in English plurals: friend/friends) can be contrasted with irregular ones (e.g., catch/caught; woman/women). Because electrophysiological measures reflect subtle processing differences between different classes of stimuli, they are well suited for determining the extent to which regular and irregular word forms are differentially processed. In three experiments, Penke et al. (1997) found that irregular past participle stems with the regular (i.e., incorrect) suffix -t elicited a left anterior negativity, whereas regular past participle stems with the irregular suffix -en did not. Weyerts et al. (1995) observed a similar-sized positivity from ~250 ms for both identity and morphological (infinitive) priming of past participles of regular verbs but a smaller and delayed morphological repetition effect relative to identity repetition for irregular verbs. In short, various ERP analyses do point to processing differences between regular and irregular morphological forms in adults, although it remains an open question exactly how distinct the neural representations of the two are.

4.2.2. Semantic relations between words

Reaction time and psychophysiological measures indicate that the processing of a single word (cat) is facilitated by the prior occurrence of a semantically related word (dog). This facilitation, known as semantic priming, is taken to reflect the way in which word representations are organized in our mental lexicon. Electrophysiological signs of semantic relations between words have been investigated primarily using the lexical decision task (Bentin, McCarthy, & Wood, 1985) and the category membership verification task (Boddy & Weinberg, 1981). In both tasks, ERPs to semantically primed words are more positive between 200 and 500 ms than are those to unprimed words, with the difference presumed to be a member of the N400 family. While the N400 effects in different modalities as well as cross-modally (Holcomb & Anderson, 1993) are similar in comprising a monophasic negative wave between 200 and 600 ms, they differ in amplitude, onset latency, and/or scalp distribution (Holcomb & Neville, 1990). Distributional differences notwithstanding, the reliability with which N400 amplitude is modulated by semantic relations has made it a useful metric for testing various hypotheses about language processing.

Among the more controversial issues in the semantic priming literature has been the relative contribution of "automatic" and "attentional" processes to the observed response facilitation (Den Heyer, Briand, & Dannenbring, 1983). This controversy grows out of the larger debate over the modularity of language abilities, with the assumption that modular processes are automatic. To determine whether the N400 indexes automatic lexical (modular) processes, or non-modular, controlled effects, researchers have examined the modulation of the N400 priming effect by factors such as the proportion of related and unrelated words (Holcomb, 1988; Chwilla, Brown, & Hagoort, 1995), the temporal interval between prime and target (Anderson & Holcomb, 1995), and subjects' attentional focus (McCarthy & Nobre, 1993). Overall, it seems that the N400 priming effect persists under conditions typically more associated with automatic processing, though it is often altered quantitatively.

Studies addressing the issue of automaticity via forward and/or backward masking likewise have found N400 priming effects either unchanged or present, albeit smaller (Brown & Hagoort, 1993; Deacon et al., 2000; Kiefer & Spitzer, 2000). Masked and unmasked words also appear to similarly *interfere* with N400 priming (Deacon et al., 2004), although some have reported the eradication of N400 effects with masking (Ruz et al., 2003). Whereas N400 priming effects generally persist under masking and in the attentional blink paradigm, in which streams of rapid input must be attended and processed for response, causing some stimuli to be behaviorally missed ("blinked"; Vogel, Luck & Shapiro, 1998), LPC priming effects (linked to explicit, as opposed to implicit, memory; Olichney et al., 2000) do not (Misra & Holcomb, 2003; Rolke et al., 2001). Taken together, the results suggest that the N400 indexes processing that is neither completely automatic, because it changes in size and timecourse with reduced attention, nor completely controlled, because it persists at least partially when conscious attentional resources are severely limited, as in stage 2 and REM sleep (Bastuji, Perrin, & Garcia-Larrea, 2002).

4.2.3. Other semantic relations

N400 responses are not limited to words. A negativity between 300 and 500 ms with a wide-spread, generally centrally-maximal distribution, which is reduced in amplitude in the presence of supportive context information, makes up part of the brain's response to *any* potentially meaningful stimulus, including line drawings and pictures (Ganis, Kutas, & Sereno, 1996), faces (Bobes, Valdes-Sosa, & Olivares, 1994), meaningful environmental sounds (Van Petten & Rheinfelder, 1995; Chao, Nielson-Bohlman, & Knight, 1995), and gestures (Kelly, Kravitz, & Hopkins, 2004). These types of stimuli, as well as odors (Castle, Van Toller, & Milligan, 2000), also serve as effective context for the N400 response to words, causing amplitude reductions when they are predictive. However, linguistic content does not seem to be necessary for eliciting an N400, which has been observed for anomalies within scenes (Ganis & Kutas, 2003), picture stories (West & Holcomb, 2002), and short video clips (Sitnikova, Kuperberg, & Holcomb, 2003).

The N400 seems to reflect access to stored information at a number of levels: certain aspects of orthography, phonology, and morphology, as well as physical featural similarity between referents of words (e.g., shared shape or size characteristics of named objects; Kellenbach, Wijers, & Mulder, 2000), and a variety of types of meaning relationships (e.g., categorical, associative, schematic), including spatial reference frames (Taylor et al., 2001). This, coupled with the fact that the N400 is sensitive to factors related to the ease with which information can be accessed from memory, has led to the suggestion that it indexes search through long-term, semantic memory. Indeed, N400-like potentials have also been observed in other domains in which memory search would seem to play a role, such as the processing of mathematical relationships among numbers (Galfano et al., 2004; Jost et al., 2003), though not all types of well-learned information elicit or influence N400s. For example, N400s are not observed to grammatical violations if these do not impact meaning, violations of melody (Besson & Macar, 1987) or prosody (Astesano, Besson, & Alter, 2004), or social expectancy (Bartholow et al., 2001) or to mismatches between faces and (recently learned) names (Huddy et al., 2003).

The N400 thus seems to index processing important for, but not limited to, language, which involves the access of relatively well-established, complex, and multidimensional representations from stimuli known from experience to be potentially meaningful. Potentials at the same latency, and sensitive to the same kind of semantic variables, are observed in the fusiform gyrus of patients with implanted electrodes (e.g., Nobre & McCarthy, 1995), although the inferotemporal cortex and superior temporal sulcus (which perform higher-order, modality-specific perceptual processing), as well as the medial temporal lobe, hippocampus, and ventrolateral prefrontal cortex (which process input from multiple modalities) are also active within this time window (Halgren et al., 1994a,b). The scalp-recorded N400 thus may reflect a set of temporally-restricted neural processes that are common to the analysis of all sensory inputs, allowing cross-modal interaction for the purposes of meaning construction (for MEG-based analysis, see Halgren et al., 2002).

4.3. Sentence comprehension

While the psychology of words is a rich field, analyses at the word level alone will not suffice to explain how meaning is derived from language, as even many aspects of words are difficult to understand without appealing to the sentence level or beyond.

4.3.1. Semantic context in sentences

The processing of words in sentences and how they are influenced by semantic and syntactic constraints have been extensively studied with ERPs. Kutas and Hillyard (1980) observed a large negativity peaking around 400 ms (N400) to a lexically semantically anomalous word at the end of a sentence; this has been replicated for written, spoken, and signed languages (see Figure 24.1). N400 elicitation, however, is not specific to semantic anomalies, and its amplitude reflects finer gradations of the contextual constraints placed on the eliciting word (Kutas & Federmeier, 2001). In fact, N400 amplitude and the cloze probability of a word (e.g., what proportion of subjects will fill in a particular word as being the most likely completion of a sentence fragment; Taylor, 1953) are inversely correlated at a level

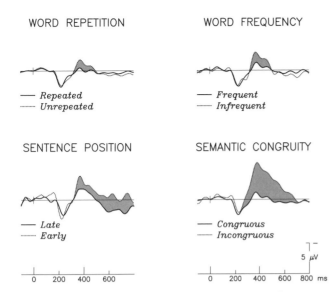

WORD REPETITION

—— *Repeated*
········· *Unrepeated*

WORD FREQUENCY

—— *Frequent*
········· *Infrequent*

SENTENCE POSITION

—— *Late*
········· *Early*

SEMANTIC CONGRUITY

—— *Congruous*
········· *Incongruous*

5 μV

0   200   400   600   0   200   400   600   800 ms

Figure 24.1. Sample N400 effects at a midline parietal site.

above 90%. Moreover, the finding that N400 amplitude to a low cloze word is the same regardless of the degree of prior contextual constraint was critical in establishing that the N400 does not index the violation of previously established expectancies for a particular word that was not presented, but rather the degree to which the sentence fragment prepares the way for the word that actually followed (Kutas & Hillyard, 1984). This effect of contextual constraint is also seen in the monotonic decrease in N400 amplitude to open class words with their ordinal position in congruent sentences, but not in random word strings of equal length. The semantic aspect of sentential context is also capable of eliminating the N400 frequency effect (Van Petten, 1995).

Contrasts of lexical/associative semantic relationships and sentence-level semantic relationships indicate that both independently influence N400 amplitude (Van Petten, 1995; see also Swaab et al., 2003, for a similar conclusion) and interact with comprehension skill (Van Petten et al., 1997). The N400 is sensitive to the relationships between a word and other words in the lexicon, its immediate sentential context, and discourse-level information, in both the auditory and visual modalities, as well as in nonverbal stories (West & Holcomb, 2002). van Berkum and colleagues (1999, 2003), for example, found that equivalent-sized N400s to the final words of isolated sentences like "Jane told her brother that he was exceptionally *quick/slow*" differed in amplitude when embedded in a discourse context like "That morning, Jane's brother finished his shower in only 5 minutes." It is important to note, however, that despite the exquisite sensitivity of the N400 to semantic relationships even outside of a sentence context and contextual expectancy (operationalized by cloze probability), it is not a good index of either sentential plausibility or meaning in terms of truth value: N400s to *white* are only marginally smaller than those to *sour* when completing sentence fragments such as "Dutch trains are —" (when they in fact yellow), are hardly present to *eat* in "For break-

fast the eggs would only *eat . . .*", and are equally small to *bird* in "A robin is/is not a *bird*" (Fischler et al., 1983; Kuperberg et al., 2003; Hagoort et al., 2004).

The N400 also has been used to examine when and how context exerts its influence on word processing. Van Petten and colleagues (1999) found that auditory ERPs to congruent and incongruent sentence completions differ within 200 ms after word onset, before the auditory signal was sufficient to uniquely identify the words (according to a gating study). Furthermore, the N400 to incongruent words (*captive*) that shared initial phonemes with the expected completions (*captain*) deviated from that to the expected item significantly later than did the N400 to incongruent words that did not share initial phonemes. Inconsistent with a bottom-up integration account, listeners do begin semantic analysis with incomplete acoustic information from contextually-derived expectations (semantic and perhaps phonological), prior to word identification and semantic access.

Such results suggest that language comprehenders may use context not only to guide the integration of the bottom-up information gleaned from a word in that context, but to actively prepare for the processing of likely upcoming – but not yet presented – words. Indeed, a number of recent studies have provided evidence that normal language comprehension involves semantic (and perhaps lexical) prediction. For example, Federmeier and Kutas (1999a) asked participants to read pairs of sentences leading to an expectation for a particular item in a particular semantic category; e.g.:

Ann wanted to treat her foreign guests to an all-American dessert. So she went out in the back yard and picked some apples.

which terminated with the expected item (*apples*), an unexpected item from the expected category (*oranges*), or an unexpected item from a different semantic category (*carrots*). Though both unexpected endings – of equal cloze probability and plausibility – elicited a large N400 relative to the expected one, those from the expected category elicited smaller N400s, even more so in high than low constraining contexts. As this pattern goes in the opposite direction from the rated plausibility of these items, N400 amplitudes to the within category items seem to be largely a function, not of the plausibility of the word itself, but of the expected (but not presented) exemplars. This constitutes clear evidence for prediction given that the featural overlap between the within category violation (*oranges*) and the contextually expected item (*apples*) could affect processing only if the features of the expected item were already activated in the comprehender's mind.

Further evidence for prediction in sentence processing has come from a series of studies in which readers' or listeners' ERPs to articles or adjectives differ according to whether they matched or mismatched the gender of an *upcoming* noun (written, spoken or in picture form) – a difference that indicates contextually-based expectation for a noun of a particular gender, or prescience

(Wicha, Moreno, & Kutas, 2004; van Berkum et al., 2005).

Alongside this evidence for predictive processing mechanisms in whole brain language comprehension is a growing realization that the brain may employ *multiple* processing strategies. Federmeier and Kutas (1999b) examined hemispheric differences in sentence comprehension by lateralizing the sentence-final words of three category types as described above. Since stimuli presented in one half of visual space are processed preferentially by the contralateral hemisphere, this procedure reveals hemispheric processing biases. Federmeier and Kutas replicated the pattern observed for normal reading when target words were preferentially processed by the left hemisphere (right visual field), but observed only a difference between expected and unexpected endings (of both types, consistent with plausibility ratings) for left visual field/right hemisphere processing. Thus, whereas left hemisphere comprehension strategies involve prediction, right hemisphere processing appears more bottom-up, focused on the *integration* of the current word with context information.

4.3.2. Syntactic investigations

Two of the most important and hotly contested debates within linguistics and psycholinguistics, namely, (1) the competence versus performance distinction (section 4.3.2.1) and (2) the modularity of language representation and language processing (section 4.3.2.2) have played out most energetically with regard to the syntactic (phrasal and sentential) levels of linguistic analysis, as detailed below.

4.3.2.1. *The role of working memory, a performance construct, in syntactic processing.* The main focus of psychophysiological investigations of working memory (WM) in syntactic processing has been structures in which one sentence element must be associated with another at a distance (often across a clause boundary) in order for both to be interpreted correctly. In English, this is true of so-called "*wh*-questions", formed from "*wh*-words" like *who*, *what*, *which*, *where*, etc., and relative clauses. Any sentence constituent – subject, object, object of a preposition, even an entire prepositional phrase – can be displaced as a question word or relative pronoun from the position it would occupy in a corresponding declarative sentence (indicated in the examples by underlining) to the left periphery of a clause, as shown here for subjects and direct objects:

Declarative sentence:	She said [the reporter criticized the senator].
Subject *wh*-question:	**Who** [did she say [__criticized the senator]]?
Subject relative clause:	The reporter [**who** [she said [__ criticized the senator]]] . . .
Object *wh*-question:	**Who** [did she say [the reporter criticized __]]?
Object relative clause:	The senator [**who** [she said [the reporter criticized __]]] . . .

The displaced element is referred to as a "filler," and the corresponding underlined position is referred to as a "gap" (Fodor, 1978), reflecting the fact that the gapped position must be "filled" with some such displaced constituent for sentence interpretation to succeed, and that the two are interdependent: fillers without gaps are illicit (*Who did she say the reporter criticized the senator?), and gaps without licensing fillers are equally ill-formed (*Did she say__ criticized the senator?). For this reason, structures of this nature are generally referred to as dependencies. Just exactly how the association of gaps with their fillers is effected in linguistic representation and processing is a long-standing unresolved issue.

Gaze duration (Holmes & O'Regan, 1981), word-by-word reading times (King and Just, 1991), and pupillary diameter measures (Just & Carpenter, 1993) have established that, in English, object relative clauses are more difficult to process than are subject relative clauses, due in part to the added load they place on working memory. Information provided earlier in the sentence (the filler) must be maintained over time in order to determine the correct identity of the corresponding gap, and in object dependencies this information must be maintained over a longer distance while the processing of additional material continues (Kluender, 1998; Gibson, 2000).

In an ERP study of English *wh*-questions, Kluender and Kutas (1993a,b) showed in word-by-word comparisons of sentence positions between filler and gap that, relative to control sentences, object questions reliably elicited greater negativity over left anterior regions of scalp between 300 and 500 ms post-word onset (left anterior negativity, or LAN), while subject questions did not, presumably due to the increased working memory load of object dependencies. Direct comparisons of subject versus object relative clauses in the visual (King & Kutas, 1995) and auditory (Müller, King, & Kutas, 1997) modalities in English over longer time windows revealed that these phasic effects were most likely time slices of slow anterior negative potentials (left-lateralized with visual but not auditory presentation; see Figure 24.2). In a related paradigm comparing biclausal structures that differed only in the first word ("After/Before the scientist submitted the paper, the journal changed its policy"), Münte, Schiltz, and Kutas (1998) showed that "before" sentences with reversed chronological order similarly elicited slow negative potentials over left anterior sites, which were directly modulated by working memory capacity. Studies of *wh*-questions in German (Kluender & Münte, 1998; Fiebach, Schlesewsky, & Friederici, 2001; Felser, Clahsen, & Münte, 2003) and objects displaced leftwards ("scrambled" in linguistic terminology) in Japanese (Ueno & Kluender, 2003) essentially replicated the English results.

Other studies have added to this overall picture. Because of the idiosyncrasies of German word order, the use of German nouns ambiguously marked for nominative (subject) versus accusative (object) case can postpone the disambiguation of subject from object relative clauses and questions until the final word of the clause. When this is the

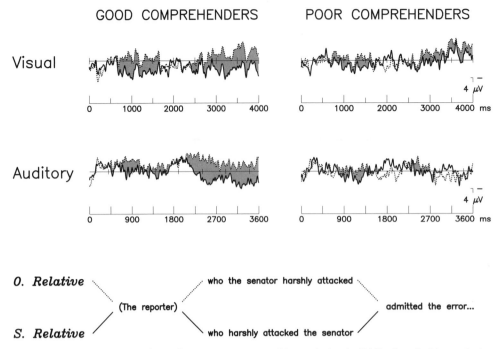

Figure 24.2. Comparison of grand average ERPs to subject relative (solid line) and object relative (dotted line) sentences from a left anterior site in good and poor comprehenders for word by word (500 ms/word) reading and natural speech. The visual data are taken from King and Kutas (1995) and the auditory data are taken from Mueller, King and Kutas (1997). Reprinted by permission of the authors.

case, readers appear to prefer and expect subject dependencies, as evidenced by the fact that the final word of object dependencies elicits a late positivity similar to that seen in response to dispreferred parses and ungrammatical stimuli – the P600 (Mecklinger et al., 1995) – though primarily in participants with high verbal working memory spans (Bornkessel et al., 2004).

Kaan et al. (2000) found that the association of a filler with its gap in English object questions similarly elicits a late positivity, which they interpreted as associated with integration rather than with storage costs of syntactic working memory (Gibson, 2000). This effect of gap-filling also has been replicated in verb-final languages like German (Fiebach, Schlesewsky, & Friederici, 2001; Felser, Clahsen, & Münte, 2003) and Japanese (Ueno & Kluender, 2003).

Overall, these studies conform to the generally accepted linguistic analysis of long-distance dependencies and point to its psychological reality with regard to the processing mechanisms involved. A related line of inquiry in the neural imaging literature has focused on the localization of such mechanisms by studying differences in activation of cortical areas in response to subject versus object dependencies. In an fMRI study, Just, Carpenter, and Keller, (1996) compared subject and object relative clauses with control sentences containing conjoined clauses, and found left-lateralized activation in both Broca's and Wernicke's areas in response to both relative clause conditions, with object relative clauses showing the greatest levels of activation. They interpreted these findings as reflecting gen-

eral working memory demands distributed across multiple cortical areas, directly or indirectly subserving lexical and syntactic processes (Keller, Carpenter, & Just 2001).

A series of PET studies by Caplan and colleagues comparing subject and object dependencies produced differing but mostly consistent results (Stromswold et al., 1996; Caplan, Alpert, & Waters, 1998, 1999; Caplan et al., 2000). Overall, this series of studies consistently elicited activation in the inferior frontal gyrus (BA 44 or 45) – and less consistently in the anterior cingulate, medial frontal gyri, and the superior parietal lobe – in response to object dependencies. These were interpreted as a measure of syntactic complexity related to syntactic integration processes. Subsequent studies, however, failed to confirm this precise picture. Caplan et al. (2001), for example, in an attempted replication of Just, Carpenter, and Keller, (1996), found that object versus subject relative clauses yielded activation of the left angular gyrus (BA 39), and marginal activation in the adjacent portion of the left superior temporal gyrus (BA 22) – essentially Wernicke's area. Ben-Shachar and colleagues (2003; 2004) reported greater activation of left inferior frontal cortex, but also of the posterior superior temporal gyrus bilaterally, when various types of object dependencies in Hebrew were compared with conditions lacking long-distance dependencies; no such effects were seen in direct comparisons with subject dependencies.

Cooke et al. (2001) manipulated the linear distance between filler and gap as well as clause type, and found that all long (relative to short) filler-gap conditions consistently elicited activation in the right posterior superior temporal gyrus. Holding filler-gap length constant, comparisons of object relative clauses with subject relative clauses produced activations in the left posterior temporal-occipital area and the right lingual and fusiform gyri, but not in inferior frontal regions. Only when object relative clauses with long filler-gap distances were compared to either subject or object relative clauses with short filler-gap distances was there activation in left inferior frontal cortex, albeit BA 47. In a similar study of German *wh*-questions, Fiebach, Schlesewsky, and Friederici (2001) likewise failed to find activation in left inferior frontal regions except when object questions with long filler-gap distances were compared to subject questions with short filler-gap distances; they linked Broca's area to syntactic working memory resources, rather than to syntactic integration costs related to syntactic complexity.

Caplan, Waters, and Alpert (2003) and Waters et al. (2003) used the Stromswold et al. (1996) stimuli to examine individual differences in the processing of relative clauses. Both studies reported correlations with processing speed rather than working memory capacity; inferior frontal areas (left-lateralized in the first study, bilaterally in the second) were activated in response to object relatives only in subjects with fast reaction times, while slow-responding subjects showed activation only in left parietal (first study) or superior temporal areas (second study).

In short, there seems to be some relation between the processing of object dependencies, particularly those with long distances between filler and gap, and the activation of left inferior frontal regions. Though consistent with the left lateralization of slow anterior negative potentials to object dependencies in ERP studies, this is unlikely a direct one-to-one mapping, but rather part of a more complex neural network, as suggested by the additional, disparate areas activated by object dependencies in most neural imaging studies (cf. Keller, Carpenter, & Just 2001).

The status of working memory processes in the processing of object dependencies remains similarly unclear at this point. While all the ERP studies cited are consistent with the hypothesis that left anterior negativity (LAN) is an index of working memory resources engaged in the processing of more difficult object dependencies, the exact correlation has not yet been conclusively established. King and Kutas (1995) showed that better relative clause comprehenders had larger LAN responses, but this can at best be taken as an indirect measure of working memory capacity. Münte, Schiltz, and Kutas (1998) showed a direct correlation between working memory capacity as measured by reading span and LAN amplitude, but not in a study of long-distance dependencies. Finally, the direct correlation in the Fiebach, Schlesewsky, and Friederici (2001) study of German *wh*-questions was not in the expected direction.

Discrepancies between ERP studies and neural imaging studies further complicate the picture. The Cooke et al.

(2001) and Fiebach, Schlesewsky, and Friederici (2001, 2002) studies both suggest that activation of left inferior frontal areas of cortex is tied to the processing of long-distance object dependencies that especially tax working memory, not object dependencies *per se*. If so, then the role of working memory in long-distance dependencies may indeed be more of a performance than competence factor. On the other hand, the corresponding Fiebach, Schlesewsky, and Friederici (2001) ERP study reported a shorter but reliable anterior negativity in object versus subject questions with short filler-gap distances, perhaps indicating a greater sensitivity of ERP measures to such transient responses. Finally, the finding of Waters et al. (2003) that working memory capacity does not differentiate localization of cortical response to object dependencies (i.e., both high- and low-capacity subjects show bilateral activation in the inferior frontal lobe), while speed of sentence processing does (i.e., only high-proficiency subjects show bilateral inferior frontal activation) points to the fact that other individual differences contributing to overall proficiency need to be taken more seriously in future investigations as well. The bilingual neural imaging literature serves as a useful reference point in this regard, as it has convincingly shown that proficiency level is also a better predictor of second-language cortical representation than age of acquisition (Perani et al., 1998). Given what we now know about the plasticity of cortical representation (Merzenich et al., 2001), this should come as no surprise.

4.3.2.2. *The role of modularity in syntactic processing.*
Within sentence processing, there are two separate but related areas of investigation with regard to modularity. One has to do with the dissociation of syntactic from semantic aspects of processing (section 4.3.2.2.2); the other has to do with the dissociation of automatic from controlled aspects of syntactic processing itself (section 4.3.2.2.1). In both cases, the intended contrast is between the automatic processes inherent in a phrase structural parsing module, and more controlled processes like semantic interpretation, which are considered to be the purview of a central processor. Since specialized modules by hypothesis feed into the central processor, which takes their output as its own input, controlled processes within the central executive are presumed to occur later within the overall processing stream than automatic, modularized processes, and to be associated with a different underlying neural system.

The fine-grained temporal resolution of ERPs together with the possibility of, at least inferentially, dissociating the neural processes associated with different types of cognitive events by examining their various parameters (polarity, latency, overall morphology, and scalp distribution) have fueled a large body of research aimed at teasing apart automatic from controlled processes, at the same time that PET and fMRI have been used to look for localization differences, as reviewed below.

GRAMMATICALITY   PROBABILITY

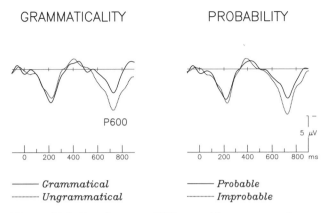

P600

5 μV

0 200 400 600 800   0 200 400 600 800 ms

—— *Grammatical*   —— *Probable*
········· *Ungrammatical*   ········· *Improbable*

Figure 24.3. Grand average ERPs to mid-sentence words at a right parietal site: ungrammatical versus grammatical continuations (left), and improbable (20%) versus probable continuations, regardless of grammaticality (right). Data from Coulson, King, and Kutas (1997).

First, it may be useful to briefly give an overview of the three main ERP components that figure in these debates: the N400, the LAN, and the P600. The N400 component is discussed at length in sections 4.1.2, 4.2.2, and 4.3.1. Kutas and Hillyard (1983) attempted a dissociation of the N400 to violations of semantic well-formedness from potentially different ERP responses to violations of grammatical (morphosyntactic) well-formedness, including violations of number agreement between subjects and verbs ("she dig") and within noun phrases ("a balloons"), as well as the use of finite and non-finite verb forms in inappropriate sentence contexts ("to stayed", "are consider"). Significant early negative differences (300–400 ms) were found in all three conditions over anterior sites, together with marginally significant late positive differences over parietal sites 300 ms post-onset of words immediately following grammatical violations (Kutas and Hillyard, 1983: p. 544, Figure 4). Kutas and Hillyard thus noted that the association of the N400 with semantic but not grammatical anomalies pointed to non-identical processing systems.

It was not until a decade later, however, that the significance of these other components became apparent when a spate of exploratory ERP studies of syntactic processing (Neville et al., 1991; Osterhout & Holcomb, 1992; Hagoort, Brown, & Groothusen, 1993; Kluender & Kutas, 1993a) confirmed the existence of both a left-lateralized anterior negativity (LAN) between 300 and 500 ms post-stimulus onset, and a later broad positive shift (500–800 ms) with a more central distribution (P600; see Figure 24.3). These ERP components were elicited in response to various manipulations of sentence structure, and contrasted with the N400s to semantic manipulations within the same experimental designs. While the polarity and latency of the LAN (or family of such negative potentials) are essentially the same as that of the N400, they differ in their eliciting conditions, scalp distribution and morphology. Both the distribution and the latency of the P600 vary

more widely: while it typically exhibits a posterior distribution, it sometimes appears over anterior regions of scalp (Osterhout & Holcomb, 1992), and it can onset as early as 200 ms (i.e., overlapping the P200 component).

After these early studies, much effort went into characterizing exactly which cognitive processes each potential might be indexing. With regard to the P600, the main debate centers on whether or not it is specific to syntactic processing (Osterhout & Hagoort, 1999), or reflects instead the engagement of a more general purpose process, reflected by a family of positive potentials known as the P3, especially the P3b (cf. Donchin & Coles, 1988), to unexpected but task-relevant anomalies of various types (Gunter, Stowe, & Mulder, 1997; Coulson et al., 1998a,b). In line with the latter view, a number of studies have demonstrated similar late positivities in response to various violations of semantics or pragmatics – either following the N400 response (Münte et al., 1998) or replacing it altogether (Shao, 1995; Kolk, Chwilla, van Herten, & Oor, 2003; Stowe, Kuperberg, Sitniknova, Caplan, & Holcomb, 2003; Hoeks, Stowe, and Doedens, 2004; van Herten, Kolk, & Chwilla, 2005) – and in response to orthographic violations that leave correct pronunciation intact (Münte et al.1998), harmonic violations in music (Patel et al., 1998), and violations of arithmetic rules (Nunez-Pena & Honrubia-Serrano, 2004). In line with the former view, it has been reported that the P600 elicited by syntactic anomalies is absent in patients with lesions of the basal ganglia (Frisch et al., 2003; Kotz et al., 2003; however, not in Friederici, von Cramon, & Kotz, 1999) and reduced in patients with Parkinson's disease (Friederici et al., 2003), though patients with basal ganglia lesions produce normal P300 responses in an auditory oddball paradigm. There is a related debate regarding the functional significance of the P600 within language contexts: should it be considered an index of syntactic processes *per se* (Hagoort, Brown, & Groothusen 1993), of late, controlled processes of reanalysis and repair once a syntactic parsing error has been detected in a multi-stage parsing model (Friederici, Hahne, & Mecklinger, 1996), of syntactic integration processes in general (Kaan et al., 2000), of the reanalysis necessitated by any kind of linguistic parsing difficulty (semantic, morphosyntactic, or orthographic; Münte et al., 1998), or of structural integration processes generally construed (Patel et al. 1998)?

With regard to the LAN, the first challenge was to tease apart the influence of (morpho)syntactic violations versus that of working memory in syntactic processing. Early studies reported LANs both to violations of syntactic well-formedness (Neville et al., 1991; Friederici, Pfeifer, & Hahne, 1993) as well as to manipulations of syntactic working memory (Kluender & Kutas, 1993a,b; King & Kutas, 1995). Kluender and Münte (1998) showed anterior negativities to manipulations of both working memory load and grammaticality within the same experimental design: the negativity elicited by WM manipulations consisted of slow frontal potentials (as in King &

Kutas, 1995), which could also be seen in individual word responses, while the negativity to syntactic violations consisted of more reliably left-lateralized phasic responses. At times, these phasic responses can be bilaterally distributed as well, under auditory (Hahne & Friederici, 2002) and visual (Hagoort, Wassenaar, & Brown, 2003) stimulus presentation.

Much discussion has also focused on the existence of a left anterior negativity that starts 150–200 ms earlier than the LAN, but usually persists into the same 300–500 ms latency window, and exhibits the same scalp distribution. This early left anterior negativity or ELAN (Neville et al., 1991; Friederici, Pfeifer, & Hahne 1993) is sometimes but not always elicited by word category violations, which occur when the parser's expectation that the next incoming word will be of a particular grammatical category (e.g., a noun following an article and adjective, such as "the red...") is violated. What remains unclear is whether the ELAN, which has been elicited only in manipulations of this kind, is a response to the presence of the unexpected word category (a verb following "the red...") or the absence of the expected category (e.g., a noun).

4.3.2.2.1. *The relationship of automatic and controlled syntactic processes.* Frazier and Fodor (1978), among others, proposed that parsing consists of at least two stages, an initial structure-building process based on hierarchical phrase structure and independent of meaning, and a later phase of syntactic reanalysis that comes into play when the initial parse fails and requires revision. Part of the motivation for such a model came from so-called "garden path" sentences (e.g., "The horse raced past the barn fell"), in which the parser is essentially led "down the [wrong] garden path." In this classic example, the parser initially attempts to analyze this sentence as containing an intransitive verb, but is stymied by the sentence-final verb "fell," which forces a reanalysis of "raced" as a passive participle within a reduced relative clause ("The horse [that was raced {by some unspecified rider} past the barn] fell"). The claim has been that the first (-pass parsing) process is automatic, not under conscious control, and impervious to non-syntactic influences, whereas the second process of revision or reanalysis is instead a conscious, controlled process that interacts with other types of information, such as that provided by semantic and/or pragmatic context.

An obvious factor contributing to the garden path phenomenon during silent reading is the lack of prosodic information or intonational contours that are superimposed on the words "raced" and "barn" to mark the (prosodic) boundaries of the reduced relative clause. Such prosodic boundaries help to avoid the garden path effect, and are reflected in the brain's responses to spoken sentences as a positive deflection in the ERP, known as the closure positive shift (Steinhauer et al., 1999); they are also elicited to a lesser degree for subvocal prosodic phrasing in written texts that include punctuation such as commas (Steinhauer, 2003).

Since the earliest studies of syntactic parsing reported both LAN and P600s to grammatically ill-formed stimuli, and since the two components have essentially complementary latency windows (300–500 ms and 500–800 ms, respectively), there has been an understandable attempt to map these components onto different stages of syntactic parsing (Friederici, Pfeifer, & Hahne, 1993; Osterhout et al., 1994). Most researchers now agree that the P600 most likely reflects either revision or integration – under either interpretation, a controlled process – despite the lack of consensus on whether the P600 is specific to syntactic processing, much less to language (see 4.3.2.2).

The existence of ERP markers of earlier, automatic stages of syntactic processing is similarly controversial. In particular, the exact relationship of the ELAN (100–300 ms), and the LAN (300–500 ms), has not been conclusively established, as in most paradigms that elicit an ELAN there is also a LAN present. In any case, the LAN is taken to precede semantic processes indexed by the N400, and dissociations of the two by factors that suppress the N400 but not the LAN have been demonstrated in normal populations (Friederici et al., 2004; Friederici, Steinhauer, & Frisch, 1999; Hahne & Friederici, 2002; Hahne & Jescheniak, 2001). Dissociations of the (E)LAN from the P600 have similarly been demonstrated in normal populations (Hahne & Friederici, 1999) and in patients with left frontal cortical lesions (Friederici, von Cramon, & Kotz, 1999).

While the imperviousness of the ELAN to experimental manipulations of this type and its suppression under degraded visual presentation suggest that it may index automatic processes, the component has to date been reliably elicited using only one general stimulus paradigm. The validity of claims made from the ELAN thus must await further research.

4.3.2.2.2. *The relationship of syntactic and semantic processes.* Although there is general agreement that comprehension requires reconciliation of semantic information about what the words in a sentence might mean and structural information about how they relate to each other, a heated debate rages as to whether or not initial syntactic analyses are modular (informationally encapsulated) and, at least initially, operate automatically, isolated from more controlled semantic/conceptual/pragmatic processes. There are fMRI data consistent with both theoretical perspectives. On the one hand, some brain areas appear to be selectively activated during semantic (e.g., BA 47 in the anterior LIFG) or syntactic processing (BA 44 in the posterior LIFG for word order processing, (Dapretto & Bookheimer, 1999; Indefrey et al., 2001), consistent with the possibility that these two levels of analysis can proceed independently. On the other hand, neuroimaging investigations offer no shortage of substrates for semantic-syntax interactions – many brain areas that are reliably activated during both semantic and syntactic tasks (Kaan & Swaab, 2002), with activation patterns that differ only in degree (Kang et al., 1998; Kuperberg et al., 2003; Ni et al., 2000), Moreover, to the extent that researchers have explicitly sought semantic-syntax interactions, such patterns have been found in Broca's area (Röder et al., 2002), the frontal operculum in the LIFG, and the left anterior STG (Friederici, Meyer, & von Cramon, 2000).

ERP data are equally equivocal on this issue. When researchers have combined semantic violations and syntactic violations and compared the brain's response to such double violations with that for each of the simple violations alone, they have consistently found that the LAN – viewed by some as an early sign of syntactic parsing operations – is insensitive to semantic manipulations (Gunter, Friederici, & Schriefers, 2000; Gunter, Stowe, & Mulder, 1997). Based on such evidence, Friederici and her colleagues argue that the earliest parsing operations proceed impervious to semantic information (see section 4.3.2.2). The results for the processes reflected in the N400 and P600, however, are less straightforward.

Several laboratories have demonstrated that N400 effects triggered by semantic manipulations are modulated by a number of different morphosyntactic factors. For example, the N400 to a semantically anomalous (versus congruent) noun in a sentence is larger when the semantic violation co-occurs with a mismatch between either the gender or the number of the noun and that of an associated article (Hagoort, Wassenaar, & Brown, 2003; Wicha, Moreno, & Kutas, 2004). Though this apparent "syntactic boost" in N400 amplitude could be a spurious consequence of overlap between an N400 and a LAN elicited by the syntactic violation (Gunter, Friederici, & Schriefers, 2000), its posterior scalp distribution favors the view that it is an increase in N400 amplitude per se. This could be an increase engendered by the additional load placed on semantic integration processes by the concomitant need to deal with the syntactic inconsistency (Hagoort, 2003). An increase in N400 amplitude triggered by verb inflection violations even in the absence of a semantic violation likewise attests to N400 sensitivity to morphosyntactic variables (Gunter & Friederici, 1999). These sorts of data thus seem to indicate an interaction of certain semantic and syntactic variables between 200 and 500 ms after word onset. However, word-category violations seem to suppress the significant N400 increase that would otherwise have been elicited by a semantically anomalous word (Friederici et al., 2004; Friederici, Steinhauer, & Frisch, 1999; Hahne & Friederici, 2002; Hahne & Jescheniak, 2001), in line with a more modular syntax-first view of sentence processing, with the breakdown in phrase-structure building due to a syntactic violation effectively shutting down any subsequent semantic analysis (Friederici et al., 2004).

Assessing semantic effects on the P600 component, typically linked to moments of syntactic ambiguity or outright violation (but see section 4.3.2.2), is complicated by the fact that it often follows close on the heels of an N400, as in double violations, leading to at least partial overlap of the two. Smaller positivity in the P600 time window to double violations might thus reflect less P600 activity per se or partial overlap with a larger preceding N400. In fact, the inference with regard to the independence versus interaction of semantic and syntactic processes hinges on how P600 amplitude is measured. Measured with respect to a pre-stimulus baseline, semantic fit and grammatical factors (gender agreement or verb inflection) seem to interact, with the P600 to double violations smaller than to pure grammatical violations (Wicha, Moreno, & Kutas, 2004), perhaps because less effort is devoted to syntactic re-analysis (smaller P600) when finding meaning is difficult (Gunter, Friederici, & Schriefers, 2000). In contrast, when P600 amplitudes are measured with reference to the immediately preceding N400 peak, the interaction between semantic and morphosyntactic factors does not reach statistical significance, perhaps reflecting independence (Hagoort, Wassenaar, & Brown, 2003; though see Wicha, Moreno, & Kutas, 2004).

Though N400s are especially sensitive to semantic manipulations, P600s fairly reliably modulated by parsing difficulties, and LANs often elicited by morphosyntactic violations, the jury is still out on whether these brain potentials reflect psychophysiological primitives that readily map onto individual linguistic processes or representations. Indeed, it may be a mistake to attempt functional brain surgery (or phrenology) according to predetermined linguistic categories. Since neither psychophysiological measures nor linguistic analyses are completely above reproach, it may ultimately prove more rewarding to investigate what functions brain circuits actually compute, and how these could yield the types of regularities that linguists and psycholinguists have uncovered over the years. It may also be useful to bear in mind that the language comprehender's main goal is not to identify or categorize linguistic errors, but to make sense – whenever possible – of the available linguistic input.

4.4. Language production

While language production has been less thoroughly investigated with neuroimaging (especially electrophysiological) techniques than language comprehension, this gap has been narrowed in the past six or so years with the development of the lateralized readiness potential (LRP) and the no go N200 effect. Both have been used to delineate the relative time course of information transmission (encoding and/or retrieval) within a two choice go/no go paradigm, typically involving tacit picture naming.

The LRP is derived from a negative-going readiness brain potential (RP) that develops around 800 or so ms prior to a voluntary movement (Kornhuber & Deecke, 1965); a few hundred ms before the actual movement, the RP becomes larger over the central scalp contralateral to the moving hand. Single cell recordings from monkey cortex indicate that the lateralized portion of the RP is generated, at least in part, in the primary motor cortex (Miller, Riehle, & Requin, 1992).

The LRP is a derived measure computed in the stimulus-locked average with respect to the correct hand (Coles, 1989). On each trial, potentials from left (C3′) and right hand (C4′) areas are subtracted from one another (equivalent to a bipolar C3′–C4′ recording), yielding the lateralized portion of the RP. These difference RPs are then averaged separately for trials where each hand was the correct response and subtracted from each other, canceling lateralized potentials unrelated to response preparation and leaving the average lateralization associated with response preparation – the LRP. Response preparation thus can be monitored a few hundred ms prior to an overt response and even when no response is given: its polarity indicates which response hand is being prepared and its amplitude indicates the degree of preparation, with overt response initiation triggered when LRP amplitude exceeds a certain threshold. The LRP is thus taken as a real-time measure of selective response preparation.

Also appearing in stimulus-locked averages within a dual choice go/no go task, when the motor response is withheld as per the cued instructions, is a fronto-central negativity (1–4 uV) with a latency that varies with task demands. This no go N200 is presumed to reflect response inhibition processes within the frontal cortex, based on single unit activity patterns in monkey frontal cortex during go/no go tasks, and suppression of the monkey's overt response on go trials by stimulation of prefrontal cortex at the time a no go N200 would have occurred if the response were withheld (Sasaki, Gemba, & Tsujimoto, 1989; see also Casey et al., 1998 for supporting fMRI evidence). The peak latency of the N200 effect (go minus no go ERPs) is typically taken as an upper estimate of the time by which the information needed for the go/no go decision must have been encoded. Overall, the N200 is larger, more robust, and more reliably elicited across individuals than is the LRP.

Essentially the same experimental paradigm (two choice go/no go paradigm) has been employed to delineate the relative time course of availability of different types of linguistic information (conceptual, semantic, word form or lemma, syntactic, phonological) during tacit picture naming. Participants view line drawings and are asked to make two decisions on the basis of the depicted item's characteristics (semantic versus phonological decisions as in van Turennout, Hagoort, & Brown, 1998; Schmitt, Münte, & Kutas, 2000; semantic versus syntactic decisions as in van Turennout, Hagoort, & Brown, 1998; Schmitt et al., 2001). Within an experimental setting, one decision maps onto the responding hand (which hand executes the response if there is one) and the other onto the go/no go choice (whether or not any overt response is given) and vice versa.

Though tacit naming in such a design is not actual language production, it is assumed that decisions (necessary for implicit as well as overt naming) made during a trial render the semantic, conceptual, syntactic and phonological properties of the depicted item available, with a time course measurable with psychophysiological measures and without the accompanying artifacts of overt speech. Moreover, it is assumed that (in may cases, even partial) information is transmitted to the response system as it becomes available. Accordingly, if the responding hand is mapped onto information that is available faster than the information that determines whether or not any response is given, then there will be some response preparation (LRP activity) on no go trials, at least until the information needed for the go/no go decision is available to halt response preparation. LRP presence on no go trials with this mapping but not the reverse thus reflects the temporal availability advantage of one information type over another. This temporal advantage is also presumably reflected in the onset and peak latencies of the N200 no go effect (no go minus go difference), as the N200 for no go trials can occur only after enough relevant information that the response is to be withheld has accrued.

Overall, the results of these electrophysiological studies of language production have been remarkably consistent. On average, following a pictured item, conceptual/semantic information is available by ~150 to 225 ms, syntactic (gender) information is available by ~225 to 275 ms, and phonological information is available by ~ 275 to 400 ms. These results then indicate that semantic processing precedes syntactic processing, which in turn precedes phonological processing. These results, however, cannot be used to distinguish between models of language production that argue for or against strict seriality wherein phonological processing is temporally contingent upon a full syntactic analysis and/or syntactic processing is contingent on a complete semantic analysis (Rahman, van Turennout, & Levelt, 2003).

5. CONCLUSIONS AND FUTURE DIRECTIONS

Psychophysiological data have thus converged with behavioral data to fashion a set of viable hypotheses about *when* and *where* language processes occupy the brain – data that in some cases also constrain accounts of *how* language processing (reading, listening, preparing to speak) must be transpiring in real time. The past few decades or so of research attest to the multifaceted nature of language. Indeed, language processing involves an astonishing array of computational and neurobiological processes that operate on a large number of representation types at a number of different time scales in much of the brain's expanse. Much research effort has gone into cataloging and understanding these differences, such that we now know something about the different information types that are typically activated, their relative order of availability, their relative importance, and their relative independence, as well as something about the brain areas involved. Even routine language processing seems to engage considerable amounts of the brain, including not only cortical but also subcortical regions, and, within the cortex, areas in every lobe and in both hemispheres, although typically not to the same extents.

Recent work has highlighted the right hemisphere's role in language comprehension, revealing that it performs functions that are arguably as critical for real understanding as those under the purview of the left hemisphere. More neuroimaging studies of nonliteral language processing in the coming years will be a welcome addition to the existing handful on metaphor, jokes, indirect speech acts, and the like, in our aim of understanding not only the right hemisphere's capacity for and involvement in language but also the nature of the differences, if any, between literal and nonliteral language processing. A relatively new approach to these issues combines neuroimaging techniques with the visual half field paradigm – an excellent way to get a sense of how each hemisphere in the intact brain reacts to input when it receives a slight processing headstart. However, ultimately, we need to face the challenge of explaining how the two hemispheres work in unison during language while making use of the different processes and representations that previous research has defined. Understanding language as an integrated, goal-directed process will moreover require elucidation of the relationships holding among language subcomponents, and between language and other cognitive abilities.

There is as of yet surprisingly little consensus on precisely which brain areas are essential for – as opposed to merely involved in – language processing, their exact computational function(s), and therefore on their specificity for language. Likewise, there is still remarkably little accord among researchers about the degree to which language representations and/or processes (if such a sharp distinction is ultimately viable) are functionally isolable from non-linguistic representations and/or processes, or, within the domain of language, whether or not any subprocesses are isolated from each other. Moreover, whatever one's stance with respect to these issues, we are all comparatively illiterate with respect to how, if at all, the answers to these questions are tempered by individual differences of any kind (age, personality, mood), the particular language or type of languages under investigation (different languages or modalities of linguistic input), and/or the specifics of the dependent measures and/or experimental paradigms with which the questions are probed.

Even experiments that go beyond the single word to include whole sentence processing, discourse, text, and nonliteral language are a far cry from the types of communicative interactions that we encounter daily outside the laboratory. And, indeed, a few researchers are breaking new ground in their inquiry into more natural language processing, so-called "language in the wild," which arrives in fits and starts with pauses, false starts, repetitions, and without a complete sentential structure. Neuroimaging researchers also have begun to explore the communicative role of gestures. Yet another direction of current research pays homage to the crucial social aspect of language acts by recording brain activity from two participants in parallel or from only one participant in the conversational presence of another. In addition, even within the sterile context of the laboratory, increasingly more neuroimaging researchers are beginning to appreciate that individual and group differences in age, working memory capacity, physical and intellectual experiences and general knowledge, psychological and emotional traits and states, as well as biological gender, all may impact the pattern of behavioral and neuroimaging results obtained, and thereby the inferences that we are likely to draw from them. One consequence of this is that researchers are sorting experimental participants into group types as a function of other criteria or subjecting the data to correlational analyses. Such an approach may help to explain the substantial variance in the neuroimaging data that seems to characterize even the best experimental designs.

Much of this variance comes from differences in what we know. And, what we know not only influences what we ultimately understand from language input but also the very processes by which we make sense of that input – determining what information is activated and in what order and with what strength, and how quickly an utterance or text is functionally stored for subsequent retrieval. Very little is known, however, about the relative importance of immediate context and longer-term background knowledge for meaning construction, and future research will need to address their interaction. It will also be important to understand just how critical it is for what is comprehended and/or how comprehension proceeds that people's experiences take place within human bodies with sensory receptors, motor effectors, and the brain betwixt. More research will be devoted to delineating how language representations are built out of both abstract, linguistic features and concrete, perceptual features.

There is also a continued need to explore connections between language processing and other cognitive feats, such as visual scene analysis, the understanding of diagrams, and the perception of music, as these activities likewise require that meaning be obtained over time from a well-structured source of information. By understanding the similarities (and differences) between these types of cognitive processes, we gain insight into the general principles underlying all of cognition, as well as an increased understanding of the defining properties of language.

In large part, psychophysiological data tend to be used either atheoretically, as findings to add to some database of what we know about when, or where any particular factor may have its influence on some brain (and/or behavioral) measure, or theoretically, as empirical evidence for (or in a few cases against) some particular point of view or hypothesis. Misguidedly, however, many instances of this latter use tend to be offered as empirical support for some position when they are just not inconsistent with it. In some cases, the authors seem to believe in their theory so strongly that almost any significant effect within the neuroimaging data constitutes support for the biological plausibility and validity of the original theory. Tempting as this may be, it is not a particularly productive approach to scientific inquiry. Nor is intentionally or unintentionally ignoring relevant data from another imaging modality. Indeed, one of the biggest challenges facing us in the next few decades will be how to make sense not only of discrepant results, but of the data from different imaging modalities, as we still know so little about the fundamental relationships among them. It should go without saying that the more we continue to learn about the physiological and physical basis of our measures and their sensitivities to external and internal energies, the better. However, even with what we know now, we can begin to use psychophysiological data not only to give body to our favorite linguistic theories, but to develop theories of brain functioning which can account for our brain's ability to understand and to produce language, the types of miscommunications and breakdowns that routinely do or could never occur, the nature and time course of language development and usage across the lifespan for a first language, a second language, or more, as well as language processing in individuals experiencing abnormal language experiences due to innate or experiential factors.

In the future, then, using the various and sundry psychophysiological tools at our disposal, we may yet come to understand how Dickinson used her brain to generate poems – which we use our brains to decipher and appreciate.

ACKNOWLEDGMENTS

This work was supported by funds from HD22614 and AG08313 to M. K. and was written while M. K. was a Lady Davis Fellow at Hebrew University of Jerusalem.

REFERENCES

Ackermann, H., & Riecker, A. (2004). The contribution of the insula to motor aspects of speech production: a review and a hypothesis. *Brain and Language*, 89(2), 320–328.

Allison, T., McCarthy, G., Nobre, A., Puce, A., & Belger, A. (1994). Human extrastriate visual cortex and the perception of faces, words, numbers, and color. *Cerebral Cortex* 4(5), 544–554.

Anderson, J. E., & Holcomb, P. J. (1995). Auditory and visual semantic priming using different stimulus onset asynchronies: an event-related brain potential study. *Psychophysiology*, 32(2), 177–190.

Anderson, J. M., Gilmore, R., Roper, S., Crosson, B., Bauer, R. M., Nadeau, S., Beversdorf, D. Q., Cibula, J., Rogish, M., III, Kortemcamp, S., Hughes, J. D., Gonzalez Rothi, L. J., & Heilman, K. M. (1999). Conduction aphasia and the arcuate fasciculus: a reexamination of the Wernicke-Geschwind model. *Brain and Language*, 70(1), 1–12.

Astesano, C., Besson, M., & Alter, K. (2004). Brain potentials during semantic and prosodic processing in French. *Cognitive Brain Research*, 18(2), 172–184.

Bartholow, B. D., Fabiani, M., Gratton, G., & Bettencourt, B. A. (2001). A psychophysiological examination of cognitive processing of and affective responses to social expectancy violations. *Psychological Science*, 12(3), 197–204.

Bastuji, H., Perrin, F., & Garcia-Larrea, L. (2002). Semantic analysis of auditory input during sleep: Studies with event related potentials. *International Journal of Psychophysiology. Special Event-related potential measures of information processing during sleep*, 46(3), 243–255.

Baum, S. R., & Dwivedi, V. D. (2003). Sensitivity to prosodic structure in left- and right-hemisphere-damaged individuals. *Brain and Language*, 87(2), 278–289.

Beeman, M., & Chiarello, C. (1998). *Right Hemisphere Language Comprehension: Perspectives from Cognitive Neuroscience.* Mahwah, NJ: Erlbaum.

Ben-Shachar, M., Hendler, T., Kahn, I., Ben-Bashat, D., & Grodzinsky, Y. (2003). The neural reality of syntactic transformations: evidence from functional magnetic resonance imaging. *Psychological Science*, 14(5), 433–440.

Ben-Shachar, M., Palti, D., & Grodzinsky, Y. (2004). Neural correlates of syntactic movement: converging evidence from two fMRI experiments. *NeuroImage*, 21, 1320–1336.

Bentin, S., McCarthy, G., & Wood, C. C. (1985). Event-related potentials, lexical decision and semantic priming. *Electroencephalography and Clinical Neurophysiology*, 60(4), 343–355.

Besson, M., & Macar, F. (1987). An event-related potential analysis of incongruity in music and other non-linguistic contexts. *Psychophysiology*, 24(1), 14–25.

Binder, J. R., Frost, J. A., Hammeke, T. A., Cox, R. W., Rao, S. J., & Prieto, T. (1997). Human brain language areas identified by functional magnetic resonance imaging. *Journal of Neuroscience*, 17(1), 353–362.

Binder, J. R., Frost, J. A., Hammeke, T. A., Bellgowan, P. S. F., Springer, J. A., Kaufman, J. N., & Possing, E. (2000). Human temporal lobe activation by speech and nonspeech sounds. *Cerebral Cortex* 10(5), 512–528.

Binkofski, F., Amunts, K., Stephan, K. M., Posse, S., Schormann, T., Freund, H.-J., Zilles, K., & Seitz, R. J. (2000). Broca's region subserves imagery of motion: A combined cytoarchitectonic and fMRI study. *Human Brain Mapping*, 11(4), 273–285.

Boatman, D. (2004). Cortical bases of speech perception: Evidence from functional lesion studies. *Cognition* 92(1–2), 47–65.

Bobes, M. A., Valdes-Sosa, M., & Olivares, E. (1994). An ERP study of expectancy violation in face perception. *Brain and Cognition*, 26(1), 1–22.

Boddy, J., & Weinberg, H. (1981). Brain potentials, perceptual mechanism and semantic categorisation. *Biological Psychology*, 12(1), 43–61.

Bookheimer, S. (2002). Functional MRI of language: New approaches to understanding the cortical organization of semantic processing. *Annual Review of Neuroscience*, 25, 151–188.

Bornkessel, I. D., Fiebach, C. J., & Friederici, A. D. (2004). On the cost of syntactic ambiguity in human language comprehension: an individual differences approach. *Cognitive Brain Research*, 21(1), 11–21.

Bottini, G., Corcoran, R., Sterzi, R., Paulesu, E., Schenone, P., Scarpa, P., Frackowiak, R. S., & Frith, C. D. (1994). The role of the right hemisphere in the interpretation of figurative aspects of language. A positron emission tomography activation study. *Brain*, 117(6), 1241–1253.

Brown, C. M., & Hagoort, P. (1993). The processing nature of the N400: Evidence from masked priming. *Journal of Cognitive Neuroscience*, 5(1), 34–44.

Brown, C. M., Hagoort, P., & ter Keurs, M. (1999). Electrophysiological signatures of visual lexical processing: Open- and closed-class words. *Journal of Cognitive Neuroscience*, 11(3), 261–281.

Buchanan, T. W., Lutz, K., Mirzazade, S., Specht, K., Shah, N. J., Zilles, K., & Jancke, L. (2000). Recognition of emotional prosody and verbal components of spoken language: an fMRI study. *Cognitive Brain Research, 9*(3), 227–238.

Buchman, A. S., Garron, D. C., Trost-Cardamone, J. E., Wichter, M. D., & Schwartz, M. (1986). Word deafness: one hundred years later. *Journal of Neurology, Neurosurgery and Psychiatry, 49*(5), 489–99.

Caplan, D., Alpert, N., & Waters, G. (1998). Effect of syntactic structure and propositional number on patterns of regional cerebral blood flow. *Journal of Cognitive Neuroscience, 10*, 541–552.

Caplan, D., Alpert, N., & Waters, G. (1999). PET studies of syntactic processing with auditory sentence presentation. *NeuroImage, 9*, 43–51.

Caplan, D., Alpert, N., Waters, G., & Olivieri, A. (2000). Activation of Broca's area by syntactic processing under conditions of concurrent articulation. *Human Brain Mapping, 9*, 65–71.

Caplan, D., Vijayan, S., Kuperberg, G., West, C., Waters, G., Greve, D., & Dale, A. M. (2001). Vascular responses to syntactic processing: Event-related fMRI study of relative clauses. *Human Brain Mapping, 15*, 26–38.

Caplan, D., & Waters, G. S. (1999). Verbal working memory and sentence comprehension. *Behavioral and Brain Sciences, 22*, 77–94; discussion 95–126.

Caplan, D., Waters, G., & Alpert, N. (2003). Effects of age and speed of processing on rCBF correlates of syntactic processing in sentence comprehension. *Human Brain Mapping, 19*, 112–131.

Casey, B. J., Trainor, R. J., Orendi, J., Schubert, A., Nystrom, L., & Giedd, J. (1998). A developmental functional MRI study of Prefrontal activation during performance of a Go-NoGo task. *Journal of Cognitive Neuroscience, 9*, 835–847.

Castle, P. C., Van Toller, S., & Milligan, G. J. (2000). The effect of odour priming on cortical EEG and visual ERP responses. *International Journal of Psychophysiology, 36*(2), 123–131.

Champagne, M., Virbel, J., Nespoulous, J. L., & Joanette, Y. (2003). Impact of right hemispheric damage on a hierarchy of complexity evidenced in young normal subjects. *Brain and Cognition, 53*, 152–157.

Chao, L. L., Haxby, J. V., & Martin, A. (1999). Attribute-based neural substrates in posterior temporal cortex for perceiving and knowing about objects. *Nature Neuroscience, 2*, 913–919.

Chao, L. L., Nielsen Bohlman, L., & Knight, R. T. (1995). Auditory event-related potentials dissociate early and late memory processes. *Electroencephalography and Clinical Neurophysiology, 96*(2) 157–168.

Chomsky, N. (1965). *Aspects of the theory of syntax*. Cambridge, MA: MIT Press.

Chomsky, N. (1980). Rules and representations. *Behavioral and Brain Sciences, 3*, 1–61.

Chwilla, D. J., Brown, C. M., & Hagoort, P. (1995). The N400 as a function of the level of processing. *Psychophysiology, 32*, 274–85.

Cohen, L., Lehericy, S., Chochon, F., Lemer, C., Rivaud, S., & Dehaene, S. (2002). Language-specific tuning of visual cortex? Functional properties of the visual word form area. *Brain, 125*, 1054–1069.

Coles, M. G. (1989). Modern mind-brain reading: psychophysiology, physiology, and cognition. *Psychophysiology, 26*(3), 251–69.

Coltheart, M., Davelaar, E., Jonasson, J. T., & Besner, D. (1977). Access to the internal lexicon. In S. Dornic (Ed.), *Attention and performance IV* (pp. 535–555). Hillsdale, NJ: Erlbaum.

Cooke, A., Zurif, E. B., DeVita, C., Alsop, D., Koenig, P., Detre, J., Gee, J., Pinango, M., Balogh, J., & Grossman, M. (2001). Neural basis for sentence comprehension: grammatical and short-term memory components. *Human Brain Mapping, 15*, 80–94.

Cornelissen, P., Tarkiainen, A., Helenius, P., & Salmelin, R. (2003). Cortical effects of shifting letter position in letter strings of varying length. *Journal of Cognitive Neuroscience, 15*(5), 731–746.

Coulson, S., King, J. W., & Kutas, M. (1998a). Expect the unexpected: Event-related brain response to morphosyntactic violations. *Language and Cognitive Processes, 1*(1), 21–58.

Coulson, S., King, J. W., & Kutas, M. (1998b). ERPs and domain specificity: beating a straw horse. *Language and Cognitive Processes, 13*(6), 653–672.

Dapretto, M., & Bookheimer, S. Y. (1999). Form and content: dissociating syntax and semantics in sentence comprehension. *Neuron, 24*, 427–432.

Deacon, D., Hewitt, S., Yang, C. M., & Nagata, M. (2000). Event-related potential indices of semantic priming using masked and unmasked words: Evidence that the N400 does not reflect a post-lexical process. *Cognitive Brain Research, 9*(2), 137–146.

Deacon, D., Dynowska, A., Ritter, W., & Grose-Fifer, J. (2004). Repetition and semantic priming of nonwords: Implications for theories of N400 and word recognition. *Psychophysiology, 41*(1), 60–74.

Demonet, J. F., Price, C., Wise, R., & Frackowiak, R. S. (1994). A PET study of cognitive strategies in normal subjects during language tasks. Influence of phonetic ambiguity and sequence processing on phoneme monitoring. *Brain, 117*, 671–682.

Den Heyer, K., Briand, K., & Dannenbring, G. L. (1983). Strategic factors in a lexical decision task: Evidence for automatic & attentional-driven processes. *Memory and Cognition, 11*, 374–381.

Dominguez, A., de Vega, M., & Barber, H. (2004). Event-related brain potentials liced by morphological, homographic, orthographic, and semantic priming. *Journal of Cognitive Neuroscience, 16*(4), 598–608.

Donchin, E., & Coles, M. G. H. (1988). Is the P300 component a manifestation of context updating? *Behavioral and Brain Sciences, 11*, 357–374.

Dronkers, N. F. (1996). A new brain region for coordinating speech articulation. *Nature, 384*, 159–161.

Dronkers, N. F., Wilkins, D. P., Van Valin, R. D., Jr., Redfern, B. B., & Jaeger, J. J. (2004). Lesion analysis of the brain areas involved in language comprehension. *Cognition, 92*, 145–177.

Elman, J. L. (2004). An alternative view of the mental lexicon. *Trends in Cognitive Sciences, 8*, 301–306.

Federmeier, K. D., & Kutas, M. (1999a). A rose by any other name: Long-term memory structure and sentence processing. *Journal of Memory and Language, 41*(4), 469–495.

Federmeier, K. D., & Kutas, M. (1999b). Right words and left words: Electrophysiological evidence for hemispheric differences in meaning processing. *Cognitive Brain Research, 8*(3), 373–392.

Federmeier, K. D., Segal, J. B., Lombrozo, T., & Kutas, M. (2000). Brain responses to nouns, verbs, and class-ambiguous words in context. *Brain, 123*(12), 2552–2566.

Felser, C., Clahsen, H., & Münte, T. F. (2003). Storage and integration in the processing of filler-gap dependencies: An ERP study of topicalization and *wh*-movement in German. *Brain and Language, 87*, 345–354.

Fiebach, C. J., Schlesewsky, M., & Friederici, A. D. (2001). Syntactic working memory and the establishment of filler-gap dependencies: insights from ERPs and fMRI. *Journal of Psycholinguistic Research, 30*, 321–338.

Fiebach, C. J., Schlesewsky, M., & Friederici, A. D. (2002). Separating syntactic memory costs and syntactic integration costs during parsing: The processing of German WH-questions. *Journal of Memory and Language, 47*(2), 250–272.

Fischler, I. S., Bloom, P. A., Childers, D. G., Roucos, S. E., & Perry, N. W. (1983). Brain potentials related to stages of sentence verification. *Psychophysiology, 20*, 400–409.

Fodor, J. A. (1983). *Modularity of mind: an essay on faculty psychology*. Cambridge, MA: MIT Press.

Fodor, J. D. (1978). Parsing strategies and constraints on transformations. *Linguistic Inquiry, 9*, 427–473.

Frazier, L., & Fodor, J. D. (1978). The sausage machine: A new two-stage model of the parser. *Cognition, 6*, 291–325.

Friederici, A. D. (2002). Towards a neural basis of auditory sensory processing. *Trends in Cognitive Science, 6*, 78–84.

Friederici, A. D., & Frazier, L. (1992). Thematic analysis in agrammatic comprehension: syntactic structures and task demands. *Brain and Language, 42*, 1–29.

Friederici, A. D., Gunter, T. C., Hahne, A., & Mauth, K. (2004). The relative timing of syntactic and semantic processes in sentence comprehension. *Neuroreport, 15*, 165–169.

Friederici, A. D., Hahne, A., & Mecklinger, A. (1996). Temporal structure of syntactic parsing: Early and late effects elicited by syntactic anomalies. *Journal of Experimental Psychology: Learning, Memory, and Cognition, 22*, 1219–1248.

Friederici, A. D., Kotz, S. A., Werheid, K., Hein, G., & von Cramon, D. Y. (2003). Syntactic comprehension in Parkinson's disease: Investigating early automatic and late intergrational processes using event-related brain potentials. *Neuropsychology, 17*, 133–142.

Friederici, A. D., Meyer, M., & von Cramon, Y. D. (2000). Auditory language comprehension: An event-related fMRI study on the processing of syntactic and lexical information, *Brain and Language, 74*(2), 289–300.

Friederici, A. D., Pfeifer, E., & Hahne, A. (1993). Event-related brain potentials during natural speech processing: Effects of semantic, morphological and syntactic violations. *Cognitive Brain Research, 2*, 183–192.

Friederici, A. D., Steinhauer, K., & Frisch, S. (1999). Lexical integration: sequential effects of syntactic and semantic information. *Memory and Cognition, 27*, 438–453.

Friederici, A. D., von Cramon, D. Y., & Kotz, S. A.(1999). Language related brain potentials in patients with cortical and subcortical left hemisphere lesions. *Brain, 122*, 1033–1047.

Friedmann, N., & Grodzinsky, Y. (1997). Tense and agreement in agrammatic production: pruning the syntactic tree. *Brain and Language, 56*, 397–425.

Frisch, S., Kotz, S. A., von Cramon, D. Y., & Friederici, A. D. (2003). Why the P600 is not just a P300: The role of the basal ganglia. *Clinical Neurophysiology, 114*, 336–340.

Gabrieli, J. D., Poldrack, R. A., & Desmond, J. E. (1998). The role of left prefrontal cortex in language and memory. *Proceedings of the National Academy of Sciences, USA, 95*, 906–913.

Galfano, G., Mazza, V., Angrilli, A., Umiltà, C. (2004). Electrophysiological correlates of stimulus-driven multiplication facts retrieval. *Neuropsychologia, 42*(10), 1370–1382.

Ganis, G., Kutas, M., & Sereno, M. I. (1996). The search for common sense: an electrophysiological study of the comprehension of words and pictures in reading. *Journal of Cognitive Neuroscience, 8*, 89–106.

Ganis, G., & Kutas, M. (2003). An electrophysiological study of scene effects on object identification. *Cognitive Brain Research, 16*(2), 123–144.

Gibson, E. (2000). The dependency locality theory: A distance based theory of linguistic complexity. In A. Marantz, Y. Miyashita, & W O'Neil (Eds.), *Image, language, brain: Papers from the first mind articulation project symposium* (pp. 94–126). Cambridge, MA: The MIT Press.

Grodzinsky, Y. (2000). The neurology of syntax: Language use without Broca's area. *Behavioral and Brain Sciences, 23*, 1–71.

Gunter, T. C., & Friederici, A. D. (1999). Concerning the automaticity of syntactic processing. *Psychophysiology, 36*, 126–137.

Gunter, T. C., Friederici, A. D., & Schriefers, H. (2000). Syntactic gender and semantic expectancy: ERPs reveal early autonomy and late interaction. *Journal of Cognitive Neuroscience, 12*, 556–568.

Gunter, T. C., Stowe, L. A., & Mulder, G. (1997). When syntax meets semantics. *Psychophysiology, 34*, 660–676.

Hagoort, P. (2003). Interplay between syntax and semantics during sentence comprehension: ERP effects of combining syntactic and semantic violations. *Journal of Cognitive Neuroscience, 15*, 883–899.

Hagoort, P., Brown, C., & Groothusen, J. (1993). The syntactic positive shift (SPS) as an ERP measure of syntactic processing. *Language and Cognitive Processes, 8*, 439–483.

Hagoort, P., Hald, L., Bastiaansen, M., & Petersson, K., (2004). Integration of word meaning and world knowledge in language comprehension. *Science, 304*, 438–440.

Hagoort, P., Wassenaar, M., & Brown, C. M. (2003). Syntax-related ERP-effects in Dutch. *Cognitive Brain Research, 16*, 38–50.

Hahne, A., & Friederici, A. D. (1999). Electrophysiological evidence for two steps in syntactic analysis: Early automatic and late controlled processes. *Journal of Cognitive Neuroscience, 11*, 194–205.

Hahne, A., & Friederici, A. D. (2002). Differential task effects on semantic and syntactic processes as revealed by ERPs. *Cognitive Brain Research, 13*, 339–356.

Hahne, A., & Jescheniak, J. D. (2001). What's left if the Jabberwock gets the semantics? An ERP investigation into semantic and syntactic processes during auditory sentence comprehension. *Cognitive Brain Research, 11*, 199–212.

Halgren, E., Baudena, P., Heit, G., Clark, M., & Marinkovic, K. (1994a). Spatio-temporal stages in face and word processing. 1. Depth-recorded potentials in the human occipital, temporal and parietal lobes [corrected] [published erratum appears in *Journal de Physiologie* (1994), 88(2), following 151]. *Journal de Physiologie, 88*(1), 1–50.

Halgren, E., Baudena, P., Heit, G., Clark, M., & Marinkovic, K. (1994b). Spatio-temporal stages in face and word processing. 2. Depth-recorded potentials in the human frontal and Rolandic cortices. *Journal de Physiologie, 88*(1), 51–80.

Halgren E., Dhond R. P., Christensen N., Van Petten C., Marinkovic K., Lewine J. D., & Dale A. M. (2002). N400-like magnetoencephalography responses modulated by semantic context, word frequency, and lexical class in sentences. *NeuroImage, 17*(3), 1101–16.

Hanakawa, T., Immisch, I., Toma, K., Dimyan, M. A., Van Gelderen, P., & Hallett, M. (2003). Functional properties of brain areas associated with motor execution and imagery. *Journal of Neurophysiology, 89*, 989–1002.

Hawkins, J. A. (1994). *A performance theory of order and constituency*. Cambridge, GB: Cambridge University Press.

Hawkins, J. A. (1999). Processing complexity and filler-gap dependencies across grammars. *Language, 75*, 244–285.

Hickok, G., & Poeppel, D. (2000). Towards a functional neuroanatomy of speech perception. *Trends in Cognitive Sciences, 4*, 131–138.

Hickok, G., & Poeppel, D. (2004). Dorsal and ventral streams: a framework for understanding aspects of the functional anatomy of language. *Cognition, 92*, 67–99.

Hillis, A. E., Work, M., Barker, P. B., Jacobs, M. A., Breese, E. L., & Maurer, K. (2004). Re-examining the brain regions crucial for orchestrating speech articulation. *Brain, 127*, 1479–1487.

Hoeks, J. C. J., Stowe, L. A., & Doedens, G. (2004). Seeing words in context: The interaction of lexical and sentence level information during reading. *Cognitive Brain Research, 19*, 59–73.

Holcomb, P. J. (1988). Automatic and attentional processing: an event-related brain potential analysis of semantic priming. *Brain and Language, 35*, 66–85.

Holcomb, P. J., & Anderson, J. E. (1993). Cross-modal semantic priming: A time-course analysis of event-related brain potentials. *Language & Cognitive Processes, 8*(4), 379–411.

Holcomb, P. J. & Anderson, J. E. (1995). Similarities and differences in comprehension processes during reading and listening. In G. Karmos, M. Molnar, V. Csepe, I. Czigler, & J. E. Desmedt (Eds.), *Perspectives of event-related potentials research* (EEG Suppl. 44, pp. 250–254). Amsterdam: Elsevier.

Holcomb, P. J., Grainger, J., & O'Rourke, T. (2002). An electrophysiological study of the effects of orthographic neighborhood size on printed word perception. *Journal of Cognitive Neuroscience, 15*(6), 938–950.

Holcomb, P. J., Kounios, J., Anderson, J. E., & West, C. (1999). Dual-coding, context-availability, and concreteness effects in sentence comprehension: An electrophysiological investigation. *Journal of Experimental Psychology: Learning, Memory, and Cognition, 25*(3), 721–742.

Holcomb, P. J., & Neville, H. J. (1990). Auditory and visual semantic priming in lexical decision: A comparison using event-related brain potentials. *Language and Cognitive Processes, 5*, 281–312.

Holmes, V. M., & O'Regan, J. K. (1981). Eye fixation patterns during the reading of relative-clause sentences. *Journal of Verbal Learning and Verbal Behavior, 20*, 417–430.

Huddy, V., Schweinberger, S. R, Jentzsch, I., & Burton, A. M. (2003). Matching faces for semantic information and names: an event-related brain potentials study. *Cognitive Brain Research, 17*(2), 314–326.

Iacoboni, M., Woods, R. P., Brass, M., Bekkering, H., Mazziotta, J. C., & Rizzolatti, G. (1999). Cortical mechanisms of human imitation. *Science, 286*, 2526–2528.

Indefrey, P., Hagoort, P., Herzog, H., Seitz, R. J., & Brown, C. M. (2001). Syntactic processing in left prefrontal cortex is independent of lexical meaning. *NeuroImage, 14*, 546–555.

Indefrey, P., & Levelt, W. J. M. (2000). The neural correlates of language production. In M. Gazzaniga (Ed.), *The new cognitive neurosciences* (2nd ed., pp. 845–865). Cambridge, MA: MIT Press.

Indefrey, P., & Levelt, W. J. M. (2004). The spatial and temporal signatures of word production components. *Cognition, 92*(1–2), 101–144.

Ivry, R., & Robertson, L. (1998). *The two sides of perception*. Cambridge, MA: MIT Press.

Joanette, Y., Goulet, P., & Hannequin, D. (Eds.). (1990). *Right Hemisphere and Verbal Communication*. New York: Springer-Verlag.

Jost, K., Beinhoff, U., Hennighausen, E., & Rösler, F. (2003). Facts, rules, and strategies in single-digit multiplication: Evidence from event-related brain potentials. *Cognitive Brain Research, 20*(2), 183–193.

Just, M. A., & Carpenter, P. A. (1993). The intensity dimension of thought: pupillometric indices of sentence processing. *Canadian Journal of Experimental Psychology, 47*, 310–339.

Just, M. A., Carpenter, P. A., & Keller, T. A. (1996). The capacity theory of comprehension: new frontiers of evidence and arguments. *Psychological Review, 103*, 773–780.

Just, M. A., Carpenter, P. A., Keller, T. A., Eddy, W. F., & Thulborn, K. R. (1996). Brain activation modulated by sentence comprehension. *Science, 274*, 114–116.

Kaan, E., Harris, T., Gibson, E., & Holcomb, P. J. (2000). The P600 as an index of syntactic integration difficulty. *Language and Cognitive Processes, 15*, 159–201.

Kaan, E., & Swaab, T. Y. (2002). The brain circuitry of syntactic comprehension. *Trends in Cognitive Sciences, 6*, 350–356.

Kan, I. P., & Thompson-Schill, S. L. (2004). Effect of name agreement on prefrontal activity during overt and covert picture naming. Cognitive, *Affective, and Behavioral Neuroscience, 4*(1), 43–57.

Kang, A. M., Constable, R. T., Gore, J. C., & Avrutin, S. (1998). An event-related fMRI study of implicit phrase-level syntactic and semantic processing. *NeuroImage, 10*(5), 555–561.

Kaplan, J. A., Brownell, H. H., Jacobs, J. R., and Gardner, H. 1990. The effects of right hemisphere damage on the pragmatic interpretation of conversational remarks. *Brain Lang, 38*, 315–333.

Kapur, S., Rose, R., Liddle, P. F., Zipursky, R. B. (1994). The role of the left prefrontal cortex in verbal processing: Semantic processing or willed action? *Neuroreport, 5*, 2193–2196.

Kellenbach, M. L., Wijers, A. A., & Mulder, G. (2000). Visual semantic features are activated during the processing of concrete words: Event-related potential evidence for perceptual semantic priming. *Cognitive Brain Research, 10*(1–2), 67–75.

Keller, T. A., Carpenter, P. A., & Just, M. A. (2001). The neural bases of sentence comprehension: a fMRI examination of syntactic and lexical processing. *Cerebral Cortex, 11*(3), 223–237.

Kelly, S. D., Kravitz, C., & Hopkins, M. (2004). Neural correlates of bimodal speech and gesture comprehension. *Brain and Language, 89*(1), 253–260.

Khader, P., Scherag, A., Streb, J., & Rösler, F. (2003). Differences between noun and verb processing in a minimal phrase context: a semantic priming study using event-related brain potentials. *Cognitive Brain Research, 17*(2), 293–313.

Kiefer, M. (2002). The N400 is modulated by unconsciously perceived masked words: Further evidence for an automatic spreading activation account of N400 priming effects. *Cognitive Brain Research, 13*(1), 27–39.

Kiefer, M. (2001). Perceptual and semantic sources of category-specific effects: Event-related potentials during picture and word categorization. *Memory and Cognition, 29*(1), 100–116.

Kiefer, M., & Spitzer, M. (2000). Time course of conscious and unconscious semantic brain activation. *Neuroreport 11*(11), 2401–2407.

King, J., & Just, M. A. (1991). Individual differences in syntactic processing: The role of working memory. *Journal of Memory and Language, 30*, 580–602.

King, J. W., & Kutas, M. (1995). Who did what and when? Using word- and clause-related ERPs to monitor working memory usage in reading. *Journal of Cognitive Neuroscience, 7*, 378–397.

King, J. W., & Kutas, M. (1998). Neural plasticity in the dynamics of human visual word recognition. *Neuroscience Letters, 13,* 244(2):61–4.

Kircher, T. T., Brammer, M., Tous Andreu, N., Williams, S. C., & McGuire, P. K. (2001). Engagement of right temporal cortex during processing of linguistic context. *Neuropsychologia, 39,* 798–809.

Kluender, R. (1998). On the distinction between strong and weak islands: a processing perspective. In P. W. Culicover and L. McNally (Eds.), *Syntax and Semantics 29: The Limits of Syntax* (pp. 241–279). San Diego, CA: Academic Press.

Kluender, R. (2005). Are subject islands subject to a processing account? In V. Chand, A. Kelleher, A. J. Rodriguez, & B. Schmeiser (Eds.), *Proceedings of the 23rd West Coast Conference on Formal Linguistics*. Somerville, MA: Cascadilla Press.

Kluender, R., & Kutas, M. (1993a). Bridging the gap: Evidence from ERPs on the processing of unbounded dependencies. *Journal of Cognitive Neuroscience, 5,* 196–214.

Kluender, R., & Kutas, M. (1993b). Subjacency as a processing phenomenon. *Language and Cognitive Processes, 8,* 573–633.

Kluender, R., & Münte, T. F. (1998, March). Subject/object asymmetries: ERPs to grammatical and ungrammatical *wh*-questions. *Poster presented at the 11th Annual CUNY Conference on Human Sentence Processing, New Brunswick, NJ.*

Koenig, T., & Lehmann, D. (1996). Microstates in language-related brain potential maps show noun-verb differences. *Brain and Language, 53,* 169–182.

Kolk, H. H. J., Chwilla, D. J., van Herten, M., & Oor, P. J. W. (2003). Structure and limited capacity in verbal working memory: A study with event-related potentials. *Brain and Language, 85,* 1–36.

Kornhuber, H. H., & Deecke, L. (1965). Hirnpotentialänderungen bei Willkürbewegungen und passiven Bewegungen des Menschen: Bereitschaftspotential und reafferente Potentiale. *Pflügers Archiv für die gesamte Physiologie, 248,* 1–17.

Kotz, S. A., Frisch, S., von Cramon, D. Y., & Friederici, A. D. (2003). Syntactic language processing: ERP lesion data on the role of the basal ganglia. *Journal of the International Neuropsychological Society, 9,* 1053–1060.

Kounios, J., & Holcomb, P. J. (1994). Concreteness effects in semantic processing: ERP evidence supporting dual-coding theory. *Journal of Experimental Psychology: Learning, Memory, and Cognition, 20,* 804–823.

Kuperberg, G. R., Holcomb, P. J., Sitnikova, T., Greve, D., Dale, A. M., & Caplan, D. (2003). Distinct patterns of neural modulation during the processing of conceptual and syntactic anomalies. *Journal of Cognitive Neuroscience, 15,* 272–293.

Kuperberg, G. R., Sitnikova, T., Caplan, D., & Holcomb, P. J. (2003). Electrophysiological distinctions in processing conceptual relationships within simple sentences. *Cognitive Brain Research, 17,* 117–129.

Kutas, M., & Federmeier, K. D. (2001). Electrophysiology reveals semantic memory use in language comprehension. *Trends in Cognitive Sciences, 4*(12), 463–470.

Kutas, M., & Hillyard, S. A. (1980). Reading senseless sentences: Brain potentials reflect semantic incongruity. *Science, 207,* 203–205.

Kutas, M., & Hillyard, S. A. (1983). Event-related brain potentials to grammatical errors and semantic anomalies. *Memory and Cognition, 11*(5), 539–550.

Kutas, M., & Hillyard, S. A. (1984). Brain potentials during reading reflect word expectancy and semantic association. *Nature, 307,* 161–163.

Leslie, K. R., Johnson-Frey, S. H., & Grafton, S. T. (2004). Functional imaging of face and hand imitation: towards a motor theory of empathy. *NeuroImage, 21,* 601–607.

Lewis, J. W., Wightman, F. L., Brefczynski, J. A., Phinney, R. E., Binder, J. R., & DeYoe, E. A. (2004). Human Brain Regions Involved in Recognizing Environmental Sounds. *Cerebral Cortex, 14,* 1008–1021.

Liotti, M., Gay, C. T., & Fox, P. T. (1994). Functional imaging and language: evidence from positron emission tomography. *Journal of Clinical Neurophysiology, 11,* 175–190.

Liu, Y., Perfetti, C. A., & Hart, L. (2003). ERP Evidence for the Time Course of Graphic, Phonological, and Semantic Information in Chinese Meaning and Pronunciation Decisions. *Journal of Experimental Psychology: Learning, Memory, and Cognition, 29*(6), 1231–1247.

Lüders, H., Lesser, R. P., Hahn, J., Dinner, D. S., Morris, H., Wyllie, E., & Godoy, J. (1991). Basal temporal language area. *Brain, 114,* 743–754.

Marcel, A. J. (1983). Conscious and unconscious perception: Experiments on visual masking and word recognition. *Cognitive Psychology, 15,* 197–237.

Martin, A., & Chao, L. L. (2001). Semantic memory and the brain: structure and processes. *Current Opinion in Neurobiology, 11,* 194–201.

McCarthy, G., & Nobre, A. C. (1993). Modulation of semantic processing by spatial selective attention. *Electroencephalography and Clinical Neurophysiology, 88,* 210–219.

McCarthy, G., Nobre, A. C., Bentin, S., & Spencer, D. D. (1995). Language-related field potentials in the anterior-medial temporal lobe: I. Intracranial distribution and neural generators. *Journal of Neuroscience, 15*(2), 1080–1089.

McKinnon, R., Mark, A., & Osterhout, L. (2003). Morphological decomposition involving non-productive morphemes: ERP evidence. *Neuroreport, 14*(6), 883–886.

McKinnon, R., & Osterhout, L. (1996). Constraints on movement phenomena in sentence processing: Evidence from event-related brain potentials. *Language and Cognitive Processes, 11*(5), 495–523.

Mecklinger, A., Schriefers, H., Steinhauer, K., & Friederici, A. D. (1995). Processing relative clauses varying on syntactic and semantic dimensions: An analysis with event-related potentials. *Memory and Cognition, 23,* 477–494.

Merzenich, M. M. Cortical plasticity contributing to child development. In J. L. McClelland & R. S. Siegler (Eds.) (2001). *Mechanisms of cognitive development: Behavioral and neural perspectives. Carnegie Mellon symposia on cognition* (pp. 67–95). Mahwah, NJ: Erlbaum.

Meyer, M., Alter, K., Friederici, A. D., Lohmann, G., & von Cramon, D. Y. (2002). FMRI reveals brain regions mediating slow prosodic modulations in spoken sentences. *Human Brain Mapping, 17,* 73–88.

Meyer, M., Friederici, A. D., & von Cramon, D. Y. (2000). Neurocognition of auditory sentence comprehension: Event related fMRI reveals sensitivity to syntactic violations and task demands. *Cognitive Brain Research, 9,* 19–33.

Miller, G. A., & Chomsky, N. (1963). Finitary models of language users. In D. Luce, R. Bush, & E. Galanter (Eds.), *Handbook of mathematical psychology* (pp. 419–492). New York, NY: John Wiley.

Miller, J., Riehle, A., & Requin J. (1992). Effects of preliminary perceptual output on neuronal activity of the primary motor cortex. *Journal of Experimental Psychology: Human Perception and Performance, 18,* 1121–1138.

Misra, M., & Holcomb, P. (2003). Event-related potential indices of masked repetition priming. *Psychophysiology, 40*(1), 115–130.

Mitchell, P. F., Andrews, S., & Ward, P. B. (1993). An event-related potential study of semantic congruity and repetition: Effect of content change. *Psychophysiology, 30*, 496–509.

Müller, H. M., King, J. W., & Kutas, M. (1997). Event-related potentials to relative clause processing in spoken sentences. *Cognitive Brain Research, 5*, 193–203.

Müller, R. A., & Basho, S. (2004). Are nonlinguistic functions in "Broca's area" prerequisites for language acquisition? FMRI findings from an ontogenetic viewpoint. *Brain and Language, 89*, 329–336.

Münte, T. F., Heinze, H. -J., Matzke, M., Wieringa, B. M., & Johannes, S. (1998). Brain potentials and syntactic violations revisited: No evidence for specificity of the syntactic positive shift. *Neuropsychologia, 36*, 217–226.

Münte, T. F., Schilz, K., & Kutas, M. (1998). When temporal terms belie conceptual order. *Nature, 395*, 71–73.

Münte, T. F., Wieringa, B. M., Weyerts, H., Szentkuti, A., Matzke, M., & Johannes, S. (2001). Differences in brain potentials to open and closed class words: Class and frequency effects. *Neuropsychologia, 39*(1), 91–102.

Neville, H. J, Nicol, J. L., Barss, A., Forster, K. I., & Garrett, M. F. (1991). Syntactically based sentence processing classes: Evidence from event-related brain potentials. *Journal of Cognitive Neuroscience, 3*, 151–165.

Newman, A. J., Pancheva, R., Ozawa, K., Neville, H. J., & Ullman, M. T. (2001). An event-related fMRI study of syntactic and semantic violations. *Journal of Psycholinguistic Research, 30*, 339–364.

Ni, W., Constable, R. T., Mencl, W. E., Pugh, K. R., Fulbright, R. K., Shaywitz, S. E., Shaywitz, B. A., Gore, J. C., & Shankweiler, D. (2000). An event-related neuroimaging study distinguishing form and content in sentence processing. *Journal of Cognitive Neuroscience, 12*, 120–133.

Nobre, A. C., & McCarthy, G. (1995). Language-related field potentials in the anterior-medial temporal lobe: II. Effects of word type and semantic priming. *Journal of Neuroscience, 15*, 1090–1098.

Noppeney, U., & Price, C. J. (2004). An FMRI study of syntactic adaptation. *Journal of Cognitive Neuroscience, 16*, 702–713.

Novick, B., Lovrich, D., & Vaughan, H. G. (1985). Event-related potentials associated with the discrimination of acoustic and semantic aspects of speech. *Neuropsychologia, 23*, 87–101.

Nunez-Pena, M. I., & Honrubia-Serrano, M. L. (2004). P600 related to rule violation in an arithmetic task. *Cognitive Brain Research, 18*, 130–141.

Olichney, J., van Petten, C., Paller, K. A., Salmon, D. P., Iragui, V. J., & Kutas, M. (2000). Word repetition in amnesia: Electrophysiological measures of impaired and spared memory. *Brain, 123*(9), 1948–1963.

Osterhout, L., & Hagoort, P. (1999). A superficial resemblance does not necessarily mean that you are part of the family: Counterarguments to Coulson, King, and Kutas (1998) in the P600/SPS-P300 debate. *Language and Cognitive Processes, 14*, 1–14.

Osterhout, L., & Holcomb, P. (1992). Event-related brain potentials elicited by syntactic anomaly. *Journal of Memory and Language, 31*, 785–806.

Osterhout, L., Holcomb, P., & Swinney, D. A. (1994). Brain potentials elicited by garden path sentences: Evidence of the application of verb information during parsing. *Journal of Experi-*

mental Psychology: Learning, Memory, and Cognition, 20(4), 786–803.

Osterhout, L., & Mobley, L. A. (1995). Event-related brain potentials elicited by failure to agree. *Journal of Memory and Language, 34*, 739–773.

Osterhout, L., Bersick, M., & McKinnon, R. (1997). Brain potentials elicited by words: Word length and frequency predict the latency of an early negativity. *Biological Psychology, 46*(2), 143–168.

Pacht, J. M., & Rayner, K. (1993). The processing of homophonic homographs during reading: Evidence from eye movement studies. *Journal of Psycholinguistic Research, 22*, 251–271.

Patel, A. D., Gibson, E., Ratner, J., Besson, M., & Holcomb, P. J. (1998). Processing syntactic relations in language and music: An event-related potential study. *Journal of Cognitive Neuroscience, 10*(6), 717–733.

Penke, M., Weyerts, H., Gross, M., Zander, E., Münte, T. F., & Clahsen, H. (1997). How the brain processes complex words: An event-related potential study of German verb inflections. *Cognitive Brain Research, 6*(1), 37–52.

Perani, D., Paulesu, E., Sebastian Galles, N., Dupoux, E., Dehaene, S., Bettinardi, V., Cappa, S., Fazio, F., & Mehler, J. (1998). The bilingual brain: proficiency and age of acquisition of the second language. *Brain, 121*, 1841–1852.

Perrin, F., & Garcia-Larrea, L. (2003). Modulation of the N400 potential during auditory phonological/ semantic interaction. *Cognitive Brain Research, 17*(1), 36–47.

Petersen, S. E., & Fiez, J. A. (1993). The processing of single words studied with positron emission tomography. *Annual Review of Neuroscience, 16*, 509–530.

Pickering, E. C., & Schweinberger, S. R. (2003). Event-related brain potentials reveal three loci of repetition priming for familiar names. *Journal of Experimental Psychology: Learning, Memory & Cognition, 29*(6), 1298–1311.

Poeppel, D. (2001). Pure word deafness and the bilateral processing of the speech code. *Cognitive Science, 25*, 679–693.

Polich, J., McCarthy, G., Wang, W. S., & Donchin, E. (1983). When words collide: orthographic and phonological interference during word processing. *Biological Psychology, 16*, 155–180.

Polk, T. A., & Farah, M. J. (2002). Functional MRI evidence for an abstract, not perceptual, word form area. *Journal of Experimental Psychology: General, 131*, 65–72.

Price, C. J., & Devlin, J. T. (2003). The myth of the visual word form area. *NeuroImage, 19*, 473–481.

Proverbio, A. M., Vecchi, L., & Zani, A. (2004). From Orthography to Phonetics: ERP Measures of Grapheme-to-Phoneme Conversion Mechanisms in Reading. *Journal of Cognitive Neuroscience, 16*(2), 301–317.

Puce, A., Allison, T., Asgari, M., Gore, J. C., & McCarthy, G. (1996). Differential sensitivity of human visual cortex to faces, letter-strings, and textures: a functional magnetic resonance imaging study. *Journal of Neuroscience, 16*(16), 5205–5215.

Pulvermüller, F. (2001). Brain reflections of words and their meaning. *Trends in Cognitive Sciences, 5*(12), 517–524.

Rahman R. A., van Turennout M., & Levelt W. J. (2003). Phonological encoding is not contingent on semantic feature retrieval: an electrophysiological study on object naming. *Journal of Experimental Psychology: Learning, Memory, and Cognition, 29*(5), 850–860.

Robertson, D. A., Gernsbacher, M. A., Guidotti, S. J., Robertson, R. R., Irwin, W., Mock, B. J., & Campana, M. E. (2000). Functional neuroanatomy of the cognitive process of mapping during discourse comprehension. *Psychological Science, 11*, 255–260.

Röder, B., Stock, O., Neville, H., Bien, S., & Rösler, F. (2002). Brain activation modulated by the comprehension of normal and pseudo-word sentences of different processing demands: a functional magnetic resonance imaging study. *NeuroImage, 15*, 1003–1014.

Rolke, B., Heil, M., Streb, J., & Hennighausen, E. (2001). Missed prime words within the attentional blink evoke an N400 semantic priming effect. *Psychophysiology, 38*(2), 165–174.

Rösler, F., Pütz, P., Friederici, A. D., & Hahne, A. (1993). Event-related brain potentials while encountering semantic and syntactic constraint violations. *Journal of Cognitive Neuroscience, 5*, 345–362.

Rugg, M. D. (1990). Event-related brain potentials dissociate repetition effects of high- and low-frequency words. *Memory and Cognition, 18*, 367–379.

Rugg, M. D., & Barrett, S. E. (1987). Event-related potentials and the interaction between orthographic and phonological information in a rhyme-judgement task. *Brain and Language, 32*, 336–361.

Ruz, M., Madrid, E., Lupianez, J., & Tudela, P. (2003). High density ERP indices of conscious and unconscious semantic priming. *Cognitive Brain Research, 17*(3), 719–731.

Sanquist, T. F., Rohrbaugh, J. W., Syndulko, K., & Lindsley, D. B. (1980). Electrocortical signs of levels of processing: Perceptual analysis and recognition memory. *Psychophysiology, 17*, 568–576.

Sapir, E. (1933). La realité psychologique des phonèmes. *Journal de Psychologie Normale et Pathologique, 30*, 247–265.

Sarter, M., Berntson, G. G., & Cacioppo, J. T. (1996). Brain imaging and cognitive neuroscience: Toward strong inference in attributing function to structure. *American Psychologist, 51*, 13–21.

Sasaki, K., Gemba, H., & Tsujimoto, T. (1989). Suppression of visually initiated hand movement by stimulation of the prefrontal cortex in the monkey. *Brain Reserach, 495*, 100–107.

Schendan, H., Ganis, G., & Kutas, M. (1998). Neurophysiological evidence for visual perceptual organization of words and faces within 150 ms. *Psychophysiology, 35*(3), 240–251.

Schmitt, B. M., Münte, T. F., & Kutas, M. (2000). Electrophysiological estimates of the time course of semantic and phonological encoding during implicit picture naming. *Psychophysiology, 37*, 473–484.

Schmitt, B. M., Schiltz, K., Zaake, W., Kutas, M., & Münte, T. F. (2001). An electrophysiological analysis of the time course of conceptual and syntactic encoding during tacit picture naming. *Journal of Cognitive Neuroscience, 13*, 510–522.

Scott, S. K., Blank, C. C., Rosen, S., & Wise, R. J. S. (2000). Identification of a pathway for intelligible speech in the left temporal lobe. *Brain, 123*, 2400–2406.

Scott, S. K., & Wise, R. J. S. (2004). The functional neuroanatomy of prelexical processing in speech perception. *Cognition, 92*, 13–45.

Sells, P. (1985). *Lectures on contemporary syntactic theories*. Stanford, CA: Center for the Study of Language and Information.

Shao, J. (1995). Analyzing semantic processing using event-related brain potentials. Unpublished manuscript, University of California, San Diego.

Sitnikova, T., Kuperberg, G., & Holcomb, P. J. (2003). Semantic integration in videos of real-world events: An electrophysiological investigation. *Psychophysiology, 40*(1), 160–164.

St. George, M., Mannes, S., & Hoffman, J. E. (1994). Global semantic expectancy and language comprehension. *Journal of Cognitive Neuroscience, 6*, 70–83.

St. George, M., Kutas, M., Martinez, A., & Sereno, M. I. (1999). Semantic integration in reading: engagement of the right hemisphere during discourse processing. *Brain, 122*(7), 1317–1325.

Steinhauer, K. (2003). Electrophysiological correlates of prosody and punctuation. *Brain and Language, 86*, 142–164.

Steinhauer, K., Alter, K., & Friederici, A. D. (1999). Brain potentials indicate immediate use of prosodic cues in natural speech processing. *Nature Neuroscience, 2*, 191–196.

Stowe, L. A., Paans, A. M. J., Wijers, A. A., Zwarts, F., Mulder, G., & Vaalburg, W. (1999). Sentence comprehension & word repetition: A positron emission tomography investigation. *Psychophysiology, 36*, 786–801.

Stromswold, K., Caplan, D., Alpert, N., & Rauch, S. (1996). Localization of syntactic comprehension by positron emission tomography. *Brain and Language, 52*, 452–473.

Swaab, T., Brown, C. M., & Hagorrt, P. (2003). Understanding words in sentence contexts: The time course of ambiguity resolution. *Brain and Language, 86*(2), 326–343.

Tarkiainen, A., Cornelissen, P. L., & Salmelin, R. (2002). Dynamics of visual feature analysis and object-level processing in face versus letter-string perception. *Brain, 125*, 1125–1136.

Taylor, W. L. (1953). "Cloze" procedure: A new tool for measuring readability. *Journalism Quarterly, 30*, 415–417.

Taylor, H. A., Faust, R. R., Sitnikova, T., Naylor, S. J., & Holcomb, P. J. (2001). Is the donut in front of the car? An electrophysiological study examining spatial reference frame processing. *Canadian Journal of Experimental Psychology, 55*(2), 175–184.

Thompson-Schill, S. L. (2003). Neuroimaging studies of semantic memory: inferring "how" from "where". *Neuropsychologia, 41*, 280–292.

Thompson-Schill, S. L., Aguirre, G. K., D'Esposito, M., & Farah, M. J. (1999). A neural basis for category and modality specificity of semantic knowledge. *Neuropsychologia, 37*, 671–676.

Thompson-Schill, S. L., D'Esposito, M., Aguirre, G. K., & Farah, M. J. (1997). Role of left inferior prefrontal cortex in retrieval of semantic knowledge: a reevaluation. *Proceedings of the National Academy of Sciences, USA, 94*, 14792–14797.

Thompson-Schill, S. L., Swick, D., Farah, M. J., D'Esposito, M., Kan, I. P., & Knight, R. T. (1998). Verb generation in patients with focal frontal lesions: a neuropsychological test of neuroimaging findings. *Proceedings of the National Academy of Sciences, USA, 95*, 15855–15860.

Ueno, M., & Kluender, R. (2003). Event-related brain indices of Japanese scrambling. *Brain and Language, 86*, 243–271.

van Berkum, J., Brown, C. M., Zwitserood, P., Kooijman, V., & Hagoort, P. (2005). Anticipating upcoming words in discourse: Evidence from ERPs and reading times. *Journal of Experimental Psychology: Learning Memory, & Cognition, 31*(3), 443–467.

van Berkum, J., Hagoort, P., & Brown, C. M. (1999). Semantic integration in sentences and discourse: Evidence from the N400. *Journal of Cognitive Neuroscience, 11*(6), 657–671.

van Berkum, J., Zwitserlood, P., Hagoort, P., & Brown, C. M. (2003). When and how do listeners relate a sentence to the wider discourse? Evidence from the N400 effect. *Cognitive Brain Research, 17*(3), 701–718.

van Herten, M., Kolk H. H. J., & Chwilla, D. J. (2005). An ERP study of P600 effects elicited by semantic anomalies. *Cognitive Brain Research, 22*, 241–255.

Van Petten, C. (1995). Words and sentences: event-related brain potential measures. *Psychophysiology, 32*, 511–525.

Van Petten, C., & Rheinfelder, H. (1995). Conceptual relationships between spoken words and environmental sounds: event-related brain potential measures. *Neuropsychologia, 33*, 485–508.

Van Petten, C., Kutas, M., Kluender, R., Mitchiner, M., & McIsaac, H. (1991). Fractionating the word repetition effect with event-related potentials. *Journal of Cognition Neuroscience, 3*, 131–150.

Van Petten, C., Coulson, S., Rubin, S., Plante, E., & Parks, M. (1999). Time course of word identification and semantic integration in spoken language. *Journal of Experimental Psychology: Learning, Memory, and Cognition, 25*(2), 394–417.

Van Petten, C., Weckerly, J., McIsaac, H. K., & Kutas, M. (1997). Working memory capacity dissociates lexical and sentential context effects. *Psychological Science, 8*, 238–242.

van Turennout, M., Hagoort, P., & Brown, C. M. (1997). Electrophysiological evidence on the time course of semantic and phonological processes in speech production. *Journal of Experimental Psychology: Learning, Memory, and Cognition, 23*, 787–806.

van Turennout, M., Hagoort, P., & Brown, C. M. (1998). Brain activity during speaking: From syntax to phonology in 40 milliseconds. *Science, 280*, 572–574.

Vogel, E. K., Luck, S. J., & Shapiro, K. L. (1998). Electrophysiological evidence for a postperceptual locus of suppression during the attentional blink. *Journal of Experimental Psychology: Human Perception and Performance, 24*, 1656–1674.

Wagner, A. D., Paré-Blagoev, E. J., Clark, J., & Poldrack, R. A. (2001). Recovering meaning: Left prefrontal cortex guides controlled semantic retrieval. *Neuron, 31*, 329–338.

Waters, G., Caplan, D., Alpert, N., & Stanczak, L. (2003). Individual differences in rCBF correlates of syntactic processing in sentence comprehension: effects of working memory and speed of processing. *NeuroImage, 19*, 101–112.

West, W. C., & Holcomb, P. J. (2002). Event-related potentials during discourse-level semantic integration of complex pictures. *Cognitive Brain Research, 13*(3), 363–375.

Weyerts, H., Münte, T. F., Smid, H. G. O. M., & Heinze, H. J. (1995). Mental representation of morphologically complex words: an event-related potential study with adult humans. *Neuroscience Letters, 206*, 125–128.

Wicha, N. Y. Y., Moreno, E. M., & Kutas, M. (2004). Anticipating words and their gender: an event-related brain potential study of semantic integration, gender expectancy, and gender agreement in Spanish sentence reading. *Journal of Cognitive Neuroscience, 16*, 1–17.

Wymer, J. H., Lindman, L. S., & Booksh, R. L. (2002). A neuropsychological perspective of aprosody: features, function, assessment, and treatment. *Applied Neuropsychology, 9*, 37–47.

Zatorre, R. J., Meyer, E., Gjedde, A., & Evans, A. C. (1996). PET studies of phonetic processing of speech: review, replication, and reanalysis. *Cerebral Cortex, 6*, 21–30.

25 Emotion and Motivation

MARGARET M. BRADLEY AND PETER J. LANG[1]

PROLOGUE

Part of the complexity in studying emotion is defining it: There are almost as many definitions as there are investigators (see Panksepp, 1982, for a representative list). An aspect of emotion upon which most agree, however, is that in emotional situations, the body acts. The heart pounds, flutters, stops and drops; palms sweat; muscles tense and relax; blood boils; faces blush, flush, frown, and smile. We note these reactions in ourselves, and make inferences about the emotional life of others based on visible bodily responses. These changes are clear and strong in what William James (1890) called the "coarser emotions: fear, rage, grief, love, in which everyone recognizes a strong organic reverberation." James, however, also thought that body was involved in subtle emotions, even though the "organic reverberation is less obvious and strong." Lange (1882), joined with James in their eponymous theory, was even more grounded in biology, defining emotion explicitly as a cardiovascular response: "We owe...the emotional side of our mental life, our joys and sorrows, our happy and unhappy hours, to our vasomotor system." (p. 80)

In the late 19th and early 20th centuries when James and Lange were speculating about the basis of affective life, emotion's "organic reverberation" was not easy to assess in a precise, quantitative way. With the advent of elec-

tronic amplifiers, however, it has become possible to measure a broad ranged of physiological reactions to emotional challenges in the laboratory. In 1958, John Lacey could confidently state: "Such measures as skin resistance, heart rate, blood pressure, blood flow, skin temperature, blood-oxygen saturation, gastric motility, pupillary diameter, muscle tension, and other variables have been shown to be remarkably sensitive and responsive measures in a variety of "emotional" states. Conflict, threat and frustration; anxiety, anger, and fear; startle and pain; embarrassment; pleasant and unpleasant stimuli; – all these produce autonomic changes." (p. 160).

In the late 19th and early 20th centuries when James and Lange were speculating about the basis of affective life, emotion's "organic reverberation" was not easy to assess in a precise, quantitative way. With the advent of electronic amplifiers, however, it has become possible to measure a broad range of physiological reactions to emotional challenges in the laboratory. In 1958, John Lacey could confidently state: "Such measures as skin resistance, heart rate, blood pressure, blood flow, skin temperature, blood-oxygen saturation, gastric motility, pupillary diameter, muscle tension, and other variables have been shown to be remarkably sensitive and responsive measures in a variety of "emotional" states. Conflict, threat and frustration; anxiety, anger, and fear; startle and pain; embarrassment; pleasant and unpleasant stimuli; – all these produce autonomic changes." (p. 160).

Despite this clear relation to bodily physiology, emotion is often considered synonymous with mental "feelings" in the popular culture, but its etymological roots are consistent with the biological imperative: the word emotion stems from the Latin *movere*, meaning to move. When emotions are intense, people move: they act, they react, sometimes dramatically, as in crimes of passion. It is instructive that the word 'motivation' stems from the same verb; a motive is, literally, 'something that moves one'. Whereas the term 'emotion' is usually reserved for describing stimuli that are felt to be moving, prompting an affective experience in humans, 'motivation' is the word more often used in interpreting the actions of animals.

[1] The International Affective Picture System (IAPS, Lang, Bradley, & Cuthbert, 2004), International Affective Digitized Sounds (IADS, Bradley & Lang, 1999a) and Affective Norms for English Words (ANEW, Bradley & Lang, 1999b) are available on CD-ROM. These stimulus sets and technical manuals can be obtained on request from the authors at the NIMH Center for the Study of Emotion and Attention, Box 100165 HSC, University of Florida, Gainesville, FL 32610–0165, USA.

This work was supported in part by National Institutes of Health Grants De 13956 and P50-MH52384, an NIMH behavioral science grant to the Center for the Study of Emotion and Attention (CSEA), University of Florida, Gainesville, send request for reprints to Margaret M. Bradley at NIMH Center for the Study of Emotion and Attention (CSEA), Box 100165 hsc, University of Florida, Gainesville, FL 32610–0165.

Not surprisingly, William James noted the conjunction of these two descriptors, and, influenced by Darwin, emphasized a close relationship between emotion and motivation. In James's view, the basic motives (which he called "instincts") of both humans and animals are obligatory actions that are elicited by specific stimuli in the environment. The organism automatically freezes, flees, or fights at the sight of a predator, depending on the environmental context. Instincts, for James, were very like what we would now call motivational systems, defined by limbic circuits, and now a major focus of neuroscience research. James further noted that any object that elicited an instinct elicited an emotion as well, and that instincts and emotions *"shade imperceptibly into each other"*. Even so, instinctive (motivated) behavior differs from the emotions: "Emotions...fall short of instincts, in that [whereas] the emotional reaction usually terminates in the subject's own body, the instinctive reaction is apt to go farther and enter into practical relations with the exciting object." That is, emotions are action dispositions, mobilizing the body for behavior, but in which the overt action itself is often delayed or totally inhibited.

CONCEPTUALIZING MOTIVATIONAL ORGANIZATION

Those studying motivated behavior in animal subjects have consistently agreed that two basic parameters of *direction* and *intensity* control action (e.g., Schneirla, 1959; Hebb, 1949). That is, in the simplest organism, stimuli that promote survival (e.g., food, nurturance) elicit behaviors towards the eliciting stimulus, whereas those that threaten the organism prompt withdrawal, escape, or avoidance. Both approach and avoidance behaviors can occur with varying strength, speed and vigor. In humans, although the specific direction of behavior (i.e., approach, avoid) is no longer completely dictated by the eliciting stimulus, the basic motivational parameters of direction (towards, away) and intensity can still be considered fundamental in organizing emotional behavior.

Biphasic motivation

For instance, most theorists agree that the primary distinction among emotional events is whether they are good or bad (Arnold, 1960), appetitive or aversive (Dickinson & Dearing, 1979) agreeable or disagreeable (MacLean, 1993), positive or negative (Cacioppo & Berntson, 1994), pleasant or unpleasant (Lang, Bradley, & Cuthbert, 1990), hospitable or inhospitable (Cacioppo, Berntson, & Crites, 1996) which clearly relates to the motivational parameter of direction in animal behavior. Moreover, all agree that hedonically valenced events differ in the degree to which they arouse or engage action – a link to motivation's intensity parameter. Based on these observations, a number of theorists have advocated a biphasic approach to emotion, which posits that emotion fundamentally stems from varying activation in centrally organized appetitive and defensive motivational systems that have evolved to mediate the wide range of adaptive behaviors necessary for an organism struggling to survive in the physical world (Konorski, 1967; Davidson et al., 1990; Lang, Bradley, & Cuthbert, 1990; Cacioppo & Berntson, 1994).

Dickinson and Dearing (1979) further proposed that these two motivational systems, (*aversive* and *attractive*) were activated by a wide range of different unconditioned stimuli, and additionally that they had *reciprocal inhibitory connections* (p. 5) which modulated learned behavior and responses to new unconditioned input. However, Miller (1959) proposed that motivation to approach and avoid could be simultaneously engaged (e.g., a stimulus could be both aversive and attractive) resulting in an inhibition of action with an intermediate state of arousal. More recently, Cacioppo and Berntson (1994) suggested a flexible conceptualization of biphasic activation, in which appetitive and defensive activation varies from being mutually reciprocal (Dickinson & Dearing, 1979), to being simultaneously active, to being separably active. Different points in bivariate space, defined by the intensity of biphasic motivational activation, identify instances when defensive and appetitive activation are highly co-active to when they reciprocally related, with the entire space representing all possible scenarios.

Discrete states

Another way to conceptualize emotion is in terms of a set of diverse, discrete emotions, such as fear, anger, sadness, happiness, and so on. Lists of basic emotions have typically varied from theorist to theorist. Descartes (discussed in Panksepp, 1982) listed wonder, love, joy, desire, hate, and sadness as fundamental; this is the last time that positive emotions outrepresented negative, and that love was included on the list. Watson (1924), observing allegiance to definitions based on observable behavior, had a short list of fear, rage, and sexual activity. More contemporary lists include surprise, enjoyment, interest, disgust, shame, distress, fear, contempt, and anger (Izard, 1972); surprise, acceptance, desire, fear, rage, panic, and disgust (Plutchik, 1980), and others.

Lists of discrete states have traditionally been the products of introspective analyses. James famously conjectured that our feelings, consciously apprehended, were in fact percepts of the bodily changes induced directly by a compelling stimulus; and furthermore, that (at least for the stronger, *coarse* emotions of anger, fear, etc.), specific emotions would have a specific physiology. This hypothesis prompted intense psychophysiological research over the last century. However, as John Lacey noted already in 1958: "The search for differential patterns of bodily response in differently named affective states was abandoned early in the history of psychophysiology, with results generally conceded to be disappointing." That is, while there were some provocative findings (e.g., Ax, 1953; Ekman, 1971; see Cacioppo et al., 1993, for a review), the stimulus contexts were generally idiosyncratic to the laboratory, participant response variability was high, and results failed to replicate. More recently, Cacioppo et al. (1993) noted additional problems including inadequate experimental designs, inappropriate comparisons, use of different dependent measures, and, importantly, comparisons across very different induction contexts. Nonetheless, Cacioppo et al. (1993) selected studies that met a number of important criteria for determining emotional specificity, and still, the data were quite disappointing, with "...little evidence for replicable autonomic differences..." (p. 125).

Physiology and action

In addition to a lack of empirical confirmation, the question of whether specific emotional states are related to specific physiological patterns neglects the important facts that physiology will vary with action, and that actions associated with the same emotional state will also often vary. That is, most, if not all, peripheral (and to some degree, central) indices of physiological activity will vary as a function of the amount and type of somatic involvement and the accompanying demand for metabolic support. Put bluntly, running (or preparing to run) will produce a very different configuration of physiological activity than sitting and observing, with activity in one system (e.g., cardiovascular) dependent, to some degree, on activity in another system (e.g., somatic). Moreover, both animal and human research indicate that a cue signaling threat, for example, can lead to fight, flight, or freezing, as well as a variety of specific idiosyncratic behaviors ("displacement" behaviors as described by Tinbergen, 1969, and other ethologists; also see Mackintosh, 1983), depending upon available contextual support and the organism's learning history. The physiology of fear in the context of headlong flight will necessarily be different from the physiology of fear in the context of freezing. From a psychophysiological standpoint, it will at least be necessary to specify whether a commonly proposed discrete emotion (e.g., "fear") occurs in a context which prompts fleeing fear or freezing fear or fighting fear.

STUDYING EMOTION IN THE PSYCHOPHYSIOLOGICAL LABORATORY: INDUCTION CONTEXT, AFFECT VARIATION & THREE SYSTEMS MEASUREMENT

Lacey (1958) noted the great variety of contexts in which emotion can be induced in the laboratory: "The threat to the organism can be real or imagined, present or recalled or anticipated, social or physical, verbalizable or totally inaccessible to verbalization at the time. In all these situations many physiological changes occur. . . . Indeed, in predisposed individuals, painful and even dangerous somatic changes – such as headache, backache . . . production of blood, bile and excessive hydrochloric acid in the stomach . . . can be precipitated by the [mere] discussion of conflictful and psychologically threatening material." (p. 160). Lacey was also cognizant of what he called "situational stereotypy" – the idea that the nature and direction of phys-

Broad Domains of Emotion Induction in the Psychophysiological Laboratory

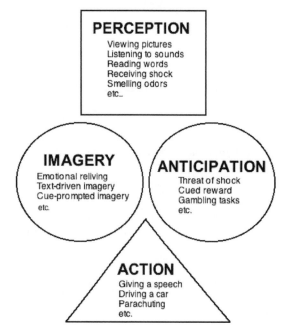

Figure 25.1. The most common induction paradigms in the psychophysiological study of emotion can be roughly classified as involving perception, imagination, anticipation, or action.

iological change is dependent, to a great extent, on the experimental context.

In the emotion literature, on the other hand, inferences regarding the physiology of fear, for example, are often made by comparing data from contexts as diverse as hearing loud noises, anticipating shock, imagining an intruder in the house, looking at a picture of an amputated leg, viewing a scary film, giving a speech, putting one's hand in cold water, or hearing an anguished scream. Conversely, responses to stimuli such as receiving money, listening to joyful music, looking at a picture of puppies, viewing an erotic film, imagining a day on the beach, receiving a good grade, thinking about winning the lottery, or anticipating a vacation are compared on the basis that they prompt a happy emotional state. The diverse sensory, cognitive, and motor processes elicited by these induction procedures may prompt quite different physiological profiles, irrespective of modulation by emotion. Moreover, the nature and direction of affect's modulatory influence can also depend on the specific induction context. Taken together, understanding the psychophysiology of emotion will depend on clearly specifying the context of the emotional induction in the laboratory.

Induction context

In the laboratory, contexts routinely used to induce affective reactions can be roughly organized into those that primarily target perception, anticipation, imagination, or action (see Figure 25.1). While clearly not mutually exclusive (e.g., most anticipatory or imagery tasks include some perceptual input), these induction domains represent broadly similar contexts with respect to psychophysiological responses that may be task, but not emotion, related. For instance, physiological reactions in perception differ both quantitatively and qualitatively from those in imagination, due to the requisite physiology of these different tasks. Moreover, both within and between broad induction contexts, specific parameters can have strong effects on the degree and nature of emotional engagement – i.e., the ease with which neural systems mediating emotional responses are activated – and the resulting pattern of physiological change that can be associated with affective engagement.

Perception. Tasks that primarily target **emotional perception** focus on measuring affective responses to sensory information that is presented in visual (e.g., pictures, words, films, etc.), acoustic (e.g., sounds, music, etc.), tactile (e.g., shock, cold pressor, etc.), olfactory, or gustatory modalities. Perceptual cues can vary in a number of ways that may influence the magnitude and likelihood of emotional engagement, including their modality (e.g., visual, acoustic, tactile, etc.) and duration, the degree to which they are unconditioned (e.g., an electric shock) or conditioned stimuli (e.g., picture of bomb exploding) and the extent to which they involve static (e.g., picture) or dynamic cues (e.g., film). For instance, it is likely that cues in different modalities have differential access to motivational circuits. In non-human primates, visual input to the amygdaloid complex, a neural structure implicated in affective reactivity, is more extensive than auditory input (Amaral et al., 1992), suggesting that modality may be important in engaging affective responses. Similarly, whereas intense physical stimuli (e.g., painful shocks, loud noises) reflexively (and unconditionally) prompt defensive reactions, symbolic (conditioned) stimuli such as the pictures, films, and language cues often used in emotion research rely on learning and association formation for motivational activation, with ramifications for the strength of emotional response.

Imagery. Many psychophysiological studies of emotion measure responses in the context of mentally created or "relived" emotional events. In the *emotional imagery* context, participants are prompted to mentally engage in imagining events that represent a wide range of emotional experiences in the world. Parameters potentially affecting the extent and strength of emotional and physiological engagement in this context include the information in the eliciting cue, and whether the events imagined are non-fictional (i.e., personally experienced) or fictional (i.e., non-experienced). For instance, Jones and Johnson (1978) demonstrated that imagery cues describing action produced more cardiac reactivity during imagery than cues describing passive scenes, and Lang and his colleagues (Miller et al., 1987; Lang et al., 1980) further

demonstrated that when information describing appropriate responses (e.g., your palms are sweaty) is included, emotional responding during imagery is enhanced. Moreover, when subjects imagine emotional events that have been personally experienced, larger skin conductance and heart rate changes occur than when events are imagined that are not personally relevant (Miller et al., 1987), suggesting that motivational and physiological activation is more successful when a specific event is episodically represented in memory. Importantly, in the experiments described above, specific texts were used to prompt imaginal experience. Because the degree of psychophysiological responding during imagery relies intimately on information in the prompting cue, those which specify *only* the image's affective quality (e.g., "imagine a happy event in your life") may fail to clearly define or control important features of the imagined event.

Anticipation. In this affective context, emotional reactions are assessed during a period in which a subject awaits the presentation of an affective stimulus. Threat of shock studies (e.g., Grillon et al., 1991), and classical conditioning paradigms (see Ohman, this volume) fall into this class. Anticipating rewards or payoffs in gambling tasks represent an appetitive anticipatory context (Skolnick & Davidson, 2002). Numerous temporal and associative parameters have been noted as critical in modulating conditioning effects (e.g., MacIntosh, 1983; Stern, 1972), and are potentially relevant when assessing emotional reactions during anticipation (see Putnam, 1990). Among these are the duration of the cuing stimulus, and the nature of the cue (i.e., a light or a picture, for example), both of which can affect the amount of orienting activity (e.g., perceptual intake) that is occurring during the anticipatory interval. The specificity of the warning cue can also affect anticipatory reactions, in terms of whether the cue provides specific (e.g., snake) or non-specific (e.g., something bad) information regarding the upcoming affective event.

Action. Emotional actions, such as giving a speech, driving a car (for a phobic), or parachuting from an airplane represent active induction contexts in which psychophysiological reactions can be measured. Contexts involving overt action are employed less often in psychophysiological investigations of emotion, and for good reason. Gross motor activity can saturate amplifiers, produce artifact in cardiovascular and electrodermal records, and generally interfere with recording the often smaller physiological effects related to emotional parameters. The main variable in an action context is the required activity: Giving a speech will obviously be more physiologically demanding than a simple button press. Ambulatory monitoring studies, which attempt to study emotional reactions (e.g., panic) as they occur in the natural environment, fall within this class, and these investigators are coping with the issues involved in trying to separate the physiology of emotion

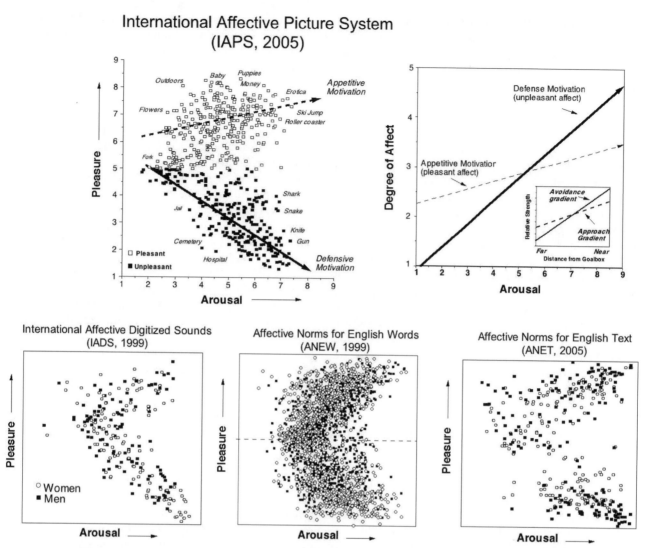

Figure 25.2. Emotional stimuli (pictures, sounds, words, text) are each plotted in the 2-dimensional space defined by the mean ratings of judged pleasure and arousal for each stimulus by a large group of participants. Regression lines drawn through the pleasant and unpleasant stimuli for affective picture ratings are similar to the approach and avoidance gradients first found by Miller (1959) when studying motivated behavior in rats. From Lang et al. (2005), Bradley & Lang (1999a), and Bradley and Lang (1999b).

from the physiology of ongoing action (e.g., see Wilhelm & Roth, 1996; Turpin, 1990; Alpers, Wilhelm, & Roth, 2005).

Affect variation

Following selection of a specific induction procedure, the emotion researcher will need to systematically vary affective features of the stimulus or task, and investigators working from a biphasic motivational perspective will be concerned with varying the degree to which the stimulus activates the defensive and/or appetitive systems. Beginning with Wundt's (1896) early studies of feeling states, it has been recognized that emotional differences among stimuli – words, objects, events – can succinctly be described by a few affective dimensions. In more current factor analyses of evaluative reports (e.g., Osgood, Suci, & Tannenbaum, 1957; see also Mehrabian & Russell, 1974; see

Russell, 1980), two dimensions of *pleasure* and *arousal* control the majority of the variance. In the biphasic view, evaluative reports of *pleasure* roughly index which motivational system is activated by the stimulus or task (i.e., appetitive "pleasant," or defensive "unpleasant"), whereas judgments of *arousal* index (again, roughly) the degree of activation in each motivation system.

Using ratings of *pleasure* and *arousal* gathered from large standardization samples, Lang, Bradley, and their colleagues have developed several sets of affective stimuli defined by these evaluative reports for use in emotion research. The stimulus sets include extensive samples of pictures (Lang, Bradley, & Cuthbert, 2004), sounds (Bradley & Lang, 1999a), words (Bradley & Lang, 1999b) and texts. The distribution of these stimuli in Cartesian space defined by their mean pleasure and arousal rating are quite similar across stimulus sets (see Figure 25.2).

Furthermore, it is noteworthy that the separate regression lines for pleasant and unpleasant pictures (Figure 25.2, top right) are consistent with the hypothesis of varying activation in two underlying appetitive or defensive motivational systems. When activation in both systems is minimal (neither pleasant nor unpleasant), emotional arousal is low and events are usually labelled Unemotional or Neutral. From a motivational perspective, this suggests only a weak tendency to approach or withdraw from the stimulus, and little energy mobilization required for what is, essentially, an absence of response. As defensive or appetitive motivation increases, arousal increases as well, presumably indexing the metabolic requirements of increased attention and anticipated actual action (e.g., approach or avoidance; appetitive incentive or defense).

The slopes and intercepts of the separate regression lines for pleasant and unpleasant pictures (Figure 25.2, top right) also recall the motivational gradients of approach and avoidance that Neal Miller described (1959) based on the strength of behavior in rodents, moving in a runway either towards a food reward or away from a punishing shock (Figure 25.2, top right, inset). Like Miller's data, the slope of the regression line for appetitive motivation is less steeply inclined than the slope for defense-activating, unpleasant stimuli, and the intercept for appetitive materials has a larger offset than does aversive material. Miller noted that the activation of approach behavior (towards food) began when the animal was relatively distant from the goal (hence the larger offset); in contrast, avoidance behavior (i.e., away from shock) began at a point more proximal to the site of the shock and showed a more rapid increase in intensity.

Broadening Miller's analysis, Cacioppo and his colleagues (Berntson, Boysen, & Cacioppo, 1993; Cacioppo, Gardner, & Berntson, 1997) suggest that weak appetitive activation is the base motivational disposition of organisms. They propose, furthermore, that this *positivity offset* of the appetitive gradient – the tendency to approach at low levels of motivation – is the foundation of orienting and exploratory reactions that mediate necessary, quotidian interactions with environmental stimuli. On the other hand, when unpleasant stimuli are proximal, the defense system is abruptly engaged, and rapidly dominates the organism's behavior. The point at which defensive motivation overcomes appetitive motivation is a function of the strength of aversive stimulation and individual differences in temperament and learning history. Survival, however, is always the bottom line and *negativity bias* and the ascendancy of defense when aversive stimuli are near is a fundamental disposition in a world full of diverse threats and dangers.

Discrete emotional states. Researchers proceeding from a discrete emotion view, on the other hand, will seek stimuli or tasks that are held to induce specific emotional states such as fear, anger, sadness, etc. Many recent efforts to study discrete emotions have used facial expressions to define discrete emotions in experimental stimuli, and Ekman and colleagues (Ekman & Friesen, 1979) have developed a coding system (Facial Action Coding System: FACS; Ekman, Friesen, & Hager, 2002) that has been widely used in the observational analysis of the human face, reacting to emotional stimuli. Based on the facial data, Ekman defined a set of primary affects (fear, anger, disgust, joy, sad, surprise), proposing that they were programmed centrally and accompanied by specific patterns of bodily reactions.

A number of facial stimulus sets that reliably vary in the discrete emotion labels people apply to them are now available to researchers that consist of photographs of models posing the basic affective expressions (Pictures of Facial Affect, Ekman & Friesen, 1979; the Karolinska Directed Emotional Face System (KDEF), Lundqvist, Flykt, & Öhman, 1998). The latter collection includes color photographs of several different male and female actors posing facial expressions in a naturalistic manner. In general, posed facial expressions communicate the intended specific emotions, as evidenced by the reliability of emotion labeling by naive observers. Furthermore, research (Ekman, 1971) suggests that at least a subset of facial expressions communicates similar emotions that are reliably labelled across different races and cultures (an issue that intrigued even Darwin, 1873).

3-system measurement

The indices that can be measured and quantified across emotional induction contexts include three systems of (1) evaluative reports, (2) physiological responses, and (3) overt actions (e.g., Lang, 1968). In much of psychological research, emotion measurement relies mainly on evaluative reports, including verbal descriptions (e.g., "I'm afraid"), ratings (e.g., ratings of fear on a scale of 1 to 10), reports of associated responses (e.g., circling or listing bodily reactions), and a variety of other methods that elicit judgments from subjects regarding their affective reactions. On the other hand, overt actions, such as running, jumping, fighting, freezing, and so on, which are used extensively in studies of motivated behavior in laboratory animals, are somewhat less commonly measured in human studies, but have included observable behaviors such as overt facial expressions. Physiological responses are those bodily events that can be assessed using psychophysiological instrumentation and methods, and are not necessarily observable. In emotion research to date, these have included responses in cardiovascular, electrodermal, somatic, reflex, gastric, respiratory, central, and neuroendocrine systems.

There are a number of possible relationships between three-system measures of emotion. Affective reactions can be assessed by measuring only overt behavior (e.g., freezing) or physiology (e.g., cardiovascular), in the absence of verbal reports, as studies of motivated behavior in animals demonstrates. Motivational systems operate independently of a link to a developed language system. In addition, when behavior is observable, changes in associated physiological measures will also tend to occur. Most obviously, if a person is overtly smiling, changes will be detected in EMG activity measured over the appropriate muscles. Because of their inter-dependence, behavioral and physiological measures will not be 'discordant' in the same sense that reports of affective experience and physiology may be.

THE PSYCHOPHYSIOLOGY OF EMOTION: AUTONOMIC AND SOMATIC MEASURES

The autonomic and somatic responses – heart, skin, and muscles – that are hallmarks of affective response are proximally controlled by the peripheral nervous system (see Guyton & Hall, 1996, for an overview), and the anatomical and functional distinctions between its parasympathetic ("homeostatic") and sympathetic ("fight or flight") branches have been important in the study of emotion. The sympathetic nervous system is characterized by post-ganglionic fibers that are quite lengthy, and which branch and divide as they make their way to specific target organs. Functionally, this means that a single sympathetic fiber activates a number of different effectors, providing an anatomical substrate for Cannon's emergency reaction, which proposed a volley of responses – heart rate and blood pressure increases, electrodermal reactions, increase in respiration rate and depth – on the basis of sympathetic activation. Conversely, the post-ganglionic fibers in the parasympathetic branch are short, and therefore more likely to quickly target a specific effector.

Most organs are innervated by nerves from both the parasympathetic and sympathetic divisions, which tend to exert opposite effects. The reciprocal effects of these two systems on different organs are mediated by the release of different neurotransmitters at the neuro-effector junction, with acetycholine released by parasympathetic fibers (cholinergic) and noradrenaline released by sympathetic fibers (adrenergic). Their subsequent action (e.g., increase or decrease in heart rate) is also temporally differentiated by the fact that noradrenaline dissipates slowly, whereas acetycholine dissipates more rapidly. Thus, parasympathetic control will tend to activate specific organs with rapid, phasic effects, whereas sympathetic control is not only more diffuse, but also somewhat longer lasting.

Cardiovascular reactions and emotion

Early investigations exploring emotion in perception assessed cardiovascular activity such as vascular changes and heart rate (e.g., Roessler, Burch, & Childers, 1966; Epstein, 1971; Turpin & Siddle, 1983) as a function of differences in stimulus intensity, as this variable was considered critical in eliciting orienting or defense responses. Low-intensity sensory stimuli were held to prompt orienting activity, mediated by parasympathetic dominance and

associated with a pattern of peripheral and cephalic vaso-constriction and heart rate deceleration, whereas intense stimuli were hypothesized to prompt defense responses, mediated by sympathetic reactivity, and associated with peripheral vasoconstriction, cephalic vasodilation, and heart rate acceleration (see Sokolov, 1963; Graham 1979; Turpin, 1986).

In this conception, sympathetic activity was associated with mobilization to respond to aversive events, whereas pleasant affect was associated with parasympathetic dominance (Arnold, 1960; Gellhorn & Loofbourrow, 1963; Schneirla, 1959). This notion suggests a mode of consistent reciprocal activation between the sympathetic and parasympathetic branches that is no longer tenable. Rather, Berntson, Cacioppo, and Quigley (1991; see also Berntson et al., 1994) have proposed a theory of autonomic control in which physiological measures of a dually-innervated end-organ (e.g., the heart) may differ as a function of the weighting of activation in the parasympathetic and sympathetic systems: systems can be independently active, reciprocally controlled, or co-active.

For instance, Quigley and Berntson (1990) demonstrated that heart rate acceleration to an aversive stimulus (in the rat) is larger than to a low-intensity stimulus not because of differential sympathetic activity, but because parasympathetic activity decreases with high-intensity stimulation. Similarly, in humans, an aversive loud noise prompts a cardiac defense response that consists of an initial acceleration (4–6 s), followed by a decelerative component (17–23 s), and a later secondary accelerative component (31–76 s). Similar to Quigley and Berntson (1990), Reyes del Paso, Godoy, and Vila (1993) concluded that the initial acceleratory component is mediated by the parasympathetic system (vagal release), as this component was not blocked by the administration of a sympathetic beta-adrenergic blockade. On the other hand, the delayed secondary acceleration *was* blocked by the drug (as was stroke volume), suggesting that the slower cardiac component was at least in part sympathetically mediated.

In a picture perception context, stimulus "intensity" has generally been implemented by varying hedonic valence, and work by the Laceys (e.g., Libby, Lacey, & Lacey, 1973), Klorman (e.g., Klorman, Weissberg, & Austin, 1975; Klorman, Weissbert, & Wiessenfeld, 1977), and Hare (e.g., Hare, 1973; Hare, Wood, Britain, & Shadman, 1971; Hare, Wood, Britain, & Frazelle, 1971) consistently found that the heart decelerated, rather than accelerated, when people viewed pictures of unpleasant emotional events, contrary to the notion that these aversive stimuli might prompt defensive heart rate acceleration. Based on these kinds of data, Lacey (1967) originally proposed the notion of *stimulus specificity* (i.e., that specific stimuli or tasks are associated with specific patterns of physiological response). Based on these data, Lacey hypothesized that cardiac deceleration was an index of perceptual processing, reflecting sensory intake, whereas cardiac acceleration was an index of mental processing, reflecting sensory rejection.

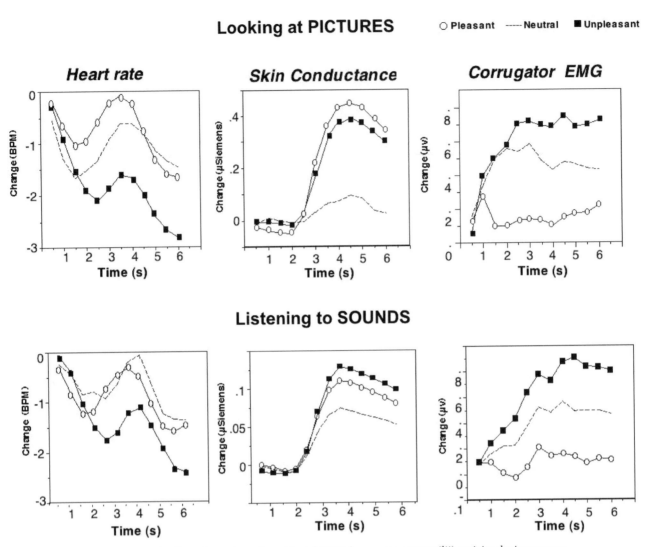

Figure 25.3. Cardiac, electrodermal, and facial EMG (corrugator supercilii) activity during perception of 6 s presentations of pleasant, neutral, or unpleasant pictures (top) and sounds (bottom) show similar affective modulation. Based on data reported in Bradley et al. (2005) and Bradley and Lang (2001).

In the aversive picture perception context, Lacey assumed people were perceptually rejecting the aversive content and turning inward, or away from the sensory display.

Many recent studies have confirmed that the cardiac response during aversive picture viewing involves significant initial deceleration. When viewing pictures, those that are rated as unpleasant typically prompt more initial deceleration than do pleasant or neutral pictures (Lang et al., 1993; see Figure 25.3, top left). When specific picture contents are explored, significant cardiac deceleration is obtained for all unpleasant contents, including highly arousing pictures of threat and mutilation, as well as relatively low arousal contents such as pollution and loss (Bradley et al., 2001a). An initial deceleratory response when viewing unpleasant pictures is reminiscent of the fear bradycardia elicited in animals to threatening stimuli. In animals, this decelerative response is vagally mediated, as atropine (a parasympathetic blockade) completely elim-

inates it, indicating release of parasympathetic control, and has been interpreted as reflecting heightened sensory intake and orienting (see Campbell, Wood, & McBride, 1996). Consistent with a hypothesis of increased sensory intake, highly arousing appetitive pictures, particularly those involving erotica, prompt significantly more initial cardiac deceleration than pleasant pictures rated as lower in arousal (Bradley et al., 2001a), suggesting that pleasant, arousing contents can also attract increased perceptual processing and sensory intake.

If cardiac deceleration during picture perception reflects sensory processing, cardiac responses in other perceptual contexts should also show decelerative differences that reflect hedonic valence. Consistent with this, heart rate also reliably decelerates when viewing films (rather than pictures) that depict bloody surgical interventions (Palomba et al., 2000), suggesting a stance of heightened attention and intake. Moreover, listening to highly arousing unpleasant sounds (e.g., bombs exploding, etc.) also prompts greater initial deceleration than listening to neutral sounds (Bradley & Lang, 2000; Figure 25.3, bottom left). On the other hand, reading sentences that describe emotional or neutral events prompts significant cardiac deceleration, but does not vary with emotion: In this perceptual context, the sensory cues (words) require equivalent processing and the cardiac response reflects sensory intake that does not differ in terms of the affective meaning of the words. Associative processes following encoding (i.e. imagery) do reflect differences in emotional arousal that are not decelerative, but accelerative, in direction (Vrana et al., 1986).

Imagery. Lacey originally proposed that heart rate acceleration indicated "sensory rejection," and was an index of internal processing on the basis of data indicating clear accelerative responses during tasks involving mentation, such as silent arithmetic calculations. Consistent with these findings, the general heart rate response during mental imagery is an acceleratory response that is often enhanced by affective features of the imagined stimulus, with a number of studies finding greater heart rate increases during text-prompted fearful, compared to neutral imagery (Bauer & Craighead, 1979; Cook et al., 1988; Grayson, 1982; Grossberg & Wilson, 1968; Haney & Euse, 1976; Lang et al., 1983; May, 1977b; Van Egeren, Feather, & Hein, 1971).

Heart rate similarly accelerates when imagining pleasant, compared to neutral, scenes (Vrana & Rollock, 2002), and the increase is even more pronounced when participants imagine emotional scenes based on their actual life experiences (Miller, Patrick, & Levenston, 2002). In general, heart rate acceleration during imagery varies most consistently with stimulus arousal – increasing for emotionally arousing (either pleasant or unpleasant) images (Cook et al., 1991; van Oyen Witvliet & Vrana, 1995; Fiorito & Simons, 1994), and these effects are more pronounced when the imagined scenes are personally relevant (Miller, Patrick, & Levenston, 2002).

In an effort to separate cardiac concomitants of mental imagery from heart rate variance associated with simply processing text, Schwartz (1971) developed a paradigm in which subjects first memorized emotionally arousing texts, then imagined the events described by these texts in a fixed sequence. Simply imagining arousing stimuli (i.e., without prior processing of the text prompt) resulted in greater heart rate acceleration than when imagining a neutral sequence (e.g., the letters ABCD). May and Johnson (1973) required subjects to memorize neutral or arousing words, and Vrana, Cuthbert, and Lang (1986) had subjects memorize sentences describing neutral and unpleasant events and then used tones to cue imagery. In all cases, heart rate acceleration was increased when imagining emotional, compared to neutral, events. A second study by May (1977b) found that actively imagining a fearful sentence produced more heart rate acceleration than either hearing the sentence, or seeing a slide depicting the same material as the sentence.

Lang (1987) has interpreted heart rate acceleration during emotional imagery as indicating that in imagery, as in an actual situation, heart rate changes reflect activation of information associated with appropriate actions. Consistent with this, Jones and Johnson (1978, 1980) obtained faster heart rate during imagery of high activity sentences (e.g., "I feel happy, and I'm jumping for joy.") than imagery of low activity relaxing sentences (e.g., "I feel happy, and I just want to relax."), and Miller et al. (1987) demonstrated that, like imagery of fear or anger scenes, imagery of active (neutral) scenes produced greater heart rate acceleration and electrodermal reactivity than neutral scenes involving low activity.

Taken together, the heart rate patterns obtained during picture perception and imagination are consistent with Lacey's (1967) early observation that deceleration is associated with sensory intake (perception), whereas acceleration is associated with mentation. On the other hand, Lacey's interpretation of heart rate acceleration during imagery as reflecting sensory rejection, has been refined: Rather than focusing on sensory processing (e.g., rejection of perceptual information), a number of theories (see Cuthbert, Vrana, & Bradley, 1991, for a review) hypothesize that cardiac acceleration during imagery reflects action engagement prompted by the imagery scene.

According to Lang's (1979) bioinformational theory of emotional imagery, affective events are represented in memory by an associative network that includes coded sensory, conceptual, and action information. Stimulus units in the associative network code information regarding specific sensory and perceptual features of the event (e.g., visual, acoustic, and tactile features of a snake and the current context), whereas meaning units code conceptual information previously learned about the stimulus (i.e., snakes are dangerous). An important feature of bio-informational theory are units that code appropriate actions in the representation of emotional events. Although many cognitive models primarily focus on stimulus and semantic information, bio-informational theory emphasizes the importance of action units, which code associated behaviors (e.g., running) and relevant autonomic support (e.g., heart rate acceleration) that are part of the associative structure of an emotional event. During mental imagery, activation of relevant action units in affective networks prompts heightened physiological engagement during emotional, compared to neutral, events, because emotion is, inherently, a disposition to act.

Electrodermal reactivity and emotion

Whereas the heart is dually innervated, and subject to modulation by either parasympathetic or sympathetic activity (or both), the electrodermal system is innervated solely by the sympathetic system, although the mechanism of its action is cholinergic, rather than adrenergic. In a variety of induction contexts, electrodermal reactivity consistently varies with emotional intensity, with larger responses elicited in either unpleasant and pleasant contexts and that are most pronounced in those that rated highly arousing.

During picture perception, for example, many studies have found increased skin conductance when people view pictures rated as emotional, compared to neutral, regardless of whether they are rated pleasant or unpleasant in hedonic valence (e.g., Lang et al., 1993; Winton, Putnam, & Krause, 1984; see Figure 25.3, top middle). Moreover, electrodermal reactions increase with increases in defensive or appetitive activation, with the most arousing pleasant and unpleasant contents (e.g., erotica, threat, and mutilation) prompting the largest responses (Bradley et al., 2001a). Similarly, when listening to affective sounds (Bradley & Lang, 2000; Verona et al., 2004) or music (Gomez & Danuser, 2004), skin conductance activity increases as the acoustic stimuli are rated higher in emotional arousal, regardless of hedonic valence (see Figure 25.3, bottom middle). Demonstrating consistent modulation by affective intensity across perceptual contexts, elevated electrodermal reactions are also clearly found when people view film clips that are either unpleasant (Kunzmann, Kupperbusch, & Levenson, 2005; Palomba et al., 2000) or pleasant (Christie & Friedman, 2004). When hedonic valence and emotional arousal of film stimuli were co-varied, skin conductance responses were largest for highly arousing films, irrespective of hedonic valence (Gomez et al., 2004), consistent with the notion that these reactions primarily reflect differences in emotional arousal, rather than hedonic valence.

Whereas the cardiac patterns seen in perception and imagery are quite different, skin conductance responses during imagery often show the same modulation by emotional arousal as perceptual contexts. For instance, Miller, Patrick, and Levenston (2002) found increased skin conductance responses when people imagined pleasant or unpleasant, compared to neutral, events, and these responses were accentuated when personally relevant scenes were imagined. Similarly, as Figure 25.4 (left panel) illustrates, anticipating the presentation of a threatening stimulus (e.g., shock; Bradley, Moulder, & Lang, 2005) or a pleasant stimulus (e.g., a picture of erotica; Sabatinelli, Bradley, & Lang, 2001) also prompts large skin conductance changes that reflect increased arousal during anticipation.

Taken together, rather than simply responding to aversive stimulation, the sympathetic nervous system, as indexed by the electrodermal reaction, is also engaged by appetitive activation, and, moreover, appears to be similarly activated in perception, imagery, and anticipation contexts. One interpretation is that this physiological measure reflects the primary nature of emotions as action dispositions that are mediated by sympathetic activity preparing the organism for fight, flight, and other appropriate appetitive and defensive behaviors. Regardless of whether the affect cue involves perceptual, imaginal, or anticipatory processing, those that activate the fundamental appetitive or defensive motivation systems engage measurable sympathetic activity, as measured by the palmar skin conductance response. Thus, whereas the cardiac response differs in emotional perception and emotional imagery, presumably reflecting differences in sensory intake in the different induction contexts, the electrodermal response in both perception and imagination indexes the preparation for action that is the hallmark of both motivation and emotion.

Facial EMG and emotion

Facial expressions of emotion, such as frowns, grimaces, smiles, and so on are often the most overt signs of emotional engagement, and are mediated by muscles that are attached to the skin of the face, all of which are innervated by the facial nerve (cranial nerve VII) via the facial motor nucleus located in the pons. The facial motor nucleus is organized into subdivisions (medial, lateral, dorsal, intermediate) that contain the motor neurons controlling different facial muscles, with the upper half of the nucleus containing neurons that generally control the lower part of the face, and neurons in the lower half innervating the upper facial muscles. Different branches of the facial nerve (temporal, zygomatic, buccal, cervical, and marginal mandibular) innervate different facial muscles, with combinations of activity in different muscles related to various facial expressions that are common in emotion.

In the Facial Action Coding System (FACS; Ekman & Friesen, 1986; Ekman, Friesen, & Hager, 2002), "action units" that correspond to observable activity in specific muscles and facial regions can be scored by an observer. In a recent study, Kohler et al. (2004) used FACS to code expressions in a set of 128 photographs that included posed and evoked faces displaying happy, sad, fearful, and angry expressions. Their primary goals were to identify the characteristic action units present in different expressions and to determine whether unique action units are related to correct recognition performance (in a sample of naive participants). For happy expressions, an action unit associated with a lip corner pull was present in all expressions, and appeared to be critical in both defining and recognizing a smile. On the other hand, expressions of sadness elicited characteristic features (e.g., furrowed eyebrows, opened mouth with raised upper lip) but no clear unique features, seeming instead to rely on a combination of features for successful recognition.

Identification of more subtle changes in facial muscle activity can be achieved by monitoring electromyographic (EMG) activity using electrodes placed over appropriate facial muscles. In fact, appropriate facial EMG activity accompanies changes in appetitive and defensive activation in a number of different induction contexts (e.g., Fridlund, Schwartz, & Fowler, 1984; Tassinary, Cacioppo, & Geen, 1989). Most commonly, measurement of activity

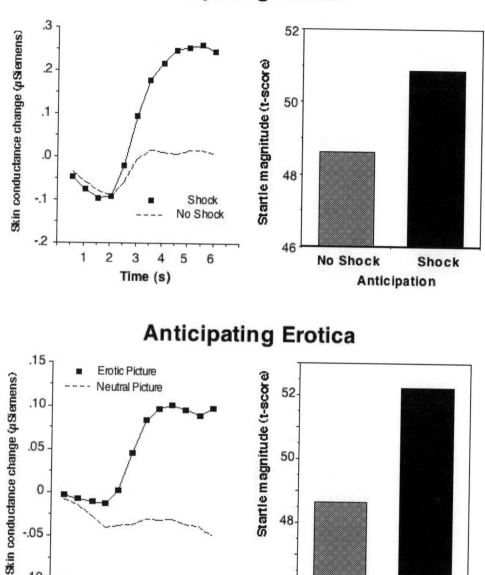

Figure 25.4. Electodermal and startle reflex magnitude when anticipating an electric shock or anticipating the presentation of an erotic picture show similar modulation. Based on data reported by Bradley et al. (2005) and Sabatinelli et al. (2001).

over the muscles associated with frowning and smiling have been used as indices of affective engagement in perception, imagery, and anticipation.

The corrugator supercilii muscles, located above and between the eyes, are responsible for lowering and contraction of the brows. This facial action is held to be an index of distress (see Ekman, Levenson, & Freissen, 1983; Fridlund & Izard, 1983, for a review) and firing of motor units in this muscle region is obtained if a stimulus is judged to be unpleasant (even if the degree of unit activity is insufficient to produce visible

brow movement). Significant contraction of the corrugator muscle occurs when viewing pictures that are rated as unpleasant, compared to neutral pictures (Cacioppo et al., 1986; Lang et al., 1993), and shows similar modulation when people listen to unpleasant, compared to neutral, sounds, as Figure 25.3 (left panel) illustrates. Moreover, activity measured over this muscle often shows relaxation below baseline activity for materials rated high in pleasure.

Larsen, Norris, and Cacioppo (2003) measured facial EMG activity in a variety of different perceptual contexts, including viewing affective pictures, listening to affective sounds, and reading affective words. In all contexts, a highly significant linear relationship was found relating corrugator supercilii EMG activity to hedonic valence, with greater corrugator supercilii activity elicited when viewing the most unpleasant stimuli. Moreover, the most highly pleasant materials prompted significant inhibition, consistent with the hypothesis that appetitive and defensive activation show reciprocal effects on this facial muscle.

When exploring specific picture contents, Bradley et al. (2001a) found that all unpleasant picture contents prompted significant increases (over neutral) in corrugator EMG activity, with pictures of mutilations and contamination (i.e., disgust) prompting slightly larger changes than other unpleasant stimuli. Although women responded with greater overall facial EMG activity than men, all participants showed significant increases in corrugator EMG reactivity when viewing unpleasant pictures (Bradley et al., 2001b), indicating that both men and women facially respond to aversive stimuli. The least corrugator EMG activity was obtained for pleasant pictures depicting babies and families, which are rated quite high in pleasure, but relatively low in arousal.

Activity measured over the *zygomaticus major* muscle occurs when the cheek is drawn back or tightened (Tassinary, Cacioppo, & Geen, 1989), and this muscle is involved in facial expressions of smiling. Because emotional expressions such as smiling have communicative function in human culture and can be initiated for instrumental effect, their connection to a reflexive psychophysiology of emotion cannot be automatically assumed. That is, a person may choose to look "happy," engaging in deceptive behavior to achieve some goal, in much the same way that individuals may, for similar reasons of social use, *say* that they are "happy"(or angry) in the absence of any confirming physiology. Ekman, Davidson, and Friesen (1980) have considered this issue, and noted an interesting observational difference between true and false smiles. Whereas an authentic "Duchenne" smile includes both action of the zygomaticus major and orbicularis oculi muscles, false "social" smiles involve only the zygomaticus major muscle.

Consistent with the hypothesis that facial EMG activity in picture perception reflects an authentic emotional reaction, Cacioppo et al. (1986) found co-activation of the zygomaticus major and orbicularis oculi muscles when participants viewed pleasant, compared to neutral, pictures. When specific picture contents were assessed (Bradley et al., 2001a), co-activation in these facial muscles was again apparent, and was most pronounced for pictures judged to be high in pleasure, but not highly arousing, including pictures of babies, families, and food. Facial EMG activity consistent with smiling at babies and families was only apparent for women (Bradley et al., 2001b), however, and neither men nor women showed any evidence that pictures of highly arousing erotica evoked facial expressions related to smiling.

Unpleasant materials that are highly arousing also prompt slight increases in activity measured over the zygomaticus major muscle. Lang et al. (1993) noted a significant quadratic trend for this zygomatic muscle in which highly unpleasant pictures prompted significant activity (although less than for highly pleasant stimuli). Larsen, Norris, and Cacioppo (2003) replicated this finding, and further found that this pattern was more representative of reactions to pictures and sounds; simply reading unpleasant words did not engage strong activity over this facial muscle. When exploring specific picture contents, Bradley et al. (2001a) found that increased zygomatic activity during unpleasant picture viewing tended to co-occur with significant changes in both the corrugator supercilii and the orbicularis oculi muscles. Co-activation in these three muscles was associated with a pattern of facial activity that was most pronounced for pictures rated as disgusting, including mutilated bodies and contamination (e.g., spoiled food, etc.) scenes. Thus, this muscle also appears to be active in a facial expression of disgust that involves both lowering of the brow and tightening of the cheek and eyes.

Studies investigating facial EMG activity during mental imagery have also consistently found that activity measured over the corrugator supercilii and zygomaticus major muscle regions index the hedonic valence of the imagined stimulus (e.g., van Oyen Witvliet & Vrana, 1995; Fiorito and Simons, 1994; Fridlund, Schwartz, & Fowler, 1984). Schwartz and his colleagues (e.g., Schwartz, Ahern, & Brown, 1979; Schwartz, Brown, & Ahern, 1980) conducted a series of studies which indicated that corrugator and zygomatic EMG activity primarily differentiated between imagery of negative (e.g., fear, sadness, anger) and positive (e.g., happy) emotions, whereas EMG activity over the masseter and lateral frontalis muscle regions did not differ. Importantly, Schwartz, Brown, and Ahern (1980) also found that women were more reactive than men, consistent with the sex differences obtained in picture perception.

Summarizing the imagery work, Cacioppo et al. (1993) conclude that covert measures of facial EMG activity in imagery may reflect "... a rudimentary bivalent evaluative disposition or *motivational tendency* rather than discrete emotions" (p. 136). Facial expressions of disgust may be an exception, however. In a recent study in our laboratory, imagining unpleasant events was, as usual, associated with increased corrugator EMG activity for scenes that people label as evoking fear, anger, and disgust. On the other hand, similar to picture perception, scenes involving disgust uniquely involved co-activation of corrugator supercillii and orbicularis oculi EMG activity, consistent with the idea that EMG activity reliably discriminates facial expressions of disgust in both perception and imagery.

Startle reflex modulation

In most mammals, an abrupt sensory event will prompt a startle response, a chained series of rapid extensor-flexor movements that cascade throughout the body (Landis &

Hunt, 1939). This reaction is a defensive reflex, facilitating escape in simpler organisms, and perhaps still serving a protective function in more complex animals (i.e., avoiding organ injury as in the eyeblink, or in retraction of the head to avoid attack from above, Yeomans, Steidl, & Li, 2000). When under threat (of pain or predation) animals show an exaggerated startle reflex. As first described by Brown, Kalish, and Farber (1951), the amplitude of the acoustically elicited startle reflex in rats is increased when elicited in the presence of a light previously paired with footshock. Humans similarly show larger startle blink reflexes when processing cues previously paired with exposure to aversive shock (Hamm et al., 1993).

Davis (1989; Davis, Hitchcock, & Rosen, 1987) and others (e.g., Koch & Schnitzler, 1997) have systematically investigated the neural circuitry underlying potentiation of the startle response during aversive learning in animals. When stimulated by an abrupt noise, the afferent path of the reflex proceeds from the cochlear nucleus to the pontine reticular formation; from there efferent connections pass through spinal neurons to the reflex effectors. This is the basic obligatory circuit, driven by the parameters of the input stimulus (e.g., stimulus intensity, frequency, steepness of the onset ramp). A secondary circuit, intersecting this primary reflex pathway, determines startle potentiation after fear conditioning. There is now overwhelming evidence that the amygdala is the critical structure mediating this effect: First, there are direct projections from the central nucleus of the amygdala to the reticular site which mediates potentiation (i.e., nucleus reticularis pontis caudalis); second, electrical stimulation of the amygdala's central nucleus enhances startle reflex amplitude; finally, and most important, lesions of the amygdala abolish fear conditioned startle potentiation (Davis, 1989).

In studies with human beings, rapid eye closure is one of the most reliable components of the behavioral sequence that constitutes the startle response, and the associated blink reflex can be measured electromyographically by placing sensors over the orbicularis oculi muscle beneath the eye (see Figure 25.5). When startle probes are administered in the context of picture perception, blink responses are reliably potentiated when viewing unpleasant pictures, and inhibited when viewing pleasant pictures, compared to neutral picture processing (see Figure 25.5; Vrana, Spence, & Lang, 1988; see Bradley, Cuthbert, & Lang, 1999 for an overview). These effects have proven highly replicable in the picture perception context (e.g., Bradley et al., 2001a; Buchanan, Tranel, & Adolphs, 2004; Cook et al., 1992; Dichter et al., 2004; Hamm et al., 1997; Vanman et al., 1996). Startle potentiation is largest for unpleasant pictures that are rated highly arousing (e.g., threat and mutilation), while the most arousing pleasant pictures evidence the largest startle inhibition (e.g., erotica and romance; Bradley et al., 2001a, Schupp et al., 2004).

The startle reflex is modulated by affective valence during picture viewing regardless of whether the startle probe is visual, acoustic, or tactile (e.g., Bradley, Cuthbert, & Lang, 1991; Hawk & Cook, 1997), indicating that modality-specific processes are not central in these modulatory effects. Affective modulation of startle is also not confined to static visual percepts: The startle reflex is modulated by affective valence when dynamic visual stimuli (i.e., affective films) are presented (Jansen and Frijda, 1994; Koukounas & McCabe, 2001), or when the sensory modality involves odors (Erlichman et al., 1995). Furthermore, when the emotional stimuli consist of short, 6 s sound clips of various affective events (e.g., sounds of love-making; babies crying; bombs bursting), and the startle probe is a visual light flash, the same pattern of affective modulation is obtained, suggesting that its mediation in perception is broadly motivational and thus consistent across affective foregrounds of different stimulus modalities (Bradley & Lang, 1998).

In the picture viewing context, a search for differences in startle potentiation when viewing different categories of unpleasant pictures have produced mixed results. Balaban and Taussig (1994) first found evidence for greater reflex potentiation when viewing pictures depicting fearful scenes than other unpleasant contents, and more recently Stanley and Knight (2004) reported greater potentiation when viewing threat, compared to mutilation, pictures. On the other hand, Yartz and Hawk (2002) found that startle reflexes elicited when viewing disgusting pictures that either involved blood or other disgusting contents (e.g., bugs, toilets, etc.) showed potentiation similar to that elicited when viewing pictures of threat. Bradley et al. (2001a), in a similar design, also found equivalent potentiation for threatening scenes involving animals (presumably eliciting fear) and disgusting contents (e.g., mutilations or others), although fearful pictures of human attack (particularly toward the viewer) prompted slightly (and significantly) larger reflexes than pictures of mutilated humans. Taken together, although there is some evidence of slightly larger reflex potentiation when viewing scenes involving threat or imminent danger (fear?), the effect is somewhat variable, possible reflecting differences in material or participant samples.

The defense cascade in picture perception. Like normal subjects, specific phobics show potentiated startles when viewing unpleasant pictures. However, startle reflexes are even more enhanced when these subjects view pictures of the objects they fear (Hamm et al., 1997). On the other hand, the typical bradycardia obtained during unpleasant picture viewing does not characterize the response of phobic subjects to pictures of objects they fear (e.g., Hamm et al., 1997; Klorman, Weissbert, & Wissenfeld, 1977): rather, when high fear subjects view pictures of the phobic object, the heart accelerates. Also unlike non-phobic subjects, they quickly terminate "looking" in a free-viewing situation. Thus, whereas reflex potentiation to aversive materials characterizes responses for highly arousing unpleasant pictures for both normal and phobic subjects, cardiac and other behavioral measures of attentive

Startle Reflex & Emotional Perception

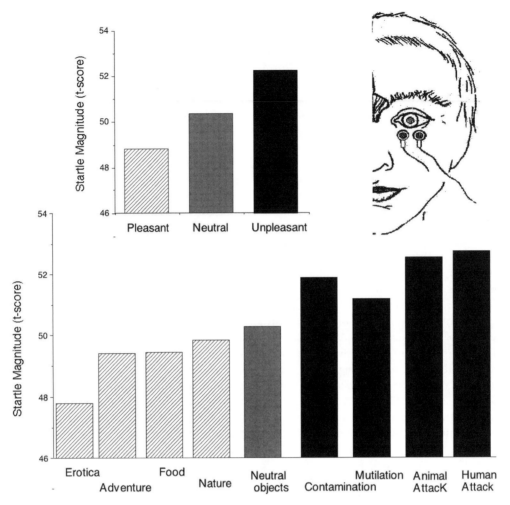

Figure 25.5. During picture perception, the startle blink reflex is modulated by hedonic valence, with potentiation during unpleasant picture viewing, and attenuation during appetitive picture viewing. Startle reflex modulation is greatest for pictures that are rated as highly arousing, including erotica, threat, and mutilation. Based on data from Bradley et al. (2001a).

orienting are absent when phobics process very highly fearful content.

These data suggest that, instead of a single response indicating activation of the defensive motivation system, one observes instead a cascade of physiological responses, changing in different ways as activation increases. The idea that defense involves stages of responding has been advocated by a number of theorists, including Tinbergen (1969), Blanchard and Blanchard (1989), and Fanselow (1994). Based on data obtained during picture perception, we have proposed a similar cascade of changing defensive reflexes, determined by increasing metabolic and neuromuscular mobilization that is paralleled by greater judged emotional arousal. Figure 25.6 illustrates the defense cascade model in picture perception.

Stimuli that moderately activate the defensive system prompt a pattern of responding that is suggestive of oriented attention, in which measurable conductance

changes are obtained, the heart decelerates under vagal control, and startle reflexes are not potentiated. In fact, at lower levels of rated arousal, the startle reflex is inhibited when viewing unpleasant, compared to neutral, pictures (Bradley et al., 2001a; Cuthbert, Bradley, & Lang, 1996). Thus, at this first stage of defensive activation, heightened attention and orienting are apparent, signaled by cardiac deceleration and dampened startle reflexes, both of which are consistent with the hypothesis of greater sensory intake and resource allocation to a meaningful foreground. (As Lacey [1958] recognized, unpleasant events are not automatically "rejected," but instead evoke a physiology consistent with sustained attention.) This reflex pattern changes dramatically, however, when danger becomes more imminent, with mobilization and active defense reflexes occurring later in the sequence. Evidence of a change in defensive posture is first seen in the startle reflex: As the stimulus becomes more threatening/arousing

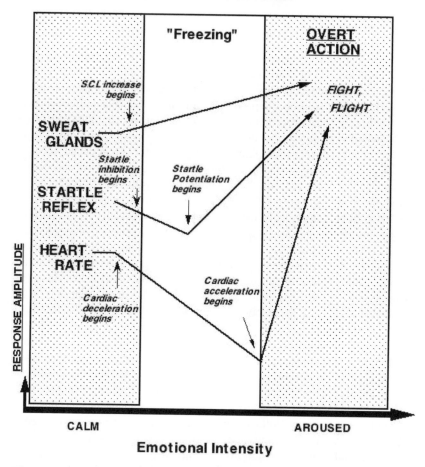

Defense Cascade
during aversive perception

Figure 25.6. Stages of defensive responding are depicted, in which different physiological systems change at different rates, based on the intensity of activation in defensive motivation (see Lang, Bradley, & Cuthbert, 1997).

(a negative outcome is more imminent), startle amplitude increases and the reflex is potentiated rather than inhibited. As defensive activation increases, just prior to action, the heart rate response is also modulated: Vagal release is followed by a sympathetically driven acceleration that is the classic cardiac defense response. Thus, when processing pictures of their feared objects, phobic subjects do not show the initial decelerative stage of defense, but instead show an immediate cardiac acceleration, accompanied by dramatically large startle reflex potentiation. In effect, phobics are more aroused by these stimuli, and thus further along in the 'defense cascade' than normal subjects processing standard unpleasant pictures.

Reflex modulation in anticipation. The defense cascade model describes defensive reactions that occur specifically concurrent with *perception* of external stimuli, i.e., when sensory stimuli are processed that vary symbolically in degree of threat (probability of harm), and thus weakly or strongly activate the defense motivational system. In the picture-viewing context, of course, pleasant stimuli (varying in arousal) do not prompt a similar change in startle probe modulation. Rather, there is a progressive augmentation of the cardiac decelerative/inhibitory startle attentive set that is maximal at the highest levels of picture arousal (most dramatically, for pleasant erotic images). Interestingly, however, and highlighting the importance of understanding the local effects of the emotion inducing context, these two physiological measures (heart rate and startle blink reflexes) show parallel responses to pleasant and unpleasant stimuli in the context of *anticipation* and *imagery.*

For instance, when men reporting high fear of snakes anticipated (during a 6 s interval) presentation of an erotic, snake or neutral picture, startle reflexes were significantly and similarly potentiated during anticipation of either type of arousing content – snakes or erotica – compared to neutral household objects (Sabatinelli, Bradley, & Lang, 2001). The same pattern of reflex potentiation was found when non-fearful participants anticipated viewing a selection of pleasant or unpleasant images, relative to anticipation of neutral pictures (Nitschke et al., 2002). Furthermore, numerous studies have demonstrated that the startle reflex is reliably enhanced during an interval when participants anticipate the possibility of receiving electric shock, compared to a "safe" period (e.g., Grillon et al., 1991; Bradley, Moulder, & Lang, 2005). Recently, reflex potentiation was consistently observed in our laboratory during an interval in which participants anticipated the possibility of winning a substantial sum of money. Similarly, Skolnick and Davidson (2002) found reliable reflex potentation when participants anticipated winning in a gambling game, as well during a period in which they anticipated the presentation of aversive noise.

Reflex modulation in imagery. Several studies (Witlviet & Vrana, 1995; Robinson & Vrana, 2000) have examined startle modulation during text-driven imagery, varying both the hedonic valence (pleasant, unpleasant) and judged arousal (low, high) of the imagery scripts. Although startle blinks were consistently larger when imagining unpleasant, compared to pleasant scenes; nevertheless, reflexes elicited when imaging pleasant, arousing scenes were potentiated relative to pleasant scenes rated lower in arousal. Bradley, Cuthbert, and Lang (1995) obtained similar results: Compared to imagining neutral scenes, the startle reflex was significantly potentiated when imagining either unpleasant or pleasant events.

In a series of imagery studies conducted in our laboratory, the pattern of startle modulation that we obtained replicated Vrana and colleagues, with low arousal scenes again prompting significantly smaller blink reflexes than high arousal scenes during both pleasant and unpleasant imagery. No differences were found among unpleasant scenes rated as highly arousing (regardless of different emotion reports of eliciting fear, anger, or disgust). However, when the participants imagined pleasant, highly arousing scenes (e.g., winning the lottery), startle reflex magnitude was substantially greater than for less arousing pleasant contents, and equivalent to blinks elicited when imagining highly arousing unpleasant scenes. Miller et al. (2000) also found that blinks elicited during pleasant (arousing) imagery were equivalent to those elicited during unpleasant (arousing) imagery, noting this particularly for imagined scenes that were personally relevant.

Thus, different from the modulatory pattern found during *perception* and attentive intake (i.e., the reflex inhibition seen during picture perception), reflex modulation during mental *imagery* is more similar to that observed in *anticipation*, that is, the startle reflex is potentiated when imagining highly arousing events, regardless of their affective valence. Overall, the startle data suggest that reflex inhibition – both during appetitive perception and early defensive vigilance – accompanies sensory processing and heightened attention to external stimulation, with a resulting inhibition of reactions to other sensory input (as is also found for non-startling reaction time probes, Bradley, Cuthbert, & Lang, 1996). However, when the perceptual stimulus is sufficiently arousing (proximal, threatening, imminently aversive), active defense mobilization ensues, priming related defensive reflexes, such as the startle blink.

During the anticipation of a future event (or during mental imagery), however, there is generally no concurrent sensory intake that competes with startle probe processing. Moreover, during mental imagery, the dominant cardiac pattern is accelerative, rather than decelerative, consistent with the hypothesis that preparation for action, rather than sensory intake, characterizes imaginal processing. It is also instructive to consider the heart rate response that can occur in an anticipatory context: Chase, Graham, and Graham (1968) noted that if the anticipated event requires vigorous motor action, the anticipatory cardiac response is a marked acceleration. Assuming that affective anticipation involves active preparation, potentiation of both autonomic (heart rate acceleration) and somatic motor responses (startle reflex potentiation) might be an expected consequence. When comparing the responses of fearful subjects in anticipation and mental imagery, Lang et al. (1983) noted that, for snake phobics, increases in both skin conductance and heart rate were found both when imagining scenes involving snakes and when anticipating an actual confrontation with an alive snake. One is tempted to conclude that similar cognitive processes, and a physiology primed for action, may characterize both anticipation and imagination of emotional events, prompting similar modulation by emotion for cardiac, electrodermal, and startle responses.

THE NEUROANATOMY OF EMOTION

Understanding the neural circuits mediating the psychophysiology of emotion will depend to some degree on determining which brain structures are important in controlling the peripheral autonomic and somatic responses that together define emotion. Not surprisingly, control systems occur at every level of the central nervous system: from the spinal cord to the brain stem to sub-cortical and cortical structures (for a more extensive discussion, see LeDoux, 1987; Gellhorn & Loofbourrow, 1963; Guyton & Hall, 1996). Thus, for instance, mechanisms in the spinal cord can affect the level of activity in sympathetic and parasympathetic fibers in the absence of supraspinal controls. Among the more important *brain stem* control structures is the medulla oblongata: Electrical stimulation of the rostral portion of this structure evokes sympathetic reactions throughout the body, including heart rate and blood pressure increases, dilation of pupil, inhibition of gastro-intestinal activity, secretion of sweat, etc. Conversely, activation of the vagal nucleus of the medulla oblongata causes a decrease in heart rate and blood pressure and an increase in gastrointestinal activity – reactions associated with parasympathetic activity. Because of its ability to control many elements of autonomic function, the medulla oblongata has been proposed as the final common pathway for autonomic responses associated with defense reactions (LeDoux, 1987).

Cannon originally advocated that key structures in the brain, particularly the hypothalamus and thalamus, were important in controlling peripheral emotional reactions, which was supported by a number of animal studies demonstrating that electrical stimulation of the hypothalamus produced physiological reactions associated with sympathetic activation, and even full motor sequences indicative of emotion, including freezing, piloerection, hissing, and attack (collectively termed the *defense reaction*, Hess & Burgger, 1943), as well as grooming, mating, and feeding/drinking. Lesions of the hypothalamus (Bard, 1934) effectively eliminated these reactions. Despite proposing a much more extensive neural circuit, Papez (1937) also focused on the hypothalamus as a central structure in mediating emotion, particularly bodily responses. Although Papez's circuit is generally considered incomplete today, mainly because it neglects to include structures currently thought important in emotion (e.g., amygdala) and includes structures that are now recognized as more important for memory (e.g., hippocampus; LeDoux, 1987) certain key structures in Papez' circuit, such as the thalamus and cingulate cortex have been implicated in recent neuroimaging explorations of emotional processing (e.g., Breiter et al., 1997; George et al., 1995; Lane, Reiman, Ahern et al., 1997; Lane, Reiman, Bradley et al., 1997).

Prior to the advent of neuroimaging techniques, information regarding the neural circuits mediating emotional experience and expression relied on data from animal studies and patients suffering different types of brain damage. New technologies for measuring brain activity during emotional processing (including PET, fMRI) now allow an investigation of cortical and subcortical activity during emotional processing in awake alert human participants. The explosion in neuroimaging studies over the past 10 years has produced a burgeoning data base in which new studies are added at an exponential rate, many of these focused on emotion and affect. Making sense of this large data base will rely, again, on careful attention to the specific context of emotional induction in the scanner.

For instance, in a recent meta-analysis of brain activation during emotional processing, data from over 100 PET and fMRI studies were aggregated across a number of different induction contexts (e.g., viewing facial expressions, listening to music, conditioned fear, anticipating pain, and so on (Murphy, Nimmo-Smith, & Lawrence, 2003). When the resulting activation clusters that reportedly varied with emotion were plotted in a 3-dimensional space defined by the Talairach-Tourneau coordinates, a figure eerily reminiscent of the entire brain emerges. Assuming that different perceptual, anticipatory, imaginal, and action contexts prompt activity in divergent and overlapping neural circuits, it may be difficult to understand the neural circuitry of emotion in the absence of making comparisons that control the specific context of emotion induction.

In another meta-analysis (Phan et al., 2004), an effort to control the specific context of the emotional induction was made by comparing neural activation in visual perception, auditory perception, or imagery contexts as they varied with fear, sadness, anger, etc. Across all studies, no specific brain region was reliably activated, suggesting that emotion is not mediated by a specific neural structure. The region most likely to be active across different induction contexts was the prefrontal cortex (medial), a structure highlighted as central in emotion by Davidson (2003), whose work on hemispheric asymmetry indicates tonic differences in resting EEG in frontal regions as a function of affect and temperament (Davidson, 2002).

Regions implicated as active in different affective induction contexts included a greater probability of anterior cingulate and insula activation during emotional imagery, with affective visual perception more likely to additionally include greater activation of occipital cortex and the amygdala. Animal and human patient studies had already noted the potential importance of the amygdala in emotional processing, based, to a large extent, on the same type of data originally invoked to support the hypothalamus as the center of the emotion system. Thus, both lesion and stimulation studies in animals indicate that specific nuclei in this structure mediate specific emotional phenomena, both appetitive and defensive (e.g., Amaral et al., 1992; Gaffen, 1992). Stimulation of the amygdala produces rage, attack and defense reactions similar to those earlier elicited by activation of the hypothalamus

and lesions of the amygdala eliminate the fear-potentiated startle response (Davis, 1986), and have been implicated in disrupting appetitive behaviors such as mating, food-getting, and reward learning (Gaffen, 1992).

The amygdala includes multiple afferent and efferent connections to cortical, subcortical, and brainstem structures that have been implicated in mediating the autonomic and somatic responses involved in emotional behaviors (see Davis & Lang, 2003). Inputs to the lateral nucleus of the amygdala include those from unimodal cortical sensory areas, including vision, audition and somatosensory (via the insula) information, as well as from polysensory association cortex. Olfactory input is relayed to the periamygdaloid nucleus (rather than lateral) and gustatory information may also be relayed to this nucleus via its thalamic input. Consistent with this, a number of neuroimaging studies have reported significant activation of the amygdala during perception of aversive visual, olfactory, auditory and gustatory stimuli (see Zald, 2003, for a review).

The outputs from the amygdala are extensive as well, and include almost all of the structures highlighted as important in emotional reactions, including direct connections to the hypothalamus, the central gray, the brain stem, the striatum, and cortical structures including the cingulate gyrus, frontal lobe, visual cortex, and more. The amygdala's central nucleus sends prominent projections to the lateral hypothalamus – a key center activating the sympathetic branch of the autonomic nervous system in emotion (LeDoux, 1987). In addition, direct projections from the lateral extended amygdala go to the dorsal motor nucleus of the vagus, the nucleus of the solitary tract, and the ventrolateral medulla. These brainstem nuclei are known to regulate heart rate and blood pressure (Schwaber et al., 1982), and may thus modulate cardiovascular responses in emotion.

Subcortical structures such as the amygdala and hypothalamus are clearly central in the expression of emotion, particularly in mediating the defensive and appetitive responses that even animal subjects clearly display when under threat or seeking sustenance. With increasing brain complexity, however, the neural circuitry of emotion increasingly includes activation in numerous cortical structures that can modulate subcortical activation, and vice versa. During picture perception, for instance, both unpleasant and pleasant pictures prompt significantly greater activation throughout the visual sensory regions, including middle occipital, inferior occipital, and fusiform cortex, as illustrated in Figure 25.7 (top left; see Lang et al., 1998; Bradley et al., 2003).

As noted by Amaral et al. (1992), the amygdala is extensively interconnected with the visual sensory system, in the primate with bidirectional connections that could promote both initial amygdaloid access as well as later perceptual modulation through its efferent connections. These projections could potentially "close the loop" with the visual system (Amaral et al., 1992), representing an amygdala feedback circuit that may be significant for the

fMRI activity during Affective Picture Perception

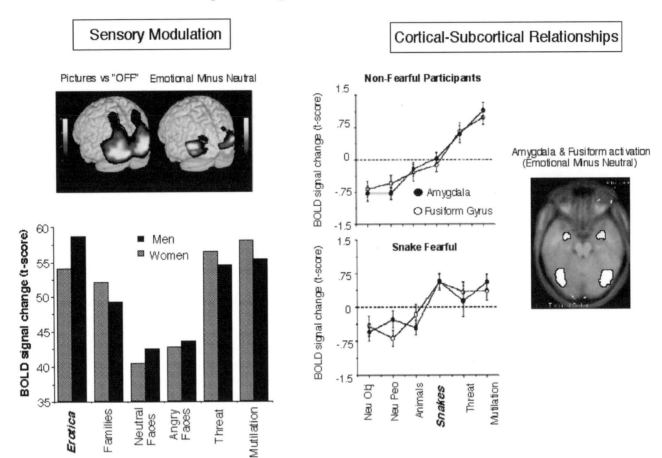

Figure 25.7. Neural activity measured during picture perception using functional magnetic resonance imaging shows greater activity in visual sensory cortex for emotional, compared to neutral, pictures, with men showing greater visual activation when viewing erotica than women. The covariation in activation for sensory fusiform cortex and the amygdala is strikingly high, with snake phobics responding with greater activation in both structures when viewing snakes than non-fearful participants. Based on data from Sabatinelli et al. (2004, 2005).

sustained perceptual evaluation seen in the early stages of emotional processing. Consistent with this, as illustrated in Figure 25.7 (top right), activation in the amygdala consistently and significantly covaries with the magnitude of activation in the fusiform areas (Sabatinelli et al., 2005). Moreover, this effect is even more apparent when snake phobics view pictures of snakes: both the amygdala and the visual fusiform areas show significantly greater activation than for those reporting no fear of snakes (Figure 25.7). These data are consistent with previous PET studies showing greater activation in the occipital cortex when phobics view pictures of phobic objects (e.g., Fredrikson et al., 1993), and furthermore, indicate that increased activity in visual cortex is paralleled by heightened activation of the amgydala as well.

It is now also clear that not only aversive stimuli activate the amygdala: Numerous studies have found significantly elevated functional activity in this structure when people view highly arousing pleasant pictures (e.g., Lane, Chua, &

Dolan, 1999; Garavan et al., 2001; see Zald, 2003). In fact, the covariation between activity in the amygdala and in visual association areas such as the fusiform cortex when people view erotica is identical to that obtained for highly aversive stimuli (see Figure 7, bottom left; Sabatinelli et al., 2005). Hamann, Herman, Nolan, and Wallen (2004) recently reported larger increases in bilateral amygdala activation (and hypothalamus) when men viewed erotica, compared to women, in a study that included pictures of erotic couples, opposite sex erotica and non-erotic couples. Relatedly, men also show greater functional activity in visual cortical regions viewing erotica, compared to women (Sabatinelli et al., 2004; see Figure 25.7, bottom left). These data are consistent with evaluative and physiological data which find that men rate erotica as more arousing than do women, and also show heightened electrodermal reactions (Bradley et al., 2001b), suggesting that visual cues depicting erotica vary in the magnitude of appetitive activation in men and women. Moreover, taken together,

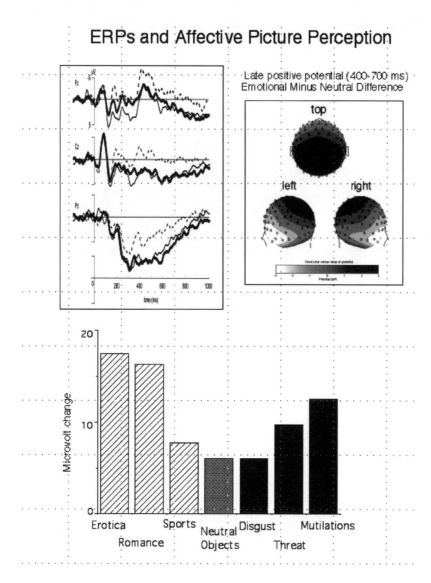

ERPs and Affective Picture Perception

Late positive potential (400-700 ms)
Emotional Minus Neutral Difference

Figure 25.8. The late positive potential elicited 300–1000 ms after picture onset is larger when viewing emotional (pleasant or unpleasant), compared to neutral, pictures, and is maximal over centro-parietal sites (based on data from Keil et al., 2002). The magnitude of the late positive potential is largest for emotional pictures that are rated as highest in arousal (based on data from Schupp et al., 2005).

these data suggest a link between the magnitude of physiological reflexes, such as electrodermal reactivity, and the magnitude of cortical and subcortical activation such as the BOLD signal in the fusiform cortex and the amygdala.

In fact, as fMRI, PET and other imaging modalities are used to explore emotion in the brain, the classic psychophysiology of bodily reflexes has an increasingly important role to play. In order to confirm that regional changes in neural activity are in fact related to affect and motivation, we will need to measure the well-established reflex physiology of emotion by simultaneously recording these, if possible, or by measuring these affective reactions in the same participants and paradigm in a simulated imaging context. As emotion researchers well know, evaluative reports are only loosely related to emotion's physiology, varying greatly in their covariation with context as well as with the personality and temperament of the participants, and can not serve as the sole measure of emotional engagement in neuroimaging explorations. (see Figure 25.8). Rather, standard practice in neuroimaging studies should be to include a coincident sample of measures

that assess hedonic valence (e.g., facial EMG or cardiac response in perceptual contexts) and emotional arousal (e.g., skin conductance; event-related potentials).

The neurophysiology of emotion

A second source of information regarding the neural activity accompanying affective processing is measurement of electrophysiological signals on the scalp, which provide excellent information regarding the timecourse of neural processing. When measuring event-related potentials during affective picture viewing, the most common finding is of a larger late positive potential (Cacioppo et al., 1994) that is elicited 300–1000 ms after picture onset and is maximal over centro-parietal sites. The late positive potential is more pronounced when viewing emotional (pleasant or unpleasant), compared to neutral, pictures (Palomba et al., 2000; Cuthbert et al., 2000), and is largest for highly arousing pictures of erotica, mutilation, and attack (Schupp et al., 2004).

On the other hand, although several studies have reported modulation of earlier ERP components, the nature and direction of the difference are quite variable across studies. For instance, Cuthbert et al. (2000) found that pleasant pictures prompted greater positivity in a 200–300 ms time window following picture onset (at frontal, central, and parietal sites) and a similar pattern of greater positivity over parietal, central, and frontal sites for pleasant pictures in this time window was reported by Palomba, Angrilli, and Mini (1997).

Using a dense sensor array, a variety of effects that are maximal over occipital sensors have also been reported in early time windows. Using a relatively slow (1.5 s) presentation, emotional pictures (pleasant or unpleasant) have prompted less positivity over occipital sensors than neutral pictures in a 200–300 ms time window following picture onset (e.g., Schupp et al., 2003). On the other hand, when pictures are presented very rapidly (e.g., 3 per second), a somewhat different pattern is obtained, with emotional pictures prompting greater negativity than neutral pictures over occipital sensors which is again is maximal 200–300 ms after picture onset (Junghofer et al., 2001).

Even earlier effects, in the neighborhood of 100 ms following picture onset have also been reported. Larsen, Norris, and Cacioppo (2003) reported an occipital P1 (about 114 ms after picture processing) that was larger for unpleasant, compared to pleasant, pictures in a design which assessed ERPs to pictures presented in varying hedonic contexts. Keil et al. (2002), on the other hand, found a larger N1 occipitally specifically for pleasant, compared to unpleasant or neutral, pictures. Taken together, the variety of modulatory patterns by hedonic valence and/or emotional arousal very early in the viewing interval suggest that characteristics of specific stimulus sets, subject samples, or task parameters may contribute at least in part to early ERP differences during affective picture viewing, as the pattern of ERP modulation varies widely even in very similar picture perception contexts.

The larger late positive potential for emotional pictures (compared to neutral) is, however, a robust and well-replicated finding. It has also been reliably observed that the amplitude of the late potential increases systematically with the judged arousal of emotional pictures (Cuthbert et al., 2000). According to a biphasic view of emotion, motivationally relevant pictures activate reentrant projections from the anterior, basal brain, naturally engaging attentional resources and enhancing processing in the secondary and tertiary centers of the visual system (e.g., Amaral, 1992; Davis & Lang, 2003). Consistent with enhanced sensory processing, dipole source localization of the late positive potential highlights occipito-temporal and parietal sites. Using a dense sensor EEG array (129 electrodes), Keil et al. (2002) reported sources over both the occipito-temporal and posterior parietal areas that differed as a function of emotion, with greater source strength over these regions when viewing emotional, compared to neutral, pictures.

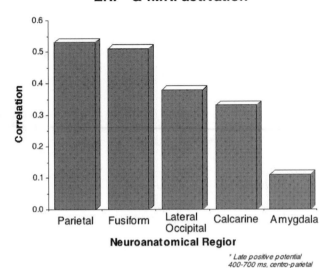

Figure 25.9. The correlation between the magnitude of the late positive potential scored in a window from 400–700 ms after picture onset over centro-parietal sites and the magnitude of BOLD activity in different brain regions, measured in the same participants viewing the same pictures in the scanner and in a simulated scanner using dense sensor (256 channels) EEG measurement.

In a recent study (Sabatinelli, Bradley, & Lang, 2005) ERPs and BOLD measures were monitored in the same experimental participants in the same picture perception paradigm, conducted once in the fMRI scanner and once in a MRI simulator (using dense sensor (256) EEG array). In the analysis of data from the fMRI session, greater BOLD activity for emotional, compared to neutral, picture viewing was found in regions that included the parietal, temporal (fusiform), lateral occipital, calcarine fissure, and amygdala. In the ERP session, the amplitude of the late positive potential recorded over centro-parietal sensors was (as seen previously) greater for emotional, compared to neutral, pictures. When correlations were performed that assessed covariation in the amplitude of the late positive potential and BOLD changes in each region (see Figure 25.9), the late positive potential correlated most strongly with activity in parietal and fusiform regions, and considerably less with either striate cortex or the deeper, more anterior amygdala. The data support the hypothesis that the emotion-related late positive potential is linked to enhanced processing in the dorsal (occipito-parietal) and ventral (occipito-temporal) processing visual streams.

EPILOGUE

Emotion and action

We have speculated that emotion and motivation are related processes, with both involving stimuli and events that move an organism towards action. Animal studies have clearly demonstrated that motivational circuits are initially activated by unconditioned stimuli – those that reflexively active appetitive and defensive systems. New, 'conditioned' stimuli come to activate the same circuits, however, through association with these primary appetitive and aversive reinforcers (e.g., Halgren, 1981). Because humans, as well as animals, learn to respond in adaptive ways to a wide variety of different environmental stimuli and events through this basic learning process, stimuli that activate appetitive and defensive systems through association can be idiosyncratic, not so clearly valenced to bystanders, as well as not obviously related to basic survival mechanisms.

The close link between motivational engagement and overt action has been loosened in humans, presumably due to the evolution of cortical control of these fundamental behaviors (i.e., inhibition and delay), and development of the ability to mentally process, off-line, events that are not currently perceptually prompted. Thus, emotions are most often reported during inhibitory states, when the body is mobilized to respond but action is restrained. Nonetheless, when a provocation is intense (e.g., the attacker threatens), action (i.e., fleeing) is evident, even in humans. Weaker affective cues (e.g., a movie of the same scene), on the other hand, may elicit only small increases in muscle tension, a mere remnant of the original defensive activity. Thus, emotional reactions in humans often involve primarily a disposition towards, or preparation for, action (Frijda, 1986; Arnold, 1970; Lang, 1987), rather than clear overt expression.

Conscious experience of emotion

If emotion is defined in terms of subjective reports, overt behaviors, and bodily responses, one might wonder which measure, if any, taps conscious feelings. The issue of the conscious experience of emotion, and how to approach it scientifically, has posed a number of problems in emotion research. As LeDoux (1995) notes, "... it is understandable why the field of emotion has had so much trouble in solving the problem of emotion – it has set as its goal the task of understanding consciousness" (p. 1059). Animal theorists, in general, balk at using the term 'emotion' in describing motivated behavior in their subjects, mainly because of the added assumption of conscious awareness. The study of motivated behavior, however, does not necessitate taking on the Goliath issue of consciousness, which, in the end, may prove to be more amenable to philosophic, rather than scientific, inquiry.

From a measurement perspective, one solution is to operationally define conscious experience on the basis of evaluative reports: People's reports (verbal or non-verbal) about their emotional experience could be used to index the private, internal state that is usually meant when one speaks of feelings. Some might argue this is unsatisfactory, due to the dependence of personal reports on cultural norms and individual differences in disclosure. In addition, feelings are often held to include the bodily reactions involved in emotional response, such as a racing heart, sweaty palms, and so on. A second solution has

been to include 'conscious awareness' as a fourth type of response system in emotion. The difficulty here is that one needs a reliable operational measure of consciousness, and, other than the three-system measures of behavior, physiology, and reports, there are currently no additional methods for directly measuring an internal feeling state. Although clearly central to the personal experience of emotion, the concept of internal states raises more questions than it answers in the scientific study of emotion, as it at can be simultaneously invoked as a cause (e.g., he ran because he felt afraid), an effect (e.g., he saw the bear and felt afraid) or, as James proposed, a consequence of the physiology (e.g., he saw the bear and ran so felt afraid).

Emotion and mood

In this chapter, the emphasis has been on discrete, phasic physiological responses to appetitive or defensive stimuli using cardiovascular, electrodermal, somatic, reflex, electrophysiological, and hemodynamic measures. Such phasic responding is representative of "emotional" reactions, whereas longer-lasting, more tonic changes in physiology are more representative of what is typically meant by "mood." In the laboratory, moods can be induced by sustained exposure to affective stimuli. Using sustained presentation of blocks of unpleasant, neutral, or pleasant pictures, for example, both corrugator EMG activity and the startle reflex increase in magnitude as the duration of aversive picture exposure increases (Bradley, Cuthbert, & Lang 1996; Smith, Bradley, & Lang 2005), indicative of a sustained and increasingly aversive mood state with the duration of exposure. Sustained exposure to pleasant stimuli, on the other hand, was less strongly associated with increasing appetitive activation in both studies.

Codispoti et al. (2003) recently explored neuroendocrine responses in the picture viewing context, using an intravenous catheter to draw blood samples during a 30-minute sustained exposure to mutilation, neutral, or erotic pictures presented in a blocked design on separate days. For unpleasant pictures, significant increases in noradrenaline, cortisol, and ACTH were found, compared to a baseline condition, consistent with previous data indicating that these neuroendocrine changes are associated with sympathetic activation mediated by sustained exposure to stress or aversive contexts (Lovallo & Thomas, 2000). For erotic pictures, these sympathetic changes were not obtained, with the main difference indicating in increase in prolactin from baseline to exposure. Taken together, whereas sustained exposure to aversive stimuli prompts tonic changes indicative of increasing defensive activation, sustained exposure to pleasant pictures is less strongly indicative of increasing appetitive activation.

Arousal and emotional intensity

The concept of arousal in the psychophysiological study of emotion has not fared well over the past thirty years, due in part to Lacey's (1967) observation that physiological responses do not uniformly, and in parallel, increase with increasing arousal. This is supported by more recent data which find that different physiological systems change at different rates, with some (such as startle potentiation) modulated at relatively lower levels of arousal than others (see Lang, 1995). Thus, while not unidirectionally resulting in an increased response in all systems arousal, or intensity is a critical factor in organizing the *pattern* of physiological responses in emotional (i.e., hedonically valenced) reactions. Emotional intensity presumably reflects the strength of activation in motivational systems subserving appetitive and defensive behaviors, and, as such, has clear ramifications for the amount and type of physiological response.

Theorists reasoning from data on motivated behavior in animals have relied on a proximity dimension to operationalize intensity: Fanselow's (1994) model is based on 'predator imminence' (the distance of the threatening stimulus from the organism), and Miller (1959) also operationalized arousal in terms of distance from an aversive or appetitive goal. Drawing parallels between emotional intensity and imminence, arousal in humans appears to reflect the degree to which a stimulus elicits appropriate appetitive or defensive behaviors. The importance of variations in arousal within separable appetitive and defensive systems points to the necessity of controlling affective intensity when making psychophysiological comparisons between pleasant and unpleasant emotion.

Revisiting discrete states: The tactics of emotion

Biphasic and discrete state views of emotion are complementary, rather than mutually exclusive positions, as many theorists recognize (e.g., Mehrabian & Russell, 1974). Not only can a specific state such as fear be categorized along a dimension of aversiveness, but a particular aversive event can be described as involving fear. The issue of how to define discrete states of emotion is central in terms of distinguishing among specific emotions. Ortony, Clore, and Collins (1988) have provided a compelling cognitive analysis detailing the features of situations and stimuli that may differentiate among events people generally label with different emotional terms. Consistent with a biphasic view, the superordinate division in their scheme is one of hedonic valence, differentiating among desirable and undesirable events. Specific features of environmental events are then proposed to control how different hedonically valenced events are labelled. For instance, whereas "distress" labels the *actual* occurrence of an undesirable event, and "joy," the actual occurrence of a desirable event, "fear" and "hope" label undesirable and desirable events that are only *anticipated*.

Although conscious feeling states are often considered synonymous with a discrete emotion perspective, this is not necessarily the case. Panksepp (1982), for instance, advocates a discrete emotion view in the rat, based on his hypothesis that four separate neural systems of expectancy, rage, fear, and panic underlie motivated behavior. In his view, these emotions stem from systems that

have evolved to deal with specific classes of environmental stimuli (i.e., positive incentives, irritation, threat, and loss). The dependence of emotional behavior on specific stimulus contexts is also clearly an issue in the psychophysiological study of emotion, and one that has been emphasized throughout this chapter. Identifying the critical features of specific induction contexts and their implications for physiological and behavioral output (e.g., freeze, flee, or fight) in investigations of emotion may help us to understand whether and when there is consistent physiological patterning as a function of contextual similarity.

Conclusion

This chapter has explored the psychophysiological study of emotion primarily from a biphasic motivational view. This view posits that human emotions are organized by neural systems of appetitive and defensive motivation that mediate a range of attentional and action reflexes presumably evolved from primitive approach and withdrawal tendencies. Discrete states of emotion, such as fear, anger, sadness, and so on are considered to be based on tactical responses (e.g., freezing, fight, flight) that are deployed by the motive systems in specific environmental circumstances. Rather than physiology being emotion-specific, as James suggested, it was emphasized throughout this chapter that understanding the psychophysiology of emotion will depend on close attention to the context of its occurrence in the laboratory and in life. Common induction paradigms in the psychophysiological study of affect, including perception, imagination, anticipation, and action, generate overlapping and divergent physiological signatures that suggest common motivational determination but which elude easy folk description and instead, demand understanding of the specific sensory, attentional, and action requirements elicited in different emotional/motivational contexts.

REFERENCES

Alpers, G. W., Wilhelm, F. H., & Roth, W. T. (2005). Psychophysiological assessment during exposure in driving phobic patients. *Journal of Abnormal Psychology*, 114(54), 126–139.

Amaral, D. G., & Price, J. L. (1984). Amygdalo-cortical connections in the monkey (Macaca fascicularis). *Journal of Comparative Neurology. 230*, 465–496.

Amaral, D. G., Price, J. L., Pitkanen, A., & Carmichael, S. T. (1992). Anatomical organization of the primate amygdaloid complex. In J. P. Aggleton (Ed.), *The amygdala: Neurobiological aspects of emotion, memory, and mental dysfunction*. (pp. 1–66). New York: Wiley.

Amrhein, C., Muhlberger, A., Pauli, P., Wiedemann, G. (2004). Modulation of event-related brain potentials during affective picture processing: a complement to startle reflex and skin conductance reponse? *International Journal of Psychophysiology*, 54, 231–240.

Arnold, M. B. (1960). *Emotion and personality* (Vols. I and II). New York: Columbia University.

Arnold, M. B. (1970). *Feelings and Emotions*. New York: Academia Press.

Ax, A. F. (1953). The physiological differentiation between fear and anger in humans. *Psychosomatic Medicine, 15*, 433–442.

Balaban, M. T., & Taussig, H. N. (1994). Salience of fear/threat in the affective modulation of the human startle blink. *Biological Psychology, 38*, 117–131.

Bard, P. (1934). The neuro-humoral basis of emotional reactions. In C. Murchinson (Ed.), *Handbook of general experimental psychology*. Worcester, MA: Clark University Press.

Bauer, R. M., & Craighead, W. E. (1979). Psychophysiological responses in the imagination of fearful and neutral situations: The effects of imagery instructions. *Behavior Therapy, 10*, 389–403.

Baum, A., Grunberg, N. E., & Singer, J. E. (1992). Biochemical measurements in the study of emotion. *Psychological Science, 3*, 56–60.

Berntson, G. G., Boysen, S. T., & Cacioppo, J. T. (1993). Neurobehavioral organization and the cardinal principle of evaluative bivalence. In F. M. Crinella & J. Yu (Eds.), *Annals of the New York Academy of Sciences: Vol. 702. Brain mechanisms: Papers in memory of Robert Thompson* (pp. 75–102). New York: New York Academy of Sciences.

Berntson, G. G., Cacioppo, J. T., & Quigley, K. S. (1991). Autonomic determinism: The modes of autonomic control, the doctrine of autonomic space, and the laws of autonomic constraint. *Psychological Review, 98*, 459–487.

Berntson, G. G., Cacioppo, J. T., Quigley, K. S., & Fabro, V. T. (1994). Autonomic space and psychophysiological response. *Psychophysiology, 31*, 44–61.

Blanchard, R. J., & Blanchard, D. C. (1989). Attack and defense in rodents as ethoexperimental models for the study of emotion. *Progress in Neuropsychopharmacological Biological Psychiatry, 13*, 3–14.

Bradley, M. M., Codispoti, M., Cuthbert, B. N., & Lang, P. J. (2001a). Emotion and motivation I: Defensive and appetitive reactions in picture processing. *Emotion, 1*, 276–298.

Bradley, M. M., Codispoti, M., Sabatinelli, D., & Lang, P. J. (2001b). Emotion and motivation II: Sex differences in picture processing. *Emotion, 1*, 300–319.

Bradley, M. M., Cuthbert, B. N., & Lang, P. J. (1991). Startle modification: Emotion or attention? *Psychophysiology, 27*(5) 513–522.

Bradley, M. M., Cuthbert, B. N., & Lang, P. J. (1995). Imagine that! Startle in action and perception. *Psychophysiology, 32*, S21.

Bradley, M. M., Cuthbert, B. N., & Lang, P. J. (1996). Picture media and emotion: Effects of a sustained affective context. *Psychophysiology, 33*, 662–670.

Bradley, M. M., Cuthbert, B. N., & Lang, P. J. (1999). Affect and the startle reflex. In M. E. Dawson, A. Schell, and A. Boehmelt (Eds.) *Startle Modification: Implications for Neuroscience, Cognitive Science and Clinical Science (pp. 157–183)*. Stanford, CA: Cambridge.

Bradley, M. M. & Lang, P. J. (2000). Affective reactions to acoustic stimuli. *Psychophysiology, 37*, 204–215.

Bradley, M. M., Moulder, M., & Lang, P. J. (2005). When good things go bad: The reflex physiology of defense. *Psychological Science, 16*, 468–473.

Bradley, M. M., Sabatinelli, D., Lang, P. J., Fitzsimmons, J. R., King, W. M., & Desai, P. (2003). Activation of the visual cortex in motivated attention. *Behavioral Neuroscience, 117*, 369–380.

Bradley, M. M. & Lang, P. J. (1999a). The international affective digitized sounds (IADS). Stimuli, instruction manual, and affective ratings. Technical Report B-2. The Center for Research in Psychophysiology, University of Florida.

Bradley, M. M. & Lang, P. J. (1999b). Affective norms for English words (ANEW): Stimuli, instruction manual, and affective ratings. Technical report C-1. The Center for Research in Psychophysiology, University of Florida.

Breiter, H. C., Gollub, R. L., Weisskoff, R. M., Kennedy, D. N., Makris, N., Berke, J. D., Goodman, J. M., Kantor, H. L., Gastfriend, D. R., Riorden, J. P., Mathew, R. T., Makris, N., Rosen, B. R., & Hyman, S. E. (1997). Acute effects of cocaine on human brain activity and emotion, *Neuron, 19*, 591–611.

Brown, J. S., Kalish, H. I., & Farber, I. E. (1951). Conditioned fear as revealed by magnitude of startle response to an auditory stimulus. *Journal of Experimental Psychology, 32*, 317–328.

Buchanan, T. W., Tranel, D., & Adolphs, R. (2004). Anteromedial temporal lobe damage blocks startle modulation by fear and disgust. *Behavioral Neuroscience, 118*, 429–437.

Cacioppo, J. T., Klein, D. J., Berntson, G. G., & Hatfield, E. (1993). The psychophysiology of emotion. In M. L. & J. M. Haviland (Eds.), *Handbook of emotions* (pp. 67–83). New York: Guilford Press.

Cacioppo, J. T., Petty, R. E., Losch, M. E., & Kim, H. S. (1986). Electromyographic activity over facial muscle regions can differentiate the valence and intensity of affective reactions. *Journal of Personality and Social Psychology, 50*, 260–268.

Cacioppo, J. T., & Berntson, G. G. (1994). Relationships between attitudes and evaluative space: A critical review with emphasis on the separability of positive and negative substrates. *Psychological Bulletin, 115*, 401–423.

Cacioppo, J. T., Berntson, G. G., & Crites, S. L. (1996). Social neuroscience: Principles of psychophysiological arousal and response. In E. T. Higgins and A. W. Kruglanski (Eds.) *Social psychology: Handbook of basic principles*. (pp. 72 –101). New York: Guilford Press.

Cacioppo, J. T., Crites, S. L., Gardner, W. L., & Berntson, Gary G. (1994). Bioelectrical echoes from evaluative categorization: I. A late positive brain potential that varies as a function of trait negativity and extremity. *Journal of Personality & Social Psychology, 67*, 115–125.

Cacioppo, J. T., Gardner, W. L., & Berntson, G. G. (1997). Beyond bipolar conceptualizations and measures: The case of attitudes and evaluative space. *Personality and Social Psychology Review, 1*, 3–25.

Campbell, B. A., Wood, G., & McBride, T. Origins of orienting and defensive responses: An evolutionary perspective. In P. J. Lang, R. F. Simons & M. T. Balaban (Eds.) *Attention and Orienting: Sensory and Motivational Processes*. (pp. 41–68). Hillsdale, NJ: Lawrence Erlbaum Associates, Inc.

Chase, W. G., Graham, F. K., & Graham, D. T. (1968). Components of heart rate response to anticipation of reaction time and exercise tasks. *Journal of Experimental Psychology, 76*, 642–648.

Christie, I. C., & Friedman, B. H. (2004). Autonomic specificity of discrete emotion and dimensions of affective space: A multivariate approach. *International Journal of Psychophysiology, 51*, 143–153.

Codispoti, M., Gerra, G., Montebarocci, O., Zaimovic, A., Raggi, M. A., & Baldaroa, B. (2003). Emotional perception and neuroendocrine changes. *Psychophysiology, 40*, 863–868.

Cook, E. W., III, Hawk, L. W., Davis, T. L., & Stevenson, V. E. (1991). Affective individual differences and startle reflex modulation. *Journal of Abnormal Psychology, 100*, 3–13.

Cook, E. W., III, Melamed, B. G., Cuthbert, B. N., McNeil, D. W., & Lang, P. J. (1988). Emotional imagery and the differential diagnosis of anxiety. *Journal of Consulting and Clinical Psychology, 56*, 734–740.

Cook, E. W., III, Davis, T. L., Hawk, L. W., Jr., Spence, E. L., & Gautier, C. H. (1992). Fearfulness and startle potentiation during aversive visual stimuli. *Psychophysiology, 29*, 633–645.

Cuthbert, B. N., Bradley, M. M., & Lang, P. J. (1996). Probing picture perception: Activation and emotion. *Psychophysiology, 33*, 103–111.

Cuthbert, B. N., Schupp, H. T., Bradley, M. M., Birbaumer, N., & Lang, P. J. (2000). Brain potentials in affective picture processing: Covariation with autonomic arousal and affective report. *Biological Psychology, 62*, 95–111.

Cuthbert, B. N., Vrana, S. R. and Bradley, M. M. (1991). Imagery: Function and physiology. In P. K. Ackles, J. R. Jennings and M. G. H. Coles (Eds.), *Advances in Psychophysiology*. (Vol. 4., pp. 1–42). Greenwich, CT: JAI.

Darwin, C. (1873). *The expression of the emotions in man and animals*. New York: Appleton. (Original work published in 1872).

Davidson, R., Ekman, P., Saron, C. D., Senulis, J. A., & Friesen, W. V. (1990). Approach/withdrawal and cerebral asymmetry: Emotional expression and brain physiology. *Journal of Personality and Social Psychology, 58*, 330–341.

Davidson, R. (2003). Affective neuroscience and psychophysiology: Toward a synthesis. *Psychophysiology, 40*, 655–665.

Davidson, R. (2002). Anxiety and affective style: Role of prefrontal cortex and amygdala. *Biological Psychiatry, 51*, 61–80.

Davis, M. (1989). The role of the amygdala and its efferent projections in fear and anxiety. In. P. Tyrer (Ed.) *Psychopharmacology of anxiety*. (pp. 52–79). Oxford: Oxford University Press.

Davis, M., Hitchcock, J., & Rosen, J. (1987). Anxiety and the amygdala: pharmacological and anatomical analysis of the fear potentiated startle paradigm. In G. H. Bower (Ed.) *Psychology of Learning and Motivation*. (Vol. 21, pp. 263–305). New York: Academic Press.

Davis, M. & Lang, P. J. (2003). Emotion. In M. Gallagher, R. J. Nelson, & I. B. Weiner (Eds). *Handbook of Psychology* (Volume 3: Biological Psychology, pp. 405–439) New Jersey: John Wiley & Sons, Inc.

Dichter, G. S., Tomarken, A. J., Shelton, R. C., & Sutton, S. K. (2004). Early and late onset startle modulation in unipolar depression. *Psychophysiology, 41*, 443–440.

Dickinson, A., & Dearing, M. F. (1979). Appetitive-aversive interactions and inhibitory processes. In A. Dickinson & R. A. Boakes (Eds.), *Mechanisms of learning and motivation* (pp. 203–231). Hillsdale, NJ: Erlbaum.

Ekman, P. (1971). Universals and cultural differences in facial expressions of emotion. In J. Cole (Ed.), *Nebraska Symposium on Motivation* (Vol. 19, pp. 207–283). Lincoln: University of Nebraska Press.

Ekman, P., Davidson, R. J., Friesen, W. V. (1990). The Duchenne smile: Emotional expression and brain physiology II. *Journal of Personality & Social Psychology, 58*, 342–353.

Ekman, P., & Friesen, W. V. (1979): *Pictures of Facial Affect*. Palo Alto, CA: Consulting Psychologists.

Ekman, P., & Friesen, W. V. (1986). FACS. *Facial Action Coding System*. Palo Alto, CA: Consulting Psychologist Press.

Ekman, P., Levenson, E. W., & Friesen, W. V. (1983). Autonomic nervous system activity distinguishes between emotions. *Science, 221*, 1208–1210.

Ekman, P. Friesen. W. V., & Hager, J. C. (2002). *The facial action coding system*. (2nd ed.). Salt Lake City:Research Nexus eBook.

Erlichman, H., Brown, S., Zhu, J. & Warrenburg, S. (1995). Startle reflex modulation during exposure to pleasant and unpleasant odors. *Psychophysiology, 32*, 150–154.

Epstein, A. N. (1971). The lateral hypothalamic syndrome. In E. Stellar & J. M. Sprague (Eds.), *Progress in physiological psychology* (Vol. 4, pp. 264–318) New York: Academic Press.

Fanselow, M. S. (1994). Neural organization of the defensive behavior system responsible for fear. *Psychonomic Bulletin & Review, 1*, 429–438.

Fiorito, E. R. & Simons, R. F. (1994). Emotional imagery and physical anhedonia. *Psychophysiology, 31*, 513–521.

Fredrikson, M., Wik, G., Greitz, T., Eriksson, L., Stone-Elander, S., Ericson, K., & Sedvall, G. (1993). Regional cerebral blood flow during experimental phobic fear. *Psychophysiology, 30*, 127–131.

Fridlund, A. J. & Izard, C. E. (1983). Electromyographic studies of facial expressions of emotion and patterns of emotion. In J. T. Cacioppo, & R. E. Petty (Eds.). *Social Psychophysiology*. (pp. 243–280).

Fridlund, A. J., Schwartz, G. E., & Fowler, S. C. (1984). Pattern recognition of self-reported emotional state from multiple-site facial EMG activity during affective imagery. *Psychophysiology, 21*, 622–637.

Frijda, N. H. (1986). *The Emotions*. New York: Cambridge.

Gaffan, D. (1992). Amygdala and the memory of reward. In J. Aggleton (Ed.), *The amygdala: Neurobiological aspects of emotion, memory, and mental dysfunction* (pp. 471–483). New York: Wiley-Liss.

Garavan, H., Pendergrass, J. C., Ross, T. J., Stein, E. A., & Risinger, R. C. (2001). *Amygdala response to both positively and negatively valenced stimuli. NeuroReport, 12*, 2779–2783.

Gellhorn, E., & Loofbourrow, N. (1963). *Emotions and emotional disorders: A neurophysiological study*. Harper and Row: New York.

George, J. S., Aine, C. J., Mosher, J. C., Schmidt, D. M., Ranken, D. M., Schlitt, H. A., Wood, C. C., Lewine, J. D., Sanders, J. A., & Belliveau, J. W. (1995). Mapping function in the human brain with magnetoencephalography, anatomical magnetic resonance imaging, and functional magnetic resonance imaging. *Journal of Clinical Neurophysiology. 12*, 406–431.

Gomez, P., & Danuser, B. (2004). Affective and psychophysiological response to environmental noises and music. *International Journal of Psychophysiology, 53*, 91–103.

Gomez, P., Zimmermann, P., Guttormsen-Schär, S., & Danuser, B. (2004). Respiratory responses associated with affective processing of film stimuli. *Biological Psychology, 68*, 223–235.

Graham, F. K. (1979). Distinguishing among orienting, defense, and startle reflexes. In H. D. Kimmel, E. H. van Olst, & J. F. Orlebeke (Eds.), *The Orienting Reflex in Humans*. (pp. 137–167) Hillsdale, N. J.: Lawrence Erlbaum Associates.

Grayson, J. B. (1982). The elicitation and habituation of orienting and defensive responses to phobic imagery and the incremental stimulus intensity effect. *Psychophysiology, 19*, 104–111.

Grillon, C., Ameli, R., Woods, S. W., Merikangas, K., & Davis, M. (1991). Fear-potentiated startle in humans: effects of anticipatory anxiety on the acoustic blink reflex. *Psychophysiology, 28*, 588–595.

Grossberg, J. M., & Wilson, H. K. (1968). Physiological changes accompanying the visualization of fearful and neutral situations. *Journal of Personality and Social Psychology, 10*, 124–133.

Grunberg, N. E., & Singer, J. E. (1990). Biochemical measurement. In J. T. Cacioppo and L. G. Tassinary (Eds.) *Principles of psychophysiology: Physical, social, and inferential elements* (pp. 149–176). New York: Cambridge University Press.

Guyton, A. C. & Hall, J. E. (1996). *Textbook of medical physiology.* (Rev. ed.). Philadelphia, PA: Saunders.

Halgren, E. (1981). The amygdala contribution to emotion and memory: Current studies in humans. In Y. Ben-Ari (Ed.), *The amygdaloid complex.* (pp. 395–408) Elsevier/North-Holland.

Hamann, S., Herman, R. A., Nolan, C. L., & Wallen, K. (2004). Men and women differ in amygdala response to visual sexual stimuli. *Nature Neuroscience, 7*, 411–416.

Hamm, A. O., Globisch, J., Cuthbert, B. N., & Vaitl, D. (1997). Fear and the startle reflex: Blink modulation and autonomic response patterns in animal and mutilation fearful subjects. *Psychophysiology, 34*, 97–107.

Hamm, A. O., Greenwald, M. K., Bradley, M. M., & Lang, P. J. (1993). Emotional learning, hedonic change, and the startle probe. *Journal of Abnormal Psychology, 102*, 453–465.

Haney, J. N., & Euse, F. J. (1976). Skin conductance and heart rate response to neutral, positive and negative imagery. *Behavior Therapy, 7*, 494–503.

Hare, R. D. (1973). Orienting and defensive responses to visual stimuli. *Psychophysiology, 10*, 453–463.

Hare, R. D. Wood, K. Britain, S. & Shadman, J. (1971). Autonomic responses to affective visual stimulation. *Psychophysiology, 7*, 408–417.

Hare, R. D., Wood, K., Britain, S., & Frazelle, J. (1971). Autonomic responses to affective visual stimulation: Sex differences. *Journal of Experimental Research in Personality, 5*, 14–22.

Hawk, L. W. & Cook, E. W. (1997). Affective modulation of tactile startle. *Psychophysiology, 34*, 23–31.

Hebb, D. O. (1949). *The organization of behavior: A neuropsychological theory.* New York: Wiley.

Izard, C. E. (1972). *Patterns of emotions.* New York: Academic Press.

James, W. (1890). *The principles of psychology.* New York: Holt.

Jansen, D. M., & Frijda, N. H.1994. Modulation of the acoustic startle response by film-induced fear and sexual arousal. *Psychophysiology, 94*, 565–571.

Jones, G. E., & Johnson, H. J. (1978). Physiological responding during self generated imagery of contextually complete stimuli. *Psychophysiology, 15*, 439–446.

Jones, G. E., & Johnson, H. J. (1980). Heart rate and somatic concomitants of mental imagery. *Psychophysiology, 17*, 339–347.

Junghofer, M., Bradley, M. M., Elbert, T. R., & Lang, P. J. (2001). Fleeting images: A new look at early emotion discrimination. *Psychophysiology, 22*, 545–560.

Keil, A., Bradley, M. M., Hauk, O., Rockstroh, B., Elbert, T., & Lang, P. J.(2002). Large scale neural correlates of affective picture processing. *Psychophysiology, 39*, 641–649.

Klorman, R., Weissberg, A. R., & Austin, M. L. (1975). Autonomic responses to affective visual stimuli. *Psychophysiology, 11*, 15–26.

Klorman, R., Weissbert, R. P., & Wiessenfeld, A. R. (1977). Individual differences in fear and autonomic reactions to affective stimulation. *Psychophysiology, 14*, 45–51.

Koch, M., & Schnitzler, H. U. (1997). The acoustic startle response in rats – circuits mediating evocation, inhibition and potentiation. *Behavioral Brain Research, 89*, 35–49.

Kohler C. G., Turner T., Stolar N. M., Bilker W. B., Brensinger C. M., Gur R. E., Gur R. C. (2004). Differences in facial expressions of four universal emotions. *Psychiatry Research, 128*, 235–44

Konorski, J. (1967). *Integrative activity of the brain: An interdisciplinary approach.* Chicago: University of Chicago Press.

Koukounas, E., & McCabe, M. P. (2001). Sexual and emotional variables influencing sexual response to erotica: A psychophysiological investigation. *Archives of Sexual Behavior, 2*, 393–408.

Kunzmann, U., Kupperbusch, C. S., & Levenson, R. W. (2005). Behavioral inhibition and amplification during emotional arousal: a comparison of two age groups. *Psychology of Aging, 20*, 144–58.

Lacey, J. I. (1958). Psychophysiological approaches to the evaluation of psychotherapeutic process and outcome. In E. A. Rubinstein & M. B. Perloff (Eds.), *Research in psychotherapy.* Washington, DC: National Publishing.

Lacey, J. I. (1967). Somatic response patterning and stress: Some revisions of activation theory. In M. H. Appley & R. Trumbull (Eds.), *Psychological stress: Issues in research* (pp. 14–38). New York: Appleton-Century-Crofts.

Landis, C., & Hunt, W. A. (1939). *The startle pattern.* New York: Farra and Rinehart.

Lane, R. D., Reiman, E. M., Bradley, M. M., Lang, P. J., Ahern, G. L., Davidson, R. J., & Schwartz, G. E. (1997). Activation of thalamus and medial prefrontal cortex during emotion. *Neuropsychologia, 35*, 1437–1444.

Lane, R. D., Chua, P. M., & Dolan, R. J. (1999). Common effects of emotional valence, arousal and attention on neural activation during visual processing of pictures. *Neuropsychologia, 37*, 989–997.

Lane, R. D., Reiman, E. M., Ahern, G. L., Schwartz, G. E., & Davidson, R. J. (1997). Neuroanatomical correlates of happiness, sadness, and disgust. *American Journal of Psychiatry, 154*, 926–933.

Lang, P. J. (1968). Fear reduction and fear behavior: Problems in treating a construct. In J. M. Schlien (Ed.), *Research in Psychotherapy.* (Vol. 3., pp. 90–103). Washington, DC: American Psychological Association.

Lang, P. J. (1979). A bio-informational theory of emotional imagery. *Psychophysiology, 16*, 495–512.

Lang, P. J. (1987). Image as action. *Cognition and Emotion, 1*, 407–426.

Lang, P. J. (1995). The emotion probe: Studies of motivation and attention. *American Psychologist, 50*, 371–385.

Lang, P. J., Bradley, M. M., & Cuthbert, B. N. (1990). Emotion, attention, and the startle reflex. *Psychological Review, 97*, 377–398.

Lang, P. J., Bradley, M. M., & Cuthbert, M. M. (1997). Motivated attention: Affect, activation and action. In P. J. Lang, R. F. Simons & M. T. Balaban (Eds.) *Attention and Orienting: Sensory and Motivational Processes.* (pp. 97–136). Hillsdale, NJ: Lawrence Erlbaum Associates, Inc.

Lang, P. J., Bradley, M. M., & Cuthbert, B. N. (2005). International affective picture system (IAPS): Instruction Manual and Affective Ratings. Technical Report A-6. Gainesville, FL. The Center for Research in Psychophysiology, University of Florida.

Lang, P. J., Bradley, M.M, Fitzsimmons, J. R., Cuthbert, B. N., Scott, J. D., Moulder, B. & Nangia, V. (1998). Emotional arousal and activation of the visual cortex: An fMRI analysis. *Psychophysiology, 35*, 199–210.

Lang, P. J. Greenwald, M. K., Bradley, M. M., & Hamm, A. O. (1993). Looking at pictures: Affective, facial, visceral, and behavioral reactions. *Psychophysiology, 30*, 261–273.

Lang, P. J., Kozak, M. J., Miller, G. A., Levin, D. N., & McLean, Jr., A. (1980). Emotional imagery: Conceptual structure and pattern of somato-visceral response. *Psychophysiology, 17*, 179–192.

Lang, P. J., Levin, D. N., Miller, G. A., & Kozak, M. J. (1983). Fear imagery and the psychophysiology of emotion: The problem of affective response integration. *Journal of Abnormal Psychology, 92*, 276–306.

Larsen, J. X., Norris, C. T., & Cacioppo, J. T. (2003) Effects of positive and negative affect on electromyographic activity over zygomaticus major and corrugator supercifii. *Psychophysiology, 40*, 776–783.

Lange, L. (1885, 1992). Om sindsbevagelser et psyko. fysiolog. studie. Lund, Jac. *The emotions.* Baltimore: Williams & Wilkins.

LeDoux, J. E. (1987). Emotion. In V. B. Mountcastle, F. Plum, & St. R. Geiger (Eds.), *Handbook of Physiology. Section 1: The nervous system* (Vol. 5, pp. 419–459). Bethesda, MD: American Physiological Association.

LeDoux, J. E. (1995). In search of an emotional system in the brain: Leaping from fear to emotion and consciousness. In M. S. Gazzaniga (Ed.), *The cognitive neurosciences* (pp. 1049–1061). Cambridge, MA: MIT Press.

Libby, W. L., Jr., Lacey, B. C., & Lacey, J. I. (1973). Pupillary and cardiac activity during visual attention. *Psychophysiology, 10*, 270–294.

Lovallo, W. R., & Thomas, T. L. (2000). Stress hormones in psychophysiological research: Emotional, behavioral, and cognitiveimplications. In J. T. Cacioppo, L. G. Tassinary, & G. Berntson (Eds.), *Handbook of psychophysiology* (pp. 342–367). New York: Cambridge University Press.

Lundqvist, D., Flykt, A., & Öhman, A. (1998). *The Karolinska Directed Emotional Faces.* Karolinska Institutet, Stockholm.

Mackintosh, N. J. (1983). *Conditioning and associative learning.* New York: Oxford.

MacLean, P. D. (1993). Cerebral evolution of emotion. In M. L. & J. M. Haviland (Eds.) *Handbook of emotions*, (pp. 67–83). New York: Guilford Press.

May, J. R. (1977b). A psychophysiological study of self and externally regulated phobic thoughts. *Behavior Therapy, 8*, 849–861.

May, J. R., & Johnson, H. J. (1973). Physiological activity to internally elicited arousal and inhibitory thoughts. *Journal of Abnormal Psychology, 83*, 239–245.

Mehrabian, A., & Russell, J. A. (1974). *An approach to environmental psychology.* Cambridge, MA: MIT Press.

Miller, G. A., Levin, D. N., Kozak, M. J., Cook, E. W., III, McLean, A., Jr., & Lang, P. J. (1987). Individual differences in imagery and the psychophysiology of emotion. *Cognition and Emotion, 1*, 367–390.

Miller, M. W., Patrick, C. J., & Levenston, G. K. (2002). Affective imagery and the startle response: Probing mechanisms of modulation during pleasant scenes, personal experiences, and discrete negative emotions. *Psychophysiology, 39*, 519–529.

Miller, N. E. (1959). Liberalization of basic S-R concepts: Extensions to conflict behavior, motivation and social learning. In: Koch, S. (Ed.): *Psychology: A study of a science* (Vol 2). New York: McGraw-Hill.

Murphy, F. C., Nimmo-Smith, I., & Lawrence, A. D. (2003). Functional neuroanatomy of emotions: a metaanalysis. *Cognitive, Affective & Behavioral Neuroscience, 3*, 207–233.

Nitschke, J. B., Larson, C. L., Smoller, M. J., Navin, S. D., Pederson, A. J. C., Ruffalo, D., Mackiewicz, K. L., Gray, S. M., Victor, E., & Davidson, R. J. (2002). Startle potentiation in aversive anticipation: evidence for state but not trait effects. *Psychophysiology, 39*, 254–258.

Ortony, A., Clore, G. L., & Collins, A. (1988). *The cognitive structure of emotions.* Cambridge: Cambridge Press.

Osgood, C., Suci, G., & Tannenbaum, P. (1957). *The measurement of meaning.* Urbana, IL: University of Illinois.

Palomba, D., Angrilli, A. & Mini, A. (1997). Visual evoked potentials, heart rate responses, and memory to emotional pictorial stimuli. *International Journal of Psychophysiology, 27*, 55–67.

Palomba, D., Sarto, M., Angrilli, A., Mini, A., & Stegagno, L. (2000). Cardiac responses associated with affective processing of unpleasant film stimuli. *International Journal of Psychophysiology, 36*, 45–57.

Panksepp, J. (1982). Toward a general psychobiological theory of emotions. *The Behavioral and Brain Sciences, 5*, 407–467.

Papez, J. W. (1937). A proposed mechanism of emotion. *Archives of Neurology and Psychiatry, 38*, 725–743.

Phan, K. L., Wager, T. D., Taylor, S. F., & Liberzon, I. (2004). *Functional neuroimaging studies of human emotions. CNS Spectrums, 9*, 258–266.

Plutchik, R. (1980). A general psychoevolutionary theory of emotion. In R. Plutchik & H. Kellerman (Eds.), *Emotion: Theory, research and experience, Volume 1: Theories of emotion.* (pp. 3–31). New York: Academic Press.

Putnam, L. E. (1990). Great expectations: Anticipatory responses of the heart and brain. In J. W. Rohrbaugh, R. Parasuraman, R. Johnson Jr. (Eds.), *Event-related brain potentials: Basic issues and applications* (pp. 109–129). New York: Oxford University Press.

Quigley, K. S., & Bertnson, G. G. (1990). Autonomic origins of cardiac responses to nonsignal stimuli in the rate. *Behavioral Neuroscience, 104*, 751–762.

Reyes del Paso, G. A., Godoy, J., & Vila, J. (1993). *Respiratory sinus arrhythmia as an index of parasympathetic cardiac control during the cardiac defense response. Biological Psychology, 35*, p. 17–35.

Robinson, J. D., & Vrana, S. R. (2000). The time course of emotional and attentional modulation of the startle reflex during imagery. *International Journal of Psychophysiology, 37*, 275–289.

Roessler, R., Burch, N. R., & Childers, H. E. (1966). Personality and arousal correlates of specific galvanic skin responses. *Psychophysiology, 3*, 115–130.

Russell, J. (1980). A circumplex model of affect. *Journal of Personality and Social Psychology, 39*, 1161–1178.

Sabatinelli, D., Bradley, M. M., & Lang, P. J. (2001). Affective startle modulation in anticipation and perception. *Psychophysiology, 38*, 719–722.

Sabatinelli, D., Bradley, M. M., & Lang, P. J. (2005). ERPs and BOLD responses to affective pictures in the same participants. Manuscript in preparation.

Sabatinelli, D., Flaisch, T., Bradley, M. M., Fitzsimmons, J. R., & Lang, P. J. (2004). Affective picture perception: Gender differences in visual cortex? *NeuroReport, 15*, 1109–1112.

Sabatinelli, D., Bradley, M. M., Fitzsimmons, J. R., & Lang, P. J. (2005). Parallel amygdala and inferotemporal activation reflect emotional intensity and fear relevance. *NeuroImage, 24*, 265–1270.

Schneirla, T. (1959). An evolutionary and developmental theory of biphasic processes underlying approach and withdrawal. In M. Jones (Ed.), *Nebraska Symposium on Motivation* (pp. 1–42) Lincoln: University of Nebraska Press.

Schupp, H. T., Cuthbert, B. N., Bradley, M. M., Hillman, C. H., Hamm, A. O., & Lang, P. J. (2004). Brain processes in emotional perception: Motivated attention. *Cognition & Emotion, 18,* 593–611.

Schupp, H. T., Junghofer, M., Weike, A. I., & Hamm, A. O. (2003). Emotional facilitation of sensory processing in the visual cortex. *Psychological Science, 14,* 7–13.

Schupp, H. T., Junghofer, M., Weike, A. I., & Hamm, A. O. (2004). The selective processing of briefly presented affective pictures: An ERP analysis. *Psychophysiology, 41,* 441–449.

Schwaber, J. S., Kapp, B. S., Higgins, G. A., & Rapp, P. R. (1982). Amygdaloid and basal forebrain direct connections with the nucleus of the solitary tract and the dorsal motor nucleus. *Journal of Neuroscience, 2,* 14141–438.

Schwartz, G. E. (1971). Cardiac responses to self-induced thoughts. *Psychophysiology, 8,* 462–466.

Schwartz, G., Ahern, G., & Bowen, S. (1979). Lateralized facial muscle response to positive and negative emotional stimuli. *Psychophysiology, 16,* 561–571.

Schwartz, G., Brown, S., & Ahern, G. (1980). Facial muscle patterning and subjective experience during affective imagery: Sex differences. *Psychophysiology, 17,* 75–82.

Selye, H. (1950). Stress and the general adaptation syndrome. *British Medical Journal,* 1383–1392.

Skolnick, A. J., & Davidson, R. J. (2002). Affective modulation of eyeblink startle with reward and threat. *Psychophysiology, 39,* 835–850.

Smith, J. C., Bradley, M. M., & Lang, P. J. (2005). State anxiety and affective physiology: Effects of sustained exposure to affective pictures. *Biological Psychology, 69,* 247–260.

Smith, N. K., Cacioppo, J. T., Larsen, J. T., & Chartrand, T. L. (2003). May I have your attention, please: Electrocortical responses to positive and negative stimuli. *Neuropsychologia, 41,* 171–183.

Sokolov, Y. N. (1963). *Perception and the Conditioned Reflex* (S. W. Waydenfeld, Trans.). New York: Macmillan. (Original work published 1958).

Stanley, J. & Knight, R. G. (2004). Emotional specificity of startle specificity during the early stages of picture viewing. *Psychophysiology, 41,* 935–940.

Stern, J. A. (1972). Physiological response measures during classical conditioning In N. S. Greenfield & P. A. Sternbach (Eds.), *Handbook of psychophysiology* (pp. 197–228). New York: Holt, Rinehart & Winston.

Tassinary, L. G., Cacioppo, J. T., & Geen, T. R. (1989). A psychometric study of surface electrode placements for facial electromyographic recording: I. The brow and cheek muscle regions. *Psychophysiology, 26,* 1–16.

Tinbergen, N. (1969). *The study of instinct.* New York: Oxford University Press.

Turpin, G. (1986). Effects of stimulus intensity on autonomic responding: The problem of differentiating orienting and defense reflexes. *Psychophysiology, 23,* 1–14.

Turpin, G. (1990) Ambulatory clinical psychophysiology: An introduction to techniques and methodological issues. *Journal of Psychophysiolog, 4,* 299–304.

Turpin, G., & Siddle, D. A. T. (1983). Effects of stimulus intensity on cardiovascular activity. *Psychophysiology, 20,* 611–624.

Van Egeren, L. F., Feather, B. W., & Hein, P. L. (1971). Desensitization of phobias: Some psychophysiological propositions. *Psychophysiology, 8,* 213–228.

van Oyen Witvliet, C. & Vrana, S. R. (1995). Psychophysiological responses as indicators of affective dimensions. *Psychophysiology, 2,* 436–443.

Vanman, E. J., Boehmelt, A. H., Dawson, M. E., & Schell, A. M. (1996). The varying time courses of attentional and affective modulation of the startle eyeblink reflex. *Psychophysiology, 33,* 691–697.

Verona, E., Patrick, CJ., Curtin, J. J., Bradley, M. M., Lang, P. J. (2004). Psychopathy and physiological response to emotionally evocative sounds. *Journal of Abnormal Psychology, 113,* 99–108.

Vrana, S. R., Cuthbert, B. N., & Lang, P. J. (1986). Fear imagery and text processing. *Psychophysiology, 23,* 247–253.

Vrana, S. & Rollock, D. (2002). The role of ethnicity, gender, emotional content, and contextual differences in physiological, expressive, and self-reported emotional responses to imagery. *Cognition and Emotion, 16,* 165–192.

Vrana, S. R., Spence, E. L., & Lang, P. J. (1988). The startle probe response: A new measure of emotion? *Journal of Abnormal Psychology, 97,* 487–491.

Watson, J. (1924). *Behaviorism.* New York: People's Institute.

Wheeler, R. E., Davidson, R. J., & Tomarken, A. J. (1993). Frontal brain asymmetry and emotional reactivity: A biological substrate of affective style. *Psychophysiology, 30,* 82–89.

Wilhem, F. H., & Roth, W. T. (1996). Ambulatory assessment of clinical anxiety. In J. Fahrenberg, and M. Myrtek (Eds.), *Ambulatory Assessment: Computer-Assisted Psychological and Psychophysiological Methods in Monitoring and Field Studies.* Gottingen: Hogrefe & Huber Publishers.

Williams, L. M., Das, P., Liddell, B., Olivieri, G., Peduto, A., Brammer, M. J., Gordon, E. (2005). BOLD, sweat and fears: fMRI and skin conductance distinguish facial fear signals. *Neuroreport, 16,* 49–52.

Winton, W. M., Putnam, L. E., & Krauss, R. M. (1984). Facial and autonomic manifestations of the dimensional structure of emotion. *Journal of Experimental Social Psychology, 20,* 195–216.

Witvliet, C. V., Vrana, S. R. (1995). Psychophysiological responses as indices of affective dimensions. *Psychophysiology. 32,* 436–43.

Wundt, W. (1896). *Grundriss der Psychologie* (Outlines of Psychology). Leipzig: Entgelmann.

Yartz, A. R., & Hawk, L. W., Jr. (2002). Addressing the specificity of affective startle modulation: Fear versus disgust. *Biological Psychology, 59,* 55–68.

Yeomans, J. S., Steidl, S., & Li, L. (2000). Conditioned brain-stimulation reward attenuates the acoustic startle reflex in rats. *Social Neuroscience Abstracts. 30,* 1252.

Zald, D. H. (2003). The human amygdala and the emotional evaluation of sensory stimuli. *Brain Research-Brain Research Review, 41,* 88–123.

26 Stress and Illness

BERT N. UCHINO, TIMOTHY W. SMITH, JULIANNE HOLT-LUNSTAD,
REBECCA CAMPO, AND MAIJA REBLIN

PROLOGUE

Life is largely a process of adaptation to the circumstances in which we exist. A perennial give-and-take has been going on between living matter and its inanimate surroundings, between one living being and another, ever since the dawn of life in the prehistoric oceans. The secret of health and happiness lies in successful adjustment to the ever-changing conditions on this globe; the penalties for failure in this great process of adaptation are disease and unhappiness. (Selye, 1956, p. vii)

Overview. It has been almost 50 years since the publication of the classic book by Hans Selye (1956) on stress, adaptation, and disease. In his formulation of the general adaptation syndrome, the role of the autonomic and endocrine systems on stress-related disease processes was highlighted. These two physiological systems continue to be the major focus of contemporary research aimed at understanding the health consequences of stress. The emergence of psychoneuroimmunology (PNI) as a discipline in the early 1970s has resulted in the immune system becoming a third major physiological perspective, which links stress to health outcomes. However, we now have a more detailed understanding of how these major stress systems are coordinated during threats and its implications for health. The major aim of this chapter is to provide a detailed overview of the links between stress and illness with an emphasis on underlying physiological and stress component processes (see Chrousos, 2006, this volume for an overview of stress physiology).

Historical background. The study of stress and disease has a rich history. The term "stress" originated from its physical analogy of strain present in materials. However, even before there was an understanding of the biological

Preparation for this chapter was generously supported by National Institute on Aging grant RO1 AG018903, and National Heart, Lung, and Blood Institute grant R01 HL68862. Correspondence concerning this article should be addressed to Bert N. Uchino, Department of Psychology, 380 S. 1530 E. RM 502, University of Utah, Salt Lake City, Utah 84112, or via e-mail (bert.uchino@psych.utah.edu).

stress process, researchers have been interested in how this "strain" might influence health. In one research program far ahead of its time, Ishigami (1918–1919) reported case studies suggesting that anxiety on the part of tuberculosis patients was associated with a poorer prognosis as a result of immune system changes. Ishigami (1918–1919) speculated that the higher tuberculosis mortality rates in Japan's occupational class might be due, in part, to the increased stress and anxiety in such individuals.

A more systematic advance in our understanding of health relevant stress processes has its roots in the writing of French physiologist Claude Bernard (1878/1974). Bernard introduced the concept of dynamic equilibrium in order to understand disease. The dynamic equilibrium was conceptualized as a constant internal milieu that was critical because any factor that threatened this consistency could potentially adversely influence health. Although the main focus of Bernard's work was on physical factors (e.g., temperature) in relation to dynamic equilibrium, this work set the stage for a generalization of this model to stress-related processes.

Perhaps the first researcher to make this leap was Walter Cannon (1929) who introduced the concept of homeostasis as an extension of Bernard's work. Homeostasis was defined as the coordinated responses that maintain the steady state of the body. One of the factors that could threaten homeostasis according to Cannon was physical stress. However, Walter Cannon (1928) also suggested that emotional stress could be an important factor in this process. In his well-known work on the "fight or flight" response, he suggested that emotional stress can lead an organism to fight or flee, both factors that if successful can help protect homeostasis. These emotional responses were seen as driven by the catabolic effects of the sympathetic nervous system (SNS) that could energize the organism in times of need.

It was also the work by Walter Cannon that set the stage for viewing the SNS as one culprit for stress-induced health problems. Of course, Cannon viewed such responses as adaptive in the service of homeostasis and applicable primarily to short-term threats. A biological perspective that directly addressed the longer-term effects of emotional distress can be traced to the classic work of Hans Selye (1956). In his model of the general adaptation syndrome (GAS), Selye found that animals exposed to more chronic stress seemed to go through a distinct sequence of behavioral and physiological changes. Initially, in what he termed the alarm stage, the SNS dominated. As more coping attempts were initiated (i.e., the resistance phase), the release of glucocorticoids (e.g., cortisol) from the hypothalamic-pituitary-adrenal (HPA) axis became important. The effects of glucocorticoids are broad and include increased glucose metabolism, increased lipolysis, and inhibition of immune processes (Munck, Guyre, & Holbrook, 1984). Although the immunosuppressive effects of cortisol was not anticipated by the GAS (Munck, Guyre, & Holbrook, 1984), the HPA axis was given special status by Selye as he suggested coping attempts that failed to terminate a stressor could result in exhaustion and compromise health.

Although more contemporary views of stress, physiological regulation, and disease (e.g., allostasis) have been proposed and are presently favored (see Berntson & Cacioppo, 2000; Sterling & Eyer, 1988), these prior perspectives provided important initial frameworks linking stress to physical health. The legacy of these perspectives is also evident in that a focus on the SNS and HPA axis continues to dominate contemporary research on stress and health. However, the emergence of PNI has resulted in the immune system as a third major physiological perspective for researchers interested in health and disease (see Solomon & Moos, 1964). More important is the fact that extensive interactions exist among the autonomic, neuroendocrine, and immune systems. Evidence for such interactions is starting to pave the way for a more integrated (but complex) view of how stress might influence health.

In the remainder of this chapter we provide a representative review of research linking stress to health outcomes. The major diseases considered here include cardiovascular disease, cancer, and infectious diseases. These diseases are perhaps the most studied in terms of links between stress and health, as well as being among the leading causes of mortality in the world. We will first cover briefly the basic epidemiology and pathophysiology of these diseases, and then review the evidence linking stress directly to these important health outcomes. Emerging evidence on the mechanisms by which stress is related to health will then be examined. We conclude by proposing a more integrative view of stress processes applied to health outcomes, as well as important future areas of research. To start, we provide a brief review of conceptual issues related to stress.

THE CONCEPTUALIZATION OF STRESS

The concept of stress is often used ubiquitously in the research literature to refer to either acute or chronic strains. The focus of researchers has historically emphasized stress as a stimulus (stressor), a response (biologi-

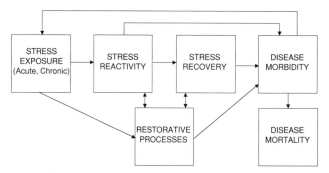

Figure 26.1. Stress-related component processes potentially related to health outcomes.

cal changes), or a transactional process in which perceptions of stress are emphasized (Lazarus & Folkman, 1984). A classic distinction is also usually drawn between more acute (or time-limited) versus chronic (long-term) stressors. Chronic stress is generally regarded as being more consequential for health and usually results from long-term exposure to stressors. However, chronic stress may also be a result of lasting perceptions of stress that are driven by ruminative thinking (Baum, O'Keefe, & Davidson, 1990). Thus, chronic stress may be defined as long-term exposure, lasting perceptions, or both (e.g., caregiving for a family member with Alzheimer's disease).

Although the time course and associated perception of stress have traditionally been emphasized in past research, more recent models are attempting to separate component processes associated with stress. This "new look" is important because a strict focus on general perceptions of stress does less to elucidate the precise mechanisms operating to influence health outcomes. Cacioppo & Berntson (in press) have argued that stress may have at least four health-related components: exposure, reactivity, recovery, and restoration. Exposure refers to the number of stressors that an individual experiences; reactivity refers to the strength of an individual's physiological reaction to any given event; and recovery refers to how long it takes an individual to return to "baseline" following stressful events. A unique aspect of this perspective is on restoration, which focuses on anabolic processes that refresh or repair the organism, because stress may directly impede our ability to perform these functions (e.g., disturbed sleep and impaired wound healing).

A simplified conceptual model based on the framework of Cacioppo & Berntson (in press) is presented in Figure 26.1. Accordingly, stress exposure may be either acute or chronic and influence reactivity. Stress reactivity may then lead to differential stress recovery, and some evidence suggests these processes are separable (Linden, Stossel, & Maurice, 1996). Stress reactivity, recovery, and exposure may also have effects on restorative processes such as sleep and wound healing. It is also predicted that these restorative processes may in turn influence stress reactivity and recovery, especially over time as insufficient restoration may be associated with changes in the set-point and response characteristics of physiological systems (Sterling & Eyer, 1988; Epel, McEwen, & Ickovics, 1998). These stress components may ultimately influence health depending on the disease context (i.e., development or exacerbation of disease). Of course, disease morbidity also entails significant psychological, behavioral, and social adjustments that can in turn be associated with greater stress exposure (Nicassio & Smith, 1995). Although there are conceptual issues related to these stress components that will be discussed later (e.g., independence of components and time course), it provides a broad and potentially unique means for evaluating and organizing current research linking stress to health outcomes.

STRESS AND CARDIOVASCULAR DISEASE

Background information. Cardiovascular disease is a broad term used to cover several diseases of the cardiovascular system, including coronary artery disease (CAD) and hypertension. It is by far the leading cause of death in the United States and most industrialized countries (American Heart Association, 2004). In fact, it accounts for about as many deaths as the next six leading causes of death combined. It is estimated that if all major forms of cardiovascular disease were eliminated, life expectancy would be raised by about seven years. This stands in comparison to a life expectancy gain of three years if all forms of cancers were eliminated (American Heart Association, 2004).

CAD is a condition in which the coronary arteries become narrowed, and ultimately results in decreased blood flow to the heart. The pathological change in the coronary arteries is due to a process called atherosclerosis, which is a progressive buildup of fatty deposits within the arterial walls. This buildup is not a passive process that simply occurs with the passage of time. Recent research suggests that inflammation (e.g., macrophage activity or cytokine release) may play a key role in the progression of CAD (Libby, 2002; Ross, 1999). The end result of this process is the formation of arterial lesions and narrowing of the arteries. These processes increase the chance that a blood clot will form thereby increasing the risk of blocking the arterial passage. Although most people think of CAD as occurring in older adults, it is important to note that this atherogenic process starts very early. For instance, the beginnings of arterial plaque can be found in children, while some young adults already show evidence of advanced lesions. Of course, only when the disease is in its later stages (as is often the case with older adults) does it result in clinical symptoms. Thus, CAD is generally considered a disease with a long-term developmental history.

Hypertension is another leading cardiovascular disorder and is a condition of elevated blood pressure (SBP $\geq$ 140 mmHg or DBP $\geq$ 90 mmHg). However, there is also increasing appreciation of the health relevance of blood pressure previously labeled as "normal." Recent guidelines suggest that both SBP between 120–139 mmHg or DBP

between 80–89 mmHg be considered "prehypertension" (American Heart Association, 2004). In about 5% to 10% of cases, the cause of high blood pressure can be determined and is labeled secondary hypertension (e.g., kidney problems). However, in the vast majority of cases the cause of elevated blood pressure is unknown and is labeled essential or primary hypertension. Because of the heightened workload within the cardiovascular system, as well as the increased pressure in various organ systems, the consequences of hypertension can be kidney damage and increased risk of MI, stroke, and heart failure.

Evidence linking stress to cardiovascular disease. The overall evidence linking stress to cardiovascular disease appears strong (Krantz et al., 2000; Linden, Stossel, & Maurice, 1996; Rozanski, Blumenthal & Kaplan, 1999; Schneiderman et al., 2001; Smith & Ruiz, 2002). In a comprehensive review, Rozanski and colleagues (1999) found that exposure to both acute and chronic stress (especially work stress) was associated with an increased risk for morbidity and mortality from cardiovascular disease. Moreover, interventions explicitly aimed at decreasing stress appear to be effective in reducing cardiovascular mortality (Dusseldorp et al., 1999; Krantz et al., 2000; Linden, Stossel, & Maurice, 1996).

Because of the pathophysiology of CAD, there are at least two ways that stress may influence cardiovascular outcomes. The influence of stress on health may be due to effects on either the development or the exacerbation of CAD in clinical patients. Importantly, research suggests that stress may play a role in both processes, although the putative physiological mechanisms appear to differ. Animal studies clearly suggest a role for stress in the development of cardiovascular disease (Manuck, Kaplan, & Clarkson, 1983). In one study from an important program of research, Manuck, Kaplan, & Clarkson (1983) examined monkeys that were high or low in heart rate reactivity to stress. The monkeys were then placed in unstable, stressful environments in which they had to reestablish their dominance. Results revealed that monkeys who were high in heart rate reactivity had greater coronary atherosclerosis upon necropsy. These results have been replicated, are eliminated by β-adrenergic blockade, and exacerbated by other risk factors such as an atherogenic diet (Kaplan et al., 1987). These data are consistent with other animal models such as the borderline hypertensive rat that develops elevated blood pressure following exposure to chronic stress (Sanders & Lawler, 1992).

Another line of evidence for the role of stress in the development of disease comes from studies utilizing non-invasive imaging of carotid arteries (Kamarck et al., 2004; Troxel et al., 2003). Measures such as carotid ultrasounds and computed tomography (CT) scans of coronary arteries assess the extent of preclinical disease and are robust predictors of future cardiovascular risk (Rumberger et al., 1999). One study found that even when statistically controlling for various risk factors (e.g., lipid profiles and resting blood pressure), a composite measure of stress was associated with higher carotid intima-media thickness in African American women (Troxel et al., 2003).

Epidemiological studies on CAD incidence in humans provide further evidence for an influence of stress on the development of cardiovascular problems. INTERHEART is a large, global case-control study aimed at understanding the risk factors for a first heart attack (Rosengren et al., 2004). Results from this huge undertaking in 52 countries showed that stress from both home and work was associated with an increased risk for a first heart attack after adjustments for age, gender, geographic region, and smoking habits (odds ratios of 1.38–2.14). These results are consistent with a recent large prospective study conducted in Japan that also found general perceptions of stress in initially healthy individuals to predict subsequent cardiovascular mortality over a seven to nine year followup in women (Iso et al., 2002). Although these two studies statistically controlled for known risk factors such as smoking, exercise, and body mass index, they may provide only a conservative estimate of the stress-disease link given it may be mediated, in part, by such health behaviors (Stetson et al., 1997). Nevertheless, these data are consistent with other prospective studies that found stress to predict the incidence of CAD in middle-aged to older adult samples (Ming et al., 2004; Rosengren, Tibblin, & Wilhelmsen, 1991).

Prospective studies further suggest a role for stress in the clinical course of diagnosed cardiovascular disease. A recent study by Sheps and colleagues (2002) examined stress-induced ischemia in the laboratory by having 196 cardiac patients perform a speech task. They found that wall motion abnormalities during the speech were predictors of mortality over the five-year followup (also see Manuck et al., 1992). These studies are consistent with work in the laboratory or daily life linking the experience of acute stress to arrhythmia/ischemia in cardiac patients (Carels et al., 1988).

It is important to note that interventions designed to decrease stress in cardiac patients also show some promise in reducing disease reoccurrence and mortality (Dusseldorp et al., 1999; Krantz et al., 2000; Linden, Stossel, & Maurice, 1996). Dusseldorp and colleagues (1999) reviewed 37 interventions consisting of health education, stress management programs, or both with cardiac patients. Results revealed that myocardial infarction reoccurrence was 20% to 29% lower in the intervention groups. Moreover, survival during the study period was about 34% greater in patients provided with such psycho-educational interventions.

Potential mechanisms linking stress to cardiovascular disease. Overall, strong evidence is available linking stress to the development and course of cardiovascular disease. One limitation, however, is that less direct evidence is available in these studies on the mechanisms responsible for such links. Furthermore, stress in these studies has usu-

ally been operationalized in its aggregate or as general perceptions. As a result, the more precise stress-related components that might be operating are unclear. There is, however, a relatively large literature linking stress to more "intermediate" cardiovascular endpoints such as reactivity, ambulatory blood pressure (ABP), or noninvasive imaging of carotid/coronary arteries. Such research can help clarify the conceptual role of stress in the development and exacerbation of cardiovascular disease.

One model linking stress to cardiovascular disease is represented by the reactivity hypothesis (Krantz & Manuck, 1984). According to this perspective, individuals or situations characterized by high levels of cardiovascular reactivity (usually indexed by blood pressure or heart rate) may be related to higher risk for the development and exacerbation of cardiovascular disease. Research linking reactivity to cardiovascular disease is still ongoing, but current evidence is consistent with this hypothesis. For instance, relatively high levels of reactivity prospectively predict increased blood pressure in adolescents (Matthews, Woodall, & Allen, 1993) and middle-aged adults (Light et al., 1992; Matthews, Woodall, & Allen, 1993). A recent review of this literature found evidence consistent with the reactivity hypothesis, although exceptions were evident (Treiber et al., 2003).

The more precise stress components responsible for these findings are unclear as the reactivity hypothesis assumes that both exposure and reactivity are important to influence disease. This assumption is important to emphasize as several studies suggest that modeling the effects of stressful environments strengthen the association between cardiovascular reactivity assessed in the lab and disease outcomes. For instance, Everson and colleagues (1997) found that workplace demands and cardiovascular reactivity assessed in the lab interacted to predict changes in carotid atherosclerosis four years later. More specifically, individuals more reactive (as indexed by anticipation of an exercise test) and with more demanding jobs had up to 40% greater progression of intima-medial-thickness and plague height (also see Lynch et al., 1998). These results echo the comments by Light (2001) who noted that prior animal models in which the reactivity hypothesis was based (e.g., borderline hypertensive rat) show that the combination of social environment and genes are critically important to model.

The mechanisms responsible for reactivity effects on CAD, however, may differ depending on the stage of disease. The role of stress reactivity in the development of disease highlights the role of endothelial injury because mechanical (e.g., shear force) or chemical (e.g., catecholamines) factors are important precipitating events (Krantz & Manuck, 1984). More recent research focuses on the possibility that following endothelial injury, inflammatory processes take center stage as a result of the migration of macrophages, T-cells, and the release of cytokines (Libby, 2002; Ross, 1999). This process may be accelerated or exacerbated for individuals who are exposed to stress, or who are high stress reactors (Bosch et al., 2003a; Goebel & Mills, 2000).

In comparison, the mechanisms linking stress to the exacerbation of disease may be related more to the induction of myocardial ischemia, arrhythmias, and thrombosis (Rozanski, Blumenthal, & Kaplan, 1999). Acute stress may precipitate ischemia because of hemodynamic changes in blood pressure (Rozanski et al., 1988), perhaps as a result of stress-induced increases in endothelial dysfunction and subsequent vasoconstriction (Goldberg et al., 1996; Yeung et al., 1991). Acute stress may cause changes in the autonomic nervous system (ANS) that lead to arrhythmia and sudden cardiac death (Kamarck & Jennings, 1991). Finally, stress may be linked to changes in endothelial function, platelet aggregation, and blood hemoconcentration that render plaques vulnerable to thrombosis (Strike et al., 2004; Veldhuijzen van Zanten et al., 2004). These data suggest that, although chronic stress increases the probability of these adverse effects, in theory, acute stressful events in and of themselves may be sufficient to induce problems in cardiac patients.

Although the prior literature has focused on stress reactivity and exposure, recent attention is also turning to indices of cardiovascular recovery from stress in predicting cardiovascular outcomes (Schuler & O'Brien, 1997). In theory, delayed recovery may be a result of the cumulative effects of stress (perhaps because of allostatic changes) or may be driven by ruminative thinking (Glynn, Christenfeld, & Gerin, 2002). Methods for calculating recovery differ and range from simple change or residualized change scores from baseline to measures of area under the curve and slope analyses (Llabre et al., 2001). Although many researchers statistically partial baseline levels from recovery indices, very few researchers control for levels of stress reactivity. Because reactivity and recovery may be correlated, it is difficult to distinguish the potential independence of recovery from the reactivity hypothesis.

There are currently few studies that examined the link between recovery and cardiovascular disease processes, and existing studies are heterogeneous in terms of its method of calculating recovery (Schuler & O'Brien, 1997). Despite this variability, a meta-analysis of recovery indices and cardiovascular risk factors showed small but significant associations between cardiovascular recovery and hypertension status, race, and lack of fitness (Schuler & O'Brien, 1997). In one study conducted over a three-year period, blood pressure and heart rate recovery indices predicted increases in ABP even when statistically controlling for corresponding reactivity levels (Rutledge, Linden, & Paul, 2000). Thus, although more data are needed, recent research suggest a role for recovery indices in shedding additional insight into how stress may be related to cardiovascular risk.

A final process that may be responsible for links between stress and cardiovascular disease is related to its effects on restorative processes (Cacioppo & Berntson, in press).

These anabolic processes are energy conserving and building, and include biological processes that help to refresh or repair the organism. Although not a main focus of prior stress research, evidence suggests the importance of such restorative processes. One important restorative process is sleep. Problems with sleep can have important consequences as it is linked to adverse changes in health (e.g., Mallon, Broman, & Hetta, 2002). Importantly, stress has been shown to have negative effects on sleep quality (Cartwright & Wood, 1991). In one study, participants were recruited for a night in a sleep lab and half of the participants were told they were to perform a stressful speech task in the morning (Hall et al., 2004). Results revealed that individuals expecting stress in the morning had less parasympathetic modulation of several sleep stages, and greater sympathovagal balance during nonrapid eye movement sleep, which in turn related to lower sleep maintenance. These data highlight the importance of stress on the restorative process of sleep and further suggest that ANS processes related to cardiovascular disease may be involved.

STRESS AND CANCER

Background information. Perhaps no diagnosis strikes more fear in people than that of cancer. Cancer is the second leading cause of death in the United States and over 1.3 million new cancer cases are expected to be diagnosed in 2004. In fact, one of every three individuals is predicted to be afflicted by cancer at some point in their lives (American Cancer Society, 2004). Cancer is a broad term used to describe many different diseases that are characterized by the uncontrolled growth and spread of abnormal cells (Abbas & Lichtman, 2003). A key to cancer appears to lie in the DNA of cells. DNA contains the genetic code that directs cell development and growth. However, carcinogens can cause damage to cells with subsequent changes in their DNA. In many cases, the body is able to repair such damages to DNA or the cell dies off before it replicates. However, in the case of cancer, uncontrolled replication of such cells leads to tumors that can ultimately result in death if not detected and treated. Cancerous tumors can also metastasize and spread cancerous cells to different parts of the body via blood or lymph.

There is no one cause of cancer and many factors seem to play a role in its initial development and progression. Research clearly suggests the importance of genetics in the risk for some forms of cancer (e.g., BRCA II gene for breast and ovarian cancer). Also important are carcinogens that include chemical factors and ionizing radiation that may damage cells and increase cancer risk. However, some of the main factors implicated in the development of cancer are behavioral or lifestyle in nature. These lifestyle factors include smoking, excessive alcohol consumption, diet, and sun exposure. In fact, several types of cancer could be almost completely eliminated (lung cancer by not smoking) or significantly reduced (skin cancer with the use of sunscreen) just by altering one's behavior (American Cancer Society, 2004).

Fortunately, the body is not defenseless against cancer (Abbas & Lichtman, 2003; Dunn et al., 2002). According to the concept of immunosurveillance, the immune system plays an important role in destroying abnormal cells before they become tumors or killing tumors in the body once they are formed (Burnett, 1970). A number of specific immune cells have been implicated in playing a role in immunosurveillance. For instance, natural killer (NK) cells have the ability to nonspecifically kill certain tumor cell lines. Cytotoxic T-cells and the cytokine interferon-γ also appear to be important mechanisms of immunosurveillance because they can target tumors that express certain peptides or viral proteins (Shankaran et al., 2001).

There is some debate about whether the immune system defends the body adequately against most cancers. Animal models provide the clearest evidence for the protective effects of the immune system, although the strength of this effect may depend on the type of cancer (Abbas & Lichtman, 2003). More recently, Dunn and colleagues (2002) have proposed the concept of cancer immunoediting as a more comprehensive framework to describe immune processes related to tumor resistance and development. According to these authors, this term better describes the role of the immune system in initially protecting against cancer, and actively selecting for cancer variants that might eventually grow in an immunocompetent individual. For instance, the immune system may select for tumor that have less immunogenicity (i.e., ability to generate an immune response) by initially killing off more immunogenic tumors. However, these less immunogenic tumors can further mutate into more aggressive variants that "carry over" their initial advantage (i.e., Darwinian selection), and could eventually provide it with an advantage over the immune system.

The processes described above refer collectively to three postulated stages of cancer immunoediting: elimination, equilibrium, and escape (Dunn et al., 2002). Elimination coincides with the initial concept of immunosurveillance and T-cells, along with the production of interferon-γ, appear critical for the detection and elimination of immunogenic tumors. In the equilibrium stage, tumors with less immunogenicity survive elimination and are at equilibrium with the immune system. At this stage, immune processes invoked by T-lymphocytes and interferon-γ can keep the tumor in check but not eliminate it. However, mutating variants of these tumor cells are constantly arising and may carry mutations that make them even more resistant to immune processes (e.g., loss of MHC molecules, interferon-γ insensitivity). Finally, the phase of escape corresponds to resulting tumors that are much less immunogenic and can thus grow in an immunocompetent individual. This later stage of escape usually corresponds to clinically diagnosed malignant disease, and the immune system is less able to control it as a result of earlier selection processes. Although the concept of immunoediting is still being refined, it provides a broad, developmental framework for interpreting prior research.

Evidence linking stress to cancer. The overall evidence linking stress to cancer outcomes is controversial. Animal models provide a stronger case for stress influencing some types of cancer (Fox; 1998, Sklar & Anisman, 1981). However, human studies have provided inconsistent findings linking stress to overall cancer outcomes (e.g., Cooper, Davies-Cooper, & Faragher, 1986; see review by Fox, 1998). As noted by others (e.g., Cohen & Herbert, 1996; Kiecolt-Glaser & Glaser, 1995), the evidence linking stress to cancer is complex and several issues are in need of greater consideration. First, past research has tended to focus on all cancers combined, or failed to consider the stage of cancer potentially impacted by stress. This is important because some cancers are more deadly than others (e.g., pancreatic cancer). It has further been suggested that psychosocial factors such as stress are less likely to influence survival from cancer in later stages of the disease (Kiecolt-Glaser & Glaser, 1995).

These points would suggest that studies examining certain types of cancers might provide a stronger test of the role of stress in the development of cancer. Of such studies most have focused on breast cancer. In a meta-analysis, McKenna, Zevon, Corn, and Rounds (1999) did find evidence of an association between stress and the development of breast cancer. Although the number of studies were not large (16 for separation/loss and 12 for stressful life events), significant stress effects on breast cancer development were found with overall mean effect sizes (Hedges's g) ranging from .25 to .29. Furthermore, these effect sizes were not moderated by various methodological factors such as type of control group and sample size.

Although there are studies that have failed to find a link between stressful life events and breast cancer development (e.g., Kvikstad et al., 1994), there is some evidence that increased stress exposure may be important to consider. In the Finnish Twin Cohort study, a comprehensive assessment of stressful life events was obtained for the five years preceding a baseline assessment (Lillberg et al., 2003). During a 15-year followup, the experience of five major life events predicted the incidence of breast cancer even after statistically controlling for social class, smoking, alcohol use, and exercise patterns. Further examination of the data suggested a cumulative effect of stress on breast cancer development as the number of life events increased.

There is also controversy about whether stress can influence subsequent survival following a cancer diagnosis (Fox, 1998). The strongest evidence for a link between stress and the course of cancer comes from intervention studies (Fawzy & Fawzy, 1998). Although the number of studies is not large, these interventions usually include an educational or stress management component and appear to have beneficial influence on health outcomes (Baum &

Posluszny, 1999). In one well-known intervention, Fawzy and colleagues (1993) evaluated the effects of a six-week structured group intervention that provided education, problem-solving skills, stress management, and social support to cancer patients. Importantly, a six-year followup revealed that only 9% of individuals in the structured group intervention had died compared to 29% of individuals in the no-intervention condition.

Potential mechanisms linking stress to cancer. The overall evidence linking stress to cancer development and survival is controversial (Fox, 1998), although studies that focus on specific cancers show some promise (Andersen, Kiecolt-Glaser, & Glaser, 1994; McKenna et al., 1999). In retrospect, these inconsistent results are not surprising given that modulation of the immune system is one of the primary proposed mechanisms linking stress to cancer, and the effectiveness of such immune processes may be dependent on the type of cancer (Abbas & Lichtman, 2003). The concept of immune system involvement in cancer is also undergoing development (Dunn et al., 2002). The emerging concept of cancer immunoediting suggests why stress may only be weakly associated with cancer outcomes later in the clinical course of disease. At this later "escape" stage, tumors with less immunogenicity have been selected and mutating variants may already have made them resistant to immune processes (Dunn et al., 2002). In such cases, stress-induced modulation of immune function may evidence little association with disease outcomes. The concept of cancer immunoediting highlights more generally the importance of modeling stress effects across the full course of cancer. In theory, by suppressing the immune system (e.g., interferon-γ production), chronic stress may hasten the progression through stages of cancer immunoediting. Of course, some cancers are more deadly than others (e.g., pancreatic cancer) and this complexity would also need to be considered in modeling the time course of stress effects on cancer outcomes.

Importantly, stress does appear to be related to early processes that in theory should be related to the development of cancer. As reviewed earlier, damaged cells may become cancerous following changes to their DNA. However, the cell is usually repaired or it dies off before it replicates (i.e., apoptosis). There is a small literature indicating that stress may influence both of these processes. In studies of medical students during high stress (i.e., exams), apoptosis of blood leukocytes in response to gamma irradiation is impaired (Tomei et al., 1990). In addition, rats exposed to rotational stress showed lower levels of a DNA repair enzyme in response to carcinogens (Glaser et al., 1985). These findings highlight the potential role of stress exposure, stress reactivity, and stress restoration in early biological events related to cancer development.

Evidence linking stress to direct changes in immune function may also have relevance for understanding the development and course of cancer. The elimination phase of cancer immunoediting is characterized by immune processes that actively prevent and eliminate tumors (Dunn et al., 2002). Importantly, there is strong evidence indicating that stress can influence aspects of both innate and adaptive immunity (Segerstrom & Miller, 2004). However, it is clear that the chronicity of the stressor is one important dimension to consider. Studies modeling how short-term laboratory stress (three minutes to half hour) influences aspects of immunity mostly show increases in cytotoxic T-cells, NK cells, NK cell activity, and decreases in the proliferative response to the mitogens PHA and Con A (Cacioppo et al. 1995; Matthews et al. 1995). These changes appear short-term, reflect changes in cell trafficking, and are mediated by activation of the SNS (Bachen et al., 1995).

Given the short-term nature of these changes, it might be argued that these alterations have little relevance for understanding disease outcomes such as cancer. However, similar to research linking acute stress to cardiovascular disease, it is assumed that these laboratory studies model stress reactions during daily life. This is important because according to the concept of allostasis such changes may be adaptive initially, but, if extended to repeated experiences of stress, may lead to changes that place an individual at risk for disease (Sterling & Eyer, 1988; McEwen, 1998). Consistent with this perspective, there is preliminary evidence for the utility of examining both laboratory stress reactions and stressor exposure in understanding immune-mediated disease risk (Boyce et al., 1995).

The concept of allostasis is consistent with research suggesting that more chronic stress (weeks to years) is associated with decrements in immune function (Segerstrom & Miller, 2004). Aspects of immune function are decreased in survivors of natural or human disasters (Ironson et al., 1997; Solomon et al., 1997); caregivers for family members with Alzheimer's disease (AD) (Kiecolt-Glaser et al., 1991; Kiecolt-Glaser et al., 1995); individuals suffering marital discord (Kiecolt-Glaser et al., 1987); and recently bereaved individuals (Bartrop et al., 1977; Kemeny et al., 1995). The effects of chronic stress on the immune system appear stronger using measures that capture the functional ability of the immune system to respond to challenge (i.e., proliferative response to mitogen) rather than cell counts (Kiecolt-Glaser & Glaser 1995). Importantly, such functional measures are generally regarded as more health relevant (Kiecolt-Glaser & Glaser, 1995).

Stress has also been directly linked to decreases in immunity in cancer patients and hence may theoretically play a role in disease progression depending on the stage and time course of disease (Kiecolt-Glaser & Glaser, 1995). In one study, investigators examined if perceptions of cancer-related stress had an influence on immune measures following surgical treatment (Andersen et al., 1998). Cancer-related stress in these patients had uniform effects on immunity as it was related to lower NK cell activity, proliferative responses to mitogens, NK cell activation via interferon-γ, and T-cell proliferation to antibody (Ab) directed at the T-cell receptor. This study is consistent with the results of interventions suggesting that stress-reduction may improve immune function in cancer patients, and has potential beneficial influences on survival (Fawzy et al., 1993). It is important to note, however, that direct evidence is still needed suggesting immune-related mediation of such effects (Cohen & Herbert, 1996), as well as the components of stress that might be impacted by such interventions.

One critically important pathway linking chronic stress to changes in immunity is through neuroendocrine activation. Cells of the immune system (e.g., lymphocytes) have functional receptors for endocrine hormones, which provide a mechanism by which stress may influence immunity (Sanders et al., 2001). It is now evident that immune cells have receptors for a variety of hormones including EPI, norepinephrine (NE), ACTH, cortisol, opioids, growth hormone, prolactin, and estrogen that provide a pharmacological basis for neuromodulation (Sanders et al., 2001).

The three major hormonal pathways linking stress to immune processes include activation of the HPA, SNS, and opioid systems. Of these, much focus has been placed on hormones of the HPA, such as cortisol, given its theoretical role in chronic stress processes (Selye, 1956). The major influence of HPA hormones on immune processes appears inhibitory (Munck, Guyre, & Holbrook, 1984). For instance, glucocorticoids inhibit aspects of antigen presentation (Baus et al., 1996) and pre-incubation of PBLs with glucocorticoids tends to decrease the proliferative response to mitogens as well as NKCA (Holbrook, Cox, & Horner, 1983; Wiegers et al., 1993). Many of these effects were blocked by the specific glucocorticoid receptor antagonist RU-486 (e.g., Wiegers et al., 1993).

HPA hormones may indirectly suppress *in vivo* cellular immune function in at least two ways. Central administration of CRH reliably decreases the proliferative response to mitogens (Johnson et al., 1994) and splenic NK cell activity (Irwin et al., 1989). Although central CRH activates the HPA axis, it also activates the ANS and the influence of central CRH on splenic NK cell activity appears mediated by activation of the ANS (Irwin et al., 1989). HPA hormones also appear to modulate cytokine production (Munck, Guyre, & Holbrook, 1984). The cytokines interferon-γ and IL-2 enhance the cytolytic activity of NK cells and cytotoxic T-cells, and appear to play an important role in the elimination phase of cancer immunoediting (Dunn et al., 2002). Importantly, HPA hormones, such as ACTH, appear to inhibit the synthesis of both interferon-γ and IL-2 (Arya, Wong-Staal, & Gallo 1984; Kelso & Munck, Guyre, & Holbrook, 1984).

Although the SNS is clearly involved in short-term changes in immunity, the longer-term consequences of SNS activation may also be significant. Sympathetic nerve fibers innervate both primary and secondary lymphoid organs (Felton et al. 1987), and provide a direct mechanism by which the SNS may influence aspects of immunity. Destruction of lymphoid sympathetic fibers via treatment with 6-hydroxydopamine appears to potentiate immune responses to antigen. These observations have led some to argue that the SNS exerts a tonic inhibitory influence on lymphoid immune processes. In a sustained program of research, Ben-Eliyahu and Shakhar (2001) have found that stress decreases NK cell activity and increases tumor growth. These effects appear mediated by the SNS because β-adrenergic blockade or adrenal demedullation eliminated these stress-induced effects, whereas β-adrenergic agonists mimicked the effects of stress on tumor growth.

Another pathway of interest is through an opioid mechanism because stress has been linked to activation of the opioid system (Wang et al., 2002). *In vivo* studies suggest that infusion of morphine or implantation of morphine pellets decreases splenic NK cell activity and the proliferative response to mitogens (Bayer et al., 1990; Shavit et al., 1986). These effects appear partially eliminated by opioid antagonists (Bayer et al., 1990), with activation of the SNS and HPA as two potential indirect mechanisms also responsible for such effects (Fecho, Dykstra, & Lysle, 1993; Freier & Fuchs, 1994). Consistent with the role of opioid hormones on immune processes and tumor growth, fentanyl (an opioid analgesic) was associated with a suppression of NK cell activity and decreased resistance to tumor metastasis in rats (Shavit et al., 2004).

The data linking stress to immune function highlights the potential role for stress-reduction interventions in enhancing aspects of immune function, with potential beneficial influences on cancer-related processes. One cognitive-behavioral stress management intervention in early stage breast cancer patients found decreases in cortisol (Cruess et al., 2000), a finding mediated by changes in patients' perceptions of benefit finding. In general, interventions in chronically stressed populations such as cancer patients appear to have beneficial influences on immunity (Fawzy et al., 1993; Lutgendorf et al., 1997). However, little evidence exists suggesting that stress management interventions can increase immunity in healthy, nonstressed populations (Miller & Cohen, 2001).

The link between chronic stress and immune processes potentially highlights the role of stress reactivity, exposure, recovery, and restoration on cancer outcomes. Very little research has separated out the effects of these stress component processes on cancer outcomes, especially in regards to stress recovery. The association between stress and immune-mediated restorative processes is just being established, however, existing evidence is promising. As noted earlier, sleep is one such restorative process and chronic stress has been linked to poorer sleep quality (Cartwright & Wood, 1991). There is also strong evidence linking sleep disruption to decrements in immunity, including NK cell activity (Irwin, 2002). Although the mechanisms responsible for these changes in immune function are not yet clear, evidence implicates sleep-mediated changes in cytokines such as IL-1, IL-2, and IL-6 (Irwin, 2002). In one study, the stress of bereavement was associated with lower circulating NK cells, and poor sleep was a mediator of this association (Hall et al., 1998).

During sleep, the release of certain hormones may play an important role in restorative processes (Epel, McEwen, & Ickovics, 1998; McEwen, 1998). Of these, growth hormone may be particularly important because most of it is released during sleep (Veldhuis & Aranmanesh, 1996). Importantly, growth hormone appears to augment aspects of immune function and hence may have a beneficial influence on tumor resistance (Koo et al., 2001). These data, however, need to be considered in light of epidemiological links between the growth promoting peptide IGF-I, which mediates the effects of growth hormone on tissue growth, and increased cancer incidence (Chan et al., 1998).

STRESS AND INFECTIOUS DISEASES

Background information. Although mortality as a result of infectious diseases has declined in industrialized countries, it nevertheless remains an important cause of morbidity and mortality. More specifically, the emergence of HIV has highlighted the importance of understanding links between stress and infectious disease processes. According to recent statistics, over 20 million people have died worldwide since the start of the epidemic in the early 1980s and an additional 40 million individuals are now living with HIV or AIDS (UNAIDS/WHO, 2004). With no known cure, it is clear that HIV and AIDS will continue to be a significant worldwide health problem. It is also important to note that infectious diseases such as influenza, even in industrialized countries, are an important cause of mortality in older adults (Effros & Walford, 1987). In addition, tuberculosis (TB) was responsible for an estimated 2 million deaths in 2002 and the incidence of new infections continues to pose major health risks in many countries (WHO, 2004).

The immune system plays an important role in the control of such infectious diseases. However, the specific effector mechanisms responsible for protection depend on the type of challenge (Abbas & Lichtman, 2003). Protection against viruses and bacteria begins with innate immunity to prevent them from entering the host (e.g., skin, mucous membranes). Innate immune processes such as complement activation, macrophage activity, and inflammation provide further protection once pathogens enter the host. For instance, some extracellular bacteria have features in their cell walls (e.g., LPS in gram-negative bacteria) that activate the alternate complement pathway that in turn can destroy the bacteria. Macrophages and NK cells may also play important roles in innate immunity because they are able to phagocytize some pathogens once they enter the host.

However, once the pathogen begins replicating inside the body, the adaptive immune response becomes the important mechanism for resolution of these infections. For extracellular pathogens such as some bacteria, the primary arm of adaptive immunity is humoral. Humoral immunity refers to the activity of B-cells that replicate and produce Ab specific to the pathogen. Antibodies can facilitate the elimination of extracellular pathogens by neutralizing them and their toxins, marking them for destruction, or both (e.g., opsonization). Helper T-cells (i.e., TH2 subset) facilitate this process by aiding in the clonal expansion of B-cells.

However, viruses and some bacteria (e.g., TB) are intracellular pathogens and the resolution of these infections is primarily T-cell mediated via the cellular arm of adaptive immunity (Abbas & Lichtman, 2003). Cytotoxic T-cells recognize viral antigen in the context of MHC class I molecules and can directly lyse infected cells. In addition, helper T-cells (i.e., TH1 subset) aid in the clonal expansion of cytotoxic T-cells and secrete cytokines (i.e., IL-2, interferon-γ) that enhance NK lysis or phagocytosis of infected cells. Helper T-cells may also stimulate B-cells to produce Ab. Antibodies and complements may then directly lyse infected cells or opsonize them for subsequent killing.

One virus of particular interest is HIV, which is found in blood, semen, vaginal fluids, and breast milk of infected individuals at biologically relevant quantities. Upon entering the body, it infects cells possessing specific surface molecules (e.g., CD4+ cells). One of the important cells infected and destroyed by HIV is the helper T-cell. As illustrated above, helper T-cells are absolutely essential to coordinate both the cellular and humoral arms of adaptive immunity. By depleting helper T-cells, HIV cuts off the ability of the immune system to effectively fight against foreign invaders. Although the body mounts a vigorous immune response, the virus can reside in a "latent stage" that can last for years. During this phase, HIV may be diminished in blood, but disease progression continues in lymphoid organs. Ultimately, HIV infection can result in the destruction of this important cell line and the subsequent development of AIDS which is a condition in which the body's immune system eventually loses its ability to fight off foreign invaders (Abbas & Lichtman, 2003). As a result, the infected person is at risk for morbidity and mortality from pathogens that a healthy person would normally have no trouble fighting off. Although no cure is presently available, recent biomedical advances have successfully extended the lives of HIV+ individuals (Kelly et al., 1998). Although significant challenges exist (e.g., ability of HIV to mutate because of encoding errors), vaccines against HIV are now being evaluated in several large clinical trials and remains a high priority for biomedical research.

Evidence linking stress to infectious diseases. The overall evidence linking stress to infectious diseases appears strong (Baum & Posluszny, 1999; Cohen & Williamson, 1991; Kiecolt-Glaser et al., 2002). There have been two general approaches to examining the links between stress and infectious diseases. One approach has been to link stress to naturally occurring infections. Recent studies suggest that life stress, and chronic stress in particular, is related to increased susceptibility to infectious disease (Dyck, Short, & Vitaliano, 1999; Kiecolt-Glaser et al., 1991). For instance, caregiving for a family member with schizophrenia was related to the risk of developing an infectious disease (Dyck, Short, & Vitaliano, 1999). Results of this study showed that patient symptoms during acute exacerbation of schizophrenia, but not more stable symptoms, was related to risk for infections in caregivers. In the context of long-term stress, these data suggest that exposure to less predictable sources of stress may be particularly important to consider.

Although the above data are consistent with the role of stress in the risk for infections, a more controlled approach has been to expose consenting adults to a viral challenge. Recent studies, which improved on the methodological limitations of prior research, provide strong evidence for a link between stress and susceptibility to infectious diseases (Cohen et al., 1998). In one study that examined different types of stressors prior to challenge, consenting adults were inoculated with the common cold virus and quarantined for five days (Cohen et al., 1998). Only stressors lasting over one month were associated with increased risk for verified colds. Of these, chronic interpersonal and work stressors were primarily responsible for the effects of chronic stress on infections. These effects were independent of prechallenge Ab status, demographic factors, personality processes, and various health practices. In another study, these investigators also reported the combination of high life stress and high cortisol responses to acute laboratory stress predicted an increase in verified upper respiratory illnesses (Cohen et al., 2002).

One of the hallmarks of immunity is memory in which pathogens that have been eradicated from the host are met with a more effective immune response upon subsequent exposure. However, some viruses (e.g., EBV) avoid elimination by going latent and "hiding" relatively inactive in certain cells. The exposed individual is infected for life, but the cellular immune response is usually successful at keeping the virus in check. However, individuals with compromised cellular immune processes (e.g., HIV+ populations or patients on immunosupressive therapies) may experience reactivation of one or more of these latent viruses. In such cases, increased Ab titers to latent viruses suggest poorer cellular immunity because the reactivation of the virus triggers the humoral arm of adaptive immunity. Importantly, there is strong evidence from both animal and human studies that stress can result in reactivation of latent viruses (Padgett et al., 1998).

A final paradigm of interest is the handful of studies examining the link between stress and the progression of HIV infection. An early meta-analysis found that stress was not reliably associated with CD4+ counts, an important marker of disease progression in HIV+ individuals (Zorrilla et al., 1996). However, evidence was found for an association between stress and lower NK cells counts and NK cell activity in HIV+ populations. Although the links between stress and NK cell function were consistent with poorer immune regulation of HIV, the lack of findings for CD4+ cells was unexpected. However, some researchers have argued that more long-term studies were needed in order to examine how stress is related to the entire course of disease. In one such study, Leserman and colleagues (1999) followed a sample of HIV+ individuals for up to seven and a half years. In their study, 37% of the sample had progressed to AIDS. Importantly, faster progression to AIDS was predicted by a total index of stressful events (i.e., number and severity). Although more research is needed, there is recent preliminary evidence linking stress to the progression of HIV infection (see Cole & Kemeny, 2001; Kopnisky, Stoff, & Rausch, 2004).

In the context of HIV it is also important to discuss how stress may influence exposure to HIV infection (Baum & Posluszny, 1999). This is salient because the primary route of HIV infection is behavioral in nature (Kelly et al., 1993). Stress is linked to changes in health behaviors, including alcohol and drug use (Testa & Collins, 1997). The use of alcohol and illicit drugs may in turn increase risky sexual behavior through processes such as disinhibition and facilitation of sexual arousal (McCarty, Diamond, & Kaye, 1982; O'Keeffe, Nesselhof-Kendall, & Baum, 1990). Thus, stress appears to influence behavioral factors that may place individuals at risk for HIV infection.

Potential mechanisms linking stress to infectious diseases. There is strong evidence linking stress to infectious disease susceptibility. The major protective mechanism in susceptibility to infectious disease is the immune system (Abbas & Lichtman, 2003). Thus, evidence linking stress to immune function can inform researchers about the stage(s) that stress influences susceptibility. One paradigm that lends clear evidence to the links between chronic stress and decreased immunity is research on caregivers of family members with AD. Caregiving for a family member with AD is characterized as a prototypic chronic stressor due to the long-term, severe, and unpredictable problems caregivers often deal with. In an important program of research, Kiecolt-Glaser and colleagues (1991) found that long-term caregiving for a family member with AD was associated with impaired adaptive immune processes (e.g., decreased proliferative response to mitogens, increased Ab titers to latent viruses) compared to demographically-matched controls. These changes did not appear to "rebound" upon termination of the chronic stressor. Caregivers whose family members had been deceased on average of two years still showed signs of a downregulated immune response (Esterling et al., 1994).

Research further suggests that these stress-induced immune changes in caregivers are biologically relevant. Caregivers are less likely to seroconvert to influenza vaccination, have higher rates of infectious diseases, and evidence poorer wound repair (Kiecolt-Glaser et al., 1995; Kiecolt-Glaser et al., 1996). Fortunately, interventions aimed at decreasing stress in caregivers have shown some initial promise in terms of decreasing distress and augmenting some immune processes (Bourgeois, Schulz, & Burgio, 1996; Hosaka & Sugiyama, 2003). It is important to note that caregiver stress paradigms implicate the role of both stress reactivity and stress exposure in infectious disease risk. Older caregivers show greater acute stress reactions, and are also exposed to a relatively high number of stressful events related to caregiving (Bourgeois, Schulz, & Burgio, 1996; Uchino, Kiecolt-Glaser, & Caciopppo, 1992). These data are consistent with the study by Cohen and colleagues (2002) that found the combination of high life stress and high cortisol reactivity predicted increases in upper respiratory illnesses (Cohen et al., 2002).

Studies examining the links between stress and vaccination provide a promising paradigm for understanding more specific biological mechanisms because increased Ab titers to such vaccines are related to lower risk for infection (Center for Disease Control, 1996). Importantly, stress predicts lower Ab production in response to influenza (Kiecolt-Glaser et al., 1996; Miller et al., 2004; Vedhara et al., 1999), hepatitis B (Jabaaij et al., 1993; Glaser et al., 1992), meningitis C (Burns et al., 2002), and Pneumococcal Pneumonia vaccinations (Glaser et al., 2000). One preliminary study also found that a stress-management intervention was associated with higher seroconversion to an influenza vaccination compared to nonintervention caregivers, although there was no evidence that changes in stress perceptions mediated such differences (Vedhara et al., 2003).

The studies linking stress to Ab titers following vaccination clearly implicate the humoral arm of adaptive immunity as one important mechanism linking stress to infectious disease susceptibility. One question, however, relates to the kinetics of the Ab response and the phase in which stress may influence susceptibility to disease. In one of the only studies that we know of to examine this question, Miller and colleagues (2004) examined daily assessments of stress and its association to Ab production to an influenza vaccination in healthy participants. Daily levels of stress were followed for three days prior to and ten days postvaccination. Results of this intriguing study found that stress prior to and on the day of the vaccination was not related to subsequent Ab production. However, from the third day postvaccination, daily stress was associated with less Ab production, with the strongest independent effect evident on the tenth day postvaccination (Miller et al., 2004). Of course, the findings regarding the kinetics of the susceptible period need to be considered in light of the healthy population because these patterns may change as a function of an individual's immune status (e.g., caregivers).

In an attempt to model biological mechanisms, several studies have examined if neuroendocrine processes were responsible for some of these stress-induced vaccination effects. Cortisol is a prime candidate given its general immunosuppressive effects (Munck, Guyre, & Holbrook, 1984). In the case of Ab production following vaccination, one study found little evidence that changes in cortisol

were responsible for such differences in healthy participants (Miller et al., 2004). However, a study looking at the chronic stress of caregiving found associations between stress, cortisol, and Ab titers that were consistent with mediation (Vedhara et al., 1999). In addition, Caciopppo and colleagues (1998) reported that cortisol reactivity to acute psychological stress predicted a decline in the T-cell response to an influenza vaccination in older adults. These data suggest that cortisol may play a relatively larger role in stress-induced immune changes during chronic stress or in populations with more compromised immune systems.

Animal models may provide a stronger test of neuroendocrine mediation because of the increased experimental control and more detailed assessments that can be obtained. In a murine model of influenza infection, restraint stress was associated with a virus-specific decrease in IL-2, IL-10, and interferon-γ production (Dobbs et al., 1996). These effects were blocked by the glucocorticoid blocker RU-486. It should be noted that although hormones of the HPA axis appear important, there are other hormonal pathways that need to be considered. For instance, in one study stress was linked to a poorer Ab response to a novel antigen in rats (Shao et al., 2003). However, significant correlations were only found between Ab titers and norepinephrine levels ($r = -.56$) but not corticosterone levels. Sheridan et al. (1998) also reported that the effects of restraint stress on lymphocyte trafficking and cytokine responses in virus-infected rats were mediated by activation of the HPA axis. However, the decreased cytolytic T-cell response to stress was not influenced by treatment with RU-486 but by β-adrenergic blockade, which suggests a sympathetic mechanism for this effect.

Although many studies have examined cortisol levels at one point, or in some cases averaged over an extended period of time, some research suggests the importance of modeling repeated exposure to cortisol. Such studies would be consistent with the role of stress exposure in these disease processes. In vitro studies suggest that cortisol can reactivate latent EBV (Glaser et al., 1995), the kinetics of such changes were recently tested by Caciopppo et al. (2002). These researchers incubated latently infected cells in varying concentrations of dexamethasone (DEX) (i.e., 10^{-5} M to 10^{-9} M every 24 hours for three days). The different concentrations of DEX were thought to model the in vivo effects of pulsatile cortisol changes that are likely to occur with acute stressors. Control cells were incubated with media only, or a single concentration of DEX for three days. Replicating prior research, it was found that the control media alone resulted in only a small (2–3%) percentage of EBV antigen positive cells, while single concentrations of DEX were associated with greater reactivation of EBV as measured by antigen positive cells after three days (5.63–8.06%). However, varying the concentration of DEX over three days resulted in a threefold or greater increase in EBV antigen positive cells. These results are consistent with the notion that pulsatile changes in HPA hormones, which covary with repeated exposure to stress, may have greater health consequences than tonic levels of these hormones.

Promising evidence for mechanism also exists regarding the neuroendocrine pathways potentially responsible for the links between stress and HIV infections (Kopnisky, Stoff, & Rausch, 2004). *In vitro* studies suggest that incubation of HIV infected cells with glucocorticoids can increase viral load in some cell lines (Markham et al., 1986). In work using a primate model of HIV infection (simian immunodeficiency virus, or SIV), Capitanio, Mendoza, Lerche, and Mason (1998) examined the influence of social stress on various outcomes. Results revealed that infected animals in stressful (unstable) social groups had lower basal cortisol and shorter survival. The investigators speculated that the lower baseline cortisol levels might indicate a dysregulation of the HPA axis as often seen with posttraumatic stress patients (e.g., Yehuda et al., 1990).

Research also suggests the importance of considering other neuroendocrine processes in HIV+ individuals. As reviewed earlier, both SNS and opioid processes appear to inhibit aspects of immune function and hence may play a role in HIV progression. *In vitro* studies suggest that NE can increase HIV replication, an effect that appeared mediated by a β-adrenergic mechanism (Cole et al., 1998). Similar *in vitro* effects of opioid hormones (e.g., morphine) on HIV replication have been found (Li et al., 2003). Moreover, opioids appear to increase macrophage susceptibility to infection, possibly by up-regulating CCR5 receptor expression which is an important coreceptor for HIV infection (Li et al., 2003).

Research also suggests the promise of modeling the coordination among the cardiovascular, neuroendocrine, and immune responses during acute stress and its association to infectious disease risk. It is assumed that these acute stress paradigms index how an individual responds to stress in their daily lives. In one study, older women participated in a combined math and speech stressor and were divided based on a median split on pre-ejection period (PEP) reactivity scores (Cacioppo et al., 2002). Consistent with the possibility that these paradigms tap into how individuals respond to stress in daily life, high PEP reactors (indicating greater sympathetic control of the heart) showed greater EBV titers than low PEP reactors. This research team also found that PEP reactivity to acute psychological stress predicted a decline in the T-cell response to vaccination three months later (Cacioppo et al., 1998). Given the association between PEP reactivity and cortisol changes during acute stress (Cacioppo et al., 1995; Uchino et al., 1995), these data suggest that individuals characterized by high cardiac sympathetic reactivity may be more at risk for infectious diseases because of co-activation of the HPA axis during daily stress. These data, again, highlight the importance of considering components of both stress reactivity and exposure in modeling infectious disease risk.

Although most research examining autonomic modulation of stress-induced immune responses has focused on the SNS, there is evidence to indicate that parasympathetic influences on immune function may also be important (Haas & Schauenstein, 1997; Tracey, 2002). Gordon, Cohen, and Wilson (1978) provided evidence that lymphocytes express muscarinic receptors. There also appears to be vagal innervation of lymphoid tissues (Najima, 1995; Rinner et al., 1994). In a preliminary study, PNS denervation resulted in a *decreased* antibody response to sheep red blood cells in mice (Alito et al., 1987). These data are opposite of those reported following SNS denervation and suggest that the PNS may potentiate lymphoid immune processes (but see discussion of methodological issues in Bellinger et al., 2001).

Although more data are needed, existing studies suggest that hormones of the PNS tend to potentiate aspects of the cellular immune response. For instance, incubation of cholinergic agonists (i.e., carbamylcholine) with T-cells resulted in greater cytotoxic activity (Strom et al., 1974; Katz, Zaytoun, & Fauci, 1982). Activation of muscarinic receptors appears responsible for the enhanced cytotoxicity because muscarinic antagonists (i.e., atropine) but not nicotinic antagonists (e.g., *d*-tubocurarine) blocked the effects of PNS agonists on cell-mediated cytotoxicity (Katz, Zaytoun, & Fauci, 1982; Strom et al., 1974). Consistent with the importance of PNS activation, one recent study found that a passive coping task, which resulted in co-activation of the SNS and PNS was associated with the largest increases in salivary proteins involved in innate immunity (Bosch et al., 2003b). These findings are important as such secretory processes serve to protect mucosal surfaces against initial infection.

The importance of not ignoring PNS influences on immune processes is further highlighted by the recently characterized "inflammatory reflex" (Tracey, 2002). In response to inflammation, activation of the PNS serves to blunt the inflammatory response in "real time." This reflex serves to limit pro-inflammatory processes that, if left unchecked, can in some cases be more dangerous than the initial pathogen (e.g., septic shock). This PNS reflex is mediated by nicotinic receptors on cytokine producing cells that decrease the synthesis of pro-inflammatory cytokines (e.g., macrophages, Tracey, 2002).

In terms of component stress processes, very little evidence exists on the role of stress recovery on immune-mediated disease processes. However, there is evidence indicating that restorative processes may play an important role in stress-induced susceptibility to infectious disease. Although critical data are just appearing, research appears consistent with the important role of sleep in immune function (Irwin, 2002). Even acute stress predicts decreased objective (e.g., rapid eye movement count) and subjective (e.g., sleep quality) aspects of sleep (Germain et al., 2003; Morin, Rodrigue, & Ivers, 2003). In one study, Lange and colleagues (2003) examined if sleep deprivation (i.e., 36 hours) following a Hepatitis A vaccination influenced subsequent Ab responses. Results showed that the immediate effects of sleep deprivation included less release of growth hormone, prolactin, and dopamine. Sleep deprivation started to have an effect on the primary immune response about 14 days after vaccination and became larger up to 28 days postvaccination. The authors speculated that early immune processes related to IL-2 production, a cytokine that enhances both T- and B-cell differentiation, may have been responsible for these effects.

Importantly, several studies have now shown that sleep disturbances mediate the effects of stress on aspects of immunity for more chronically stressed participants (Cruess et al., 2003; Hall et al., 1998; Ironson et al., 1997). These studies have reported mediation of stress effects on aspects of immune function in victims of natural disasters (Ironson et al., 1997), bereaved participants (Hall et al., 1998), and HIV-infected patients (Cruess et al., 2003). For instance, researchers examined the impact of Hurricane Andrews one to four months after the disaster. The stress of Hurricane Andrew was associated with posttraumatic symptoms that in turn were related to lower NK cell activity. Importantly, the onset of new sleep problems statistically mediated the posttraumatic symptoms – NK cell activity relationship.

More recent evidence also implicates stress in the restorative process of wound healing (Kiecolt-Glaser et al., 1998). Following tissue injury, early immune responses play a key role in the wound healing process (Abbas & Lichtman, 2003). For instance, inflammatory cytokines (e.g., IL-1, IL-6) play an initial role in the recruitment of phagocytes (e.g., neutrophils) that then protect and prepare the wound for healing (Barbul, 1990). In one study, Kiecolt-Glaser and colleagues (1995) examined if the chronic stress of caregiving was associated with delayed wound healing following a punch biopsy. Results showed that caregivers produced less IL-1β and took significantly longer to heal (also see Broadbent et al., 2003). These findings are consistent with animal models of stress and wound repair (Padgett et al., 1998). Such findings are important as delayed wound healing may be related to increased infections (Kiecolt-Glaser et al., 1998). Consistent with this possibility, researchers found that restraint stress in mice was associated with delayed wound healing, and greater levels of opportunistic bacteria compared to control animals (Rojas et al., 2002). These effects were significantly reduced by treating mice with the glucocorticoid blocker RU-486.

TOWARDS AN INTEGRATIVE ANALYSIS OF STRESS AND HEALTH

The research reviewed in this chapter suggests that stress may play a role in the leading causes of death worldwide. There appears to be a reliable link between stress and cardiovascular disease, as well as infectious illnesses. Evidence linking stress to cancer outcomes is controversial,

but progress regarding the concept of cancer immunoediting may be important for future progress by describing the more precise role of immune processes across the full course of the disease. Research linking stress to HIV progression is preliminary, but some evidence exists on such a link.

Because the complexity of these health outcomes, most research linking stress to health, or its underlying pathways, has focused on one disease. However, recent research is painting in broad strokes, a more integrative picture of how these stress-related health outcomes may be coordinated. This view highlights the linkages among the major biological stress systems, and how these processes unfold in the context of specific diseases. An integrative understanding of such processes may be important to identify common (potentially modifiable) pathways, as well as reconcile inconsistencies in prior research (e.g., protective or damaging effects). This more integrative approach is highlighted by research on (a) the role of inflammation in cardiovascular disease (Black & Garbutt, 2002; Libby, 2002; Ross, 1999), (b) coordinated central nervous system (CNS) involvement in the stress response (Chrousos & Gold, 1992; Dunn & Berridge, 1990), and (c) multilevel perspectives on stress and health (Cacioppo & Berntson, 1992).

The role of immune processes in cardiovascular disease. Traditionally, the immune system has been linked to infectious diseases and cancer. Cardiovascular disease can now be added to that list of disease processes with an immunologic component (Libby, 2002; Ross, 1999). Immune processes are implicated in just about every stage of atherogenesis (Libby, 2002). In fact, inflammatory processes have been linked to more widespread health problems including diabetes, some cancers, and frailty more generally (Coussens & Werb, 2002; Kiecolt-Glaser et al., 2002; Papanicolaou et al., 1998).

One of the earliest events in the atherogenic process is endothelial damage (Ross, 1999). Factors such as differential shear stress at vessel walls, elevated low-density lipoproteins (LDLs), and some infectious organisms (e.g., Chlamydia Pneumoniae) may precipitate endothelial damage (Ross, 1999; Worthley et al., 2001). Although the specific mechanisms linking such triggers to damage are still under investigation, modified LDLs that undergo oxidization (or form immune complexes) can be trapped in vessel walls and injure the vascular endothelium, smooth muscle, or both (Steinberg, 1997). Oxidized LDL is in itself a direct and indirect chemoattractant for monocytes and T-cells via the release of monocyte chemoattractant protein-1 (MCP-1) from endothelial cells (Young & McEneny, 2001).

At early stages of damage, the endothelium begins to express adhesion molecules such as vascular adhesion molecule-1 that help in the binding of immune cells to the vasculature. Monocytes and T-lymphocytes are then recruited to sites of inflammation and migrate into vessel walls via various chemokines (e.g., MCP-1) that are released from vascular cell walls (Charo & Taubman, 2004). Once inside of vessel walls, these immune cells proliferate and release a variety of growth factors (e.g., platelet-derived growth factors) and cytokines (e.g., IL-1) characteristic of the inflammatory response (Libby, 2002). The release of cytokines from these cells, as well as from vessel walls, further up-regulates the expression of adhesion molecules, while increasing the proliferation of smooth muscles cells (SMC). Macrophages expressing scavenger receptors begin to ingest lipids (e.g., oxidized LDL) to form the foam cell that is characteristic of the advancing lesion.

Of course, inflammation can be beneficial under "normal" conditions. For instance, the inflammatory response appears to play a role in the enlargement of existing vessels and the healing of plaque following thrombosis (Charo & Taubman, 2004; Libby, 2002). However, if the source of damage is not removed, these processes can lead to a vicious cycle of inflammation as cytokines further increase LDL binding to endothelial and smooth muscle walls (Ross, 1999). The resulting advanced lesion has a fibrous cap that protrudes into the lumen and contains elements of the inflammatory response including macrophages, T-cells, foam cells, and lipids (Ross, 1999). Vulnerable plaques have a large ratio of lipids to fibrotic components and such plaques may be responsible for as much as 75% of complications leading to acute coronary events (Worthley et al., 2001). Immune events at later stages can lead to the rupture of such plaques. For instance, macrophages are common in vulnerable plaques and can produce enzymes (e.g., metalloproteinases) that degrade the fibrous cap, while T-lymphocytes release interferon-γ that can impede collagen formation by SMC (Libby, 2002).

Importantly, stress can directly lead to the release of cytokines, which are crucial mediators of the cardiovascular inflammatory response (Black & Garbutt, 2002; Kop & Cohen, 2001). Animal models show that stress increases the release of inflammatory cytokines such as IL-1, IL-6, and tumor necrosis factor-α (TNF-α), as well as subsequent acute phase proteins such as C-reactive proteins (CRP) (Black & Garbutt, 2002). In a meta-analysis of human studies, Segerstrom and Miller (2004) found that IL-6 was significantly increased during both laboratory and brief real world stressors. Less data in humans exists on cytokine production during more chronic stressors (Segerstrom & Miller, 2004). However, existing studies do suggest that chronic stress is associated with increased inflammatory cytokine release (Brydon et al., 2004; Kiecolt-Glaser et al., 2002; Lutgendorf et al., 1999). For instance, Kiecolt-Glaser et al. (2003) examined age-related differences in IL-6 in caregivers of AD patients. These investigators found that the predicted rate of change in IL-6 for caregivers was almost fourfold higher than that of controls and not explained by various demographic factors or health behaviors (e.g., exercise or alcohol consumption).

Stress-induced cytokine production may be mediated by the release of neuroendocrine hormones that influ-

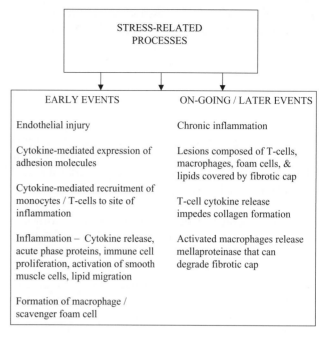

Figure 26.2. The potential role of stress-related immune processes in cardiovascular disease.

ence cytokine release and macrophage or T-cell function more generally (Sanders et al., 2001). However, it is important to note that inflammatory cytokines are not just produced from cells of the immune system (Papanicolaou et al., 1998). For instance, IL-6 is produced by bone marrow stromal cells, epithelial cells, SMCs, and cells of the anterior pituitary (Papanicolaou et al., 1998). When released, such cytokines can cause an increase in adhesion molecules that promote the migration of monocytes and T-lymphocytes characteristic of early endothelial damage (Libby, 2002). Moreover, Bosch and colleagues (2003a) found that acute psychological stress was associated with a selective increase in T-cells that express chemokine receptors. These changes were most pronounced in high cardiac sympathetic reactors and further highlight the importance of a more integrative analysis of stress effects across systems.

Illustrative steps in which stress can influence inflammation and cardiovascular disease risk are provided in Figure 26.2. As detailed above, stress-induced cytokine release can influence early inflammatory processes that are related to cardiovascular disease. Cytokine release during stress may also influence cardiovascular disease processes as the lesion advances. The cytokine macrophage colony-stimulating factor (M-CSF) is implicated in the development of the foam cell as it can augment scavenger receptor expression on macrophages (Libby, 2002). M-CSF, as well as IL-1 and TNF-α, can also increase the binding of LDL to vessel walls, and up-regulate the LDL-receptor gene (Libby, 2002; Ross, 1999). At later stages of the lesion, plaque disruption can be influenced by cytokines (Libby, 2002). Activated T-cells produce interferon-γ that can decrease collagen production by SMC. Cytokines such as IL-1 and

TNF-α can increase the production of the protein metalloproteinase that in turn can degrade the fibrotic cap of advanced lesions (Rajavashisth et al., 1999). The result is a weaker fibrotic cap that is susceptible to rupture due to factors such as increased hemodynamic stress (Libby, 2002).

An additional pathway by which stress-induced inflammatory cytokine release can influence cardiovascular disease is via the subsequent release of acute-phase proteins (Papanicolaou et al., 1998). IL-6 is a potent stimulator of CRP and fibrinogen production from the liver. CRP has received much recent attention as it has been shown in a number of large prospective studies to predict future coronary risk, even in participants with normal levels of cholesterol (Libby, 2002). Although CRP can be thought of as a clinical marker of inflammatory processes, recent research is showing that CRP may play a direct pro-inflammatory role in the atherogenic process (Khreiss et al., 2004; Verma, Szmitko, & Yeh, 2004). For instance, CRP may decrease nitric oxide production and increase cytokine production (Verma, Szmitko, & Yeh, 2004). These factors can up-regulate adhesion molecules and increase monocyte recruitment (Khreiss et al., 2004; Verma, Szmitko, & Yeh, 2004). Although the release of CRP via IL-6 seems to be an important factor in inflammation and cardiovascular disease, consistent with the crucial role of cytokines in all phases of the atherogenic process, IL-6 continues to predict cardiovascular risk even after statistically controlling for CRP (Ridker et al., 2000).

The more precise mechanisms responsible for cytokine release during stress, and its implications for health more generally, are actively being investigated (Black & Garbutt, 2002; Kiecolt-Glaser et al., 2002). One cytokine of recent interest is IL-6 given its diverse physiological role in inflammation as well as the adaptive immune response (Hawkley et al., in press; Kiecolt-Glaser et al., 2002). IL-6 predicts a range of health problems including cardiovascular disease, diabetes, osteoporosis, and some autoimmune disorders (Papanicolaou et al., 1998).

The links between stress, IL-6, and other health-relevant physiological changes are starting to be understood. A key first step in this process appears to be stress-induced changes in SNS processes (Papanicolaou et al., 1998). Both stress and SNS agonists increase the production of IL-6 (Soszynski et al., 1996), and β_2-adrenegic blockade eliminates these effects (Soszynski et al., 1996; van Gool et al., 1990). Importantly, the mechanism of action appears to be central β_2-adrenergic receptors as agonist more selective to such central processes (e.g., L-propanolol), but not more peripheral processes reduce the stress-induced increase in IL-6 (Soszynski et al., 1996).

Following SNS release, IL-6 is a potent stimulator of the HPA axis (Papanicolaou et al., 1998; Webster et al., 1998). Administration of IL-6 is associated with an increase in glucocorticoids that can occur through a CRH-dependent or independent mechanism (Kariagina et al., 2004). For instance, Bethin, Vgot, and Muglia (2000) found IL-6 receptors on both pituitary and adrenalcortical cells. These investigators also found that knockout mice deficient in IL-6 produced less corticosterone during stress. However, knockout mice deficient in both CRH and IL-6 produced the lowest levels of corticosterone (also see Kariagina et al., 2004). Under normal conditions, the subsequent increase in glucocorticoids serves as a negative feedback mechanism to down-regulate the inflammatory response (Papanicolaou et al., 1998). However, high levels of stress can decrease the sensitivity of immune cells to the inhibitory effects of glucocorticoids (Miller, Cohen, & Ritchey, 2002; Stark et al., 2001). One mechanism for this effect may be high or prolonged cytokine release that can directly modulate important isoforms of glucocorticoid receptors on cytokine producing cells (Webster et al., 2001).

Although IL-6 can influence the release of CRH, there is good evidence that the links between IL-6 and CRH are bidirectional. CRH plays an important role in the *in vitro* and *in vivo* regulation of IL-6 (Webster et al., 1998). Incubation of LPS-challenged macrophages with CRH leads to an increase in inflammatory cytokines, including IL-6 (Agelaki et al., 2002). Similar findings were demonstrated *in vivo* as mice given antalarmin (a CRH-receptor antagonist with both central and peripheral effects) showed decreased inflammatory cytokine responses to LPS. Moreover, the biological significance of these CRH-induced processes was shown as antalarmin prolonged survival in mice challenged with LPS-induced septic shock (Agelaki et al., 2002). Thus, IL-6 can activate and be activated by CRH, and CRH is in turn a major coordinator of the biologic and behavioral responses seen following stress (Habib et al., 2000; Webster et al., 1998).

Despite links between stress and inflammation, there are several complexities in these associations that require further discussion. First, although evidence does exist on the pro-inflammatory influences of IL-6 (e.g., via induction of CRP, see Verma, Szmitko, & Yeh, 2004); the ability of IL-6 to activate the HPA axis suggests that it may also have important anti-inflammatory properties. In fact, Hawkley and colleagues (in press) have argued that the primary function of IL-6 may be anti-inflammatory. Consistent with this view, IL-6 in itself does not appear to up-regulate inflammatory mediators (e.g., prostagladins) or the expression of adhesion molecules (Barton, 1997). IL-6 can also down-regulate the synthesis of pro-inflammatory cytokines (i.e., IL-1, TNF-α), and increase the synthesis of IL-1ra and the soluble TNF receptor factor p55 (Tilg et al., 1994). IL-6 knockout mice also produced higher levels of TNF-α in response to endotoxin challenge, and administration of IL-6 in these knockout mice eliminated the observed differences in TNF-α production (Xing et al., 1998). These IL-6 knockout mice also had a 50% lower survival rate in response to endotoxin challenge. Interestingly, levels of IL-10 were not different in the IL-6 knockout mice suggesting that IL-10 could not compensate for the deficiency in IL-6 (Xing et al., 1998). As a result of existing data, Hawkley and colleagues (in press) caution researchers in interpreting the results of correlational studies because it is possible that elevated levels of IL-6 may be co-activated in an attempt to control inflammation. Future research will be necessary to determine the disease-relevant contexts in which IL-6 has pro- or anti-inflammatory effects.

A second complexity related to links between stress and inflammation that requires increased attention relates to the conditions under which normal control points can be disrupted (Hawkley et al., in press). One important control mechanism is activation of the HPA axis that tends to suppress immunity (Munck, Guyre, & Holbrook, 1984). However, chronic stress can also lead to a state of glucocorticoid resistance (Miller, Cohen & Ritchey, 2002; Hawkley et al., in press). For instance, pro-inflammatory cytokines such as TNF-α can modulate important isoforms of glucocorticoid receptors on cytokine producing cells (Webster et al., 2001). The cytokine macrophage migration inhibitory factor (MIF) is also receiving attention as an important mechanism of glucocorticoid resistance (Hawkley et al., in press). MIF is a pro-inflammatory cytokine that is released from the anterior pituitary, as well as from macrophages during glucocorticoid release (see reviews by Baugh & Donnelly, 2003; Hawkley et al., in press). It has been shown to override the suppressive effects of glucocorticoids and may control the "set-point" of the inflammatory response (e.g., via modulation of NF-κB activity).

CNS coordination of the stress response. Evidence for co-ordinated central pathways involved in the stress response provides further impetus for a more integrative view of the association between stress and health. Of course, the central pathways involved in the stress response are complex and moderated by a number of factors including the duration of exposure, prior experience, and the social environment. These moderational influences are not surprising given the role of multiple brain structures (e.g., hippocampus, amygdala) with reciprocal connections that are crucial to interpreting, responding to, and receiving feedback about potential threats (Chrousos, this volume, Dunn & Berridge, 1990; Gray, 1993). However, there are identifiable brain structures and pathways that appear critically important in the coordinated stress response.

One promising integrating mechanism linking stress to health outcomes may involve the activation and release of central CRH (Dunn & Berridge, 1990). Central administration of CRH mimics many of the physiological and behavioral states seen during stress. For instance, central CRH activates both the ANS and HPA axis (Irwin et al., 1989) and stimulates the release of β-endorphins (Rivier et al., 1982). Increased CRH in brain regions involved in emotional responses, such as the amygdala, paraventricular nucleus, locus coeruleus, and cortex, mediate many behavioral responses to stress (Dunn & Berridge, 1990). These include increased freezing behavior (Swiergiel, Takahashi, & Kalin, 1993), decreased appetitive behavior (Krahn et al., 1986), decreased sexual behavior (Sirinaths-inghji et al., 1983), increased grooming behavior (Holahan, Kalin, & Kelly, 1997), and an enhanced startle response (Lee & Davis, 1997). In fact, the CRH receptor antagonist antalarmin attenuates both biological and behavioral responses during stress (Habib et al., 2000).

A simplified version of central stress pathways is depicted in Figure 26.3. CRH containing neurons and receptors are prevalent in the amygdala, hypothalamus, and the locus coeruleus (Gray, 1993; Menzaghi et al., 1993; Valentino, Foote, & Page, 1993). Subsequent efferent pathways provide one mechanism by which stress may be coordinated to influence health. For instance, the amygdala has direct projections to the hypothalamus (Gray, 1993). Release of CRH from the hypothalamus activates the HPA axis. As reviewed earlier, cortisol has been linked to some of the stress-related changes in immune function. Prolonged stress can down-regulate hippocampal glucocorticoid receptors that are responsible for turning off the cortisol response, which is a process postulated to play a role in the biological aging process (Sapolsky, 1996). The hypothalamus also has efferent projections to the ANS via the sympathetic preganglionic neurons of the intermediolateral cell column, the ventral lateral medulla, and the nucleus tractus solitarus (Menzaghi et al., 1993). In combination, the release of HPA hormones and activation of the ANS may account for many of the stress-induced changes in health detailed earlier in this review.

Although CRH activates the noradrenergic system, it is also apparent that reciprocal interactions exist (Chrousos & Gold, 1992; Dunn & Berridge, 1990). For instance, catecholaminergic inputs are evident to hypothalamic cell regions containing CRH and appear to stimulate central CRH release via an α_1-adrenergic mechanism (Al-Damluji et al., 1987; Cunningham & Sawchenko, 1988). As discussed earlier, central adrenergic mechanisms are also implicated in the release of IL-6 (Soszynski et al., 1996; van Gool et al., 1990) and IL-6 can activate the HPA axis (Papanicolaou et al., 1998). The central coordination of these stress-related inflammatory processes may further explain variance in the links between stress and health (Papanicolaou et al., 1998).

It is also important to emphasize that there are critical afferent (ascending) pathways to brain structures that may be activated in stressful circumstances. Vagal afference appears to play an important role in the immune response to infection that may then have implications for stress processes (Maier & Watkins, 1998). Berntson, Sarter, and Cacioppo (2003) also reviewed evidence for the role of these afferent pathways in modulating anxiety-related physiological reactions. According to their model, these ascending pathways provide an opportunity for anxiety or stress-induced physiological reactions to influence cortical information processing (e.g., attentional functions). For instance, activation of the locus coeruleus via afferent pathways is linked to increased EEG arousal and vigilance to significant stimuli (Aston-Jones et al., 1996). Many of these "bottom-up" processes appear mediated by the basal

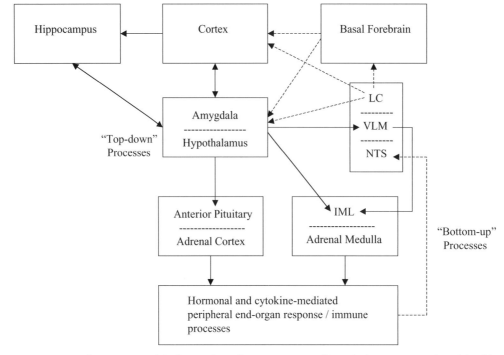

Figure 26.3. Illustrative model of central mechanisms potentially underlying stress-induced health links, including efferent (solid lines) and afferent (broken lines) projections. Abbreviations: IML = sympathetic preganglionic neurons of the intermediolateral cell column, LC = locus coeruleus, NTS = nucleus tractus solitarus, and VLM = ventral lateral medulla.

forebrain cholinergic system that has (a) reciprocal connections with the amygdala, and (b) widespread projections to the cerebral cortex (Berntson, Sarter, & Cacioppo, 2003). As a result it is well situated to participate in the potentiation of stress-related responses.

Multilevel analyses of stress and health. Although not a focus of this review, a more integrative view of stress and health will also need to consider diverse but complementary levels of analyses. Although most of the emphasis has been on biological mechanisms, understanding stress effects on disease may require similar attention to the social, personologic, psychological, and behavioral levels of analyses (Cacioppo & Berntson, 1992). In many cases, these different functional levels are embedded; hence, processes at more macrolevels can influence the more microlevel processes and vice versa (Cacioppo & Berntson, 1992).

Integrative research on the mechanisms linking stress to health across functional levels of analyses is in its infancy. However, the prior literature does provide some data on these processes. At a more macrolevel of analysis, there is evidence that social stressors may be particularly important sources of stress explaining variations in health outcomes (e.g., Kiecolt-Glaser et al., 1996; Padgett et al., 1998). For instance, Padgett and colleagues (1998) exposed latently infected HSV rats to either social stress (i.e., social group reorganization) or physical stress (i.e., restraint stress). Results revealed that only social stress was associated with significant reactivation of HSV (i.e.,

over 40% of socially stressed animals). These findings are consistent with research indicating that social stressors appear to have relatively large and lasting effects on mood (Bolger et al., 1989) and immunity in humans (Cohen et al., 1998) and nonhuman primates (Coe, 1993).

There are also potential personality factors that may influence the links between stress and health. Personality factors such as neuroticism are linked to greater subjective stress and hence may be responsible for the results of stress on some health outcomes (Bolger & Eckenrode, 1991). Cohen and colleagues (1998) reported that self-esteem and the big-five personality factors could not account for the effects of stress on susceptibility to the common cold. However, a likely role for personality factors is in the moderation of stress-induced health processes. Prime candidates for examination include trait hostility and optimism that appear to influence physiological processes and health-related outcomes (Scheier & Bridges, 1995; Smith & Gallo, 2001).

Stress has been linked to changes in health behaviors such as exercise and alcohol consumption (Ng & Jeffrey, 2003). Therefore, it is also important to evaluate the effects of health behaviors as pathways responsible for the effects of stress on health outcomes. In most of the studies detailed earlier, health behaviors including exercise and alcohol did not explain much of the variance in the effects of stress on health (Cohen et al., 1998; Kiecolt-Glaser et al., 1995, 1996). However, it is clear that stress influences health behaviors, and health behaviors are tied to similar physiological processes that are linked to health risks (Kiecolt-Glaser et al., 2002). Better measurement and conceptualization of health behaviors in light of more integrative mechanisms may allow a clearer test of their mediational role in explaining links between stress and health.

One discussion that bears on these different levels of analyses involves the stress components reviewed in this chapter. These components linking stress to health include exposure, reactivity, recovery, and restoration (Cacioppo & Berntson, in press). Of these components, relatively little research exists on stress recovery, especially in regards to immune-mediated disease processes. Although the components of stress reactivity and stress exposure were often confounded, there was good evidence for links to disease outcomes, with interactive effects apparent when modeling both processes (e.g., Cohen et al., 2002). Research on chronic stress and sleep disturbances also highlights the potential direct role of reactivity and exposure on restorative processes (Figure 26.1). Beyond this, little empirical evidence exists in these studies on how these stress components may have cascading or reciprocal effects as depicted in Figure 26.1. Future research will need to take a more integrative approach to modeling these stress components and clarify their related (mediated), independent, or interactive effects on disease processes.

Of these components, restorative processes are particularly interesting given their potential unique association with health outcomes. Indeed, preliminary evidence exists linking restorative processes such as sleep and wound healing to health-related stress outcomes (Irwin, 2002; Kiecolt-Glaser et al., 1998). Although the concept of restorative processes is promising, several questions will be important for future research to address. One question relates to what indices or outcomes are most relevant to restorative processes. Restoration is linked to anabolic (energy conserving) processes and a number of potential indicators seem relevant such as growth hormone release and PNS processes (see Hawkley & Cacioppo, 2004). Integrating measurement and conceptual issues related to restorative processes at different functional levels would provide more guidance to future research. A second question concerns the balance of anabolic to catabolic processes that is health relevant (Epel et al., 1998). Anabolic processes play an important role in physiological regulation, but direct research on how it counteracts harmful catabolic processes is needed. A final, related question is how anabolic and catabolic processes unfold over time in ways that are health relevant. Epel and colleagues (1998) have argued that one process relates to having sufficient time following catabolic processes to recuperate. In general, research on restorative processes as they relate to stress and health is just beginning, but process questions will soon begin to take on added importance.

CONCLUSIONS

In this chapter, we reviewed evidence linking stress to illness. These diseases include the leading causes of morbidity and mortality: cardiovascular disease, cancer, and infectious illnesses. There was strong evidence linking stress to cardiovascular and infectious diseases. The literature linking stress to cancer was controversial, but future research guided by the emerging concept of cancer immunoediting may prove informative. Importantly, impressive evidence exists on the biological mechanisms potentially linking stress to these disease processes. Of these, immune processes (e.g., inflammation) appear to play a critical role across these diseases and, along with an examination of CNS processes, may provide the impetus for an integrative approach to the study of stress and health. The time is ripe for such an approach. Research that elucidates the complex links outlined in this chapter at different functional levels of analyses may play a crucial role in helping us better understand, in Selye's (1956) words, the "secrets of health and happiness" and the "penalties for failure in this great process of adaptation."

REFERENCES

Abbas, A. K. & Lichtman, A. H. (2003). *Cellular and molecular immunology*. Philadelphia, PA: Saunders.

Agelaki, S., Tsatsanis, C., Gravanis, A., & Margioris, A. N. (2002, November). Corticotropin-releasing hormone augments proinflammatory cytokine production from macrophages in vitro and in lipopolysaccharide-induced endotoxin shock in mice. *Infection and Immunity, 70,* 6068–6074.

Al-Damluji, S., Perry, L., Tomlin, S., Bouloux, P., Grossman, A., Rees, L. H., & Besser, G. M. (1987). Alpha-adrenergic stimulation of corticotrophin secretion by a specific central mechanism in man. *Neuroendocrinology, 45,* 68–76.

Alito, A. E., Romeo, H. E., Baler, R., Chuluyan, H. E., Braun, M., & Cardinali, D. P. (1987). Autonomic nervous system regulation of murine immune responses as assessed by local surgical sympathetic and parasympathetic denervation. *Acta Physiol. Pharmacol. Latinoam., 37,* 305–319.

American Cancer Society. (2004). *Cancer facts and figures 2004.* Atlanta, Ga.: American Cancer Society.

American Heart Association. (2004). *2004 Heart and stroke statistical update.* Dallas, Tex.: American Heart Association.

Andersen, B. L., Farrar, W. B., Golden-Kreutz, D., Kutz, L. A., MacCallum, R., Courtney, M. E., & Glaser, R. (1998, January). Stress and immune responses after surgical treatment for regional breast cancer. *Journal of the National Cancer Institute, 90,* 30–36.

Andersen, B. L., Kiecolt-Glaser, J. K., & Glaser, R. (1994). A biobehavioral model of cancer stress and disease course. *American Psychologist, 49,* 389–404.

Arya, S. K., Wong-Staal, F., and Gallo, R. C. 1984. Dexamethasone-mediated inhibition of human T cell growth factor and γ-interferon messenger RNA. *Journal of Immunology 133,* 273–276.

Aston-Jones, G., Rajkowski, J., Kubiak, P., Valentino, R. J., & Shipley, M. T. (1996). Role of the locus coeruleus in emotional activation. In G. Holstege, R Bandler, C. B. Saper (Eds.), *Progress in Brain Research* (pp. 379–402). New York: Elsevier.

Bachen, E. A., Manuck, S. B., Cohen, S., Muldoon, M. F., Raible, R., Herbert, T. B., & Rabin, B. S. (1995). Adrenergic blockade ameliorates cellular immune responses to mental stress in humans. *Psychosomatic Medicine, 57,* 366–372.

Barbul, A. (1990). Immune aspects of wound repair. *Clinical Plastic Surgery, 17*, 433–442.

Baugh, J. A. & Donnelly, S. C. (2003). Macrophage migration inhibitory factor: A neuroendocrine modulator of chronic inflammation. *Journal of Endocrinology, 179*, 15–23.

Barton, B. E. (1997). Molecule of the month: IL-6: Insights into novel biological activities. *Clinical Immunology and Immunopathology, 85*, 16–20.

Bartrop, R. W., Luckhurst, E., Lazarus, L., Kiloh, L. G., & Penny, R. (1977, April). Depressed lymphocyte function after bereavement. *The Lancet, 1*, 834–836.

Baum, A., O'Keefe, M. K., & Davidson, L. M. (1990). Acute stressors and chronic response: The case of traumatic stress. *Journal of Applied Social Psychology, 20*, 1643–1654.

Baum, A., & Posluszny, D. M. (1999). Health psychology: Mapping biobehavioral contributions to health and illness. *Annual Review of Psychology, 50*, 137–163.

Baus, E., Andris, F., Dubois, P. M., Urbain, J., & Leo, O. (1996). Dexamethasone inhibits the early steps of antigen receptor signaling in activated T lymphocytes. *Journal of Immunology, 156*, 4555–4561.

Bayer, B. M., Daussin, S., Hernandez, M., and Irvin, L. (1990). Morphine inhibition of lymphocyte activity is mediated by an opioid dependent mechanism. *Neuropharmacology, 29*, 369–374.

Bellinger, D. L., Lorton, D., Lubahn, C., & Felton, D. L. (2001). Innervation of lymphoid organs-association of nerves with cells of the immune system and their implications in disease. In R. Ader, D. L. Felten and N. Cohen (Eds.), *Psychoneuroimmunology*, Vol. 1, 3rd edition (pp. 55–112). New York: Academic Press.

Ben-Eliyahu, S., & Shakhar, G. (2001). The impact of stress, catecholamines, and the menstrual cycle on NK activity and tumor development: From in vitro studies to biological significance. In R. Ader , D. L. Felten and N. Cohen (Eds.), *Psychoneuroimmunology*, Vol. 2, 3rd edition (pp. 545–563). New York: Academic Press.

Bernard, C. (1878/1974). *Lectures on the phenomena of life common to animals and plants*. Springfield, IL: Thomas.

Berntson, G. G., & Cacioppo, J. T. (2000). From homeostatsis to allodynamic regulation. In J. T. Cacioppo, L. G. Tassinary, & G. G. Berntson (Eds.), *Handbook of psychophysiology* (2nd ed., pp. 459–481). Cambridge University Press.

Berntson, G. G., Sarter, M., & Cacioppo, J. T. (2003). Ascending visceral regulation of cortical affective information processing. *European Journal of Neuroscience, 18*, 2103–2109.

Bethin, K. E., Vgot, S. K., & Muglia, L. J. (2000, August). Interleukin-6 is an essential, corticotropin-releasing hormone-independent stimulator of the adrenal axis during immune system activation. *PNAS, 97*, 9317–9322.

Black, P. H., & Garbutt, L. D. (2002). Stress, inflammation and cardiovascular disease. *Journal of Psychosomatic Research, 52*, 1–23

Bolger, N., DeLongis, A., Kessler, R. C., & Schilling, E. A. (1989). Effects of daily stress on negative mood. *Journal of Personality and Social Psychology, 57*, 808–818.

Bolger, N. & Eckenrode, J. (1991). Social relationships, personality, and anxiety during a major stressful event. *Journal of Personality and Social Psychology, 61*, 440–449.

Bosch, J. A., Berntson, G. G., Cacioppo, J. T., Dhabhar, F. S., & Marucha, P. T. (2003a). Acute stress evokes selective mobilization of T cells that differ in chemokine receptor expression: A potential pathway linking immunologic reactivity to cardiovascular disease. *Brain, Behavior, and Immunity, 17*, 251–259.

Bosch, J. A., de Geus, E. J. C., Veerman, E. C. I., Hoogstraten, J., & Nieuw Amerongen, V. (2003b). Innate secretory immunity in response to laboratory stressors that evoke distinct patterns of cardiac autonomic activity. *Psychosomatic Medicine, 65*, 245–258.

Boyce, W. T., Chesney, M., Alkon, A., Tschann, J. M., Adams, S., Chesterman, B., Cohen, F., Kaiser, P., Folkman, S., & Wara, D. (1995). Psychobiologic reactivity to stress and childhood respiratory illnesses: Results of two prospective studies. *Psychosomatic Medicine, 57*, 411–422,

Bourgeois, M. S., Schulz, R., and Burgio, L. (1996). Interventions for caregivers of patients with Alzheimer's disease: A review and analysis of content, process, and outcomes. *International Journal of Aging and Human Development, 43*, 35–92.

Broadbent, E., Petrie, K. J., Alley, P. G., & Booth, R. J. (2003). Psychological stress impairs early wound repair following surgery. *Psychosomatic Medicine, 65*, 865–869.

Brydon, L., Edwards, S., Mohamed-Ali, V., & Steptoe, A. (2004). Socioeconomic status and stress-induced increases in interleukin-6. *Brain, Behavior, and Immunity, 18*, 281–290.

Burnett, F. M. (1970). The concept of immunological surveillance. *Prog. Exp. Tumor Res., 13*, 1–27.

Burns, V. E., Drayson, M., Ring, C., & Carroll, D. (2002). Perceived stress and psychological well-being are associated with antibody status after Meningitis C conjugate vaccination. *Psychosomatic Medicine, 64*, 963–970.

Cacioppo, J. T., & Berntson, G. G. (1992). Social psychological contributions to the decade of the brain: Doctrine of multilevel analysis. *American Psychologist, 47*, 1019–1028.

Cacioppo, J. T., & Berntson, G. G. (in press). *Balancing demands of the internal and external milieu*. To appear in H. S. Friedman & R. Cohen Silver (Eds.), Oxford Handbook of health psychology.

Cacioppo, J. T., Berntson, G. G., Malarkey, W. B., Kiecolt-Glaser, K. G., Sheridan, J. F., Poehlmann, K. M., Burleson, M. H., Ernst, J. M., Hawkley, L. C., & Glaser, R. (1998). Autonomic, neuroendocrine, and immune responses to psychological stress: The reactivity hypothesis. *Annals of the New York Academy of Sciences, 840*, 664–673.

Cacioppo, J. T., Kiecolt-Glaser, J. K., Malarkey, W. B., Laskowski, B. F., Rozlog, L. A., Poehlmann, K. M., Burleson, M. H., & Glaser, R. (2002). Autonomic and glucocorticoid associations with the steady-state expression of latent Epstein-Barr virus. *Hormones and Behavior, 42*, 32–41.

Cacioppo, J. T., Malarkey, W. B., Kiecolt-Glaser, K. G., Uchino, B. N., Sgoutas-Emch, S. A., Sheridan, J. F., Berntson, G. G., & Glaser, R. (1995). Heterogeneity in neuroendocrine and immune responses to brief psychological stressors as a function of autonomic cardiac activation. *Psychosomatic Medicine 57*, 154–164.

Cannon, W. B. (1928). The mechanism of emotional disturbance of bodily functions. *New England Journal of Medicine, 198*, 877–884.

Cannon, W. B. (1929). Organization for physiological homeostasis. *Physiological Reviews, IX*, 399–431.

Capitanio, J. P., Mendoza, S. P., Lerche, N. W., & Mason, W. A. (1998, April). Social stress results in altered glucocorticoid regulation and shorter survival in simian acquired immune deficiency syndrome. *Proc. National Academy of Sciences: Neurobiology, 95*, 4714–4719.

Carels, R. A., Cacciapaglia, H., Perez-Benitez, C. I., Douglass, O., Christie, S., & O'Brien, W. H. (2003). The association between emotional upset and cardiac arrhythmia during daily life. *Journal of Consulting and Clinical Psychology, 71*, 613–618.

Cartwright, R. D., & Wood, E. (1991). Adjustment disorders of sleep: The sleep effects of a major stressful event and its resolution. *Psychiatry Research, 39*, 199–209.

Center for Disease Control (1996). Prevention and control of influenza: Recommendations of the advisory committee on immunization practices (ACIP). *MMWR, 45*, 1–24.

Chan, J. M., Stampfer, M. J., Giovannucci, E., Gann, P. H., Ma, J., Wilkinson, P., Hennekens, C. H., & Pollak, M. (1998). Plasma insulin-like growth factor-I and prostate cancer risk: A prospective study. *Science, 279*, 563–566.

Charo, I. F., & Taubman, M. B. (2004). Chemokines in the pathogenesis of vascular disease. *Circulation Research, 95*, 858–866.

Chrousos, G. P., & Gold, P. W. (1992). The concepts of stress and stress system disorders: Overview of physical and behavioral homeostasis. *JAMA, 267*, 1244–1252.

Coe, C. L. (1993). Psychosocial factors and immunity in nonhuman primates: A review. *Psychosomatic Medicine, 55*, 298–308.

Cohen, S., Frank, E., Doyle, W. J., Skoner, D. P., Rabin, B. S., & Gwaltney, Jr., J. M. (1998). Types of stressors that increase susceptibility to the common cold in healthy adults. *Health Psychology, 17*, 214–223.

Cohen, S., Hamrick, N., Rodriguez, M. S., Feldman, P. J., Rabin, B. S., & Manuck, S. B. (2002). Reactivity and vulnerability to stress-associated risk for upper respiratory illness. *Psychosomatic Medicine, 64*, 302–310.

Cohen, S., & Herbert, T. B. (1996). Health Psychology: Psychological factors and physical disease from the perspective of human psychoneuroimmunology. *Annual Review of Psychology, 47*, 113–142.

Cohen, S., & Williamson, G. M. (1991). Stress and infectious disease in humans. *Psychological Bulletin, 109*, 5–24.

Cole, S. W., & Kemeny, M. E. (2001). Psychosocial influences on the progression of HIV infection. In R. Ader, D. L. Felten and N. Cohen (Eds.), *Psychoneurommunology*, vol. 2, 3rd edition (pp. 583–612). New York: Academic Press.

Cole, S. W., Korin, Y. D., Fahey, J. L., & Zack, J. A. (1998). Norepinephrine accelerates HIV replication via protein kinase A-dependent effects on cytokine production. *Journal of Immunology, 161*, 610–616.

Cooper, C. L., Davies-Cooper, R. F., & Faragher, E. B. (1986). A prospective study of the relationship between breast cancer and life events, type A behavior, social support and coping skills. *Stress Medicine, 2*, 271–278.

Coussens, L. M., & Werb, Z. (2002, December). Inflammation and cancer. *Nature, 420*, 860–867.

Cruess, D. G., Antoni, M. H., Gonzalez, J., Fletcher, M. A., Klimas, N., Duran, R., Ironson, G., & Schneiderman, N. (2003). Sleep disturbance mediates the association between psychological distress and immune status among HIV-positive men and women on combination antiretroviral therapy. *Journal of Psychsomatic Research, 54*, 185–189.

Cruess, D. G., Antoni, M. H., McGregor, B. A., Kilbourn, K. M., Boyers, A. E., Alferi, S. M., Carver, C. S., & Kumar, M. (2000). Cognitive-behavioral stress management reduces serum cortisol by enhancing benefit finding among women being treated for early stage breast cancer. *Psychosomatic Medicine, 62*, 304–308.

Cunningham, Jr., E. T., & Sawchenko, P. E. (1988). Anatomical specificity of noradrenergic inputs to the paraventricular and supraoptic nuclei of the rat hypothalamus. *The Journal of Comparative Neurology, 274*, 60–76.

Dobbs, C. M., Feng, N., Beck, F. M., & Sheridan, J. F. (1996). Neuroendocrine regulation of cytokine production during experimental influenza viral infection. *The Journal of Immunology, 157*, 1870–1877.

Dunn, A. J., & Berridge, C. W. (1990). Physiological and behavioral responses to corticotropin-releasing factor administration: Is CRF a mediator of anxiety or stress responses? *Brain Research Reviews, 15*, 71–100.

Dunn, G. P., Bruce, A. T., Ikeda, H., Old, L. J., & Schreiber, R. D. (2002). Cancer immunoediting: From immunosurveillance to tumor escape. *Nature Immunology, 3*, 991–998.

Dusseldorp, E., van Elderen, T., Maes, S., Meulman, J., & Kraaij, V. (1999). A meta-analysis of psychoeducational programs for coronary heart disease patients. *Health Psychology, 18*, 506–519.

Dyck, D. G., Short, R., & Vitaliano, P. P. (1999). Predictors of burden and infectious illness in schizophrenia caregivers. *Psychosomatic Medicine, 61*, 411–419.

Effros, R. B., & Walford, R. L. (1987). Infection and immunity in relation to aging. In E. A. Goidl (Ed.), *Aging and the immune response* (pp. 45–65). N.Y.: Marcel Dekker.

Epel, E. S., McEwen, B. S., & Ickovics, J. R. (1998). Enbodying psychological thriving: Physical thriving in response to stress. *Journal of Social Issues, 54*, 301–322.

Esterling, B. A., Kiecolt-Glaser, J. K., Bodnar, J. C., and Glaser, R. (1994). Chronic stress, social support, and persistent alterations in the natural killer cell response to cytokines in older adults. *Health Psychology*, 13: 291–299.

Everson, S. A., Lynch, J. W., Chesney, M. A., Kaplan, G. A., Goldberg, D. E., Shade, S. B., Cohen, R. D., Salonen, R., & Salonen, J. T. (1997). Interaction of workplace demands and cardiovascular reactivity in progression of carotid atherosclerosis: Population based study. *BMJ, 314*, 553–558.

Fawzy, F. I., & Fawzy, N. W. (1998). Psychoeducational interventions. In J. C. Holland (Ed.), *Psycho-oncology* (pp. 676–693). New York: Oxford University Press.

Fawzy, F. I., Fawzy, N. W., Hyun, C. S., Gutherie, D., Fahey, J. L., & Morton, D. (1993). Malignant melanoma: Effects of an early structured psychiatric intervention, coping, and affective state on recurrence and survival six years later. *Archives of General Psychiatry, 50*, 681–689.

Fecho, K., Dykstra, L. A. and Lysle, D. T. (1993). Evidence for beta adrenergic receptor involvement in the immunomodulatory effects of morphine. *Journal of Pharmacology and Experimental Therapeutics, 265*, 1079–1087.

Freier, D. O., & Fuchs, B. A. (1994). A mechanism of action for morphine-induced immunosuppression: Corticosterone mediates morphine-induced suppression of natural killer cell activity. *Journal of Pharmacology and Experimental Therapeutics, 270*, 1127–1133.

Felton, D. L., Ackerman, K. D., Wiegand, S. J., & Felton, S. Y. (1987). Noradrenergic sympathetic innervation of the spleen: I. Nerve fibers associate with lymphocytes and macrophages in specific compartments of the splenic white pulp. *Journal of Neuroscience Research, 18*, 28–36.

Fox, B. H. (1998). Psychosocial factors in cancer incidence and prognosis. In J. C. Holland (Ed.), *Psycho-oncology* (pp. 110–124). New York: Oxford University Press.

Germain, A., Buysse, D. J., Ombao, H., Kupfer, D. J., & Hall, M. (2003). Psychophysiological reactivity and coping styles influence the effects of acute stress exposure on rapid eye movement sleep. *Psychosomatic Medicine, 65*, 857–864.

Glaser, R., Kiecolt-Glaser, J. K., Bonneau, R. H., Malarkey, W., Kennedy, S., & Hughes, J. (1992). Stress-induced modulation of the immune response to recombinant Hepatitis B vaccine. *Psychosomatic Medicine, 54*, 22–29.

Glaser, R., Sheridan, J., Malarkey, W. B., MacCallum, R. C., & Kiecolt-Glaser, J. K. (2000). Chronic stress modulates the immune response to a pneumococcal pneumonia vaccine. *Psychosomatic Medicine, 62*, 804–807.

Glaser, R., Thorn, B. E., Tarr, K. L., Kiecolt-Glaser, J. K., & D'Ambrosio, S. M. (1985). Effects of stress on methyltransferase synthesis: An important DNA repair enzyme. *Health Psychology, 4*, 403–412.

Glaser, R., Kutz, L. A., MacCallum, R. C., & Malarkey, W. B. (1995). Hormonal modulation of Epstein-Barr virus replication. *Neuroendocrinology, 62*, 356–361.

Glynn, L. M., Christenfeld, N., & Gerin, W. (2002). The role of rumination in recovery from reactivity: Cardiovascular consequences of emotional states. *Psychosomatic Medicine, 64*, 714–726.

Goebel, M. U., & Mills, P. J. (2000). Acute psychological stress and exercise and changes in peripheral leukocyte adhesion molecule expression and density. *Psychosomatic Medicine, 62*, 664–670.

Goldberg, A. D., Becker, L. C., Bonsall, R., Cohen, J. D., Ketterer, M. W., Kaufman, P. G., Krantz, D. S., Light, K. C., McMahon, R. P., Noreuil, T., Pepine, C. J., Raczynski, J., Stone, P. H., Strother, D., Taylor, H., & Sheps, D. S. (1996). Ischemic, hemodynamic, and neurohormonal responses to mental and exercise stress: Experience from the psychophysiological investigations of myocardial ischemia study (PIMI). *Circulation, 94*, 2402–2409.

Gordon, M. A., Cohen, J. J., & Wilson, I. B. (1978). Muscarinic cholinergic receptors in murine lymphocytes: Demonstration by direct binding. *Proceedings of the National Academy of Sciences, 75*, 2902–2904.

Gray, T. S. (1993). Amygdaloid CRF pathways: Role in Autonomic, neuroendocrine, and behavioral responses to stress. *Annals of the New York Academy of Sciences, 697*, 53–60.

Haas, H. S. & Schauenstein, K. (1997). Neuroimmunomodulation via limbic structures – The neuroanatomy of psychoimmunology. *Progress in Neurobiology, 51*, 195–222.

Habib, K. E., Weld, K. P., Rice, K. C., Pushkas, J., Champoux, M., Listwak, S., Webster, E. L., Atkinson, A. J., Schulkin, J., Contoreggi, C., Chrousos, G. P., McCann, S. M., Suomi, S. J., Higley, J. D., & Gold, P. W. (2000, May). Oral administration of a corticotropin-releasing hormone receptor antagonist significantly attenuates behavioral, neuroendocrine, and autonomic responses to stress in primates. *PNAS, 97*, 6079–6084.

Hall, M., Baum, A., Buysse, D. J., Prigerson, H. G., Kupfer, D. J., & Reynolds, C. F. (1998). Sleep as a mediator of the stress-immune relationship. *Psychosomatic Medicine, 60*, 48–51.

Hall, M., Vasko, R., Buysse, D., Ombao, H., Chen, Q., Cashmere, J. D., Kupfer, D., & Thayer, J. F. (2004). Acute stress affects heart rate variability during sleep. *Psychosomatic Medicine, 66*, 56–62.

Hawkley, L. C., Bosch, J. A., Engeland, C. G., Marucha, P. T., & Cacioppo, J. T. (in press). Loneliness, dysphoria, stress and immunity: A role for cytokines. In N. P. Plotnikoff, R. E. Faith,

& A. J. Murgo (Eds.), *Cytokines: Stress and immunity* (2nd ed.). Bocan Raton, LA: CRC Press.

Hawkley, L. C., & Cacioppo, J. T. (2004). Stress and the aging immune system. *Brain, Behavior, and Immunity, 18*, 114–119.

Holbrook, N. J., Cox, W. I., & Horner, H. C. (1983). Direct suppression of natural killer activity in human peripheral blood leukocyte cultures by glucocorticoids and its modulation by interferon. *Cancer Research, 43*, 4019–4025.

Holahan, M. R., Kalin, N. H., & Kelley, A. E. (1997). Microinfusion of corticotropin-releasing factor into the nucleus accumbens shell results in increased behavioral arousal and oral motor activity. *Psychopharmacology, 130*, 189–196.

Hosaka, T., & Sugiyama, Y. (2003). Structured intervention in family caregivers of the demented elderly and changes in their immune function. *Psychiatry and Clinical Neurosciences, 57*, 147–151.

Irwin, M. (2002). Effects of sleep and sleep loss on immunity and cytokines. *Brain, Behavior, and Immunity, 16*, 503–512.

Irwin, M., Hauger, R. L., Brown, M., and Britton, K. T. (1989). CRF activates autonomic nervous system and reduces natural killer cytotoxicity. *American Journal of Physiology, 255*: R744–R747.

Ironson, G., Wynings, C., Schneiderman, N., Baum, A., Rodriguez, M., Greenwood, D., Benight, C., Antoni, M., LaPerriere, A., Huang, H.-S., Klimas, N., & Fletcher, M. A. (1997). Posttraumatic stress symptoms, intrusive thoughts, loss and immune function after Hurricane Andrew. *Psychosomatic Medicine, 59*, 128–141.

Ishigami, T. (1918–1919). The influence of psychic acts on the progress of pulmonary tuberculosis. *American Review of Tuberculosis, 2*, 470–484.

Iso, H., Date, C., Yamamato, A., Toyoshima, H., Tanabe, N., Kikuchi, S., Kondo, T., Watanabe, Y., Wada, Y., Ishibashi, T., Suzuki, H., Koizumi, A., Inaba, Y., Tamakoshi, A., Ohno, Y., & JACC Study Group. (2002). Perceived mental stress and mortality from cardiovascular disease among Japanese men and women: The Japan collaborative cohort study for evaluation of cancer risk sponsored by Monbusho (JACC Study). *Circulation, 106*, 1229–1236.

Jabaaij, L., Grosheide, P. M., Heijtink, R. A., Duivenvoorden, H. J., Ballieux, R. E., & Vingerhoets, A. J. J. M. (1993). Influence of perceived psychological stress and distress on antibody response to low dose fDNA Hepatitis B vaccine. *Journal of Psychosomatic Research, 37*, 361–369.

Johnson, R. W., von Borell, E. H., Anderson, L. L., Kojic, L. D., & Cunnick, J. E. (1994). Intracerebroventricular injection of corticotropin-releasing hormone in the pig: Acute effects on behavior, adrenocorticotropin secretion, and immune suppression. *Endocrinology, 135*, 642–648.

Kamarck, T., & Jennings, J. R. (1991). Biobehavioral factors in sudden cardiac death. *Psychological Bulletin, 109*, 42–75.

Kamarck, T. W., Muldoon, M. F., Shiffman, S., Sutton-Tyrrell, K., Gwaltney, C., & Janicki, D. L. (2004). Experiences of demand and control in daily life as correlates of subclinical carotid atherosclerosis in a healthy older sample. *Health Psychology, 23*, 24–32.

Kaplan, J. R., Manuck, S. B., Adams, M. R., Weingand, K. W., & Clarkson, T. B. (1987). Inhibition of coronary atherosclerosis by propanolol in behaviorally predisposed monkeys fed an atherogenic diet. *Circulation, 76*, 1365–1372.

Kariagina, A., Romanenko, D., Ren, S.-G., & Chesnokova, V. (2004). Hypothalamic-pituitary cytokine network. *Endocrinology, 145*, 104–112.

Katz, P., Zaytoun, A. M., & Fauci, A. S. (1982). Mechanisms of human cell-mediated cytotoxicity I. Modulation of natural killer cell activity by cyclic nucleotides. *Journal of Immunology, 129,* 287–296.

Kelly, J. A., Murphy, D. A., Sikkema, K. J., & Kalichman, S. C. (1993). Psychological interventions to prevent HIV infection are urgently needed: New priorities for behavioral research in the second decade of AIDS. *American Psychologist, 10,* 1023–1034.

Kelly, J. A., Otto-Salaj, L. L., Sikkema, K. J., Pinkerton, S. D., & Bloom, F. R. (1998). Implications of HIV treatment advances for behavioral research on AIDS: Protease inhibitors and new challenges in HIV secondary prevention. *Health Psychology, 17,* 310–319.

Kelso, A., & Munck, A. (1984). Glucocorticoid inhibition of lymphokine secretion by alloreactive T lymphocyte clones. *Journal of Immunology, 133,* 784–791.

Kemeny, M. E., Weiner, H., Duran, R., Taylor, S. E., Visscher, B., & Fahey, J. L. (1995). Immune system changes after the death of a partner in HIV-positive gay men. *Psychosomatic Medicine, 57,* 547–554.

Khreiss, T., Jozsef, L., Potempa, L. A., & Filep, J. G. (2004). Conformational rearrangement in C-reactive protein is required for proinflammatory actions on human endothelial cells. *Circulation, 109,* 2016–2022.

Kiecolt-Glaser, J. K., Dura, J. R., Speicher, C. E., Trask, O. J., & Glaser, R. (1991). Spousal caregivers of dementia victims: Longitudinal changes in immunity and health. *Psychosomatic Medicine, 53,* 345–362.

Kiecolt-Glaser, J. K., & Glaser, R. (1995). Psychoneuroimmunology and health consequences: Data and shared mechanisms. *Psychosomatic Medicine, 57,* 269–274.

Kiecolt-Glaser, J. K., Glaser, R., Gravenstein, S., Malarkey, W. B., & Sheridan, J. (1996). Chronic stress alters the immune response to influenza virus vaccine in older adults. *Proc. National Academy of Science, 93,* 3043–3047.

Kiecolt-Glaser, J. K., Marucha, P. T., Malarkey, W. B., Mercado, A. M., & Glaser, R. (1995). Slowing of wound healing by psychological stress. *The Lancet, 346,* 1194–1196.

Kiecolt-Glaser, J. K., McGuire, L., Robles, T. F., & Glaser, R. (2002). Emotions, morbidity, and mortality: New perspectives from psychoneuroimmunology. *Annual Review of Psychology, 53,* 83–107.

Kiecolt-Glaser, J. K., Page, G. G., Marucha, T., MacCallum, R. C., & Glaser, R. (1998). Psychological influences on surgical recovery: Perspectives from psychoneuroimmunology. *American Psychologist, 53,* 1209–1218.

Kiecolt-Glaser, J. K., Preacher, K. J., MacCallum, R. C., Atkinson, C., Malarkey, W. B., & Glaser, R. (2003). Chronic stress and age-related increases in the proinflammatory cytokine IL-6. *Proc. National Academy of Science, 100,* 9090–9095.

Kiecolt-Glaser, J. K., Fisher, L. D., Ogrocki, P., Stout, J. C., Speicher, C. E., & Glaser, R. (1987). Marital quality, marital disruption, and immune function. *Psychosomatic Medicine, 49,* 13–34.

Koo, C. K., Huang, C., Camacho, R., Trainor, C., Blake, J. T., Sirotina-Meiser, A., Schleim, K. D., Wu, T. J., Cheng, K., Nargund, R., & McKissick, G. (2001). Immune enhancing effect of a growth hormone secretagogue. *The Journal of Immunology, 166,* 4195–4201.

Kop, W. J., & Cohen, N. (2001). Psychological risk factors and immune system involvement in cardiovascular disease. In R. Ader, D. L. Felten, & N. Cohen (Eds.), *Psychoneuroimmunology,* (Vol. 2, 3rd edition, pp. 525–544). New York: Academic Press.

Kopnisky, K. L., Stoff, D. M., & Rausch, D. M. (2004). Workshop report: The effects of psychological variables on the progression of HIV-1 disease. *Brain, Behavior, and Immunity, 18,* 246–261.

Krahn, D. D., Gosnell, B. A., Grace, M., & Levine, A. S. (1986). CRF antagonist partially reverses CRF- and stress-induced effects on feeding. *Brain Research Bulletin, 17,* 285–289.

Krantz, D. S., & Manuck, S. B. (1984). Acute physiologic reactivity and risk of cardiovascular disease: A review and methodologic critique. *Psychological Bulletin, 96,* 435–464.

Krantz, D. S., Sheps, D. S., Carney, R. M., & Natelson, B. H. (2000). Effects of mental stress in patients with coronary artery disease: Evidence and clinical implications. *Journal of the American Medical Association, 283,* 1800–1802.

Kvikstad A., Vatten L. J., Tretli S., Kvinnsland S. (1994). Widowhood and divorce related to cancer risk in middle-aged women. A nested case-control study among Norwegian women born between 1935 and 1954. *Int J Cancer, 58,* 512–516.

Lange, T., Perras, B., Fehm, H. L., & Born, J. (2003). Sleep enhances the human antibody response to Hepatitis A vaccination. *Psychosomatic Medicine, 65,* 831–835.

Lazarus, R. S., & Folkman, S. (1984). *Stress, appraisal, and coping.* New York: Springer.

Lee, Y., & Davis, M. (1997). Role of the hippocampus, the bed nucleus of the stria terminalis, and the amygdala in the excitatory effect of corticotropin-releasing hormone on the acoustic startle reflex. *Journal of Neuroscience, 17,* 6434–6446.

Leserman, J., Jackson, E. D., Petitto, J. M., Golden, R. N., Silva, S. G., Perkins, D. O., Cai, J., Folds, J. D., & Evans, D. L. (1999). Progression to AIDS: The effects of stress, depressive symptoms, and social support. *Psychosomatic Medicine, 61,* 397–406.

Li, Y., Merrill, J. D., Mooney, K., Song, L., Wang, X., Guo, C.-J., Savani, R. C., Metzger, D. S., Douglas, S. D., & Ho, W.-Z. (2003). Morphine enhances HIV infection of neonatal macrophages. *Pediatric Research, 54,* 282–288.

Libby, P. (2002). Inflammation in atherosclerosis. *Nature, 420,* 868–874.

Light, K. C. (2001). Hypertension and the reactivity hypothesis: The next generation. *Psychosomatic Medicine, 63,* 744–746.

Light, K. C., Dolan, C. A., Davis, M. R., & Sherwood, A. (1992). Cardiovascular responses to an active coping challenge as predictors of blood pressure patterns 10 to 15 years later. *Psychosomatic Medicine, 54,* 217–230.

Lillberg, K., Verkasalo, P. K., Kaprio, J., Teppo, L., Helenius, H., & Koskenvuo, M. (2003). Stressful life events and risk of breast cancer in 10,808 women: A cohort study. *American Journal of Epidemiology, 157,* 415–423.

Linden, W., Stossel, C., & Maurice, J. (1996). Psychosocial interventions for patients with coronary artery disease: A meta-analysis. *Arch Intern Med, 156,* 745–752.

Llabre, M. M., Spitzer, S. B., Saab, P. G., & Schneiderman, N. (2001). Piecewise latent growth curve modeling of systolic blood pressure reactivity and recovery from the cold pressor test. *Psychophysiology, 38,* 951–960.

Lutgendorf, S. K., Antoni, M. H., Ironson, G., Klimas N., Starr, K., Schneiderman, N., McCabe, P., Kumar, M., Cleven, K., & Fletcher, M. A. (1997). Cognitive behavioral stress management intervention decreases dysphoria and herpes simplex virus-Type 2 antibody titers in symptomatic HIV seropositive gay men. *Journal of Consulting and Clinical Psychology, 65,* 31–43.

Lutgendorf, S. K., Garand, L., Buckwalter, K. C., Reimer, T. T., Hong, S. Y., & Lubaroff, D. M. (1999). Life stress, mood disturbance, and elevated interleukin-6 in healthy older women. *Journals of Gerontology, 54*, M434–M439.

Lynch, J. W., Everson, S. A., Kaplan, G. A., Cohen, R. D., Salonen, R., & Salonen, J. T. (1998). Does low socioeconomic status potentiate the effects of heightened cardiovascular responses to stress on the progression of carotid atherosclerosis? *American Journal of Public Health, 88*, 389–394.

Maier, S. F., & Watkins, L. R. (1998). Cytokines for psychologists: Implications of bidirectional immune-to-brain communication for understanding behavior, mood, and cognition. *Psychological Review, 105*, 83–107.

Mallon, L., Broman, J. E., & Hetta, J. (2002). Sleep complaints predict coronary artery disease mortality in males: A 12-year follow-up study of a middle-aged Swedish population. *Journal of Internal Medicine, 251*, 207–216.

Manuck, S. B., Kaplan, J. R., & Clarkson, T. B. (1983). Behaviorally induced heart rate reactivity and atherosclerosis in cynomolgus monkeys. *Psychosomatic Medicine, 45*, 95–108.

Manuck, S. B., Olsson, G., Hjemdahl, P., & Rehnqvist, N. (1992). Does cardiovascular reactivity to mental stress have prognostic value in postinfarction patients? A pilot study. *Psychosomatic Medicine, 54*, 102–108.

Markham, P. D., Salahuddin, S. Z., Veren, K., Orndorff, S., & Gallo, R. C. (1986). Hydrocortisone and some other hormones enhance the expression of HTLV-III. *International Journal of Cancer, 37*, 67–72.

Matthews, K. A., Caggiula, A. R., McAllister, C. G., Berga, S. L., Owens, J. F., Flory, J. D., & Miller, A. L. (1995). Sympathetic reactivity to acute stress and immune response in women. *Psychosomatic Medicine, 57*, 564–571.

Matthews, K. A., Woodall, K. L., & Allen, M. T. (1993). Cardiovascular reactivity to stress predicts future blood pressure status. *Hypertension, 22*, 479–485.

McCarty, D., Diamond, W., & Kaye, M. (1982). Alcohol, sexual arousal, and the transfer of excitation. *Journal of Personality and Social Psychology, 42*, 977–988.

McEwen, B. S. (1998, January). Protective and damaging effects of stress mediators. *The New England Journal of Medicine, 338*, 171–179.

McKenna, M. C., Zevon, M. A., Corn, B., & Rounds, J. (1999). Psychosocial factors and the development of breast cancer: A meta-analysis. *Health Psychology, 18*, 520–531.

Menzaghi, F., Heinrichs, S. C., Pich, E. M., Weiss, F., & Koob, G. F. (1993). The role of limbic and hypothalamic corticotropin-releasing factor in behavioral responses to stress. *Annals of the New York Academy of Sciences, 697*, 142–154.

Miller, G. E., & Cohen, S. (2001). Psychological interventions and the immune system: A meta-analytic review and critique. *Health Psychology, 20*, 47–63.

Miller, G. E., Cohen, S., & Ritchey, A. K. (2002). Chronic psychological stress and the regulation of pro-inflammatory cytokines: A glucocorticoid-resistance model. *Health Psychology, 21*, 531–541.

Miller, G. E., Cohen, S., Pressman, S., Barkin, A., Rabin, B. S., & Treanor, J. J. (2004). Psychological stress and antibody response to influenza vaccination: When is the critical period for stress, and how does it get inside the body? *Psychosomatic Medicine, 66*, 215–223.

Ming, E. E., Adler, G. K., Kessler, R. C., Fogg, L. F., Matthews, K. A., Herd, J. A., & Rose, R. M. (2004). Cardiovascular reactivity to work stress predicts subsequent onset of hypertension:

The air traffic controller health change study. *Psychosomatic Medicine, 66*, 459–465.

Morin, C. M., Rodrigue, S., & Ivers, H. (2003). Role of stress, arousal, and coping skills in primary insomnia. *Psychosomatic Medicine, 65*, 259–267.

Munck, A., Guyre, P. M., & Holbrook, N. J. (1984). Physiological functions of glucocorticoids in stress and their relation to pharmacological actions. *Endocrine Reviews, 5*, 25–44.

Nicassio, P. C., & Smith, T. W. (1995). *Psychosocial management of chronic illness*. Washington, DC: American Psychological Association.

Najima, A. (1995). An electrophysiological study of the vagal innervation of the thymus in the rat. *Brain Research Bulletin, 38*, 319–323.

Ng, D. M., & Jeffery, R. W. (2003). Relationships between perceived stress and health behaviors in a sample of working adults. *Health Psychology, 22*, 638–642.

O'Keeffe, M. K., Nesselhof-Kendall, S., & Baum, A. (1990). Behavior and prevention of AIDS: Bases of research and intervention. *Personality and Social Psychology Bulletin, 16*, 166–180.

Padgett, D. A., Sheridan, J. F., Dorne, J., Berntson, G. G., Candelora, J., & Glaser, R. (1998, June). Social stress and the reactivation of latent herpes simplex virus type 1. *Proc. National Academy of Science, 95*, 7231–7235.

Papanicolaou, D. A., Wilder, R. L., Manolagas, S. C., & Chrousos, G. P. (1998). The pathophysiologic roles of interleukin-6 in human disease. *Annals of Internal Medicine, 128*, 127–137.

Rajavashisth, T. B., Liao, J. K., Galis, Z. S., Tripathi, S., Laufs, U., Tripathi, J., Chai, N.- N., Xu, X.-P., Jovinge, S., Shah, P. K., & Libby, P. (1999). Inflammatory cytokines and oxidized low density lipoproteins increase endothelial cell expression of membrane type 1-matrix metalloproteinase. *The Journal of Biological Chemistry, 274*, 11924–11929.

Ridker, P. M., Rifai, N., Stampfer, M. J., & Hennekens, C. H. (2000). Plasma concentration of interleukin-6 and the risk of future myocardial infarction among apparently healthy men. *Circulation, 101*, 1767–1772.

Rinner, I., Kukulansky, T., Felsner, P., Skriener, E., Globerson, A., Kasai, M., Hirokawa, K., Korsatko, W., & Schauenstein, K. (1994). Cholinergic stimulation modulates apoptosis and differentiation of murine thymocytes via a nicotinic effect on thymic epithelium. *Biochemical and Biophysical Research Communications, 203*, 1057–1062.

Rivier, C., Brownstein, M., Speiss, J., Rivier, J., & Vale, W. (1982). In vivo corticotropin-releasing factor-induced secretion of adrenocorticotropin, β-endorphin, and corticosterone. *Endocrinology, 110*, 272–278.

Rojas, I.-G., Padgett, D. A., Sheridan, J. F., & Marucha, P. T. (2002). Stress-induced susceptibility to bacterial infection during cutaneous wound healing. *Brain, Behavior, and Immunity, 16*, 74–84.

Rosengren, A., Hawken, S., Ounpuu, S., Sliwa, K., Zubaid, M., Almahmeed, W. A., Ngu Blackett, K., Sitthi-amorn, C., Sato, H., & Yusuf, S. (2004, September). Association of psychosocial risk factors with risk of acute myocardial infarction in 11 119 cases and 13 648 controls from 52 countries (the INTERHEART study): Case-control study. *The Lancet, 364*, 953–962.

Rosengren A., Tibblin G., Wilhelmsen L. (1991). Self-perceived psychological stress and incidence of coronary artery disease in middle-aged men. *American Journal of Cardiology, 68*, 1171–1175.

Ross, R. (1999, January). Atherosclerosis – an inflammatory disease. *The New England Journal of Medicine, 340*, 115–126.

Rozanski, A., Bairey, C. N., Krantz, D. S., Friedman, J., Resser, K. J., Morell, M., Hilton-Chalfen, S., Hestrin, L., Bietendorf, J., & Berman, D. S. (1988). Mental stress and the induction of silent myocardial ischemia in patients with coronary artery disease. *The New England Journal of Medicine, 318*, 1005–1012.

Rozanski, A., Blumenthal, J. A., & Kaplan, J. (1999). Impact of psychological factors on the pathogenesis of cardiovascular disease and implications for therapy. *Circulation, 99*, 2192–2217.

Rumberger, J. A., Brundage, B. H., Rader, D. J., and Kondos, G. (1999). Electron beam computed tomographic coronary calcium scanning: A review and guidelines for use in asymptomatic persons. *Mayo Clinic Proceedings, 74*, 243–252.

Rutledge, T., Linden, W., & Paul, D. (2000). Cardiovascular recovery from acute laboratory stress: Reliability and concurrent validity. *Psychosomatic Medicine, 62*, 648–654.

Sanders, B. J., & Lawler, J. E. (1992). The borderline hypertensive rat (BHR) as a model for environmentally induced hypertension: A review and update. *Neuroscience and Biobehavioral Reviews, 16*, 207–217.

Sanders, V. M., Kasprowicz, D. J., Kohm, A. P., & Swanson, M. A. (2001). Neurotransmitter receptors on lymphocytes and other lymphoid cells. In R. Ader, D. L. Felten, & N. Cohen (Eds.), *Psychoneuroimmunology*, (Vol. 1, 3rd edition, pp. 161–196). New York: Academic Press.

Sapolsky, R. M. (1996). Why stress is bad for your brain. *Science, 273*, 749–750.

Scheier, M. F., & Bridges, M. W. (1995). Person variables and health: Personality predispositions and acute psychological states as shared determinants for disease. *Psychosomatic Medicine, 57*, 255–268.

Schneiderman, N., Antoni, M. H., Saab, P. G., & Ironson, G. (2001). Health psychology: Psychosocial and biobehavioral aspects of chronic disease management. *Annual Review of Psychology, 52*, 555–580.

Schuler, J. L., & O'Brien, W. H. (1997). Cardiovascular recovery from stress and hypertension risk factors: A meta-analytic review. *Psychophysiology, 34*, 649–659.

Segerstrom, S. C., & Miller, G. E. (2004). Psychological stress and the human immune system: A meta-analytic study of 30 years of inquiry. *Psychological Bulletin, 130*, 601–630.

Selye, H. (1956). *The stress of life*. New York: McGraw-Hill.

Shao, F., Lin, W., Wang, W., Washington, W. C., & Zheng, L. (2003). The effects of emotional stress on the primary humoral immunity of rats. *Journal of Psychopharmacology, 17*, 179–183.

Shankaran, V., Ikeda, H., Bruce, A. T., White, J. M., Swanson, P. E., Old, L. J., & Schreiber, R. D. (2001). INF-γ and lymphocytes prevent primary tumour development and shape tumour immunogenicity. *Nature, 410*, 1107–1111.

Shavit, Y., Ben-Eliyahu, W., Zeidel, A., & Beilin, B. (2004). Effects of fentanyl on natural killer cell activity and on resistance to tumor metastasis in rats: Dose and timing study. *Neuroimmunomodulation, 11*, 255–260.

Shavit, Y., Depaulis, A., Martin, F. C., Terman, G. W., Pechnick, R. N., Zane, C. J., Gale, R. P., & Liebeskind, J. C. (1986). Involvement of brain opiate receptors in the immune-suppressive effect of morphine. *Proceedings of the National Academy of Sciences, 83*, 7114–7117.

Sheps, D. S., McMahon, R. P., Becker, L., Carney, R. M., Freedland, K. E., Cohen, J. D., Sheffield, D., Goldberg, A. D., Ketterer, M. W., Pepine, C. J., Raczynski, J. M., Light, K., Krantz, D. S., Stone, P. H., Knatterud, G. L., & Kaufmann, P. G. (2002). Mental stress-induced ischemia and all-cause mortality in patients with coronary artery disease: Results from the psychophysiological investigations of Myocardial Ischemia study. *Circulation, 105*, 1780–1784.

Sheridan, J. F., Dobbs, C., Jung, J., Chu, X., Konstantinos, A., Padgett, D., & Glaser, R. (1998). Stress-induced neuroendocrine modulation of viral pathogenesis and immunity. *Annals of the New York Academy of Sciences, 840*, 803–808.

Sirinathsinghji, D. J. S., Rees, L. H., Rivier, J., & Vale, W. (1983). Corticotropin-releasing factor is a potent inhibitor of sexual receptivity in the female rat. *Nature, 305*, 232–235.

Sklar, L. S., & Anisman, H. (1981). Stress and cancer. *Psychological Bulletin, 89*, 369–406.

Smith, T. W., & Gallo, L. C. (2001). Personality traits as risk factors for physical illness. In A. Baum, T. Revenson, & J. Singer (Eds.), *Handbook of health psychology*. (pp 139–172). Hillsdale, N. J.: Lawrence Erlbaum.

Smith, T. W., & Ruiz, J. M. (2002). Psychosocial influences on the development and course of coronary heart disease: Current status and implications for research and practice. *Journal of Consulting and Clinical Psychology, 70*, 548–567.

Solomon, G. F., & Moos, R. H. (1964). Emotions, immunity, and disease: A speculative theoretical integration. *Archives of General Psychiatry, 11*, 657–674.

Solomon, G. F., Segerstrom, S. C., Grohr, P., Kemeny, M., & Fahey, J. (1997). Shaking up immunity: Psychological and immunologic changes after a natural disaster. *Psychosomatic Medicine, 59*, 114–127.

Soszynski, D., Lozak, W., Conn, C. A., Rudolph, K., & Kluger, M. J. (1996). Beta-adrenoceptor antagonists suppress elevation in body temperature and increase in plasma IL-6 in rats exposed to open field. *Neuroendocrinology, 63*, 459–467.

Stark, J. L., Avitsur, R., Padgett, D. A., Campbell, K. A., Beck, F. M., & Sheridan, J. F. (2001). Social stress induces glucocorticoid resistance. *American Journal of Physiol Regulatory Integrative Comp Physiol, 280*, R1799–R1805.

Steinberg, D. (1997). Oxidative modification of LDL and atherogenesis. *Circulation, 95*, 1062–1071.

Sterling, P., & Eyer, J. (1988). Allostasis: A new paradigm to explain arousal pathology. In S. Fisher & J. Reason (Eds.), *Handbook of life stress, cognition and health* (pp. 629–649). John Wiley & Sons.

Stetson, B. A., Rahn, J. M., Dubbert, P. M., Wilner, B. I., & Mercury, M. G. (1997). Prospective evaluation of the effects of stress on exercise adherence in community-residing women. *Health Psychology, 16*, 515–520.

Strike, P. C., Magid, K., Brydon, L., Edwards, S., McEwan, J. R., & Steptoe, A. (2004). Exaggerated platelet and hemodynamic reactivity to mental stress in men with coronary artery disease. *Psychosomatic Medicine, 66*, 492–500.

Strom, T. B., Sytkowski, A. J., Carpenter, C. B., & Merrill, J. P. (1974). Cholinergic augmentation of lymphocyte-mediated cytotoxicity. A study of the cholinergic receptor of cytotoxic T lymphocytes. *Proceedings of the National Academy of Sciences, 71*, 1330–1333.

Swiergiel, A. H., Takahashi, L. K., & Kalin, N. H. (1993). Attenuation of stress-induced behavior by antagonism of corticotropin-releasing factor receptors in the central amygdala in the rat. *Brain Research, 623*, 229–234.

Testa, M. & Collins, R. L. (1997). Alcohol and risky sexual behavior: Event-based analyses among a sample of high-risk women. *Psychol. Addict. Beh., 11*, 190–201.

Tilg, H., Trehu, E., Atkins, M. B., Dinarello, C. A., & Mier, J. W. (1994, January 1). Interleukin-6 (IL-6) as an anti-inflammatory cytokine: Induction of circulating IL-1 receptor antagonist and soluble tumor necrosis factor receptor p55. *Blood, 83*, 113–118.

Tomei, L. D., Kiecolt-Glaser, J. K., Kennedy, S., & Glaser, R. (1990). Psychological-stress and phorbol ester inhibition of radiation-induced apoptosis in human peripheral blood leukocytes. *Psychiatry Research, 33*, 59–71.

Tracey, K. J. (2002). The inflammatory reflex. *Nature, 420*, 853–859.

Treiber, F. A., Kamarck, T., Schneiderman, N., Sheffield, D., Kapuku, G., & Taylor, T. (2003). Cardiovascular reactivity and development of preclinical and clinical disease states. *Psychosomatic Medicine, 65*, 46–62.

Troxel, W. M., Matthews, K. A., Bromberger, J. T., & Sutton-Tyrrell, K. (2003). Chronic stress burden, discrimination, and subclinical carotid artery disease in African American and Caucasian women. *Health Psychology, 22*, 300–309.

Uchino, B. N., Kiecolt-Glaser, J. K., & Cacioppo, J. T. (1992). Age-related changes in cardiovascular response as a function of a chronic stressor and social support. *Journal of Personality and Social Psychology, 63*, 839–846.

Uchino, B. N., Cacioppo, J. T., Malarkey, W., & Glaser, R. (1995). Individual differences in cardiac sympathetic control predict endocrine and immune responses to acute psychological stress. *Journal of Personality and Social Psychology, 69*, 736–743.

UNAIDS/WHO (2004). *Aids epidemic update: 2004.* Geneva, Switzerland. Retrieved from www.unaids.org/wad2004/report_pdf.html.

Valentino, R. J., Foote, S. L., & Page, M. E. (1993). The locus coeruleus as a site for integrating corticotropin-releasing factor and noradrenergic mediation of stress responses. *Annals of the New York Academy of Sciences, 697*, 173–188.

Van Gool, J., van Vugy, H., Helle, M., & Aarden, L. A. (1990). The relation among stress, adrenalin, interleukin 6 and acute phase proteins in the rat. *Clinical Immunology and Immunopathology, 57*, 200–210.

Vedhara, K., Bennett, P. D., Clark, S., Lightman, S. L., Shaw, S., Perks, P., Hunt, M. A., Philip, J. M. D., Tallon, D., Murphy, P. J., Jones, R. W., Wilcock, G. K., & Shanks, N. M. (2003). Enhancement of antibody responses to influenza vaccination in the elderly following a cognitive-behavioural stress management intervention. *Psychotherapy and Psychosomatics. 72*, 245–252.

Vedhara, K., Cox, N. K. M., Wilcock, G. K., Perks, P., Hunt, M., Anderson, S., Lightman, S. L., & Shanks, N. M. (1999). Chronic stress in elderly carers of dementia patients and antibody response to influenza vaccination. *Lancet, 353*, 627–631.

Veldhuijzen van Zanten, J. J. C. S., Ring, C., Burns, V. E., Edwards, K. M., Drayson, M., & Carroll, D. (2004). Mental stress-induced haemoconcentration: sex differences and mechanisms, *Psychophysiology, 41*, 541–551.

Veldhuis, J. D., & Aranmanesh, A. (1996). Physiological regulation of the human growth hormone (GH)-insulin-like growth factor I (IGF-I) Axis: Predominant impact of age, obesity, gonadal function, and sleep. *Sleep, 19*, S221–S224.

Verma, S., Szmitko, P. E., & Yeh, E. T. H. (2004). C-reactive protein: Structure affects function. *Circulation, 109*, 1914–1917.

Wang, J., Charboneau, R., Barke, R. A., Loh, H. H., & Roy, S. (2002). u-opioid receptor mediates chronic restraint stress-induced lymphocyte apoptosis. *Journal of Immunology, 169*, 3630–3636.

Webster, E. L., Torpy, D. J., Elenkov, I. J., & Chrousos, G. P. (1998, May). Corticotropin-releasing hormone and inflammation. *Annals of the New York Academy of Sciences, 840*, 21–32.

Webster, J. C., Oakley, R. H., Jewell, C. M., & Cidlowski, J. A. (2001, June). Proinflammatory cytokines regulate human glucocorticoid receptor gene expression and lead to the accumulation of the dominant negative B isoform: A mechanism for the generation of glucocorticoid resistance. *PNAS, 98*, 6865–6870.

WHO. (2004). Tuberculosis. Geneva, Switzerland. Retrieved at www.who.int/mediacentre/factsheets/fs104/en/.

Wiegers, G. J., Croiset, G., Reul, J. M. H. M., Holsboer, F., & De Kloet, E. R. (1993). Differential effects of corticosteroids on rat peripheral blood T-lymphocyte mitogenesis in vivo and in vitro. *American Journal of Physiology, 265*, E825–E830.

Worthley, S. G., Osende, J. I., Helft, G., Badimon, J. J., & Fuster, V. (2001, May). Coronary artery disease: Pathogenesis and acute coronary syndromes. *The Mount Sinai Journal of Medicine, 68*, 167–181.

Xing, Z., Gauldie, J., Cox, G., Baumann, H., Jordana, M., Lei, X-F., & Achong, M. K. (1998, January). IL-6 is an anti-inflammatory cytokine required for controlling local or systemic acute inflammatory responses. *Journal of Clinical Investigation, 101*, 311–320.

Yehuda, R., Southwick, S. M., Nussbaum, G., Wahby, V., Giller, E. L., & Mason, J. W. (1990). Low urinary cortisol excretion in patients with posttraumatic stress disorder. *The Journal of Nervous and Mental Disorder, 178*, 366–369.

Yeung, A. C., Vekshtein, V. I., Krantz, D. S., Vita, J. A., Ryan, Jr., T. J., Ganz, P., & Selwyn, A. P. (1991). The effect of atherosclerosis on the vasomotor response of coronary arteries to mental stress. *New England Journal of Medicine, 325*, 1551–1556.

Young, I. S., & McEneny, J. (2001). Lipoprotein oxidation and atherosclerosis. *Biochemical Society Transactions, 29*, 358–362.

Zorrilla, E. P., McKay, J. R., Luborsky, L., & Schmidt, K. (1996). Relation of stressors and depressive symptoms to clinical progression of viral illness. *American Journal of Psychiatry, 153*, 626–635.

27 Sleep and Dreaming

R. T. PIVIK

INTRODUCTION

The majority of our behavioral and cognitive lives are spent in the waking state – a time during which activities viewed as essential to personal existence and continuation of the species is accomplished. It is, therefore, to be expected that for many the waking state is likely to be considered "the sole portion of . . . existence that 'counts' in any way, sleep appearing as 'time out' from the game of living" (Kleitman, 1963, p. 3). However, although sleep may appear to constitute an interruption of the critical activities of wakefulness, it is indisputable that the alternation between sleep and wakefulness is essential to "normal" existence in higher life forms. The importance of sleep to normal waking activities can be immediately appreciated when the well-documented adverse effects of sleep reduction on waking behavioral and psychological functions are considered – effects extending from decreased alertness and impaired performance (Gillberg & Akerstedt, 1994; Monk, 1991) to death (Bentivoglio & Grassi-Zucconi, 1997; Everson, 1995; Horne, 1988; Rechtschaffen et al., 2002). There is gathering evidence as well that specific aspects of learning and memory during wakefulness may benefit from, or require, sleep-dependent processes (Fischer et al., 2002; Born 2002; Mölle et al., 2004; Stickgold, James, & Hobson, 2000). Clearly, these two states interact in a complementary and synergistic relationship to maintain and extend life, and although the precise nature of this codependence has, to a great extent, been obscured by a lack of detailed knowledge regarding the physiology and psychology of sleep, recent advances in these areas have provided significant insights into these puzzling within- and between-state variations and relationships.

It is at the same time surprising and revealing that sleep should support any form of cognitive activity – surprising because at first glance it is difficult to imagine the purpose of mental activity during such sustained periods of disengagement from the environment, and revealing because of the unexpected psychophysiological relationships the presence of such activity implies. Still, if concepts subscribing to the interaction or psychophysi-ological parallelism of mind-body relationships are even closely approximated, then it would be expected that the marked behavioral and physiological sleep-wakefulness differences would be reflected in equally marked differences in the characteristics of associated cognitive activity. In this instance, state-dependent expectations are apparently reinforced because, unlike the generally more organized, rational, and self-directed nature of waking cognition, cognitive activity during sleep is seemingly disorganized, distorted, and subject to little volitional control. This distinctive cognitive behavior – not associated with an abnormal-state or condition, yet so apparently different from waking mental activity – has been provided with an appropriately distinctive name: dreaming.

HISTORICAL BACKGROUND

The relative inaccessibility of processes underlying sleep and dreaming fostered wide-ranging speculation regarding the nature and function of these activities. Early theories attributed sleep to various changes in the distribution, temperature, or constitution of blood, and many considered the difference between sleep and death simply a matter of degree (Kleitman, 1963; Nitz, 1993). Later concepts extending into the early twentieth century localized sleep to the brain and ascribed many functions to this state, including enhancing digestion, creating new "animal spirits" required for waking behavior, and eliminating potentially harmful "humors" from the body (Wittern, 1989). Paralleling these notions were beliefs that dreams contained messages foretelling the future, revealed cures for illnesses, or provided unique access to the unconscious (Kramer, 1994; Webb, 1993). These various conceptualizations had in common a view of sleep as a unimodal state, and dreams as sporadic, relatively rare events.

Although sleep and dreaming have long been sources of fascination and speculation, scientific interest in these behaviors significantly intensified in the twentieth century. In the second edition of his classic text summarizing information regarding sleep and wakefulness Kleitman (1963) listed over 4,000 references – less than 2% of which referred to publications before the twentieth century. However, the most marked acceleration of experimental studies into the nature of sleep physiology and psychology can be traced to the mid-twentieth century when Eugene Aserinsky, a physiology doctoral student at the University of Chicago, observed episodes of eye movement activity during sleep in what were the first whole-night polygraphical recordings of such activities (Aserinsky, 1953). Although slower than waking eye movements of comparable amplitude, and more impressed with the "jerkiness" than the velocity of these eye movements, Aserinsky nevertheless elected to characterize this as Rapid Eye Movement (REM) activity in large part to avoid "the anticipated taunts relative to the popular slang meaning of 'jerk'" (Aserinsky, 1996; p. 218).

This observation, utilizing a newly emerging technology that made possible longterm recordings of electrophysiological activities, led to a series of publications that revolutionized and redirected thinking regarding both the nature of sleep and the occurrence of dreaming (Aserinsky & Kleitman, 1953, 1955; Dement, 1955; Dement & Kleitman, 1957a, 1957b; Dement & Wolpert, 1958a, 1958b). The finding of recurring episodes of physiological activation embedded within sleep that were unlike either wakefulness or the remainder of sleep flew in the face of existing concepts of sleep as a unitary, passive state. So unique were these rapid eye movement periods, that they prompted investigators to consider REM sleep as a third state of existence (Dement, 1969; Snyder, 1966; Steriade & McCarley, 1990). Not only did these REM periods deviate in their physiological characteristics from other normal states, but upon awakening from these episodes subjects commonly reported dreaming – suggesting that an objective index had been identified for determining "the incidence and duration of periods of dreaming" (Aserinsky & Kleitman, 1953, p. 274).

Although electrographic recordings of brain wave and oculomotor activities assisted in the discovery of REM sleep and its association with dreaming, these observations did not require such technologic assistance. Determination of whether an individual is asleep can be made subjectively with reasonable reliability, and movements of the eyes are readily apparent from associated displacements of the corneal bulge under the eyelids. Furthermore, because of the prominence of visual images in dream reports, it had long been speculated that dreams would be accompanied by eye movements (Griesinger, 1868; Ladd, 1892). Given such considerations, why had these remarkable periods of physiological and cognitive activation – which occur nightly, are distributed across the night, and may last 20 minutes or longer – not been previously discovered? In a publication in which he chronicles the discovery of REM sleep, Aserinsky (1996) considered this question, with the following observations:

the obvious answer must lie in human behavior. Since the first REM period is not obvious during the first couple of hours of sleep, and cyclicity would require a still longer period of observation, the discovery of REM would have required an

obsessive, highly motivated individual to peer continually for hours at a sleeper's eyes. This would explain the failure of the layman to discover REM, but what about scientists who are infamous for both obsessiveness and motivation, and thus should have looked for the eye movements? My guess is that no one was sufficiently driven to spend an inordinate amount of time to fill in the gaps of sleep studies in which the position of the eyes was noted by occasional lifting of the sleeper's eyes. (pp. 226–227)

The technologic capability of recording physiological measures over long periods of time may not have been required for the discovery of REM sleep, but it was essential for the subsequent exploration and detailing of the general physiology of sleep. Although Aserinsky (1996) considered the relationship of rapid eye movements in sleep to dreaming as "almost incidental with respect to its import in understanding brain function" (p. 226), it was the linkage of sleep-state physiology to sleep-state cognitive activity that provided the major impetus for the next two decades of sleep and dream research, and established the foundation for what could be considered the "new sleep research." Furthermore, this focus on psychophysiological relationships during sleep presented an opportunity to determine if such relationships are maintained across states and, consequently, to provide a broader understanding of mind-body relationships. Even before specific physiological sleep-wakefulness differences were determined it was apparent that these states differed along significant dimensions, among which was the profound change in level of consciousness. Relative to wakefulness, there is a dramatic decrease in awareness of both the external and internal physical environments during sleep as reflected by increased sensory thresholds to external and internal stimulation, as well as by an absence of appreciation of significant physiological variations, for example, galvanic skin response activation during slow wave sleep or breathing cessation associated with sleep apnea (Guilleminault, 1994; Johnson, 1973). With few exceptions (e.g., lucid dreaming), this decrease in awareness is accompanied by a general loss of volitional control over physiological and psychological processes. The relative inaccessibility of sleep processes, together with the associated greatly diminished awareness and control, created both real and apparent obstacles to the scientific study of these behaviors. Still, the very factors that complicated the study of these processes also removed or attenuated potentially confounding variables commonly associated with investigations during wakefulness (e.g., stress, expectations, and undefined variations in level of arousal), raising the possibility that relationships either obscured by or absent during wakefulness would be unmasked during sleep.

PHYSICAL CONTEXT

Questions concerning why and how wakefulness-sleep state alternations occur have motivated speculation and inquiry into the mechanisms of these variations. Early views of sleep as the passive behavioral default which results when wakefulness-maintaining activities from specific sensory (Bremer, 1937, 1938) or nonspecific brainstem reticular pathways (Moruzzi & Magoun, 1949) were withdrawn, had to be modified to incorporate evidence of active sleep promoting processes. This evidence was provided by brainstem and cortical stimulation and lesion studies (reviewed in Jones, 2000; Steriade & McCarley, 1990) as well as by indications of active control processes effecting and modulating sleep, such as recurring periods of activated (REM) sleep and predictable sleep pattern variations across the night (i.e., the sleep cycle). The separation of sleep promoting mechanisms into passive and active categories provided a conceptual framework within which studies could be formulated and interpreted. However, technologic advances permitting more discerning anatomical and neurophysiological evaluations of systems and processes underlying sleep and waking behavior made it apparent that the passive-active dichotomy was too simplistic, and that sleep initiation and maintenance most likely involved cascading effects and interactions resulting from both the passive effects of functional deafferentation as well as activation of structures with hypnogenic properties. The search for specific brain regions or centers, the activation of which are essential to the occurrence or promotion of sleep, identified several candidates, for example, the solitary tract nucleus in the medulla, the preoptic basal forebrain area, the anterior hypothalamus, and the brain stem raphe nuclei for nonrapid eye movement (NREM) sleep, and the pons for REM sleep (for reviews see Jones, 2000; McCarley, 2004; Steriade & McCarley, 1990).

Paralleling and complementing these studies were those capitalizing on developments in the detection and localization of biochemicals in the peripheral and central nervous systems and how these compounds were related to state determination. Although the notion of a chemical hypnogenic factor had been hypothesized early in the twentieth century (Pieron, 1913), the technology necessary to effectively pursue this line of inquiry did not begin to become available until the 1950s and 1960s, and since that time this technology has become increasingly sensitive and sophisticated. Studies using these techniques have implicated interactions among a wide range of chemicals that exert sleep or wakefulness promoting influences, and have reinforced research focused on anatomical or neurophysiological aspects of sleep in demonstrating the complexity of systems involved in sleep-wakefulness state determination. These compounds, produced centrally and peripherally and acting as neurotransmitters, neuromodulators or neurohormones, have been variously localized to neurons, cerebrospinal fluid, and blood (see Basheer et al., 2004; Jones, 2000; Krueger & Kamovsky, 1995; Steriade & McCarley, 1990 for reviews). These quests for sleep centers and chemical sleep factors have proven to be highly informative and heuristically beneficial, and the outcomes of these studies have been summarized as follows: "no sleep or wake state *in toto* can be said to have a center and . . . few,

if any, components of waking-sleep states have 'a center'" (Steriade & McCarley, 1990, pg. 21), and "no single chemical neurotransmitter, neuromodulator, or neurohormone has been identified that is necessary or sufficient for the generation and maintenance of sleep or waking. Instead, multiple factors and systems are involved in the onset and maintenance of these states" (Jones, 2000, pg. 149). The idea of distributed and interacting systems is being increasingly utilized in theoretical formulations integrating neuronal and neurochemical processes that attempt to explain state determination (Krueger & Karnovsky, 1995; McCarley & Hobson, 1975). Ultimately, understanding the mechanisms responsible for state determination and the relationship of these mechanisms to behavior will provide insights into the function of sleep – an enigma that continues to elude resolution (Greene & Siegel, 2004; Rechtschaffen, 1998).

SOCIAL CONTEXT

It requires little reflection to appreciate that scientific investigations may be unintentionally influenced by aspects of the experimental process such as the laboratory environment, measurement apparatus, experimental demands, and the presence of investigators. These factors may exert what has been termed "reactive measurement effects" (Campbell, 1957) on study outcome measures. Recognizing that the sleeping environment, sleep behavior, and associated personal thoughts (dreams) of individuals are usually considered among the most private of behavioral domains, attempts to study these behaviors would seem to require obtrusive intervention and present multiple opportunities for reactive measurement effects. In attempts to control for or at least minimize such effects, investigators have applied several techniques or procedures. For example, in addition to assuring subject confidentiality with respect to study results, it has proven helpful to introduce subjects to the laboratory environment, procedures and personnel prior to undertaking sleep recordings, or to minimize the number of sensors (e.g., Stickgold & Hobson, 1996). Still, in view of the apparent intrusiveness of procedures necessary to evaluate sleep physiology, statements referring to such procedures as "noninvasive" and "minimally sleep disturbing" would seem to underestimate the sleep disturbance expected under these conditions. However, studies of sleep in populations across the pediatric to geriatric age range during the past half-century have clearly established that most subjects can, and do, sleep well under these circumstances. Commonly, the initial nights in the laboratory are accompanied by sleep disturbance in the form of increased latencies to sleep onset, more body movements, and fragmentation of sleep patterns. Because sleep patterns normally stabilize subsequent to this initial period, these variations have been considered to be transient responses to the novel sleeping environment and instrumentation. This adaptation phenomenon has been termed the "first night effect" (Agnew, Webb, & Williams, 1966). Once adaptation has occurred, the night-to-night stability of many sleep measures is remarkable. This consistency is expressed across several variables, including the amounts and cyclic characteristics of sleep stages (Figure 27.3), autonomic measures (heart rate and variability: Pivik et al., 1996; Figures 27.5 and 27.6), and specific electrographic events (K-complexes: Johnson, 1973; ponto-geniculo-occipital spike activity: Jouvet, 1972). The development of portable instrumentation to record physiological parameters necessary for sleep-wakefulness differentiation and sleep staging has allowed the comparison of results from recordings made in subjects' home environments with those obtained from the same subjects studied in the laboratory. The fact that such comparisons have revealed minimal between-condition differences (Sewitch & Kupfer, 1985) attests to the general robustness of sleep processes and the adaptability of subjects.

Concerns regarding the influence of experimental factors on sleep mentation reports have focused on possible confabulation by subjects in the interest of pleasing the investigator, and the extent to which the laboratory environment may directly affect the content in these reports. The potential for experimental confounds because of confabulation is always of concern in situations where other measures, such as those provided by physiological or performance variables, cannot provide corroborative indexes. This issue, of long-standing concern to investigators studying sleep mentation, was effectively addressed by Rechtschaffen (1967) in a series of logical considerations to be used as guidelines for evaluating the acceptance of such reports as true representations of sleep experiences. These guidelines have been summarized as follows:

1. *Parsimony* – interpretations requiring the fewest assumptions are favored.

2. *Prevalence* – phenomena known to occur most frequently are favored over those of rare occurrence. For example, in the absence of indications of impaired memory in the recall processes in wakefulness, the subject's postarousal report is accepted as a valid representation of his or her experience, rather than questioned on the grounds of cognitive impairment.

3. *Plausibility* – an extension of the prevalence guideline, which, however, "gives special emphasis to frequency and occurrence in given situations" (Rechtschaffen & Kales, 1968, p. 7). For example, although it could be assumed that subjects are lying when questioned about the presence and details of dream experiences, one would consider it unlikely that subjects would lie so consistently about dream reports, given the current understanding of the motivational factors promoting lying.

4. *Private experience* – "in the absence of objective indices, there is a strong tendency to accept the existence of phenomena if they have been part of one's own experience." (Pivik, 1986, p. 393).

As might be expected, elements of the experimental environment or procedures may be incorporated into dream reports (Domhoff & Kamiya, 1964; Okuma, Fukuma, & Kobayashi, 1975) and, although some content differences may exist between dreams collected at home relative to those collected in the laboratory (Lloyd & Cartwright, 1995; Stickgold, Pace-Schott, & Hobson, 1994; Weisz & Foulkes, 1970), these differences are minor. A more major issue relates to whether dreams collected in the laboratory are so influenced by the experimental conditions that they provide an unfaithful representation of the subject's dreamlife, depicting it as more mundane, realistically oriented, and coherent than it may be (Dorus, Dorus, & Rechtschaffen, 1971; Snyder, 1970). The studies cited above indicating content similarities between home and laboratory dreams when collected under similar sampling conditions suggest that reports collected in the laboratory do not provide an unrepresentative view of dream content and processes. Furthermore, it has been argued (Foulkes & Cavalerro, 1993) that spontaneous recall of dreams in the home environment may, in fact, present an atypical view of dream content because laboratory dreams are better sampled and home dreams that are remembered may be so because of bizarre, emotional, or vivid characteristics.

INFERENTIAL CONTEXT

Every area of scientific endeavor is confronted with unique methodological challenges, but for sleep research the usual challenges (e.g., satisfying criteria fundamental to the reliable and valid measurement of physiological and cognitive processes) are compounded by the need to obtain these measures from the sleeping organism while maintaining state integrity and continuity. This state maintenance is, and continues to be, critical to the recognition of physiological indices that may be used as more discrete and objective correlates of sleep behaviors, and to the valid assignment of behaviors to their proper state domain.

In this regard, it is instructive to consider how demand characteristics differ between studies conducted during wakefulness and sleep, the methodological challenges these differences create, and how some of these challenges have been resolved. During waking investigations, which generally extend for a few minutes up to perhaps two hours, subjects are aware of physiological transducers attached to their bodies and can comply with instructions to avoid or minimize behaviors, such as body movements and eye blinks, which might compromise the quality of the recordings. By comparison, sleep recordings normally last at least six to eight hours, and while asleep subjects do not have volitional control over biological sources of artifact, such as frequent adjustments in body position which take place during the course of a normal night of sleep (Altshuler & Brebbia, 1967; DeKoninck, Lorrain, & Gagnon, 1992; Kleitman, w1963). Accordingly, procedures have had to be developed to more securely attach transducers for reliable recordings over these extended periods

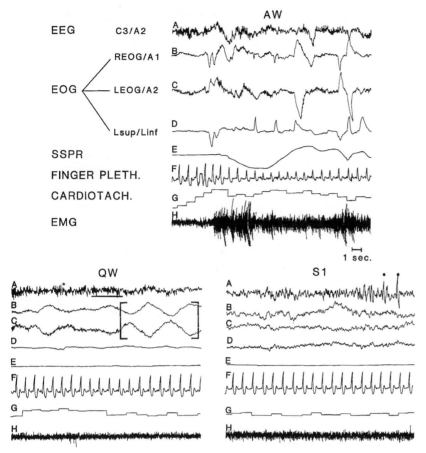

Figure 27.1. Polygraphical tracings of physiological measures associated with sleep-wakefulness state variations. Eight channels of activity (A-H) are depicted during active and quiet wakefulness (AW and QW, respectively) and the first stage of sleep (NREM Stage 1, or S1). The recorded variables include the electroencephalogram (EEG; C3/A2, channel A), the electrooculogram [EOG; horizontal (right and left outer canthi) and vertical (placements superior and inferior to right eye orbit), channels B, C, and D, respectively], autonomic activity [spontaneous skin potential response, (SSPR), channel E); finger plethysmogram (channel F); cardiotachometer recordings (channel G)] and the facial (orbicularis oris) electromyogram (EMG; channel H). In these examples the passive decrease in EMG activity, which commonly occurs at sleep onset (S1), does not become evident until slow wave sleep (Figure 27.2, S3 and S4). Electrophysiological features of note are alpha activity (underscored, channel A) and slow rolling eye movements (channels B and C) preceding sleep onset in QW, and vertex sharp waves in Stage 1 (see dots, channel A). See text for discussion of sleep stage definitions and electrophysiological composition. (Reprinted with permission from Pivik, 1986, © The Guilford Press.)

of time, and it has often been necessary to design special devices or techniques to access measures of interest while minimizing sleep disturbance. For example, electrodes used to record the electrooculogram (EOG) also detect brain waves or electroencephalographic (EEG) signals (see Figures 27.1 and 27.2; S1-S4), and to obtain eye movement recordings not contaminated by these signals required transducers which could be applied to the eyelids to register mechanical movements of the eye (Baldridge, Whitman, & Kramer, 1963; Conduit, Crewther, & Coleman, 2004; Gross, Byrne, & Fisher, 1965). Although such crosstalk is diminished when low amplitude, fast frequency EEG activity predominates (e.g., during waking and REM sleep) and does not generally compromise

state identification, even at these times EEG events may influence EOG recordings (Iacono & Lykken, 1981) and EOG events may influence EEG recordings (see chapters 3 and 4 of this volume). To investigate variations in spinal monosynaptic reflex activity recorded from leg musculature, a method of leg restraint was devised which maintains the positions of stimulating and recording electrodes without altering reflex responses or disturbing sleep as a result of excessive restraint (Mercier & Pivik, 1983; Pivik & Dement, 1970; Pivik, 1971). A variety of devices, which can be comfortably inserted into the external auditory canal, have been developed for controlling stimulus delivery in sleep auditory arousal threshold (Busby, Mercier, & Pivik 1994) or evoked potential (Campbell & Bartoli, 1986) studies, providing measures of middle ear muscle activity by converting changes in sound pressure level to variations in impedance (Pessah & Roffwarg, 1972), or measuring core body temperature by means of a thermistor positioned near the ear drum (Palca, Walker, & Berger, 1981). In addition to these examples, the field of sleep disorders medicine has developed many novel approaches to assess physiological functioning during sleep (see Kryger, Roth, & Dement, 1994, 2000).

The amount of data collected in even the most fundamental of sleep studies using electrographic techniques is formidable. Over an eight-hour period, a single channel of EEG recording (at the recommended paper speed of 10 mm/sec) will trace a trail on paper extending .2 miles or, if digitized, will require approximately 25 megabytes of computer storage space. When it is considered that multiple channels of physiological information are commonly recorded for two to five nights, the magnitude of the associated information acquisition, processing, and storage requirements can be appreciated. Increasingly, sleep investigations are utilizing new developments in computer technology, which make these challenges more manageable and greatly facilitate associated data analysis (Armitage, 1995a; Kubicki & Herrmann, 1996). Examples of the application of computerized methods of analysis to an autonomic measure (heart rate) and EEG are presented in Figures 27.4–27.6 and 27.7–27.8, respectively.

The organizing principle, which imposed meaning on these extensive data and was key to the recognition of REM

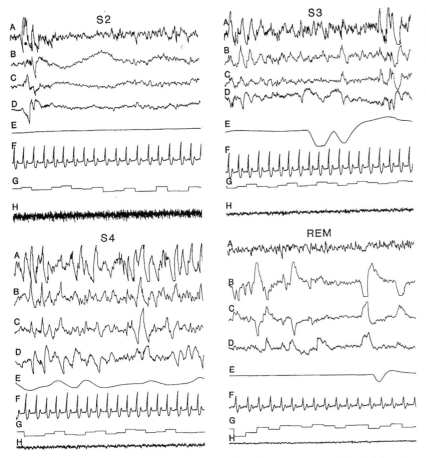

Figure 27.2. Polygraphical tracings of physiological measures associated with variations in sleep stages [NREM Stages 2–4 (S2-S4) and REM]. For explanation of channels A-H, see Figure 27.1. Of note is the occurrence of Stage 2 K-complexes (see dot, channel A). See text for discussion of sleep stage definitions and electrophysiological composition. (Reprinted with permission from Pivik, 1986, © The Guilford Press.)

and which seem to repeat themselves" (Prechtl et al., 1968, p. 200). According to these criteria, existence in mammals may be partitioned into three general states: wakefulness, REM sleep, and NREM sleep.

If a state may be likened to the gestalt that emerges from associated, defining attributes, then a stage represents the identification of progressive within-state changes in these attributes. These component stages are defined by relatively precise, but nevertheless arbitrary, criteria. Referring again to the different states H_2O may assume, it is possible to define stages of transition bridging these states as a function, for example, of precise temperature and pressure variations. By analogy, NREM sleep in the human beings has been divided into four stages based on EEG criteria. Although REM sleep has been differentially examined on the basis of the presence or absence of various activities (e.g., eye movements or autonomic activation), further fragmentation of REM sleep into stages has not been proposed.

To arrive at valid and enduring state and stage criteria necessitates the development of an adequate and reliable descriptive database from which such criteria can be derived. The initial set of such criteria for sleep states and stages was proposed within five years of the discovery of REM sleep and the use of all-night polygraphical recordings of sleep electrophysiology (Dement & Kleitman, 1957a), but it would be more than another decade before standardized scoring manuals would be developed. These manuals defined criteria for the reliable scoring and interpretation of electrophysiological sleep recordings based on the evaluation of 20–30 second epochs (Anders, Emde, & Parmelee, 1971; Rechtschaffen & Kales, 1968), and provided a reasonable solution for managing the large datasets associated with such studies. The choice of the specific scoring epochs for chunking sleep behavior, although not specifically rationalized, did not reflect a validated 20–30 second behavioral sleep unit. Instead, it was most likely based on several practical factors, including discriminability of recordings, reduction of an extensive database to more manageable dimensions, and providing the best fit between physiological data and technical parameters of recording instrumentation. It is of historical interest in this regard that the early electrographic recordings of human sleep were conducted using a recorder that cut a moving strip of paper on which variations in brain potentials were traced every 20 or 30 seconds (Loomis, Harvey, & Hobart, 1938).

sleep as a discrete entity, involved discerning and clustering patterns of activity into larger blocks of behavior termed "states and stages." These concepts, often loosely applied, are important to differentiate because of the significantly different implications they carry for the conceptualization and understanding of behavior. In the physical world the differentiation between state and stage is often quite distinct, for example, the defining state characteristics of H_2O when it exists in a liquid, frozen, or gaseous form are clearly evident. However, in living organisms where behaviors are based on complex interactions among a variety of systems, state definition is often more equivocal and more judgmental. Still, as indicated by the following definitions, even under these more complex conditions there is common agreement regarding criteria for state determination. That is, a state may be defined as "a cluster of attributes whose simultaneous and repeated occurrence is highly unique" (Dement & Mitler, 1974, p. 278); "a recurring temporally enduring constellation of values of a set of indicator variables of the organism" (Steriade & McCarley, 1990, p. 8,); or "constellations of functional patterns and physiological variables which may be relatively stable

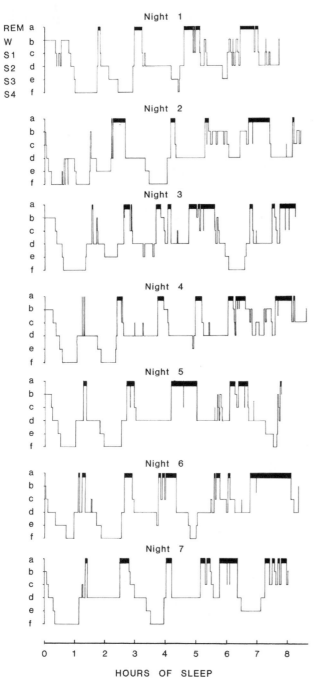

REM a
W b
S1 c
S2 d
S3 e
S4 f

Night 1

Night 2

Night 3

Night 4

Night 5

Night 6

Night 7

HOURS OF SLEEP

Figure 27.3. Sleep profiles depicting variations in sleep stages (ordinate) as a function of time asleep (abscissa). These profiles, based on seven consecutive nights of baseline sleep in a young adult, illustrate the stability of sleep patterns across nights, the presence of patterned oscillations between REM (darkened rectangles) and NREM sleep (i.e., sleep cycle), and the decrease in Stage 4 and increase in REM sleep as a function of sleep time within a given night. (Reprinted with permission from Pivik, 1986, © The Guilford Press.)

A caveat to the use of such relatively long scoring epochs is the resultant smoothing of the dynamic flux of physiological changes that occurs within briefer time intervals, which gives the impression that sleep states are played out in a very stable and continuous manner and

that state and stage transitions are relatively abrupt. The extent to which the duration of the scoring epoch contributes to this impression was underscored in an investigation in which 24-hour recordings of sleep in the cat were analyzed using a three-second scoring interval (Ferguson et al., 1969). With this procedure it was found that uninterrupted intervals of either wakefulness or NREM sleep were quite brief, in the range of one to two minutes. Briefer scoring intervals have also been applied in humans to provide more precise assessments of variations in normal (Ogilvie & Wilkinson, 1984; Pivik, Busby, & Brown, 1993) or disruptive physiological processes during sleep (ASDA, 1992). However, obtaining information of such temporal precision presents additional data processing and conceptual demands. For example, in terms of data processing, using three-second scoring intervals in the 24-hour animal recordings increases the number of individual data samples to be analyzed tenfold (i.e., from 2,880 to 28,800). Focusing on increasingly briefer intervals also requires determining valid and reliable scoring criteria for these intervals and, most importantly, raises the question of what is the smallest meaningful unit of sleep behavior that can be practically determined. Although the feasibility of analyzing extended datasets using more discrete time intervals has been significantly facilitated by computer technology, when such technology has been applied to studies of sleep the convention of reporting computerized results based on 20–30 second or longer intervals has generally been maintained (Armitage, 1995b; Itil, 1970; Sussman et al., 1979).

Microepoch analyses of physiological variables during sleep not only provide a more faithful representation of the actions and interactions of these variables, but the resulting enhanced microstructural view of sleep variables may help resolve questions relating to sleep-wakefulness interactions which continue to go unanswered. For example, the basis for what constitutes a refreshing night of sleep remains undetermined, but there is growing emphasis on sleep continuity as an important contributing factor (Carskadon, Brown, & Dement, 1982; Stepanski et al., 1984). In this regard, it has been shown that discrete interruptions of sleep, either spontaneously occurring or resulting from external stimulation, can be associated with enhanced daytime sleepiness and reports of significantly reduced sleep quality, even though these disturbances may not effect a significant reduction in total sleep time (Roehrs et al., 1994; Stepanski et al., 1987).

As new methods of data acquisition and analysis have developed, the descriptive picture of sleep physiology has become increasingly detailed and has provided information relevant to the study of psychophysiological relationships during sleep. Still, accounts of thought processes can be directly accessed or confirmed only by means of verbal communication. Although verbalization may occur during both REM and NREM sleep, intelligent dialogue with a sleeping subject has not been initiated or maintained, and attempts to provide subjects with posthypnotic suggestions to relate ongoing mentation without awakening

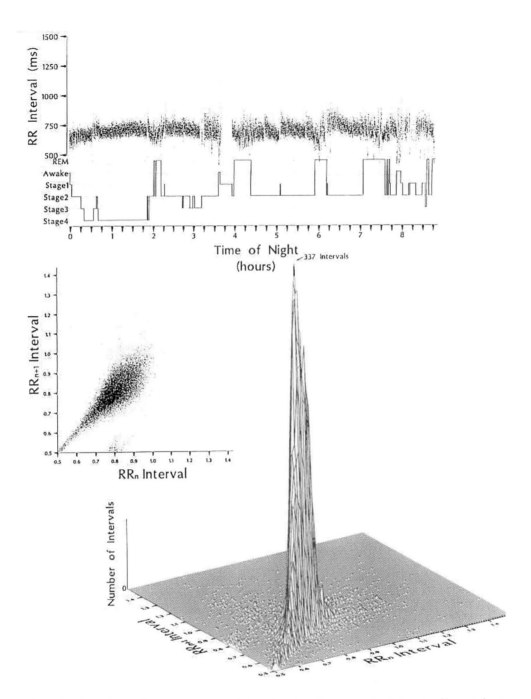

Figure 27.4. Analyses of heart rate across a night of sleep based on computer-determined beat-to-beat (RR) intervals. The upper graph depicts a sleep histogram with associated RR interval plots. In the middle graph, each RR interval (RRn) is plotted against the subsequent interval (RRn + 1) to produce a graph known as a Poincaré plot reflecting the beat-to-beat dispersion for specific heart rate intervals as well as inter-beat interval variability as heart rate changes. Expanding the two dimensional Poincaré plot into three dimensions (lower figure) more clearly illustrates the density distribution of graphed values. In this Poincaré plot and those in Figures 27.5 and 27.6, RR interval values (both axis) extend from 0 to 1.4 seconds in 100 millisecond intervals.

have been unsuccessful (Arkin et al., 1970; Arkin, 1978). Inferences can be made about thought processes from nonverbal measures, for example, motor (Berger & Oswald, 1962b; Dement & Wolpert, 1958b; Shimizu & Inoue, 1986) or autonomic responses (Hobson, Goldfrank, & Snyder, 1965; Laberge, Greenleaf, & Kedzierski, 1983), but such inferences are most reliably determined during wakeful-

ness in the context of a controlled experiment (see Chapters 4, 7, 8, and 10 of this volume), as opposed to sleep in which directional control over subjects' behavior and associated thought processes is minimal if not absent. Although some variation in state can be said to occur when subjects are required to provide a verbal report of immediately preceding experiences, this shift is much greater for

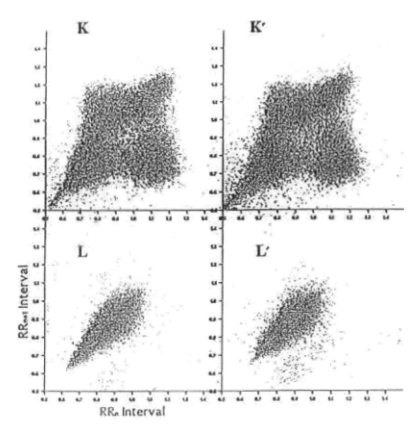

Figure 27.5. Whole-night Poincaré plots for two subjects (K and L) on two consecutive baseline nights (night 3: left column; night 4: right column). In these graphs, the within-subject consistency and between-subject variability across nights are notable. (Reprinted with permission from Pivik et al. 1996, p. 124, © American Sleep Disorders Association and Sleep Research Society.)

the reporting of sleep mentation where a major between-state change must occur (sleep to wakefulness) compared to the relatively minor within-state change associated with reports of waking experiences in wakefulness. Furthermore, this state-change is a gradual process (Balkin et al., 2002). The more extreme nature of the state change required to access reports of sleep cognition distinguishes studies of sleep mentation from others not characterized by such marked differences between conditions at the time of the experience relative to those at the time of reporting. The inability to more directly and immediately access cognitive activity in the sleeping subject, coupled with aspects of sleep physiology that differ remarkably from those commonly associated with cognitive activity during wakefulness, has prompted skepticism regarding whether postawakening reports reflected cognitive activity occurring during sleep. Alternative explanations considered included suggestions that the reports reflected hypnopompic experiences generated in the process of waking up (Goblot, 1896) or were intentionally contrived in the interest of pleasing the experimenter. Experimental data addressing these concerns will be presented once fundamental attributes of sleep physiology and psychology have been considered.

SLEEP PHYSIOLOGY AND PSYCHOLOGY: DESCRIPTIVE ASPECTS

Nearly two decades before the discovery of REM sleep, Loomis, Harvey, and Hobart, (1937, 1938) recorded EEG activity in sleeping subjects and described five sequential brain potential patterns, which they referred to as "stages or states of sleep" (Loomis, Harvey, & Hobart, 1938, p. 421). These patterns, designated A, B, C, D, and E, generally similar across subjects and occurring reliably across recording sessions in the same subjects, were characterized as follows: A: intermittent alpha activity; B: low voltage potentials (theta); C: the occurrence of 14 Hz spindles; D: spindles in conjunction with 1 Hz delta waves; and E: increased delta activity with less conspicuous spindling (Loomis, Harvey, & Hobart, 1938). It was noted that "during the night of sleep a sleeper continually shifts back and forth from one state to another, either spontaneously or as the result of stimuli." (p. 422). These investigators did not comment on the remarkable implication of their findings that sleep was not the unitary phenomenon it had been traditionally considered to be. Two decades passed before a more comprehensive differentiation of EEG patterns during sleep appeared – using numbers rather than letters to designate stage and including the newly discovered state of REM sleep (Dement & Kleitman, 1957a). It was also at this time that a second fundamental characteristic of sleep was recognized, namely, that sleep stage pattern variations across the night were largely predictable from night-to-night, indicating the existence of the sleep cycle (Dement & Kleitman, 1957a; Figure 27.3).

The discovery of REM sleep and the sleep cycle had far-reaching implications for both biological and psychological processes during sleep. Physiologically, in contrast to previous thinking that sleep occurred passively in response

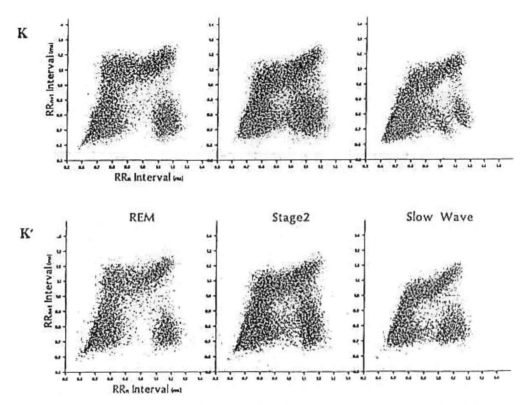

Figure 27.6. Sleep-stage Poincaré plots illustrating night-to-night similarities for subject K (upper and lower plots derived, respectively, from whole-night plots). (Reprinted with permission from Pivik et al 1996, p. 126, © American Sleep Disorders Association and Sleep Research Society.)

to the absence of wakefulness, these findings indicated that sleep was governed by active mechanisms. Furthermore, since the extended time intervals involved in stage and cycle variations could not be explained by short-term neurophysiologic processes, it was necessary to invoke neurochemical mechanisms with longer time constants. In terms of concepts of sleep cognition, these discoveries had equally dramatic effects. Now that dreaming could be associated with a physiological state recurring predictably across each night and which, in the adult, normally accounted for one quarter of each night of sleep, beliefs that dreams occurred only sporadically and under special conditions had to be rejected.

Although the scoring criteria in the Dement & Kleitman (1957a) publication provided descriptions of EEG frequency, amplitude, and waveform characteristics associated with sleep stages, a study by Monroe (1969) revealed an unacceptable level of scoring differences across laboratories. Monroe's findings were instrumental in the development of guidelines for scoring human sleep (Rechtschaffen & Kales, 1968), which presented more precise definitions of sleep states and stages, and provided the standardized criteria since used for the recording and reliable analysis of adult human sleep. Figures 27.1 and 27.2 provide examples of physiological variations characteristic of sleep-wakefulness and within-sleep stage differentiations described in that manual. These figures illustrate basic measures required for sleep evaluation (EEG, EOG, and

EMG; channels A, B, C, and H), but also include optional measures, such as recordings of vertical eye movements (channel D) and autonomic activity (channels E, F, and G). In these tracings, wakefulness (AW and W) is associated with a low-voltage, mixed frequency EEG, which may contain varying amounts of alpha (8–12 Hz) activity. Wakefulness is also usually associated with blinking, rapid eye movements, and variations in the levels of tonic facial EMG activity.

As accurately described 30 years previously (Davis et al., 1938), alpha activity is attenuated in the transition from wakefulness to sleep. Concurrently, there is a slowing of EEG activity with an increase in 4–7 Hz theta activity coupled with the sporadic occurrence of vertex sharp waves (see Figure 27.1, S1). The transition from wakefulness to Stage 1 is also accompanied by slow horizontal eye movements (see Porte, 2004 for a systematic evaluation of this activity), and facial muscle tonus is usually decreased relative to that of relaxed wakefulness (Figure 27.1). Stage 2 is characterized by the intermittent occurrence of K-complexes and 12–14 Hz spindle activity against relatively low amplitude, mixed frequency background (Figure 27.2). Stages 3 and 4, which together constitute "slow-wave sleep," differ from Stage 2 and from each other in the amount of delta activity (.5–4 Hz) present in each scoring epoch. Stage 3 epochs must contain 20–50%, and Stage 4 epochs more than 50%, of this activity (Figure 27.2). Defining characteristics of REM sleep include a relatively

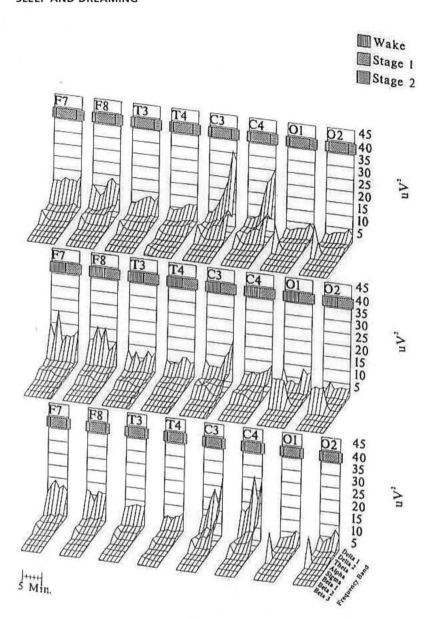

Figure 27.7. Variations in sleep onset EEG and as reflected in computerized analysis of activity from eight homologous scalp placements (frontal: F; temporal: T; central: C; and occipital: O) across three nights in the same subject. The graphs display these data in absolute (μV^2) values following FFT and power spectral analysis. These figures show within-subject differences as a function of recording site and night. (Reprinted with permission from Pivik, 1991 © John Wiley & Sons, Ltd.)

low-voltage, mixed-frequency EEG without K-complexes or spindles, sporadic eye movements, and reduced levels of submental and facial EMG activity (Figure 27.2). Although not required for REM sleep determination, other distinctive EEG features that may be present include bursts of theta activity (sawtooth waves) preceding clusters of eye movements (Berger, Olley, & Oswald, 1962), and alpha activity which is 1–2 Hz slower than subjects' waking alpha frequency (Johnson et al., 1967).

The above criteria underscore the emphasis on EEG activity for discriminating state and stages – an emphasis, which for NREM sleep, is absolute, but for REM sleep includes a requirement of relatively reduced EMG activity. Paradoxically, REM sleep can occur in the relative (i.e., epochs within REM periods without eye movement) or absolute (as in the congenitally blind; Berger et al., 1962) absence of the very parameter for which the state was initially named (i.e., rapid eye movements).

The following statements place the Rechtschaffen and Kales scoring criteria in broader physiological context. Note the fundamental ways in which these criteria describe sleep-wakefulness differences:

1. The presence of waveforms unique to sleep – for example, endogenously determined K-complexes, 12–14 Hz spindle activity, vertex sharp waves, and frontal sawtooth waves.

2. The prevalence and concentration of activities – for example, the enhancement of slower EEG frequencies (delta and theta), and the concentration of these and other activities, such as eye movements or galvanic skin responses (GSRs), at specific times of the night. With respect to EEG activity, computerized analyses have shown that in only rare instances is the EEG composed of a single frequency. Even in the desynchronized low-voltage EEG of wakefulness in normal individuals there

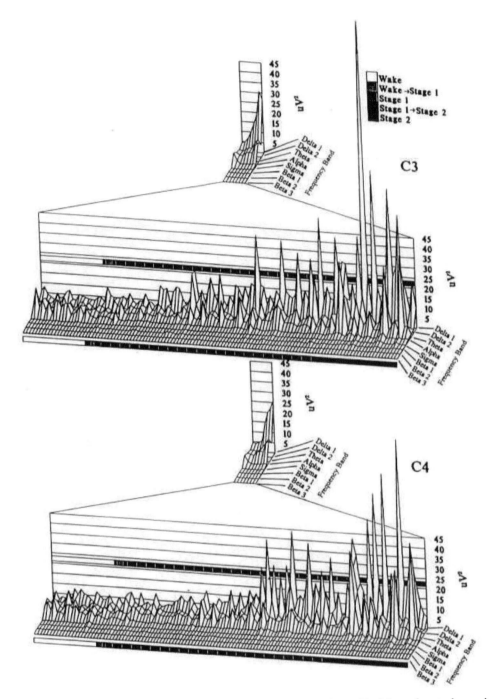

Figure 27.8. These illustrations expand the eight minute time base charted for bilateral central recordings depicted in the upper and middle panels in Figure 27.7 and present absolute power data in four-second bins. Using modified Rechtschaffen and Kales (1968) criteria, each four-second bin was classified into state categories as indicated in the legend. These figures demonstrate the complexities in EEG variations across hemispheres and nights in a single subject during the transition from wakefulness to sleep. (Reprinted with permission from Pivik, 1991, © John Wiley & Sons, Ltd.)

is a small but nonetheless real component of delta activity present (Lubin, Johnson, & Austin, 1969; Hoffman et al., 1979). The shift away from the higher frequencies associated with arousal during wakefulness and the concentration on slower activities are what make sleep unique.

3. The predictable constellations of physiological patterns that occur – for example, concentrations of delta

activity are associated with high GSR activation during slow-wave sleep, and indices of cortical, ocular-motor, and autonomic arousal are associated with sustained muscular inhibition during REM sleep (Pivik, 1986, p. 384).

Sleep profiles (Figure 27.3) are useful for representing general sleep characteristics, such as latencies, cyclicity, stage distribution, and relative amounts of sleep disturbance. However, these graphs do not communicate more rapid physiological variations that occur as sleep patterns play out across the night and which are often most frequent during shifts between states and stages. These transitional periods reflect shifting physiological priorities for which the determinants are not well understood. Among these state transitions one has been the focus of great interest: the sleep onset period. Although most investigators identify sleep onset with the presence of Stage 1 EEG patterns, because of inconsistencies in the covariation of psychological and behavioral measures with EEG criteria for sleep, others have argued for considering initial Stage 2 as sleep onset (Agnew & Webb, 1972; Johnson, 1973; Ogilvie, Wilkinson, & Allison, 1989). It is clear that the EEG changes that take place at sleep onset (Figures 27.1, 27.7, and 27.8) do not occur in physiological isolation. For example, several measures, including oculomotor activity (slow horizontal eye movements: Foulkes & Vogel, 1965; Rechtschaffen & Kales, 1968), variations in skin potential (Hori, 1982), decreased ventilation (Naifeh & Kamiya, 1981; Tinder et al., 1992), and decreased heart rate (Pivik & Busby, 1996; Zemaityte, Varonockas, & Sokolov, 1984), may accompany or even anticipate Stage 1 EEG changes by several seconds. Furthermore, distinctive variations in cerebral blood flow differentiate relaxed wakefulness and Stage 1 sleep (Kjaer et al., 2002). Such systematic and coordinated changes across systems are consistent with concepts of physiological state. However, the relationship between these physiological changes and the point of perceptual disengagement from the waking environment is imperfect, as indicated both by studies of sleep onset mentation (Foulkes & Vogel, 1965; Rowley, Stickgold, & Hobson, 1998; Vogel, Foulkes, & Trosman, 1966) and the ability to elicit behavioral responses to external stimulation in some individuals in Stage 1 and, to a lesser extent, in the initial moments of Stage 2 (Ogilvie & Wilkinson, 1984; Ogilvie, Wilkinson, & Allison, 1989). Another indication that transitions between states or stages are commonly not achieved abruptly is reflected in the practice of many investigators to require several consecutive epochs of Stage 1 or Stage 2 for sleep onset determination (Born, Muth, & Fehm, 1988; Mercier, Pivik, & Busby, 1993; Reynolds et al., 1983).

Associated with global patterns of state change across the night are predictable variations in the presence and distribution of physiological activity within sleep stages. For example, Stage 4 occurs predominantly in the first third of the night, and REM sleep in the last third (Williams, Agnew, & Webb, 1964, 1966; Figure 27.3). These observations are reflected in the exponential decrease in delta activity across the night as determined from more recent computerized analyses of EEG sleep data (Feinberg, Fein, & Floyd, 1980). Other notable stage-related physiological variations include: increases in body movements and K-complexes just prior to REM periods (Dement & Kleitman, 1957a; Halasz et al., 1977; Pivik & Dement, 1968);

reduced incidence of K-complexes and increased spindle activity in the few minutes subsequent to REM periods (Azumi, Shirakawa, & Takabashi, 1975; Pivik & Dement, 1968); the relative difficulty in engaging REM mechanisms early in the night, as indicated by the brevity or even omission of a REM period within the first two hours of sleep (Berger & Oswald, 1962a; Dement & Kleitman, 1957a; Roffwarg, Muzio, & Dement, 1966); and increased density of eye movements as a function both of time within individual REM periods and within REM periods across the night (Aserinsky, 1969, 1971).

It might be expected that state and stage distinctions made in the 1950s would undergo significant modification when subjected to the scrutiny of intense investigation over several decades. However, those definitions have been preserved and the ensuing research has detailed characteristics of physiological measures which, although not integral to stage determination, have nevertheless served to reinforce and extend our understanding of state physiology. Prominent among these is the presence of generalized physiological activation during REM sleep, including increases in the rate and irregularity in respiratory (Aserinsky, 1965; Snyder et al., 1964) and cardiovascular (Pivik et al., 1996; Snyder, Hobson, & Goldfrank, 1963; Snyder et al., 1964) activities. Electrodermal activity in REM sleep is limited in incidence and more similar in form to responses of this system during wakefulness (Broughton, Poire, & Tassinari, 1965; Hauri & Van de Castle, 1973b). These variations occur against a background of centrally mediated inhibition of facial and submental musculature and spinal monosynaptic reflexes (Berger, 1961; Hodes & Dement, 1964; Jacobson et al., 1964; Jouvet & Michel, 1959; Pompeiano, 1966).

Relative to REM sleep, physiological activation in the majority of NREM sleep is unremarkable. Exceptions to this generalization are the unusual levels of autonomic, hormonal, and motor activation present during slow wave sleep, particularly during Stage 4. During Stage 4, there is commonly a dramatic increase in electrodermal activity (Broughton, Poire, & Tassinari, 1965; Johnson & Lubin, 1966; Figure 27.2,) which, in its extreme, has been referred to as "GSR storms" (Burch, 1965). Normally, electrodermal activation of this intensity would suggest an enhanced level of arousal, yet arousal threshold during Stage 4 is the highest of all sleep stages (Bonnet & Moore, 1982; Busby, Mercier, & Pivik, 1994; Goodenough et al., 1965; Lammers & Badia, 1991). Consequently, the excessive electrodermal activity during Stage 4 has been considered to result from the release of subcortical brain areas involved in the production of these responses from inhibition by higher centers rather than indexing enhanced physiological arousal (Johnson, 1973; Johnson & Lubin, 1966; see Chapter 7 of this volume). Slow-wave sleep is also the time when approximately 80% of the total daily secretion of growth hormone is released (Born, Muth, & Fehm, 1988; Sassin et al., 1969) and during which a variety of arousal disorders termed "parasomnias" occur (Roffwarg, 1979).

The latter disorders are characterized by varying degrees of motor and autonomic activity, and include such behaviors as sleep-walking, sleep-talking, enuresis, night terrors, and confusional arousals. For the interested reader more detailed considerations of the nosology, description, and treatment of these and other sleep-related disorders are available (ICSD, 1990; Kryger et al., 1994, 2000).

The initial wave of psychophysiological studies of sleep following the discovery of REM sleep was driven by the emphatic physiological distinctions between REM and NREM sleep and were essentially studies of state relationships. They were significantly influenced by the belief that REM sleep provided an objective measure of dreaming, and that dreaming occurred only during these periods. For the most part, these studies reported a high incidence of recall following arousals from REM sleep (approximately 80%) – although subsequent investigations also detected subjects who typically fail to recall dreams (Goodenough, 1978; Goodenough et al., 1959) – and a relative mental void in NREM sleep (less than 10% recall). However, reports suggesting that mental activity was present during NREM sleep (Goodenough et al., 1959) continued to accumulate, and by 1967 Foulkes reviewed data from nine studies reporting NREM recall values ranging from 23–74%. To some extent, the apparent discrepancy between the early and later studies regarding the presence of NREM mentation can be attributed to differences in what investigators were willing to accept as a dream. The early studies relied on an intuitive and implicit understanding of the nature of the dream and consequently did not provide an operational definition of this variable. The first study to provide some clarification in this regard was published in 1957, and entitled "The Relation of Eye Movements During Sleep to Dream Activity: An Objective Method for the Study of Dreaming" (Dement & Kleitman, 1957b). In this study, upon awakening subjects were queried as to "whether or not they had been dreaming," and only those reports which related a "coherent, fairly detailed description" (p. 341) of the sleep mental experience qualified as dreams. Reports of having dreamt "without recall of content, or vague fragmentary impressions of content" (p. 341) were considered negative and disregarded. Based on these criteria, the commonly reported REM-NREM recall differentiation (80% recall in REM and 7% from NREM) was observed. These early studies, restrictive as they were with respect to dream definition, nevertheless provided an important insight into the nature of the dreaming process, namely, that in most individuals this process occurred with its greatest intensity during REM sleep.

It became obvious that a systematic and effective evaluation of mental activity during sleep would require a more detailed operational definition of what would be accepted as a dream, and a variety of such definitions has been advanced. For example, the dream has been variously characterized as a "verbal report describing an occurrence involving multisensory images and sensations, frequently of a bizarre and unreal nature and involving the narrator himself" (Berger, 1967, p. 16); "the presence of any sensory imagery with development and progression of mental activity" (Kales et al., 1967, p. 556); "any occurrences with visual, auditory, or kinesthetic imagery (Foulkes, 1962, p. 17); a "multidimensional conglomerate of a hallucinatory belief in the actual occurrence of an imagined experience which, in turn, tends to be an extended visual, sometimes bizarre, drama" (Antrobus et al., 1978, p. 40); or simply "thinking" (Foulkes, 1978, p. 3).

The range of definitions represented by these examples places various constraints on which reports would be accepted into the "dreaming" dataset, consequently tailoring the perception of the general nature of cognitive activity during sleep and more profoundly affecting the incidence of acceptable reports of dreaming occurring outside the confines of REM sleep. However, when reports elicited from arousals during sleep were examined using more permissive criteria that allow more fragmentary and less perceptual reports to be accepted as data, the presence of a much more extensive mental life during sleep was revealed. Lifting these definitional restrictions primarily affected the amounts of recall from NREM sleep arousals, with observations of more than 50% recall not being uncommon (Foulkes, 1962; Goodenough et al., 1959; Herman, Ellman, & Roffwarg, 1978; Molinari & Foulkes, 1969; Pivik & Foulkes, 1968; Zimmerman, 1970). As suggested by the substantial increase in amounts of NREM recall, which become apparent when a more relaxed definition of sleep mentation is allowed, there are qualitative distinctions that differentiate REM and NREM reports. The major differences that have been repeatedly observed (Antrobus, 1983; Foulkes & Rechtschaffen, 1964; Pivik, 1971; Rechtschaffen, Verdone, & Wheaton, 1963) have been summarized as follows:

> reports obtained in periods of REM activity showed more organismic involvement in affective, visual and muscular dimensions and were more highly elaborated than non-REMP reports. REMP reports showed less correspondence to the waking life of the subjects than did reports from spindle and delta sleep. The relatively frequent occurrence of thinking and memory processes in spindle and delta sleep was an especially striking result. (Foulkes, 1962, pp. 24–25)

REM-NREM distinctions in amounts of recall and associated qualitative characteristics of reports seemed to imply a fundamental difference in cognitive activity during these states, with more complex, vivid and bizarre "dreaming" during REM sleep and less developed, more mundane "thinking" during NREM sleep. However, NREM reports of dreaming have been observed to be as common (Goodenough et al., 1965) or more common (Bosinelli et al., 1968; Foulkes, 1960, 1962; Pivik, 1971; Pivik & Foulkes, 1968; Rechtschaffen, Vogel, & Shaikun, 1963) than NREM thinking reports. Still, when reports from the two kinds of sleep are contrasted directly using a method of paired comparison, judges are generally able to reliably discriminate REM from NREM reports (Bosinelli et al., 1968; Monroe et al., 1965). An exception to this discriminability is the NREM mentation elicited following arousals during sleep onset. Reports of mental activity at this time share many features with REM sleep reports that make it difficult to discriminate between them, including incidence, hallucinatory dramatic quality, and report length (Foulkes, Spear, & Symonds, 1966; Foulkes & Vogel, 1965; Vogel, 1978; Vogel, Foulkes, & Trosman, 1966), as well as perceptual and emotional qualities (Vogel, Barrocough, & Giesler, 1972). Recognition that dream-like mentation occurred outside REM sleep implied that REM sleep deprivation could not be equated with dream deprivation (Dement, 1960) and called into question claims that REM sleep dreams were vital to psychological normality during wakefulness (Sampson, 1965, 1966; Vogel et al., 1975).

The characteristics of NREM mentation outlined in cognitive sleep studies conducted during the initial 15 years following the discovery of REM sleep have been confirmed by subsequent research. Yet, despite the weight and persistence of such evidence, there was substantial reluctance to acknowledge the validity of mental activity during sleep occurring outside REM sleep. Although it was necessary to consider other plausible explanations for reports of NREM mentation – such as viewing them as artifacts of arousal generated in the process of waking up, confabulating in an effort to please the investigators, or reflecting recall of mental activity from previous REM periods – even when such possibilities had been effectively countered (Foulkes, 1967) skepticism remained. Foulkes (1967) offered several probable reasons for this persisting unwillingness to accept the authenticity of NREM mentation despite convincing arguments to the contrary:

a) while the low-voltage random EEG of REM sleep is compatible with the existence of ongoing thought processes, the high-voltage, low-frequency EEG of NREM is not;

b) a report of a mental experience is not credible unless supported by public behavioral or physiological observation; and,

c) REM sleep is so vastly different physiologically from NREM sleep that there must also be a vast psychological difference between the two, such as vivid dreaming versus. little or no mental activity (p. 31).

These statements are consistent with the emphasis on physiological correlates as validating indices of psychological experience. Although providing useful guidelines, the dependence on such physiological correlates can, in the extreme, demand an unsupportable degree of mind-body isomorphism. The points outlined by Foulkes serve to illustrate the extent to which prevailing theoretical thinking can promote expectations that interfere with scientific objectivity. The concept of NREM mentation was no more iconoclastic than that of recurrent phases of physiological activation occurring during sleep, yet the latter reports were not met with the same degree of skepticism as

reports of NREM mentation. Even though the association between REM sleep and dreaming dramatically altered existing views regarding the nature of dreaming, dreaming was already accepted as a sleep-related cognitive event. Furthermore, because visual experiences are perhaps the most common and compelling components of dreams, the finding that the experience of dreaming appeared to be associated with these periods of rapid eye movements during sleep simply confirmed prior expectations. Aserinsky (1996) explicitly refers to this situation when he notes that "the prospect that these eye movements may be associated with dreaming did not arise as a lightening stroke of insight" (p. 217) because the notion of "an association of the eyes with dreaming is deeply engrained in the unscientific literature and can be categorized as common knowledge" (p. 218). Although not extensive, there was evidence of the kind of linkage between NREM reports and pre-awakening events, which provided precisely the kind of "public evidence" demanded to validate NREM mentation, for example, spontaneously occurring activity, such as sleep talking (Arkin et al., 1970; Rechtschaffen, Goodenough, & Shapiro, 1962) or experimentally induced incorporations (Foulkes, 1967; Foulkes & Rechtschaffen, 1964; Rechtschaffen, Verdone, & Wheaton, 1963).

It is likely that a detailed search for observable physiological events that correlate with, validate, and perhaps explain psychological activity during sleep would have occurred regardless of the REM-NREM mentation controversy. However, if the presence of cognitive activity during NREM sleep had been dismissed these studies would have focused exclusively on REM sleep, and our appreciation of the physiological conditions and requirements underlying cognitive activity would have been significantly diminished. In this search for psychophysiological measures which might best predict the presence of mental activity during sleep, it is not surprising that EEG activity, despite limitations in understanding the precise nature and origin of such activity (Niedermeyer & Lopes da Silva, 1993), would be a primary focus.

The similarity between EEG activity during waking and REM sleep has been previously noted, and Dement and Kleitman (1957a) suggested that generally this pattern was a better correlate of dreaming than eye movements. Subsequent research has supported this impression, and indicates that as EEG activity becomes more desynchronized there is greater recall and the reports obtained contain more vivid and bizarre dream-like material. Accordingly, arousals from sleep with low-voltage, mixed-frequency EEG patterns (Stage 1 and REM) produced the highest incidence of recall and recall of the most vivid, bizarre, and emotional nature (Dement, 1955; Dement & Kleitman, 1957b; Foulkes & Vogel, 1965; Vogel, Foulkes, & Trosman, 1966) relative to that obtained from arousals where the sleep EEG is characterized by slower and higher amplitude patterns (Armitage, 1980; Pivik, 1971; Pivik & Foulkes, 1968). The positive relationship between levels of EEG activation and the quantity and quality of recall is consistent with findings of increased recall of more dream-like material across the night (Foulkes, 1960; Goodenough et al., 1959; Pivik & Foulkes, 1968; Verdone, 1963, 1965) because there is marked reduction in slower EEG activity and a greater presence of faster frequencies in the second half of the night. As indicated in Figure 27.3, these variations reflect a concentration of slow wave sleep early in the night and more Stage 2 and REM sleep later. This confounding of sleep stage and time of night frustrates attempts to determine independent relationships between these variables and aspects of sleep cognition. One approach to circumventing this confound has been to focus on Stage 2, which, although more prevalent later in the night, nevertheless normally occurs throughout the night. When Stage 2 mentation is sampled across the night, increases in both recall and dream-like quality in reports elicited later in the night have been observed (Arkin et al., 1978; Pivik & Foulkes, 1968). Although these findings suggest a time of night rather than background EEG influence on sleep mentation, computer analyses of all-night sleep EEG recordings have shown a covariation between EEG activity and time of night – for example, linear decreases across the night in alpha (Harman & Pivik, 1996) and delta (Feinberg, Fein, & Floyd, 1980) bands – which indicates that Stage 2 early in the night contains greater amounts of slow EEG activity relative to that occurring later in the night. These observations underscore the importance of supplementing, where possible, standard analyses with procedures that may provide additional information. In this case, computer analysis more precisely quantifies not only the above-threshold delta activity (scoring criteria for Stage 2 allow up to 20% per epoch of $\geq 75\ \mu V$ delta activity), but includes activity occurring below the criterion level and thereby provides a more faithful representation of the amount of this activity within each epoch (Armitage, 1995b).

Recently, attention has been drawn to the occurrence of synchronized fast EEG rhythms (20–40 Hz) during both wakefulness and sleep in animals and humans (Cantero et al., 2004; Franken et al., 1994; Llinás & Ribary, 1993; Steriade, Amzica, & Confreres, 1996). These rhythms are most prevalent during wakefulness and REM sleep, but have been detected as well during NREM sleep. The involvement of this activity in state- and event-related aspects of consciousness and cognition is still being defined (Behrendt, 2003; Hobson et al., 1998; Kahn, Pace-Schott, & Hobson, 1997).

The global time-of-night, EEG-sleep mentation relationships noted above indicate variations in mental activity over relatively long periods of time, but short-term temporal relationships between recall and physiological events have also been reported. For example, recall of REM sleep mentation is reduced if awakenings are made soon after a gross body movement (Dement & Wolpert, 1958b; Wolpert & Trosman, 1958). Duration of time in a sleep stage prior

to arousal may also influence the amount and quality of recalled material. Arousals made early in REM periods produce fewer reports and reports of less dream-like quality relative to those obtained from arousals later in REM (Foulkes, 1962; Kramer, Roth, & Czaya, 1975; Whitman, 1969), and although arousals from Stage 4 generally produce less recall and recall that is less dream-like than that from other sleep stages, such differences between Stage 4 and Stage 2 are minimized when the amount of within-stage time prior to awakening is controlled (Tracy & Tracy, 1974). Furthermore, recall rates between REM and slow wave sleep (SWS) are not as widely discrepant when temporal factors (time of night and time into stage) are regulated (REM: 89%; SWS: 65%; Cavallero et al., 1992).

The general differences in incidence and qualitative aspects of REM and NREM mentation favor the more "awake-like" Stage 1 pattern as a reasonable predictor of dream-like cognitive activity, but the fact that NREM sleep stages with quite different EEG patterns also support an extensive amount of cognitive activity – often dream-like – forces the conclusion that these tonic background patterns are at best only global correlates of mental activity during sleep. This conclusion is further underscored by observations of within-state variations and between-state similarities in the frequency and characteristics of recalled material. Clearly, the psychophysiological relationship between sleep cognition and EEG activity is imperfect.

The characterization by early sleep cognition studies of REM sleep mentation as visual, bizarre experiences and NREM mentation as more thought-like and mundane seemed to fit well with an extensive and developing literature in waking subjects indicating cortical hemispheric specialization for different features of cognitive activity. Neurophysiological and psychophysiological studies in waking subjects assigned linguistic and analytical processes to the left hemisphere, and visuospatial and holistic processes to the right hemisphere (Geschwind & Galaburda, 1987). Accordingly, global REM-NREM variations suggested differential cerebral hemispheric involvement, with the visuomotor loading of REM sleep dreams suggesting greater right hemisphere involvement during REM sleep (Broughton, 1975; Goldstein, Stolzfus, & Gardocki, 1972).

At a strictly electrophysiological level using the amount of alpha activity as a primary index of differential hemispheric EEG activation (because alpha increases have been related to decreases in attention or effort), findings with respect to REM-NREM hemispheric activation have been inconsistent in supporting the right hemispheric nature of REM sleep (Armitage, Hoffman, & Moffitt, 1992; Bertini & Violani, 1992; Doricchi & Violani, 1992). The few studies documenting the extent of EEG lateralization in conjunction with concomitant sleep mentation have, with few exceptions (e.g., Angeleri, Scarpino, & Signorino, 1984), not supported the REM right-hemisphere, NREM left-hemisphere dichotomy (Armitage, Hoffman, & Moffitt,

1992; Cohen, 1977; Guevara et al., 1995; Moffitt et al., 1982; Pivik et al., 1982). It should be emphasized, however, that interpretation of interhemispheric EEG sleep data is complicated by variations in subject characteristics, scalp recording sites, EEG frequency bands considered, and the analytical procedures used (Armitage, Hoffman, & Moffitt, 1992; Pivik et al., 1982; see Chapter 3 of this volume), as well as by the fact that the sleep EEG sleep may vary dynamically with specific features of ongoing mentation (Bertini & Violani, 1992; Doricchi & Violani, 1992).

In addition to EEG variables, efforts to determine physiological correlates of mental activity during sleep have also examined autonomic and motor variables. Among autonomic measures investigated in this respect are heart and respiratory rates, electrodermal activity, and penile erections. In general, robust relationships between tonic levels of autonomic activity and either the incidence or qualitative aspects of recalled mentation have not been observed. Furthermore, when positive correlations have been observed, they have often been in association with transient changes in these measures (for reviews see Rechtschaffen, 1973; Pivik, 1991).

Perhaps most remarkable are the apparent dissociations between certain autonomic measures and cognitive activity during sleep. Prominent in this regard is the "storm-like" occurrence of electrodermal activity during Stages 3 and 4 (Burch, 1965). It would be expected that these high rates of electrodermal activity would impact on associated mental activity, either in terms of enhanced recall or qualitative aspects of recalled mentation, but such relationships have not been observed (Hauri & Rechtschaffen, 1963; Pivik, 1971, Tracy & Tracy, 1974). Similarly, the increased blood flow to the genitalia during REM sleep resulting in penile erections (Fisher, Gross, & Zuch, 1965; Karacan et al., 1966) or clitoral engorgement (Cohen & Shapiro, 1970) would suggest that the great majority of REM reports would contain overt sexual content. However, with the exception of lucid dreaming (LaBerge, 1985; LaBerge, Greenleaf, & Kedzierski, 1983), REM reports with manifest sexual features are relatively uncommon (Fisher, 1966; Hall & Van de Castle, 1966). Interestingly, lucid dreams containing sexual activity are associated with expected variations in some (e.g., respiration and skin conductance), but not all (e.g., heart rate) autonomic measures (LaBerge 1985, 1992).

To the casual observer, with the exception of occasional twitches and body movements, sleep would appear to be a state of general motor quiescence – an impression physiologically documented for trunk and limb musculature (Jacobson et al., 1964). Not apparent to the observer would be the previously noted tonic inhibition of face and neck muscles that accompany, and may slightly anticipate the onset of, REM sleep (Berger, 1961; Jacobson et at., 1964). Because tonically reduced EMG activity is a defining characteristic of REM sleep, it is not possible to determine the relationship between this variable and ongoing mentation

independent of that in other systems also tonically active at this time, for example, EEG. However, because of the variability in the timing of EMG inhibition and EEG desynchronization signaling REM sleep onset, it has been possible to systematically examine characteristics of NREM sleep mentation (generally Stage 2) immediately preceding REM sleep as a function of the presence or absence of tonic EMG inhibition. It was expected that the preREM decrease in facial and submental muscle activity might signal a shift to more REM-like mental activity, but instead these lowEMG, preREM periods yielded fewer reports and reports which were less dream-like than those from awakenings with high EMG levels (Larson & Foulkes, 1969; Pivik, 1971).

TONIC-PHASIC DISTINCTIONS

As indicated by the above review and commented upon by others (Antrobus & Bertini, 1992), the relationship between tonic physiological activation and cognitive activity is complex, with the strongest psychophysiological association to emerge being that between the presence of a Stage 1 EEG pattern and recall of dream-like mentation. Although the psychophysiological sleep studies conducted during the decade and a half following the discovery of REM sleep emphasized general state relationships, it had been apparent that, though sleep stages were defined primarily in terms of tonic physiological criteria, these stages were nevertheless characterized by transient variations in these measures. In fact, a closer psychophysiological correspondence was generally obtained when reports were elicited following such abrupt variations. This improved relationship was reflected both in increased recall and qualitative variations in recalled material and was observed across EEG, autonomic, and motor systems (Pivik, 1986, 1991). Among such phasically occurring activity, the relationship of one type of discrete motor activity (namely, eye movements) to REM sleep mentation has been most intensively investigated. These studies have evaluated this relationship in terms of both general associations as well as trying to determine if a strict relationship existed between eye movements and dream images. In terms of the more nonspecific approach, although increased eye movement activity is commonly associated with enhanced recall, the magnitude of this relationship is not particularly remarkable (Pivik, 1991). Similarly, reports obtained in association with increased eye movement are often, but not consistently, more vivid and emotional (Ellman et al., 1974; Hobson, Goldfrank, & Snyder, 1965). Interestingly, increased eye movement density may not always be a good predictor of the amount of activity reported in the dream (Berger & Oswald, 1962a; Firth & Oswald 1975; Hauri & Van de Castle, 1973a; Pivik & Foulkes, 1968).

The discovery of the association between REM sleep and dreaming not only confirmed the expectation that visual

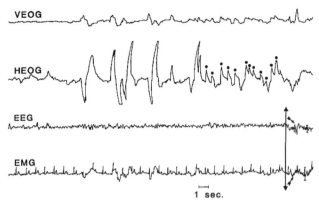

VEOG

HEOG

EEG

EMG

1 sec.

Figure 27.9. An example of the correspondence between eye movements and dream content. Immediately following a series of horizontal nystagmoid eye movements (designated by dots) during REM sleep, the subject was awakened (vertical line, lower channels) and related a dream experience (viewing parallel parking lines while riding by in a car) that provided the precise perceptual conditions required to elicit optokinetic nystagmus. In this example, the EMG recordings contain EKG artifact made more prominent by the tonic EMG inhibition during REM sleep. However, this artifact does not interfere with the general purpose of EMG recordings during sleep (i.e., stage differentiation). (Reprinted with permission from Pivik, 1986, © The Guilford Press.)

dreams would be accompanied by eye movements, but suggested the corollary hypothesis that these eye movements were not random but were functioning as they would during wakefulness to view the perceived images – in this case dream images. This precise relationship between the eye movements and dream imagery of REM sleep has come to be known as the scanning hypothesis (Roffwarg et al., 1962). Although intuitively appealing and appearing to provide an ideal opportunity for demonstrating the extent to which psychophysiological isomorphism can occur during sleep, attempts to substantiate this relationship have met with mixed success. Examples of highly specific correspondence have been noted (Figure 27.9), but demonstrating this relationship as a general feature of REM sleep has been largely unsuccessful (reviewed in Pivik, 1991; Rechtschaffen, 1973). However, interpretation of these generally negative results needs to be tempered with an appreciation of the experimental demands inherent in these studies. These include having investigators highly skilled in interviewing procedures and techniques with a detailed understanding of head-eye movement relationships and highly motivated subjects who can awaken quickly and provide high quality detailed recall of dream imagery and associated gaze shifts. Insight into the difficulty in determining whether, or the extent to which, eye movements during REM sleep are scanning dream images was provided by an investigation conducted during wakefulness (Bussel, Dement, & Pivik, 1972) in which eye movements were recorded and subjects were periodically interviewed and requested to detail their eye movements in the few seconds prior to the interview. These reports were then

correlated with the associated eye movement recordings. It was observed that subjects' reports during wakefulness could not be related to polygraphically recorded eye movement activity with any greater reliability than has been possible in the REM dream-eye movement studies. More positive eye movement-dream imagery associations have been reported in lucid dreams (LaBerge, 1992), and indirect support for these associations is suggested by studies using imaging technology indicating involvement of the same cortical areas in the control of both waking and REM sleep eye movements (Hong et al., 1995), as well as studies using more nonspecific, correlational techniques associating numbers of eye movements with the amount of visual imagery in dream reports (Hong et al., 1997).

Interest in the association between more discrete variations in physiological activity during sleep and concurrent mentation became part of a more general shift in focus from state to event relationships that impacted significantly on both physiological and psychophysiological sleep studies. The critical differentiation which was made focused on the duration and temporal clustering of events with sustained or tonic activities lasting several seconds or minutes (e.g., background and EEG and EMG stage correlates) being contrasted with sporadic or phasic activities lasting less than a second (e.g., muscle twitches, rapid eye movements, or K-complexes) or, at most, a few seconds (e.g., isolated transient autonomic variations). Initially based on such events during REM sleep in the cat (Moruzzi, 1963), this reconceptualization was soon extended to NREM sleep events as well (Grosser & Siegal, 1971). Notable influences of this tonic-phasic distinction on psychophysiological studies of sleep included: 1) providing a structured physiological framework within which to consider these studies, 2) the suggestion that REM-NREM physiological differences were quantitative and not absolute, and 3) providing what came to be considered a prototypic phasic event which served as a model in the search for the human analogue of such activity (namely, the PGO spike). This event is named for the brain regions from which it was most readily recorded – the pons, lateral geniculate bodies, and occipital cortex – and acquired psychophysiological prominence in part because of the anatomical and sleep stage distribution of this activity. Consistent with both the visual emphasis in dreams and the high incidence of dream reports from REM sleep, PGO spikes were most prominent in the visual system during REM sleep (Brooks, 1967, 1968; Jouvet, 1972). Furthermore, the occurrence of this activity during NREM sleep, most intensely just prior to REM onset and less frequently at other times in the NREM cycle, held out promise that this activity might provide a physiological correlate of NREM mentation.

This tonic-phasic distinction provided the theoretical orientation which dominated the field for many years and which continues to influence psychophysiological sleep studies (Antrobus & Bertini, 1992; Conduit, Crewther, &

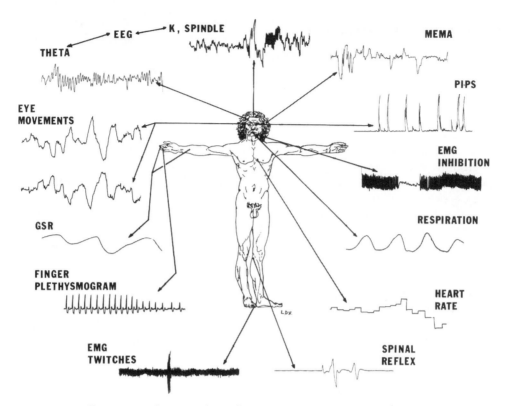

Figure 27.10. Illustrations of various phasically occurring electrophysiological measures that have been investigated in the context of psychophysiological studies of sleep. These variables, with approximate designations of anatomical areas from which they are recorded, include the following: EEG measures (K-complex, spindle, and theta activity); expressions of muscle activity from auditory middle ear muscle activity (MEMA)], visual [eye movements, periorbital integrated potentials (PIPS)], and skeletal musculature (facial EMG inhibition, spinal reflexes, and EMG twitches) systems; and autonomic activity [galvanic skin response (GSR), finger plethysmogram, respiration, and heart rate]. (Reprinted with permission from Pivik, 1986, © The Guilford Press.)

Coleman, 2004; Pivik, 1991; Rechtschaffen, 1973). This model prompted increasing numbers of studies comparing reports obtained from awakenings following episodes of tonic or phasic physiological activation during sleep, stimulated the search for physiological measures which might reflect activity of the phasic event system proposed by Moruzzi (1963; see Figure 27.10 for examples of events examined in these studies), and led to the formulation of new proposals regarding the relationship between phasic events and sleep mentation (Hobson, 1992; Hobson & McCarley, 1977). These investigations provided new insights into sleep physiology and psychophysiology, but failed to indicate either that phasic events were a prerequisite for the presence of cognitive activity during sleep or that these events could be reliably related to specific qualitative measures of sleep mentation, for example, the degree of cognitive processing of dream-experiences (Foulkes & Pope, 1973; Molinari & Foulkes, 1969) or the presence of discontinuity and bizarreness within reports (Antrobus, 2000; Foulkes & Pope, 1973; Ogilvie et al., 1982; Reinsel, Antrobus, & Wollman, 1985; Watson, 1972). Furthermore, there are unusual features differentiating sleep from waking cognitive activity, which have received little attention in

terms of either general or tonic-phasic physiological sleep correlates. Among these are what has been termed the "single-mindedness" and "nonreflectiveness" of dreams. Single-mindedness refers to "the strong tendency for a single train of related thoughts and images to persist over extended periods without disruption or competition from other simultaneous thoughts and images" (Rechtschaffen, 1978, p. 97). It has been suggested that this attribute is a reflection of a combination of increased sensory thresholds and cortical activation during sleep (Reinsel, Antrobus, & Wollman, 1992). Nonreflectiveness refers to the attenuation or arrest of judgmental processes during dreaming (Kleitman, 1967; Rechtschaffen, 1978), that is, the general acceptance of events or images during dreaming without the critical evaluation that normally takes place during waking. This characteristic may reflect the possibility that an inherent feature of dreaming is the absence of the need for "a constant regulating function of self-evaluation" (Meier, 1993, p. 64). The apparent limited use of evaluative information from waking cognitive experiences in this context implies either restricted access to such information during sleep or a discontinuity between selective waking and sleeping cognitive processes (Foulkes, 1993).

SLEEP COGNITION: RECONCEPTUALIZATIONS

For the first 25 years following the discovery of the REM sleep-dreaming relationship investigations into the psychology of sleep were largely physiologically driven. There were, nevertheless, concurrent lines of research which provided information regarding more general issues concerning both the circumstances under which dreaming occurs and the nature of dreams, observations from which is emerging a significantly modified view of dreaming. In the process of documenting the apparent pervasiveness of mental activity across sleep stages, investigators provided insights into what may generally be considered necessary and sufficient conditions for dreaming to occur. Studies of variations in mental activity during the transition from waking to sleep were particularly revealing in this regard. Early investigations identified four stages of EEG-EOG patterns occurring sequentially during this sleep onset period and studied the variations in mental activity associated with these stages (Foulkes & Vogel, 1965). These stages defined a progression of decreases in alpha, which could be accompanied by eye movements (rapid in the initial stage, and slow in later stages), and included initial epochs of Stages 1 and 2 EEG patterns. Mental activity – much of it dream-like – was reported on 90–98% of arousals from these stages. The similarities between these reports and those from REM sleep were later emphasized (Foulkes, Spear, & Symonds, 1966; Vogel, Barrowclough, & Giesler, 1972). Furthermore, the reports of mental activity changed in a systematic way as subjects progressed from the alpha REM stage to Stage 2. These variations began with subjects initially relinquishing control over the course of mental activity, then becoming unaware of the environment, and finally losing reality orientation and having hallucinatory experiences (Vogel, Foulkes, & Trosman, 1966). These results suggested reduced sensory input and subsequent abrogation of voluntary ideational control are essential for dream production. it is notable that when these conditions have been established in waking subjects, either in the context of classic sensory deprivation studies (e.g., Freedman, Grunebaum, & Greenblatt, 1971) or under more benign conditions (Foulkes & Fleischer, 1975; Foulkes & Scott, 1973; Reinsel, Antrobus, & Wollma, 1992; Singer, 1978), dream-like, bizarre, and hallucinatory experiences have occurred. These observations, coupled with accumulating evidence that REM and NREM reports were not so qualitatively dissimilar (Antrobus, 1983; Cavallero et al., 1992; Foulkes & Schmidt, 1983), have led to the proposition of a single dream system or process which functions across states at different levels of activation (Cavallero & Cicogna, 1993; Cicogna et al., 2000; Foulkes & Cavallero, 1993). This conceptualization identifies REM sleep as one condition among many which would be expected to accompany dreaming, and thereby minimizes the expectation that REM sleep physiology will provide an explanation for dreaming (Foulkes & Cavallero, 1993).

However, just as brain injury may impact on the characteristics of cognitive activity during both wakefulness and sleep (Kerr, 1993), so too must characteristics of sleep cognition be influenced by alterations of the functional architecture of the sleeping relative to the waking brain. Brain imaging studies in humans (Braun et al., 1997, 1998; Hong et al., 1995; Kjaer et al., 2002; Maquet, 2000; Maquet et al., 1996) are beginning to document similarities and differences in cortical and subcortical activation between the waking and sleeping brain that may offer new possibilities for understanding specific dream characteristics. For example, the reported deactivation during REM sleep of areas of the frontal cortex known to be involved in integration of sensory information during wakefulness (Braun et al., 1997; Maquet, 2000), may be consistent with the absence of reflectiveness which is characteristic of REM dream reports.

In addition to the findings indicating qualitative similarities between REM and NREM mentation, there have been additional reports contradicting the generally accepted view of dreams as characteristically bizarre, unusual, and dramatic experiences that differ significantly from waking thought (Dorus et al., 1971; Foulkes et al., 1967; Snyder, 1970). On the basis of these reports and others comparing, for example, the nature of dreams collected in home or laboratory environments, Foulkes (1996) concluded that "representatively sampled dream experiences, in both content and form, have a texture not so vastly different from, or unfamiliar to, waking experience." (p. 615). These observations effectively demystify the dreaming process but, while acknowledging variations that occur as a consequence of state differences, nevertheless suggest fundamental cross-state similarities between waking and sleeping cognitive systems. Although the determinants of waking-life representation in sleep mentation are still not well understood (Nielsen et al., 2004; Schredl & Hofmann, 2003), support for cross-state commonality of cognitive systems has been provided by studies indicating that individuals with waking cognitive or sensory defects (e.g., resulting from brain damage) show deficits consistent with these impairment in dream experiences (Doricchi & Violani, 1992; Kerr, 1993). Another source of support comes from developmental studies of dreaming. The latter are particularly relevant, not only because of their normative nature, but because features of the ontogeny of physiological aspects of sleep offer unusual opportunities to investigate the development of dreaming. Many of the physiological characteristics of sleep in the adult are not present in the newborn, but perhaps the most dramatic difference is the predominance of REM sleep at this time (40–70% of total sleep time) with an approximation of adult levels of REM sleep not occurring until after the first year (Louis et al., 1997; Pivik, 1983; Roffwarg, Muzio, & Dement 1966; but see Frank & Heller, 2003 for a modified view of sleep ontogeny). The presence of large amounts of this state at a time in development when neuronal processes underlying CNS maturation are highly active prompted

Roffwarg, Muzio, and Dement (1966) to suggest that REM-associated activity provided a source of endogenous stimulation important for aspects of normal CNS development. This hypothesis, which is consistent with the influence of activity dependent factors on neural development, has received support from animal studies demonstrating that interruption of REM sleep phasic influences early in the postnatal period, either by REM sleep deprivation or suppression of PGO spike activity, impairs the course of visual system development (Marks et al., 1995; Oksenberg et al., 1996). However, to expect that the REM sleep-dreaming association, which is so prominent in adults, would be present in early development when waking sensory and cognitive skills are only beginning to form requires ascribing extraordinary psychological functions to the REM state. At what point does the REM sleep-dreaming relationship become evident, and with what implications for the relationship between cognitive processes during wakefulness and sleep? Given the emphasis in early postREM discovery sleep research on sleep physiology and psychology in adults, it is not surprising that answers to these questions were not immediately forthcoming. When the results of studies of dreaming in early childhood were presented (Foulkes, 1982; Foulkes et al., 1990, 1991) they revealed that reports of REM dreams with formal properties of adult dreams only became evident by the age of eight or nine, and that the processes required for imagery during waking and sleep develop in parallel. It was concluded that dreaming "is a symbolic process with strong cognitive prerequisites and with a developmental history much like that of waking symbolic thought [and waking consciousness]" (Foulkes, 1996, p. 19). Consistent with this parallelism between waking and sleeping cognitive processes is the observation that visual imagery is absent in the dreams of the congenitally blind or those blinded before the age of five (i.e., before dreaming can be demonstrated), but present in those blinded at or after this time when dreaming with properties essentially similar to those in adults occurs (Foulkes, 1993; Kerr, 1993).

CONCLUSIONS, UNANSWERED QUESTIONS, AND FUTURE DIRECTIONS

Overviews of research fields too often emphasize unresolved issues or areas of contention and neglect to emphasize accomplishments. In little more than one generation, research into the related topics of sleep and dreaming has produced remarkable achievements and revelations. These areas, once almost exclusively the topic of anecdotal and speculative discussion, have been redefined by the application of rigorous scientific investigation with resulting significant empirical revelation regarding the physiological and psychological nature of these ubiquitous human experiences. At the physiological level, enough has been discovered about sleep mechanisms, influences on these mechanisms, and normative aspects of sleep (McGinty et

al., 1985; Montplaisir & Godbout, 1990 Steriade & McCarley, 1990) to permit the extensive differentiation of a variety of sleep abnormalities, many of which can now be effectively treated (ICDS, 1990; Kryger et al., 1994, 2000). Nevertheless, questions remain regarding the processes underlying virtually every aspect of sleep control, including the initiation, maintenance and termination of sleep as a state, as well as between- and within-sleep stage variations. These are truly complex questions, but the coupling of new molecular and genetic methods with those of anatomy, neurophysiology, and biochemistry (Cirelli, Pompeiano, & Tononi, 1996; Pack & Mackiewicz, 1996; Thakkar, 1996) to address these issues offers real promise that they may be resolved.

Unmasking the mechanisms underlying these sleep-specific processes will undoubtedly provide information essential to understanding an equally challenging and important mystery, namely how the states of sleep and wakefulness, which together constitute the entirety of normal human existence, are effectively interfaced to determine our physiological and cognitive status and capabilities. In this regard, studies related to sleep debt are particularly relevant. Sleep debt – a construct inferred from influences of "inadequate sleep" on neurobehavioral and metabolic measures during wakefulness – ultimately relates to an ideal, but likely individualized (Van Dongen et al., 2004), balance between optimal daily amounts of sleep and wakefulness (Dinges, 2004; Horne, 1988; Van Dongen et al., 2003). Whether current society suffers from a debilitating curtailment of sleep amount continues to be debated (Dinges, 2004; Horne, 2004). However, negative effects of sleep reduction on neurocognitive (Belenky et al., 2003; Drake et al., 2001; Van Dongen et al., 2003), metabolic (Spiegel, Leproult, & Van Cauter, 1999), and health-related variables, including appetite control (Spiegel et al., 2004), cardiovascular modulation (Ayas et al., 2003; Spiegel et al. 2004), socioeconomic status (Van Cauter & Spiegel, 1999), loneliness (Cacioppo et al., 2002), and longevity (Kripke et al., 2002), continue to be documented. There is evidence of compensatory adaptive mechanisms that function to counter sleep restriction effects (Drake et al., 2001; Spiegel et al., 2000), but these adaptive changes may persist beyond the period of sleep restriction, thereby maintaining performance at reduced, but stabilized levels, and effectively delaying recovery (Belenky et al., 2003).

Studies of sleep cognition have produced results that are no less remarkable than those of sleep physiology. These investigations have broadened our understanding not only of the organization and formal characteristics of dreams, but have demonstrated that dreaming is a pervasive behavior that is not restricted to a particular sleep stage or even to sleep (Antrobus & Bertini, 1992; Cavallero & Foulkes, 1993; Ellman & Antrobus, 1991; Foulkes, 1985). Furthermore, the evidence showing that this behavior requires cognitive abilities, which normally are not developed until well into the first decade of life (Foulkes, 1982; 1993), indicates that dreaming is not an automatic and inevitable consequence of REM sleep. The many empirical accomplishments resulting from years of research into sleep cognition have significantly informed us regarding many aspects of dreams and the dreaming process, but have also raised new questions (e.g., what features and processes are common to, or distinguish between, cognitive activity during wakefulness and sleep) and left us still contemplating fundamental questions such as why dreams are so readily forgotten or whether dreaming has an adaptive function.

Of relevance to this question of possible adaptive consequences of sleep cognition is a recent resurgence of interest into relationships between sleep and learning. Although the function(s) of sleep remain a matter of debate and research, it seems highly improbable that the biological and behavioral costs associated with maintaining such a state would be tolerated without the realization of significant benefits essential to normal functioning. Given the basic dependence on learning and memory for daily functioning and survival, it would seem judicious to allocate resources associated with these processes to a protected time, such as sleep, when interactions with the environment and the related need for online processing of new information are minimized. Consistent with this sleep-related reduction in sensory appreciation, sleep learning, or at least the memory for materials presented to the sleeping subject, has been shown to be generally impaired (Goodenough, 1978). The new emphasis on sleep, learning, and memory focuses rather on the enhanced consolidation of learning processes set in motion during wakefulness. Evidence is gathering indicating an important facilitating effect of sleep processes on learning and memory [see special issues of *Science* (294, 2001) and *Learning and Memory* (11, 2004) for current reviews]. A basic premise underlying these studies is the reactivation and extended processing during sleep of waking memories. Animal studies have provided support for this reactivation process by showing the replay, during sleep, of ensemble activity patterns of neuronal activity observed during specific waking experiences (Pennartz et al., 2004; Skaggs & McNaughton, 1996).

Among the many questions about memory processes and sleep to be addressed by future research are those related to possible functions of dreams beyond the reported memory enhancement by strengthening old memories and forming new memory connections. Is the dream narrative simply epiphenomenal to the memory functions being accomplished, or does the matrix of associations generating the specific dream experience also reflect the operation of adaptive processes involved for example, in the formulation of basic behavior strategies used to deal with daily problems (Cartwright, 2004)? An example of the failure of mental activity during sleep to provide a psychological adaptive resolution of an existing problem can be found in the dreams of posttraumatic stress disorder patients. Dreams of this group are atypical in two important respects: first, whereas dreams are generally composed of the integration of new and old memory fragments (Fosse et al., 2003; Paller & Voss, 2004), these consist of the replay of intact episodic memories; and secondly, these dreams may occur repetitively over long periods of time (Van der Kolk et al., 1984). These recurrent anxiety dreams may reflect the disruption of adaptive memory-modulating mechanisms (Wiedenmayer, 2004). When taken together with the effects of sleep restriction on waking neurobehavior, these indications of an important involvement of sleep with memory processes suggest an even more profound effect of sleep deprivation on behavior because it compromises both the effective processing of recent information as well as the acquisition of new information.

REM sleep remains the state from which dreaming is most likely to be reported but, except for the general association between REM sleep state physiology and dreaming, attempts to determine reliable links between sleep physiology and sleep cognition have been largely unsuccessful. Perhaps, as suggested by Rosenlicht and Feinberg (1997) for REM sleep, but probably applicable to any situation where dreaming occurs, this apparent "gross psychophysiological mismatch" may reflect an inherent dissociation during dreaming which relates to both physiological and psychological state function at this time. If, as Foulkes (1997) suggests for "minds capable of conscious representational and self-representational intelligence" (p. 4) that "dreaming is the form assumed by consciousness whenever there is residual but somewhat dissociated cognitive/cerebral activation in the relative absence of direction either from the person's environment or from voluntary self-control" (p. 3), then perhaps these dissociations may be better understood in terms of the functional activation of various brain areas and systems at the time of the dream relative to that during nondream experiences. Promising indications that such relationships may indeed be the case can be found in the application of sophisticated EEG analyses (Cantero et al., 2004; De Gennaro et al., 2004; Mölle et al., 2004) and functional imaging technology to the study of physiological and cognitive processes during sleep (Balkin et al., 2002; Braun et al., 1997, 1998; Hong et al., 1995; Kjaer et al., 2002; Maquet, 2000; Maquet et al., 1996), in the array (Domhoff, 2000, 2003) and refinement of instruments and procedures to evaluate such features of these cognitive experiences as bizarreness (Reinsel et al., 1992) and sensory qualities (Antrobus et al., 1987; Rechtschaffen & Buchignani, 1992), and in the development of heuristic theoretical models that integrate these complex data (Antrobus, 1993; Kahn et al., 1997). The continuing development of such technologic and methodological procedures and their combined application in the same subjects at times associated with the occurrence of sleep mentation, as well as during wakefulness under conditions where levels of perceptual processing and symbolic cognition are controlled, will facilitate the identification of similarities and differences in cross-state processes. Such studies will most likely reveal that the sleep-wakefulness state barrier is more permeable than once thought, and the biological and cognitive processes defining these states are more meaningfully related than many previously imagined.

ACKNOWLEDGMENTS

The author gratefully acknowledges the assistance of Ralph Nevins and Jane Buttrum in the preparation of figures. This work was supported by USDA CRIS 6251–51000–002–03S.

GLOSSARY

dreaming A manifestation of human consciousness consisting of the symbolic representation of knowledge that occurs when appreciation and processing of environmental stimuli are minimal and voluntary control of thought processes is lost.

nonrapid eye movement (NREM) sleep includes all sleep other than REM and collectively refers to sleep stages 1–4.

ponto-geniculo-occipital (PGO) spikes as reported from animal studies, this activity consists of monophasic potentials, most readily recorded during sleep from the pons, lateral geniculate bodies, and occipital cortex just prior to and during REM sleep, which are considered to be a primary source of phasic activity during REM sleep.

rapid eye movement (REM) sleep a periodically occurring sleep stage characterized by low voltage, mixed frequency EEG, rapid eye movements, autonomic variability, motor inhibition, and commonly associated with frequent dream recall.

scanning hypothesis the proposition that eye movements during REM sleep are examining dream images as they would visual images during wakefulness.

sleep cycle the recurrent alternation of REM and NREM sleep occurring across the night with a periodicity of approximately 60 minutes in infants and 90 minutes in adults.

slow wave sleep (SWS) sleep characterized by low frequency EEG activity, particularly in the delta band (0.5–4 Hz), and generally refers to sleep stages 3 and 4 combined.

REFERENCES

Agnew, H. W., Jr., and Webb, W. B. (1972). Measurement of sleep onset by EEG criteria. *Am. J. EEG Technol., 12,* 127–134.

Agnew, H. W., Jr., Webb, W. B., and Williams, R. L. (1966). The first night effect: An EEG study of sleep. *Psychophysiology, 2,* 263–266.

Altshuler, K. Z., and Brebbia, D. R. (1967). Body movement artifact as a contaminant psychophysiological studies of sleep. *Psychophysiology, 3,* 86–91.

Anders, T., Emde, R., and Parmelee, A. (Eds.). (1971) *A Manual of Standardized Terminology, Techniques and Criteria for Scoring of States of Sleep and Wakefulness in Newborn Infants.* Los Angeles: UCLA Brain Information, NIMDS Neurological Information Network.

Angeleri, F., Scarpino, O., and Signorino, M. (1984). Information processing and hemispheric specialization: Electrophysiological study during wakefulness, stage 2 and stage REM sleep. *Res. Commun. Psychol., Psychiatry, Behav., 9,* 121–138.

Antrobus, J. (2000). Theories of dreaming. In M. H. Kryger, T. Roth, W. C. Dement (Eds.), *Principles and Practice of Sleep Medicine, 3rd Edition,* (pp. 472–481), Philadelphia, PA: W. B. Saunders Company.

Antrobus, J., Hartwig, P., Rosa, D., Reinsel, R., and Fein, G. (1987). Brightness and clarity of REM and NREM imagery: Photo response scale. *Sleep Res., 16,* 240.

Antrobus, J. S. (1983). REM and NREM sleep reports: Comparison of word frequencies by cognitive classes. *Psychophysiology, 20,* 562–568.

Antrobus, J. S. (1993). The dreaming mind/brain: understanding its processes with connectionist models. In C. Cavallero, D. Foulkes (Eds.), *Dreaming as Cognition* (pp. 77–92). New York: Harvester Wheatsheaf.

Antrobus, J. S., and Bertini, M. (Eds.) (1992). *The Neuropsychology of Sleep and Dreaming,* Hillsdale, NJ: Lawrence Erlbaum Associates, Inc.

Antrobus, J., Ehrlichman, H., and Wiener, M. (1978). EEG asymmetry during REM and NREM Failure to replicate. *Sleep Res., 7,* 24 (Abstract).

Antrobus, J. S. and Ellman, S. J. (Eds.) (1991). *The Mind in Sleep (2nd Edition),* Hillsdale, NJ: Lawrence Erlbaum Associates, Inc.

Antrobus, J. S., Fein, G., Jordan, L., Ellman, S. J., and Arkin, A. M. (1978). Measurement and design in research on sleep reports. In A. M. Arkin, J. S. Antrobus and S. J. Ellman (Eds.), *The Mind in Sleep* (pp. 19–55). Hillsdale, NJ: Lawrence Erlbaum Associates, Inc.

Arkin A. M. (1978). Sleeptalking. In A. M. Arkins. J. S. Antrobus. and S. J. Ellman (Eds.), *The Mind in Sleep* (pp. 513–532). Hillsdale, NJ: Lawrence Erlbaum Associates, Inc.

Arkin, A. M., Antrobus, J. S., Ellman, S. J., and Farber, J. (1978). Sleep mentation as affected by REMP deprivation. In A. M. Arkin, J. S. Antrobus and S. J. Ellman (Eds.), *The Mind in Sleep* (pp. 459–484). Hillsdale, NJ: Lawrence Erlbaum Associates, Inc.

Arkin, A. M., Toth, M., Baker, J., and Hastey, J. M. (1970). The frequency of sleep-talking in the laboratory among chronic sleep-talkers and good dream recallers. *J. Nerv. Ment. Dis., 15*(1), 369–374.

Armitage, R. (1980). *Changes in dream content as a function of time of night, stage of awakening and frequency of recall,* master's thesis, Carleton University, Ottawa.

Armitage, R. (1995a). Microarchitectural findings in sleep EEG in depression: Diagnostic implications. *Biol. Psychiatry, 37,* 72–84.

Armitage, R. (1995b). The distribution of EEG frequencies in REM and NREM sleep stages in healthy young adults. *Sleep, 18,* 334–341.

Armitage, R., Hoffmann, R., and Moffitt, A. (1992). Interhemispheric EEG activity in sleep and wakefulness: Individual differences in the basic rest-activity cycle (BRAC). In Antrobus, J. S., Bertini, M. (Eds.), *The Neuropsychology of Sleep and Dreaming* (pp. 17–45). Hillsdale, NJ: Lawrence Erlbaum Associates, Inc.

ASDA (American Sleep Disorders Association and Sleep Research Society). (1992). Atlas Task Force Report. EEG Arousals: Scoring rules and examples. *Sleep, 15,* 173–184.

Aserinsky, E. (1953). *Ocular motility during sleep and its application to the study of rest-activity cycles and dreaming.* Thesis, Univ. Chicago.

Aserinsky, E. (1965). Periodic respiratory pattern occurring in conjunction with eye movements during sleep. *Science, 150,* 763–766.

Aserinsky, E. (1969). The maximal capacity for sleep: rapid eye movement density as an index of sleep satiety. *Biol. Psychiatry, 1,* 147–159.

Aserinsky, E. (1971). Rapid eye movement density and pattern in the sleep of normal young adults. *Psychophysiology, 8*, 361–375.

Aserinsky, E. (1996). The discovery of REM sleep. *J. Hist. Neurosci.*, 5(3), 213–227.

Aserinsky, E., and Kleitman, N. (1953). Regularly occurring periods of eye motility and concomitant phenomena during sleep. *Science, 118*, 273–275.

Aserinsky, E., and Kleitman, N. (1955). Two types of ocular motility occurring during sleep. *J. Appl. Physiol., 8*, 1–10.

Ayas, N. T., White, D. P., Manson, J. E., Stampfer, M. J., Speizer, F. E., Malhotra, A., and Hu F. B. (2003). A prospective study of sleep duration and coronary heart disease in women. *Arch. Intern. Med., 163*, 205–209.

Azumi, K., Shirakawa, S., and Takahashi, S. (1975). Periodicity of sleep spindle appearance in normal adults. *Sleep Res., 4*, 263 (Abstract).

Baldridge, B. J., Whitman, R. M., and Kramer, M. (1963). A simplified method for detecting eye movements during dreaming. *Psychosomatic Med., 25*, 78–82.

Balkin, T. J., Braun, A. R., Wesensten, N. J., Jeffries, K., Varga, M., Baldwin, P., Belenky, G., and Herskovitch, P. (2002). The process of awakening: a PET study of regional brain activity patterns mediating the re-establishment of alertness and consciousness. *Brain, 125*, 2308–2319.

Basheer, R., Strecker, R. E., Thakkar, M. M. and McCarley, R. W. (2004) Adensoine and sleep-wake regulation. *Prog. Neurobiol., 73*, 379–396.

Behrendt, R. P. (2003). Hallucinations: Synchronization of thalamocortical γ oscillations underconstrained by sensory input. *Concsious Cogn., 12*, 413–451.

Belenky, G., Wesensten, N. J., Thorne, D. R., Thomas, M. L., Sing, H. C., Redmond, D. P., Russo, M. B., and Balkin, T. J. (2003). Patterns of performance degradation and restoration during sleep restriction and subsequent recovery: a sleep dose-response study. *J Sleep Res., 12*, 1–12.

Bentivoglio, M., and Grassi-Zucconi, 0. (1997). The pioneering experimental studies on sleep deprivation. *Sleep, 20*, 570–576.

Berger, R. J. (1961). Tonus of extrinsic laryngeal muscles during sleep and dreaming. *Science, 134*, 840.

Berger, R. J. (1967). When is a dream is a dream is a dream? *Exp. Neurol.*, 19(4), 15–28.

Berger, R. J., Olly, P., and Oswald, L. (1962). The EEG, eye movements, and dreams of the blind. *Quarterly J. Exp. Psychol., 14*, 183–186.

Berger, R. J., and Oswald, I. (1962a). Effects of sleep deprivation on behavior, subsequent sleep and dreaming. *J. Ment. Sci., 108*, 457–465.

Berger, R. J., and Oswald, I. (1962b). Eye movements during active and passive dreams. *Science, 137*, 601.

Bertini, M., and Violani, C. (1992). The postawakening testing technique in the investigation of cognitive asymmetries during sleep. In J. S. Antrobus, M. Bertini (Eds.), *The Neuropsychology of Sleep and Dreaming*. (pp. 47–62). Hillsdale, N J: Lawrence Erlbaum Associates, Inc.

Bonnet, M. H., and Moore, S. E. (1982). The threshold of sleep: Perception of sleep as a function of time asleep and auditory threshold. *Sleep, 5*, 267–276.

Born, J., Muth, S., and Fehm, H. L. (1988). The significance of sleep onset and slow wave sleep for nocturnal release of growth hormone (GH) and cortisol. *Psychoneuroendocrinology, 13*, 233 243.

Bosinelli, M., Molinari, S., Bagnaresi, G., and Salzarulo, P. (1968). Caratteristiche dell attiva psycofisiologica durante il sonno: Un

contributo alle technique di valutazion. *Riv. Speriment.Freiatria, 92*, 128–150.

Braun, A. R., Balkin, T. J., Wesensten, N. L., Carson, R. E., Varga, M., Baldwin, P. S., Selbie, J., Belenky, G., Herscovitch, P. (1997). Regional cerebral blood flow throughout the sleep-wake cycle; An $H_2^{15}O$ PET study. *Brain, 120*, 1173–1197.

Braun, A. R., Balkin, T. J., Wesensten, N. L., Carson, R. E., Varga, M., Baldwin, P. S., Selbie, J., Belenky, G., Herscovitch, P. (1998). Dissociated pattern of activity in visual cortices and their projections during human rapid eye movement sleep. *Science, 279*, 91–95.

Bremer, F. (1937). L'activité cérébrale au cours du sommeil et de la narcose. Contribution a l'étude lu mécanisme du sommeil. *Bull. Acad. R. Med. Belg., 4*, 68–86.

Bremer, F. (1938). L'activité électrique de l'écorce cérébrale et le probleme physiologique du sommeil. *Boll. Soc. Ital. Biol. Sper., 13*, 271–290.

Brooks, D. C. (1967). Localization of the lateral geniculate nucleus monophasic waves associated with eye movements in the cat. *Electroencephalogr. Clin. Neurophysiol., 23*, 123–133.

Brooks, D. C. (1968). Localization and characteristics of the cortical waves associated with eye movements in the cat. *Exp. Biol., 22*, 603–163.

Broughton, R. J. (1975). Biorhythmic variations in consciousness and psychological function. *Can. Psychological Rev., 16*, 2 17–239.

Broughton, R. J., Poire, R., and Tassinari, C. A. (1965). The electrodermogram (Tarchanoff effect) during sleep. *Electroencephalogr. Clin. Neurophysiol., 18*, 691–708.

Burch, N. (1965). Data processing of psychophysiological recordings. In L. D. Proctor and W. R. Adey (Eds.), *Symposium on the analysis of central nervous system and cardiovascular data using computer methods*. (pp. 165–180). Washington, DC: National Aeronautics and Space Administration.

Busby, K. A., Mercier, L., and Pivik, R. T. (1994). Ontogenetic variations in auditory arousal threshold during sleep. *Psychophysiology, 31*, 182–188.

Bussell, J., Dement, W., and Pivik, R. T. (1972). The eye movement-imagery relationship in REM sleep and waking. *Sleep Res., 1*, 100 (Abstract).

Cacioppo, J. T., Hawkley, L. C., Crawford, E., Ernst, J. M., Burleson, M. H., Kowalewski, R. B., Malarkey, W. B., Van Couter, E., and Berntson, G. G. (2002). Loneliness and health: Potential mechanisms. *Psychosom. Med., 64*, 407–417.

Campbell, D. T. (1957). Factors relevant to the validity of experiments in social settings. *Psych. Bull., 54*, 297–312.

Campbell, K., and Bartoli, E. (1986). Human auditory evoked potentials during natural sleep: The early components. *Electroencephal. Clin. Neurophysiol., 65*, 149–149.

Cantero, J. L., Atienza, M., Madsen, J. R., and Stickgold, R. (2004). Gamma EEG dynamics in neocortex and hippocampus during human wakefulness and sleep. *Neuroimage, 22*, 1271–1280.

Carskadon, M. A., Brown, E. D., and Dement, W. C. (1982). Sleep fragmentation in the elderly: Relationship to daytime sleep tendency. *Neurobiology of Aging, 3*, 321–327.

Cartwright, R. D. (2004). The role of sleep in changing our minds: A psychologist's discussion of papers on memory reactivation and consolidation in sleep. *Learn. Mem., 11*, 660–663.

Cavallero, C., and Cicogna, P. (1993). Memory and dreaming. In C. Cavallero and D. Foulkes (Eds.), *Dreaming as Cognition* (pp. 38–57). New York: Harvester Wheatsheaf.

Cavallero, C., Cicogna, P., Natale, V., Occhionero, M., and Zito, A. (1992). Slow wave sleep dreaming. *Sleep, 15*, 562–566.

Cavallero, C. and Foulkes, D.(Eds.) (1993). *Dreaming as Cognition*. New York: Harvester Wheatsheaf.

Cicogna, P., Natale, V., Occhionero, M., and Bosinelli, M. (2000). Slow wave and REM sleep mentation. *Sleep Res. Online, 3*, 67–72.

Cirelli, C., Pompeiano, M., and Tononi, G. (1996). New perspectives on sleep and gene expression *SRS Bull.*, 2(1–2), 12–17.

Cohen, D. B. (1977). Changes in REM dream content during the night: Implications for a hypothesis about changes in cerebral dominance across REM periods. *Percept. Mot. Skills*, 44, 1267–1277.

Cohen, H. D., and Shapiro, A. (1970). Vaginal blood flow during sleep. *Psychophysiology*, 1, 338 Abstract).

Conduit, R., Crewther, S. G., and Coleman, G. (2004). Spontaneous eyelid movements (ELMS) during sleep are related to dream recall on awakening. *J. Sleep Res.*, *13*, 137–144.

Davis, H., Davis, P. A., Loomis, A. L., Harvey, E. N., and Hobart, G. (1938). Human brain potentials during the onset of sleep. *J. Neurophysiol., 1*, 24–38.

De Gennaro, L., Vecchio, F., Ferrara, M., Curcio, G., Rossini, P. M., and Babiloni, C. (2004). Changes in fronto-posterior functional coupling at sleep onset in himans. *J. Sleep Res.*, *13*, 209–217.

DeKoninck, 1., Lorrain, D., and Gagnon, P. (1992). Sleep positions and position shifts in five age groups: An ontogenetic picture. *Sleep*, 15, 143–149.

Dement, W. C. (1955). Dream recall and eye movement during sleep in schizophrenics and normal *J. Nerv. Ment. Dis.*, 122, 263–269.

Dement, W. C. (1960). The effect of dream deprivation. *Science*, 131, 1705–1707.

Dement, W. C. (1969). A new look at the third state of existence. *Stanford Medical Alumi Association*, 8, 2–8.

Dement, W. C., and Kleitman, N. (1957a). Cyclic variations in EEG during sleep and their relation eye movements, bodily motility and dreaming. *Electroencephalogr. Clin. Neurophysiol.*, 9, 673–690.

Dement, W.C, and Kleitman, N. (1957b). The relation of eye movements during sleep to dream activity: An objective method for the study of dreaming. *J. Exp. Psychol.*, 53, 339–346.

Dement, W. C., and Mitler, M. M. (1974). An introduction to sleep. In O. Petre-Quadens, J. D. Schlag (Eds.), *Basic Sleep Mechanisms* (pp. 271–296). New York: Academic Press.

Dement, W., and Wolpert, E. (1958a). Interrelations in the manifest content of dreams occurring on the same night. *J. Nerv. Ment. Dis.*, *126*, 568–578.

Dement, W., and Wolpert, E. (1958b). The relation of eye movements, body motility, and external stimuli to dream content. *J. Exp. Psychol.*, 55, 543–554.

Dinges, D. F. (2004). Sleep debt and scientific evidence. *Sleep*, 27, 1050–1052

Domhoff. G. W. (2000). Methods and measures for the study of dream content. In M. H. Kryger, T. Roth, W. C. Dement (Eds.), *Principles and Practice of Sleep Medicine, 3rd Edition* (pp. 463–471), Philadelphia, PA: W. B. Saunders Company.

Domhoff, G. W. (2003). *The scientific study of dreams: Neural networks, cognitive development, and content analysis*. Washington, DC: American Psychological Association.

Domhoff, G. W. and Kamiya, J. (1964). Problems in dream content study with objective indicators: 1 A comparison of home and laboratory dream reports. *Arch. Gen. Psychiatry, 11*, 519–524.

Doricchi, F., and Violani, C. (1992). Dream recall in brain-damaged patients: A contribution to the neuropsychology of dreaming through a review of the literature. In J. S. Antrobus,

M. Bertini (Eds.), *The Neuropsychology of Sleep and Dreaming* (pp. 99–140). Hillsdale, NJ: Lawrence Erlbaum Associates, Inc.

Dorus, E., Dorus, E., and Rechtschaffen, A. (1971). The incidence of novelty in dreams. *Arch. Gen.Psychiatry, 25*, 364–368.

Drake, C. L., Roehrs, T. A., Burduvali, E., Bonahoom, A., Rosekind, M., and Roth, T. (2001). Effects of rapid versus slow accumulation of eight hours of sleep loss. *Psychophysiology, 38*, 979–987.

Ellman, S. J., and Antrobus, J. S. (Eds.) (1991) *The Mind in Sleep (2nd ed.)*. New York, Wiley.

Ellman, S. J., Antrobus, J. S., Arkin, A. M., Farber, J., Luck, D., Bodnar, R., Sanders, K., and Nelson, W. J. Jr. (1974). Sleep mentation in relation to phasic and tonic events – REMP and NREM. *Sleep Res., 3*, 115 (Abstract).

Everson, C. A. (1995). Functional consequences of sustained sleep deprivation in the rat. *Behav. Brain Res., 69*, 43–54.

Feinberg, I., Fein, G., and Floyd, T. C. (1980). Period and amplitude analysis of NREM EEG in sleep: repeatability of results in young adults. *Electroencephalogr. Clin. Neurophysiol., 48*, 2 12–221.

Ferguson, J., Cohen, H., Barchas, J., and Dement, W. (1969). Sleep and wakefulness: A closer look. Presented at a meeting of the Federation of Amer. Soc. for Exp. Biol. Symp. on "Neurohumoral aspects of sleep and wakefulness". Atlantic City, New Jersey.

Firth, H., and Oswald, I. (1975). Eye movements and visually active dreams. *Psychophysiology, 12*, 602–605.

Fischer, S. Hallschmidt, M., Elsner, A. L., and Born, J. (2002). Sleep forms memory for finger skills. *Proc. Natl. Acad. Sci., 99*, 11987–11991.

Fisher, C. (1966). Dreaming and sexuality. In R. Lowenstein, L. Newman, M. Shur and A. Solnit (Eds.), *Psychoanalysis: A general psychology*. New York: International Universities Press.

Fisher, C., Gross, J., and Zuch, J. (1965). Cycles of penile erection synchronous with dreaming (REM) sleep. *Arch. Gen. Psychiatry, 12*, 29–45.

Fosse, M. J., Fosse, R., Hobson, J. A., and Stickgold, R. J. (2003). Dreaming and episodic memory: A functional dissociation? *J. Cog. Neurosci. 15*, 1–9.

Foulkes, D. (1960). *Dream reports from different stages of sleep*. Unpublished doctoral dissertation, University of Chicago.

Foulkes, D. (1962). Dream reports from different stages of sleep. *J. Abn. Soc. Psychol. 65*, 14–25.

Foulkes, D. (1967). Nonrapid eye movement mentation. *Exp. Neurol., 19(4)*, 28–38.

Foulkes, D. (1978). *A grammar of dreams*. New York: Basic Books.

Foulkes, D. (1982). *Children's dreams: Longitudinal studies*. New York: Wiley.

Foulkes, D. (1985). *Dreaming: A cognitive-psychological analysis*. Hillsdale, N.J.: Lawrence Erlbaum Associates.

Foulkes, D. (1993). Children's dreaming. In C. Cavallero, D. Foulkes (Eds.), *Dreaming as Cognition* (pp. 114–132). New York: Harvester Wheatsheaf.

Foulkes, D. (1996). Dream research: 1953–1993. *Sleep*, 19(8), 609–624.

Foulkes, D. (1997). A contemporary neurobiology of dreaming. *SRS Bull.*, 3(1), 2–4.

Foulkes, D., and Cavallero, C. (1993). Introduction. In C. Cavallero and D. Foulkes (Eds.), *Dreaming as Cognition* (pp. 1–17). New York: Harvester Wheatsheaf.

Foulkes, D., and Fleisher, S. (1975). Mental activity in relaxed wakefulness. *J. Abnorm. Psychol.*, 4, 66–75.

Foulkes, D., Hollifield, M., Bradley, L., Terry, R., and Sullivan, B. (1991). Waking self-understanding, REM-dream self representation, and cognitive ability variables at ages 5–8. *Dreaming, 1*, 41–51.

Foulkes, D., Hollifield, M., Sullivan, B., Bradley, L., and Terry, R. (1990). REM dreaming and cognitive skill at ages *5–8*: a cross-sectional study. *Int. J. Behav. Devel. 13*, 447–465.

Foulkes, D., Pivik, T., Steadman, H. S., Spear, P. S., and Symonds, J. D. (1967). Dreams of the male child: An EEG study. *J. Abnorm. Psychology, 72*, 457–467.

Foulkes, D., and Pope, R. (1973). Primary visual experience and secondary cognitive elaboration in stage REM: A modest confirmation and an extension. *Percept. Mot. Skills, 37*, 107–118.

Foulkes, D., and Rechtschaffen, A. (1964). Presleep determinants of dream content: Effects of two films. *Percept. Mot. Skills, 19*, 983–1005.

Foulkes, D., and Schmidt, M. (1983). Temporal sequence and unit composition in dream reports from different stages of sleep. *Sleep, 6*, 265–280.

Foulkes, D., and Scott, E. (1973). An above-zero waking baseline for the incidence of momentarily hallucinatory mentation. *Sleep Res., 2*, 108 (Abstract).

Foulkes, D., Spear, P. S., and Symonds, J. (1966). Individual differences in mental activity at sleep onset. *J. Abnorm. Psychol., 71*, 280–286.

Foulkes, D., and Vogel, G. (1965). Mental activity at sleep onset. *J. Abnorm. Psychol., 70*, 231–243.

Frank, M. G., and Heller, H. C. (2003). The ontogeny of mammalian sleep: a reappraisal of alternative hypotheses. *J. Sleep Res., 12*, 25–34.

Franken, P., Dijk, D. J., Tobler, I., and Borbely, A. A. (1994). High-frequency components of the rat electrocorticogram are modulated by the vigilance states. *Neurosci. Lett., 167*, 89–92.

Freedman, S. J., Grunebaum, H. U., Greenblatt, M. (1971). Perceptual and cognitive changes in sensory deprivation. In P. Solomon, P. E. Kubzansky, P. Herbert Leiderman, J. H. Mendelson, R. Trumbull, D. Wexler (Eds.), *Sensory Deprivation. A symposium held at Harvard Medical School* (pp. 58–71). Cambridge, MA: Harvard University Press.

Geschwind, N., and Galaburda, A. M. (Eds.) (1987). *Cerebral Lateralization: Biological Mechanisms, Associations, and Pathology*. Cambridge, Massachusetts: The MIT Press.

Gillberg, M., and Akerstedt, T. (1994). Sleep restriction and SWS-suppression: Effects on daytime alertness and night-time recovery. *J. Sleep Res., 3*, 144–151.

Goblot, E. (1896). Sur le souvenir des rêves. *Revue Philosophique, 42*, 288.

Goldstein, L., Stolzfus, N., and Gardocki, J. (1972). Changes in interhemispheric amplitude relations in EEG during sleep. *Physiological Behav., 8*, 811–815.

Goodenough, D. R. (1978). Dream recall: History and current status of the field. In A. M. Arkin, J. S. Antrobus, and S. J. Ellman (Eds.), *The Mind in Seep* (pp. 113–140). Hillsdale, NJ: Lawrence Erlbaum Associates, Inc.

Goodenough, D. R. Lewis, H. B., Shapiro, A., and Sleser, I. (1965). Some correlates of dream reporting following laboratory awakenings. *J. Nerv. Ment Dis., 140*, 365–373.

Goodenough, D. R., Shapiro, A., Holden, M., and Steinschriber, L. (1959). A comparison of "dreamers" and "nondreamers": Eye movements, electroencephalograms and the recall of dreams. *J. Abnorm. Psychol., 59*, 295–302.

Greene, R., and Siegel, J. (2004). Sleep: A functional enigma. *Neuromolecular Med., 5*, 59–68.

Griesinger, X. X. (1868). Physio-psychologische Selbstbeobachtungen. *Arch. Psychiatr Nervenkr, 1*, 200–204.

Gross, J., Byrne, J., and Fisher, C. (1965). Eye movements during emergent stage I EEG in subjects with life-long blindness. *J. Nerv. Ment. Dis., 141*, 365–370.

Grosser, G., and Siegal, A. (1971). Emergence of a tonic-phasic model for sleep and dreaming: Behavioral and physiological observations. *Psychol. Bull., 75*, 60–72.

Guevara, M. A., Lorenzo, I., Arce, C., Ramos, M., and Corsi-Cabrera, M. (1995). Inter-and intrahemispheric EEG correlation during sleep and wakefulness. *Sleep, 18*, 257–265.

Guilleminault, C. (1994). Clinical features and evaluation of obstructive sleep apnea. In M. H. Kryger, T. Roth, W. C. Dement (Eds.), *Principles and Practice of Sleep Medicine, 2nd Edition* (pp. 667–677). Philadelphia, PA: W. B. Saunders Company.

Halasz, P., Rajna, P., Pal, I. Kundra, 0., Vargha, A., Balogh, A., and Kemeny, A. (1977). K-complexes and micro-arousals as functions of the sleep process. In W. P. Koella and P. Levin (Eds.), *Sleep* (pp. 292–294). Basel: S. Karger.

Hall, C., and Van de Castle, R. L. (1966). *The Content Analysis of Dreams*. New York: Appleton Century-Crofts.

Harman, K., and Pivik, R. T. (1996). Site-specific variations in alpha activity across sleep cycles in normal adults. *Sleep Res, 25*, 127, 1996 (Abstract).

Hauri, P., and Van de Castle, R. L. (1973a). Psychophysiological parallelism in dreams. *Psychosomatic Med., 35*, 297–308.

Hauri, P., and Van de Castle, R. L. (1973b). Psychophysiological parallels in dreams. In U. J. Jovanovic (Ed.), *The nature of sleep* (pp. 140–142). Stuttgart: Fischer.

Hauri, P., and Rechtschaffen, A. (1963). An unsuccessful attempt to find physiological correlates of NREM recall. Paper presented at the meeting of the Association for the Psychophysiological Study of Sleep, New York.

Herman, J. H., EIlman, S. J., and Roffwarg, H. P. (1978). The problem of NREM dream recall reexamined. In A. M. Arkin, J. S. Antrobus and S. J. Ellman (Eds.), *The Mind in Sleep* (pp. 59–92). Hillsdale, NJ: Lawrence Erlbaum Associates, Inc.

Hobson, J. A. (1992). A new model of brain-mind state: Activation level, input source, and mode of processing (AIM). *In* J. S. Antrobus and M. Bertini (Eds.), *The Neuropsychology of Sleep and Dreaming* (pp. 227–245). Hillsdale, NJ: Lawrence Erlbaum Associates, Inc.

Hobson, J. A., Goldfrank, F., and Snyder, F. (1965). Respiration and mental activity in sleep. *J. Psychiatric Res., 3*, 79–90.

Hobson, J. A., and McCarley, R. W. (1977). The brain as a dream state generator: An activation-synthesis hypothesis of the dream process. *Am. J. Psychiatry. 134*, 1335–1348.

Hobson, J. A., Pace-Schott, E. F., Stickgold, R., and Kahn, D. (1998). To dream or not to dream? Relevant data from new neuroimaging and electrophysiological studies. *Curr. Opin. Neurobiol. 8*, 239–244.

Hodes, R., and Dement, W. C. (1964). Depression of electrically induced reflexes ("H"-reflexes) in man during low voltage EEG "sleep". *Electroencephalogr. Clin. Neurophysiol., 17*, 617–629.

Hoffman, R. F., Moffit, A. R., Shearer, J. C., Sussman, P. S., and Wells, R. B. (1979). Conceptual and methodological considerations towards the development of computer-controlled research on the electro-physiology of sleep. *Waking and Sleeping, 3*, 1–16.

Hong, C. C-H., Gillin, J. C., Dow, B. M., Wu, J., and Buchsbaum, M. S. (1995). Localized and lateralized cerebral glucose metabolism associated with eye movements during REM sleep and wakefulness: A positron emission tomography (PET) study. *Sleep*, 18(7), 570–580.

Hong, C. C-H., Potkin, S. G., Antrobus, J. S., Dow, B. M., Callaghan, G. J., and Gillin, J. C. (1997). REM sleep eye movement counts correlate with visual imagery in dreaming: A pilot study. *Psychophysiology, 34*, 377–381.

Hori, T. (1982). Electrodermal and electro-oculographic activity in a hypnagogic state. *Psychophysiology, 19*, 668–672.

Horne, J. (1988). *Why we sleep. The functions of sleep in humans and other mammals*. Oxford: Oxford University Press.

Horne, J. (2004). Is there a sleep debt? *Sleep, 27*, 1047–1049.

Iacono, W. G. and Lykken, D. T. (1981). Two-year retest stability of eye tracking performance and a comparison of electro-oculographic and infrared recording techniques: Evidence of EEG in the electro-oculogram. *Psychophysiology, 18*, 49–55.

ICSD – *International classification of sleep disorders: Diagnostic and coding manual*. (1990). Diagnostic Classification Steering Committee, Thorpy, M. J., Chairman. Rochester, Minnesota: American Sleep Disorders Association.

Itil, T. (1970). Digital computer analysis of the electroencephalogram during eye movement sleep state in man. *J. Nerv. Ment. Dis., 150*, 20 1–208.

Jacobson, A., Kales, A., Lehmann, D., and Hoedemaker, F. S. (1964). Muscle tonus in human subjects during sleep and dreaming. *Exp. Neurol., 10*, 418–424.

Johnson, L. C. (1973). Are stages of sleep related to waking behavior? *Am. Scientist, 61*, 326–338.

Johnson, L. C., and Lubin, A. (1966). Spontaneous electrodermal activity during waking and sleeping. *Psychophysiology, 3*, 8–17.

Johnson, L. C., Nute, C. Austin, M. J., and Lubin, A. (1967). Spectral analysis of the EEG during waking and sleeping. *Electroencephalogr. Clin. Neurophysiol., 23*, 80.

Jones, B. E. (2000). Basic mechanisms of sleep-wake states. In M. H. Kryger, T. Roth, W. C. Dement (Eds.), *Principles and Practice of Sleep Medicine, 3rd Edition* (pp. 134–154). Philadelphia, PA: W. B. Saunders Company.

Jouvet, M. (1972). The role of monoamines and acetylcholine-containing neurons in the regulation of the sleep-waking cycle. *Ergeb. Physiol., 64*, 166–307.

Jouvet, M., and Michel, F. (1959). Correlations electromyographiques du sommeil chez le chat elecortique et mesencephalique chronique. *Compte Rendu Sociologie et Biologie, (Paris) 153*, 422–425.

Kahn, D., Pace-Schott, E. F., and Hobson, J. A. (1997). Consciousness in waking and dreaming: The roles of neuronal oscillation and neuromodulation in determining similarities and differences. *Neuroscience, 78(1)*, 13–38.

Kales, A., Hoedmaker, F., Jacobson, A., Kales, J., Pawlson, M., and Wilson, T. (1967). Mentation during sleep: REM and NREM recall reports. *Percept. Mot. Skills, 24*, 556–560.

Karacan, I., Goodenough, D. R., Shapiro, A., and Starker, S. (1966). Erection cycle during sleep in relation to dream anxiety. *Arch. Gen. Psychiatry, 15*, 183–189.

Kerr, N. H. (1993). Mental imagery, dreams and perception. In C. Cavallero, D. Foulkes (Eds.), *Dreaming as Cognition* (pp. 18–37). New York: Harvester Wheatsheaf.

Kjaer, T. W., Law, I., Wiltschiøtz, G., Paulson, O. B., and Madsen, P. L. (2002). Regional cerebral blood flow during light sleep – a H_2^{15}O-PET study. *J. Sleep Res., 11*, 201–207.

Kleitman, N. (1963). *Sleep and wakefulness* (2nd ed.). Chicago: University of Chicago Press.

Kleitman, N. (1967). The basic rest-activity cycle and physiological correlates of dreaming. *Exp. Neurol., 19*, 2–4.

Kramer, M. (1994). The scientific study of dreaming. In M. H. Kryger, T. Roth, W. C. Dement (Eds.), *Principles and Practice of Sleep Medicine, 2nd Edition*, (pp. 394–399). Philadelphia, P.A.: W. B. Saunders Company.

Kramer, M., Roth, T., and Czaya, J. (1975). Dream development within a REM period. In P. Levin and W. P. Koella (Eds.), *Sleep*, (pp. 406–409). Basel: S. Karger.

Kripke, D. F., Garfinkel, L., Wingard, D. L., Klauber, M. R., and Marler, M. R. (2002). Mortality associated with sleep duration and insomnia. *Arch. Gen. Psychiatry, 59*, 131–136.

Krueger, J. M., Karnovsky, M. L. (1995). Sleep as a neuroimmune phenomenon: A brief historical perspective. *Adv. Neuroimmunol., 5*, 5–12.

Kryger, M. H., Roth, T., and Dement, W. C. (Eds.). (1994). *Principles and Practice of Sleep Medicine, 2nd Edition*. Philadelphia, PA: W. B. Saunders Company.

Kryger, M. H., Roth, T., and Dement, W. C. (Eds.). (2000). *Principles and Practice of Sleep Medicine, 3rd Edition*. Philadelphia, PA: W. B. Saunders Company.

Kubicki, S., and Herrmann, W. M. (1996). The future of computer-assisted investigation of the polysomnogram: Sleep microstructure. *J. Clin. Neurophysiol., 13*, 285–294.

LaBerge, S. (1985). *Lucid Dreaming*. Los Angeles: J. P. Tarcher.

LaBerge, S. (1992). The postawakening testing technique in the investigation of cognitive asymmetries during sleep. In J. S. Antrobus, M. Bertini (Eds.), *The Neuropsychology of Sleep and Dreaming* (pp. 289–303). Hillsdale, NJ: Lawrence Erlbaum Associates, Inc.

LaBerge, S., Greenleaf, W., and Kedzierski, B. (1983). Physiological responses to dreamed sexual activity during lucid REM sleep. *Psychophysiology, 20*, 454–455.

Ladd, G. T. (1892). Contributions to the psychology of visual dreams. *Mind, 1*, (New Series), 299–304.

Lammers, W. J., and Badia, P. (1991). Motor responsiveness to stimuli presented during sleep: The influence of time-of-testing on sleep stage analyses. *Physiology and Behavior, 50*, 867–868.

Larson, J. D., and Foulkes, D. (1969). Electromyogram suppression during sleep, dream recall and orientation time. *Psychophysiology, 5*, 548–555.

Llinás, R., and Ribary, U. (1993). Coherent 40-Hz oscillation characterized dream state in humans. *Proc. Natl. Acad. Sci. USA, 90*, 2078–2081.

Lloyd, S. R., Cartwright, R. D. (1995). The collection of home and laboratory dreams by means of an instrumental response technique. *Dreaming: J. Assoc. Study Dreams, 5*, 63–73.

Loomis, A. L., Harvey, E. N., and Hobart, G. A. (1937). Cerebral states during sleep as studied by human brain potentials. *J. Exp. Psychol., 21*, 127–144.

Loomis, A. L., Harvey, E. N., and Hobart III, G. A. (1938). Distribution of disturbance-patterns in the human electroencephalogram, with special reference to sleep. *J. Neurophysiol., 1*, 413–430.

Louis, J., Cannard, C., Bastuji, H., and Challamel, M.-J. (1997). Sleep ontogenesis revisited: longitudinal 24-hour home polygraphic study on 15 normal infants during the first two years of life *Sleep, 20*, 323–333.

Lubin, A., Johnston, L. C., and Austin, M. J. (1969). Discrimination among states of consciousness using EEG spectra. *Psychophysiology, 6*, 122–132.

Maquet, P. (2000). Functional neuroimaging of normal human sleep by positron emission tomography. *J. Sleep Res., 9*, 207–231.

Maquet, P., Peters, J.-M., Aerts, J., Delfiore, G., Degueldre, C., Luxen, A., and Granck, G. (1996). Functional neuranatomy of human rapid-eye-movement sleep and dreaming. *Nature, 383*, 163–166.

Marks, G. A., Shaffery, J. P., Oksenberg, A., Speciale, S. G., and Roffwarg, H. P. (1995). A functional role for REM sleep in brain maturation. *Behav. Brain Res., 69*, 1–11.

McCarley, R. W. (2004). Mechanisms and models of REM sleep control. *Arch. Ital. Biol., 142*, 429–467.

McCarley, R. W., and Hobson, J. A. (1975). Neuronal excitability modulation over the sleep cycle: a structural and mathematical model. *Science, 189*, 58–60.

McGinty, D. J., Drucker-Colin, R., Morrison, A., and Parmeggiani, P. L. (Eds.) (1985). *Brain Mechanisms of Sleep*. New York: Raven Press.

Meier, B. (1993). Speech and thinking in dreams. In C. Cavallero, D. Foulkes (Eds.), *Dreaming as Cognition* (pp. 58–76). New York: Harvester Wheatsheaf.

Mercier, L., and Pivik, R. T. (1983). Spinal motoneuronal excitability during wakefulness and non-REM sleep in hyperkinesis. *J. Clin. Neurophysiology, 5*, 321–336.

Mercier, L., Pivik, R. T., and Busby, K. (1993). Sleep patterns in reading disabled children. *Sleep, 16*, 207–215.

Moffitt, A., Hoffmann, R., Wells, R., Armitage, R., Pigeau, R., and Shearer, J. (1982). Individual differences among pre- and post-awakening EEG correlates of dream reports following arousals from different stages of sleep. *Psych. J. Univ. Ottawa, 7*, 111–125.

Molinari, S., and Foulkes, D. (1969). Tonic and phasic events during sleep: Psychological correlates and implications. *Percept. Mot. Skills, 29*, 343–368.

Mölle, M., Marshall, L., Gais, S., and Born, J. (2004). Learning increases human electroencephalographic coherence during subsequent slow sleep oscillations. *Proc Natl Acad Sci., 101*, 13963–13968.

Monk, T. H. (1991). *Sleep, Sleepiness and Performance*. New York: John Wiley & Sons.

Monroe, L. J. (1969). Inter-rater reliability and the role of experience in scoring EEG sleep records: Phase I. *Psychophysiology, 5*, 376–384.

Monroe, L. J., Rechtschaffen, A., Foulkes, D., and Jensen, J. (1965). Discriminability of REM and NREM reports. *J. Pers. Soc. Psychol., 2*, 45 6–460.

Montplaisir, J., and Godbout, R. (Eds.) (1990). *Sleep and Biological Rhythms*. New York, Oxford University Press.

Moruzzi, G. (1963). Active processes in the brain stem during sleep. *Harvey Lecture Series, 58*, 233–297.

Moruzzi, G., and Magoun, H. W. (1949). Brain stem reticular formation and activation of the EEG *Electroencephalogr. Clin. Neurophysiol., 1*, 455–473.

Naifeh, K. H., and Kamiya, J. (1981). The nature of respiratory changes associated with sleep onset. *Sleep, 4*, 49–59.

Niedermeyer, E., and Lopes Da Silva, F. (Eds). (1993). *Electroencephalography: Basic Principles, Clinical Applications, and Related Fields* (3rd ed.). Baltimore: Williams & Wilkins.

Nielsen, T. A., Kuiken, D., Alain, G., Stenstrom, P., and Powell, R. A. (2004). Immediate and delayed incorporations of events into dreams: further replication and implications for dream function. *J. Sleep Res., 13*, 327–336.

Nitz, D. (1993). Early sleep theories. In M. A. Carskadon (Ed.), *Encyclopedia of Sleep and Dreaming* (pp. 200–201). New York, Macmillan Publishing Company.

Ogilvie, R., Hunt, H., Sawicki, C., and McGowan, K. (1978). Searching for lucid dreams. *Sleep Res., 7*, 165 (Abstract).

Ogilvie, R. D., Hunt, H. T., Sawicki, C., and Samahalskyi, J. (1982). Psychological correlates of spontaneous middle-ear muscle activity during sleep. *Sleep, 5*, 11–27.

Ogilvie, R. D., and Wilkinson, R. T. (1984). The detection of sleep onset: Behavioral and physiological convergence. *Psychophysiology, 21*, 510–520.

Ogilvie, R. D., Wilkinson, R. T., and Allison, S. (1989). The detection of sleep onset: Behavioral physiological, and subjective convergence. *Sleep, 12*, 458–474.

Oksenberg, A., Shaffery, J. P., Marks, G. A., Speciale, S. G., Mihailoff, G., and Roffwarg, H. P. (1996). Rapid eye movement sleep deprivation in kittens amplifies LGN cell-size disparity induced by monocular deprivation. *Dev. Brain Res., 97*, 5 1–61.

Okuma, T., Fukuma, E., and Kobayashi, K. (1976). "Dream detector" and comparison of laboratory and home dreams collected by REMP-awakening technique. *Adv. Sleep Res., 2*, 223–231.

Pack, A. I., and Mackiewicz, M. (1996). Potential molecular biological approaches to the study of sleep. *SRS Bull., 2*(1–2), 2–7.

Palca, J. W., Walker, J. M., and Berger, R. J. (1981). Tympanic temperature and REM sleep in cold exposed humans. *Acta Universitatis Carolinae-Biologica 1979*, 225–227.

Paller, K. A. and Voss, J. L. (2004). Memory reactivation and consolidation during sleep. *Learn. Mem., 11*, 664–670.

Pennartz, C. M. A., Lee, E., Verheul, J., Lipa, P., Barnes, C. A., and McNaughton, B. L. (2004). The ventral striatum in off-line processing: Emsemble reactivation during sleep and modulation by hippocampal ripples. *J. Neurosci., 24*, 6446–6456.

Pessah, M., and Roffwarg, H. (1972). Spontaneous middle ear muscle activity in man: A rapid eye movement phenomenon. *Science, 178*, 773–776.

Pieron, H. (1913). *Le problème physiologique du sommeil*. Paris: Masson.

Pivik, R. T. (1971). *Mental activity and phasic events during sleep*. Unpublished docton dissertation, Stanford University.

Pivik, R. T. (1978). Tonic states and phasic events in relation to sleep mentation. In A. M. Arkin, J. S. Antrobus, and S. J. Ellman (Eds.), *The Mind in Sleep* (pp. 245–271). Hillsdale, NJ: Lawrence Erlbaum Associates, Inc.

Pivik, R. T. (1983). Order and disorder during sleep ontogeny: A selective review. In P. Firestone, P. J. McGrath, and W. Feldman (Eds.), *Advances in Behavioral Medicine for Children and Adolescents* (pp. 75–102). Hillsdale, NJ: Lawrence Erlbaum Associates, Inc.

Pivik, R. T. (1986). Sleep: Physiology and Psychophysiology. In G. H. Coles, E. Donchin, and S. W. Porges (Eds.), *Psychophysiology* (pp. 378–406). New York: The Guilford Press.

Pivik, R. T. (1991). Tonic states and phasic events in relation to sleep mentation. In J. S. Antrobus, and S. J. Ellman (Eds.), *The Mind in Sleep (2nd ed.)*, (pp. 2 14–247). Hillsdale, NJ: Lawrence Erlbaum Associates, Inc..

Pivik, R. T., & Busby, K. (1996). Heart rate associated with sleep onset in preadolescents. *J. Sleep Res., 5*, 33–36.

Pivik, R. T., Busby, K., & Brown, M. (1993). Characteristics of sleep onset in adolescents: Temporal relationships among cardiovascular and EEG power spectral measures. Presented at the conference on Sleep Onset Mechanisms: Normal and Abnormal Processes, Niagara-on-the-Lake, Ontario.

Pivik, R. T., Busby, K. A., Gill, E., Hunter, P., and Nevins, R. (1996). Heart rate variations during sleep in preadolescents. *Sleep, 19,* 117–135.

Pivik, R. T., Bylsma, F., Busby, K., Sawyer, S. (1982). Interhemispheric EEG changes: Relationship to sleep and dreams in gifted adolescents. *Psychiat. J. Univ. Ottawa, 7,* 56–76.

Pivik, T., and Dement, W. (1968). Amphetamine, REM deprivation and K-complexes. *Psychophysiology, 5,* 241 (Abstract).

Pivik, T., and Dement, W. C. (1970). Phasic changes in muscular and reflex activity during non REM sleep. *Exp. Neurol., 27,* 115–124.

Pivik, T., and Foulkes, D. (1968). NREM mentation: Relation to personality, orientation time and time of night. *J. Consult. Clin. Psychol., 37,* 144–151.

Pompeiano, O. (1966). Muscular afferents and motor control during sleep. In R. Granit (Ed.), *Muscular Afferents and Motor Control* (pp. 4 15–436). Stockholm: Almquist & Siksell.

Porte, H. S. (2004). Slow horizontal eye movement at human sleep onset. *J. Sleep Res., 13,* 239–249.

Prechtl, H. F. R., Akiyama, Y., Zinkin, P., and Grant, D. K. (1968). Polygraphic studies of the full term newborn. Technical aspects and qualitative analysis. In M. C. Bax and R. C. MacKeith (Eds.), *Studies in Infancy* (pp. 1–21). London: Heinemann.

Rechtschaffen, A. (1967). Dream reports and dream experiences. *Exp. Neurol., 19 (Suppl. 4),* 4–15.

Rechtschaffen, A. (1973). The psychophysiology of mental activity during sleep. In F. J. McGuigan, and R. A. Schoonover (Eds.), *The Psychophysiology of Thinking* (pp. 153–205). New York: Academic Press.

Rechtschaffen, A. (1978). The single-mindedness and isolation of dreams. *Sleep, I,* 97–109.

Rechtschaffen, A. (1998). Current perspectives on the function of sleep. *Perspect. Biol. Med., 41,* 359–390.

Rechtschaffen, A., Bergmann, B. M., Everson, C. A., Kushida, C. A., and Gilliland, M. A. (2002). Sleep deprivation in the rat: X. Integration and discussion of the findings. 1989. *Sleep, 25,* 68–87.

Rechtschaffen, A., and Buchignani, C. (1992). The visual appearance of dreams. In J. S. Antrobus, and M. Bertini (Eds.), *The Neuropsychology of Sleep and Dreaming* (pp. 143–155). Hillsdale, NJ: Lawrence Erlbaum Associates.

Rechtschaffen, A., Goodenough, D., and Shapiro, A. (1962). Patterns of sleep talking. *Arch. Gen. Psychiatry, 7,* 418–426.

Rechtschaffen, A., and Kales, A. (Eds.) (1968). *A manual of standardized terminology, techniques and scoring system for sleep stages of human subjects* (NIM Publ. No. 204). Washington, DC: U. S. Government Printing Office.

Rechtschaffen, A., Verdone, P., and Wheaton, J. (1963). Reports of mental activity during sleep. *Can. Psychiat. Assoc. J., 8,* 409–414.

Rechtschaffen, A., Vogel, G., and Shaikun, G. (1963). Interrelatedness of mental activity during sleep. *Arch. Gen. Psychiatry, 9,* 536–547.

Reinsel, R., Antrobus, J., and Wollman, M. (1985). The phasic-tonic difference and the time-of-night effect. *Sleep Res., 14,* 115.

Reinsel, R., Antrobus, J., and Wollman, M. (1992). Bizarreness in sleep and waking mentation. In J. Antrobus, M. Bertini (Eds.), *TheNeuropsychology of Dreaming Sleep* (pp. 157–186). Hillsdale, NJ: Erlbaum Associates.

Reynolds, C. F., Taska, L. S., Jarrett, D. B., Coble, P. A., and Kupfer, D. J. (1983). REM latency in depression: Is there one best definition? *Biol. Psychiatry, 18,* 849–863.

Roehrs, T., Merlotti, L., Petrucelli, N., Stepanski, E., and Roth, T. (1994). Experimental sleep fragmentation. *Sleep, 17,* 438–443.

Roffwarg, H. P. (1979). Association of sleep disorders centers (Diagnostic classification of sleep and arousal disorders, first edition, prepared by the Sleep Disorders Classification Committee, H. P. Roffwarg, Chairman). *Sleep, 2,* 1–137.

Roffwarg, H., Dement, W., Muzio, J., and Fisher, C. (1962). Dream imagery: relationship to rapid eye movements of sleep. *Arch. Gen. Psychiatry, 7,* 235–258.

Roffwarg, H., Muzio, J. N., and Dement, W. C. (1966). Ontogenetic development of the human sleep. dream cycle. *Science, 152,* 604–619.

Rosenlicht, N., and Feinberg 1. (1997). REM sleep=dreaming: only a dream. *SRS Bull., 3,* 10–12.

Rowley, J. T., Stickgold, R., and Hobson, J. A. (1998). Eyelid movements and mental activity at sleep onset. *Conscious. Cogn., 7,* 67–84.

Sampson, H. (1965). Deprivation of dreaming sleep by two methods: 1. Compensatory REM time. *Arch. Gen. Psychiatry, 13,* 79–86.

Sampson, H. (1966). Psychological effects of deprivation of dreaming sleep. *J. Nerv. Ment. Dis., 143,* 305–317.

Sassin, J. F., Parker, D. C., Mace, J. W., Gotlin, R. W., Johnson, L. C., and Rossman, L. G. (1969). Human growth hormone release: Relation to slow-wave sleep and sleep-waking cycles. *Science, 165,* 513–515.

Schredl, M., and Hofmann, F. (2003). Continuity between waking activities and dream activities. *Conscious Cogn., 12,* 298–308.

Sewitch, D. E., and Kupfer, D. J. (1985). A comparison of the Telediagnostic and Medilog systems of recording normal sleep in the home environment. *Psychophysiology, 22,* 7 18–726.

Shimizu, A., and Inoue, T. (1986). Dreamed speech and speech muscle activity. *Psychophysiology,* 23(2), 210–214.

Singer, J. L. (1978). Experimental studies of daydreaming and the stream of thought. In K. S. Pope, and J. L. Singer (Eds.), *The Stream of Consciousness* (pp. 187–223). New York: Plenum Press.

Skaggs, W. E., and McNaughton, B. L. (1996). Replay of neuronal firing sequences in rat hippocampus during sleep following spatial experience. *Science, 272,* 1870–1873.

Snyder, F. (1966). Toward an evolutionary theory of dreaming. *Am. J. Psychiatry, 123,* 121–142.

Snyder, F. (1970). The phenomenology of dreaming. In H. Madow, and L. H. Snow (Eds.), *The Psychodynamic Implications of the Physiological Studies on Dreams* (pp. 124–151). Springfield, IL: Thomas.

Snyder, F., Hobson, J., and Goldfrank, F. (1963). Blood pressure changes during human sleep. *Science, 142,* 1313–1314.

Snyder, F., Hobson, J., Morrison, D., and Goldfrank, F. (1964). Changes in respiration, heart rate, and systolic blood pressure in human sleep. *J. Appl. Physiol., 19,* 417–422.

Spiegel, K., Leproult, R., Colecchia, E. F., L'Hermite-Baleriaux, M., Nie, Z. Copinschi, G., and Van Cauter, E. (2000). Adaptation of the 24-h growth hormone profile to a state of sleep debt. *Am. J. Physiol. Regul. Integr. Comp. Physiol., 279,* R874–R883

Spiegel, K., Leproult, R., L'Hermite-Baleriaux, M., Copinschi, G., Penev, P. D., and Van Cauter, E. (2004). Leptin levels are dependent on sleep duration: Relationships with sympathovagal balance, carbohydrate regulation, cortisol and thyrotropin. *J. Clin. Endocrinol. Metab., 89,* 5762–5771.

Spiegel, K., Leproult, R., and Van Cauter, E. (1999). Impact of sleep debt on metabolic and endocrine function. *The Lancet, 354* 1435–1439.

Stepanski, E., Lamphere, J., Badia, P., Zorick, F., and Roth, T. (1984). Sleep fragmentation and daytime sleepiness. *Sleep, 7,* 18–26.

Stepanski, E., Lamphere, J., Roehrs, T., Zorick, F., and Roth, T. (1987). Experimental sleep fragmentation in normal subjects. *Intern. J. Neurosci., 33,* 207–214.

Steriade. M., Amzica. F., and Contreras. D. (1996). Synchronization of Fast (30–40 Hz) spontaneous cortical rhythms during brain activation. *J. Neurosci., 16,* 392–417.

Steriade, M., and McCarley, R. W. (1990). *Brainstem control of wakefulness and sleep.* New York: Plenum Press.

Stickgold, R. and Hobson, J. A. (1996). On-line vigilance monitoring with the Nightcap. *Sleep Res., 25,* 533.

Stickgold, R., James, L., and Hobson, J. A. (2000). Visual discrimination learning requires sleep after training. *Nature Neurosci., 3,* 1237–1238.

Stickgold, R., Pace-Schott, E., and Hobson, J. A. (1994). A new paradigm for dream research: Mentation reports following spontaneous arousal from REM and NREM sleep recorded in a home setting. *Conscious Cogn., 3,* 16–29.

Sussman, P., Moffitt, A., Hoffman, R., Wells, R., and Shearer, J. (1979). The description of structural and temporal characteristics of tonic electrophysiological activity during sleep. *Waking and Sleeping, 3,* 279–290.

Thakkar, M. (1996). REM sleep: A biochemical perspective. *SRS Bull., 2*(1–2), 22–28.

Tracy, R. L., and Tracy, L. N. (1974). Reports of mental activity from sleep stages 2 and 4. *Percept. Motor Skills, 38,* 647–648.

Trinder, J., Whitworth, F., Kay, A., and Wilkin, P. (1992). Respiratory instability during sleep onset *J. Appl. Physiol., 73,* 2462–2469.

Van Cauter, E., and Spiegel, K. (1999) Sleep as a mediator of the relationship between socioeconomic status and health: A hypothesis. *Ann. N. Y. Acad. Sci., 896,* 254–261.

Van der Kolk, B., Blitz, R., Burr, W., Sherry, S., and Hartmann, E. (1984). Nightmares and trauma: A comparison of nightmares after combat with lifelong nightmares in veterans. *Am. J. Psychiatry., 141,* 187–190.

Van Dongen, H. P. A., Baynard, M. D., Maislin, G., and Dinges, D. F. (2003). The cumulative cost of additional wakefulness: Dose-response effects on neurobehavioral functions and sleep physiology from chronic restriction and total sleep deprivation. *Sleep, 2,* 117–126.

Van Dongen, H. P. A., Maislin, G., Mullington, J. M., and Dinges, D. F. (2004). Systematic interindividual differences in neurobehavioral impairment from sleep loss: Evidence of trait-like differential vulnerability. *Sleep, 27,* 423–433.

Verdone, P. (1963). *Variables related to the temporal reference of manifest dream content.* Unpublished doctoral dissertation, University of Chicago.

Verdone, P. (1965). Temporal reference of manifest dream content. *Percept. Mot. Skills, 20,* 1253–1268.

Vogel, G. W. (1975). Review of REM sleep deprivation. *Arch. Gen. Psychiatry, 32,* 749–761.

Vogel, G. W. (1978). Sleep-onset mentation. In A. Arkin, J. Antrobus, and S Ellman (Eds.), *The Mind in Sleep* (pp. 97–108). Hillsdale, NJ: Lawrence Erlbaum Associates, Inc.

Vogel, G. W., Barrowclough, B., and Giesler, D. (1972). Limited discriminability of REM and sleep onset reports and its psychiatric implications. *Arch. Gen. Psychiatry, 26,* 449–455.

Vogel, G. W., Foulkes, D., and Trosman, H. (1966). Ego functions and dreaming during sleep onset *Arch. Gen. Psychiatry, 14,* 238–248.

Vogel, G. W., Thurmond, A., Gibbons, P., Sloan, K., Boyd, M., and Walker, M. (1975). REM sleep reduction effects on depression syndromes. *Arch. Gen. Psychiatry, 32,* 765–777.

Watson, R. K. (1972). *Mental correlates of periorbital potentials during REM sleep.* Unpublished doctoral dissertation, University of Chicago.

Webb WB. (1993). Dream theories of the ancient world. In M. A. Carskadon (Ed.), *Encyclopedia of Sleep and Dreaming* (pp. 192–194). New York: Macmillan Publishing Company.

Weisz, R., and Foulkes, D. (1970). Home and laboratory dreams collected under uniform sampling conditions. *Psychophysiology, 6,* 588–596.

Whitman, R. (1969). A summary. In M. Kramer (Ed.), *Dream Psychology and the New Biology of Sleep* (pp. 405–442). Springfield, Ill.: Charles C. Thomas.

Wiedenmayer, C. P. (2004). Adaptations or pathologies? Long-term changes in brain and behavior after a single exposure to severe threat. *Neurosci. Biobehav. Rev., 28,* 1–12.

Williams, R. L., Agnew, H. W., Jr., and Webb, W. B. (1964). Sleep patterns in young adults: An EEG study. *Electroencephalogr. Clin. Neurophysiol., 17,* 376–381.

Williams, R. L., Agnew, H. W., Jr., and Webb, W. B. (1966). Sleep patterns in the young adult female: An EEG study. *Electroencephalogr. Clin. Neurophysiol., 20,* 264–266.

Wittern, R. (1989). Sleep theories in antiquity and the Renaissance. In J. A. Horne (Ed.), *Sleep '88,* (pp. 11–22). Stuttgart/New York: Fischer-Verlag.

Wolpert, E. A., and Trosman, H. (1958). Studies in the psychophysiology of dreams. I: Experimental evocation of sequential dream episodes. *Am. Assoc. Arch Neurol. Psychiatry, 79,* 603–606.

Zemaityte, D., Varoneckas, G., and Sokolov, E. (1984). Heart rhythm control during sleep. *Psychophysiology, 21,* 279–289.

Zimmerman, W. B. (1970). Sleep mentation and auditory awakening thresholds. *Psychophysiology, 6,* 540–549.

Applications

SECTION EDITOR: LOUIS G. TASSINARY

28 Psychophysiology in Research on Psychopathology

J. CHRISTOPHER EDGAR, JENNIFER KELLER, WENDY HELLER,
AND GREGORY A. MILLER

Psychophysiological measures such as hemodynamic imaging, electromagnetic source imaging, startle blink, eye movement, and autonomic responses provide diverse and sometimes unique views of an individual's functioning. Psychophysiological findings can corroborate (or contradict) findings from more traditional psychological measures of functioning, including self-report scales, behavioral performance, informant data, and diagnostic interviews as well as complement traditional biological measures spanning endocrine, genetic, and other domains. Psychophysiological findings are also useful in monitoring the time course of mental processes involved in task performance, in measuring mental processes the individual does not report, and in assessing behavior when the production of an overt response is undesired or unavailable (Coles, 1989). In psychopathology research psychophysiological measures are increasingly used as endophenotypes, and researchers increasingly examine the use of psychophysiological measures rather than subjective symptoms to define diagnostic subtypes.

A goal of this chapter is to consider some of the theoretical and practical issues associated with the use of psychophysiological techniques to study psychopathology. The chapter provides a discussion of several theoretical concepts underpinning early psychophysiology studies and some philosophical issues that currently confront psychophysiology researchers, a selective review of psychophysiological studies examining three disorders (anxiety, depression, and schizophrenia), and proposals for how to handle some of the practical difficulties associated with psychophysiological research. The review is necessarily limited, largely ignoring some types of psychopathology and some psychophysiological measures. However, most of the practical problems discussed are not specific to studies discussed below.

HISTORICAL CONTEXT OF PSYCHOPHYSIOLOGICAL STUDY OF PSYCHOPATHOLOGY

Theories of psychopathology often explicitly encompass physiological phenomena, and psychophysiology has been a useful tool for the investigation of clinical phenomena. Much of the best psychophysiological work on psychopathology has been driven by prevailing theory. In order to gain insight into the history of psychophysiological investigation of psychopathology it is important to consider the work in the context of the theoretical concepts of the time.

The concept of nonspecific reactivity was an early influence in psychophysiological research on psychopathology. Individuals with schizophrenia and depression were often noted to appear withdrawn and to exhibit blunted affect. Much early work attempted to account for this behavioral hypoactivity by looking for physiological hyporeactivity. This was consistent with the James-Lange theory of emotion, which defined emotions not merely as correlates of but actually as being peripheral physiological changes. In an attempt to understand emotional abnormalities in psychopathology researchers sought abnormal physiology (e.g., Malmo & Shagass, 1949).

Landis (1932) conducted an extensive review of electrodermal studies looking for a consistent pattern of abnormal physiology in schizophrenia, but none was apparent. Cohen and Patterson (1937) found that changes in pulse rate tended to be larger in patients than controls. Malmo and Shagass (1949, 1952) examined heart rate, electrodermal activity, respiration, and blood pressure in patients with acute or chronic schizophrenia. First-episode patients showed greater reactivity to stressors than either chronic patients or controls, who were similar. These findings were taken as evidence against the notion that behavioral hyporesponsiveness can be attributed to physiological hyporesponsiveness.

Lang and Buss (1968) reviewed the literature on physiological responsivity and found evidence that some individuals with psychopathology were physiologically hyporesponsive to particular stressors. The fact that the hyporesponsiveness was limited to certain types of stressors argued against a generalized deficit in physiological responsivity and accounted for the pervasive deficits seen in psychopathology. Overall, early studies of physiological reactivity in psychopathology suggested that hyporeactivity is more prevalent in more chronic individuals, but that generally patients react normally under higher levels of stimulus intensity.

Many early studies examining reactivity did not provide critical methodological information, such as an adequate description of the patient sample or the stimuli. Diagnostic criteria were not uniform and have evolved considerably. In addition, poor description of stimuli, tasks, or data analysis is problematic given that comparing physiological reactions across groups can be a challenge because differences in basal levels can complicate interpretation of the response (Lacey, 1956).

Over time, the concept of nonspecific physiological reactivity proved not to be broadly viable as a central organizing principle. Lacey (1967), Lang (1968), and others (see Miller & Kozak, 1993) argued convincingly that different response systems too often diverge for the concept to be of general use. Remarkably, to this day the overwhelming evidence for that conclusion is not widely appreciated, and vague concepts of generalized arousal are still invoked all too often in studies of psychopathology and psychophysiology. This usage should be distinguished from arousal concepts applied more defensibly in domains such as in self-report measurement of the dimensions of emotion or theories of region-specific brain activity in emotion and psychopathology (reviewed below) for which "arousal" is more narrowly defined and operationalized.

Another theoretical concept guiding early research was physiological activation. Clinical observations suggested that some psychiatric groups differ from controls in baseline level of physiological activity as opposed to responses to specific stressors. Muscle tension was a common measure of activation, and the general finding was that some patients demonstrated greater skeletal tension than controls (Duffy, 1962). EEG was also used to assess activation, on the assumption that brain activity is inversely and monotonically related to activity in the 8–13 Hz range (alpha band). Davis and Davis (1939) found that patients demonstrated less alpha than did control subjects. Other studies found less resting alpha and more activity in higher and lower bands in anxious subjects (see Duffy, 1962, for review of early EEG findings in psychopathology). Although finding group differences in EEG has not been uncommon in subsequent studies, the functional significance of such differences is often unclear. Global EEG activity as a measure of resting, nonspecific activation has not proven very useful in psychopathology research. For example, more recent work on region-specific alpha has rendered the nonspecific activation concept obsolete (e.g., Salmelin & Hari, 1994), like what had happened to the related but distinct concept of nonspecific arousal.

A third concept that has received substantial psychophysiological attention is physiological dysregulation in psychopathology. In contrast to traditional concepts of arousal and activation, dysregulation has often been conceptualized narrowly rather than as a nonspecific phenomenon operating more or less indiscriminately across peripheral physiological systems or brain regions. Perhaps as a result, the concept of physiological dysregulation has remained a prominent focus in psychopathology research. The early work investigated not only how physiological patterns were disrupted but circumstances that could influence the regulation. Buck, Carscallen, and Hobbs (1950, 1951) reported lower and less variable body temperature in schizophrenia. Ax (1962) analyzed physiological regulation in schizophrenia and suggested that dysregulation was best observed when comparing multiple systems that typically operate together (such as heart rate and respiration). The dysregulation appeared between multiple systems that were not coordinating properly rather than within a single system. Because respiration affects heart rate by means of proprioceptive signals from the chest, diaphragm, and lungs, Ax (1962) suggested that such signals are impaired in schizophrenics. A more recent view of schizophrenia suggested that an impairment of proprioceptive information is involved in the development of positive symptoms (Frith, 1992). These findings on dysregulation are a few of many that reinforce the approach of examining multiple systems. This theme recurs in the review of modern work on psychopathology presented below.

CURRENT PHILOSOPHICAL ISSUES IN PSYCHOPHYSIOLOGICAL RESEARCH

The potential of psychophysiology to contribute to the study of psychopathology has been undermined historically by two common, problematic assumptions. First, naively reductionistic conceptualizations of the relationship between psychological and physiological phenomena have been a consistent embarrassment in psychopathology research for decades. Approaches that aim to identify either the biological or the psychological phenomena "underlying" psychopathology fail to recognize that psychopathology must be understood in terms of both biological and psychological factors. Indeed, it is not clear whether biology underlies psychology, whether psychology underlies biology, or whether the concept "underlie" is even a valid representation of the relationships among psychological and biological phenomena (for further discussion see Miller, 1996; Miller & Keller, 2000; Miller, in press).

A second problematic assumption is grounded in the psychological realm but has implications for the selection and interpretation of biological measures. Phenomena of interest in psychopathology (and in psychology more generally) are often dichotomized into emotion and cognition. In psychophysiology, this dichotomy often plays out as an implicit assumption that central nervous system measures are appropriate for the study of cognition, whereas peripheral nervous system measures are better suited to the study of emotion. Yet there is very little theoretical need or empirical support for this dichotomy or for limiting which physiological measures to associate with which psychological events. A common misstep in research on psychopathology, especially research emphasizing cognitive processes, is to seem to differentiate emotion from cognition without carefully articulating the distinction and then to invoke "emotion" as some qualitatively distinct phenomenon or process that drives or is driven by (and in any case is quite distinct from) cognition. It is far more parsimonious to assume that emotion processing involves the same types of psychological and biological computations that accomplish cognition and to employ emotion in one's model accordingly (for further discussion see Miller, 1996; Miller & Keller, 2000; Miller, Engels, & Herrington, in press).

The growing appeal of psychophysiological measures in research on psychopathology reflects their specificity to the operation of mental processes associated with symptoms of psychopathology. An exclusive focus on behavioral symptoms can be a frustrating basis for identification of related mental events. Similar disturbances in mental processing can be associated with different symptoms, just as disturbances of different mental processes can lead to similar symptoms. By studying mental processes as opposed to symptoms or traditional diagnoses alone, it is possible to determine diverse manifestations of a disease process in cognitive and emotional function. Although the present chapter reflects the historical emphasis on psychological processes in psychophysiology, psychophysiological measures are equally valuable for research questions emphasizing physiological processes (Miller, 2000; Miller & Ebert, 1988). Thus, for example, psychopathology is by definition a disorder of psychological functioning and not of biological function (Miller & Keller, 2000; Kozak & Miller, 1982; Miller, 1996). However, the value of understanding the neurobiology of normal and abnormal psychological functioning is now widely appreciated. Because of its noninvasive technology and its sophistication in psychological theory and experimental design, psychophysiology remains at the forefront of the increasingly biological agenda in psychopathology research.

PSYCHOPHYSIOLOGICAL STUDIES OF PSYCHOPATHOLOGY: SELECTED EXAMPLES

There is an ongoing debate in the psychopathology literature about whether to view psychological disorders as discrete categories or within a dimensional framework (Clark, Watson, & Reynolds, 1995; Millon, 1991; Widiger & Samuel, 2005), but the bulk of psychophysiological research has assumed a categorical approach. The present focus on three diagnostic categories that have received the most attention from psychophysiological studies (anxiety disorders, depression, and schizophrenia) is not intended as an endorsement of a categorical approach over a dimensional approach or a judgment that standard categories are most appropriate for psychophysiological study.

For each disorder, rather than a cursory overview of the many different psychophysiological techniques that have been used to examine each disorder, a detailed review of

the use of psychophysiological measures to examine particular constructs (e.g., selective attention) or brain regions (e.g., hippocampus) is provided. In providing an in-depth examination of particular research areas – comparing and contrasting findings across studies – conceptual and pragmatic difficulties associated with research in each area are highlighted. As will become evident, the difficulties discussed (e.g., dealing with patients with comorbid disorders) are common to all psychophysiological studies of psychopathology.

Anxiety disorders

Fourteen anxiety disorders are listed in the Diagnostic and Statistical Manual of Mental Disorders (DSM-IV-TR; American Psychiatric Association, 2000, pp. 754–755). That list does not take into account potential dimensions of anxiety suggested in the literature (e.g., Barlow, 1988, 1991; Heller et al., 1997; Koven et al., 2003), subclinical forms, or degrees of anxiety studied in the personality literature and probably of great clinical relevance. The debate about whether mental disorders should be seen as discrete categories or as points on a continuum of normal behavior is prominent in the anxiety literature because it is unclear whether subclinical anxiety and the various anxiety disorders are best conceptualized in terms of one or more dimensions or as qualitatively distinct phenomena. Even if healthy and pathological anxiety represents distinct phenomena, there may be some overlap between them including their physiology. Thus, it is useful to study nonclinical individuals under stressful and anxiety-provoking conditions as well as individuals with pathological anxiety.

When studying psychopathology with psychophysiological measures, one issue that arises is whether the focus of study is mechanisms of the psychopathology itself or the consequences of the psychopathology. Physiological differences are often discussed as if they are due to anxiety rather than being part of anxiety. Such a view may misrepresent the role of physiology in anxiety or in any emotion. Lang (1968, 1978) addressed the study of emotions by proposing the "three-systems" model, which suggests that emotions are expressed in three observable domains: verbal, physiological, and behavioral activity. Thus, a complete picture of normal and pathological emotion requires assessment of all three. Although the three-systems model is widely cited, a more subtle but equally fundamental recommendation in Lang's work is less widely appreciated (see Miller & Kozak, 1993, for discussion). Lang suggested that the activity of all three systems is part of anxiety, and not due to anxiety. For example, elevated heart rate or lateralized EEG patterns are not responses to an anxious state, but part of what it means to be in an anxious state. Similarly, physiological events during fear-provoking imagery are not responses to imagery stimuli but part of the process of imagery.

Psychophysiological approaches to anxiety long focused on autonomic measures (see Zahn, 1986). Interest has grown in modulation of the startle reflex (Blumenthal et al., 2005; Bradley, in press; Cuthbert, in press) and in brain regions (Bradley, in press; Davidson, Jackson, & Larson, 2000) that become more or less active during periods of anxiety. Although some early studies found no relationship between anxiety and cerebral metabolism (Giordani et al., 1990), most have suggested that one hemisphere is more active during anxiety than the other. However, the direction of this effect has been inconsistent (for reviews see Nitschke et al., 1999; Heller et al., 1997; Heller et al., 2002).

In light of these inconsistencies, Gruzelier (1989) and Heller and colleagues (Heller, Etienne, & Miller, 1995; Heller et al., 1997; Heller, Koven, & Miller, 2003; Nitschke et al., 1999) suggested that anxiety can favor either hemisphere, and the direction is dependent on the severity and type of anxiety. They suggested that left-hemisphere involvement is associated with anxious apprehension, which is reflected in cognitive processes such as worry, rumination, and obsessional thinking, whereas right-hemisphere involvement is associated with anxious arousal, which is reflected in sympathetic nervous system activity and cognitive processes such as vigilance and enhanced hemispatial attention. These types reflect lateralized EEG findings and behavioral data from lateralized tasks, although evidence using autonomic measures also suggests that subtypes of anxiety can be dissociated (Zahn, 1986). Studies of both central and autonomic measures associated with anxiety will be necessary to develop a more complete theory of these dimensions and how they relate to DSM subtypes (Keller, Hicks, & Miller, 2000).

Diagnostic categories of anxiety are distinguished in part by whether there is a specific eliciting event. Research on anxiety disorders in which specific stressors or circumstances are found to elicit anxiety, such as simple phobias, social phobia, and post-traumatic stress disorder (PTSD), has noted a number of psychophysiological changes during exposure to anxiety-eliciting stimuli. When anxiety has a specific prompt, the individual generally responds with increased sympathetic autonomic activity (see Hugdahl, 1989, and Öst, 1989, for reviews on simple phobias and panic disorder, agoraphobia, and social phobia). However, an unusually large clinical case series documented considerable differential somatic physiology as a function of type of anxiety (Cuthbert et al., 2003). Importantly, the pattern of self-reported symptoms did not align well with the differential physiology, which suggests distinct and somewhat complex relationships of various observable indicators of anxiety to underlying processes that may speak to the responsiveness of different types of anxiety to various types of therapy.

Whereas research on generalized anxiety has used central nervous system measures such as EEG and rCBF, the vast majority of research on stimulus-specific anxiety disorders employed autonomic measures until recently. This emphasis on autonomic measures in the study of emotion may reflect two arguable assumptions. The first assumption is that anxiety is an emotional disorder as opposed to a disorder of cognition. As discussed above, it is unnecessary to assume that a given psychological phenomenon should be understood in exclusively emotional or exclusively cognitive terms. The second problematic assumption is that, if anxiety is a disorder of emotion, it is more appropriate to study it using physiological measures historically associated with emotion rather than those typically associated with cognition. As noted above, this historically common assumption is unnecessary. Anxiety can be investigated with either central or peripheral measures.

Posttraumatic stress disorder (PTSD). To illustrate roles for both central and peripheral measures when researching anxiety disorders, psychophysiological findings for PTSD will be selectively reviewed. This is a rapidly growing research area, and the number of reviews of psychophysiological studies on PTSD continues to grow (McNally, 2003; Shin, Rauch, & Pitman, in press; Shin et al., 2004a; Karl, Malta, & Maercker, 2006).

In autonomic studies, PTSD patients have consistently been found more reactive to trauma-related stimuli than a variety of groups, including nonPTSD trauma victims, nonpsychiatric controls, and other anxiety-disordered patients. This has been observed across a variety of experimental contexts, including paradigms using auditory and visual traumatic stimuli and script-driven imagery (e.g., Pitman et al., 1987; Prins, Kaloupek, & Keane, 1995).

With PTSD patients clearly hyperresponsive to trauma-related stimuli, it is important to determine whether the hyperresponsiveness is limited to trauma-related stimuli. Some studies have found that PTSD patients are not hyperresponsive in trauma-neutral contexts, such as mental arithmetic (e.g., Blanchard et al., 1996; Gerardi, Blanchard, & Kolb, 1989; Pallmeyer, Blanchard, & Kolb, 1986), whereas others have found an exaggerated startle response to neutral auditory stimuli (see Prins, Kaloupek, & Keane, 1995).

EEG studies examining PTSD patients' responses to nontrauma stimuli have found differences in various ERP components. P50 auditory sensory gating, augmenting-reducing P200, and P300 in target detection oddball tasks are the most frequently studied ERP components. For example, employing a paired-click task to examine auditory gating processes, Gillette et al. (1997) observed impaired P50 gating in individuals with combat-related PTSD, with gating ratios correlating with intensity of PTSD re-experiencing symptoms (e.g., trauma-related nightmares and flashbacks). Although the finding of abnormal P50 gating in subjects with PTSD has been replicated (e.g., Ghisolfi et al., 2004, Neylan et al., 1999, Skinner et al., 1999), the relationship between PTSD symptoms and impaired gating is unclear. For example, Metzger et al. (2002), examining female Vietnam nurse veterans with and without current PTSD, observed that reduced P50 suppression was associated with increased severity of general psychopathology, but not with a PTSD diagnosis. In addition, as described below, atypical P50 gating ratios are observed in many patient populations. Research is needed to determine the significance of impaired auditory gating in PTSD and to examine auditory gating differences between patient groups. In any case, the P50 findings are clearly indicative of abnormal brain activity in response to nontrauma stimuli.

Perhaps the most commonly studied ERP component is the P300, a positive voltage shift in the EEG time-locked to an infrequent or significant event. McFarlane, Weber, & Clark (1993) examined midline ERPs in a three-tone auditory oddball task in controls and patients with PTSD. For the PTSD group, N200, a negative-going ERP component that typically occurs following the recognition of a change in the stimulus series, occurred later. P300 amplitude was smaller and did not distinguish the infrequent tones, whereas controls demonstrated larger P300 to targets than to distracters. McFarlane, Weber and Clark (1993) suggested that patients spent more time on stimulus discrimination, reflected in N200 latency, which leaves fewer resources available for subsequent processing, as evidenced by decreased P300 amplitude.

P300 abnormalities in PTSD have been replicated by some investigators (e.g., Charles et al., 1995; Metzger et al., 1997a; Metzger et al., 1997b), but not others (e.g., Metzger et al., 2002, observed increased target P3b amplitudes in female Vietnam nurse veterans with PTSD). It appears that some differences across studies may be attributable to a more variable P300 in individuals with PTSD (see Neylan et al., 2003). At present, P300 findings suggest the importance of examining measures of variability as well as measures of central tendency, and highlight the need to consider the role of comorbid diagnoses and medication effects when interpreting results.

Difficulty in trauma-related recall is a cardinal feature of PTSD, and several studies have reported impaired performance on tests of verbal and visual memory (e.g., Bremner et al., 1993; Bustamante et al., 2001; Gilbertson et al., 2001). Given the role of the hippocampus in memory processes, researchers have become interested in hippocampal structure and function in PTSD subjects. Interest in the hippocampus also comes from theories about the effect of stress on the hippocampus. Nadel and Jacobs (1998) proposed that some symptoms of PTSD reflect hippocampal damage secondary to stress-related steroid exposure. A number of subsequent authors have endorsed this view, but McNally (2003) argued that having a small hippocampus is a risk factor for, rather than a result of, clinically significant PTSD. Although several studies have observed reduced hippocampal volume in individuals with PTSD (e.g., Bremner et al., 1995; Bremner et al., 2003; Gilbertson et al., 2002; Gurvits et al., 1996; Lindauer et al., 2004; Villarreal et al., 2002a), these findings have not been consistently replicated (e.g., DeBellis et al., 1999, DeBellis et al., 2001; Bonne et al., 2001; Schuff et al., 2001). Aside from reduced hippocampal volume, magnetic resonance spectroscopy (MRS) studies have reported decreased neu-

ronal integrity in hippocampus, as measured by decreased N-acetylaspartate (NAA) levels (e.g., Schuff et al., 2001; Villarreal et al., 2002b).

Although there is clear evidence for structural hippocampal abnormalities in at least a subset of individuals with PTSD, the significance of these abnormalities is uncertain. For example, examining bilaterally reduced hippocampal volume in abused women with PTSD and without PTSD, Bremner et al. (2003) reported that in abused women with PTSD measures of symptoms of dissociation were correlated with smaller left hippocampal volume, and measures of PTSD symptoms were correlated with smaller right hippocampal volume. Bremner et al. (2003) additionally noted that smaller hippocampal volume was not seen in all subjects with a history of childhood abuse, but only in subjects with both a history of abuse and a diagnosis of PTSD. In an earlier study, Gurvits et al. (1996) reported that hippocampal volume is negatively correlated with amount of combat exposure, and suggested that repeated traumatic stress damages the hippocampus. However, in contrast to these studies, examining hippocampal volume in controls, trauma-exposed subjects with PTSD, and trauma-exposed subjects without PTSD, Winter and Irle (2004) found significantly smaller volumes of the right hippocampus in both trauma-exposed groups (severe burn subjects both with and without PTSD). In addition, larger total areas of burned body surface were significantly related to smaller left hippocampal volumes, and the use of analgesic/sedative treatment of the N-methyl-D-aspartic acid (NMDA) antagonist ketamine was significantly related to larger right hippocampal volumes and to stronger PTSD symptoms. Winter and Irle concluded that small hippocampal size may not be associated with PTSD, but instead reflects the result of traumatic stress. In addition, although the application of NMDA antagonists may protect against hippocampal damage induced by traumatic stressors, this treatment strategy increases the patient's risk of developing PTSD symptoms. Additional studies examining trauma subjects with and without PTSD are needed to replicate and interpret these recent findings.

In addition to structural abnormalities, several studies have observed abnormal hippocampal activation (Semple et al., 1993; Bremner et al., 2003; Osuch et al., 2001; Shin et al., 2004; although see Rauch et al., 1996). In a PET study examining hippocampal rCBF during an explicit memory recall task, Shin et al. (2004) took findings of generally elevated hippocampal activity in firefighters with PTSD as indicative of both reduced efficiency of hippocampus during the performance of a memory task or impaired integrity of inhibitory interneurons within the hippocampus. They further observed that symptom severity was positively associated with rCBF in hippocampus and parahippoampal gyrus. These findings are similar to the positive correlation between flashback intensity during symptom provocation and perihippocampal rCBF observed by Osuch et al. (2001).

Although both structural and functional hippocampal abnormalities are consistently observed in subjects with PTSD, research examining the relationship between functional and structural abnormalities is needed, which is a point underscored by Shin et al. (2004). Noting that rCBF abnormalities in the hippocampus might reflect a functional compensation for reduced hippocampal volumes, Shin et al. (2004) hypothesized that hippocampal rCBF changes should correlate with hippocampal volumes and that statistically controlling for hippocampal volumes should eliminate the group differences in rCBF increases (see Roadblocks and Recommendations section for a discussion on methods for controlling for group differences). However, they found neither to be true, and noting a small sample size (N = 8 per group) they indicated the need for further research in this area with larger samples.

As with other physiological measures, studies examining the relationship between hippocampal structure and function, state/trait factors, and premorbid risk factors are of interest, especially with regard to etiological theories of PTSD. Whereas one line of research suggests that stress-induced neurotoxicity causes hippocampal damage (glucocorticoids secreted during stress), a separate line of research suggests hippocampal abnormalities predate trauma exposure (see Sapolsky, 2002 for a succinct overview of these findings). Given that hippocampal abnormalities are sometimes observed in other disorders (e.g., depression, Steffens et al., 2000; Frodl et al., 2002), the clinical implications of hippocampal abnormalities in subjects with PTSD have yet to be determined.

Summary. Autonomic measures had been the predominant psychophysiological tool in anxiety research, but it is becoming clear that central nervous system measures provide valuable information about the nature of anxiety. Aside from examining differences in stimulus, paradigm, and data analysis methods, an examination of the relationship of state/trait factors and premorbid risk factors to psychophysiological measures is clearly of interest. Also warranting attention is the high rate of comorbidity in PTSD, including major depression, other anxiety disorders, and substance abuse. Bremner (2003) and Friedman and Yehuda (1995) cautioned against the exclusion of patients with comorbid depression and anxiety from PTSD because excluding subjects with these comorbid disorders would in many cases result in an unrepresentative selection of subjects with PTSD. Additionally, a history of early life stress (such as early parental loss or childhood physical or sexual abuse) can confound some of the psychophysiological findings in PTSD (e.g., Heim & Nemeroff, 2002). Successful investigations of PTSD will need to deal with comorbidity issues. Heller and Nitschke (1998), Miller (in press), Miller, Engels, and Herrington (in press), and Mineka, Watson, and Clark (1998) discussed this issue for anxiety and related disorders more generally.

Mood disorders

Research on mood disorders and research on anxiety disorders share some critical elements (Heller & Nitschke, 1998; Heller et al., 2002). Mood and anxiety are both broad constructs, and diagnostic criteria designed to provide discrete boundaries for each disorder may leave much ambiguity. DSM-IV recognizes several mood disorders, including major depression, dysthymia, bipolar disorder, and several subtypes. Additional distinctions within depression have been utilized, including endogenous/exogenous and agitated/retarded as well as a depressive personality subtype. This range of depressive syndromes can complicate the comparison and interpretation of findings. A second issue is the problem of comorbidity. Depression often co-occurs with anxiety, substance abuse, and other disorders. Isolated or subsyndromal symptoms of depression and anxiety are found in other psychological disorders, and symptoms of other disorders may occur in individuals whose primary disorder is depression or anxiety. Research based on well defined theoretical models and well characterized subject groups can help address these issues, but to date such efforts are too rare to permit much integration. This area is especially in need of the improved delimitation of homogeneous endophenotypes (whether defined categorically or dimensionally) that psychophysiology may foster, as discussed above.

Functional asymmetries in depression. One emphasis that has received increasing attention in psychophysiological research is the relationship between asymmetric activity in specific brain regions, affective factors such as valence, and approach versus defensive withdrawal motivation, and specific aspects of cognition. Recent research examining the central circuitry of depression has identified abnormal activity patterns in the dorsolateral prefrontal cortex (DLPFC) during resting states (for review, see Nitschke et al., 2004). A number of positron emission tomography (PET) studies have reported bilateral DLPFC decreases in blood flow and glucose metabolism (for a recent review see Davidson, 2004). Decreased DLPFC activity has also been observed during task performance. Depressed patients showed less DLPFC activity bilaterally on a complex planning task than nonpsychiatric controls in a PET study measuring blood flow (Elliott et al., 1997).

Other evidence suggests that right DLPFC figures importantly in the negative memory bias accompanying depression. An extensive literature has implicated right PFC mechanisms in withdrawal-related negative emotions and in threat perception. Activity in this region under such circumstances is likely to contribute to a negative memory bias (for reviews, see Davidson, 1998; Heller & Nitschke, 1997; Nitschke & Heller, 2002). Furthermore, numerous electroencephalography (EEG) studies have reported more right than left PFC activity in depression (for reviews, see Davidson & Henriques, 2000; Davidson et al., 2002;

Heller & Nitschke, 1997, 1998). A similar pattern of asymmetry has also been observed in a number of the above-mentioned PET studies showing bilateral DLPFC decreases, in which hypoactivity was more pronounced on the left.

Although these findings indicate an asymmetry in favor of the right PFC in depression, investigation into the brain mechanisms contributing specifically to the negative explicit memory bias in depressed subjects has only recently begun. An ERP study revealed no evidence of a negative memory bias in depressed patients, including no topographical differences for P300 between patients and nonpsychiatric controls during encoding or recognition of negative words or faces (Deldin, Keller, Gergen, & Miller, 2001). Another ERP study examining the slow-wave component for negative adjectives in a delayed-match-to-sample paradigm primarily implicated left parietal irregularities in depressed patients with some right PFC abnormalities observed for correlations with depression severity (Deldin, Deveney, Kim, Casad, & Best, 2001). However, behavioral data indicated that the paradigm was not successful in eliciting an overt negative working memory bias in depressed patients. A fMRI study (Elliott et al., 2002) examined another type of processing bias via an emotional go/no-go task previously shown to result in a bias toward sad stimuli in depressed patients. They reported greater right DLPFC activity for sad stimuli in patients than nonpsychiatric controls. Finally, an earlier blood flow study using PET assessing attentional biases did not report DLPFC abnormalities in depressed patients for a standard Stroop paradigm or an emotional Stroop task (George et al., 1997). Thus, although results from studies examining the brain's instantiation of negative memory biases in depression have thus far been mixed, other research on emotion, depression, and anxiety leads to predictions of right prefrontal engagement.

Psychophysiological studies of memory bias in depression are beginning to make sense of a conflicted literature. Nitschke et al. (2004) measured EEG immediately prior to and during the auditory presentation of a sad narrative in a sample of college students with extreme levels (low and high) of depression and anxiety. Bilateral activity recorded over PFC during a preparatory period immediately preceding the sad narrative was associated with better memory performance in participants reporting low levels of depression but not in those with high levels of depression. This finding is consistent with behavioral studies (for reviews, see Hertel, 1994, 2000) suggesting that depressed individuals do not initiate task-relevant cognitive processes unless concrete strategies are provided. Corroborating other research implicating the right PFC in withdrawal-related negative emotions and threat perception, factors that may play a role in negative cognitive biases (Heller & Nitschke, 1997; Nitschke & Heller, 2002), high depression participants showed an association between right PFC activity when exposed to the sad narrative and improved subsequent recognition of words used in that narrative.

These right PFC findings are highly consistent with prior studies investigating various forms of withdrawal-related negative emotions (Davidson et al., 2002, Davidson et al., 2003; Heller & Nitschke, 1997; Nitschke & Heller, 2002). On the other hand, the bilateral frontal effect supporting Hertel's model was particularly pronounced on the left, as indicated by an analysis on asymmetry scores. Such a pattern would be expected to the extent that initiating cognitive strategies is approach-related (e.g., Davidson et al., 2003) or involves verbal processing. In addition, the analyses for EEG data (regardless of memory performance) replicated previous findings. During preparation for the sad narrative, there was a trend for high-depression subjects to show relatively less left than right frontal activity compared to the low depression subjects (for review, see Davidson et al., 2002).

The associations between brain activity and subsequent memory performance in this study are consistent with two seemingly conflicting literatures, one which documents memory deficits in depression and another which reports better memory performance for negative material. Those studies finding memory deficits in depressed samples either have not used negative stimuli or have not systematically assessed the emotional content of the material tested. These findings provide a neurocognitive account for why memory performance in depression might be impaired in some circumstances and enhanced in others. Furthermore, the confluence of the cognitive-initiative deficit producing memory impairment and the negative memory bias producing selective memory enhancement may result in no apparent memory effects in depressed individuals under certain circumstances.

A more longstanding lateralization literature in depression has developed around EEG alpha as an (inverse) measure of emotion-related regional brain activity. Although controversial with regard to methodology and interpretation (Allen et al., 2004), a considerable number of studies point to important differences in cortical activity as a function of emotion and as a function of depression (Davidson, 2004). Surprisingly, until Herrington et al. (2005) the hemodynamic imaging literature was unable to observe the effects long seen with EEG. This study focused on DLPFC activation during an emotional Stroop task. Whereas the EEG literature has invariably included hemisphere as a factor in the analysis, in the cognitive fMRI literature this has been remarkably rare because the analysis tradition unfortunately has tended not to include brain region as a factor. Davidson (1998) argued that explicit laterality tests are essential in most such cases. Herrington et al. (2005) included hemisphere and obtained a Valence × Hemisphere interaction reflecting a highly significant enhancement of left-DLPFC activity for pleasant stimuli relative to unpleasant stimuli versus a small and nonsignificant enhancement in the homologous right-DLPFC region. Using the same fMRI paradigm, Mohanty et al. (2005) demonstrated differential DLPFC lateralization in response to emotional words as a function of trait schizotypy. Thus, the fMRI literature is beginning to come into line with the large EEG literature on frontal laterality and emotion. A next step will be studying depression with these methods.

Although less studied than frontal asymmetries, abnormal asymmetries in activity for posterior regions have also been described in depression. Heller (1993) suggested that autonomic activity related to emotion is modulated by right-posterior cortex activity. Reduced right-posterior activity is associated with depressed mood, whereas increased right-posterior activity is associated with anxiety characterized by autonomic hyperarousal. Support came from studies showing that depressives have a selective deficit on right-hemisphere tasks (e.g., Rubinow & Post, 1992; Silberman, Weingartner, & Post, 1983). Depressives have also shown a right-hemisphere deficit in paradigms using lateralized stimulus presentation (Bruder, 1995). This abnormal lateralization has been linked to clinical features of depression, such as subtype and treatment outcome. Furthermore, depressives have been reported to show an attentional bias reflecting underutilization of the posterior right hemisphere (Heller, Etienne, & Miller, 1995; Jaeger, Borod, & Peselow, 1987) on the Chimeric Faces Task, a free-vision facial affect processing test (Levy et al., 1983). Keller, Hicks, and Miller (2000) directly addressed this issue in studies of patients and nonpatients with varying amounts of comorbid depression and anxiety. Two experiments, one using patients and a community control group and another using questionnaire-selected nonpatients with controlled amounts of comorbidity, showed the same pattern of more right-posterior activity in anxiety, less in depression, and a nonadditive combined effect associated with comorbidity.

Right-parietal involvement in depression has also been supported by EEG studies reporting decreased brain activity near right-posterior areas in major depressives during tasks of dichotic listening (Bruder et al., 1995), nonlateralized emotional face presentation (Deldin et al., 2000), and verbal memory (Henriques & Davidson, 1995), though not in language processing (Deldin et al., 2006). Neuropsychological findings and theoretical perspectives of Heller and colleagues (e.g., Heller, Etienne, & Miller, 1995) emphasizing the importance of comorbidity in identifying right posterior involvement have been firmly supported by Bruder's research with clinical populations (Bruder, 1995; Bruder et al., 1997; Bruder et al., 2002; Bruder et al., 1999). Decreased right-posterior activity has been found in individuals with remitted depression (Henriques & Davidson, 1990), which suggests that the relationship reflects trait and not state characteristics of depression. Blood-flow studies have reported similar findings (e.g., Flor-Henry, 1979; Post et al., 1987; Uytdenhoef et al., 1983), but with some exceptions (see Davidson & Tomarken, 1989). Extensive reviews are available from Mayberg and Fossati (in press) and Shestyuk and Deldin (in press).

Amygdalar abnormalities in depression. Numerous studies have examined the structure and function of the amygdala, although findings in depression have been mixed. Increased amygdala volumes have been observed in first-episode major depression patients (Frodl et al., 2002) and patients with dysthymia (Tebartz van Elst et al., 1999). However, amygdala atrophy has also been associated with chronic depression (Sheline et al., 1999), and it has been suggested that depressed individuals have smaller core amygdala nuclei than never-depressed individuals. Potentially this is due to hypercortisolemia, which facilitates excitotoxic effects of glutamate (Sheline et al., 1999). Other studies have not observed altered amygdala volumes in depression (Mervaala et al., 2000; Frodl et al., 2002).

Studies examining blood flow in depression suggest increased activation in limbic and paralimbic areas, such as the amygdala, hippocampus, and basal ganglia (for review, see Mayberg & Fossati, in press). In the amygdala, both increased activity during a resting state (e.g., Abercrombie et al., 1998; Drevets et al., 2002) and reduced activity during an experimental task (e.g., Kimbrell et al., 2002; Thomas et al., 2001) have been observed. Depressed patients (both unipolar and bipolar) have also demonstrated increased left amygdala metabolism correlated with depression severity and plasma cortisol levels (Drevets et al., 2002), and elevated amygdala metabolism during remission has also been associated with a risk for relapse (Bremner et al., 1997). Increased resting amygdala metabolism may be specific to primary mood disorders because increased amygdala metabolism has not been observed in anxiety disorders (Drevets, 2003).

Several studies have examined amygdala activation in response to emotionally valenced stimuli. Thomas et al. (2001) found that, although healthy subjects showed increased left amygdala activity in response to fear pictures, this response was blunted in depressed adults. Similarly, Thomas et al. (2001) found a decreased amygdala response in depressed children and an increased response with anxious children. However, other researchers have observed exaggerated left amygdala responses in major depression in response to fearful stimuli (Sheline et al., 2001). Although the available data show some inconsistencies, this relatively new work on cognitive and emotional processing in mood disorders is an exciting area that has potential to integrate theories of depression and psychophysiology.

Summary. For some time, there has been considerable focus on the role of attentional resources or cognitive workload and on whether resource allocation is deficient in depression. Research strongly suggests that the psychological deficits seen in depression reflect reduced initiative and strategic information processing associated with deficient prefrontal activity, especially the left hemisphere. This work remains to be systematically integrated with the extensive literature on asymmetric activity in specific brain regions, affective valence, and cognitive processing. Recent research examining the central circuitry of depression has identified abnormal activity patterns in DLPFC and in posterior brain regions. Functional and structural abnormalities have also been observed in limbic and paralimbic areas. Across all areas of study, research based on well-defined theoretical models and well-characterized subject groups is needed to clearly interpret findings obtained in studies examining subjects with mood disorders.

Schizophrenia

Across the enormous psychophysiological literature on schizophrenia, findings are varied and an integrated model of pathology in schizophrenia remains elusive. Schizophrenia is thought of as primarily a disorder of cognition, although a variety of other symptoms are frequently present as well. Psychophysiology studies of schizophrenia point to several broad areas of disturbance, including abnormalities in primary auditory processes, attention, working memory, language, and emotional processing. Across psychophysiological methods, no single abnormality has been found to be present in all individuals with schizophrenia and the degree of overlap between patient and control distributions is typically so extensive that only a minority of patients is distinguishable from healthy research participants (Heinrichs, 2004).

The good news for psychophysiology researchers is that effect sizes across the biological methods commonly used to study schizophrenia (e.g., neurochemical, cytoarchitectural, and neurotransmitter receptor densities) indicate that the most powerful and robust patient and control differences pertain to cognitive and psychophysiological aspects of brain function (Heinrichs, 2004). For example, saccadic frequency scores from eye-tracking tests and reduced frontal brain metabolism and blood flow during mental activity produce average effect sizes large enough to describe abnormalities that probably occur in half of the schizophrenia patient population. The review below examines a few of the psychophysiological measures commonly used to study schizophrenia, organized around issues in primary auditory processes and attention.

Primary auditory processes. Numerous neuroimaging studies have reported auditory processing abnormalities in schizophrenia, involving both basic tasks, such as listening to simple tones or clicks without overt performance demands, and more complex tasks. Reviewed below are auditory studies using either MEG source localization methods or spectral analysis techniques.

N100 (EEG) and N100m (MEG) are the most prominent deflections of the auditory event-related potential or field, evolving with a peak latency of about 100 ms after stimulus onset (for a review see Hari, 1990). Examining auditory evoked fields (AEFs) in a nonpatient population, Pantev et al. (1998) observed lateralized latency differences

for the processing of tones with shorter N100m latencies in temporal areas contralateral to the stimulated ear. Similar findings were reported in Picton et al. (1999). These studies replicated findings previously obtained in single-hemisphere MEG studies (Elberling et al., 1980; Mäkelä, 1988; Rogers et al., 1990) as well as whole-cortex MEG studies (Mäkelä et al., 1993; Nakasato et al., 1995). Results were taken to correspond to the anatomical differences of the auditory ascending pathways, which were shorter after the inferior colliculi on the contralateral than on the ipsilateral side (Evans, 1982). Pantev et al. (1998) also observed that the root mean square (rms) value of the measured field strength and the absolute value of the estimated dipole moment were larger for the contralateral hemisphere. These results were interpreted as in line with the fact that most of the fibers of the auditory pathway cross to the contralateral side, where a large cortical response is evoked. Eulitz et al. (1995) observed similar lateralized differences for the processing of phonetic stimuli, and these findings were later replicated (Gootjes et al., 1999).

Extending this line of research to examine basic auditory processes in patients with schizophrenia, hemispheric lateralization has been examined using MEG source localization methods. In the first of a series of studies examining atypical structural and functional laterality, Rockstroh et al. (1998) presented tone stimuli to the right ear in control subjects and in patients with schizophrenia. N100m occurred earlier over the contralateral (left) hemisphere in both controls and patients with schizophrenia, but N100m source strength showed a larger contralateral magnitude only in controls. It was suggested that the symmetry in patients with schizophrenia may reflect a developmental failure in structural brain asymmetry. Rockstroh et al. (2001) extended their investigation to include verbal stimuli (/ba/) as well as tones (1000 Hz) and obtained measures from both unilateral left- and right-ear stimulation. All control subjects showed the expected contralateral predominance of N100m strength, whereas asymmetry in was reversed for left-ear tones in 47% of the patient subjects and for right-ear tones in 76% of patient subjects. No group differences were observed using syllable stimuli. Examining the relationship between N100m strength asymmetry scores and patient symptoms, negative correlations indicated that smaller asymmetry scores were associated with more pronounced negative symptoms, longer overall hospitalization, and a higher daily dosage of neuroleptic medication. Examining N100m latency scores, pronounced differences between left and right syllable stimulation were found in patients, and differences were less in control subjects. These results suggest that interhemispheric conduction velocity is similar in control subjects and not in patients with schizophrenia. Rockstroh et al. (2001) concluded that deviation from the normal functional lateralization in schizophrenia appears in a proportion of patients at a basic stage of auditory processing but may be compensated for at higher levels such as the processing of syllables.

In addition to examining temporally discrete components of the auditory event-related potential or field a literature is beginning to study oscillatory phenomena in schizophrenia. The interest in examining time-frequency domain activity arises from the belief that frequency domain information may provide a more accurate measure of neuronal activity. In particular, it is hypothesized that auditory stimuli generate evoked-potentials by reorganizing the phase spectra of the existing ongoing EEG/MEG. Early work by Pantev and his colleagues (Pantev et al., 1991) showed that the overlapping auditory components (e.g., 50 ms and 100 ms) energies belong to different spectral regions and can be separated in the frequency domain. However, in addition to examining the amount of activity in specific frequencies at different times, time-frequency analyses allow for a wide range of additional analyses. Thus, besides the frequency and site of activity, other parameters, such as enhancement, time-locking, phase locking, delay of the oscillation, and prolongation of oscillation can be examined, and are of interest because they are strongly related to brain function.

As previously mentioned, investigators frequently have observed a decreased N100 response in individuals with Sz (e.g., Boutros et al., 2004), and a few studies have employed time-frequency-domain analyses to examine this finding. Winterer et al. (2000) concluded that the decreased N100 amplitude commonly observed in individuals with schizophrenia is the result of an increased amount of EEG background noise and an impaired stimulus-induced phase locking of background EEG. In a related study, Gilmore, Clementz, & Buckley (2004) examined the ability of patient's with schizophrenia to increase N100 amplitude. Noting that N100 amplitude is increased by presenting bursts of steady-state stimuli with frequencies greater than 30 to 40 Hz (suggesting that N100 indexes information integration over time) they hypothesized that although a single transient stimulus conveys insufficient information for efficient processing by patients with schizophrenia, bursts of steady-state stimuli, to a point, would reduce or eliminate patient-control N100 differences. However, they also hypothesized that there is a low ceiling on the ability of patients to handle high-density auditory information and that this would result in a decrease in N1 at high (>40 Hz) burst rates. At 10 Hz patients showed the expected decreased N1 response. The N1 amplitude in controls increased as a function of increased rate of stimulation. At 20 Hz no group differences were observed. However, patients were unable to manage stimulation rates above 20 Hz, and at 40 and 80 Hz low frequency activity decreased. They concluded that patients have a limited capacity for processing high-density auditory information.

The investigation of high frequency activity has been of particular interest as brain activity in the 40 Hz range is thought to be critical for feature binding, allowing functionally and spatially separate brain systems processing distinct stimulus features to cooperate in object perception (Singer, 1993). Abnormality in 40 Hz synchronization could result in a variety of perceptual and cognitive abnormalities, including abnormal perceptions and hallucinations, in schizophrenia. A few studies have examined entrainment of the EEG to trains of clicks presented at constant frequencies (including 40 Hz). In patients with schizophrenia, Kwon et al. (1999) observed a decrease in the ability of auditory neural networks to support synchronous neural activity at 40 Hz, but not at lower click train frequencies (20 and 30 Hz). Hong et al. (2004) observed that the relatives of individuals with schizophrenia-spectrum personality symptoms had reduced power at 40 Hz compared to controls. In addition, although Hong et al. (2004) failed to replicate Kwon et al.'s (1999) findings, they observed that patients taking new-generation antipsychotics had enhanced 40 Hz synchronization compared to patients taking conventional antipsychotics.

Research examining the integrity of the auditory system in schizophrenia is in its infancy. However, given the STG structural abnormalities and auditory functional impairments observed in schizophrenia, research in this area is of great importance. More research is needed examining the relationship between impaired low and high frequency activity and the symptoms and neurocognitive deficits associated with schizophrenia. Particularly promising would be studies exploring interregional synchrony or other types of functional connectivity.

Filtering in schizophrenia. Problems with attention and perception are often noted to be core features of schizophrenia and have been hypothesized to result from defects in filtering or gating of afferent sensory input. In the 1970s and 1980s a large number of studies examined information processing and attentional deficits in schizophrenia subjects. As Braff (1993) noted, "The fundamental focus of these studies and reviews is that schizophrenia patients have critical deficiencies in information processing abilities that are revealed and enhanced when high processing loads, multiple tasks, distraction, or other stressors demand the rapid and efficient processing of information" (p. 56).

Braff (1993) presented a simple framework for understanding information-processing abnormalities in schizophrenia patients. In this framework, attentional and information processing abilities are hypothesized to rely on intact psychophysiological function, normal neurotransmitter and hormonal balance, and an intact neuroanatomic substrate. When these systems are intact and function properly, normal cognition, emotion, and overt function are observed. When these systems are damaged, abnormalities occur manifested in psychiatric symptoms.

Deficient processing in patients with schizophrenia has been hypothesized to result from such factors as excess stimulation as a result of sensory flooding, a smaller pool of resources, an inability to mobilize and allocate resources, or excess resource allocation to task-irrelevant stimuli

(Braff, 1993). Many paradigms have been developed to examine information processing and attention dysfunction in patients with schizophrenia. These include oculomotor function (smooth pursuit eye movement), visual backward masking, continuous performance tasks, latent inhibition, and sensorimotor gating (prepulse inhibition, P50 gating). Poor performance has been observed in patients with schizophrenia on each of these tasks. It is important to note that poor performance is not necessarily slowed performance. In a latent inhibition task, in which the subject is asked to count meaningless syllables while the stimulus of interest (e.g., a 30 ms burst of white noise) is presented concurrently, acute schizophrenia patients identify the target stimuli more rapidly than do control subjects, indicating a failure of inhibitory function. Thus, in this task, normal performance consists of increased levels of inhibition, and the latent inhibition paradigm induces a situation in which failure of inhibition causes "better" performance in patients with schizophrenia.

Across the above tasks, many of the variables under study appear to be fundamental, trait-linked markers for schizophrenia. Antipsychotic medications do not fully normalize these information-processing functions, and many of the observed deficits in schizophrenia patients are not medication-induced artifacts. In addition, subjects at the boundaries of schizophrenia show a pattern of trait-linked information-processing deficits similar to those of schizophrenia patients (Braff, 1993).

It has long been thought that some schizophrenia symptoms, such as hallucinations and delusions of reference, may result from an impaired attentional filter (Kisley, Noecker, & Guinther, 2004; McGhie & Chapman, 1961). The purpose of such a filter is to protect limited-capacity systems from being overloaded with incoming information. An impaired filter could lead to the inability to process optimally the most important information, as well as a tendency to attribute special or inappropriate significance to other information.

Disturbed filtering is frequently examined in schizophrenia using a simple paired-click gating paradigm. In the paired-click paradigm subjects are presented two clicks separated by 500 ms, and the P50 component of the ERP to each click is scored, typically at electrode Cz. In normal subjects suppression of P50 to the second click occurs when the interstimulus interval is less than 1 s. However, in patients with schizophrenia the response to S2 shows less suppression. The larger S2 response in patients is interpreted as a gating deficit. Methodological issues and inconsistencies undermined the early P50 gating literature, including evidence of poor reliability of the P50 ratio measure (Smith, Boutros, & Schwarzkopf, 1994). However, sufficient replications now exist that the deficit can be considered well established. Indeed, recent meta-analyses have found that P50 abnormality is one of the most powerful and reliable neuroscience findings in the schizophrenia literature (Bramon et al., 2004, Heinrichs, 2004).

Uncertainty remains as to relationships of P50 amplitude and P50 suppression to diagnostic subtypes, task demands, and experimental conditions (for review, see Bramon et al., 2004). Issues such as posture of the subject during recording, P50's sensitivity to attentional and stress factors, and selection of valid trials have yet to be resolved. Measurement of P50 can be compromised by the fact that several components (e.g., P30, N40, N100, Nd) occur during or adjacent to P50. Further study of these issues is needed before the nature of P50 suppression and its suitability as a measure of disturbed filtering in schizophrenia-spectrum disorders can be fully determined.

Recently, MEG source localization methods have been used as a means to explore the circuitry of P50 gating and identify the locus of the abnormality in schizophrenia. Huang et al. (2003) showed that bilateral superior temporal gyrus (STG) generators contribute virtually all of the variance in Cz P50. Noting significant between-subject and within-hemisphere differences in the strength, orientation, and latency of the STG generators, Edgar et al. (2003) suggested that a better understanding of the paired-click gating deficit observed schizophrenia could be obtained if activity from the individual 50 ms STG generators was examined rather than the aggregate P50 score at Cz. Thoma et al. (2003) observed a gating deficit for a schizophrenia group in the left- but not right-hemisphere for 50 ms STG activity and also found that left- but not right-hemisphere M50 gating correlated with behavioral measures of sustained attention and working memory. Thoma et al. (2004) reported that, although there were no relationships between EEG P50 sensory gating and positive or negative symptoms, negative symptoms correlated positively with right-hemisphere M50 gating ratio. In contrast, positive symptoms correlated with left M50 gating ratio when a subgroup of patient subjects characterized by particularly good gating and atypical lateralization was removed from the analysis. Together, these studies established the potential of MEG source localization in furthering understanding of dysfunctional sensory gating mechanisms in schizophrenia.

As with the N100/M100m studies, P50/M50 time-frequency domain studies are increasingly common. In a series of studies, Clementz, Blumenfeld, and colleagues used EEG and MEG techniques to examine P50/M50 Low Frequency Responses (LFRs: 1–20 Hz) and Gamma Band Responses (GBR: 20–40 Hz) in patients with schizophrenia. Using multichannel EEG and spatial Principle Component Analysis (PCA) to integrate information over all channels, Clementz and Blumenfeld (2001) observed that groups differed on LFR measures to S1 but not S2. In a similar study examining MEG auditory evoked fields (AEFs), Blumenfeld and Clementz (2001) applied spatial generalized eigenvalue (GEV) decompensation techniques to 148 MEG channels. Controls had larger amplitude LFRs to the first stimulus than did patients. Discussing the results obtained across multiple studies, Blumenfeld and Clementz concluded that controls and patients with schizophrenia do not differ on initial sensory registration as the patients and controls did not differ on first or second click GBR activity. In addition, they suggested that the abnormally small S1 LFR is inconsistent with a basic stimulus filtering theory for explaining normal-schizophrenia group differences on gating. They speculated that patients have difficulty encoding stimuli after long time delays and that attention effects may be influencing group differences on AER suppression. Results from Johannesen et al. (2005) generally support this claim. Johannesen et al. (2005) observed that both nonparanoid and paranoid schizophrenia patients had a smaller S1 response and spectral analyses revealed smaller S1 and normal S2 responses in schizophrenia across both the GBR and LFR. Poor attention was inversely related to both S1 and S2 values. Given both the smaller LFR and S1 values, they concluded that the low S1 amplitude in schizophrenia reflects a diminished capacity to gate-in relevant signals.

Much more work is needed before the auditory gating abnormalities observed in patients with schizophrenia are fully understood. A greater understanding of the abnormality has been obtained using source localization techniques to study source rather than scalp activity. Whereas previous studies employing time-frequency analyses have provided a way to study activity in particular frequency ranges, recent time-frequency studies have focused on examining the time-frequency profile of the scalp recorded activity. Studies applying time-frequency analyses to the localized STG sources are now needed to more completely investigate normal and abnormal primary and secondary auditory processes. Finally, studies that simultaneously examine activity in different nodes in the auditory system (e.g., prefrontal and perhaps hippocampal areas) are needed to examine the integrity of the entire auditory system.

Selective attention in schizophrenia. According to Braver, Barch, and Cohen (1999), the most consistently reported attentional impairments in schizophrenia involve the exertion of attention in a selective and controlled manner to facilitate processing of task-relevant information and/or to inhibit the processing of task-irrelevant information. Recently, the Stroop task has been used to examine selective attention impairments in patients with schizophrenia. The traditional Stroop (1935) task requires subjects to respond to stimuli that vary in two dimensions, only one of which is task relevant. Thus, it is a means to study the subjects' ability to select or ignore task dimensions and parameters of task interference. Macleod (1991, 1992) provided a comprehensive review of behavioral studies of the Stroop task, and called it the "gold standard" of selective attention phenomena.

Stroop interference is commonly associated with enhanced activity in anterior cingulate cortex (ACC; e.g., Banich et al., 2001). Abnormal ACC activation during Stroop has been frequently observed in schizophrenia, but both the direction (hypoperfusion or hyperperfusion) and the laterality of the findings have been inconsistent. It has been hypothesized that abnormal ACC activity fosters or reflects deficits in selective attention by disturbing a network of brain areas important in selective attention tasks. Yucel et al. (2002) suggested that schizophrenia is "a disorder of connectivity with specific involvement of the limbic anterior cingulate" (p. 253). Carter et al. (1997), noting that areas other than the ACC showed abnormal activation during the Stroop task, suggested that "patients with schizophrenia fail to modulate cortical activity in distributed networks in a task-appropriate manner" (p. 1677). As Carter et al. (1997) and Yücel et al. (2002) went on to note (see also David, Cosmelli, & Friston, 2004), the development of methods to examine functional connectivity would be a boon to the study of selective attention in schizophrenia, providing investigators with methods to investigate hypotheses about the dynamic operation of the brain.

Aside from abnormalities in ACC, DLPFC has also been implicated in theories of selective attention and schizophrenia. DLPFC appears to play an important role in active maintenance of contextual information (e.g., Braver, Barch, & Cohen, 1999; Banich et al., 2000; Banich et al., 2001), particularly in the face of interference (Miller, Erickson, & Desimone, 1996). It has been proposed that a deficit in the ability to maintain contextual information in patients with schizophrenia involves a disturbance in DLPFC (e.g., Barch et al., 2001). Studies integrating neuropsychological performance with hemodynamic neuroimaging data show that individuals with schizophrenia or at risk for schizophrenia do not activate DLPFC normally when performing a task that places demands on relevant processing resources (e.g., Andreasen et al., 1992; Barch et al., 2001; Gold, Goldberg, & Weinberg, 1992; MacDonald et al., 2003; Mohanty et al., 2004; Weinberger, Berman, & Zec, 1986). This finding has contributed to the concept of 'hypofrontality' in schizophrenia. However, there is increasing evidence that the traditional concept of hypofrontality is incomplete (Ramsey et al., 2002; Weiss et al., 2003). For example, increased task-related activity in either right (Callicott et al., 2000; Callicott et al., 2003; Weiss et al., 2003) or left (Manoach et al., 1999; Manoach et al., 2000; Weiss et al., 2003) DLPFC has been reported in individuals with schizophrenia or at risk for developing it. These apparent inconsistencies might be attributed to many factors, including experimental design and behavioral task complexity, presence of reward (Manoach et al., 2000), and analytic issues such as examining group-averaged data (thus underestimating DLPFC activation due to heterogeneity of location within DLPFC) versus single-subject data (Manoach et al., 2000). In addition, despite considerable evidence demonstrating DLPFC dysfunction in schizophrenia, it remains uncertain whether this dysfunction arises from neural abnormalities primarily in DLPFC or from abnormal dysregulation of DLPFC by other structures (Callicott et al., 2000; Manoach et al., 2000). Again, the development of methods to study functional brain connectivity is needed to explore these different possibilities.

Summary. Current psychophysiology research on schizophrenia has focused on abnormalities in processing auditory information, filtering deficits, and selective attention impairments. Comparing psychophysiological findings across studies is difficult because of differences in schizophrenia patient subtypes, differences in syndrome-dimensions (e.g., psychomotor poverty, disorganization, and reality distortion), and in medications. Heterogeneous results may also arise from differences in experimental design. In particular, studies that do not employ a within-subjects design may fail to observe between-group differences because they lack the power to detect such changes. In addition, group differences are generally small, making it difficult to observe patient-control differences without large sample sizes. Such reasons are thought to explain the inconsistent findings of slightly enlarged cerebral ventricles and subtle anatomical abnormalities in the region of the anterior hippocampus (Suddath et al., 1990). Overall, study designs that employ adequate Ns, that reduce within-group variability, and that examine medication effects systematically will generally have greater success at identifying subtle electrophysiological changes.

Schizophrenia has long been a focus of psychophysiological research, first emphasizing autonomic, then electrocortical, and most recently hemodynamic measures and MEG. Neuropathology and neuroimaging studies have identified abnormalities in multiple brain regions in schizophrenia, including hippocampus, thalamus, frontal lobes, temporal lobes, and parietal lobes. Given this widespread pathology, it is often hypothesized that the symptoms associated with schizophrenia are the product of distributed abnormalities rather than focal pathology. Several theorists have proposed that functional disconnections between brain regions account for many of the symptoms and impairments in schizophrenia. As researchers continue to examine brain activity in schizophrenia-spectrum disorders, the development of methods to assess communication between multiple brain regions will be of considerable interest.

ROADBLOCKS AND RECOMMENDATIONS

The past decade has seen growing faith in psychophysiology as a means of understanding psychopathology, especially via hemodynamic neuroimaging. A number of challenges must be faced, however.

Problems comparing populations

The study of psychopathology often involves the comparison of groups of individuals in an attempt to understand what is specific to a given population. Such comparisons face a host of problems related to the interpretation of group differences. Because clinical groups typically dif-

fer prior to the experiment, it is difficult to determine whether measured differences are the result of experimental manipulations or to pre-existing differences. Because psychopathology studies cannot rely on random assignment to avoid such differences, alternative approaches must be considered.

Two approaches that appear useful, but are ineffective as general solutions, are matching of samples and analysis of covariance (ANCOVA). Researchers often attempt to match patient and control groups on the basis of pre-experimental scores on various measures, such as intelligence or physiological responsiveness. A central problem with matching samples on one measure is that if the populations from which the samples are drawn do in fact differ on the measure, neither sample is representative of its respective population. Thus, matching subjects on one variable tends to unmatch the groups systematically on other variables (Meehl, 1970, 1971). Furthermore, such matching based on pretesting can foster regression to the mean in the main experimental test (Chapman & Chapman, 1973). These vulnerabilities of the matched-samples strategy have long been known but are frequently overlooked. The implication is not that matching is always unwise but that these vulnerabilities must be taken into account in designing and interpreting between-group studies.

The second approach involves ANCOVA and hopes to remove the effect of differences in scores on one measure from scores on a second measure. Unfortunately, when the question at hand involves group differences, this is not generally a valid use of ANCOVA. Score differences may reflect real differences between groups. It has long been established that no statistical technique can "correct" for a real difference between groups (Benjamin, 1967; Chapman & Chapman, 1973; Fleiss & Tanur, 1973; Miller & Chapman, 2001). Indeed, "correcting" for such a difference is not even an appropriate goal. When a potential covariate is related to the grouping variable, removing variance associated with the covariate necessarily means that the (residual) grouping variable is altered. ANCOVA is properly employed to remove noise variance, but not systematic variance. Studies of psychopathology that examine group differences are typically inappropriate for candidates for ANCOVA (for extended discussion, see Miller & Chapman, 2001).

There are better ways to compare groups that deal with preexisting differences. One way is to employ multiple measures of performance on the same task. Measures might be carefully selected in order to tap distinct subsets of the mental operations involved in task performance. Evaluation of the pattern of results obtained from the different measures may isolate specific operations which are affected or unaffected by psychopathology. Psychophysiological approaches are particularly well suited for this type of approach because they can often provide multiple measures of aspects of task performance (Coles, 1989).

A second generally sound approach involves the use of the same or similar measures across several tasks in order to determine to what extent a deficit on one task may exceed a deficit on another task. Measures may be considered similar based on their being matched on administration format, difficulty, and reliability. Even when one group of subjects scores below another across all tasks measured, the difference on one task may be substantially larger than the difference on another task. Such a pattern would suggest that the larger deficit involves mental processes that are especially deficient in one group (Chapman & Chapman, 1973). However, it can be difficult to identify or develop tasks and measures that are equated in terms of difficulty and reliability across groups. Differences in difficulty or reliability can produce artifactual findings that misrepresent the importance of a specific deficit. Davidson et al. (1990) and Hanlon et al. (in press) are rare examples of a psychophysiological study that handled them explicitly.

A third approach to address pre-existing differences is to manipulate task difficulty such that each group performs an equally difficult task. A common implementation of this approach is to adjust task difficulty until each group attains accuracy scores approximating 50% (Chapman & Chapman, 1989). A more sophisticated and flexible version of this approach is to employ a task in which each group's performance is equally distant from 50% (Miller, Chapman, Chapman, & Collins, 1995). However, the difficulty of tasks of interest is not always readily adjustable.

A fourth approach to address pre-existing differences is related to ANCOVA, but does not require that the groups be equal on the covariate. Rather than treating the apparently tangential variable on which the groups differ as a covariate, the analysis incorporates it and attempt to understand its substantive role. Procedurally, this can be accomplished in a standard hierarchical regression analysis by treating the variable simply as another predictor of interest, especially if its interaction with other variables of interest is included in the analysis. Leutner and Rammsayer (1995) discussed this approach in a personality/self-report context, but their examples generalize well to psychopathology and psychophysiology.

A final approach attempts to sidestep the problem of group differences by using groups that exhibit some characteristics of psychopathology, but are sufficiently well functioning that their performance is substantially equal to the functioning of the controls. One way to accomplish this is to study individuals at risk for developing psychopathology but fully functional (Miller, 1995). Such at-risk individuals may include relatives of patients, demographically similar individuals, or individuals with subthreshold or few symptoms. Because onset of psychopathology is presumably determined by numerous factors, it is not necessary for at-risk individuals to develop full-blown psychopathology for data from them to be useful. They provide the opportunity to study processes that are important in psychopathology while avoiding many of the complications that result from studying manifest psychopathology.

Problems studying affected populations

The benefits of working with at-risk samples notwithstanding, much of the work has to be carried out with fully affected samples. A common challenge in such studies is differentiating the effects of psychotropic medications (Blanchard & Neale, 1992). Conflicting findings and limited data have made it difficult to draw firm conclusions about the effects of medications on various physiological measures. Self-medication (including tobacco, alcohol, and illicit drugs) can cause similar problems. Another challenge is the ability to provide informed consent for participation in clinical research. Individuals with psychopathology will vary in their ability to understand the research protocol, its risks, and its implications. This topic is receiving increasing attention and more systematic empirical research, including increased priority at NIH.

Despite difficulties in working with psychiatric populations, there are ways to address many of these problems. Although medication is often not under the control of the research team, nor is random assignment normally possible, researchers can obtain information about the medication of the participants and employ this information when analyzing the data. Research-specific diagnostic screening is often necessary to ensure adequate characterization of patients because treatment and research staff may use diagnoses for different purposes. Careful screening procedures may also address such problems of substance abuse and comorbidity (see discussion below).

Yet another challenge in studying psychopathology is identifying appropriate control or comparison groups. Patient groups may offer a population that is perhaps comparably medicated and hospitalized. Nonpsychiatric groups provide a basis for comparison to nonpsychopathology research, but can be surprisingly difficult to find given the high rate of subthreshold and undiagnosed disorders in the general population. Researchers need to choose comparison groups based on their experimental questions, but an underutilized strategy is to involve multiple control groups of which none may be ideal but in aggregate can address a number of issues (Miller & Chapman, 2001).

An alternative to studying diagnosed patients is studying nonpatients at risk for developing diagnosable psychopathology or already showing certain symptoms. As noted above, there are well-established advantages to using at-risk groups to examine psychopathology. First, the use of at-risk groups generally avoids problems associated with patient status such as medication effects, informed consent, and tolerance for research protocols. Second, if a deficit in a particular mental function is fundamental to the development of a disorder, then indications of that deficit will often be manifest prior to the actual onset of the disorder. Third, premorbid studies allow researchers to identify possible compensatory mechanisms that at-risk individuals could employ to delay or avoid the onset of more severe psychopathology. Information gained from such studies of at-risk individuals would be useful for understanding the process of the disorder as well as developing preventive or ameliorative interventions.

Problems of heterogeneity

The heterogeneity of symptom patterns allowed in DSM-IV can be problematic for psychopathology research. Within-group variance can be considerable for both the clinical manifestations that drive diagnosis and the psychophysiological phenomena one tries to identify. It is particularly important to consider the prevalence and theoretical significance of particular physiological symptoms in order to select appropriate psychophysiological measures. Because traditional diagnostic categories rely heavily on verbal and behavioral symptoms, they typically fail to consider the role of physiological symptoms or nonsymptomatic physiological manifestations of relevant processes. It is quite striking that the operationalization of diagnoses in DSM-IV includes virtually no physiological criteria (not to be confused with self-reports of physiological symptoms), despite the increasing claims for biological factors in psychopathology. Starting points for psychophysiological research are often not obvious. However, though little utilized, the option of defining abnormality in terms of a specific physiological phenomenon may be a very promising strategy as a means of reducing diagnostic heterogeneity.

Problems of comorbidity

Another problem that complicates psychopathological research is comorbidity of different mental disorders in the same individual (Cuthbert, in press; Heller & Nitschke, 1998; Mineka, Watson, & Clark, 1998). Because each diagnosis is associated with different clusters of verbal, physiological, and behavioral symptoms, comorbidity becomes particularly problematic when co-occurring disorders have divergent effects on the same measure. For example, if depression and anxiety have divergent effects on EEG alpha suppression, then the co-occurrence of these disorders will confound interpretation of this physiological variable. This problem is particularly challenging when an individual meets criteria for one diagnosis and is subthreshold for another diagnosis.

Investigators have a choice of describing psychopathology in terms of a diagnosis (e.g., schizophrenia), an observed symptom (e.g., disorganized speech, depressed mood, or exaggerated startle response), or an inferred mental process (e.g., impaired working memory, hallucinations). Although genetic and other biological phenomena are a growing focus of research on psychopathology, they do not themselves constitute psychopathology. The investigator's choice depends on many considerations, including the level of resolution needed to answer the research question (Cacioppo & Berntson, 1992), which is in turn dependent on (too often only implicit) value judgments about what is most important or most promising. Psychophysiological methods have often been applied haphazardly, which has caused the literature to be spread rather thinly, with relatively little conclusive evidence.

Problems comparing neuroimaging methods

For researchers interested in studying psychopathology, neuroimaging approaches can be especially enticing, which is evidenced by the rapid growth of this literature in recent years. Electromagnetic measures offer a noninvasive method for monitoring physiological activity with excellent temporal resolution and in most cases provides direct assessment of aggregate neural activity. In many cases EEG is relatively limited in the spatial resolution that it can provide, although aggressive research programs are underway that are improving spatial localization (e.g., Baillet, Mosher, & Leahy, 2001; Dale & Halgren, 2001; Grave de Peralta et al., 2004; Hoechstetter et al., 2004; Huang et al., 1998, Huang et al., 2004, under review; Michel et al., 2004; Scherg & Berg, 1996). MEG is noninvasive, provides excellent temporal resolution, and is often better suited for studying neural events in that they are not distorted by conductivity differences between bone and other tissue separating the sensor from neuronal activity (Hämäläinen et al., 1993; Lewine & Orrison, 1995). Hemodynamic methods such as fMRI and PET, based on blood flow, blood oxygenation, etc., offer less direct information about the location and timing of neural events. Hemodynamic methods are also far more expensive and less widely available than electrophysiological measures. However, in many circumstances fMRI offers spatial resolution equal to that of MEG for most of cortex and superior for deeper structures, yet under some circumstances MEG can reach deep structures such as hippocampus (Hanlon et al., 2003).

Not widely appreciated is the recent revolution in EEG and MEG research methods and, as a consequence, the rich potential of combining them with MRI (e.g., Ahlfors et al., 1999; Dale et al., 2000; Dale & Halgren, 2001; Korvenoja et al., 1999). A widespread misperception of EEG (and to a lesser degree MEG) as substantially inferior to fMRI in spatial localization is based on a failure to appreciate the respective histories of these methods. EEG evolved long prior to the availability of subject-specific brain anatomy information such as is now increasingly available via structural MRI (sMRI). Furthermore, for most of the long history of EEG the norm was to record from no more than a few widely spaced electrodes. Low electrode density, poor coverage of the entire head, and absence of subject-specific anatomical information precluded generally acceptable source localization. Although much valuable research on cognition does not require dense-array recordings or source localization, such methods are becoming common.

In contrast, fMRI is in its infancy. Much of its literature is primitive by comparison to EEG. For example, what in the fMRI literature is often called an "event-related design" is not a feature of the experimental design but a data-analysis strategy. The event-related design was introduced into the fMRI literature with much fanfare and much-deserved impact, but has been routine in event-related brain potential (ERP) studies of EEG phenomena for 35 years. It must be appreciated that new methods are almost invariably primitive and not immediately infused with expertise available in more developed traditions. Thus, fMRI methods are improving rapidly. Furthermore, it should be anticipated that, as a relatively new method, fMRI will see profound improvements in the near term in directions not presently obvious.

More germane to the issue of the relative spatial localization ability of EEG and fMRI is that the horserace has often been set up inappropriately. Taken very literally, essentially no one conducts fMRI research. Virtually every study examines a combination of fMRI with sMRI. Even superficial familiarity with fMRI data analysis would make one reluctant to place much faith in inferences about localization obtained from fMRI data in the absence of carefully coregistered sMRI data. A separate but very practical consideration is that the marginal cost of obtaining sMRI data given fMRI data is trivial, whereas in general the marginal cost of obtaining sMRI data given EEG data is quite high. Given that inclusion of sMRI is essentially universal in fMRI studies, but that the vast majority of EEG studies (even those with dense-array electrode montages) do not have sMRI information available, any comparison of fMRI (with sMRI) and EEG (without sMRI) is uninformative and even systematically misleading.

As a result, the common perception of EEG (and MEG) as inherently unsatisfactory for spatial localization of functional activity is unfounded. On the contrary, a number of demonstrations of successful spatial localization have been available for some time, most impressively when sMRI data are brought to bear (e.g., Sanders, Lewine, & Orrison, 1996). It should also be noted that, in many research contexts, localization within a few millimeters is of little interest or consequence. Rather, the source localization solutions are valuable primarily as a systematic means of reducing the dimensionality of the data. Particularly of value in studies of psychopathology, the structure of the solution (e.g., number of generators, hemispheric symmetry of generators, and the relative time courses of their activity) may be more important that anatomic specificity.

Much work remains to be done, and will be done, to advance electromagnetic and hemodynamic methods. One can anticipate that spatial localization will continue to improve for electromagnetic methods and that temporal localization will continue to improve for hemodynamic methods. Yet each will retain certain advantages. A pressing need is for research that identifies the linkages and diverges of these two classes of methods.

An even newer development is optical neuroimaging (see papers in special section of *Psychophysiology*; Gratton et al., 2003). It shows promise as a means to bridge the gap between hemodynamic and electromagnetic neuroimaging. To date, it appears to have been used just once in psychopathology research (Matsuo et al., 2003).

A growing consensus in the psychophysiology/cognitive neuroscience community is that the various established and emerging electromagnetic, hemodynamic, and optical measures are mutually complementary and individually essential. Some of the most exciting work since the original draft of this chapter (Keller et al., 2000) integrates multiple psychophysiological measures in this way. Psychophysiological approaches that combine several measures can provide a rich view of biological systems associated with psychopathology. Particularly promising is the ability of psychophysiology to define the endophenotype in psychopathology, the manifestation of a disorder via anomalies not observable by diagnostic interview or observation of overt behavior. This may prove to be crucial, for example, for identification of affected individuals in genetic linkage studies (Iacono, 1998).

Suggestions for future psychophysiological research on psychopathology

This chapter has argued that findings that are particularly meaningful share a common feature: the integration of good psychological with good physiological theory. Unfortunately, the modal report is simply one more empirical demonstration that individuals with psychopathology differ from controls. The field should ask more of itself.

Perhaps the greatest current challenge facing psychophysiological research on psychopathology is the development of tools to evaluate functional connectivity among brain regions. This need is arguably greater than the considerable and ongoing improvements in spatial localization underway in EEG and MEG research. As David et al. (2004) recently noted, functional connectivity analysis strategies are growing but in most cases are new and diverse, "making research in this area exciting but quite confusing" (p. 659). Broad progress in this domain will challenge researchers in psychophysiology and in psychology more generally to upgrade their quantitative skills (Miller, Elbert, Sutton, & Heller, in press).

This chapter has also emphasized the importance of a number of issues that arise in psychopathology research and are crucial, though not specific, to psychophysiological measurement. Thorough, reliable diagnostic screening is essential for clear characterization of subject samples. Careful strategies for addressing and interpreting group differences on tangential variables are critical. Consideration of diagnostic comorbidity as well as delineation and evaluation of relevant symptom or diagnostic subtypes is necessary.

Psychophysiology has a tradition of innovation and as a result an increasingly powerful set of tools that provide valuable information in understanding psychopathology. A number of considerations have been outlined here that influence the utility, significance, and impact of psychophysiological research on psychopathology. Research in this area will be most beneficial when strong theories of the fundamental psychological disturbance are integrated with solid theories of related physiological processes.

REFERENCES

Abercrombie, H. C., Schaefer, S. M., Larson, C. I., Oakes, T. R., Lindgren, K. A., Holden, J. E., et al. (1998). Metabolic rate in the right amygdala predicts negative affect in depressed patients. *Neuroreport, 9*, 3301–3307.

Ahlfors, S. P., Simpson, G. V., Dale, A. M., Belliveau, J. W., Liu, A. K., Korvenoja, A. et al. (1999). Spatiotemporal activity of a cortical network for processing visual motion revealed by MEG and fMRI. *Journal of Neurophysiology, 82*, 2545–2555.

Allen, J. B., Urry, H. L., Hitt, S. L., & Coan, J. A. (2004). The stability of resting frontal electroencephalographic asymmetry in depression. *Psychophysiology, 41*, 269–280.

American Psychiatric Association. (2000). *Diagnostic and statistical manual of mental disorders (4th ed.)*. Washington, DC: American Psychiatric Association.

Andreasen, N. C., Rezai, K., Alliger, R., Swayze, V. W., Flaum, M., Kirchner, P., et al. (1992). Hypofrontality in neuroleptic–naïve and chronic schizophrenic patients: Assessment with xenon-133 single-photon emission computed tomography and the Tower of London. *Archives of General Psychiatry, 49*, 943–958.

Ax, A. F. (1962). Psychophysiological methodology for the study of schizophrenia. In R. Roessler & N. S. Greenfield (Eds.), *Physiological correlates of psychological disorder*. Madison: University of Wisconsin Press.

Baillet, S., Mosher, J. C., & Leahy, R. M. (2001). Electromagnetic brain mapping. *IEEE Signal Processing Magazine, November*, 14–30.

Banich, M. T., Milham, M. P., Atchley, R. A., Cohen, N. J., Webb, A., Wszalek, T., et al. (2000). Prefrontal regions play a predominant role in imposing an attentional 'set': Evidence from fMRI. *Cognitive Brain Research, 10*, 1–9.

Banich, M. T., Milham, M. P., Jacobson, B. L., Webb, A., Wszalek, T., Cohen, N. J., et al. (2001). Attentional selection and the processing of task-irrelevant information: Insights from fMRI examinations of the Stroop task. *Progress in Brain Research, 134*, 459–470.

Barch, D. M., Carter, C. S., Braver, T. S., Sabb, F. W., MacDonald, A., III, Noll, D. C., et al. (2001). Selective deficits in prefrontal cortex function in medication-naive patients with schizophrenia. *Archives of General Psychiatry, 58*, 280–288.

Barlow, D. H. (1988). *Anxiety and its disorders: The nature and treatments of anxiety and panic*. New York: Guilford.

Barlow, D. H. (1991). Disorders of emotion. *Psychological Inquiry, 2*, 58–71.

Benjamin, L. S. (1967). Facts and artifacts in using analysis of covariance to "undo" the law of initial values. *Psychophysiology, 4*, 187–206.

Blanchard, E. B., Kickling, E. J., Buckley, T. C., Taylor, A. E., Vollmer, A., & Loos, W. R. (1996). Psychophysiology of posttraumatic stress disorder related to motor vehicle accidents: Replication and extension. *Journal of Consulting and Clinical Psychology, 64*, 742–751.

Blanchard, J. J., & Neale, J. M. (1992). Medication effects: Conceptual and methodological issues in schizophrenia research. *Clinical Psychology Review, 12*, 345–361.

Blumenfeld, L. D., & Clementz, B. A. (2001). Response to the first stimulus determines reduced auditory evoked response suppression in schizophrenia: Single trials analysis using MEG. *Clinical Neurophysiology, 112*, 1650–1659.

Blumenthal, T. D., Cuthbert, B. N., Filion, D. L., Hackley, S., Lipp, O. V., & van Boxtel, A. (2005). Committee report: Guidelines for human startle eyeblink electromyographic studies. *Psychophysiology, 42*, 1–15.

Bonne, O., Brandes, D., Gilboa, A., Gomori, J. M., Shenton, M. E., Pitman, R. K., et al. (2001). Longitudinal MRI study of hippocampal volume in trauma survivors with PTSD. *American Journal of Psychiatry, 158*, 1248–1251.

Boutros, N. N., Korzyukov, O., Jansen, B., Feingold, A., & Bell, M. (2004). Sensory gating deficits during the mid-latency phase of information processing in medicated schizophrenia patients. *Psychiatry Research, 126*, 203–215.

Bradley, M. M. (In press). Natural selective attention: Emotion in perception. *Psychophysiology, 42*.

Braff, D. L. (1993). Information processing and attention dysfunctions in schizophrenia. *Schizophrenia Bulletin, 19*, 233–259.

Bramon, E., Rabe-Hesketh, S., Sham, P., Murray, R. M., & Frangou, S. (2004). Meta-analysis of the P300 and P50 waveforms in schizophrenia. *Schizophrenia Research, 70*, 315–329.

Braver, T. S., Barch, D. M., & Cohen, J. D. (1999). Cognition and control in schizophrenia: A computational model of dopamine and prefrontal function. *Biological Psychiatry, 46*, 312–328.

Bremner, J. D. (2003). Long-term effects of childhood abuse on brain and neurobiology. *Child and Adolescent Psychiatric Clinics of North America, 12*, 271–292.

Bremner, J. D., Randall, P., Scott, T. M., Bronen, R. A., Seibyl, J. P., Southwick, S. M., et al. (1995). MRI-based measurement of hippocampal volume in patients with combat-related posttraumatic stress disorder. *American Journal of Psychiatry, 152*, 973–981.

Bremner, J. D., Innis, R. B., Salomon, R. B., Staib, L. H., Ng, C. K., et al. (1997). Positron emission tomography measurement of cerebral metabolic correlates of tryptophan depletion-induced depressive relapse. *Archives of General Psychiatry, 54*, 364–374.

Bremner, J. D., Scott, T. M., Delaney, R. C., Southwick, S. M., Mason, J. W., Johnson, D. R., et al. (1993). Deficits in short-term memory in posttraumatic stress disorder. *American Journal of Psychiatry, 150*, 1015–1019.

Bremner, J. D., Vythilingam, M., Vermetten, E., Southwick, S. M., McGlashan, T., Nazeer, et al. (2003). MRI and PET study of deficits in hippocampal structur and function in women with childhood sexual abuse and posttraumatic stress disorder. *American Journal of Psychiatry, 160*, 924–932.

Bruder, G. E. (1995). Cerebral laterality and psychopathology: Perceptual and event-related potential asymmetries in affective and schizophrenic disorders. In K. W. Spence & J. T. Spence (Eds.), *Brain Asymmetry* (pp. 661–691). Cambridge: MIT Press.

Bruder, G. E., Fong, R., Tenke, C. E., Leite, P., Towey, J. P., Stewart, J. E., et al. (1997). Reginal brain asymmetry in major depression with and without an anxiety disorder: a quantitative electroencephalographic study. *Biological Psychiatry, 41*, 939–948.

Bruder, G. E., Kayser, J., Tenke, C. E., Leite, P., Schneier, F. R., Stewart, J. W., et al. (2002). Cognitive ERPs in depression and anxiety disorders during tonal and phonetic oddball tasks. *Clinical Electroencephalography, 33*, 119–124.

Bruder, G. E., Wexler, B. E., Stewart, J. W., & Price, L. H. (1999). Preceptual asymmetry differences between major depression with or without comorbid anxiety disorder: a dichotic listening study. *Journal of Abnormal Psychology, 108*, 233–239.

Buck, C. W., Carscallen, H. B., & Hobbs, G. E. (1950). Temperature regulation in schizophrenia: I. Comparison of schizophrenic and normal subjects. II. Analysis of duration of psychosis. *Archives of Neurology and Psychiatry, 64*, 828–842.

Buck, C. W., Carscallen, H. B., & Hobbs, G. E. (1951). Effect of prefrontal lobotomy on temperature regulation in schizophrenic patients. *Archives of Neurology and Psychiatry, 65*, 197–205.

Bustamante, V., Mellman, T. A., David, D., & Fins, A. I. (2001). Cognitive functioning and the early development of PTSD. *Journal of Traumatic Stress, 14*, 791–797.

Cacioppo, J. T., & Berntson, G. G. (1992). Social psychological contributions to the Decade of the Brain: Doctrine of multilevel analysis. *American Psychologist, 47*, 1019–1028.

Callicott, J. H., Bertolino, A., Mattay, V. S., Langheim, F. J. P., Duyn, J., Coppola, R., et al. (2000). Physiological dysfunction of the dorsolateral prefrontal cortex in schizophrenia revisited. *Cerebral Cortex, 10*, 1078–1092.

Callicott, J. H., Egan, M. F., Mattay, V. S., Bertolino, A., Bone, A. D., Verchinski, et al. (2003). Abnormal fMRI response of the dorsolateral prefrontal cortex in cognitively intact siblings of patients with schizophrenia. *American Journal of Psychiatry, 160*, 709–719.

Carter, C. S., Mintun, M., Nichols, T., & Cohen, J. D. (1997). Anterior cingulated gyrus dysfunction and selective attention deficits in schizophrenia: [^{15}O]H$_2$O PET study during single-trial Stroop task performance. *American Journal of Psychiatry, 154*, 1670–1675.

Chapman, L. J., & Chapman, J. P. (1973). Problems in the measurement of cognitive deficit. *Psychological Bulletin, 79*, 380–385.

Chapman, L. J., & Chapman, J. P. (1989). Strategies for resolving the heterogeneity of schizophrenics and their relatives using cognitive measures. *Journal of Abnormal Psychology, 98*, 357–366.

Charles, G., Hansenne, M., Anssea, M., Pitchot, W., Machowski, R., Schittecatte, M., et al. (1995). P300 in posttraumatic stress disorder. *Neuropsychobiology, 32*, 72–74.

Clark, L. A., Watson, D., & Reynolds, S. (1995). Diagnosis and classification of psychopathology: Challenges to the current system and future directions. *Annual Review of Psychology, 46*, 121–153.

Clementz, B. A., & Blumenfeld, L. D. (2001). Multichannel electroencephalography assessment of auditory evoked response suppression in schizophrenia. *Experimental Brain Research, 139*, 377–390.

Cohen, L. H., & Patterson, M. (1937). Effect of pain on the heart rate of normal and schizophrenic individuals. *Journal of General Psychology, 17*, 273–289.

Coles, M. G. H. (1989). Modern mind-brain reading: Psychophysiology, physiology, and cognition. *Psychophysiology, 26*, 251–269.

Cuthbert, B. N. (In press). Brain motivational systems: Toward 'standard models' for co-occurring anxiety and mood symptoms. *Psychophysiology, 42*.

Cuthbert, B. N., Lang, P. J., Strauss, C., Drobes, D., Patrick, C., & Bradley, M. (2003). The psychophysiology of anxiety disorder: Fear memory imagery. *Psychophysiology, 40*, 407–422.

Dale, A. M., & Halgren, E. (2001). Spatiotemporal mapping of brain activity by integration of multiple imaging modalities. *Current Opinions in Neurobiology, 11*, 202–208.

Dale, A. M., Liu, A. K., Fischl, B. R., Buckner, R. L., Belliveau, J. W., Lewine, J. D. et al. (2000). Dynamic statistical parametric mapping: combining fMRI and MEG for high- resolution imaging of cortical activity. *Neuron, 26*, 55–67.

David, O., Cosmelli, D., & Friston, K. J. (2004). Evaluation of different measures of functional connectivity using a neural mass model. *NeuroImage, 21*, 659–673.

Davidson, R. J. (1998). Affective style and affective disorders: Perspectives from affective neuroscience. *Cognition & Emotion, 12*, 307–330.

Davidson, R. J. (2004). What does the prefrontal cortex "do" in affect: Perspectives on frontal EEG asymmetry research. *Biological Psychology, 67*, 219–233.

Davidson, R. J., Chapman, J. P., Chapman, L. J., & Henriques, J. B. (1990). Asymmetrical brain electrical activity discriminates between psychometrically matched verbal and spatial cognitive tasks. *Psychophysiology, 27*, 528–543.

Davidson, R. J., & Henriques, J. B. (2000). Regional brain function in sadness and depression. In J. C. Borod (Ed), *The Neuropsychology of Emotion* (pp. 269–297) New York: Oxford University Press.

Davidson, R. J., Jackson, D. C., & Larson, C. L. (2000). Human electroencephalography. In J. T. Cacioppo, L. G. Tassinary, & G. G. Berntson (Ed.), *Handbook of psychophysiology, second edition* (pp. 27–52). Cambridge, UK: Cambridge University Press.

Davidson, R. J., Pizzagalli, D., Nitschke, J. B., & Kalin, N. H. (2003). Parsing the subcomponents of emotion and disorders of emotion: perspectives from affective neuroscience. In R. J. Davidson, K. R. Scherer, H. H. Goldsmith, (Eds.), *Handbook of as* (pp. 8–24) New York: *Affective Science*. Oxford University Press.

Davidson, R. J., Pizzagalli, D., Nitschke, J. B., & Putnam, K. (2002). Depression: perspectives from affective neuroscience. *Annual Review of Psychology, 53*, 545–574.

Davidson, R. J., & Tomarken, A. J. (1989). Laterality and emotion: An electrophysiological approach. In F. Boller, & J. Grafman (Eds.), *Handbook of Neuropsychology* (pp. 419–441). Amsterdam: Elsevier.

Davis, P. A., & Davis, H. (1939). The electroencephalograms of psychotic patients. *American Journal of Psychiatry, 95*, 1007–1025.

DeBellis, M. D., Keshavan, M. S., Clark, D. B., Casey, B. J., Giedd, J. N., Boring, A. M., et al. (1999). Developmental traumatology, II. Brain development. *Biological Psychiatry, 45*, 1271–1284.

DeBellis, M. D., Hall, J. Boring, A. M., Frustaci, K, & Moritz, G. (2001). A pilot longitudinal study of hippocampal volumes in pediatric maltreatment-related posttraumatic stress disorder. *Biological Psychiatry, 50*, 305–309.

Deldin, P. J., Deveney, C. M., Kim, A. S., Casas, B. R., & Best, J. L. (2001). A slow wave investigation of working memory biases in mood disorders. *Journal of Abnormal Psychology, 110*, 267–281.

Deldin, P. J., Keller, J., Gergen, J. A., & Miller, G. A. (2001). Cognitive bias and emotion in neuropsychological models of depression. *Cognition and Emotion, 15*, 787–802.

Deldin, P., Keller, J., Casas, B. R., Best, J., Gergen, J., & Miller, G. A. (2006). Normal N400 in mood disorders. *Biological Psychology, 71*, 74–79.

Deldin, P. J., Keller, J., Gergen, J. A., & Miller, G. A. (2000). Right-posterior face-processing anomaly in depression. *Journal of Abnormal Psychology, 109*, 116–121.

Drevets, W. C., Price, J. L., Bardgett, M. E., Reich, T., Todd, R.D, et al. (2002). Glucose metabolism in the amygdala in depression:

relationship to diagnostic subtype and plasma cortisol levels. *Pharmacol Biochem Behav, 71*, 431–47.

Drevets, W. C. (2003). Neuroimaging abnormalities in the amygdala in mood disorders. *Annals of the New York Academy of Sciences, 985*, 420–44.

Duffy, E. (1962). *Activation and behavior* (pp. 277–321). New York: John Wiley & Sons.

Edgar, J. C., Huang, M. X., Weisend, M. P., Sherwood, A., Miller, G. A., Adler, L. E., et al. (2003). Interpreting abnormality: An EEG and MEG study pf P50 and the auditory paired-stimulus paradigm. *Biological Psychology, 65*, 1–20.

Elberling, C., Bak, C., Kofoed, B., Lebech, J., & Saermark, K. (1980). Magnetic auditory responses from the human brain. A preliminary report. *Scand Audiol, 9*, 185–190.

Elliott, R., Baker, S. C., Rogers, R. D., O'Leary, D. A., Paykel, E. S., Frith, C. D., et al. (1997). Prefrontal dysfunction in depressed patients performing a complex planning task: a study using positron emoission tomography. *Psychological Medicine, 27*, 931–942.

Elliott, R, Rubinszein, J. S., Sahakian, B. J., & Dolan, R. J. (2002). The neural basis of mood-congruent processing biases in depression. *Archives of General Psychiatry, 59*, 597–604.

Eulitz, C., Diesch, E., Pantev, C., Hampson, S., & Elbert, T. (1995). Magnetic and electric brain activity evoked by the processing of tone and vowel stimuli. *Journal of Neuroscience, 15*, 2748–2755.

Evans, E. F. (1982). Functional anatomy of the auditory system. In H. B. Barlow, J. D. Mollon (E., eds). *The Senses* (pp. 255–306). Cambridge University Press.

Fleiss, J. L., & Tanur, J. M. (1973). The analysis of covariance in psychopathology. In M. Hammer, K. Salzinger, & S. Sutton (Eds.), *Psychopathology: Contributions from the social, behavioral, and biological sciences* (pp. 509–527). New York: Wiley.

Flor-Henry, P. (1979). On certain aspects of the localization of the cerebral systems regulating and determining emotion. *Biological Psychiatry, 14*, 677–698.

Friedman, M. J., & Yehuda, R. (1995). Posttraumatic stress disorder and co-morbidity: psychobiological approaches to differential diagnosis. In M. J. Friedman, D. S. Charney, and A. Y. Deutch (Eds.), *Neurobiological and ccClinical Consequences of sfnaStress: From Normal Adaptation to PTSD* (pp. 429–446). New York, Raven Press.

Frith, C. D. (1992). *The cognitive neuropsychology of schizophrenia.* Hove, UK: L. Erlbaum Associates.

Frodl, T., Meisenzahl, E. M., Zetzsche, T., Born, C., Groll, C., Jager, M., et al. (2002). Hippocampal changes in patients with a first episode of major depression. *American Journal of Psychiatry, 159*, 1112–1118.

George, M. S., Ketter, T. A., Parekh, P. I., Rosinsky, N., Ring, H. A., Pazzaglia, P. J., et al. (1997). Blunted left cingulate activation in mood disorder subjects during a response interference task (the Stroop). *Journal of Neuropsychiatry and Clinical Neuroscience, 9*, 55–63.

Gerardi, R. J., Blanchard, E. B., & Kolb, L. C. (1989). Ability of Vietnam veterans to dissimulate a psychophysiological assessment for post-traumatic stress disorder. *Behavior Therapy, 20*, 229–243.

Ghisolfi, E. S., Margis, R., Becker, J., Zanardo, A. P., Strimitzer, I. M., & Lara, D. R. (2004). Impaired P50 sensory gating in posttraumatic stress disorder secondary to urban violence. *International Journal of Psychophysiology, 51*, 209–214.

Gilbertson, M. W., Gurvits, T. V., Lasko, N. B., Orr, S. P., & Pitman, R. K. (2001). Multivariate assessment of explicit memory func-

tion in combat veterans with posttraumatic stress disorder. *Journal of Traumatic Stress, 14*, 413–432.

Gilbertson, M. W., Shenton, M. E., Ciszewski, A., Kasai, K., Lasko, N. B., Orr, S. P., & Pitman, R. K. (2002). Smaller hippocampal volume predicts pathologic vulnerability to psychological trauma. *Nature Neuroscience, 5*, 1242–1247.

Gillette, G. M., Skinner, R. D., Rasco, L. M., Rielstein, E. M., Davis, D. H., Pawelak, J. E., et al. (1997). Combat veterans with posttraumatic stress disorder exhibit decreased habituation of the P1 midlatency auditory evoked potential. *Life Sciences, 61*, 1421–1434.

Gilmore, C. S., Clementz, B. A. & Buckley, P. F. (2004). Rate of stimulation affects schizophrenia-normal differences on the NI auditory-evoked potential. *Neurological Report, 15*, 2713–2717.

Giordani, B., Boibin, M. J., Berent, S., Betley, A. T., Kieppe, R. A., Rothley, J. M., et al. (1990). Anxiety and cerebral cortical metabolism in normal persons. *Psychiatry Research: Neuroimaging, 35*, 49–60.

Gold, J. M., Goldberg, T. E., & Weinberger, D. R. (1992). Prefrontal function and schizophrenic symptoms. *Neuropsychiatry, Neuropsychology, and Behavioral Neurology, 5*, 253–261.

Gootjes, L., Raij, T., Salmelin, R., & Hari, R. (1999). Left-hemisphere dominance for processing of vowels: a whole-scalp neuromagnetic study. *Neuroreport, 10*, 2987–2991.

Gratton, G., Fabiani, M., Elbert, T., & Rockstroh, B. (2003). Seeing right through you: Applications of optical imaging to the study of the human brain. *Psychophysiology, 40*, 487–491.

Grave de Peralta, R., Murray, M. M., Michel, C. M., Martuzzi, R., & Gonzalez Andino, S. (2004). Electrical neuroimaging based on biophysical constraints. *Neuroimage, 21*, 527–539.

Gruzelier, J. H. (1989). Lateralization and central mechanisms in clinical psychophysiology. In G. Turpin (Ed.), *Handbook of clinical psychophysiology* (pp. 135–174). New York: Wiley.

Gurvits, T. V., Shenton, M. E., Hokama, H., & Ohta, H. (1996). Magnetic resonance imaging study of hippocampal volume in chronic, combat-related posttraumatic stress disorder. *Biological Psychiatry, 40*, 1091–1099.

Hämäläinen, M., Hari, R., Ilmoniemi, R. J., Knuutila, J., & Lounasmaa, O. V. (1993). Magnetoencephalography- theory, instrumentation, and applications to the studies of the working human brain. *Rev Mod Phys, 65*, 413–498.

Hanlon, F. M., Weisend, M. P., Huang, M., Lee, R. R., Moses, S. N., Paulson, K. M., et al. (2003). A noninvasive method for observing hippocampal function. *NeuroReport, 14*, 1957–1960.

Hanlon, F. M., Weisend, M. P., Yeo, R. A., Huang, M., Thoma, R. J., Lee, R. R., et al. (2005). A specific test of hippocampal deficit in schizophrenia. *Behavioral Neuroscience, 119*, 863–875.

Hari, R. (1990). The Neuromagnetic method in the study of the human auditory cortex. In F. Grandori, M. Hoke, and G. Romani (Eds.). *Auditory Evoked Magnetic Fields and Potentials. Advances in Audiology* (vol. 6. pp. 222–282). Basel, Seitzerland: Karger.

Heinrichs, R. W. (2004). Meta-analysis and the science of schizophrenia: variant evidence or evidence of variants? *Neurosciences and Biobehavioral Reviews, 28*, 379–394.

Heim, C, & Nemeroff, C. B. (2002). Neurobiology of early life stress: clinical studies. *Semin Clinical Neuropsychiatry, 7*, 147–159.

Heller, W. (1993). Neuropsychological mechanisms of individual differences in emotion, personality, and arousal. *Neuropsychology, 7*, 476–489.

Heller, W., Etienne, M. A., & Miller, G. A. (1995). Patterns of perceptual asymmetry in depression and anxiety: Implications for neuropsychological models of emotion. *Journal of Abnormal Psychology, 104,* 327–333.

Heller, W., Isom, J., Nitschke, J. B., Koven, N., Mohanty, A., Fisher, J. E., et al. (2002). States, traits, and symptoms: Investigating the neural correlates of emotion, personality and psychopathology. In D. Cervone & W. Mischel (Eds.), *Advances in Personality Science* (pp. 106–126). New York: Guilford Press.

Heller, W., Koven, N., & Miller, G. A. (2003). Regional brain activity in anxiety and depression, cognition/emotion interaction, and emotion regulation. In K. Hugdahl & R. J. Davidson (Eds.), *The asymmetrical brain* (pp. 533–564). Cambridge, MA: MIT Press.

Heller, W., & Nitschke, J. B. (1997). The puzzle of regional brain activity in depression and anxiety: The importance of subtypes and comorbidity. *Cognition and Emotion, 12,* 421–428.

Heller, W., & Nitschke, J. B. (1998). Regional brain activity in emotion: A framework for understanding cognition in depression. *Cognition and Emotion, 11,* 637–661.

Heller, W., Nitschke, J. B., Etienne, M. A., & Miller, G. A. (1997). Patterns of regional brain activity differentiate anxiety subtypes. *Journal of Abnormal Psychology, 106,* 375–385.

Henriques, J. B., & Davidson, R. J. (1990). Regional brain electrical asymmetries discriminate between previously depressed and healthy control subjects. *Journal of Abnormal Psychology, 99,* 22–31.

Herrington, J. D., Mohanty, A., Koven, N. S., Fisher, J. E., Stewart, J. L., Banich, M. T., et al. (2005). Emotion-modulated performance and activity in left dorsolateral prefrontal cortex. *Emotion, 5,* 200–207.

Hertel, P. T. (1994). Depression and memory: Are impairments remediable through attentional control? *Current Directions in Psychological Science, 3,* 190–193.

Hertel, P. T. (2000). The cognitive–initiative account of depression-related impairments in memory. In D. L. Medin (Ed.), *Psychology of Learning and Motivation: Advances in Research and Theory* (pp. 47–71). San Diego: Academic Press.

Hoechstetter, K. Bornfleth, H. Weckesser, D., Ille, N., Berg, P., & Scherg, M. (2004). BESA source coherence: A new method to study cortical oscillatory coupling. *Brain Topography, 16,* 233–238.

Hong, L. E., Summerfelt, A., McMahon, R., Adami, H., Francis, G., Elliott, A., et al. (2004). Evoked gamma band synchronization and the liability for schizophrenia. *Schizophrenia Research, 70,* 293–302.

Huang, M., Dale, A. M., Song, T., Halgren, E., Harrington, D. L., Podgorny, I., et al. (Under review). Vector based spatial temporal minimum L1-norm for MEG.

Huang, M. X., Edgar, J. C., Thoma, R. J., Hanlon, F. M., Moses, S. N., Lee, R. R., et al. (2003). Predicting EEG responses using MEG sources in superior temporal gyrus reveals source asynchrony in patients with schizophrenia. *Clinical Neurophysiology, 114,* 835–850.

Huang, M. X., Shih, J., Lee, R. R., Harrington, D. L., Thoma, R. J., Weisend, M. P., et al. (2004). Commonalities and differences among vectorized beamformers in electromagnetic source imaging. *Brain Topography, 16,* 139–158.

Hugdahl, K. (1989). Simple phobias. In G. Turpin (Ed.), *Handbook of Clinical Psychophysiology* (pp. 283–308). New York: Wiley.

Iacono, W. G. (1998). Identifying psychophysiological risk for psychopathology: Examples from substance abuse and schizophrenia research. *Psychophysiology, 35,* 621–637.

Jaeger, J., Borod, J. C., & Peselow, E. (1987). Depressed patients have atypical hemispace biases in the perception of emotional chimeric faces. *Journal of Abnormal Psychology, 96,* 321–324.

Johannesen, J. K., Kieffaber, P. D., O'Donnel, B. F., Shekhar, A., Evans, J. D., & Hetrick, W. P. (in press). Contributions of subtype and spectral frequency analyses to the study of P50 ERP amplitude and suppression in schizophrenia. *Schizophrenia Research.*

Karl, A., Malta, L. S., & Maercker, A. (2006). Meta-analytic review of event-related potential studies in post-traumatic stress disorder. *Biological Psychology, 71,* 123–147.

Keller, J., Hicks, B. D., & Miller, G. A. (2000). Psychophysiology in the study of psychopathology. In L. G. Tassinary, J. T. Cacioppo, & G. G. Berntson (Eds.), *Handbook of psychophysiology, 2nd edition* (pp. 719–750). New York: Cambridge University Press.

Kisley, M. A., Noecker, T. L., & Guinther, P. M. (2004). Comparison of sensory gating to mismatch negativity and self-reported perceptual phenomena in healthy adults. *Psychophysiology, 41,* 604–612.

Korvenoja, A., Huttunen, J., Salli, E., Pohjonen, H., Martinkauppi, S., Palva, J. M., et al. (1999). Activation of multiple cortical areas in response to somatosensory stimulation: combined magnetoencephalographic and functional magnetic resonance imaging. *Human Brain Mapping, 8,* 13–27.

Koven, N. S., Heller, W., Banich, M. T., & Miller, G. A. (2003). Relationships of distinct affective dimensions to performance on an emotional Stroop task. *Cognitive Therapy and Research, 27,* 671–680.

Kozak, M. J., & Miller, G. A. (1982). Hypothetical constructs versus intervening variables: A re-appraisal of the three-systems model of anxiety assessment. *Behavioral Assessment, 4,* 347–358.

Kimbrell, T. A., Ketter, T. A., George, M. S., Little, J. T., Benson, B. E., et al. (2002). Regional cerebral glucose utilization in patients with a range of severities of unipolar depression. *Biological Psychiatry, 51,* 237–52.

Kwon, J. S, O'Donnell, B., Wallenstein, G., Greene, R., Hirayasu, Y., Nestor, P. G., et al. (1999). Gamma frequency-range abnormalities to auditory stimulation in schizophrenia. *Archives of General Psychiatry, 56,* 1001–1005.

Lacey, J. I. (1956). The evaluation of autonomic responses: Toward a general solution. *Annals of the New York Academy of Sciences, 67,* 123–164.

Lacey, J. I. (1967). Somatic response patterning and stress: Some revisions of activation theory. In M. H. Appley & R. Trumbull (Eds.), *Psychological stress: Issues in research* (pp. 14–38). New York: Appleton-Century-Crofts.

Landis, C. (1932). Electrical phenomena of the skin. *Psychological Bulletin, 29,* 693–752.

Lang, P. J. (1968). Fear reduction and fear behavior: Problems in treating a construct. In J. M. Shlien (Ed.), *Research in psychotherapy, Volume 3* (pp. 90–102). Washington, D. C.: American Psychological Association.

Lang, P. J. (1978). Anxiety: Toward a psychophysiological definition. In H. S. Akiskal, & W. L. Webb (Eds.), *Psychiatric diagnosis: Exploration of biological criteria* (pp. 265–389). New York: Spectrum.

Lang, P. J., & Buss, A. H. (1968). Psychological deficit in schizophrenia: II. Interference and activation. In D. S. Holmes (Ed.), *Reviews of research in behavior pathology.* (pp. 400–452). New York: Wiley.

Leutner, D., & Rammsayer, T. (1995). Complex trait-treatment-interaction analysis: a powerful approach for analysing individual differences in experimental designs. *Personality and Individual Differences, 19*, 493–511.

Levy, J., Heller, W., Banich, M. T., & Burton, L. A. (1983). Asymmetry of perception in free viewing of chimeric faces. *Brain and Cognition, 2*, 404–419.

Lewine, J. D., & Orrison, W. W. (1995). Magnetoencephalography and magnetic source imaging. In W. W. Orrison, J. D. Lewine, J. A. Sanders & M. Hartshorne (Eds.), *Functional brain imaging* (pp. 369–417). Boston: Mosby.

Lindauer, R. J., Vlieger, E. J., Jalink, M., Olff, M., Carlier, I. V., Majoie, C. B., et al. (2004). Smaller hippocampal volume in Dutch police officers with posttraumatic stress disorder. *Biological Psychiatry, 56*, 356–363.

MacDonald, A. W., III., Johnson, M. K., Becker, T. M., & Carter, C. S. (2003, March). Context processing deficits associated with hypofrontality in the healthy relatives of schizophrenia patients: An event related fMRI study. Paper presented at the IXth meeting of International Congress of Schizophrenia Research, Colorado Springs, Colorado.

MacLeod, C. M. (1991). Half a century of research on the Stroop effect: An intergrative review. *Psychological Bulletin, 109*, 163–203.

MacLeod, C. M. (1992). The Stroop task: The "gold standard" of attentional measures. *Journal of Experimental Psychology: General, 121*, 12–14.

Mäkelä J. P. (1988). Contra- and ipsilateral auditory stimuli produce different activation patterns at the human auditory cortex: a neuromagnetic study. *Pflugers Arch, 412*, 12016.

Mäkelä J. P., Ahonen, A., Hämäläinen, M., Hari, R., Ilmoniemi, R., Kajola, M., et al. (1993). Functional differences between auditory corticies of the two hemispheres revealed by whole-head Neuromagnetic recordings. *Human Brain Mapping, 1*, 48–56.

Malmo, R. B., & Shagass, C. (1949). Physiological studies of reaction to stress in anxiety states and early schizophrenia. *Psychosomatic Medicine, 11*, 9–24.

Malmo, R. B., & Shagass, C. (1952). Studies of blood pressure in psychiatric patients under stress. *Psychosomatic Medicine, 14*, 82–93.

Manoach, D. S., Press, D. Z., Thangaraj, V., Searl, M. M., Goff, D. C., Halpern, E., et al. (1999). Schizophrenic subjects activate dorsolateral prefrontal cortex during a working memory task, as measured by fMRI. *Biological Psychiatry, 45*, 1128–1137.

Manoach, D. S., Gollub, R. L., Benson, E. S., Searl, M. M., Goff, D. C., Halpern, E., et al. (2000). Schizophrenic subjects show aberrant fMRI activation of dorsolateral prefrontal cortex and basal ganglia during working memory performance. *Biological Psychiatry, 48*, 99–109.

Matsuo, K., Kata, T., Taneichi, K., Matsumoto, A., Ohtani, T., Hamamoto, T., et al. (2003). Activation of the prefrontal cortex to trauma-related stimuli measured by near-infrared spectroscopy in posttraumatic stress disorder due to terrorism. *Psychophysiology, 40*, 492–500.

Mayberg, H., & Fossati, P. (In press). Dysfunctional limbic-cortical circuits in major depression: A functional neuroimaging perspective. In D. Barch (Ed.), *Cognitive and affective neuroscience of psychopathology*.

McFarlane, A. C., Weber, D. L., & Clark, C. R. (1993). Abnormal stimulus processing in posttraumatic stress disorder. *Biological Psychiatry, 34*, 311–320.

McGhie, A., & Chapman, J. (1961). Disorders of attention and perception in early schizophrenia. *British Journal of Medical Psychology, 34*, 103–116.

McNally, R. J. (1992). Psychopathology of post-traumatic stress disorder PTSD: Boundaries of the syndrome. In M. Basoglu (Ed.), *Torture and its consequences: Current treatment approaches* (pp. 229–252). Cambridge, England: Cambridge University Press.

McNally, R. J. (2003). Progress and controversy in the study of posttraumatic stress disorder. *Annual Review of Psychology, 54*, 229–252.

Meehl, P. E. (1970). Nuisance variables and the ex post factor design. In M. Radner & S. Winokur (Eds.), *Minnesota studies in the philosophy of science (volume 4): Analyses of theories and methods of physics and psychology* (pp. 373–402). Minneapolis: University of Minnesota Press.

Meehl, P. E. (1971). High school yearbooks: A reply to Schwartz. *Journal of Abnormal Psychology, 77*, 143–148.

Mervaala, E., Fohr, J., Kononen, M., Valkonen-Korhonen, M., Vainio, P., Partanen, K., et al. (2000). Quantitative MRI of the hippocampus and amygdala in severe depression. *Psychological Medicine, 30*, 117–125.

Metzger, L. J., Carson, M. A., Paulus, L. A., Lasko, N. B., Paige, S. R., Pitman, R. K., et al. (2002). Event-related potentials to auditory stimuli in female Vietnam nurse veterans with posttraumatic stress disorder. *Psychophysiology, 39*, 49–63.

Metzger, L. J., Orr, S. P., Lasko, N. B., & Pitman, R. K. (1997a). Auditory event-related potentials to tone stimuli in combat-related posttraumatic stress disorder. *Biol Psychiatry, 42*, 1006–1015.

Metzger, L. J., Orr, S. P., Lasko, N. B., Berry, N. J., & Pitman, R. K. (1997b). Evidence for diminished P3 amplitudes in PTSD. In R. Yehuda & A. C. McFarlane (Eds.), *Psychobiology of posttraumatic stress disorder* (pp. 499–503). New York: Annals of the New York Academy of Sciences.

Michel, C. M., Murray, M. M., Lantz, G., Gonzalez, S., Spinelli, L., & de Peralta, R. G. (2004). EEG source imaging. *Clinical Neurophysiology, 115*, 2195–2222.

Miller, G. A. (Ed.) (1995). *The behavioral high-risk paradigm in psychopathology*. New York: Springer-Verlag.

Miller, G. A. (1996). Presidential address: How we think about cognition, emotion, and biology in psychopathology. *Psychophysiology, 33*, 615–628.

Miller, G. A. (2000). Editorial. *Psychophysiology, 37*, 1–4.

Miller, G. A. (In press). Clinical science: How psychological and biological convergence can and can't work. In T. Treat, R. Bootzin, & R. Leveson (Eds.), *Festschrift for Richard McFall: Papers in honor of clinical psychological science*.

Miller, G. A. (In press). Mood disorders section editor commentary. In D. Barch (editor), *Cognitive and affective neuroscience of psychopathology*.

Miller, G. A., & Chapman, J. P. (2001). Misunderstanding analysis of covariance . . . *Journal of Abnormal Psychology, 110*, 40–48.

Miller, G. A., & Ebert, L. (1988). Conceptual boundaries in psychophysiology. *Journal of Psychophysiology, 2*, 13–16.

Miller, G. A., Elbert, T., Sutton, B. P., & Heller, W. (Accepted pending revision). Invited paper: Innovative clinical assessment technologies: Challenges and opportunities in neuroimaging. *Psychological Assessment*.

Miller, G. A., Engels, A. S., & Herrington, J. D. (In press). The seduction of clinical science: Challenges in psychological and biological convergence. In T. Treat, R. Bootzin, & R. Levenson (Eds.), *Psychological clinical science: Papers in honor of Richard McFall*.

Miller, E. K., Erickson, C. A., & Desimone, R. (1996). Neural mechanisms of visual working memory in prefrontal cortex of the macaque. *Journal of Neuroscience, 16,* 5154–5167.

Miller, G. A., & Keller, J. (2000). Psychology and neuroscience: Making peace. *Current Directions in Psychological Science, 9,* 212–215.

Miller, G. A., & Kozak, M. J. (1993). Three-system assessment and the construct of emotion. In N. Birbaumer, & A. Öhman (Eds.), *The structure of emotion: Psychophysiological, cognitive and clinical aspects* (pp. 31–47). Seattle: Hogrefe & Huber Publishers.

Miller, M. B., Chapman, J. P., Chapman, L. J., & Collins, J. (1995). Task difficulty and cognitive deficits in schizophrenia. *Journal of Abnormal Psychology, 104,* 251–258.

Millon, T. (1991). Classification in psychopathology: Rationale, alternatives, and standards. *Journal of Abnormal Psychology, 100,* 245–261.

Mineka, S., Watson, D., & Clark, L. A. (1998). Comorbidity of anxiety and unipolar mood disorders. *Annual Review of Psychology, 49,* 377–412.

Mohanty, A., Herrington, J. D., Koven, N. S., Wenzel, E. A., Webb, A. G., Heller, W., et al. (2005). Neural mechanisms of affective interference in schizotypy. *Journal of Abnormal Psychology, 114,* 16–27.

Nadel, L., & Jacobs, W. J. (1998). Traumatic memory is special. *Current Directions in Psychological Science, 7,* 154–157.

Nakasato, N, Fujita, S., Seki, K., Kawamura, T., Matani, A., Tamura, I., et al. (1995). Functional localization of bilateral auditory cortices using an MRI-linked whole head magnetoencephalography (MEG) system. *Electroencephalography and Clinical Neurophysiology, 94,* 183–190.

Neylan, T. C., Fletcher, D. J., Lenoci, M., McCallin, K., Weiss, D. S., Schoenfeld, F. B., Marmar, C. T., & Fein, G. (1999). Sensory gating in chronic posttraumatic stress disorder: reduced auditory P50 suppression in combat veterans. *Biological Psychiatry, 46,* 1656–1664.

Neylan, T. C., Jasiukaitis, P. A., Lenoci, M., Scott, J. C., Metzler, T. J., Weiss, D. S., Schoenfeld, F. B., & Marmar, C. R. (2003). Temporal instability of auditory and visual event-related potentials in posttraumatic stress disorder. *Biological Psychiatry, 53,* 216–225.

Nitschke, J. B., Heller, W., Etienne, M., & Miller, G. A. (2004). Prefrontal cortex activation differentiates processes affecting memory in depression. *Biological Psychology, 67,* 125–243.

Nitschke, J. B., Heller, W., Miller, G. A. (2000). Anxiety, stress, and cortical brain function. In J. C. Borod, J. C. (Ed.), *The Neuropsychology of Emotion* (pp. 298–319). New York: Oxford University Press.

Nitschke, J. B., Heller, W., Palmieri, P. A., & Miller, G. A. (1999). Contrasting patterns of brain activity in anxious apprehension and anxious arousal. *Psychophysiology, 36,* 628–637.

Nitschke, J. B., & Heller, W. (2002). The neuropsychology of anxiety disorders: affect, cognition, and neural circuitry. In H. D'Haenen, J. A. den Boer, P. Willner (Eds.), *Biological Psychiatry* (pp. 975–988) Chichester: Wiley.

Öst, L. (1989). Panic disorder, agoraphobia, and social phobia. In G. Turpin (Ed.), *Handbook of clinical psychophysiology* (pp. 309–328). New York: Wiley.

Osuch, E. A., Benson, B., Geraci, M., Podell, D., Herscovitch, P., McCann, U. D., et al. (2001). Regional cerebral blood flow correlated with flashback intensity in patients with posttraumatic stress disorder. *Biological Psychiatry, 50,* 246–253.

Pallmeyer, T., Blanchard, E., & Kolb, L. (1986). The psychophysiology of combat induced post-traumatic stress disorder in Vietnam veterans. *Behaviour Research and Therapy, 24,* 645–652.

Pantev, C., Ross, B., Berg, P., Elbert, T., & Rockstroh, B. (1998). Study of the human auditory cortices using whole-head magnetometer: left vs. right hemisphere and ipsilateral vs. contralateral stimulation. *Audiology and Neuro-Otology, 3,* 183–190.

Pantev, C., Markeig, S., Hoke, M., Galambos, R., Hampson, S., & Gallen, C. (1991). Human auditory evoked gamma-band magnetic fields. *Proceedings of the National Academy of Science of the United States of America, 88,* 8986–9000.

Picton, T. W., Alain, C., Woods, D. L., John, M. S., Scherg, M., Valdes-Sosa, P., et al. (1999). Intracerebral sounces of human auditory-evoked potentials. *Audiology Neuro-Otology, 4,* 64–79.

Pitman, R. K., Orr, S. P., Forgue, deJong, J., & Claiborn, J. (1987). Psychophysiologic assessment of posttraumatic stress disorder imagery in Vietnam combat veterans. *Archives of General Psychiatry, 44,* 970–975.

Post, R. M., DeLisi, L. E., Holcomb, H. H., Uhde, T. W., Cohen, R., & Buchsbaum, M. (1987). Glucose utilization in the temporal cortex of affectively ill patients: Positron emission tomography. *Biological Psychiatry, 22,* 545–553.

Prins, A., Kaloupek, D. G., & Keane, T. M. (1995). Psychophysiological evidence for autonomic arousal and startle in traumatized adult populations. In M. J. Friedman, D. S. Charney, & A. Y. Deutch (Eds.), *Neurobiological and clinical consequences of stress: From normal adaption of PTSD* (pp. 291–314). Raven Press: New York.

Ramsey, N. F., Koning, H. A., Welles, P., Cahn, W., Van Der Linden, J. A., & Kahn, R. S. (2002). Excessive recruitment of neural systems subserving logical reasoning in schizophrenia. *Brain, 125,* 1793–1807.

Rauch, S. L., van der Kolk, B. A., Fisler, R. E., Alpert, N., Orr, S. P., Savage, C. R., et al. (1996). A symptom provocation study of posttraumatic stress disorder using positron emission tomography and script-driven imagery. *Archives of General Psychiatry, 53,* 380–387.

Rockstroh, B., Clementz, B. A., Pantev, C., Blumenfeld, L. D., Sterr, A., & Elbert, T. (1998). Failure of dominant left-hemispheric activation to right-ear stimulation in schizophrenia. *Neuro Report, 19,* 3819–3822.

Rockstroh, B., Kissler, J., Mohr, B., Eulitz, C., Lommen, U., Wienbruch, C., et al. (2001). Altered hemispheric asymmetry of auditory magnetic fields to tones and syllables in schizophrenia. *Biological Psychiatry, 49,* 694–703.

Rogers, R. L., Papanicolaou, A. C., Baumann, S. B., Eisenberg, H. M., & Saydjari, C. (1990). Spatially distributed cortical excitation patterns of auditory processing during contralateral and ipsilateral stimulation. *Journal of Cognitive Neuroscience, 2,* 44–50.

Rubinow, D. R., & Post, R. M. (1992). Impaired recognition of affect in facial expression in depressed patients. *Biological Psychiatry, 31,* 947–953.

Salmelin, R., & Hari, R. (1994). Characterization of spontaneous MEG rhythms in healthy adults. *Electroencephalograhy and Clinical Neurophysiology, 91,* 237–248.

Sanders, J. A., Lewine, J. D., & Orrison, W. W. (1996). Comparison of primary motor localization using functional magnetic resonance imaging and magnetoencephalography. *Human Brain Mappging, 4,* 47–57.

Sapolsky, R. M. (2002). Chickens, eggs and hippocampal atrophy. *Nature Neuroscience, 5,* 1111–1112.

Scherg, M., & Berg, P. (1996). New concepts of brain source imaging and localization. *Electroencephalography & Clinical Neurophysiology – Supplement, 46*, 127–137.

Schuff, N., Neylan, T. C., Lenoci, M. A., Du, A. T., Weiss, D. S., Marmar, C. R., et al. (2001). Decreased hippocampal N-acetylaspartate in the absence of atrophy in posttraumatic stress disorder. *Biological Psychiatry, 50*, 952–959.

Semple, W. E., Goyer, P., McCormick, R., Morris, E., Compton, B., Muswick, G., et al. (1993). Preliminary report: Brain blood flow using PET in patients with posttraumatic stress disorder and substance-abuse histories. *Biological Psychiatry, 34*, 115–118.

Sheline, Y. I., Sanghavi, M., Mintum, M. A., & Gado, M. H. (1999). Depression duration but not age predicts hippocampal volume loss in medically healthy women with recurrent major depression. *Journal of Neuroscience, 19*, 5034–43.

Sheline, Y. I., Barch, D. M., Donnelly, J. M., Ollinger, J. M., Snyder, et al., (2001). Increased amygdala response to masked emotional faces in depressed subjects resolves with antidepressant treatment: an fMRI study. *Biological Psychiatry, 50*, 651–8.

Shestyuk, A.Y, & Deldin, P. J. (In press). The neurobiology of cognitive deficits in major depression: Perspectives from functional neuroimaging and event-related potential research. In D. Barch (Ed.), *Cognitive and affective neuroscience of psychopathology.*

Shin, L. M., Rauch, S. L., & Pitman, R. K. (In press). Structural and functional anatomy of PTSD. In J. J. Vasterling & C. R. Brewin (Eds.). *Neuropsychology of PTSD: Biological, clinical, and cognitive perspectives.* New York: Guilford Press.

Shin, L. M., Shin, P. S., Heckers, S., Krangel, T. S., Macklin, M. L. et al. (2004). Hippocampal function in posttraumatic stress disorder. *Hippocampus, 14*, 292–300.

Silberman, E. K., Weingartner, H., & Post, R. M. (1983). Thinking disorder in depression: Logic and strategy in an abstract reasoning task. *Archives of General Psychiatry, 40*, 775–780.

Singer, W. (1993). Synchronization of cortical activity and its putative role in information processing and learning. *Annu Rev Physiol., 55*, 349–374.

Skinner, R. D., Rasco, L. M., Fitzgerald, J., Karson, C. N., Matthew, M., Williams, D. K., et al. (1999). Reduced sensory gating of the P1 potential in rape victims and combat veterans with posttraumatic stress disorder. *Depression and Anxiety, 9*, 122–130.

Smith, D. A., Boutros, N. N., & Schwarzkopf, S. B. (1994). Reliability of P50 auditory event-related potential indices of sensory gating. *Psychophysiology, 31*, 495–502.

Steffens, D. C., Byrum, C. E., McQuoid, D. R., Greenberg, D. L., Payne, M. E., Blitchington, T. F., et al. (2000). Hippocampal volume in geriatric depression. *Biological Psychiatry, 48*, 301–309.

Stroop, J. (1935). Studies of interference in serial verbal reactions. *Experimental Psychology, 18*, 643–662.

Suddath, R. L., Christison, G. W., Torrey, E. F., Casanova, M. F., & Weinberger, D. R. (1990). Anatomical abnormalities in the brains of monozygotic twins discordant for schizophrenia. *New England Journal of Medicine, 322*, 789–794.

Thoma, R., Hanlon, F., Moses, S., Edgar, J. C., Huang, M. X., Weisend, M., et al. (2003). Lateralization of auditory sensory gating and neuropsychological dysfunction in schizophrenia. *American Journal of Psychiatry, 160*, 1595–1605.

Thoma, R., Hanlon, F., Moses, S., Ricker, D., Huang, D., Edgar, C., et al. (2005). M50 sensory gating predicts negative symptoms in schizophrenia. *Schizophrenia Research, 73*, 311–318.

Thomas, K. M., Drevets, W. C., Dahl, R. E., Ryan, N. D., Birmacher, B., et al. (2001). Amygdala response to fearful faces in anxious and depressed children. *Archives of General Psychiatry, 58*, 1057–63.

Tebartz van Elst, L., Woermann, F. G., Lemieux, L., & Trimble, M. R. (1999). Amygdala enlargement in dysthymia – a volumetric study of patients with temporal lobe epilepsy. *Biological Psychiatry, 46*, 1614–1623.

Uytdenhoef, P., Portelange, P., Jacquy, J., Charles, G., Linkowshi, P., & Mendlewicz, J. (1983). Regional cerebral blood flow and lateralized hemispheric dysfunction in depression. *British Journal of Psychiatry, 143*, 128–132.

Villarreal, G., Hamilton, D. A., Petropoulos, H., Driscoll, I., Rowland, L. M., Griego, J. A., et al. (2002a). Reduced hippocampal volume and total white matter volume in posttraumatic stress disorder. *Biological Psychiatry, 52*, 119–125.

Villarreal, G., Petropoulos, H., Hamilton, D. A., Rowland, L. M., Horan, W. P., Griego, et al. (2002b). Proton magnetic resonance spectroscopy of the hippocampus and occipital white matter in PTSD: preliminary results. *Canadian Journal of Psychiatry, 47*, 666–670.

Weinberger, D. R., Berman, K. F., & Zec, R. F. (1986). Physiological dysfunction of dorsolateral prefrontal cortex in schizophrenia I: Regional cerebral blood flow (rCBF) evidence. *Archives of General Psychiatry, 43*, 114–124.

Weiss, E. M., Golaszewski, S., Mottaghy, F. M., Hofer, A., Hausmann, A., Kemmler, G., et al. (2003). Brain activation patterns during a selective attention test – a functional MRI study in healthy volunteers and patients with schizophrenia. *Psychiatry Research: Neuroimaging, 123*, 1–15.

Widiger, T. A., & Samuel, D. B. (2005). Diagnostic categories or dimensions: A question for the Diagnostic and Statistical manual of mental Disorders – fifth edition. DSM-II. *Journal of Abnormal Psychology, 114*, 494–504.

Winter, H., & Irle, E. (2004). Hippocampal volume in adult burn patients with and without posttraumatic stress disorder. *American Journal of Psychiatry, 161*, 2194–2200.

Winterer, G., Ziller, M., Dorn, H., Frick, K., Mulert, C. & Wuebben, Y., et al. (2000). Schizophrenia: reduced signal-to-noise ratio and impaired phase-locking during information processing. *Clinical Neurophysiology, 111*, 837–849.

Yücel, M., Pantelis, C., Stuart, G. W., Wood, S. J., Maruff, P., Velakoulis, D., et al. (2002). Anterior cingulated activation during Stroop task performance: A PET to MRI coregistration study of individual patients with schizophrenia. *American Journal of Psychiatry, 159(2)*, 251–254.

Zahn, T. P. (1986). Psychophysiological approaches to psychopathology. In M. G. H. Coles, E. Donchin, & S. W. Porges (Eds.), *Psychophysiology: Systems, processes, and applications* (pp. 508–610). New York: Guilford Press.

29 Detection of Deception

WILLIAM G. IACONO

INTRODUCTION

Relying on their listening and observational skills, people can detect liars with about 54% accuracy, which is only slightly better than chance (DePaulo et al., 2003). Given the ease with which we are deceived and the often high cost of being taken in by a liar, it is little wonder that security and law enforcement agencies, corporations striving to maintain a competitive edge, and private individuals concerned about the trustworthiness of friends and relatives would like to have an accurate "lie detector." However, there is no foolproof technique for detecting lies or liars, although efforts to develop and improve procedures to do so have been around since Harvard psychologist William Marston (1917) introduced his systolic blood pressure test for detecting lying in the early part of the last century.

In this chapter, I will provide an overview of psychophysiological techniques used to detect deception, how well they work, and a critical appraisal of the science underlying these methods. Besides highlighting issues of continuing importance, my focus will be on recent developments, especially those spanning the time elapsing since the second edition of this *Handbook* was published in 2000. Readers wishing for a broader account of the development of deception detection techniques are urged to consult the second edition (Iacono, 2000).

APPLICATIONS

Lie detection techniques have been developed to detect two types of liars: criminals and untrustworthy employees. Forensic procedures are primarily used by law enforcement to detect criminals. These techniques are often referred to as specific incident tests because the examiner is attempting to resolve a known criminal incident under investigation. In contrast, screening procedures are typically employed by government and private agencies to detect security risks. For these procedures, it is not known whether a particular incident has taken place, so the questions deal with the likelihood that the examinee has engaged in past behaviors that would make that individual a security risk. Forensic and security screening tests measure autonomic nervous system reactions to questions put to the examinee. Modern field polygraphs are computer based, and are accompanied by proprietary software that scores test outcomes to yield a probability estimate of a subject's truthfulness. However, as sophisticated as these devices have become, they are designed to monitor the same types of physiological reactions recorded by field polygraphs of the 1940s (electrodermal, blood pressure, and respiratory responses), and hand scoring of charts remains the preferred method of reaching a verdict.

Forensic applications

Control question technique (CQT)

The so-called control question test and its many variants are by far the procedures most widely used by law enforcement. A typical test contains 10 questions that are repeated two or more times in somewhat different order each time. All variants of the CQT include two types of questions, designated control and relevant, which are used to evaluate the outcome. For a typical CQT, there are three pairs of such questions (six questions total; the other four questions are not scored). Relevant questions deal with involvement in the specific incident under investigation (e.g., "Did you rob the bank?"). Control questions deal with assumed transgressions that everyone taking the test is likely to have committed (e.g., "Did you ever take something from a person who trusted you?"). Examinees are led to believe that it is important to tell the truth about both the control and relevant questions. The polygraph operator tells the examinees that the subject is expected to be able to answer all the questions truthfully with a "no." In this way, the examiner implies that failing a control question would lead to a failed test outcome, which is a psychological manipulation that is intended to make it appear as though control questions are as important as the relevant questions.

The CQT is scored by comparing the magnitude of responses to these two types of questions. Guilty individuals are assumed to be unconcerned by their answers to the control questions, and thus are expected to give substantially larger responses to the lies elicited by the relevant queries. Innocent people are presumed to not care about the accusation embedded in the relevant question. Instead, CQT theory requires that they be more concerned about the transgression tapped by the control question, which causes it to elicit stronger physiological responses than relevant questions. Proponents of the CQT argue accuracy rates exceeding 90%. For instance, the American Polygraph Association (2005) asserts that its review of polygraph studies involving almost 2,200 real life examinations points to an average accuracy of 98%. Psychologists trained in psychophysiology have also argued an average of 98% accuracy for field examiners (Honts, Raskin, & Kircher, 2002; see Table 29.5 and accompanying text).

Criticisms of the CQT focus on the likelihood that guilty and innocent examinees respond as predicted often enough to ensure the claimed high accuracy. Innocent examinees who have a lot at stake, especially if they have misgivings about validity, may be more reactive to their denial of the false but important accusation contained in the relevant question than by their possibly truthful but presumed lie to whatever misdeed is covered by the control question. Innocent people taking a CQT are not likely to attach the same consequences to "failing" control and relevant questions despite the polygraph operators' efforts to convince them otherwise. In other words, the control question does not provide a true scientific control for the emotional impact of being asked the accusatory relevant question. To blunt this criticism, in 1999 the American Polygraph Association elected to abandon the use of the term "control question." Now proponents of polygraphy refer to the CQT as the *comparison* question technique (Raskin & Honts, 2002), arguing in effect that it does not matter whether the question provides a true scientific control because the (claimed) high accuracy of the CQT speaks to the appropriateness of the control question irrespective of its theoretical rationale.

Although there are various reasons why guilty individuals may respond more to relevant questions (Iacono & Lykken, 2002), prime among them concerns the likelihood that they can learn simple countermeasures (e.g., carrying out mental arithmetic exercises) to boost their response to control questions enough to overwhelm reactions to relevant questions. Various readily accessed sources explain CQT methods and countermeasure techniques (e.g., www.polygraph.com, www.antipolygraph.org), and studies have shown that guilty mock crime participants provided with this type of information (in the form of a half hour tutorial) can defeat the CQT while going undetected by skilled examiners (Honts, Hodes, & Raskin, 1985; Honts, Raskin, & Kircher, 1994).

Directed lie technique (DLT)

The DLT differs from the CQT in one respect: The "probable lie" control questions of the CQT are replaced with "directed lies." In effect, the polygraph examiner develops a set of questions with the examinee that both individu-

als agree elicit lies (e.g., "Have you ever made even one mistake?"). Subjects are told to think of a specific instance of a lie covered by the directed lie question. Those taking the DLT are told that the purpose of the question is to determine what a lie response looks like. In this way, the DLT attempts to remedy the shortcomings associated with the CQT assumption that control questions elicit actual lies and real concern when in fact they may not.

The DLT has stimulated little research while generating the same criticisms as the CQT. The DLT has the additional shortcoming of making transparent the purpose of the directed lie, thereby facilitating the application of countermeasures.

Guilty knowledge test (GKT)

The GKT (also referred to as the concealed information test or CIT) has been developed and promoted by Lykken as a scientifically based alternative to the CQT (Lykken, 1959, 1981). The GKT is a psychophysiological examination designed to uncover whether a suspect possesses crime-specific knowledge that the perpetrator of a crime, but not uninvolved individuals, would be expected to have. Questions take the form of multiple-choice items. However, rather than the examinee choosing the correct alternative to each question, physiological reactions to each alternative are monitored to see if the guilty knowledge alternative elicits a stronger reaction than the others. For instance, a suspect might be asked: "If you committed this bank robbery, then you would know how much cash you took. Was it about $3000...$7000...$11000...$13000? You would also know what you wrote on your holdup note. Was it Don't sound the alarm?; Do as I say and you won't get hurt?; This is a robbery? Listen closely I have a gun pointed at you? An innocent suspect taking such a test would respond randomly to the various options, but the recognition of correct alternatives by the perpetrator would elicit stronger physiological reactions to the guilty knowledge options by likely reflecting an orienting response to the concealed information (Verschuere et al., 2004). The orienting response, a phasic autonomic reaction first identified by Pavlov and studied extensively by Sokolov (Sokolov, 1963), arises when a person is first presented with a discrete stimulus. The orienting response reflects the degree to which the stimulus has significance, in this case, the degree to which it reflects incriminating knowledge. With repeated presentations, eventually a stimulus loses its significance, and the orienting response and its associated autonomic accompaniments habituate. For this reason, GKT question lists are typically presented only once as habituation eventually diminishes the ability to differentiate responses between the meaningful guilty knowledge and meaningless alternative options (Iacono, Boisvenu, & Fleming, 1984).

A properly administered GKT with a sufficient number of items has almost no chance of producing a false positive outcome. Unfortunately, there is no similar built-in mechanism to protect against false negative outcomes. Anyone can develop a GKT that even a perpetrator would pass by choosing material for items that is obscure or easily forgotten. Indeed, the major challenge facing widespread acceptance of the GKT in forensic settings is the lack of research concerning how to develop good items that are likely to be recalled by criminals. Most laboratory GKT studies require participants to commit to memory relevant crime details, and then administer the GKT immediately after the mock crime, ensuring minimal forgetting. When crimes are made more realistic and a delay is introduced between crime commission and GKT administration detection accuracy drops with GKT questions involving peripheral crime details (e.g., the contents of a wall hanging in the room where the crime takes place) less effective than those dealing with features more central to the crime (Carmel et al., 2003). Hence, the method followed to develop items is a key aspect of the evaluation of any GKT administration. Unfortunately, it is not always apparent what constitutes a good item, but premeditated crimes that are well thought out and sex crimes that are executed following a distinct ritual would be examples of crimes that may be productively addressed with the GKT.

Although these problems undermine the confidence that can be placed in passed GKTs, similar problems do not exist for failed GKTs. For instance, for a 10 item GKT each with five alternatives, an innocent person has one chance in ten million of responding most strongly to all the guilty alternatives (Lykken, 1998, p. 302). Depending how the threshold is set for what constitutes a failure, a carefully administered but failed GKT can be highly incriminating (Iacono, 1985; Iacono, 2000; Iacono et al., 1984; Lykken, 1981). Thus, compared to the CQT which is biased against innocent individuals and, therefore, apt to be prejudicial when failed, the GKT is likely to have probative value when failed.

Despite the apparent strengths of the GKT, the complexity of the procedure coupled with the belief of the polygraph profession that the simpler-to-administer CQT is nearly infallible has led to its being largely ignored by practitioners. Although the GKT is used extensively in Japan (Hira & Furumitsu, 2002; Nakayama, 2002; Suzuki, Nakayama, & Furedy, 2004), virtually all forensic polygraph tests administered in the U.S., Canada, and Israel, are CQTs.

Security screening

Most polygraph tests are administered by the U.S. federal government, and most of these tests are for security screening. There are about two-dozen federal agencies using polygraph procedures, and their use has escalated over the last decade as concerns about security and terrorism have heightened. These tests are used to screen prospective employees, such as FBI and CIA agents, as part of the hiring evaluation process. They are also used to check whether current employees, such as those responsible for protecting government secrets and national safety, warrant their security clearances.

Because those undergoing screening procedures are not known to have committed any wrongdoing, for these tests, the relevant questions resemble CQT control questions as they cover possible past misdeeds over the lifetime of the examinee. Hence, ambiguity surrounds what constitutes an appropriate "control" question on a screening test. This introduces greater subjectivity in how these tests are constructed and interpreted. The evidence available from various government reports indicates that examiners giving these tests alter the threshold for diagnosing deception depending on the expected base rate of deception in the population they are testing as well as the perceived consequences of false positive outcomes (Barland, Honts, & Barger, 1989; Honts, 1991; Iacono & Lykken, 2002). That is, when testing rigorously screened and currently employed individuals with high-level security clearances, few of whom are apt to be spies and all of whom may be difficult to replace given their esoteric training and expertise, only a tiny fraction (1–2%) are deemed to fail a polygraph test. But when screening employee prospects, who exceed the number of available positions and have not undergone expensive training, a third or more are likely to fail.

An issue that is unique to screening government employees is the cumulative likelihood of failing a test over the employee's lifetime. The tests are administered repeatedly, with government programs advocating the retesting of employees both aperiodically and periodically at intervals spanning 3–5 years. Little attention has been paid to the likelihood of these tests eventually generating a false positive outcome for an employee with a career spanning decades who may have to take the test a half dozen or more times.

Relevant/irrelevant technique (RIT)

Although there are many different screening test formats, these procedures are descendants of the relevant/irrelevant technique (RIT), a forerunner of the CQT that was commonly used in criminal investigations. In the original RIT, relevant questions like those on the CQT were intermixed with irrelevant questions (e.g., "Do you now live in Minneapolis?"). Consistently stronger reaction to relevant questions is considered presumptive evidence of guilt.

Even staunch proponents of polygraphy acknowledge the inadequacy of irrelevant questions as legitimate controls. Thus, modern screening tests include such questions largely to provide a type of psychological refuge from the stream of relevant questions covering topics like drug use, alcoholism, work habits, trustworthiness, and rule compliance. After presenting multiple questions tapping each of these themes, examiners attempt to identify question categories (e.g., concerning drug use) that elicit stronger reactions than other content areas (Ferguson, 1966). Having identified a topic that appears to elicit strong responses, the examiner probes the examinee for an explanation. This explanation may in turn provoke the development of additional questions and the running of more charts to test the truthfulness of the clarification. Examinees adept at impression management and capable of "explaining away" their reactions (e.g., "I was bothered by your questions about irresponsible drinking because my alcoholic father died of cirrhosis last year.") may be those most likely to pass these tests (Thurber, 1981).

The premises on which screening techniques are based are no more sound than those of the CQT. Heightened reactions to certain types of questions can occur for reasons other than deceptiveness, and there is no reason why these reactions should dissipate once an explanation for them is presented to a polygraph examiner. At one time, these tests were used routinely by private corporations to screen the integrity of their employees. A Congressionally mandated study carried out in the 1980s raised serious concerns about these tests (Saxe, Dougherty, & Cross, 1985), which led to their being banned under the Employee Polygraph Protection Act (Public Law 100–347). Ironically, Congress exempted government agencies from this law, and subsequent to its passage expanded polygraph testing programs (Krapohl, 2002).

Test for espionage and sabotage (TES)

U.S. national security agencies have recently introduced the Test for Espionage and Sabotage (TES). The TES is typically administered periodically to government employees with top-secret security clearances as a response to concerns that some of these individuals may be spies. Questions such as "Have you committed espionage?" are compared to directed lie control questions (e.g., "Did you ever violate a traffic law?"). The TES can be scored using the same procedures followed for the CQT and DLT and is vulnerable to the same criticisms.

EVALUATION

Before considering how well these procedures work, it is important to highlight several points critical to their evaluation.

Research has focused on forensic applications

Very little research has addressed the accuracy of security screening tests. Only the GKT and CQT have received extensive research attention, and the CQT is by far the most studied polygraph procedure.

Polygraph tests are investigative tools

Field examiners using polygraph tests and the government agencies that sponsor them have been largely unconcerned about what scholars conclude regarding polygraph accuracy. True for decades, this is no less true today, because it is the perceived utility of polygraph testing that sustains its use in the face of stiff criticism regarding accuracy.

Good polygraph examiners are expert interrogators skilled at using the polygraph as a tool to extract admissions of wrongdoing as well as outright confessions. Confronted by an examiner who uses the polygraph to justify skepticism over an examinee's account of the facts, many examinees will divulge information in an attempt to get the examiner to back down. Government agents are happy to collect this information, much of which could either not be obtained in any other way or would be prohibitively expensive to obtain through other investigative means. In security screening, this information might include acknowledging procedure violations or eliciting suspicions about other employees who then become the focus of investigation. In criminal investigations, suspects may correct inaccuracies in their statements, confess to other wrongdoings, or confess to the matter under investigation. A common forensic application of polygraph tests is a sex crime where there is skimpy physical evidence and the case is reduced to the credibility of those involved. In the hands of a skilled examiner, one of the involved parties may "come clean," not only solving the case, but avoiding the expense and uncertain outcome of a protracted trial.

Despite the widespread acceptance of polygraph testing utility, empirical data indicating how often admissions and confessions lead to investigative breakthroughs is unavailable. This is especially so in national security investigations where it has been noted that no spy has ever been identified as a result of a polygraph test, while false negatives, such as the failure to catch notorious CIA spy Aldrich Ames despite repeated polygraph tests, are known (Iacono & Lykken, 2002). Having such data would be especially useful given the accumulating evidence that individuals often make false admissions during stressful interrogations (Kassin, 2005; Kassin & Gudjonsson, 2004). In particular, data are needed to show how often a confession is corroborated (e.g., by the confession leading to the uncovering of other investigation-relevant information).

Legal status of polygraph testing

By federal law, government agencies and certain private corporations where security is important are allowed to evaluate employees using screening tests. New Mexico is the only state allowing routine admittance of polygraph test results in criminal cases, although about half the states allow the admission of stipulated tests, i.e., those that the prosecution and defense agree will be admissible in advance of test administration. Otherwise, polygraph test results seldom find their way into state or federal courts (Faigman et al., 2002).

Scientific opinion

Psychologists and psychophysiologists have been surveyed repeatedly regarding their opinions of polygraph testing, in part because the consensus opinion of the scientific community has been used by courts as one of the criteria to consider in determining whether the results of a technique are acceptable as scientific evidence. The most favorable surveys (Amato, 1993; Gallup, 1984), both polling members of the Society for Psychophysiological Research (SPR), have found that approximately 60% indicated that a polygraph test is "a useful diagnostic tool when considered with other available information." However, these surveys did not ask directly about accuracy; diagnostic usefulness could be equated as easily with utility as with accuracy. They also did not distinguish among types of polygraph tests. Thus, these surveys left it unclear to what degree they refer to the CQT as opposed to, for instance, the GKT, which most scientists view as on a more solid footing than the CQT. David Lykken and I (Iacono & Lykken, 1997) carried out surveys of members of both SPR and the American Psychological Association, and were careful to make clear when questions addressed the CQT, DLT, or GKT. The opinions of members of both groups were quite similar, and indicated strong skepticism about the CQT and DLT but not about the GKT. For instance, these scientists did not believe the CQT: (a) is based on sound theory, (b) could be as accurate as polygraph professionals claim, (c) should be used in court, (d) is standardized, (e) is objective, or (f) is immune to countermeasures.

What is needed to evaluate accuracy

A second reason why polygraph testing continues despite persisting accuracy concerns is that it has proved impossible to provide anything approaching a definitive validity test. Although the nature of social science research seldom provides for definitive conclusions, there are only two meaningful outcomes for a polygraph test, and those taking it are either truthful or lying. Hence, many of the measurement and criterion problems that complicate psychological study in general are not applicable to polygraph validity studies. So why, then, has the validity question remained intractable?

Laboratory studies

The simplest way to ensure criterion validity is to conduct a mock crime study where participants are assigned to guilty or innocent groups. The criterion (guilt or innocence) can be unambiguously established by ensuring that subjects follow the experimenter's programmed instructions, and criterion validity can be estimated by the degree to which programmed guilty subjects fail and innocent subjects pass their polygraph tests. The generally acknowledged problem using this approach to evaluate validity is that it is unrealistic. In real life, those undergoing polygraph exams face serious consequences if they fail, and are living under the veil of a serious accusation. Under these circumstances the emotional impact of the relevant questions is likely to be heightened, as is the motivation to beat the test. In the laboratory situation, innocent subjects have little to fear if they are diagnosed "guilty." When tested with the CQT, they are more apt than in real life to find the privacy invading control questions emotionally troubling. This outcome

is likely because control questions are potentially more psychologically bothersome than relevant questions that deal with a "crime" carried out only to satisfy study requirements. Moreover, a recent study from scientists at the Department of Defense Polygraph Institute attempted to evaluate the generalizability of the data from laboratory mock crime investigations by comparing the physiological responses obtained from mock crime and real life cases (Pollina et al., 2004). The results indicated that electrodermal, cardiovascular, and respiratory responses were more pronounced in field polygraph applications. Following Sokolov's orienting theory (Sokolov, 1963), the authors interpreted these findings as possibly reflecting defensive responses motivated by fear during field polygraph tests, and orienting responses reflecting "fascination with the process and a desire to 'win the game'" (p. 1104) in laboratory situations.

For the GKT, a major limitation of laboratory investigations relates to item development. Mock crime studies are typically set up to ensure both that subjects pay attention to crime details and that the examiner knows what the relevant details are. In real life, neither of these circumstances is likely. Laboratory studies are useful for examining factors that may moderate outcomes, such as personality characteristics or drug effects, but there is no way to tell how well their hit rates generalize to real-life settings.

Field studies

Field studies effectively address the realism issue because they are designed to evaluate accuracy in real-life criminal cases that have involved polygraph tests. However, criterion validity presents a problem. Confessions have become the accepted standard for establishing ground truth because they unambiguously identify the guilty and clear the innocent when a suspect in a multisuspect case confesses. Having established ground truth, polygraph charts can be blindly scored to see how closely the polygraph verdicts match the confession criterion. However, confessions are almost always obtained by the original examiner who, working in the field, has concluded the psychophysiological record is indicative of deception. When this occurs, the confession is not independent of the outcome of the polygraph test, and the charts that ultimately are chosen for study are only likely to be those where the original examiner was correct. As I have illustrated elsewhere (Iacono, 1991), under these circumstances, a test with no better than chance accuracy can be made to look virtually infallible.

The problems inherent to the use of confessions to establish ground truth are highlighted in Figure 29.1. Cases where guilty individuals appear truthful on their polygraph charts will not lead to confessions because the examiner, who believes the suspect to be innocent, will not seek a confession (see Figure 29.1, flowchart A). Likewise, cases where the original examiner erroneously scored the charts deceptive would not be selected for field study because the innocent victims of such an outcome would not be

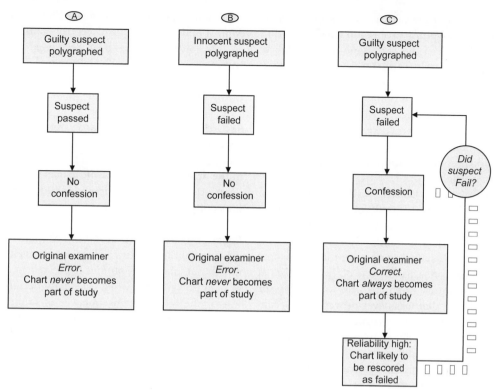

Figure 29.1. Flowcharts indicating how cases are selected for field studies of polygraph validity when confessions are used to verify ground truth. In these studies, the original examiner establishes ground truth if it is possible to obtain a confession of guilt from a suspect who fails a polygraph. Flowchart A indicates that guilty suspects whom the examiner passes will not be asked to confess, and their false negative chart thus does not become part of the validity study. Flowchart B illustrates that innocent suspects who fail also do not become part of such a study because their false positive result does not yield a confession. Only cases represented in Flowchart C become part of field validity studies. This flowchart illustrates the circularity of a case selection method that forces biased selection of only cases that the original examiner scored correctly, which results in a re-scored deceptive chart that almost always matches the confession criterion. Not represented is how confirmed innocent cases become part of such a study. When flowchart C applies to multiple suspect cases, charts from individuals who pass a polygraph are included because they are confirmed as innocent by the confession of the guilty party.

expected to confess (see Figure 29.1, flowchart B). Hence, studies that select cases using a confession to confirm ground truth systematically eliminate all of the original examiner's false positive and false negative errors. The only cases included for study are those where the original examiner was correct (see Figure 29.1, flowchart C). In these cases, a guilty individual must both fail the polygraph and confess. When this occurs, the selected charts are rescored and then compared to ground truth (i.e., the confession). Because chart scoring is highly reliable, blindly rescoring the charts can be expected to result in the same failed polygraph verdict that led to the confession in the first place. As a consequence, field studies overestimate accuracy.

The solution to these problems with laboratory and confession-based field studies is to carry out a field study where the criterion for ground truth is independent of test outcome. Christopher Patrick and I (Patrick & Iacono, 1991) conducted such a study with the Royal Canadian Mounted Police (RCMP). We identified cases where individuals had undergone a polygraph test and a confession was obtained not by the polygraph operator, but as part of

the ongoing detective work accompanying the case. When these independently obtained confessions were compared to the blindly rescored polygraph charts, the hit rate for innocent examinees was 57%. Unfortunately, the corresponding hit rate could not be determined for guilty examinees. This difficulty establishing independent evidence of ground truth for the guilty reflected the fact that the confessions obtained, while frequently clearing the innocent, seldom also originated with a guilty person who had taken a polygraph test.

Reviews of the deception detection literature

Reviews of CQT studies carried out by those who themselves administer polygraph tests have concluded that the CQT is highly accurate (Honts, Raskin, & Kircher, 2002; Raskin & Honts, 2002). Reviews of the same CQT investigations carried out by those not affiliated with the polygraph profession have concluded these claims are indefensible (Ben-Shakar, 2002; Fiedler, Schmod, & Stahl, 2002; Iacono & Lykken, 2002; Oskol & O'Donohue, 2003). Although polygraph proponents are generally skeptical that the GKT offers any advantage over the CQT, reviews of the GKT by those outside of the polygraph profession have pointed to the under-realized value of this technique (Ben-Shakar & Elaad, 2003; Ben-Shakhar, Bar-Hillel, & Kremnitzer, 2002; Iacono & Lykken, 2002). The most recent and comprehensive review of this literature was published as a book by the National Research Council (NRC) of the National Academy of Sciences (2003). Given the extensiveness of this report and the prestige of its authors, I will highlight in some detail the circumstances surrounding this review as well as its main conclusions.

As part of the National Defense Authorization Act of 2000, Public Law 106–65 required scientists at nuclear weapons laboratories (such as New Mexico's Sandia and Los Alamos Laboratories) to submit to security screening tests to maintain their top-secret clearances. This law was passed following concerns that one of the scientists at the Los Alamos laboratory (Wen Ho Lee) was spying for the Chinese – a charge that was never proved (see Greenberg, 2002). Confronted with the prospect that they would have to undergo these security tests, a panel of Sandia's senior weapons scientists and engineers conducted their own evaluation of the polygraph literature (Sandia's Senior Scientists & Engineers, 1999). These scientists often provide evaluations of technical issues of concern to weapons lab management. They concluded that there were no adequate studies to support screening, and that it was impossible to predict what error rates might be expected. They also expressed concern that the implementation of this program might reduce the likelihood that talented scientists would choose a career at these labs if they knew their employment future depended on polygraph test outcomes. Against this backdrop, as part of the National Defense Authorization Act for 2002, Congress instructed the U.S. Department of Energy (DOE), which oversees the labs, to evaluate their use of lie detectors. DOE in turn asked the National Academy to examine the validity of polygraph testing.

The NRC panel was composed of 14 distinguished scholars with diverse backgrounds in psychophysiology, psychology, statistics, law, and medicine. Aided by a scientific support staff, this panel conducted the most far-reaching and thorough evaluation of polygraph testing ever undertaken. Their work spanned almost two years and included public hearings, visits to polygraph facilities, and access to unpublished government reports, including classified material. Although security screening was a primary concern of the panel, because there is little available research on this topic, most of the research the panel had to evaluate was derived from specific incident polygraph testing (disproportionately CQT studies), so their conclusions apply to polygraph testing broadly. The following key NRC findings address the scientific basis of polygraph testing.

Regarding polygraph theory. The NRC panel noted that the theoretical rationale for CQT polygraph testing is quite weak. Little is known about the psychological states or specific factors purported to cause differential responses to control and relevant questions. By contrast, the theoretical basis of the GKT has been developed and linked to orienting response theory. The NRC panel concluded that "in short, the bulk of polygraph research . . . can be accurately characterized as atheoretical" (p. 94).

Regarding polygraph research. Research on polygraph testing was characterized as similarly weak. The studies themselves were found to be of generally low quality. Taken in the aggregate, there was little evidence of accumulated knowledge that had strengthened the scientific underpinnings of polygraph testing.

Regarding laboratory studies. The panel characterized existing validity studies as having serious limitations, and noted that laboratory studies fail to reflect critical aspects of field polygraph testing, especially because they do not mirror the real-life consequences of failing a polygraph. The panel concluded that laboratory studies "are likely to overestimate accuracy in field practice, but by an unknown amount" (p. 210).

Regarding field studies. The panel commented that "virtually all of the observational field studies have been focused on specific incidents and have been plagued by measurement biases that favor overestimation of accuracy, such as examiner contamination, as well as biases created by the lack of a clear and independent measure of truth" (p. 214). This led them to conclude that "the available field studies are also likely to overestimate the accuracy achieved in actual practice" (p. 210).

Regarding accuracy. The panel was clearly dubious of the accuracy claims of the polygraph profession: "What is remarkable, given the large body of relevant research, is that claims about the accuracy of the polygraph made today parallel those made throughout the history of the polygraph: practitioners have always claimed extremely high levels of accuracy, and these claims have rarely been reflected in empirical research (p. 107) . . . almost a century of research in scientific psychology and physiology provides little basis for the expectation that a polygraph test could have extremely high accuracy" (p. 212). Accuracy cannot be established because "the evidence does not allow any precise quantitative estimate of polygraph accuracy or provide confidence that accuracy is stable across personality types, sociodemographic groups, psychological and medical conditions, examiner and examinee expectancies, or ways of administering the test and selecting questions" (p. 214).

Summary. Despite this clear indictment of polygraph testing, this report has had little effect on the practice of polygraphy even in the DOE laboratories (Malakoff, 2003). Possible reasons for this include the fact that the report did not challenge strongly claims regarding utility. Rather, the authors concluded that polygraph tests might be useful when they "elicit admissions and confessions, deter undesired activity, and instill public confidence" (p. 214). As noted previously, belief in the utility of polygraph testing has always been used to justify its use in the face of scientific criticism. In addition, the NRC noted that no alternative method for detecting deception appears to outperform the polygraph even for security screening. Given the current salience of concerns over security, there is little incentive to drop or substantially modify polygraph practice.

Finally, despite the panel's lack of confidence in the quality of the existing polygraph research, the panel identified 57 specific incident studies (combining both CQT and GKT formats) that met "minimal criteria" (p. 107) for inclusion in a signal detection analysis. This analysis was based on receiver operating curves (ROC) calculated for each of the 57 studies. The area under the ROC curve yields an "accuracy index" (designated A). The ROC analysis demonstrated high variability across studies in the value of A by yielding a median value $A = .86$. A does not translate directly into hit rate estimates, such as those provided in other reviews of this literature, primarily because the ROC analysis takes into account inconclusive outcomes as well as differences across studies in the rules followed to identify passed and failed tests. Because none of the 57 investigations generated ROC curves indicating less than chance or near perfect accuracy, the panel concluded that for those untrained in countermeasures, "specific incident polygraph tests for event-specific investigations can discriminate lying from truth telling at rates well above chance, though well below perfection" (p. 214). This ambiguous statement is not seen as inconsistent with proponents' claims that the CQT may have better than 90% accuracy. Of course, it is also not inconsistent with critic's claims that accuracy is substantially lower.

RECENT ADVANCES

In this section, I will review deception detection research that relies on measures other than autonomic measures to infer deceptive behavior. Some of this research was covered by the NRC report, so my focus will be to briefly highlight progress in this area with an eye toward future developments. Without exception, this area of investigation fails to grapple successfully with the many problems that have plagued lie detection research for the last half-century. This research is laboratory based and fails to tackle seriously the problem associated with the low levels of jeopardy experienced by laboratory subjects.

Computer voice stress analyzer (CVSA)

Voice stress analysis has been around for over 30 years, and was evaluated (and largely dismissed as invalid) based on research in the 1970s and 1980s (Lykken, 1998). However, it has experienced a renaissance with heightened U.S. concerns about terrorism and the purchase of CVSA equip-

ment by many police departments across the country (see the National Institute of Truth Verification web page at www.cvsa1.com/product.php). Basically, the CVSA revival has involved packaging old voice stress technology with a computer and marketing the package as an unobtrusive method to catch liars. The theoretical foundation for voice stress analysis is weak because it is based on the unsubstantiated, although perhaps plausible, notion that the human voice produces inaudible microtremors associated with lying that can be analyzed from a voice recording. The assumptions on which voice stress is based are similar to those on which conventional lie detection is founded, and require the ability to discriminate between stress associated with lying from stress associated with any other human emotion that might be associated with accusations, denials, and other forms of highly charged speech. However, there is little evidence that voice stress analyzers do an adequate job of reliably assessing voice stress (Brenner, Branscomb, & Schwartz, 1979; Horvath, 1978; Lynch & Henry, 1979; Waln & Downey, 1987), let alone its causes. The NRC panel reviewed five unpublished government studies of the CVSA conducted between 1994 and 2000, and found no evidence that it worked much better than chance (NRC, 2003).

Thermal imaging

This technology made a big splash when a paper published in *Nature* was covered by the media as a possible method to screen airline passengers who might have terroristic intent (Pavlidis, Eberhardt, & Levine, 2002). Like the CVSA, thermal imaging can be carried out unobtrusively, without attaching sensors to the subject. Thermography relies on a high-speed motion picture camera sensitive to changes in facial blood flow. In a mock-crime study, Pavlidis, Eberhardt, and Levine (2002) correctly identified 6/8 guilty and 11/12 innocent participants based on thermal characteristics of blood flow around the eyes. Although the original report of this research resembled more a news article than a scientific paper, a more detailed presentation of the methodology has since become available (Pavlidis & Levine, 2002). Nevertheless, much more work would be required to determine whether facial temperature monitoring has potential as a lie detection procedure.

P300 event related potential GKT

Most GKT research has been based on the recording of autonomic reactions, especially skin conductance. In the 1980s (for reviews, see Allen & Iacono, 2001; Iacono & Patrick, 2005; Rosenfeld, 2002), this technique was adapted to an oddball event-related potential (ERP) paradigm designed to elicit P300 ERPs. Many hundreds of studies have demonstrated that the P300 response is sensitive to the probability of stimulus occurrence and relevance. Because the guilty knowledge alternatives of GKT multiple-choice questions are both uncommon (compared to the nonguilty knowledge foils) and highly relevant to the guilty, there is a strong prima facie basis to expect the GKT paradigm to lend itself well to ERP adaptations.

Unlike the traditional autonomic GKT, an ERP extension of the GKT is now being pushed for forensic applications. Larry Farwell (see www.brainwavescience.com) has patented aspects of this technology and marketed it under the trademark "Brain Fingerprinting." He has also applied it in legal appeals of convicted felons who have maintained their innocence, most notably in the case of Terry Harrington, an Iowan convicted of murder, who passed Farwell's test and ultimately won his appeal. The publicity surrounding this case led to a review of this technique by the General Accounting Office (GAO, 2001). Farwell has started a company devoted to developing forensic and medical applications of "brain fingerprinting," making it possible that this technique will grow in significance in the near future. Farwell's procedure involves analysis of the P300 waveform and another aspect of the ERP termed the memory and encoding related multifaceted electroencephalographic response, or MERMER (Farwell & Smith, 2001). The MERMER appears to include P300 and other aspects of the ERP, but exactly what constitutes the MERMER is considered proprietary. Consequently, the criteria used to identify it are unspecified in the one publication that describes it (Farwell & Smith, 2001).

P300-GKTs can be tailored to include validity-enhancing novel elements not typically part of a conventional GKT that allow each subject to serve as his or her own control. In P300 adaptations of the GKT, three types of stimuli may be presented to a suspect on a computer monitor. "Target" stimuli reflect information that is known to all examinees. In a bank robbery, this might be generally available information about the robbery (e.g., the name of the bank). "Probe" stimuli reflect guilty knowledge (e.g., the phrasing of the holdup note). Targets and probes are presented relatively infrequently such that each has the potential to elicit a P300 response. "Irrelevant" stimuli are similar to alternatives on a conventional GKT that serve as foils (e.g., other bank names, made-up phrasing). Because these stimuli have no special meaning and they are abundant, they are not expected to elicit a strong P300 response. All examinees are expected to show a pronounced P300 wave to targets and a diminished wave to irrelevants. If an examinee did not show this result, the particular test administration would be invalid. For the innocent, probes and irrelevants are equivalent in their (lack of) significance, so the probes would not be expected to generate a P300 response. For the guilty, the probe and target both have relevance, so the probe should elicit a P300 response that makes the probe ERP more like the target ERP than the irrelevant ERP. Hundreds of probe, target, and irrelevant stimuli can be presented, yielding reliable representations of the brain response to these stimuli, and their resulting ERPs averaged. By statistically computing the degree to which the average probe ERP resembles the average target versus the irrelevant ERPs, it is possible to determine whether the examinee possesses guilty knowledge. The statistical comparison can be conducted such that strong resemblance of the probe ERP to either the target or the irrelevants is required for a verdict to be issued; otherwise, the outcome is inconclusive.

A conventional GKT could in principle be developed following the ERP-GKT format. Doing so requires overcoming the sensitivity of autonomic nervous system measures like electrodermal reactivity to order and habituation effects, which could become pronounced in an extended GKT with many questions and additional item alternatives to cover targets (Iacono, Boisvenu, & Fleming, 1984). Groundwork for overcoming these problems has been laid by Lim et al. (Lim et al., 1999) who showed that skin conductance responses could be effectively recorded to targets using an oddball paradigm with 287 stimuli (40 targets) presented every 1.3 seconds. In addition, Ben-Shakar and colleagues (Ben-Shakar, Gronau, & Elaad, 1999) have shown that the introduction of a target stimulus into a conventional GKT may reduce the likelihood of false positive outcomes.

An additional enhancement of this procedure is the requirement that the subject respond manually to each stimulus presentation and that a target presentation requires a different key response than all nontargets. This requirement forces subjects to attend to the stimuli, and makes it possible to deem invalid any test administration associated with unusually slow reaction times or frequent target errors. A test like this can be presented with the simple instruction to press a "yes" key every time a crime relevant detail is presented and a "no" key for all crime irrelevant details. For a guilty person who recognizes probes as crime relevant, the natural tendency to press "yes" to the recognition of crime relevant stimuli must be suppressed before responding with the "no" key, thus lengthening reaction times to probe stimuli. Analysis of reaction time data has the potential to usefully complement the P300 analysis. Whether reaction time alone may itself lead to highly accurate classification of guilty and innocent test takers remains to be determined (Allen & Iacono, 1992; Gronau, Ben-Shakhar, & Cohen, 2005; Seymour et al., 2000). Like the autonomically based GKT, P300 adaptations have generally produced high hit rates, including studies showing perfect classification accuracy for both innocent and guilty subjects when inconclusive outcomes were removed from the analyses (Allen & Iacono, 1997; Farwell & Donchin, 1991; Farwell & Smith, 2001).

While aggregating results across studies is often a useful way to evaluate the effectiveness of a technique, the important question to ask is how well the procedure works when optimally applied? This question has been asked in a meta-analysis of the conventional GKT, and has led to both the identification of validity enhancing features and a substantial boost in the GKT's estimated accuracy (Ben-Shakhar & Elaad, 2003). However, this question also needs to be addressed when considering the effectiveness of event related potential GKTs. A P300-based GKT study could be carried out *without* the inclusion of a target condition, the need to respond manually to each stimulus presentation, or the inclusion of decision-making rules that allow for inconclusive outcomes. Omitting one or more of these features, as many studies have, would make the test more like a traditional GKT, but may not optimize classification accuracy.

For both types of GKT, it is probably better to use the equivalent of multiple-choice alternatives that are easily perceived as different in order to minimize response generalization across similar stimuli. A GKT item that lists as murder weapon options "hammer-ice pick-rope-poison" is more likely to register a distinct recognition response than one that lists types of hammers. Likewise, a test with multiple items may generally be more effective than one with only a few items (assuming the items have equivalent psychometric properties). Although this was shown in a meta-analysis of the autonomic GKT literature (Ben-Shakhar & Elaad, 2003), questions have been raised about its appropriateness in P300-GKTs because of the added complexity of this type of GKT (Rosenfeld et al., 2004). Tests should be reviewed with a prospective subject to determine if any of the items or alternatives have personal significance that could elicit a recognition response even if the individual was not involved in the crime. A plumber who works with ball peen hammers should not be asked a question that includes this type of hammer as one of the multiple choice alternatives.

In the previous edition of this *Handbook*, I posited that P300 adaptations of the GKT might be difficult to beat. This speculation was premised on the supposition that introducing countermeasures would lengthen ERP latencies and manual reaction times, introduce more variability into these measures, and possibly produce atypical manual response errors. These results might be expected as the guilty individual strains to introduce an effective manipulation into a procedure that depends on millisecond timing to ensure the validity of an individual test. Hence, the important question is not whether ERPs and associated behavioral data can be altered by countermeasures, but whether countermeasures can be used easily without being detected or generating an inconclusive result.

Using a mental countermeasure in which participants carried out a serial subtraction task, Sasaki and colleagues (Sasaki, Hira, & Matsuda, 2002) found little evidence of countermeasure effectiveness. A more thorough evaluation of countermeasure effects was recently published by Rosenfeld and colleagues (Rosenfeld et al., 2004). This ambitious study had many components making it difficult to summarize thoroughly, so the interested reader should consult the original paper.

These investigators taught mock-crime guilty subjects to use countermeasures to appear innocent on a P300-GKT. The countermeasures involved pressing a finger against a leg, wiggling a toe, and imagining being slapped following the appearance of irrelevant stimuli. Because it used small samples (group size averaged 11 subjects), it was not possible to reach firm conclusions for many interesting hypotheses (e.g., the classification hit rate difference between guilty and countermeasure subjects was not statistically significant). Nevertheless, the study provided evidence indicating that countermeasures could be effective for some subjects. ERPs were altered in a way that compromised accurate classification of those using countermeasures, and the reaction time data of some of these individuals appeared relatively unaffected by their use.

However, this study had a number of features that did not allow for a thorough evaluation of the likelihood that countermeasures would be both effective and go undetected. No inconclusive category was included. To the extent that a probe ERP resembled an irrelevant ERP more than a target ERP, the subject was classified as nondeceptive without considering the magnitude of the similarity between the probe and irrelevant stimuli or the magnitude of the differences in similarity between the ERP pairings. The use of countermeasures directed at irrelevant stimuli is likely to blur distinction between these stimuli and both targets and probes. To the extent all three types of stimuli produce similar P300 responses, this should lead to a test administration being dismissed as invalid; *no test should be accepted as valid if the irrelevant and target stimuli cannot be easily differentiated*. This problem was noted by the authors in one of their analyses when they commented that "all three stimulus types generated a small P300, probably because all were meaningful. The reduced size is probably due to the loss of unique oddball probability for probe and target" (p. 214).

Manual response data could have also been used more effectively either to identify guilty subjects or to render evaluations inconclusive. Guilty subjects, especially in the countermeasure group, were significantly more likely to give a "yes" response to probe stimuli. This information was dismissed as of no value because the rates of such error were low. However, there is no reason for any innocent person to respond disproportionately with "yes" responses to probe stimuli, so such a pattern should at least cast doubt on the validity of the test administration if not be used to indict participants as guilty. Although as many as 9 of the 11 subjects in the countermeasure group were deemed to beat the test in certain ERP analyses, only three subjects in this group produced manual reaction times to probe and irrelevant stimuli that were as fast as those of even the slowest innocent subjects. Again, such discrepant behavioral data should at least cast doubt on the validity of the ERP analyses. Finally, questions can be raised about the salience of the probes used in this study, even for guilty subjects, because they did not elicit responses as large as the targets. This led to these subjects being erroneously classified 46% of the time when using Farwell's method which has yielded high accuracy with guilty subjects in three different studies (Allen & Iacono, 1992; Farwell & Donchin, 1991; Farwell & Smith, 2001) even when counting inconclusive outcomes in these three studies as errors. Coincidentally, this error rate matched that of Rosenfeld et al.'s countermeasure group when analyzed using the same method. Despite these qualifications, the report of Rosenfeld et al. (2004) is important because it is the first to explore how countermeasures might affect this type of GKT, and it suggests that those using this methodology cannot be confident that it is immune to countermeasure effects.

In this regard, it is also useful to consider enhancements that might improve the accuracy of P300-GKTs in the face of countermeasures. In this study, subjects used one hand to manipulate both the "yes" and "no" response buttons while the other hand was used for leg self-stimulation. Subjects could be given pushbuttons for each hand, a modification that would probably eliminate this countermeasure and provide reaction time data that is more sensitive to the expected delays caused by the effortful use of countermeasures. If sufficient numbers of subjects were examined using a standardized version of the P300-GKT, behavioral and ERP norms could be developed that might be used profitably to identify outliers whose test results could be treated with skepticism.

Physical countermeasures can be detected through electromyographic (EMG) recordings when used with conventional polygraph tests (Honts et al., 1994), but the field instrumentation used by polygraphers does not lend itself to adding sensors that might detect them. Although movement sensors that can be attached to examinee chairs are available for monitoring countermeasure attempts, they are seldom used by field polygraphers. A similar problem does not exist for ERP-GKTs, which depend on multichannel laboratory instruments. These devices can easily be adapted to record EMG from muscles anywhere on the body. In addition, extra scalp electrodes positioned over the sensorimotor cortex have the potential to detect repeated muscle manipulations such as the finger and toe countermeasure movements used in Rosenfeld et al. (2004).

Finally, it is noteworthy that countermeasures only affect the confidence that can be placed in passed tests. As noted previously, the great value of these procedures in forensic applications may eventually lie with the incriminating nature of a failed test.

Other electrocortical research

Other brain electrocortical measures besides P300 also have been used to study deception. Unfortunately, each of these methods has been examined in a single report, thus rendering difficult an evaluation of their potential.

Taking advantage of the N400 ERP's sensitivity to semantic incongruity, Boaz et al. (Boaz, Perry, Raney, Fieschler, & Shuman, 1991) employed a GKT design to determine how subjects responded to crime relevant phrases that terminated with endings that were either true or false. Although the average observed hit rate exceeded 70%, this technique does not appear to offer any advantage over the P300-GKT, which yields higher accuracy.

More recently, Fang and associates (Fang, Liu, & Shen, 2003) evaluated the utility of the contingent negative variation (CNV) for detecting deception. Their design required subjects to evaluate whether pictures of faces presented to them were novel or familiar. Compared to trials on which subjects responded truthfully, CNV was augmented when participants were preparing to lie. Taking a slightly different tack, Lo et al. (Lo, Fook-Chong, & Tan, 2003) used transcranial magnetic stimulation to examine motor control mechanisms potentially associated with lying. Their participants either silently lied or told the truth when asked 80 different questions. The amplitude of motor evoked potentials (MEP) to magnetic pulses presented before and after each question was significantly greater after a question associated with lying. MEP amplitudes were no different when responding truthfully to questions. In addition, MEPs preceding a question that elicited a lie were elevated. These results suggest that cortical excitability is increased both following a lie and in anticipation of deceiving. Because neither Fang et al. nor Lo et al. estimated hit rates using these methods, their results cannot be compared easily to those of other ERP investigations.

Johnson and colleagues (Johnson, Barnhardt, & Zhu, 2003, 2004) have moved beyond evaluating applications to isolate brain processes that underlie deception. Using multichannel EEG recording, they have introduced tasks that are designed to separate the different psychological processes involved in lying. Their results suggest that lying is associated with medial frontal negativities reflecting anterior cingulate (ACC) processes. These processes are related to the response conflict associated with having to inhibit the prepotent truthful response prior to lying. A second process, associated with parietal cortex late positivity, appears to be related to recollection and episodic memory of past truthfulness, which reflects a guilty knowledge effect.

Brain mechanisms

Deception detection research has been driven largely by applied considerations. The result has been a collection of box scores indicating how well physiological measures differentiate lying from truth telling in one paradigm or another. As Furedy et al. (Furedy, Davis, & Gurevich, 1988) have noted, research on deception detection has done little to shed light on underlying processes, in part because lie detection methods, even if they work, provide few clues as to why they might work. This problem is well illustrated with the CQT because differential responding to control and relevant questions may stem from any of the many psychological attributes, which vary across these two question types. They confound cognitive and emotional processes. They do not differ in the likelihood that they elicit lies, nor do they differ along the same dimensions for guilty and innocent examinees. CQT theory presumes that both questions elicit lies for the guilty, but the relevant question elicits a more significant lie. For the innocent, only the control question is expected to elicit a lie, but this is merely plausible and not known to be the case. Fear of detection, guilt, cognitive processes associated with both the intent to lie and the act of lying, and social behavior associated with lying all confound the ability to interpret the psychological significance of responses to control and relevant questions. To varying extents, similar problems exist with other deception detection formats. Until research moves substantially beyond evaluating applications, we will miss the opportunity for insightful discoveries that have potential to inform the development of improved deception detection techniques.

Recently, a number of investigators have begun to move beyond empirical evaluation to isolate brain structure and processes that underlie deception. As noted above, Johnson et al. (Johnson, Barnhardt, & Zhu, 2003, 2004) have extended EEG research along these lines. In a structural imaging study, Yang et al. (2005) found differences in prefrontal white and grey matter when pathological liars were compared to antisocial and normal controls. Other investigators, taking advantage of recent developments in functional magnetic resonance imaging (fMRI), have also investigated processes and brain regions involved with deception. In the first of these studies (Spence et al., 2001), subjects were presented with autobiographical questions to which they responded manually with a "yes" or "no" button press. Every question was answered once truthfully and once with a lie. The task was characterized as requiring the suppression of the prepotent response (the truth) in favor of its alternative, a lie. Consistent activation of the bilateral ventrolateral prefrontal cortex was observed. The authors noted that their design did not allow them to differentiate between two possible interpretations for the brain activation, one associated with answering with a lie and the other associated with the withholding of the truth in order to lie.

Langleben et al. (2002) employed a GKT in which subjects tried to conceal their possession of a playing card as different cards were presented to them. The guilty knowledge card and the cards serving as foils were presented along with the question "Do you have this card?" To ensure that subjects paid attention and did not simply answer every question with an automatic "no," occasionally the question "Is this the 10 of spades?" appeared together with the 10 of spades (to which they responded "yes"). The key finding involved activation of the ACC, but not the dorsolateral prefrontal cortex (DLPFC) during lying. Because other studies have shown that ACC activation is proportional to the degree of response conflict and inversely related to DLPFC activation, the results suggested that a conflict with the prepotent response (truth) and eventually its inhibition took place. Activation of right frontal motor and premotor and adjacent anterior parietal cortex was also observed and attributed to the increased demand for motor control involved in directing the left hand to the appropriate response button. Although this GKT paradigm seems fairly straightforward, even this simple manipulation confounded lying to the guilty knowledge card with recognition memory, as this was apparently the only card presented to subjects before they entered the scanner. This illustrates the difficulty conducting these types of experiments in a way that leads to unambiguous conclusions, which is a problem that looms even larger in some of the other imaging-deception studies.

Adopting a different approach, Lee et al. (2002) evaluated brain activation when subjects lied to feign memory impairment in what were referred to as two "forced choice" tasks designed to assess short and longterm memory impairment. The first task required them to decide whether two three-digit numbers presented about two seconds apart were the same or different. The second task asked an autobiographical question followed two seconds later by an answer. The brain activation from these two memory tests was contrasted with that of each subject when doing the same task answering all the questions truthfully. Participants were given a description of the nature of the memory tests they were about to take, and told "your goal is to fake well, do it with skill, and avoid detection." Presumably participants understood that this meant they should not answer every single question with a lie. Doing so would make them detectable because their response pattern would suggest a significant departure from the chance responding that those with memory impairment would be expected to display. Subjects were, however, left on their own to decide how to respond when given the two different memory tasks. Results common to both tasks revealed bilateral prefrontal (including DLPFC), frontal, parietal, and caudate activation. From this, the authors concluded that feigned memory impairment involves a prefrontal-parietal-caudate circuit reflecting memory processes (frontal), calculations regarding how often to respond with a lie versus the truth so as to look impaired but escape detection (parietal), and the inhibition of typical responding coupled with performance monitoring (caudate).

Two types of lies were examined by Ganis et al. (Ganis et al., 2003). One involved answering questions about a prepared but made-up autobiographical account of a vacation or work experience. These lies were thus rehearsed and elaborate. The other lies were spontaneously created in the scanner and dealt with single facts about these same experiences (rather than the coherent set of rehearsed, integrated facts characteristic of the prepared lies). Brain responses to the two types of lies were compared to each other as well as to those associated with truthful answers to questions that were designed to stimulate the two types of lies. Rehearsed, elaborate lies were more likely to activate right frontal cortex than spontaneous, isolated lies, whereas the latter evoked more ACC and posterior visual cortex responses than the well-prepared lies. Compared with truth telling, both types of lies activated prefrontal cortex and the parahippocampal gyrus, right precuneus, and left cerebellum. Hence, different patterns of brain activation were associated with different types of lies.

These activations were interpreted as likely to reflect cognitive processes involving semantic and episodic knowledge, visual imagery, working memory, and response conflict.

In the only imaging research on deception to involve a constructive replication, Kozel and colleagues (Kozel, Padgett, & George, 2004; Kozel et al., 2004) contrasted truthful and false answers to questions concerning under which objects money was hidden. Somewhat different protocols were followed in each study, but prior to scanning, subjects searched a room to determine under which objects $50 was concealed. They then viewed pictures and indicated whether the money was under the pictured object. As most of the pictured objects did not have money under them, this procedure was like a GKT. Because participants had been exposed to all the objects in advance, memory was not confounded with lying. Each study included pictures that required a truthful response as well as pictures that required a lie. Results indicated that for lying, there was more activation in the right ACC; right inferior, middle, and orbitofrontal cortex; and left middle temporal areas. Given that fear of detection is likely to be present when one lies, of special interest were possible amygdala effects. In one of the studies (Kozel et al., 2004), a specific effort was made to test for amygdala activation, but the result was negative. In the other report (Kozel, Padgett, & George, 2004), a special effort was made to determine whether data from each individual subject could be analyzed to detect lying on a person by person basis. Consistent activation patterns were not evident.

Two recent studies have extended fMRI technology to the identification of individual lies and liars. Langleben et al. (2005) extended the GKT paradigm of Langleben et al. (2002) and obtained a classification accuracy of 78% in their ability to discrimnate lie from truth. Kozel et al. (2005) had subjects particpate in a mock theft where either a ring or a watch was stolen. During the fMRI recording, participants denied stealing both items, thus lying about their involvemnt with one of them. Truthful and deceptive responses were differentited from each other with accuracies ranging from 90–93%. Based on the results of these laboratory studies, patents have been filed and two startup companies have been formed (see www.cephoscorp.com and www.noliemri.com) with the intent of offerring fMRI-based lie detection services.

This collection of imaging studies is illuminating in several important respects. Thus far, the research has not been programmatic and a diversity of deception protocols has been used, and render difficult any interpretation of the inconsistencies in brain activation evident across studies. These investigations did little to take advantage of the accumulated knowledge regarding the methodological pitfalls associated with the last 50 years of deception detection research. None of the investigations was designed well enough to tease apart the many processes involved in lying. Instead, patterns of brain activation were generally interpreted post hoc as consistent with the likely role of various cognitive processes (and the unlikely role of other processes, like emotion, that was not considered seriously in the simple, constrained paradigms employed). Although the prefrontal cortex and ACC emerged as activated regions in most of the studies, on balance, this collection of investigations has thus far provided little insight into the neural circuitry underlying lying.

Although fMRI technology is now being advertised as ready for field applications, the use of these techniques in real-life situations requires a much more substantial research foundation, one that comes to grips with the many methodological problems that have been identified in attempts to validate the CQT and GKT. These studies used fairly simple paradigms, yet a diversity of brain activation patterns was observed. None of the investigations included anything approaching the circumstances one would encounter in a real-life application. Had they done so, there is a good chance the results would be even more complex because emotion would play a more prominent role in brain activation, which is likely true even for the GKT (Suzuki, Nakayama, & Furedy, 2004). It is not unreasonable to imagine brain activation associated with lying to vary according to the type of crime (or criminal). For instance, how reasonable would it be to expect a sex offender's brain activation during a lie to resemble that of a burglar's or of someone making a false accusation? This is an empirical question, and many such issues would have to be resolved to advance an fMRI-based lie detector.

fMRI holds obvious promise over autonomic measures, in part because it taps more directly brain processes involved in lying. In theory, a pattern of brain activation that is uniquely associated with lying could exist; no such pattern is ever likely to be found for autonomic measures. Because the research conducted to date is quite preliminary, it is unrealistic to expect great headway to this point in time. For now, perhaps basic science fMRI research focused on elucidating the neural and cognitive mechanisms associated with deceit has the greatest potential to contribute to the eventual development of an improved lie detector regardless of the technology ultimately used.

CONCLUSION

Professional polygraph testing has gone through many changes over the last 20 years, which have been advertised as improvements by the polygraph profession. These changes have included renaming the CQT, substituting the measurement of skin conductance for resistance, switchig to computerized recording and scoring, better examiner training, more attention to standardization, and elimination of the most widespread abuses of polygraphy associated with employee screening by private corporations. Nevertheless, the forensic and screening tests used today are on no surer scientific footing than they were at their inception. This state of affairs persists because no matter what remedies are introduced to improve the output of polygraph tests, the psychological premises on which they are based remain weak. There is no way to know how a given person, whether guilty or innocent, will respond to the different types of questions on these tests or why they respond as they do. Countermeasures remain a serious threat. Research on polygraph testing has failed to grapple successfully with the vexing methodological issues that have plagued it since evaluative research was begun in earnest 40 years ago. How a polygraph test is conducted and the outcome obtained remains highly dependent on who gives it. It remains an investigative tool that assists information gathering. Simply put, it is unscientific (Iacono, 2001), and there is no simple way to adjust current practices to change this fact.

The GKT, by contrast, has a reasonable scientific foundation. Innovations in GKT methodology, especially P300-based modifications, have at least the potential to lead to improved applications. However, these techniques beg for research designed to identify what constitutes good material for developing GKT items. In particular, what are criminals likely to pay attention to and remember that is related to the crime they commit? Until this question is seriously tackled, law enforcement is unlikely to embrace GKT techniques because of concern over false negatives. While laboratory research can help refine the GKT, ultimately field studies or investigations with excellent external validity need to be conducted to place the development of GKT items on a solid footing.

Most detection deception research has focused on applications in the absence of any sound theoretical foundation regarding the psychological and neurobiological underpinnings of lying. Recent psychophysiological and fMRI studies have begun to fill this void, but clearly much remains to be done. In the absence of any significant breakthroughs, it is unlikely that forensic and security screening applications of lie detection can be improved or that these techniques will give way to better methods with proven validity.

REFERENCES

Allen, J. J. B., & Iacono, W. G. (1992). The identification of concealed memories using the event-related potential and implicit behavioral measures: A methodology for prediction in the face of individual differences. *Psychophysiology, 29*, 504–522.

Allen, J. J. B., & Iacono, W. G. (1997). A comparison of methods for the analysis of event-related potentials in deception detection. *Psychophysiology, 34*, 234–240.

Allen, J. J. B., & Iacono, W. G. (2001). Assessing the validity of amnesia in dissociative identity disorder: A dilemma for the DSM and the courts. *Psychology, Public Policy, & Law, 7*, 311–344.

Amato, S. L. (1993). *A survey of the Society for Psychophysiological Research regarding the polygraph: Opinions and interpretations.* University of North Dakota.

American Polygraph Association. (2005). Validity and reliability of polygraph testing. *Retrieved May 19, 2005, from http://www.polygraph.org/validityresearch.htm.*

Barland, G. H., Honts, C. R., & Barger, S. D. (1989). *Studies of the accuracy of security screening polygraph examinations.*
Fort McClellan, AL: Department of Defense Polygraph Institute.

Ben-Shakar, G. (2002). A critical review of the control questions test (CQT). In M. Kleiner (Ed.), *Handbook of polygraph testing* (pp. 103–126). San Diego: Academic Press.

Ben-Shakar, G., & Elaad, E. (2003). The validity of psychophysiological detection of information with the guilty knowledge test: A meta-analytic review. *Journal of Applied Psychology, 88*, 131–151.

Ben-Shakar, G., Gronau, N., & Elaad, E. (1999). Leakage of relevant information to innocent examinees in the GKT: An attempt to reduce false-positive outcomes by introducing target stimuli. *Journal of Applied Psychology, 84*, 651–660.

Ben-Shakhar, G., Bar-Hillel, M., & Kremnitzer, M. (2002). Trial by polygraph: reconsidering the use of the guilty knowledge technique in court. *Law and Human Behavior, 26*, 527–541.

Ben-Shakhar, G., & Elaad, E. (2003). The validity of psychophysiological detection of information with the Guilty Knowledge Test: a meta-analytic review. *Journal of Applied Psychology, 88*, 131–151.

Boaz, T. L., Perry, N. W., Raney, G., Fieschler, I. S., & Shuman, D. (1991). Detection of guilty knowledge with event related potentials. *Journal of Applied Psychology, 76*, 788–795.

Brenner, M., Branscomb, H. H., & Schwartz, G. E. (1979). Psychological Stress Evaluator – Two tests of a vocal measure. *Psychophysiology, 16*, 351–357.

Carmel, D., Dayan, E., Naveh, A., Raveh, O., & Ben-Shakhar, G. (2003). Estimating the validity of the guilty knowledge test from simulated experiments: the external validity of mock crime studies. *Journal of Experimental Psychology: Applied, 9*, 261–269.

DePaulo, B. M., Lindsay, J. J., Malone, B. E., Muhlenbruck, L., Charlton, K., & Cooper, H. (2003). Cues to deception. *Psychological Bulletin, 129*, 74–118.

Faigman, D. L., Kaye, D. H., Saks, M. J., & Sanders, J. (2002). The legal relevance of scientific research on polygraph tests. In D. L. Faigman, D. Kaye, M. J. Saks & J. Sanders (Eds.), *Modern scientific evidence: The law and science of expert testimony* (Vol. 2, pp. 427–446). St. Paul, MN: West Publishing.

Fang, F., Liu, Y., & Shen, Z. (2003). Lie detection with contingent negative variation. *International Journal of Psychophysiology, 50*, 247–255.

Farwell, L. A., & Donchin, E. (1991). The truth will out: Interrogative polygraphy ("lie detection") with event related brain potentials. *Psychophysiology, 28*, 531–547.

Farwell, L. A., & Smith, S. S. (2001). Using brain MERMER testing to detect knowledge despite efforts to conceal. *Journal of Forensic Sciences, 46*, 1–9.

Fergusse, R. J. (1966). *The polygraph in private industry.* Springfield, IL: Charles c. Thomas.

Fiedler, K., Schmod, J., & Stahl, T. (2002). What is the current truth about polygraph lie detection? *Basic & Applied Social Psychology, 24*, 313–324.

Furedy, J. J., Davis, C., & Gurevich, M. (1988). Differentiation of deception as a psychological process: A psychophysiological approach. *Psychophysiology, 25*, 683–688.

Gallup, O. (1984). Survey of members of the American Society for Psychophysiological Research concerning their opinion of polygraph test interpretation. *Polygraph, 13*, 153–165.

Ganis, G., Kosslyn, S. M., Stose, S., Thompson, W. L., & Yurgelun-Todd, D. A. (2003). Neural correlates of different types of deception: An fMRI investigation. *Cerebral Cortex, 13*, 830–836.

GAO, G. A. O. (2001). *Federal agency views on "Brain Fingerprinting"* (No. GAO-02–22). Washington, D.C.: General Accounting Office.

Greenberg, D. S. (2002). Polygraph fails scientific review in the USA. *Lancet, 360*(9342), 1309.

Gronau, N., Ben-Shakhar, G., & Cohen, A. (2005). Behavioral and physiological measures in the detection of concealed information. *Journal of Applied Psychology, 90,* 147–158.

Hira, S., & Furumitsu, I. (2002). Polygraphic examinations in Japan: Application of the guilty knowledge test in forensic investigations. *International Journal of Police Science and Management, 4.*

Honts, C. R. (1991). The emperor's new clothes: Application of polygraph tests in the American workplace. *Forensic Reports, 4,* 91–116.

Honts, C. R., Hodes, R. L., & Raskin, D. C. (1985). Effects of physical countermeasures on the physiological detection of deception. *Journal of Applied Psychology, 70,* 177–187.

Honts, C. R., Raskin, D., & Kircher, J. (1994). Mental and physical countermeasures reduce the accuracy of polygraph tests. *Journal of Applied Psychology, 79,* 252–259.

Honts, C. R., Raskin, D., & Kircher, J. (2002). The scientific status of research on polygraph techniques: The case for polygraph tests. In D. L. Faigman, D. H. Kaye, M. J. Saks & J. Sanders (Eds.), *Modern scientific evidence: The law and science of expert testimony* (Vol. 2, pp. 446–483). St. Paul, MN: West Publishing.

Horvath, F. (1978). An experimental comparison of the Psychological Stress Evaluator and the galvanice skin response in the detection of deception. *Journal of Applied Psychology, 63,* 338–344.

Iacono, W. G. (1985). Guilty knowledge. *Society, 22,* 52–54.

Iacono, W. G. (1991). Can we determine the accuracy of polygraph tests? In J. R. Jennings, P. K. Ackles & M. G. H. Coles (Eds.), *Advances in psychophysiology* (pp. 201–207). London: Jessica Kingsley Publishers.

Iacono, W. G. (2000). The detection of deception. In J. T. Cacioppo, L. G. Tassinary & G. Berntson (Eds.), *Handbook of Psychophysiology. 2nd Ed.* (pp. 772–793). New York: Cambridge.

Iacono, W. G. (2001). Forensic "lie detection:" Procedures without scientific basis. *Journal of Forensic Psychology Practice, 1,* 75–86.

Iacono, W. G., Boisvenu, G. A., & Fleming, J. A. (1984). The effects of diazepam and methylphenidate on the electrodermal detection of guilty knowledge. *Journal of Applied Psychology, 69,* 289–299.

Iacono, W. G., & Lykken, D. T. (1997). The validity of the lie detector: Two surveys of scientific opinion. *Journal of Applied Psychology, 82,* 426–433.

Iacono, W. G., & Lykken, D. T. (2002). The scientific status of research on polygraph techniques: The case against polygraph tests. In D. L. Faigman, D. H. Kaye, M. J. Saks & J. Sanders (Eds.), *Modern scientific evidence: The law and science of expert testimony* (Vol. 2, pp. 483–538). St. Paul, MN: West Publishing.

Iacono, W. G., & Patrick, C. J. (2005). Polygraph ("lie detecdtor") testing: Current status and emerging trends. In A. K. Hess & I. B. Weiner (Eds.), *Handbook of forensic psychology* (3rd ed., pp. 552–588). New York: Wiley.

Johnson, R., Jr., Barnhardt, J., & Zhu, J. (2003). The deceptive response: Effects of response conflict and strategic monitoring on the late positive component and episodic memory-related brain activity. *Biological Psychology, 64,* 217–253.

Johnson, R., Jr., Barnhardt, J., & Zhu, J. (2004). The contribution of executive processes to deceptive responding. *Neuropsychologia, 42,* 878–901.

Kassin, S. M. (2005). On the psychology of confessions: does innocence put innocents at risk? *American Psychologist, 60,* 215–228.

Kassin, S. M., & Gudjonsson, G. H. (2004). The Psychology of Confessions: A review of the literature and issues. *Psychological Science in the Public Interest, 5,* 33–67.

Kozell, A. F., Johnson, K. A., Mu, Q., Grenesko, E. L., Laken, S. J., & George, M. S. (2005). Detecting deception using functional magnetic resonance imaging. *Biological Psychiatry, 58,* 605–613.

Kozel, F. A., Padgett, T. M., & George, M. S. (2004). A replication study of the neural correlates of deception. *Behavioral Neuroscience, 118,* 852–856.

Kozel, F. A., Revell, L. J., Lorberbaum, J. P., Shastri, A., Elhai, J. D., Horner, M. D., et al. (2004). A pilot study of functional magnetic resonance imaging brain correlates of deception in healthy young men. *Journal of Neuropsychiatry & Clinical Neuroscience, 16,* 295–305.

Krapohl, D. J. (2002). The polygraph in personnel screening. In M. Kleiner (Ed.), *Handbook of polygraph testing* (pp. 217–236). San Diego: Academic Press.

Langleben, D. D., Loughead, J. W., Bilker, W. B., Ruparel, K., Childress, A. R., Busch, S. I., & Gur, R. C. (2005). Telling truth from lie in individual subjects with fast event-related fMRI. *Human Brain Mapping, 26,* 262–272.

Langleben, D. D., Schroeder, L., Maldjian, J. A., Gur, R. C., McDonald, S., Ragland, J. D., et al. (2002). Brain activity during simulated deception: An event-related functional magnetic resonance study. *Neuroimage, 15,* 727–732.

Lee, T. M., Liu, H. L., Tan, L. H., Chan, C. C., Mahankali, S., Feng, C. M., et al. (2002). Lie detection by functional magnetic resonance imaging. *Human Brain Mapping, 15,* 157–164.

Lim, C. L., Gordon, E., Rennie, C., Wright, J. J., Bahramali, H., Li, W. M., et al. (1999). Dynamics of SCR, EEG, and ERP activity in an oddball paradigm with short interstimulus intervals. *Psychophysiology, 36,* 543–551.

Lo, Y. L., Fook-Chong, S., & Tan, E. K. (2003). Increased cortical excitability in human deception. *Neuroreport, 14,* 1021–1024.

Lykken, D. T. (1959). The GSR in the detection of guilt. *Journal of Applied Psychology, 43,* 385–388.

Lykken, D. T. (1981). *A tremor in the blood: Uses and abuses of the lie detector.* New York: McGraw-Hill.

Lykken, D. T. (1998). *A tremor in the blood: Uses and abuses of the lie detector* (2nd ed.). New York: Plenum.

Lynch, B. E., & Henry, D. R. (1979). A validity study of the Psychological Stress Evaluator. *Canadian Journal of Behavioral Science, 11,* 89–94.

Malakoff, D. (2003). Polygraph testing. DOE says fewer workers will face the machine. *Science, 301*(5639), 1456.

Marston, W. M. (1917). Systolic blood pressure symptoms of deception. *Journal of Experimental Psychology, 2,* 117–163.

Nakayama, M. (2002). Practical use of the concealed information test for criminal investigations in Japan. In M. Kleiner (Ed.), *Handbook of polygraph testing* (pp. 49–86). San Diego: Academic Press.

NRC, N. R. C. (2003). *The polygraph and lie detection.* Washington, DC: National Academies Press.

Oskol, E. M., & O'Donohue, W. T. (Eds.). (2003). *A critical analysis of the polygraph.* San Diego: Academic Press.

Patrick, C. J., & Iacono, W. G. (1991). Validity of the control question polygraph test: The problem of sampling bias. *Journal of Applied Psychology, 76*, 229–238.

Pavlidis, I., Eberhardt, N. L., & Levine, J. A. (2002). Seeing through the face of deception: Thermal imaging offers a promising hands-off approach to mass security screening. *Nature, 415*, 35.

Pavlidis, I., & Levine, J. (2002). Thermal imaging analysis for polygraph testing. *IEEE Engineering in Medicine & Biology Magazine 21*, 56–64.

Pollina, D. A., Dollins, A. B., Senter, S. M., Krapohl, D. J., & Ryan, A. H. (2004). Comparison of polygraph data obtained from individuals involved in mock crimes and actual criminal investigations. *Journal of Applied Psychology, 89*, 1099–1105.

Raskin, D. C., & Honts, C. R. (2002). The comparison question test. In M. Kleiner (Ed.), *Handbook of polygraph testing* (pp. 1–47). San Diego: Academic Press.

Rosenfeld, J. P. (2002). Event-related potentials in the detection of deception, malingering, and false memories. In M. Kleiner (Ed.), Handbook of Polygraph Testing. New York: Academic Press.

Rosenfeld, J. P., Soskins, M., Bosh, G., & Ryan, A. (2004). Simple, effective countermeasures to P300-based tests of detection of concealed information. *Psychophysiology, 41*, 205–219.

Sandia's Senior Scientists & Engineers. (1999). Polygraphs and security. Retrieved at *http://www.fas.org/sgp/othergov/polygraph/sandia.html on May* 19, 2005.

Sasaki, M., Hira, H., & Matsuda, T. (2002). Effects of a mental countermeasure on the physiological detection of deception using P3. *Studies in the Humanities & Sciences, 42*, 73–84.

Saxe, L., Dougherty, D., & Cross, T. (1985). The validity of polygraph testing: Scientific analysis and public controversy. *American Psychologist*, 355–366.

Seymour, T. L., Seifert, C. M., Shafto, M. G., & Mosmann, A. L. (2000). Using response time measures to assess "guilty knowledge". *Journal of Applied Psychology, 85*, 30–37.

Sokolov, E. (1963). *Perception and the conditioned reflex*. New York: Macmillan.

Spence, S., Farrow, T., Herford, A., Wilkinson, I., ZHENG, Y., & Woodruff, P. (2001). Behavioural and functional anatomical correlates of deception in humans. *Neuroreport, 12*, 2433–2438.

Suzuki, R., Nakayama, M., & Furedy, J. J. (2004). Specific and reactive senstivies of skin resistance response and respiratory apnea in a Japanese concealed information test (CIT) of criminal guilt. *Canadian Journal of Behavioural Science, 36*, 202–209.

Thurber, S. (1981). CPI variables in relation to the polygraph performance of police officer candidates. *Journal of Social Psychology, 113*, 145–146.

Verschuere, B., Crombez, G., De Clercq, A., & Koster, E. H. (2004). Autonomic and behavioral responding to concealed information: differentiating orienting and defensive responses. *Psychophysiology, 41*, 461–466.

Waln, R. F., & Downey, R. G. (1987). Voice stress analysis: Use of telephone recordings. *Journal of Business & Psychology, 1*, 379–389.

Yang, Y., Raine, A., Lencz, T., Bihrle, S., Lacasse, L., & Colletti, P. (2005). Prefrontal white matter in pathological liars. *British Journal of Psychiatry, 187*, 320–325.

30 Neuroergonomics: Application of Neuroscience to Human Factors

ARTHUR F. KRAMER AND RAJA PARASURAMAN

The main goal of this chapter is to illustrate how human neuroscience techniques, as well as scientific theories that integrate behavioral and neuroscientific levels of description, can be used to address problems and concerns in the field of human factors and ergonomics. In order to accomplish this goal we begin with a brief discussion of the field of human factors and describe a limited but important subset of current questions and issues. Next we describe some of the criteria that must be met for human neuroscience measures to serve a useful function in assisting human factors researchers and practitioners to enhance the functionality, efficiency, and safety of current and future human-machine systems. We then provide a brief history of the role of neuroscience methods and theories as applied to the field of human factors. This is followed by a description of some recent developments in methods and a discussion of their potential application to questions of relevance to human factors. We then briefly describe a few illustrative examples of human factors issues that have been addressed with a series of converging operations, which include neuroscience measures and models. These topics include: the study of mental workload and multitask processing, the examination of individual differences in performance and information processing strategies, and the use of neuroscience techniques and theory to develop brain-computer interfaces. This discussion is followed by a brief conclusions and future directions section.

I. A BRIEF INTRODUCTION TO HUMAN FACTORS

Human factors has been defined as the study of human capabilities and limitations that affect the design of human-machine systems (Wickens, 2000). However, the field of human factors extends beyond the theoretical and empirical study of human behavior and cognition in complex systems to the formulation of guidelines, principles, and models that can be used to design systems that accommodate human users and operators (Meister, 1989). In other words, human factors is neither a domain that resides solely in the laboratory nor one that focuses exclusively on the engineering of new (or the retrofitting of old) human-machine systems. That is, the field of human factors endeavors to provide a bridge between (1) the study of human behavior and cognition in laboratory and other relatively well-controlled, specified simulated environments, and (2) the design and evaluation of human-machine systems. These systems range from (purportedly) simple consumer products such as TVs, VCRs, PDAs, and cell phones to complex systems such as automobiles, aircraft, process control plants, medical equipment and systems, and the World Wide Web.

Over the years, the core topics of interest within the human factors community have changed with the development of technology. Specifically, the change has occurred in technologies that have reduced the need for humans to serve as manual laborers and controllers, and has shifted the role of humans to that of system managers and supervisors. Although such developments in technology have generally been advantageous for the humans who have participated in the operation of complex systems and products, there have also been a number of costs associated with the transition of humans from the role of manual controller to that of supervisor, who is occasionally a more active participant, especially when an unexpected problem occurs in semi-automated and automated systems.

For example, one recurrent problem has been referred to as automation-induced complacency. This occurs when human operators are expected to perform a series of manual tasks while also monitoring automated systems. Under such conditions monitoring performance often decreases precipitously rather quickly, often within 30 minutes. However, such performance decrements occur less often when the human operator's only task is to monitor the automated systems (Parasuraman, Molloy, & Singh, 1993). Thus, if human operators are expected to perform multiple

The preparation of this chapter was supported by grants from the Office of Naval Research, the Defense Advanced Research Projects Agency, and the National Institute on Aging.

tasks, some of which require active intervention and manual control, then the monitoring of automated systems may suffer. Of course, one solution to such a problem might be to automate the manual tasks and thereby unburden the operator from the dual tasks of manual control and supervisory management. However, such a change is often technically impractical and may also overwhelm the human operator with excessive monitoring demands. Even when highly automated systems are a practical alternative, operators have been shown to overestimate the reliability of the automated systems and succumb to automation-induced complacency even in the absence of manual control demands (Riley, 1994).

Another problem associated with highly automated systems has been referred to as out-of-the-loop unfamiliarity or, more generally, as a lack of situation awareness (Endsley 1994; Wickens 1992). This occurs when human operators must suddenly, and often without warning, get back into the control loop and perform manual control duties, detect and diagnose problems with automated systems, or both. In such cases the human operators are slower and more error-prone in carrying out these duties than if they had been an active participant in the operation of the system rather than a passive system monitor (Metzger & Parasuraman, 2001). Important questions regarding this problem include how to keep the operator continuously aware of the state of important systems and how best to monitor (human) operator readiness to take over important duties should automation fail (Scerbo, 1994).

There is still another set of important issues that arises in the context of complex semi-automated and automated systems. How should the overwhelming amounts of multimodal information be presented to human operators, and how should we assess whether mission-critical information has been adequately extracted and retained by the operators? These general issues include questions of a sensory and perceptual nature. Is critical information sufficiently distinct from background information? Is critical information displayed long enough for operators to note and extract task-critical components? There are also important cognitive concerns. Is the information presented to the operator in a format that is consistent with his or her mental representation of the system? Do the working memory requirements exceed operator capacity? Given the rapid development of virtual and augmented reality technology for operator training and system control, the sensory, perceptual, and cognitive issues associated with information presentation and multimodal integration have become more than an academic exercise. These issues are now on the verge of becoming a serious bottleneck for the effective use of this technology.

The issues raised here (and many others) have been and continue to be addressed through the application of a variety of traditional human factors methodologies. For example, the questions of whether and when to automate system functions have been addressed with several different methods, including (1) the use of both engineering and psychologically-inspired models of human performance and cognition to predict the situations in which human performance is likely to degrade, (2) the continuous assessment of human performance via measurement of overt actions and responses, and (3) the use of self-report procedures and questionnaires such as the NASA-TLX workload scale and a variety of different scales that assess attentiveness or error-proneness. Indeed, the model-based and assessment-based procedures have also been combined into a hybrid approach to enhance the efficiency of adaptively automated systems (Byrne & Parasuraman, 1996). Similar techniques have been employed to evaluate new display concepts and to ensure the information is presented in formats consistent with the perceptual capabilities and cognitive representations of human operators (Stanny et al., 2004).

II. ROLE OF NEUROSCIENCE IN HUMAN FACTORS

Traditionally, human factors and ergonomics have not paid much attention to neuroscience or to the results of studies concerning brain mechanisms underlying human perceptual, cognitive, affective, and motor processes. This relative neglect of human brain function is understandable given that this discipline had its roots in a psychology of the 1940s, which was firmly in the behaviorist camp. The rise of cognitive psychology in the 1960s influenced the field, but while the cognitive approach is a major feature of modern human factors, neuroscience is ignored for the most part. Currently, however, our understanding of human cognitive functions has been considerably enriched by neuroscience research. It is, therefore, natural to seek applications of this knowledge to problems of cognition in relation to technology and work. This intersection of neuroscience and human factors (ergonomics) has been termed neuroergonomics (Parasuraman, 2003).

Given that there are a multitude of techniques available to address human factors problems and issues, one must ask what novel and important role neuroergonomics might play in human factors research and application. Certainly, to the extent that information gained through neuroscience measurement is redundant with that obtained from other measures and models employed by the human factors community, neuroergonomics measures will be unlikely to gain wide acceptance. This is likely to be the case for a number of the human neuroscience measures when compared with the subjective rating and performance-based measurement techniques traditionally employed by human factors practitioners and researchers, in light of the relatively high cost and substantial amount of expertise required for collecting, analyzing, and interpreting neuroergonomic measures when compared with the subjective rating and performance-based measurement techniques traditionally employed by human factors practitioners and researchers.

Thus, for neuroergonomic measurement techniques to gain acceptance in the human factors research and applications community, these measures must:

1. prove to be more valid and/or reliable indices of relevant psychological (or, in some cases, physiological) constructs than traditional behavioral and subjective measures; or

2. enable the measurement of psychological constructs that are difficult or impossible to measure with traditional measures; or

3. enable the measurement of relevant psychological or physiological constructs in situations where other types of measures are unavailable or difficult to obtain.

Indeed, there is evidence (to be discussed shortly) that each of these three criteria has been or can be met within a human factors context with measures obtained via models inspired by neuroscience.

Another important consideration is the temporal sensitivity of neuroergonomic measures. In many human factors contexts – for example, the evaluation of new display concepts, the examination of the effects of different environmental conditions (e.g., differences in ambient temperature, humidity, or lighting) on human performance and information processing, the evaluation of training proficiency, and the assessment of fitness for duty – data can be collected and then analyzed and interpreted offline (i.e., at a later time that can, depending on circumstances, range from minutes to days). In such situations, enough time and effort can often be allocated to ensure adequate signal-to-noise ratios and to deal adequately with potential artifacts in the neuroscience data. On the other hand, there are also a number of human factors contexts that demand almost instantaneous data processing and interpretation. For example, given the increasing trend toward adaptive automation in systems, such as aircraft and process control, it has become important to develop measures that can both describe and predict changes in psychological constructs in or near real-time such as mental workload, alertness, and information processing strategies. Such information could then serve, in addition to inferences about human information processing capacities extracted from dynamic models of the interaction between humans, tasks, and environment, as input to algorithms that determine the dynamic task allocation policy between humans and automated systems. Of course, such situations pose technical problems for neuroergonomic measures that are not encountered in offline contexts such as rapid data collection, processing, artifact rejection, and interpretation. Additionally, the bandwidth of some systems (e.g., high-performance aircraft) may be high enough to preclude collecting sufficient amounts of (at least some types of) neuroer-

gonomic data to ensure adequate reliability or signal-to-noise ratios.

One additional issue that merits some discussion is the applicability of neuroergonomic measurement techniques to extralaboratory environments. Most human neuroscience research has focused on explicating the functional significance of different measures and components with relatively simple tasks in well-controlled laboratory environments. Even so, a great deal of effort has been expended on the elimination of potential artifacts (e.g., from ambient electrical fields, contamination from other physiological signals that may mask the signal of interest, individual differences in baselines, or a measure's morphology or topography). When such artifacts are difficult or impossible to eliminate during data recording, the focus has been on adjusting the physiological measures in order to minimize the impact of artifacts on data interpretation. Given the diversity and magnitude of the artifacts encountered in such well-controlled settings, is it a reasonable expectation to collect valid and reliable neuroergonomics data in less well-controlled environments such as high-fidelity (and sometimes motion-based) simulators or operational environments? Although collecting neuroscience data in such environments clearly provides a considerable technical challenge, there have been a number of promising developments in the design of miniaturized recording equipment that can withstand the rigors of operational environments (Berka et al., 2004; Hoover & Muth, 2004; Miller, 1995; Sterman & Mann, 1995). There have also been developments in pattern recognition and signal analysis techniques that enhance the detection, recognition, and processing of a number of physiological signals in noise (Bostanov, 2004; Wolpaw et al., 2002), as well as development of automated artifact rejection procedures (Berka et al., 2004; Du, Leong, & Gevins 1994). For example, Gevins et al. (1995; see also Berka et al., 2004) reported the development of a "smart helmet" system in flight helmets, which incorporates a combination of 32 EEG and EOG electrodes along with miniaturized preamplifiers. Barring technological roadblocks, such developments should continue to increase the potential for recording psychophysiological signals in a number of complex environments.

In summary, each of the issues discussed so far needs to be carefully considered when human neuroscience theory and measures are to be used in addressing human factors issues. Indeed, it is likely that some measures will be appropriate for only a subset of situations in which human factors issues are examined, for example, Positron Emission Tomography (PET) and functional Magnetic Resonance Imaging, (fMRI), whereas other measures may be more widely applicable. At the same time, neuroscience theory may be used to inform human factors issues, even though no neural measures are used (Parasuraman, 2003). In an effort to make some of these considerations more concrete, we now turn to a critical review of current applications of psychophysiological measurement issues in the human factors field.

III. NEUROERGONOMICS AND HUMAN FACTORS: A BRIEF HISTORY

Human factors developed as a unique discipline in response to human performance questions that arose around the time of World War II. For the first time, systems such as military aircraft, ships, and ground vehicles were becoming sufficiently complex that more numerous (and sometimes catastrophic) errors were observed, even though the systems were functioning as designed from a mechanical standpoint. That is, human operators either could not execute their assigned functions as expected or they did not have sufficient training to do so. As a consequence of these system problems and the well-founded suspicion that systems were not being designed to ensure adequate human performance, experimental psychologists were called upon to evaluate the human-machine interface and training regimes, to diagnose problems, predict problems not yet observed, and suggest system improvements and training modifications to ensure safe and efficient system operation (Fitts & Jones, 1947; Mackworth, 1948).

It is interesting to note that psychophysiological measures, principally measures of gaze direction, played an important role in the examination of human performance in complex systems during the early years of human factors. Fitts and colleagues (Fitts, Jones, & Milton, 1950; Jones, Milton, & Fitts, 1950) used measures of gaze direction, gaze duration, and the sequence of eye movements to examine the information extraction strategies employed by novice and experienced aircraft pilots during instrument flight. Data acquired from these studies were used to reconfigure instrument panels to optimize the speed and accuracy with which pilots could locate and extract flight-relevant information. Eye scan measures continue to be used today, in conjunction with measures of pilot and automobile driver performance, to assess strategies for extracting information as well as mental workload and skill acquisition in a variety of different transportation systems (Bellenkes et al., 1997; McCarley et al., 2004; Strayer, Drews, & Johnston, 2003).

The use of other neuroscience and psychophysiological measures to examine issues of interest to the human factors community soon followed the pioneering research of Fitts and co-workers. For example, Sem-Jacobsen and colleagues (Sem-Jacobsen 1959, 1961; Sem-Jacobsen & Sem-Jacobsen 1963) recorded electroencephalographic (EEG) activity from pilots as they flew missions of varying difficulty during simulated and actual flight in an effort to examine the utility of this psychophysiological measure for assessing the deleterious effects of high-G environments and mental and emotional workload. It was also speculated that psychophysiological measures, in particular measures of the EEG, would prove useful for the selection and evaluation of pilots for high-performance aircraft and for adaptively automated systems (see also Gomer, 1981). Although Sem-Jacobsen's visions for applications have not yet been realized, our review of the current literature will indicate that at least some of these applications soon will be realized.

Finally, measures of heart rate and heart rate variability have long been used to provide a continuous record of the cardio-respiratory function and mental workload of operators in complex simulated and real-world systems. Heart rate measures have been recorded as aircraft pilots execute a number of maneuvers in simulated and actual aircraft such as landing (Ruffel-Smith, 1967), refueling during long-haul flights (Brown et al., 1969), performing steep descents (Roscoe, 1975), and flying combat missions (Roman, Older, & Jones, 1967). Such measures continue to be used today, often in the context of other psychophysiological measures and along with a more sophisticated appreciation for the underlying physiology.

In summary, although the application of neuroscience techniques to issues of human factors has a relatively recent history, these measures have provided useful insights into human performance and cognition in and outside of the laboratory. In the following section of the chapter we provide a brief discussion of neuroscience techniques, of a relatively recent vintage, that have not yet been widely applied to human factors questions and issues, but have the potential to provide important insights into human performance in and outside of the laboratory.

IV. A BRIEF DISCUSSION OF SOME RECENT DEVELOPMENTS IN HUMAN NEUROSCIENCE TECHNIQUES OF RELEVANCE FOR HUMAN FACTORS

Electroencephalographic activity and event-related brain potentials. As briefly discussed above (and in more detail in the Applications sections below), event-related brain potentials (ERP) and EEG activity have served as the main central nervous systems measures in Human Factors research to date. These techniques provide a measure of the electrical fields of simultaneously active neurons that are recorded at the scalp. EEG data is analyzed in the frequency domain and entails the derivation of differences in power across different individuals or experimental conditions in frequency bands that have been empirically related to perceptual, cognitive, and motor constructs. On the other hand, the ERP is a transient series of voltage oscillations in the brain, which can be recorded from the scalp in response to discrete stimuli and responses. Specific ERP components, usually defined in terms of polarity and minimum latency with respect to a discrete stimulus or response, have been found to reflect a number of distinct perceptual, cognitive, and motor processes and prove useful in decomposing the processing requirements of complex tasks (Fabiani, Gratton, & Coles, 2000).

An important advantage of EEG measures is that they can be recorded in the absence of discrete stimuli or responses that make them useful in situations in which an operator is monitoring slowly changing displays that require little intervention. Indeed, as a result of this characteristic EEG measures have been employed as an index of vigilance in a variety of different simulated and real-world settings encountered in human factors research including flying (Gundel, Drescher, & Turowski, 2000), driving (Miller, 1995), and performance of rotating shift work in power plants (Gillberg et al., 2003). Additionally, EEG measures have served as the basis for online alertness predictors (Makeig, Elliot, & Postal, 1994). However, although EEG measures can be employed to provide a somewhat precise temporal index of changes in alertness and attention, ERPs can be used to decompose, in a temporally precise manner, the information processing activities that transpire between the time stimuli impinge on sensory receptors until an individual produces an action, whether it is an eye movement, vocalization, or skilled movement of the hands or feet. Another important advantage of ERPs is that for a number of ERP components the brain regions from which a component is generated are known. This knowledge enables the researcher to capitalize on the extensive neuropsychological literature that maps particular cognitive functions to neuroanatomical circuits.

However, as is the case with all of the measures discussed in this chapter, there are also constraints and potential difficulties in using EEG and ERP measures in different situations. Given problems with motion artifacts and electrical noise it is preferable to record EEG and ERPs from individuals who are not ambulatory. This clearly reduces the number of situations in which these can be utilized. In any event, there are still ample professions and settings or from which ERP and EEG recording is possible (e.g., pilots, drivers, office workers, process control operators, etc). However, as discussed above the increasingly rapid development of noise detection and signal processing algorithms will continue to increase the feasibility of recording EEG and ERP measures in a wider range of simulated and real-world environments (e.g., Berka et al., 2004). ERPs, unlike EEG, require a discrete stimulus or response. Therefore, some situations are not easily amenable to ERP recording, for instance, situations in which it is difficult to record ERPs from discrete stimuli or responses in a closed system (e.g., a system in which it is difficult to acquire precise timing of new stimuli and responses) or when it is unfeasible to introduce signals from which ERPs can be recorded (e.g., in a secondary task). Finally, ERP and EEG recording, analysis and interpretation require relatively substantial training both in terms of the recording procedures as well as in the relevant psychological and physiological literatures.

Positron emission tomography and function magnetic resonance imaging.

The field of cognitive neuroscience has benefited tremendously from the utilization of relatively noninvasive in vivo neuroimaging techniques. However, given the constraints of these techniques and the fact that thus far the focus has been on elucidating patterns of brain activation in relatively simple tasks in an effort to isolate specific cognitive processes, the field of human factors has yet to reap substantial benefits.

Both PET and fMRI utilize biophysiological correlates of neural activity to infer the involvement of cortical regions in a given task. One of the clear advantages of PET is the ability to translate detected signals into biologically meaningful units (e.g., glucose metabolism or regional cerebral blood flow; e.g., Brickman et al., 2003). In contrast, the signal changes detected by fMRI methods vary along arbitrary units that do not directly translate into an absolute metric of biological function. Another advantage of PET is the ability for researchers to design isotope-tagged molecules that bind to specific biologically relevant elements, such as dopamine receptors. This allows one to map out brain function and other important individual differences in brain chemistry that can potentially be linked to gene expression (see the Applications section for further discussion of molecular genetic studies of individual differences). Perhaps the most obvious disadvantage of PET is that the participants must be injected with or inhale a radioactive substance, whereas fMRI uses the native contrast of naturally occurring biological processes to infer function. fMRI also has the advantage of improved temporal resolution, which allows the researchers to resolve inferred neural activity from rapidly presented stimuli (e.g., Burock et al., 1998) or even self-paced events (e.g., Maccotta, Zacks & Buckner, 2001) on a trial-by-trial basis. This allows the researcher to separate and compare, for example, correct responses from errors (Hester, Fassbender, & Garavan, 2004), remembered versus forgotten events or objects (Morcom et al., 2003), or intermixed conditions of varying difficulty (Olson et al., 2004). In contrast, given the slow evolution of the signal changes, PET studies must utilize blocked designs, where the participant responds to repeated trials of a given type. This precludes the use of more standard cognitive experimental designs in which trials of each type are often intermixed and balanced for order of presentation. Additionally, it is not possible to resolve neural activity to individual trials (e.g., errors), and the neural activity from all trials within the block becomes averaged together. Furthermore, compared to electrophysiological and optical methods (see Optical Imaging section below), both fMRI and PET cannot easily resolve activity within a trial because of the intrinsically slow course of hemodynamic and metabolic phenomena that follow neuronal activity. Nonetheless, PET and fMRI studies have contributed substantially to our understanding of cortical and cognitive function.

As mentioned above, the great majority of studies that have employed PET and fMRI have done so in relatively simple tasks in an effort to isolate specific perceptual, cognitive, motor, and affective processes. However, even the investigation of patterns of brain activation in relatively simple tasks has provided insights that are potentially relevant to performance outside of the laboratory. For example, the use of fMRI and PET to investigate executive control processes, which include planning, scheduling, working memory, resolving conflicts between stimuli and responses, and multi-tasking, has provided insights which enable both the testing of theories of relevance to the design of displays and information presentation strategies (e.g., Jiang, Saxe, & Kanwisher, 2004; Smith & Jonides, 1999) as well as the understanding of the nature of individual differences in performance (Scarmeas et al., 2003). Investigators have also begun to use PET and fMRI measures to address other issues of relevance to human factors. For example, Chee and Choo (2004) examined changes in performance and fMRI activation in both short-term and working memory tasks before and after 24 hours of sleep deprivation. They found a pattern of both deactivations and, presumably, compensatory activations following sleep loss that were predictive of changes in memory performance. Whether such changes can be used to predict performance deficits in specific individuals, which enable the implementation of effective countermeasures, is an interesting and important question for future research. Finally, a number of investigators have begun to tackle the examination of changes in brain activation in components of complex real-world tasks such as the inspection of static and dynamic real-world scenes (Bartels & Zeki, 2003; Huettel, Guzeldere, & McCarthy, 2001) and automobile driving (Calhoun et al., 2002). While the constraints of PET and fMRI recording will likely preclude the recording of data in extra-laboratory environments, the continued development of Virtual Reality systems and technology will enable investigators to bring high fidelity simulations of real-world tasks into the laboratory by capitalizing on the benefits of these neuroimaging techniques for exploring the interface between brain and mind.

Optical imaging of brain activity. Noninvasive optical imaging represents a relatively recent addition to the neuroimaging tools available for human research. It has been known for over 50 years that the activity of neurons are associated with changes in optical as well as chemical and electrical properties (Hill & Keynes, 1949). Since this time optical properties of brain cells have been examined in cell cultures and within intact brains (Villringer & Chance, 1997), either from recordings on the exposed cortex or with indwelling optical sensors.

However, more recently a class of optical techniques has been developed that enable the noninvasive measurement of functional activity of the brain. These techniques capitalize on the absorption and scattering properties of near-infrared light (between 700 and 1000 nm) in biological tissue. Light within this range can penetrate and diffuse several cm into tissue because water and other substances present in tissue do not absorb much of the light within this part of the spectrum. Indeed an optical measurement approach referred to as photon migration has enabled the reliable and non-invasive recording of functional brain activity in humans to depths of approximately 2.5 cm (Gratton et al., 2003). This optical measurement procedure is based on the assessment of the intensity or delay of photons as they travel from a source to a detector along a mathematically well-described path in the brain.

The photon migration technique, which is based on the measurement of the delay in photons between a source and detector (generally referred to as the time-resolved optical method), has a number of distinct advantages including the ability to separately quantify the scattering and absorption coefficients in the tissue through which the photons travel and provides good spatial resolution similar to that obtained with fMRI.

The use of the photon migration technique has enabled the measurement of a number of different signals: (1) relatively slow signals which enable the quantification of changes in oxy- and deoxy-hemoglobin in selective regions of the cortex (Villinger & Chance, 1997), and (2) faster stimulus or response locked signals, referred to as the event-related optical signal (EROS), that reflect neuronal activity (Gratton & Fabiani, 2001). As in fMRI, the slower signals provide an index of changes in hemodynamic activity that may differ over experimental conditions and individuals. However, unlike fMRI, the slower signals have the advantage of providing separate estimates of oxy- and deoxy-hemoglobin. The faster signal is quite similar, in many ways, to the ERP with the additional advantage of superior spatial resolution. Thus, the measurement of optical activity can enable the concurrent collection of hemodynamic and neuronal activity, which capitalizes on the relative strengths of both of these neuroimaging techniques.

However, as with any measurement procedure there are also several disadvantages, some of which can likely be overcome with the development of new signal analysis techniques, software, and hardware that are associated with optical imaging. For example, unlike fMRI, spatial resolution is limited to approximately 2.5 cm from the scalp. It is also the case that, at present, the fast neuronally based optical signal has a relatively low signal-to-noise ratio. This requires the collection of a substantial amount of data, more so than for ERPs, to reliably resolve optical components. However, there have been a number of recent proposals, which include new data filters and hardware, that have the potential to substantially improve signal to noise ratio (Mackin, Gratton, & Fabiani, 2003).

Early studies of both the slow hemodynamic and fast neuronal optical signals focused on validating these measures against ERP, PET, and fMRI indices of different sensory and motor processes. That is, these early studies demonstrated the selective recording of optical parameters in motor (Gratton et al., 1995), somatosensory (Steinbrink et al., 2000), visual (Gratton, Goddman-Wood, & Fabiani, 2001), and auditory (Rinne et al., 1999) cortexes with appropriate task stimulation.

More recent studies have gone beyond establishing the reliability and validity of optical measures and have begun to utilize them to address important theoretical and practical issues for which they are well suited. For example, DeSoto et al. (2001) examined whether conflict between two different dimensions of a stimulus can result in the simultaneous activation of multiple motor responses.

Previous studies using the lateralized readiness potential (LRP) of the ERP, a component that provides an index of motor activation, have already been used to track motor activation during the performance of a variety of different tasks (e.g., Osman & Moore, 1993). However, because the LRP is a measure of the differential activation between the left and right motor cortices, it cannot provide information about their simultaneous activation. Given the appropriate placement of sensors, activation of multiple responses in different hemispheres can be measured with optical imaging. Using EROS, DeSoto and colleagues measured activation in a Stroop experiment in which subjects either were to pay attention to the meaning or the spatial position of words such as above and below. When the responses to these two dimensions (i.e., one task relevant and one task irrelevant dimension on each trial) conflicted evidence of activation of motor responses was obtained for both the dimensions. Such data suggests, in agreement with parallel but inconsistent with serial models of information processing, that priming of multiple responses can indeed occur concurrently. The ability to simultaneously measure the activation of multiple responses could be, in principle, invaluable in future brain-computer interfaces (see discussion below).

In summary, while noninvasive optical imaging of human brain activity is still in its infancy, the research conducted to date suggests great promise for this technique given its ability to tap both hemodynamic and neuronal activity, thereby capitalizing on both good spatial and temporal resolution without the physical constraints of other neuroimaging measures (e.g., PET and fMRI). Clearly additional research is necessary to successfully address the signal-to-noise issue, but given the rapid development of new signal processing techniques and multiple channel optical recording devices this would appear to be a solvable problem in the near future.

Assessing brain structure. The topic of brain structure or anatomy might seem out of place in a chapter on the application of neuroscience techniques to the field of Human Factors. However, it has recently become acknowledged, in the scientific literature, that human brain structure can, and indeed does, change as a function of a variety of experiences. It has also become increasingly clear that individual differences in anatomy, often measured as differences in cortical volume, density, or both can be related to performance on a variety of perceptual and cognitive tasks. Therefore, it is conceivable that in the near future that the nonintrusive measurement of brain structure might be a useful converging measure of both individual differences in components of neural circuits that support performance and a reflection in the efficacy of training induced cortical plasticity.

Both hand tracing and automated segmentation techniques have been used for a number of years to characterize change in brain volume in regionally specific fashion, during development and aging, and to relate changes

in volume to selective aspects of cognition. For example, hand-traced estimates of prefrontal gray matter volume in cross-sectional samples significantly predict age-correlated reductions in performance on frontally mediated executive tasks such as the Wisconsin Card Sorting Test (Gunning-Dixon & Raz, 2003) and verbal working memory (Head et al., 2002). Another set of studies linked the hippocampal volume of older adults to their long-term memory performance (across several weeks) and even accounted for the effects of age on memory (Walhovod, et al., 2004).

However, perhaps more exciting, are a couple of recent studies that have used automated segmentation techniques to track within individual changes in human brain structure over time in response to environmental interventions. Draganski et al. (2004) examined change in the cortical volume of 24 young adults, half of whom were taught to juggle over a three-month period. Compared to the non-training controls, those individuals who were taught to juggle displayed bilateral increases in the volume of the medial-temporal region of cortex, which is a brain region responsible, in part, for the processing of motion. Interestingly, when the study participants were scanned again three months after training (in which no further juggling practice was received), there were slight reductions in the volume of medial-temporal cortex. Colcombe et al. (submitted) used automated segmentation techniques to assess longitudinal changes in the brain structure of older adults who were randomly assigned to participate in either a six-month cardiovascular fitness-training program or a nonexercise control group. They found that older adults who participated in the exercise group showed a significant increase in gray matter volume in regions of the frontal and superior temporal lobe than the control group. And exercising older adults showed a significant increase in the volume of the anterior white matter tracts that allow the frontal lobes of the brain to communicate. Thus, these two studies, when viewed together, suggest that an analysis of high resolution MRI data has the potential to reflect changes in anatomy that may be related to human performance in and outside the laboratory. However, it should be noted that the limitations of the automated segmentation techniques do not allow one to infer precisely what mechanism(s) results in these changes (e.g., increase in cell body size, increased dendritic connections, increased capillary bed volume, and increased glial size or number, etc.). Clearly, more research is needed, including animal studies and human magnetic imaging spectroscopy, to further delineate the nature of the volume changes.

Transcranial doppler sonography. Ultrasound techniques have long been used for various medical applications, including fetal heart rate monitoring and assessment of blood flow in the carotid arteries in stroke patients. More recently, Transcranial Doppler Sonography (TCD) has been used in neuropsychological research to measure dynamic changes in cerebral blood perfusion that occur during the performance of a wide variety of mental tasks (Duschek & Schandry, 2003; Stroobant & Vingerhoets, 2001). Accordingly, there has also been recent interest in using TCD in the examination of issues relevant to human factors and ergonomics (Tripp & Warm, in press; Wilson, Finemore, & Estepp, 2003; Zinni & Parasuraman, 2004).

TCD offers the advantages over PET and fMRI of low cost, does not require participants to be immobile, and good temporal resolution (Aaslid, 1986). The TCD technique capitalizes on the well-known Doppler effect, which refers to the modulation of the frequency of optical or acoustic waves between a source and a receiver that are moving relative to one another. TCD uses a transducer mounted on the participant's head that directs ultrasound waves toward an artery within the brain. A Doppler shift in frequency occurs when the ultrasound waves are reflected back by red blood cells moving through the cerebral arteries, and the sign of the shift depends on whether the blood is flowing away from or towards the transducer. Blood flow velocity can then be measured in the middle (MCA), anterior (ACA), or the posterior cerebral arteries (PCA). The MCA carries over 75% of the blood flow within each cerebral hemisphere and, hence, is usually the artery that is imaged in the majority of TCD studies.

Assessments of the reliability of TCD have focused both on baseline and activation-related values of blood flow. Several investigations have reported moderate to high reliability (>.7) for baseline blood flow values (Baumgartner et al., 1994). With respect to task-induced blood flow changes Knecht et al. (1998) reported a test-retest reliability coefficient of .9 for blood flow in a linguistic (word-fluency) task. Stroobant and Vingerhoets (2001) also reported moderate to high reliability values for several verbal and visuospatial tasks. The validity of TCD blood flow changes has been compared to those obtained with PET and fMRI. Most studies report high correlations between techniques with respect to overall blood flow changes in each cerebral hemisphere (Duschek & Schandry, 2003). Knake et al. (2003) also reported a correlation between TCD-based assessment of hemispheric laterality for language and the Wada test, which is generally considered the gold standard.

Gaze contingent displays

Although the measurement of eye movements, and more specifically saccades have long been used as a technique to elucidate information extraction strategies from visual displays, for example, the pioneering research of Fitts and colleagues, which used eye movements to understand instrument scanning by pilots (Fitts, Jones, & Milton 1950; Jones, Milton, & Fitts 1950.) new saccade measurement procedures have further enhanced the utility of eye movements in both basic and applied research.

The moving window technique, first developed to examine peripheral information utilization in reading (McConkie & Rayner, 1975), has proven useful in the study of visual search and, in particular, in the study of the size of the visual field from which individuals can effectively extract information within a fixation (referred to as the perceptual span). This technique entails providing a window, centered around fixation, in which information is presented normally (i.e., how it would be perceived in the absence of a viewing window). Information outside of the window is either removed or degraded. The critical aspect of the technique is the manipulation of the size of the eye-movement contingent window and the comparison of search performance with different window sizes to search to performance with normal, unobstructed viewing (see Reingold et al., 2003, for a recent detailed review of this technique). Visual span is defined in terms of the window size that yields search performance equivalent to that obtained via normal viewing.

Bertera and Rayner (2000) used the moving window technique to examine average visual span size in the search of cluttered displays. They found that window sizes of five degrees and larger yielded search performance equivalent to that obtained through normal viewing. Based on the number, size, and separation of letter stimuli used in their study they estimated that individuals were able to extract between three and six items within each fixation. Loschky and McConkie (2002) found that by manipulating the size of the high resolution window centered on fixation they could actually speed search among the items in the window, but at a cost for inspecting objects outside of the high resolution window. Pomplun, Reingold, and Shen (2001) examined the impact of processing load, both within the search task and from other tasks, on visual span using the moving window technique. They discovered that both the difficulty of the search task as well as the introduction of and increase in difficulty of an auditory secondary task decreased the effective visual span. Such a result is interesting in that it suggests that nonvisual processing can detrimentally impact our ability to efficiently extract information from a visual display.

A variation of the moving window technique that is referred to as the gaze contingent technique has been used to examine the memory representations that underlie visual search. In the version of the contingent search paradigm developed by McCarley and colleagues (2003; see also Boot et al., 2004), a subject is initially presented with a fixation cross and one search item on a computer display. At this point, there is only one possible search item to examine. During the initial saccade to the first search item, a second search item is presented. By presenting new search items during saccades, saccadic suppression prevents the new items from acting as abrupt onsets and capturing attention. If the fixated item is the target the individual is to respond with the appropriate keypress and the trial is terminated. If the fixated item is a distractor search continues until the target is found or all of the items have been presented.

After the first saccade, the subject still has only one potential saccade target. As the subject makes the next saccade, a new item is added to the display and the first item remains on the screen. From this point on, three items will always be present in the display: the currently fixated item and two potential saccade targets. One of the potential saccade targets is always a *new* item that has not yet been identified, and the other is an *old* item that has already been examined (the *decoy*). Decoys always reappear in the same location and same orientation as originally presented, and except for the third event, where there is only one previously examined item, decoys are randomly chosen from the list of examined items.

Critical to this paradigm is that the subject is forced to choose between making a saccade to a new item or a decoy. If visual search is guided by a memory that is perfect, then a new item will always be chosen. If there is no memory, or memory has failed, the subject will chose to make a saccade to a decoy half the time. McCarley and colleagues (2003) examined how long memory lasts during visual search by looking at the probability that a decoy was reexamined based on the number of intervening fixations since the decoy was first examined (*lag*). Memory for the last two previously fixated items is quite good with most of the saccades going to the new item. However, with additional lags, performance eventually reaches chance levels (generally by the 4th or 5th lag), providing an estimate of the size of the memory buffer that supports memory for previously visited locations in search. Followup studies with this gaze contingent paradigm have revealed that (1) the memory representations that underlie visual search are largely implicit (Boot et al., 2004), (2) background layout and landmarks boost memory for previously inspected locations (Peterson et al., 2004), and (3) substantial individual differences exist in the size of the memory buffer that supports efficient visual search (Becic, Kramer, & Boot, in press). It is important to note, however, that thus far this technique has been used with relatively simple visual search displays in well-controlled laboratory settings. Clearly, an important question for the future is whether this gaze contingent technique can be "scaled-up" and perhaps also combined with other eye movement monitoring and neuroimaging techniques to enable the assessment of the role of memory in search and information extraction in more realistic and varied environments. For example, Belopolsky and Kramer (in preparation) have recently combined eye movement and ERP recording techniques to examine the nature of error processing when the eyes are misdirected away from an intended goal.

V. APPLICATION AREAS

A. Workload/multi-task processing

Assessment of mental workload continues to be an important topic in human factors research and practice. This is primarily because the design of an efficient human-machine system does not simply involve assessing operator performance, but also evaluating how well operators can meet the workload demands imposed on them by the system. A major question that must be addressed in any human-machine system is whether the human operators are overloaded and can meet additional unexpected demands if they arise during system operations. Behavioral measures such as accuracy and speed of response to probe events have been widely used to assess mental workload, but measures of brain function offer some unique advantages that can be exploited in particular applications (Kramer & Weber 2000; Parasuraman, 2003). Such measures can also be linked to emerging cognitive neuroscience knowledge, thereby, allowing for the development of neuroergonomic theories of mental workload.

There are many approaches to the study of mental workload and a variety of definitions (Wickens & Hollands, 2000). From a neuroergonomic perspective, mental workload can be considered to be a composite set of brain/mind states that modulate human performance of perceptual, cognitive, and motor tasks (Parasuraman & Caggiano, 2002). Workload can be driven exogenously ("bottom-up") by environmental sources (task load) or endogenously (or "top-down") by the voluntary application of attentional resources (Wickens, 1984). Both sources of workload are presumably reflected in changes in regional patterns of brain activation. The challenge for neuroergonomic research is to be able to characterize these patterns in a theoretically meaningful way.

Cerebral blood flow measures of mental workload and dual-task interference. Although mental workload has been viewed in a number of different ways, the notion that it can be linked to the brain has a long history. The British physiologist Charles Sherrington first demonstrated the close relationship between neuronal activity, the energy demands of the associated cellular processes, and regional cerebral blood flow (Roy & Sherrington, 1890). His pioneering work suggested that, in principle, increased neuronal activity associated with mental processing could be assessed by measuring the blood flow responses of the brain. The development of noninvasive techniques for measuring cerebral blood flow in humans, such as TCD, PET, and fMRI, has paved the way for testing his suggestion.

Several TCD studies have shown that cerebral blood flow increases in response to the requirement to engage in mental activities. In general, an increase in cerebral blood flow from a baseline condition to one requiring cognitive processing can be demonstrated reliably (Stroobant & Vingerhoets, 2001). To be useful as a measure of mental workload, however, TCD measures of blood flow need to be linked to manipulations of task difficulty. Despite the large literature on TCD and neuropsychological task performance, only a few such studies have been carried out.

Serrati et al. (2000) examined changes in blood flow in a mental rotation task. They found that the increase in blood flow from baseline to task performance was greater for more difficult mental rotations. Wilson, Finomore, and Estepp (2003) also found that blood flow associated with performance of the Multi-Attribute Task Battery, a simple flight simulation task, varied with task difficulty. However, Zinni and Parasuraman (2004) could not find reliable changes in cerebral blood flow with within-task changes in difficulty in a working memory task and in a tracking task. More such studies involving parametric variations in difficulty must be conducted before the use of TCD can be validated to assess mental workload. However, the major drawback of TCD is that it cannot provide any information on localization of blood flow changes associated with cognitive processing within a hemisphere. Accordingly, understanding the brain systems of mental workload requires other neuroimaging methods with better spatial localization capability, such as PET and fMRI.

Studies of mental workload often compare performance on two concurrent tasks (dual-task) to single-task performance. A major issue is whether dual-task decrements result from activation of a distinct, resource-consumptive, multitask coordination module or whether they result from interference in functionally independent modules or resource pools (Wickens, 2002). Can neuroimaging studies localize such a general-purpose module or provide evidence for multiple resource pools? D'Esposito et al. (1995) reported that the dorsolateral prefrontal cortex was activated preferentially during the performance of concurrent tasks compared to single-task performance. However, subsequent studies have not provided consistent support for the overadditivity of activation in this brain region, and have had some failures in replicating the original finding (Adcock et al., 2000; Bunge et al., 2000). One problem may be that these studies used dual tasks with interspersed blank-time intervals (to enable fMRI analysis), so that task switching rather than dual tasking might have occurred. Dreher and Grafman (2003) examined patterns of activation in prefrontal cortex in a comparison of dual-task (concurrently performing two tasks) and task-switching (alternatively performing each of the two tasks alone) conditions. They reported that dual-task processing selectively activated the anterior cingulate region of the medial frontal cortex, whereas task switching activated the dorsolateral prefrontal cortex.

Another group of studies have used the psychological refractory period (PRP) paradigm, which allows for the partitioning of dual-task interference to discrete processing stages (Pashler, 1994). Herath et al. (2001) found that the superior frontal gyrus and the intraparietal sulcus were activated to a greater extent in the PRP task compared to single task conditions. Moreover, they found that activation in the right inferior frontal gyrus was positively associated with individual differences in the degree of dual-task interference. The results of this and other PRP studies (e.g., Schubert & Szameitat, 2003) indicate that, consistent with behavioral studies, the source of dual-task interference in the PRP paradigm lies primarily in the response selection and response execution stages. However, Jiang (2004) compared the standard PRP task to conditions in which the two overlapping tasks were either both presented in the periphery or one was presented centrally and the other peripherally. The first condition imposed a greater competitive demand on spatial attention than the second condition or the standard PRP task (for which both tasks were presented centrally). The right inferior frontal gyrus was differentially activated when the overlapping tasks were presented peripherally, which indicates that in addition to response selection, competition for spatial attention also limits dual-task performance.

These studies indicate that dual-task performance is associated with the activation of prefrontal cortex, which is consistent with the general view that this brain region is critically involved in executive control processes. Such control processes are likely to be involved in dual-task performance and in other conditions, for instance, resolving conflict between competing responses. There is also some evidence that regions of the inferior and middle frontal gyrus may be specifically implicated in dual-task performance, at least in the PRP paradigm, but additional work with other dual-task pairings, including continuous (as opposed to discrete) and more complex tasks, needs to be conducted to assess the generality of this finding.

Event-related brain potentials. The neuroimaging studies discussed previously have been informative with regard to the identification of a global hemispheric measure of mental workload, as well as the possible localization of brain systems underlying dual-task performance. However, in general, such studies have not been informative with respect to the temporal locus of dual-task interference. This is a natural consequence of the limited temporal resolution of fMRI. (but see Jiang, 2004). Event-related potentials offer good temporal resolution in assessing neural activity. Accordingly, it is instructive to examine ERP studies of dual-task performance.

Most such ERP studies have examined the P3 or P300 component, which was first described by Sutton et al. (1965). P300 is characterized by a slow positive wave with a mean latency following stimulus onset of about 300 ms, depending on stimulus complexity, probability, and other factors (Polich, 1987). The P300 is thought to reflect postperceptual or postcategorical processes prior to response selection and execution stages. For example, increasing the difficulty of identifying the target stimulus increases the latency of P300 (Kutas, McCarthy, & Donchin, 1977), whereas increasing the difficulty of response selection does not (Magliero et al., 1984). This has led to the view that the latency of the P300 provides a relatively pure measure of perceptual processing and categorization time that is independent of response selection and execution stages (Kutas, McCarthy, & Donchin, 1977).

It has also been proposed that the amplitude of P300 is proportional to the amount of central processing resources allocated to the P300 eliciting stimulus (Johnson, 1986). Thus, any diversion of processing resources away from target discrimination in a dual-task situation will lead to a reduction in P300 amplitude. Isreal et al. (1980) showed that the amplitude of P300 decreased when a primary task, tone counting, was combined with a secondary task of visual tracking. However, increases in the difficulty of the tracking task (by increasing the bandwidth of the forcing function) did not lead to a further reduction in P300 amplitude. This pattern of findings was taken to support the view that the P300 reflects processing resources associated with perceptual processing and stimulus categorization, but not response-related processes, which was manipulated in the tracking task.

These and other related studies (Kramer, Wickens, & Donchin, 1983, 1985) have clearly established that P300 amplitude provides a reliable index of resource allocation related to perceptual and cognitive processing in dual-task situations. Similar results have been obtained when P300 has been used in conjunction with performance in flight simulators (Kramer, Sirevaag, & Braune, 1987; Sirevaag et al., 1993). P300, therefore, provides a reliable and valid index of mental workload, to the extent that perceptual and cognitive aspects of information processing are major contributors to workload in a given performance setting. Response-related contributions to workload, however, are not reflected in P300 amplitude.

A more recent human factors study exploited these characteristics of P300 to assess cognitive workload during simulated driving (Baldwin, Freeman, & Coyne, 2004). P300 in a visual, color-discrimination task was recorded while participants engaged in driving conditions of normal and reduced visibility (fog). P300 amplitude, but not discrimination accuracy or reaction time (RT), was reduced when participants drove in fog compared to driving with normal visibility. However, P300 did not vary significantly with changes in traffic density, while RT measures were sensitive to this manipulation of driving difficulty. Baldwin, Freeman, and Coyne (2004) concluded that neither neural nor behavioral measures alone are sufficient for assessing cognitive workload during different driving scenarios, but that multiple measures may be needed.

A unique feature of the P300 is that it is simultaneously sensitive to the allocation of attentional resources (P300 amplitude) and to the timing of stimulus identification and categorization processes (P300 latency). These features allow not only for assessing the workload associated with dual- or multitask performance, but also for identifying the sources that contribute to workload and dual-task interference. These features were further elegantly exploited in a dual-task study by Luck (1998) using the PRP paradigm. The typical finding in this paradigm is that RT to the second target is substantially delayed when the interval between the two targets is short. Luck (1998) identified the source of this interference by recording the P300 to the second target stimulus, which was either the letter X or the letter O, with one of the letters being presented only 25% of the time (the odd ball). Whereas RT was significantly increased when the interval between the two stimuli was short, P300 latency was only slightly increased. This suggested that the primary source of dual-task interference was the

response selection stage, which affected RT but not P300 latency.

Despite the large body of evidence confirming the sensitivity of P300 to perceptual and cognitive workload, the issue of whether P300 can be used to track dynamic variation in workload, in real-time or near real-time, has not been fully resolved. On the one hand, P300 is a relatively large ERP component, so that its measurement on single (or a few) trials is easier than for other ERP components. However, the question remains whether P300 amplitude computed on the basis of just a few trials can reliably discriminate between different levels of cognitive workload. Humphrey and Kramer (1994) provided important information relevant to this issue. They had participants perform two complex, continuous tasks, a gauge-monitoring and mental arithmetic, and recorded ERPs to discrete events from each task. The difficulty of each was manipulated to create low and high workload conditions. The amplitude of the ERP, which was averaged over many samples, was sensitive to increased processing demands in each task. Humphrey and Kramer then used a stepwise discriminant analysis to ascertain how the number of ERP samples underlying P300 affected accuracy of classification of the low and high workload conditions. They found that classification accuracy increased monotonically with the number of ERP samples, but that high accuracy (~90%) could be achieved with relatively few samples (5–10). Such a small number of samples can be collected relatively quickly, say in about 25–50 seconds, assuming a 20% oddball target frequency and a one-second interstimulus interval. These results are encouraging with respect to the use of single-trial P300 for dynamic assessment of workload.

The early N1 component of the ERP, which has a peak latency of about 100 ms in audition and about 160 ms in vision (Naataanen, 1992), has also been shown to be resource sensitive. Parasuraman (1985) had participants perform a visual and an auditory discrimination concurrently, and systematically varied the priority to be placed on one task relative to the other, from 0% to 100%. The amplitudes of the visual N160 and the auditory N100 components varied directly and in a graded manner with task priority. The auditory N100 component is known to consist of both an exogenous N100 component and an endogenous Nd component that is modulated by attention (Naataanen, 1992). It is of interest to note that the Nd component is also resource sensitive. Singhal, Doerfling, and Fowler (2002) had participants perform a dichotic listening task while engaged in a simulated flight task of varying levels of difficulty. The amplitudes of both Nd and P300 were reduced at the highest level of difficulty.

In conclusion, the sensitivity of ERPs to temporal aspects of neural activation has been put to good use in dissecting sources of dual-task interference. Furthermore, as illustrated by the research of Humphrey and Kramer (1994), there has also been some success in using ERP components as near real-time measures of mental workload. Furthermore, flight and driving simulation studies have shown the added value that ERPs can provide in assessment of workload in complex tasks. However, additional work is needed with single-trial ERPs to further validate the use of ERPs for real-time workload assessments.

B. Brain-computer interfaces

If EEG and ERP signals can be obtained reliably in real-time in order to assess and, perhaps, modulate operator mental workload, then it is a logical to ask about other applications of these signals. Another neuroergonomic application involves using such brain signals to directly control devices, an area of research and development that has come to be known as brain-computer interfaces (BCI). The basic idea behind BCIs is to use brain signals to control external devices without the need for motor output, which would be advantageous for individuals who either have only limited motor control or, as in the case of "locked-in" patients with amyotrophic lateral sclerosis (ALS), virtually no motor control.

The idea of BCIs follows naturally from the work on "biocybernetics" in the 1980s pioneered by Donchin and others (Donchin, 1980; Gomer, 1981). The goal of biocybernetics was to use EEG and ERPs as an additional communication channel for use in human-machine interaction. Similarly, BCI researchers hope to provide those with limited communication abilities additional means of communicating with and interacting with the world. Farwell and Donchin (1988) characterized the BCI as a "mental prosthesis" which could assist individuals with little or no motor function. The BCI allows a user to interact with the environment without engaging in any muscular activity, for example, without the need for hand, eye, foot, or mouth movement. Instead, the user is trained to engage in a specific type of mental activity that is associated with a unique brain electrical "signature." The resulting brain potentials are recorded, processed and classified in such a way as to provide a control signal in real-time for an external device. A reliable BCI requires considerable technical development and "tailoring" a system to a specific individual. Effective use of BCIs may also require extensive training on the part of the user. BCI applications have used a variety of different measures of brain electrical activity. Invasive methods include recording of field potentials and multi-unit neuronal activity from implanted electrodes. Success has been reported in controlling robotic arms with both intracortical electrode grids (Nicolelis, 2003) and subdural electrode strips (Levine et al., 2000). Such invasive recording techniques have superior signal to noise ratio but are obviously limited to use in animals or patients with no motor functions in whom electrode implantation is clinically justified.

Noninvasive BCIs have used a variety of brain signals derived from scalp EEG recordings. These include quantified EEG from different frequency bands, such as beta and mu waves (Pfurtscheller & Neuper, 2001). BCIs based on ERPs have included P300 (Donchin, Spencer, & Wijesinghe, 2000), steady state evoked potentials (McFarland, Sarnacki, & Wolpaw, 2003), and contingent negative variation and other slow potentials (Birbaumer et al., 1999). The BCIs based on these signals have been used to operate voice synthesizers, control cursor movements on a computer display, and move robotic arms. Pfurtscheller and Neuper (2001), for example, have created a "virtual keyboard" based on EEG mu rhythms that can be operated by the user, following extensive training, by imagining movements.

Currently many of the noninvasive BCIs suffer from poor signal-to-noise ratio (compared to the invasive BCIs) and slow throughput. Extensive training is also required, and the need for periodic recalibration can be a hindrance to routine usage. However, researchers in the area think that further technical refinements will allow for faster interaction times and reduced training. They also envisage promising new applications in areas such as control of virtual reality and multimedia systems (Pfurtscheller, Scherer, & Neuper, in press).

C. Individual differences: genetics, selection, and training

The importance of methods for assessing and quantifying individual differences in human performance has long been recognized in human factors (Matthews, Davies, & Stammers, 2000). Traditionally, individual differences have been assessed using the psychometric approach in which questionnaire measures of intelligence, personality, specific cognitive abilities, and other individual attributes have been linked to measures of task or job performance. More recently, alternative approaches to characterizing individual differences have begun to emerge. Some involve the neuroimaging techniques such as fMRI, ERPs, and EEG that we have discussed previously in this chapter. The most recent of these new approaches to the study of individual differences involves the application of molecular genetic methods, a trend that is a direct result of the stunning success of the Human Genome Project.

It is widely understood that both genetic and environmental factors contribute to individual differences in cognitive ability. In the past, identifying the genetic component required comparing identical and fraternal twins for a particular ability or trait, a paradigm that has been widely used in behavioral genetics research for over a century. For example, such studies have shown convincingly that general intelligence, or g, is highly heritable, and that the degree of heritability for g and for other psychological traits can be quantified (Plomin & Crabbe, 2000). However, this approach cannot identify the particular genes involved in intelligence or the cognitive components of g. Recent advances in molecular genetics now allow a different, complementary approach to behavioral genetics: *allelic association*. This method has been recently applied to the study of individual differences in cognition in healthy individuals and reveals evidence of modulation of cognitive task performance by specific genes (Diamond et al., 2004; Fan et al., 2003; Greenwood et al., 2000; Parasuraman et al., 2005).

Molecular genetics of human performance: A framework. Parasuraman and Greenwood (2004) have outlined a framework for examining the molecular genetics of cognition that combines cognitive neuroscience with the cognitive, or information-processing, approach. The framework involves several steps, beginning with the identification of *candidate* genes – genes deemed likely to influence a given cognitive ability or trait because of the functional role of protein product of the gene in the brain. The vast majority (>99%) of individual DNA sequences in the human genome do not differ between individuals. The remainder, which still amount to several million sequences, is of primary interest to those investigating individual differences in normal cognition.

DNA sequences involve combinations of four nucleotides (bases): adenine (A), cytosine (C), guanine (G), and thymine (T). Some of the DNA base pairs (bp) occur in different forms or *alleles*. Many types of allelic variation result from the substitution of one nucleotide for another, which is known as a single nucleotide polymorphism (SNP). For example, a particular gene may have variants involving a T to C substitution at a particular location within the gene sequence. Accordingly, the bp at that location may be TT (no substitution), TC (one of the T bases replaced), or CC (both T bases replaced). TT, TC, and CC define the three different alleles of the SNP. Variation can also occur because some small parts of the DNA sequence are repeated more or less often in different individuals. SNPs and other allelic variations are estimated to occur at a rate of about 1 every 1000 bp in unrelated individuals. There are several web sites that list currently known human SNPs, and the databases being updated regularly. Because they are so numerous, some constraint on a search through the SNP databases is necessary. In the Parasuraman and Greenwood (2004) framework, SNPs are selected if they are likely to influence neurotransmitter activity and are expressed in brain regions that are known (e.g., from neuroimaging studies) to be involved in networks that control a particular cognitive function. For example, visual attention, lesion, and electrophysiological studies in animals (Everitt & Robbins, 1997) and neuroimaging and pharmacological studies in humans (Posner & Petersen, 1990) indicate the key role of acetylcholine in posterior parietal cortex in the control of spatial attention. Hence, SNPs that can be linked to cholinergic pathways that include parietal cortex would represent candidate genes for examining individual differences in spatial attention. Similarly, dopaminergic (Sawaguchi & Goldman-Rakic, 1991) and noradrenergic (Arnsten, 1998) pathways converging in prefrontal cortex have been implicated in the control of working memory (Jiang et al., 2000), which suggest that SNPs linked to

dopamine or norepinephrine would be good candidates for assaying individual differences in this cognitive function.

The limitations of the combined allelic association/cognitive neuroscience approach to the genetics of cognition should also be considered. No component of human performance, no matter how microscopic, is likely to be modified by only one gene, and the interpretation of individual differences in a particular cognitive function will ultimately involve specification of the role of many genes as well as environmental factors (Plomin & Crabbe, 2000). It is also important that SNPs or other candidate genes are chosen in a theory-based manner for their functional significance for cognition, so as to minimize the probability of type I error. Nevertheless, several investigators have been able to demonstrate single gene-cognition links using this basic approach.

Genetics of spatial attention and working memory. A recent study of spatial attention and working memory by Parasuraman et al. (2005) illustrates this approach. These authors examined a SNP in the dopamine hydroxylase (DBH) gene, which involves a G to A substitution at a specific location (444, exon 2; G444A) within chromosome 9. DBH is a functional polymorphism – the A allele is associated with lower levels of the enzyme dopamine beta hydroxylase in blood and in spinal fluid, and the G allele with higher levels (Cubells et al., 1998). A group of healthy adults were genotyped for the G444A polymorphism of the DBH gene and tested on tasks of working memory and visuospatial attention. The genotyping resulted in three sub-groups, the GG, GA, and AA genotypes. The working memory task involved maintaining a representation of up to three target locations over a period of time, and at the end of the taskof memory for the location(s) was tested with a probe. Working memory accuracy declined as the number of locations to be remembered increased from one to two to three. Accuracy was equivalent for all three genotypes at the lowest memory load, but increased with higher gene dose of the G allele, particularly for the highest (3 target) load. Memory accuracy for the group with the GG allele (G gene dose = 2) was significantly greater than that for both the AG (G gene dose = 1) and AA alleles (G gene dose = 0).

A simple visuospatial attention task involving cued letter discrimination with little or no working memory component was also administered to the same group of participants. Individual differences in performance of this task were not significantly related to allelic variation in the DBH gene. Furthermore, working memory accuracy at the highest memory load was not correlated with performance on the attention task. In sum, these findings point to a reliable association between the DBH gene and working memory performance. Increasing gene dose of the G allele of the DBH was associated with better working memory performance. This effect was most apparent when the number of target locations to be retained was high. Thus, the association between the DBH gene and working memory was particularly marked under conditions that most taxed the working memory system.

Parasuraman et al. (2005) also examined a cholinergic receptor gene, CHRNA4, and found that it was significantly associated with performance on the spatial attention task, but not with the same working memory task that was associated with the DBH gene. These findings are consistent with a double dissociation between the effects of CHRNA4 and DBH on spatial attention and working memory. In addition, another study that used a cued visual search task confirmed the association between CHRNA4 and spatial attention (Greenwood, Fossella, & Parasuraman, in press).

These results, and those of other groups (Diamond et al., 2004; Egan et al., 2001) using similar approaches, are indicative of the progress that is being made on establishing a molecular basis for normal individual variation in cognitive functions. It is also encouraging that the effect sizes in cognitive studies have been moderate to large (Parasuraman et al., 2005), in contrast to genetic studies of disease in which, they are often very low (Ioannidis et al., 2001). In future research, cognitive phenotypes will need to be supplemented by those derived from electrophysiological and neuroimaging measures (e.g., Fan et al., 2003). PET studies using neurotransmitter ligands may also permit new genetic associations to be discovered. All these methods will lead to better understanding of sources of individual differences in cognition.

Implications for selection and training. Reliable quantification of individual differences in cognitive function will have obvious implications for selection of operators for high-workload demanding occupations. The molecular genetic approach to cognition does not have immediate applications to personnel selection, but further programmatic research on more complex cognitive tasks will undoubtedly lead to progress in such an endeavor. The postgenomic era has clearly demonstrated that inheritance of a particular genotype only sets a range for the phenotypic expression of that genotype with the exact point within that range being determined by other genetic and environmental factors. What genomic analysis allows is for a much more precise specification of that range for any phenotype, and for linking phenotypic variation to specific genetic polymorphisms. To the extent that selection for a particular skill or job can be linked to a desired range of cognitive ability, molecular genetic analysis will have implications for selection for high-performance skills.

Molecular genetic research on cognition can be complemented by additional work on the influence of environmental factors on brain plasticity and cognitive performance. It has become increasingly clear that genetic studies, far from downplaying the importance of environmental factors for the development of adult cognitive skills, have pointed to new ways in which environmental variables can be identified and their effects on behavior quantified. Moreover, gene-environment interactions may be nonlinear, so that genetic effects need to be examined

over a wide range of environmental factors. For example, the effects of environmental factors on the development of intelligence in children may be substantial in low socioeconomic groups compared to that in middle and upper class children, even given the high heritability of intelligence (Turkheimer et al., 2003). Thus, additional gene-environment interaction studies are needed for a complete understanding of individual differences in cognition.

Recent studies on the effects of training on neural activation provide some exciting pointers for future work in this area. For example, Scalf et al., (2005) found that performance on multiple tasks activated some of the same prefrontal cortex regions involved in executive control that were reviewed earlier. More importantly, Scalf et al. (2005) examined how cognitive training improved attentional capacity and whether such training altered neural activation patterns. They found that training-related alterations in activation in brain regions that were sensitive to the effects of cognitive load. Relative to a control group, the training group showed decreased sensitivity to cognitive load (effect of a secondary task on the functional field of view in a primary task) in inferior frontal gyrus. Recall that this brain region has been shown to be differentially activated during dual-task performance (e.g., Jiang, 2004). This important finding regarding brain plasticity suggests that cognitive training improved the computational efficiency of this brain region under attentional demanding conditions. Scalf et al. also found similar task-related deactivations in a number of different task paradigms, indicating that cognitive training improved the efficiency of neural systems that were involved in the performance of each task. The improved efficiency is most probably the result of increased selectivity and specificity of the neural populations recruited to support task performance. It may be profitable in future research to combine the neuroimaging and genetic studies that have been discussed in this chapter with training/brain plasticity studies to examine the interactions of selection and training on brain function and performance. Selection and training have traditionally been considered together in human factors research and practice (e.g., Sanders & McCormick, 1983), but rarely in terms of a common biological framework. The examination of cortical activation in relation to molecular genetics and plasticity provides such a framework.

VI. CONCLUSIONS AND FUTURE DIRECTIONS

In this chapter we have provided a brief synopsis of several current issues in the field of human factors that have benefited from the theoretically based application of neuroergonomic techniques. In discussing each of these potential application areas, we have endeavored, whenever possible, to describe studies in which neuroergonomic measures have been used to address issues of concern to the human factors community in complex tasks, simulated environments, or, to a lesser extent, operational environments. Indeed, if neuroergonomics is to make a lasting contribution to the field of human factors, it is important that we "transition" our measurement techniques from the relatively sterile yet well-controlled environment of the laboratory to the much richer but less controlled, simulated (including the increasingly richer virtual reality environments), and operational settings. Clearly, as evidenced by our critical review of the literature, such transitions are beginning to take place, at least, in selective research domains such as the characterization of skill development in driving and flying and in the development of brain-computer interfaces for handicapped individuals and for other potential uses.

In each of the research and application domains that we discussed – the assessment of mental workload and multitask performance and processing, assessment of individual differences through converging operations from the fields of neuroscience and molecular genetics, and the development of brain-computer interfaces – there have been demonstrations of successful applications of neuroergonomic techniques. In these cases, neuroergonomic measurement has either (1) provided converging support, along with performance and subjective measures, of important changes in information processing strategies, attention, or memory; or (2) provided insights that were not available with other measures, for example, by indicating changes in resource allocation and attentional strategies with implications for multitask performance, revealing the role and nature of memory representations that support visual search, and providing an index of attention or motor processes in individuals who are unable to communicate through traditional channels. Clearly, given the continued development of semi-automated and automated systems in which human operators monitor rather than actively control system functions, there will be numerous additional opportunities for the use of neuroergonomic measures and theories to provide insights into the covert processes of the mind.

However, in each of the research domains that we have discussed, there remain a number of important challenges for neuroergonomic measurement. These challenges include:

1. the development and further refinement of signal extraction, pattern recognition, and artifact rejection and compensation algorithms that can be employed in relatively noisy environments and in situations in which the available data is relatively sparse;

2. the continued development of neurophysiological and psychological models of processes of relevance to human performance and information processing of interest to the human factors community;

3. the mapping of important psychological and neurophysiological constructs to neuroergonomic measures and models; and

4. the continued development of converging measures from cognitive psychology, ergonomics, industrial engineering, and other fields that can, when used together, provide a rich and relatively comprehensive view of human performance and cognition in a variety of different environments and tasks.

Indeed, there appears to be activity on each of these fronts and in particular on the integration of neuroergonomics, neuroscience, cognition, and emotion in the development of both micro- and macromodels of human psychological function, both inside and outside the laboratory.

REFERENCES

Aaslid, R. (Ed.). (1986). Transcranial Doppler sonography. New York: Springer-Verlag.

Adcock, R. A., Constable, R. T., Gore, J. C., & Goldman-Rakic, P. S. (2000). Functional neuroanatomy of executive processes involved in dual-task performance. Proceedings of the National Academy of Sciences USA, 97, 3567–3572.

Arnsten, A. F. T. (1998). Catecholamine modulation of prefrontal cortical cognitive function. *Trends in Cognitive Sciences, 11*, 436–447.

Baldwin, C. L., Freeman, F. G., & Coyne, J. T. (2004). Mental workload as a function of road type and visibility: Comparison of neurophysiological, behavioral, and subjective measures. In Proceedings of the Human Factors and Ergonomics Society 48th Annual Meeting, pp. 2309–2313.

Bartels, A., & Zeki, S. (2003). Functional brain mapping during free viewing of natural scenes. *Human Brain Mapping, 21*, 75–85.

Bartels, A. & Zeki, S. (2004). Functional brain mapping during free viewing of natural scenes. (2003). *Human Brain Mapping, 21*, 75–85.

Baumgartner, R. W., Mathis, J., Sturzenegger, M., & Mattle, H. P. (1994). A validation study on the intraobserver reproducibility of transcranial color-coded duplex sonography velocity measurements. *Ultrasound in Medicine and Biology, 20*, 233–237.

Becic, E., Kramer, A. F. & Boot, W. R. (in press). Age-related differences in the use of background layout in visual search. *Aging, Neuropsychology, and Cognition*.

Bellenkes, A. H., Wickens, C. D., & Kramer, A. F. (1997). Visual scanning and pilot expertise: The role of attentional flexibility and mental model development. *Aviation, Space and Environmental Medicine, 68*, 869–879.

Berka, C., Levendowski, D., Cventinovic, M., Petrovic, M., Davism G., Lumicao, M., Zivkovic, V., Popovic, M. & Olmstead, R. (2004). Real-time analysis of EEG indices of alertness, cognition, and memory acquired with a wireless EEG headset. *International Journal of Human-Computer Interaction, 17*, 151–170.

Bertera, J. H. and Rayner, K. (2000). Eye movements and the span of the effective stimulus in visual search. *Perception and Psychophysics, 62*, 576–585.

Birbaumer, N., Ghanayim, N., Hinterberger, T., Iversen, I., Kotchoubey, B., Kubler. A., Perelmouter, J., Taub, E., & Flor, H. (1999). A spelling device for the paralysed. *Nature, 398*, 297–298.

Boot, W. R., McCarley, J. S., Kramer, A. F. & Peterson, M. S. (2004). Automatic and intentional memory processes in visual search. *Psychonomic Bulletin and Review*, 11(5), 854–861.

Bostanov, V. (2004). BCI competition 2003 – Data sets IB and IC: Feature extraction from event-related brain potentials with the continuous wavlet transform and t-value scalogram. *IEEE Transactions on Biomedical Engineering, 51,* 1057–1061.

Brickman AM. Buchsbaum MS. Shihabuddin L. Hazlett EA. Borod JC. & Mohs RC. (2003). Striatal size, glucose metabolic rate, and verbal learning in normal aging. *Cognitive Brain Research,* 17(1), 106–116.

Bunge, S. A., Klingberg, T., Jacobsen, R. B., & Gabrieli, J. D. (2000). A resource model of the neural basis of executive working memory. *Proceedings of the National Academy of Sciences USA, 97,* 3573–3578.

Byrne, E. A., & Parasuraman, R., (1996). Psychophysiology and adaptive automation. *Biological Psychology, 42,* 361–377.

Burock MA. Buckner RL. Woldorff MG. Rosen BR. & Dale AM. (1998). Randomized event-related experimental designs allow for extremely rapid presentation rates using functional MRI. *Neuroreport,* 9(16), 3735–3739.

Calhoun, V. D., Pekar, J. J., McGinty, V. B., Adali, T., Watson, T. D. & Pearlson, G. D. (2002). Different activation dynamics in different neural systems during simulated driving. *Human Brain Mapping, 16,* 158–167.

Chee, M. W. L. & Choo, W. C. (2004). Functional imaging of working memory after 24 HR of total sleep deprivation. *The Journal of Neuroscience, 24,* 4560–4567.

Colcombe, S. J., Kramer, A. F., Erickson, K. I., & Scalf, P. (in press). The implications of cortical recruitment and brain morphology for individual differences in cognitive performance in aging humans. *Psychology and Aging.*

Cubells, J. F., van Kammen, D. P., Kelley, M. E., Anderson, G. M., O'Connor, D. T., Price, L. H., Malison, R., Rao, P. A., Kobayashi, K., Nagatsu, T., Gelernter, J. (1998). Dopamine beta-hydroxylase: two polymorphisms in linkage disequilibrium at the structural gene DBH associate with biochemical phenotypic variation. *Human Genetics,* 102(5), 533–40.

DeSoto, M. C., Fabiani, M., Geary, D. C., & Gratton, G. (2001). When in doubt, do it both ways: Brain evidence of the simultaneous activation of conflicting responses in a spatial Stroop task. *Journal of Cognitive Neuroscience,* 13(4), 523–536.

D'Esposito, M., Detre, J. A., Alsop, D. C., Shin, R. K., Atlas, K., & Grossman, M. (1995). The neural basis of the central executive system of working memory. *Nature, 378,* 279–281.

Diamond, A., Briand, L., Fossella, J., & Gehlbach, L. (2004). Genetic and neurochemical modulation of prefrontal cognitive functions in children. *American Journal of Psychiatry,* 161(1), 125–132.

Donchin, E. (1980). Event-related potentials: inferring cognitive activity in operational settings. In F. E. Gomer (Ed.), *Biocybernetic applications for military systems.* (Technical Report MDC EB1911, pp. 35–42). Long Beach, CA: McDonnell Douglas.

Donchin, E, Spencer K. M, & Wijesinghe, R. (2000). The mental prosthesis: assessing the speed of a P300-based brain-computer interface. *IEEE Transactions on Rehabilitation Engineering* 8(2), 174–179.

Draganski, B, Gaser, C, Busch, V, Schuirer, G, Bogdahn, U & May, A. (2004). Changes in grey matter induced by training. *Nature,* 427(22), 411–412.

Dreher, J. C., Grafman, J. (2003). Dissociating the roles of the rostral anterior cingulate and the lateral prefrontal cortices in performing two tasks simultaneously or successively. *Cerebral Cortex, 13,* 329–339.

Du, W., Leong, H., & Gevins, A. (1994). *Ocular artifact rejections by adaptive filtering.* Paper presented at the 7th IEEE SP Workshop on Statistical Signal and Array Processing (Quebec City, CA).

Duschek, S. & Schandry, R. (2003). Functional transcranial Doppler sonography as a tool in psychophysiological research. *Psychophysiology, 40,* 436–454.

Egan, M. F., Goldberg, T. E., Kolachana, B. S., Callicott, J. H., Mazzanti, C. M., Straub, R. E., Goldman, D., & Weinberger, D. R. (2001). Effect of COMT Val108/158 Met genotype on frontal lobe function and risk for schizophrenia. *Proceedings of the National Academy of Sciences U S A,* 98(12), 6917–6922.

Everitt, B. J., & Robbins, T. W. (1997). Central cholinergic systems and cognition. *Annual Review of Psychology, 48,* 649–684.

Fabiani, M., Gratton, G. & Coles, M. G. H. (2000). Event-related brain potentials. In J. Cacioppo, L. G. Tassinary (Eds.), *Handbook of Psychophysiology* (pp. 53–84). New York: Cambridge University Press.

Fan, J., Fossella, J. A., Sommer, T., Wu, Y., & Posner, M. I. (2003). Mapping the genetic variation of attention onto brain activity. *Proceedings of the National Academy of Sciences USA,* 100(12), 7406–7411.

Farwell, L. A., & Donchin, E. (1988). Talking off the top of your head: Toward a mental prosthesis utilizing event-related potentials. *Electroencephalography and Clinical Neurophysiology, 70,* 510–523.

Fitts, P., Jones, R., & Milton, J. (1950). Eye fixations of aircraft pilots III: Frequency, duration and sequence of fixations while flying Air Force Ground Controlled Approach System (GCA). Air Material Command Technical report no. USAF TR-5967.

Frackowiak, R. S. J., Friston, K. J., Frith, C., Dolan, R., Price, P., Zeki, S., Ashburner, J. & Penny, W. D. (2003). *Human Brain Function.* New York: Academic Press.

Gevins, A., Leong, H., Du, R., Smith, M., Le, J., DuRousseau, D., Zhang, J., & Libove, J. (1995). Towards measurement of brain function in operational environments. *Biological Psychology, 40,* 169–186.

Gillberg, M., Kecklund, G., Goransson, B. & Ackerstedt, T. (2003). Operator performance and signs of sleepiness during day and night work in a simulated thermal power plant. *International Journal of Industrial Ergonomics, 31,* 101–109.

Gomer, F. (1981). Physiological systems and the concept of adaptive systems. In J. Moraal & K. F. Kraiss (Eds.), *Manned systems design.* (pp. 257–263). New York: Plenum Press.

Gundel, A. Drescher, J. & Turowski, J. (2000). Alertness in airline pilots during night flights: Assessment of alertness using EEG measures. In R. W. Backs & W. Boucsein (Eds.), *Engineering psychophysiology: Issues and applications* (pp. 177–187). Mahwah, NJ: Lawrence Erlbaum.

Gratton, G., Corballis, P. M., Cho, E., Fabiani, M., & Hood, D. (1995). Shades of gray matter: Noninvasive optical images of human brain responses during visual stimulation. *Psychophysiology, 32,* 505–509.

Gratton, G. & Fabiani, M. (2001). Shedding light on brain function: The event-related optical signal. *Trends in Cognitive Science,* 5(8), 357–363.

Gratton, G., Fabiani, M., Elbert, T. & Rockstroh, B. (2003). Seeing right through you: Applications of optical imaging to the study of the human brain. *Psychophysiology, 40,* 487–491.

Gratton, G., Goddman-Wood, M. R. & Fabiani, M. (2001). Comparison of neuronal and henodynamic measures of the brain response to visual stimulation: an optical imaging study. *Human Brain Mapping, 13,* 13–25.

Greenwood, P. M., Fossella, J., & Parasuraman, R. (in press). Specificity of the effect of a nicotinic receptor polymorphism on individual differences in visuospatial attention. *Journal of Cognitive Neuroscience.*

Greenwood, P. M., Sunderland, T., Friz, J. L., & Parasuraman, R. (2000). Genetics and visual attention: Selective deficits in healthy adult carriers of the varepsilon 4 allele of the apolipoprotein E gene. *Proceedings of the National Academy of Sciences U S A, 97*(21), 11661–11666.

Gunning-Dixon FM., & Raz N. (2003). Neuroanatomical correlates of selected executive functions in middle-aged and older adults: a prospective MRI study. *Neuropsychologia.* 41(14), 1929–1941.

Head, D., Raz, N., Gunning-Dixon, F., Williamson, A. & Acker, J. D. (2002). Age-related differences in the course of cognitive skill acquisition: The role of regional cortical shrinkage and cognitive resources. *Psychology and Aging, 17,* 72–84.

Herath, P., Klingberg, T., Young, J., Amunts, K., & Roland, P. (2001). Neural correlates of dual-task interference can be dissociated from those of divided attention: an fMRI study. *Cerebral Cortex, 11,* 796–805.

Hester R. Fassbender C. & Garavan H. (2004). Individual differences in error processing: A review and reanalysis of three event-related fMRI studies using the Go/NoGo task. *Cerebral Cortex.* 14(9), 986–994.

Hill, D. K. & Keynes, R. D. (1949). Opacity changes in a stimulated nerve. *Journal of Physiology, 108,* 278–281.

Hoover, A. & Muth, E. (2004). A real-time index of vagal activity. *International Journal of Human-Computer Interaction, 17,* 197–210.

Huettel, S., Guzeldere, G. & McCarthy, G. (2001). Dissociating the neural mechanisms of visual attention in change detection using functional MRI. *Journal of Cognitive Neuroscience, 13,* 1006–1018.

Humphrey, D., & Kramer, A. F. (1994). Towards a psychophysiological assessment of dynamic changes in mental workload. *Human Factors, 36,* 3–26.

Ioannidis, J. P., Ntzani, E. E., Trikalinos, T. A., & Contopoulos-Ioannidis, D. G. (2001). Replication validity of genetic association studies. *Nature Genetics, 29,* 306–309.

Isreal, J., Chesney, G., Wickens, C. D., & Donchin, E. (1980). P300 and tracking difficulty: Evidence for multiple resources in dual-task performance. *Psychophysiology, 17,* 259–273.

Isreal, J., Wickens, C. D., Chesney, G., & Donchin, E. (1980). The event-related brain potential as an index of display monitoring workload. *Human Factors, 22,* 211–224.

Jiang, Y. (2004). Resolving dual-task interference: an fMRI study. *Neuroimage, 22,* 748–754.

Jiang, Y., Haxby, J. V., Martin, A., Ungerleider, L. G., & Parasuraman, R. (2000). Complementary neural mechanisms for tracking items in human working memory. *Science, 287,* 643–646.

Jiang, Y., Saxe, R. & Kanwisher, N. (2004). Functional magnetic resonance imaging provides new constraints on theories of the psychological refractory period. *Psychological Science, 15,* 390–396.

Johnson (1986). A triarchic model of P300 amplitude. *Psychophysiology, 23,* 367–384.

Jones, R., Milton, J., & Fitts, P. (1950). Eye fixations of aircraft pilots IV: Frequency, durations and sequence of fixations during routing instrument flight. Technical report no. 5795, Wright-Patterson AFB, Ohio.

Knake, S., Haag, A., Hamer, H. M, Dittmer, C., Bien, S., Oertel, W. H., Rosenow, F. (2003). Language lateralization in patients with temporal lobe epilepsy: a comparison of functional transcranial Doppler sonography and the Wada test. *Neuroimaging, 19,* 1228–1232.

Knecht, S., Deppe, M., Ebner, A., Henningsen, H., Huber, T., Jokeit, H., & Ringelstein, E. B. (1998). Noninvasive determination of language lateralization by functional transcranial Doppler sonography: A comparison with the Wada Test. *Stroke, 29,* 82–86.

Kramer, A. F., Sirevaag, E. J., & Braune, R. (1987). A psychophysiological assessment of operator workload during simulated flight missions. *Human Factors, 29,* 145–160.

Kramer. A. F., & Weber, T. (2000). Applications of psychophysiology to human factors. In J. T. Cacioppo, L. G. Tassinary, and G. G. Berntson (Eds.), *Handbook of psychophysiology* 2nd ed. (pp. 794–814). New York: Cambridge University Press.

Kramer, A. F., Wickens, C. D., & Donchin, E. (1983). An analysis of the processing demands of a complex perceptual-motor task. *Human Factors, 25,* 597–622.

Kramer, A. F., Wickens, C. D., & Donchin, E. (1985). The processing of stimulus attributes: Evidence for dual-task integrality. *Journal of Experimental Psychology: Human Perception and Performance, 11,* 393–408.

Kutas, M., McCarthy, G. & Donchin, E. (1977). Augmenting mental chronometry: The P300 as a measure of stimulus evaluation time. *Science, 197,* 792–795.

Levine, S. P., Huggins J. E., BeMent, S. L., et al. (2000). A direct brain interface based on event-related potentials. *IEEE Transactions on Rehabilitation Engineering, 8*(2), 180–185.

Loschky, L. & McConkie, G. W. (2002). Investigating spatial vision and dynamic attentional selection using a gaze contingent multiresolutional display. *Journal of Experimental Psychology: Applied, 8,* 99–117.

Luck, S. J. (1998). Sources of dual-task interference: Evidence from human electrophysiology. *Psychological Science, 9,* 223–227.

Maccotta, L., Zacks, J. M., Buckner, R. L. (2001). Rapid self-paced event-related functional MRI: Feasibility and implications of stimulus-versus response-locked timing. *Neuroimage, 14*(5), 1105–1121.

Mackin, E., Gratton, G. & Fabiani, M. (2003). Optimum filtering for EROS measurements. *Psychophysiology, 40,* 542–547.

Magliero, A., Bashore, T. R., Coles, M. G. H. & Donchin, E. (1984). On the dependence of P300 latency on stimulus evaluation processes. *Psychophysiology, 21,* 171–186.

Makeig, S., Elliot, F. S. & Postal, M. (1994). First demonstration of an alertness monitoring – management system. U.S. Naval Health Research Center Report. Rpt. Mo 93–36. US: US Naval Health Research Center.

Matthews, G., Davies, D. R., & Stammers, R. B. (2000) Human performance: Cognition, stress and individual differences. London: Routledge.

McCarley, J. S., Wang, R., Kramer, A. F., Irwin, D. E. & Peterson, M. S. (2003). How much memory does oculomotor search have? *Psychological Science, 14,* 422–426.

McCarley, J. S., Vais, M., Pringle, H., Kramer, A. F., Irwin, D. E. & Strayer, D. L. (2004). Conversation disrupts change detection in complex driving scenes. *Human Factors, 46,* 424–436.

McConkie, G. W. and Rayner, K. (1975). The span of the effective stimulus during a fixation in reading. *Perception and Psychophysics, 17,* 578–586.

McFarland, D. J., Sarnacki, W. A. & Wolpaw, J. R. (2003). Brain computer interface (BCI) operation: optimizing information transfer rates. *Biological Psychology, 63,* 237–251.

Meister, D. (1989). *Conceptual Aspects of Human Factors*. Baltimore: Johns Hopkins University Press.

Metzger, U., & Parasuraman, R. (2001). The role of the air traffic controller in future air traffic management: An empirical study of active control versus passive monitoring. *Human Factors, 43,* 519–528.

Miller, J. C. (1995). Batch processing of 10,000 hours of truck driver EEG data. *Biological Psychology, 40,* 209–222.

Morcom, A. M., Good, C. D., Frackowiak, R. S., & Rugg, M. D. (2003). Age effects on the neural correlates of successful memory encoding. *Brain, 126(Pt 1),* 213–229.

Naataanen, R. (1992). Attention and brain function. Mahwah, NJ: Erlbaum.

Nicolelis MA. (2003). Brain-machine interfaces to restore motor function and probe neural circuits. *Nature Reviews Neuroscience, 4(5),* 417–422.

Olson IR. Zhang JX. Mitchell KJ. Johnson MK. Bloise SM. & Higgins JA. (2004). Preserved spatial memory over brief intervals in older adults. *Psychology and Aging.* 19(2), 310–317.

Osman, A. & Moore, K. (1993). The locus of dual-task interference: Psychological refractory effects on movement related brain potentials. *Journal of Experimental Psychology: Human Perception and Performance, 19,* 1292–1312.

Parasuraman, R. (1985). Event related brain potentials and intermodal divided attention. Proceedings of the Human Factors Society, Baltimore, MD.

Parasuraman, R. (2003). Neuroergonomics: Research and practice. *Theoretical Issues in Ergonomics Science, 4,* 5–20.

Parasuraman, R., & Caggiano, D. (2002). Mental workload. In V. S. Ramachandran (Ed.), *Encyclopedia of the human brain*. Volume 3. (pp. 17–27). San Diego: Academic Press.

Parasuraman, R., & Greenwood, P. M. (2004). Molecular genetics of visuospatial attention and working memory. In M. I. Posner (Ed.), *Cognitive neuroscience of attention*. (pp. 245–259). New York: Guilford.

Parasuraman, R., Greenwood, P. M, Kumar, R., & Fossella, J. (2005). Beyond heritability: Neurotransmitter genes differentially modulate visuospatial attention and working memory. *Psychological Science,* 16(3), 200–207.

Pashler, H. (1994). Dual-task interference in simple tasks: data and theory. *Psychological Bulletin, 116,* 220–244.

Peterson, M. S., Boot, W. R., Kramer, A. F. & McCarley, J. S. (2004). Landmarks help guide attention during visual search. *Spatial Vision, 17,* 497–510.

Pfurtuscheller, G. & Neuper, C. (2001). Motor imagery and direct brain-computer communication. *Proceedings of the IEEE* 89(7) 1123–1134, 2001.

Pfurtscheller, G., Scherer, R. & Neuper, C. (in press). EEG-based brain computer interface. In R. Parasuraman & M. Rizzo (Eds.), *Neuroergonomics: The brain at work*. New York: Oxford University Press.

Phelps, M. E., Mazziotta, J. C. & Schelbert, H. (1986). Positron EmissionTomography and Autoradiography: Principles and Applications for the Brain and Heart. New York: Raven.

Plomin, R., & Crabbe, J. (2000). DNA. *Psychological Bulletin,* 126(6), 806–828.

Polich, J. (1987). Task difficulty, probability, and inter-stimulus interval as determinants of P300 from auditory stimuli. *Electroencephalography and Clinical Neurophysiology, 68,* 311–320.

Pomplun, M., Reingold, E. M. & Shen, J. (2001) Investigating the visual span in comparative search: the effects of task difficulty and divided attention. *Cognition, 81,* 57–67.

Posner, M. I. & Petersen, S. E. (1990). The attention system of the human brain. 13, 25–42.

Pouratian, N., Sheth, A. A., Martin, N. A. & Toga, A. W. (2003). Shedding light on brain mapping: advances in human optical imaging. *Trends in Neurosciences, 26,* 277–282.

Reingold, E. M., Loschky, L., McConkie, G. W. & Stampe, D. M. (2003). Gaze-contingent multiresolutional displays: An integrative review. *Human Factors, 45,* 307–328.

Rinne, T., Gratton, G., Fabiani, M., Cowan, N., Maclin, E., Stinard, A., Sinkkonen, J., Alho, K. & Naatanen, R. (1999). Scalp recorded optical signals make sound processing from the auditory cortex visible. *Neuroimage, 10,* 620–624.

Roman, J., Older, H., & Jones, W. L. (1967). Flight research program. VII: Medical monitoring of Navy Carrier pilots in combat. *Aerospace Medicine, 38,* 133–139.

Roscoe, A. H. (1975). Heart rate monitoring of pilots during steep gradient approaches. *Aviation, Space and Environmental Medicine, 46,* 1410–1415.

Roy, C. S., & Sherrington, C. S. (1890). On the regulation of the blood supply of the brain. *Journal of Physiology (London), 11,* 85–108.

Ruffel-Smith, H. P. (1967). Heart rate of pilots flying aircraft on scheduled airlines routes. *Aerospace Medicine, 38,* 1117–1119.

Sanders, M. S., & McCormick, E. F. (1983). Human factors in engineering and design. New York: McGraw-Hill.

Sawaguchi, T., & Goldman-Rakic, P. S. (1991). D1 dopamine receptors in prefrontal cortex: involvement in working memory. *Science,* 251(4996), 947–950.

Scalf, P., Erickson, K., Kramer, A. F., & Colcombe, S. (2005). Influence of training on attentional control and multi-task processing: An event-related fMRI study. Paper to be presented the International Conference on Augmented Cognition, Las Vegas, NV.

Scarmeas, N., Zarahn, E., Anderson, K. E., Hilton, J., Flynn, J., Van Heertum, R. L., Sackeim, H. A. & Stern, Y. (2003). Cognitive reserve modulates functional brain responses during memory tasks: a PET study in health young and elderly subjects. *Neuroimage, 19,* 1215–1227.

Schubert, T., & Szameitat, A. J. (2003). Functional neuroanatomy of interference in overlapping dual tasks: an fMRI study. *Cognitive Brain Research, 17,* 733–746.

Sem-Jacobsen, C. W. (1959). Electroencephalographic study of pilot stress. *Aerospace Medicine, 30,* 797–803.

Sem-Jacobsen, C. W. (1961). Black-out and unconsciousness revealed by airborne testing of fighter pilots. *Aerospace Medicine, 32,* 247–253.

Sem-Jacobsen, C. W., & Sem-Jacobsen, J. E. (1963). Selection and evaluation of pilots for high performance aircraft and spacecraft by in-flight EEG study of stress tolerance. *Aerospace Medicine, 34,* 605–609.

Serrati, C., Finocchi, C., Calautti, C., Bruzzone, G. L., Colucci, M., Gandolfo, C., Del Sette, M., Lantieri, P. B., & Favale, E. (2000). Absence of hemispheric dominance for mental rotation ability: A transcranial Doppler study. *Cortex, 36,* 415–425.

Singhal, A., Doerfling, P. & Fowler, B. (2002). Effects of a dual-task on N100-P200 complex and the early and late Nd attention waveforms. *Psychophysiology, 39*, 236–245.

Sirevaag, E., Kramer, A. F., Wickens, C. D., Reisweber, M., Strayer, D., & Grenell, J. (1993). Assessment of pilot performance and workload in rotary wing helicopters. *Ergonomics, 37*, 1121–1140.

Shin E., Fabiani M. & Gratton G. (2004). Evidence of partial response activation in a memory-search task. *Cognitive Brain Research*, 20(2), 281–93.

Smith, E. E. & Jonides, J. (1999). Storage and executive control processes in the frontal lobes. *Science, 283*, 1657–1661.

Stanny, K., Samman, S., Reeves, L., Hale, K., Buff, W., Bowers, C., Goldiez, B., Nicholson, D. & Lackey, S. (2004). A paradigm shift in interactive computing: Deriving multimodal design principles from behavioral and neurological foundations. *International Journal of Human-Computer Interaction, 17*, 259–274.

Steinbrink, J., Kohl, M., Obrig, H., Curio, G., Syre, F., Thomas, F., Wabnitz, H., Rinneberg, H. & Villringer, A. (2000). Somatosensory evoked fast optical intensity changes detected non-invasively in the adult human head. *Neuroscience Letters, 291*, 105–108.

Sterman, B., & Mann, C. (1995). Concepts and applications of EEG analysis in aviation performance evaluation. *Biological Psychology, 40*, 115–130.

Strayer, D. L., Drews, F. A. & Johnston, W. A. (2003). Cell phone induced faiulures of visual attention during simulated driving. *Journal of Experimental Psychology: Applied, 9*, 23–52.

Stroobant, N., Vingerhoets, G. (2000). Transcranial Doppler ultrasonography monitoring of cerebral hemodynamics during performance of cognitive tasks: A review. *Neuropsychology Review, 10*, 213–231.

Stroobant, N. & Vingerhoets, G. (2001). Test-retest reliability of functional transcranial Doppler ultrasonography. *Ultrasound in Medicine and Biology, 27*, 509–514.

Sutton, S., Braren, M., Zubin, J. & John, E. R. (1965). Evoked potential correlates of stimulus uncertainty. *Science, 150*, 1187–1188.

Tripp, L. D. & Warm, J. S. (in press). Transcranial Doppler Sonography. In R. Parasuraman & M. Rizzo (Eds.), *Neuroergonomics: The brain at work*. New York: Oxford University Press.

Turkheimer, E., Haley, A., Waldron, M., D'Onofrio, B., & Gottesman, I. (2003). Socioeconomic status modifies heritability of IQ in young children. *Psychological Science, 14*, 623–628.

Walhovd K. B., Fjell A. M., Reinvang I., Lundervold A., Fischl B., Quinn B. T. & Dale A. M. (2004). Size does matter in the long run – Hippocampal and cortical volume predict recall across weeks. *Neurology*, 63(7), 193–1197.

Wickens, C. D. (1984). Processing resources in attention. In R. Parasuraman & D. R. Davies (Eds.), *Varieties of attention*. (pp. 63–101). San Diego, CA: Academic.

Wickens, C. D. (2000). Multiple task performance. In A. E. Kazdin (Ed.), *Encyclopedia of Psychology* (pp. 352–354). London: Oxford University Press.

Wickens, C. D. (2002). Multiple resources and performance prediction. *Theoretical Issues in Ergonomics Science*, 3(2), 159–177.

Wickens, C. D., & Hollands, J. G. (2000). *Engineering psychology and human performance* (3rd ed.). Upper Saddle River, NJ: Prentice Hall.

Wickens, C. D., Kramer, A. F., Vanasse, L., & Donchin, E. (1983). The performance of concurrent tasks: A psychophysiological analysis of the reciprocity of information processing resources. *Science, 221*, 1080–1082.

Wilson, G., Finomore, Jr., V., & Estepp, J. (2003). Transcranial Doppler oximetrey as a potential measure of cognitive demand. Proceedings of the 12th International Symposium on Aviation Psychology Dayton, OH: pp. 1246–1249.

Wolpaw, J. R., Birbaumer, N., McFarland, D. J., Pfurtscheller, G. & Vaughan, T. M. (2002). Brain-computer interfaces for communication and control. *Clinical Neurophysiology, 113*, 767–791.

Zinni, M., & Parasuraman, R. (2004). The effects of task load on performance and cerebral blood flow velocity in a working memory and a visuomotor task. Proceedings of the 48th Annual Meeting of the Human Factors and Ergonomics Society. Santa Monica, CA, pp. 1890–1894.

31 Psychophysiological Contributions to Behavioral Medicine and Psychosomatics

ANDREW STEPTOE

INTRODUCTION

Behavioral medicine first emerged in the 1970s as interest developed in the application of behavioral treatments, such as biofeedback and relaxation training, to alleviate physical health problems, and the role of learning in physical disease etiology. Later, behavioral medicine expanded to become defined as the interdisciplinary field concerned with the development and integration of social, behavioral, and biomedical science, the knowledge and techniques relevant to health and illness, and the application of this knowledge to prevention, diagnosis, treatment, and rehabilitation (Slater, Steptoe, Weickgenant, & Dimsdale, 2003). Psychosomatics has a longer history and originated in the middle decades of the twentieth century as an application of psychodynamic psychotherapy to physical illness. Researchers and therapists in the psychosomatic tradition primarily focused on a small number of psychosomatic conditions such as hypertension (high blood pressure), peptic ulcer, rheumatoid arthritis, and bronchial asthma.

Behavioral and psychosomatic medicine were once polar opposites, the first concerned with behavior and the relevance of experimental psychological concepts such as operant conditioning to illness, and the second concentrating on intrapsychic and interpersonal influences. However, there has long been reconciliation such that the research described in behavioral medicine and psychosomatic conferences and journals is virtually interchangeable. The field has also moved beyond the small group of illnesses prioritized by psychosomatic medicine to a broader concept in which psychosocial and social factors are deemed to be relevant across the entire spectrum of physical illnesses. Modern research and practice views psychosocial factors as part of the broader biomedical and behavioral risk profile for disease, and operates to a variable extent in different cases, which depends on individual characteristics and on the disorder being investigated (Steptoe, 1998).

Other contributions to the *Handbook* have described many of the psychophysiological processes relevant to behavioral medicine and psychosomatics, including specific autonomic, neuroendocrine and immunological pathways, emotional influences on physiology, and stress and illness. The purpose of this chapter is to outline how this psychophysiological knowledge is applied in behavioral medicine and psychosomatics and focuses on two broad issues. First is the application of psychophysiology to understanding the etiology of physical illnesses such as coronary heart disease, hypertension, infectious illness, immune-related diseases, and musculoskeletal disorders. This is the field in which psychophysiological methods have deepened our understanding of physical disease development and maintenance. The second general issue is the application of psychophysiology to the management of physical illnesses, and the evaluation of treatment effects. Additionally, I will explain how psychophysiology provides a powerful set of tools for research and clinical practice in behavioral medicine and psychosomatics. Researchers in this field have developed particular approaches to psychophysiology that differ to some extent from those that are commonly used in experimental research. The chapter, therefore, begins with a summary of methodological issues relevant to the application of psychophysiology to behavioral medicine and psychosomatics.

METHODS OF STUDYING PSYCHOPHYSIOLOGICAL PROCESSES

Much of nonpsychiatric clinical medicine involves the measurement of biological functions. As psychophysiology has expanded beyond traditional measures such as heart rate and electrodermal activity to include hormonal, immunological, and even molecular variables, the dividing line between where clinical measurement ends and psychophysiology begins has become increasingly opaque. It is, however, important to recognize that in behavioral medicine and psychosomatics, the psychophysiological measures studied fall into three categories (Steptoe, 2005):

1. Biological indicators of disease states, such as blood pressure in hypertension, blood glucose in diabetes, or

airways resistance in bronchial asthma. These measures are direct measures of the physiological dysfunctions constituting the disease state, are used in research on the role of psychophysiological processes in the etiology of disease, and in evaluating the impact of psychosocial interventions.

2. Biological markers of processes involved in the etiology of disease. Examples include measures of vascular endothelial function and fibrinogen in coronary heart disease, the concentration of circulating lymphocyte subsets in HIV/AIDS, and the measurement of gut hormones in obesity. The biological parameters assessed in such studies are more distal to disease states than those assessed in category 1, but nevertheless provide objective information concerning the impact of psychophysiological factors on precursors of disease, which underlie pathological dysfunctions, and on treatment effects.

3. Nonspecific biological markers of activation or resistance to disease that are influenced by stress and other psychosocial factors. Psychophysiological measures in this category include heart rate, blood pressure, electrodermal activity, stress hormones such as cortisol and catecholamines, circulating lymphocyte numbers and activity, and concentrations of inflammatory cytokines and immunoglobulins. These variables are not assessed as markers of specific disease states, but as more general indicators of biological activation and host resistance.

These distinctions are important because the implications of responses in these categories of measure can be quite different.

Strategies of psychophysiological measurement

Psychophysiology is traditionally a laboratory-based science involving measurement of physiological function under carefully controlled conditions and the application of experimental research designs, such as the random allocation of participants to different experimental conditions or the comparison of biological responses to different patterns of behavioral stimulation. Psychophysiological applications in behavioral medicine and psychosomatics are broader, frequently moving outside the laboratory to clinical situations in which environmental conditions are less tightly controlled.

Within the laboratory, the major method of investigation is psychophysiological or mental stress testing. This involves monitoring biological responses to standardized psychological or social stimuli, often comparing groups such as people with and without a specific illness or people at low and high risk for a particular condition. A wide range of behavioral challenges is employed including cognitive and problem solving tasks, simulated public speaking, upsetting films, and interpersonal conflict tasks. Although most tasks involve cognitive processing, experimental conditions are commonly selected for their stress-

fulness and not because they mobilize particular cognitive processes.

A psychophysiological stress testing session typically involves a period of rest so that baseline levels of physiological function can be established. Many studies now include blood sampling as well as traditional psychophysiological measures, so baseline periods may be prolonged in order to allow the impact of the blood taking or cannulation to dissipate before exposure to challenges that may last anywhere from five minutes to three hours. Further biological measures are obtained during the challenge period and for some time afterwards, depending on the dynamics of the measure under investigation. For example, blood pressure and heart rate respond within minutes of onset of behavioral tasks, while cortisol in saliva and blood may not peak for 30 minutes, and inflammatory cytokines such as interleukin (IL) 6 continue to rise for at least two hours.

The value of psychophysiological stress testing is that responses to psychosocial stimuli can be monitored under environmentally controlled conditions, which reduces many of the sources of bias and individual difference that might otherwise be present. Experimental designs can be used with randomization to different conditions (such as low and high stress controllability), and sophisticated biological measures are possible. There are two major limitations to this type of study. The first is that the stimuli used are often arbitrary and divorced from everyday life. After all, few people spend much of their lives carrying out mirror tracing, though this is a popular research task. Studies using more ecologically valid challenges such as interpersonal conflict tasks remain in the minority. Second, the stimuli used are brief and only acute biological responses are recorded. Chronic challenges may elicit different response patterns because of habituation and adaptation. The generalizability of biological adjustments, therefore, remains uncertain in many cases and has led to great interest in the correlations between psychophysiological responses in the laboratory and field as well as in the predictive power of individual differences in acute response.

The second major setting for psychophysiology in behavioral medicine and psychosomatics is naturalistic or ambulatory monitoring. These studies take many forms, from recordings during challenging tasks, such as speaking in public, to repeated measures of blood pressure or salivary cortisol over an ordinary day. Some of these techniques are extensions of methods used in clinical investigation, as in the use of ambulatory blood pressure monitors for evaluating hypertension, or *Holter*, monitoring of the electrocardiogram (EKG) in patients with coronary heart disease (CHD). The purpose of these psychophysiological methods is to assess biological activity under natural conditions, and to examine the covariation between everyday activities, emotions, and biology. For example, one study of patients with bronchial asthma and a nonasthmatic comparison group involved repeated spirometric measurements and mood assessments several times a day for three weeks. Naturally occurring negative mood states were found to relate to reduced forced expiratory volume in asthmatic participants but not in controls (Ritz & Steptoe, 2000). Measurements of muscle tension from surface electrodes have been made in supermarket checkout clerks, and have shown heightened trapezius muscle tension during work that is associated with complains of neck and shoulder pain (Lundberg et al., 1999).

Naturalistic monitoring methods have the advantage of ecological validity because psychophysiological activity is measured in real life rather than the artificial conditions of laboratory or clinic. Associations between psychosocial factors and biological responses may be observed that are not detectable when measures are taken in a single situation such as a physician's office. Unfortunately, naturalistic methods have several limitations. First, the range of biological markers that can be assessed is relatively small in comparison with the more sophisticated possibilities available in the laboratory or clinic. Second, measurement techniques need to be relatively unobtrusive, so as not to interfere with ongoing activities. Some techniques, such as repeated blood sampling or esophageal pH probes, are very stressful in themselves, so associations with psychosocial factors may be obscured. Third, several extrinsic factors that influence biological function must be taken into account, which includes cigarette smoking, time of day, food and caffeine intake, sleep, and physical activity. This raises complex statistical issues and techniques such as multilevel modeling may be required in analyzing the data (Schwartz & Stone, 1998).

The third setting in which psychophysiological methods are used is in epidemiological surveys. Observational epidemiology is the core technique for establishing the contribution of psychosocial factors to the development of physical disease. A typical study involves measuring a range of potential biological and behavioral risk factors for the disease under investigation (e.g., breast cancer, diabetes, or CHD) in a large sample of healthy individuals. The cohort is tracked, often for years, until a sufficient number of clinical cases have accrued to allow multivariate analysis of associations between risk factors and health outcomes. Physiological measures can be introduced so as to identify the biological mediators of the associations observed. For instance, lower socioeconomic status (SES) is consistently associated with increased risk of CHD (Mensah, Mokdad, Ford, Greenlund, & Croft, 2005). It has been found by adding biological measures to epidemiological surveys that plasma fibrinogen and C-reactive protein are elevated in lower SES individuals, while the incidence of the metabolic syndrome (characterized by abdominal adiposity, high blood pressure, and elevated lipid levels) is also raised (Brunner et al., 1996; Wamala et al., 1999). In mediational analyses, these physiological variables account for a proportion of the variance in CHD attributable to SES, so it is probable that they are on the pathway linking SES with CHD.

Epidemiological studies have the advantage that prospective study designs can be employed and objective disease endpoints studied. Biological measures can be obtained from large samples at relatively low cost, and potential confounders can be taken into account statistically. However, the biological measures in epidemiological studies are generally recorded on a single occasion under resting conditions (in a screening clinic or medical office) that are not typical of everyday life. Such studies therefore provide limited information about the dynamics of psychophysiological responses.

All these approaches are valuable in the investigation of psychophysiological processes in behavioral medicine and psychosomatics, but an integrated strategy is required to exploit these methods to the full. The later sections of this chapter therefore present findings derived from all these different settings.

PSYCHOPHYSIOLOGY IN THE ETIOLOGY AND PROGRESSION OF PHYSICAL ILLNESS

There is an extensive literature relating psychosocial factors with physical illness. Acute and chronic life stress, social support and social networks, psychological distress, and emotions like anger and depression have been associated with a range of health outcomes. In some cases, psychosocial factors are thought to contribute to the development of disease in initially healthy individuals, while in others these factors may influence the progression of preexisting disorders. In a condition like CHD, psychosocial factors may affect both the development of the underlying pathology (atherosclerosis) and the triggering of acute clinical events in people with existing disease.

Psychophysiology is central to understanding the pathways and processes through which psychosocial factors influence disease risk and health outcomes. However, the way in which psychophysiological processes are involved differs markedly across medical conditions (Steptoe & Ayers, 2004). This is illustrated in the following sections that focus on some of the major health problems studied in behavioral medicine and psychosomatics. In each case, the disorder is briefly described and the evidence linking its development or maintenance with psychosocial factors is summarized. Particular emphasis is placed on prospective observational epidemiological studies on population samples because these provide more robust data than cross-sectional and clinical studies on selected populations. I then review the ways in which psychophysiological studies have helped us understand how these effects are mediated.

Space prevents an exhaustive review of literature related to all health conditions. I have not, therefore, included discussion of a number of outcomes including stroke, gastrointestinal illness, HIV/AIDS, cancer, and gynecological conditions. Some of these disorders are described in detail elsewhere in the *Handbook*, while others follow similar principles to the conditions that are discussed – namely

CHD, hypertension, metabolic disorders, infectious illness, autoimmune conditions, and musculoskeletal problems.

Two issues are critical to understanding the contribution of psychophysiological investigations to disease etiology. The first is that individual differences in the duration and magnitude of psychophysiological responses appear to be relevant to risk of many adverse health outcomes. In some diseases, heightened responsivity is associated with increased risk, but in other conditions reduced responsivity may be problematic. Either way, individual differences are crucial. The second pivotal concept is exposure. Disturbances of psychophysiological responsivity are only likely to contribute to disease etiology if they are elicited in the person's ordinary life and not just in a laboratory test. Repeated or continued exposure to adverse psychosocial conditions will, therefore, moderate whether or not an individual difference in responsivity is actually relevant to etiology.

Coronary heart disease

Coronary heart disease is the single largest cause of death in men and women in the USA, United Kingdom, and many other countries. In the USA, 38% of deaths in 2002 were caused by cardiovascular disease, of which 53% were CHD fatalities (American Heart Association, 2005). The estimated prevalence of CHD in 2002 was 8.4% of men and 5.6% of women, and the average number of years lost as a result of a heart attack was 11.5. Although CHD is a disease of old age, it also afflicts many younger people. In the UK, it accounted for 22% of male and 13% of female deaths in people under 75 years old (British Heart Foundation, 2004). The major risk factors are high blood cholesterol levels, high blood pressure, smoking, diabetes, and family history. These are in turn affected by behaviors such as physical inactivity, food choice, and alcohol consumption. The INTERHEART study has shown that the potentially modifiable risk factors for CHD are similar across genders, ethnic groups, and geographical regions of the world (Yusuf et al., 2004).

The process underlying CHD is coronary atherosclerosis, a condition starting early in life and developing progressively through adulthood. Coronary atherosclerosis typically comes to clinical attention with angina pectoris, sudden cardiac death, or an acute coronary syndrome. Conceptualization of coronary atherosclerosis has changed in the last two decades, and it is now considered to be a chronic inflammatory condition rather than a passive lipid storage disease (Libby & Theroux, 2005; Ross, 1999). Coronary atherosclerosis develops at a variable rate in the population, but by middle age a substantial proportion of men and women will have definite coronary artery disease.

Understanding of advanced CHD and acute coronary syndromes has also changed over recent years. Acute coronary syndrome constitutes a spectrum of clinical conditions, including ST elevation myocardial infarction (MI), non-ST elevation MI and unstable angina. The notion that acute coronary syndromes are caused simply by progressive narrowing of coronary arteries until blood flow is blocked is inconsistent with angiographic findings that culprit lesions are mostly not flow limiting. Rather, coronary events occur when atherosclerotic plaques either rupture or erode, leading to direct contact between the blood and the lipid-rich plaque core and the formation of a thrombus (Davies, 1996). The most angiographically severe lesions are not necessarily at highest risk of rupture, and rupture does not always result in acute coronary syndromes (Libby & Theroux, 2005; Monaco, Mathur, & Martin, 2005). Other factors are involved, notably "vulnerable blood," in which blood platelets are prone to activation, the coagulation system is in a prothrombotic rather than fibrinolytic state, and high levels of circulating inflammatory factors are present. During an acute coronary syndrome, there is a marked inflammatory response with increases in IL-6, IL-1 receptor antagonist (IL-1Ra), tumor necrosis factor (TNF) α, and C-reactive protein. These inflammatory markers predict poor prognosis.

The implication of this pathological sequence is that psychophysiological processes may be relevant both to the longterm development of atherosclerosis, and to the acute events that initiate an acute coronary syndrome in the vulnerable patient. The important variables include vascular endothelial function, lipids, proinflammatory cytokines, C-reactive protein and hemostatic variables. Cardiovascular responses including raised blood pressure, heart rate, and total peripheral resistance are important in that they may heighten shear stress across arterial plaques, which increases risk of rupture.

Psychosocial risk factors

There is a large literature using observational population-based prospective designs that has examined psychosocial factors predicting future CHD. Systematic reviews of this work are in agreement that chronic stressors, social factors, and certain psychological characteristics are associated with future CHD independently of standard risk factors (Everson-Rose & Lewis, 2005; Kuper, Marmot, & Hemingway, 2005). Among chronic stressors, there is particularly strong evidence for work-related factors such as job strain (high demand/low control) and effort-reward imbalance, though other sources of stress such as financial strain, informal caregiving, and marital conflict are also relevant (Iso et al., 2002; Lee, Colditz, Berkman, & Kawachi, 2003). The social factors that have been associated with increased CHD risk include social isolation, small social networks, and low levels of emotional support. Research on psychological factors has highlighted depressive mood and anger/hostility with more limited but still consistently positive results for anxiety as a risk factor (Steptoe, in press; Suls & Bunde, 2005). Additionally, there is a pronounced socioeconomic gradient in CHD with higher levels among less privileged groups as defined by educational attainment, occupational status, and income (Mensah et al., 2005). Low SES is in turn associated with greater work, financial and neighborhood stress, greater social isolation, and increased ratings of depression and hostility, so the psychosocial risk factors for CHD are more prevalent in low SES groups.

The impact of psychosocial factors on underlying disease can be investigated using noninvasive measures of subclinical atherosclerosis. Carotid ultrasound scans detect carotid plaque and the intima-medial thickness (IMT) of the carotid artery wall, while a more direct scanning technique, electron beam computed tomography (EBCT), can image advanced plaque in the coronary arteries themselves. Associations have been described between carotid artery atherosclerosis and low SES, job strain, poor marital quality, and hostility (Diez-Roux, Nieto, Tyroler, Crum, & Szklo, 1995; Everson et al., 1997a; Gallo et al., 2003). At least 10 population studies have been published relating carotid IMT or coronary artery calcification with depression, hopelessness, and psychological distress (Steptoe, in press). For instance, in the Work Site Blood Pressure Study, depressed mood at baseline predicted carotid plaque 10 years later, after adjustment for cardiovascular risk factors including age, gender, ethnicity, education, cholesterol, body mass index (BMI), diabetes, smoking, blood pressure, and family history (Haas et al., 2005). Another study tracked a cohort of 726 French men and women aged 59–71 years with no history of CHD (Paterniti et al., 2001). Men with higher anxiety scores showed greater progression in carotid IMT over a four-year period than did less anxious individuals with a similar but weaker effect among women.

Psychosocial factors can also act more acutely, triggering cardiac events in people with advanced underlying coronary artery disease, as has been found in studies of natural disasters and acts of war and terrorism and in clinical investigations of patients admitted to hospital with acute MI (Strike & Steptoe, 2005). For example, on the day of the Northridge earthquake in the Los Angeles area in January 1994, there was an abrupt rise in the number of sudden cardiac deaths, total CHD mortality and hospital admission for acute MI (Leor, Poole, & Kloner, 1996). Interviews with patients in hospital who have survived acute cardiac events have shown an increased risk following acute episodes of anger and stress (Mittleman et al., 1995; Moller, Theorell, de Faire, Ahlbom, & Hallqvist, 2005). A study in which the relatives of 100 men who suffered a sudden cardiac death were interviewed showed that victims were more likely to have experienced moderate or severe stress in the 30 minutes prior to onset than had patients admitted to hospital with an acute MI (Myers & Dewar, 1975). Factors like depression, work stress, social isolation, and low social support also predict future cardiac morbidity in patients following hospital admission for acute coronary syndrome (Kuper et al., 2005; van Melle et al., 2004). Thus, there is evidence for a contribution of psychosocial adversity to many stages of the CHD disease process.

Psychophysiological processes

Psychophysiological methods are used extensively to investigate the ways in which social, emotional, and behavioral factors impact on the development of CHD. The literature is extensive and fast moving, so this chapter will highlight some important themes rather than providing a comprehensive review.

Pathological responses and psychosocial factors. Psychophysiological studies of CHD began in the 1950s when the principle physiological measures were blood pressure, heart rate, and corticosteroid metabolites. In the past decade, interest has focused on whether psychological stimulation affects physiological parameters that are more directly involved in the pathogenesis of CHD, and whether the magnitude and duration of these responses are related to psychosocial risk factors.

One of the earliest stages of atherogenesis is vascular endothelial dysfunction. The healthy endothelium maintains vascular tone and inhibits cell adhesion and migration into the subendothelial layer. Ghiadoni and coworkers (2000) demonstrated that endothelial function was impaired following acute stress induced by simulated public speaking. Interestingly, responses were maintained up to 90 minutes poststress, long after the 3-minute speech task had terminated, which indicates that brief psychological stimulation can have extended effects. The effect can be blocked by metyrapone, a drug that inhibits cortisol production, and suggests that the hypothalamic-pituitary-adrenocortical (HPA) axis is involved (Broadley et al., 2005). Impaired endothelial function has also been described in depressed patients without other cardiovascular risk factors (Broadley, Korszun, Jones, & Frenneaux, 2002).

As noted earlier, inflammatory cytokines such as IL-6 and TNFα, and acute phase reactants like C-reactive proteins are also implicated in atherogenesis. Blood levels of C-reactive protein are elevated in population studies of depression and depressed mood (Ford & Erlinger, 2004), and associations between proinflammatory cytokines and hostility have been described (Suarez, Lewis, Krishnan, & Young, 2004). Chronic stressors such as caring for a dementing relative stimulate heightened plasma IL-6 with accelerated increases over time in caregivers (Kiecolt-Glaser et al., 2003). Low SES is associated with heightened levels of several markers of inflammation, including von Willebrand factor, C-reactive protein, and fibrinogen (Brunner et al., 1996; Kumari, Marmot, & Brunner, 2000). Psychophysiological studies have demonstrated that these inflammatory markers respond acutely to psychological stimulation, and responses are greater in individuals with psychosocial CHD risk factors. Thus, the acute stress-induced increase in IL-6 is larger in people of lower SES (Brydon, Edwards, Mohamed-Ali, & Steptoe, 2004), while acute fibrinogen responses are elevated in people experiencing low control at work (Steptoe, Kunz-Ebrecht, Owen, et al., 2003), and in lonely individuals (Steptoe, Owen, Kunz-Ebrecht, & Brydon, 2004).

Closely linked with inflammatory processes are hemostatic factors involved in the development of thrombotic states. Hemostatic factors are highly sensitive to psychological stimulation with a combination of procoagulant (or prothrombotic) and anticoagulant responses (von Kanel, Mills, Fainman, & Dimsdale, 2001). The magnitude and duration of stress-induced responses appears to be greater in more depressed people (von Kanel et al., 2004) and in lower SES groups (Steptoe, Kunz-Ebrecht, Rumley, & Lowe, 2003).

Another mechanism linked both with the longterm development of atherosclerosis and with acute cardiac events is autonomic balance in cardiac control with greater parasympathetic activation being protective. Heart rate variability is often used as an index of parasympathetic activity, and it is notable that lower SES, greater job stress, and depressed mood are characterized by reduced heart rate variability (Hemingway et al., 2005; Kim et al., 2005).

Longitudinal significance of psychophysiological responses.

Biological responses relevant to CHD can be elicited by behavioral stimulation, and responsivity is related to psychosocial risk factors. However, these cross-sectional effects do not demonstrate that response profiles are causally significant. Fortunately, over recent years, longitudinal results have begun to emerge, which indicate that individual differences in responsivity do predict acceleration of risk profiles or subclinical disease progression. A good example is the discovery by Jennings et al. (2004) that blood pressure stress responses predict increases in carotid IMT. The study involved 756 Finnish men who were administered a battery of psychophysiological stress tests. Individual differences in systolic pressure reactivity were positively related to changes in carotid IMT over a seven-year period independently of baseline IMT and other risk factors. Prospective effects relating individual differences in stress responsivity in other CHD risk factors such as blood cholesterol concentration with subsequent levels have also been described (Steptoe & Brydon, in press). These individual differences in psychophysiological stress responsivity will be relevant if they are representative of the individual's experience during daily life. As noted earlier, heightened responsivity per se is not likely to increase risk of CHD. Psychophysiological factors will contribute to CHD risk if reactive individuals are exposed over months or years to environments that elicit damaging patterns of intense response. Thus, in addition to evaluating the impact of cardiovascular stress responsivity, it is necessary to monitor exposure to life stress. Thus far, there has been comparatively little work of this kind. However, one example is from the Kuopio study in Finland, in which an interaction between blood pressure

stress reactivity and exposure to chronic life stress (in this case, work place demands) was observed (Everson et al., 1997b). These two factors interacted in predicting progression of carotid IMT; over a four-year period, the increase in subclinical atherosclerosis was greatest in men who were stress reactive and had been exposed to high work demands.

The model underlying these psychophysiological processes in CHD and some other health problems is outlined in Figure 31.1. Heightened or prolonged psychophysiological stress responsivity is sustained by individual differences or propensities, arising from genetic, early life, and adult psychological factors. Various types of psychosocial adversity, including low SES, chronic life stress, and social isolation, not only elicit this heightened or prolonged responsivity, but also increase responsivity over the long term. The impact of this process on disease risk depends on continuing exposure to adverse psychosocial conditions that not only stimulates repeated activation, but also serves further to increase the responsivity of the vulnerable individual. The impact of this pathway is set against a background of constitutional and biological risk and lifestyle factors that independently contribute to CHD risk.

Psychophysiological responses in people with CHD.

The summary of psychophysiological processes given above applies primarily to the etiology of CHD and the development of subclinical disease. Psychophysiological methods also throw light on the mechanisms triggering clinical events such as MI in people with established disease. Research with clinical groups is difficult to conduct, partly because of ethical concerns about patient safety, and partly because the medication status of patients can obscure psychophysiological responsivity. For instance, there is good evidence that sympathovagal imbalance, indexed by low heart rate variability and suppressed cardiac baroreceptor reflex sensitivity, predicts negative clinical outcomes in CHD (La Rovere, Bigger, Marcus, Mortara, & Schwartz, 1998). This has lead to the clinical recommendation in most countries that CHD patients are medicated with β-blockers. In turn, this reduces the opportunities for assessing heart rate variability in relation to psychosocial factors. Although depression in CHD patients has been associated with low heart rate variability in some studies (Carney et al., 2001), this effect has proved difficult to replicate, in part because of medication problems (Gehi, Mangano, Pipkin, Browner, & Whooley, 2005). However, a secondary analysis of postmyocardial patients in the Enhancing Recovery in Coronary Heart Disease (ENRICHD) study compared 24-hour electrocardiograms in 311 depressed and 367 nondepressed patients (Carney et al., 2005). Heart rate variability was reduced in the depressed patients, and partly accounted for the increased mortality in the depressed group over a 30-month followup period.

Psychophysiological studies using conventional measures such as blood pressure and heart rate to compare

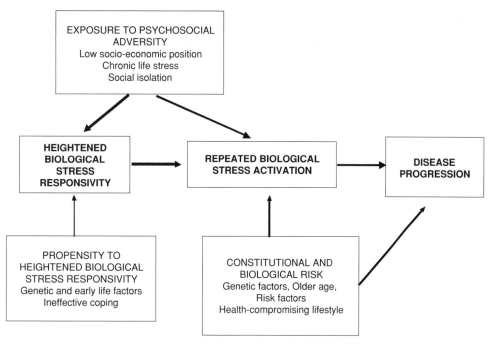

Figure 31.1. Schematic summary of the contribution of psychophysiological processes to disease development.

coronary artery disease patients with controls have also been conducted. Sundin, Ohman, Palm, and Strom (1995) showed that patients exhibited greater total peripheral resistance responses to stress than did controls with no poststress return to baseline. A similar pattern was observed by Strike and coworkers (Strike et al., 2004), who reported that peripheral resistance continued to rise up to 75 minutes poststress in coronary artery disease patients but not in controls. This group also recorded more sustained stress-induced activation of platelets in cardiac patients.

The most extensive psychophysiological research of the past decade has focused on stress-induced transient myocardial ischemic responses (Strike & Steptoe, 2003). Transient ischemia occurs when there is a temporary interruption of blood supply to the working muscle of the heart because of supply not keeping up with demand. This may be a result of the reduced capacity of the diseased coronary vessels to supply sufficient blood (as in exercise-induced ischemia), abnormal responses in the epicardial coronary arteries and microvasculature, or aberrant α-adrenergic vasoconstrictive responses. More than 50 studies have been published assessing stress-induced ischemia with a variety of measures including EKG assessments, radionuclide imaging, and coronary angiography. Psychophysiological stress tests such as mental arithmetic and simulated speech tasks appear to induce transient ischemic responses in 35–50% of patients with coronary artery disease (Strike & Steptoe, 2003). Most of these episodes are not accompanied by pain, and occur at lower levels of oxygen demand than ischemia induced by physical exertion. Stress-induced hemodynamic changes, particularly increases in systemic vascular resistance and coronary

artery vasoconstriction may also contribute. Importantly, it has been demonstrated in at least four prospective studies that mental stress-induced myocardial ischemia is of prognostic significance, which predicts further cardiac events such as myocardial infarction (e.g., Krantz et al., 1999; Sheps et al., 2002).

Ambulatory psychophysiological techniques can also be used to investigate cardiac ischemic responses. Results from 24 or 48h Holter EKG monitoring records can be analyzed for the presence of transient myocardial ischemia by detecting changes in the ST segment of the EKG. These episodes are more likely under conditions of increased mental stress or tension (Gabbay et al., 1996). Gullette et al. (1997) investigated 132 patients with coronary artery disease, of whom 45% showed transient ischemia during ambulatory monitoring. Patients also completed mood and activity diaries, and it was found that episodes of sadness, frustration, and tension were associated with a two to five-fold increase in risk of ischemia. In another study, ischemic episodes during ambulatory monitoring were shown to be preceded by a reduction in high frequency heart rate variability spectral power, indicative of vagal withdrawal (Kop et al., 2001). It is notable that this association between depressed high frequency variability and ischemia was present when patients reported engaging in high but not low levels of mental activity, which suggests that parasympathetic influences on the myocardium mediated the impact of psychological activation.

A novel field of psychophysiological cardiac research has emerged in recent years with the study of patients with implantable cardioverter-defibrillators (ICDs). These devices are implanted in individuals at high risk of serious arrhythmias as a result of CHD and other cardiac diseases.

By combining monitoring of the times at which the ICD administered shocks with diary ratings of mood and activity, Lampert et al. (2002) demonstrated an increased risk of shocks following episodes of anger. More recently, it has been found that depression is a risk factor for greater numbers of shocks from ICDs for preventing dangerous ventricular arrhythmias (Whang et al., 2005). In animal models of depression, reduced heart rate variability and increased susceptibility to ventricular arrhythmias have been described (Grippo et al., 2004). Taken together, this evidence suggests that disturbances in autonomic function are probably responsible for the impact of psychosocial factors on cardiac arrhythmia, and potentially sudden cardiac death.

Hypertension

Hypertension, or high blood pressure, is a major health problem worldwide. The definition of hypertension is somewhat arbitrary because the distribution of blood pressure level in the population is continuous and not bimodal. Nonetheless, the current definition of hypertension is a systolic blood pressure ≥ 140 mmHg and diastolic pressure ≥ 90 mmHg. Most authorities regard a blood pressure in the range 130–139/85–89 mmHg as high-normal, although the Joint National Committee on Prevention, Detection, Evaluation, and Treatment of High Blood Pressure has defined levels of 120–139/80–89 mmHg as prehypertensive (Chobanian et al., 2003). It has also concluded that risk of cardiovascular disease begins with blood pressures greater than 115/75 mmHg, indicating that levels previously regarded as benign may carry some health risk. Between 1999 and 2002, 28.7% of men and 30.5% of women in the United States were hypertensive (National Center for Health Statistics, 2004). However, blood pressure tends to rise with age, so these overall figures disguise a substantial increase in hypertension in middle age. Thus in the USA, prevalence increased from 8.1% men and 2.7% women aged 20–34 years, to 44.9% and 53.9% of those aged 55–64 years. There are also striking ethnic variations with high rates in African Americans and in African Caribbean people in the UK.

Blood pressure is moderately heritable, so family history is a major risk factor for hypertension. It also shows tracking through life; individuals with higher pressures within the normal range being at increased risk for hypertension in the future. In addition, factors such as body weight, diet (in particular salt consumption), sedentary lifestyle, and alcohol intake contribute to its development.

White coat hypertension

Hypertension is typically diagnosed in the physician's office. But there is one diagnostic problem that has psychophysiological origins. This is *white coat hypertension*, the phenomenon of having a high blood pressure when it is measured in the clinic by a physician but lower blood pressure levels in everyday life. White coat hypertension

has become increasingly recognized because of the development of ambulatory blood pressure instruments that allow everyday levels to be recorded as well as the growing popularity of blood pressure self-monitoring. The clinical significance of white coat hypertension remains unclear despite several years of investigation. Some studies have shown an increased risk of cardiovascular disease intermediate between that of normotensives and hypertensives (Gustavsen, Hoegholm, Bang, & Kristensen, 2003), while others have not (Verdecchia et al., 2005).

Because white coat hypertension depends on the measurement situation, it can be seen as a psychophysiological stress response to the circumstances and implications of assessments in the physician's office or clinic. There is little evidence for an unusual psychological profile in people showing white coat effects (Siegel, Blumenthal, & Divine, 1990). However, a number of studies have shown that white coat effects are associated with heightened cardiovascular stress responses (Lantelme, Milon, Gharib, Gayet, & Fortrat, 1998). White coat effects are also correlated with cortisol output (Nystrom, Aardal, & Ohman, 1998) and disturbances of autonomic balance with greater low-to-high frequency ratio in the heart rate variability spectrum (Neumann, Jennings, Muldoon, & Manuck, 2005).

Psychosocial factors

Hypertension was one of the classic psychosomatic disorders studied in the heyday of psychodynamic research with the belief that high blood pressure emerged because of inhibition of emotional conflict and other intrapsychic forces. A major problem with the early research is that studies were carried out with individuals known to be hypertensive. High blood pressure is generally asymptomatic, so a substantial proportion of hypertension is undetected in the population. Clinical samples may not be representative of people with hypertension in general, and awareness of high blood pressure in itself may lead to psychological distress (Rostrup, Mundall, Westheim, & Eide, 1991).

The most convincing evidence for psychosocial contributions to hypertension derives from population-based epidemiological studies rather than clinical investigations. Many studies have documented associations between work stress as defined by the demand/control model and blood pressure with elevated levels among individuals who work in high demand/low control jobs (Schnall, Landsbergis, & Baker, 1994). In the Work Site Blood Pressure Study in New York City, job strain (high demand/low control) was an independent predictor of hypertension after controlling for age, body mass index, Type A behavior, 24-h sodium excretion, physical activity at work, education, smoking, and alcohol consumption (Schnall et al., 1990). Longitudinally, individuals exposed to more years of high job strain had higher blood pressure (Landsbergis, Schnall, Pickering, Warren, & Schwartz, 2003).

Exposure to other types of chronic stress has been linked with hypertension as well. In elderly spousal caregivers for dementing relatives, caregiver burden predicts increases in blood pressure over a seven-year period (Shaw et al., 2003). Individuals with a lack of cohesion in their marriages have higher ambulatory blood pressure, as do people who report poor marital role quality (Barnett, Steptoe, & Gareis, 2005). The experience of racism may contribute to high blood pressure in African Americans (Williams, Neighbors, & Jackson, 2003), while factors such as acculturation stress and status incongruity are relevant. Perhaps one of the most elegant illustrations of the impact of psychosocial experience has been a study of a cohort of Italian nuns living in a secluded order who have been compared with lay women from the same region over a 30-year period (Timio et al., 1997). The blood pressure of the nuns has remained low and stable throughout adult life, compared with the usual rise with age that was observed in the comparison group. There was also a difference in cardiovascular morbidity with fewer fatal and nonfatal cardiac events among the nuns. The predictable, peaceful, and socially supportive lifestyle of the nuns may be responsible for this difference.

A range of psychological characteristics has been associated with hypertension, including anger inhibition, anxiety, and depressive traits (Rutledge & Hogan, 2002). Early research in this field highlighted anger coping styles, and developed the notion that the inhibition of anger expression in people living or working under stressful conditions was a potent stimulus to hypertension (Jorgensen, Johnson, Schreer, & Kolodziej, 1996). Subsequent prospective studies have provided further support for the influence of psychological traits. Jonas and Lando (2000) analyzed data from 3310 initially normotensive adults tracked for up to 22 years, and found that negative affect predicted hypertension after adjusting for other risk factors such as baseline blood pressure and adiposity. In a follow-up of the Framingham cohort, anxiety but not anger was an independent predictor (Markovitz, Matthews, Kannel, Cobb, & D'Agostino, 1993), while hostility was associated with future hypertension over a 15-year period in the CARDIA study (Yan et al., 2003).

Psychophysiological processes

Psychophysiological studies can help to define the pathways through which psychosocial factors influence blood pressure. However, it should be recognized that adverse psychosocial experience might also stimulate behavior patterns that influence blood pressure levels directly. In the Air Traffic Controllers Health Change study, an accelerated rate of development of hypertension was found in controllers. This was found to be mediated in part by increased alcohol consumption, rather than direct sympathoadrenal responses (DeFrank, Jenkins, & Rose, 1987). The increases in blood pressure recorded among young adults from the Luo tribe in western Kenya who migrated to Nairobi are not primarily attributable to the strain of moving to a stressful urban environment, but to higher salt intake and greater body weight (Poulter et al., 1990).

Nonetheless, disturbed psychophysiological responsivity also appears to contribute to hypertension. As in the case of CHD, the disturbance may take the form of heightened stress reactivity or impaired recovery. The hypothesis governing much of this research is that heightened reactivity or impaired recovery not only stimulate acute increases in blood pressure, but lead to progressive vascular remodeling and dysregulation of autonomic, endocrine, and renal regulatory mechanisms, so that more responsive individuals are at increased risk. Acute psychophysiological stress testing has been the main method of investigation, which has been supplemented over recent years by ambulatory monitoring techniques.

Within this paradigm, several different types of study have been conducted. The simplest is the comparison of stress responses in hypertensives and normotensives. Since the work of Jan Brod in the 1950s, it has been known that hypertensives tend to show enhanced blood pressure responses to acute behavioral stress accompanied by greater renal vasoconstriction and increased norepinephrine turnover. However, it is possible that this exaggerated cardiovascular responsivity is the result of the complex physiological adjustments that occur in hypertension, and is secondary rather than primary. Additionally, awareness of high blood pressure influences cardiovascular, neuroendocrine and hemostatic responses, so studies of clinical samples may be compromised (Rostrup et al., 1991).

A second approach that attempts to overcome these problems is the study of people with normal blood pressure who are at increased risk for the development of hypertension in the future. Two risk factors, a family history of hypertension and raised blood pressure within the normal range, have been investigated. The principle underlying these studies is that if disturbed psychophysiological responsivity precedes the onset of the condition, then it should be present in people who have a raised risk. Many studies comparing young adults with and without these risk factors were carried out in the 1970s and 1980s, and were reviewed by Muldoon, Terrell, Bunker, and Manuck (1993) and more recently by Pierce, Grim, and King (2005). About one third of studies found that individuals with a positive family history showed greater blood pressure or heart rate stress reactivity than negative history groups. Much of this work has been criticized for the weak evaluation of family history, which often relies on reports by young people on their parents' medical condition, and classification on the basis of a single parent's history. Unfortunately, more recent studies that have involved more rigorous assessment of hypertension in both parents have continued to generate somewhat inconsistent results (de Visser et al., 1995; Gerin & Pickering, 1995; Manuck et al., 1996).

A number of factors may account for this inconsistency. First, the emphasis in most of the literature has been on heightened reactivity. Delayed recovery may be as important as an indicator of disturbances of normal physiological regulatory processes, and several studies indicate that young normotensives at raised risk for future hypertension show impaired post-stress cardiovascular recovery (de Visser et al., 1995; Gerin & Pickering, 1995). Second, the psychological characteristics of participants may be important. In the light of the epidemiological literature outlined earlier, Vögele and Steptoe (1993) hypothesized that psychophysiological responsivity might be especially important among people who inhibit anger expression. They studied adolescent boys whose parents' blood pressure had previously been measured, and found heightened reactivity among those with high parental blood pressure who were also anger inhibitors. Third, it appears that differences in cardiovascular responsivity are more likely to emerge with actively demanding tasks eliciting sympathoadrenal activation, rather than other types of challenge. Pierce et al. (2005) have also argued that differences between positive and negative history groups are likely to emerge when the responses of negative history group are small, rather than there being a clear pattern of exaggerated reactivity in the positive history groups.

There is in addition an important limitation to the use of both family history and raised normal blood pressure to determine whether disturbances of psychophysiological responsivity precede the development of hypertension. That is, in both groups, there are already detectable changes in vascular physiology, including changes in cardiac morphology, increased end organ responsivity, and minimal arteriolar resistance, which may mean that disturbed responsivity is secondary rather than primary.

Longitudinal studies

Stronger evidence concerning the role of psychophysiological responsivity in the evolution of hypertension emerges from prospective studies. These test the possibility that high reactivity or impaired recovery predicts future rises in blood pressure. Early work on this topic was based primarily on the cold pressor test as a stimulus, and produced mixed results. Subsequent studies have assessed responses to actively challenging tasks; several large-scale investigations show that cardiovascular reactivity is an independent predictor of future elevated blood pressure (Carroll, Ring, Hunt, Ford, & Macintyre, 2003; Carroll et al., 2001; Markovitz, Raczynski, Wallace, Chettur, & Chesney, 1998). Impaired poststress recovery is also relevant. In a recent three-year followup of 209 middle-aged men and women, we found that increases in resting blood pressure were predicted by poor poststress recovery in systolic and diastolic blood pressure and in total peripheral resistance independently of baseline blood pressure, age, gender, socioeconomic status, hypertensive medication, body mass, and smoking (Steptoe & Marmot, 2005). The adjusted odds of an increase in systolic pressure ≥ 5 mmHg were 3.50 (95% confidence interval 1.19 to 10.8) for individuals with poor compared with effective post-stress recovery.

Nonetheless, findings have been somewhat inconsistent, primarily because of limitations in study design. Again the issue of exposure to adverse experiences in everyday life is relevant, so in addition to evaluating cardiovascular responsivity, it is necessary to monitor exposure to life stress. Thus, Light et al. (1999) demonstrated that high stress reactivity predicted increases in blood pressure over a 10-year period only if it was associated both with family history and with high levels of daily stress. In the same vein, a 20-year followup of the Air Traffic Controller Health Change Study sample reported that risk of hypertension was increased among those who showed raised blood pressure reactions to chronic work stress (Ming et al., 2004). Including assessments of exposure to situations likely to provoke psychophysiological responses is likely to increase the strength of associations with future hypertension.

Inflammatory stress responses and hypertension

Psychophysiological investigations of hypertension have largely been limited to the measurement of cardiovascular and autonomic processes, but recent research has linked hypertension with inflammatory responses. Cross-sectionally, blood pressure is correlated with C-reactive protein, IL-6, sICAM-1, TNFα, and fibrinogen in population studies (Chae, Lee, Rifai, & Ridker, 2001; Chrysohoou, Pitsavos, Panagiotakos, Skoumas, & Stefanadis, 2004). These inflammatory markers could be involved in hypertension pathogenesis in several ways, including stimulation of sympathoadrenal and HPA axes, effects on hemostasis, and direct influences on vascular remodeling (Intengan & Schiffrin, 2001; Pasceri, Willerson, & Yeh, 2000).

Psychophysiological studies of inflammation and hypertension are in their infancy. There is evidence that stress induced leukocyte adhesion is heightened in hypertensives compared with normotensives (Mills et al., 2003). Brydon and Steptoe (2005) found that individual differences in the acute stress responses of plasma IL-6 and fibrinogen predict 3-year changes in ambulatory blood pressure. The fact that these effects were independent of any association between future elevated blood pressure and cardiovascular responsivity suggests that there may be separate stress-related inflammatory pathways to hypertension. The challenge over the next decade is to discover whether these psychophysiological processes mediate the impact of psychosocial factors on hypertension.

Metabolic disorders

The metabolic disorders discussed here are diabetes and the metabolic syndrome. Diabetes mellitus is a heterogeneous metabolic disease, the central feature of which is high blood glucose (hyperglycemia). It is the leading cause of nontraumatic limb amputation, new cases of end stage renal disease, and blindness in adults (World Health Organization, 2002). It is a major cause of death in itself, while also contributing to CHD and stroke. The prevalence in the USA in 2002 has been estimated at 8.7% of adults aged 20 and over, of whom more than a quarter are undiagnosed and, therefore, unaware of their condition. Prevalence rises to more than 18% of people aged 60 and over, and is lower in people of white European than African American or Hispanic descent.

There are two forms of diabetes, of which Type 2 is much the more common, accounting for some 90% of cases. Type 1 (insulin dependent diabetes) is due to failures in insulin secretion which result in there being insufficient insulin action on peripheral target tissues, while in Type 2 diabetes there is a diminished tissue response to insulin. Type 1 diabetes typically occurs in early life, and is an autoimmune condition in which the body's immune system destroys insulin-synthesizing beta cells in the pancreas. Type 2 diabetes is more likely of adult onset, and begins with insulin resistance, in which cells in tissues such as muscle, liver, and adipose tissue are not able to use insulin effectively. The need for insulin consequently rises, and the pancreas progressively loses its ability to produce insulin. Diabetes is associated with disturbances in protein, carbohydrate, and fat metabolism as well as hyperglycemia, and there is a hereditary component to both forms.

The metabolic syndrome is a constellation of cardiovascular risk factors that includes abdominal adiposity (a large waist circumference or waist/hip ratio), elevated blood pressure, high fasting glucose (hyperglycemia), and triglyceride levels, and low fasting high-density lipoprotein (HDL) cholesterol. It is strongly related to insulin resistance and, thus, to risk of Type 2 diabetes, so has a similar demography. Behavioral factors are relevant both to the development of Type 2 diabetes and the metabolic syndrome in which physical inactivity and eating habits lead to excessive energy intake and obesity being critical.

Several psychosocial factors apparently increase risk for diabetes and the metabolic syndrome. At least three prospective epidemiological studies have documented associations between depressive symptoms and future Type 2 diabetes that were independent of other risk factors (Musselman et al., in press). Diabetic individuals in turn have an elevated risk of depression, and depressed diabetics are prone to poor glycemic control and a high prevalence of diabetes complications (de Groot, Anderson, Freedland, Clouse, & Lustman, 2001). The relationship between insulin resistance and depression is less consistent with both positive and negative associations being described (Everson-Rose et al., 2004; Lawlor, Smith, & Ebrahim, 2003). In the Whitehall II epidemiological study, low SES, depression, and work stress (effort-reward imbalance) were related to future Type 2 diabetes and impaired glucose tolerance (Kumari, Head, & Marmot, 2004). Components of the metabolic syndrome have been associated with psychosocial factors such as low social support, hostility, and marital conflict (Horsten, Mittleman, Wamala, Schenck-Gustafsson, & Orth-Gomer, 1999; Knox, Weidner, Adelman, Stoney, & Ellison, 2004; Troxel, Matthews, Gallo, & Kuller, 2005). An analysis from the Normative Aging Study indicated that the metabolic syndrome when combined with hostility predicted a fourfold increase in odds of developing a myocardial infarction over a 13-year follow-up period (Todaro et al., 2005).

Evidence concerning psychosocial factors and the development of Type 1 diabetes is more controversial, but Sepa, Wahlberg, Vaarala, Frodi, and Ludvigsson (2005) recently reported a study of 4,400 infants in which diabetes-related autoantibodies were more likely to be present in the blood of infants whose mothers experienced high parenting stress, life events and low education independently of family history of diabetes. By contrast, studies of stressful life events in adult life show no convincing association with onset of Type 1 diabetes (Cosgrove, 2004). Nonetheless, it has been found that psychosocial factors modulate glycemic control in type 1 diabetes with impaired control in individuals experiencing personal life stressors (Lloyd et al., 1999).

Psychophysiological processes

There has been relatively little conventional psychophysiological research in relation to Type 1 diabetes. Some investigators have investigated whether Type 1 diabetics show hyperglycemic responses to acute laboratory stress, but results have been inconsistent (Kemmer et al., 1986; Moberg, Kollind, Lins, & Adamson, 1994). Naturalistic studies involving simultaneous measures of everyday stress and blood glucose have shown positive associations only in a minority of individuals (Riazi, Pickup, & Bradley, 2004). Nevertheless, this is a topic that merits further investigation. A recent analysis of 188 Type 1 diabetics assessed whether associations between hyperglycemia and depression were mediated by poor self-care behaviors such as failure to monitor glucose, eat and exercise appropriately (Lustman, Clouse, Ciechanowski, Hirsch, & Freedland, 2005). It was found that these behaviors did not account for the relationship of depression to poor glycemic control, and suggested that more direct psychophysiological processes might be responsible.

There has been more work related to the Type 2 diabetes, metabolic factors, and obesity. One approach has been to assess acute lipid responses to stress. The concentration in the blood of total and low density lipoprotein (LDL) cholesterol increase following acute laboratory stressors, but there has been controversy about whether these effects represent increased lipids in the bloodstream or are secondary to reductions in blood volume (Muldoon et al., 1995; Stoney, Bausserman, Niaura, Marcus, & Flynn, 1999). The significance of individual differences in cholesterol responsivity is uncertain, but Steptoe and Brydon (2005) have recently found that raised fasting LDL-cholesterol and total/HDL-cholesterol ratio were predicted by heightened cholesterol stress responses measured three years earlier.

Psychophysiological studies of abdominal adiposity in behavioral medicine and psychosomatics have explored both neuroendocrine and autonomic function. Abdominal adiposity is associated with disturbances of glucocorticoid function (Björntorp, 2001). A number of studies have demonstrated that cortisol responses to acute stress are positively correlated with waist/hip ratio, although effects have been observed more consistently in women than men (Epel et al., 2000; Ljung et al., 2000). Naturalistic monitoring studies have shown that waist/hip ratio in men is correlated with the cortisol awakening response, which is a measure of cortisol secretion in everyday life that is regarded as a marker of stress-induced HPA dysregulation (Steptoe, Kunz-Ebrecht, Brydon, & Wardle, 2004).

There is also a relationship between obesity and cardiovascular stress responsivity. Both adults and adolescents with higher central adiposity exhibit heightened blood pressure responses during psychophysiological stress testing, which may be sustained by increased peripheral vascular resistance (Barnes, Treiber, Davis, Kelley, & Strong, 1998; Jern, Bergbrant, Bjorntorp, & Hansson, 1992). We recently assessed the relationship between cardiovascular reactivity and recovery and changes in waist/hip ratio over three years in a sample of 225 middle-aged men and women (Steptoe & Wardle, 2005). It was found that increases in waist/hip ratio were predicted by impaired poststress recovery of systolic blood pressure and cardiac output in men independently of baseline waist/hip ratio, age, SES, alcohol intake, and baseline cardiovascular function. It, therefore, appears that individual differences in psychophysiological responses may reflect patterns of dysregulation that contribute to the development of abdominal adiposity.

Psychophysiological research on the metabolic syndrome and insulin resistance is sparse to date. Certainly it appears that the metabolic syndrome is associated with increased excretion of cortisol and norepinephrine metabolites, raised levels of IL-6 and C-reactive protein, and reduced heart rate variability (Brunner et al., 2002). Abnormal vascular reactivity to stress has also been described (Sung, Wilson, Izzo, Ramirez, & Dandona, 1997), while studies of cortisol output in everyday life suggest that stress-related alterations in HPA function are also present (Rosmond, 2005). One study has demonstrated an association between cortisol/testosterone ratio and future CHD over a 16-year followup period that was independent of smoking, social class, and other confounders (Davey Smith et al., 2005). This relationship was markedly attenuated when insulin resistance was taken into account, suggesting that HPA effects may be mediated through metabolic pathways.

Infectious illness

Scientific research on the influence of psychosocial factors on risk of infections illness has been in progress for more than 40 years (Cohen & Williamson, 1991). In an early study, Meyer and Haggerty (1962) took throat swabs every three weeks from families over several months to assess the presence of streptococcal infection. An increased likelihood of both infection and overt illness was recorded during periods following acute life stress or daily hassles. Life

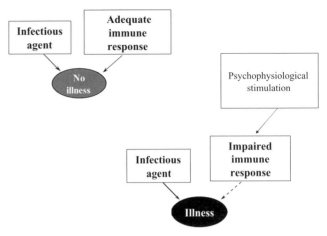

Figure 31.2. Schematic illustration of the interaction between host resistance, exposure to infection, and psychophysiological processes. The upper panel represents effective host resistance to infection, whereas in the lower panel, psychosocial stimulation has induced down-regulation of immune defenses, so that the infectious challenge leads to illness.

event stress was also found to predict upper respiratory tract infection in a later longitudinal family study as well, though effects were moderated by coping style (Turner Cobb & Steptoe, 1996). Associations between psychosocial factors and recurrent infections have also been described. Cohen, Kemeny, et al. (1999) studied 58 women with a history of genital herpes on a weekly basis over a six-month period. There were frequent herpes recurrences during the study period, and these were predicted by persistent stress (continuing for more than one week), after other factors had been taken into account.

It is plausible that these associations are mediated by psychophysiological processes, particularly impairment of host resistance. The immune system is responsible for defending the person against infectious agents such as bacteria, viruses, and fungi. There is ample evidence, as noted in other chapters in the *Handbook*, for stress and other psychosocial factors promoting downregulation of protective immune responses (Segerstrom & Miller, 2004). Figure 31.2 summarizes the possible sequence of events. The upper panel illustrates the pattern of healthy normal response to minor infections in which the individual mounts an adequate defense that excludes the infection and prevents illness. In the lower panel, exposure to the infectious agent takes place against a backdrop of impaired immune function because of psychosocial stimulation, and this is not sufficient to prevent illness from developing.

However, alternative pathways might be involved. First, there may be changes in exposure. Because infectious diseases are caused by pathogens, any changes in exposure that are stimulated by psychosocial factors may influence the chances of becoming ill. Some people respond to distressing events in their lives by seeking social support and mobilizing social networks, and this might have the unwanted effect of exposing the individual to more respiratory infections. Alternatively, people may withdraw socially and reduce contact with airborne pathogens. Exposure to pathogens is a key issue in HIV/AIDS, and in the prevention of outbreaks of serious waterborne, airborne, and sexually transmitted infections in the developing world.

Second, health behaviors and lifestyle have an influence on infectious disease. Smoking, alcohol consumption, and physical exercise all influence vulnerability to infection and the duration of symptoms. Malnutrition is probably the principle cause of diminished immunity and susceptibility to infection across the world. Although severe protein energy malnutrition is rare in developed countries, undernutrition is common among the elderly and impairs immune resistance. The pattern of health behavior can be altered in response to psychosocial factors, such as work stress, so the acquisition and course of infectious disease may be modified. Behaviors can have direct effects on infectious disease, for example, when sexual behavior stimulates the reactivation of latent herpes virus, the acquisition of human papilloma virus, and subsequent risk of cervical cancer (Waller, McCaffery, Forrest, & Wardle, 2004).

Third, variations in symptom reporting may be involved. People differ in the extent to which they attend to physical sensations and recognize them as symptoms of illness. Illness behavior research has shown that the same infection, depending on levels of psychosocial stress, may elicit quite different levels of complaint, work absence, and health service utilization. Negative affect can influence symptom reporting and illness behavior with more symptoms being reported in distressed individuals independently of objective illness.

There are also plausible sequences of events that differ from the two possibilities outlined in Figure 31.2. One is that immune downregulation may occur in the absence of exposure to an active infection. Under these circumstances, a change in host resistance may have no adverse consequences. Another is that the infection is very severe and leads to illness, despite the mounting of a vigorous immune response. When this happens, it is not necessary to postulate any psychophysiologically mediated alteration in immune function.

It is for these and other reasons that some research groups have turned to experimental studies as a means of understanding psychosocial influences. This approach has been championed by Sheldon Cohen, and has involved healthy volunteers being inoculated with standard doses of virus (Miller & Cohen, 2005). If an appropriate dose is administered, not everyone will become ill; thus, differences in the subsequent rates of infection and illness must then be due to differences in vulnerability. Social activities are limited by quarantine in these studies, and health behaviors such as smoking are controlled. Cohen, Tyrrell, and Smith (1991) demonstrated with this paradigm that susceptibility to common cold viruses was directly asso-

ciated with a psychological stress index created through an amalgam of measures of major life events over the past 12 months, perceived stress, and negative affect. The dose-response association was independent of age, allergic status, and other risk factors. Later work established that chronic stressors such as longterm work problems and relationship difficulties are particularly relevant. By contrast, social networks have a protective effect in which there is lower susceptibility to experimental infection among volunteers with more extensive and diverse social networks (Cohen et al., 1997). Associations with psychological characteristics such as negative emotional style and sociability have also been established (Cohen, Doyle, Turner, Alper, & Skoner, 2003).

Psychophysiological processes
This work clearly demonstrates that psychosocial factors can influence vulnerability to infectious disease. There has been less success in identifying psychophysiological mediators because susceptibility is not related to catecholamines, cortisol, or various markers of immune function. However, one study from Cohen's group showed that associations between psychological stress and the severity of symptoms were related to the levels of IL-6 production in the nasal passages following influenza virus administration. More severe symptoms were experienced by participants who reported higher perceived stress which was accompanied by raised IL-6 (Cohen, Doyle, & Skoner, 1999). This suggests that inflammatory mediators may be involved in symptom production in stressed individuals.

Another method of investigating psychophysiological processes in infectious illness is to study responses to vaccines and immunization. This approach is based on the fact that immunizations such as those for influenza, rubella, and hepatitis B involve injecting antigen (a foreign substance), which elicits an antibody response. The effectiveness of the immunization is indexed by the quantity of antigen-specific antibody that is produced over subsequent days and weeks. Although the literature is somewhat inconsistent, several studies have shown that antibody responses are impaired by psychosocial adversity. Two studies have shown that antibody responses following influenza vaccination are reduced in informal caregivers for dementing relatives compared with controls (Kiecolt-Glaser, Glaser, Gravenstein, Malarkey, & Sheridan, 1996; Vedhara et al., 1999). In one, concomitant disturbances in inflammatory cytokine production was observed, while in the other study, caregivers had heightened cortisol levels in the morning.

Laboratory-based psychophysiological studies can be used to understand these processes, though findings to date have been inconsistent. Marsland, Cohen, Rabin, and Manuck (2001) tested cardiovascular and immune responses to a stress test (simulated public speaking) in undergraduates who were undergoing a course of hepatitis B immunization. Lower antibody responses to the vaccine were predicted by a diminished stress-induced lymphoproliferative response to phytohemagglutinin. Another smaller study of students found that poorer antibody responses were associated with low cortisol responses coupled with heightened cardiac output responses to acute stress (Burns, Ring, Drayson, & Carroll, 2002). Individual differences in corticosteroid responsivity have also been implicated in the expression and reactivation of latent viruses such as Epstein-Barr (Cacioppo et al., 2002). Phillips, Carroll, Burns, and Dryson (2005) reported that antibody responses to influenza vaccination were negatively associated with cortisol responses to mental arithmetic stress, and also with neuroticism. Findings of this type suggest that differences in cardiovascular, immune, and neuroendocrine regulation in response to stress are involved in impaired resistance to infectious illness. However, it remains to be seen whether these psychophysiological pathways mediate the links between life stress and infection.

Allergic and atopic conditions

The allergic disorders that have been investigated in behavioral medicine and psychosomatics include bronchial asthma and atopic skin conditions. Bronchial asthma is characterized by reversible airway obstruction, increased airway responsiveness to a range of stimuli, and airway inflammation. Atopic dermatitis is a chronic inflammatory skin disease characterized by eczematous inflammation of the skin, recurrent episodes, and severe pruritus (itchiness). These allergic conditions involve activation of allergen-specific T and B cells which produce allergen-specific immunoglobulins (i.e., IgE). There are thought to be distinct immediate and delayed phases of allergic conditions. Immediate responses result from the release of mast cell products, such as histamine, that have a variety of effects including smooth muscle contraction, mucus release, and increased capillary permeability. Different symptoms arise depending on the site of antigen contact. Delayed responses may occur after several hours and result from the synthesis of other mediators that stimulate the accumulation of eosinophils and basophils. The immune system, and in particular balance between Th1 and Th2 immune responses is critical, while in asthma autonomic control of airways caliber is also involved.

The National Health Interview Survey in 2001 in the USA estimated that more than 31 million (11.3%) Americans had been diagnosed with asthma at some point in their lives with around 20 million currently having asthma. There is a higher rate (14.4%) in children aged 5–17 years. The number of physician office visits for asthma is around 10.8 million annually. Women and African Americans have higher rates than men and white Europeans. There are ethnic variations in other atopic conditions as well, and African Americans more likely to seek medical care for dermatitis than people of white European origin (Janumpally,

Feldman, Gupta, & Fleischer, 2002). The economic cost of asthma in direct health costs and lost productivity has been estimated at $14 billion annually.

Quality of life is adversely affected by many atopic conditions, and anxiety and depression are frequent. In allergic dermatitis, associations between depression and the extent of body surface affected have been found, and depression is closely linked with the perception of pruritis (Gupta & Gupta, 2003). A recent review concluded that in both child or adolescent and adult groups, about one third of people with asthma meet the criteria for a comorbid anxiety disorder (Katon, Richardson, Lozano, & McCauley, 2004). These psychological difficulties may have an impact on self-care and functional status. In a followup conducted among asthmatic patients admitted for emergency care, elevated anxiety or depression was associated with an increased risk of relapse (Dahlen & Janson, 2002). However, a study of risk factors associated with asthma death in a large representative sample in the UK showed no association with a number of psychosocial factors including family problems, domestic abuse, or social isolation. Financial difficulties and psychosis did increase risk, while prescription of antidepressant medications was protective (Sturdy et al., 2002). There have been few prospective studies of infants and young children susceptible to atopic disorder. But in work on newborns at elevated genetic risk of atopy, Wright, Cohen, Carey, Weiss, and Gold (2002) found that stress reported by caregivers over the first three months of the infants' lives was associated with wheeze at 14 months independently of other risk factors such as smoking, low SES, and parental asthma. A direct psychophysiological link between psychosocial experience and atopy is therefore plausible (Wright, Cohen, & Cohen, 2005).

Psychophysiological processes

Atopic conditions are especially interesting from the psychophysiological point of view because processes that are thought to be potentially pathological for other health problems are beneficial for this group of disorders. In particular, corticosteroids have a positive anti-inflammatory effect on asthma and atopic skin conditions and are widely used therapeutically. Medications that mimic sympathetic nervous system activation have favorable effects on bronchial asthma, while heightened activity in the vagus causes bronchoconstriction. Thus the psychophysiological pathways that are implicated in mediating risk in many other conditions appear to have positive effects in atopic disorders.

Early psychophysiological studies of asthma focused on the responses of the airways to challenge and showed that asthmatics display bronchoconstrictive responses while healthy individuals do not (Steptoe, 1998). Subsequently, Ritz, Steptoe, DeWilde, and Costa (2000) found that increased airways resistance emerged not only with stressful tasks but also in response to emotional stimuli with both positive and negative valence. Interestingly, airways responses to negative emotional stimuli in the laboratory were associated with alterations in airways function that occurred with negative mood states in everyday life, which indicates some generalizability of responses to standardized testing (Ritz & Steptoe, 2000).

There is growing evidence that atopic individuals display inhibited stress-related HPA responsiveness. For example, Buske-Kirschbaum et al. (1997) reported that children with atopic dermatitis produced lower cortisol responses to standardized challenges than nonatopic controls, and a similar pattern was observed in asthmatics (Buske-Kirschbaum et al., 2003). This pattern was replicated in a larger sample of adolescents with a range of atopic conditions including allergic rhinitis (Wamboldt, Laudenslager, Wamboldt, Kelsay, & Hewitt, 2003). Interestingly, this pattern may not be present from birth, but evolve during the early years of life. A recent study tested the stress responsivity of newborn babies by assessing cortisol responses to a standard heel prick (Buske-Kirschbaum, Fischbach, Rauh, Hanker, & Hellhammer, 2004). The offspring of parents with atopic conditions showed larger rather than smaller cortisol responses than controls, the opposite of the pattern observed in people with established atopy. It may be that this early hyperreactivity is followed by downregulation of the HPA axis in later years with a corresponding increase in allergic responses.

As noted earlier, acute inflammation in atopic conditions is controlled by activated T lymphocytes and the Th1/Th2 balance. Th2-type cytokines promote the production of IgE. It is possible that the neuroendocrine responses manifest in atopic individuals shift the immune balance towards Th2 responses. Consistent with this hypothesis, Wright et al. (2004) observed in their birth cohort that family stress when the infant was 6–18 months old was correlated with increased IgE expression and with levels of the Th2 cytokine TNFα. This is an area of research in which psychophysiological methods are poised to make a major contribution to behavioral medicine through helping to tease out the complex interaction between psychosocial experience, neuroendocrine, and immune function.

Autoimmune conditions

Autoimmune conditions are a disparate collection of chronic medical disorders in which the immune system attacks the body's own biology instead of alien material, which leads to inflammation and other problems. Because hormones and neurotransmitters regulate the activity of the immune system, it is possible that psychophysiological processes are involved in the development and progression of autoimmune conditions. Most research has focused on neuroendocrine and inflammatory processes in autoimmune conditions, though work on autonomic function is becoming more prominent. Several autoimmune

conditions have been investigated, but this chapter will highlight two topics – rheumatoid arthritis and multiple sclerosis.

Rheumatoid arthritis

Rheumatoid arthritis is a systemic disease involving inflammation of the synovial membrane that lubricates joints, which leads to erosion of cartilage and bone. T cells, B cells, cytokines, and macrophages are produced locally by these cells and contribute to joint deformation. Inflammation and deformation of joints are responsible for the pain in rheumatoid arthritis. The disease affects multiple organs and is associated with increased risk of CHD and other health outcomes. No specific cause has been identified that initiates the autoimmune response, but this becomes self-perpetuating. Prevalence is around 1–3% of the adult population with peak occurrence between the ages of 30 and 55 years, and the condition is more common in women than men. Incidence is higher in Native Americans, African Caribbean, and Asian groups than in Caucasians. A particularly distressing form is juvenile idiopathic arthritis, an inflammatory joint disease of childhood, some forms of which are irreversible.

There is an extensive literature concerning the role of life stress in the etiology of rheumatoid arthritis (Herrmann, Scholmerich, & Straub, 2000). Almost all studies have been retrospective and results have been mixed, although findings have been more consistently positive for juvenile forms. The evidence is stronger for psychosocial factors exacerbating the course of rheumatoid arthritis. More than a dozen prospective studies have shown that minor life stress predicts future disease activity (Herrmann et al., 2000). The presence of depression, a common concomitant of rheumatoid arthritis, amplifies the effect of interpersonal stress on disease activity (Zautra et al., 2004). There is also some evidence that emotional support is protective, although at least one large study has found cross-sectional but not longitudinal associations between social support or networks and functional limitations and distress in rheumatoid arthritis (Demange et al., 2004).

An interesting feature of autoimmune conditions shared with atopic conditions is that corticosteroids, normally released during emotional stress, are immunosuppressive. Indeed, they are widely used in the treatment of rheumatoid arthritis. Norepinephrine is also immunomodulatory. It might, therefore, be hypothesized that psychosocial adversity stimulates an impaired HPA response, so that inflammatory reactions are not inhibited. Animal studies certainly indicate that blunted HPA activity is associated with increased susceptibility to arthritis (Sternberg, 2001). Unfortunately, experimental psychophysiological studies of humans are very limited. However, Jacobs et al. (2001) found that acute stress induced a blunted interferon-γ response in rheumatoid patients, while increased C-reactive protein responses to stress have also been described (Veldhuijzen van Zanten, Ring, Carroll, & Kitas, 2005). An increase in IL-6 production following acute stress is present in juvenile rheumatoid arthritis patients but not age-matched controls, despite comparable norepinephrine responses (Roupe van der Voort, Heijnen, Wulffraat, Kuis, & Kavelaars, 2000). The time course of neuroendocrine and inflammatory responses following behavioral change is clearly crucial, and sympathetic stimulation may have both pro and anti-inflammatory effects (Straub, Dhabhar, Bijlsma, & Cutolo, 2005). For example, Viswanathan and Dhabhar (2005) have demonstrated how acute stress induces increased trafficking of leukocytes to the site of immune activation in animals. This may enhance immunoprotection during infection or surgery, but exacerbate pathology in autoimmune conditions.

Multiple sclerosis

Multiple sclerosis involves inflammatory damage to the myelin sheath of neurons in the central nervous system. It is a relapsing-remitting illness with many clinical manifestations including double vision, unsteady gait, poor coordination, weakness of the limbs, and slurred speech. It is fortunately relatively rare, and preferentially affects people of Caucasian origin. One reason why it may be particularly relevant to psychophysiological investigation is that disease exacerbations and relapses may be triggered by emotional factors (Brown, Tennant, Dunn, & Pollard, 2005). A meta-analysis of 14 studies relating stressful life events with disease exacerbation was published by Mohr, Hart, Julian, Cox, and Pelletier (2004). A consistent positive association was observed with a medium effect size ($d = 0.53$). An increased risk of onset of multiple sclerosis following the very severe trauma of the death of a child has been seen in one large study (Li et al., 2004), but otherwise data concerning psychosocial factors and disease onset are limited.

As with the psychophysiological research on other autoimmune conditions, it appears that immune responses to standardized behavioral challenge are disturbed in multiple sclerosis. Heesen et al. (2005) compared 23 patients with 25 controls in their responses to a 40-minute cognitive challenge. The multiple sclerosis patients had a reduced heart rate response to the task and showed a blunted interferon-γ response, which suggests autonomic dysfunction coupled with impaired TH-1 stress responsivity. Blood pressure and heart rate stress responses were assessed at the start of a year-long study of multiple sclerosis disease exacerbation by Ackerman et al (2003). Over the year, exacerbations of disease state were more likely in periods following the experience of stressful life events than at other times, while greater cardiovascular stress reactivity also predicted the number of disease flares. In multiple regression analysis, disability level, medication use, cardiovascular reactivity, baseline heart rate, and life events together explained 30%

of the variance in the proportion of weeks during which patients were ill. The results of these studies are, therefore, somewhat mixed, but suggest that further psychophysiological investigation of multiple sclerosis will prove fruitful.

Musculoskeletal conditions

Musculoskeletal disorders constitute a range of syndromes including low back pain, neck and shoulder pain, repetitive strain injury, carpal tunnel syndrome, tendonitis, and others. Many musculoskeletal disorders are work related and a major pubic health problem. According to the National Institute for Occupational Safety and Health in the USA, musculoskeletal disorders affect 7% of the population, and account for 19% of hospital says. It has been estimated that nearly 70 million physician office visits occur annually because of musculoskeletal disorders, and that in 1999 around one million Americans were off work because of treatment for or recovery from work-related musculoskeletal pain (Institute of Medicine, 2001). The annual cost is a staggering $50 billion as a result of compensation, lost earnings, and lost productivity. These conditions differ from many other major health problems in that symptoms can appear early in life and after a relatively short exposure to adverse environmental conditions. In repetitive work, for example, pain syndromes may be reported after only 6–12 months on the job.

The role of bad ergonomic conditions at work, heavy lifting, and physically monotonous or repetitive work in the development of neck, shoulder, and lower back pain problems is well established (Institute of Medicine, 2001). What is remarkable, however, is that the considerable ergonomic improvements of the work environment over recent decades have not resulted in a reduced incidence of musculoskeletal disorders, and that musculoskeletal disorders are frequent not only in physically demanding jobs but also in light physical work (Lundberg, in press). This indicates that other factors are involved.

There is substantial evidence linking psychosocial aspects of work with upper extremity musculoskeletal problems (Sauter & Moon, 1996). Factors such as low autonomy, lack of role clarity, low job satisfaction, and high work pressure, have all been associated with pain in the neck and shoulder regions, and with hand or wrist problems. A recent systematic review confirmed these observations, but also pointed to evidence relating upper extremity problems with psychosocial factors outside work such as low social support and general stress (Bongers, Kremer, & ter Laak, 2002). For example, a large survey of working people in Finland showed that the prevalence of nonspecific shoulder pain was 12% and was positively associated with burnout and depression (Miranda, Viikari-Juntura, Heistaro, Heliovaara, & Riihimaki, 2005). Prospectively, a study of workers in diverse occupations initially assessed near the beginning of their employment revealed that the onset of new pain conditions over the following year was predicted by initial psychological distress, job demands, and low social support at work (Nahit et al., 2003). In a 12-month investigation of car mechanics, low job control and low social support were the best predictors of new cases of neck and low back pain after adjustment for baseline measures (Torp, Riise, & Moen, 2001). Nor are these problems confined to workers in Western countries. Recent work with nurses in China has documented a high prevalence of musculoskeletal complaints that were associated with high mental pressure, boring, repetitive tasks, and low social support at work (Smith, Wei, Zhao, & Wang, 2004). Work-related upper extremity disorders are particularly common in jobs with a static load involving monotonous and repetitive tasks, even when physical demands are only low or moderate. Computer data entry, cashier work in supermarkets and other outlets, routine scientific bench work, and traditional assembly line work all have these characteristics. Musculoskeletal problems are particularly common among women, partly because they are likely to work in these lower status jobs, and partly because much ergonomic design is still based on male stature and physique (Klumb & Lampert, 2004).

Psychophysiological processes

Much research on musculoskeletal disorders is based on self-report or physical examination. However, direct measurement of muscle tension using surface electromyography (EMG) provides valuable additional information. Miniaturized transducers and telemetric equipment are available that allow readings to be obtained from free-moving individuals. Positive correlations have been reported between objectively assessed muscle tension and feelings of stress and exhaustion during work, but correlations with pain are often not obtained (e.g., Rissen, Melin, Sandsjo, Dohns, & Lundberg, 2000). Studies of this kind indicate that the perception and appraisal of muscle tension may be important as well as objective differences in tension.

Laboratory experiments provide clues about how psychosocial factors might contribute to the development of musculoskeletal problems by interacting with physical demands. Marras, Davis, Heaney, Maronitis, and Allread (2000) monitored trunk motion and EMG while 25 volunteers carried out lifting tasks with different degrees of trunk extension. The tasks were carried out under stressed and unstressed conditions. In the stress condition, feedback to participants about their movement and speed was manipulated to indicate that they were failing task demands, which led to verbal criticism from the experimenters. It was found that stress increased spine compression and lateral shear because of increased activity of several trunk muscles. Similar effects have been observed in response to mental processing tasks being performed at the same time as lifting tasks with substantial increases in spine loading and compression coupled with less controlled movements and greater muscle coactivation (Davis,

Marras, Heaney, Waters, & Gupta, 2002). Such patterns could increase risk for low back pain.

Musculoskeletal disorders are also common among people engaged in light physical work with effects on muscle tension that can be very subtle. Even computer work using a mouse elicits increases in EMG in the forearm, shoulder and neck, and there is greater tension when people are performing more mentally demanding tasks (Laursen, Jensen, Garde, & Jorgensen, 2002). Interestingly, these differences are also associated with shifts in heart rate variability towards sympathetic activation and vagal withdrawal (Garde, Laursen, Jorgensen, & Jensen, 2002). It is possible that sustained or repeated low-level muscle activity induced by psychological demands may initiate a pathogenic mechanism resulting in muscle pain.

Lundberg (in press) has pointed out that unlike the physical demands of work that stop with the end of the work period or during breaks, psychosocial issues are persistent. Concern about job satisfaction, low income, work-home conflict, and interpersonal relationships at work are experienced on a more sustained basis, both before and after work. A psychophysiological concept that may be relevant to this difference is that of EMG silence or "gaps." These are episodes in which muscular electrical activity is very low. It has been hypothesized that short periods during which muscle tension is very low are essential to avoid shoulder and neck problems. Hägg and Astrom (1997) compared medical secretaries with and without musculoskeletal complains during their work, and found that the former had fewer EMG gaps during the day. A prospective study of industrial workers found that women who developed trapezius myalgia over the first year of employment had higher muscle activity during breaks at work but not during actual work than those who remained healthy, and had fewer EMG gaps (Veiersted, Westgaard, & Andersen, 1993). Such findings indicate that lack of relaxation during breaks at work and after work may be an important risk factor for musculoskeletal disorders.

Commonalities

It will be apparent from this discussion of psychophysiological contributions to understanding the etiology and maintenance of physical illnesses that quite different types of relationship operate with different health outcomes. In conditions such as CHD, hypertension, and some metabolic and musculoskeletal disorders, the psychosocial evidence suggests that causal relationships may be present, and aberrant psychophysiological responses may contribute to the primary etiology of the condition. Such effects are best studied in longitudinal, population-based studies, which inevitably involve larger samples and longer time frames than are typically implemented in psychophysiology. In health problems related to infection, psychophysiological processes do not play a direct etiological role, but may have a permissive function in modulating host resistance so that the primary pathogen has a greater or lesser chance of causing disease. The research designs required to study these processes are quite different and involve experimental infection or more intense longitudinal tracking of the covariation between psychophysiological factors, exposure to pathogens, and illness. In a third set of health conditions including atopic and autoimmune illnesses, it is likely that the primary role of psychophysiological processes is in modulating disease course and mediating acute exacerbations in people with pre-existing illnesses. Investigations of these pathways require a clinical research approach and intensive studies of patients, so as to assess their psychophysiological responses to different life experiences and subsequent effects on health status.

Nevertheless, there are a number of commonalities across health problems in psychophysiological studies of disease etiology and progression in behavioral medicine and psychosomatics. The first is the importance of the interplay between background psychosocial conditions (e.g., life stress, social factors, and psychological characteristics), the acute or immediate psychosocial environment (e.g., momentary demands) and biological responses. These relationships must be understood if psychophysiological factors are to be put in context. Second, it is apparent that recent research in behavioral medicine and psychosomatics emphasizes the balance of responses in different physiological systems, rather than simple hyperreactivity. Some health conditions are associated with reduced physiological activity and some with heightened activity, but the complex interplay between biological systems always needs to be taken into account. Finally, it is striking how little research there has yet been into the manipulation of psychophysiological responses in order to understand disease etiology. A key tool in the armory of biomedical research is to interrupt postulated causal pathways in order to see whether this has the anticipated effect on the health outcome. There is of course extensive work on treatment in behavioral medicine, but little intervention with pharmacological, behavioral, or psychosocial methods in order to understand mechanisms. As these disciplines become more mature, it is essential that this approach be developed.

PSYCHOPHYSIOLOGY AND THE MANAGEMENT OF PHYSICAL ILLNESS

Much of the original impetus for behavioral medicine came from the promise of psychophysiological methods for managing physical illness. In the 1970s and 1980s, there was hope that biofeedback would revolutionize the treatment of chronic illness, allowing patients to become responsible for their own care by self-regulation of physiological functions that had not previously been regarded as amenable to voluntary control. Biofeedback was developed for the management of conditions such as epilepsy, hypertension, migraine, tension headache, asthma, and incontinence. Other psychophysiological techniques like progressive muscle relaxation and autogenic training were also brought into play and were advocated for the management of stress, tension, and psychosomatic problems.

The optimism surrounding these direct applications of psychophysiological techniques dissipated for a number of reasons: limited efficacy in randomized controlled trials, the immense amount of intervention required to generate effects (often incompatible with the constraints of managed care), the growth in clinical psychology of the cognitive-behavioral movement, and the introduction of more effective pharmaceutical agents. Biofeedback and allied methods have never joined the mainstream of medical care, but flourish in the complementary and alternative medicine sector. For example, the Association for Applied Psychophysiology and Biofeedback recommends the use of these methods for more than 30 conditions, including various types of pain, psychological, and behavioral problems such as anxiety, insomnia, and substance abuse as well as number of chronic medical conditions.

Nevertheless, the development of integrated stress management methods has led to psychophysiology retaining an important role in the management of physical illness. In this section, I will summarize evidence for the effects of direct psychophysiological therapies such as biofeedback and relaxation in the treatment of physical illness, then outline ways in which psychophysiological methods illuminate broader behavioral treatments such as cognitive-behavioral stress management.

Direct psychophysiological therapies

Direct psychophysiological therapies are treatments or interventions in which physiological monitoring plays a central role. The archetypal direct therapy is biofeedback, and this is applied in two different ways. First, biofeedback can involve the monitoring and provision of a feedback signal from the physiological measure, which is disturbed in a clinical condition, such as blood pressure in hypertension, blood flow in Raynaud's syndrome, and airways resistance in asthma. Second, biofeedback may involve learning voluntary control over a physiological system that is not a direct index of the disorder, but a correlate of it; two examples are the use of heart rate variability biofeedback in asthma and skin conductance biofeedback for hypertension. Biofeedback used in this way is often an adjunct to other direct physiological self-regulation therapies such as muscle relaxation and meditation techniques.

Hypertension

Direct blood pressure feedback was difficult to develop when biofeedback first emerged because conventional measures of blood pressure with a sphygmomanometer provide a reading every 30–60 seconds at best. If patients were provided with feedback of these readings, they would receive information about fewer than 5% of cardiac cycles, as well as ending up with rather sore arms through repeated squeezing. Imaginative adaptations of standard sphygmomanometry and indirect measures of blood pressure were devised, but curiously little research has used the continuous finger blood pressure measurement instruments based on vascular unloading such as the Finapres and Portapres. More research has been carried out with other psychophysiological methods like relaxation, thermal feedback, and meditation.

The methodological quality of research in this area has been limited with small samples, nonrandomized designs, inadequate comparison conditions, and poor characterization of participants (Blumenthal, Sherwood, Gullette, Georgiades, & Tweedy, 2002). A recent meta-analysis of studies using Transcendental Meditation, for example, was only able to locate one randomized trial that had involved documented hypertensives, even though the method has been advocated for this condition (Canter & Ernst, 2004). Another major difficulty lies in the establishment of an adequate baseline blood pressure against which to assess changes. Even if patients are not white coat hypertensives, levels tend to diminish with repeated testing, so treatments might apparently have effects that actually are due to adaptation. This was evident in Johnston et al.'s (1993) comparison of relaxation-based stress management with control procedures in 96 hypertensive patients. The intervention was preceded by a 12-week baseline period, during which blood pressure continued to fall, so that stress management generated no additional effect. Meta-analysis of relaxation and biofeedback studies in hypertension indicates that effects are no greater than those stimulated by nonspecific behavioral treatment comparisons (Nakao, Yano, Nomura, & Kuboki, 2003). It is notable that in evidence-based guidelines, direct psychophysiological approaches such as relaxation and biofeedback are given little attention compared with behavioral methods such as weight reduction through physical activity and dietary change, restriction of salt intake, control of alcohol intake, and methods of improving adherence to medication (Chobanian et al., 2003).

Bronchial asthma

Asthma might be considered a more promising target for psychophysiological treatments because direct noninvasive measures of lung function and airways resistance are available. However, the implementation of direct biofeedback of airways function has proved difficult with only limited effects after prolonged training (Ritz, Dahme, & Roth, 2004). One difficulty is that patients often resort to active respiratory maneuvers to reduce airways resistance, for example, increasing functional residual capacity, and these are not therapeutic in the long run. Indirect feedback of frontalis EMG has generated more positive effects, but studies have suffered from various design flaws (Ritz et al., 2004).

A promising application of heart rate variability biofeedback was recently developed by Lehrer and coworkers (2004). Ninety-four adult asthmatics were randomized to heart rate variability feedback coupled with abdominal breathing training, heart rate variability feedback alone, placebo biofeedback (EEG training), and waiting list control. The study involved extensive respiratory assessments and monitoring of medication by a physician blinded to treatment allocation. The two heart rate variability feedback groups showed significant reductions in medication over the 10-week treatment in comparison with controls. This result is intriguing, not least because it appears to be contrary to the known effects of autonomic regulation on asthma. As noted on page 736, increases in parasympathetic or vagal activity stimulate bronchoconstriction. Heart rate variability biofeedback is intended to increase parasympathetic control, so precisely how it may promote bronchodilation is puzzling (Ritz et al., 2004).

Epilepsy

One of the earliest applications of biofeedback involved the monitoring of EEG and provision of feedback to epileptics of rhythms considered to be incompatible with seizure activity (Sterman, 2000). Despite the efforts of pioneers in this field, the approach has remained experimental and has been little used outside a few centers. Promising results have been reported for the self-regulation of slow cortical potentials with substantial reductions of seizure activity in about a third of patients who adhere to training (Strehl, Kotchoubey, Trevorrow, & Birbaumer, 2005). However, few clients and physicians have the patience and resources to persist with the prolonged training over months that appear to be required.

Pain conditions

Behavioral medicine approaches to the management of pain in arthritis and cancer have not been psychophysiological in orientation, but have emphasized coping skills training, emotional disclosure and pain education (Keefe, Abernethy, & Campbell, 2005). The pain conditions in which psychophysiological methods have been more prominent are in migraine and tension-type headache. The early applications of psychophysiological methods were based on pathophysiology models that emphasized the role of contraction of muscles in the head and neck in the etiology of tension-type headache and the effects of paroxysmal vasodilation of the cranial circulation in migraine headache (Holroyd, 2002). Thus, thermal feedback, relaxation, and EMG biofeedback were applied to migraines, while EMG feedback and relaxation were the main methods used with tension-type headaches.

These pathophysiological models have been revised substantially over recent years. Tension-type headaches are now thought to result from central nervous system (CNS) dysfunction rather than heightened peripheral nerve input with sensitization of pain pathways and reduced thresholds for transmission to higher centers (Ashina, 2004). Migraine is thought to be a CNS rather than vascular problem in which there are disturbances in activation of the trigeminal innervation of the vascular system and CNS modulation of trigeminal pain (Goadsby, 2005). Nevertheless, meta-analyses indicate that behavioral treatments are efficacious, with effect sizes of 0.75 to 1.25 for relaxation, biofeedback, and other psychophysiological methods (Holroyd, 2002). The explanation may be that these techniques work through cognitive-attributional pathways rather than directly through regulating physiological dysfunction, although it should be pointed out that many studies have involved small samples of nonrepresentative participants with weak control conditions and limited evidence of generalisability (Rains, Penzien, McCrory, & Gray, 2005). These problems need to be rectified if psychophysiological methods are to gain widespread acceptance as therapies.

Psychophysiological aspects of behavioral treatments

As noted earlier, many of the interventions and treatments used in behavioral medicine and psychosomatics are not psychophysiological in orientation, but involve techniques such as cognitive-behavioral therapy, attitude change, coping skills training, behavioral modification, and social support intervention (Slater et al., 2003). The emphasis even in the management of disorders such as hypertension, diabetes, and arthritis is not on psychophysiological methods, but lifestyle modification, self-monitoring, education, and skill training (Astin, Beckner, Soeken, Hochberg, & Berman, 2002; Blumenthal et al., 2002; Ismail, Winkley, & Rabe-Hesketh, 2004). Nevertheless, psychophysiology has a role to play in the broader remit of behavioral medicine, even when it is not the primary intervention modality.

Objective indicators of physiological change

The first role of psychophysiology is to provide objective information about the impact of cognitive-behavioral methods on biological function. It has been known for many decades that the effect of relaxation training and other behavioral arousal control methods is the reverse of stress activation, which result in reduced muscle tension, lower heart rate and blood pressure, and increases in alpha wave activity in the EEG. These effects of stress management on biological function have been confirmed with measures of neuroendocrine and autonomic activity. For instance, Antoni and colleagues (2000; 2000) randomized HIV+ men to group-based cognitive-behavioral stress management or a waiting list control condition. After the 10-week training period, there were significantly lower levels of anxiety and perceived stress following stress management coupled with reduced 24-hour excretion of norepinephrine and cortisol. The reduction in cortisol correlated with decreases in depressed mood, while anxiety changes correlated with norepinephrine responses. The evaluation of other behavioral interventions also benefits from psychophysiological assessment. An example is the effect of exercise training on resting heart rate, which is thought to be due partly to enhanced vagal modula-

tion. Sandercock, Bromley, and Brodie (2005) have carried out a meta-analysis of heart rate variability measures in response to exercise training. In 13 studies assessing heart rate variability by spectral analysis, there was a consistent increase in high frequency power with a medium effect size of 0.48.

The impact of behavioral intervention on disease markers

The psychophysiological measures described in the last section were employed as nonspecific indicators of physiological activation. A more interesting use of psychophysiology is in evaluating the impact of behavioral interventions on processes that are directly related to disease. In these applications, psychophysiology provides information about the effects of treatments on the putative biological targets of therapeutic effects. At its simplest, this merely involves the measurement of a biological marker of disease state. For instance, the majority of psychological interventions for the management of Type 2 diabetes have involved assessments of blood glucose level or glycated hemoglobin as markers of glycemic control (Ismail et al., 2004). But nuanced evaluations are also possible.

An instance is the assessment of the effects of emotional disclosure. The idea that the written expression of emotional material might be therapeutic was formulated by Pennebaker in the 1980s. Since then, numerous studies have reported potential benefits in relatively healthy groups in terms of physician visits, mood, and self-rated health (Smyth, 1998). Effects have also been recorded on symptom levels in conditions such as rheumatoid arthritis and fibromyalgia (Broderick, Junghaenel, & Schwartz, 2005; Smyth, Stone, Hurewitz, & Kaell, 1999). One problem with such findings is that they might reflect effects on symptom reporting and subjective status only and not on objective function. Psychophysiological methods have, therefore, been used to corroborate these results and discover whether effects are present at the biological level as well. Smyth et al. (1999) randomized asthmatic patients to write about stressful events or emotionally neutral topics, and found four months later that lung function assessed spirometrically had improved by more than 15% in the emotional disclosure group. Unfortunately, this effect has not been replicated in a more recent trial (Harris, Thoresen, Humphreys, & Faul, 2005). Petrie, Booth, Pennebaker, Davison, and Thomas (1995) examined the impact of emotional expression on antibody responses to vaccination. Forty medical students wrote about personal traumatic experiences or neutral topics for four consecutive days. They were then vaccinated against hepatitis B and antibodies were assessed at four and six months. The antibody levels were greater in the emotional expression group, and are indicative of more effective immune responses to the vaccination. Favorable effects on immune function in HIV+ individuals have also been observed (Petrie, Fontanilla, Thomas, Booth, & Pennebaker, 2004).

A more elaborate use of psychophysiological methods to evaluate behavioral intervention is found in a recent study of the effects of physical activity training and stress management in CHD patients (Blumenthal et al., 2005). One hundred thirty-four patients with documented CHD were randomized to routine care, 16 weeks of supervised aerobic training or 16 weekly sessions of stress management, which involved education, coping skills training, relaxation training, and social support. The evaluation included assessments of mental stress-induced myocardial ischemia and cardiac wall motion abnormalities (see page 729), vascular endothelial function, and heart rate variability. It was found that after training, both the aerobic and stress management groups showed reduced myocardial ischemia in response to mental stress, and improved endothelial function. Additionally, heart rate variability and baroreceptor reflex sensitivity were enhanced in the stress management condition but not the aerobic training group. These findings suggest that the behavioral interventions had positive effects on markers of clinical risk, even though the study was not large enough to detect differences in hard clinical endpoints.

Combining psychophysiological with medical interventions

One of the principal methods of determining causality in biomedical research is to modify putative causal pathways and assess impact on outcome. Unfortunately, psychophysiological methods have not yet been used extensively to test causal models in this way, for example, by blocking physiological responses to determine whether they are the mediators of psychosocial influence on disease. Such an approach has been used in animal research, for example, by using beta-adrenergic blockade to assess whether sympathetic activation mediates the impact of social stress on atherosclerosis development in primates (Kaplan, Pettersson, Manuck, & Olsson, 1991). At present intervention approaches have yet to be exploited fully in psychophysiological research in many health care settings.

Nevertheless, a limited amount of research has combined psychophysiological with pharmacological methods in disease management. A good example is the combination of relaxation-based stress management and antidepressants in the treatment of tension-type headaches reported by Holroyd et al. (2001). Two hundred three chronic headache patients were randomized to tricyclic antidepressants, antidepressants combined with brief stress management training, stress management plus placebo medication, or placebo medication only. Both antidepressants and stress management stimulated larger reductions in headache activity, disability, and analgesic use than did placebo, but the effects of antidepressants were more rapid. Interestingly, a higher proportion of patients in the combined treatment group showed clinically significant ($\geq$50%) reductions in headache index scores than did those in the antidepressant only condition

(64% versus 38%), and suggests that a combined approach may be fruitful.

CONCLUSIONS

Psychophysiology is a pivotal discipline in behavioral medicine and psychosomatics, and complements work in the psychosocial, behavioral, and cognitive domains. Psychophysiology plays a central role in understanding how life experiences and psychological characteristics relevant to health get under the skin and affect the development and management of physical health problems. The panoply of psychophysiological methods has still not been fully exploited in behavioral medicine. Techniques such as CNS imaging, genetic analysis, and molecular biological approaches to gene expression will become more prominent in this field over the next decade. We are also likely to see greater integration of behavioral medicine work on systemic diseases with studies of behavioral and psychiatric problems. Already there are commonalities emerging, for example, in research linking central serotonergic function both with problems of depression and aggression as well as with cardiovascular and metabolic disease (Manuck, Flory, Muldoon, & Ferrell, 2002; Muldoon et al., 2004). At the same time, behavioral medicine and psychosomatics must prompt psychophysiologists to take a broader conceptualization of their discipline. Population-based approaches to study sampling, as opposed to the psychophysiological tradition of convenience sampling, is becoming mandatory in this context. The integration of psychophysiological techniques into biomedical etiological studies requires larger samples and prospective designs. The evolution of clinical trials methodology embodied in consensus documents such as the CONSORT guidelines means that psychophysiologists need to attend to a wider set of design issues if they wish their work to become part of evidence-based medicine (Moher, Schulz, & Altman, 2001). Psychophysiologists working in behavioral medicine and psychosomatics are taking up these challenges and this is likely to result in a new era of research in which psychophysiological methods have an even greater impact on health and health care.

ACKNOWLEDGMENT

The preparation of this chapter was supported by the British Heart Foundation.

REFERENCES

Ackerman, K. D., Stover, A., Heyman, R., Anderson, B. P., Houck, P. R., Frank, E., et al. (2003). Relationship of cardiovascular reactivity, stressful life events, and multiple sclerosis disease activity. *Brain, Behavior and Immunity, 17,* 141–151.

American Heart Association. (2005). *Heart and Stroke Statistical – 2005 Update.* Dallas: American Heart Association.

Antoni, M. H., Cruess, D. G., Cruess, S., Lutgendorf, S., Kumar, M., Ironson, G., et al. (2000). Cognitive-behavioral stress management intervention effects on anxiety, 24-hr urinary norepinephrine output, and T-cytotoxic/suppressor cells over time among symptomatic HIV-infected gay men. *Journal of Consulting and Clinical Psychology, 68*, 31–45.

Antoni, M. H., Cruess, S., Cruess, D. G., Kumar, M., Lutgendorf, S., Ironson, G., et al. (2000). Cognitive-behavioral stress management reduces distress and 24-hour urinary free cortisol output among symptomatic HIV-infected gay men. *Annals of Behavioral Medicine, 22*, 29–37.

Ashina, M. (2004). Neurobiology of chronic tension-type headache. *Cephalalgia, 24*, 161–172.

Astin, J. A., Beckner, W., Soeken, K., Hochberg, M. C., & Berman, B. (2002). Psychological interventions for rheumatoid arthritis: a meta-analysis of randomized controlled trials. *Arthritis and Rheumatism, 47*, 291–302.

Barnes, V. A., Treiber, F. A., Davis, H., Kelley, T. R., & Strong, W. B. (1998). Central adiposity and hemodynamic functioning at rest and during stress in adolescents. *International Journal of Obesity, 22*, 1079–1083.

Barnett, R. C., Steptoe, A., & Gareis, K. C. (2005). Marital-role quality and stress-related psychobiological indicators. *Annals of Behavioral Medicine, 30*, 36–43.

Björntorp, P. (2001). Do stress reactions cause abdominal obesity and comorbidities? *Obesity Reviews, 2*, 73–86.

Blumenthal, J. A., Sherwood, A., Babyak, M. A., Watkins, L. L., Waugh, R., Georgiades, A., et al. (2005). Effects of exercise and stress management training on markers of cardiovascular risk in patients with ischemic heart disease: a randomized controlled trial. *Journal of the American Medical Association, 293*, 1626–1634.

Blumenthal, J. A., Sherwood, A., Gullette, E. C., Georgiades, A., & Tweedy, D. (2002). Biobehavioral approaches to the treatment of essential hypertension. *Journal of Consulting and Clinical Psychology, 70*, 569–589.

Bongers, P. M., Kremer, A. M., & ter Laak, J. (2002). Are psychosocial factors, risk factors for symptoms and signs of the shoulder, elbow, or hand/wrist?: A review of the epidemiological literature. *American Journal of Industrial Medicine, 41*, 315–342.

British Heart Foundation. (2004). *Coronary Heart Disease Statistics*. London: British Heart Foundation.

Broadley, A. J., Korszun, A., Abdelaal, E., Moskvina, V., Jones, C. J., Nash, G. B., et al. (2005). Inhibition of cortisol production with metyrapone prevents mental stress-induced endothelial dysfunction and baroreflex impairment. *Journal of the American College of Cardiology, 46*, 344–350.

Broadley, A. J., Korszun, A., Jones, C. J., & Frenneaux, M. P. (2002). Arterial endothelial function is impaired in treated depression. *Heart, 88*, 521–523.

Broderick, J. E., Junghaenel, D. U., & Schwartz, J. E. (2005). Written emotional expression produces health benefits in fibromyalgia patients. *Psychosomatic Medicine, 67*, 326–334.

Brown, R. F., Tennant, C. C., Dunn, S. M., & Pollard, J. D. (2005). A review of stress-relapse interactions in multiple sclerosis: important features and stress-mediating and -moderating variables. *Multiple Sclerosis, 11*, 477–484.

Brunner, E., Davey Smith, G., Marmot, M., Canner, R., Beksinska, M., & O'Brien, J. (1996). Childhood social circumstances and psychosocial and behavioral factors as determinants of plasma fibrinogen. *Lancet, 347*, 1008–1013.

Brunner, E. J., Hemingway, H., Walker, B. R., Page, M., Clarke, P., Juneja, M., et al. (2002). Adrenocortical, autonomic, and inflammatory causes of the metabolic syndrome: nested case-control study. *Circulation, 106*, 2659–2665.

Brydon, L., Edwards, S., Mohamed-Ali, V., & Steptoe, A. (2004). Socioeconomic status and stress-induced increases in interleukin-6. *Brain, Behavior, and Immunity, 18*, 281–290.

Brydon, L., & Steptoe, A. (2005). Stress-induced increases in interleukin-6 and fibrinogen predict ambulatory blood pressure at 3-year follow-up. *Journal of Hypertension, 23*, 1001–1007.

Burns, V. E., Ring, C., Drayson, M., & Carroll, D. (2002). Cortisol and cardiovascular reactions to mental stress and antibody status following hepatitis B vaccination: a preliminary study. *Psychophysiology, 39*, 361–368.

Buske-Kirschbaum, A., Auer, K. von, Krieger, S., Weis, S., Rauh, W., & Hellhammer, D. (2003). Blunted cortisol responses to psychosocial stress in asthmatic children: a general feature of atopic disease? *Psychosomatic Medicine, 65*, 806–810.

Buske-Kirschbaum, A., Fischbach, S., Rauh, W., Hanker, J., & Hellhammer, D. (2004). Increased responsiveness of the hypothalamus-pituitary-adrenal (HPA) axis to stress in newborns with atopic disposition. *Psychoneuroendocrinology, 29*, 705–711.

Buske-Kirschbaum, A., Jobst, S., Wustmans, A., Kirschbaum, C., Rauh, W., & Hellhammer, D. (1997). Attenuated free cortisol response to psychosocial stress in children with atopic dermatitis. *Psychosomatic Medicine, 59*, 419–426.

Cacioppo, J., Kiecolt-Glaser, J., Malarkey, W., Laskowski, B., Rozlog, L., Poehlmann, K., et al. (2002). Autonomic and glucocorticoid associations with the steady-state expression of latent Epstein-Barr virus. *Hormones and Behavior, 42*, 32.

Canter, P. H., & Ernst, E. (2004). Insufficient evidence to conclude whether or not Transcendental Meditation decreases blood pressure: results of a systematic review of randomized clinical trials. *Journal of Hypertension, 22*, 2049–2054.

Carney, R. M., Blumenthal, J. A., Freedland, K. E., Stein, P. K., Howells, W. B., Berkman, L. F., et al. (2005). Low heart rate variability and the effect of depression on post-myocardial infarction mortality. *Archives of Internal Medicine, 165*, 1486–1491.

Carney, R. M., Blumenthal, J. A., Stein, P. K., Watkins, L., Catellier, D., Berkman, L. F., et al. (2001). Depression, heart rate variability, and acute myocardial infarction. *Circulation, 104*, 2024–2028.

Carroll, D., Ring, C., Hunt, K., Ford, G., & Macintyre, S. (2003). Blood pressure reactions to stress and the prediction of future blood pressure: effects of sex, age, and socioeconomic position. *Psychosomatic Medicine, 65*, 1058–1064.

Carroll, D., Smith, G. D., Shipley, M. J., Steptoe, A., Brunner, E. J., & Marmot, M. G. (2001). Blood pressure reactions to acute psychological stress and future blood pressure status: a 10-year follow-up of men in the Whitehall II study. *Psychosomatic Medicine, 63*, 737–743.

Chae, C. U., Lee, R. T., Rifai, N., & Ridker, P. M. (2001). Blood pressure and inflammation in apparently healthy men. *Hypertension, 38*, 399–403.

Chobanian, A. V., Bakris, G. L., Black, H. R., Cushman, W. C., Green, L. A., Izzo, J. L., Jr., et al. (2003). The Seventh Report of the Joint National Committee on Prevention, Detection, Evaluation, and Treatment of High Blood Pressure: the JNC 7 report. *Journal of the American Medical Association, 289*, 2560–2572.

Chrysohoou, C., Pitsavos, C., Panagiotakos, D. B., Skoumas, J., & Stefanadis, C. (2004). Association between prehypertension status and inflammatory markers related to atherosclerotic disease: The ATTICA Study. *American Journal of Hypertension, 17*, 568–573.

Cohen, F., Kemeny, M. E., Kearney, K. A., Zegans, L. S., Neuhaus, J. M., & Conant, M. A. (1999). Persistent stress as a predictor of genital herpes recurrence. *Archives of Internal Medicine, 159*, 2430–2436.

Cohen, S., Doyle, W. J., & Skoner, D. P. (1999). Psychological stress, cytokine production, and severity of upper respiratory illness. *Psychosomatic Medicine, 61*, 175–180.

Cohen, S., Doyle, W. J., Turner, R. B., Alper, C. M., & Skoner, D. P. (2003). Emotional style and susceptibility to the common cold. *Psychosomatic Medicine, 65*, 652–657.

Cohen, S., Line, S., Manuck, S. B., Rabin, B. S., Heise, E. R., & Kaplan, J. R. (1997). Chronic social stress, social status, and susceptibility to upper respiratory infections in nonhuman primates. *Psychosomatic Medicine, 59*, 213–221.

Cohen, S., Tyrrell, D. A. J., & Smith, A. P. (1991). Psychosocial stress and susceptibility to the common cold. *New England Journal of Medicine, 325*, 606–612.

Cohen, S., & Williamson, G. M. (1991). Stress and infectious disease in humans. *Psychological Bulletin, 109*, 5–24.

Cosgrove, M. (2004). Do stressful life events cause type 1 diabetes? *Occupational Medicine (London), 54*, 250–254.

Dahlen, I., & Janson, C. (2002). Anxiety and depression are related to the outcome of emergency treatment in patients with obstructive pulmonary disease. *Chest, 122*, 1633–1637.

Davey Smith, G., Ben-Shlomo, Y., Beswick, A., Yarnell, J., Lightman, S., & Elwood, P. (2005). Cortisol, testosterone, and coronary heart disease: prospective evidence from the Caerphilly study. *Circulation, 112*, 332–340.

Davies, M. J. (1996). Stability and instability: two faces of coronary atherosclerosis. The Paul Dudley White Lecture 1995. *Circulation, 94*, 2013–2020.

Davis, K. G., Marras, W. S., Heaney, C. A., Waters, T. R., & Gupta, P. (2002). The impact of mental processing and pacing on spine loading: 2002 Volvo Award in biomechanics. *Spine, 27*, 2645–2653.

DeFrank, R. S., Jenkins, C. D., & Rose, R. M. (1987). A longitudinal investigation of the relationships among alcohol consumption, psychosocial factors, and blood pressure. *Psychosomatic Medicine, 49*, 236–249.

de Groot, M., Anderson, R., Freedland, K. E., Clouse, R. E., & Lustman, P. J. (2001). Association of depression and diabetes complications: a meta-analysis. *Psychosomatic Medicine, 63*, 619–630.

de Visser, D. C., van Hooft, I. M., van Doornen, L. J., Hofman, A., Orlebeke, J. F., & Grobbee, D. E. (1995). Cardiovascular response to mental stress in offspring of hypertensive parents: the Dutch Hypertension and Offspring Study. *Journal of Hypertension, 13*, 901–908.

Demange, V., Guillemin, F., Baumann, M., Suurmeijer, T. P., Moum, T., Doeglas, D., et al. (2004). Are there more than cross-sectional relationships of social support and support networks with functional limitations and psychological distress in early rheumatoid arthritis? *Arthritis and Rheumatism, 51*, 782–791.

Diez-Roux, A. V., Nieto, F. J., Tyroler, H. A., Crum, L. D., & Szklo, M. (1995). Social inequalities and atherosclerosis. The atherosclerosis risk in communities study. *American Journal of Epidemiology, 141*, 960–972.

Epel, E. S., McEwen, B., Seeman, T., Matthews, K., Castellazzo, G., Brownell, K. D., et al. (2000). Stress and body shape: stress-induced cortisol secretion is consistently greater among women with central fat. *Psychosomatic Medicine, 62*, 623–632.

Everson, S. A., Lynch, J. W., Chesney, M. A., Kaplan, G. A., Goldberg, D. E., Shade, S. B., et al. (1997a). Interaction of workplace demands and cardiovascular reactivity in progression of carotid atherosclerosis: population based study. *British Medical Journal, 314*, 553–558.

Everson, S. A., Lynch, J. W., Chesney, M. A., Kaplan, G. A., Goldberg, D. E., Shade, S. B., et al. (1997b). Interaction of workplace demands and cardiovascular reactivity in progression of carotid atherosclerosis: population based study. *British Medical Journal, 314*, 553–558.

Everson-Rose, S. A., & Lewis, T. T. (2005). Psychosocial factors and cardiovascular diseases. *Annual Review of Public Health, 26*, 469–500.

Everson-Rose, S. A., Meyer, P. M., Powell, L. H., Pandey, D., Torrens, J. I., Kravitz, H. M., et al. (2004). Depressive symptoms, insulin resistance, and risk of diabetes in women at midlife. *Diabetes Care, 27*, 2856–2862.

Ford, D. E., & Erlinger, T. P. (2004). Depression and C-reactive protein in US adults: data from the Third National Health and Nutrition Examination Survey. *Archives of Internal Medicine, 164*, 1010–1014.

Gabbay, F. H., Krantz, D. S., Kop, W. J., Hedges, S. M., Klein, J., Gottdiener, J. S., et al. (1996). Triggers of myocardial ischemia during daily life in patients with coronary artery disease: physical and mental activities, anger and smoking. *Journal of the American College of Cardiology, 27*, 585–592.

Gallo, L. C., Troxel, W. M., Kuller, L. H., Sutton-Tyrrell, K., Edmundowicz, D., & Matthews, K. A. (2003). Marital status, marital quality, and atherosclerotic burden in postmenopausal women. *Psychosomatic Medicine, 65*, 952–962.

Garde, A. H., Laursen, B., Jorgensen, A. H., & Jensen, B. R. (2002). Effects of mental and physical demands on heart rate variability during computer work. *European Journal of Applied Physiology, 87*, 456–461.

Gehi, A., Mangano, D., Pipkin, S., Browner, W. S., & Whooley, M. A. (2005). Depression and heart rate variability in patients with stable coronary heart disease: findings from the Heart and Soul Study. *Archives of General Psychiatry, 62*, 661–666.

Gerin, W., & Pickering, T. G. (1995). Association between delayed recovery of blood pressure after acute mental stress and parental history of hypertension. *Journal of Hypertension, 13*, 603–610.

Ghiadoni, L., Donald, A., Cropley, M., Mullen, M. J., Oakley, G., Taylor, M., et al. (2000). Mental stress induces transient endothelial dysfunction in humans. *Circulation, 102*, 2473–2478.

Goadsby, P. J. (2005). Migraine pathophysiology. *Headache, 45* (Suppl. 1), S14–24.

Grippo, A. J., Santos, C. M., Johnson, R. F., Beltz, T. G., Martins, J. B., Felder, R. B., et al. (2004). Increased susceptibility to ventricular arrhythmias in a rodent model of experimental depression. *American Journal of Physiology, 286*, H619–626.

Gullette, E. C., Blumenthal, J. A., Babyak, M., Jiang, W., Waugh, R. A., Frid, D. J., et al. (1997). Effects of mental stress on myocardial ischemia during daily life. *Journal of the American Medical Association, 277,* 1521–1526.

Gupta, M. A., & Gupta, A. K. (2003). Psychiatric and psychological co-morbidity in patients with dermatologic disorders: epidemiology and management. *American Journal of Clinical Dermatology, 4,* 833–842.

Gustavsen, P. H., Hoegholm, A., Bang, L. E., & Kristensen, K. S. (2003). White coat hypertension is a cardiovascular risk factor: a 10-year follow-up study. *Journal of Human Hypertension, 17,* 811–817.

Haas, D. C., Davidson, K. W., Schwartz, D. J., Rieckmann, N., Roman, M. J., Pickering, T. G., et al. (2005). Depressive symptoms are independently predictive of carotid atherosclerosis. *American Journal of Cardiology, 95,* 547–550.

Hagg, G. M., & Astrom, A. (1997). Load pattern and pressure pain threshold in the upper trapezius muscle and psychosocial factors in medical secretaries with and without shoulder/neck disorders. *International Archive of Occupational and Environmental Health, 69,* 423–432.

Harris, A. H., Thoresen, C. E., Humphreys, K., & Faul, J. (2005). Does writing affect asthma? A randomized trial. *Psychosomatic Medicine, 67,* 130–136.

Heesen, C., Koehler, G., Gross, R., Tessmer, W., Schulz, K. H., & Gold, S. M. (2005). Altered cytokine responses to cognitive stress in multiple sclerosis patients with fatigue. *Multiple Sclerosis, 11,* 51–57.

Hemingway, H., Shipley, M., Brunner, E., Britton, A., Malik, M., & Marmot, M. (2005). Does autonomic function link social position to coronary risk? The Whitehall II study. *Circulation, 111,* 3071–3077.

Herrmann, M., Scholmerich, J., & Straub, R. H. (2000). Stress and rheumatic diseases. *Rheumatic Disease Clinics of North America, 26,* 737–763.

Holroyd, K. A. (2002). Assessment and psychological management of recurrent headache disorders. *Journal of Consulting and Clinical Psychology, 70,* 656–677.

Holroyd, K. A., O'Donnell, F. J., Stensland, M., Lipchik, G. L., Cordingley, G. E., & Carlson, B. W. (2001). Management of chronic tension-type headache with tricyclic antidepressant medication, stress management therapy, and their combination: a randomized controlled trial. *Journal of the American Medical Association, 285,* 2208–2215.

Horsten, M., Mittleman, M. A., Wamala, S. P., Schenck-Gustafsson, K., & Orth-Gomer, K. (1999). Social relations and the metabolic syndrome in middle-aged Swedish women. *Journal of Cardiovascular Risk, 6,* 391–397.

Institute of Medicine. (2001). *Musculoskeletal Disorders in the Workplace: Low Back and Upper Extremities.* Washington, D.C.: National Academy Press.

Intengan, H. D., & Schiffrin, E. L. (2001). Vascular remodeling in hypertension: roles of apoptosis, inflammation, and fibrosis. *Hypertension, 38,* 581–587.

Ismail, K., Winkley, K., & Rabe-Hesketh, S. (2004). Systematic review and meta-analysis of randomized controlled trials of psychological interventions to improve glycemic control in patients with type 2 diabetes. *Lancet, 363,* 1589–1597.

Iso, H., Date, C., Yamamoto, A., Toyoshima, H., Tanabe, N., Kikuchi, S., et al. (2002). Perceived mental stress and mortality from cardiovascular disease among Japanese men and women: the Japan Collaborative Cohort Study for Evaluation of Cancer Risk Sponsored by Monbusho (JACC Study). *Circulation, 106,* 1229–1236.

Jacobs, R., Pawlak, C. R., Mikeska, E., Meyer-Olson, D., Martin, M., Heijnen, C. J., et al. (2001). Systemic lupus erythematosus and rheumatoid arthritis patients differ from healthy controls in their cytokine pattern after stress exposure. *Rheumatology (Oxford), 40,* 868–875.

Janumpally, S. R., Feldman, S. R., Gupta, A. K., & Fleischer, A. B., Jr. (2002). In the United States, blacks and Asian/Pacific Islanders are more likely than whites to seek medical care for atopic dermatitis. *Archives of Dermatology, 138,* 634–637.

Jennings, J. R., Kamarck, T. W., Everson-Rose, S. A., Kaplan, G. A., Manuck, S. B., & Salonen, J. T. (2004). Exaggerated blood pressure responses during mental stress are prospectively related to enhanced carotid atherosclerosis in middle-aged Finnish men. *Circulation, 110,* 2198–2203.

Jern, S., Bergbrant, A., Bjorntorp, P., & Hansson, L. (1992). Relation of central hemodynamics to obesity and body fat distribution. *Hypertension, 19,* 520–527.

Johnston, D. W., Gold, A., Kentish, J., Smith, D., Vallance, P., Shah, D., Leach, G., et al. (1993). Effect of stress management on blood pressure in mild primary hypertension. *British Medical Journal, 306,* 963–966.

Jonas, B. S., & Lando, J. F. (2000). Negative affect as a prospective risk factor for hypertension. *Psychosomatic Medicine, 62,* 188–196.

Jorgensen, R. S., Johnson, B. T., Schreer, G. E., & Kolodziej, M. E. (1996). Elevated blood pressure and personality: a meta-analytic review. *Psychological Bulletin, 120,* 293–320.

Kanel, R. von, Dimsdale, J. E., Adler, K. A., Patterson, T. L., Mills, P. J., & Grant, I. (2004). Effects of depressive symptoms and anxiety on hemostatic responses to acute mental stress and recovery in the elderly. *Psychiatry Research, 126,* 253–264.

Kanel, R. von, Mills, P. J., Fainman, C., & Dimsdale, J. E. (2001). Effects of psychological stress and psychiatric disorders on blood coagulation and fibrinolysis: a biobehavioral pathway to coronary artery disease? *Psychosomatic Medicine, 63,* 531–544.

Kaplan, J. R., Pettersson, K., Manuck, S. B., & Olsson, G. (1991). Role of sympathoadrenal medullary activation in the initiation and progression of atherosclerosis. *Circulation, 84,* VI23–32.

Katon, W. J., Richardson, L., Lozano, P., & McCauley, E. (2004). The relationship of asthma and anxiety disorders. *Psychosomatic Medicine, 66,* 349–355.

Keefe, F. J., Abernethy, A. P., & Campbell, L. C. (2005). Psychological approaches to understanding and treating disease-related pain. *Annual Review of Psychology, 56,* 601–630.

Kemmer, F. W., Bisping, R., Steingruber, H. J., Baar, H., Hardtmann, F., Schlaghecke, R., et al. (1986). Psychological stress and metabolic control in patients with type I diabetes mellitus. *New England Journal of Medicine, 314,* 1078–1084.

Kiecolt-Glaser, J. K., Glaser, R., Gravenstein, S., Malarkey, W. B., & Sheridan, J. (1996). Chronic stress alters the immune response to influenza virus vaccine in older adults. *Proceedings of the National Academy of Sciences of the United States of America, 93,* 3043–3047.

Kiecolt-Glaser, J. K., Preacher, K. J., MacCallum, R. C., Atkinson, C., Malarkey, W. B., & Glaser, R. (2003). Chronic stress and age-related increases in the proinflammatory cytokine IL-6. *Proceedings of the National Academy of Sciences of the United States of America, 100,* 9090–9095.

Kim, C. K., McGorray, S. P., Bartholomew, B. A., Marsh, M., Dicken, T., Wassertheil-Smoller, S., et al. (2005). Depressive symptoms and heart rate variability in postmenopausal women. *Archives of Internal Medicine, 165,* 1239–1244.

Klumb, P. L., & Lampert, T. (2004). Women, work, and well-being 1950–2000: a review and methodological critique. *Social Science and Medicine, 58*, 1007–1024.

Knox, S. S., Weidner, G., Adelman, A., Stoney, C. M., & Ellison, R. C. (2004). Hostility and physiological risk in the National Heart, Lung, and Blood Institute Family Heart Study. *Archives of Internal Medicine, 164*, 2442–2448.

Kop, W. J., Verdino, R. J., Gottdiener, J. S., O'Leary, S. T., Bairey Merz, C. N., & Krantz, D. S. (2001). Changes in heart rate and heart rate variability before ambulatory ischemic events. *Journal of the American College of Cardiology, 38*, 742–749.

Krantz, D. S., Santiago, H. T., Kop, W. J., Merz, C. N. B., Rozanski, A., & Gottdiener, J. S. (1999). Prognostic value of mental stress testing in coronary artery disease. *American Journal of Cardiology, 84*, 1292–1297.

Kumari, M., Head, J., & Marmot, M. (2004). Prospective study of social and other risk factors for incidence of type 2 diabetes in the Whitehall II study. *Archives of Internal Medicine, 164*, 1873–1880.

Kumari, M., Marmot, M., & Brunner, E. (2000). Social determinants of von Willebrand factor: the Whitehall II study. *Arteriosclerosis, Thrombosis and Vascular Biology, 20*, 1842–1847.

Kuper, H., Marmot, M., & Hemingway, H. (2005). Systematic review of prospective cohort studies of psychosocial factors in the etiology and prognosis of coronary heart disease. In P. Elliott & M. Marmot (Eds.), *Coronary Heart Disease Epidemiology*, (2nd ed., pp. 363–413). Oxford: Oxford University Press.

Lampert, R., Joska, T., Burg, M. M., Batsford, W. P., McPherson, C. A., & Jain, D. (2002). Emotional and physical precipitants of ventricular arrhythmia. *Circulation, 106*, 1800–1805.

Landsbergis, P. A., Schnall, P. L., Pickering, T. G., Warren, K., & Schwartz, J. E. (2003). Life-course exposure to job strain and ambulatory blood pressure in men. *American Journal of Epidemiology, 157*, 998–1006.

Lantelme, P., Milon, H., Gharib, C., Gayet, C., & Fortrat, J. O. (1998). White coat effect and reactivity to stress: cardiovascular and autonomic nervous system responses. *Hypertension, 31*, 1021–1029.

La Rovere, M. T., Bigger, J. T. J., Marcus, F. I., Mortara, A., & Schwartz, P. J. (1998). Baroreflex sensitivity and heart-rate variability in prediction of total cardiac mortality after myocardial infarction. *Lancet, 351*, 478–484.

Laursen, B., Jensen, B. R., Garde, A. H., & Jorgensen, A. H. (2002). Effect of mental and physical demands on muscular activity during the use of a computer mouse and a keyboard. *Scandinavian Journal of Work and Environmental Health, 28*, 215–221.

Lawlor, D. A., Smith, G. D., & Ebrahim, S. (2003). Association of insulin resistance with depression: cross sectional findings from the British Women's Heart and Health Study. *British Medical Journal, 327*, 1383–1384.

Lee, S., Colditz, G. A., Berkman, L. F., & Kawachi, I. (2003). Caregiving and risk of coronary heart disease in U.S. women: a prospective study. *American Journal of Preventive Medicine, 24*, 113–119.

Lehrer, P. M., Vaschillo, E., Vaschillo, B., Lu, S. E., Scardella, A., Siddique, M., et al. (2004). Biofeedback treatment for asthma. *Chest, 126*, 352–361.

Leor, J., Poole, W. K., & Kloner, R. A. (1996). Sudden cardiac death triggered by an earthquake. *New England Journal of Medicine, 334*, 413–419.

Li, J., Johansen, C., Bronnum-Hansen, H., Stenager, E., Koch-Henriksen, N., & Olsen, J. (2004). The risk of multiple sclerosis in bereaved parents: A nationwide cohort study in Denmark. *Neurology, 62*, 726–729.

Libby, P., & Theroux, P. (2005). Pathophysiology of coronary artery disease. *Circulation, 111*, 3481–3488.

Light, K. C., Girdler, S. S., Sherwood, A., Bragdon, E. E., Brownley, K. A., West, S. G., et al. (1999). High stress responsivity predicts later blood pressure only in combination with positive family history and high life stress. *Hypertension, 33*, 1458–1464.

Ljung, T., Holm, G., Friberg, P., Andersson, B., Bengtsson, B. A., Svensson, J., et al. (2000). The activity of the hypothalamic-pituitary-adrenal axis and the sympathetic nervous system in relation to waist/hip circumference ratio in men. *Obesity Research, 8*, 487–495.

Lloyd, C. E., Dyer, P. H., Lancashire, R. J., Harris, T., Daniels, J. E., & Barnett, A. H. (1999). Association between stress and glycemic control in adults with type 1 (insulin-dependent) diabetes. *Diabetes Care, 22*, 1278–1283.

Lundberg, U. (in press). Workplace stress. In G. Fink (Ed.), *Encyclopedia of Stress, 2nd Edition*. Oxford: Elsevier.

Lundberg, U., Dohns, I. E., Melin, B., Sandsjo, L., Palmerud, G., Kadefors, R., et al. (1999). Psychophysiological stress responses, muscle tension, and neck and shoulder pain among supermarket cashiers. *Journal of Occupational Health Psychology, 4*, 245–255.

Lustman, P. J., Clouse, R. E., Ciechanowski, P. S., Hirsch, I. B., & Freedland, K. E. (2005). Depression-related hyperglycemia in type 1 diabetes: a mediational approach. *Psychosomatic Medicine, 67*, 195–199.

Manuck, S. B., Flory, J. D., Muldoon, M. F., & Ferrell, R. E. (2002). Central nervous system serotonergic responsivity and aggressive disposition in men. *Physiology and Behavior, 77*, 705–709.

Manuck, S. B., Polefrone, J. M., Terrell, D. F., Muldoon, M. F., Kasprowicz, A. L., Waldstein, S. R., et al. (1996). Absence of enhanced sympathoadrenal activity and behaviorally evoked cardiovascular reactivity among offspring of hypertensives. *American Journal of Hypertension, 9*, 248–255.

Markovitz, J. H., Matthews, K. A., Kannel, W. B., Cobb, J. L., & D'Agostino, R. B. (1993). Psychological predictors of hypertension in the Framingham Study. Is there tension in hypertension? *Journal of the American Medical Association, 270*, 2439–2443.

Markovitz, J. H., Raczynski, J. M., Wallace, D., Chettur, V., & Chesney, M. A. (1998). Cardiovascular reactivity to video game predicts subsequent blood pressure increases in young men: The CARDIA study. *Psychosomatic Medicine, 60*, 186–191.

Marras, W. S., Davis, K. G., Heaney, C. A., Maronitis, A. B., & Allread, W. G. (2000). The influence of psychosocial stress, gender, and personality on mechanical loading of the lumbar spine. *Spine, 25*, 3045–3054.

Marsland, A. L., Cohen, S., Rabin, B. S., & Manuck, S. B. (2001). Associations between stress, trait negative affect, acute immune reactivity, and antibody response to hepatitis B injection in healthy young adults. *Health Psychology, 20*, 4–11.

Mensah, G. A., Mokdad, A. H., Ford, E. S., Greenlund, K. J., & Croft, J. B. (2005). State of disparities in cardiovascular health in the United States. *Circulation, 111*, 1233–1241.

Meyer, R., & Haggerty, R. J. (1962). Streptococcal infections in families. *Pediatrics, 29*, 539–549.

Miller, G. E., & Cohen, S. (2005). Infectious disease and psychoneuroimmunology. In K. Vedhara & M. Irwin (Eds.), *Human Psychoneuroimmunology* (pp. 219–242). Oxford: Oxford University Press.

Mills, P. J., Farag, N. H., Hong, S., Kennedy, B. P., Berry, C. C., & Ziegler, M. G. (2003). Immune cell CD62L and CD11a expression in response to a psychological stressor in human hypertension. *Brain, Behavior and Immunity, 17*, 260–267.

Ming, E. E., Adler, G. K., Kessler, R. C., Fogg, L. F., Matthews, K. A., Herd, J. A., et al. (2004). Cardiovascular reactivity to work stress predicts subsequent onset of hypertension: the Air Traffic Controller Health Change Study. *Psychosomatic Medicine, 66*, 459–465.

Miranda, H., Viikari-Juntura, E., Heistaro, S., Heliovaara, M., & Riihimaki, H. (2005). A population study on differences in the determinants of a specific shoulder disorder versus nonspecific shoulder pain without clinical findings. *American Journal of Epidemiology, 161*, 847–855.

Mittleman, M. A., Maclure, M., Sherwood, J. B., Mulry, R. P., Tofler, G. H., Jacobs, et al. (1995). Triggering of acute myocardial infarction onset by episodes of anger. *Circulation, 92*, 1720–1725.

Moberg, E., Kollind, M., Lins, P. E., & Adamson, U. (1994). Acute mental stress impairs insulin sensitivity in IDDM patients. *Diabetologia, 37*, 247–251.

Moher, D., Schulz, K. F., & Altman, D. G. (2001). The CONSORT statement: revised recommendations for improving the quality of reports of parallel-group randomized trials. *Lancet, 357*, 1191–1194.

Mohr, D. C., Hart, S. L., Julian, L., Cox, D., & Pelletier, D. (2004). Association between stressful life events and exacerbation in multiple sclerosis: a meta-analysis. *British Medical Journal, 328*, 731.

Moller, J., Theorell, T., de Faire, U., Ahlbom, A., & Hallqvist, J. (2005). Work related stressful life events and the risk of myocardial infarction. Case-control and case-crossover analyses within the Stockholm heart epidemiology program (SHEEP). *Journal of Epidemiology and Community Health, 59*, 23–30.

Monaco, C., Mathur, A., & Martin, J. F. (2005). What causes acute coronary syndromes? Applying Koch's postulates. *Atherosclerosis, 179*, 1–15.

Muldoon, M. F., Herbert, T. B., Patterson, S. M., Kameneva, M., Raible, R., & Manuck, S. B. (1995). Effects of acute psychological stress on serum lipid levels, hemoconcentration, and blood viscosity. *Archives of Internal Medicine, 155*, 615–620.

Muldoon, M. F., Mackey, R. H., Williams, K. V., Korytkowski, M. T., Flory, J. D., & Manuck, S. B. (2004). Low central nervous system serotonergic responsivity is associated with the metabolic syndrome and physical inactivity. *Journal of Clinical Endocrinology and Metabolism, 89*, 266–271.

Muldoon, M. F., Terrell, D. F., Bunker, C. H., & Manuck, S. B. (1993). Family history studies in hypertension research. Review of the literature. *American Journal of Hypertension, 6*, 76–88.

Musselman, D. L., Bowling, A., Gilles, N., Larsen, H., Betan, E., & Phillips, L. S. (in press). The interrelationship of depression and diabetes. In A. Steptoe (Ed.), *Depression and Physical Illness*. Cambridge: Cambridge University Press.

Myers, A., & Dewar, H. A. (1975). Circumstances attending 100 sudden deaths from coronary artery disease with coroner's necropsies. *British Heart Journal, 37*, 1133–1143.

Nahit, E. S., Hunt, I. M., Lunt, M., Dunn, G., Silman, A. J., & Macfarlane, G. J. (2003). Effects of psychosocial and individual psychological factors on the onset of musculoskeletal pain: common and site-specific effects. *Annals of Rheumatic Disease, 62*, 755–760.

Nakao, M., Yano, E., Nomura, S., & Kuboki, T. (2003). Blood pressure-lowering effects of biofeedback treatment in hypertension: a meta-analysis of randomized controlled trials. *Hypertension Research, 26*, 37–46.

National Center for Health Statistics. (2004). *Health, United States, 2004*. Hyattsville, MD: US Department of Health and Human Services.

Neumann, S. A., Jennings, J. R., Muldoon, M. F., & Manuck, S. B. (2005). White-coat hypertension and autonomic nervous system dysregulation. *American Journal of Hypertension, 18*, 584–588.

Nystrom, F., Aardal, E., & Ohman, K. P. (1998). A population-based study of the white-coat blood pressure effect: positive correlation with plasma cortisol. *Clinical and Experimental Hypertension, 20*, 95–104.

Pasceri, V., Willerson, J. T., & Yeh, E. T. (2000). Direct proinflammatory effect of C-reactive protein on human endothelial cells. *Circulation, 102*, 2165–2168.

Paterniti, S., Zureik, M., Ducimetiere, P., Touboul, P. J., Feve, J. M., & Alperovitch, A. (2001). Sustained anxiety and 4-year progression of carotid atherosclerosis. *Arteriosclerosis Thrombosis and Vascular Biology, 21*, 136–141.

Petrie, K. J., Booth, R. J., Pennebaker, J. W., Davison, K. P., & Thomas, M. G. (1995). Disclosure of trauma and immune response to a hepatitis B vaccination program. *Journal of Consulting and Clinical Psychology, 63*, 787–792.

Petrie, K. J., Fontanilla, I., Thomas, M. G., Booth, R. J., & Pennebaker, J. W. (2004). Effect of written emotional expression on immune function in patients with human immunodeficiency virus infection: a randomized trial. *Psychosomatic Medicine, 66*, 272–275.

Phillips, A. C., Carroll, D., Burns, V. E., & Drayson, M. (2005). Neuroticism, cortisol reactivity, and antibody response to vaccination. *Psychophysiology, 42*, 232–238.

Pierce, T. W., Grim, R. D., & King, J. S. (2005). Cardiovascular reactivity and family history of hypertension: a meta-analysis. *Psychophysiology, 42*, 125–131.

Poulter, N. R., Khaw, K. T., Hopwood, B. E., Mugambi, M., Peart, W. S., Rose, G., et al. (1990). The Kenyan Luo migration study: observations on the initiation of a rise in blood pressure. *British Medical Journal, 300*, 967–972.

Rains, J. C., Penzien, D. B., McCrory, D. C., & Gray, R. N. (2005). Behavioral headache treatment: history, review of the empirical literature, and methodological critique. *Headache, 45* (Suppl. 2), S92–109.

Riazi, A., Pickup, J., & Bradley, C. (2004). Daily stress and glycemic control in Type 1 diabetes: individual differences in magnitude, direction, and timing of stress-reactivity. *Diabetes Research and Clinical Practice, 66*, 237–244.

Rissen, D., Melin, B., Sandsjo, L., Dohns, I., & Lundberg, U. (2000). Surface EMG and psychophysiological stress reactions in women during repetitive work. *European Journal of Applied Physiology, 83*, 215–222.

Ritz, T., Dahme, B., & Roth, W. T. (2004). Behavioral interventions in asthma: biofeedback techniques. *Journal of Psychosomatic Research, 56*, 711–720.

Ritz, T., & Steptoe, A. (2000). Emotion and pulmonary function in asthma: reactivity in the field and relationship with laboratory induction of emotion. *Psychosomatic Medicine, 62*, 808–815.

Ritz, T., Steptoe, A., DeWilde, S., & Costa, M. (2000). Emotions and stress increase respiratory resistance in asthma. *Psychosomatic Medicine, 62*, 401–412.

Rosmond, R. (2005). Role of stress in the pathogenesis of the metabolic syndrome. *Psychoneuroendocrinology, 30,* 1–10.

Ross, R. (1999). Atherosclerosis – an inflammatory disease. *New England Journal of Medicine, 340,* 115–126.

Rostrup, M., Mundall, H. H., Westheim, A., & Eide, I. (1991). Awareness of high blood pressure increases arterial plasma catecholamines, platelet noradrenaline and adrenergic responses to mental stress. *Journal of Hypertension, 9,* 159–166.

Roupe van der Voort, C., Heijnen, C. J., Wulffraat, N., Kuis, W., & Kavelaars, A. (2000). Stress induces increases in IL-6 production by leucocytes of patients with the chronic inflammatory disease juvenile rheumatoid arthritis: a putative role for alpha(1)-adrenergic receptors. *Journal of Neuroimmunology, 110,* 223–229.

Rutledge, T., & Hogan, B. E. (2002). A quantitative review of prospective evidence linking psychological factors with hypertension development. *Psychosomatic Medicine, 64,* 758–766.

Sandercock, G. R., Bromley, P. D., & Brodie, D. A. (2005). Effects of exercise on heart rate variability: inferences from meta-analysis. *Medicine and Science in Sports and Exercise, 37,* 433–439.

Sauter, S. L., & Moon, S. D. (Eds.). (1996). *Beyond Biomechanics: Psychosocial Factors and Musculoskeletal Disorders in Office Work.* New York: Taylor & Francis.

Schnall, P. L., Landsbergis, P. A., & Baker, D. (1994). Job strain and cardiovascular disease. *Annual Review of Public Health, 15,* 381–411.

Schnall, P. L., Pieper, C., Schwartz, J. E., Karasek, R. A., Schlussel, Y., Devereux, R. B., et al. (1990). The relationship between "job strain," workplace diastolic blood pressure, and left ventricular mass index. Results of a case-control study. *Journal of the American Medical Association, 263,* 1929–1935.

Schwartz, J. E., & Stone, A. A. (1998). Strategies for analyzing ecological momentary assessment data. *Health Psychology, 17,* 6–16.

Segerstrom, S. C., & Miller, G. E. (2004). Psychological stress and the human immune system: a meta-analytic study of 30 years of inquiry. *Psychological Bulletin, 130,* 601–630.

Sepa, A., Wahlberg, J., Vaarala, O., Frodi, A., & Ludvigsson, J. (2005). Psychological stress may induce diabetes-related autoimmunity in infancy. *Diabetes Care, 28,* 290–295.

Shaw, W. S., Patterson, T. L., Semple, S. J., Dimsdale, J. E., Ziegler, M. G., & Grant, I. (2003). Emotional expressiveness, hostility and blood pressure in a longitudinal cohort of Alzheimer caregivers. *Journal of Psychosomatic Research, 54,* 293–302.

Sheps, D. S., McMahon, R. P., Becker, L., Carney, R. M., Freedland, K. E., Cohen, J. D., et al. (2002). Mental stress-induced ischemia and all-cause mortality in patients with coronary artery disease: Results from the Psychophysiological Investigations of Myocardial Ischemia study. *Circulation, 105,* 1780–1784.

Siegel, W. C., Blumenthal, J. A., & Divine, G. W. (1990). Physiological, psychological, and behavioral factors and white coat hypertension. *Hypertension, 16,* 140–146.

Slater, M. A., Steptoe, A., Weickgenant, A. L., & Dimsdale, J. E. (2003). Behavioral medicine. In A. Tasman & J. Kay & J. A. Leiberman (Eds.), *Psychiatry, Second Ed.* (pp. 1838–1852). Chichester: John Wiley.

Smith, D. R., Wei, N., Zhao, L., & Wang, R. S. (2004). Musculoskeletal complaints and psychosocial risk factors among Chinese hospital nurses. *Occupational Medicine (London), 54,* 579–582.

Smyth, J. M. (1998). Written emotional expression: effect sizes, outcome types, and moderating variables. *Journal of Consulting and Clinical Psychology, 66,* 174–184.

Smyth, J. M., Stone, A. A., Hurewitz, A., & Kaell, A. (1999). Effects of writing about stressful experiences on symptom reduction in patients with asthma or rheumatoid arthritis: a randomized trial. *Journal of the American Medical Association, 281,* 1304–1309.

Steptoe, A. (1998). Psychophysiological bases of disease. In M. Johnston & D. Johnston (Eds.), *Comprehensive Clinical Psychology Volume 8: Health Psychology* (pp. 39–78). New York: Elsevier Science.

Steptoe, A. (2005). Tools of psychosocial biology in health care research. In A. Bowling & S. Ebrahim (Eds.), *Handbook of Health Research Methods* (pp. 471–493). Maidenhead: Open University Press.

Steptoe, A. (2006). Depression and the development of coronary heart disease. In A. Steptoe (Ed.), *Depression and Physical Illness.* (pp. 53–86). Cambridge: Cambridge University Press.

Steptoe, A., & Ayers, S. (2004). Stress, health and illness. In S. Sutton & A. Baum & M. Johnston (Eds.), *Sage Handbook of Health Psychology* (pp. 169–196). London: Sage.

Steptoe, A., & Brydon, L. (2005). Associations between acute lipid stress responses and fasting lipid levels three years later. *Health Psychology, 24,* 601–607.

Steptoe, A., Feldman, P. M., Kunz, S., Owen, N., Willemsen, G., & Marmot, M. (2002). Stress responsivity and socioeconomic status: A mechanism for increased cardiovascular disease risk? *European Heart Journal, 23,* 1757–1763.

Steptoe, A., Kunz-Ebrecht, S., Owen, N., Feldman, P. J., Rumley, A., Lowe, G. D., et al. (2003). Influence of socioeconomic status and job control on plasma fibrinogen responses to acute mental stress. *Psychosomatic Medicine, 65,* 137–144.

Steptoe, A., Kunz-Ebrecht, S., Rumley, A., & Lowe, G. D. (2003). Prolonged elevations in haemostatic and rheological responses following psychological stress in low socioeconomic status men and women. *Thrombosis and Haemostasis, 89,* 83–90.

Steptoe, A., Kunz-Ebrecht, S. R., Brydon, L., & Wardle, J. (2004). Central adiposity and cortisol responses to waking in middle-aged men and women. *International Journal of Obesity, 28,* 1168–1173.

Steptoe, A., & Marmot, M. (2005). Impaired cardiovascular recovery following stress predicts 3-year increases in blood pressure. *Journal of Hypertension, 23,* 529–536.

Steptoe, A., Owen, N., Kunz-Ebrecht, S., & Brydon, L. (2004). Loneliness and neuroendocrine, cardiovascular, and inflammatory stress responses in middle-aged men and women. *Psychoneuroendocrinology, 29,* 593–611.

Steptoe, A., & Wardle, J. (2005). Cardiovascular stress responsivity, body mass and abdominal adiposity. *International Journal of Obesity, 29,* 1329–1337.

Sterman, M. B. (2000). Basic concepts and clinical findings in the treatment of seizure disorders with EEG operant conditioning. *Clinical Electroencephalography, 31,* 45–55.

Sternberg, E. M. (2001). Neuroendocrine regulation of autoimmune/inflammatory disease. *Journal of Endocrinology, 169,* 429–435.

Stoney, C. M., Bausserman, L., Niaura, R., Marcus, B., & Flynn, M. (1999). Lipid reactivity to stress. II. Biological and behavioral influences. *Health Psychology, 18,* 251–261.

Straub, R. H., Dhabhar, F. S., Bijlsma, J. W., & Cutolo, M. (2005). How psychological stress via hormones and nerve fibers may exacerbate rheumatoid arthritis. *Arthritis and Rheumatism, 52,* 16–26.

Strehl, U., Kotchoubey, B., Trevorrow, T., & Birbaumer, N. (2005). Predictors of seizure reduction after self-regulation of slow cortical potentials as a treatment of drug-resistant epilepsy. *Epilepsy and Behavior, 6,* 156–166.

Strike, P. C., Magid, K., Brydon, L., Edwards, S., McEwan, J. R., & Steptoe, A. (2004). Exaggerated platelet and hemodynamic reactivity to mental stress in men with coronary artery disease. *Psychosomatic Medicine, 66,* 492–500.

Strike, P. C., & Steptoe, A. (2003). Systematic review of mental stress-induced myocardial ischemia. *European Heart Journal, 24,* 690–703.

Strike, P. C., & Steptoe, A. (2005). Behavioral and emotional triggers of acute coronary syndromes: a systematic review and critique. *Psychosomatic Medicine, 67,* 179–186.

Sturdy, P. M., Victor, C. R., Anderson, H. R., Bland, J. M., Butland, B. K., Harrison, B. D., et al. (2002). Psychological, social and health behavior risk factors for deaths certified as asthma: a national case-control study. *Thorax, 57,* 1034–1039.

Suarez, E. C., Lewis, J. G., Krishnan, R. R., & Young, K. H. (2004). Enhanced expression of cytokines and chemokines by blood monocytes to in vitro lipopolysaccharide stimulation are associated with hostility and severity of depressive symptoms in healthy women. *Psychoneuroendocrinology, 29,* 1119–1128.

Suls, J., & Bunde, J. (2005). Anger, anxiety, and depression as risk factors for cardiovascular disease: the problems and implications of overlapping affective dispositions. *Psychological Bulletin, 131,* 260–300.

Sundin, O., Ohman, A., Palm, T., & Strom, G. (1995). Cardiovascular reactivity, Type A behavior, and coronary heart disease: comparisons between myocardial infarction patients and controls during laboratory-induced stress. *Psychophysiology, 32,* 28–35.

Sung, B. H., Wilson, M. F., Izzo, J. L., Jr., Ramirez, L., & Dandona, P. (1997). Moderately obese, insulin-resistant women exhibit abnormal vascular reactivity to stress. *Hypertension, 30,* 848–853.

Timio, M., Lippi, G., Venanzi, S., Gentili, S., Quintaliani, G., Verdura, C., et al. (1997). Blood pressure trend and cardiovascular events in nuns in a secluded order: a 30-year follow-up study. *Blood Pressure, 6,* 81–87.

Todaro, J. F., Con, A., Niaura, R., Spiro, A., III, Ward, K. D., & Roytberg, A. (2005). Combined effect of the metabolic syndrome and hostility on the incidence of myocardial infarction (the Normative Aging Study). *American Journal of Cardiology, 96,* 221–226.

Torp, S., Riise, T., & Moen, B. E. (2001). The impact of psychosocial work factors on musculoskeletal pain: a prospective study. *Journal of Occupational and Environmental Medicine, 43,* 120–126.

Troxel, W. M., Matthews, K. A., Gallo, L. C., & Kuller, L. H. (2005). Marital quality and occurrence of the metabolic syndrome in women. *Archives of Internal Medicine, 165,* 1022–1027.

Turner Cobb, J. M., & Steptoe, A. (1996). Psychosocial stress and susceptibility to upper respiratory tract illness in an adult population sample. *Psychosomatic Medicine, 58,* 404–412.

van Melle, J. P., de Jonge, P., Spijkerman, T. A., Tijssen, J. G., Ormel, J., van Veldhuisen, D. J., et al. (2004). Prognostic association of depression following myocardial infarction with mortality and cardiovascular events: A meta-analysis. *Psychosomatic Medicine, 66,* 814–822.

Vedhara, K., Cox, N. K. M., Wilcock, G. K., Perks, P., Hunt, M., Anderson, S., et al. (1999). Chronic stress in elderly carers of dementia patients and antibody response to influenza vaccination. *Lancet, 353,* 627–631.

Veiersted, K. B., Westgaard, R. H., & Andersen, P. (1993). Electromyographic evaluation of muscular work pattern as a predictor of trapezius myalgia. *Scandinavian Journal of Work and Environmental Health, 19,* 284–290.

Veldhuijzen van Zanten, J. J., Ring, C., Carroll, D., & Kitas, G. D. (2005). Increased C reactive protein in response to acute stress in patients with rheumatoid arthritis. *Annals of Rheumatic Disease.*

Verdecchia, P., Reboldi, G. P., Angeli, F., Schillaci, G., Schwartz, J. E., Pickering, T. G., et al. (2005). Short- and long-term incidence of stroke in white-coat hypertension. *Hypertension, 45,* 203–208.

Viswanathan, K., & Dhabhar, F. S. (2005). Stress-induced enhancement of leukocyte trafficking into sites of surgery or immune activation. *Proceedings of the National Academy of Sciences of the United States of America, 102,* 5808–5813.

Vögele, C., & Steptoe, A. (1993). Anger Inhibition and family history as modulators of cardiovascular responses to mental stress in adolescent boys. *Journal of Psychosomatic Research, 37,* 503–514.

Waller, J., McCaffery, K. J., Forrest, S., & Wardle, J. (2004). Human papillomavirus and cervical cancer: issues for biobehavioral and psychosocial research. *Annals of Behavioral Medicine, 27,* 68–79.

Wamala, S. P., Lynch, J., Horsten, M., Mittleman, M. A., Schenck-Gustafsson, K., & Orth-Gomer, K. (1999). Education and the metabolic syndrome in women. *Diabetes Care, 22,* 1999–2003.

Wamboldt, M. Z., Laudenslager, M., Wamboldt, F. S., Kelsay, K., & Hewitt, J. (2003). Adolescents with atopic disorders have an attenuated cortisol response to laboratory stress. *Journal of Allergy and Clinical Immunology, 111,* 509–514.

Whang, W., Albert, C. M., Sears, S. F., Jr., Lampert, R., Conti, J. B., Wang, P. J., et al. (2005). Depression as a predictor for appropriate shocks among patients with implantable cardioverter-defibrillators: results from the Triggers of Ventricular Arrhythmias (TOVA) study. *Journal of the American College of Cardiology, 45,* 1090–1095.

Williams, D. R., Neighbors, H. W., & Jackson, J. S. (2003). Racial/Ethnic discrimination and health: findings from community studies. *American Journal of Public Health, 93,* 200–208.

World Health Organization. (2002). *Diabetes: the cost of diabetes.* Geneva: World Health Organization.

Wright, R. J., Cohen, R. T., & Cohen, S. (2005). The impact of stress on the development and expression of atopy. *Current Opinion in Allergy and Clinical Immunology, 5,* 23–29.

Wright, R. J., Cohen, S., Carey, V., Weiss, S. T., & Gold, D. R. (2002). Parental stress as a predictor of wheezing in infancy: a prospective birth-cohort study. *American Journal of Respiratory Critical Care Medicine, 165,* 358–365.

Wright, R. J., Finn, P., Contreras, J. P., Cohen, S., Wright, R. O., Staudenmayer, J., et al. (2004). Chronic caregiver stress and IgE expression, allergen-induced proliferation, and cytokine profiles in a birth cohort predisposed to atopy. *Journal of Allergy and Clinical Immunology, 113,* 1051–1057.

Yan, L. L., Liu, K., Matthews, K. A., Daviglus, M. L., Ferguson, T. F., & Kiefe, C. I. (2003). Psychosocial factors and risk of hypertension: the Coronary Artery Risk Development in Young Adults (CARDIA) study. *Journal of the American Medical Association, 290,* 2138–2148.

Yusuf, S., Hawken, S., Ounpuu, S., Dans, T., Avezum, A., Lanas, F., et al. (2004). Effect of potentially modifiable risk factors associated with myocardial infarction in 52 countries (the INTERHEART study): case-control study. *Lancet, 364,* 937–952.

Zautra, A. J., Yocum, D. C., Villanueva, I., Smith, B., Davis, M. C., Attrep, J., et al. (2004). Immune activation and depression in women with rheumatoid arthritis. *Journal of Rheumatology, 31,* 457–463.

32 Environmental Psychophysiology

RUSS J. PARSONS

1. INTRODUCTION

Every scientific psychology must take into account whole situations, i.e., the state of both person and environment. (Lewin, 1936, p. 12)

In this chapter we examine how psychophysiological constructs and methods can be used to understand human transactions with the physical environment. Although psychophysiologists appreciate the power of changing physical contexts to influence human behavior and often hold aspects of the physical environment constant in their research, they do not typically focus on human-environment transactions per se. Conversely, environmental psychologists (and other environment and behavior researchers), whether through limited resources, lack of expertise, or ignorance, rarely use psychophysiology in their work. Despite these trends, a good deal of work is being done where these two broad research areas meet, which reflects, perhaps, a natural tendency to see "embodied" humans as intimately related to their environments (Atran, 1998). This work has been called *environmental psychophysiology*, and is formally defined as "the study of relationships between organism-place transactions and physiological events" (Tassinary, 1995). The conceptualization of environment and methodological approaches used in environmental psychophysiology derive largely from three disciplines within the life sciences: *environmental psychology*, in which relationships between human behavior, and sociophysical environments are studied (Stokols & Altman, 1987); *psychophysiology*, in which psychological phenomena related to and revealed through physiological principles and events are studied (Cacioppo & Tassinary, 1990); and *environmental physiology*, in which the study of animal-environment relationships with particular attention given to the biological effects of changes in the geophysical environment are studied (Schmidt-Nielsen, 1997). Environmental psychophysiology can also be distinguished from the related subdisciplines of cognitive psychophysiology and social psychophysiology. The former is concerned with *intra-organismic* information processing, while the latter focuses on *inter-organismic* information

processing (see Cacioppo, Tassinary, & Berntson, this volume).[1] This fairly broad disciplinary heritage implies an extensive purview for this new field. However, we will limit the scope of our coverage of environmental psychophysiology in this chapter to minimize overlap with other chapters in this volume, especially those in the social processes section. The focus of this chapter will be the physical aspects of environments ordinarily encountered, and the level of analysis will emphasize the psychological import of the physical environments of daily life.

The research in environmental psychophysiology has focused on relatively discrete physical environmental dimensions and features, especially those features that can be conceived of as environmental stressors. Although some studies have considered whole environments or situations, most have examined particular environmental dimensions, such as light or sound. This follows in part from a desire to understand the effects of different environmental stressors, but some research has also been motivated to discover information that can inform the design and management of environments in which we live, work, and relax. This is the second noteworthy characteristic of the research to be reviewed: its applied orientation. From examinations of traffic congestion to the design of lighting for work environments and the effects of overflight noise in elementary school districts, research in environmental psychophysiology has generated information of direct relevance for policy and decision makers who can

---

[1] Readers familiar with Andreassi's (1995) psychophysiology text will recognize that "environmental psychophysiology" is not being minted here. Andreassi's use of the term, however, is somewhat more restricted than ours, though his definition obscures the fact. He maintains that environmental psychophysiology refers to "the effects of physical environments on the physiology of a behaving person" (p. 360). This seemingly broad consideration of potential effects belies the narrowly focused content of his environmental psychophysiology chapter. The physical environment of interest is the *internal* physical environment, primarily as it is influenced by changing hormone levels, the ingestion of drugs and exposure to neurotoxic chemicals. As indicated in the introduction, our understanding of the physical environment is conceived more broadly so to keep with Lewin's and other psychologists' longstanding admonitions to consider "whole situations."

influence the design and management of everyday environments.

The pages that follow cover work in three broad areas: (1) environmental stress, (2) palliative environments, and (3) topographic cognition. These areas both exemplify existing work and suggest the broad potential for the application of psychophysiological constructs and methods to the study of human transactions with the physical environment. The research ranges from commonly encountered psychophysiological applications in environmental stress, through more recent applications of similar constructs and methods to examine the restorative and analgesic potential of large-scale outdoor environments, to the emerging use of functional brain imaging and other psychophysiological techniques to draw inferences about the neural substrates of wayfinding and related spatial behaviors. In keeping with the major themes of this volume, an appropriate historical context for the material covered in each of these sections is provided, as well as discussions of relevant biological (i.e., anatomical, neural, or hormonal substrates) and experimental (e.g., research setting and individual differences) contexts.

2. ENVIRONMENTAL STRESS: HUMAN TRANSACTIONS WITH NOISE

The term *environmental stress* is typically construed broadly to include both social and physical environmental stressors, though socially-oriented daily life events are often of primary interest.[2] Here, however, we examine what is perhaps the quintessential physical environmental stressor, noise. Stress is a psychophysiological state arising from one of two general types of suboptimal person-environment transactions: 1) the environment presents demands that a person is ill-prepared to meet, or 2) environmental opportunities for goal attainment are either absent or thwarted. Most environmental psychologists (see Evans & Cohen, 1987) advocate a relational concept of stress wherein appraisal of the fit between the environment (demands and opportunities) and oneself (capacities and goals) is central to the stress that is experienced and the coping that is engaged. Despite this interactive or relational perspective, we must acknowledge the possibility of normative environmental stressors, such as noisome odors or nociceptive sounds, which are widely experienced as noxious (see Moos & Swindle, 1990). We must acknowledge as well the possibility that chronic environmental stressors may go largely unnoticed and yet contribute to the stress that is experienced over the course of a day. What these and other limitations of the relational perspective suggest is that there is more to the stressor-appraisal-coping process than can be learned from self-

reports of daily life events. Thus, knowledge of individual differences, psychophysiological assessments of situational experience, and objective measurements of physical conditions can all help to understand a process that is unlikely to be completely available to or accurately represented by conscious recollection.

2.1. Noise

Noise, n. A stench in the ear. Undomesticated music. The chief product and authenticating sign of civilization. (Bierce, 1911/1993, p. 85)

In antiquity there was only silence. In the nineteenth century, with the invention of the machine, Noise was born. Today, Noise triumphs and reigns supreme over the sensibility of men. (Russolo, 1913/1971, p. 166)

As these epigrams suggest, noise has long been regarded as an Industrial Age phenomenon with untoward psychological consequences. Much of the early research on the effects of noise, however, focused on establishing dose-response curves for potential hearing loss as a function of stimulus intensity and duration of exposure (see Kryter, 1994, for a review). Our primary concern here will be with the *nonauditory* effects of noise, which are all those effects not directly related to hearing loss (DeJoy, 1984). The modal definition of noise in this literature is "unwanted sound" (Belojevic, Jakovljevic, & Slepcevic, 2003; Kryter, 1994; Evans & Cohen, 1987; McLean & Tarnopolsky, 1977; Ward & Suedfeld, 1973), a definition that clearly implies the importance of cognitive interpretations and the psychological meaning of sound independent of its physical characteristics. In particular, the controllability and predictability of sound are critically important to understanding the nonauditory effects of noise. And, as we shall see, personality and other individual differences also can be used to predict psychophysiological responsiveness and the performance effects of noise, as can nonauditory situational attributes (e.g., effort) of transactions with the sociophysical environment. We begin with brief overviews of occupational epidemiology and human laboratory work on the nonauditory effects of noise, and highlight inferential issues pertinent to the conduct of field research. We then examine two areas of field research (noise in sleep and school environments) that exemplify the application of psychophysiological constructs and methods to human transactions with the physical environment.

2.2. Epidemiological research

Extensive research on the nonauditory effects of noise is a relatively recent phenomenon, arising 25–30 years ago out of public concern for possible health effects of noise pollution in industrial and other workplace environments (DeJoy, 1984). Reviewers of the epidemiological research on industrial noise exposure have generally

---

[2] This is especially true of the clinical literature. See, for instance, the "Environmental Perspective" section of a recent book on measuring stress (Cohen, Kessler, & Gordon, 1995) in which all four chapters are heavily slanted towards measuring socially-oriented life events, such as problems on the job and marital conflicts.

concluded that the strongest evidence for potential health effects is from long-term (3–5 years) exposure to noise at or above 85dB(A) (Stansfeld & Haines, 1997; Welch, 1979). Under these conditions, cardiovascular effects are typically reported (e.g., Parvizpoor, 1976; Zhao, Zhang, Selvin, & Spear, 1993), with peripheral vasoconstriction (e.g., Jansen, 1969) and elevated blood pressure (e.g., Anticaglia & Cohen, 1970; Tomei et al., 2000) being the symptoms most commonly associated with occupational noise (see DeJoy, 1984; McLean & Tarnopolsky, 1977; Smith, 1991; Thompson, 1996 for reviews). Occupational noise has also been associated with higher rates of cardiovascular disease (Knipschild, 1977; 1980) and myocardial infarction (Ising et al., 1996). It has been difficult to draw conclusions about health effects based on this work, however, because not all of the epidemiological studies suggest that there are deleterious effects (e.g., Cohen, Taylor, & Tubbs, 1980; Lees, Romeril, & Wetherall, 1980; van Dijk, Verbeek, & De Vries, 1987), while others indicate that harmful effects only accrue after very long exposures on the job (≥ 25 years; Lang, Fouriaud, & Jacquinet-Salord, 1992). Many of the studies that do show effects have not included adequate control groups, and others that do not show effects have often used inappropriate thresholds for high versus low noise exposure [85dB(A)], failed to account for the use of ear protection, or used dubious estimates of noise exposure rather than onsite measurements (Babisch, 1998; Ising & Kruppa, 2004). A meta-analysis of the relationship between noise exposure and cardiovascular disease reflects this ambiguity in the literature (van Kempen et al., 2002). The authors examined 43 epidemiological studies published from 1970–1999 and estimated that per 5 dB(A) increase in noise the relative risk of hypertension is 1.14 for occupational noise and 1.26 for aircraft noise, though the data were inconclusive for a relationship between noise and myocardial infarction.

Recent epidemiological and quasi-experimental field research efforts have begun to address some of these methodological concerns by more carefully measuring noise exposures, accounting for hearing protection, and using ambulatory psychophysiological instruments. A retrospective study of 27,464 lumber mill workers, for instance, used onsite visits and extensive personal dosimetry measurements to estimate noise exposures and found (marginally significant) elevated standardized mortality ratios (SMRs) for deaths from myocardial infarction for the full cohort, and significant SMRs for a subgroup without hearing protection, ranging from 1.3–1.5 for increasing exposures (Davies et al., 2005). The importance of incorporating methodological or statistical controls for hearing protection is underscored by field research in industrial work settings, which indicates that elevated postshift fatigue, irritability, cortisol (Melamed & Bruhis, 1996) and resting blood pressure levels (Lusk, Hagerty, Gillespie, & Caruso, 2002) can be lowered by using hearing protection. Other field researchers have paired personal dosime-

try with 24 hr ambulatory blood pressure and heart rate measurements to examine the extent to which occupational noise is associated with acute versus more chronic influences on cardiovascular functioning. These studies indicate that workers exposed to >85dB(A) during the work shift experience significant work period increases in SBP (6–19mmHg), DBP (3–7mmHg; Chang, Jain, Wang, & Chan, 2003; Fogari et al., 2001), and heart rate (3 bpm; Fogari et al., 2001) relative to workers in quieter environments. There were also indications of possible chronic effects in this work, as both studies reported sustained cardiovascular effects in the evening (5pm–11pm) and night time (11pm–8am) hours, albeit not for all measures; and Fogari et al. (2001) found that noise-exposed workers had elevated 24 hr heart rates even when measured on a nonwork day. The Fogari et al. data are particularly interesting because they controlled not only for typical cardiovascular risk factors (e.g., smoking, body mass, and age) but also for the physical exertion required of noise-exposed and nonexposed workers, something that is not routinely done; these data are interesting as well because 94% of the noise-exposed workers wore hearing protection. Taken together, these studies suggest that the cardiovascular effects of industrial noise extend beyond the 8-hr period when workers are exposed to noise. And, because these effects occur even when hearing protection is used, it appears that they can be elicited at levels far below the 85dB(A) threshold typically regarded as the dividing line between harmless and harmful exposures.[3]

Although the combined use of personal dosimetry and ambulatory psychophysiology is still rare in field research on occupational noise, the few studies that have used these techniques clearly illustrate the methodological power of densely measuring both halves of the putative cause and effect relationship between noise and health. First, the continuous measurement of sound and physiology allows for the discovery of relationships that might otherwise be missed. In both the Chang et al. (2003) and the Fogari et al. (2001) studies, differences in blood pressure and HR between noise-exposed and nonexposed workers only emerged when data were integrated over fairly long periods (8 hrs), both on and off the job; preshift, single point comparisons of resting blood pressure and HR did not discriminate these groups.

Second, continuous measurements of noise that extend beyond the work shift can be used to isolate the effects of occupational noise vis-á-vis evening and late night noise exposures, which can interfere with home life and sleep and may also have deleterious health effects. Chang et al.

---

[3] Further evidence that the 85dB(A) threshold is outmoded comes from field research in much quieter office environments [<65 dB(A)], where there are indications that noise can elevate stress-related hormones (Evans & Johnson, 2000) and interact with psychosocial variables such as job strain to influence self-reported well being, job satisfaction, and organizational commitment (Leather, Beale, & Sullivan, 2003).

(2003) were able to confirm that workers who were exposed to high and low noise conditions on the job experienced similar sound intensities during the early evening hours at home. Thus they were able to ascribe the cardiovascular effects to occupational noise more confidently; they did not measure noise during the sleep period, however, and consequently their assertion of a cause and effect relationship is not as strong as it might have been. Using personal dosimetry to parse varying environmental noise exposures would be useful in non-occupational settings too. Research on the ill effects of noise at school, for instance, often fails to examine the potential cumulative or interactive effects of noise at home, even though as many as a third of the students may be cross-classified with respect to noise at home versus noise at school (e.g., noisy home environment, quiet school, or vice versa; Haines, Stansfeld, Job, Berglund, & Head, 2001a).

Finally, when noise and psychophysiological endpoints are both measured continuously, it is possible to track physiological responding to peak noise events, which can be useful in isolating specific sources of trouble in a given environment and assessing their relative value as pollutants. This would be especially useful in home environments, where road noise has been associated with increased risk of myocardial infarction (Babischet et al., 2005) and overnight catecholamine excretion (Babisch, Fromme, Beyer, & Ising, 2001), and aircraft over flights have been associated with increased risk of hypertension (Rosenlund et al., 2001). Although the current trend in the literature is to examine the health effects of these noise sources separately, and there is evidence that noise from aircraft, road, and rail traffic can be ranked from high to low in terms of annoyance (Miedema & Vos, 1998), it is by no means clear that individual analyses are to be preferred over cumulative or interactive models. Further research that pairs personal dosimetry with ambulatory psychophysiology could help to assess the relative merits of such models.

Thus, though it has been difficult to make causal inferences based on this literature, with continuing methodological improvements in epidemiological and field research, there is increasing evidence that longterm exposure to occupational noise at or above 85dB(A) compromises cardiovascular health. There are indications, as well, that this threshold is likely too high (see below), especially when the cumulative effects of nonoccupational noise are considered and other health effects are examined. Indeed, throughout this work the presumed mechanism of the cardiovascular effects of occupational noise is that noise is a stressor, and as such, this implicates a broad range of possible health effects. In the following sections we briefly review complementary laboratory work and highlight quasi-experimental research on the nonauditory effects of noise in sleep and school environments, all of which has emphasized the physiological concomitants of stress and coping.

2.3. Human laboratory research

With the exception of the effects of noise on sleep, much of the human laboratory research on the nonauditory effects of noise has emphasized effects on the performance of cognitive and psychomotor tasks. Very often, complete factorial designs (i.e., those including noise-only conditions) are not used, and thus it becomes difficult to assess the physiological effects of noise independent of the physiological activation required to perform the task. Those laboratory studies that have examined the effects of noise independent of task performance have generally found mild cardiovascular effects, including peripheral vasoconstriction (Kryter & Poza, 1980), increased diastolic BP, decreased systolic BP and sinus arrhythmia (Mosskov & Ettema, 1977a; 1977b), and a reduction in cardiac output (Andren, Hansson, Bjorkman, & Jonsson, 1980; Andren, Hansson, Bjorkman, Jonsson, & Borg, 1979). Many of these same cardiovascular effects emerge under task performance, and they are exacerbated when task performance is accompanied by noise (Carter & Beh, 1989; Conrad, 1973; Kryter & Poza, 1980; Millar & Steels, 1990; Mosskov & Ettema, 1977a; 1977b). Some sympathoadrenal and adrenocortical endocrine effects associated with task performance and noise have been found as well, including increased epinephrine (Evans & Johnson, 2000; Frankenhauser & Lundberg, 1977, aftereffects only) and elevated cortisol responding (Brandenberger et al., 1980; Follenius, Brandenberger, Lecornu, Simeoni, & Reinhardt, 1980; Persson-Waye et al., 2002), but the effects for these systems are less consistent.

Although laboratory research on the nonauditory effects of noise on humans has emphasized the ergonomics of performance, some of the findings from this work can be used to help interpret field studies of noise exposure in which the emphasis has been on the potential health effects of environmental noise. There are several reasons for this. First, laboratory work focusing on transient exposures to noise in the context of cognitive performance can offer a reasonable model for the effects of environmental noise in school and occupational settings. Though the specific tasks used in laboratory noise research typically do not have direct analogs in school and occupational settings, noise effects on the general psychological processes central to their performance (e.g., attention and short-term memory) likely do generalize to these environments (see Anderson & Bushman, 1997, for a fuller exposition of this point). The focus on *transient* noise in laboratory research is also relevant to nonlaboratory settings because much of the noise experienced in school, occupational, and other nonlaboratory settings is transient in nature (e.g., oscillating traffic volumes, airplane overflights, aperiodic neighborhood noise).

Laboratory research can also be used to isolate different aspects of human-environment transactions that can mediate the effects of environmental stressors. For instance, experimental work indicates that task performance and psychophysiological responding can be influenced by the perceived predictability and controllability of the stimulus source. Though many laboratory studies have failed to find performance effects of noise exposures (e.g., Conrad, 1973; Millar & Steels, 1990), careful reviews of this varied and complex body of work have repeatedly concluded that noise can have definite effects on performance that depend upon both the nature of the noise and the nature of the task (see Broadbent, 1979; Kjellberg, 1990; Smith, 1991 for reviews). To the extent that environmental noise is uncontrollable, aperiodicor experienced for extended periods, as may well be the case in many occupational and school settings, then tasks requiring concentration and sustained attention are likely to suffer.

Several classic psychophysiological studies have found that autonomic responsiveness to noise is decreased when participants are given control over the noise, even when control is not exercised (Glass, Singer, & Friedman, 1969). Lundberg and Frankenhauser (1978), for instance, reported significantly elevated heart rates for students performing math under uncontrollable noise relative to those who could set noise levels. Breier et al. (1987) found significant increases in skin conductance during uncontrollable noise relative to controllable noise, as well as increased levels of epinephrine and adrenocorticotropic hormone during performance of a postnoise anagram task among those who had experienced uncontrollable noise. And in a recent study focusing on uncontrollable open-office noise, Evans and Johnson (2000) reported elevated urinary epinephrine among experienced office workers exposed to low intensity noise [55dB(A)]. Although their performance of a simple typing task did not suffer relative to nonexposed participants, the noise-exposed group did exhibit postural invariance (a risk factor for musculoskeletal disorders), and they averaged fewer attempts at an unsolvable postnoise puzzle. Other, more lingering postnoise effects may also be associated with on-the-job noise exposures, as reported above for ambulatory field measures (Chang et al., 2003; Fogari et al., 2001) and as occasionally seen in experimental work. Gitanjali and Ananth (2003) found that 8 hr exposures to industrial noise [>75 dB(A)] were associated with disturbed sleep, elevated sleeping heart rates, and increases in morning-after serum cortisol. Thus, there is good experimental evidence that the actual and perceived stimulus characteristics of noise can influence both task performance and stress-related psychophysiological responding.

Other laboratory work suggests that an understanding of situational characteristics could be critical to the interpretation of potential health and other effects of environmental noise exposures in the field. Several studies relying on self-report measures indicate that exposure to noise can elicit negative changes in mood when noise interferes with ongoing activities (Aniansson, Pettersson, & Peterson, 1983; Jones & Broadbent, 1979; Öhrström & Rylander, 1982). Dimberg (1990) monitored facial EMG activation during exposures to loud [95 dB(A)] and moderate

(75 dBA) 1000 Hz tones, and found that activity recorded from *corrugator supercilii* and *zygomaticus major* muscle regions was congruent with the negative and positive emotional responses participants reported for the loud and soft tones, respectively. And, recent work on noise exposures and mood suggests that serotonin may moderate negative moods associated with uncontrollable noise (Richell, Deakin, & Anderson, 2005), a finding that may have implications for morning moods, as evidence indicates that the overnight serotonin profile changes significantly when slow wave sleep is disturbed by noise, trending down rather than up towards awakening (Rao et al., 1996). In both the shortterm and the longterm, noise-induced changes in mood could potentially have deleterious health effects (Stone, Cox, Valdimarsdottir, Jandorf, & Neale, 1987; Stone et al., 1994). Such changes could also have important implications in school and occupational settings, where changes in mood could influence self-imposed performance standards (Cervone, Kopp, Schaumann, & Scott, 1994), and possibly increase the stress of maintaining performance standards in challenging working conditions. A study by Tafalla and Evans (1997), which examined an "adaptive costs" model of physiological activation and performance under stress, highlights this possibility.

The autonomic effects of noise (and other stressors) in the laboratory coupled with reports of minimal negative performance effects for many tasks has prompted several research groups to propose the adaptive costs model of stress to account for both sets of findings (Cohen, Evans, Krants, & Stokols, 1980; Cohen, Evans, Stokols, & Krants, 1986; Frankenhaeuser, 1980; Glass & Singer, 1972). According to this model, adequate or superior performance levels are maintained under noise through dint of increased effort, which is reflected in increased autonomic responding. Thus, though performance may be maintained in the face of environmental noise, health costs are ultimately thought to accrue through repeated or sustained increases in autonomic activation, such as sustained increases in cardiovascular responding (Krantz, Contrada, Hill, & Friedler, 1988). Consistent with the adaptive costs hypothesis, there is good evidence in the psychophysiological literature that cardiovascular activation is greatest when effort and active coping are high (Lovallo et al., 1985; Obrist et al., 1978). Coping and sustained effort to perform in the face of noise in particular have been shown to elicit sustained increases in heart rate, blood pressure (Carter & Beh, 1989), and peripheral vasoconstriction (Millar & Steels, 1990).

Building on work by Frankenhaeuser and her colleagues (Lundberg & Frankenhaeuser, 1978; Frankenhaeuser & Lundberg, 1977) suggesting that there may be a trade-off between performance under noise and psychophysiological responding, Tafalla and Evans (1997) explicitly manipulated effort and environmental noise while participants performed mental arithmetic. The presence of uncontrollable noise did not impair performance when increased effort was encouraged, but these conditions did elicit increases in heart rate, norepinephrine, and cortisol. Conversely, when increased effort was not induced, performance declined under uncontrollable noise but cardiovascular and neuroendocrine responding did not change from levels observed during task performance in quiet surroundings. These findings have direct implications for those occupational settings where workers are exposed to uncontrollable noise and yet have strong incentives to maintain performance levels (e.g., exacting quality standards or high productivity requirements). Such conditions may obtain in a wide range of occupations from blue collar industrial workers to white collar office employees, and they may also occur in urban school settings where various kinds of transportation noise are often unavoidable. An appropriate assessment of human-environment transactions in noisy (and other stressful) environments, then, should include an examination of sociophysical aspects of environments, such as controllability of potential physical stressors and psychosocial incentives to perform (see Evans, Johansson, & Carrere, 1994).

Apart from stimulus properties, situational characteristics and state-dependent individual responding, personality characteristics have also been examined in the laboratory. Perhaps the most pertinent personality characteristic is sensitivity to noise, though the evidence for sensitivity as a stable trait that accounts for variability in performance and physiological responding is somewhat checkered (see Kjellberg, 1990). Recent work indicates that sensitivity to noise is an evaluative construct that has no relationship to auditory functioning (e.g., auditory thresholds, intensity discriminations, or auditory reaction time; Ellermeier, Eigenstetter, & Zimmer, 2001), though several reviews have confirmed that self-reported sensitivity increases the annoyance associated with noise (Miedema & Vos, 2003; van Kamp et al., 2004). Noise-sensitive individuals may also be especially attuned to low frequency noise, even at low intensity [40 dB(A)], as they release more cortisol relative to nonsensitive participants when performing cognitively challenging tasks under these conditions (Persson-Waye et al., 2002).

Anxiety and neuroticism have been popularly linked to noise sensitivity, and a classic study by Bennett (1945) indicated that questions regarding annoyance with noise were useful in discriminating normals from those diagnosed as neurotic. More recent evidence, however, has been mixed. Several studies suggest that there is no relationship between self-reported sensitivity to noise and scores on the Eysenck Personality Inventory (EPI), Cattell's 16 PF or the MMPI (Griffiths & Delauzun, 1977; Moreira & Bryan, 1972). Conversely, those with an internal locus of control who believe they have control over a noise stressor exhibit lower cortisol in response to the stressor (Bollini, Walker, Hamann, & Kestler, 2004). And, introverts have been found to prefer lower environmental noise levels (Standing, Lynn, & Moxness, 1990) and lower laboratory noise stimulation levels (Hockey, 1972), findings that hold when scores for neuroticism are controlled (Geen, 1984). Geen (1984) also

reported greater cardiovascular and electrodermal reactivity among introverts compared to extraverts at moderate noise exposure levels [55–75 dB(A)], but in a second study, cardiovascular responding did not differ at very low [40 dB(A)] or very high [85 dB(A)] noise levels. Interestingly, there was no difference in physiological reactivity between introverts and extroverts when participants from each group were exposed to preferred noise stimulation levels (55 dB(A) and 72 dB(A), respectively), regardless of whether exposure levels were chosen or assigned.

Several researchers have suggested that inconsistencies in the evidence for noise sensitivity as a stable trait reflect the fact that putative measures of noise sensitivity may actually measure general annoyance with environmental stimuli (Kjellberg, 1990; Weinstein, 1980). Consistent with this, Thomas and Jones (1982) have reported that 35% of the variability in noise annoyance scores can be accounted for by responses to a general annoyance questionnaire. However, though discomfort thresholds for noise, light, heat, and cold are moderately related (pairwise r values range from .25–.52), sensitivity to below-discomfort-threshold noise seems to be unrelated to sensitivities to these other physical environmental stimuli (Öhrström, Björkman, & Rylander, 1988). This finding would not be predicted if noise sensitivity were simply an indication of a more general underlying sensitivity to environmental conditions. Thus, researchers have yet to conclusively determine the extent to which noise sensitivity and general environmental sensitivity overlap, or even whether either type of sensitivity constitutes a stable individual characteristic.

2.4. Field research

Except for epidemiological research on the effects of noise in occupational settings, much of the field research on noise has examined effects in sleep environments and the deleterious effects of noise on children in school and home environments. We will consider each of these broad areas in turn.

Sleep environments. Sleep environments research is conducted both in field and laboratory settings, with reasonably good evidence suggesting that laboratory methods and findings can generalize to nonlaboratory environments (Coates et al., 1979; Johns, 1977). Although noise-induced *awakenings* tend to be more likely in laboratory studies (see review by Pearsons, Barber, & Tabachnick, 1990), various sleep *disturbances* have been found in both field and laboratory settings. These disturbances often take the form of increases in cortical arousal or changes in sleep stages that do not lead to awakenings. For instance, early laboratory research suggested that relatively loud aircraft flyovers (peak intensities of [65–80 dB(A)] reliably elicit increases in cortical arousal (LeVere & Davis, 1977) and are associated with performance decrements on reaction time (RT) tasks administered upon awakening, despite the absence of noise-induced awakenings during the night (LeVere, Bartus, & Hart, 1972). These results parallel findings in the field, which indicate that body movements (Öhrström & Björkman, 1983), transient electroencephalographic (EEG) fluctuations (Vallet, Gagneux, Blanchet, Favre, & Labiale, 1983a), shifts to lighter sleep levels (Stevenson & McKellar, 1988; Vallet et al., 1983a) and phasic cardiovascular responding (Tulen, Kumar, & Jurriëns, 1986; Vallet et al., 1983a,b) are linearly related to dB(A) levels of noise events. Such linear relationships are often established by recording all instances of a particular class of outdoor noise event (e.g., automobile passbys or airplane overflights) and correlating peak SPLs for these events with various physiological measures. Apart from correlational analyses, these data sets lend themselves to more detailed examinations of transient physiological responding to nocturnal noise events. Heart rates of sleeping field participants, for example, tend to increase momentarily when cars or airplanes pass by, followed by a deceleration that mimics the receding noise level of the sound source (Muzet & Ehrhart, 1980).

In part because there are difficulties associating specific noise events with specific sleep disturbances (e.g., when there are multiple, simultaneous automobile passbys), many researchers have examined the quality of sleep in noisy versus quiet field settings. Sleep quality is typically inferred from sleep stage analyses based on EEG and electrooculogram (EOG) recordings in which the duration, distribution, and latency-to-onset of sleep stages are examined. Studies using quasi-experimental designs to manipulate noise exposure provide the strongest evidence for deleterious effects of noise on sleep quality. Manipulations of noise exposures in the field comprise the introduction of double-glazed windows (Öhrström & Björkman, 1983; Tulen et al., 1986; Wilkinson & Campbell, 1984), the use of sound-dampening insulation on single-glazed windows (Eberhardt & Akselsson, 1987), open versus closed windows (Griefahn & Gros, 1986; Tulen et al., 1986), earplugs verus none (Griefahn & Gros, 1986), and moving participants' sleep location from noisy to quiet parts of their homes (Vallet et al., 1983a). Two prominent findings emerge from this work indicating that both slow wave sleep (SWS), stages 3 and 4 (Bergamasco, Benna, & Gilli, 1976; Eberhardt & Akselsson, 1987; Griefahn & Gros, 1986; Wilkinson & Campbell, 1984) and rapid eye movement (REM) sleep (Jurriëns, 1981; Vallet et al., 1983a) can be adversely impacted by noise. Researchers have repeatedly found that latency-to-onset increases and duration decreases for both SWS and REM sleep as peak SPLs increase. Interestingly, these effects of noise are rarely observed for both types of sleep in the same study, an occurrence that Eberhardt and Akselsson (1987) attribute to the inhibition that each sleep stage exerts on the other. They suggest that the particular deleterious effects observed in any given study are a result of the distribution of peak noise events relative to the occurrence of sleep stages.

Several researchers have reported that peak characteristics of nocturnal noise events are more closely related to sleep quality (Eberhardt & Akselsson, 1987; Tulen et al., 1986) and transient sleep disturbances (Vallet et al., 1983a) than measures that integrate acoustic energy over protracted periods (e.g., Leq_8). There is some consistency among researchers who report peak SPLs suggesting that noise events producing indoor peak SPLs of 45–55 dB(A) and above are more likely to both cause transient disturbances or influence sleep stage parameters than noise events with lower peak SPLs (Eberhardt & Akselsson, 1987; Öhrström & Björkman, 1983; Vallet et al., 1983a). Despite some consensus regarding peak thresholds of noise that will cause disturbances, other peak characteristics have been much less carefully studied in field settings. Both the rise time (Tulen et al., 1986) and the duration (Lukas, 1976; Tulen et al., 1986) of peak noise events have been suggested as important stimulus parameters, though neither is reported with sufficient regularity to warrant a reasonable assessment of their respective contributions to sleep disturbances. Despite limited data about peak characteristics, the sharp rise times of aircraft noise have been used to explain the greater annoyance associated with aircraft relative to road or rail noise (Spreng, 2004). And, certain situational characteristics of peak noise events may also influence the likelihood and nature of sleep disturbances. For instance, the likelihood that a given peak SPL will elicit a sleep disturbance depends in part upon the background noise level (Vallet et al., 1983a; Vallet, Gagneux, & Simonnet, 1980). Thus, although there may be difficulties in obtaining data regarding the specific characteristics of each noise event over the course of a night's sleep, information such as time of occurrence, rise time, and relative magnitude may well be critical to understanding the potential deleterious effects of nighttime noise.

This conclusion is underscored by research concerning habituation to environmental noise after years of exposure. Sleep researchers have repeatedly found that the sleep quality of those who have slept in noisy environments for one or more years improves significantly when changes are introduced (sound insulation, double-glazed windows) to reduce indoor peak SPLs (Eberhardt & Akselsson, 1987; Griefahn & Gros, 1986; Vallet et al., 1983a; Wilkinson & Campbell, 1984). Laboratory and field research indicate that although behavioral habituation to nocturnal noise events does occur (e.g., awakenings decline; Thiessen & Lapointe, 1978), EEG arousals (Townsend, Johnson, & Muzet, 1973), shifts in sleep level (Thiessen & Lapointe, 1978), and phasic cardiovascular responding (Vallet, Gagneux, Clairet, et al., 1983) are much more resistant to habituation. These findings are consistent with animal research, which suggests that cells in the dorsal Raphe nuclei are responsible for regulating ultradian sleep cycles (e.g., Lydic, McCarley, & Hobson, 1987; Shima, Nakahama, & Yamamoto, 1986), and that these cells do not habituate to auditory and visual stimuli during sleep while other cells in the classical reticular formation do (Heym, Trulson, & Jacobs, 1982). These findings are consistent as well with a recently presented model of subcortical stress responding to noxious auditory stimuli. Relying on animal and human literature showing the fear-conditioned plasticity of the amygdala, Spreng (2004) suggests that, once negative assessments have been associated with particular noise events, the amygdala becomes tuned to the event type (e.g., dominant frequencies and peak characteristics) and recruits fast-reacting neurons to subcortically trigger vegetative responses (stress hormone release) to future occurrences of the event. Thus, rather than habituating to environmental noise, this model suggests that we become hypersensitive to those noise events we have evaluated negatively. It seems unlikely, then, that complete adaptation to nocturnal noise events ordinarily occurs in field settings, highlighting the need to carefully characterize the potential health effects of chronic exposure to noise in sleep environments.

Several sleep researchers interested in sleep quality and the health effects of noise have examined endocrine responses to both acute and chronic noise exposures. Endocrine responses are interesting in part because certain patterns are seen as indicative of stress and have implications for stress-related disorders. Recent English-language reviews of German research over the past 10–15 years concur that night time (air and road) traffic noise are positively associated with stress-related hormone levels and negatively related to sleep quality (Maschke & Hecht, 2004; Ising & Kruppa, 2004). Babisch et al. (2001), for instance, reported that women whose bedrooms faced heavily traveled Berlin roads had elevated overnight urinary noradrenaline relative to those whose bedrooms faced quiet environments. However, perceived sleep disturbances were only related to noradrenaline for those women who failed to get relief from the traffic noise by closing their windows. Neither of these effects was found for women whose living rooms (rather than bedrooms) faced the noisy street, suggesting that night time noise per se elicited the negative responses. Sleep researchers have also begun to monitor endocrines during sleep as a way to help identify noise-related disruptions of ultradian, circadian, and circaseptan cycles of responding because such disruptions may diminish sleep quality (and thereby the functions of sleep) and ultimately have health effects. In particular, a distinction between SWS and REM sleep disturbances is gaining currency in the literature, with several researchers suggesting that increased cortisol during its circadian trough (first half of the sleep period, when SWS predominates) constitutes a biological marker for chronic stress (Born & Fehm, 2000; Maschke & Hecht, 2004). Although biological markers for chronic stress have yet to be substantiated (others have been suggested; see, e.g., Clow, 2004), given the evidence for nonhabituation to overnight noise and the slow metabolic rate of cortisol (60–130 mins; Spreng, 2004), chronically elevated night time cortisol is highly plausible for people sleeping in noisy environments, which puts them at risk for a broad range of disorders.[4]

Children in home and school environments. The effects of chronic exposure to noise have also been the focus of research on children in home and school environments. Although noise in both environments can have deleterious effects on school performance and health, noise research with children has tended to focus on one or the other setting, and often on a particular type of noise (air or road traffic). And unlike research in sleep environments, there have been few quasi-experimental studies of children in which noise levels have been manipulated by the investigators.

Researchers have been able to capitalize on nonexperimental changes or differences in existing noise levels, however. In an early classic study, noise levels in apartment buildings that spanned a busy highway were associated with impaired auditory discrimination and reading abilities of children who lived in the apartments (Cohen, Glass, & Singer, 1973). Several early researchers highlighted cardiovascular and other stress-related physiological responding to examine the potential health effects of chronic noise exposure on school-age children. Studies examining aircraft (Karogodina, 1969) and road traffic (Karsdorf & Klappach, 1968) noise, for instance, suggested that children in noisy schools had higher resting blood pressure than their counterparts in quiet schools, and this has generally been confirmed by more recent work (see review by Evans & Lepore, 1993). Cohen and his colleagues (Cohen, Evans et al., 1980) reported cross-sectional data from an oftcited study of children attending noisy schools underneath busy air corridors (one flight every 2.5 mins.) surrounding Los Angeles International airport. Compared to matched children from quiet schools, children attending schools under the noisy air corridors had higher resting SBP and DBP, measured in a quiet environment. Subsequent longitudinal data did not support habituation of these effects over time (Cohen et al., 1981). Regecová and Kellerová (1995) reported similar results when traffic noise was the focus of a large-scale study (n = 1542) in Bratislava. Children attending schools in noisy urban areas (>60 dB(A) Leq_{24}) showed elevated resting SBP and DBP relative to that of matched children attending schools in quiet urban areas (<60 dB(A) Leq_{24}), and in both the Los Angeles and Bratislava studies, noise at home had little or no relationship to the cardiovascular measures.

Two research groups have published much of the recent nonauditory noise research on children, Haines and her colleagues focusing on the cognitive effects of aircraft noise in school environments, and Evans and his colleagues, who have examined stress-related and cognitive

---

[4] Including cardiovascular diseases (e.g., hypertension and myocardial infarction), diabetes, osteoporosis, gastric ulcer and immunosupression (see Spreng, 2000).

effects of noise in both home and school environments. Both groups have repeatedly found that noise is associated with less proficient reading (Evans, Hygge, & Bullinger, 1995; Haines et al., 2001b; Haines et al., 2001c; Stansfeld et al., 2005) and pre-reading skills (Maxwell & Evans, 2000), though occasionally these effects only occur for the most difficult reading items (Haines et al., 2001a; Hygge, Evans, & Bullinger, 2002), and the effects may disappear altogether when socioeconomic status is controlled (Haines, Stansfeld, Head, & Job, 2002) or if road noise is considered independently of aircraft noise (Stansfeld et al., 2005). Thus, as with the early research, negative effects on reading have been the most consistent finding in the recent literature, but there is still enough variability in the results to raise questions about the nature of any cause and effect relationships that might be responsible for these findings. Other negative psychological effects reported include decreased attention and social adaptability (Ristovska, Gjorgiev, & Jordanova, 2004), increased self-reported stress (Haines et al., 2001c; Evans et al., 2001), and behavioral problems in class (Lercher, Evans, Meis, & Kofler, 2002; Ristovska et al., 2004). These cognitive and other psychosocial effects are complemented by several reports of stress-related physiological effects, but these are not consistently found either. Evans and colleagues, for instance, have reported increased resting blood pressure for noise exposed children, but these have mostly been marginally significant effects (Evans, Hygge, & Bullinger, 1995; Evans et al., 1998; Evans et al., 2001). They have also collected overnight urinary endocrines in these studies, with epinephrine and norepinephrine discriminating between noise and quiet groups in two studies (Evans et al., 1995; Evans et al., 1998), and cortisol in one (Evans et al., 2001). Finally, Haines and her colleagues have not found noise-related cortisol or catecholamine effects in the two studies where they collected these data (Haines, Stansfeld, Brental, et al., 2001; Haines, et al., 2001b), but Ising and his colleagues have reported increased cortisol associated with low frequency night time road traffic noise (Ising & Ising, 2002; Ising et al., 2004).

Thus, the recent literature on noise and children presents a hodge-podge of somewhat contradictory findings. Though we might begin to interpret these contradictions by parsing the many differences among the studies (e.g., type and intensity of noise events, age of students, control of confounds, etc.), it may be more fruitful to examine some of their common weaknesses. First, and perhaps most important, is how sound is measured in these studies. Sound intensities are typically estimated for areas (e.g., neighborhoods, schools, communities) based on civil aviation and other transport-related contour maps and models, rather than measured on site.[5] The accuracy of these estimates is only as good as that of the models, which is rou-

tinely not reported, and thus the error variance that sound estimates contribute to the relationship between noise and dependent variables is largely unknown.[6] The accuracy of these estimates is clouded as well by the time period used to estimate exposures at school – usually 16 or 24 hours – which presumes either that the students are at school for the period in question (clearly unlikely), or that noise exposures at home and school are essentially the same. Though few of the recent studies have measured noise at home and school, those that have cast doubt on the suitability of this latter assumption. As mentioned above, Haines and her colleagues have found that roughly one third of students' have school noise exposures that do not match their home noise exposures (Haines, Stansfeld, Brentnall et al., 2001; Haines et al., 2001b), a mismatch that will contribute error variance to the extent that noise at home impacts the stress-related physiological and cognitive performance variables typically examined in these studies. As for physiological variables, we saw in the review of occupational literature above that noise experienced during working hours can clearly be associated with increased resting cardiovascular and endocrine levels measured at other times of the day. This suggests that mismatched home and school noise environments may add considerable error variance to the noise/stress-variable relationships examined in the child noise literature. As for the effects of noise at home on cognitive performance variables, we need to examine the effects of noise on learning, and this brings us to the second common weakness in recent research on children and noise: the understanding and measurement of learning.

Learning is usually not formally defined in the child noise literature. However, implicit in the focus on school environments and cognitive performance variables is the hypothesis that noise can disrupt learning. In particular, much of the recent work has focused on whether (and to what extent) noise disrupts the acquisition of knowledge in school settings. The effects of noise on knowledge retrieval are either methodologically controlled (Evans and colleagues) or regarded as a confounding factor (Haines and colleagues), and the effects of noise in other settings are interpreted vis-à-vis knowledge acquisition in school. For example, when the effects of noise at home are considered, the emphasis is on stress and other health-related outcomes that might impact both in-class motivation or overgeneralized "tuning out" strategies that can interfere with knowledge acquisition. There is little acknowledgement in this work that learning is an ongoing psychophysiological process that extends beyond the school setting. A process that involves interim processes between acquisition and retrieval, processes that are closely tied to circadian and ultradian rhythms of endocrines and neurotransmitters,

---

[5] Evans and colleagues have measured noise on site in two recent studies (Evans et al., 1998; Hygge et al., 2002), but they used 24 hr measurements at school, which may or may not reflect noise exposures at home.

[6] And, even if the models are very accurate for reasonably small areas (e.g., neighborhoods), local conditions within these areas will always add noise to the data, as in the Babisch et al. (2001) study reported above, in which the difference between significant and nonsignificant effects of road noise hinged on whether or not bedrooms faced the busy street.

and thus they may also be vulnerable to the effects of noise. Learning, of course, relies heavily on memory, and the longterm retention of information requires that memories be stabilized, enhanced, and often reorganized to optimally integrate with existing knowledge and skills (Stickgold, 2005). A common umbrella term for these postencoding, interim processes is "consolidation," and it has long been held that sleep is critical to memory consolidation. If this is true, it may be just as important to study children's sleep environments as it is to study school settings if we want to fully understand the effects that noise can have on learning.

In the past 10–15 years, the sleep and memory research communities have shown a renewed interest in sleep-dependent memory consolidation, and this work has direct implications for the effects of noise on learning. Researchers have found that, relative to similarly long waking periods, sleep enhances memory for recently acquired knowledge and skills (for reviews, see Gais & Born, 2004a; Payne & Nadel, 2004; Stickgold, 2005), and may even inspire insight into problems encountered during the day (Wagner et al., 2004). And, there is increasing evidence that the consolidation of certain types of learning may be associated with different aspects of sleep. The primary distinction has been between SWS and REM sleep, which predominate in the first and second halves of the night, respectively. Consolidation of memory for declarative (episodic and semantic) information is associated with SWS periods, while the consolidation of memory for nondeclarative (procedural) information is associated with REM sleep periods. Researchers have also proposed two-step models of consolidation for procedural information that implicate both the early phase of SWS and the latter phase of REM sleep (Power, 2004; Stickgold et al., 2000).

One especially interesting aspect of this work (with respect to the effects of noise on children) is the relationship between circadian endocrine rhythms and sleep-dependent memory consolidation. In particular, increases in cortisol during its nighttime trough have been shown to eliminate the enhancement of memory for declarative information that is associated with SWS (Plial & Born, 1997, 1999).[7] This result suggests a possible explanation for the contradictory or weak cognitive performance findings in the recent child noise literature. If noise experienced at home raises cortisol during its circadian trough, it may compromise learning (by disrupting consolidation) independently of noise experienced at school, which interferes with the acquisition of knowledge. Ising and Ising (2002) recently reported just such a finding with children, showing that cortisol during the first half of the night was correlated with low frequency road traffic noise levels, as well as with impaired sleep, memory, and ability to concentrate. These relationships were not found for cortisol levels during the latter half of the night, which

suggests that the noise-related increase in cortisol during SWS per se was responsible for the negative impacts on cognitive performance. In contrast to this work, studies that focus narrowly on noise at school and its effects on knowledge acquisition, as much of the recent research has, may well be mischaracterizing the potential that noise has to disrupt learning. This is because the reported cognitive performance effects reflect not only noise exposures during knowledge acquisition but noise exposures during consolidation as well. If noise exposures at home and school are substantially different (as we have seen they can be), it is virtually impossible to interpret the effects of noise measured only at school because many of the students will have been misclassified with respect to noise at home.

Perhaps the most important way, then, to address the apparent contradictions in the child noise literature is to more carefully measure noise, first by relying on onsite measurements rather than estimates,[8] and second by measuring noise in those environments where children spend most of their time, not just in one environment to make assumptions about the others. Although the practical constraints of working with children may make the use of personal noise dosimetry impossible, more densely measuring exposures in multiple environments would vastly improve the power of research in the child noise literature. And, as illustrated above by some of the recent occupational noise research, when densely measured noise events are paired with densely measured physiological responding, relationships can be found that might otherwise go undetected. This is important not only for establishing possible health-related stress responses associated with noise in different environments, but dense measurements of both halves of this putative cause and effect relationship can also help us understand how noise experienced outside the school setting can negatively impact cognitive processes central to learning.

We turn now from our examination of this quintessential environmental stressor to a review of more positively toned transactions with the physical environmental, those that are thought to reduce psychological stress and restore cognitive functioning.

3. PALLIATIVE ENVIRONMENTS

the enjoyment of scenery employs the mind without fatigue and yet exercises it; tranquilizes it and yet enlivens it; and thus, through the influence of the mind over the body, gives the effect of refreshing rest and reinvigoration to the whole system. (F. L. Olmsted, 1865).

Beliefs in the beneficial effects of nature are as old as urban civilization itself (Ulrich & Parsons, 1992), and they have been a consistent theme in historical accounts of human relationships with the natural world (Eisenberg,

---

[7] This is true of acetylcholine as well, which also reaches its nadir during SWS (Gais & Born, 2004b; Power, 2004).

[8] Or, at the very least, report the accuracy of the models that are used to make estimates.

1998; Glacken, 1967). Typically, people cite unique opportunities to relax or unwind in natural environments as being key to their benefits. They usually attribute salutary psychological and physical effects to transactions with nature, transactions that are as engaging as a wilderness adventure trip, or as fleeting as a glance out the window. Beliefs such as these are currently very strong and very popular among laypersons (Korpela, Hartig, Kaiser, & Fuhrer, 2001; Ogunseitan, 2005), but also among a broad range of academics and policymakers, especially those in the design and healthcare fields (Frumkin, 2001; Schweitzer, Gilpin, & Frampton, 2004; St. Leger, 2003). In fact, confidence in these beliefs is such that Berry and colleagues recently told healthcare administrators that "healing gardens" can routinely be incorporated into hospital design because the estimated cost they add to a typical new hospital ($1,000,000) can be more than offset by savings attributable to environmental distracters (see Berry et al., 2004, exhibits 1 & 2). Prudent readers may wonder what (beyond beliefs) justifies such claims, and as we shall see, the evidence for actual health effects of contact with nature is surprisingly thin, albeit growing. Although there is a broad empirical base of self-reports indicating that nature has beneficial effects, and some psychophysiological evidence that nature transactions reduce sympathetic arousal associated with stressful and other negative emotional states, there is almost no epidemiological data on health effects. In the following sections we will briefly review some of this evidence, describe two major theories that have been used to account for the findings, and then examine how psychophysiological constructs might be used to sharpen distinctions between these theories.

3.1. Empirical evidence for the beneficial effects of nature

The notion that certain environmental features are stress-reducing and thereby salutary is the obverse of the idea that environmental stressors have deleterious health effects. Unlike the environmental stress literature, however, epidemiologists have not examined the question of restorative natural environments, except for one research group in Japan. Takano, Nakamura, and Watanabe (2002) analyzed the five year survival data (1992–1997) of 3144 people born from 1903–1918 in two cities in the Tokyo metropolitan area. Independent of several control variables (age, sex, functional status, SES, environmental noise, etc.), those with nearby parks, tree-lined streets, and walkable areas were 14% more likely to survive than those without these environmental features. In an earlier study, Tanaka, Takano, Nakamura, and Takeuchi (1996) reported a negative correlation between mortality rates and land area devoted to woodland and/or farmland in cities with more than 4000 people per km^2, but not in less densely populated cities. Other researchers examining the relationship between urban green space and health have used self-reported health and quality of life mea-

sures rather than mortality or morbidity statistics, and they have reported similar outcomes. In a large and well-controlled Dutch study (10,000+ survey), for example, the amount of green space in urban living environments was positively related to self-reported physical and mental health, and negatively related to number of symptoms recently reported (de Vries, Verheij, Groenewegen, & Spreeuwenberg, 2003). Apart from being well-controlled, this study is also impressive because of the effect size reported: if the correlations reflect a true cause and effect relationship, then a 10% increase in urban green space would lead to a decrease in symptoms comparable to a five year decrease in age. The frequency of visits to and amount of time spent in urban green spaces have also been related to both self-reported restorative and preventative health benefits (Grahn & Stigsdotter, 2003), as has the presence of a garden or other greenery adjacent to one's dwelling (Stigsdotter & Grahn, 2004; Wells & Evans, 2003). Even the mere access to a window with a "green" view has been found to be beneficial (Kaplan, 2001; Ulrich, 1984).

While suggestive, especially when considered in toto, these studies are correlational in nature and thus it is difficult to infer cause and effect relationships between urban green space and health. In most studies, either exposure to nature or health effects are estimated by respondents, and in other studies respondents estimate both types of variables, which makes demand characteristics plausible if not likely alternative explanations. And, even in those cases where exposures to nature (e.g., the proximity of parks) are independently verified by geographic data and health status is gleaned from medical records or public health sources, there are still plausible alternative explanations, such as the beneficial effects of walking (Murphy, Nevill, Neville, Biddle, & Hardman, 2002; Osei-Tutu & Campagna, 2005),[9] that preclude definitive statements about the effects of nature per se. Thus, we turn next to some experimental work that emphasizes the stress-reducing qualities of nature, the presumptive mechanism implicit in the epidemiological and other urban research on the beneficial effects of nature.

Perhaps the most influential study of the potential health effects of natural environments was not an experimental study at all, but a retrospective examination of patients recovering from gall bladder surgery under different environmental conditions. Matching patients on pertinent control variables, Ulrich (1984) found that those patients with a window view of a small wooded area recovered more quickly, used fewer potent analgesics and were generally easier to handle (according to chart notes) than those whose view was of a brick wall. In subsequent experimental work, Ulrich and colleagues (1991) explicitly tested the stress-reducing quality of natural environments

---

[9] In fact, when public open spaces are nearby, large and attractive, people are 50% more likely to engage in high levels of walking than when these circumstances do not obtain (Giles-Corti et al., 2005).

by monitoring psychological and physiological recovery from a brief laboratory stressor. Following the stressor, participants viewed a videotaped traffic intersection, an urban pedestrian mall, or one of several natural environments. Those who viewed the natural environments showed quicker and more complete recovery from elevated frontalis, skin conductance, and pulse transit time measures. Psychological responding echoed these results, as well as those from an earlier study of psychological restoration (Ulrich, 1979), as the natural environment groups reported less anger and fear and more happiness following the environmental exposures than did the urban environment groups. Several conceptual replications followed, one assessing the relative importance of water as an element in restorative environments (Parsons, 1991a), and the other examining whether fairly minimal views of nature (as seen through the windshield of a moving car) would have restorative effects (Parsons et al., 1998). In both studies, nature-dominated environments elicited a greater reduction in sympathetic arousal following a stressor than urban environments did, although in the former study an urban scene with a substantial natural element (a river) elicited similar restorative effects. One interesting finding in the latter study was that exposure to a natural environment helped participants handle a subsequent stressor, which is consistent with recent data from Cackowski and Nasar (2003), who found that participants who viewed videotaped drives though tree-lined parkways showed greater tolerance for postdrive frustration than those who viewed more urbanized drives. Finally, a recent field study of inpatients in a cardiopulmonary rehabilitation program found that those who participated in a one hour introductory horticulture therapy session had lower heart rates and improved moods relative to those who attended a one hour patient education class (Wichrowski et al., 2005). Although the authors attributed these effects to the horticulture therapy session, which included a brief lecture, a tour of the garden/greenhouse, and repotting a plant, the therapy session also was more physically active than the patient education class, and this alternative explanation cannot be ruled out.

The research reviewed thus far has emphasized stress-reduction and other positive emotions people feel in response to natural environments. Other researchers have emphasized more cognitively oriented benefits, especially the restoration of voluntary or "directed" attention (see Kaplan & Kaplan, 1989). Ottosson and Grahn (2005), for instance, examined the focal attention of nonstressed elderly participants after spending a leisure hour indoors and an hour in an outdoor green area, and found that the latter intervention improved their concentration abilities but had no effect on HR or blood pressure. Hartig, Mang, and Evans (1991, study 2) found that after performing a demanding cognitive task, participants who walked through a natural environment performed better on a subsequent proofreading task than did those who walked through an urban environment or those who sat quietly in a research room listening to music and reading magazines; there were no differences, however, in post-walk blood pressure or heart rate.[10] In a recently reported similar study, Hartig and colleagues (2003) had participants drive to an urban or a natural research field site, after which half of the people in each setting performed cognitively demanding tasks for one hour to deplete directed attention capacity. Following their arrival (and tasks, if assigned), all participants then sat for 10 mins in either a windowless room (urban setting) or a room with a view of some trees (natural setting) before taking a 50 min walk in their respective environments. Regardless of whether they performed the cognitive tasks, participants who sat in the room with the nature view had lower diastolic blood pressure than those in the windowless room; and, lower systolic BP and diastolic BP also discriminated the nature group from the urban group during the subsequent walk. The two measures of directed attention capacity yielded conflicting results, however, with one indicating greater attentional capacity for the natural environment group, regardless of whether they had performed the depleting tasks, and the other showing no differences. Given the conflicting nature of the cognitive results, and the fact that both the physiological and cognitive effects occurred regardless of whether participants had performed the hour long, attention-depleting task, these effects might be more appropriately labeled "exposure" rather than "restorative" effects. That is, it may be that nature ordinarily elicits attention (as reflected in physiological responding) regardless of one's current capacity to direct attention and in direct proportion to its aesthetic value. Consider some conceptually related work in which natural stimuli appear to capture attention involuntarily, do not have the expected cognitive effects, yet the results are readily interpreted in terms of the environments' affective qualities.

Laumann, Gärling, and Stormark (2003) found that participants recovering from a cognitively demanding task had slower heart rates while viewing a nature video than participants who viewed an urban video, though the nature group performed worse on a subsequent selective attention task. Following Lacey and Lacey (1974), they interpreted the slower heart rates for the nature group as indicative of greater attentional or sensory intake for natural versus urban stimuli. They attributed the nature group's poorer performance on the cognitive task to the broader attentional set (reduced selectivity) that accompanies reduced physiological arousal (Easterbrook, 1959). However, the nature group only had slower heart rates while viewing the nature video, not during the subsequent cognitive task, so it seems unlikely that reduced physiological arousal accounts for the difference in performance between the two groups. Alternatively, had they measured emotional responding, they might well have found that the nature group's mood improved following the video, and, given

---

[10] This may have been due to the delay involved in re-instrumenting participants after the walk (see Parsons & Hartig, 2000).

numerous reports by Isen and her colleagues (see Isen, 1999, for a review) showing that positive moods facilitate broad or inclusive thinking, they could reasonably have attributed poorer performance on the focal attention task to the moods elicited by the environments rather than to arousal. Larsen and colleagues (1998), for instance, have reported data on natural stimuli that suggest such an effect. They found that as the number of houseplants in an office environment increases, the mood of the occupants increases as well, though their performance on a narrowly focused cognitive task decreases.

Another group of studies on the cognitive effects of nature-dominated environments is also more readily interpreted when affective responding is considered, though most of the authors involved were not specifically studying emotions or the benefits of natural environmental stimuli. Researchers and clinicians interested in nonpharmocological adjuncts to pain relief have long used various distraction techniques, such as hypnosis (Rainville et al., 1999) music, (Good et al., 1999), and humor (Cogan, Cogan, Waltz, & McCue, 1987) to draw attention away from painful treatments and medical procedures. There is good evidence that painful stimuli monopolize attention in the absence of compelling non-painful stimuli (Eccleston & Crombez, 1999), and recent research suggests that certain classes of natural environmental stimuli constitute compelling distractions from pain. Clinicians performing various painful medical procedures have found that patients randomly assigned to view natural environment surrogates report reduced pain (Diette et al., 2003), or reduced pain and anxiety (Lembo et al., 1998; Miller, Hickman, & Lemasters, 1992) relative to control conditions, with some case study evidence suggesting that greater interactivity with environmental stimuli leads to greater pain reduction (Hoffman et al., 2001). Experimental studies with healthy volunteers support these clinical data, indicating that both pain thresholds and pain tolerance increase when viewing nature-dominated stimuli (Tse, Ng, Chung, & Wong, 2002), and that more compelling environmental surrogates are more effective analgesics than less compelling ones (Hoffman et al., 2004). Finally, recent fMRI research indicates that, in addition to self-reports of reduced pain, nature-dominated environmental stimuli also elicit reduced activation of several brain areas associated with the perceived intensity and unpleasantness of pain (Hoffman et al., 2004).

These data on reduced anxiety and the unpleasantness of pain are especially interesting, as they suggest that the pain relief attributable to nature-dominated stimuli may be a function not only of the cognitive distraction they provide but also of their valence. Indeed, though only one of the pain studies cited above explicitly tested the effectiveness of positively toned environmental stimuli (Diette et al., 2003), the authors of the other studies seem to have intuitively concluded that valence is important, as they have all used pleasant environmental scenes as *cognitive* distracters. Their successful use of pleasant environmen-

tal distracters (whether intentional or not) complements the results of other pain research, which suggests that valence mediates the effect of cognitive distracters, generally lessening perceived pain when distracters are positive and increasing it when they are negative (de Wied & Verbaten, 2001; Meagher, Arnau, & Rhudy 2001; Rhudy & Meagher, 2001; Villemure & Bushnell, 2002). Although it is still unclear how affect mediates pain perception, there is recent evidence that affect can influence the perceived unpleasantness of pain independent of its perceived intensity (Rainville, Duncan, Price, Carrier, & Bushnell, 1997; Villemure, Slotnick, & Bushnell, 2003), and that affect can also influence the attention that is paid to pain (Keogh, Ellery, Hunt, & Hannent 2001; see also, Dolan, 2002, on the pre-attentive processing of emotion-laden stimuli). Thus, the emotional distress caused by pain seems to be somewhat dissociable from the attention paid to its sensory qualities (e.g., intensity, quality, or location), and both components of pain perception appear to be vulnerable to the influence of pre-existing or competing emotions, including the positive emotions elicited by nature-dominated environments.[11]

We have seen, then, that stressful, cognitively draining and painful states of mind all find succor in the pleasant diversion that nature-dominated environments provide. We have seen, as well, that the effects reported from both affectively-oriented (stress-reduction) and cognitively-oriented (attention restoration or distraction from pain) lines of research are best understood via significant affective mediation. That is, pleasant natural environments that have long been regarded as restorative cannot be adequately described either as involuntary-attention sinks or mere cognitive distracters: the positive emotions they elicit are central to the beneficial effects they produce. In the next section, we will see that the two dominant restorative environment theories emphasize affective and cognitive components of restoration, respectively, though neither of them integrates these aspects well enough to account for the empirical data reviewed here.

3.2. Restorative environments theory

Kaplan and Kaplan (1982, 1989) and Ulrich (1983, 1993) have proposed similar evolution-based explanations for restorative effects of natural environments, and in both cases the explanations grow out of their respective theories of environmental aesthetics. The evolutionary focus of these theories can be traced to numerous environmental aesthetics studies in the 1970s and 1980s showing overwhelming visual preferences for nature-dominated versus more urbanized environments, preferences that have been found in many cultures. The features of preferred environments include both certain types of natural contents (primarily water and green vegetation) and

---

[11] Whether this is true, as well, of negative emotions elicited by environmental stimuli is an open question: it has not been tried.

structural characteristics (open fore- and mid-ground, relatively low and even groundcovers, undulating topography, and occasional clumps of trees). These features represent the major empirical findings that must be accounted for in any theory of environmental aesthetics, and though the Kaplans and Ulrich both incorporate these findings in their models, they treat them somewhat differently.

Reasoning from the structural characteristics that predict preference, the Kaplans proposed that humans have two basic information processing needs that are central to functional capacity and health, exploration and understanding. People need to explore to acquire information from their surroundings, and they need to be able to quickly interpret the functional value of that information. The structural characteristics listed above are thought to facilitate both processes, and that is why they predict environmental preferences: they help to fulfill two basic human information processing needs. When opportunities for exploration and understanding are not immediately forthcoming (as they are in preferred environments), people must use directed (rather than involuntary) attention to acquire information and understand it. In developing their Attention Restoration Theory (ART), the Kaplans argue that the sociophysical environments of modern life present far fewer opportunities for ready exploration and understanding than our pre-urban environments did, and thus we rely on directed attention much more so than did our ancestors (Kaplan & Kaplan, 2003). However, because directed attention is a limited resource, it becomes depleted with both frequent and extended use and must be replenished before effective information acquisition and understanding (and thus, effective functioning) can resume. Discontinued use of directed attention (via *soft fascination*, which is involuntary attention to inherently interesting and positively toned environmental features and activities) is necessary though not sufficient for its restoration. We must also escape (either physically or psychologically) the sociophysical circumstances that depleted directed attention, to a place of sufficient scope and coherence as to be compatible with our psychological needs and behavioral inclinations. To the extent that environments embody these four components – fascination, being away, coherence and compatibility – they will restore directed attention, and the Kaplans maintain that nature-dominated environments are more likely than urban environments to have these features.

Although research indicates that these components predict the perceived restorativeness of environments (see Herzog, Maguire, & Nebel, 2003, for a review), there is relatively little evidence that they are related to actual restoration. In fact, there is a certain circularity to the work on perceived restorativeness, as the Kaplans derived these components in part from self-reports of the benefits of natural environments (e.g., Kaplan & Talbot, 1983). It is not surprising, then, that the reputed benefits of natural environments (passed through an information-processing filter) are related to the perceived benefits of natural environments as measured by various perceived-restorativeness scales. Whether perceived restorativeness is a useful construct, however, is still unclear. Recent research indicates that perceived restorativeness may be little more than a proxy for visual environmental preferences (Herzog et al., 2003), and this suggests that the reputed benefits of natural environments are closely tied to their attractiveness – That is, to their capacity to elicit liking, which is the focus of Ulrich's model.

In contrast to the Kaplans, Ulrich emphasizes the contents of aesthetically preferred environments as much as their structural charcteristics in his functional-evolutionary model of restorative environments. Thus, the potential safety and sustenance that elements such as water, trees, and flowering plants provide are as important as the promise of information gleaned from their spatial configuration. In more recent formulations of the model, Ulrich (1993) has adopted Orians' savanna hypothesis (Orians, 1980; 1986; Orians & Heerwagen, 1992) and Appleton's prospect and refuge notions (1975) to account for the positive regard we have for the structural features listed above. In particular, he emphasizes the feelings of safety and well-being that supportive savanna configurations engender, suggesting that opportunities to avoid harm and regain composure after threatening or challenging episodes are as important as the sustenance preferred elements in such environments provide. He also maintains that the positive emotions elicited by such supportive environments serve to block negative emotions and thoughts, facilitate restoration. This *opponent process* conception of emotions is congruent with current dynamic theories of emotion, which suggest that positive and negative emotions may occur simultaneously (and somewhat independently) under quiescent conditions, but tend to be negatively correlated under conditions of uncertainty or stress (Davis, Zautra, & Smith, 2004). Ulrich's notion of restoration, then, is considerably broader than the Kaplans' specific focus on attention restoration, encompassing all those situations that might elicit stress, including phasic episodes (e.g., encounters with predators or hostile conspecifics) and more tonic periods (e.g., extended vigilance during a hunt or while crafting a tool), as well as all the psychological and physiological effects that might accompany those situations. As befits a stress recovery model of restoration, and as evidenced by the review of research above, Ulrich has incorporated psychophysiological constructs and methods into his investigations of the restorative effects of nature-dominated environments. And, though the Kaplans and their colleagues have not emphasized psychophysiological investigations of attention restoration, there is no conceptual reason why more such studies could not be done. In fact, psychophysiological constructs and methods might help us sharpen the distinction between two theories that have a great deal of conceptual overlap.

3.3. Conceptual and methodological issues

There are a number of interrelated conceptual and methodological issues in the foregoing overviews of research and theory that warrant closer inspection. First, we will consider whether a distinction can be made between stress recovery and directed attention restoration, an issue with implications for choices regarding the selection, frequency, and timing of measures in studies of environmental restorativeness. As suggested above, there is a fair degree of conceptual overlap between these models. Ulrich et al. (1991), for instance, have suggested that the directed attention fatigue (DAF) construct can be accommodated by existing models of environmental stress, such as information overload models (e.g., Cohen, 1978; Cohen & Spacapan, 1978). Kaplan and Kaplan (1982), however, maintain that DAF can be experienced independently of stressful conditions, and that consequently it represents a distinct psychological state. Though several operationalizations of DAF have appeared in the literature (e.g., Cimprich, 1993; Hartig et al., 2003), they have not been adequately distinguished from stress manipulations (Kaplan, 1995), and thus the construct validity of DAF has yet to be empirically verified. As we have described, psychophysiological constructs and methods have been central to the development of the stress recovery model and only incidental to the directed attention restoration model. However, we see an opportunity for these psychophysiological tools to help determine the relative utility of DAF as a construct and, by extension, the ultimate heuristic value of distinguishing between stress recovery and directed attention restoration (cf. Hartig & Evans, 1993).

As an example, consider the problem of determining whether DAF can be experienced independently of stress. DAF is thought to occur through prolonged bouts of focal attention, and has been operationalized in terms of performance on tasks that require vigilance. The experience of stress is typically described as resulting from a perception of threat, harm, or frustrated goal attainment, and it is often operationalized in terms of autonomic reactivity, such as changes in blood pressure and skin conductance. Thus, to determine whether procedures thought to produce DAF were also stressful, we might monitor a measure such as skin conductance during administration of vigilance tasks. This approach is problematic, however, to the extent that our measure of stress is also responsive to manipulations of attention, which is the case for many autonomic measures, including skin conductance (Strube, 1990, p. 49). Clearly what we need is a pair of measures, one that indexes stress but is relatively nonresponsive to focal attention, and one that indexes focal attention but is relatively nonresponsive to stress. Tasks that lead to increases in the latter and quiesence (or decreases) in the former would be likely candidates for DAF procedures.

Though there may be no ideal measures that uniquely index stress and focal attention, psychophysiological measures that might be used to assess the suitability of DAF tasks can be found among the growing number of components identified in event-related brain potentials (ERPs). Over the last 30 years, extensive evidence in the psychophysiological literature has established that the amplitude of negative ERPs occurring 100–150 ms (N100) after a target stimulus is related to selective attention (see Coles, Gratton, & Fabiani, 1990, for a review). Attended stimuli elicit larger (more negative) N100s relative to nonattended stimuli. Because the onset latency of a variant of the N100, *processing negativity*, has been associated with the allocation of attentional resources (see Coles et al., 1990; Hansen & Hillyard, 1983), this class of ERP may well be useful in tracking deteriorating attentional capacity (i.e., DAF). A more recently identified ERP component, the P50 (positive deflection, $\approx$50 ms peak latency), has been shown to be insensitive to changes in directed attention under certain circumstances, yet it is influenced by stress manipulations (White & Yee, 1997).

Apart from ERPs, there are other measures that might help environmental researchers discriminate between DAF and more stressful psychological states. One interesting example comes from research on tonic electromyographic (EMG) activity recorded from task-irrelevant musculature during the performance of protracted vigilance and other cognitive tasks. Rising EMG gradients during such tasks are often found in task-irrelevant muscles, and they have repeatedly been related to task difficulty, subjective effort, and stress elicited by the task (see Tassinary, Cacioppo, & Vanman, this volume). Because EMG gradients unfold over similar time courses as those used for putative DAF tasks, they appear well-suited to track the potential stressfullness of such tasks. Another measure that might be useful in this regard comes from the pain perception and related literatures in which numerous researchers have found that activations of the rostral and caudal portions of the anterior cingulate cortex (ACC) are associated with affectively- and cognitively-oriented tasks, respectively (see Bush et al., 1998; Whalen et al., 1998, for reviews). Interestingly, there is some evidence that the affective and cognitive divisions of the ACC are reciprocally inhibitory (Bantick et al., 2002), and that the cognitive division is part of a distributed attentional network activated by cognitively demanding tasks (Devinsky, Morrel, & Vogt, 1995). If we monitor the ACC, then, during the performance of a candidate DAF task, we would expect to see increased caudal activation throughout the task if it truly elicits DAF independently of stress. However, if we see initial activation in the caudal ACC giving way to more rostral activation, we would have to suspect that the task was becoming stressful. In fact, given the inhibitory relationship between the rostral and caudal ACC and the attentional focus of caudal activation, we could propose that rising activation in the rostral ACC contributes to DAF.[12] Of course, the timing of the change in ACC activation relative

---

[12] Note how this comports with Ulrich's contention that DAF can be incorporated into existing models of environmental stress.

to decreasing performance on the attentional task would be critical in making such a causal attribution.

Thus, in these three measures – ERP components, EMG gradients, and rostral versus caudal ACC activation – we have the beginnings of an analytical toolkit that may help us determine the construct validity of DAF and, more broadly, the relative utility of a distinction between the stress recovery and directed attention restoration models of environmental restorativeness.

A set of issues related to the conceptualization of DAF (i.e., its stressful/nonstressful character) concern operationalizations of restoration, which have been inadequately addressed in the literature on restorative environments. Restoration has not been consistently defined in the environmental literature, nor has recovery been consistently defined in the stress recovery literature. Haynes, Gannon, Orimoto, O'Brien, and Brandt (1991) have defined recovery from stress as "changes in stressor-induced responses following stressor termination" (p. 356). This broad definition incorporates both nonlinear and bidirectional changes in variables following stressor offset, which allows for "recovery" that does not necessarily reflect a return to prestressor response levels. In particular, however, if the word "stimulus" is used in place of "stressor" in this definition, then the simple notion of "changes following stimulus offset" is broad enough to capture the presumed depletion/replenishment cycle of DAF and restored attentional capacity as well as the experience of stress and the return to autonomic equanimity. "Stress recovery" would no longer be appropriate for the term being defined, though "restoration" is suitable, as it could be applied both to the replenishment of a capacity and to the return to physiological homeostasis.

Under this conceptualization, then, if restoration can involve the replenishment of a capacity, then the operationalization of restoration does not necessarily imply the measurement autonomic (and other) stress-related variables. For instance, just as the N100 ERP component may prove useful in determining the construct validity of DAF, the onset latency of processing negativity also may be useful in assessing the restoration of directed attentional capacity. The onset latency of processing negativity increases as the difficulty in discriminating between attended and unattended channels increases. And, presumably, the difficulty of a given attentional discrimination is related to the available directed attentional capacity, and as this capacity is depleted attentional discriminations become more difficult. Thus, the onset latency of processing negativity might be expected to increase as directed attentional capacity is depleted. That is, as DAF increases, discriminations among attended and unattended channels should be more difficult. Conversely, as directed attentional capacity is restored, the onset latency of processing negativity might be expected to decrease because attentional discriminations should become easier.

If DAF is eventually resolved to be a stressful psychological state, however, it may still be useful to distin-guish it from other stressors, in part because of the complex nature of physiological mechanisms that underlie stress responses and stress recovery. As typically conceived (Kaplan, 1995) and induced (Hartig et al., 2003), DAF unfolds over a protracted period of focused cognitive activity. The slowly developing nature of DAF has direct implications for the stress-related physiological mechanisms that may be engaged by this psychological state and, ultimately, for any health-related consequences that may be inferred, which has been a prime concern in the restorative environments literature (see Parsons, 1991b). As Haynes et al. (1991) have noted, the duration of a stressor has important influences on patterns of physiological responding. Relatively brief, acute stressors (such as the math tasks, extemporaneous speeches, and iced appendages that abound in the stress literature) engage the sympathetic adrenomedullary system, which quickly leads to increased levels of immune activity and circulating epinephrine and norepinephrine. More long-lived stressors engage the hypothalamic-pituitary-adrenocortical system, leading to the release of cortisol, which has immunosuppressive effects. Thus, the physiological parameters that may be useful in assessing DAF and the associated restoration of directed attention, ERPs, corticosteroids, and immunocompetence, differ from the primarily cardiovascular and sympathetically-mediated (e.g., SCR) measures that have characterized empirical investigations of the stress recovery model of environmental restorativeness.

Finally, in closing this section we examine in passing methodological issues related to environmental sampling and representativeness, which have also been inadequately addressed in this relatively young field. Environmental psychologists have often been concerned with the representativeness of the environments under study. For our purposes here, this concern refers not only to the sampling of environments across the effective range of the physical variables of interest, but also to the restorative implications of sociophysical changes in environments over time, as was suggested by the Frankenhaeuser and colleagues (1989) study described above. In the empirical examinations of restorative environments thus far, environmental classes such as "natural" or "urban" have too often been represented by very small numbers of exemplars, leaving the interpretation of results open to attributions to particular environmental instantiations rather than to the environmental classes or variables of interest. While this particular problem in environmental sampling can be easily resolved (at least conceptually), others are less tractable, such as the selection of appropriate comparison or "control" conditions. Because people are never encountered outside of an environment, the concept of a "no-environment" control condition has no meaning (see Fredrickson & Levenson, 1998). Lastly, we raise the difficult issue of the ecological validity of environmental surrogates. Psychophysiological research on environmental restorativeness is more conveniently conducted in the laboratory than in the field, and thus a reliance on environmental surrogates is a primary concern. If the restorative qualities of environments can be adequately represented visually, then high-quality photography and videography may well produce adequate surrogates. However, to the extent that the environmental qualities of interest (restorative or otherwise) are not well represented by visually-oriented technologies, then the adequacy of environmental surrogates is called into question. This issue, in the guise of adequately represented movement through space, receives more careful consideration in the final section of this chapter, on topographic cognition.

4. TOPOGRAPHIC COGNITION

Don't know where I am and got no mother to guide me home. (Chariton, 1990, p. 141)

One can define spatial cognition broadly as any aspect of an organism's behavior that involves space and is informed by cerebral activity (Kritchevsky, 1988). Topographic cognition refers to a subset of these behaviors wherein cerebral activity guides an organism's movement through the molar environment. For purposes of this discussion, and as is typically conceived in studies of topographic cognition (e.g., Aguirre, Zarahn, & D'Esposito, 1998; Allen, 1985; Kuipers, 1982; Maguire, 1997), the molar environment is both large in scale or visually occluded so that it cannot be completely perceived from a single vantage point. Thus, walking a maze in a laboratory room, navigating a building, or exploring a city all constitute transactions with molar environments that engage topographic cognition.

Though we do it every day, mostly without thinking about it, finding our way through the world is both a critically important and quite complex behavior. Common animal behaviors that are crucial to survival, such as gathering food, finding mates or shelter, hunting prey, avoiding predators, and caching of young, all depend on an organism's ability to understand and navigate its physical surroundings (Spencer, Blades, & Morsley, 1989). While few of us still rely on our hunting skills for survival, case study evidence from clinical neuropsychology suggests that topographic disorientation can nevertheless be quite devastating (e.g., Cammalleri et al., 1996; Habib & Sirigu, 1987; Landis, Cummings, Benson, & Palmer, 1986; Whiteley & Warrington, 1978). Wayfinding is a complex behavior as well, as it requires the coordination of spatial perception, memory and attention, and often involves dynamic spatial processes, such as mental rotation and the construction of spatial imagery (Kritchevsky, 1988). In the last section of this chapter, we examine the contributions that psychophysiology can make to our understanding of these processes. We briefly review historical and recent work in clinical neuropsychology, psychobiology, and cognitive psychology, which suggests the importance of multimodal integration of perceptual information for topographic cognition. We then highlight some very interesting work that exploits recent advances in functional brain imaging techniques to investigate wayfinding. The reliance on transactions with environmental surrogates in this research prompts a discussion of how representations of large-scale environments can be assessed in psychophysiology, which is still largely a laboratory science.

4.1. Origins and recent research on topographic cognition

The origins of our current understanding of topographic cognition can be traced to late nineteenth century Europe, when clinical reports of spatial disorders associated with topographic disorientation began appearing in the medical literature. There were reports of impaired wayfinding in familiar environments (Badal, 1888/1982; Jackson, 1876/1958), and the inability to recognize familiar places (Meyer, 1900/1996), as well as reports of retained spatial knowledge accompanied by the inability to apply it (Wilbrand, 1892/1982). Although most researchers during this period distinguished these spatial deficits from more common aphasias, they typically did not acknowledge a commonality among reports – that many of these problems were associated with posterior lesions in the right hemisphere (Morrow & Ratcliff, 1988). In an influential series of papers, Zangwill and his colleagues (Ettlinger, Warrington, & Zangwill, 1957; McFie, Piercy, & Zangwill, 1950; Paterson & Zangwill, 1944, 1945) documented the importance of the posterior right hemisphere for spatial behavior (DeRenzi, 1982), and, in particular, Paterson and Zangwill (1945) identified a key distinction between two visuospatial deficits (topographic agnosia and amnesia) that continues to inform the bulk of latter day theory and research on topographic cognition. Topographic agnosics have difficulty recognizing familiar buildings and landmarks, while topographic amnesics cannot readily specify routes within or draw maps of familiar territory.

Echoing these neuropsychological findings, complementary strands of research in psychobiology and cognitive and environmental psychology have developed similar distinctions between topographic recognition and memory abilities. Early Hullian stimulus-response accounts of spatial behavior and learning in nonhuman animals have been supplanted by "cognitive mapping" explanations (Tolman, 1948), which assume that animals use allocentric[13] representations of the spatial relationships among environmental features to navigate their surroundings (see Allen, 1985, 1987; Schacter & Nadel, 1991). In particular, work with

---

[13] The terms *allocentric* and *egocentric* are used in the general literature on spatial cognition to refer to types of frames of reference, environment-centered and person-centered, respectively. Egocentric frames of reference include retinocentric, craniocentric, and somatocentric, while allocentric frames of reference may include any (usually stable) element or set of elements in the environment other than the self. Developmentally, egocentric frames of reference emerge first, followed by simple allocentric reference frames focusing on proximal elements in the environment, progressing through allocentric frames focused on more distal elements including those beyond the immediate perceptual horizon.

animals suggests a clear maturational distinction between landmark learning ability (early onset) and map learning ability (later onset; see Schacter & Nadel, 1991), and this is echoed by work with humans (Pine et al., 2002). Neural localization studies with animals (primarily the rat) have also been important in isolating the hippocampal formation as central to cognitive mapping functions (see O'Keefe & Nadel, 1978 for a review and seminal theoretical account of this work). Cognitive and environmental psychologists have devoted much of their research efforts to identifying and understanding types of topographic knowledge. Following Shemyakin's (1962) early theoretical account, researchers have generally identified three types of topographic knowledge: landmark knowledge, route knowledge, and configural or survey knowledge (Allen, 1985; Golledge & Stimson, 1997; Schacter & Nadel, 1991; Siegel & White, 1975; Thorndyke, 1981). Landmark knowledge confers the ability to recognize previously encountered, distinctive environmental features, and to use them as reference points for locomotion through the environment. Route knowledge comprises spatiotemporal relations among sequentially ordered environmental features coordinated with motor actions required to traverse set paths through an environment. And, possession of the most complex form of topographic knowledge, configural or survey knowledge, implies the ability to infer spatial relations among multiply interconnected environmental features from an allocentric frame of reference (see Allen, 1987; Schacter & Nadel, 1991; and Thorndyke, 1981 for variations on these basic definitions). More colloquially, configural knowledge refers to the possession of a "cognitive" or "mental" map, which allows one to flexibly interact with the environment to recognize short cuts, generate new routes when existing ones are blocked, judge distance to and direction of occluded elements, etc.

Although most researchers acknowledge these three basic types of topographic knowledge and regard both the microgenetic acquisition and the ontogenetic development of landmark, route, and configural knowledge and abilities to be sequential (Allen, 1985; Golledge, 1987; Siegel & White, 1975), the consensus is not absolute (see Golledge & Stimson, 1997, Ch. 5; Spencer et al., 1989, Ch. 1). Some have questioned the evidentiary basis of configural knowledge (e.g., Pick, 1993) or suggested that true configural knowledge cannot develop independently of exposure to symbolic representations of the environment (Moeser, 1988), while others have questioned the sequential microgenetic acquisition of topographic knowledge types (Montello, 1998). What these questions suggest is that the simple description of an orderly development of topographic knowledge and abilities is likely overly simple, and perhaps wrong in several respects, as others have noted (e.g., Magliano, Cohen, Allen, & Rodrigue, 1995; Mandler, 1988; Montello, 1998; Pick, 1993; Spencer et al., 1989). In particular, two distinctions regarding the manner in which topographic information is acquired have important implications for the brain imaging research described below.

First, topographic information about the environment can be gained through direct experience with the world or through interaction with symbolic representations of the environment, such as maps or verbal descriptions of routes. Presson and Hazelrigg (1984) have labeled the former *primary* and the latter *secondary spatial learning*, and many researchers have found that performance on topographic tasks can depend upon this distinction (Howard & Kerst, 1981; Scholl, 1987; Thorndyke & Hayes-Roth, 1982). Evans and Pezdek (1980), for example, reported that latencies to judge the accuracy of spatial relations among triads of buildings are linearly related to rotational disparity from typical Cartesian presentation (i.e., $0° =$ North) for students who learned the building locations from a map, though latencies are unrelated to Cartesian coordinates for those who learned the locations in situ.

Second, evidence suggests that a distinction between *passive* and *active* primary spatial learning may be important (see Cohen & Cohen, 1985, for a review). In general, active engagement with the environment is thought to produce more flexible cognitive maps (Cohen & Cohen, 1985; Siegel & White, 1975), whereas passive interactions tend to produce orientation-specific representations (e.g., Hintzman, O'Dell, & Arndt, 1981). Both correlational (Acredolo, 1988; Appleyard, 1970; Beck & Wood, 1976; Golledge & Spector, 1978) and experimental work (Cohen & Weatherford, 1980, 1981; Klatzky, Loomis, Beall, Chance, & Golledge, 1998; Richardson, Montello, & Hegarty, 1999; Simons & Wang, 1998; Wang & Simons, 1999) support this distinction, and the importance of active engagement seems not to lie with movement through the environment per se, but with the opportunity to monitor the environment that movement affords (e.g., Acredolo, Adams, & Goodwyn, 1984; Böök & Gärling, 1980a, 1980b, 1981). Many researchers have suggested that the integration of perceptual information during locomotion is central to maintaining orientation in and constructing representations of environments (e.g., Caplan et al., 2003; Evans & Pezdek, 1980; Gärling, Böök, & Lindberg, 1985; Montello, 1998; Spencer et al., 1989). Although some researchers have emphasized the importance of integrating multiple visual perceptions over time (e.g., Heft, 1983), others have suggested that periodic attention to retinal flow information in the environment can be used to calibrate orientation estimates gleaned from biomechanical and proprioceptive afferents (e.g., Pick, 1993).[14] Rieser and his colleagues (Rieser, Pick, Ashmead, & Garing, 1995) have shown that the accuracy of biomechanical estimates of distance (i.e., walking to a target with eyes closed) can be manipulated when prior biomechanical and visual

---

[14] Pick (1993, p. 36) actually used the term *optical flow*, though the context suggests that the intended meaning was retinal flow. Retinal flow is motion as it is presented to the retina, and it comprises both rotational flow and optical flow. The former is due to motion produced by eye movements, while the latter is produced by movement of the observer through the environment (see Cutting, Springer, Braren, & Johnson, 1992).

feedback regarding rate of travel are mismatched. Rieser et al. (1995) observed similar inaccuracies for orientation judgments after participants experienced a rotational visual/biomechanical discontinuity. Scene recognition also suffers following a change in perspective that disrupts vestibular and proprioceptive feedback (Simons & Wang, 1998). These findings suggest that biomechanical actions (and associated kinesthetic afferents) performed during self-locomotion are important sources of information regarding course and distance knowledge, and that the accuracy of this knowledge is periodically updated by the opportunity to integrate visual and nonvisual information sources.

In sum, it seems clear that movement through the environment has the potential to influence the manner in which topographic information is acquired and used, and as we will see next, this has implications for the use of functional brain imaging techniques to study topographic cognition.

4.2. Topographic cognition, functional brain imaging and virtual reality

Researchers have used several functional brain imaging techniques to study topographic cognition in humans, including EEG, fMRI, and positron emission tomography (PET). Although interesting work on hippocampal theta rhythms associated with navigational movement is being done with intracranial EEG recordings (Caplan et al., 2003), most of the brain imaging research on topographic cognition has relied on the latter techniques in which inferences about brain activation are made based on magnetic or radioisotope evidence for regional cerebral blood flow (rCBF). Because of the restrictive nature of brain imaging equipment, research participants' transactions with environments are limited to either recollections of actual environments, or interactions with environmental surrogates, with the latter approach predominating. Environmental surrogates have included videotaped "walk-throughs," modified versions of commercially available computer games, and other computer-generated virtual environments that allow participants to control apparent movement through maze-like or town-like settings. Topographic tasks have included imagined point-to-point (PTP) traversals of previously learned actual environments, exploration of novel computer-represented environments, learning of videotaped environments, and traversals and directional judgments in previously learned computer environments. Despite these differences in environmental representations and tasks, as well as differences in specific research questions, the primary focus among researchers using functional brain imaging to study topographic cognition has been to localize neural substrates involved in the learning and retrieval of topographic information. They have found that learning and retrieval of topographic information activate many of the same structures in the medial temporal, posterior parietal

and occipitotemporal regions, including the hippocampus, parahippocampus, posterior cingulate (retrosplenial) cortex, fusiform and lingual gyri, precuneus, and the inferior and superior parietal lobules.

Activations of the hippocampus, parahippocampus, posterior cingulate, and precuneus, in particular, have consistently been associated with more complex topographic tasks, including those putatively requiring allocentric representations of the environment. Activation of these structures for complex topographic behavior is consistent with animal models of navigation, which suggest that egocentric (head- and body-centered) reference coordinates (based in part on externally acquired landmark information) are integrated with an internally generated sense of direction (based on vestibular, proprioceptive and motor afferents) to produce allocentric reference coordinates used to navigate complex environments (McNaughton, Knierim, & Wilson, 1995; Taube, Goodridge, Golob, Dudchenko, & Stackman, 1996). Evidence suggests that posterior parietal regions, including the precuneus, are important for generating egocentric coordinates (Andersen, Snyder, Li, & Stricanne, 1993), whereas several models have focused on the hippocampal formation for processing of idiothetic (internally generated) heading information used to produce allocentric coordinates (Burgess, Recce, & O'Keefe, 1994; McNaughton, Chen, & Markus, 1991). The contribution of the posterior cingulate to this process has alternatively been represented as the starting point for the transformation of coordinates from egocentric to allocentric (Vogt, Finch, & Olson, 1992), or as processing parietal coordinate information to update idiothetic position signals, which tend to drift independent of external verification (McNaughton et al., 1991; McNaughton et al., 1995).

This broad consistency between structures implicated in topographic cognition of intact humans with those structures being delineated as integral to navigational neural circuits in animals is encouraging. However, several important caveats must be raised regarding interpretation of the brain imaging work, and these caveats in turn have important implications for the ultimate utility of brain imaging methods for the study human topographic cognition. We will briefly mention three issues that are common inferential concerns in functional brain imaging research, regardless of the psychological phenomena of interest, after which we will concentrate on a fourth issue that has specific import for those studying topographic cognition. First, with respect to fMRIs and PET scans, there are issues associated with the functional significance of neural activation inferred from rCBF. Though increased blood flow to a particular region may be associated with increased neural activity, the functional significance of that activity is difficult to determine in the absence of any information regarding the specific nature (e.g., excitatory/inhibitory) or patterns of neuronal firing (see Posner & Raichle, 1994; Sarter, Berntson, & Cacioppo, 1996, for discussion of similar concerns).

Second, though recent advances in brain imaging techniques have dramatically improved the spatial resolution of both PET and fMRI scans, the temporal resolution of these techniques is still rather limited (Brodal, 1998). Although the temporal resolution of fMRI can be as small as just a few seconds, brain scans of topographic tasks are often integrated over anywhere from 30–90 s, a long period of time during which participants may engage in both task-focused and off-task processing. While researchers may assume that off-task processing is randomly distributed among experimental conditions (though it is not clear how one could convincingly test this assumption), when cerebral localization of cognitive functioning is the primary purpose of the research, attempts should be made to limit the likelihood of off-task processing. Participants may also engage in *unexpected task-focused* processing, which may also limit the attribution of functional significance to particular brain regions when data from rCBF are integrated over long epochs. Aguirre and D'Esposito (1997), for example, trained participants to a 90% accuracy criterion for topographic knowledge of a computer-simulated town, and then gave them prescanning practice on two tasks that putatively discriminated landmark cognitive processing from survey (allocentric) cognitive processing. Importantly, these tasks were administered within subjects and were self-paced during (separate) 60 s scanning blocks. Given the prior training to a knowledge criterion (i.e., acquisition of both landmark and survey knowledge), exposure to both tasks beforehand, and the time to implement any desired strategies during scanned task performance, participants may well have used both types of knowledge for both tasks, regardless of the instructions and the presumed task requirements. That participants will adopt navigational strategies they are most comfortable with is clear from research that allows participants to learn environments without specific navigational instructions (e.g., explore the environment, find targets, and remember the environment for subsequent use). Under these conditions, some participants will spontaneously adopt route-learning strategies (memorizing left- and right-turn sequences), others will acquire allocentric knowledge based on relationships among landmarks, and still others will change strategies in mid stream (Bohbot, Iaria, & Petrides, 2004; Iaria et al., 2003). In this research, only those participants using allocentric landmark knowledge showed the expected hippocampal activation for wayfinding, and thus, a specific mapping of function to structure depends critically upon some measure of navigational strategies actually used, regardless of task instructions.[15]

These examples help to illustrate the third general caveat to the interpretation of brain imaging research: there are limitations associated with the *subtractive logic*, which is routinely used to draw inferences about the functional significance of regional neural activity. In a continuously active system such as the human brain, observed activations at a particular period of time under a given set of conditions are only meaningful relative to activations observed under a comparison set of conditions. When observed activations associated with comparison conditions are subtracted from those associated with the experimental conditions of interest, the remaining activations are assumed to be functionally significant that is, selectively associated with the cognitive processes engaged by the experimental conditions. For a number of reasons (see Sarter et al., 1996), however, when such subtractions are made it is possible that information is lost regarding the neural substrates subserving the functions of interest. For example, regions that are active to a similar extent for both experimental and control tasks may be active for different reasons (i.e., they subserve different functions), and thus experimentally relevant, interpretable activations would be lost to subtraction. Andersen et al. (1993), for instance, report evidence for posterior parietal cell assemblies that contribute to the representation of space in both head-centered and body-centered coordinates, depending upon the conditions under which activation is elicited. In a situation where activations associated with both sets of conditions were directly compared, the subtractive logic of imaging techniques could well lead to a discounted role for this parietal region in both functions.

Given these concerns, it is important that brain imaging evidence for the localization of cognitive functions be interpreted in light of pertinent evidence from related disciplines, such as psychobiological work with animals and neuropsychological research with impaired human populations. Inferences for the localization of cognitive function to candidate neural structures based on brain imaging data become much stronger if it can also be shown that lesions of the same structures in animals and humans lead to deficits in behaviors that (putatively) require the function in question. To their credit, researchers using functional brain imaging of topographic cognition have usually marshaled psychobiological and neuropsychological evidence to support the neural localization inferences they have made.

However, there is one last set of concerns specific to the study of topographic cognition that requires further interpretational caution, and may suggest a modification of typical experimental procedures. This fourth set of concerns is related to a critical assumption that is often made when environmental surrogates are paired with brain imaging techniques to study topographic cognition, namely, that participants' interactions with environmental surrogates engage the same cognitive processes that encounters with actual environments engage (Aguirre et al., 1998). To illustrate the nature of these concerns, we will focus on conflicting evidence from recent brain imaging work regarding the relative contribution of the hippocampus to human topographic cognition.

---

[15] See also Jordan, Schadow, Wuestenberg, Heinze, & Jänke (2004), in which navigation through a simple virtual maze elicited bilateral parahippocampal and left hippocampal activation among those reporting an allocentric strategy.

As briefly mentioned in the review above, there is good evidence from the animal literature that the hippocampus is central to processing that requires allocentric spatial representations. Much of this evidence comes from work with rodents (for reviews, see McNaughton et al., 1995; O'Keefe & Nadel, 1978), though research with avian species also supports the importance of the hippocampus for complex spatial behavior (e.g., Biegler, McGregor, Krebs, & Healy, 2001; Bingman & Jones, 1994; Sherry, Jacobs, & Gaulin, 1992). There has been some work with nonhuman primates that is supportive as well (e.g., Feigenbaum & Rolls, 1991; Rolls, Robertson, & Georges-François, 1995), though the issue of topographic cognition has been less intensively explored with these animals than with rodents. Finally, the evidence from clinical neuropsychology has been much less clearcut, in large part because focal damage to the hippocampus proper is a relatively rare event.[16] There has been some neuropsychological evidence, however, that parahippocampal damage can lead to topographic disorientation (with primarily spatial location deficits rather than landmark agnosia; e.g., Habib & Sirigu, 1987). Aguirre et al. (1998) have cited this evidence of parahippocampal involvement in topographic cognition to support findings in their brain imaging work that also implicate the parahippocampus. They suggest that neural substrates for allocentric representations of space may differ in primates and rats, with the parahippocampus being more important in the former and the hippocampus in the latter. In two studies they collected fMRI data while participants explored either a computer-simulated maze (Aguirre, Detre, Alsop, & D'Esposito, 1996) or a computer-simulated town (Aguirre & D'Esposito, 1997). Although the specific research questions were slightly different in these two studies (acquisition versus retrieval of topographic information in one, and place identity versus topographic location, in the other), activations in the medial temporal regions implicated the parahippocampus in both studies, while the hippocampus proper was not recruited in either study.

In contrast, Maguire and her colleagues have reported three PET scan studies in which the right hippocampus was activated for both learning (Maguire, Frakowiak, & Frith, 1996) and retrieval (Maguire, Frakowiak, & Frith, 1997; Maguire, Burgess, et al., 1998) of complex topographic information relative to activations observed for less complex topographic and non-topographic tasks. Ghaëm et al. (1997) have also reported hippocampal activation using PET scan imaging during recall of complex environmental information learned on site. Considering possible reasons for this conflicting evidence regarding

the contribution of the hippocampus proper to complex topographic cognition, we can quickly dispatch two possibilities by referring to a fourth study by Maguire and her colleagues. Although separate laboratories using different brain imaging techniques have reported this conflicting evidence (Aguirre et al. using fMRI, Maguire et al. and Ghaëm et al. using PET), Maguire, Frith, Burgess, Donnett, & O'Keefe (1998b) found that medial temporal activation for topographic tasks was limited to the right parahippocampal gyrus. Thus, the cross-study differences in implicated neural substrates do not appear to be attributable to differences in laboratories or imaging techniques per se, as Maguire, Frith et al. (1998) again used PET but this time failed to find activation of the hippocampus proper. Beyond the conflicting evidence from these research groups, others have found that allocentric navigation tasks recruit both hippocampal and parahippocampal activation, muddying the waters even further (Mellet et al., 2000; Parslow et al., 2004).

A possible explanation for the conflicting evidence across studies regarding the contribution of the hippocampus to topographic cognition lies in the specific nature of the participants' environmental transactions. The three studies that failed to find hippocampal activation for complex topographic cognition all used relatively simple computer simulations of either mazes (Aguirre et al., 1996; Maguire, Frith et al., 1998), or a town with distinctly maze-like characteristics (Aguirre & D'Esposito, 1997).[17] On the other hand, the three studies by Maguire and colleagues, in which the hippocampus was implicated in topographic cognition, all relied on much more complex environmental transactions. Maguire et al. (1997) scanned participants while they described routes through London based on their intimate first-hand knowledge of the city from years of driving taxis; Maguire et al. (1996) scanned participants while they viewed information-rich videotaped urban "walks"; and, although Maguire, Burgess, et al. (1998) did use a computer-simulated town, the published depictions and verbal descriptions of the town suggest that it was substantially more sophisticated than previously used simulations.[18]

Whether these differences in environmental transactions can account for the differential activation of the hippocampus across imaging studies is difficult to determine. At the very least, given the evidence from these initial imaging studies, it is probably premature to assume that all simulated environmental transactions engage the

---

[16] Morris and his colleagues (Morris, Pickering, Abrahams, & Feigenbaum, 1996), however, have published a short report on the spatial abilities of temporal lobe resection (TLR) patients suffering from focal temporal lobe epilepsy. Resections, which were confined to the amygdala and the anterior two thirds of the hippocampus, impaired both egocentric and allocentric spatial performance of right TLR patients relative to left TLR patients and controls.

[17] The town is laid out in a 4 × 4 grid of named places, and though the presence of a background skyline suggests the possibility of using distal features for orientation within the immediate environment, the authors claimed that this was not possible (Aguirre & D'Esposito, 1997, p. 2513, figure 2). In other respects, the published map and first-person views of the environment are strongly suggestive of a maze.

[18] The town comprised four streets with shops, bars, a cinema, church, bank, train station, and a video-game arcade, and the buildings were accessible and navigable, lending considerable complexity to environmental transactions.

same cognitive processes (or engage them to the same degree) as those engaged for transactions with actual environments. Although the environmental transactions in those studies that elicit hippocampal activation differ from the simple computer-simulated transactions in those that do not, the nature of those differences is not uniform. In one case we might focus on the visual complexity of videotaped environments (Maguire et al., 1996), in others on the visual and interactive richness of recalled actual environments (Maguire et al., 1997; Mellet et al., 2000), and in still others on visually and navigationally complex perceptual interactions with computer-simulated environments (Maguire, Burgess, et al., 1998; Parslow et al., 2004). The common thread among these environmental transactions is not obvious, other than a vague notion that each is more compelling or complex than transactions with computer-simulated mazes. However, recent work by Maguire and her colleagues (Hartley, Maguire, Spiers, & Burgess, 2003) suggests that a compelling or complex environmental transaction is not simply a matter of interacting with a reasonably complex environment. If the nature of the interaction is a simple one (e.g., route following), then complex environments do not elicit activation of the hippocampus proper. Furthermore, in this particular study, as in an earlier one (Maguire, Burgess et al., 1998), hippocampal activation was also tied to performance: good navigators, and other participants when navigating well, show hippocampal activation during wayfinding in a complex environment, but not during route following. Thus, a compelling human-environment transaction appears to be necessary to recruit hippocampal involvement in topographic cognition, where "compelling" comprises wayfinding (i.e., use of allocentric knowledge) in a reasonably complex environment. Whether accuracy of navigation should be included in the definition of compelling transactions is an open question in this inchoate research area, as others have reported hippocampal activation that was not tied to performance (Mellet et al., 2000; Parslow et al., 2004). Indeed, many factors that might bear on this question, such as preferences for navigational strategies (allocentric vs. egocentric, see above) and facility/familiarity with virtual environments (McNamara & Shelton, 2003), are not routinely assessed and thus it is impossible to determine the relative importance of accurate wayfinding for hippocampal activation.

Despite this uncertainty, we can speculate that more compelling environmental transactions are more likely to recruit hippocampal activation because they simulate movement through the environment more convincingly. As we have seen in the review above, active engagement with the environment may well influence the way people represent space and perform spatial tasks and, in particular, the opportunity to integrate visual and kinesthetic inputs when people move through space may play a key role in the cognitive processing of topographic information. Prominent animal models of hippocampal involvement in navigation have also identified movement through the environment as being requisite for the generation of allocentric referents and the calibration of an idiothetic sense of direction (Burgess et al., 1994; McNaughton et al., 1991; McNaughton et al., 1995). These models were developed based on research with freely moving animals, and this work has provided abundant evidence, such as hippocampal "place" cells,[19] for the involvement of the hippocampus in the performance of complex navigational tasks (see O'Keefe, 1991). Work with animals also indicates that the firing rate of hippocampal place cells is linked to the speed and direction of an animal's movement (Wiener, Paul, & Eichenbaum, 1989). Interestingly, hippocampal place cells cease firing almost completely when animals are passively restrained (Foster, Castro, & McNaughton, 1989), and, though video simulations of movement through the environment do not elicit place cell responding in primates, actual movement through the environment does (Froehler & Duffy, 2002).[20]

Thus, information gleaned from movement through the environment appears to be an important component of topographic cognition, at least in animal models.[21] This is a potential stumbling block for brain imaging studies of topographic cognition, as "wearable" brain scanning devices have yet to be developed and environmental simulations are likely to play an important role in this research for the foreseeable future. Thus, to the extent that environmental simulations can convincingly mimic the perceptual experiences of movement, they may be more apt to engage the cognitive processes central to topographic cognition, and thereby help to improve the internal validity of brain imaging studies. There is, therefore, a critical need for a conceptual framework that specifies criteria by which researchers can discriminate stronger from weaker environmental simulations, especially with respect to the simulation of movement, and we will briefly examine one framework that borrows heavily from concepts in the communications literature.

In developing a definition of virtual reality (VR), Steuer (1992) has proposed a set of criteria for assessing the *telepresence* of VR systems. Telepresence refers to a feeling of being in a physical environment that is both spatially and temporally removed from one's immediate physical surroundings, and the feeling is produced by mediated rather than direct perceptual experience. In Steuer's model, mediation is through any indirect form of communication, and thus even relatively simple technologies (e.g., letters or telephones) can function as VR systems. This expansive potential for VR is felicitous for examining the simulated environmental transactions used in brain

---

[19] These are hippocampal cells selectively tuned for an animal's location in space, regardless of its orientation (i.e., its egocentric perspective).

[20] Monkeys, presumably, have little familiarity with egocentric video movement, and such simulations are unlikely to convincingly mimic movement through the environment for them.

[21] For a full consideration of hippocampal and parahippocampal involvement in spatial cognition, see Burgess, Maguire, and O'Keefe (2002).

imaging research because it allows us to assess such media as maps, videotape, and sophisticated three-dimensional computer animations within the same conceptual framework. The criteria Steuer presents are similar in content to those developed by others in the communications field (e.g., Zeltzer, 1992), and focus on two dimensions of presentation media that are presumed to elicit a feeling of telepresence: *vividness* and *interactivity*. Vividness refers to the representational richness of a simulated environment and can be judged in terms of the *breadth* and *depth* of the sensory information presented. Breadth refers to the range of perceptual systems simultaneously addressed by a presentation medium. Redundant information contained in multimodal sensory presentations is thought to eliminate competing perceptual interpretations and thereby enhance a given perceptual experience. Depth is determined individually for each sensory channel and is gauged according to its resolution, or density of data. The second media dimension determining telepresence, interactivity, is the extent to which users can manipulate the content and form of a simulated environment. Interactivity can be assessed in terms of the speed (real-time or slower) and range of available manipulations, as well as the fidelity of actions required to manipulate simulated environments (often referred to as *mapping*). Using a steering wheel to control simulated driving, for instance, constitutes a more veridical VR interaction than would button presses or keypad-controlled motion.

This model is for illustrative purposes only, as the dimensions and underlying variables of telepresence mentioned above have not been empirically verified, nor are they likely to be the only relevant factors (see Biocca & Levy, 1995; Cutting, 1996, 1997). However, this model does give us a vocabulary and initial conceptual framework within which the simulated environmental transactions used in brain imaging research can be evaluated. For example, video game systems routinely trade-off visual depth and, thereby, vividness to retain real-time motion in the service of interactivity. If we compare Maguire et al.'s (1996) videotaped environmental simulation, which did activate the hippocampus, and the two simulated maze-environments used by Aguirre and colleagues (Aguirre et al., 1996; Aguirre & D'Esposito, 1997), which did not, we may reach the tentative conclusion that visually vivid simulations are more apt to recruit hippocampal involvement than are more visually impoverished (though) interactive simulations. Comparing Maguire, Burgess et al.'s (1998) more complex VR town with Aguirre's and D'Esposito's (1997) maze-like VR town, we can begin to parse the differences in complexity in terms of the former simulation's (apparently) greater visual depth and broader range of interactivity (provided by building accessibility and functioning doors). Comparisons with the remaining PET study eliciting hippocampal activation (Maguire et al., 1997) are problematic within this conceptual framework because the taxi drivers' environmental transactions were with recalled actual environments. This presents two problems. First,

the definition of telepresence specifies a mediated perception of being in a physical environment other than one's immediate spatiotemporal surroundings, but recalled (and imagined) environments are internally generated, not perceived. Thus, we need a term (and definition) similar to telepresence, yet broad enough to incorporate recalled and imagined source stimuli for simulated environmental transactions. As the growing community of virtual reality researchers has gravitated towards the term *presence*, we will use that term here to refer to a perceptual, mnestic, or imaginal feeling of being in a physical environment that is either spatially or temporally removed from one's immediate physical surroundings. This definition is essentially the same as that for telepresence, yet it allows for mediated perception rather than requiring it and is expanded to include internally generated environmental transactions.

A second problem presented by a conceptual framework that must accommodate both internally and externally generated source material for simulated environmental transactions is the need for person-centered assessment dimensions to complement vividness and interactivity, which are technology- or medium-centered. As an example, consider *familiarity*, which can take at least two forms. *Environmental familiarity* refers to one's personal knowledge of the specific environments to be simulated. Given the behavioral evidence described above regarding the microgenetic and ontogenetic development of topographic knowledge and abilities, we might expect a shift in the cognitive processes used to perform spatial tasks as one's familiarity with a particular environment increases, a shift that may be reflected in patterns of recruited neural activation. There is minimal evidence of this in the topographic brain imaging research conducted thus far. Aguirre et al. (1996) did report greater parahippocampal activation for maze-environment acquisition relative to retrieval, but the issue largely has not been addressed. One interesting exception is Maguire's work with London taxi drivers, which suggests that extensive reliance on navigational skills can alter the shape and size of one's hippocampus, in direct relation to years on the job (Maguire et al., 2000), and seemingly independent of initial navigational ability (Maguire et al., 2003).

The importance of assessing environmental familiarity can also be illustrated by examining the critical (yet commonly made) assumption that transactions with virtual environments engage the same cognitive processes as transactions with actual environments. Heretofore, computer simulations used in brain imaging studies of topographic cognition have depicted nonexistent environments. Simulations of existing environments, however, would allow researchers to directly compare the behavior and neural activity of individuals who had acquired topographic information in actual environments versus those acquiring the same information through simulations. Similar regional patterns of neural activations across groups under these circumstances (e.g., during a topographic recall task) would help to support the assumption of similar engagement of cognitive processes for simulated and real-world transactions. Mellet et al. (2000) conducted a study along these lines, having participants learn a novel environment either through actual exploration of the environment or via examination of a map. In terms of the framework above, a map likely elicits an anemic sense of presence because it engages a single sense modality, with relatively little information, the content and form of which cannot be manipulated. In short, the breadth, depth, and interactivity of a map are all rather limited. However, it does afford an immediate allocentric perspective, something that must be built up over time through actual engagement with the environment. After learning their respective environments, participants in both groups performed a series of imagined point to point navigations through the environment, based on memorized landmarks. PET scans during the imagined navigations indicated that both groups engaged the right hippocampus to perform this task, while those who learned the environment in situ also recruited the parahippocampus bilaterally. The latter result likely reflects the established finding of parahippocampal involvement in object and scene recognition (Aguirre et al., 1996; Epstein & Kanwisher, 1998), including recent evidence that the parahippocampus automatically stores navigationally relevant object locations after one pass through an environment, irrespective of attentional demands and subsequent memory for the objects (Janzen & van Turrenout, 2004). The fact that the map learners did not engage the parahippocampus to perform the imagined navigations suggests that the colored dots and verbal labels used to designate landmarks on the map were insufficient to trigger object/scene encoding. As these research examples suggest, the study of environmental familiarity, and the means by which it is acquired, can help us address some of the methodological concerns of using functional brain imaging to study topographic cognition.

We might also expect the cognitive processes engaged by topographic behavior to differ as a function of one's *simulation familiarity* – familiarity with the means of environmental simulation. With respect to internally generated source stimuli, individual differences in experience generating environmental imagery, route information, relative spatial locations, etc., may lead people to develop different ways of processing topographic information. Cab drivers, for instance, routinely generate complex point-to-point route information, while bus drivers (with well-learned, set routes) would likely have less experience generating novel route information, as would those who are not professional drivers. With respect to externally generated source stimuli, there may be perceptual learning curves associated with the emergent technologies used to create and display environmental simulations, and individual differences in familiarity with such technologies could influence the cognitive processes they engage. Over the past 200 years, one psychologically interesting by-product of industrialization has been the continual creation of novel

sensory phenomena, the perceptual mastery of which has occasionally been physically unpleasant for members of our species (Schivelbusch, 1986). To use an example cited by Cutting et al. (1992), the advent of widespread train travel in the mid-nineteenth century was accompanied by clinical reports of eye fatigue, back strain, and overall body stress. The eye fatigue was presumably due to novice train travelers' inexperience in engaging the visual environment at previously unknown speeds.[22] More recently, reports of "side-effects" associated with immersive VR environments include dizziness, headaches, eyestrain, and nausea (Regan & Price, 1994), symptoms that increase steadily with time spent in an immersive VR environment (Murata, 2004), but which can be reduced with the prior administration of antimotion-sickness drugs (e.g., scopolamine hydrobromide; Regan & Ramsey, 1996). Although it is not yet clear whether symptoms such as these would subside with increasing VR experience, their relatively common occurrence (e.g., upwards of 60% of participants experiencing at least one symptom, Regan & Price, 1994) represents prima facie evidence that VR environmental simulations may not engage the same cognitive processes as those engaged by actual environments. Indeed, one reason why videotaped environmental simulations elicit increased hippocampal activations while many computer simulations do not may be broad familiarity with the former medium relative to the latter, especially with respect to the perception of motion.

In sum, the brain imaging studies reviewed here represent a promising initial psychophysiological foray into the investigation of human topographic cognition. Serious concerns regarding the interpretation of neural substrates recruited during topographic behavior have been met with felicitous reference to pertinent theory and converging lines of evidence from neuropsychology, psychobiology, and cognitive and environmental psychology. Inferential concerns regarding the comparability of cognitive processing engaged by transactions with simulated versus actual environments, however, have been less well met. The importance of these concerns is thrown into sharp relief by the research described above regarding the distinction between primary and secondary acquisition of topographic information, the importance of active relative to passive engagement with environments, and reports of perceptual maladies associated with immersive VR environments. Because brain imaging techniques have the potential to make important contributions to our understanding of human topographic cognition, the assumption regarding transactional comparability between simulated and actual environments deserves careful scrutiny, and we have outlined a conceptual framework that can facilitate comparisons among simulated environmental transactions. Additional psychophysiological measures might

---

[22] Scanning patterns that are appropriate at pedestrian speeds – roughly equal numbers of fixations on proximal and distal cues – are extremely difficult to maintain at high speeds, and attempts to do so should lead to eye strain.

also be used, however, to examine comparability among environmental simulations. If some simulations are substantially better than others, for instance, at depicting self-locomotion through the environment, then EMG recordings from muscle groups involved in locomotion may reveal increased activations associated with those more immersive simulations.

Beyond examinations of the comparability among simulations, there are other techniques (as well as constructs and research) within psychophysiology that can be brought to bear on the inferential issues raised by the use of brain imaging to investigate topographic cognition. For example, interpretation of the localization of neural substrates associated with the performance of various topographic tasks could benefit from an analysis of task-related activations in terms of both cortical and autonomic arousal. Some of the structures activated by topographic tasks in these brain imaging studies (and interpreted solely in terms of the cognitive processes engaged) have also been implicated in the production of skin conductance responses elicited by non-topographic tasks (Tranel & Damasio, 1994). Thus, increased activation in the right inferior parietal region may reflect cognitive processes associated with a survey-oriented relative to a landmark-oriented task (Aguirre & D'Esposito, 1997), but it may also reflect the relative difficulty of the tasks, independent of the specific cognitive processes engaged. To date, only one of the reviewed brain imaging studies (Ghaëm et al., 1997) has measured autonomic or other psychophysiological concomitants of rCBF during topographic cognition. Thus, it seems that there are broad opportunities here for the application of psychophysiological methods and constructs that could help brain imaging researchers address some of the inferential concerns inherent in laboratory studies of topographic cognition.

5. CONCLUDING REMARKS

As intimated at the beginning of this chapter, environmental psychophysiology is not an established field as such. However, the existing work regarding the significant effects that ordinary transactions with the physical environment can have on individuals argues strongly for the psychophysiological study of human-environment transactions. As the reviews of environmental noise, palliative environments, and topographic cognition indicate, psychophysiological constructs and methods have already been used profitably in this regard over a wide range of transactions. There are other areas as well, not reviewed here, where psychophysiology has contributed to our knowledge of how people engage the physical environment. These include other areas of environmental stress, such as thermal extremes and crowding (Taylor, Allsopp, & Parkes, 1995; Baum & Paulus, 1987), less obviously oppressive environmental transactions, including chronobiological and other effects of light (Küller & Laike, 1998; Küller & Mikellides, 1993), as well as emerging fields of

investigation regarding the effects of environmental elements such as negative air ions and olfactory stimuli (Morton & Kershner, 1987; Miltner et al., 1994).

Although considerable work has been done in environmental psychophysiology as described above, more explicit recognition of this subdiscipline may well have advantages. The coordinated development and use of shared methodological approaches, for instance, would arguably be more easily accomplished with the institutional infrastructure (e.g., conferences and journal outlets) of a more formal discipline. In particular, given the repeated references in this chapter to the ecological validity of simulating large-scale environmental conditions in the laboratory, further development of lightweight, affordable ambulatory psychophysiological recording systems is a prime concern. Institutional imprimatur of this fledgling field could also facilitate the acquisition of research support and help to set research agendas that are responsive to needs in the field. For instance, as indicated in the section on topographic cognition, some psychophysiological methods (such as brain imaging techniques) that are ill-suited to field research must rely on environmental simulations and thus research questions regarding human transactions with various kinds of simulations will have to be addressed (e.g., to what extent and under what conditions do immersive VR systems elicit nausea?).

Thus, we present the material in this chapter in part to exemplify the application of psychophysiology to human transactions with the physical environment, but also to foster the recognition and nurture the development of environmental psychophysiology as a subdiscipline.

ACKNOWLEDGMENTS

Special thanks to Lou Tassinary and Phyllis Sanchez, who each in their own way have made this chapter possible. This work represents a revision and update of a previous chapter by Parsons & Hartig (2000).

REFERENCES

Acredolo, L. P. (1988). Infant mobility and spatial development. In J. Stiles-Davis, M. Kritchevsky & U. Bellugi (Eds.), *Spatial cognition: Brain bases and development* (pp. 157–166). Hillsdale, NJ: Lawrence Erlbaum Associates.

Acredolo, L. P., Adams, A., & Goodwyn, S. W. (1984). The role of self-produced movement and visual tracking in infant spatial orientation. *Journal of Experimental Child Psychology*, 38, 312–237.

Aguirre, G. K., & D'Esposito, M. (1997). Environmental knowledge is subserved by separable dorsal(ventral neural areas. *The Journal of Neuroscience*, 17 (7), 2512–2518.

Aguirre, G. K., Detre, J. A., Alsop, D. C., & D'Esposito, M. (1996). The parahippocampus subserves topographic learning in man. *Cerebral Cortex*, 6, 823–829.

Aguirre, G. K., Zarahn, E., & D'Esposito, M. (1998). Neural components of topographical representation. *Proceedings of the National Academy of Sciences*, 95, 839–846.

Allen, G. L. (1985). Strengthening weak links in the study of the development of macrospatial cognition. R. Cohen (Ed.), *The development of spatial cognition* (pp. 301–322). Hillsdale, NJ: Lawrence Erlbaum Associates.

Allen, G. L. (1987). Cognitive influences on the acquisition of route knowledge in children and adults. In P. Ellen & C. Thinus-Blanc (Eds.), *Cognitive processes and spatial orientation in animal and man* (pp. 274–283). Boston: Martinus Nijhoff.

Andersen, R. A., Snyder, L. H., Li, C. S., & Stricanne, B. (1993). Coordinate transformations in the representation of spatial information. *Current Opinion in Neurobiology, 3,* 171–176.

Anderson, C. A., & Bushman, B. J. (1997). External validity of "trivial" experiments: The case of laboratory aggression. *Review of General Psychology, 1* (1), 19–41.

Andreassi, J. L. (1995). *Psychophysiology: Human behavior and physiological response* (3rd ed.). Hillsdale, NJ: Lawrence Erlbaum Associates.

Andren, L., Hansson, L., Bjorkman, M., & Jonsson, A. (1980). Noise as a contributory factor in the development of elevated arterial pressure. *Acta Medica Scandinavica, 207,* 493–498.

Andren, L., Hansson, L., Bjorkman, M., Jonsson, A., & Borg, K. O. (1979). Haemodynamic and hormonal changes induced by noise. *Acta Medica Scandinavica, 625* (Suppl.), 13–18.

Aniansson, G., Pettersson, K., & Peterson, Y. (1983). Traffic noise annoyance and noise sensitivity in persons with normal and impaired hearing. *Journal of Sound and Vibration, 88* (1), 85–97.

Anticaglia, J. R., & Cohen, A. (1970). Extra-auditory effects of noise as a health hazard. *American Industrial Hygiene Association Journal, 31,* 277–281.

Appleton, J. (1975). *The experience of landscape.* Hoboken, NJ: John Wiley & Sons.

Appleyard, D. (1970). Styles and methods of structuring a city. *Environment and Behavior, 2,* 100–117.

Atran, S. (1998). Folk biology and the anthropology of science: Cognitive universals and cultural particulars. *Behavioral and Brain Sciences, 21,* 547–609.

Babisch, W. (1998). Epidemiological studies of the cardiovascular effects of occupational noise: A critical appraisal. *Noise & Health, 1,* 24–39.

Babisch, W., Beule, B., Schust, M., Kersten, N., & Ising, H. (2005). Traffic noise and risk of myocardial infarction. *Epidemiology, 16* (1), 33–40.

Babisch, W., Fromme, H., Beyer, A., & Ising, H. (2001). Increased catecholamine levels in urine in subjects exposed to road traffic noise: The role of stress hormones in noise research. *Environment International, 26,* 475–481.

Badal, J. (1888/1982). Contribution a l'étude des cécités psychiques. Alexie, agraphie, hémianopsie inférieure, trouble du sens d'l'espace. *Arch. Ophthalmol., 140,* 97–117. (As cited in DeRenzi, 1982, chap. 1)

Bantick, S. J., Wise, R. G., Ploghaus, A., Clare, S., Smith, S. M., & Tracey, I. (2002). Imaging how attention modulates pain in humans using MRI. *Brain, 125,* 310–319.

Baum, A., & Paulus, P. (1987). Crowding. In D. Stokols & I. Altman (Eds.), *Handbook of environmental psychology* (Vol. 1, pp. 533–570). New York: Wiley.

Beck, R. J., & Wood, D. (1976). Cognitive transformation of information from urban geographic fields to mental maps. *Environment and Behavior, 8,* 199–238.

Belojevic, G., Jakovljevic, B., & Slepcevic, V. (2003). Noise and mental performance: Personality attributes and noise sensitivity. *Noise & Health, 6* (21), 3–34.

Bennett, E. (1945). Some tests for the discrimination of neurotic from normal subjects. *British Journal of Medical Psychology, 20,* 271–277.

Bergamasco, B., Benna, P., & Gilli, M. (1976). Human sleep modifications induced by urban traffic noise. *Acta Oto-Laryngology, 339* (Suppl.), 33–36.

Berry, L. L., Parker, D., Coile, R. C., Hamilton, D. K., O'Neill, D. D., & Sadler, B. L. (2004). The business case for better buildings. *Frontiers of Health Services Management, 21* (1), 3–24.

Biegler, R., McGregor, A., Krebs, J. R., & Healy, S. D. (2001). A larger hippocampus ia associated with longer-lasting spatial memory. *Proceedings of the National Academy of Sciences of USA, 98,* 6941–6944.

Bierce, A. (1911/1993). *The devil's dictionary.* Toronto: Dover Publications. First published as Volume VII of *The collected works of Ambrose Bierce,* 1911, by the Neale Publishing Co., New York.

Bingman, V. P., & Jones, T. J. (1994). Sun compass-based spatial learning impaired in homing pigeons with hippocampal lesions. *Journal of Neuroscience, 14,* 6687–6694.

Biocca, F., & Levy, M. R. (Eds.). (1995) *Communication in the age of virtual reality.* Hillsdale, NJ: Lawrence Erlbaum Associates.

Bohbot, V. D., Iaria, G., & Petrides, M. (2004). Hippocampal function and spatial memory: Evidence from functional neuroimaging in healthy participants and performance of patients with medial temporal lobe resections. *Neuropsychology, 18* (3), 418–425.

Bollini, A. M., Walker, E. F., Hamann, S., & Kestler, L. (2004). The influence of perceived control and locus of control on the cortisol and subjective responses to stress. *Biological Psychiatry, 67,* 245–260.

Böök, A., & Gärling, T. (1980a). Processing of information about location during locomotion: Effects of a concurrent task and locomotion patterns. *Scandinavian Journal of Psychology, 21,* 185–192.

Böök, A., & Gärling, T. (1980b). Processing of information about location during locomotion: Effects of amount of visual information about the locomotion pattern. *Perceptual and Motor Skills, 51,* 231–238.

Böök, A., & Gärling, T. (1981). Maintenance of orientation during locomotion in unfamiliar environments. *Journal of Experimental Psychology: Human Perception and Performance, 7,* 995–1006.

Born, J., & Fehm, H. L. (2000). The neuroendocrine recovery function of sleep. *Noise & Health, 7,* 25–37.

Brandenberger, G., Follenius, M., Wittersheim, G., Salame, P., Siméoni, M., & Reinhardt, B. (1980). Plasma catecholamines and pituitary adrenal hormones related to mental task demand under quiet and noise conditions. *Biological Psychology, 10,* 239–252.

Breier, A., Albus, M., Pickar, D., Zahn, T. P., Wolkowitz, O. M., & Paul, S. M. (1987). Controllable and uncontrollable stress in humans: Alterations in mood, neuroendocrine and psychophysiological function. *American Journal of Psychiatry, 144,* 1419–1425.

Broadbent, D. E. (1979). Human performance and noise. In C. S. Harris (Ed.), *Handbook of noise control,* (pp. 2066–2085). New York: McGraw-Hill.

Brodal, P. (1998). *The central nervous system: Structure and function.* New York: Oxford University Press.

Burgess, N., Maguire, E. A., & O'Keefe, J. (2002). The human hippocampus and spatial and episodic memory. *Neuron, 35,* 625–641.

Burgess, N., Recce, M., & O'Keefe, J. (1994). A model of hippocampal function. *Neural Networks, 7* (6/7), 1065–1081.

Bush, G., Whalen, P. J., Rosen, B. R., Jenike, M. A., McInerney, S. C., & Rauch, S. L. (1998). The counting Stroop: An interference task specialized for functional neuroimaging – Validation study with functional MRI. *Human Brain Mapping, 6,* 270–282.

Cacioppo, J. T., & Tassinary, L. G. (1990). Psychophysiology and psychophysiological principles. In J.T Cacioppo & L. G. Tassinary (Eds.), *Principles of psychophysiology: Physical, social and inferential elements* (pp. 3–33). New York: Cambridge University Press.

Cackowski, J. M., & Nasar, J. L. (2003). The restorative effects of roadside vegetation: Implications for automobile driver anger and frustration. *Environment and Behavior, 35* (6), 736–751.

Cammalleri, R., Gangitano, M., D'Amelio, M., Raieli, V., Raimondo, D., & Camarda, R. (1996). Transient topographical amnesia and cingulate cortex damage: A case report. *Neuropsychologia, 34* (4), 321–326.

Caplan, J. B., Madsen, J. R., Schulze-Bonhage, A., Aschenbrenner-Scheibe, R., Newman, E. L., & Kahana, M. J. (2003). Human θ oscillations related to sensorimotor integration and spatial learning. *The Journal of Neuroscience, 23* (11), 4726–4736.

Carter, N. L., & Beh, H. C. (1989). The effect of intermittent noise on cardiovascular functioning during vigilance task performance. *Psychophysiology, 26* (5), 548–559.

Cervone, D., Kopp, D. A., Schaumann, & Scott, W. D. (1994). Mood, self-efficacy and performance standards: Lower moods induce higher performance standards. *Journal of Personality and Social Psychology, 67,* 499–512.

Chang, T. Y., Jain, R. M., Wang, C. S., & Chan, C. C. (2003). Effects of occupational noise exposure on blood pressure. *Journal of Occupational and Environmental Medicine, 45* (12), 1289–1296.

Chariton, W. O. (1990). *This dog'll hunt: An entertaining Texas dictionary.* Plano, TX: Wordware Publishing.

Cimprich, B. (1993). Development of an intervention to restore attention in cancer patients. *Cancer Nursing, 16,* 83–92.

Clow, A. (2004). Cortisol as a biomarker of stress. *Journal of Holistic Healthcare, 1* (3), 10–14.

Coates, T. J., Rosekind, M. R., Strossen, R. J., Thoresen, C. E., & Kirmil-Gray, K. (1979). Sleep recordings in the laboratory and home: A comparative analysis. *Psychophysiology, 16,* 339–346.

Cogan, R., Cogan, D., Waltz, W., & McCue, M. (1987). Effects of laughter and relaxation on discomfort thresholds. *Journal of Behavioral Medicine, 10,* 139–144.

Cohen, A., Taylor, W., & Tubbs, R. (1980). Occupational exposures to noise, hearing loss and blood pressure. In J. V. Tobias, G. Jansen & W. D. Ward (Eds.), *Noise as a public health problem: Proceedings of the third international congress,* (ASHA Reports 10, pp. 322–326). Rockville, MD: The American Speech-Language-Hearing Association.

Cohen, R., & Weatherford, D. L. (1980). Effects of route traveled on the distance estimates of children and adults. *Journal of Experimental Child Psychology, 29,* 403–412.

Cohen, R., & Weatherford, D. L. (1981). The effect of barriers on spatial representations. *Child Development, 52,* 1087–1090.

Cohen, S. (1978). Environmental load and the allocation of attention. In A. Baum, J. E. Singer & S. Valins (Eds.), *Advances in environmental psychology*: Vol. 1 (pp. 1–29). Hillsdale, NJ: Lawrence Erlbaum Associates.

Cohen, S., & Spacapan, S. (1978). The aftereffects of stress: An attentional interpretation. *Environmental Psychology and Nonverbal Behavior, 3,* 43–59.

Cohen, S., Evans, G. W., Krants, D. S., & Stokols, D. (1980). Physiological, motivational and cognitive effects of noise on children: Moving from the laboratory to the field. *American Psychologist, 35,* 231–243.

Cohen, S., Evans, G. W., Krantz, D. S., Stokols, D., & Kelly, S. (1981). Aircraft noise and children: Longitudinal and cross-sectional evidence on adaptation to noise and the effectiveness of noise abatement. *Journal of Personality and Social Psychology, 40* (2), 331–345.

Cohen, S., Evans, G. W., Stokols, D., & Krants, D. S. (1986). *Behavior, health and environmental stress.* New York: Plenum Press.

Cohen, S., Glass, D. C., & Singer, J. E. (1973). Apartment noise, auditory discrimination, and reading ability in children. *Journal of Experimental Social Psychology, 9,* 407–422.

Cohen, S., Kessler, R. C., & Gordon, L. U. (1995). *Measuring stress: A guide for health and social scientists.* New York: Oxford University Press.

Cohen, S. L., & Cohen, R. (1985). The role of activity in spatial cognition. In R. Cohen (Ed.), *The development of spatial cognition* (pp. 199–223). Hillsdale, NJ: Lawrence Erlbaum Associates.

Coles, M. G. H., Gratton, G., & Fabiani, M. (1990). Event-related brain potentials. In J.T Cacioppo & L. G. Tassinary (Eds.), *Principles of psychophysiology: Physical, social and inferential elements* (pp. 413–455). New York: Cambridge University Press.

Conrad, D. W. (1973). The effects of intermittent noise on human serial decoding performance and physiological response. *Ergonomics, 16* (6), 739–747.

Cutting, J. E. (1996). Wayfinding from multiple sources of local information in retinal flow. *Journal of Experimental Psychology: Human Perception and Performance, 22* (5), 1299–1313.

Cutting, J. E. (1997). How the eye measures reality and virtual reality. *Behavior Research Methods, Instruments and Computers, 29,* 27–36.

Cutting, J. E., Springer, K., Braren, P. A., & Johnson, S. H. (1992). Wayfinding on foot from information in retinal, not optical, flow. *Journal of Experimental Psychology: General, 121* (1), 41–72.

Davies, H. W., Teschke, K., Kennedy, S. M., Hodgson, M. R., Hertzman, C., & Demers, P. A. (2005). Occupational exposure to noise and mortality from acute myocardial infarction. *Epidemiology, 16* (1), 25–32.

Davis, M. C., Zautra, A. J., & Smith, B. W. (2004). Chronic pain, stress, and the dynamics of affective differentiation. *Journal of Personality, 72* (6), 1133–1160.

de Vries, S., Verheij, R. A., Groenewegen, P. P., & Spreeuwenberg, P. (2003). Natural environments – healthy environments? An exploratory analysis of the relationship between greenspace and health. *Environment and Planning A, 35,* 1717–1731.

de Wied, M., & Verbaten, M. N. (2001). Affective pictures processing, attention and pain tolerance. *Pain, 90,* 163–172.

DeJoy, D. M. (1984). The nonauditory effects of noise: Review and perspectives for research. *The Journal of Auditory Research, 24,* 123–150.

DeRenzi, E. (1982). *Disorders of space exploration and cognition.* New York: John Wiley & Sons.

Devinsky, O., Morrel, M. J., & Vogt, B. A. (1995). Contributions of anterior cingulate to behavior. *Brain, 118,* 279–306.

Diette, G. B., Lechtzin, N., Haponik, E., Devrotes, A., & Rubin, H. R. (2003). Distraction therapy with nature sights and sounds reduces pain during flexible bronchoscopy. *Chest, 123* (3), 941–948.

Dimberg, U. (1990). Facial electromyographic reactions and autonomic activity to auditory stimuli. *Biological Psychology, 31,* 137–147.

Dolan, R. (2002). Emotion, cognition and behavior. *Science, 298,* 1191–1194.

Easterbrook, J. A. (1959). The effect of emotion on cue utilization and the organization of behavior. *Psychological Review, 66,* 183–201.

Eberhardt, J. L., & Akselsson, K. R. (1987). The disturbance by road traffic noise of the sleep of young male adults as recorded in the home. *Journal of Sound and Vibration, 114* (3), 417–434.

Eccleston, C., & Crombez, G. (1999). Pain demands attention: A cognitive -affective model of the interruptive function of pain. *Psychological Bulletin, 125,* 356–366.

Eisenberg, E. (1998). *The ecology of Eden.* New York: Alfred A. Knopf, Inc.

Ellermeier, W., Eigenstetter, M. & Zimmer, K. (2001). Psychoacoustic correlates of individual noise sensitivity. *Journal of the Acoustical Society of America, 109* (4), 1464–1473.

Epstein, R., & Kanwisher, N. (1998). Cortical representation of the local visual environment. *Nature, 392,* 598–601.

Ettlinger, G., Warrington, E. K., & Zangwill, O. L. (1957). A further study of visual-spatial agnosia. *Brain, 80,* 335–361.

Evans, G. W., & Cohen, S. (1987). Environmental stress. In D. Stokols & I. Altman (Eds.), *Handbook of environmental psychology,* (Vol. 1, pp. 571–610). New York: John Wiley & Sons.

Evans, G. W., & Johnson, D. (2000). Stress and open-office noise. *Journal of Applied Psychology, 85* (5), 779–783.

Evans, G. W., & Lepore, S. J. (1993). Nonauditory effects of noise on children: A critical review. *Children's Environments, 10* (1), 31–51.

Evans, G. W., & Pezdek, K. (1980). Cognitive mapping: Knowledge of real world distance and location information. *Journal of Experimental Psychology: Human Learning and Memory, 6,* 13–24.

Evans, G. W., Bullinger, M., & Hygge, S. (1998). Chronic noise exposure and physiological response: A prospective study of children living under environmental stress. *Psychological Science, 9* (1), 75–77.

Evans, G. W., Hygge, S., & Bullinger, M. (1995). Chronic noise and psychological stress. *Psychological Science, 6* (6), 333–338.

Evans, G. W., Johansson, G., & Carrere, S. (1994). Psychosocial factors and the physical environment: Inter-relations in the workplace. In C. L. Cooper & I. T. Robertson (Eds.), *International review of industrial and organizational psychology* (Vol. 9, pp. 1–29). Chichester, England: Wiley.

Evans, G. W., Lercher, P., Meis, M., Ising, H., & Kofler, W. W. (2001). Community noise exposure and stress in children. *Journal of the Acoustical Society of America, 109* (3), 1023–1027.

Feigenbaum, J., & Rolls, E. T. (1991). Allocentric and egocentric spatial information processing in the hippocampal formation of the behaving primate. *Psychobiology, 19,* 21–40.

Fogari, R., Zoppi, A., Corradi, L., Marasi, G., Vanasia, A., & Zanchetti, A. (2001). Transient but not sustained blood pressure increments by occupational noise: An ambulatory blood pressure measurement study. *Journal of Hypertension, 19,* 1021–1027.

Follenius, M., Brandenberger, G., Lecornu, C., Simeoni, M., & Reinhardt, B. (1980). Plasma catecholamines and pituitary adrenal hormones in response to noise exposure. *European Journal of Applied Physiology, 43,* 253–261.

Foster, T. C., Castro, C. A., & McNaughton, B. L. (1989). Spatial selectivity of rat hippocampal neurons is dependent upon is dependent on preparedness for movement. *Science, 244,* 1580–1582.

Frankenhaeuser, M. (1980). Psychoneuroendocrine approaches to approaches to the study of person-environment transactions. In H. Selye (Ed.), *Selye's guide to stress research* (Vol. 1, pp. 46–70.) New York: Van Nostrand Reinhold Company.

Frankenhaeuser, M., & Lundberg, U. (1977). The influence of cognitive set on performance and arousal under different noise loads. *Motivation and Emotion, 1* (2), 139–149.

Frankenhaeuser, M., Lundberg, U., Fredrikson, M., Melin, B., Tuomisto, M., Myrsten, A.-L., et al. (1989). Stress on and off the job as related to sex and occupational status in white-collar workers. *Journal of Organizational Behavior, 10,* 321–346.

Fredrickson, B. L., & Levenson, R. W. (1998). Positive emotions speed recovery from the cardiovascular sequelae of negative emotions. *Cognition and Emotion, 12,* 191–220.

Froehler, M. T., & Duffy, C. J. (2002). Cortical neurons encoding path and place: Where you go is where you are. *Science, 295,* 2462–2465.

Frumkin, H. (2001). Beyond toxicity: Human health and the natural environment. *American Journal of Preventive Medicine, 20* (3), 234–240.

Gais, S., & Born, J. (2004a). Declarative memory consolidation: Mechanisms acting during human sleep. *Learning & Memory, 11,* 679–685.

Gais, S., & Born, J. (2004b). Low acetylcholine during slow-wave sleep is critical for declarative memory consolidation. *Proceedings of the National Academy of Sciences, 101* (7), 2140–2144.

Gärling, T., Böök, A., & Lindberg, E. (1985). Adults' memory representations of the spatial properties of their everyday physical environment. In R. Cohen (Ed.), *The development of spatial cognition.* Hillsdale, NJ: Lawrence Erlbaum Associates.

Geen, R. (1984). Preferred stimulation levels in introverts and extraverts: Effects on arousal and performance. *Journal of Personality and Social Psychology, 46* (6), 1303–1312.

Ghaëm, O., Mellet, E., Crivello, F., Tzourio, N., Mazoyer, B., Berthoz, A. et al. (1997). Mental navigation along memorized routes activates the hippocampus, precuneus and insula. *Neuroreport, 8* (3), 739–744.

Giles-Corti, B., Broomhall, M. H., Knuiman, M., Collins, C., Douglas, K., Ng, K., et al. (2005). Increasing walking: How important is distance to, attractiveness, and size of public open space? *American Journal of Preventive Medicine, 28* (2S2), 169–176.

Gitanjali, B., & Ananth, R. (2003). Effect of acute exposure to loud occupational noise during daytime on the nocturnal sleep architecture, heart rate, and cortisol secretion in healthy volunteers. *Journal of Occupational Health, 45,* 146–152.

Glacken, C. J. (1967). *Traces on the Rhodian shore.* Berkeley, CA: University of California Press.

Glass, D. C., & Singer, J. E. (1972). *Urban stress: Experiments in noise and social stressors.* New York: Academic Press.

Glass, D. C. Singer, J. E., & Friedman, L. N. (1969). Psychic cost of adaptation to an environmental stressor. *Journal of Personality and Social Psychology, 12,* 200–210.

Golledge, R. G. (1987). Environmental cognition. In D. Stokols and I. Altman (Eds.), *Handbook of environmental psychology* (pp. 131–174). New York: John Wiley & Sons.

Golledge, R. G., & Spector, A. N. (1978). Comprehending the urban environment: Theory and practice. *Geographical Analysis, 10*, 401–426.

Golledge, R. G., & Stimson, R. J. (1997). *Spatial behavior: A geographical perspective*. New York: The Guilford Press.

Good, M., Stanton-Hicks, M., Grass, J. A., Cranston Anderson, G., Choi, C., Schoolmeesters, L. J. et al. (1999). Relief of postoperative pain with jaw relaxation, music and their combination. *Pain, 81* (1), 163–172.

Grahn, P., & Stigsdotter, U. A. (2003). Landscape planning and stress. *Urban Forestry & Urban Greening, 2*, 1–18.

Griefahn, B., & Gros, E. (1986). Noise and sleep at home: A field study on primary and after-effects. *Journal of Sound and Vibration, 105* (3), 373–383.

Griffiths, I. D., & Delauzun, F. R. (1977). Individual differences in sensitivity to traffic noise: An empirical study. *Journal of Sound and Vibration, 55* (1), 93–107.

Habib, M., & Sirigu, A. (1987). Pure topographical disorientation: A definition and antaomical basis. *Cortex, 23*, 73–85.

Haines, M. M., Stansfeld, S. A., Brentnall, S., Head, J., Berry, B., Jiggins, M., et al. (2001a). The West London Schools Study: the effects of chronic aircraft noise exposure on child health. *Psychological Medicine, 31*, 1385–1396.

Haines, M. M., Stansfeld, S. A., Head, J., & Job, R. F. S. (2002). Multilevel modelling of aircraft noise on performance tests in schools around Heathrow Airport London. *Journal of Epidemiology and Community Health, 56*, 139–144.

Haines, M. M., Stansfeld, S. A., Job, R. F. S., Berglund, B., & Head, J. (2001c). A follow-up study on the effects of chronic aircraft noise exposure on child stress responses and cognition. *International Journal of Epidemiology, 30*, 839–845.

Haines, M. M., Stansfeld, S. A., Job, R. F. S., Berglund, B., & Head, J. (2001b). Chronic aircraft noise exposure, stress responses, mental health and cognitive performance in school children. *Psychological Medicine, 31*, 265–277.

Hansen, J. C., & Hillyard, S. A. (1983). Selective attention to multidimensional auditory stimuli in man. *Journal of Experimental Psychology: Human Perception and Performance, 9*, 1–19.

Hartig, T., & Evans, G. W. (1993). Psychological foundations of nature experience. In T. Gärling & R. G. Golledge (Eds.), *Advances in psychology: Vol. 96: Behavior and environment: Psychological and geographical approaches* (pp. 427–457). Amsterdam: North-Holland.

Hartig, T., Evans, G. W., Jamner, L. D., Davis, D., & Gärling, T. (2003). Tracking restoration in natural and urban field settings. *Journal of Environmental Psychology, 23*, 109–123.

Hartig, T., Mang, M., & Evans, G. W. (1991). Restorative effects of natural environment experiences. *Environment and Behavior, 23*, 3–26.

Hartley, T., Maguire, E. A., Spiers, H. J., & Burgess, N. (2003). The well-worn route and the path less traveled: Distinct neural bases of route following and wayfinding in humans. *Neuron, 37*, 877–888.

Haynes, S. N., Gannon, L. R., Orimoto, L., O'Brien, W. H., & Brandt, M. (1991). Psychophysiological assessment of post-stress recovery. *Psychological Assessment, 3*, 356–365.

Heft, H. (1983). Way-finding as the perception of information over time. *Population and Environment: Behavioral and Social Issues, 6*, 133–150.

Herzog, T. R., Maguire, C. P., & Nebel, M. B. (2003). Assessing the restorative components of environments. *Journal of Environmental Psychology, 23*, 159–170.

Heym, J., Trulson, M. E., & Jacobs, B. L. (1982). Raphe unit activity in freely moving cats: Effects of phasic auditory and visual stimuli. *Brain Research, 232*, 29–39.

Hintzman, D. L., O'Dell, C. S., & Arndt, D. R. (1981). Orientation in cognitive maps. *Cognitive Psychology, 13*, 149–206.

Hockey, G. R. J. (1972). Effects of noise on human efficiency and some individual differences. *Journal of Sound and Vibration, 20*, 299–304.

Hoffman, H. G., Patterson, D. R., Carrougher, G. J., Nakamura, D., Moore, M., Garcia-Palacios, A. et al. (2001). The effectiveness of virtual reality pain control with multiple treatments of longer durations: A case study. *International Journal of Human-Computer Interaction, 13* (1), 1–12.

Hoffman, H. G., Richards, T. L., Coda, B., Bills, A. R., Blough, D., Richards, A. L., et al. (2004). Modulation of thermal pain-related brain activity with virtual reality: Evidence from fMRI. *Neuroreport, 15*, 1245–1248.

Howard, J. H., & Kerst, S. M. (1981). Memory and perception of cartographic information for familiar and unfamiliar environments. *Human Factors, 23*, 495–504.

Hygge, S., Evans, G. W., & Bullinger, M. (2002). A prospective study of aircraft noise on cognitive performance in school children. *Psychological Science, 13* (5), 469–474.

Iaria, G., Petrides, M., Dagher, A., Pike, B., & Bohbot, V. D. (2003). Cognitive strategies dependent upon the hippocampus and caudate nucleus in human navigation: Variability and change with practice. *The Journal of Neuroscience, 23* (13), 5945–5952.

Isen, A. (1999). Positive affect. In T. Dalgleish & M. Power (Eds.), *The handbook of cognition and emotion* (pp. 521–539). New York: Wiley.

Ising, H., Babisch, W., Kruppa, B., Lindthammer, A. & Wiens, D. (1996). Subjective work noise – A major risk factor in myocardial infarction. In *Proceedings of the International Congress on Noise Control Engineering*, (Vol. 4, pp. 2159–2164). St. Albans, U. K.: Institute of Acoustics.

Ising, H., & Ising, M. (2002). Chronic cortisol increases in the first half of the night caused by road traffic noise. *Noise & Health, 4* (16), 13–21.

Ising, H., & Kruppa, B. (2004). Health effects caused by noise: Evidence in the literature from the past 25 years. *Noise & Health, 6*, 5–13.

Ising, H., Lange-Asschenfeldt, H., Moriske, H-J., Born, J., & Eilts, M. (2004). Low frequency noise and stress: Bronchitis and cortisol in noise in children exposed chronically to traffic noise and exhaust fumes. *Noise & Health, 6* (23), 21–28.

Jackson, J. H. (1876/1958). Case of large cerebral tumor without optic neuritis and with left hemiplegia and imperception. Reprinted in J. Taylor (Ed.), *Selected Writings of John Hughlings Jackson* (pp. 146–152). New York: Basic Books.

Jansen, G. (1969). Effects of noise on physiological state. In W. D. Ward & J. E. Fricke (Eds.), *Noise as a public health problem* (pp. 89–98). Washington, D. C.: American Speech and Hearing Association.

Janzen, G., & van Turrenout, M. (2004). Selective neural representation of objects relevant for navigation. *Nature Neuroscience, 7* (6), 673–677.

Johns, M. W. (1977). Validity of subjective reports of sleep latency in normal subjects. *Ergonomics, 20*, 683–690.

Jones, D., & Broadbent, D. E. (1979). Side-effects of interference with speech by noise. *Ergonomics*, *22*, 1073–1081.

Jordan, K., Schadow, J., Wuestenberg, T., Heinze, H., & Jänke, L. (2004). Different cortical activations for subjects using allocentric or egocentric strategies in a virtual navigation task. *NeuroReport*, *15* (1), 135–140.

Jurriëns, A. A. (1981). Noise and sleep in the home: Effects on sleep stages. In W. P. Koella (Ed.), *Sleep 1980: Fifth European Congress on Sleep Research* (pp. 217–220). Basel, Switzerland: Karger.

Kaplan, R. (2001). The nature of the view from home: Psychological benefits. *Environment and Behavior*, *33* (4), 507–542.

Kaplan, R., & Kaplan, S. (1989). *The experience of nature: A psychological perspective*. New York: Cambridge University Press.

Kaplan, S. (1995). The restorative benefits of nature: Toward an integrative framework. *Journal of Environmental Psychology*, *15*, 169–182.

Kaplan, S., & Kaplan, R. (1982). *Cognition and environment: Functioning in an uncertain world*. New York: Praeger.

Kaplan, S., & Talbot, J. F. (1983). Psychological benefits of a wilderness experience. In I. Altman & J. F. Wohlwill (Eds.), *Human behavior and environment: Advances in theory and research. Vol. 6: Behavior and the natural environment* (pp. 163–203). New York: Plenum.

Karogodina, I. L. (1969). Effect of aircraft noise on population near airports. *Hygiene and Sanitation*, *34*, 182–187.

Karsdorf, G., & Klappach, H. (1968). The influence of traffic noise on the health and performance of secondary school students in a large city (Literature Research Company, Trans.). *Zeitschrifte fur die Gesempte Hygiene*, *14*, 52–54. (As cited in Evans & Lepore, 1993)

Keogh, K., Ellery, D., Hunt, C., & Hannent, I. (2001). Selective attentional bias for pain-related stimuli amongst pain fearful individuals. *Pain*, *91*, 91–100.

Kjellberg, A. (1990). Subjective, behavioral and psychophysiological effects of noise. *Scandinavian Journal of Work Environments and Health*, *16* (Suppl. 1), 29–38.

Klatzky, R. L., Loomis, J. M., Beall, A. C., Chance, S. S., & Golledge, R. G. (1998). Spatial updating of self-position and orientation during real, imagined and virtual locomotion. *Psychological Science*, *9* (4), 293–298.

Knipschild, P. (1977). Medical effects of aircraft noise: Community cardiovascular survey. *International Archives of Occupational and Environmental Health*, *40*, 185–190.

Knipschild, P. (1980). Aircraft noise and hypertension. In J. V. Tobias, G. Jansen, & W. D. Ward (Eds.), *Noise as a public health problem: Proceedings of the third international congress*, (ASHA Reports 10, pp. 283–287). Rockville, MD: The American Speech-Language-Hearing Association.

Korpela, K. M., Hartig, T., Kaiser, F. G., & Fuhrer, U. (2001). Restorative experience and self-regulation in favorite places. *Environment and Behavior*, *33* (4), 572–589.

Krantz, D. S., Contrada, R. J., Hill, D. & Friedler, E. (1988). Environmental stress and biobehavioral antecedents of coronary heart disease. *Journal of Consulting and Clinical Psychology*, *56*, 333–341.

Kritchevsky, M. (1988). The elementary spatial functions of the brain. In J. Stiles-Davis, M. Kritchevsky, & U. Bellugi (Eds.), *Spatial cognition: Brain bases and development* (pp. 111–140). Hillsdale, NJ: Lawrence Erlbaum Associates.

Kryter, K. D. (1994). *The handbook of hearing and the effects of noise: Physiology, psychology and public health*. San Diego: Academic Press.

Kryter, K. D., & Poza, F. (1980). Effects of noise on some autonomic system activities. *Journal of the Acoustical Society of America*, *67* (6), 2036–2044.

Kuipers, B. (1982). The "map in the head" metaphor. *Environment and Behavior*, *14*, 202–220.

Küller, R., & Laike, T. (1998). The impact of flicker from fluorescent lighting on well-being, performance, and physiological arousal. *Ergonomics*, *41* (1), 433–447.

Küller, R., & Mikellides, B. (1993). Simulated studies of color, arousal, and comfort. In R. W. Marans & D. Stokols (Eds.), *Environmental simulation: Research and policy issues* (pp. 163–190). New York: Plenum Press.

Lacey, B. C., & Lacey, J. I. (1974). Studies of heart rate and other bodily processes in sensorimotor behavior. In P. A. Obrist, A. H. Black, J. Brenner, & L. V. DiCara (Eds.), *Cardiovascular psychophysiology* (pp. 538–564). Chicago: Aldine.

Landis, T., Cummings, J. L., Benson, F., & Palmer, P. (1986). Loss of topographic familiarity: An environmental agnosia. *Archives of Neurology*, *43*, 132–136.

Lang, T., Fouriaud, C., & Jacquinet, M. C. (1992). Length of occupational noise exposure and blood pressure. *International Archives of Occupational and Environmental Health*, *63*, 369–372.

Larsen, L., Adams, J., Deal, B., Kweon, B. S., & Tyler, E. (1998). Plants in the workplace: The effects of plant density on productivity, attitudes and perceptions. *Environment and Behavior*, *30* (3), 261–281.

Laumann, K., Gärling, T., & Stormark, K. M. (2003). Selective attention and heart rate responses to natural and urban environments. *Journal of Environmental Psychology*, *23*, 125–134.

Leather, P., Beale, D., & Sullivan, L. (2003). Noise, psychosocial stress and their interaction in the work environment. *Journal of Environmental Psychology*, *23*, 213–222.

Lees, R. E. M., Romeril, C. S., & Wetherall, L. D. (1980). A study of stress indicators in workers exposed to industrial noise. *Canadian Journal of Public Health*, *71*, 261–265.

Lembo, T., Fitzgerald, L., Matin, K., Woo, K., Mayer, E. A., & Naliboff, B. D. (1998). Audio and visual stimulation reduces patient discomfort during screening flexible sigmoidoscopy. *The American Journal of Gastroenterolgy*, *93*, 1113–1116.

Lercher, P., Evans, G. W., Meis, M., & Kofler, W. W. (2002). Ambient neighborhood noise and children's mental health. *Occupational Environmental Medicine*, *59*, 380–386.

LeVere, T. E., & Davis, N. (1977). Arousal from sleep: The physiological and subjective effects of a 15 dB(A) reduction in aircraft flyover noise. *Aviation, Space and Environmental Medicine*, *48* (7), 607–611.

LeVere, T. E., Bartus, R. T., & Hart, F. D. (1972). Electroencephalographic and behavioral effects of nocturnally occurring jet aircraft sounds. *Aerospace Medicine*, *43* (4), 384–389.

Lewin. K. (1936). *Principles of topological psychology*. (F. Heider & G. M. Heider, Trans.). New York: McGraw-Hill Book Company.

Lovallo, W. R., Wilson, M. F., Pincomb, G. A., Edwards, G. L., Tompkins, P., & Brackett, D. J. (1985). Activation patterns to aversive stimulation in man: Passive exposure versus effort to control. *Psychophysiology*, *22* (3), 283–291.

Lukas, J. S. (1976). Noise and sleep: A literature review and a proposed criterion for assessing effect. *Journal of the Acoustical Society of America*, *58* (6), 1232–1242.

Lundberg, U., & Frankenhaeuser, M. (1978). Psychophysiological reactions to noise as modified by personal control over noise intensity. *Biological Psychology*, *6*, 51–59.

Lusk, S. L., Hagerty, B. M., Gillespie, B., & Caruso, C. C. (2002). Chronic effects of workplace noise on blood pressure and heart rate. *Archives of Environmental Health*, *57* (4), 273–281.

Lydic, R., McCarley, R. W., & Hobson, J. A. (1987). Serotonin neurons and sleep: II. Time course of dorsal raphe discharge, PGO waves, and behavioral states. *Archives Italiennes de Biologie*, *126* (1), 1–28.

Magliano, J. P., Cohen, R., Allen, G. L., & Rodrigue, J. R. (1995). The impact of a wayfinder's goal on learning a new environment: Different types of spatial knowledge as goals. *Journal of Environmental Psychology*, *15*, 65–75.

Maguire, E. A. (1997). Hippocampal involvement in human topographical memory: Evidence from functional imaging. *Philosophical Transactions of the Royal Society, London B*, *352*, 1475–1480.

Maguire, E. A., Burgess, N., Donnett, J. G., Frakowiak, R. S. J., Frith, C. D., & O'Keefe, J. (1998). Knowing where and getting there: A human navigation network. *Science*, *280*, 921–924.

Maguire, E. A., Frakowiak, R. S. J., & Frith, C. D. (1996). Learning to find your way: A role for the human hippocampal formation. *Proceedings of the Royal Society, London B*, *263*, 1745–1750.

Maguire, E. A., Frakowiak, R. S. J., & Frith, C. D. (1997). Recalling routes around London: Activation of the right hippocampus in taxi drivers. *The Journal of Neuroscience*, *17* (18), 7103–7110.

Maguire, E. A., Frith, C. D., Burgess, N. Donnett, J. G., & O'Keefe, J. (1998). Knowing where things are: Parahippocampal involvement in encoding object locations in virtual large-scale space. *Journal of Cognitive Neuroscience*, *10* (1), 61–76.

Maguire, E. A., Gadian, D. G., Johnsrude, I. S., Good, C. D., Ashburner, J., Frackowiak, R. S. J. et al. (2000). Navigation-related structural change in the hippocampi of taxi drivers. *Proceedings of the National Academy of Sciences*, *97* (8), 4398–4403.

Maguire, E. A., Spiers, H. J., Good, C. D., Hartley, T., Frackowiak, R. S. J. & Burgess, N. (2003). Navigation expertise and the human hippocampus: A structural brain imaging analysis. *Hippocampus*, *13*, 250–259.

Mandler, J. M. (1988). The development of spatial cognition: On topological and Euclidean representation. In J. Stiles-Davis, M. Kritchevsky, & U. Bellugi (Eds.), *Spatial cognition: Brain bases and development* (pp. 423–432). Hillsdale, NJ: Lawrence Erlbaum Associates.

Maschke, C., & Hecht, K. (2004). Stress hormones and sleep disturbances: Electrophysiological and hormonal aspects. *Noise & Health*, *6* (22), 49–54.

Maxwell, L. E., & Evans, G. W. (2000). The effects of noise on preschool children's pre-reading skills. *Journal of Environmental Psychology*, *20*, 91–97.

McFie, J., Piercy, M. F., & Zangwill, O. L. (1950). Visual-spatial agnosia associated with lesions of the right cerebral hemisphere. *Brain*, *73*, 167–190.

McLean, E. K., & Tarnopolsky, A. (1977). Noise, discomfort and mental health: A review of the socio-medical implications of disturbance by noise. *Psychological Medicine*, *7*, 19–62.

McNamara, T. P., & Shelton, A. L. (2003). Cognitive maps and the hippocampus. *Trends in Cognitive Sciences*, *7* (8), 333–335.

McNaughton, B. L., Chen, L. L., & Markus, E. J. (1991). "Dead reckoning," landmark learning and sense of direction: A neuro-physiological and computational hypothesis. *Journal of Cognitive Neuroscience*, *3* (2), 190–202.

McNaughton, B. L., Knierim, J. J., & Wilson, M. A. (1995). Vector encoding and vestibular foundations of spatial cognition: Neurophysiological and computational mechanisms. In M. S. Gazzaniga (Ed.), *The cognitive neurosciences* (pp. 585–595). Cambridge, MA: MIT Press.

Meagher, M. W., Arnau, R. C., & Rhudy, J. L. (2001). Pain and emotion: Effects of affective picture modulation. *Psychosomatic Medicine*, *6363*, 79–90.

Melamed, S., & Bruhis, S. (1996). The effects of chronic industrial noise exposure on urinary cortisol, fatigue, and irritability: A controlled field experiment. *Journal of Occupational and Environmental Medicine*, *38* (3), 252–256.

Mellet, E., Bricogne, S., Tzuorio-Mazoyer, N., Ghaëm, O., Petit, L., Zago, L., et al. (2000). Neural correlates of topographic mental exploration: The impact of route versus survey perspective learning. *NeuroImage*, *12*, 588–600.

Meyer, O. (1900/1996). Ein- und doppelseitige homonyme hemianopsie mit orient-irrungsstören. *Monatsschrift für psychiatrie und neurologie*, *8*, 440–456. (As cited in Farrel, 1996)

Miedema, H. M., & Vos, H. (1998). Exposure-response relationships for transportation noise. *Journal of the Acoustical Society of America*, *104*, 3432–3445.

Miedema, H. M., & Vos, H. (2003). Noise sensitivity and reactions to noise and other environmental conditions. *Journal of the Acoustical Society of America*, *113* (3), 1492–1504.

Millar, K., & Steels, M. J. (1990). Sustained peripheral vasoconstriction while working in continuous intense noise. *Aviation, Space and Environmental Medicine*, *61*, 695–698.

Miller, A. C., Hickman, L. C., & Lemasters, G. K. (1992). A distraction technique for control of burn pain. *Journal of Burn Care and Rehabilitation*, *13*, 576–580.

Miltner, W., Matjak, M., Braun, C., Diekmann, H., & Brody, S. (1994). Emotional qualities of odors and their influence on the startle reflex in humans. *Psychophysiology*, *31*, 107–110.

Moeser, S. D. (1988). Cognitive mapping in a complex building. *Environment and Behavior*, *20*, 21–49.

Montello, D. R. (1998). A new framework for understanding the acquisition of spatial knowledge in large-scale environments. In M. J. Egenhofer & R. G. Golledge (Eds.), *Spatial and temporal reasoning in geographic information systems* (pp. 143–154). New York: Oxford University Press.

Moos, R. H., & Swindle, R. W. (1990). Person-environment transactions and the stressor-appraisal-coping process. *Psychological Inquiry*, *1* (1), 30–32.

Moreira, N. M., & Bryan, M. E. (1972). Noise annoyance susceptibility. *Journal of Sound and Vibration*, *21* (4), 449–462.

Morris, R. G., Pickering, A., Abrahams, S. & Feigenbaum, J. D. (1996). Space and the hippocampal formation in humans. *Brain Research Bulletin*, *40*, 487–490.

Morrow, L., & Ratcliff, G. (1988). The neuropsychology of spatial cognition. In J. Stiles-Davis, M. Kritchevsky, & U. Bellugi (Eds.), *Spatial cognition: Brain bases and development* (pp. 5–32). Hillsdale, NJ: Lawrence Erlbaum Associates.

Morton, L. L., & Kershner, J. R. (1987). Negative ion effects on hemispheric processing and selective attention in the mentally retarded. *Journal of Mental Deficiency Research*, *31*, 169–180.

Mosskov, J. I., & Ettema, J. H. (1977a). Extra-auditory effects in short-term exposure to aircraft and traffic noise. II. *International Archives of Occupational and Environmental Health*, *40*, 165–173.

Mosskov, J. I., & Ettema, J. H. (1977b). Extra-auditory effects in short-term exposure to aircraft and traffic noise. IV. *International Archives of Occupational and Environmental Health*, *40*, 177–184.

Murata, A. (2004). Effects of duration of immersion in a virtual reality environment on postural stability. *International Journal of Human-Computer Interaction*, *17* (4), 463–477.

Murphy, M., Nevill, A. Neville, C., Biddle, S., & Hardman, A. (2002). Accumulating brisk walking for fitness, cardiovascular risk and psychological health. *Medicine and Science in Sports and Exercise*, *34* (9), 1468–1474.

Muzet, A., & Ehrhart, J. (1980). Habituation of heart rate and finger pulse responses to noise in sleep. In J. V. Tobias, G. Jansen & W. D. Ward (Eds.), *Noise as a public health problem: Proceedings of the third international congress*, (ASHA Reports 10, pp. 401–404). Rockville, MD: The American Speech-Language-Hearing Association.

Obrist, P. A., Gaebelein, C. J., Teller, E. S., Langer, A. W., Grignolo, A., Light, K. et al. (1978). The relationship among heart rate, carotid dP/dt, and blood pressure in humans as a function of the type of stress. *Psychophysiology*, *15*, 102–115.

Ogunseitan, O. A. (2005). Topophilia and the quality of life. *Environmental Health perspectives*, *113* (2), 143–148.

Öhrström, E. & Björkman, M. (1983). Sleep disturbance before and after traffic noise attentuation in an apartment building. *Journal of the Acoustical Society of America*, *73* (3), 877–879.

Öhrström, E., & Rylander, R. (1982). Sleep disturbance effects of noise – a laboratory study on after effects. *Journal of Sound and Vibration*, *84* (1), 87–103.

Öhrström, E., Björkman, M. & Rylander, R. (1988). Noise annoyance with regard to neurophysiological sensitivity, subjective noise sensitivity and personality variables. *Psychological Medicine*, *18*, 605–613.

O'Keefe, J., & Nadel, L. (1978). *The hippocampus as a cognitive map*. Oxford: Clarendon Press.

O'Keefe, J. (1991). The hippocampal cognitive map and navigational strategies. In J. Paillard (Ed.), *Brain and space* (pp. 273–295). Oxford: Oxford University Press.

Olmsted, F. L. (1865). The Yosemite Valley and the Mariposa Big Trees: A preliminary report. With an introductory note by L. W. Roper (1952). *Landscape Architecture*, *43*, 12.

Orians, G. H., & Heerwagen, J. H. (1992). Evolved responses to landscapes. In J. H. Barkow, L. Cosmides, & J. Tooby (Eds.), *The adapted mind: Evolutionary psychology and the generation of culture*. New York: Oxford University Press.

Orians, G. H. (1980). Habitat selection: General theory and applications to human behavior. In J. S. Lockard (Ed.), *The evolution of human social behavior*. New York: Elsevier North-Holland.

Orians, G. H. (1986). An ecological and evolutionary approach to landscape aesthetics. In E. C. Penning-Rowsell & D. Lowenthal (Eds.), *Meanings and values in landscape*. London: Allen & Unwin.

Osei-Tutu, K. B., & Campagna, P. D. (2005). The effects of short- vs. long-bout exercise on mood, VO$_2$ max and percent body fat. *Preventive Medicine*, *40* (1), 92–98.

Ottosson, J., & Grahn, P. (2005). A comparison of leisure time spent in a garden with leisure time spent indoors: On measures of restoration in residents in geriatric care. *Landscape Research*, *30* (1), 23–55.

Parslow, D. M., Rose, D., Brooks, B., Fleminger, S., Gray, J. A., Giampietro, V., et al. (2004). Allocentric spatial memory activation of the hippocampal formation measured with fMRI. *Neuropsychology*, *18* (3), 450–461.

Parsons, R. (1991a). *Recovery from stress during exposure to videotaped outdoor environments*. Unpublished doctoral dissertation, Psychology Department, University of Arizona, Tucson, AZ.

Parsons, R. (1991b). The potential influences of environmental perception on health. *Journal of Environmental Psychology*, *11*, 1–23.

Parsons, R., & Hartig, T. (2000). Environmental psychophysiology. In J. T. Cacioppo & L. G. Tassinary (Eds.), *Handbook of psychophysiology (2nd ed.)* (pp. 815–846). New York: Cambridge University Press.

Parsons, R., Tassinary, L. G., Ulrich, R. S., Hebl, M. R., & Grossman-Alexander, M. (1998). The view from the road: Implications for stress recovery and immunization. *Journal of Environmental Psychology*, *18*, 113–140.

Parvizpoor, D. (1976). Noise exposure and prevalence of high blood pressure among weavers in Iran. *Journal of Occupational Medicine*, *18*, 730–731.

Paterson, A., & Zangwill, O. L. (1944). Disorders of visual space perception associated with lesions of the right cerebral hemisphere. *Brain*, *67*, 331–358.

Paterson, A., & Zangwill, O. L. (1945). A case of topographical disorientation associated with unilateral cerebral lesion. *Brain*, *68*, 188–211.

Payne, J. D., & Nadel, L. (2004). Sleep, dreams, and memory consolidation: The role of the stress hormone cortisol. *Learning & Memory*, *11*, 671–678.

Pearsons, K. S., Barber, D. S. & Tabachnick, B. G. (1990). *Analyses of the predictability of noise-induced sleep disturbance*. Report no. HSD-TR-*(-029. Ohio: Wright-Patterson Air Force Base.

Persson-Waye, K., Bengtsson, J., Rylander, R., Hucklebridge, F., Evans, P., & Clow, A. (2002). Low frequency noise enhances cortisol among noise sensitive subjects during work performance. *Life Sciences*, *70*, 745–758.

Pick, H. L. (1993). Organization of spatial knowledge in children. In N. Eilan, R. McCarthy & B. Brewer (Eds.), *Spatial representation: Problems in philosophy and psychology* (pp. 31–42). Cambridge, MA: Blackwell.

Pine, D. S., Grun, J., Maguire, E. A., Burgess, N., Zarahn, E., Koda, V., et al. (2002). Neurodevelopmental aspects of spatial navigation: A virtual reality fMRI study. *NeuroImage*, *15*, 396–406.

Plial, W., & Born, J. (1997). Effects of early and late nocturnal sleep on declarative and procedural memory. *Journal of Cognitive Neuroscience*, *9*, 534–547.

Plial, W., & Born, J. (1999). Memory consolidation in human sleep depends upon inhibition of glucocorticoid release. *NeuroReport*, *10*, 2741–2747.

Posner, M. I., & Raichle, M. E. (1994). *Images of mind*. New York: Freeman.

Power, A. E. (2004). Slow-wave sleep, acetylcholine, and memory consolidation. *Proceedings of the National Academy of Sciences*, *101* (7), 1795–1796.

Presson, C. C., & Hazelrigg, M. D. (1984). Building spatial representations through primary and secondary learning. *Journal of Experimental Psychology: Learning, Memory and Cognition*, *10*, 716–722.

Rainville, P., Carrier, B., Hofbauer, R. K., Bushnell, M. C., & Duncan, G. H. (1999). Dissociation of pain sensory and affective dimensions using hypnotic modulation. *Pain*, *82*, 159–171.

Rainville, P., Duncan, G. H., Price, D. D., Carrier, B., & Bushnell, M. C. (1997). Pain affect encoded in human anterior cingulate but not in somatosensory cortex. *Science*, 277, 968–971.

Rao, M. L., Pelzer, E., Papassotiropoulos, A., Tiemeier, H., Jönck, L., & Möller, H. J. (1996). Selective slow-wave sleep deprivation influences blood serotonin profiles and serum melatonin concentrations in healthy subjects. *Biological Psychiatry*, 40, 664–667.

Regan, E. C., & Price, K. R. (1994). The frequency of occurrence and severity of side-effects of immersion virtual reality. *Aviation Space and Environmental Medicine*, 65, 527–530.

Regan, E. C., & Ramsey, A. D. (1996). The efficacy of hyoscine hydrobromide in reducing side-effects during immersion in virtual reality. *Aviation Space and Environmental Medicine*, 67, 222–226.

Regecová, V., & Kellerová, E. (1995). Effects of urban noise pollution on blood pressure and heart rate in preschool children. *Journal of Hypertension*, 13, 405–412.

Rhudy, J. L., & Meagher, M. W. (2000). Fear and anxiety: Divergent effects on human pain thresholds. *Pain*, 84, 65–75.

Richardson, A. E., Montello, D. R. & Hegarty, M. (1999). Spatial knowledge acquisition from maps and from navigation in real and virtual environments. *Memory & Cognition*, 27 (4), 741–750.

Richell, R. A., Deakin, J. F. W., & Anderson, I. M. (2005). Effect of acute tryptophan depletion on the response to controllable and uncontrollable noise stress. *Biological Psychiatry*, 57, 295–300.

Rieser, J. J., Pick, H. L., Ashmead, D. H., & Garing, A. E. (1995). Calibration of human locomotion and models of perceptual-motor organization. *Journal of Experimental Psychology: Human Perception and Performance*, 21 (3), 480–497.

Ristovska, G., Gjorgjev, D., & Jordanova, N. P. (2004). Psychosocial effects of community noise: Cross-sectional study of school children in urban center of Skopje, Macedonia. *Croatian Medical Journal*, 45 (4), 473–476.

Rolls, E. T., Robertson, R. G. & Georges-François, P. (1995). The representation of space in the primate hippocampus. *Society for Neuroscience Abstracts*, 21, 1492.

Rosenlund, M., Berglind, N., Pershagen, G., Järup, L., & Bluhm, G. (2001). Increased prevalence of hypertension in a population exposed to aircraft noise. *Occupational and Environmental Medicine*, 58, 769–773.

Russolo, L. (1913/1971). *The art of noise*. (Futurist manifesto, transl. and reprinted in M. Kirby). *Futurist performance*. New York: E. P. Dutton & Co.

Sarter, M., Berntson, G., & Cacioppo, J. T. (1996). Brain imaging and cognitive neuroscience: Toward strong inference in attributing function to structure. *American Psychologist*, 51 (1), 13–21.

Schacter, D. L., & Nadel, L. (1991). Varieties of spatial memory: A problem for cognitive neuroscience. In R. G. Lister & H. J. Weingartner (Eds.), *Perspectives on cognitive neuroscience*. New York: Oxford University Press.

Schivelbusch, W. (1986). *The railway journey*. Berkeley: University of California Press.

Schmidt-Nielsen, K. (1997). *Animal physiology: Adaptation and environment* (5th ed.). New York: Cambridge University Press.

Scholl, M. J. (1987). Cognitive maps as orienting schemata. *Journal of Experimental Psychology: Learning, Memory and Cognition*, 13, 615–628.

Schweitzer, M., Gilpin, L., & Frampton, S. (2004). Healing spaces: Elements of environmental design that make an impact in health. *The Journal of Alternative and Complementary Medicine*, 10 (S1), S71–S83.

Shemyakin, F. N. (1962). General problems of orientation in space and space representations. In B. G. Anan'yev *et al.* (Eds.), *Psychological science in the USSR* (Vol. 1), NTIS Report No. TT62–11083 (pp. 184–225). Washington, DC: Office of Technical Services. (As cited in Golledge & Stimson, 1997).

Sherry, D. F., Jacobs, L. F., & Gaulin, S. J. (1992). Spatial memory and adaptive specialization of the hippocampus. *Trends in Neuroscience*, 15, 298–303.

Shima, K., Nakahama, H., & Yamamoto, M. (1986). Firing properties of two types of nucleus raphe dorsalis neurons during the sleep-waking cycle and their responses to sensory stimuli. *Brain Research*, 399 (2), 317–326.

Siegel, A. W., & White, S. H. (1975). The development of spatial representation of large-scale environments. In H. W. Reese (Ed.), *Advances in child development and behavior* (Vol. 10, pp. 9–55). New York: Academic Press.

Simons, D. J., & Wang, R. F. (1998). Perceiving real-world viewpoint changes. *Psychological Science*, 9 (4), 315–320.

Smith, A. (1991). A review of the nonauditory effects of noise on health. *Work and Stress*, 5 (1), 49–62.

Spencer, C., Blades, M., & Morsley, K. (1989). *The child in the physical environment: The development of spatial knowledge and cognition*. New York: John Wiley & Sons.

Spreng, M. (2000). Possible health effects of noise induced cortisol increase. *Noise & Health*, 7, 59–63.

Spreng, M. (2004). Noise induced nocturnal cortisol secretion and tolerable overhead flights. *Noise & Health*, 6 (22), 35–47.

St. Leger, L. (2003). Health and nature: New challenges for health promotion. *Health Promotion International*, 18 (3), 173–175.

Standing, L., Lynn, D., & Moxness, K. (1990). Effects of noise upon introverts and extroverts. *Bulletin of the Psychonomic Society*, 28 (2), 138–140.

Stansfeld, S. A., & Haines, M. (1997). *Environmental noise and health: A review of nonauditory effects*. Report for the Department of Health, London, U. K.

Stansfeld, S. A., Berglund, B., Clark, C., Lopez-Barrio, L., Fischer, P., Öhrström, E., Haines, M. M., Head, J., Hygge, S., van Kamp, I., & Berry, B. F. (2005). Aircraft and road traffic noise and children's health and cognition. *The Lancet*, 365 (Jun 4), 1942–1949.

Stansfeld, S. A., Clark, C. R., Turpin, G., Jenkins, L. M., & Tarnopolsky, A. (1985). Sensitivity to noise in a community sample: II. Measurement of psychophysiological variables. *Psychological Medicine*, 15, 255–263.

Steuer, J. (1992). Defining virtual reality: Dimensions determining telepresence. *Journal of Communications*, 42 (4), 73–93.

Stevenson, D. C., & McKellar, N. R. (1988). The effect of traffic noise on sleep of young adults in their home. *Journal of the Acoustical Society of America*, 85 (2), 768–771.

Stickgold, R. (2005). Sleep-dependent memory consolidation. *Nature*, 437, 1272–1278.

Stigsdotter, U. A., & Grahn, P. (2004). A garden at your doorstep may reduce stress: Private gardens as restorative environments in the city. Paper presented at *Open Space/People Space Conference*, Edinburgh, Scotland, Oct. 30th, 2004.

Stokols, D., & Altman, I. (Eds.)(1987). *Handbook of environmental psychology*. New York: John Wiley & Sons.

Stone, A. A., Cox, D. S., Valdimarsdottir, H., Jandorf, L., & Neale, J. M. (1987). Secretory IgA as a measure of immunocompetence. *Journal of Human Stress*, 13, 136–140.

Stone, A. A., Neale, J. M., Cox, D. S., Napoli, A., Valdimarsdottir, H., & Kennedy-Moore, E. (1994). Daily events are associated with a secretory immune response to an oral antigen in men. *Health Psychology, 13* (5), 440–446.

Strube, M. J. (1990). Psychometric principles: From physiological data to psychological constructs. In J. T. Cacioppo & L. G. Tassinary (Eds.), *Principles of psychophysiology: Physical, social and inferential elements* (pp. 34–57). New York: Cambridge University Press.

Tafalla, R. J. & Evans, G. W. (1997). Noise, physiology and human performance: The potential role of effort. *Journal of Occupational Helath Psychology, 2* (2), 148–155.

Takano, T., Nakamura, K., & Watanabe, M. (2002). Urban residential environments and senior citizens' longevity in megacity areas: the importance of walkable green spaces. *Journal of Epidemiology and Community Health, 56*, 913–918.

Tanaka, A., Takano, T., Nakamura, K., & Takeuchi, S. (1996). Health levels influenced by urban residential conditions in a megacity – Tokyo. *Urban Studies, 33* (6), 879–894.

Tassinary, L. G. (1995). Unpublished lecture notes.

Taube, J. S., Goodridge, J. P., Golob, E. J., Dudchenko, P. A., & Stackman, R. W. (1996). Processing the head direction cell signal: A review and commentary. *Brain Research Bulletin, 40* (5/6), 477–486.

Taylor, N. A. S., Allsopp, N. K., & Parkes, D. G. (1995). Preferred room temperature of young vs. aged males: The influence of thermal sensation, thermal comfort and affect. *Journal of Gerentology: Medical Sciences, 50A*, M216–M221.

Thiessen, G. J., & Lapointe, A. C. (1978). Effect of intermittent truck noise on percentage of deep sleep. *Journal of the Acoustical Society of America, 64* (4), 1078–1080.

Thomas, J. R., & Jones, D. M. (1982). Individual differences in noise annoyance and the uncomfortable loudness level. *Journal of Sound and Vibration, 82* (2), 289–304.

Thompson, S. (1996). Non-auditory health effects of noise: An updated review. In *Proceedings of the International Congress on Noise Control Engineering*, (Vol. 4, pp. 2177–2182). St. Albans, U. K.: Institute of Acoustics.

Thorndyke, P. W., & Hayes-Roth, B. (1982). Differences in spatial knowledge acquired from maps and navigation. *Cognitive Psychology, 14*, 560–589.

Thorndyke, P. W. (1981). Spatial cognition and reasoning. In J. H. Harvey (Ed.), *Cognition, social behavior and the environment* (pp. 137–149). Hillsdale, NJ: Lawrence Erlbaum Associates.

Tolman, E. C. (1948). Cognitive maps in rats and men. *Psychological Review, 55*, 189–208.

Tomei, F., Fantini, S., Tomao, E., Baccolo, T. P., & Rosati, M. V. (2000). Hypertension and chronic exposure to noise. *Archives of Environmental Health, 55* (5), 319–325.

Townsend, R. E., Johnson, L. C., & Muzet, A. (1973). Effects of the long term exposure to tone pulse noise on human sleep. *Psychophysiology, 10* (4), 369–376.

Tranel, D., & Damasio, H. (1994). Neuroanatomical correlates of electrodermal skin conductance responses. *Psychophysiology, 31* (5), 427–438.

Tse, M. M. Y., Ng, J. K. F., Chung, J. W. Y., & Wong, T. K. S. (2002). The effect of visual stimuli on pain threshold and tolerance. *Journal of Clinical Nursing, 11*, 462–469.

Tulen, J. H. M., Kumar, A., & Jurriëns, A. A. (1986). Psychophysiological acoustics of indoor sound due to traffic noise during sleep. *Journal of Sound and Vibration, 110* (1), 129–141.

Ulrich, R. S. (1979). Visual landscapes and psychological well-being. *Landscape Research, 4*, 17–23.

Ulrich, R. S. (1983). Aesthetic and affective response to natural environment. In I. Altman & J. F. Wohlwill (Eds.), *Human behavior and environment: Advances in theory and research. Vol. 6: Behavior and the natural environment* (pp. 85–125). New York: Plenum.

Ulrich, R. S. (1984). View through a window may influence recovery from surgery. *Science, 224*: 420–421.

Ulrich, R. S. (1993). Biophilia, biophobia and natural landscapes. In S. R. Kellert & E. O. Wilson (Eds.), *The Biophilia Hypothesis* (pp. 73–137). Washington, D. C.: Island Press.

Ulrich, R. S., & Parsons, R. (1992). The influences of passive experiences with plants on human well-being and health. In D. Relf (Ed.), *The Role of Horticulture in Human Well-Being and Social Development* pp. 93–105). Portland, OR: Timber Press.

Ulrich, R. S., Simons, R., Losito, B. D., Fiorito, E., Miles, M. A., & Zelson, M. (1991). Stress recovery during exposure to natural and urban environments. *Journal of Environmental Psychology, 11*, 201–230.

Vallet, M., Gagneux, J. M., & Simonnet, F. (1980). Effects of aircraft noise on sleep: An *in situ* experience. In J. V. Tobias, G. Jansen, & W. D. Ward (Eds.), *Noise as a public health problem: Proceedings of the third international congress*, (ASHA Reports 10, pp. 391–396). Rockville, MD: The American Speech-Language-Hearing Association.

Vallet, M., Gagneux, J. M., Blanchet, V., Favre, B., & Labiale, G. (1983a). *Journal of Sound and Vibration, 90* (2), 173–191.

Vallet, M., Gagneux, J. M., Clairet, J. M., Laurens, J. F., & Letisserand, D. (1983b). Heart rate reactivity to aircraft noise after a long-term exposure. In *The 4th International Congress on Noise as a Public Health Problem* (pp. 965–971). Milan: Centro Richerche E Studi Amplifon.

van Dijk, F. J. H., Verbeek, J. H. A. M., & De Vries, F. F. (1987). Nonauditory effects of noise in industry, V: A field study in a shipyard. *International Archives of Occupational and Environmental Health, 59*, 55–62.

van Kamp, I., Job, R. F. S., Hatfield, J., Haines, M., Stellato, R. K., & Stansfeld, S. A. (2004). The role of noise sensitivity in the noise-response relationship: A comparison of three international airport studies. *Journal of the Acoustical Society of America, 116* (6), 3471–3479.

van Kempen, E. E. M. M., Kruize, H., Boshuizen, H. C., Ameling, C. B. Staatsen, B. A. M., & de Hollander, A. E. M. (2002). The association between noise exposure and blood pressure and ischemic heart disease: A meta-analysis. *Environmental Health Perspectives, 110*, 307–317.

Villemure, C., & Bushnell, M. C. (2002). Cognitive modulation of pain: How do attention and emotion influence pain processing? *Pain, 95*, 195–199.

Villemure, C., Slotnick, B. M., & Bushnell, M. C. (2003). Effects of odors on pain perception: Deciphering the roles of emotion and attention. *Pain, 106*, 101–108.

Vogt, B. A., Finch, D. M., & Olson, C. R. (1992). Functional heterogeneity in cingulate cortex: The anterior executive and posterior evaluative regions. *Cerebral Cortex, 2*, 435–443.

Wagner, U., Gais, S., Haider, H., Verleger, R., & Born, J. (2004). Sleep inspires insight. *Nature, 427*, 352–355.

Wang, R. F., & Simons, D. J. (1999). Active and passive scene recognition across views. *Cognition, 70* (2), 191–210.

Ward, L. M., & Suedfeld, P. (1973). Human responses to highway noise. *Environmental Research, 6,* 306–326.

Weinstein, N. D. (1980). Individual differences in critical tendencies and noise annoyance. *Journal of Sound and Vibration, 68* (2), 241–248.

Welch, B. L. (1979). *Extra-auditory health effects of industrial noise: Survey of foreign literature.* Aerospace Medical Research Laboratory Technical Report, AMRL-TR-79–41. Dayton, OH: Wright Patterson Air Force Base.

Wells, N. M., & Evans, G. W. (2003). Nearby nature: A buffer of life stress among rural children. *Environment and Behavior, 35* (3), 311–330.

Whalen, P. J., Bush, G., McNally, R. J., Wilhelm, S., McInerney, S. C., Jenike, M. A., & Rauch, S. L. (1998). The emotional counting Stroop paradigm: A functional magnetic imaging probe of the anterior cingulate affective division. *Biological Psychiatry, 44,* 1219–1228.

White, P. M., & Yee, C. M. (1997). Effects of attentional and stressor manipulations on the P50 gating response. *Psychophysiology, 34,* 703–711.

Whiteley, A. M., & Warrington, E. K. (1978). Selective impairment of topographic memory: A single case study. *Journal of Neurology, Neurosurgery and Psychiatry, 41,* 575–578.

Wichrowski, M., Whiteson, J., Haas, F., Mola, A., & Rey, M. J. (2005). Effects of horticulture therapy on mood and heart rate in patients participating in an inpatient cardiopulmonary rehabilitation program. *Journal of Cardiopulmonary Rehabilitation, 25,* 270–274.

Wiener, S. I., Paul, C. A., & Eichenbaum, H. (1989). Spatial and behavioral correlates of hippocampal neuronal activity. *Journal of Neuroscience, 9,* 2737–2763.

Wilbrand, H. (1892/1982). Ein fall von seelenblindheit und hemianopsie mit sections-befund. *Deutsch. Z. Nervenheilk., 2,* 361–387. (As cited in DeRenzi, 1982, chap. 8).

Wilkinson, R. T., & Campbell, K. B. (1984). Effects of traffic noise on quality of sleep: Assessment by EEG, subjective report, or peformance the next day. *Journal of the Acoustical Society of America, 75* (2), 468–475.

Zeltzer, D. (1992). Autonomy, interaction and presence. *Presence: Teleoperators and Virtual Environments, 1* (1), 127–132.

Zhao, Y., Zhang, S., Selvin, S., & Spear, R. (1993). A dose-response relationship between cumulative noise exposure and hypertension among female textile workers without hearing protection. In M. Vallet (Ed.), *Noise as a Public Health Problem: Proceedings of the 6th International Congress,* (Vol. 3, pp. 274–279). Arcuil Cedex, France: l'INRETS.

Experimental Design, Data Representation, and Data Analysis Issues

SECTION EDITOR: HOWARD C. NUSBAUM

33 Psychometrics

MICHAEL J. STRUBE AND LAUREL C. NEWMAN

All scientists grapple with the limitations of faulty observations. Rarely are the concepts that are embedded in theories easily revealed or conveniently available with little error. This is especially true in psychophysiology in which an attempt is made to link physical processes to psychological constructs. The ability to make these linkages rests on attention to important psychometric principles. After all, physiological measurement, like all other forms of measurement, is the replicable assignment of numbers to represent properties (Campbell, 1957). Accordingly, basic psychometric principles are as relevant to psychophysiological assessment as they are to the measurement of intelligence, assessment of job performance, or self-reports of emotion. Our goal in this chapter is to provide a guide to the issues requiring attention when inferences about psychological constructs are based on the collection of physiological data. In the discussion that follows, we will outline the core psychometric issues relevant to measurement in any area, but with an emphasis on their psychophysiological application.

A topic that is as broad as psychometrics cannot be covered comprehensively in a single chapter. It ranges widely and includes topics and issues that overlap with research design, statistics, and philosophy of science.[1] There is a danger that a chapter attempting to summarize this broad topic could devolve into a selective listing of formulas and facts. To avoid that problem, we will attempt to emphasize and illustrate a very simple theme that has wide-reaching implications: Science is essentially an error-correcting enterprise. The ability to uncover "truth" hinges on the ability to identify, estimate, and remove error from fallible observations. We will show how this theme underlies traditional psychometric principles and why psychophysi-

ologists should be concerned about these principles. We will emphasize general principles rather than problems specific to particular modes of physiological measurement. The number of physiological systems now measured is so numerous and the technological advances are so rapid (e.g., Cacioppo and Tassinary, 1990b; Cacioppo, Tassinary, & Berntson, 2000; Coles, Donchin, & Porges, 1986; Druckman & Lacey, 1989) that a discussion of particular measurement problems would be highly selective and not particularly educational. Other chapters in this volume amply document the measurement nuances and idiosyncrasies for particular problem areas, and are reminders that inadequate technical knowledge and inadequate statistical representation can hinder inference for particular physiological measures (see Cacioppo and Tassinary, 1990a; Sarter, Berntson, & Cacioppo, 1996). We will focus instead on principles that are general to all psychophysiological measurement.

THE BASIC INFERENTIAL TASK

The behavioral sciences encompass a staggering number of topics and narrowing the focus to psychophysiology does not do much to reduce the impression of amazing diversity. Fortunately, all scientists attempt to solve the same basic problem depicted in Figure 33.1. The basic task of science is to make inferences about *hypothetical constructs* (e.g., stress, compliance, reactivity, attention, and memory) that cannot be observed directly. That requires operationalizing those constructs so that numbers can be attached to them in a meaningful way that can be replicated by others.[2] Once operational definitions are created, the logic and power of research design and statistics can be brought to bear on the problem. It is this operationalization stage that also makes necessary careful attention to psychometric principles because the quality of the

---

[1] We will not attempt to provide a comprehensive coverage of psychometric principles in this chapter; that task is ably accomplished in numerous book-length treatments (e.g., Ghiselli, Campbell, & Zedeck, 1981; Nunnally & Bernstein, 1994). Instead, the discussion will focus on key issues and their application. Similarly, discussion of closely related issues in research design and statistics can be found in numerous sources (e.g., Cohen & Cohen, 1983; Maxwell & Delaney, 1990; Myers & Well, 1991; Shadish, Cook, & Campbell, 2001; Whitley, 2002; Winer, 1971).

[2] To be sure, the "distance" from constructs to operations varies greatly and for some topics the leap is not all that great. For most areas in the behavioral sciences, however, the constructs are not isomorphic with their measurements and require careful attention to psychometric principles to avoid leaps of faith.

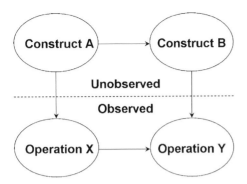

Figure 33.1. The basic inferential task in science.

inferences about constructs and construct relations will depend on the quality of the measurements, which will stand for or represent those constructs. The ability to make accurate and complete descriptive statements about the constructs (e.g., how much stress a sample is experiencing) and the ability to make logically justified inferences about construct relations (e.g., stress is caused by control loss) rests on the extent to which the observations that represent those constructs possess desirable psychometric qualities.

The problem is illustrated by a simple example shown in Figure 33.2. Suppose that a researcher posed the hypothesis that control loss is stressful. This implies a causal relation between two constructs. This hypothesis would presumably be derived from some carefully developed conceptual model. These constructs, however, cannot be observed directly. Instead, clear, specific, and measurable operational definitions must be defined that will "stand for," or represent, the underlying constructs. Control loss, for example, might be operationally defined as the number of daily frustrations from a list of 40 possible frustrations that a person claims to have experienced on a given day. Stress might be defined by a physiological measure of reactivity such as systolic blood pressure. Two inferential problems are immediately obvious. First, under what conditions can we safely infer that a causal relation exists between number of daily frustrations and systolic blood pressure? Second, given that such an empirical inference is warranted, under what conditions can we make

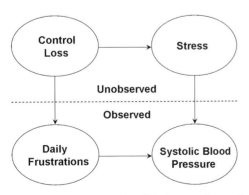

Figure 33.2. An example of the basic inferential task.

the more important inference that control loss is causally antecedent to the experience of stress? The answers to both questions rely on relatively error-free operational definitions. Psychometric principles guide the development of operational definitions that are (relatively) error free.

Before proceeding, it is important to emphasize another feature embedded in Figures 33.1 and 33.2 and assumed throughout this chapter: Scientific progress is guided by clear and carefully derived statements about constructs and construct relations. The ability to plan quality research and the ability to make clear inferences from that research depend on the clarity of the guiding conceptual model. The most conscientious attention to the psychometric principles, which we will discuss, will be wasted if those principles are applied to poorly defined conceptual hypotheses. Psychometric principles, then, are aids to, but not replacements for, creative thought and logical analysis.

With this basic view of the scientific inference process in mind, we can now turn to a discussion of the psychometric principles that guide the identification, estimation, and control of error in measurement.

RELIABILITY

The ability to make inferences about constructs depends upon the ability to "see" those constructs clearly, that is, to have relatively error-free representations of them. Estimating and controlling error in measurement requires a theory about measurement that defines the nature of error in operational definitions. In the sections that follow, two measurement theories will be described. The first, known as *classical theory*, is very simple and provides a convenient vehicle for introducing some important ideas about measurement. It also is the view of measurement upon which many common reliability estimates are based. The classical view of reliability, however, has two important limitations: It views error as entirely random and it views error as being a unitary entity. A more complex and more realistic view of measurement, called *generalizability theory*, overcomes these limitations and provides a very general and far-reaching approach to measurement.[3]

---

[3] Another prominent measurement model – item response theory (IRT) will not be discussed in this chapter. The model has much to recommend it as a general approach to measurement. It focuses on individual item responses and estimates item parameters apart from the particular samples that may eventually complete a test composed of those items. When successful, IRT avoids features of classical theory that many measurement specialists find unrealistic or undesirable (e.g., item and test characteristics in classical theory can be sample dependent and test dependent). But, IRT is also impractical for many psychophysiological measurement problems because they are difficult to conceptualize in the latent trait or ability framework of the model and because the development of "items" in IRT requires very large samples of items and respondents in order to develop good estimates of item parameters. Interested readers can consult Hambleton, Swaminathan, and Rogers (1991) for an introduction to the topic.

The classical theory of reliability[4]. The classical theory of reliability assumes that an observation (x) is composed of a *true score* (t) and an *error score* (e), which are related in a very simple way:

$$X = t + e \qquad (33.1)$$

The true score (t) is assumed to represent the standing of a given individual (or other *object of measurement*) on the construct of interest, that is, the score that would be obtained under ideal (i.e., error-free) conditions. The observed score deviates from the true score because of the influence of error, which in the classical view of reliability is assumed to be random. Random error is the noise against which the signal of the true score is detected, and large amounts of random error obscure the scientist's ability to see the true score clearly.

According to the classical view, if an obtained score is composed of a true score and random error, then the variability of a sample of obtained scores (symbolized as σ_x^2) will likewise be composed of true score variance (σ_t^2) and error variance (σ_e^2):

$$\sigma_x^2 = \sigma_t^2 + \sigma_e^2 \qquad (33.2)$$

This view of obtained score variability provides the basis for the classical theory definition of reliability. A relatively error-free measure will produce scores that vary because they contain more true score variance than error variance. In other words, the obtained scores will vary because the objects of measurement are truly different on the construct being measured and not because of random differences. An intuitively appealing way to represent this idea is the proportion of obtained score variance that is due to true score variance:

$$\frac{\sigma_t^2}{\sigma_t^2 + \sigma_e^2} \qquad (33.3)$$

This, in fact, is the classical theory definition of reliability, symbolized r_{xx} (e.g., Nunnally & Bernstein, 1994). The square root of the reliability coefficient estimates the correlation of obtained scores with true scores:

$$r_{xt} = \sqrt{r_{xx}} \qquad (33.4)$$

and emphasizes quite clearly that as reliability increases, obtained scores are better estimates of true scores. Stated differently, as reliability increases people (or other objects of measurement) are more likely to get the scores they deserve. This definition also makes clear why the reliability of a measure is often described with such terms as *consistency*, *repeatability*, and *dependability*. If a measure is reliable, then similar obtained score distributions should emerge on different measurement occasions provided the

true score component does not change over those measurement occasions. That latter assumption is critical – if the construct being measured moves out from under the measurement, reliability cannot be estimated.

Classical theory also allows for a more formal statement of the way random error obscures the ability to detect relationships between two operational definitions, and, thus, may thwart the goal of identifying causal relations (see Figures 33.1 and 33.2):

$$r_{xy} = \rho_{xy} \sqrt{r_{xx} r_{yy}} \qquad (33.5)$$

in which r_{xy} is the obtained correlation between two different operational definitions (x and y), ρ_{xy} is their correlation under conditions of perfect measurement, and r_{xx} and r_{yy} are the reliabilities associated with the measurement of x and y, respectively. Equation 33.5 makes one point quite clear: Low reliability in either measure can impair the ability to detect relationships.[5]

Because classical theory assumes that error is random, it provides a convenient way to estimate reliability: the correlation between "parallel" measures over different measurement "occasions." The logic is simple. If two measures of the same true score are correlated, that correlation can only be due to their shared true score variability; the random error components by definition cannot correlate with anything. By definition, a correlation is equal to a covariance between two measures divided by the standard deviations of those measures:

$$r_{xy} = \frac{\sigma_{xy}}{\sigma_x \sigma_y} \qquad (33.6)$$

If x and y are in deviation score form and are measures of the same true score (i.e., parallel forms), then their covariance takes on a familiar form:

$$\sigma_{xy} = \frac{1}{n} \sum_1^n (t_i + e_{x_i})(t_i + e_{y_i})$$
$$= \frac{\sum_1^n t_i^2}{n} + \frac{\sum_1^n t_i e_{x_i}}{n} + \frac{\sum_1^n t_i e_{y_i}}{n} + \frac{\sum_1^n e_{x_i} e_{y_i}}{n}$$
$$= \frac{\sum_1^n t_i^2}{n} = \sigma_t^2 \qquad (33.7)$$

because true scores cannot correlate with the random error components nor can different random error components (e_{x_i} and e_{y_i}) correlate with each other. Furthermore,

---

[4] There are actually several classical views of reliability that make slightly different assumptions. Those differences are not important here but are described in detail elsewhere (e.g., Ghiselli et al., 1981; Feldt & Brennan, 1989; Nunnally & Bernstein, 1994).

[5] Another point is more subtle, but also important. One of the variables in Equation 5 could be a manipulated independent variable in an experiment. It is easy to imagine that this variable will have perfect reliability. After all, everyone in a particular experimental condition gets the same score. But, the crucial question is whether everyone in an experimental condition is brought to the same psychological state (Strube, 1989). For example, an experiment that uses mental arithmetic to examine the physiological consequence of a cognitive challenge assumes that the experimental manipulation is equally challenging to all participants in that condition. This may not be true, however. Subtle variations in the delivery of the challenge act like random variability because all participants in a condition get the same score but not necessarily the score they deserve.

because the two measures are assumed to be parallel measures, σ_x and σ_y are assumed to be equal (at least in the population) so the denominator of Equation 33.6 can be assumed to equal the variance of either measure. The correlation between two measures of the same true score is equal to true score variance divided by obtained score variance according to the classical theory definition of reliability.[6] Thus, if two parallel measures are correlated, those measures must each be composed of shared true score variance and the higher the correlation, the more true score variance (relative to error variance) they contain. This idea gives rise to three popular reliability estimates: *test-retest reliability*, *alternative forms reliability*, and *internal consistency reliability*.

Test-retest reliability is simply the correlation between the same measure on two different occasions. Alternative forms reliability is the correlation between two different measures, each assumed to measure the same true score, administered on different occasions. Internal consistency reliability is based on the correlations among multiple items of one test or measure given during a single administration. In each case, the different measurement occasions (i.e., different times, different forms, or different items) are assumed to differ only in their random components so that the correlation between occasions reveals the relative amounts of true score variance that the measures contain. Of course, as we pointed out earlier, if the true score has changed between measurement occasions (i.e., the construct is unstable), then the reliability estimate is ambiguous as an indicator of measurement error. These different estimates of reliability need not agree, which highlights a key problem with the classical view – error can come from many sources, but those multiple sources are not formally documented in the classical approach. Later, we describe generalizability theory as a remedy to this problem.

In addition to providing a means of estimating reliability, the classical theory also suggests an important way to reduce error and make measures more reliable: *aggregation*. If multiple observed scores of the same construct are combined, the random sources of error that contaminate each observed score have a chance to cancel out and leave standing a better estimate of the true score. If a measure of a construct is based on a single observation, then the obtained score for a given individual will be biased up or down to some extent because of the random error. If we have a second observation that is also a measure of the same true score, it also has an error component, but the direction in which this error influences the obtained score is likely be different than the first item because error is random in the classical view. If we average the two observations, that average might provide a better measure because the two error components might partly cancel out

each other. They will not completely cancel out each other unless their influences are directly opposite, but if we average more and more observations, each with its own random error source but measuring the same true score, then the odds of the error canceling out keep improving. This is a fundamental idea in measurement. Aggregating items or observations that measure the same true score will allow the random error components to cancel out and provide a more reliable measure (e.g., Kamarck, Debski, & Manuck, 2000). In fact, the well known Spearman-Brown prophecy formula is based on this idea (see Nunnally & Bernstein, 1994).

Although we have emphasized r_{xx} as a measure of reliability, there is another way to view reliability. We could just as easily think about reliability of measures in terms of the amount of error those measures contain (σ_e^2). The square root of this variance, the *standard error of measure* (σ_{meas}), gauges the uncertainty inherent in an obtained score by providing an estimate of how much obtained scores would be expected to vary on subsequent measurement occasions even though the true score has remained constant:

$$\sigma_{\text{meas}} = \sigma_x \sqrt{1 - r_{xx}} \qquad (33.8)$$

The σ_{meas} communicates reliability in terms of the original scale of measurement, which can be very revealing. Furthermore, the σ_{meas} can be used to form confidence intervals around true scores to provide an even clearer sense of the error inherent in a measurement application and the degree to which score differences are meaningful.

Although the classical view is very popular and widely used, it suffers from an important flaw: It views error as a unitary entity. That flaw is apparent by considering closely the different ways that reliability can be estimated. Each defines error in slightly different ways and consequently the different estimates need not reach the same conclusions about reliability. For example, the internal consistency approach to reliability construes error as random fluctuations that vary across responses to multiple items given at the same time. Sources of error that might change from one day to another do not have any opportunity to show up as error. Indeed, on any one-measurement occasion, such sources masquerade as true score because they impose a constant influence on the observed scores for all items for a particular individual. For example, a bad headache could impair a person's concentration and influence responses to all items on a cognitive abilities test. Consequently, that person would not get the score he or she truly deserves. On a different day the headache might be better and so too would performance, but not because of any change in underlying cognitive abilities. On a given measurement occasion, a person's health is not variable so it does not have an opportunity to emerge as a source of error on a measure of internal consistency reliability. Instead, its constant status makes it act like true score. On the other hand, test-retest reliability would count the health changes and other changes for individuals over time as error. The major point here is that a source of error

---

[6] The measures need not be strictly parallel. Classical models that relax this assumption (e.g., domain sampling) merely assume parallelism or similarity in the random sampling sense, yet still arrive at similar conclusions and definitions of reliability (e.g., Nunnally & Bernstein, 1994).

only "counts" in classical theory if it can show variability for a particular individual across measurement occasions. Clearly, then, error is multidimensional and a means of capturing this multidimensionality provides a more powerful approach to estimating and controlling error. Generalizability theory provides that means.

Generalizability theory. The major advantage of generalizability theory (Brennan, 1992, 2001; Cronbach, Gleser, Nanda, & Rajaratnam, 1972; Shavelson & Webb, 1991; Shavelson, Webb, & Rowley, 1989) over the traditional classical approach is the ability to specify and estimate more precisely the multiple sources of error that can contaminate obtained scores. This is accomplished by specifying carefully the conditions of measurement and estimating the influence of those conditions of measurement as sources of error variance in the obtained scores. In generalizability theory the conditions of measurement are known as *facets*. A facet is simply a clearly defined way that measurement occasions can vary and so represents a potential source of influence on obtained scores in addition to true score variance. Different days on which a measure could be collected, for example, are a facet of measurement. Measures collected on one day could vary systematically from those collected on another day (an overall effect for everyone) or the relative standing of participants might differ across days (an effect that varies by person). In either case, scores could vary by day so that any one obtained score would not necessarily provide a dependable indication of a person's standing on the construct being measured. Multiple items on a test, multiple recordings on the same day, and multiple judges of the same behavior are all examples of measurement conditions (facets) that could introduce variability into obtained scores and obscure the ability to detect true score differences. The list of possible facets of measurement potentially is very long and depends on the specific measurement problem. Accordingly, a key challenge in generalizability theory is the identification of important measurement facets for a particular problem or application.

Generalizability theory gets its name from the idea that the ability to generalize obtained scores across conditions of measurement requires explicitly specifying and testing the conditions of measurement that might affect obtained score variability. Unlike classical theory in which assumptions about the importance of measurement conditions are often handled with a wink and a prayer, in generalizability theory such assumptions are put to an empirical test. Generalizability theory links conclusions about reliability to well-defined measurement facets. Collectively these measurement facets define what is considered an acceptable measurement and identify the boundaries within which the investigator considers observations potentially to be interchangeable. That exchangeability, however, is an empirical question.

Using generalizability theory to solve measurement problems can be thought of as a two-step process that requires specifying two kinds of measurement boundaries, or "universes," of measurement. In the first step, a *universe of admissible observations* is defined, which identifies explicitly the facets of measurement and the particular way those facets are defined. For example, a researcher interested in measurement of systolic blood pressure might define the universe of admissible observations to include an examiner facet and a time of day facet. This would reflect the belief by the researcher that these two aspects of measurement are potentially important sources of obtained score variability that need to be taken into account when measuring systolic blood pressure. The magnitudes of these contributions are important to know so that claims about generalization can be made with confidence or qualified appropriately. Furthermore, if any pairing of examiner and time of the day in which a measurement is taken was deemed an acceptable measurement, then the universe would be *completely crossed* (other possible arrangements of facets, such as nested facets, will be described later). Implicit in the definition of the universe of admissible observations is a population of respondents. Indeed, the nature of the respondents (e.g., healthy children or college students performing a stressful experimental task) quite often guides the definition of measurement facets (e.g., the characteristics of acceptable examiners or the times of day that are considered appropriate for measurement). Once the universe of admissible observations is defined, the specific contributions of the facets of measurement to obtained score variability – called *variance components* – need to be estimated. This is accomplished in what is called a *Generalizability Study* (or *G study*), in which particular instances of the facets are selected, a sample from the population is evaluated, and the obtained score variability is decomposed into variance component estimates. These estimates then indicate the relative size of true score and error components.

The second major step in the application of generalizability theory uses the variance components from a G study to explore specific intended applications. In an application, multiple measurements across facet levels will be combined (e.g., averaged) to produce more reliable composites. The characteristics of these composites are the focus of this second step and require defining a second universe – *the universe of generalization*. This universe represents the particular facets and their arrangements, which will be used in a particular application. For example, a researcher may want to know how well systolic blood pressure is measured if the assessments of two randomly selected examiners each collecting measurements at three randomly selected times of the day are averaged. Using the variance components from the G study, this question can be addressed in what is called a *Decision Study* (or *D study*). Different D studies can explore the consequences for reliability of different measurement protocols (e.g., using a nested measurement design, difference in numbers of instances of the facets, or assuming a facet is fixed rather than random). According to generalizability theory, then, there is no single reliability for a measure. Reliability depends on the conditions of measurement and there are potentially as many reliabilities for a measure as there are unique uses or conditions of measurement. Generalizability theory provides a systematic framework for exploring these multiple reliabilities.

Generalizability theory essentially defines true score and error more carefully than the traditional classical view. The somewhat nebulous idea of a true score is replaced in generalizability theory with the *universe score*, the expected value of all observations in the universe of generalization. This universe represents the particular arrangement of measurement conditions defined by the particular interest or problem of the investigator. Although this too is a hypothetical value, it at least is bounded by well-specified measurement conditions and no claims about reliability are made outside those boundaries. The unitary error score of the classical view is replaced by several error scores, which are defined by the conditions of measurement. Generalizability theory is designed to estimate these multiple components of obtained score variability and to use those components to explore the consequences of different sources of measurement error. In the discussion that follows, we will take a closer look at the two major parts of generalizability theory via some examples in order to highlight the substantial advantages this approach has over the traditional classical approach (for other examples, see Burgess & Gruzelier, 1996; Di Nocera, Ferlazzo, & Borghi, 2001; Wohlgemuth, Edinger, Fins, & Sullivan 1999).

As an initial example, suppose that a researcher wished to explore the reliability of systolic blood pressure (SBP) measurement, perhaps because SBP is to be used in research on the cardiovascular effects of cognitive and physical challenges. The ability to detect changes in SBP relies on knowing a person's "true" or typical blood pressure, but that true value might be obscured by several kinds of error (e.g., Garćia-Vera & Sanz, 1999; Llabre et al., 1988). The universe of admissible observations must be defined to include facets of measurement that could create variability in blood pressure readings such that those sources of variability can be estimated separately in a G study. Of course, one source of variability will be characteristics of the participants in the study. In generalizability theory, this component of variability is known as the *object of measurement*, and is not usually referred to as a facet. Variability for this component is desirable and corresponds to true score variance in classical theory. This is referred to as the *p* component for *persons* or *participants*. Another source of variability might be called *observer* (*o*) and represents fluctuations that depend on the person recording the blood pressure. Variability in the obtained scores that are due to observer differences would be an undesirable source because it obscures the underlying universe score. If this were the only facet of interest, if any observer meeting an appropriately specified definition (e.g., regarding training in blood pressure measurement)

	Observer 1	Observer 2
Person 1		
Person 2		
Person 3		
Person 4		
Person 5		

Figure 33.3. Data collection design for a simple Person × Observer G study.

were considered interchangeable with any other qualified observer, and if any observer could assess any member of the population, then we have defined a one-facet Person × Observer universe of admissible observations. To estimate the variance components in this universe, we might have two observers record blood pressures from five people. The data collection design would look like that depicted in Figure 33.3. In practice, of course, many more people would be sampled and more observers would be desirable so that sources of variance are estimated with higher precision.

Figure 33.4 displays a Venn diagram depicting the unique sources of variance in this *po* design. The sources indicate an expanded view of obtained score variability:

$$\sigma_x^2 = \sigma_p^2 + \sigma_o^2 + \sigma_{po}^2 \tag{33.9}$$

The variance components in a G study are estimated from the mean squares provided by *analysis of variance*, which in this case, yields three distinct sources of variance: Person (*p*), Observers (*o*), and Person × Observers (*po*) (for details on variance component estimation see Brennan, 2001; Cronbach et al., 1972; Shavelson & Webb, 1991). With one exception, the mean squares in analysis of variance are not themselves pure variance component estimates. For the simple *po* design, the mean squares have the following expected values:

$$\text{EMS}(P) = \sigma_{po}^2 + n_o \sigma_p^2 \tag{33.10}$$

$$\text{EMS}(O) = \sigma_{po}^2 + n_p \sigma_o^2 \tag{33.11}$$

$$\text{EMS}(PO) = \sigma_{po}^2 \tag{33.12}$$

where n_o is the number of observers in the study and n_p is the number of people whose blood pressure has been measured. These expected mean squares allow the following

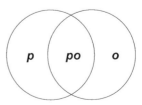

Figure 33.4. Sources of variance for a Person (*p*) × Observer (*o*) G study.

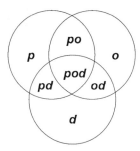

Figure 33.5. Sources of variance for a Person (p) × Observer (o) × Day (d) G study.

algebraic manipulation of mean squares to obtain variance component estimates:

$$\hat{\sigma}_p^2 = [MS_p - MS_{po}]/n_o \qquad (33.13)$$

$$\hat{\sigma}_o^2 = [MS_o - MS_{po}]/n_p \qquad (33.14)$$

$$\hat{\sigma}_{po}^2 = MS_{po} \qquad (33.15)$$

Rules for generating variance components from more complicated designs are described by Cronbach et al. (1972), Shavelson and Webb (1991), and Brennan (2001).

The Person (p) component represents real differences in the systolic blood pressures of the participants. It is interpreted like any other variance, but in this case refers to the variance of scores representing the average of all recordings in the universe of admissible observations. The Observer (o) component represents systematic differences between the observers. For example, if readings were systematically lower for one observer, perhaps because of that person's calmer demeanor, then that would show up in the o component of variance and would affect scores for all individuals equally. The Person × Observer (po) component reflects differences in the relative standing of participants for the two observers, plus any unaccounted for random sources of variability. The Person × Observer interaction might represent, for example, systematically different ways that particular individuals react to particular observers. These effects, however, cannot be separated from the random errors of measurement in this design.[7]

It should by now be clear that the classical theory and generalizability theory view error in fundamentally different ways. In the classical view, random error is the only source of error. In generalizability theory, random error is a default category that represents error that could not be defined by conditions of measurement. Conditions of measurement reflect systematic ways that obtained scores can vary besides the object of measurement, that is, systematic error. Stated more strongly, in generalizability theory the presence of random error signals a relatively poor understanding of how measurement conditions affect obtained score variability.

Of course, the universe of admissible observations can be more complex. It might, for example, be completely

crossed and contain two facets: observers and days. On any given day, a person's blood pressure might be depressed or elevated for idiosyncratic reasons (e.g., a person attended a yoga class or had an extra cup of coffee). Those influences could obscure the detection of the person's true or typical blood pressure. The influence would be constant for a particular person on that day and so would be confused as true score, but from the standpoint of identifying typical blood pressure, a person would not get the value he or she deserves. The only way to separate this source of error is to include it explicitly in the measurement design. Adding a Day (d) component to the previous design and crossing it with the other components produces a completely crossed Person × Observer × Day design. A completely crossed random effects G study might then be conducted with two Observers and four Days. The analysis of variance for that design produces seven sources of variation (see Figure 33.5) that are estimated by mean squares. The expected values for those mean squares are listed in Table 33.1. As can be seen, each mean square (with one exception) is a linear combination of variance components. Accordingly, some simple algebraic manipulation can isolate each variance component for the generalizability theory analysis. Some hypothetical variance components are listed in Table 33.2. Also listed in Table 33.2 are the proportions of the total variance (the sum of all the variance components) accounted for by each component so that their relative size can be gauged more easily. The largest source of variance is for the Person (p) component indicating that much of the total variability is due to real differences in systolic blood pressure, at least as defined within this universe of

---

Table 33.1. Expected mean squares and variance component estimation for a completely crossed design (persons × observers × days design)

Expected Mean Squares

$$EMS(P) = \sigma_{pod}^2 + n_o \sigma_{pd}^2 + n_d \sigma_{po}^2 + n_o n_d \sigma_p^2$$

$$EMS(O) = \sigma_{pod}^2 + n_p \sigma_{od}^2 + n_d \sigma_{po}^2 + n_p n_d \sigma_o^2$$

$$EMS(D) = \sigma_{pod}^2 + n_p \sigma_{od}^2 + n_o \sigma_{pd}^2 + n_p n_o \sigma_d^2$$

$$EMS(PO) = \sigma_{pod}^2 + n_d \sigma_{po}^2$$

$$EMS(PD) = \sigma_{pod}^2 + n_o \sigma_{pd}^2$$

$$EMS(OD) = \sigma_{pod}^2 + n_p \sigma_{od}^2$$

$$EMS(POD) = \sigma_{pod}^2$$

Estimated Variance Components

$$\hat{\sigma}_p^2 = (MS_p - n_o \hat{\sigma}_{pd}^2 - n_d \hat{\sigma}_{po}^2 - \hat{\sigma}_{pod}^2)/(n_o n_d)$$

$$\hat{\sigma}_o^2 = (MS_o - n_p \hat{\sigma}_{od}^2 - n_d \hat{\sigma}_{po}^2 - \hat{\sigma}_{pod}^2)/(n_p n_d)$$

$$\hat{\sigma}_d^2 = (MS_d - n_p \hat{\sigma}_{od}^2 - n_o \hat{\sigma}_{pd}^2 - \hat{\sigma}_{pod}^2)/(n_p n_o)$$

$$\hat{\sigma}_{po}^2 = (MS_{po} - \hat{\sigma}_{pod}^2)/n_d$$

$$\hat{\sigma}_{pd}^2 = (MS_{pd} - \hat{\sigma}_{pod}^2)/n_o$$

$$\hat{\sigma}_{od}^2 = (MS_{od} - \hat{\sigma}_{pod}^2)/n_p$$

$$\hat{\sigma}_{pod}^2 = MS_{pod}$$

---

[7] In general, the highest order effect is confounded with random error.

Table 33.2. Hypothetical variance components for a completely crossed G study of systolic blood pressure measurement

Source of variance	Component of variance	Proportion of total variance
Person (*p*)	180.00	.40
Observer (*o*)	25.00	.06
Day (*d*)	15.00	.03
po	40.00	.09
pd	75.00	.17
od	10.00	.02
pod	105.00	.23

admissible observations. The remaining sources of variability are error, some of which are relatively large. For example, the Person × Day (*pd*) component accounts for 17% of the total variability. This component reflects a shift in the relative differences of individuals over days. By contrast, the *o* effect is rather modest (only 6% of the variance) and indicates little variation across observers.

There is one other design variation that arises frequently in generalizability studies: *nested designs*. In the simple design with Observers as the only condition of measurement, it might not be possible to have the same observers test each participant. Instead, a different pair of observers might test each participant (perhaps this would occur if participants were patients being seen in different physicians' offices). In this case, observers are no longer crossed with persons, but are nested within persons. The universe of admissible observations is now defined differently than for completely crossed universe. The data collection design is shown in Figure 33.6 and is sometimes symbolized as *o: p* to indicate that observers (*o*) are nested (:) within persons (*p*). The major consequence of nesting is that some variance components, which can be estimated separately in a crossed design, are confounded in a nested design. As the Venn diagram in Figure 33.7 shows, the Person × Observer (*po*) interaction cannot be separated from the Observer (*o*) effect. The overlap of the Observer component and the Person component (which defines the interaction *po*) is completely contained in the Observer (*o*) component. Only two components of variance can be estimated in this design: a *p* component and a combined component that contains both the *o* source of variance and the *po* source of variance.

Designs can have both crossed and nested features. For example, the Person × Observer × Day design might not be realistic. Although it might be possible to assess all participants on each day (Person and Day are crossed), it might not be possible for each observer to record the blood pressures of all participants. This creates a partially nested design (see Figure 33.8). With observers nested within persons, the Observer (*o*) source of variance is confounded with the Person × Observer (*po*) interaction. As Figure 33.8 indicates, the *od* and *pod* sources of variance are also con-

founded. Consequently, only five sources of variance can be estimated from this design.

Generalizability theory makes one additional important distinction: *random effects* versus *fixed effects*. An effect is random if the facet levels are considered random samples from the population of all levels in the universe of admissible observations.[8] By contrast, an effect is fixed if the levels used are the only ones of interest. When an effect is fixed, there is no intent to generalize to some larger population, either because there is no larger population (i.e., all facet levels are included) or because the ones included in the study are the only ones that the researcher cares about. This distinction between fixed and random effects is important for appropriate estimation of variance components (for a thorough discussion see Brennan, 2001). Two approaches have been recommended (see Shavelson & Webb, 1991). First, separate generalizability analyses can be carried out at each level of the fixed effect. This makes sense if each level of the fixed effect was selected because there was particular interest in that level. Second, if a researcher wants an overall average of the generalizability of the measure, then averaging across the fixed effects is another option (see Brennan, 2001; Cronbach et al., 1972; Shavelson & Webb, 1991). Large variance components for the fixed effect, however, would dictate caution using the averaging approach because it obscures an important source of variance.

Generalizability theory clearly provides a powerful way to determine the multiple sources of error in a measure. It provides an equally powerful way to estimate the consequences of those error sources so that future measurement efforts can be planned carefully. In generalizability theory, these forecasting and planning efforts are known as D studies. A D study uses the variance components from the G study to pose "what if" questions about future possible ways to collect data. Different D Studies can estimate the consequences of changing the number of facet levels (i.e., the aggregation principle), the way those facets are arranged (e.g., crossed versus nested designs), and the type of decision about the objects of measurement that the data will guide (e.g., whether an external criterion or cut-off score is used).

The essential difference between a G study and a D study is that data are collected and variance components are estimated in a G study; those variance components are then used in D studies to pose questions about alternative measurement and decision options. These latter questions exist within the universe of generalization. The difference between the two universes might be thought of as the

---

[8] Ideally, effects would be randomly sampled from the population of possible levels. In theory this population would be infinite, but in practice it is usually very large. Furthermore, the levels actually used in a generalizability study may not be truly random samples; it is sufficient to assume that they are if there is no particular interest in the levels used and any other levels would work equally well. The distinction between random effects and fixed effects is crucial, affecting the estimation of variance components and estimates of reliability (see Brennan, 2001).

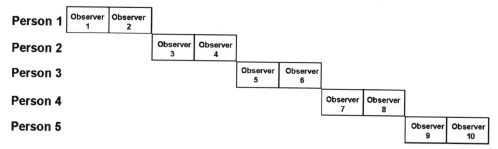

Figure 33.6. Data collection design with Observers (*o*) nested within Persons (*p*).

difference between defining what constitutes a meaningful or acceptable individual score (i.e., universe of admissible observations) and defining what constitutes a meaningful or acceptable aggregate (i.e., universe of generalization). In a D study, the number of facet levels and their arrangements are modified to determine how reliability of averages changes with different kinds of designs. It is important to recognize the critical link between the two universes. By using the variance components from a G study, any given D study is a commitment to the way individual scores and their facets are defined in the universe of admissible observations. If a researcher is unwilling to make that commitment for an intended application, then a new universe of admissible observations must be defined and a new G study must be conducted.

A key distinction in a D study is the kind of decision that will be made about the objects of measurement – a distinction that defines the nature of error and the estimation of reliability coefficients. There are two kinds of decisions that can be made. The first, known as a *relative decision*, reflects only the relative standing of the objects of measurement. The second, known as an *absolute decision*, takes the absolute value of the scores into account as well. In applied testing, these differences correspond to norm-referenced and criterion-referenced tests, respectively. Using a simple Person × Observer design, Figures 33.9 and 33.10 display the nature of these two decisions and the influence of different error components on them.

The top panel of Figure 33.9 shows that the two observers provide the same relative rank ordering for the participants. If we wanted to identify the participants with the three highest blood pressures, we would get the same answer from either observer. This occurs despite the fact that all recordings are systematically lower for the second observer. This reflects an observer effect (i.e., the *o* com-

ponent would be large), but this source of error does not affect the relative decision. The bottom panel of Figure 33.9 depicts a different pattern. In this case, the relative standing of the participants is different for the two observers. This Person × Observer interaction obscures our ability to identify the three people with the highest blood pressures. The *po* component then is a source of error for a relative decision. More generally, any interaction that involves the object of measurement will be a source of error for relative decisions. Such interactions indicate that across facet levels the differences between the objects of measurement shift in magnitude, making it difficult to consistently identify their relative standing.

Figure 33.10 displays the same two data patterns but now with reference to a criterion score. This criterion might represent an established cut-off score for defining high blood pressure. In other words, rather than defining high blood pressure as the three highest scores, an external criterion is used. Now the absolute values of the recordings are important. As the top panel indicates, the overall observer differences (i.e., the *o* component) influence whether a given participant exceeds the criterion. The bottom panel indicates that interactions involving the object of measure affect absolute decisions as well. Absolute decisions are influenced by any source of variance that influences the value of the obtained score. That means that all sources other than the object of measurement will be a source of error for absolute decisions.

These rules generalize to other designs. Consider again, for example, the Person × Observer × Day design depicted

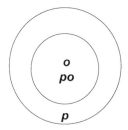

Figure 33.7. Sources of variance for a design with Observers (*o*) nested within Persons (*p*).

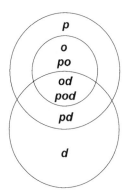

Figure 33.8. Sources of variance for a partially nested design in which Observers (*o*) are nested within Persons (*p*) and both are crossed with Days (*d*).

in Figure 33.5. For relative decisions, the *po*, *pd*, and *pod* sources all make it difficult to know with confidence the relative standing of participants. The *pd* component reflects changes in the relative standing of the participants between the different days on which recordings are made. The *pod* component reflects changes in relative blood pressure that vary simultaneously by observer and day. This component also contains other random sources of error. All of the variance sources other than *p* would contaminate absolute decisions.

Knowing the nature of the decision to be made is crucial for estimating reliability in generalizability theory. Just like classical theory, generalizability theory provides coefficients that gauge the reliability of measures defined by the universe of generalization. These coefficients, however, are calculated differently depending on the kind of decision that will be made about the objects of measurement. Reliability estimates for relative decisions, called *generalizability coefficients*, represent the proportion of obtained score variance that is due to universe score variance:

$$E\rho^2 = \frac{\sigma_p^2}{\sigma_p^2 + \sigma_\delta^2} \qquad (33.16)$$

The term, σ_δ^2, refers to the error variance for a relative decision and varies according to the type of design used

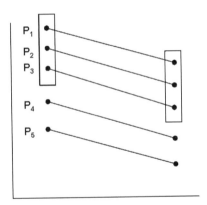

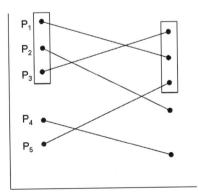

Figure 33.9. Sources of error for a relative decision.

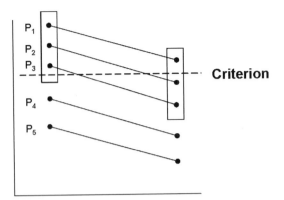

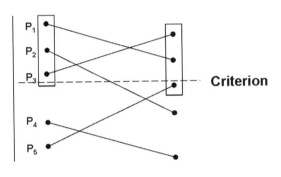

Figure 33.10. Sources of error for an absolute decision.

in the D study.[9] For the examples described previously, the error terms would be:

$$\text{Person} \times \text{Observer (po):} \; \sigma_\delta^2 = \frac{\sigma_{po}^2}{n_o'} \qquad (33.17)$$

$$\text{Person} \times \text{Observer} \times \text{Day (pod):} \; \sigma_\delta^2 = \frac{\sigma_{po}^2}{n_o'} + \frac{\sigma_{pd}^2}{n_d'} + \frac{\sigma_{pod}^2}{n_o' n_d'} \qquad (33.18)$$

$$\text{Days} \times \text{(Observers within Persons) (d[o : p]):}$$

$$\sigma_\delta^2 = \frac{\sigma_{o,po}^2}{n_o'} + \frac{\sigma_{pd}^2}{n_d'} + \frac{\sigma_{od,pod}^2}{n_o' n_d'} \qquad (33.19)$$

in which n_o' and n_d' refer to the number of facet levels for observers and days respectively and the accent marks indicate that these numbers can vary and need not be the

[9] Several links to the classical view should be noted. $E\rho^2$ is defined in the same general way as a ratio of "true" score variance to "error" variance (see Equation 33.3) and the symbol denotes a squared correlation between obtained scores and universe scores (cf. Equation 33.4). Also, for a simple one-facet design involving multiple items, $E\rho^2$ resembles Cronbach's coefficient alpha (Cronbach, 1951). Finally, Equation 33.16 can be thought of as a generalized Spearman-Brown formula, allowing the same kind of forecasting but for a much wider range of designs. Other links are described by Brennan (2001) who notes some surprising results when traditional reliability estimates are considered within the generalizability theory perspective.

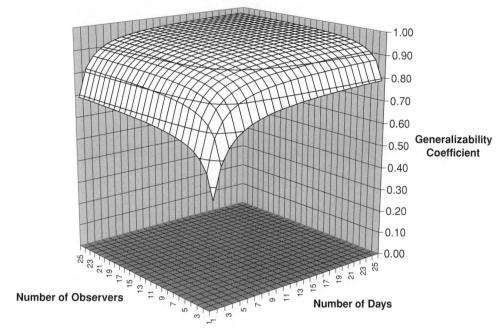

Figure 33.11. D study results for a completely crossed design using variance components from Table 33.2.

same as those that might have been used in a G study.[10] The first term and the last term in Equation 33.19 reflect the fact that some variance components cannot be estimated separately in nested designs. For the example in Table 33.2, the generalizability coefficient is:

$$E\rho^2 = \frac{\sigma_p^2}{\sigma_p^2 + \dfrac{\sigma_{po}^2}{n_o^r} + \dfrac{\sigma_{pd}^2}{n_d^r} + \dfrac{\sigma_{pod}^2}{n_o^r n_d^r}}$$

$$= \frac{180}{180 + \dfrac{40}{2} + \dfrac{75}{4} + \dfrac{105}{2(4)}} = .77 \qquad (33.20)$$

Using the variance components from Table 33.2, Figure 33.11 illustrates the impact on the generalizability coefficient for a crossed design of varying the numbers of observers and days of observation. As expected, reliability increases as the number of observers and days increase, but the rate of increase is different for the two facets; increasing the number of days has a larger influence. This could have been anticipated from Table 33.2 in which the *pd* component is the largest source of error; that component will show the largest effect of aggregation. Nonetheless, Figure 33.11 also shows that aggregation over both days and observers will be necessary to achieve a modest reliability with modest cost.

[10] D studies forecast expected results but are limited by the precision of the variance components from the G study. Confidence intervals can be placed around variance components (and around other parameter estimates) to provide an appropriate level of caution (e.g., Cronbach et al., 1972; Brennan, 1992, 2001). Sampling variability can be reduced by using large samples (e.g., people or facet levels). Also note that D studies can only investigate designs for which separate variance component estimates are available in a G study. A nested G study precludes D studies that require separate variance components that are confounded because of nesting.

Figure 33.12 represents the same information as Figure 33.11, but with reference to the standard error of measure (i.e., the square root of the error variance). The same conclusions would be drawn from this figure, but it represents reliability in the metric of the measure that will be used. This allows a better sense of the uncertainty researchers will have about a person's systolic blood pressure for different combinations of observers and days of observation.[11] For example, with two observers and two days of observation, the standard error for a relative decision will be 9.15. Using this to set confidence intervals reveals that the same universe score would be consistent with obtained scores that differ by as much as 37 points with 95% confidence (see Feldt & Brennan, 1989; Nunnally & Bernstein, 1994). This might be quite sobering and more informative to a researcher or practitioner than knowing that the generalizability coefficient under these conditions is .68.

The design is free to vary too, provided the appropriate variance components are available from the G study. For example, the G study might have been a completely crossed design, but different D studies could explore partially nested (e.g., *d[o:p]*) or completely nested (e.g., *o:d:p*) options. This allows careful planning that can optimize reliability while taking design cost into account (Marcoulides & Goldstein, 1990). If two designs produce essentially the same reliability the researcher can choose the one that is easier or is less costly to conduct. Alternatively, for a fixed cost a researcher can identify the

[11] Measurement error may not be equivalent for all score levels. Recent work has attempted to overcome this problem by providing conditional standard errors of measurement (Brennan, 1996, 2001; Feldt & Qualls, 1996; Kolen, Hanson, & Brennan, 1992). An extensive discussion is provided by Brennan (2001).

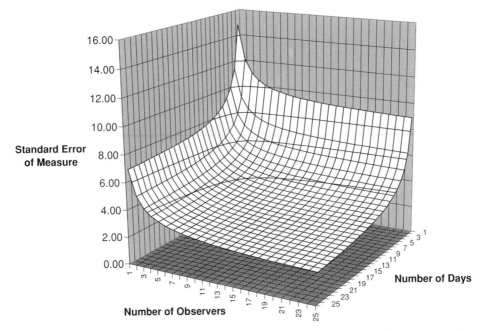

Figure 33.12. Projected standard errors of measure for a completely crossed design using variance components from Table 33.2.

design that maximizes reliability. It is usually fairly easy to specify costs on a "per observation" basis and to estimate any training or equipment costs. These can be linked to appropriate facet level indicators in the D study calculations, providing total cost estimates along with reliability estimates.

D studies can be used to ask "trade-off" questions within designs as well. We can ask, for example, what numbers of observers and days of observation will produce a reliability or standard error of a given amount. Figure 33.13 displays the results of asking this question for the design in Table 33.2 and a generalizability coefficient of .80, which is a common reliability benchmark. Clearly more than one day of observation will be necessary and the trade-off to limiting the number of days is a larger number of observers. Depending on the costs of training observers and collecting data over multiple days, a sensible combination of observers and days can be determined. If no combination will produce the desired reliability at a reasonable cost, then a different arrangement of facets (e.g., partially nested) might be considered. Also, efforts might be made to reduce error in other ways (e.g., standardization) or through inclusion of additional measurement facets. Nonetheless, any change in the measurement protocol that introduces new facets must be accompanied by a new G study to estimate new variance components.

The results in Figures 33.11, 33.12, and 33.13 assume that a relative decision will be made. If the blood pressure readings will be used to identify "at risk" individuals, then an external criterion will be used; the decision is then absolute rather than relative and subject to more sources of error. For absolute decisions, the reliability coefficient is called the *index of dependability* (symbolized as ϕ in Brennan & Kane, 1977) and is defined as follows:

$$\phi = \frac{\sigma_p^2}{\sigma_p^2 + \sigma_\Delta^2} \qquad (33.21)$$

The term, σ_Δ^2, refers to the error variance for absolute decisions. For the designs described previously, those error terms are:

$$\text{po: } \sigma_\Delta^2 = \frac{\sigma_o^2}{n_o'} + \frac{\sigma_{po}^2}{n_o'} \qquad (33.22)$$

$$\text{pod: } \sigma_\Delta^2 = \frac{\sigma_o^2}{n_o'} + \frac{\sigma_d^2}{n_d'} + \frac{\sigma_{od}^2}{n_o' n_d'} + \frac{\sigma_{po}^2}{n_o'} + \frac{\sigma_{pd}^2}{n_d'} + \frac{\sigma_{pod}^2}{n_o' n_d'}$$
$$(33.23)$$

$$\text{d(o:p) } \sigma_\Delta^2 = \frac{\sigma_d^2}{n_d'} + \frac{\sigma_{o,po}^2}{n_o'} + \frac{\sigma_{pd}^2}{n_d'} + \frac{\sigma_{od,pod}^2}{n_o' n_d'} \qquad (33.24)$$

Using Equation 33.23, the example in Table 33.2 yields an index of dependability of .72, smaller than the generalizability coefficient because of the additional sources of error that hinder absolute decisions (*o*, *d*, and *od*).

Several aspects of the reliability estimates provided by generalizability theory are clear from Equations 33.16 through 33.24:

1. Reliability estimates are design dependent.

2. Reliability depends on the number of facet levels (i.e., the aggregation principle).

3. Reliability depends on the type of decision that will be made.

4. Reliability depends as much on the universe score variance (σ_p^2) as it does on error variance.

This last point is especially important. Inadequate sampling of the objects of measurement can distort reliability estimates. This can occur because a restricted sample

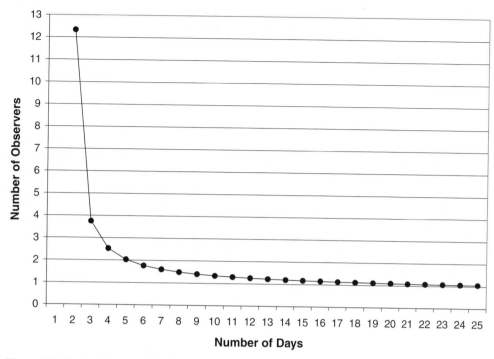

Figure 33.13. Combinations of observers and days that produce a generalizability coefficient of .80 (based on variance components from Table 33.2).

does not fairly capture the natural variation in the objects of measurement or because intentional sampling inflates the apparent variability of the objects of measurement. A fair sample represents a random sample from the population to which inferences will be made. All of these points underscore a comment made earlier that there are as many reliabilities for a measure as there are applications or conditions of measurement. In other words, there is an external validity to reliability estimation that is quite explicitly modeled by generalizability theory.[12]

Identifying and controlling error. Generalizability theory emphasizes the estimation of separate error components, but that estimation hinges on correctly identifying those error components in the first place (for an excellent discussion of the general problem of error identification and correction see Schmidt & Hunter, 1996). One common problem is to ignore "hidden" facets (Brennan, 2001). For example, a researcher might administer multiple items to a group of respondents on one occasion and forget that occasion is a constant in the study, though it will be a likely source of variability and considered as error in application. The problem is that occasion variance, which Schmidt and Hunter (1996) call *transient error*, acts like a constant for each individual on a given occasion, and is counted as true score or universe score for each individual. For example, the systolic blood pressure of participants could be temporarily elevated or depressed on any give occasion in ways that are idiosyncratic (e.g., one person meditated that day and another person nearly had a traffic accident) or constant for all (e.g., a tornado warning was in effect on the day of examination). These sources exert a systematic effect that cannot be distinguished from the universe score on a single measurement occasion. Their status as error is only revealed through their variability over multiple measurement occasions. Brennan (2001) provides an excellent discussion of hidden facets and the complex problems they can create for interpretation of reliability.

Similarly, error specific to a particular test condition or mode of measurement, which Schmidt and Hunter (1996) refer to as *specific error*, can masquerade as universe score variance unless test condition or measurement mode is explicitly included in the measurement design and its

[12] There are additional features of generalizability theory that cannot be described in detail here, but expand its potential range of application. For example, any facet can take on the role of objects of measurement (Cardinet, Tourneur, & Allal, 1976, 1981). A familiar example makes this clear. In a typical experimental design, persons are nested within groups (*p:g*) and groups are the objects of measurement. That is, decisions will be made about groups (e.g., are they different?). The generalizability coefficient then refers to the reliability of group means (Brennan, 1995) and the standard error of measure is the familiar standard error of the mean (also see Brennan, 2001; Kane & Brennan, 1977). Generalizability theory does not apply to ranked data without modification (Vanleeuwen & Mandabach, 2002), which is a reminder that, like other statistical models, generalizability theory has assumptions that must be kept in mind. There is also a multivariate extension of generalizability theory that allows examining the influence of measurement conditions on the covariances between multiple outcome measures and exploring the generalizability of protocols or multiple measures (Brennan, Gao, & Colton, 1995; Cronbach et al., 1972; Hoyt, 2000; Marcoulides,1994; Nussbaum, 1984; Webb & Shavelson, 1981; Webb, Shavelson, & Maddahian, 1983). Finally, some applications of generalizability theory may require an unbalanced design, with some facets varying in number of levels across other facets. This creates estimation complexities that are described well by Brennan (2001).

contribution to error is estimated (Llabre et al., 1988; Llabre, Spitzer, Saab, Ironson, & Schneiderman, 1991). The G study in the example could be expanded to include a standard mercury sphygmomanometer, a Dynamap automatic blood pressure monitor, and an ambulatory blood pressure monitor (Llabre et al., 1988). Variability because of measurement mode could then be estimated, although in this example it might be argued that measurement mode is a fixed effect.

A related problem is ignoring facets. Here the problem is not that a facet is held constant, but that a facet exists in a measurement problem and is not included in the statistical analyses. For example, in the blood pressure study, a time-of-day facet would exist if blood pressures were taken at various times throughout the day. Failure to include this source of variance could distort estimates of reliability. The general principle here is simple: Universe score variability, error variability, and estimates of reliability depend on the conditions of measurement and the conditions of application. Very careful attention must be given to what should count as error and, then, the measurement design must be constructed so all sources of error are given a fair opportunity to emerge and be estimated correctly. Stated differently, the measurement model must be defined correctly or the resulting measurement characteristics will be estimated incorrectly.

There is, of course, another option for the control of error other than aggregation: *standardization*. Rather than letting an error source be free to vary and harnessing that error through aggregation, the error source can be controlled effectively through standardization. Standardization is simply the attempt to control the measurement conditions carefully so that no extraneous sources of error are allowed to influence scores. For example, the same instructions delivered in the same way should precede a measure. Otherwise individuals' obtained scores might vary slightly in response to differences in instructions and that would be an additional source of error that obscures the ability to detect the true score. Similarly, environmental conditions should be the same for all respondents otherwise respondents' scores could vary depending on temperature, humidity, or ambient noise. The important point about standardization is that when measurement conditions are standardized, potential sources of variance become constants and cannot influence the variability of obtained scores. When is an error source a constant and when is it a hidden facet? It depends on the intended application. Conditions that will be free to vary in an application must be free to vary and their influence estimated in a generalizability study. Indeed, generalizability theory underscores the responsibility of a researcher to carefully mimic the intended application parameters when modeling variance components in G studies and D studies. This might seem to fly in the face of conventional wisdom that all sources of error should be controlled. If D studies are to provide informative forecasts, however, the conditions likely to be present in the application need to be present in the forecasting model.

Three additional points about error are pertinent. First, reliability of measurement does not ensure sensitivity of measurement. A poor choice of measurement instrument may preclude detecting the phenomenon of interest even though what is detected is done so reliably. For example, verbal reports of physical symptoms may be quite reliable, but they are notoriously insensitive to specific visceral reactions (Pennebaker, 1982). Second, reliable measurement alone will not insure a correct causal inference. Reliability increases the maximum possible correlation that can be detected between two operational definitions (Equation 33.5), but this does not imply that a causal relation exists between those operational definitions. Additional requirements for inferring causality must be considered (i.e., internal validity, see Shadish et al., 2001). In fact, reliable measures may fail to reveal associations between variables because other statistical assumptions are not met (i.e., statistical conclusion validity, see Cook & Campbell, 1979). Finally, standards of reliability should be recognized as arbitrary and crude benchmarks for the control of error in measurement. To be sure, with reliability, higher is better. However, attempting to achieve a particular reliability value may provide only a crude approximation to the real goal of keeping measurement error at a known level or achieving an acceptably sensitive test for an effect of known size. Accordingly, concerns about statistical power (see Bollen, 1989; Fleiss & Shrout, 1977; Humphreys & Dasgrow, 1989; Kopriva & Shaw, 1991; Williams & Zimmerman, 1989; Zimmerman & Williams, 1986) and the setting of confidence intervals should guide the choice of a reliability value to achieve.

VALIDITY

Validity is defined traditionally as the extent to which a measure assesses what it purports to measure (Kelley, 1927). Perhaps a better way to think about validity is the appropriateness of the label that is applied to a given application for a measure (Messick, 1989). This reminds us that, as was true with reliability, there are as many validities for a measure as there are applications for it. State differently, numbers are just numbers until they are put to some use.

The basic problem of invalidity can be viewed as an extension of our previous discussion of reliability. In classical theory an obtained score is conceptualized as being composed of a true score plus a random error score. In generalizability theory, this idea was expanded to include multiple error sources in which some of them are systematic. That is, in generalizability theory, some components of variance exert a predictable influence on the scores of individuals, but those variance sources have nothing to do with the true or universe score. If those sources (e.g., observers) influence the obtained variability to a great extent, then the labeling of the measure as an indication of stress could be inappropriate, particularly if the universe score variability is quite small. In this sense, generalizability theory is appropriately described as blending the concepts of reliability and validity (Shavelson & Webb, 1991; Brennan, 2001). It suggests as well that the two concerns of psychometrics – reliability and validity – each addresses aspects of measurement error. Invalidity represents the erroneous labeling of an operational definition.

More generically, the conceptualization of an obtained score might be displayed simply as:

$$X = t_1 + t_2 + e \qquad (33.25)$$

in which t_1 represents the true score of primary interest and t_2 represents the true score for another construct (e, as before, represents random error). If the variability in x is due to t_1 being substantial, then a label (based on t_1) applied to x is appropriate, that is, it is valid. If, however, the variability in x is primarily due to t_2, then a label based on t_1 will be invalid. For example, heart rate would be a relatively poor measure of sympathetic nervous system influence because it is affected by both sympathetic (t_1) and parasympathetic (t_2) systems.

Strictly speaking, then, a measure is not validated; rather the interpretation or purpose for which the measure will be used is validated. Accordingly, the number of validities for a measure can vary considerably (Fahrenberg et al., 1986). The ways that measures can be validated can vary widely. Indeed, it could be accurately said that most of science is a process of validation. Nonetheless, there are several well-defined approaches to validation that emphasize some useful points.

Content validation. Content validation is a consensual approach that relies on expert agreement about the content universe or domain, the degree to which a given indicator or item represents that domain, and the degree to which a collection of indicators adequately represents all facets of the domain. Representation here might include issues about the appropriate measurement circumstances and the particular profile or patterning of responses over time or situation (cf. Cacioppo & Tassinary, 1990). The question is essentially whether a given operational definition is a good proxy for the underlying construct, that is, the extent to which most experts agree that it "stands for" the construct. Broadly speaking, content validity refers to consensus on the universe of admissible observations.

There are two distinct types of content validation. The first and more common approach is to assess expert agreement about representativeness after the measure has been developed. For example, if the intent were to assess cardiovascular function, the researchers could propose a set of indicators (e.g., systolic blood pressure, diastolic blood pressure, pulse transit time, forearm blood volume, and heart rate) and measure expert agreement concerning suitability of each indicator and the representativeness of any set of indicators. This might be accomplished by having a group of experts rate each indicator, indicator profile, and their measurement circumstances (e.g., on a seven-point scale) according to their appropriateness given the construct definition and then assessing expert agreement

using generalizability theory (see Crocker, Llabre, & Miller, 1988).[13]

A second, more preferred, approach is to use expert opinion in the measurement development phase. Each expert would generate indicators or measurement conditions believed to be appropriate given the construct definition. Then those indicators or measurement conditions generated by a sizeable majority of the experts would be selected for inclusion (e.g., parallel-panels approach, see Ghiselli et al., 1981). For example, experts could be queried about the times of day, testing conditions, and other situational influences that should be covered to insure adequate sampling of the blood pressure domain (cf. Pickering et al., 1982). These facets of measurement can affect the obtained scores and potentially challenge the preferred labeling of those obtained scores. Similarly, expert opinion can be sought about the appropriate response dimensions to use (e.g., amplitude or frequency), the correct profile to construct, or the appropriate ways to represent a measure statistically. Accordingly, it is more appropriate to speak of content-oriented measurement development than of content validation (Guion, 1978).

Not surprisingly, content validation is easiest when constructs are simple and well defined. In this case the body of content is clear and there is a greater likelihood of agreement among experts. But even for relatively concrete constructs the content validation approach is not without problems. One crucial decision is selection of experts. They should possess technical competence, have adequate knowledge of the field, and be unbiased in their research and theoretical orientations. An aggressive attempt should be made to prevent the kind of confirmatory bias that can so easily enter into validation attempts as a function of the critical choices made in structuring the research setting (Greenwald 1975; Greenwald, Pratkanis, Leippe, & Baumgardner, 1986).

Content validation is easiest when the "distance" from the construct to the operation is fairly short. When the construct is more abstract, the identification of an adequate sample of operational definitions is more difficult. In this case, the content validation approach can be thought of as an initial quality check on the operational definitions with the need for additional construct validation.

Criterion-related validation. A second approach to validation – the criterion-related approach – is essentially based on the desire for a measure that can be substituted for the criterion. In other words, there is an agreed upon "gold standard," but (a) the criterion is too difficult or costly to assess, (b) the criterion has not yet occurred but a measure that can predict its likely occurrence is desired, or (c) the criterion has occurred in the past but is no longer

---

[13] Agreement in categorical judgments could be assessed using Cohen's kappa to guard against capitalization on chance agreement (Cohen, 1960, 1968; Conger, 1980; Fleiss, 1971; Hsu & Field, 2003; Janson & Olson, 2001, 2004; Kraemer, 1980; Li & Lautenschlager, 1997; Schuster, 2004; Schuster & Smith, 2005; Uebersax, 1982, 1987, 1988).

directly accessible. These three conditions are referred to respectively as *concurrent validity*, *predictive validity*, and *postdictive validity*. An example of concurrent validity is the substitution of x-rays for the more costly but more accurate surgical detection of tumors. An example of predictive validity is the search for cardiovascular markers of future hypertension and coronary disease. An example of postdictive validation is the use of electrocardiography to determine past occurrence of myocardial infarction.

Criterion-related validation is common in psychophysiology because of the cost, invasiveness, and difficulty of measuring physiological variables for certain samples or under specific conditions. Examples include the substitution of self-reported sleep for physiologically documented sleep (Hoch et al., 1987), development of an efficient measure of sleep parameters for use in the home (Helfand, Lavie, & Hobson, 1986) or in clinical studies (Huupponen, Himanen, Hasan, & Värri, 2004), investigation of an indirect measure of beat-to-beat change in blood pressure (Shapiro, Greenstadt, Lane, & Rubinstein, 1981) or heart period (Giardino, Lehrer, & Edelberg, 2002), examination of practical means for assessing psychophysiological markers of stress (Diaz, Vallejo, & Comeche, 2003), and development of a measure of neonate blood pressure (Hall, Thomsas, Friedman, & Lynch, 1982). In other cases, it may be easier to standardize the administration of an alternative measure or protocol compared to the gold standard (Moretti et al., 2003) or to use an alternative measure as an efficient screening device (Kovatchev et al., 2001; Yamada et al., 2000).

In choosing the criterion-related approach to validation, researchers need to be aware of some potential dangers. First, selection of a criterion may be quite arbitrary and no more representative of the construct than the proposed predictor. The criterion is ideally the most appropriate operational definition from a theoretical standpoint that has itself been validated rigorously. Accordingly, the criterion-related approach should not become a mindlessly empirical effort in which any measure is correlated with the criterion in order to find a suitable substitute but without regard for the theoretical appropriateness or meaning of the predictor. To be sure, for some applied problems there is often little interest in the nature of the predictor so long as it provides a statistically reliable means of assessing the past, current, or future presence of the criterion. This is not necessarily inappropriate if one's interests are purely functional. More care is necessary, however, if advances in conceptual understanding are to be gained. Note, as well, that a purely empirical search for predictors places one at the mercy of correlations that are inflated because of chance or dependent on unknown moderator variables.

A second danger is the assumption of an isomorphic relation between the criterion and the proxy. Their consistent and perhaps high association does not necessarily warrant the conclusion that they have a one-to-one relation (see Cacioppo &, Tassinary 1990). Although a proxy variable might be highly associated with a criterion, the proxy could well have a different pattern of relations with other constructs and these relations would alter the meaning of the proxy. This problem highlights that, although linking a measure to an existing criterion is a valuable validation tool, it is not a complete validation exercise. Additional evidence is needed to establish firmly the correct label for the measure.

The practical utility of the criterion-related approach is limited in that it presupposes that a carefully validated and reliable criterion has already been established (cf. Cole, Howard, & Maxwell, 1981). In one sense, then, the criterion-related approach to validation represents a somewhat later phase in a complete validation program: (a) an important construct is identified and defined, (b) an operational definition of that construct is developed (perhaps via content validation), (c) the link between construct and operational definition is validated (via construct validation), and (d) a decision is made to find additional operational definitions that are easier to obtain than the original and that can be used in future theory-based and applied research. The validity of these additional operational definitions is examined via the criterion-related approach with the original operational definition as the criterion (see Ghiselli et al., 1981 for a discussion of additional statistical issues that can arise with the criterion-related approach), and the validity of that criterion-based label is verified further via construct validation. A good example of a criterion-related substitute measure is the use of glycosylated hemoglobin (HbA_1) as an indicator of recent compliance with a blood glucose control regimen (e.g., Bann, 1981; Kennedy & Merimec, 1981; for comments about the validity of a biochemical index of smoking behavior see Bliss & O'Connell, 1984).

Construct validation. Although content validation and criterion-related validation are important parts of the measurement labeling process, more convincing evidence for an interpretation of an operational definition derives from *construct validation*. The hallmark of the construct validation process is the placement of a construct within a network of logically and theoretically justified constructs and construct relations with specifications as to how these translate into observable operational definitions (i.e., a nomological network, Cronbach & Meehl, 1955; Messick, 1981; Westen & Rosenthal, 2003). The validation of a construct then entails the validation of the multiple operation-level relations that are derived. The network or theory surrounding the constructs informs and guides the researcher as to the operational definitions that should and should not be related as well as to the direction and magnitude of those relations. For example, if we were attempting to validate systolic blood pressure as a measure of stress, our theory might dictate that stress occurs in response to control loss (i.e., Figure 33.2). Accordingly, establishing an empirical relation between control loss and systolic blood pressure provides *partial* validation of systolic

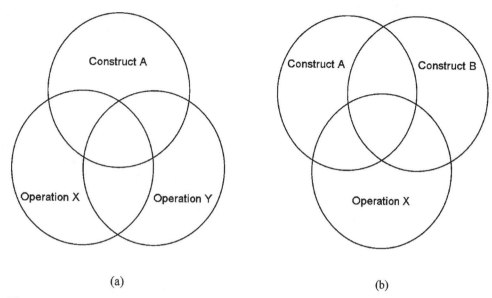

(a)

(b)

Figure 33.14. Two problems with operational definitions: (a) incomplete representation of a single construct and (b) representation of multiple constructs.

blood pressure as a measure of stress. Other empirical relations (e.g., correlations with other validated measures of stress) would add to or detract from our confidence in this interpretation depending on their magnitude and the conditions under which they are obtained. So too would relations with nonstress-related measures; these relations would challenge the appropriateness of the label.

Demonstrating construct validity is typically hampered by two common characteristics of operational definitions: (a) any one operational definition may capture only part of the underlying construct and (b) operational definitions are multidimensional and may represent two or more constructs. These relations are depicted in Figure 33.14 (see also Shadish et al., 2001; Fiske, 1987). Note that the claim that a construct is poorly represented at the operation level assumes that the construct is clearly defined in the first place. Consequently, construct invalidity can be seen to arise from problems with methods or operations (this point is argued in a very compelling fashion by Fiske, 1987; but see Shadish et al., 2001).

The dangers of incomplete representation are two-fold. First, it is possible that a particularly crucial aspect of the construct has been missed. For example, the full range of a construct may not be included in an experimental manipulation. Failure to find an empirical relation between the operational definitions might then lead to the inference that the constructs are not related when in fact an adequate test has not been performed. In psychophysiology, exclusive use of verbal reports to measure stress or emotion may lead to the conclusion that a stimulus has no long lasting effects on behavior. But this may be incorrect, as Zillmann (1978) demonstrated in his work on excitation transfer. Zillmann found that residual arousal from a prior stimulus (e.g., physical exercise) can influence later behavior (e.g., aggression) despite reports by participants that they are no longer aroused. Second, if only part of

the construct has been tested and an empirical relation is found, there is no guarantee that the results generalize to the more complete construct. Additional work may, in fact, suggest the need for a narrower construct (Fiske, 1987).

Operational definitions may also represent more than one construct (Figure 33.14). This situation often reflects the actual state of affairs: Most behaviors are multiply-determined and can be expected to be influenced by more than one source of variance. Indeed the ease with which researchers can come up with alternative explanations for internally valid empirical relations speaks to the complex and multiple constructs tapped to varying degrees by incomplete or inaccurate operational definitions. An example is the skin conductance response, which has long been recognized as being affected by widely varying stimulus conditions, across sense modalities, with interpretations including an index of specific emotions, a measure of motivation, a measure of attention, and a personality index. A not so obvious danger to multiple construct representation is the assumption that obtained relations between operational definitions imply an isomorphic relation, a point to which we will return.

The construct representation problems indicate that reliance on any one operational definition could lead to seriously distorted conclusions and that the validity of any one operational definition depends on convergent and discriminant evidence. The solution to both problems is *multiple operationism*, that is, to specify a set of correspondence rules that serve to associate a single concept with multiple operations. Only when empirical relations replicate across multiple operations can any confidence in construct relations be attained and the proper interpretation of an operational definition be made confidently. The logic of multiple operationism, depicted in Figure 33.15, is based on the simultaneous collection of convergent

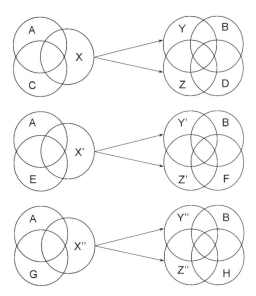

Figure 33.15. The consequences of multiple operationism.

and discriminant validation evidence. Each hypothetical study in Figure 33.15 tests the same conceptual hypothesis: A → B. In each study, however, a different set of operations is used. Across studies, the "excess" representation varies, whereas the relation between constructs A and B is constant. Likewise, across studies, the incomplete construct coverage in any one study is compensated for by different coverage in other studies. Based on supportive and consistent empirical relations, the most parsimonious explanation for the entire set of results is that Construct A is causally related to Construct B. Although it is not possible to rule out entirely the conclusion that, for example, Construct C caused Construct D in Study 1, Construct E caused Construct F in Study 2, and Construct G caused Construct H in Study 3, such a complex model is less parsimonious and becomes less plausible as additional supportive studies are added. Ordinarily, of course, many more such conceptual replications are necessary to establish firmly the appropriate label for a measure.

Multiple operationism actually refers to two distinct tasks. First, any one construct will give rise to many possible operational definitions (e.g., the many ways that arousal can be operationalized physiologically). The relations among these operations must be examined for their internal consistency. This *monoconstruct* multiple operationism provides information about the validity of interpreting any given operation as representing the construct. Second, relations between constructs must be tested by examining the interrelatedness of different sets of operations. For example, if researchers investigate the hypothesis that arousal increases vigilance, they would want to examine relations between multiple measures of arousal (e.g., heart rate and skin conductance) and multiple measures of vigilance (e.g., reaction time and event-related potentials). This *multiconstruct* multiple operationism speaks to the validity of the proposed construct linkages.

Both validation tasks are crucial to model testing and both are represented in Figure 33.15 in which monoconstruct multiple operationism is represented within each study for dependent variables and multiconstruct multiple operationism occurs across studies.

An additional word of caution regarding multiple operationism is in order. The power of using multiple operations is greatest when they diverge substantially from each other. There is little to be gained from using two self-report measures, or two nearly identical modes of physiological assessment. Any correlation between the operations might reflect their similarity in method rather than any common underlying construct. Stated differently, a construct should not be method bound, unless one is taking a particularly narrow view of a construct. The only way to demonstrate the independence of method and construct is through multiple operationism. The importance of avoiding method artifact has led to the development of the multiattribute-multimethod matrix procedure (Campbell & Fiske, 1959; Fiske, 1987; Hammond, Hamm, & Grassia, 1986; Kenny, 1995), a technique for identifying the degree to which operational relations are contaminated by method variance. This approach can be combined with structural equation modeling to provide concomitant control of measurement error (Marsh & Grayson, 1995; Wothke, 1996).

An example might make some of the preceding discussion clearer. Expanding the previous example in Figure 33.2, we might propose that the following conditions are representative of *control loss* and will bring about an increase in *stress*: (a) failing a driving test, (b) unexpectedly losing a job, (c) getting caught in a traffic jam, (d) having someone cut in line just as you near the ticket counter, and (e) getting caught in the rain without an umbrella. In successive investigations we could devise operational definitions and examine their relation to our operational definition of stress: systolic blood pressure (perhaps measured using an ambulatory monitor). We could also include in each study additional measures of stress. Taken together, this type of evidence would provide convergent validation that systolic blood pressure measures stress. On the other hand, our model might also predict that stress is not related to (f) simple physical exertion or (g) chemical stimulation. Accordingly we would not predict empirical relations between operational definitions of these variables (e.g., treadmill test, ingestion of caffeine) and systolic blood pressure. That these relations would most assuredly be found would indicate a lack of discriminant validity.

In our previous discussion of reliability we noted that aggregation is an important principle for the suppression of error. Over repeated measurement occasions, random errors have an increasing chance of canceling out and leaving true score more apparent. A similar aggregation principle operates for validation via multiple operationism. Over repeated studies using multiple operations, errors because of construct mislabeling can be identified and corrected.

The process of construct validation. As might be clear by now, construct validation is an iterative, evolving, programmatic process, which can be highlighted by examining the logic involved in making inferences based on data-level relations more closely (see Nunnally & Bernstein, 1994). Consider again the original diagram of the basic inferential task (Figure 33.1). All that we have to base our inferences on is a relation between operational definitions X and Y; perhaps this is a causal relation, $X \rightarrow Y$. Any inference that we make, however, involves three other relations: (a) the extent to which X is a valid representation of construct A, (b) the extent to which Y is a valid representation of construct B, and (c) the extent to which A is causally related to B. In any one study we cannot simultaneously make inferences about all three of these relations. Rather, we must first assume two of them to be true, and then allow the empirical relation $X \rightarrow Y$ to inform us about the plausibility of the remaining relation. For example, if our intent were to make inferences about $A \rightarrow B$, then we have to assume that X and Y are valid representations of constructs A and B, respectively. In other words, if we wish to make inferences about construct relations, then we must assume that the operational definitions have construct validity. Likewise, if we wish to make inferences about the construct validity of Y, then we must assume A and B are causally linked and that X is a valid representation of A. Our assumptions about the truth of the relations in our conceptual model is based on research (our own or previous research conducted by others). If our ultimate goal is making causal inferences, then we must proceed by first generating empirical evidence for the construct validity of our measures. This is a necessary first step because we must assume construct validity is present when causal hypotheses are tested and without such evidence, lack of empirical support for the causal hypothesis is uninterpretable. Furthermore, past research must be able to support considerable confidence in such assumptions because the appropriate interpretation of positive or negative empirical results hinges on the validity of those assumptions. An incorrect assumption can alter the direction of subsequent research and make the construct validation process inefficient if not completely misleading. This incremental view of construct validation returns us to a point made at the beginning of this chapter: Research must be guided by a very clear view of what one intends to infer from the data.

Several final comments about construct validation are in order. First, the construct validity of both the independent and dependent variables require careful attention. Psychophysiological research tends to emphasize the construct validity of physiological signals as dependent measures. But the construct validity of the eliciting conditions for those signals is equally important. For example, work on the physiological markers of stress has used a wide variety of stressors (e.g., physically demanding tasks, mental arithmetic, and cold pressor task). The conceptual equivalence of those tasks is an important consideration that influences the labeling of the physiological signal. Second, conceptual models should be responsive to empirical findings. A conceptual hypothesis is only an educated guess about how things work. If the evidence indicates a need for revision, it behooves researchers to let their models evolve rather than fall prey to confirmatory bias. Although it may be obvious, it is important that model revisions be tested on new samples. In a similar fashion, researchers should test their models aggressively, that is, provide empirical tests of hypotheses that are not immune to falsification. Researchers should assume that their measures and models contain errors and then set out aggressively to find and correct those errors rather than assuming measures and models are true and finding ways to protect that fragile perception. Finally, researchers should realize that construct validation is a slow, methodical process. The building of a conceptual model should be taken one sure-footed step at a time.

Psychological labels for physiological signals. Whenever labels are attached to numbers there is a danger of assuming an isomorphic relation between the measures on which the labeling is based. This is particularly a problem in psychophysiology, in which the "label" attached to a physiological signal is quite frequently a psychological state or process (Cacioppo & Tassinary, 1990; Sarter et al., 1996). As Cacioppo and Tassinary point out, an important goal of psychophysiological research is to specify the functional relation between elements in the psychological domain (Ψ) and elements in the physiological domain (Θ): $\Psi = f(\Theta)$. Often this functional relation is investigated by manipulating some element in the psychological domain and measuring the consequent response in the physiological domain. It is tempting to conclude that corresponding signal differences can be labeled with the psychological element that produced them. As Cacioppo and Tassinary (1990) remind us, however, "simply knowing that manipulating a particular psychological element such as emotional arousal leads to a particular physiological response such as electrodermal activation does not logically enable inferences about the former based on observations of the latter" (p. 24). The problem here is that the relations between elements in the psychological domain and elements in the physiological domain may not be one-to-one. Consequently, the probability of a physiological response given a psychological event, $P(\Theta|\Psi)$, is not necessarily equal to the probability of the psychological event given the physiological signal, $P(\Psi|\Theta)$. More than one distinct psychological event could produce the same physiological signal, for example (what Cacioppo and Tassinary call a many-to-one relation). The problem is perhaps clearest in cognitive neuroscience (Sarter et al., 1996). Cognitive operations are manipulated (e.g., using memory tasks or naming tasks) to determine the effect on brain images in order to isolate brain structures that may be responsible for the psychological process. Finding such associations (e.g., $P[\Theta|\Psi] > 0$) does not justify labeling the structure a particular cognitive center in the brain and inferring that a change in that structure would produce the psychological event (e.g., $P[\Psi|\Theta] > 0$). It certainly does not justify the isomorphic inference that $P(\Psi|\Theta) = P(\Theta|\Psi)$. Such invariant relations are a noble goal, but they require more evidence than is usually gathered in any single investigation.

The lessons to be learned from the inferential pitfalls identified by Cacioppo and Tassinary (1990) and Sarter et al. (1996) are that (a) strong inferences should not be assumed when the empirical relations do not justify them, and (b) one's research strategy should be planned to achieve strong inference when possible. The latter goal can be achieved through careful attempts to transform many-to-one, one-to-many, and many-to-many relations between the psychological and physiological domains into one-to-one relations. This may require thinking of the "elements" in those domains as sets or profiles of responses, that may have a temporal nature to them, and that might require restricting the circumstances under which they are measured. This brings us back to a theme that has been emphasized throughout this chapter: the characteristics of operations (e.g., reliability, validity, and relations) are not ordinarily invariant. They depend on the circumstances of measurement, broadly defined. Striving for such invariance requires increasing specification that might seem to limit the utility of the measures and defeat the goal of broad generalizability. It is, in fact, in the spirit of the kind of error-reduction that has been emphasized throughout this chapter.

A return to theory. We began this chapter by noting that measurement starts with a clear conceptual model that describes causal relations among constructs and operational definitions. This causality-based view of measurement is common in discussions of measurement (e.g., Boorsboom, Mellenbergh, & van Heerden, 2003; Edwards & Bagozzi, 2000; Embretson, 1983;), but its full implications are often lost, and as a consequence, efforts to develop good measures can get sidetracked. The point is perhaps made most forcefully by Boorsboom, Mellenbergh, and van Heerden (2004), who argue that current validation work emphasizes correlation over causality and often amounts to little more than seeking validity after the fact rather than building validity into measurement. As they put it, "the problem of validity cannot be solved by psychometric techniques or models alone. On the contrary, it must be addressed by substantive theory" (p. 1062). We would not paint as stark a picture as Boorsboom et al. (2004) regarding the current state of affairs in measurement nor would we dispense with some of the approaches in common use (e.g., criterion-related validation and the nomological network) that they find objectionable. Used properly, these validation tools can help refine measurement considerably. We are in complete agreement, however, with their statement that "no amount of empirical data can fill a theoretical gap" (p. 1068). In our opinion, science and measurement will always be a winnowing process that seeks to strip away error to reveal some meaningful truth. That process is streamlined considerably when informed by clearly reasoned theory.

CONCLUSION

The psychometric principles discussed in this chapter lie at the very heart of scientific progress. Although most researchers have a rudimentary understanding of these principles, their importance and specific application are often ignored. This arises, perhaps, because psychometric principles are most often associated with the classic psychometric traditions of intelligence, ability, and personality assessment. Yet, as has been stressed throughout this chapter, attention to psychometric principles is crucial no matter what form measurement takes. Whether one is attempting to map the physiological structure of mood, to identify stable physiological markers of future disease risk, to develop procedures for determining the physiological concomitants of cognitive function, or to demonstrate the practical utility of physiologically based lie detection, psychometric principles provide essential "rules of evidence" that are used to judge the adequacy of our conceptual and applied conclusions.

Science is aptly described as a truth-seeking enterprise, but it perhaps is best described as an error-correction enterprise. After all, scientists rarely find the truth staring them in the face. Instead, it emerges grudgingly after careful trimming and winnowing of the numerous error sources that obscure the view. Careful attention to psychometric principles can make that winnowing process more efficient and effective.

REFERENCES

Bann, H. F. (1981). Evaluation of glycosylated hemoglobin in diabetic patients. *Diabetes*, 30, 613–617.

Bliss, R. E., & O'Connell, K. A. (1984). Problems with thiocyanate as an index of smoking status: A critical review with suggestions for improving the usefulness of biochemical measures in smoking cessation research. *Health Psychology*, 3: 563–581.

Bollen, K. A. (1989). *Structural equations with latent variables.* New York: Wiley.

Boorsboom, D., Mellenbergh, G. J., & van Heerden, J. (2003). The theoretical status of latent variables. *Psychological Review*, 110, 203–219.

Boorsboom, D., Mellenbergh, G. J., & van Heerden, J. (2004). The concept of validity. *Psychological Review*, 111, 1061–1071.

Brennan, R. L. (1992). *Elements of generalizability theory* (rev. ed.). Iowa City, IA: American College Testing.

Brennan, R. L. (1995). The conventional wisdom about group mean scores. *Journal of Educational Measurement*, 32, 385–396.

Brennan, R. L. (1996). *Conditional standard errors of measurement in generalizability theory.* (ITP Occasional Paper No. 40). Iowa City: Iowa Testing Programs, University of Iowa.

Brennan, R. L. (2001). *Generalizability theory*. New York: Springer.

Brennan, R. L., Gao, X., & Colton, D. A. (1995). Generalizability analyses of work keys listening and writing tests. *Educational and Psychological Measurement*, 55, 157–176.

Brennan, R. L., & Kane, M. T. (1977). An index of dependability for mastery tests. *Journal of Educational Measurement*, 14, 277–289.

Burgess, A. P., & Gruzelier, J. H. (1996). The reliability of event-related dsynchronisation: A generalizability study analysis. *International Journal of Psychophysiology*, 23, 163–169.

Cacioppo, J. T., & Tassinary, L. G. (1990a). Inferring psychological significance from physiological signals. *American Psychologist*, 45, 16–28.

Cacioppo, J. T., & Tassinary, L. G. (Eds.) (1990b). *Principles of psychophysiology. Physical, social and inferential elements*. New York: Cambridge University Press.

Cacioppo, J. T., Tassinary, L. G., & Berntson, G. G. (Eds.) (2000). *Handbook of psychophysiology* (2nd ed.). New York: Cambridge University Press.

Campbell, D. T., & Fiske, D. W. (1959). Convergent and discriminant validation by the multitrait-multimethod matrix. *Psychological Bulletin*, 56, 81–105.

Campbell, N. R. (1957). *Foundations of science: The philosophy of theory*. New York: Dover.

Cardinet, J., Tourneur, Y., & Allal, L. (1976). The symmetry of generalizability theory: Application to educational measurement. *Journal of Educational Measurement*, 13, 119–135.

Cardinet, J., Tourneur, Y., & Allal, L. (1981). Extension of generalizability theory and its application in educational measurement. *Journal of Educational Measurement*, 18, 183–204.

Cohen, J. (1960). A coefficient of agreement for nominal scales. *Educational and Psychological Measurement*, 20, 37–46.

Cohen, J. (1968). Weighted kappa: Nominal scale agreement with provision for scaled disagreement or partial credit. *Psychological Bulletin*, 70, 213–220.

Cohen, J., & Cohen, P. (1983). *Applied multiple regression/correlation analysis for the behavioral sciences*. Hillsdale, NJ: Erlbaum.

Cole, D. A., Howard, G. S., & Maxwell, S. E. (1981). Effects of mono- versus multiple-operationalization in construct validation efforts. *Journal of Consulting and Clinical Psychology*, 49, 395–405.

Coles, M. G. H., Donchin, E., & Porges, S. W. (1986). *Psychophysiology: Systems, processes, and applications*. New York: Guilford.

Conger, A. J. (1980). Integration and generalization of kappa for multiple raters. *Psychological Bulletin*, 88, 322–328.

Cook, T. D., & Campbell, D. T. (1979). *Quasi-experimentation: Design and analysis issues for field settings*. Chicago, IL: Rand McNally.

Crocker, L., Llabre, M., & Miller, M. D. (1988). The generalizability of content validity ratings. *Journal of Educational Measurement*, 25, 287–299.

Cronbach, L. J. (1951). Coefficient alpha and the internal structure of tests. *Psychometrika*, 16, 292–334.

Cronbach, L. J., Gleser, G. C., Nanda, H., & Rajaratnam, N. (1972). *The dependability of behavioral measurements: Theory of generalizability of scores and profiles*. New York: Wiley.

Cronbach, L. J., & Meehl, P. E. (1955). Construct validity in psychological tests. *Psychological Bulletin*, 52, 281–302.

Diaz, M. I., Vallejo, M. A., & Comeche, M. I. (2003). Development of a multi-channel exploratory battery for psychophysiological assessment: The stress profile. *Clinical Neurophysiology*, 114, 2487–2496.

Di Nocera, F., Ferlazzo, F., & Borghi, V. (2001). G theory and the reliability of psychophysiological measures: A tutorial. *Psychophysiology*, 38, 796–806.

Druckman, D., & Lacey, J. I. (1989). *Brain and cognition*. Washington, DC: National Academy Press.

Edwards, J. R., & Bagozzi, R. P. (2000). On the nature and direction of relationships between constructs and measures. *Psychological Methods*, 5, 155–174.

Embretson, S. (1983). Construct validation: Construct representation versus nomothetic span. *Psychological Bulletin*, 93, 179–197.

Fahrenberg, J., Foerster, F., Schneider, H. J., Müller, W., & Myrtek, M. (1986). Predictability of individual differences in activation processes in a field setting based on laboratory measures. *Psychophysiology*, 23, 323–333.

Feldt, L. S., & Brennan, R. L. (1989). Reliability. In R. L. Linn (Ed.), *Educational measurement* (3rd ed., pp. 105–146). New York: Macmillan.

Feldt, L. S., & Qualls, A. L. (1996). Estimation of measurement error variance at specific score levels. *Journal of Educational Measurement*, 33, 141–156.

Fiske, D. W. (1987). Construct invalidity comes from method effects. *Educational and Psychological Measurement*, 47, 285–307.

Fleiss, J. L. (1971). Measuring nominal scale agreement among many raters. *Psychological Bulletin*, 76, 378–382.

Fleiss, J. L., & Shrout, P. E. (1977). The effect of measurement error on some multivariate procedures. *American Journal of Public Health*, 67, 1184–1189.

Garćia-Vera, M., & Sanz, J. (1999). How many self-measured blood pressure readings are needed to estimate hypertensive patients' "true" blood pressure? *Journal of Behavioral Medicine*, 22, 93–113.

Ghiselli, E. E., Campbell, J. P., & Zedeck, S. (1981). *Measurement theory for the behavioral sciences*. New York: Freeman.

Giardino, N. D., Lehrer, P. M., & Edelberg, R. (2002). Comparison of finger plethysmograph to ECG in the measurement of heart rate variability. *Psychophysiology*, 39, 246–253.

Greenwald, A. (1975). Consequences of prejudice against the null hypothesis. *Psychological Bulletin*, 82, 1–20.

Greenwald, A., Pratkanis, A. R., Leippe, M. R., & Baumgardner, M. H. (1986). Under what conditions does theory obstruct research progress? *Psychological Review*, 93, 216–229.

Guion, R. M. (1978). Scoring of content domain samples. *Journal of Applied Psychology*, 63, 449–506.

Hall, P. S., Thomas, S. A., Friedman, E., & Lynch, J. J. (1982). Measurement of neonatal blood pressure: A new method. *Psychophysiology*, 19, 231–236.

Hambleton, R. K., Swaminathan, H., & Rogers, H. J. (1991). *Fundamentals of item response theory*. Newbury Park, CA: Sage.

Hammond, K. R., Hamm, R. M., & Grassia, J. (1986). Generalizing over conditions by combining the multitrait-multimethod matrix and the representative design of experiments. *Psychological Bulletin*, 100, 257–269.

Helfand, R., Lavie, P., & Hobson, J. A. (1986). REM/NREM discrimination via ocular and limb movement monitoring: Correlation with polygraphic data and development of a REM state algorithm. *Psychophysiology*, 23, 334–339.

Hoch, C. C., Reynolds, C. F. III, Kupfer, D. J., Berman, S. R., Houck, P. R., et al. (1987). Empirical note: Self-report versus recorded sleep in healthy seniors. *Psychophysiology*, 24, 293–299.

Hoyt, W. T. (2000). Rater bias in psychological research: When is it a problem and what can we do about it? *Psychological Methods*, 5, 64–86.

Hsu, L. M., & Field, R. (2003). Interrater agreement measures: Comments on Kappa-sub(n), Cohen's kappa, Scott's π, and Aickin's α. *Understanding Statistics*, 2, 205–219.

Humphreys, L. G., & Drasgow, F. (1989). Some comments on the relation between reliability and statistical power. *Applied Psychological Measurement*, 13, 419–425.

Huupponen, E., Himanen, S., Hasan, J., & Värri, A. (2004). Automatic quantification of light sleep shows differences between apnea patients and healthy subjects. *International Journal of Psychophysiology*, 51, 223–230.

Janson, H., & Olsson, U. (2001). A measure of agreement for interval or nominal multivariate observations. *Educational and Psychological Measurement*, 61, 277–289.

Janson, H., & Olsson, U. (2004). A measure of agreement for interval or nominal multivariate observations by different sets of judges. *Educational and Psychological Measurement*, 64, 62–70.

Kamarck, T. W., Debski, T. T., & Manuck, S. B. (2000). Enhancing the laboratory-to-life generalizability of cardiovascular reactivity using multiple occasions of measurement. *Psychophysiology*, 37, 533–542.

Kane, M. T., & Brennan, R. L. (1977). The generalizability of class means. *Review of Educational Research*, 47, 267–292.

Kelley, T. L. (1927). *Interpretation of educational measurements*. New York: Macmillan.

Kennedy, A. L., & Merimec, P. J. (1981). Glycosylated serum protein and hemoglobin A_1 levels to measure control of glycemia. *Annals of Internal Medicine*, 95, 56–58.

Kenny, D. A. (1995). The multitrait-multimethod matrix: Design, analysis, and conceptual issues. In. P. E. Shrout & S. T. Fiske (Eds.), *Personality, research, methods, and theory: A festschrift honoring Donald W. Fiske* (pp. 111–124). Hillsdale, NJ: Lawrence Erlbaum Associates, Inc.

Kolen, M. J., Hanson, B. A., & Brennan, R. L. (1992). Conditional standard errors of measurement. *Journal of Educational Measurement*, 29, 285–307.

Kopriva, R. J., & Shaw, D. G. (1991). Power estimates: The effect of dependent variable reliability on the power of one-factor ANOVAs. *Educational and Psychological Measurement*, 51, 585–595.

Kovatchev, B., Cox, D., Hill, R., Reeve, R., Robeva, R., et al. (2001). A psychophysiological marker of attention deficit/hyperactivity disorder (ADHD) – Defining the EEG consistency index. *Applied Psychophysiology and Biofeedback*, 26, 127–140.

Kraemer, H. C. (1980). Extension of the kappa coefficient. *Biometrics*, 36, 207–216.

Li, M. F., & Lautenschlager, G. (1997). Generalizability theory applied to categorical data. *Educational and Psychological Measurement*, 57, 813–822.

Llabre, M. M., Ironson, G. H., Spitzer, S. B., Gellman, M. D., & Weidler, D. J., et al. (1988). How many blood pressure measurements are enough? An application of generalizability theory to the study of blood pressure reliability. *Psychophysiology*, 25, 97–106.

Llabre, M. M., Spitzer, S. B., Saab, P. G, Ironson, G. H., & Schneiderman, N. (1991). The reliability and specificity of delta versus residualized change as measures of cardiovascular reactivity to behavioral challenges. *Psychophysiology*, 28, 701–711.

Marcoulides, G. A. (1994). Selecting weighting schemes in multivariate generalizability studies. *Educational and Psychological Measurement*, 54, 3–7.

Marcoulides, G. A., & Goldstein, Z. (1990). The optimization of generalizability studies with resource constraints. *Educational and Psychological Measurement*, 50, 761–768.

Marsh, H. W., & Grayson, D. (1995). Latent variable models of multitrait-multimethod data. In R. H. Hoyle (Ed.), *Structural equation modeling: Concepts, issues, and applications* (pp. 117–198). Thousand Oaks, CA: Sage.

Maxwell, S. E., & Delaney, H. D. (1990). *Designing experiments and analyzing data: A model comparison perspective*. Belmont, CA: Wadsworth.

Messick, S. (1981). Constructs and their vicissitudes in educational and psychological measurement. *Psychological Bulletin*, 89, 575–588.

Messick, S. (1989). Validity. In R. L. Linn (Ed.), *Educational measurement* (3rd ed.). New York: Macmillan.

Moretti, D. V., Babiloni, F., Carducci, F., Cincotti, F., & Remondini, E., et al. (2003). Computerized processing of EEG-EOG-EMG artifacts for multi-centric studies in EEG oscillations and event-related potentials. *International Journal of Psychophysiology*, 47, 199–216.

Myers, J. E., & Well, A. D. (1991). *Research design & statistical analysis*. New York: HarperCollins.

Nunnally, J. C, & Bernstein, I. H. (1994). *Psychometric theory* (3rd ed.). New York: McGraw-Hill.

Nussbaum, A. (1984). Multivariate generalizability theory in educational measurement: An empirical study. *Applied Psychological Measurement*, 8, 219–230.

Pennebaker, J. W. (1982). *The psychology of physical symptoms*. New York: Springer-Verlag.

Pickering, T. G., Harshfield, G. A., Kleinert, H. D., Blank, S., & Laragh, J. H. (1982). Blood pressure during normal daily activities, sleep, and exercise. *Journal of the American Medical Association*, 247, 992–996.

Sarter, M., Berntson, G. G., & Cacioppo, J. T. (1996). Brain imaging and cognitive neuroscience. Toward strong inference in attributing function to structure. *American Psychologist*, 51, 13–21.

Schmidt, F. L., & Hunter, J. E. (1996). Measurement error in psychological research: Lessons from 26 research scenarios. *Psychological Methods*, 1, 199–223.

Schuster, C. (2004). A note on the interpretation of weighted kappa and its relations to other rater agreement statistics for metric scales. *Educational and Psychological Measurement*, 64, 243–253.

Schuster, C., & Smith, D. A. (2005). Dispersion-weighted kappa: An integrative framework for metric and nominal scale agreement coefficients. *Psychometrika*, 70, 1–12.

Shadish, W. R., Cook, T. D., & Campbell, D. T. (2001). *Experimental and quasi-experimental designs for generalized causal inference*. Boston: Houghton Mifflin.

Shapiro, D., Greenstadt, L., Lane, J. D., & Rubinstein, E. (1981). Tracking-cuff system for beat-to-beat recording of blood pressure. *Psychophysiology*, 18, 129–136.

Shavelson, R. J., & Webb, N. M. (1991). *Generalizability theory: A primer*. Newbury Park, CA: Sage.

Shavelson, R. J., Webb, N. M., & Rowley, G. L. (1989). Generalizability theory. *American Psychologist*, 44, 922–932.

Strube, M. J. (1989). Assessing subjects' construal of the laboratory situation. In N. Schneiderman, S. M. Weiss & P. Kaufman

(Eds.), *Handbook of research methods in cardiovascular behavioral medicine*. New York: Plenum.

Uebersax, J. S. (1982). A generalized kappa coefficient. *Educational and Psychological Measurement*, 42, 181–183.

Uebersax, J. S. (1987). Diversity of decision-making models and the measurement of interrater agreement. *Psychological Bulletin*, 101, 140–146.

Uebersax, J. S. (1988). Validity inferences from interobserver agreement. *Psychological Bulletin*, 104, 405–416.

Vanleeuwen, D. M., & Mandabach, K. H. (2002). A note on the reliability of ranked items. *Sociological Methods & Research*, 31, 87–105.

Webb, N. M., & Shavelson, R. J. (1981). Multivariate generalizability of general educational development ratings. *Journal of Educational Measurement*, 18, 13–22.

Webb, N. M., Shavelson, R. J., & Maddahian, E. (1983). Multivariate generalizability theory. In L. J. Fyans (Ed.), *New directions for testing and measurement: Generalizability theory: Inferences and practical application* (No. 18, pp. 67–82). San Francisco: Jossey-Bass.

Westen, D., & Rosenthal, R. (2003). Quantifying construct validity: Two simple measures. *Journal of Personality and Social Psychology*, 84, 608–618.

Whitley, B. E. Jr. (2002). *Principles of research in behavioral science* (2nd ed.). Mountain View, CA: Mayfield.

Williams, R. H., & Zimmerman, D. W. (1989). Statistical power analysis and reliability of measurement. *Journal of General Psychology*, 116, 359–369.

Winer, B. J. (1971). *Statistical principles in experimental design*. New York: McGraw-Hill.

Wohlgemuth, W. K., Edinger, J. D., Fins, A. I., & Sullivan, R. J. Jr. (1999). How many nights are enough? The short-term stability of sleep parameters in elderly insomniacs and normal sleepers. *Psychophysiology*, 36, 233–244.

Wothke, W. (1996). Models for multitrait-multimethod matrix analysis: In G. A. Marcoulides & R. E. Schumacker (Eds.), *Advanced structural equation modeling: Issues and techniques* (pp. 7–56). Mahwah, NJ: Lawrence Erlbaum Associates, Inc.

Yamada, S., Yamauchi, K., Yajima, J., Hisadomi, S., & Maeda, H., et al. (2000). Saliva level of free 3-methoxy-4-hydroxyphenylglycol (MHPG) as a biological index of anxiety disorders. *Psychiatry Research*, 93, 217–223.

Zillmann, D. (1978). Attribution and misattribution of excitatory reactions. In J. H. Harvey, W. Ickes, & R. F. Kidd (Eds.), *New directions in attribution research* (Vol. 2, pp. 335–368). Hillsdale, NJ: Lawrence Erlbaum Associates, Inc.

Zimmerman, D. W., & Williams, R. H. (1986). Note on the reliability of experimental measures and the power of significance tests. *Psychological Bulletin*, 100, 123–124.

34 Methodology

J. RICHARD JENNINGS AND PETER J. GIANAROS

Science is a method. We observe and then compare observations to find regularities in nature. The method of observation determines what we see and should determine how we interpret our observations. Consider two hypothetical experiments on the same topic. Both ask whether the pupil of the eye dilates during exposure to loud white noise (80 dbA). The first exposes six research participants to five minutes of relative quiet (40 dbA white noise) followed by five minutes of loud noise. The second experiment exposes six participants to five minutes of relative quiet and a different six participants to five minutes of noise. Both experiments measure pupil size and compare data collected under conditions of relative quiet and relative noise. Analyses show that noise influences pupil size, in one experiment, but not in the other. Why the discrepancy? We should suspect that the difference in the method of observation caused the discrepancy. We will discuss this particular discrepancy below when we suggest that the sensitivity of measuring the same subject under different conditions is typically higher for psychophysiological measures than sensitivity of measuring different participants under different conditions.

This chapter addresses salient issues that occur more frequently in psychophysiology than in psychological research in general. General treatments of methodology can be found in Keppel (1991), Kirk (1995), Kerlinger and Lee (2000), and Maxwell and Delaney (2004). Abelson (1995) offers an enjoyable and wise perspective on statistics and methodology, which we recommend highly.

Our emphasis will be on experimental design and its relationship to statistical analysis, although we shall also discuss issues of data collection and response representation. Methodological issues that are specific to particular measures will not be covered. Such coverage is available in measurement-oriented handbooks, for example, Martin and Venables (1980) and Hugdahl (1995). A series of publication guidelines on specific measures have been published in the journal *Psychophysiology*: skin conductance (Fowles et al., 1981), heart rate (Jennings et al., 1981), electromyography (Fridlund & Cacioppo, 1986), EEG (Pivik et al., 1993), impedance cardiography (Sherwood et al., 1990), blood pressure (Shapiro et al., 1996), respiration (Ritz et al., 2002), event-related potentials (Picton et al., 2000), startle blink (Blumenthal et al., 2005), and assessment of heart rate variability (Berntson et al., 1997). Loewenfeld (1993) covers measures of the pupil of the eye. Further information on event-related potential methodology is in a special issue of *Behavioral Research Methods* (van Boxtel, 1998). Basic issues of experimental control are addressed in chapters by Johnson and Lubin (1972) and Stemmler and Fahrenberg (1989).

PLANNING THE RESEARCH

Designing the observations

The key principle of methodology is as simple to state as it is difficult to implement. The methods must be chosen to answer the primary question posed by the research. Implementing this principle requires stating the experimental question concretely, assessing the means available for response measurement, identifying factors that could confuse the answer of the question, and employing statistics that answer the question precisely.

The psychophysiologist typically starts with a psychological concept of interest, assesses the concept with a physiological measure, and observes the correlation between the measure and the concept across an experimental manipulation or across a relevant dimension of individual differences. We will leave the choice of psychological concept to the reader. The choice of a physiological measure typically poses the first major challenge to the apparent simplicity of fitting the methods to the question. Often the experiment is conducted to see if measure x acts like a measure of a psychological concept. The basis for this expectation must be carefully reviewed. If a good basis exists, then it may also be possible to identify measures that are similar to measure x that either should or

(in preparation). Salient Method, Design, and Analysis Concerns. Chapter to appear in Cacioppo, J. T., Berntson, G. G., & Tassinary, L. G. (Eds.), *Handbooks of Psychophysiology, 3rd Edition*. New York: Cambridge University Press.

should not covary with variation in the psychological process. Drawing a complete picture of the expected mapping between concept and physiological measures should yield optimum convergent and discriminant validity for the measurement methodology. Cacioppo and Tassinary (1990), as well as Jennings (1986), provide a detailed, more formal discussion of how psychological and physiological concepts can be appropriately related to each other. Once this conceptual exercise is completed, then a number of practical concerns must be weighed against the value of obtaining convergent and divergent measures.

An example should clarify the conceptual and pragmatic issues that must be addressed. Consider an investigator interested in impulsive behavior in children. She wishes to show that positive reward induces greater impulsive behavior in children classified as impulsive on a scale of impulsivity. Positive reinforcement (a nickel) is contrasted with negative reinforcement (loss of a nickel). A visual, two choice reaction-time task is presented requiring a left hand response to the appearance of a left pointing arrow and a right hand response to the appearance of a right pointing arrow. A hundred ms before each arrow stimulus, however, a tone is presented to one of the two ears. Seventy-five percent of the time the tone is presented on the same side of the body as the side of the correct response to the upcoming arrow. On the remaining 25% of the trials a miscue is presented (i.e., a tone is presented on the side of the body opposite to the direction that the upcoming arrow is pointed).

How is the investigator to use psychophysiological measures? First, note that the investigator seems to have the modest, but hardly simple, goal of validating a scale/dimension of impulsivity. Impulsivity is operationalized as responding prior to the receipt of complete information. Behaviorally, responding is pushing a button. However, physiologically, responding includes preparatory adjustment of posture and competing motor activity, activation of motor cortex of the appropriate laterality, transmission to peripheral motor units, and electrochemical activation of the myofibrils resulting in flexion sufficient to make the button switch closure. The question of what is responding now appears more complicated. After considering the possible sources of variance in the button press initiation (e.g., nerve conduction differences and motor strength) the investigator begins to wonder how many measures could possibly be required. Some reading may convince the investigator that conduction time and motor strength differences are not likely to be a major contributor to the reaction speed, but that inhibition can stop a response even after activation of the motor cortex. At this point, the investigator may decide that impulsivity may arise both from aberrant central processing and the coupling of this with peripheral response mechanisms. Measures of motor cortex would seem useful as would measures of different aspects of the peripheral response.

At this stage, pragmatic measurement factors may be appropriate to consider. Without losing the fit between the measures and concept of impulsivity, it would be preferable that the measure is simple to use and analyze, inexpensive, not prone to noise, acceptable and ethical to apply to human participants, and capable of being understood from previous experience (or, at least, can be understood in the time one has during pilot work). Such considerations might push us, for example, toward the use of surface electrodes for electromyography rather than needle electrodes, or toward electroencephalography rather than magnetic resonance imaging.

Investigators can weigh pragmatic factors too much or too little in their considerations. The investigator who places too much weight on practicality may choose a measure already operational in the laboratory (e.g., electrocardiography), rather than a conceptually relevant measure that may not yet be operational (e.g., electromyography). The investigator who places too little weight on pragmatic factors will waste time and money, and may also incur more subtle costs. Most seasoned investigators believe that it is easier to collect data than to analyze and interpret data. Collecting 64 channels of EEG when the conceptual question only requires 4 channels may mean that each channel will receive some 1/16th of the analytic and interpretive time that the investigator would have placed on one of four channels. Although this numerical argument is specious, it seems reasonable to ask the investigator to consciously consider the trade off between understanding a small number of variables quite well and understanding a large number of variables less well. The tradeoff can also occur during data collection if too many technically difficult measures are attempted. Most investigators would not purposefully violate such common sense considerations, but most have collected data that were not analyzed or lost data from an entire measure because of an unforeseen technical failure. Some problems may be avoided if the investigator collects and completely analyzes pilot data from a few participants, which might include the investigator as a participant.

In the case of our hypothetical experiment on impulsivity, a practical set of response measures might be the lateralized readiness potential, surface electromyography, and response initiation, force, and completion measures. Briefly, a rationale can be cited, although it is not necessarily the best rationale – this is, after all, a hypothetical experiment. With surface cortical electrodes over bilateral motor sites and bilateral comparison sites, the degree of motor activation related to a response on one hand can be identified (see review; Coles, 1989; Coles, Gratton, & Donchin, 1988). Surface electromyography over muscles subserving a selected response, in this case each hand, can detect activation that may not result in an overt response (Lippold, 1967; van Boxtel, van den Boogaart, & Brunia, 1993). Finally, initiation of a response, the force of that response, and time of completion (standard RT) provide converging information on the intensity of any impulsive response (cf., Zahn & Kreusi, 1993). Our measurement choices would not be adequate if the investigator had different goals. If, for example, the investigator wished to explain impulsivity as a result of heightened midbrain activation, then convergent measures of cortical and autonomic activation indices might be required.

Design: Repeated measures versus between subject

Should we compare the influence of a variable between different groups of participants or use a single group and expose them to all levels of the variable? Our initial example of the influence of noise on pupil size compared exposing the same participants to noise and quiet with exposing different subject groups to noise and to quiet. In the first design the mean of pupil size under the noise condition is compared to the mean in the quiet condition; and in the second, the mean of one group in noise is compared to the second group in noise. Most psychophysiologists use some form of within-subject design. Why? And what problems does this create?

Similar to most psychophysiological measures the range of differences between individuals in pupil diameter is larger than the range of expected changes as a result of stimulation. The result is that pre- and postmeasures of, for example, pupil diameter, will be highly correlated. For example, three participants could have pupil diameters of 3, 4, and 5 mm. A dilation for each might yield diameters of 3.2, 4.3, and 5.1. The correlation between pre- and post-stimulation values is high despite the variability among the subject in the size of change, .2, .3, and .1 mm. Consider the statistical result if identical values for pupil size were obtained from one group of subjects for the baseline values and another for the stimulated values. Such values would be independently collected in the two groups (uncorrelated). A t-test can be computed for illustrative purposes using a t-test for dependent values for the within-subject comparison and an independent groups t-test for the other (see statistics text, e.g., Hays, 1994) (Kerlinger & Lee, 2000; Maxwell & Delaney, 2004). In both cases the mean difference between baseline and stimulated pupil is .2 mm. This value is divided by the estimate of the standard error of the mean for the between-participants design (.52) or for the within participants design (.01). The t-value of .4 for the between-subject comparison is dramatically smaller than the 20.0 for the within-subject comparison. Because of the strong correlation between baseline and test values within subject, the within-subject test statistic is markedly more sensitive than the between-subject test (Hays, 1994; Keppel, 1991). This difference in sensitivity is the primary argument for use of a within-subject design in psychophysiological research.

The primary problem of within subject designs is dependency (carryover) between conditions (see below for discussion of temporal dependency within the response measure). Serial dependency is created when our participants behave differently depending upon the condition they initially (or previously) received, for example, performing

differently in a quiet condition when it has been preceded by a noise condition rather than being the initial session of an experiment. Serial dependency seriously challenges the interpretation of research results. This problem has been discussed most thoroughly by Poulton (1973, 1982; Poulton & Freeman, 1966; Poulton & Edwards, 1979).

A recent set of experiments directly assessing carryover effects may illustrate the issue well. Altmann (2004; see also Loftus 1994), was interested in how preparatory time influenced the ability to shift efficiently from one task to another (e.g., switching from responding based on the height of objects to responding based on widths). He was concerned that if the same subject experienced both a longer and shorter preparatory time that learning to prepare with one time interval would alter how participants prepared during the other time interval (i.e., a carryover effect). To test this possibility he ran the same experiment manipulating preparatory time from trial to trial (within subject) and by having one group of participants exposed to the shorter preparatory period and one exposed to the longer (between subject). The results were strikingly different. When the manipulation was performed within subject, the longer interval enhanced the efficiency of switching between tasks; when the manipulation was performed between participants, no evidence of such an effect was found at all, despite careful attention to the statistical power of the experiments.

This demonstration and Poulton's methodological arguments, clearly warn the investigator that a validity check is important when using a within-subject design (see Osterhout, Bersick, and McKinnon (1997) for a psychophysiology example). Investigators should first adhere to the general methodological advice to avoid within-subject designs when differential carryover between conditions is likely, and to isolate conditions experimentally as much as possible. We also share Poulton's recommendation: ideally, a study would be run with both within- and between-subject designs. More practically, within-subject designs should vary the order of treatments so that the first treatment received can be analyzed as a between-participants comparison. If the design per se is not altering the results, then the mean difference is due to the treatment and should be comparable regardless of whether the comparison is between- or-within subject. If the direction or magnitude of the mean difference is inconsistent, then diagnostics should be initiated to understand any carryover effect present in the experiment.

The number of participants, power and determining effect size

Studies should be large enough to detect the differences that are sought (if present), but not significantly larger; studies should have adequate power. Power is the probability of rejecting the null hypothesis when it is false, and it complements the more familiar probability of accepting the null hypothesis when it is false, often termed alpha. Power is determined by the ratio of the expected mean differences as a result of the independent variable (the effect) and the error variance. Therefore, any parameter affecting the effect size or the error variance plays a role in increasing the power of an experimental design. This means that power can be increased not only by increasing the number of participants, but also by using the appropriate design, planning specific contrasts (Abelson & Prentice, 1997), using covariates or blocking factors, and selecting the most appropriate statistical analysis. Power analysis has been introduced in some degree to psychology by Cohen (1977, 1992).

General power computation software is now commercially available as part of program packages such as Statistica, SPSS, and SAS (Borenstein, Cohen, & Rothstein, 1997), but most do not specifically address repeated-measures designs. A general linear model approach for computing power has been successfully applied to repeated measures (Muller & Barton, 1989, 1991; Muller, LaVange, Ramey, & Ramey, 1992). The PASS program provides specific routines to calculate the power of repeated-measures designs based on the Muller approach (Hintze, 2004). A means for using SPSS to compute power for a number of complex designs has also been presented (D'Amico, Neilands, & Zambarano, 2001). See Algina and Keselman (1997) and O'Brien and Muller (1993) for further discussions of approaches to power for repeated measures.

Measurement scales

The novitiate to psychophysiology is often impressed with the technical equipment and the continuous data flowing from this equipment in objective units such as volts and siemens. This impression can conceal the important measurement issues that psychophysiology shares with the rest of psychology (and most of science). Glancing at a polygraph or computer screen, four signals might be displayed: EEG, EKG, blood pressure, and photoplethysmograph. All have been translated to voltages so they can drive a polygraph or computer display, but each is very different. Despite common appearance, these signals do not share any underlying measurement characteristic.

Common metrics with appropriate scale properties that permit the direct comparison of individuals are desired. We will consider here only scale properties of individual measures that may permit comparison between and within individuals rather than scaling techniques that compare individuals using more than a single measure. Physical measures, such as time, have equally spaced units and ratio properties so that arithmetic operations performed on the measures are meaningful (e.g., an interbeat interval of 1200 ms is twice as long as one of 600 ms) (see Stevens, 1951). Often we are, however, not really interested in the observed measure. Voltage measures have good properties. Assume that the investigator is interested in blood flow, and does not know how a voltage output from a photoplethysmograph is related to blood flow. A photoplethys-

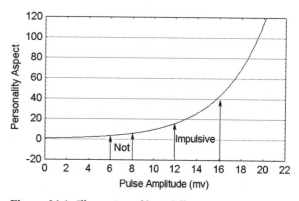

Figure 34.1. Illustration of how difference scores fail to resolve scaling issues that arise because our scaling is not linearly related to the true scaling. The x-axis is our scaling mv, of a photoplethysmograph signal, and the y-axis is the true scale value on the dimension of interest, sympathetic nervous system influences on the vasculature as driven by impulsivity. Mean data from impulsive and nonimpulsive groups under rest and task conditions are shown and the continuing distortion of the difference scores illustrated.

mographic output of 5 mv is half of one of 10 mv. If one does not know the translation to blood flow, however, the blood flow associated with the higher voltage could be 10 or 1.1 times as large as that associated with the lower voltage.

Taking this point further, physical measures with excellent scale properties do not necessarily support psychological inferences. If one is interested in impulsivity and a person has a mean pulse amplitude of 3 mv and another an amplitude of 9 mv, it can be said that the amplitude of the former is one-third less than that of the latter. It cannot be said, though, that the former has one-third more (or less) impulsivity than the latter because the investigator does not know how impulsivity alters pulse amplitude. Difference scores do not necessarily help. Assume that the mean pulse amplitude of the impulsive participants goes from 16 to 12 mv during mental arithmetic, while the mean of the nonimpulsive participants goes from 8 to 6 mv. It is tempting to think a difference score may adjust for the basal differences and put the individuals on the same scale. The difference score is −4 mv for impulsive participants and −2 mv for nonimpulsive participants. Presume, though, that pulse amplitude has a nonlinear relationship to the personality aspect relevant to the mental arithmetic response. Figure 34.1 depicts the relationship of the true scale for this aspect relative to the millivolt scoring used. If the change is read in "true" units from the graph, the impulsive change is from 42 to 17 (−25 units); while the nonimpulsive change is from 8 to 3 (−5 units). The difference scores clearly did not resolve the nonlinearity of the scaling, although the influence of the difference in pulse amplitude levels between groups was reduced.

One solution for assessing measures with unknown properties is to abandon statistical procedures based on the assumption of ratio measurement and use statistics based on ordinal or categorical scaling (Siegal 1956), or use bootstrapping to either check the significance of obtained statistics or to provide the key test statistic (Efron & Tibshirani, 1991; Wasserman, 1989). The cost of using nonparametric (ordinal or categorical) tests is a loss of power (i.e., less likelihood of detecting differences that are truly present) for specific comparisons and loss of other advantages of parametric statistical tests, for example, use of covariates and testing of the whole design of an experiment. Incurring this cost may be appropriate if scaling is truly ordinal or less, but in the case of psychophysiological measures most might argue that the scaling is more than ordinal even if ratio, equal-interval scaling has not been established. Short of conducting the considerable work to prove that appropriate scale properties are present, the best procedure may be to use parametric statistics to identify potentially significant effects and then use nonparametric statistics to confirm the statistical significance of the identified effects. Applying bootstrapping involves a slightly more complex statistical procedure. Bootstrapping may, however, not impact power as much as the application of nonparametric tests and would not require application of both parametric and nonparametric tests. The most important concern though with either method is interpretation. For example, statements of magnitude about impulsivity require a conceptual or empirical scaling that accurately places individuals on an equal interval continuum. In the absence of such scaling, only ordinal conclusions are appropriate, i.e., statements similar to "individuals with higher impulsivity scores are more likely to show earlier EMG response onsets."

Sampling: Time is sample in within subject designs

Prior to the initiation of the research, consideration should be given to data scoring and analysis. Psychophysiologists invariably sample physiological signals that are always present. An experimental psychologist must convince a subject to emit a reaction, but living participants continually produce brain potentials, heart rate, and skin conductance in the absence of volition. To collect psychophysiological data we must sample an ongoing signal extracting a time series of data points spanning the course of the time the subject is in the laboratory. Care must be taken to sample these time points without bias and in a fashion that can be replicated by other scientists. As with any sampling, the measures will be more stable and less susceptible to random error if the investigator can collect more time samples from periods sharing the characteristics of interest to us. If the investigator asks a person to do mental arithmetic for five minutes, then blood pressure collected from that period will be estimated better by three samples at 90 s intervals than by a single sample. Samples should be spaced at equal intervals unless there are good reasons to sample differently. A psychometric rationale can be offered for this advice. If one assumes that blood pressure measures have a true component, random

error component, and that the same true component is being sampled throughout the measurement period, then the true variance in the measure will increase n times as fast as the error variance when the number of measures is increased, where n is defined as the ratio of the increased number of measures taken over the original number, or in other words, the Spearman-Brown prophecy formula (see Guilford 1954). Kamarck and colleagues (1992) provide an example of increased measurement stability resulting from applying sampling ideas to the study of cardiovascular reactivity.

An important, but simple, consideration in sampling is whether the research hypothesis refers to the tonic level of a variable (e.g., heart rate levels throughout a five-minute task), or the phasic response of a variable (e.g., transient increase in heart rate following a specific stimulus). Counting r-wave spikes for the five-minute task period is an excellent sampling strategy for heart rate level, but will not be adequate to resolve the response of the heart in the five seconds following a stimulus. The count of heartbeats uses all the data available in the interval, and is more reliable than sampling the counts for only a portion of the time period. Sampling must differ for detecting the response to an environmental stimulus. The timing of each individual heart beat relative to the preceding heart beat must be saved (ideally, to millisecond accuracy), for example, five seconds preceding and following the stimulus. Tonic and phasic are relative terms, but exhaustive sampling within those timeframes should yield the most reproducible data, despite differences in sampling time frames.

Some scoring practices are questionable when viewed from the perspective of sampling. Samples of equal length should be compared to ensure the central tendency and variability of the samples are likely to be estimated equally between samples. For example, consider the response at the surface of the cortex to a flash of light. The EEG is sampled for 2 s surrounding the flash and ensemble averages are computed across multiple flashes. The event-related potential following the flash could be analyzed and graphed solely for the 1 s following the flash. This would not, however, establish that a cortical response occurred that differed from ongoing EEG activity. The 1 s prior to the stimulus should be considered. The ensemble averaging of this time sample should not yield a waveform comparable to the 1 second following the light flash. Statistical comparison could verify the existence of a waveform, and graphical presentation of pre- as well as poststimulus activity can illustrate the presence of a waveform not present in ongoing EEG.

The scoring of complex waveforms can also be biased from a sampling perspective. A biphasic heart rate response (e.g., deceleration followed by acceleration) can be scored as the difference between the heart rate at stimulus onset and the minimum heart rate following the stimulus within a 10 s window. Could the score be used to say that a reliable response to the event occurred? Not really, the scoring scheme is highly biased toward a positive difference, and significant "responses" would likely be found in the majority of random samples of heart rate. A further problem is that the minimum heart rate is a single, extreme sample value that is likely to be an unstable estimate of the size of any response and this minimum is compared to a single heart rate at stimulus onset. Stability could be increased by comparing response values to a prestimulus mean of, for example, 10 seconds of heart rate. Such a measure would remain biased though as single points are differenced from a mean value. Adequate scoring requires that the sampling be comparable for pre- and poststimulus periods. This can be done by including all heart rate values per- and poststimulus for 10 s in a single analysis (see Wilson, 1967), or by scoring maximum and minimum from smoothed data for equivalent samples of pre- and poststimulus heart rate and using these in analyses.

Response definition and intermeasure dependencies

Many psychophysiological investigations are directed at the responsivity of the person to an environmental event or a psychological process initiated by such events. Responsivity should be defined objectively prior to starting the study. What is our primary measure of responsivity? How will the onset of the response be defined? How will electrical noise influence these definitions? In our example we chose as one response measure the lateralized readiness potential of impulsive children. This measure requires bilateral (usually over C3 and C4) scalp electrodes subject to electrical noise, which is likely to obscure the readiness potential on any single trial. This will force us to use multiple trials so that the results can be ensemble averaged by aligning time samples with the stimuli and then averaging over trials to yield a mean waveform. The obtained potentials must then be assessed in some way. Are potentials examined from stimulus onset to 100 ms poststimulus? From 100 ms before the stimulus to 299 ms after? From the stimulus to when maximum negativity is reached within 500 ms? Answers to these questions define the response for your research and can also guide the design of filters and software scoring systems. An efficient, accurate, and ideally automated response scoring procedure can save hours of tedious work. As our example implies, response identification and scoring issues are largely specific to the psychophysiological measure studied. Law, Levey, and Martin (1980) provide a relatively general orientation to response scoring. After reading this chapter, more recent measure-specific articles should be consulted.

Psychophysiological responses must typically be defined by exclusion criteria as well as inclusion criteria. Physiological measures respond to many events, not only the events that are the subject of our research. A cortical negativity just after stimulus onset may meet most criteria for a readiness potential, but still be suspect if it is associated with eye movement, which could elicit an electrical nega-

tivity in the absence of any stimulus, or a particularly high voltage at an occipital (or other sensory) site. Note that these possible exclusion criteria require the investigator to collect additional measures, for instance, an eye movement index and additional scalp sites. Adequate experimental design requires the identification of all factors other than the factor we seek to manipulate that may influence our dependent measure.

The application of this dictum is not always clear. Our scientific question determines what is "artifact" and what are relevant data. In the case of the impulsive children we are examining the lateralized readiness potential to find out whether premature responses occurred more frequently in these children than in controls. However, eye movements might also index impulsivity. An eye movement toward the source of the irrelevant stimulation may reliably precede a (inappropriate) response to that stimulation. The eye movement may even produce a frontal negativity that contributes to negativity at central electrodes. The eye movement in this scenario can be seen as an index of impulsivity, and not as an "artifact." The eye movement negativity will summate with any readiness potential yielding an "amplification" of the lateralized readiness potential. In this case we may have a very sensitive index of impulsivity, but a contaminated measure of the readiness potential.

Signal processing. Psychophysiological investigations typically use some form of instrumentation to isolate, amplify, and record physiological changes. The typical choice is a combination of electronic amplifiers designed for biological signals and a personal computer with components for analog to digital conversion. This results in a measurement system that flexibly meets a variety of needs.

Physiological signals collected noninvasively result in an electrical signal that is amplified, filtered, and digitized. Amplification poses few problems with current equipment, but frequently students are concerned with the influence of filtering and the rate of sampling. Thorough and elegant treatments of these topics can be found elsewhere (Cook & Miller, 1992; Kamen, 1987; Stearns & David, 1993; Thede, 1996), but here a few very elementary points may be useful. Biological signals should be collected without distorting the features of primary interest to the investigator. Any system used to collect biological signals and digitize them for computer processing will have a sampling rate and filter characteristics. Filtering and sampling can, however, distort the signal of interest to the investigator. Filtering refers to the electronic or analytic selection of the signal of interest as typically defined by a frequency range. Frequency is the number of times per second (i.e., hertz) that a signal cycles around its mean value. In the United States the voltage in a typical house cycles around a mean of zero volts 60 times per second or 60 Hz (50 Hz is the voltage in a typical house in other countries). When delivered to a home the voltages will contain not only variation at 60 Hz, but also very small voltages at other frequencies

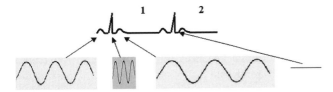

Figure 34.2. Diagram of how different segments of a physiological signal can be conceptualized as portions of a sine-cosine wave of a particular frequency.

(e.g., frequencies used by radio transmitters. An electrical filter could be designed to 'purify' the frequency). Typically this filter would taper, the amplitude of variations away from 60 Hz (i.e., reducing the amplitude of frequencies close to 60 Hz more than those at greater distance).

Filtering of biological signals works in the same way, but the change of voltages over time is not as symmetrical or continuous as household voltage, and investigators almost always want to reject or filter out 60 Hz 'noise.' Figure 34.2 shows two complexes of an electrocardiogram signal. It varies over time, but it is flat much of the time and then a complex waveform appears. Filter electronics or software views the waveform as if it were a set of simple, continuously varying waveforms. The figure illustrates this by extracting four portions of the electrocardiogram waveform and then imagining that they continued to vary in the same way over time. When this is done, the sharp (r-wave) portion of the electrocardiogram might produce a waveform with a frequency of about 30 Hz, the p-wave that precedes it will yield a waveform with a slower frequency of around 10 Hz, and the t-wave following it at an even slower frequency. The portion of the waveform between the s- and t-wave may be essentially flat (i.e., yield a frequency of less than .001 Hz).

What will happen to this signal when a low-pass filter is applied,[1] that reduces voltages in the signal with frequencies above 25 Hz? The result will be a reduction in amplitude of the r-wave. Given that the r-wave is typically used to determine the time between heartbeats, the investigator may want to shift from a 25 Hz low-pass filter to a 50 Hz low-pass filter. What will happen when a high-pass filter is applied that reduces signals below 1 Hz? The very slow frequencies will be damped, which will likely eliminate any change in the segment between S and T. This will be fine if the investigator is only measuring interbeat interval, but not when trying to see if heart disease has altered the voltage level of the segment of the signal between the s- and t-waves. The prudent investigator should estimate the interesting frequency components in the signal and then ensure that filtering via either the amplifier settings (hardware filtering) or computer programming (software filtering) does not influence the signal components. An empirical way of doing this prior to an experiment is to run an artificial signal through the entire measurement system

from a waveform generator similar to the signal of interest and note whether particular frequencies are attenuated by the system.

An analog to digital converter transforms a continuous signal into a series of numbers corresponding to the voltages sensed at a particular instant. The investigator will likely re-represent the signal as if it were continuous. The converter will make the continuous signal a series of discrete dots of voltage that hopefully will be sufficient to re-create the signal when the investigator "connects the dots." The sampling rate of an analog to digital converter, under ideal conditions, must be at least twice the frequency of the highest frequency of interest in your signal. In practice sampling at four or more times the highest frequency is advisable. The signal is missed or distorted when the sample rate is too low. This is illustrated in the top of Figure 34.3.

An EEG signal is shown and the result of sampling at two frequencies is illustrated graphically. On the left, the analog to digital converter is shown as sampling at a rate of 100 Hz and,on the right, sampling at a rate of .5 Hz. The data on the left does a reasonable job of recreating the signal, whereas the data on the right loses the waveform. When the dots are connected an apparent signal is formed, which appears to be a slowly decreasing voltage, the original signal has been distorted (i.e., aliased). The bottom of Figure 34.3 shows a complication arising from oversampling. A slow respiratory-like signal is shown with a good signal-to-noise ratio (i.e., the slowly changing component of the signal is visually very clear and does not contain much noise). On the left the signal is sampled at an appropriate low rate (e.g., 5 Hz), and the signal is recreated accurately. On the right, one breath is diagrammed as sampled at a high rate, 1000 Hz, which results in about 300 sample points for a 300 ms interval and incidentally creates large data files. The resulting data is amplified to show that the result of the high sampling rate for the 300 ms segment and reveals a fine structure of peaks and valleys in the signal (i.e., noise from the investigator's perspective). Computer programs designed for respiratory detection may find cyclic high and low points in the data

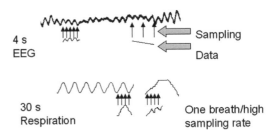

Figure 34.3. Illustration of how sampling rate will alter the obtained signal. The upper portion illustrates how distortion can occur from sampling a relatively high frequency signal with too low a sampling rate. The bottom portion of the figure illustrates how a relatively high frequency sampling rate may emphasize high frequency noise in a signal potentially obscuring the low frequency component of interest.

---

[1] This wording frequently confuses students: a low-pass filter rejects or filters out frequencies above its cutoff point and passes frequencies below its cutoff point.

for this small segment and call them "respiratory breaths." It will find about 3 breaths in this noise. This problem can be circumvented by creating "smarter" software and filtering the signal. Sampling at a lower frequency and filtering may be easier on a computer program, and permit it to do an adequate scoring job with less data storage required of the computer. A frequent, practical approach to filtering and sampling is to low-pass filter the signal electronically and sample the signal at five times the frequency of the filter cutoff frequency (Stearns & David, 1993). Further software and digital filtering may also be useful for noise that is close in frequency to the signal of interest.

The choice of gain, sampling rate, and filtering rate should be checked throughout the experiment by visually monitoring the output of the hardware and software collection system. Ideally, this would be done as the data are collected by displaying the signal at one or more points in processing as well as displaying the digitized data as it is stored. A display that shows a relatively "raw" signal and concurrently shows the digitized, processed signal will show how sampling and filtering have altered the signal. Filtering also can cause time delays; so, a comparison of when an event occurs relative to the signal in raw and processing displays is also important. Some software programs will alter the data by excluding points assumed to be invalid. For example, cardiac interbeat intervals shorter than 300 ms or greater than 1750 ms might be coded as missing data. It is useful to know immediately or, at least, after individual participants have completed their session whether such automatic editing has been done for a large or small amount of the data. The investigator should know when and how data are being transformed, and ideally be able to control such transformations (e.g., adjust the high cutoff for interbeat interval duration to 2000 ms for an athlete with average interbeat intervals in the range of 1750 ms). When hardware data displays are not available, software can be written to check on data transformations in a number of ways (e.g., box plots or stem and leaf displays on raw and less raw data) (Tukey, 1977). Also, see statistical issues concerning transformations below. Any time spent is worthwhile if it ensures that data collection is functioning as the investigator planned. Typically, psychophysiological data requires as much or more processing time as collection time. Collecting good data will make the processing time worthwhile and usually considerably shorter.

We undertook a survey of instrumentation available to psychophysiologists to see how available systems meshed with our technical needs. A questionnaire was developed that asked about the characteristics of data collection in hardware and software, analysis software, and customer service. Eleven instrumentation suppliers participated out of the 18 that had been exhibited at the annual meetings of the Society of Psychophysiological Research between 2000 and 2004. Exact comparability is not present because some suppliers emphasized EEG and ERP measures, others autonomic measures, or ambulatory data collection or analysis.

Table 34.1 lists features that varied between suppliers and the reason why the user might be interested in this feature. We have chosen to only report on items that showed considerable variation among suppliers. We queried other areas (e.g., gain control and number of data channels available) but do not report the items that were essentially invariant across suppliers. The tables are intended to provide users with a set of items to check on as they decide upon systems. The results are from December 2004 and changes to the systems described are likely to have occurred already. For this reason, we did not specifically table characteristics of specific suppliers or cost comparisons. Both the requirements of the individual psychophysiologist and the specific features of the systems that might fit individual needs are too complex and variable to pick an ideal vendor for all applications. Readers may find useful a recent chapter by Curtin et al. (in press) on design of a psychophysiological laboratory system.

DATA COLLECTION AND REDUCTION

Data quality control

Once the design is set the experiment should be run exactly as designed. Nonetheless, the results from the first few participants should be scrutinized carefully to ensure that the assumptions made in designing the study are reasonable (e.g., the investigator should examine whether a ten minute baseline truly permitted a return of blood pressure to the approximate normal values. If data from the design based on the researcher's original assumptions indicate that the assumptions are flawed, then redesigning the experiment at this early point is more efficient than completing research with an inappropriate design.

The other task that continues during data collection is data quality control. Psychophysiological data are characteristically fallible, large in quantity, individualistic in quality, and low in intrinsic interest (in their raw form). Studies of the event-related potential, for example, would typically sample data at 100 Hz and might, in a small study, accumulate 100,000 data points per subject. Although averaged electroencephalographic data presented graphically may hold some fascination, the 100,000 numbers constituting the raw data are likely to be low in intrinsic interest. Editing irrelevant values that result from head and eye movement is necessary to maintain the integrity of the data. The massiveness and low interest value of the data pose a severe challenge to visual data editing. Graphical and statistical techniques combined with human judgment are generally required for appropriate editing. Editing techniques are somewhat specific to different measures and have been discussed by others (Cheung, 1981; Bernston, Quigley, Lang, & Boysen, 1990; Gratton, Coles, & Donchin, 1983). We will provide a brief overview of approaches in order to emphasize the importance of editing for data integrity.

Table 34.1. Features varying among suppliers of psychophysiological data collection and analysis systems

Varying item	Reason for possible concern
Data collection	
Availability of direct current recording	Level of signals, e.g, S-T segment of electrocardiogram, can be important.
Filtering: analog vs digital and pre- vs post-collection	All configurations offered are functional, but you may have a preference.
Sampling rates differ by channel	Can be important if you study signals with varying frequency characteristics.
View data pre- and post-filtering	Checks on what filtering does to your data.
Specific amplifiers required	Primarily an issue if you already own amplifiers.
Direct data output from system available to user	Important if standard data processing by packages is not acceptable.
Ability to add code/routines to software	Important if your needs don't fit the collection/analysis stream of software.
Data scoring	
Amplify post-collection	Accurate visual checking may be facilitated.
Aspects of waveform scored	Slight variations in whether slopes or other features are scored may be important to certain applications.
Artifact rejection/replacement choices	User may prefer flexibility or a particular technique not offered.
Facilitated outlier detection	Graphical/coloring schemes can aid identification.
Intermediate files directly available to user	Further specific processing may be aided.
Limited to specific hardware	Important if you already own amplifiers.
Routines may be added by user	Facilitates specific/novel analyses.
SUPPORT	
On-site support	On-site support at purchase and later can be useful.
Charges for support	Most phone/email/web support free, but a few suppliers charge.
Staff devoted to support	Ratio of support to other staff varied between 11 and 50%. Check with other users to ensure satisfaction.

Note: Participating suppliers were: AD Instruments Pty Ltd., Biopac Systems, Inc., Contac Precision Instruments, Cortech Solutions, LLC, Coulbourn Instruments, EGI, Mindware Technologies, Source Signal Imaging, Thought Technologies, UFI, and Vivo Metrics, Inc. Questionnaire and spreadsheet of responses are available on website www.pghmbc.org under the Biological and Biomedical Measurement Core.

A number of useful books are available to assist in the graphical presentation of raw data. These will assist the investigator in presenting individual data so that outliers can readily be detected. Tukey's classic volume (1977), *Exploratory Data Analysis*, is a useful starting point in that graphical techniques are presented that permit rapid assessment of entire data sets; also see Greenhouse and Junker (1992). Techniques of particular relevance are box plots and stem and leaf displays, as well as the usual plotting of the frequency distribution of the data. Box plots, for example, typically display the data as a box centered on the median and extending to the first and third quartiles. Extending beyond the box are lines to the minimum and maximum values present in the data set. The investigator can quickly assess whether the data show the appropriate range of value, central tendency, and balance around the median. Fortunately, many statistical package programs (e.g., Statistica and SPSS) provide programs to efficiently display raw data in box plot and stem and leaf formats.

Once outliers, or unusually distributed data, are detected, what is to be done? Data can be transformed, outliers can be eliminated, or nothing can occur. Levey (1980) provides a thorough, well-written discussion of the various options. Little absolute advice can be offered except that the investigator should first try to understand why a data point is an outlier or why a distribution is distorted. An examination of laboratory notes might lead, for example, to an investigator finding out that a low heart rate outlier was from a child with impulsive behavior who did not meet study inclusion criterion because medications had been administered just before the study. Such data should be deleted, as it is an error that it was collected and analyzed at all. More typically, heart rate values (e.g., 10 beats per minute) or changes (e.g., an 85 beat per minute change between heartbeats) will have occurred that are physiologically impossible. Investigation may reveal computer software "bugs" or data collection errors that might be correctable or require data deletion. Similarly, distributional characteristics can identify factors, such as sampling bias, which initially escaped detection by the investigator. The investigator would then have to judge whether interpretation is possible given the bias. If not, then the data set must be discarded, as transforming data that are systematically biased will not render data interpretable. If no reasons are apparent for the outliers and the sampling or manipulations cannot be faulted, then transformation can be considered.

Transformation is indicated when outliers or the distributional pattern will inappropriately lead to a disproportionate effect on the results because of a small percentage of the observations. Appropriateness and disproportionateness are difficult to define; they remain dependent on the investigators judgment. The disproportionate influence of outliers or clusters of points can be checked by calculating descriptive statistics with and without these points. Distributions can be examined before and after a transformation to ensure that the rescaling produces conceptually reasonable results. For some investigations outliers may be theoretically expected and the most interesting outcome of the study. The weight that is given to these outliers by the original metric may be appropriate. Given the robustness of common statistics to moderate departures from assumed statistical distributions (for a discussion see Levey, 1980), transformation may frequently not be necessary if little disproportionate influence exists. As with many statistical problems, outliers and distributional problems are frequently solved by increasing the sample size.

It is necessary to be cautious when transformations are applied. Transformations necessarily make it more difficult to understand how the original measures responded to manipulations or individual differences. This problem is particularly acute when data are scaled on an individual-by-individual basis, for example, for range scores in which a skin conductance response is scored as a proportion of the individual's range of responses (Lykken, 1972). A reader interested in the size of skin conductance change in microsiemens will likely be unable to find out this number unless the investigators have taken care to provide this information.

Transformations can change the mean results more than many investigators would expect. Levey (1980), as well as Cacioppo, Tassinary, and Fridlund (1990), have provided numerical examples in which a usual transformation changes the mean difference from favoring one condition to favoring another condition. A brief excursion into sympathetic and vagal effects on the heart can illustrate the influence of the metric. Assume that interbeat interval increases 60 ms (because of a fixed vagal activation) from a baseline during which the heart beats once every 1000 ms as well as 60 ms from a baseline during which the heart beats every 500 ms (with the same vagal stimulation and with the baseline altered because of sympathetic stimulation). There is no interaction; the vagal change is identical despite a difference in sympathetic level. Transforming to the reciprocal measure, heart rate, there is a change from 60 bpm to 56.6 bpm and a change from a 120 bpm baseline to 107.1 bpm. A 3.4 bpm change compared to a 12.9 bpm change is consistent with accentuated antagonism between vagal and sympathetic systems. Statistically, an interaction is present: heart rate changes more from a higher level of sympathetic background than from a lower level. Note, however, that no interaction or "accentuated antagonism" exists if we use interbeat interval scaling.

Which transformation is correct? Berntson and colleagues (Quigley & Berntson, 1990; Berntson, Cacioppo, Quigley, & Fabro, 1994; Berntson, Uchino, & Cacioppo, 1994) have used the interbeat interval metric as well as developed and provided supporting data for model in which no accentuated antagonism exists. Levey and colleagues (Levey, 1977; Levey & Martin, 1984) used heart rate and animal stimulation data, and developed a detailed physiological model that predicts accentuated antagonism. The metric is intertwined with the theoretical views of these investigators. The correct metric may be revealed once one completely understands the detailed mechanisms of how vagal and sympathetic stimulation combine to alter heart rate (or interbeat interval).

We have already advocated the limited use of a transformation (moving to nonparametric statistics to check parametric results) when the scale properties of the measures are unknown or suspect. Nonparametric statistics convert the original scale to either rank orders or categories. The rescaling of the data to ordinal or nominal categories does provide the investigator some insight into whether the original scale may give disproportionate weight to certain observations. Significant discrepancies between parametric and nonparametric tests are a signal to the investigator to look closely at the scaling and distribution of the data. Another rescaling is frequently done but rarely discussed: a continuous measure, for example, weight, is converted to an analysis of variance factor by splitting values at the mean or median. Scale values have been converted to a nominal scale (e.g., greater weight and lesser weight). The potential loss of information relative to using a statistically equivalent testing procedure (e.g., regression analysis) has been argued elsewhere thoroughly (Cohen & Cohen, 1975; Levey, 1980).

Bush, Hess, and Wolford (1993) have provided an interesting simulation study that addresses the influence of certain transformations as well as outliers on the power of statistical outcomes. These investigators specifically examined within-subject transformations using randomly generated normal and skewed distributions. Varying sample sizes were drawn per subject (i.e., samples within a condition) as well as varying the number of participants and effect sizes. One thousand or more "experiments" were carried out for each set of parameters tested. All experiments involved a single baseline condition and a single treatment condition with the baseline-to-treatment manipulation done within each subject. Transformations examined were the arithmetic mean of a subject's data within condition (i.e., averaged over observations within that condition for that subject), log of that mean, a Z score based on the mean and standard deviations for all observations of that particular subject, a range-corrected score, and a ratio score, which expresses score as a fraction of the highest score of that subject. The Z score measure performed the best overall across variations in sample size, number of observations per subject, skewness, and percentage of data with outliers.

The Z score continued to do well relative to using medians as well as the other scores across different methods of eliminating outliers. The combination of Z scores and trimming (i.e., eliminating an equal percentage of extreme scores from all participants) performed the best when outliers were added to the simulation data. Performed "best" was defined by the ability to detect the real difference in conditions that had been added by the experimenters. Very few instances were found in which transformation yielded anomalous results (e.g., baselines higher than treatment that differed from the original data). Overall this simulation study suggests that transformations are useful when subjects vary in the degree of variability across observations.

REPRESENTATION OF RESULTS

The results of the research must be presented such that their meaning is evident not only to investigators, but one's peers, students, and, ideally, the general public. A number of books on scientific graphics are available. Most of these are rightfully critical of the modal scientific illus-

tration. Cleveland (1985), for example, found that 30% of the graphs presented in *Science* in 1980 had significant problems: features that were not explained, data points or lines that could not be discriminated, errors in construction, or reproduction so poor that the graph was illegible. Even in the absence of such significant problems it is common for graphs to obscure rather than highlight the primary feature of the results, have gridlines that overpower the results, axis numbers or legends that obscure data points, or to be excessively complex. The history of graphical presentation is used to derive principles for good graphing in the richly illustrated contributions of Tufte (1983, 1990, 1997). A number of excellent guides focusing more closely on the illustration of typical scientific data are also available (Cleveland, 1985; Wainer & Thissen, 1981, 1993). We found the Cleveland volume to be a particularly useful "hands-on" guide for graphical representation. His volume, like a number of others, provides ample illustrations of poor graphic representation with the correction of the identified faults. A recent book by Jacoby (1997) offers a pocketbook-sized condensation of graphic advice. Specific information on the plotting and analysis of residuals in regression illustrates the importance of graphing techniques for analyzing as opposed to representing results (Cook & Weisberg, 1994).

Graphical presentation of statistical results raises a specific issue. Medical and biological journals frequently ask that error bars be included in graphs so that the statistical differences between groups or conditions can be visualized. Typically, standard deviation or standard error of the mean provides the error bar for each group or condition plotted. One issue with such plots is that parametric analyses typically estimate error from the entire experiment rather than for individual groups or conditions. Furthermore, the presentation of standard deviation or standard errors for a condition varied within subject presents an estimate that is computed across participants when the analysis examined the condition effect within subject. Presentation of confidence intervals based on the statistical error term used to test an effect is an alternative. Loftus and Masson (1994) suggest this and provide a guideline for using appropriate error bars in graphs portraying within subject effects.

ANALYZING DATA

The methods that a psychophysiologist uses to analyze data should be those that are best suited to the research design and the characteristics of the dependent measures. For better or worse, however, the most common method of data analysis in psychophysiology is some form of analysis of variance. To illustrate this point, we reviewed every journal article published in *Psychophysiology* from 2000 to 2004, excluding review articles and computer simulation studies. By reading the Methods and Results sections of each article, we categorized the primary data analysis method of the article under one of the headings as listed

Table 34.2. Percentage of articles in Psychophysiology that used different methods of data analysis

Analysis method	Year				
	2000	2001	2002	2003	2004
Analysis of variance or covariance	71.1	76.7	72.1	75.8	84.4
T-tests	17.1	19.8	23.3	22.0	31.3
Multiple regression/correlation	15.8	27.9	25.6	19.8	27.1
Multivariate analysis of variance	26.3	26.7	22.1	9.9	13.5
Nonparametric analysis	6.6	9.3	5.8	7.7	8.3
Factor analysis, Principle components analyses, Multidimensional scaling, Path analysis, or Structural equation modeling	3.9	4.7	7.0	4.4	3.1

Note: Other methods of data analysis (e.g., add-mixture analyses, statistical parametric mapping of functional neuroimaging data, signal detection methods, and partial least squares tests) were not included in the above percentages because they comprised less than 1% of the approaches used in Psychophysiology from 2000–2004. The percentages for each year do not sum to 100% because the same study may have used more than one method of data analysis.

in Table 34.2. We then tallied the total number of journal articles using data analysis method in a given year, and divided this number by the total number of articles appearing in *Psychophysiology* that year. As shown, psychophysiologists, like other behavioral scientists, continue to use analysis of variance as the dominant method of data analysis – most likely at the expense of not using other methods of analysis that may prove more appropriate to the research designs and types of data that are most common to psychophysiology. As researchers, rather than statisticians, we will review the analysis of variance approach in addition to other approaches to data analysis.

Sequential time samples are statistically dependent

Most psychophysiological data take the form of sequential observations in time from the same subject. The methods that are used to analyze such repeated observations must take the correlation between observations into account. We have already discussed the enhanced power of repeated-measures designs for psychophysiological data and their inherent concerns. A remaining issue is the degree to which available methods of data analysis for such designs provide valid statistical inferences. Unfortunately, the characteristics that make repeated measures desirable are precisely those that make analyzing such data a challenge. Namely, most psychophysiological measures do not typically meet the requirements of a standard repeated-measures analysis: Correlations occurring between the successive measurements of each subject reduce error variance, but violate assumptions of unre-

lated errors and homogeneity of the variance/covariance matrix (Huynh & Feldt, 1970; Jennings & Wood, 1976; Keselman, Rogan, Mendoza, & Breen, 1980).

The repeated-measures ANOVA assumes that differences between the correlations of any set of pairs of the within-subject treatment are due to chance and there is an underlying constant correlation (Lavori, 1990). Violation of this assumption leads to using a critical test statistic that is too small or to Type I error inflation (Box, 1954). A conservative correction for the violation was developed by Greenhouse and Geisser (1959) and a more liberal one by Huynh and Feldt (1976). These adjusted (reduced) degrees of freedom work well as long as the design employs equal group sizes (Greenhouse & Geisser, 1959; Keselman & Keselman, 1990; Keselman, Keselman, & Lix, 1995). Both of these procedures are available in most statistical software packages (e.g., Statistica, BMDP, SAS, SPSS).

Multivariate tests do not carry the assumption of equivalent correlations among measures, and thus they do not require the epsilon correction factor. They do, however, carry assumptions of normality and independence of observations across subjects. Furthermore, certain situations do not favor multivariate analyses. For example, multivariate analyses can be less robust than corrected univariate analyses for unbalanced designs (Keselman et al., 1995). And, if the number of variables exceeds the number of subjects, or the study is designed with a small sample size, then the repeated-measures univariate approach with the corrected degrees of freedom may be the more appropriate choice. However, with designs that incorporate large sample sizes, a multivariate analysis is more sensitive than the univariate test (Algina & Keselman, 1997; Davidson, 1995). Because repeated-measures observations are correlated, they can essentially be viewed as a multivariate design (Cole and Grizzle, 1966). The MANOVA estimates all possible correlations of pairs of the within-subject treatment, does not assume they are equal, and, therefore, allows the influence of the covariation of the pairs to act on the analysis rather than calling it unexplained variability and increasing the error term. The MANOVA test of differences does not say how the multiple dependent measures may differ, just that they differ. Additional close examination of planned contrasts is still required (Lavori, 1990). As Russell (1990) notes, these subsequent contrasts are not completely protected from inflated experiment-wise error.

Other test statistics for repeated-measures designs are available in addition to the two salient choices: univariate or multivariate analyses. The Welch-James test for completely randomized designs (James, 1951, 1954; Welch, 1947, 1951) has been extended to work with unbalanced multivariate designs by Keselman, Carriere, and Lix (1993). This statistic employs nonpooled variance techniques and corrected degrees of freedom. Lix and Keselman (1995) also provide an easy to use SAS (Cary, 1989, 1996) and IML program. We recommended that this be the statistic of choice when there is an unbalanced design and unequal group covariances. This procedure does require a relatively large sample size: three to four times the number of within treatments minus one for main effects, and five or six times the number of within treatments minus one for interaction effects (Keselman, Kowalchuk, Algina, Lix, & Wilcox, 2000).

Analysis of covariance

An analysis of covariance is applied in psychophysiology for many reasons. A common reason is to control for factors that are not central to an experiment, but that might modify the results. For example, a characteristic of the individual, such as trait anxiety, may not be of primary interest, but may influence a psychophysiological variable. In a separate section below we discuss the use of analysis of covariance as a means to "correct for" baseline effects. To treat covariates accurately, the psychophysiologist must ask whether each subject has a single covariate value or multiple values and whether the covariate terms will be pooled across groups. If the analysis of covariance is being applied to "correct for" differences between groups, it most likely is inappropriate as clearly explained by Miller and Chapman (2001). In addition, most covariate approaches assume homogeneity among covariate relationships across treatments. In other words, across treatments all extraneous variables covary in the same way and to the same degree with the dependent variable.

Two examples that differ in their analytic approach illustrate the covariate assumptions that are unique to these approaches. In the first, a single covariate is used for each subject. In psychophysiology, this would correspond to the common design in which values from a single baseline period are used as a covariate in the assessment of values obtained from one or more tasks, for example, mental arithmetic. The covariate in this situation is a between-subjects variable. In the second situation, the covariate is measured multiple times within each subject. For example, a brief baseline period might be used prior to each of a number of tasks. The value for each of these baselines could be paired (as a covariate) with the value from the task immediately following the baseline. The covariate in this situation is a within-subject variable. In the first case, a between subject covariate results in three computational alternatives that yield comparable power, but that vary in the assumptions about error variance. The simplest approach may be to use a regression approach, which can be implemented readily in SAS (Khattree & Naik, 1995). In the second situation different approaches yield markedly different results. No simple analytic approach can be offered, but Judd, McClellland, and Smith (1996) provide guidance for analyzing such designs.

Regression alternatives to ANOVAS for repeated measures

Analysis of variance can be considered as a special case of regression analysis by using dummy variables to express the factor levels. Cohen and Cohen (1975) have developed this approach, and it is used frequently in the general linear model programs. The regression approach provides considerable flexibility that ideally would help model the data with the desired statistical approach. At a basic level, serial measurements (e.g., a repeated-measures time series) can be analyzed as a univariate regression analysis of responses with correlated errors (Ware, 1985). This is discussed further below. At the other end of the spectrum are autoregressive approaches, such as ARIMA, which essentially fit periodic components to the data (Box & Jenkins, 1970). The strength of the regression approach can also be considered as disadvantageous. A regression model that closely fits a particular set of sample data may be fitting the variance specific to the quirks of that sample. Thus, the population parameters could be estimated inaccurately. This concern makes independent replication of regression models particularly important.

Regression analyses can be a useful tool for psychophysiological studies as they allow for specific modeling of the inherent correlations of a repeated-measures design. It provides an intra-individual look at data, as well as an inter-individual perspective, that is provided by repeated-measures ANOVA. Conducting these analyses using several different regression analysis strategies leads to the construction of a more accurate picture of the data. These strategies include individual regression analysis, hierarchical and stepwise regression techniques, and random regression analysis. Appropriately applied, regression techniques can resolve problems that result from missing data or unbalanced designs, serial correlations, and time-varying covariates (Gibbons et al., 1993; Petrinovich & Widaman, 1984).

A primary concern with regression analysis techniques is the problem of colinearity. If alternative predictors of the dependent variable are highly correlated, then the one chosen by the analysis as the primary predictor will be dependent on the particular sample in use. In other words, it is governed by the quirks of the samples. Particularly in this situation, the investigator must guard against a literal acceptance of a statistical outcome, believing, for instance, that depression predicts school grades, but that anxiety does not because of the initial selection of depression by the analysis. For a more complete description of benefits and cautions of these techniques see Cohen and Cohen (1983) and Hays (1994).

We will briefly discuss two forms of regression analysis that may prove most applicable to psychophysiology: individual regression analysis and random effects analysis. Individual regression analysis, also known as growth curve analysis, is a statistical technique that detects a pattern of change in a variable across time within a particular treatment or condition (Sidani & Lynn, 1993). The temporal pattern detected by regression analysis provides a qualitative look at relationships that would otherwise be represented as difference scores at different time points by a repeated-measures ANOVA. An individual unit of analysis can be a single subject, group, or condition. The linear model, employed in the regression technique, assumes that a subject's score on one measure is a function of the score on another level, and subsequently results in a trend line for each individual, unlike a repeated-measures ANOVA that assumes one common intercept of a trend line for the within-subject variable at each time point (Gibbons et. al., 1993). When an individual regression approach is applied to a repeated-measures design, the variable of interest is regressed on the time variable. The functional relationship is depicted in the form of a regression line and the slope of this line provides the magnitude and the direction of change over time. A t-test of the slope compared to a slope of zero tests the difference. This method is useful for describing and evaluating individual differences. Furthermore, comparisons between groups can be examined by finding the regression line for each individual in the sample and testing for group differences with a t-test or an ANOVA of the intercept or slope. A significant difference between groups on the intercept indicates a baseline difference, and a significant difference between groups in slope indicates different patterns of change among the groups. Gianaros and colleagues (Gianaros et al., 2003) illustrate an application of this analysis. Gianaros et al. fit linear regression models to each individual's minute-by-minute level of respiratory sinus arrhythmia while they were exposed to a rotating optokinetic drum, a stimulus that provokes nausea. The authors found that those individuals who showed greater decreases in respiratory sinus arrhythmia over time, as defined by more negative respiratory sinus arrhythmia-by-time slopes, also reported more severe nausea. We encourage other investigators to use such individual-level approaches to quantify their psy-

chophysiological data because the approaches offer opportunities to assess experimental effects at the individual and group levels of analysis.

There are also some advantages of using an individual regression analysis over a repeated-measures analysis of variance. First, individual regression analyses clearly delineate patterns of change across time in terms of magnitude and direction, and they allow for the examination of individual change while still permitting group analysis. In addition, required assumptions are kept to a minimum. Missing data are not as crucial to the identification of the pattern and, when a nonlinear relationship is suspected, polynomial or logistic functions can be added to the regression equation to allow an accurate description. There are two practical limitations to consider before adopting individual regression analysis, however. If the variable under study, such as EEG frequency, reacts differently over time, (e.g., in different sleep stages regression will not be valid because the differences cannot be depicted in a single line. Also, values that change drastically and in different directions require a technique other than linear regression. For a more detailed description of individual regression analysis see Rogosa, Brandt, and Zimowski (1982).

Random regression models (Gibbons, Hedeker, Waternaux, & Davis, 1988), also known as random effects models (Laird & Ware, 1982; Ware, 1985), or hierarchical general linear models (Bryk & Raudenbush, 1987), provide an estimation of random person-specific effects similar to individual regression analysis. Random regression analysis goes a step beyond individual regression analysis by incorporating information about the population trend across time and providing an estimate of within-subject time trends given the individual's data (Gibbons et al., 1993). In other words, information about other subjects with similar characteristics provides support or reinforcement for a better estimate of an individual's trend. Similarly, missing data estimation in random regression models is derived from the trends of all other like-individuals in the study. These missing data points are not simply interpolated data. They are produced by the model and are consistent with the observed data of the subject, but they also differentiate between treatments to the same extent as do individuals with complete data. In addition, measurement at the same time points or for the same number of times is not required of each subject (Gibbons et al., 1993). Examples of random regression-produced estimates of missing data are depicted in Gibbons et al. (1993). A more detailed discussion of this handling is available in Ware (1985).

In random regression modeling, person-specific estimations are achieved through the use of empirical Bayesian procedures (Casella, 1985). These procedures use a weighted average based on the individual data and data from the entire sample. A subject with the most data receives a weight that is mostly influenced by the individual data. Weights of subjects with less information are more influenced by the group mean. In addition, the variance around a single person's trend is available, resulting in an estimation of the population variance-covariance matrix of person-specific effects. This is not possible with other repeated-measures analyses (Bryk & Raudenbush, 1987; Gibbons et al., 1993).

Covariates also receive distinctive treatment within a random regression model. While in repeated-measures models time-varying covariates can be a problem (as opposed to time-invariant variables that are adequately handled with a repeated-measures approach), they are easily included in a random regression model. The covariance relationships assessed by this model include (a) the overall relationship between the variable of interest and the covariate across time, (b) how this relationship changes over time, and (c) how within-subject change of interest is related to the within-subject change of the covariate (Gibbons et al., 1993).

Related to the issue of covariance is the treatment of unexplained nonrandom errors. Some examples of nonrandom errors, such as autocorrelated errors, are allowed in the random regression model; in particular, first-order nonstationary autoregressive errors (Chi & Reinsel, 1989). As this is the process in which a subject's response at one time point is influenced by the immediately preceding response, it is especially important for psychophysiological data. Repeated-measures analyses typically employed by psychophysiologists are biased when this is the situation.

Several weaknesses of the random regression modeling technique are evident. The theory from which random regression is derived requires large sample size. This creates an area of caution for psychophysiologists. In addition, a linear trend is assumed, which may not always be the case. Assumption of a linear trend also influences the estimation of missing data points used in the analysis because missing data would not occur in a linear fashion. Also, as in most other statistics, a normal distribution, to some extent, is expected. Lastly, these models are not appropriate for dichotomous variables, including transformed dummy variables (Stiratelli, Laird, & Ware, 1984).

As with any decision researchers must make, the influence of positive and negative factors are present. To decide which is the preferable analysis, a regression approach or an analysis of variance approach, ask two questions: 1. What aspect of change is of interest? (That is, do you want to know if there is change or how big a change there is or what does the change look like and what is the rate of change?) and 2. What is the unit of change that will be analyzed? (Or is it important to look at individual differences?). For general guides that include understanding and selecting regression as the analysis of choice please refer to Schroeder, Sjoquist, and Stephan (1986) and Hays (1994).

Other time series approaches

Spectral analyses of time-series data have been introduced to psychophysiology largely through their application to the analysis of heart rate variability by Porges and others (see Porges & Bohrer, 1990). The rhythmic, usually sine-cosine, functions present in a sequence of second by second heart rate values are identified using frequency (Fourier) or period (ARIMA) analyses. For example, if a sample of five minutes of heart rate per second values is examined, then rhythmic fluctuations might be identified at the frequency of respiration (about .2 Hz), which is around a frequency related to vascular fluctuations (about .1 Hz) as well as less well-defined lower frequency fluctuations (See Porges & Bohrer, 1990; Jennings & McKnight, 1994). Porges (1995) has related the power (variance at these frequencies) of these components to normal and abnormal early development; while later in life the power in these components is related to vulnerability to heart attack (see review; van Ravenswaaij-Arts et al., 1993).

Interpreting interactions

The interpretation and testing of interaction effects often puzzles students. Psychophysiologists cannot afford to be confounded by interactions because their primary interest is often in the interaction term of an analysis of variance. Typically, responses are represented within an analysis of variance by a Time factor with levels corresponding to the time series representing the response, which is often a mean value for a baseline and one for a response level. We expect this Time factor to be statistically significant. That is, we expect a response level to differ from a base level. Here, our primary interest is in the interaction of this Time factor with another factor in the experiment, such as impulsivity group or item content.

Although there are multiple ways to depict interactions, typically interactions are interpreted as cell means reflecting a difference between the differences, which is a simple effects test (Keppel, 1991). Figure 34.4 illustrates the difference-between-differences interpretation and contrasts the residual interpretation, which is discussed next.

With difference-between-difference approaches, Note that different means occur for a particular factor when utilizing difference-between-difference approaches, but this difference depends on the concurrent level of an additional factor. When interactions are examined with this approach, a meaningful interaction requires qualifying the meaning of the main effects (Kirk, 1995). For example, EMG onset could be earlier for affectively charged items than neutral items, but only among the impulsive group of the earlier example. This difference-between-differences approach would suggest that the Item Content-by-Impulsivity grouping interaction could be interpreted as EMG onset times being dependent on the affective content of an item, but only for children who are impulsive. Simple effects of task could then be analyzed. That is, investigators could statistically compare affect and neutral items only for children with impulsive behavior and

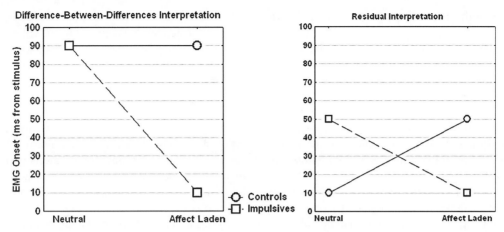

Figure 34.4. Contrast between difference between differences and residual interpretation of an interaction term. Mean results are shown either with the mean of the individual main effects removed (residual) or without this adjustment (difference between differences).

separately from children in the control group (Meyers, 1991).

An alternative approach to interpreting interactions emphasizes removing main effects so that the residuals representing the interaction can be directly examined (Rosnow & Rosenthal, 1989a, 1989b, 1991, 1995). This approach is supported by the fact that a cell mean representing an interaction also contains the influence of all lower level factors (i.e., potential main effects) (Rosenthal & Rosnow, 1991; Zuckerman, Hodgins, Zuckerman, & Rosenthal, 1993). Therefore, interpretation of the cell mean also reflects main effects. To continue with the above example, a residual representation of the Item Content × Impulsivity interaction for EMG onset could be interpreted as showing that children in the impulsive and control groups react in an exactly opposite directions for affectively laden and neutral items.

Both of these approaches, difference-between-differences and residual, result in the same interaction variance (Keppel, 1991; Rosnow & Rosenthal, 1989b), but they lead to different and, sometimes, conflicting conclusions (Petty, Fabrigar, Wegener, & Priester, 1996). The difference-between-differences approach interprets children with impulsive behavior have a different EMG onset, which is dependent on the content of the stimuli, and the residual approach interprets the children in the control group and children in the impulsive group have completely opposite reactions to the content of the stimuli in terms of EMG onset. By subtracting the main effects from the means forming the interaction, the residual approach can be compared to the difference-between-difference approach to see if one of the interpretations fits better with the conceptual issue addressed by the research.

Planned contrasts and multiple regression: Analyzing the interaction

Up to this point only the interpretation of an interaction has been discussed. Another issue is the consideration for the best statistical test. Alternatives to interaction

terms from standard analysis of variance packages exist. Contrasts are comparisons of two or more cell means, and seem to be an appropriate choice. When constructing contrasts, cell means are orthogonally weighted to correspond to the hypothesized order of their effect. This allows a focused examination of the data (Rosenthal & Rosnow, 1985; Abelson & Prentice, 1997), which is more focused than an interaction term from a standard omnibus F test. For example, the investigator could predict that the children in the impulsive group would only respond prior to a stimulus for which there is an affective item content. The investigators would then have more and less children with impulsive behavior performing under high and neutral affective content conditions with proportion of early responses as the dependent measure. A contrast could be constructed and tested by assigning equal weights to less and more impulsive children in the neutral affect condition: for example, -2, -2, and weights of 1, 3, to the children with less or more impulsive behavior in the high affect condition. The weights would directly test the hypothesis rather than depend upon the standard weighting that is assigned for an interaction in an omnibus F test. Indeed, the interaction term could be significant even if the groups differed under neutral affect conditions, but not high affect – an outcome directly opposed to the hypothesis.

Note that in the contrast test of the "interaction," the variance of the main effect was combined with the interaction variance, while the standard ANOVA F statistic would use only the interaction variance. Therefore, different results could be obtained. A match between the hypothesis and the statistic is required for appropriate testing. If an interaction is expected, a contrast may not be appropriate because the statistic will include the variance of the main effect. If there is an expectation that both a main effect and an interaction effect will be present in the data, then a contrast reflecting this is appropriate because it can incorporate the variance of each. However, if only the main effect contributes a meaningful variance, it will not be identified with the contrast because an interaction did not occur.

A multiple regression approach can also be used to implement the testing of specific patterns of interaction. First, nonorthogonal contrasts can simultaneously be tested (with the orthogonal contrast) via a multiple regression analysis. Second, several orthogonal contrasts could be specified and simultaneously entered into a regression analysis to determine the partial variance that the alternative contrasts account for (Aiken & West, 1991; Rosenthal & Rosnow, 1991).[2]

Explaining interactions with an ANOVA model is appropriate when the variables under study are discrete or if the expected relationship between the independent and dependent variable appears as stepped (Kenny, 1979), but even these instances (e.g., impulsivity groupings above) can be handled with multiple regression techniques (Aiken & West, 1991; Cohen and Cohen, 1975). Multiple regression interactions are critical when predictor variables are continuous. An interaction, as described by a multiple regression equation, states that variable Y regressed on X will have a particular slope for each individual value of Z. This provides a regression line for every point of Z. Each member of this family of regression lines is a simple regression line and the effect of X on Y is a conditional effect (Darlington, 1990).

To examine the interaction once it has been identified as such, then plotting the interaction and conducting posthoc tests are the appropriate steps. Aiken and West (1991) thoroughly discuss ways to interpret multiple regression interactions. An example of this approach to analyzing and presenting interactions within the context of a regression analysis is available in the Study 4 analysis in Graziano, Smith, Tassinary, Sun, and Pilkington (1996).

Debatable statistical issues in psychophysiology
The principle of initial values. Baseline activity in a given physiological function (e.g., heart rate) could be related to the degree, and sometimes direction, of change in that function in response to experimental manipulations. More precisely, higher baseline levels of a given function (e.g., of heart rate) might result in a limited increase in that function and lower baseline levels might result in a limited decrease in that function. A response system might well be built so that it will respond less when it is operating at a higher output level than at a lower output level. If this were true, then the investigators should certainly take baseline level of function into account when measuring change from that level. This is the so-called "law of initial

---

[2] Contrasts are especially useful when a relationship between more than two factors or levels has to be explained, for example, in a main effect composed of 4 levels. In addition, they are useful in providing further ways to discuss a linear contrast when the residuals are not significant. Significant residuals would imply the linear explanation was not an adequate one. Further contrasts can be performed on the residuals to identify quadratic trends (Abelson, 1995; Abelson & Prentice, 1997).

values" (Wilder, 1958). However, it is probably more appropriately termed the "principle of initial values" (Stern, Ray, & Quigley, 2001). Does such a principle exist? When a baseline level or change correlation does appear, what should be done? Levey (1980) suggests that baseline level dependency and data transformation are two issues akin to a bit of sand inside the shell of psychophysiology. At the time of his writing, a lustrous pearl should have formed or the irritation should have killed the area, but he notes that neither has occurred. Rather these issues, along with arousal and inverted U functions, seem to haunt the field: psychophysiologists do not believe in ghosts, but cannot stop thinking about them.

Myrtek and Foerster (1986) analyzed widely used correlation techniques to see if change was related to baseline level. They pointed out that the calculations were biased toward finding the negative correlation expected by the law of initial values. They proposed a test to eliminate this bias and found that baseline to change, if it showed anything, it showed a positive not a negative correlation. Greenen and van de Vijver (1993) arrived at the same conclusion, but provided a simpler test statistic that was largely equivalent to the Myrtek and Foerster (1986) statistic. Conceptually, the baseline to change relationship can be accurately assessed as negative (e.g., the law of initial values) if baseline variance is substantially larger than response level variance. Myrtek and Foerster found it more likely that a positive relationship is present if baseline variance is smaller than response level variance. Interestingly, Bush, Hess, and Wolford (1993) tested the sensitivity of baseline-adjusted scores in the simulation study previously discussed. The Z-score difference scores performed well when baselines changed over time within a subject's data. This Z-score difference performed slightly better than the range score, which was designed to address law of initial values issues. However, covariance adjusted scores were not tested. The primary point, however, is that statistical reasons, as well as empirical reasons, exist to discard the law of initial values.

We summarize our review by suggesting that investigators interested in psychophysiological responses carefully assess how response values might be conceptually and empirically related to basal values for their measures. A statistical or conceptual model of the relation of change and basal state should provide the best response measurement (cf. Stemmler & Fahrenberg, 1989). The conceptual assessment should consider the original design decision on choice of baseline and the degree of baseline stability present in the results. Jennings, Kamarck, Stewart, Eddy, and Johnson (1992) review the importance of baselines and suggest procedures for designing and assessing baselines. As a statistical part of this assessment the presence of an association between baseline and response could be assessed following the Greenen and van de Vijver (1993) technique. If a significant relationship does not exist, no correction should be done. If a relationship exists, then another attempt should be made to conceptualize the relationship. Lacking this conceptualization, covariance adjustments for baseline influences could be done, analyzed, and compared to either raw or transformed difference scores. Reporting only the noncorrected results is preferable, if there are not differences in outcome between corrected and noncorrected. Presentation of both analyses may be wise if corrected and noncorrected measures yield different results (see similar guidelines in Stemmler & Fahrenberg, 1989). Llabre and colleagues (1991) provide a nice overview of the statistical issues involved in using difference scores versus covariance corrected scores, which provides further depth on the issues we have just discussed and extends them to the reliability and ability to generalize results.

The null hypothesis debate. Most journals publishing psychophysiological work will review statistical results to see if they are "significant." The analysis of variance approach as well as the testing of regression coefficients implies the use of the null hypothesis to test hypotheses using a fixed probability (e.g., $p < .05$) to reject the hypothesis. This approach has been criticized widely for its arbitrariness, blindness to the size of the effect assessed, and failure to estimate the likelihood of an empirical claim (Chow, 1996; Kline, 2004; Cohen, 1977, 1994; Harris, 1991; Loftus, 1994; Loftus & Masson, 1994; Rozeboom, 1960; and a special section in *Psychological Science*, 1997 vol. 8 (1)). Alternative approaches to statistical testing have not, however, supplanted null hypothesis testing. Frick (1996) and Greenwald, Gonzalez, Harris, and Guthrie (1996) have argued that the continued popularity of null hypothesis testing is due to the appropriate fit between much of our research and the answers provided by this statistical approach. In practice, null hypothesis testing has proved rather robust in the face of critiques. The critics of the null hypothesis also have sound advice, however, which we also recommend following (Rosenthal, Rosnow, & Rubin, 2000). Cohen (1994) advises, for example, close attention to measurement, careful understanding of data using graphical techniques, attention to effect sizes, reporting of confidence intervals, use of replication of experiments, and employment of meta-analytic techniques when possible. As the critics point out, null hypothesis testing cannot establish the validity of hypotheses, null or alternative. Null hypothesis testing only estimates the chance that your findings would have occurred, given that the null hypothesis is true. In reality the conclusions must be based on thoughtful interpretation in the context of the empirical literature, available concepts, reliability within and across experiments, and available statistical indicants (see Abelson, 1995).

CLOSING COMMENT

We have attempted to highlight methodological concerns relevant at different stages of a psychophysiological research project. Psychophysiology has a traditional and continuing interest in methodology, most immediately in the technology of noninvasively acquiring physiological signals, but also in the general methodology of performing research and drawing appropriate inferences from the research. We have detected no signs of declining interest or flagging of expertise in methodology and statistics. Psychophysiologists remain methodologically sophisticated. Nonetheless, we share methodological problems with other areas of psychology, for example, a relatively blind reliance on null hypothesis testing and a rapidly expanding number of statistically significant results that fail to coalesce into conceptual advances.

The major obstacles to the use of appropriate scientific methodology may be societal rather than intellectual. An initial stage in working with a conceptual problem is exploring different measures, trying out manipulations, and generally spending time to explore methods that both follow from the conceptual question and have good measurement properties. Good hypothesis generation should precede the hypothesis testing around which much of the science is structured. A number of factors have led to a virtual disappearance of exploratory laboratory time: (a) competition among peers for positions and promotions based on research productivity, which is often defined numerically; (b) research grants awarded on a similar basis and evaluated in terms of power to confirm existing hypotheses; (c) bureaucratization of human use procedures making it impractical to vary any aspect of a research project; and (d) greater rewards for producing research articles rather than reading them. In general, the current system seems designed to produce data and reports rather than concepts and explanations. In addition to instilling greater idealism in peers and editors, a solution may be to incorporate exploratory measures and manipulations into larger hypothesis testing research. This procedure, called "leap-frogging" by some, permits the authors to get necessary exploration done while continuing to comply with current societal requirements. In the long run, exploratory results should provide the basis of solid hypothesis testing research.

Having recognized the pressures against good methodology, we would nonetheless urge psychophysiologists to use the best methods. In particular, we would urge greater time spent on the conceptualization, initial design, and piloting of projects. Care must be taken to ensure that response definitions, measures, and planned statistical analyses follow directly from the concept of the research. The almost universal dependence of psychophysiological research on within subject designs implies that we should be particularly wary of carry over effects, which are defined as the influence of one assessment upon other assessments. Designs should counter and check such effects. Once a design is established, care should be taken to use adequate sample sizes. Our success in conceptually replicating our work has not been borne out of the hope that principles can be uncovered with sample sizes of single digits per cell. Pilot work may help investigators decide whether they need double or triple digits per cell of their designs. Results should be examined graphically and numerically until the investigator understands the characteristics of the data and how the statistical analyses are expressing those characteristics. Ideally, a graphical presentation and corresponding analysis would be found that would convey the same understanding to a reader. Such a presentation should convey the amplitude and conceptual importance of a finding as well as its statistical significance. The process of analyzing the data may reveal that a "hypothesis-testing" outcome is, in fact, a poor representation of the results. It seems likely that most reports in psychophysiology should show a mixture of hypothesis testing and hypotheses generating outcomes in the process of data analysis. Ideally, our standards would change toward quality over quantity and replications of hypotheses- generating results would occur prior to publication. In practice, the field should be advanced by acknowledging the quasi-hypothesis testing of much of our work and evaluating this work, not on its post hoc value, but on the conceptual importance of the finding.

REFERENCES

Abelson, R. P. (1995). *Statistics as principled argument*. Hillsdale, NJ: Erlbaum.

Abelson, R. P., & Prentice, D. A. (1997). Contrast tests of interaction hypotheses. *Psychological Methods*, 2 (4), 315–328.

Aiken, L. S., & West, S. G. (1991). *Multiple regression: Testing and interpreting interactions*. Newbury Park, CA: Sage Publications.

Algina, J., & Keselman, H. J. (1997). Detecting repeated measures effects with univariate and multivariate statistics. *Psychological Methods*, 2 (2), 208–218.

Altmann, E. M. (2004). Advance preparation in task switching: What work is being done? *Psychological Science*, 15 (9), 616–622.

Berntson, G. G., et al. (1997). Heart rate variability: Origins, methods, and interpretive caveats. *Psychophysiology*, 34 (6), 623–648.

Berntson, G. G., Cacioppo, J. T., Quigley, K. S., & Fabro, V. T. (1994). Autonomic space and physiological response. *Psychophysiology*, 31, 44–61.

Berntson, G. G., Quigley, K. S., Lang, J. F., & Boysen, S. T. (1990). An approach to artifact identification: Application to heart period data. *Psychophysiology*, 27, 586–598.

Berntson, G. G., Uchino, B. N., & Cacioppo, J. T. (1994). Origins of baseline variance and the law of initial value. *Psychophysiology*, 31, 204–210.

Blumenthal, T. D., Cuthbert, B. N., Gilion, D. L., Hackley, S., Lipp, O. V., & van Boxtel, A. (2005). Committee report: Guidelines for human startle, eyeblink, electromyographic studies. *Psychophysiology*, 42 (1), 1–15.

Borenstein, M., Cohen, J., & Rothstein, H. (1997). *Power and precision*. Mahwah, NJ: Lawrence Erlbaum Associates.

Box, G. E. P. (1954). Some theorems on quadratic forms applied in the study of analysis of variance problems: I. Effects of inequality of variance in the one-way classification. *Annals of Mathematical Statistics*, 25, 290–302.

Box, G. E. P., & Jenkins, G. M. (1970). *Time series analysis*. San Francisco, CA: Holden Day.

Bryk, A. S., & Raudenbush, S. W. (1987). Application of hierarchical linear models to assessing change. *Psychological Bulletin*, 101, 147–158.

Bush, L. K., Hess, U., & Wolford, G. (1993). Transformations for within-subject designs: A Monte Carlo investigation. *Psychological Bulletin*, 113, 566–579.

Cacioppo, J. T., & Tassinary, L. G. (1990). Inferring psychological significance from physiological signals. *American Psychologist*, 45, 16–28.

Cacioppo, J. T., Tassinary, L. G., & Fridlund, A. J. (1990). The skeletomotor system. In J. T. Cacioppo & L. G. Tassinary (Eds.), *Principles of psychophysiology: Physical, social, and inferential elements* (pp. 325–384). New York: Cambridge University Press.

Cary, N. C. (1989). *SAS/IML software: Usage and reference, Version 6*: SAS Institute.

Cary, N. C. (1996). *SAS/STAT software: Changes and enhancements through release 6.11*: SAS Institute.

Casella, G. (1985). An introduction to empirical Bayesian data analysis. *American Statistician*, 39, 83–87.

Cheung, M. N. (1981). Detection of and recovery from errors in cardiac interbeat intervals. *Psychophysiology*, 18, 341–346.

Chi, E. M., & Reinsel, G. C. (1989). Models of longitudinal data with random effects and AR-1 errors. *Journal of the American Statistical Association*, 84, 452–459.

Chow, S. L. (1996). *Statistical significance: Rationale, validity, and utility*. Thousand Oaks, CA: Sage Publications.

Cleveland, W. S. (1985). *The elements of graphing data*. Monterey, CA: Wadsworth Publishing.

Cohen, J. (1977). *Statistical power analysis for the behavioral sciences* (rev. ed.). Hillsdale, NJ: Lawrence Erlbaum Associates.

Cohen, J. (1992). A power primer. *Psychological Bulletin*, 112 (1), 155–159.

Cohen, J. (1994). The earth is round (p < .05). *American Psychologist*, 49, 997–1003.

Cohen, J., & Cohen, P. (1975). *Applied multiple regression/ correlation analysis for the behavioral sciences*. Hillsdale, NJ: Lawrence Erlbaum Associates.

Cohen, J., & Cohen, P. (1983). *Applied multiple regression/ correlation analysis for the behavioral sciences* (2nd ed.). Hillsdale, NJ: Lawrence Erlbaum Associates.

Cole, J. W. L., & Grizzle, J. E. (1966). Application of multivariate analysis of variance to repeated measures experiments. *Biometrics*, 22, 810–828.

Coles, M. G. H. (1989). Modern mind-brain reading: Psychophysiology, physiology, and cognition. *Psychophysiology*, 26, 251–269.

Coles, M. G. H., Gratton, G., & Donchin, E. (1988). Detecting early communication: Using measures of movement-related potentials to illuminate human information processing. *Biological Psychology*, 26 (1–3), 69–89.

Cook, E. W., & Miller, G. A. (1992). Digital filtering: Background and tutorial for psychophysiologists. *Psychophysiology*, 29 (3), 350–367.

Cook, R. D., & Weisberg, S. (1994). *An introduction to regression graphics*. New York: Wiley-Interscience.

Curtin, J. J., Lozano, D. L., & Allen, J. J. B. (in press). The psychophysiology laboratory. In J. A. Coan and J. J. B. Allen (Eds.), *The Handbook Of Emotion Elicitation And Assessment*, New York: Oxford University Press.

D'Amico, E. J., Neilands, T. B., & Zambarano, R. (2001). Power analysis for multivariate and repeated measures designs: A flexible approach using the SPSS MANOVA procedure. *Behavior Research Methods, Instruments, & Computers*, 33 (4), 479–484.

Darlington, R. B. (1990). *Regression and linear models*. New York: McGraw-Hill.

Davidson, R. J. (1995). Cerebral asymmetry, emotion, and affective style. In R. J. Davidson & K. Hugdahl (Eds.), *Brain asymmetry* (pp. 361–388). Cambridge, MA: MIT Press.

Efron, B., & Tibshirani, R. (1991). Statistical data analysis in the computer age. *Science*, 253, 390–395.

Fowles, D. C., Christie, M. J., Edelberg, R., Grings, W. W., Lykken, D. T., & Venables, P. H. (1981). Publication recommendations for electrodermal measurements. *Psychophysiology*, 18, 232–239.

Frick, R. W. (1996). The appropriate use of null hypothesis testing. *Psychological Methods*, 1 (4), 379–390.

Fridlund, A. J., & Cacioppo, J. T. (1986). Guidelines for human electromyographic research. *Psychophysiology*, 23, (567–589).

Gianaros, P. J., Quigley, K. S., Muth, E. R., Levine, M. E., Vasko, R. C. J., & Stern, R. M. (2003). Relationship between temporal changes in cardiac parasympathetic activity and motion sickness severity. *Psychophysiology*, 40, 39–44.

Gibbons, R. D., et al. (1993). Some conceptual and statistical issues in analysis of longitudinal psychiatric data: Application to the NIMH Treatment of Depression Collaborative Research Program Dataset. *Archives of General Psychiatry*, 50, 739–750.

Gibbons, R. D., Hedeker, D., Waternaux, C., & Davis, J. M. (1988). Random regression models: A comprehensive approach to the analysis of longitudinal psychiatric date. *Psychopharmacological Bulletin*, 24, 438–443.

Gratton, G., Coles, M. G. H., & Donchin, E. (1983). A new method for off-line removal of ocular artifact. *Electroencephalography and Clinical Neurophysiology*, 55, 468–484.

Graziano, W. G., Smith, S. M., Tassinary, L. G., Sun, C. R., & Pilkington, C. (1996). Does imitation enhance memory for faces? Four converging studies. *Journal of Personality and Social Psychology*, 7, 874–887.

Greenen, R., & van de Vijver, F. J. R. (1993). A simple test of the law of initial values. *Psychophysiology*, 30, 525–530.

Greenhouse, J. B., & Junker, B. W. (1992). Exploratory statistical methods, with applications to psychiatric research. *Psychoneuroendocrinology*, 17 (5), 423–441.

Greenhouse, S. W., & Geisser, S. (1959). On methods in the analysis of profile data. *Psychometrika*, 24, 95–112.

Greenwald, A. G., Gonzalez, R., Harris, R. H., & Guthrie, D. (1996). Effect sizes and p-values: What should be reported and what should be replicated? *Psychophysiology*, 33, 175–183.

Guilford, J. P. (1954). *Psychometric methods* (chap 13). New York: McGraw-Hill.

Harris, R. J. (1991). Significance tests are not enough: The role of effect size estimation in theory corroboration. *Theory and Psychology*, 1, 375–382.

Hays, W. L. (1994). *Statistics*. Orlando, FL: Rinehart and Winston, Inc.

Hintze, J. (2004). NCSS PASS: http://www.ncss.com/pass.html.

Hugdahl, K. (1995). *Psychophysiology: The mind-body perspective*. Cambridge, MA: Harvard University Press.

Huynh, H., & Feldt, L. S. (1970). Conditions under which mean square ratios in repeated measurement designs have exact F distributions. *Journal of American Statistical Association*, 65, 1582–1589.

Huynh, H., & Feldt, L. S. (1976). Estimation of the Box correction for degrees of freedom from sample data in randomized block and split-plot designs. *Journal of Educational Statistics*, 1, 69–82.

Jacoby, W. G. (1997). *Statistical graphics for univariate and bivariate data: Quantitative applications in social sciences*. Thousand Oaks, CA: Sage Publications.

James, G. S. (1951). The comparison of several groups of observations when the ratios of the population variances are unknown. *Biometrika*, 38, 324–329.

James, G. S. (1954). Tests of linear hypotheses in univariate and multivariate analysis when the ratios of the population variances are unknown. *Biometrika*, 41, 19–43.

Jennings, J. R. (1986). Bodily changes during attending. In M. G. H. Coles, E. Donchin, & S. W. Porges (Eds.), *Psychophysiology: Systems, processes and applications* (pp. 268–289). New York: Guilford.

Jennings, J. R., Berg, W. K., Hutcheson, J. S., Obrist, P., Porges, S. W., & Turpin, G. (1981). Publication guidelines for heart rate studies in men. *Psychophysiology*, 18, 226–231.

Jennings, J. R., Kamarck, T., Stewart, C., Eddy, M., & Johnson, P. (1992). Alternate cardiovascular baseline assessment techniques: Vanilla or resting baseline? *Psychophysiology*, 29 (6), 742–750.

Jennings, J. R., & McKnight, J. D. (1994). Inferring vagal tone from heart rate variability. *Psychosomatic Medicine*, 56, 194–196.

Jennings, J. R., & Wood, C. C. (1976). The epsilon-adjusted procedure for repeated measures analyses of variance. *Psychophysiology*, 13, 277–278.

Johnson, L. C., & Lubin, A. (1972). On planning psychophysiological experiments: Design, measurement, and analysis. In N. S. Greenfield & R. A. Sternbach (Eds.), *Handbook of Psychophysiology* (pp. 125–158). New York: Rinehart and Wilson.

Judd, C. M., McClelland, G. H., & Smith, E. R. (1996). Testing treatment by covariate interactions when treatment varies within participants. *Psychological Methods*, 1, 366–378.

Kamarck, T., Jennings, J. R., Debski, T. W., Glickman-Weiss, E., Eddy, M. J., & Manuck, S. B. (1992). Reliable measures of behaviorally-evoked cardiovascular reactivity from a PC-based test battery: Results from student and community samples. *Psychophysiology*, 29 (1), 17–28.

Kamen, R. (1987). *Introduction to signals and systems*. New York: MacMillan.

Kenny, D. A. (1979). *Correlation and causality*. New York: John Wiley.

Keppel, G. (1991). *Design and analysis: A researcher's handbook* (3rd ed.). Englewood Cliffs, NJ: Prentice-Hall.

Kerlinger, F. N., & Lee, H. B. (2000). *Foundations of behavioral research* (4th ed.). New York: Harcourt College.

Keselman, H. J., Carriere, K. C., & Lix, L. M. (1993). Testing repeated measures hypotheses when covariance matrices are heterogeneous. *Journal of Educational Statistics*, 18, 305–319.

Keselman, J. C., & Keselman, H. J. (1990). Analyzing unbalanced repeated measures designs. *British Journal of Mathematical and Statistical Psychology*, 43, 265–282.

Keselman, H. J., Keselman, J. C., & Lix, L. M. (1995). The analysis of repeated measurements: Univariate tests, multivariate tests, or both? *British Journal of Mathematical and Statistical Psychology*, 48, 319–338.

Keselman, H. J., Kowalchuk, R. K., Algina, J., Lix, L. M., & Wilcox, R. R. (2000). Testing treatment effects in repeated measures designs: Trimmed means and bootstrapping. *British Journal of Mathematical and Statistical Psychology*, 53 (2), 175–191.

Keselman, H. J., Rogan, J. C., Mendoza, J. L., & Breen, L. J. (1980). Testing the validity conditions of repeated measures F tests. *Psychological Bulletin*, 87, 479–481.

Khatree, R., & Naik, D. N. (1995). *Applied multivariate statistics with SAS software*. Cary, NC: SAS Institute.

Kirk, R. E. (1995). *Experimental design: Procedures for the behavioral sciences* (3rd ed.). Monterey, CA: Brooks/Cole.

Kline, R. B. (2004). *Beyond significance testing: Reforming data analysis methods in behavioral research*. Washington, DC: American Psychological Association.

Laird, N. M., & Ware, J. H. (1982). Random effects models for longitudinal data. *Biometrics*, 38, 963–974.

Lavori, P. (1990). ANOVA, MANOVA, my black hen: Comments on repeated measures. *Archives of General Psychiatry*, 47, 775–778.

Law, L. N., Levey, A. B., & Martin, I. (1980). Response detection and measurement. In I. Martin & P. H. Venables (Eds.), *Techniques in psychophysiology*. Chichester, UK: Wiley.

Levey, A. B. (1980). Measurement units in psychophysiology. In I. Martin & P. H. Venables (Eds.), *Techniques in psychophysiology* (pp. 597–628). Chichester, UK: Wiley.

Levey, M. N. (1977). Parasympathetic control of the heart. In W. C. Randall (Ed.), *Neural regulation of the heart* (pp. 95–130). New York: Oxford University Press.

Levey, M. N., & Martin, P. (1984). Parasympathetic control of the heart. In W. C. Randall (Ed.), *Nervous control of cardiovascular function*. New York: Oxford University Press.

Lippold, O. C. J. (1967). Electromyography. In P. H. Venables & I. Martin (Eds.), *A manual of psychophysiological methods* (pp. 246–297). New York: Wiley.

Lix, L. M., & Keselman, H. H. (1995). Approximate degrees of freedom tests: A unified perspective on testing for mean equality. *Psychological Bulletin*, 117, 547–560.

Llabre, M. M., Spitzer, S. B., Saab, P. G., Ironson, G. H., & Schneiderman, N. (1991). The replicability and specificity of delta versus residualized change as measures of cardiovascular reactivity to behavioral challenges. *Psychophysiology*, 28, 701–711.

Loewenfeld, I. E. (1993). *The pupil: Anatomy, physiology, and clinical applications*. Ames, IA: Iowa State University Press.

Loftus, G. R. (1994). *Why psychology will never be a real science until we change the way that we analyze data*. Paper presented at the 102nd Annual Convention of the American Psychological Association. Los Angeles, California.

Loftus, G. R., & Masson, M. E. J. (1994). Using confidence intervals in within-subject designs. *Psychonomic Bulletin and Review*, 1, 476–490.

Lykken, D. T. (1972). Range correction applied to heart rate and GSR data. *Psychophysiology*, 9, 373–379.

Martin, I., & Venables, P. H. (1980). *Techniques in psychophysiology*. Chichester, UK: Wiley.

Maxwell, S. E., & Delaney, H. D. (2004). *Designing experiments and analyzing data: A model comparison approach* (2nd ed.). Mahway, NJ: Lawrence Erlbaum Associates.

Meyers, D. L. (1991). Misinterpretation of interaction effects: A reply to Rosnow and Rosenthal. *Psychological Bulletin*, 110, 571–573.

Miller, G. A., & Chapman, J. P. (2001). Misunderstanding analysis of covariance. *Journal of Abnormal Psychology*, 110 (1), 40–48.

Muller, K. E., & Barton, C. N. (1989). Approximate power for repeated measures ANOVA lacking sphericity. *Journal of the American Statistical Association*, 87, 549–555.

Muller, K. E., & Barton, C. N. (1991). Correction to "Approximate power for repeated measures ANOVA lacking sphericity". *Journal of the American Statistical Association*, 86, 255–256.

Muller, K. E., LaVange, L. M., Ramey, S. L., & Ramey, C. T. (1992). Power calculations for general linear multivariate models including repeated measures applications. *Journal of the American Statistical Association*, 87, 1209–1226.

Myrtek, M., & Foerster, F. (1986). The law of initial value: A rare exception. *Biological Psychology*, 22, 227–237.

O'Brien, R. G., & Muller, K. E. (1993). Unified power analysis for t-tests through multivariate hypotheses. In L. K. Edwards (Ed.), *Applied analysis of variance in the behavioral sciences* (pp. 297–344). New York: Marcel Dekker.

Osterhout, L., Bersick, M., & McKinnon, R. (1997). Brain potentials elicited by words: Word length and frequency predict the latency of an early negativity. *Biological Psychology*, 46 (2), 143–168.

Petrinovich, L., & Widaman, K. F. (1984). An evaluation of statistical strategies to analyze repeated-measures data. In H. V. S. Peeke & L. Petrinovich (Eds.), *Habituation, sensitivation, and behavior* (pp. 105–201). Orlando, FL: Academic Press.

Petty, R. E., Fabrigar, L. R., Wegener, D. T., & Priester, J. R. (1996). Understanding data when interactions are present or hypothesized. *Psychological Science*, 7 (4), 247–252.

Picton, T. W., et al. (2000). Guidelines for using human event-related potentials to study cognition: Recording standards and publication criteria. *Psychophysiology*, 37 (2), 127–152.

Pivik, R. T., Broughton, R. J., Coppola, R., Davidson, R. J., Fox, N., & Nuwer, M. R. (1993). Guidelines for the recording and quantitative analysis of electroencephalographic activity in research contexts. *Psychophysiology*, 30(6), 547–548.

Porges, S. W. (1995). Orienting in a defensive world. Mammalian modifications of our evolutionary heritage. A polyvagal theory. *Psychophysiology*, 32, 301–318.

Porges, S. W., & Bohrer, R. E. (1990). The analysis of periodic processes in psychophysiological research. In J. T. Cacioppo & L. G. Tassinary (Eds.), *Principles of psychophysiology* (pp. 708–753). Cambridge, MA: Cambridge University Press.

Poulton, E. C. (1973). Unwanted range effects from using within-subject experimental designs. *Psychological Bulletin*, 80, 113–121.

Poulton, E. C. (1982). Influential companions: Effects of one strategy on another in the within-subjects designs of cognitive psychology. *Psychological Bulletin*, 91, 673–690.

Poulton, E. C., & Edwards, R. S. (1979). Assymetric transfer in within-participants experiments on stress interaction. *Ergonomics*, 22, 945–961.

Poulton, E. C., & Freeman, P. R. (1966). Unwanted assymetrical transfer effects with balanced experimental designs. *Psychological Bulletin*, 66, 1–8.

Quigley, K. S., & Berntson, G. G. (1990). Autonomic interactions and chronotopic control of the heart: Heart period versus heart rate. *Psychophysiology*, 33, 605–611.

Ritz, T., et al. (2002). Guidelines for mechanical lung function measurements in psychophysiology. *Psychophysiology*, 39 (5), 546–567.

Rogosa, D., Brandt, D., & Zimowski, M. (1982). A growth curve approach to the measurement of change. *Psychological Bulletin*, 92, 726–748.

Rosenthal, R., & Rosnow, R. L. (1985). *Contrast analysis: Focused comparisons in the analysis of variance*. New York: Holt, Rinehart, & Wilson.

Rosenthal, R., & Rosnow, R. L. (1991). *Essentials of behavioral research: Explanation and prediction* (2nd ed.). New York: McGraw-Hill.

Rosenthal, R., Rosnow, R. L., & Rubin, D. B. (2000). *Contrasts and effect sizes in behavioral research: A correlational approach*. New York: Cambridge University Press.

Rosnow, R. L., & Rosenthal, R. (1989a). Definition and interpretation of interaction effects. *Psychological Bulletin*, 105, 143–146.

Rosnow, R. L., & Rosenthal, R. (1989b). Statistical procedures and the justification of knowledge in psychological science. *American Psychologist*, 44, 1276–1284.

Rosnow, R. L., & Rosenthal, R. (1991). If you're looking at the cell means, you're not looking at only the interaction (unless all main effects are zero). *Psychological Bulletin*, 110, 574–576.

Rosnow, R. L., & Rosenthal, R. (1995). Some things you learn aren't so: Cohen's paradox, Asch's paradigm, and the interpretation of interaction. *Psychological Science*, 6, 3–9.

Rozeboom, W. W. (1960). The fallacy of the null hypothesis significant test. *Psychological Bulletin*, 57, 416–428.

Russell, D. W. (1990). The analysis of psychophysiological data: Multivariate approaches. In J. T. Cacioppo & L. G. Tassinary (Eds.), *Principles of psychophysiology* (pp. 775–801). New York: Cambridge University Press.

Schroeder, L. D., Sjoquist, D. L., & Stephan, P. E. (1986). *Understanding regression analysis: An introductory guide*. Newbury Park, CA: Sage Publications.

Shapiro, D., Lane, J. D., Light, K. C., Myrtek, M., Suwada, Y., & Steptoe, A. (1996). Blood pressure publication guidelines. *Psychophysiology*, 33, 1–12.

Sherwood, A., Allen, M. T., Fahrenberg, J., Kelsey, R. M., Lovallo, W. R., & van Doornen, L. J. P. (1990). Methodological guidelines for impedance cardiography. *Psychophysiology*, 27, 1–23.

Sidani, S., & Lynn, M. R. (1993). Examining amount and pattern of change: Comparing repeated measures ANOVA and individual regression analysis. *Nursing Research*, 42 (5), 283–286.

Siegal, S. (1956). *Nonparametric statistics*. New York: McGraw Hill.

Stearns, S. D., & David, R. A. (1993). *Signal processing algorithms in Fortran and C*. Englewood Cliffs, NJ: Prentice-Hall.

Stemmler, G., & Fahrenberg, J. (1989). Psychophysiological assessment: Conceptual, psychometric, and statistical issues. In Graham & G. Turpin (Eds.), *Handbook of clinical psychophysiology* (pp. 633). Chichester, UK: John Wiley & Sons.

Stern, R. M., Ray, W. J., & Quigley, K. S. (2001). *Psychophysiological recording*. New York: University Press (2nd ed.).

Stevens, S. S. (1951). Mathematics, measurement, and psychophysics. In S. S. Stevens (Ed.), *Handbook of experimental psychology* (pp. 1–49). New York: Wiley.

Stiratelli, R., Laird, N. M., & Ware, J. H. (1984). Random-effects models for serial observations with binary response. *Biometrics*, 40, 961–971.

Thede, L. (1996). *Analog and digital filter design using C Les Thede*. Upper Saddle River, NJ: Prentice Hall.

Tufte, E. R. (1983). *The visual display of quantitative information*. Cheshire, CT: Graphics Press.

Tufte, E. R. (1990). *Envisioning information*. Cheshire, CT: Graphics Press.

Tufte, E. R. (1997). *Visual explanations: Images and quantities, evidence and narrative*. Cheshire, CT: Graphics Press.

Tukey, J. W. (1977). *Exploratory data analysis*. Reading, MA: Addison-Wesley Publishing Company.

van Boxtel, G. J. M. (1998). Computational and statistical methods for analyzing event-related potential data. *Behavior Research Methods, Instruments & Computers*, 30 (1), 87–102.

van Boxtel, G. J. M., van den Boogaart, B., & Brunia, C. H. M. (1993). The contingent negative variation in a choice reaction time task. *Journal of Psychophysiology*, 7, 11–23.

van Ravenswaaij-Arts, C. M. A., Kolle'e, L. A. A., Hopman, J. C. W., Stoelinga, G. B. A., & van Geijn, H. P. (1993). Heart rate variability. *Annals of Internal Medicine*, 118, 463–447.

Wainer, H., & Thissen, D. (1981). Graphical data analysis. *Annual Review of Psychology*, 32, 191–241.

Wainer, H., & Thissen, D. (1993). Graphical data analysis. In G. Keren & C. Lewis (Eds.), *A handbook for data analysis in the behavioral sciences: Statistical issues* (pp. 391–457). Hilladale, NJ: Lawrence Erlbaum Associates.

Ware, J. H. (1985). Linear models for the analysis of longitudinal studies. *The American Statistician*, 39 (2), 95–101.

Wasserman, S., & Bockenholt, U. (1989). Bootstrapping: Applications to psychophysiology. *Psychophysiology*, 26 (2), 208–221.

Welch, B. L. (1947). The generalization of student's problem when several different population variances are unequal. *Biometrika*, 29, 350–362.

Welch, B. L. (1951). On the comparison of several mean values: An alternative approach. *Biometrika*, 38, 330–336.

Wilder, J. (1958). Modern psychophysiology and the law of initial value. *American Journal of Psychotherapy*, 12, 199–221.

Wilson, R. S. (1967). Analysis of autonomic reaction patterns. *Psychophysiology*, 4, 125–142.

Zahn, T. P., & Kreusi, M. J. P. (1993). Autonomic activity in boys with disruptive behavior disorders. *Psychophysiology*, 30, 605–614.

Zuckerman, M., Hodgins, H. S., Zuckerman, A., & Rosenthal, R. (1993). Contemporary issues in the analysis of data. *Psychological Sciences*, 4, 49–53.

Biosignal Processing

GABRIELE GRATTON

1. INTRODUCTION

This chapter reviews issues related to the analysis of psychophysiological data. It focuses on general questions, which are relevant to a variety of techniques, rather than specific issues related to individual methods. Another chapter in this book (Jennings & Stine, this volume) also deals with statistical issues in psychophysiology, and focuses on issues of inference and data interpretation.

1.1. Stages of data processing

In describing the procedures used in analyzing psychophysiological data, it is useful to distinguish among different stages of analysis. The **first stage** is *signal-enhancement* and elimination of observations that are artifactual or can be considered outliers. This stage, sometimes called "signal-conditioning," involves, at least in part, techniques that are specific to each type of physiological measure.

The **second stage** involves *data reduction* (sometimes called "quantification" or "parameter extraction"). Most psychophysiological experiments include a large number of observations per subject (i.e., dependent variables). Whereas this provides data sets that are rich in information content, it also increases the probability of spurious or noisy observations. In general, one of the main objectives of signal processing is maximizing the signal-to-noise ratio. A large number of observations may contain many different signals to study, but may also contain a large amount of noise. It is advantageous, therefore, to select information that is relevant and to minimize redundancy between the dependent variables entered in the statistical analysis. Redundant dependent variables will not necessarily increase the signal, yet they may generate additional opportunities for noise to be present. An important step in signal processing is to reduce the data set to the smallest possible number of dependent variables (each variable affected by the smallest possible amount of noise) while preserving the information content of the original data set as much as possible. However, a moderate degree of redundancy may be useful in distinguishing random noise from systematic noise, thus making it possible to derive a valid and reliable estimate of the "signal."

The **third stage** of data processing is *statistical analysis*, which may include hypothesis testing, model fitting, parameter estimation, and so forth. As mentioned earlier most psychophysiological experiments are multivariate in nature – that is, they involve repeated observations from the same subjects. The multivariate nature of psychophysiological measures is one of their greatest assets: it allows for the experimenters to view phenomena from different "points of view," thus affording a more complete and detailed picture of bodily phenomena. However, it often introduces special types of problems in the statistical evaluation of data sets. Two general approaches can be considered: the *univariate approach*, which considers one dependent variable at a time, and the *multivariate approach*, which considers all dependent variables, as well as their covariation, together (see Huberty & Morris, 1989). Each of these approaches has advantages and disadvantages. In general, when there is a limited number of subjects in the study (relative to the number of dependent variables), and the dependent variables tend to be correlated with each other across conditions (or groups) in the same manner as within conditions (or groups), the univariate approach is more powerful. The multivariate approach is preferable when there is a large number of subjects in the study (relative to the number of dependent variables), and the within- and between-condition (or group) correlations among dependent variables add important information, as it is the when the dependent variables tend to go in opposite directions. (The statistical analysis stage is treated in the chapter by Jennings and Stine, and will not be considered in detail here).

In concluding this section, it is important to remind the reader that the output of an analysis is only as good as its input (this is captured by the well-known aphorism "garbage in, garbage out"). Complex and sophisticated data analyses in no way can be substituted for clear experimental hypotheses, elegant experimental designs, or accurate data collection procedures. However, they can complement these steps by providing clear and convincing data.

1.2. General issues

Psychophysiological data vary along a number of dimensions, and different types of data propose different types of analytical problems and solutions to the investigator. However, there are a few overarching themes that are valid for most types of measurements. Some general issues are particularly important and worth mentioning early in this chapter. **First**, *psychophysiological measures are typically indirect*. In other words, they are measures of events occurring outside the human body, which are related to events that occur inside the body. For instance, measures of the electrical activity produced by the body (such as the electrocardiogram (EKG) or the electroencephalogram (EEG)) are in fact measures of the difference in potential between two electrodes located on the surface of the body. Another example is positron emission tomography (PET), which measures the arrival of high-energy (gamma) photons to particular detectors located at some distance from the body, which, in turn, is related to the concentration of radioactive substances in various areas of the body. In general, psychophysiological measures are subject to some transformation with respect to the original signal generated within the body because of physical, physiological, or psychological reasons. This transformation may partially distort the signal (as well as its statistical properties) and may occasionally generate artifacts that need to be recognized and eliminated from the data before the statistical analysis is performed.

Second, most of the *data are sampled in a discrete fashion* both temporally and spatially. The transformation of analog parameters into discrete measures may distort the signal and require specific solutions to statistical problems. One of the major problems is obtaining a representative sample of the variable of interest, both over time and space. In addition, some techniques (e.g., measures of heart rate acceleration or deceleration) may be based on the observation of internal events (e.g., the occurrence of an R-wave in the EKG) whose spacing is variable (and, in the case of heart rate changes, is a function of the variable of interest). This may make it more difficult to compare observations across trials and subjects. Investigators using these measures have developed special approaches to address this problem (see the chapter on autonomic measures).

Third, most *psychophysiological measures are "multiply determined."* In other words, measures are determined by the interaction of a variety of factors. Some of these factors may be extraneous to, and uncorrelated with, the experimental manipulations and, therefore, will contribute to the statistical noise On the other hand, other factors may be related to the experimental manipulations in ways that are different from those intended by the researcher, which will contribute to both the statistical noise and the systematic effects. The latter type of factors are particularly insidious

and difficult to eliminate. One of the most important characteristics of good experimental methodology is the use of appropriate control procedures that distinguish between signal and systematic noise.

Fourth, most *psychophysiological measures are inherently noisy*, which make it difficult to distinguish between signal and noise in raw (single trial) observations. Several techniques have been developed to extract the signal from the noise. One of the simplest is signal averaging: a measure is repeated several times and the individual responses are then averaged together. Signal averaging is based on the central limit theorem, and can, therefore, be expected to provide reasonable estimates of the expected central tendency of the population in a large number of situations, provided that enough trials are used. Note that for signal averaging to work appropriately, it is important that the expected value of the noise be equal to zero across trials. Although this is a reasonable assumption in many cases, there are certainly situations in which it is not true. For instance, as we will see in section 3.2.2, frequency analysis (such as the Fourier transform) can be used to estimate the "power," or variance, associated with a particular frequency. Because this value cannot be less than zero, the average of the power values for a particular frequency obtained in different trials (or in different subjects) will always be greater than zero, even if no systematic activity exists at that frequency.

A problem with signal averaging is that it eliminates potentially relevant information about the trial-to-trial (and in some cases subject-to-subject) variability of the signal. This variability is entirely attributed to stochastic phenomena. However, in most cases the variability of the signal is not entirely random, but depends on the influence of intervening variables. For instance, in an experiment that evaluates the size of the visual evoked potential as a function of stimulus intensity, the size of the response may also be influenced by subjects' variables (e.g., allocation of attention or emotional factors), contextual conditions (e.g., stimulus sequence or noise in the environment), or other factors. When signal averaging is used, all of these intervening variables are treated as contributors to stochastic noise and are ignored. This may lead to loss of information or to systematic errors when contingencies exist between the experimental manipulations of interest and any of the intervening variables. Similar problems have been described with respect to other types of measures (see Estes, 1956; Siegler, 1987).

Another problem with signal averaging is that the signal may vary along dimensions other than intensity. In some cases, the latency of the phenomenon or its spatial location may vary from trial to trial (partly because of the reasons outlined above). In these cases signal averaging may produce systematic distortions, the most typical of which is a "smearing" of the response across different data points (or spatial locations). The effect of smearing is more intense for signals with a steep gradient. In cases of electrophysiological signals that vary quickly over

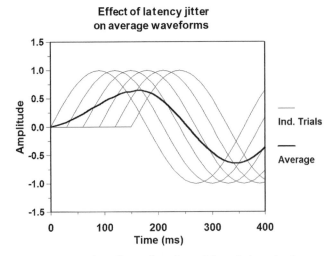

Figure 35.1. The effect of trial-to-trial variations in latency (latency jitter) on the amplitude of a an averaged psychophysiological activity. In this example, the latency of the first positive peak varies systematically in latency between 90 and 270 ms. Although the amplitude of the peak on single trials (indicated by thin lines) is always equal to one, the amplitude of the peak of the average waveform (indicated by the thick line) is considerably smaller (slightly larger than 0.5). The duration of the activity also appears prolonged.

time, smearing leads to the phenomenon of "latency jitter": the size of an evoked electrophysiological activity may be underestimated when using signal averaging because the activity "peaks" at different latencies on individual trials. A similar problem exists when data from different subjects are pooled together (for a discussion of this problem and some solutions, see Möcks, Köhler, Gasser, & Pham, 1988). Interestingly, the development of brain imaging methods, which have strong gradients in the spatial domain, has led to the recognition of a similar smearing problem in which average spatial maps are computed across subjects because of intersubject variability in brain anatomy. The effect of latency jitter is illustrated in Figure 35.1. Note that this problem is not specific to psychophysiological measures. For instance, investigators in psychology have long recognized that apparently smooth, speed-accuracy functions may result from the mixture of distributions of fast responses with a low level of accuracy and slow responses with a high level of accuracy in which the two distributions have some degree of partial overlap in response time (Yantis, Meyer, & Smith, 1991).

In order to address the smearing problem, several investigators have proposed to measure psychophysiological phenomena on single trials (or subjects). A critical step of this procedure is the development of techniques for identifying target features on single trial records. These techniques, although quite varied, can be grouped under the label of "pattern-recognition" algorithms. Some of them are based on visual inspection of individual data, and are most useful when the target features are much larger than the noise. Other techniques are "computer-controlled," and based on statistical approaches such as

cross-correlation, auto-correlation methods, as well as other automatic methods. The individual records may then be aligned along the target feature and averaged together. Alternatively, some measure of the single record distribution other than the mean can be used. An example of an alignment methodology in the time domain is the Woody filter (Woody, 1967), which is a general-purpose statistical method; an example in the spatial domain is the alignment method proposed by Talairach and Tournoux (1988), a special purpose approach, which has become standard practice in brain imaging.

2. GENERAL CLASSIFICATIONS

Psychophysiological measures are usually defined as noninvasive measures of bodily functions taken with the intent of addressing issues that are relevant to psychologists and cognitive neuroscientists. This broad definition encompasses a large variety of measures that differ along a number of dimensions. Of these dimensions, some are important for the purposes of the present chapter because they result in different types of signal processing problems. I will pay particular attention to three of these dimensions.

2.1. Fast versus slow measures

As mentioned above, psychophysiological measures reflect bodily changes that are related to psychological phenomena. These changes occur over time. Some of them evolve very quickly (within a few milliseconds) and others quite slowly (over seconds, minutes, or even longer times). Indeed, it is possible to consider a parameter that will indicate the speed at which the activity evolves for each type of psychophysiological measure used. We can refer to this parameter as the "time constant" of a particular physiological measure. This time constant depends on three factors: (a) the rate of change of the relevant psychological phenomenon; (b) the time required by the physiological event being measured to track changes in the underlying psychological phenomenon; and (c) the time required for the measurement.

By and large, it is possible to consider individual time-delay functions for each of these steps, although in some cases interaction terms should also be considered. Note that each step may itself comprise several substeps. Each step can be considered as having an input, which comes from the previous step, and an output, which influences the next step. However, a delay will usually occur in the operation of translating an input into an output. An example of a function expressing this delay can be the following:[1]

$$O_t - O_{t-1} = (I_t - OI_{t-1})^*(1 - e^{-1/tc}) \qquad (35.1)$$

[1] Note that this formula may not apply to all cases, and is only provided as an example of the typical influence of delaying factors on the time course of physiological measures. In fact, not only the time course but also the intensity of the output with respect to the input may vary from case to case.

Effect of intervening steps

on the time course of measures

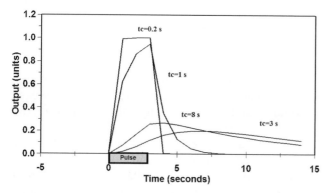

Figure 35.2. Simulated example of a series of individual steps between an input (pulse) and a final output measure. The input is a 3 second pulse (this may simulate a short duration stimulation). Each step introduces a delay, which is described by a parameter called time constant (see text). Four steps were simulated, with time constants, respectively, of 0.2, 1, 8, and 3 seconds.

In this function, the change in the output ($O_t - O_{t-1}$) of a particular step is a delayed function of the difference between its input I_t and its previous level O_{t-1}. The delay is determined by an exponential function whose critical parameter is tc, which is the *time constant* of that particular step. When several steps are involved, the total time-delay function is determined by a convolution of the individual functions. That is, the total time constant of a measurement is related to the integration of the time constants of each individual step. An example of this cascade, and of its effect on the final output measure, is illustrated in Figure 35.2. In this example, the initial input is a 3 second pulse (which is intended to simulate a brief stimulation). Four steps were simulated, with time constants of 0.2, 1, 8, and 3 seconds, respectively (for each step, the output serves as the input for the next step). Note that the final output is substantially delayed with respect to the input, and actually peaks well after the termination of the pulse (i.e., of the stimulation).

The steps contributing most to the total time constant are called "rate limiting" steps (step 3 and, to a smaller extent, step 4 in the example). Although all factors determining the measurement time constant (i.e., rate of change of the psychological event, delay of the physiological phenomena, and measurement time) are always present to some extent, there is often one (or a few) "rate limiting" factor. The nature of the rate limiting factor and the measurement time constant vary between different physiological measures. I will label measures with a long time constant "slow" measures and measures with a short time constant "fast" measures.

The following can be considered examples of slow measures: (a) measures of the electrodermal activity (EDA) in which the psychological or the physiological phenomena evolve slowly over time; (b) functional magnetic resonance imaging (fMRI) in which the physiological event

under study (e.g., a change in blood oxygenation) evolves slowly; and (c) PET (in which, in addition to a delay in the hemodynamic or metabolic response with respect to the triggering event, the actual measurement time is also relatively slow. Fast measures include (a) event-related brain potentials (ERPs); the magnetoencephalogram (MEG); (c) the electromyogram (EMG); and (d) the event-related optical signal (EROS). In all these cases, all three factors mentioned above are fast measures. Some other measures, for instance, heart rate and pupil diameter, are intermediate between these two extremes.

Measures with a short time constant have a good temporal resolution (i.e., the effects of two different psychological or physiological events occurring in rapid succession can be distinguished), whereas measures with a long time constant have a poor temporal resolution (i.e., events in rapid succession cannot be separated easily). This is illustrated in Figure 35.3 in which the time courses of the effect of two stimuli presented in rapid succession on measures with short and long time constants are compared.

Measures with a slow time constant provide few independent observations per unit time. In contrast, measures with a fast time constant provide a large number of independent observations over the same time unit. The processing of psychophysiological data usually requires transformation of the data into a series of numbers sampled over time (i.e., a time series). Then an issue arises: what is the optimal temporal sampling strategy for each type of measure? This sampling strategy must preserve the information contained in the signal as much as possible.

Comparison between measures

with short and long time constants

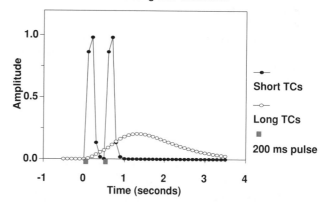

Figure 35.3. Simulated example of the response of output measures with short and long time constant to two stimulations in rapid succession. Two 200 ms stimulation pulses were presented, separated by an interval of 300 ms. This is intended to simulate two independent psychological events. The closed-circle line is obtained by assuming a cascade of three intervening steps between the stimulation and the measurement system, each introducing a delay characterized by a time constant of 200 ms. The open circle line is obtained by assuming a cascade of three intervening steps with time constants of 5 seconds. Note that short time-constant measure affords easy separation of the two pulses (i.e., psychological events), whereas the effects of the two pulses on the long time-constant measures are lumped together.

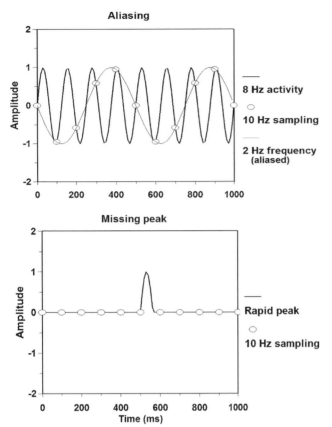

Figure 35.4. *Top:* The effect of sampling at a frequency lower than the Nyquist frequency (aliasing). The signal (indicated by the thick line) is sampled at 10 Hz (indicated by the open circles), which is less than the Nyquist frequency of 16 Hz. The result is an apparent 2 Hz signal (indicated by the thin line). *Bottom:* A rapid activity (duration = 62.5 ms) is measured using a 10-Hz sampling rate. In this particular case, the activity occurs in between two sampling points (open circles) and the peak is not detected by the measurement system.

The minimum sampling frequency at which information is maintained is twice the frequency of the signal, which is called the "Nyquist frequency." At sampling rates slower than the Nyquist frequency, aliasing causes a high frequency signal to manifest itself as a lower frequency signal. This phenomenon is illustrated in the top portion of Figure 35.4. Also, a sampling frequency that is too slow may completely miss the occurrence of a very fast, transient phenomenon. This is illustrated in the lower portion of Figure 35.4. To avoid the risk of aliasing, investigators may wish to sample at the highest possible frequency. However, it should be remembered that, because each observation will contain both signal and noise, it is important to minimize the number of data points (i.e., dependent variables) entered into the statistical analysis. This may be achieved conveniently at the data reduction stage. Finally, some recording systems impose limitations on the maximum sampling rate. However, the issue of aliasing should always be considered when studying physiological variables. This problem is likely to occur when fast phenomena are studied using a relatively slow sampling rate (e.g.,

when EEG is measured at <20 Hz, EKG at <2 Hz, and respiration at <0.5 Hz).

2.2. Direct versus indirect measures

Psychophysiological measures also differ in the number of intervening steps that occur between the physiological phenomenon, which is the "real" target of the study (e.g., neuronal activity, sympathetic, or parasympathetic activation), and the actual physiological measure that is taken (e.g., scalp electrical activity, increased blood flow, increased heart rate, or increased EDA). The "indirect" nature of these measures may have several consequences. **First**, as we mentioned earlier, it may introduce a lag between the psychological event of interest and the observed changes. **Second**, each of the intervening steps may introduce distortions in the size or shape of the observations compared with the original signal.

A particularly important issue related to the indirect nature of psychophysiological measures is that of the "linearity" of the relationship between the measure and the underlying phenomenon of interest. A measure M is linearly related to an inferred psychophysiological variable θ if the following formula is valid:

$$M = k^*\theta + \textit{offset} \qquad \textit{with } k \neq 0 \qquad (35.2)$$

For all practical purposes, it may be sufficient that this formula is valid (at least approximately) for an interval of values of M and θ, provided that this interval contains the typically observed values of the measure and the expected range of the psychophysiological factor. Note that in order for the linearity assumption to be valid, two terms must remain constant across conditions in this formula: the proportionality factor k and the measurement *offset*. The proportionality factor k depends on variables such as the relationship between the psychophysiological phenomenon of interest and the physical phenomenon actually measured, which includes the propagation of the physiological measure to the surface, the recording and analysis procedures employed, and so forth. An example of a potential change in the proportionality factor is a change in the way neuronal signals are transformed into a hemodynamic phenomenon in young and old adults, which depends on the health of the subject's cardiovascular system. Similarly, increases in neuronal activity at occipital and frontal locations may result in different increases in the scalp electrical signal measured over these areas because of different thickness of the skull in frontal and occipital regions. The offset factor may also depend on the effect of variables other than the physiological phenomenon of interest. For instance, an apparent increase in the amplitude of the ERP at frontal electrodes may be the consequence of an increase in the ocular artifact. Similarly, head movements may result in apparent large changes in the fMRI signal.

Another interesting example for psychophysiologists is the difference between measures of EDA. Two such measures are possible: (a) measures of the electrical *conductivity* between two locations on the skin, and (b) measures of the electrical *resistance* between the same locations. These two measures are inversely related to each other. However, the physiological phenomenon of interest (e.g., increase in conductivity associated with the activity of the sweat glands) is directly proportional to conductivity and inversely proportional to resistance. Therefore, in this example, conductivity is a linear measure of the physiological phenomenon, whereas resistance is not. Quigley and Berntson (1996) have pointed out that a similar case can be made for measures of heart rate compared to heart period, which are reciprocal to each other. Heart period, but not heart rate, appears to vary linearly with basic autonomic activation.

Linearity is useful because it allows for linear transformations of measure *M* (such as additions, subtractions, multiplications by a constant, and averaging), as well as the physiological variable θ, to be considered valid. Linear manipulations of the observed measures are commonly performed in the analysis of psychophysiological data. However, if the relationship between *M* and θ is nonlinear (i.e., if *k* or the offset are not constant), these types of operations, which are performed on the dependent variable, may not be valid with respect to the psychophysiological variable. Therefore, inferences should not be drawn because they may be misleading.

Lack of linearity may occur whenever any of the intervening steps between the observed measure and the psychophysiological construct of interest involve some form of nonlinear transformations. For example, consider the steps occurring between the onset of neuronal activity in response to a stimulus and the subsequent increased O_2^{15}-PET response. These steps may include the release of some chemical by the active neurons, subsequent local vasodilation, increased regional blood flow, and, if a radioactive tracer is introduced in the blood flow, increased radioactivity in a particular volume of the head. In principle, the relationships between causes and effects that exist at each step may be nonlinear or even nonmonotonic. In other words, it is not necessarily the case that a certain percent increase in neuronal activity is followed by an equal percent increase in vasodilation. Therefore linearity needs to be assessed on a case-by-case basis. In the case of PET responses, Fox and Raichle (1984) observed a nearly linear relationship between frequency of visual stimulation (within a range between 0 and 7.8 Hz) and changes in blood flow in primary visual cortex as estimated using O_2^{15}-PET method (see Figure 35.5). The presence of linearity was considered critical for the application of "subtraction" methods during the analysis of hemodynamic responses.

If the linearity assumption is not met, it is still possible that the relationship between the dependent variable and the physiological phenomenon is monotonic. Although a monotonic relationship may limit the use of linear transformations and of parametric statistics,

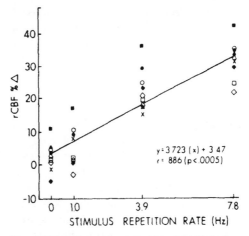

Figure 35.5. From Fox & Raichle (1984): the linearity of the relationship between stimulation frequency and blood flow measures obtained with O_2^{15}-PET.

it is still sufficient for the application of nonparametric statistics based on qualitative judgments about effect sizes. Finally, relationships that are nonlinear, but follow a more complex function, are susceptible of transformations that can make them linear (e.g., the transformation of electrodermal resistance measures into conductance measures).

So far I have discussed the linearity of the relationship between the observed measures and the physiological parameter they intend to measure. To the extent that psychophysiological measures are used to make psychological inferences, it is also important to consider the type of relationship that exists between the physiological parameter and the underlying psychological concept being investigated. For instance, the purpose of measuring neuronal activity in a certain brain area may be the investigation of memory or attention phenomena, and the purpose of measuring blood pressure may be the investigation of the effect of psychological stressors on the cardiovascular system. Clearly, the issue of linearity (or at least of monotonicity) of the relationship is just as important here as in the case of the relationship between the observed measure and the physiological variable.

2.3. Continuous versus discrete measures

The distinction between continuous and discrete measures refers to the time at which information about the status of the physiological system under study is in principle available. Some psychophysiological measures can provide information at any time with no particular restriction. For instance, the diameter of the pupil can be monitored continuously, and provide a more or less continuous measure of the level of activation for particular subcomponents of the autonomic system. The EMG and EEG are continuous measures of the electric potentials produced by muscle and brain tissue, respectively. However, other physiological measures, such as measures of the heart rate and respiration rate, reflect modification of parameters of cyclic events that occur at some intervals within the body. For these measures, information about psychological phenomena may be available only at discrete times. For instance, the state of activation of some subcomponents of the autonomic system can be studied using changes in heart rate, but information is available only when the heart beats (or when a particular EKG wave, e.g., the R-wave, is produced). Still other measures can only be obtained by using particular maneuvers that elicit special responses in the body. For instance, parameters of the blink reflex can only be measured by eliciting the blink reflex itself. Therefore, if the interest is in using the blink reflex to monitor changes in the status of a particular physiological system (e.g., one related to emotion), information may only be available at specific times (see Bradley, Cuthbert, & Lang, 1991). A similar situation is obtained when the P300 component of the ERP elicited by secondary task probes is used to monitor the level of attention of subjects to primary task stimuli (see Wickens, Kramer, Vanasse, & Donchin, 1983).

I will label those measures that can provide information about the state of a physiological system at any time "continuous," and those measures that provide information only at specific times "discrete." An advantage of continuous measures is that information about the time course of psychological phenomena is readily available on single trial records. Discrete measures can also provide information about the time course of psychological events, but their effective sampling rate is limited by the interval between the successive measurement windows. Finer sampling rates require pooling information obtained across trials, and are more complicated to obtain. An additional problem with some discrete measures is that the time at which information is available may not be completely under experimental control. For instance, certain measures related to circadian rhythms can only be obtained unobtrusively when the subject is awake. This may result in a "variable" sampling rate that may complicate the analysis. For example of solutions to this problem see Monk and Fookson (1986) and Monk (1987). Measures of heart interbeat interval changes as a function of the time at which the stimulus is shown during a cycle can also present special problems of identification because the time at which measures are available (i.e., the next heart beat) varies depending on the phenomenon under study. Appropriate representation of the effects requires special techniques (see Jennings, van der Molen, Somsen, & Ridderinkhof, 1991).

3. SIGNAL EXTRACTION AND ENHANCEMENT

3.1. Domains of analysis

Psychophysiological data can be considered as elements of a multidimensional matrix. We can consider the following dimensions specific to psychophysiological measures:

(a) type of measure, (b) time of sampling (or time with respect to some anchoring event), and (c) location in space (comprising one, two, or three subdimensions). Other dimensions may also be considered, such as experimental condition, subject, group, and so forth, but these dimensions are not specific to psychophysiological measures. Because some of the dimensions are typically grouped together (such as the three spatial axes) it is useful to talk about domains of analysis (such as temporal domain and spatial domain).

For some, and perhaps most, experiments some of these dimensions may have only one cell and are, therefore, fixed. For instance, we may record only data from one location or for one psychophysiological measure. It is important, however, to consider that different values on each of these dimensions all refer to the same individual case, and, as a consequence, possibly may be correlated. Thus, psychophysiological data can be expressed as elements of a multidimensional measurement matrix:

$$M_{m,t,x,y,z,c,s} \tag{35.3}$$

Note that each element of the measurement matrix $\nu \chi \xi M \nu H \chi \xi$ has several indices corresponding to the type of measure used (m), the time of observation (t), the spatial coordinates of the observation (x, y, and z), the conditions of observation (c), and the subject from whom the measure is recorded (s). A graphic representation of the multidimensionality of psychophysiological data is presented in Figure 35.6.

The fundamental multidimensionality of psychophysiological data creates special problems in the statistical analysis. In fact, the probability of spurious observations (i.e., alpha error) increases with the number of observations, although typically not linearly. Whereas it is essential that appropriate controls are made to reduce the probability of reaching conclusions on the basis of spurious observations (i.e., rejecting the null hypothesis when it is true), it is also equally important to maintain an acceptable probability of reaching some conclusion in the presence of noisy data (i.e., to maintain adequate power).

An additional problem is that the large number of qualifiers (i.e., indices) used for each observation may sometimes make it difficult to generalize the results. For instance, if an ERP peak is observed at a latency of 400 ms in condition A and at a latency of 600 ms in condition B, should it be concluded that the same ERP peak is delayed in condition B compared to condition A or that an altogether different type of ERP activity occurs in the two conditions?

To address these issues it is usually convenient to perform some intermediate analytical (or signal processing) steps between the level of observation of the raw data and the inferential statistical analysis *per se*, in which the data are used to provide support for or against theoretical arguments. These preliminary steps were previously labeled "data reduction" or "quantification." A consequence of

Multivariate nature of psychophysiological data

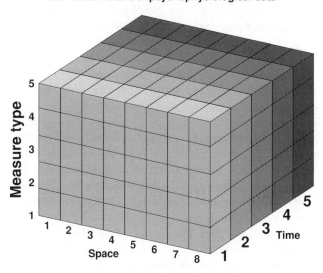

Figure 35.6. Graphic representation of the multidimensional nature of psychophysiological measures. Only three dimensions, specific to psychophysiological measures, are represented here (space, time, and type of measure). However, space itself may comprise several dimensions, and other dimensions (such as subject and experimental condition) are not represented. Note that the combination of different dimensions generates a large number of different observations for each subject. Because these are all observations from the same subjects, they may reflect different facets of the same phenomenon. Changes along one dimension may therefore be correlated to changes on another dimension.

these preliminary analysis steps is that the data should be no longer considered as "raw" observations, but as quantifications of parameters of some intermediate hypothetical construct that has heuristic value and is usually thought of as corresponding to some anatomical or physiological "entity" (e.g., activity in a particular brain structure in response to a particular stimulation condition or the blink response). In all cases, the data reduction implies some "interpretation" of the data. In other words, an analytical model is applied that makes more or less explicit assumptions about the underlying structure of the observed phenomenon, and involves some mathematical or logical transformation of the original "raw" data in order to estimate the value of some parameter of the underlying structure. The quality of the conclusions drawn from an experiment depends critically on the validity of these assumptions.

3.2. Temporal domain

3.2.1. Time domain and frequency domain

The time factor can be analyzed according to one of two basic models. According to the first model, the physiological events in the period under study evolve in a temporally ordered series that exhibits nonstationary properties (i.e., the basic structure of the activity changes over time). An example of data that fit this model well is the sequence of responses that occur in the brain after the presentation

of an individual stimulus. Another example is the changes in heart rate before and after the presentation of a critical stimulus. In these cases, it is profitable to use time as the main dimension of analysis (i.e., "time domain" analysis). Usually, particular aspects of the time series (such as maximum, minimum, integrated amplitude over an interval or a particular wave shape) are considered target features, and parameters of these features (such as amplitude, latency, or similarity with a particular template) are quantified and entered in the statistical analysis. In addition, time series can be averaged together (with or without alignment with respect to particular features) in order to increase the signal-to-noise ratio. This approach provides for a substantial data reduction, and data can be expressed in terms of properties of the target features. Averaging of ERP single trial waveforms and subsequent measurements of specific aspects of the waveforms (such as peaks) are exemplifications of this analytic approach.

The second model assumes that the basic structure of the activity does not vary over time and, therefore, exhibits stationary properties in which events repeat in a cyclical fashion. An example of data that appear to fit this model is the consistent response of the brain to a regular train of similar stimuli when habituation is not expected to play a role, and the oscillation in heart rate associated with respiration (sinus arrhythmia). When this model is appropriate, physiological activity can be analyzed by means of a set of tools that are able to extract the basic periodic structure of the activity – collectively referred to as "frequency domain" methods. In this case a new data series is built in which frequency replaces time as the ordering dimension, and data are expressed in terms of how much of the total variability over time is accounted for by fluctuations occurring at particular frequencies. Distinctive features of this new series can then be considered for quantification purposes (e.g., the "dominant" or most represented frequency in the data can be determined) in the same manner as time domain analyses. Frequency analyses may also provide information about the relative delay (or phase) at which particular rhythmic oscillations occur with respect to a reference time (such as the time of stimulation).

Recently, research has focused on mixed models, which assume that the presentation of a stimulus may lead to the *perturbation* of a basic oscillatory phenomenon. As a very simple example of this phenomenon, we may consider the change in the amplitude of the alpha rhythm (8–12 Hz) of the EEG that occurs when subjects open or close their eyes. Similarly, recent work has emphasized changes in gamma (approximately 40 Hz) and theta (4–8 Hz) rhythms that may accompany particular psychological processes (see Basar et al., 1999). Because it is assumed that a temporal event influences a specific rhythmic event, a mixed time-frequency model is required for the analysis.

3.2.2. Fourier analysis and autoregressive methods

Two types of analytic methods are most commonly used in the frequency domain: the Fourier transform and autoregressive methods. Both approaches express the original time series in terms of how much certain frequencies are present in the data. However, the Fourier transform is based on a "deterministic" approach. That is, it represents all of the information (variance) contained in the original data in terms of the independent contributions of equally spaced frequencies. Autoregressive methods (of which there are actually different varieties) are instead based on a "modeling" approach. That is, they impose some constraints on the way in which individual frequencies contribute to the original time series and do not necessarily represent all of the variance in the data. This modeling approach reduces the number of "free" parameters in the data (i.e., it reduces the dimensionality of the data). This may allow the investigator to separate signal from noise.

The Fourier transform is a numerical method commonly used in engineering and other disciplines. A prerequisite for its application is that the sampling rate is constant across a given epoch (for an example of frequency analysis techniques with irregular sampling see Monk, 1987). The basic logic of this method is that any given time series (e.g., a recording epoch) can be expressed equivalently (i.e., without loss of information or interpolation/extrapolation) in the time and frequency domains. In the frequency domain a time series can be expressed as the sum of several time series, each characterized by the equal-amplitude oscillations of sinusoidal functions with frequencies equal to a multiple of the inverse of the length of the time series (e.g., if the recording epoch is one second long, then the frequencies used to describe it will be 1 Hz, 2 Hz, 3 Hz, etc.), plus an offset term related to the mean value across data points (usually called "0 frequency" or "DC value"). The number of frequencies is equal to the number of elements in the time series divided by two. So, if we are sampling a one second epoch at 128 Hz, the Fourier decomposition will be based on one DC value and 64 basic frequencies (1 Hz, 2 Hz, 3 Hz,..., 64 Hz). Each basic frequency is associated with an *amplitude* value, related to how large the oscillation is at that particular frequency, and a *phase* value, related to the relative timing of the peak of the first oscillation with respect to the beginning of the time series. Derivation of the Fourier transform is numerically complex, and requires a number of exponential operations proportional to the square of the number of elements in the time series. Therefore, application of the Fourier transform to long time series may be cumbersome. Fortunately, when the number of elements in a time series is a power of 2 (e.g., 4, 8, 16, 32, 64, 128) the numeric problem simplifies and can be carried out using a procedure called the Fast Fourier Transform (FFT).

The outcome of the Fourier transform is a complex number associated with each frequency, in which the real and imaginary parts both contain information associated with the amplitude and phase of the basic oscillations. The real and imaginary components can be thought of as corresponding to the coordinates of a vector in a com-

plex plane. However, it is most convenient to express the results in terms of the polar coordinates of this vector (i.e., length and angle or orientation). This transformation separates the *amplitude* (equivalent to the length of the vector) and *phase* (equivalent to the orientation of the vector) associated with each frequency. Although informative, it should be remembered that this transformation is not linear. Therefore, data averaging (or other linear operations) are appropriately performed prior to this transformation.

These operations yield a set of phase and amplitude values for each frequency. In most cases, the attention of the investigators focuses on the amplitude data, although there are exceptions, such as in the study of visual evoked potentials (Tomoda, Celesia, & Taleikis, 1991). A common way of displaying the results is by plotting amplitude as a function of frequency (also known as the "periodogram"). In some cases, instead of the amplitude of each oscillation frequency, the data are expressed in terms of the square of this amplitude. This is called the "power" of a particular frequency. Amplitude and power are the frequency domain equivalents of the standard deviation and variance in the time domain. Indeed, the sum of the power values for all frequencies is related to the total variance in the data. For this reason, the Fourier transform can also be used as a method for partitioning the variance observed in a time series into subcomponents with different frequencies. As a consequence, it is possible to apply some of the standard tools used for analyzing variance (e.g., chi square test and analysis of variance) to power frequency analysis. Finally, it is a common practice to pool together the power for an interval of frequencies within a certain range (i.e., a frequency band). For example, in an EEG study we may be interested in quantifying the total power for frequencies ranging between 8 and 12 Hz (usually called the alpha band) and in a heart rate study on sinus arrhythmia we may wish to quantify the power for frequencies between 0.2 and 0.5 Hz (i.e., the respiration frequency range).

As mentioned above, the Fourier transform is based on the observation that any time series can be decomposed in a number of sinusoidal waves that extend with equal amplitude across the entire time series. Although mathematically valid in all cases, this way of describing the data may, in some cases, produce results that require further interpretation. This occurs for several reasons.

First, there may be cases in which the oscillations in the time series can be best described by functions other than a sinusoid. For instance, the pressure waves that propagate through the arteries after a heart beat are, at first approximation, triangular in shape (see the upper portion of Figure 35.7). When the shape of the oscillations departs from sinusoidal, the Fourier transform will decompose each wave into subcomponents (called "harmonics"), with each subcomponent having a frequency that is a multiple of the basic frequency (called "fundamental") at which the wave repeats. As an example of this decomposition, the periodogram of the saw-tooth arterial pressure waves is reported at the bottom of Figure 35.7. Note that the

Peripheral pulse measurement
obtained with optical measures

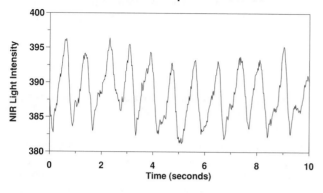

Periodogram of pulse data

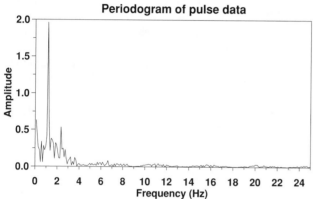

Figure 35.7. Top: Recording of the peripheral pulse from one subject during a psychological experiment obtained with near-infrared (NIR) optical methods (see Gratton, 1997). Note that intensity of the NIR light drops rapidly approximately every 0.8 seconds. The drops correspond to the times at which the arterial blood is pushed into the blood vessels by the beating of the heart. Each drop is followed by a slower increase in the light intensity, which reflects the flow of the arterial blood out of the blood vessels. The quick drop in light intensity, followed by the slow increase, generates a triangular shaped ("saw-tooth") wave that repeats approximately every 0.8 seconds. **Bottom:** Amplitude spectrum ("periodogram") corresponding to the data reported in the top portion of the figure is obtained using an FFT method (the DC component is omitted). Note that the spectrum is dominated by a 1.2 Hz frequency, which corresponds to the heart beat frequency. However, activity is also evident at 2.4 Hz and at 3.6 Hz, which are the first and second harmonics of the fundamental 1.2 Hz frequency. The presence of activity at these frequencies reflects the fact the cyclical pattern is not sinusoidal.

periodogram indicates activity not only at the basic frequency (around 1.2 Hz) but also at some of its harmonics (such 2.4 Hz). The pattern of harmonics is related to the particular wave shape of the basic, cyclical pattern. Given that in most psychophysiological measures the basic wave shape is not a sinusoid, psychophysiologists are often interested in the patterns of the harmonics as much as in the fundamental frequency.

A second way in which data may depart from the description underlying the Fourier transform is when the type of activity observed in one part of the epoch differs substantially from activity in another part of the epoch. An

extreme case is that of "phasic" features, which appear only once in a time series. Phenomena of this type, which are observed frequently in psychophysiological data, may be difficult to study using Fourier-transformed data because the variance associated with them will be distributed in a very complex manner between the DC component and various frequencies. However, this variance will still be represented in some form in the Fourier transform. In other words, the partitioning of the variance obtained using Fourier transforms is best suited for phenomena that repeat cyclically along the time series (i.e., "stationary" waves).

3.2.3. Mixed time-frequency models

3.2.3.1. Joint time-frequency domain analysis. In recent years, combinations of time-domain and frequency-domain approaches have been introduced (see Stiber & Sato, 1997). The major justification for these hybrid techniques is the assumption that the way in which the brain processes information involves the rapid modulation of basic frequencies of activity. A frequency that has been considered as particularly important in brain activity is approximately 40 Hz (also called the "gamma" band; see Gray, Engel, Konig, & Singer, 1989). According to this view, information processing may involve the amplitude modulation of a 40-Hz activity. When a new stimulus is presented, the oscillations at this frequency increase in size. A converse phenomenon is in some cases observed for the alpha band ("alpha blocking" or "enhancement"; see Pfurtscheller & Neuper, 1992). Other examples include (a) the analysis of the modulation of sinus arrhythmia over time as a method for studying the time course of vagal activity, and (b) the analysis of EMG activity, which often involves the occurrence of a brief series of high-frequency oscillations (typically above 30 Hz).

In all these cases, although the psychological events are transient (and therefore evolve over time), their physiological manifestations involve the modulation of a cyclic phenomenon. To represent appropriately this modulatory phenomenon it is necessary to study the change over time of the amplitude of specific frequencies. This involves a segmentation of the time series in shorter epochs, the determination of the amplitude of the frequency of interest in each epoch (the analysis of which is performed in the frequency domain), and the analysis of the time course of modulation of the amplitude of the frequency of interest (the analysis of which is performed in the time domain). This procedure is labeled Joint Time-Frequency Analysis (or JTFA; see Tallon-Buadry, Bertrand, Delpnech, & Pernier, 1996). In the case of EMG, the response is often analyzed entirely in the time domain, and involves: (a) recording EMG data using a relatively high-frequency band-pass (10–100 Hz), (b) rectification of the waveforms (i.e., transformation of the negative values into positive values), and (c) low-pass filtering (typically below 20 Hz). This process is adequate for determination of latency measures, but requires recordings with low noise levels.

3.2.3.2. *Wavelet decomposition.* Another method combining features from both time- and frequency-domain analyses is the wavelet decomposition method (Samar et al., 1999). Similarly to the Fourier and autoregressive methods, this procedure is also based on decomposing a complex waveform into subcomponents (called wavelets), which when added together form the original waveform. However, different from the frequency-domain methods, it is not assumed that these basic wavelets are cyclic or stationary. Rather, they are allowed to vary in duration and latency as well as amplitude. This "modeling" effort can be used to reduce the dimensionality of the data and fit an underlying structure to a particular waveform. This approach can be particularly useful for single-trial analysis of EEG data.

3.2.4. Amplitude domain measures

All of the temporal-domain data processing steps outlined so far result in descriptions of the observed activity as a function of time, frequency, or a combination of both. However, in some cases, it is preferable to analyze the overall "amount" of observed activity, without expressing it as a function of time or frequency (Cacioppo & Dorfman, 1987). This may be appropriate when the time or frequency variable is considered irrelevant, or when variations of the measurement over time depend on factors that are not related to the physiological (or psychological) variable of interest. For instance, when the stimulation condition cannot be conveniently subdivided into specific time epochs or periodic events, it may be advantageous to consider the overall physiological response observed during an experiment, rather than considering the individual responses. An example of this is the number of electrodermal responses during the presentation of a particular videotape that is not characterized by clearly identifiable time markers. Another case is when measures cannot be taken repeatedly, or whose time of acquisition is longer than the time during which the experimental manipulations are performed. An example of this is deoxyglucose-PET data, in which measures of the amount of radioactive material accumulated in various brain areas are taken at the end of the experiment (Cherry & Phelps, 1996). The temporal dimension in this case is reduced to one data point, and absolute amplitude measures are taken. Finally, there are cases in which there is interest in summarizing a unique number for all the variability of observations obtained across an extended epoch (e.g., Elui, 1969; Dorfman & Cacioppo, 1990).

3.3. Spatial domain

3.3.1. Spatial dimensions

In recent years there has been a substantial growth of interest in the spatial characteristics of psychophysiological measures because they may correspond to the anatomy of the human body, particularly to the brain. A particular impulse for this enterprise has been given by the intro-

duction of functional neuroimaging methods, for example, single-photon emission computerized tomography (SPECT), near-infrared spectroscopy (NIRS), PET, fMRI, and EROS. Brain anatomy is not conveniently expressed using frequency-domain methods because of the fundamental uniqueness of the various structures, thus other methods of analysis are most commonly used. An exception, though, is given by the use of the Fourier transform approach in the decoding of spatial information in MRI. (see Cohen, 1996).

Psychophysiological measures differ in the number of spatial dimensions used, and in their relationship with underlying anatomy. Some measures refer to brain activity (e.g., EEG, ERPs, MEG, fMRI, PET, NIRS, and EROS), whereas others refer to the activity of other body structures (e.g., EKG and heart rate, EMG, pupillary diameter, measures of the blink response, measures of EDA, blood pressure, and respiration). Although measures of both brain activity and bodily functions can be taken at different locations, usually the second group is less directly dependent on brain anatomy than the first.[2]

All measures of brain activity produce substantially different results depending on the location at which they are taken. Some of these measures provide data that can be localized to specific brain volumes (e.g., PET, fMRI, NIRS, and EROS). For these measures any recorded value will have three indices, which refer to the x, y, and z spatial coordinates of the observed value. Other measures (e.g., ERPs and MEG) provide data that refer to surface observations and have, therefore, only x and y coordinates. For these measures algorithms have been proposed that allow for the reconstruction of depth information, and thus pinpoint brain structures that are responsible for the activity observed at the surface. However, these reconstruction algorithms require a modeling effort that, for both ERPs and MEG, has multiple solutions, which are equally valid from a statistical point of view. Therefore, limited confidence must be placed on the results.

Maps and tri-dimensional (3D) reconstructions obtained with various techniques can be evaluated on the basis of two major properties: (a) localization power (i.e., the ability to attribute a particular activity to a particular location), and (b) resolution (i.e., the ability to distinguish activity coming from two closely located points). These two properties are different and should not be confused. Some techniques may possess a very good spatial localization power, but limited spatial resolution. This occurs because, as is often the case, the larger the activity, the greater the space over which it can be detected

---

[2] There are, however, notable exceptions to this rule, in particular in the area of the study of reflexes. For instance, Hackley and Johnson (1996) have used properties of the blink response (a peripheral measure) to determine whether a particular phenomenon (pre-pulse inhibition) is under the control of cortical or sub-cortical structures (which is clearly an issue of localization of function within the brain). This indicates that, if appropriate experimental designs are used, peripheral measures can provide some information about the localization of function within the brain.

(even from outside of the location at which it is generated). Therefore, two closely spaced sources may end up being fused in one single "blob."

3.3.2. Analysis of surface data: Surface maps and 3D inference

As previously mentioned, some psychophysiological measures (ERPs and MEG) can be used to generate maps of the distribution of a particular physical parameter at the surface of the scalp. Usually, these maps are generated using a process of interpolation: a reduced number of surface observations, usually less than 50, but in some cases as many as 256, are used to derive representations of the activity over the whole head, or a segment of it. The interpolation procedure requires the assumption that the spatial sampling used represents the surface distribution of the underlying phenomenon in a satisfactory way.

When considering the time domain, an issue arises concerning the minimum spatial sampling required for producing representative electrical (and magnetic) maps of brain activity. In general, information theory indicates that the spatial resolution, but not necessarily the localization, is limited to twice the distance between two adjacent measurement locations. This is called the "spatial Nyquist frequency." At first glance, it may appear that a greater spatial sampling will result in maps with superior quality. Some investigators have shown that the information content increases with the number of recording locations (Srinivasan et al., 1996). Their results make intuitive sense. However, practical and theoretical problems may limit the advantage of increasing spatial sampling of ERP and MEG data. One limiting factor is the cost of the devices required to record and analyze data from a large number of channels. Another limiting factor is that measurement errors are likely to increase with the number of recording channels, which may effectively decrease the signal-to-noise ratio.

To illustrate this problem, let us suppose that an experimenter is interested in running an ERP study to determine where a potential reaches its maximum over the scalp. Let us also suppose that, in this experiment, there exists a .01 probability that a large, inaccurate value (i.e., an artifact) may influence the measures at any given electrode location, and if such an artifact occurs, the maps may identify a maximum at an erroneous location. If only a small number of electrodes are used (e.g., <10), the probability of a "false" maximum is relatively small (p < .10). Some confidence can be attributed to the results, although the spatial resolution will be very low. However, as the number of recording locations increases, the probability that at least at one location there will be an artifactual value also increases. Therefore, the probability of incorrectly localizing the maximum will also increase, and, if enough electrode locations are used (e.g., over 100) the probability of an incorrect localization would become very high (p > .63). In this case, little confidence could be attributed to the results. This emphasizes the need of using the "appropriate" number of recording locations. It also emphasizes the difference between spatial resolution and localization – procedures that enhance spatial resolution do not necessarily enhance localization, and vice versa.

As mentioned earlier, most maps are constructed using an interpolation process. There are various algorithms for interpolations. A relatively simple procedure involves using a linear interpolation to derive the values in between the observed locations. A problem with this method is that the maximum of activity in the maps is bound to be at one of the locations at which the recordings were obtained. However, more sophisticated techniques are now commonly used. Some of them are based on fitting polynomial surfaces, or other types of surfaces obtained with some form of smoothing function, through the various observed data points (e.g., spline interpolation; Perrin et al., 1987). These interpolations may increase the localization of activity in surface maps, but at the cost of a reduced spatial resolution. In addition, assumptions need to be made about the spatial frequencies contained in the data.

Some transformations of the surface maps may be useful for counteracting some limitations of the original observations. For instance, limitations of surface maps of the electrical potential over the scalp include: (a) the absolute value at each data point is dependent on the choice of reference, and (b) activity tends to be spread out across extended areas. This may make it difficult to appreciate differences between conditions. A way of addressing both of these issues is transforming the measures mapped from voltage difference into electric currents ("current source density," or CSD, maps). According to Ohm's law, currents flowing between two points are directly related to the differences in potential and inversely related to the resistance between the points. If the resistance is assumed to be constant, then current maps can be easily computed from voltage maps. In the case of the scalp, the current can be considered to flow almost exclusively along the skin, which is a path of lower resistance than the skull underneath. The flow of current in two dimensions can then be described as a current density, which is computed using the 2D spatial derivative of the voltage map. In practice, this provides a measure of a local gradient, which is independent of the definition of the reference level because a local reference system is used, and highlights local details of the maps. However, phenomena that extend across large areas become less visible. Furthermore, small error variance may be amplified by this method.

Whereas CSD maps (and other transformed maps) of surface potentials may be useful for highlighting differences between conditions, they should not be interpreted as 3D reconstructions of the activity inside the head. Such a reconstruction requires a model of (a) how the signal is generated inside the head, and (b) how it is transferred from interior sources to the surface. Both problems require different solutions depending on the type of measure adopted. For electrical activity (EEG and ERPs), the propagation of the potential to the scalp requires information about the conductive properties of various media interposed between the sources and the surface electrodes (such as gray and white matter, cerebrospinal fluid, bones, and skin). Furthermore, because of the relatively low frequency of the data, impedance is typically not considered an issue here. The transmission of magnetic fields is less influenced by departures from homogeneity in the media than that of electric fields. Until recently, all source analysis algorithms were based on abstract models of the head (e.g., the "three-sphere model"), which modeled the head as a simple geometric shape. In the last few years, realistic head models, which are derived by using MRI or computerize axial tomography (CAT) scans, have been adopted, and the propagation of activity to the surface has been computed using finite computation methods. However, knowledge about the *in vivo* conductive properties of head tissues is still imperfect and may create substantial errors in the computation.

Notwithstanding these problems, substantial developments have been made in the modeling of the sources of electrical and magnetic activity in the last 20 years. Three types of approaches can now be used:

1. *Regional source models.* This approach models the propagation of potentials or fields within the head, rather than their generation. It produces results that tend to be quite robust (i.e., it converges to similar results if small variations in the observed activities are compared), but has low spatial resolution (up to several cm; Pascual-Marqui, Michel, & Lehmann, 1994).

2. *Diffuse source models.* With this approach, it is usually assumed that activity is generated by a large number of sources, for instance, the entire cortical surface. To reduce the number of free parameters, some assumptions can be made, for example, that sources are normal to the cortical surface, have overall as little activity as possible (i.e., minimum norm), and are spatially smooth. Diffuse source models may possess intermediate spatial resolution, but their accuracy is difficult to evaluate because they are typically largely overdetermined or the number of free parameters to estimate is several orders of magnitude greater than the number of observations (Dale & Halgren, 2001).

3. *Point-dipole models.* These models can be taken at a particular time point, or combine information accrued over time, which generates "spatiotemporal" dipoles (Scherg & von Cramon, 1986). This approach has greater spatial resolution and localization power, but also a greater level of uncertainty about the number of modeled sources. By and large, source modeling of electrical activity and, to some degree, magnetic activity still requires external validation.

The problem of how to derive 3D reconstruction of data from data with lower dimensionality is not restricted to EEG, ERPs, and MEG, but is true for all imaging techniques. Each of these imaging methods solves the problem in a different way. CAT and PET scans use a large number of surface detectors to infer activity inside the brain. Both of them are based on high-energy radiation (photons) with minimum scattering. They use a form of 3D reconstruction that is based on inferring the distribution of activity inside the head from surface activity, which ignores variations in the local anatomy, but is entirely based on geometric and statistical principles.

Optical imaging methods (e.g., EROS) use light wavelengths at which scattering is the dominant phenomenon; further diffusion parameters (scattering and absorption coefficients) vary conspicuously between tissue types. Thus, a 3D reconstruction of optical imaging data needs to take into account these properties of the medium, similarly to EEG and ERPs. However, because the movement of photons inside the head is strongly limited by the scattering and absorption properties of the head, the spatial resolution of optical imaging is inherently much higher than that of methods based on electric potentials and magnetic fields.

Magnetic resonance imaging methods use a completely different approach to 3D reconstruction. Different from the instruments for electrophysiological, optical, and PET recordings, MR machines typically have one, or very few, detectors. In this case, to provide spatial information, the magnetic fields used to induce and measure the magnetization of individual nuclei are varied over time and space in a very special manner so to provide "tags" indicating where the signal originated. Whereas this technology provides, in principle, a very high spatial resolution, it generates a few problems: (a) there are limitations in how quickly the signal can be acquired, and (b) it is essential that the local variations in the magnetic fields are accurately predictable. To partially address this second issue, it is customary to "shim" the magnets before recording data. Nevertheless, characteristic artifacts are present when distortions in the magnetic fields occur because of, for example, the presence of metal prosthesis and dental work.

3.3.3. Analysis of 3D spatial data

Imaging methods provide 3D descriptions of how the signal is generated inside the body. If the data refer to changes in the strength of the signal as a consequence of the functioning of a particular organ, they are called "functional imaging methods." Examples of functional imaging methods include fMRI and PET. Functional imaging methods vary in terms of spatial resolution and localization power, as well as other dimensions (e.g., how direct the measures are and how much temporal resolution they possess). The localization power of some of these techniques constitutes their major advantage, but it also requires attention to a number of methodological issues. One of these issues is that the anatomy of some organs – the brain in particular – varies across individuals. Therefore, a signal that may appear at a particular location in one person may appear at another location in a different person. In order to generalize conclusions across people it is indispensable to "align" the data obtained in different individuals. This process requires re-scaling the various features of the anatomy of each single person to a "standard" anatomy, so that phenomena observed in different people can be directly compared.

A commonly used procedure to align different brain anatomies to a standard anatomy was introduced by Talairach and Tournoux (1988). According to this procedure, structural scans of brains of different individuals, which can be obtained using MRI or CAT scans, are first aligned using a set of basic anatomical features. The brain is then subdivided into regions, and each region is re-scaled independently to the dimensions of a standard provided by the Talairach and Tournoux atlas. This allows researchers to compare data across different subjects, in order to examine the reliability of findings, and compute "average" brain maps across subjects. Using the standard atlas, it is then possible to associate specific functional data to particular anatomical structures of the brain (e.g., the Brodmann cytoarchitectonic areas of the cortex). This procedure is likely to introduce small distortions because the large subdivisions used in the Talairach and Tournoux system may not capture all of the individual differences in anatomy. Furthermore, the subdivisions are based on subcortical, rather than cortical landmarks. Because the cortex is the most variable part of the human brain, the Talairach and Tournoux system can sometimes lead to significant alignment problems. Furthermore, the Talairach and Tournoux method is based on a single "model" brain. A variation of this approach is the Montreal Neurological Institute (MNI) model, which is based on a statistical average of a large number of brains. However, the Talairach and Tournoux transformation is a standard method that can provide useful approximations in a number of cases, and allows scientists to compare results obtained in different experiments and labs.

More recently, other alignment methodologies have been introduced, which take into account cortical features. Some of these methods preserve the 3D structure of the brain, whereas others generate flattened images of the cortical surface (Van Essen et al., 1998). These methods are generally based on complex warping algorithms in which each location on the surface of the cortex of a particular brain is associated, because of its relative position with respect to local landmarks, with a point in a standard 3D or flat representation of the cortex.

An additional problem with 3D spatial data is the huge number of dependent variables used. A 3D scan of the brain based on voxels (i.e., the small volumes used for sampling a large volume) with a 1.5–3 mm side may generate more than 100,000 data points, each of which should be considered as a dependent variable. This has two major consequences. First, multivariate techniques are difficult to apply to these data, unless a strong reduc-

tion in the number of points is considered. Second, even univariate analyses need to take into account the problem of multiple comparisons (i.e., the inflated probability of alpha error when a large number of comparisons are carried out). There are various solutions to this problem. One is to carry out analyses only for selected points, or regions, labeled regions-of-interest (ROIs). This, however, restricts the analysis to small portions of the brain. A second, simple solution to this problem is to apply the Bonferroni inequality, which consists in setting the criterion of alpha error for each comparison to *crit/nc*, where *crit* is the criterion normally used (e.g., .05) and *nc* is the number of comparisons (in this case, data points). This guarantees that the overall probability of alpha error is less than the original criterion. However, if the number of data points, or voxels, is large (e.g., 100,000) only data points whose statistical values are associated with extremely low probability values will be significant. Although this analysis would protect against alpha error, it would reduce the power of the study as to make it virtually useless.

A solution to this problem has been proposed by Friston (1996). This solution is based on the application to neuroimaging of random field theory (also called "blob" analysis), which was developed to deal with similar problems in other disciplines. Blob analysis is based on the idea that the observations obtained at different locations are not independent from each other – close voxels are likely to be similar to each other. This confers some level of "spatial smoothness" to the imaging data, and implies that the number of independent comparisons is in fact much smaller than the number of voxels recorded. In other words, although there may be 100,000 voxels recorded, there may be 1,000 or fewer independent comparisons. To determine what statistical level is needed to reach significance, it is important to establish the spatial smoothness of the data. A critical point is to establish the *spatial smoothness of the error term* and not that of the effect to be studied. This can be achieved in various ways. The most effective is based on the computation of the spatial derivative of the error term. This approach to the analysis protects against alpha errors and still maintains a reasonable power.

An interesting consequence of the use of spatial smoothness in the estimation of the statistical significance of the data is that the greatest power is obtained for data with high spatial smoothness. However, spatial smoothness can be considered as the reciprocal of spatial resolution – the higher the spatial resolution of the data, the smaller the spatial smoothness. Thus, in order to increase the power of a particular brain imaging technique it may be advantageous to reduce its spatial resolution. This may be easily achieved by "spatially filtering" the data (see section 3.4), so that data contain only relatively low spatial frequencies. In fact, most brain imaging studies use spatial filters that reduce spatial resolution to the order of 1 cm or less.

3.4. Filtering and artifact problems

One of the major issues in processing any type of data, in particular psychophysiological data, is that of distinguishing the signals of interest from noise. Noise can be broadly defined as any other phenomena observed in the data apart from the signal(s) of interest for the investigator. In general, the ability to distinguish signals from noise can be quantified using a construct called the "signal-to-noise" ratio, which is the amplitude ratio between the signal and the noise. The larger the signal-to-noise ratio, the easier it is to identify the signal. As a consequence, more reliance can be attributed to the observations. One of the major tasks of signal processing is to increase the signal-to-noise ratio. This can be achieved by amplifying the signal, reducing the noise, or both. In general, procedures or devices that reduce the amount of noise present in the data are called filters.

By and large, filters are based on the principle that the signal can be distinguished from the noise on the basis of some characteristic features. For instance, the signal may have a particular frequency that is different from that of the noise. Therefore, by amplifying the frequencies carrying the signal and dampening the frequencies carrying the noise, it is possible to increase greatly the signal-to-noise ratio. This is common practice in psychophysiological recording, and can be achieved while the data are recorded by the use of online, usually analog, filters or at any stage of data analysis with offline, usually digital, filters.

Generally filters are described in terms of the frequency at which they attenuate the signal. High-pass filters cut off activity with a frequency lower than a designated frequency, whereas low-pass filters cut off activity with a frequency higher than a designated frequency. Other types of filters, called notch filters, only cut off a very specific frequency (e.g., 60 Hz), and leave activity with lower or higher frequencies unaltered. Usually, the cut-off point of a filter indicates that at that point activity is reduced by 3 dB (approximately 70%). However, other parameters are important in describing the performance of a filter. Specifically, the performance of a filter is described by a "performance operating characteristic" (POC) function, which describes the proportional attenuation of the signal at different frequencies. Ideally, a filter should maintain all of the activity up (for low-pass filters) or down (for high-pass filters) to the cut-off frequency and eliminate all of the frequency above or below the cut-off frequency.

Most psychophysiological recordings involve online analog filters. The advantage of these filters is that they can reduce high frequencies before digitization occurs. This may reduce the possibility of aliasing high frequencies. As already mentioned, aliasing occurs when digitization is performed at a rate that is less than twice that of a frequency present in the data. In this case, activity at a high frequency will be reflected into activity at a lower frequency. Because aliasing cannot be eliminated once it occurs, it is very important to prevent it by filtering high frequencies before digitization. Another advantage of online filters is that they can be used to cut-off large noise oscillations, which usually occur at very low frequencies. These large oscillations may generate signals that are outside the operating range of the analog-to-digital converter, which will "saturate" (i.e., it will provide an output that corresponds to the maximum or minimum value allowed by the converter, but not to the actual value).

Online frequency filters, however, are usually recursive: filtering is based on the activity that has already occurred and not on the activity that has yet to occur. Therefore, they introduce a phase distortion in the data – phenomena may appear to peak at different times from when they actually do, or their shape may be distorted.[3] Online low-pass filters, which cut off high frequencies, tend to displace peaks to a later time than when they really occur. Online high-pass filters, which cut off low frequencies, tend to displace peaks to an earlier time than when they really occur. Offline filters can be designed to be nonrecursive and, therefore, do not necessarily produce phase distortion. The extents to which these displacements occur depend on the frequencies that are cut off by the filters. It is, therefore, preferable that data be recorded online using a wide band-pass, and that filtering used for signal enhancement be mostly carried out offline using nonrecursive filters.

Various types of offline digital filters are available. Because they do not need to be analog, it is relatively simple to produce filters with very good performance (i.e., with very sharp cut-off points). Whereas filters with such characteristics may be built using a frequency-domain transformation of the data, the operations required are complex and may slow down the data processing exceedingly. It is possible to construct filters that work in the time domain that approximate the performance of these filters. Cook and Miller (1992), as well as Farwell, Martinerie, Bashore, Rapp, and Goddard (1993), present a review of some of these filters.

Wiener (1964) introduced the concept of "optimal" filter. This is a filter whose POC function is optimized to increase the signal maximally compared to the noise. For instance, a filter may be built to maximize the between-condition variance with respect to the within-condition variance. To build such a filter it is necessary to define the signal in some manner, so that the frequency carrying the signal can be identified a priori. In addition, an optimal filter is practical only if it is designed in the frequency domain. However, as already mentioned, filtering in the frequency domain may actually reduce the speed of signal processing considerably. These problems have limited the use of optimal filters.

---

[3] This phenomenon can be minimized by using a special type of filter (e.g., elliptical and/or Bessel filters).

In certain cases the investigator is interested in studying activity that is characterized by very specific frequencies. For instance, if the investigator is interested in the response to stimuli presented at regular intervals, the investigator may assume that the response also should be observed at regular intervals. In this case, the frequency of the signal is well known – either the frequency of stimulation or one of its harmonics – and activity at all other frequencies may be discarded as noise. An "inverted-notch" filter (also called a "band-pass" filter) may be used to selectively analyze the response, and may enhance greatly the signal-to-noise ratio. Procedures of this type are used to analyze "steady-state" evoked responses (Tomoda et al., 1991).

So far, this discussion has focused on filters used in the temporal domain to eliminate activity at undesirable frequencies. However, filters can also be built in the spatial domain in order to amplify activity with certain, particular spatial properties with respect to other types of activities. An example of this is the Vector Filter procedure proposed by Gratton, Coles, and Donchin (1989). The Vector Filter procedure can be considered as analogous to a planned contrast executed in the space domain. Gratton, Kramer, Coles, and Donchin (1989) and Fabiani, Gratton, Karis, and Donchin (1987) showed that this procedure could help in ERP component identification. This notion has been recently re-introduced with the label of "virtual channel," which refers to a particular EEG channel constructed by appropriately weighting a number of different channels. The weights can be selected on the basis of specific procedures, for example, Principal Component Analysis (PCA; Spencer, Dein, & Donchin, 1999), independent component analysis (ICA; Makeig et al., 1997), or other methods.

A special type of noise, present in most psychophysiological data, is referred to as an "artifact." This term is normally used to indicate large, isolated noise activities that originate outside the system of interest. Examples of artifacts include (a) the potentials associated with blinks and other types of eye movements during the recording of brain electrical activity, (b) susceptibility and movement artifacts during MRI and PET recordings, (c) missed heartbeats in measures of heart rate, and (d) pulse artifacts in the EROS and NIRS data. Artifacts may be very large – several times larger than the signal – and could, therefore, completely obliterate the signal. Furthermore, they may occur in a systematic fashion (i.e., the frequency of artifacts may be consistently greater in one experimental condition than another). However, artifacts are often easy to recognize because they have specific "signatures" that are clearly distinguishable from regular data. For instance, blinks generate electrical potentials with a characteristic spatial distribution over the scalp, and missed heartbeats in heart rate measures can produce exceedingly long intervals that are outside of the normal variability.

A number of manual and automatic procedures have been developed to detect, eliminate, or compensate for the effects of artifacts. These procedures vary from a particular physiological measure to another and, therefore, will not be reviewed here. It is important, however, to remember that appropriate procedures for dealing with artifacts are an essential step in the processing of any physiological signal.

4. DATA REDUCTION AND QUANTIFICATION

4.1. Quantification

Practically all analyses of physiological measures require a step in which a small number of numerical values are extracted from the large amount of data recorded, and are then used for inferential statistics. This step may be called quantification. Quantification usually involves two steps: (a) identification of a particular feature considered to represent a given physiological event, and (b) measurement of some parameter of this feature.

4.1.1. Feature identification

The procedures used to identify the feature of interest are quite variable. In some cases the feature can be easily identified by visual inspection of the data. This occurs when the signal-to-noise ratio is so large (e.g., >3:1) that the feature of interest can easily be distinguished from sources of noise or from other signals (e.g., blinks in electrooculographic (EOG) recordings, and R-waves in the EKG). In other cases the features of interest are buried under variable, and sometimes large, amounts of noise or other signals. An example of this is given by various components of the ERP, especially when measured from single trials, or from averages of a small number of trials. In this case, identification of the component of interest may be very complex, and require sophisticated pattern recognition algorithms, filtering procedures, or a combination of both. Thus, identification of the P300 component of the ERP on single trial recordings may require using a relatively heavy low-pass filter (band-pass 0–6 Hz or less) and pattern recognition algorithms such as cross-correlation methods (Fabiani et al., 1987; Gratton, Kramer et al., 1989). A step that is often required for identifying ERP components is the definition of a particular "time window" in which the component is expected to appear. Thus, it is possible to define P300 as a positive peak in the ERP waveform appearing in an interval between 300 and 700 ms, whereas a peak appearing earlier or later may be classified as a different component. Other attributes may also be considered important, for example, the particular location at which the activity is observed.

4.1.2. Measurement

The second step of the procedure is the measurement of a particular parameter of the feature of interest. Again, parameters vary along different dimensions. By and large, three dimensions are considered in most cases: (a) a temporal dimension, (b) a spatial dimension, and (c) the intensity or frequency of occurrence.

4.1.2.1. Temporal dimensions. In the case of temporal dimensions, activity can be considered as having a particular latency, frequency, or phase. Measures include onset, peak, center-of-gravity, and fitting of particular functions to the data. The two measures that are most commonly used are onset and peak latency.

Onset measures may be very informative because they may define the latency of a particular physiological event as well as the maximum latency of the psychological phenomenon that is intended to signal. Onset can be measured as the first data point in the time series exceeding a preset value. This value can be obtained from previous work or from statistical computations of the variability in the measurements (Miller, Patterson, & Ulrich, 1998). However, the exact onset time of physiological measures can be difficult to determine when the measures contain even low levels of noise. In case of noisy measures (e.g., ERP activity measured on single trials or on a small number of trials), onset of a particular activity can be estimated by fitting regression lines to different segments of the data (Barrett, Shibasaki, & Neshige, 1986), and by determining the point at which the regression line corresponding to the pre- and post-onset periods meet. An alternative procedure is to consider the "half-amplitude" latency, which is the latency required for the signal to reach half of its maximum peak; other proportions of the maximum value can also be used (Smulders, Kenemans, & Kok, 1996). Whereas the latter approach is quite reliable (Smulders et al., 1996), the determination of which proportion of the maximum value to use is arbitrary, and the measure may not correspond to any particular psychological (or physiological) phenomenon. In addition, if the maximum value is systematically different across conditions, determination of the latency of half-amplitude measures may be misleading. An example is presented in Figure 35.8.

Peak measures are obtained by selecting the data point (in the time or frequency domain) of the time series at which the measure reaches its maximum value. If several peaks are present, the peak point can be defined as the maximum value within a certain interval, or as the "n-th" peak in the waveform (i.e., the first peak, the second peak, and so on). Peak measures tend to be more reliable than onset measures. However, they may be very sensitive to high-frequency noise. It is, therefore, often advisable to apply a low-pass filter before estimating the peak. The main advantage of peak latency measures is that they are easy to take even on noisy data. A disadvantage, in comparison to onset measures, is that they do not necessarily identify a point in time that is of theoretical importance. Thus, although from the onset of a particular activity we may infer that a given psychological process must

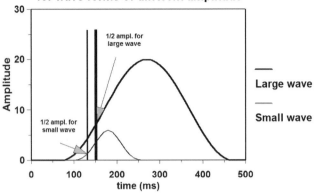

Figure 35.8. Half-amplitude onset measures for waves of large (thick curve) and small (thin wave) amplitude. The half-amplitude latency of the large wave (thick vertical line) was 170 ms, whereas that of the small wave (thin vertical line) was 147 ms. If half-amplitude measures are used to estimate onset latency, it may lead to the incorrect conclusion that the onset of the large wave occurred after the onset of the small wave.

have been carried out for the activity to occur, the peak of the physiological response may occur some time later and have no specific meaning. An extreme example is given by the time course of the hemodynamic response (measured with fMRI) and following the presentation of a train of stimuli. The time at which the fMRI response reaches its peak may provide little information about the time course of psychological events. The onset of the fMRI activity in a particular brain area, however, can be considered as the upper limit for the latency of activation of that area. It should be noted, of course, that activity in the area might in fact begin some time before it is detected. A similar situation exists for the latency of the peak of the skin conductance response. Note, however, that although for both types of signals the peak latency may provide little information about the timing of psychological events, the onset and the amplitude of either response may provide useful information about the nature of psychological events.

In general, temporal dimensions are considered as interval measures and are most commonly analyzed using parametric statistical approaches. However, temporal measures have usually a limited range. Additionally, in some cases, the distribution of the measurement error departs substantially from normality and both skewness and platykurtosis may be present (Fabiani et al., 1987). Both of these problems may lead to reduced power for statistical analysis.

4.1.2.2. Spatial dimension. The spatial dimension is most commonly analyzed in terms of the correspondence of the location of a physiological response to a particular anatomical structure, for example, it can be hypothesized that the blood-oxygenation-level-dependent (BOLD) fMRI response was observed in proximity of the calcarine fissure. In brain imaging techniques, analysis is often carried out in parallel for different voxels. Then, the voxels showing a response are identified and compared with anatomical maps. The methodologies used to determine which voxels (or set of voxels) show signs of functional activation (i.e., changes in blood flow or BOLD signal) vary conspicuously. In most cases, some type of statistic is derived for each voxels (or group of voxels). For methods based on hemodynamic or metabolic phenomena, this statistic often involves comparisons across conditions. In this case, the voxels identified are those that show differences between conditions exceeding some criterion, often expressed in terms of probability of alpha error.

In most cases the response is observed over several contiguous voxels. Indeed, given the high probability of false positive in brain imaging studies, it is often the case that only responses extending over a number of voxels are considered meaningful. In this case, the exact location of the activity may be more difficult to identify. One procedure is to consider the geometrical center of the region (or group of voxels) that shows significant effects. An alternative solution is to interpret the data as indicating a response that extends over the whole area where a significant response was observed. There are two possible problems with the latter interpretation.

First, the size of the area where a significant response is observed depends on the criterion used for considering an effect as significant and on the power of the measurements. Therefore, the activated area may depend on the number of trials or number of subjects used in the study. Paradoxically, if enough trials were collected (or the signal-to-noise ratio was sufficiently high), larger areas of the brain could show signs of activation and the response would become less localized.

Second, for some measures, such as BOLD-fMRI measures, a very large activity in one voxel may actually cause other voxels (both contiguous and noncontiguous) to show activity. For this reason a strong activity localized to a very small volume in space produces effects that are difficult to distinguish from those of a weaker response localized to a larger area.

The statistical analysis of spatial information is sometimes carried on considering location as a categorical independent variable (or a factor). For instance, analysis of ERP scalp distribution is often carried out using electrode location as a factor in a factorial ANOVA design. Effects of experimental variables on scalp distribution would then be visible as interaction between these factors. Although quite popular, this approach has been criticized for two reasons.

First, the ANOVA model is an additive model, so that the contribution of electrode location as a factor to the overall variance is considered as independent from other factors. However, because ERPs always reflect the difference in voltage between locations, if a phenomenon influences the voltage of an ERP activity, it is likely to influence different electrode locations in a different manner. Therefore, an interaction between electrode location and any experimental factor may be due to a change in the overall size of a particular ERP activity, change in its spatial distribution (or scalp distribution), or interaction between these factors. McCarthy and Wood (1985) have proposed that, before submitting ERP data to an ANOVA, the values obtained at different electrodes be re-scaled by a factor related to the absolute size of the activity (e.g., the range of values or the standard deviation across all electrode locations). This "standardization" process is intended to eliminate variance across conditions or subjects due to changes in component amplitude, so that any effects observed as a function of electrode location can be interpreted as a change in the spatial distribution of the ERP activity. This approach is useful in those cases in which the ERP observed at the scalp (at all scalp locations) is determined by a single component. However, as shown in Figure 35.9, in the case of overlapping components, the standardization procedure does not eliminate the confounding between differences in scalp distribution and differences in component amplitude.

Second, the ERP values measured at different electrode locations are in fact observations of the same phenomenon from different vantage points. For this reason, both the signal and the noise can be correlated. The correlation of the noise observed at different electrode locations (or at different data points) generates a problem in the ANOVA model that is commonly known as "lack-of-sphericity" problem (Jennings & Wood, 1976). A solution to this problem is to use a multivariate approach to the analysis of scalp distribution data. Several multivariate approaches have been proposed. They include: MANOVA (Vasey & Thayer, 1987); multiple regression (Gratton, Coles et al., 1989); principal component analysis or single-value decomposition (Lamothe & Stroink, 1991); and independent component analysis (Makeig et al., 1997).

Other investigators have considered using nonparametric statistics to evaluate location information. One such example is the use of bootstrapping procedures for studying the location of the peak of surface distribution of ERPs or optical activity (Fabiani, Gratton, Friedman, & Corballis, 1998). The purpose of the bootstrap method proposed by Fabiani and colleagues is to estimate the reliability of maxima of maps of ERP or EROS activity obtained on average data. The bootstrap method involves analysis of a large number of samples of individual trials (bootstrap replications). Each bootstrap replication is obtained by extracting at random (and with replacement, so that a given trial can occur more than once) a number of trials from the original data set equal to the number of trials used to compute the regular average. For each new bootstrap replication, an average map is computed and the location of maximum is determined. The distribution of the maxima across a large number of different bootstrap replications is then obtained. The location of a maximum is reliable if it is obtained in a large proportion (e.g., 95%) of the bootstrap replications. This bootstrap method does not require assumptions about the distribution of

Effect of standardization on
ERP scalp distribution data

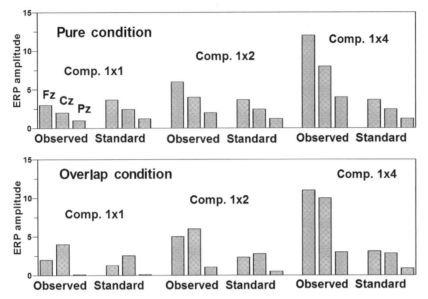

Figure 35.9. Effect of standardizing ERP scalp distribution data in conditions with different component amplitude and component overlap. *Top row:* data from a condition in which there is no component overlap (i.e., all the activity obtained at all electrode location can be attributed to one component). On the left are plots of the observed and standardized scalp distribution data from a condition in which the component is small. Standardization is obtained by dividing the data by the standard deviation across electrode locations. In the middle are similar plots for a condition in which the component has medium size. On the right are plots for a condition in which the component has large size. Note that plots of the standardize scalp distributions are identical for all component sizes. *Bottom row*: plot from conditions with component overlap. A component with central-maximum scalp distribution and fixed amplitude was added to the observed data presented on the top row. Note that the scalp distribution appears to change from a frontal to a central maximum as a function of component amplitude. Also note that the difference in scalp distribution is not eliminated by standardization.

maxima in the population, and is therefore quite robust. The method can be modified to consider the probability that the maximum is within a certain area. A limitation of the method is that it is "ad hoc," though other bootstrap procedures can be used for different applications (Wasserman & Bockenholt, 1989). Other investigators have proposed other "distribution-free" methods for the analysis of spatial distribution data (Karniski, Blair, & Snider, 1994).

4.1.3. Intensity
Intensity is usually quantified using one of four approaches: (a) peak amplitude, (b) integrated activity over time (also called "area measure"), (c) covariance with a template (Fabiani et al., 1987), and (d) frequency of response. These measures are illustrated in Figure 35.10.

Peak and area measures are heavily dependent on the definition of a "baseline" level (i.e., these measures are taken by computing the difference between the peak, or the sum of the individual values, and the baseline; see section 4.3.1 for a discussion of baseline levels in psychophysiological measures), whereas the covariance measure requires some hypotheses about the shape of the response to be

studied. The response shape can also be obtained with statistical methods such as PCA or ICA. Area measures are less sensitive to high frequency noise than peak measures. However, empirical studies have shown that if a low-pass filter is applied before the peak measurement, the latter can be at least as reliable as area measures (Fabiani et al., 1987). Covariance measures can be used to separate the contribution of overlapping physiological responses, in which case a multiple regression approach can be used, and is quite reliable. Examples of covariance measures are given by estimates of the amplitude of different components of the ERP obtained with PCA (Donchin & Heffley, 1978) or with step-wise discriminant analysis (SWDA; Donchin, 1969; Donchin & Herning, 1975; Squires & Donchin, 1976). In these cases the covariance measures are taken with respect to a "weighting" function that has been optimized on the basis of statistical properties of the data (see the next section). Multiple regression approaches have been used to analyze hemodynamic data in complex, factorial designs (e.g., fMRI and PET). An advantage of this approach, compared to the more traditional "subtraction" methods used to analyze these data, is that it is possible to identify the effects associated with interaction terms on the brain image maps. However, the assumptions underlying these methods – linearity and additivity – are as critical for these measures as they are for subtraction methods (see Sections 2.2 and 4.3.2).

All these measures are assumed to prove results along interval scales, which can be analyzed using parametric statistics. The error distribution tends to be skewed because of the fact that the range is usually limited at the lower end, but platykurtosis is not a problem as it was for latency measures. Amplitude measures may therefore be more reliable than latency measures (Fabiani et al., 1987).

Measures of the frequency of response are used for signals that are quite stereotyped and easily recognizable, but occur on a certain proportion of the trials or at irregular intervals. Note that, in many cases (e.g., blink or electrodermal responses), response frequency will not follow a normal distribution, and the distributions will be heavily positively skewed with some subjects exhibiting a large number of responses and others very few or none. Experimental variables will generally produce larger effects for the subjects exhibiting a greater base-rate of responses than for those exhibiting a smaller base-rate. For instance,

Measurement of the amplitude of a psychophysiological response

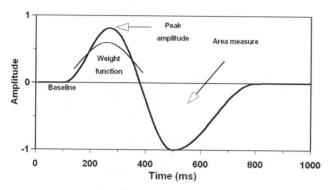

Figure 35.10. Different measures of the intensity of a psychophysiological response. Three measures are illustrated: peak amplitude, area measure, and weighted amplitude. Note that peak amplitude and area measures require a definition of the baseline value. Weighted amplitude measures can be made independent of the definition of the baseline.

all subjects may double their response frequency as a function of experimental manipulations. However, for those with a low base-rate this may generate a very small effect, whereas for those with a high base-rate the effect may be very large. This results in a large "subject by manipulation" interaction with a consequent reduced statistical power. In such cases, a logarithmic transformation of the response frequency may help increase the statistical power of the analysis. Alternatively, inferential analysis also can be conducted using a log-linear approach (Kennedy, 1984). For a discussion of other approaches, including standardization and re-scaling, see Ben-Shakhar (1985) and Stemmler (1987).

4.2. Statistical approaches to data reduction

As mentioned above, psychophysiological data are essentially multivariate. One of the major steps in the analysis is the reduction of the number of dependent variables, the number of which is often bewildering, to a smaller number appropriate for inferential analysis. Statisticians have developed a number of procedures to deal with the problem of data reduction on the basis of the statistical properties of the data. One of the simplest and most popular approaches is PCA (Donchin & Heffley, 1977). PCA is a statistical procedure for grouping dependent variables in a smaller subset of underlying (or "latent") variables that possess the following properties: (a) they explain the variance and covariance of the original set of dependent variables as much as possible, and (b) are orthogonal to each other or, in other words, are uncorrelated. PCA components can be rotated (e.g., by using the procedure of VARIMAX) to facilitate interpretability. PCA components are interpreted in terms of their correlations (or covariances) with the original variables, which are also called "component loadings." Donchin and collaborators wrote a

series of papers outlining the application of PCA to the analysis of ERP data. In this approach, ERP data are viewed as a data matrix in which data points are viewed as variates (i.e., dependent variables in a multivariate approach) and different subjects, conditions, and electrode locations are viewed as individual observations. A standard PCA is then run on the covariance matrix obtained from this data matrix. In most cases, a VARIMAX rotation is run on the results of the PCA. The component loadings are used to describe different components of the ERPs. These loadings are then used as sets of weights to compute component scores for each subject, condition, and location. The component scores are used as estimates of the amplitude of each component for each of the original waveforms, and submitted to inferential analysis (such as ANOVA). This approach has been used in a number of studies (McCallum & Curry, 1984; Karis, Fabiani, & Donchin, 1984; Squires, Squires, & Hillyard, 1975; Ruchkin, Sutton, & Stega, 1980), mostly because it provides separate estimates of the amplitude of individual components even when they overlap in time.

This PCA/VARIMAX/ANOVA approach has been subsequently criticized (Wood & McCarthy, 1984; Möcks, 1986; Möcks & Verleger, 1985) on the grounds that variance is misattributed to different components. Indeed, in principle, the subdivision of the variance into different components as obtained with PCA is entirely arbitrary, and there exist an infinite number of other ways of subdividing the variance on the basis of the same number of components. Therefore, it is unjustified to consider the components obtained with PCA as if they were physiological entities. Further problems with the use of PCA in the analysis of ERPs include the difficulty of incorporating latency shifts within the PCA model (Möcks, 1986) and possible correlations between components. However, PCA remains an interesting attempt at a principled way for data reduction, in which the original variance is retained as much as possible while the number of independent variables is minimized. This, as already mentioned, is one of the major goals of signal processing.

Recently, similar approaches have been proposed to address the issue of data reduction. For instance, Maier, Dagnelie, Spekrejse, and van Dijk (1987) have used a "spatial" PCA, in which the dependent variables used are spatial locations rather than data points, as a preliminary step for source analysis of ERPs. Spatial PCA has also been used to determine the number of active components at a certain moment in time, as a preliminary step for dipole analysis (see BESA; Scherg & von Cramon, 1986). A sequence of spatial and temporal PCAs have been recently employed by Spencer, Dien, and Donchin (1997), whereas Möcks (1988) has proposed a multivariate approach that also combines spatial and temporal information. Singular-value decomposition has also been proposed as an alternative to PCA (see EMSE; Greenblatt, 1996). A problem with most of these alternative approaches, just as for PCA, is that the results are not "unique" because an infinite number of alternative descriptions of the data are possible. Furthermore, it is often difficult to interpret the results of the various data reduction procedures used and to compare results obtained in different experiments.

Independent component analysis (Makeig et al., 1997) has also become a popular method for data reduction. As with PCA, ICA is method to decompose the variance of a set of data in a set of underlying components. It is often associated with the problem of "blind source separation," which refers to the issue of separating simultaneous signals from a time series, for example, two speech signals occurring at the same time. This problem may be considered similar to separating different concomitant psychophysiological signals. However, in contrast to PCA, components are not selected by hierarchically maximizing the amount of variance they account for. Rather, the components are selected so as to maximize their statistical independence. The extraction procedure is more complex than in PCA. Several methods are available, which typically involve a stepwise procedure. ICA has been applied to many psychophysiological studies, with two major purposes: (a) separating signals from noise (e.g., ERP from eye-movement artifacts); (b) separating different types of brain activities from each other.

4.3. Other quantification issues

4.3.1. Absolute versus relative effects: The problem of baseline and reference

In a number of cases, psychophysiological measures are intended to reflect a change in a physiological variable from a level that exists prior to the introduction of an experimental manipulation (e.g., the presentation of a stimulus or the administration of a drug) to a level that exists after the manipulation. The level of the physiological variable before the manipulation begins is called the "rest," or "baseline," level. For some variables, this level is characterized by the absence of any measurable activity (e.g., there may be little EMG activity in a muscle at rest). However, most commonly, the targeted physiological systems are already active prior to the experiment, and remain active during the experiment, which is clearly the case for the heart and the brain. In these cases, the baseline level may change as a function of subject, location, and time of measurement. For this reason, most physiological measures are expressed as changes with respect to a baseline level. Determination of an appropriate baseline level is not always simple because it is not necessarily possible to induce a pure "rest" condition. In most cases, even when the experimental condition does not require a measurable overt response, the subject may be actively predicting and evaluating situations from both a cognitive and an emotional standpoint. In addition, the subject may be paying attention to internal or external stimuli that are not experimentally controlled. All of these psychological activities may influence the measurements obtained during the baseline period. If they do so in a manner that is systematically different from that observed at the time of

the experimental measurement, or in different ways in different experimental conditions, there is the possibility that systematic effects may influence the measurements. For instance, in most experiments using ERPs, measurements are taken as differences compared with a prestimulus baseline level. However, if subjects can anticipate certain properties of the stimulus during the prestimulus period, it is possible that an anticipation component of the ERP, for example, the contingent negative variation (CNV) may be elicited during this interval (Walter et al., 1964). The differential measures taken at a later time will then be affected by the presence of a CNV during the baseline period. The same may occur if the dependent variable is heart rate. In this case, expectation for an external stimulus may induce heart rate deceleration (Lacey, Kagan, Lacey, & Moss, 1963). Note, however, that if the interest is in comparing conditions in which anticipation can be expected to be the same, this is not necessarily a critical problem because a similar value is subtracted from both conditions. Because of this and other similar reasons, it is generally easier to compare activity observed in different experimental conditions than to draw conclusions from the activity observed in a single condition alone. In other words, it is much easier to consider relative than absolute effects.

Whereas the problem of the baseline or rest level is common to most physiological measures, some measures (e.g., ERPs) entail the problem of the reference. The term "reference" is used to indicate a comparison value that is valid for all points in space and is in contrast with the term "baseline," which is used to indicate a comparison value that is valid for all points in time. In some cases, physiological measures are obtained by considering the difference in electric potential between two locations. Electric potentials do not possess absolute values, but are defined as differences between two energy levels. Therefore, measures of electric potentials should be considered with respect to the locations that are involved. It is, however, possible to compare the difference in potential that exists between point A and point B and between point C and point B. If the first difference is more positive than the second, it can be concluded that point A has a more positive voltage level than point C. In this case point B will be used as a common reference point. If measures were taken only at a single point in time, then the point that is used as a common reference makes little difference. However, voltage measures often are taken at different times, and points of maximum difference (or peak values) are identified. The point at which A is most different from B may not be the same point at which A is most different from C. Therefore, the time of the occurrence of the peak on A may differ depending on whether B or C is used as a reference. For this reason, appropriate selection of a reference location is a critical aspect of recording electrical activity.

Historically, there have been three approaches to the problem of reference selection. The first approach is to consider measurements obtained between selected pairs of electrode locations; the measurement is labeled "bipolar." Bipolar measurements are common practice in the study of EMG, EKG, and EOG. In some cases, bipolar derivations are used to study local phenomena, as in the cases of EMG and EOG. In these cases, the two electrodes are placed very close to each other, so that activity generated far away is likely to influence the electrodes equally, (i.e. to cancel out each other), whereas activity generated locally is more likely to generate differences. This approach is adequate when the interest is in studying the time course of activity of relatively simple electric field configuration, such as for EMG and EOG, and, to some extent, EKG. For EEG studies, the bipolar approach fails to account for the complexities of the fields generated by the brain, and is only used in some clinical applications or special cases, for example, the recording of auditory brainstem averaged evoked potentials (BAEPs).

A second approach is to consider measurements from a number of locations as differences with respect to the same location (or to a common value). This approach is called a "common reference system." There are a number of choices for the location of the reference value, including the ears, mastoids, nosetip, forehead, or locations outside the head (i.e., extracephalic reference). The latter may pick up electrical activity from the heart (EKG) and, therefore, require special compensation procedures (Fortgens & de Bruin, 1983). Finally, some researchers have advocated the use of an average reference, which is obtained by subtracting or adding a value to all of the observed locations, so that the algebraic sum of all of the potential values observed at different locations is equal to zero. Although arguments in favor of one or another of these systems have been proposed (Skrandies & Lehmann, 1982), there appears to be no clear advantage in using one reference system over another – the choice is arbitrary. However, because the selection of the reference may alter the shape of waveforms, including both the amplitude and the latency of the peaks, it is very important that the selection of the reference is made explicit and the same reference system is used when comparing across different data sets. The common reference system is the one most used in ERP research. Its greatest advantages are ease of computation and possibility of comparing values obtained at different locations. Its major drawback is the arbitrariness of the choice of the reference.

A third approach is that of using a transformation of the data, so that the data are expressed in terms of absolute dimensions (e.g., current flow) instead of relative dimensions (e.g., difference in potential). As seen above (Section 3.3.2), this can be achieved by computing the local gradient in potential instead of the difference with a common reference, but this requires the assumption of constant resistance between electrode locations.

4.3.2. Subtraction, comparisons, and linearity of the measures

In most cases, psychophysiologists are interested in comparing physiological responses in two (or more) condi-tions. The comparison process usually involves a study of the statistical reliability of differences between measures. This, in turn, involves computing several differences across subjects, time points, and locations. Data obtained in different conditions can be interpreted either along ordinal scales, which require using less powerful nonparametric statistics, or along interval scales, which may be analyzed using more powerful parametric statistics. The basic assumption of interval scales is that differences between intervals at any level of the scale are directly comparable. For example, the difference between the values 2 and 4 in some scale has the same significance as the difference between the values 22 and 24. This allows the investigator to subtract common terms and to compare data directly. We have previously considered a similar property called "linearity" (see Section 2.2).

Most psychophysiological measures, however, depart from linearity to some extent. One of the reasons is that the measures often have a limited range because physiological systems have feedback mechanisms that counteract extreme values in order to maintain homeostasis. For example, heart rate is very unlikely to drop below 40 beats per minute even under strong vagal activation. There are also other limitations because of the number of units (e.g., neurons) that can respond to particular stimuli. However, for most psychophysiological measures, there exists an interval of values for which linearity is valid. For practical purposes, it is advantageous that, if at all possible, measurements be taken in conditions in which the psychophysiological measures are within the range in which they exhibit linearity.

Range and scale differences may also vary as a function of subject or location on the body. For example, certain subjects may exhibit higher variability in a psychophysiological variable than others. Similarly, measures of a psychophysiological variable may have a greater range at a location than another. This will make it more difficult to compare data across subjects or locations. To counteract this problem, standardized measures in which the data are transformed, so to have equal means and standard deviations, are often used in these types of comparisons.

For a number of psychophysiological variables, it has been found that variability is correlated with the average level of the variable itself for a particular subject or condition. This relationship some time takes the form of "ceiling" or "floor" effects, which in psychophysiology often have been considered as examples of the "law of initial value" (Wilder, 1967). This would produce departure from linearity. Psychologists have often used special transformations (such as "logit" or "probit" transformations) to correct these forms of departures from linearity. In other cases, effects are proportional to the original value. In these cases, a logarithmic transformation of the data (or the division by the average value) may equalize variances (and differences) across conditions, and produce a scale that has linear properties. For a discussion of several procedures for comparing conditions with different base rates see Wainer (1991).

5. CONCLUDING REMARKS

This chapter has reviewed several issues related to the analysis of psychophysiological data. In most cases, procedures used in data analysis can be viewed as an effort to extract meaningful information from the data that are often under conditions in which the data are noisy. In these cases, the majority of the data-analyst efforts are devoted to increasing the signal-to-noise ratio. Although there are procedures that increase this ratio under all conditions, it is often the case that a priori hypotheses about what types of signals to expect will help in the design of appropriate analysis procedures. These a priori hypotheses do not necessarily have to be very specific (i.e., activity at a particular latency and at a particular location is determined by factor A or factor B). Even simple hypotheses, for example, that some activity should be observed somewhere during a particular latency interval or at a particular location, will help design appropriate analytical methods. However, in general, the power of the analytical procedure increases with the specificity of the hypotheses that are entertained.

It is often the case that psychophysiological phenomena are quite complex and unpredicted effects are obtained in a number of studies. In some cases, discovery of these new effects is what affords the greatest scientific advancements. This generates a dilemma for the data analyst – how can maximum power be obtained, while still maintaining a wide focus in the analysis? In most cases the answer is in alternating studies conducted with an "exploratory" attitude, which enables the investigators to detect unexpected findings, with other more "hypothesis-driven" studies, which provide more rigorous tests of specific hypotheses. This problem emphasizes that data analysis needs to be integrated with experimental design in a bidirectional fashion.

ACKNOWLEDGMENTS

I thank Monica Fabiani for her comments on a previous version of this manuscript. Preparation of this chapter was supported in part by NIBIB grant #R01 EB002011–08 to Gabriele Gratton. Please send all correspondence to: Gabriele Gratton, University of Illinois, Beckman Institute, 405 N. Mathews Ave., Urbana, IL 61801; E-mail: grattong@uiuc.edu.

REFERENCES

Barrett, G., Shibasaki, H., & Neshige, R. (1986). Cortical potentials preceding voluntary movement: Evidence for three periods of preparation in man. *Electroencephalography & Clinical Neurophysiology*, 63 (4), 327–339.

Basar, E., Basar-Eroglu, C., Karakas, S., & Schurmann, M. (1999). Are cognitive processes manifested in event-related gamma, alpha, theta and delta oscillations in the EEG? *Neuroscience Letters*, 259, 165–168.

Ben-Shakhar, G. (1985). Standardization within individuals: A simple method to neutralize individual differences in skin conductance. *Psychophysiology*, 22 (3), 292–299.

Bradley, M. M., Cuthbert, B. N., & Lang, P. J. (1991). Startle and emotion: Lateral acoustic probes and the bilateral blink. *Psychophysiology*, 28 (3), 285–295.

Cacioppo, J. T., & Dorfman, D. D. (1987). Waveform moment analysis in psychophysiological research. *Psychological Bulletin*, 102 (3), 421–438.

Cherry, S. R., & Phelps, M. E. (1996). Imaging brain function with positron emission tomography. In A. W. Toga & J. C. Mazziotta (Eds.), *Brain mapping: The methods* (pp. 191–222). San Diego, CA: Academic Press.

Cohen, M. S. (1996). Rapid MRI and functional applications. In A. W. Toga & J. C. Mazziotta (Eds.), *Brain mapping: The methods* (pp. 223–258). San Diego, CA: Academic Press.

Cook, E. W., & Miller, G. A. (1992). Digital filtering: Background and tutorial for psychophysiologists. *Psychophysiology*, 29 (3), 350–367.

Dale, A. M., & Halgren, E. (2001). Spatiotemporal mapping of brain activity by integration of multiple imaging modalities. *Current Opinions in Neurobiology*, 11, 202–208.

Donchin, E. (1969). Discriminant analysis in average evoked response studies: The study of single trial data. *Electroencephalography & Clinical Neurophysiology*, 27 (3), 311–314.

Donchin, E., & Herning, R. I. (1975). A simulation study of the efficacy of stepwise discriminant analysis in the detection and comparison of event related potentials. *Electroencephalography & Clinical Neurophysiology*, 38 (1), 51–68.

Donchin, E., & Heffley, E. (1978). Multivariate analysis of event-related potential data: A tutorial review. In D. Otto (Ed.), *Multidisciplinary perspectives in event-related brain potential research (EPA-600/9–77–043)* (pp. 555–572). Washington, DC: US Government Printing Office.

Dorfman, D. D., & Cacioppo, J. T. (1990). Waveform moment analysis: Topographical analysis of nonrhythmic waveforms. In L. G. Tassinary & J. T. Cacioppo (Eds.), *Principles of psychophysiology: Physical, social, and inferential elements* (pp. 661–707). New York: Cambridge University Press.

Elui, R. (1969). Gaussian behavior of the EEG: Changes during performance of mental tasks. *Science*, 164, 328.

Estes, W. K. (1956). The problem of inference from curves based on group data. *Psychological Bulletin*, 53, 133–140.

Fabiani, M., Gratton, G., Karis, D., & Donchin, E. (1987). Definition, identification, and reliability of measurement of the P300 component of the event-related brain potential. In P. K. Ackles, J. R. Jennings, & M. G. Coles (Eds.), *Advances in Psychophysiology* (Vol. 2, pp. 1–78). Greenwich, CT: JAI Press.

Fabiani, M., Gratton, G., Corballis, P., Cheng, J., & Friedman, D. (1998). Bootstrap assessment of the reliability of maxima in surface maps of brain activity of individual subjects derived with electrophysiological and optical methods. *Behavior Research Methods, Instruments, & Computers*, 30, 78–86.

Farwell, L. A., Martinerie, J. M., Bashore, T. R., Rapp, P. E., & Goddard, P. H. (1993). Optimal digital filters for long-latency components of the event-related brain potential. *Psychophysiology*, 30 (3), 306–315.

Fortgens, C., & de Bruin, M. P. (1983). Removal of eye movement and ECG artifacts from the non-cephalic reference EEG. *Electroencephalography & Clinical Neurophysiology*, 56 (1), 90–96.

Fox, P. T., & Raichle, M. E. (1984). Stimulus rate dependence of regional cerebral blood flow in human striate cortex, demonstrated by positron emission tomography. *Journal of Neurophysiology*, 51 (5), 1109–1120.

Friston, K. J. (1996). Statistical parametric mapping and other analyses of functional imaging data. In A. W. Toga & J. C. Mazziotta (Eds.), *Brain mapping: The methods* (pp. 363–388). San Diego, CA: Academic Press.

Gratton, G., Coles, M. G., & Donchin, E. (1989). A procedure for using multi-electrode information in the analysis of components of the event-related potential: vector filter. *Psychophysiology*, 26 (2), 222–232.

Gratton, G., Kramer, A. F., Coles, M. G., & Donchin, E. (1989). Simulation studies of latency measures of components of the event-related brain potential. *Psychophysiology*, 26 (2), 233–248.

Gratton, G. (1997). Attention and probability effects in the human occipital cortex: an optical imaging study. *NeuroReport*, 8 (7), 1749–1753.

Gray, C. M., Konig, P., Engel, A. K., & Singer, W. (1989). Oscillatory responses in cat visual cortex exhibit inter-columnar synchronization which reflects global stimulus properties. *Nature*, 338 (6213), 334–337.

Greenblatt, R. (1996). *Electromagnetic source estimation*. San Diego, CA: Source/Signal Imaging.

Huberty, C. J., & Morris, J. D. (1989). Multivariate analysis versus multiple univariate analyses. *Psychological Bulletin*, 105 (2), 302–308.

Jennings, J. R., & Wood, C. C. (1976). Letter: The epsilon-adjustment procedure for repeated-measures analyses of variance. *Psychophysiology*, 13 (3), 277–278.

Jennings, J. R., van der Molen, M. W., Somsen, R. J., & Ridderinkhof, K. R. (1991). Graphical and statistical techniques for cardiac cycle time (phase) dependent changes in interbeat interval. *Psychophysiology*, 28(5), 596–606.

Karis, D., Fabiani, M. & Donchin, E. (1984). "P300" and memory: Individual differences in the von Restorff effect. *Cognitive Psychology*, 16, 177–216.

Karniski, W., Blair, R. C., & Snider, A. D. (1994). An exact statistical method for comparing topographic maps, with any number of subjects and electrodes. *Brain Topography*, 6(3), 203–210.

Kennedy, J. J. (1983). *Analyzing qualitative data: Introductory loglinear analysis for behavioral research*. New York: Praeger.

Lacey, J. I., Kagan, J., Lacey, B. C., & Moss, H. A. (1963). The visceral level: Situational determinants and behavioral correlates of autonomic response patterns. In P. H. Knapp (Ed.), *Expression of the emotions in man*. New York: International Universities Press.

Lamothe, R., & Stroink, G. (1991). Orthogonal expansions: their applicability to signal extraction in electrophysiological mapping data. *Medical & Biological Engineering & Computing*, 29(5), 522–28.

Maier, J., Dagnelie, G., Spekreijse, H., & van Dijk, B. W. (1987). Principal components analysis for source localization of VEPs in man. *Vision Research*, 27 (2), 165–177.

Makeig, S., Jung, T. P., Bell, A. J., Ghahremani, D., & Sejnowski, T. (1997). Blind separation of auditory event-related brain responses into independent components. *Proceedings of the National Academy of Sciences USA*, 94 (20), 10979–10984.

McCallum, W. C., & Curry, S. H. (1984). A comparison of early event-related potentials in two target detection tasks. Sixth International Conference on Event-Related Slow Potentials of the Brain (EPIC VI): Cognition, information processing, and language (1981, Lake Forest/Chicago, Illinois). *Annals of the New York Academy of Sciences*, 425, 242–249.

McCarthy, G., & Donchin, E. (1978). Brain potentials associated with structural and functional visual matching. *Neuropsychologia*, 16 (5), 571–585.

McCarthy, G., & Wood, C. C. (1985). Scalp distributions of event-related potentials: An ambiguity associated with analysis of variance models. *Electroencephalography & Clinical Neurophysiology*, 62 (3), 203–208.

Miller, J., Patterson, T., & Ulrich, R. (1998). Jackknife-based method for measuring LRP onset latency differences. *Psychophysiology*, 35 (1), 99–115.

Möcks, J., & Verleger, R. (1985). Nuisance sources of variance in principal components analysis of event-related potentials. *Psychophysiology*, 22 (6), 674–688.

Möcks, J. (1986). The influence of latency jitter in principal component analysis of event-related potentials. *Psychophysiology*, 23 (4), 480–484.

Möcks, J. (1988). Decomposing event-related potentials: a new topographic components model. *Biological Psychology*, 26(1–3), 199–215.

Möcks, J., Köhler, W., Gasser, T., & Pham, D. T. (1988). Novel approaches to the problem of latency jitter. *Psychophysiology*, 25 (2), 217–226.

Monk, T. H., & Fookson, J. E. (1986). Circadian temperature rhythm power spectra: Is equal sampling necessary? *Psychophysiology*, 23 (4), 472–479.

Monk, T. H. (1987). Parameters of the circadian temperature rhythm using sparse and irregular sampling. *Psychophysiology*, 24 (2), 236–242.

Pascual-Marqui, R. D., Michel, C. M., & Lehmann, D. (1994). Low resolution electromagnetic tomography: A new method for localizing electrical activity in the brain. *International Journal of Psychophysiology*, 18 (1), 49–65.

Perrin, F., Pernier, J., Bertrand, O., Giard, M. H., & Echallier, J. F. (1987). Mapping of scalp potentials by surface spline interpolation. *Electroencephalography & Clinical Neurophysiology*, 66 (1), 75–81.

Pfurtscheller, G., & Neuper, C. (1992). Simultaneous EEG 10 Hz desynchronization and 40 Hz synchronization during finger movements. *NeuroReport*, 3 (12), 1057–1060.

Quigley, K. S., & Berntson, G. G. (1996). Autonomic interactions and chronotropic control of the heart: Heart period versus heart rate. *Psychophysiology*, 33 (5), 605–611.

Ruchkin, D. S., Sutton, S., & Stega, M. (1980). Emitted P300 and slow wave event-related potentials in guessing and detection tasks. *Electroencephalography & Clinical Neurophysiology*, 49 (1–2), 1–14.

Samar, V. J., Bopardikar, A., Rao, R., & Swartz, K. (1999). Wavelet analysis of neuroelectric waveforms: A conceptual tutorial. *Brain and Language*, 66 (1), 7–60.

Scherg, M., & von Cramon, D. (1986). Evoked dipole source potentials of the human auditory cortex. *Electroencephalography & Clinical Neurophysiology*, 65 (5), 344–360.

Siegler, R. S. (1987). The perils of averaging data over strategies: An example from children's addition. *Journal of Experimental Psychology: General*, 116 (3), 250–264.

Skrandies, W., & Lehmann, D. (1982). Spatial principal components of multichannel maps evoked by lateral visual half-field stimuli. *Electroencephalography & Clinical Neurophysiology*, 54 (6), 662–667.

Smulders, F. T., Kenemans, J. L., & Kok, A. (1996). Effects of task variables on measures of the mean onset latency of LRP depend on the scoring method. *Psychophysiology*, 33 (2), 194–205.

Spencer, K. M., Dien, J., & Donchin, E. (1997). Temporal-spatial analysis of the late positive components of the ERP. *Psychophysiology*, 34, S6.

Spencer, K. M., Dien, J., & Donchin, E. (1999). Componential analysis of the ERP elicited by novel events using a dense electrode array *Psychophysiology*, 36, 409–414.

Squires, N. K., Squires, K. C., & Hillyard, S. A. (1975). Two varieties of long-latency positive waves evoked by unpredictable auditory stimuli in man. *Electroencephalography & Clinical Neurophysiology*, 38 (4), 387–401.

Squires, K. C., & Donchin, E. (1976). Beyond averaging: The use of discriminant functions to recognize event related potentials elicited by single auditory stimuli. *Electroencephalography & Clinical Neurophysiology*, 41 (5), 449–459.

Srinivasan, R., Nunez, P. L., Tucker, D. M., Silberstein, R. B., & Cadusch, P. J. (1996). Spatial sampling and filtering of EEG with spline laplacians to estimate cortical potentials. *Brain Topography*, 8(4), 355–366.

Stemmler, G. (1987). Standardization within subjects: A critique of Ben-Shakhar's conclusions. *Psychophysiology*, 24 (2), 243–246.

Stiber, B. Z., & Sato, S. (1997). Visualization of EEG using time-frequency distributions. *Methods of Information in Medicine*, 36 (4–5), 298–301.

Talairach, J., & Tournoux, P. (1988). *Co-planar stereotactic atlas of the human brain: 3-dimensional proportional system: An approach to cerebral imaging.* Stuttgart, Germany: Thieme.

Tallon-Buadry, C., Bertrand, O., Delpuech, C., & Pernier, J. (1996). Stimulus specificity of phase-locked and non-phase-locked 40 Hz visual responses in human. *Journal of Neuroscience*, 16 (13), 4240–4249.

Tomoda, H., Celesia, G. G., & Toleikis, S. C. (1991). Effect of spatial frequency on simultaneous recorded steady-state pattern electroretinograms and visual evoked potentials. *Electroencephalography & Clinical Neurophysiology: Evoked Potentials*, 80 (2), 81–88.

Van Essen, D. C., Drury, H. A., Joshi, S., & Miller, M. I. (1998). Functional and structural mapping of human cerebral cortex: Solutions are in the surfaces. *Proceedings of the National Academy of Sciences USA*, 95 (3), 788–795.

Vasey, M. W., & Thayer, J. F. (1987). The continuing problem of false positives in repeated measures ANOVA in psychophysiology: A multivariate solution. *Psychophysiology*, 24 (4), 479–486.

Wainer, H. (1991). Adjusting for differential base rates: Lord's Paradox again. *Psychological Bulletin*, 109(1), 147–151.

Walter, W. G., Cooper, R., Aldridge, V. J., McCallum, W. C., & Winter, A. L. (1964). Contingent negative variation: An electrical sign of sensorimotor association and expectancy in the human brain. *Nature*, 203, 380–384.

Wasserman, S., & Bockenholt, U. (1989). Bootstrapping: Applications to psychophysiology. *Psychophysiology*, 26 (2), 208–221.

Wickens, C. D., Kramer, A. F., Vanasse, L., & Donchin, E. (1983). Performance of concurrent tasks: A psychophysiological analysis of the reciprocity of information-processing resources. *Science*, 221(4615), 1080–1082.

Wiener, N. (1964). *Extrapolation, interpolation, and smoothing of stationary time series.* Cambridge, MA: MIT Press.

Wilder, J. (1967). *Stimulus and response. The law of initial value.* Bristol, UK: John Wright & Sons.

Wood, C. C., & McCarthy, G. (1984). Principal component analysis of event-related potentials: simulation studies demonstrate misallocation of variance across components. *Electroencephalography & Clinical Neurophysiology*, 59 (3), 249–260.

Woody, C. D. (1967). Characterization of an adaptive filter for the analysis of variable latency neuroelectrical signal. *Medical and Biological Engineering*, 5, 539–553.

Yantis, S., Meyer, D. E., & Smith, J. K. (1991). Analyses of multinomial mixture distributions: New tests for stochastic models of cognition and action. *Psychological Bulletin*, 110 (2), 350–374.

36 Data-Storage Formats in Neuroimaging: Background and Tutorial

JOHN D. HERRINGTON, BRADLEY P. SUTTON, AND GREGORY A. MILLER

The growth and development of spatially multidimensional electromagnetic, hemodynamic, and optical data analysis methods in psychophysiology over the past two decades have been substantial but also fragmented. This fragmentation is partly attributable to the diversity of backgrounds of researchers using positron emission tomography (PET), magnetic resonance imaging (MRI), and dense-array MEG and EEG (in few if any other research contexts do psychologists, chemists, engineers, psychiatrists, radiologists, neurologists, and physicists so regularly work alongside one another), as well as competition between commercial interests to develop or protect proprietary standards, methods, and software. Although the parallel distributed nature of psychophysiological analysis methods development can foster creativity, it sometimes comes at the cost of clarity and comparability of methods and data across research laboratories. With an estimated 1500 new functional MRI (fMRI) studies per year producing an estimated 30–50 terabytes of data per year (Kupfer, First, & Regier, 2002), issues of data storage, data access, and transparency of methods have become critical. Most urgently, the recent development of fMRI methods as a sort of multinational cottage industry complicates the development of shared expertise and increases the risk that home-grown methods from one laboratory may be underutilized or incorrectly applied by others.

Furthermore, as the applications of functional imaging techniques cross disciplines, the consequences of misunderstanding these techniques increase. Whereas clinical applications of fMRI and MEG are presently rare, they will certainly be common within a few years, especially in applications such as presurgical planning. The use of functional imaging in clinical settings requires an awareness of data formats and spatial coordinate systems both within and across modalities (as in, e.g., the coregistration of structural MR images with EEG data). A failure to understand something like the orientation or spatial localization of imaging data could have tragic consequences for individual patients. Clearly, it is the responsibility of professionals who use this technology to take every precaution to avoid these types of errors.

Fortunately, despite the fragmentation of brain-imaging methods in research and clinical settings, in most cases their foundational principles are quite consistent. This includes the format in which MR data are stored, which may differ across research groups and software packages, but follows some basic principles. The present paper is intended as a tutorial on some of these principles and emphasizes critical concepts of data formatting and storage, differences across computer platforms, and techniques for representing and documenting multidimensional data in the unidimensional space of computer RAM and storage media. Although the formatting of MRI data in the spatial frequency domain (e.g., k-space) is considered briefly, the paper focuses on data in the image intensity domain – the domain typically preferred in fMRI data analysis. Two of the most common data formats used in fMRI research, Analyze and DICOM, are used as examples of how these principles are operationalized. In general, the presentation is geared toward structural and functional MRI as typically used by researchers in psychophysiology and cognitive neuroscience (the terms are synonymous for present purposes). However, most of it is equally applicable to other typically multidimensional data in psychophysiology such as PET, EEG, and MEG.

THE STORAGE OF MRI IMAGE INTENSITY VALUES

Common storage formats share a few basic principles related to how the intensity data are represented. The signal intensity in each voxel of a MR image depends on the number of protons in that voxel, the particular imaging sequence used (and the timings intrinsic to that sequence), the relaxation times of the protons, and proton transport properties such as flow and diffusion. MRI scanners generally record the spatial frequency (k-space) of the voltages these protons induce in the receiver coils. As described below, either for initial data storage or later in the analysis path, an inverse Fourier transform is used to convert values in k-space to per-voxel magnitude values.

The value of each point in k-space is recorded as two numbers, referred to as "real" and "imaginary" components, respectively. Therefore, when MR scanners save k-space data to disk, two integers must be saved for every sampled frequency. As a result k-space data files tend to be very large. The format of k-space data files depends on a variety of factors, including the type of imaging sequence and MRI console software used. To date, there appear to be few if any standards for k-space file formats; this information typically has to be obtained directly from scanner manufacturers. This lack of consistency is highly unfortunate because it complicates the development of new algorithms and software to manipulate and convert k-space data.

With the exception of flow-encoding sequences, the k-space data are converted from spatial frequency to spatial location via a complex manipulation of the real and imaginary components of the spatial frequency signals. After this conversion, the data are generally ordered in a manner that reflects spatial organization, in which values represent the intensity of the MR signal at each location (i.e., each voxel, for "volume element"). MRI raw data files store voxel values as binary integers. However, the number of binary digits (bits) comprising the data values (often referred to as "bit depth" and determining precision) varies depending on the type of image and software used. Analysis software must know the storage precision of a given MRI data file for the data in that file to be interpretable. This information is typically stored in the header for a given image (see the section below on headers).

Storage precision. The precision and bit depth of the integers comprising a MRI data file dictate the range of numbers that can be represented by that integer.[1] For example, if a file uses 16-bit integers, and all 16 bits are used to represent a value, the range of numbers that that integer can represent is 0000000000000000 to 1111111111111111 in base 2, which is 0 to 65535 in base 10. (This range contains 2^{16} values. Zero counts as one of the 65536 values, so the last value is $2^{16}-1$.) Integers that use all of their bits

to represent a number are called "unsigned" because they do not contain any information to indicate whether the number is positive or negative. In practice, the number is assumed to be positive. "Signed" integers, on the other hand, reserve one of the bits to indicate whether the integer is positive or negative (e.g., a bit value of zero represents a positive integer, and one represents a negative integer), which leaves one less bit available to indicate the absolute value of that integer. A signed 16-bit integer therefore has a range of -2^{15} or $+2^{15}$, or -32768 to $+32767$. (Zero counts as one of the values, so there are still $2^{16} = 65536$ possible values.) This example illustrates that the choice to use a signed or unsigned integer does not affect the resolution that can be achieved – both signed and unsigned 16-bit integers can represent up to $2^{16} = 65536$ different values.

The choice of signed versus unsigned integers for MRI data rests largely on whether negative values have a sensible interpretation.[2] The desired signal for most MR studies relies on a relationship between the magnitude of the voxel intensity and other properties, such as the number of protons in the voxel, contrast from acquisition timing, and hemodynamics. For that reason, in MRI only magnitude information is retained routinely in raw the MRI image files. Because of the illogic of obtaining a negative MRI image intensity, raw MRI files use unsigned integers. However, for subsequent data files in the analysis path that are structured like MR volumes but whose values represent the results of scaling or demeaning operations or statistical comparisons such as z-scores or correlations, the values could be negative as well as positive. In this case signed integers are the straightforward choice. Such values may be stored as floating-point numbers rather than integers and commonly consume 32 or 64 bits per value as discussed below.

The selection of storage precision. The MR machine will observe some range of voltages measured from the receiver coil, amplify these voltages and digitize them with an analog-to-digital converter (ADC). The ADC has a range of voltages (its input) that it maps linearly onto a range of integer values (its output). The storage precision in the raw data is a function of the number of different values the ADC can output, which is determined by the number of bits in each integer. As discussed above and in footnote 1, an n-bit ADC can represent 2^n distinct values. This degree of granularity must provide sufficient resolution to capture the smallest variation in signal that one hopes to find and interpret. In principle, the choice of signed versus unsigned integers has no bearing on resolution. It is bit depth of an integer that critically impacts the range of values (and, therefore, the intensity resolution) that can be represented.

[1] Binary (base-2) numbers are readily convertible to base-10 numbers by multiplying each bit by two, raising the resulting number to a certain power in base 10, and then adding up the results for the bits. The power to which each binary digit is raised is dictated by the ordinal position of that number within the number and by the endian format of the number (discussed in the main text). The 8-bit binary number 11111111 interpreted in little-endian format will serve as an example. The first step in the conversion, multiplying each of these numbers by two, results in the number 22222222. In the second step, each 2 is raised to a power corresponding to its position among the eight digits, beginning from the right-most position, here denoted position zero. Moving across the numbers from right to left, the second number is therefore in position 1, the third number is in position 2, and so on. Raising each digit to a power corresponding to its position, the set of eight 2s becomes $2^7\ 2^6\ 2^5\ 2^4\ 2^3\ 2^2\ 2^1\ 2^0$. Summing these eight values produces the value 255 in base 10. I.e., $11111111_2 = 255_{10}$. Given that at the other extreme the binary number 00000000 has the value 0 and that an eight-bit binary number can have any combination of 0s and 1s, the eight binary digits can represent $2^8 = 256$ different values, from 0 to 255.

[2] In addition to the representation of integers as unsigned or signed as described above, a third method is available. This method uses an implicit offset implemented as one's-complement or two's-complement. This method is not typically used in MRI data formats and will not be considered further.

In the fMRI literature, researchers often find statistically significant differences between signals that change little – usually less than 5% of the actual signal, often less than 1%. In order for an integer to be able to represent a difference of 1%, it must be able to represent at least 100 values. If the bit depth is 8, which allows representation of 2^8 or 256 different values, even the smallest binary integer representation would typically suffice to contain adequately detailed numeric information for calculating robust statistics on differences in MR signal. However, this would be workable only in an ideal case, in which there is no quantization noise from the ADC process, and every voxel of the image uses the full extent of the available range of values without overranging. In practice one needs more resolution. Furthermore, in addition to resolution, one needs to consider the dynamic range of potential values over both spatial and temporal dimensions. For example, there may be slow drift during a recording session, on top of which one wants to be able to observe a 1% change. One might need far more than 100 values to accommodate both the change in baseline and the more rapid changes of interest. At least 12 bits (i.e., the DICOM standard for file storage and transfer) and often 16 bits are commonly used to represent fMRI signal intensity data in the hope that small variations in signal can be captured despite sampling error and other issues, such as a wide range of absolute magnitudes seen across tissue types and subjects. It should be noted that the actual resolution depends not only on the bits allocated to store a value but on how that value was obtained in the conversion from frequency to spatial intensity values. For example, a given processing step might use only 12 bits of information, while storing values in 16-bit integers. Resolution cannot be added: the 16-bit value would still have 12 bits of information.

Floating-point representation.

Statistical operations with fMRI data are generally computed via floating-point arithmetic conceived in base-10 numbers. This is often done on a voxel-by-voxel basis with computational results stored in the same structure as the raw data. That result is referred to as a statistical parametric map (SPM) or a "stat map." Although fractional numbers can be represented in fixed-point integers by adjusting the implicit decimal place, floating-point arithmetic allows for the storage of a varying number of decimal places and a wide range of magnitudes. As with bit depth, the preference for floating-point numbers is largely a matter of how those numbers will be directly interpreted. In fMRI statistics it is often meaningful to interpret fractional numbers. For example, in a "normal" distribution, only 5% of values fall outside +/−1.96 standard deviations from the mean and exceed the conventional p-value threshold of 0.05 (two-tailed) in statistical hypothesis testing.

Floating-point number storage in computers is typically implemented and interpreted in terms of standard scientific notation. The bits storing each value typically are allocated among three elements: the sign, the mantissa (a number between 0.0 inclusive and 1.0 exclusive with some finite resolution based on number of bits allocated to it), and the exponent (the power to which 10 is raised, also with some finite number of bits allocated, thus limiting the range of exponents). Any 32-bit representation can take on 2^{32} values (i.e., approximately 4 billion). A 32-bit floating-point number typically allocates one bit to indicate the sign of the number, with some of the other 31 bits representing the mantissa, and the remainder representing the exponent. The balance between these allocations depends on hardware and software choices that affect the resolution and range of numbers that can be represented. A 64-bit floating-point number provides additional resolution, range of mantissa and exponent, or both. Knowing whether the numbers are 32- or 64-bit and how many bits are allocated to the mantissa versus the exponent can be imperative when writing one's own analysis software and, in some cases, when using others' software.

Big-endian and little-endian representation.

For binary numbers that are longer than 8 bits, modern computers usually allocate space in multiples of 8 bits referred to as bytes. Most numbers in RAM or on disk are stored in adjacent storage units that each consume more than one byte. For example, 16-bit or 32-bit fixed-point (integer) values and 32-bit or 64-bit floating-point (real) values consuming 2, 4, or 8 bytes are now common, and 64-bit integers will become common as 64-bit central processing units (CPUs) become widespread.

Importantly, the way that multibyte values are stored is not identical across brands of CPUs. In a manner analogous to the difference between written languages that are read left to right versus right to left, CPUs differ in whether the high-order byte is stored in the first- or last-addressed byte within a multibyte storage unit. As a result, problems may arise in transferring binary data between computing platforms. It may be that the bit order within a byte, the bit order within a multibyte storage unit, or the byte order within a multibyte storage unit should be inverted to accommodate the way the target machine processes binary values. Failure to adjust the storage format appropriately could produce arbitrarily corrupted data. The details of this issue depend not only on the storage format for each CPU but on whether ASCII, integer, or real values are used and whether, for real values, the source and target CPUs use the same conventions for allocation of bits to the sign, fraction, and exponent. Besides these hardware differences, software may assume different sizes of storage unit assigned to a given type of data, for example 32 bits versus 64 bits for real numbers. Software may read a data file as if it is composed of 32-bit values when it is actually written with 16-bit values.

In evaluating how these issues are dealt with in different CPUs investigators may encounter inconsistent terminology. "Endian-ness" is sometimes used to refer to the standard storage order for a given model of CPU, but typically refers to whether the lowest or highest addressed byte contains the least significant portion of a number. (See http://www.rdrop.com/~cary/html/endian_faq.html for a detailed discussion of endian-ness.) Endian-ness is important to consider in MRI analysis, given that many research groups regularly move data between machines running Windows or versions of Unix (e.g., Mac OS, Linux, or Solaris) because the transfer may involve a mix of "big-" and "little-endian" machines. Most CPUs in the traditional Unix world (e.g., Sun SPARC) are big-endian and interpret the highest addressable byte as containing the least significant byte (LSB), whereas x86 CPUs common in the Microsoft Windows world (e.g., Pentium, Xeon, Athlon, Opteron) are little-endian and interpret the lowest addressable byte as containing the LSB. The Linux variant of Unix is available for all of these and other platforms. At the hardware level, the IBM/Motorola/Apple POWER CPU architecture used in most Apple Macintosh PCs can handle either order, depending on software settings. Apple recently began to migrate the Macintosh operating system to x86 CPUs, and Sun now sells x86-based machines as well as SPARC-based machines. Thus, the endian issue can arise within a brand of computer. It can also arise at the very beginning of the data path. For example, in recent years the manufacturer has changed the console of the Siemens Allegra 3T system from a big-endian to a little-endian CPU.

Another source of inconsistency is that endian-ness may refer to how bytes within a storage unit are processed versus how bits within a byte are processed. LSB may stand for "least significant bit" rather than "least significant byte" (and MSB for "most significant . . ."). The common practice of referring to this storage issue in terms of "left-to-right" versus "right-to-left" addressing can be confusing because there is no left or right in RAM, there are only ascending or descending addresses. Generally, data stored in ASCII format are immune to this cross-platform storage-order issue, but transfer of data written in binary should be done with an understanding of the formats on both ends.

Fortunately, converting between little- and big-endian representations of binary data is straightfoward. However, users may not know when this conversion is needed, especially if data have been moved across several machines. There may be no way to tell from a data file containing binary integers whether it was written in big- or little-endian format, except when, examining the numbers, one way of reading the integers makes more sense superficially (e.g., the numbers fall within the range that one would predict given that one is examining an MR intensity image, statistical map, etc.).

Rather than relying on such a fallible judgment call, users have three choices: (1) stay on a single platform and confine analyses to software explicitly designed for that platform, which ensures invariant (if unknown) endianness at the cost of limiting one's analysis options; (2) construct a data set with known values designed to test the storage-order properties of the cross-platform data path and run appropriate comparisons; or (3) rely on unambiguous documentation. Often in MRI work, such documentation is stored in a file header, which may be part of the same file containing the image data or may be an associated but separate file. Thus, information is usually stored in the file header specifying whether the data are in big- or little-endian format. One notable exception to this is the header file of images that are in Analyze 7.5 format, which is one of the most widely used formats in the MRI literature. According to the Analyze 7.5 standard (see http://www.mayo.edu/bir/PDF/ANALYZE75.pdf), in the header there is no specific information regarding whether that header and its corresponding integer data were written in big- or little-endian format. The developers of MRI analysis software packages SPM (http://www.fil.ion.ucl.ac.uk/spm) and FSL (http://www.fmrib.ox.ac.uk/fsl/) have adopted various solutions to this problem. FSL software capitalizes on the fact that the first field within an Analyze format header contains an integer representing the size of that header file, which is typically 348 bytes. FSL programs read the first entry in the header in the endian format native to the machine running the program and check to make sure that the first integer represents the number 348. If it does not, the software converts the number to the complement endian format and checks whether the result is 348. If this is the case, the FSL software assumes that conversion is necessary for the image data as well and converts to the proper endian format when reading the data.

The issue of endian format is a prime example of a potential problem for MRI analyses that can go undetected during the analysis process unless particular care is taken. It is also an important consideration for researchers writing their own software to work with MRI data, especially if they intend to use the software across platforms or on data that have crossed platforms. To take one example, using a programming language common in the MRI, EEG, and MEG literatures, the syntax for some Matlab functions that read and write binary data (e.g., fread and fwrite) differs when working with big-endian versus little-endian byte-order formats and must be modified accordingly. Even the pervasive Matlab function that opens a file (fopen) allows the user to specify whether the contents are to be interpreted in big- or little-endian formats.

THE STORAGE OF MR DATA FILES: IMAGE FILE FORMATS

Commercial MRI manufacturers provide more or less integrated systems for acquiring, viewing, and storing MR data at the console, but these systems are often incompatible across manufacturers and models and are often not designed to anticipate the ever-growing variety of research applications for MRI because their primary market is routine clinical scanning. This market relies primarily on (from a research perspective) a very limited analysis, which is rapid and standardized. The native file storage format of manufacturers differs is not an issue in the clinical market because clinical users rely on processed output. Nevertheless, MRI data formats have converged sufficiently to share a number of common design elements. These elements apply equally to MR images (functional or structural) and statistical maps based on those images. Although the two forms of data may differ in integer size and precision (as noted above, more bytes are often required for statistical maps), they typically use similar file formats. The following is a description of the major common elements of MRI image files in terms of two storage-format standards, Analyze and DICOM.

Image data and headers. The header of an MR image is a file or a portion of a file that contains descriptive information about the image. MRI header information may be stored with the intensity data in the same file (as in the DICOM standard) or in a separate file (as in the Analyze 7.5 standard). The header information may be stored as simple ASCII text, as binary integers, or as a combination of the two.

A critical aspect of writing software to work with MRI data is having detailed documentation of the precise format and content of the image header. Depending on the standard in question and how it is licensed, this information may be more or less accessible by individual researchers and software developers. On one hand, the format of an image file and its header may be publicly unavailable, necessitating the purchase of and reliance on software developed by the company creating the standard. On the other hand, detailed information for some image formats is considered open-source and can be acquired easily via the internet or from the group responsible for the standard.

MRI file headers typically contain at least two types of information that describe the data they represent: scan parameters and details regarding the layout of the intensity data in the file. Some headers also contain information regarding the individual from whom the MR data were collected. This information as well as the scan information often represents an important historical record, but the information related to data layout may also be critical for working with the actual image data. Misunderstanding the relationship of the layout of integers in an image file, which is inherently 1D in computer storage, to the 3D structure of the object imaged can result in a variety of misinterpretations of MRI data and thorough compromise of research findings.

Image orientation. In order to understand how headers can describe the multidimensional layout of imaging data, it is critical to be familiar with a few basic principles of how MRI data are organized. The storage of MRI data starts with a fundamental problem: how to represent 3D spatial information (and 4D, when 3D volumes are acquired repeatedly over time) stored in a file that is essentially a 1D vector of data? This problem applies equally to 3D k-space data and 3D or 4D intensity data in real-world space. With k-space data, each point is typically saved to disk in the temporal order it was sampled during data acquisition. The order in which k-space values are saved therefore reflects the particular scanning trajectory used (e.g., rectilinear, spiral, or radial spoke).

The general solution to this problem with respect to image intensity data is to start with intensity values from one corner of 3D (or 4D) space, moving through each dimension in succession, and save them to the file on disk. The nesting order of the traversal of these dimensions and the direction in which each dimension is traversed are critical. Taking a single axial 3D structural MR volume as an example, one may chose to store intensity values by beginning with the inferior, posterior, leftmost corner of the volume and proceeding one voxel at a time toward the anterior end of the head. Then, moving one row of data to the right, one proceeds again anteriorly until that slice is completed, and then moving one slice superior repeats this procedure until the entire volume is stored. If multiple volumes are obtained over time, the temporal dimension is likely written as the slowest moving dimension (although it may not be slowest moving in subsequent analysis). Two important decisions were made in this example: the nesting order of the dimensions and what end of each dimension to start from. (In the standard of Talairach and Tournoux (1988) X refers to the dimension from left to right in the brain, Y from back to front, and Z from bottom to top. However, the convention in some of the EEG and MEG literature interchanges X and Y.) Given these two considerations, there are 48 ways in which a 3D array of data can be stored in a 1D vector (i.e., 3! possible dimension nesting orders $* 2^3$ possible direction combinations). In the case of 3D functional MRI data acquired over time (i.e., 4D), there are 384 possibilities ($4! * 2^4$), although it is unlikely that initial data storage formats would intersperse the time dimension with the space dimensions or reverse the ordering in the time dimension. These principles are fundamentally quite simple, but their consistency and salience are essential if the detailed spatial information of MRI is to be treated correctly.

One of the most significant potential problems in processing MRI data is the failure to adequately document the translation between 1D computer storage and the multidimensional image. A number of terms and coding systems have emerged to represent this correspondence – terms that fall in and out of favor over time. Confusion about this is a frequent topic on MRI email discussion lists. One of the most common ways of characterizing the layout of MR data is to refer to the "orientation" of the data. The MRI research literature has adopted from medicine the terms "neurological" or "radiological" orientation, which are rooted in metaphors referring to where a caregiver might choose to stand while observing a patient. The metaphor is based on the assumption that a radiologist would view a patient lying face-up on a table while standing at that patient's feet. Thus, the left side of the patient's body (and brain) would appear to the radiologist's right side, and the patient's right side would appear to the radiologist's left side. Metaphorically, in the case of neurological orientation, the neurologist stands at the patient's head, and thus the patient's left side appears to the neurologist's left side.

As initially conceived, these terms refer specifically to how one identifies which side of the body (or brain) one is looking at. The left/right dimension is the most difficult to determine by visual inspection because of the body's gross lateral symmetry. In recent MRI research the meaning of these two terms has been extended to refer to how spatially organized data are written in an inherently unidimensional data file. Thus, a file may be described as storing data in radiological or neurological orientation. These terms should be used cautiously because the degree to which there is agreement on these meanings is unclear, and in any case they do not completely specify the mapping of 3 or 4D space into the 1D space of a data file.

Another orientation coding system, which has become more common in MRI research, uses a sequence of three letters to indicate both the nesting order of and direction along which the three spatial dimensions are stored in a 1D vector. The letters L, R, A, P, S, and I refer to each pole of the three dimensions corresponding in brain space to Left and Right in the X dimension, Anterior and Posterior in the Y dimension, and Superior and Inferior in the Z dimension. The selection of and order in which the letters are combined dictates the order in which the dimensions are written. For example, in an image file described as RAS, the order in which each dimension is stored as a 1D vector is unambiguously X, then Y, then Z. In addition, these letters indicate that, when moving from the beginning of the 1D vector of data toward its end, one is moving *toward* or *away* from that pole (as *toward* that pole is more common, we will adopt this convention here). For example, if one of the letters in the code is R, the data are ordered from the left to the right side of the brain. Thus, this coding system efficiently conveys the mapping of 3D data into a 1D vector. Although the time dimension is not represented in this system, it is assumed that 3D images are stored in forward temporal order with time being the slowest moving dimension. When researchers refer to neurological and radiological orientation as aspects of the storage layout of image files, according to the above letter coding system, neurological orientation is coded as RAS and radiological orientation is coded as LAS. Though, as mentioned above, the use of the terms neurological and radiological in reference to anything other than how images are displayed should be avoided.

The Analyze 7.5 standard. "Analyze" refers to a program for examining medical imaging data as well as the default data format program's (see http://www.mayo.edu/bir and http://www.mayo.edu/bir/PDF/ANALYZE75.pdf for Ana-

lyze software and format information). Although newer versions of the Analyze file format have been developed, Analyze version 7.5 remains the most used standard and has been the native format for a large number of MRI programs including SPM and FSL.

The Analyze 7.5 standard associates two separate files for each image – one contains the intensity data, the other a header. Names for these files typically have .img and .hdr extensions, respectively. The header for Analyze 7.5 contains basic information about the scan, including some information pertaining to the orientation of multidimensional images in the 1D file. Table 36.1 is an example of the contents of an Analyze 7.5 header output by the FSL program avwhd (for FSL software see http://www.fmrib.ox.ac.uk/fsl/). The number of blank fields in the table suggests that not all software alters or uses every field in the header.

The header specifies six numeric values that can be used to identify a specific 1D orientation for the image (see the orient field in Table 36.1):

0 = transverse unflipped	3 = transverse flipped
1 = coronal unflipped	4 = coronal flipped
2 = sagittal unflipped	5 = sagittal flipped

The orientation term (transverse, coronal, or sagittal) specifies the nesting order of the 3D in the 1D vector. Using the Talairach and Tournoux (1988) meaning of X, Y, and Z, the "transverse" format nests X within Y within Z, the "sagittal" format nests Y within Z within X, and the "coronal" format nests X within Z within Y. "Unflipped" data move from right to left, posterior to anterior, and inferior to superior. "Flipped" data move in the opposite directions.

This system unambiguously specifies the organization of 3D data in an image file, but it does not allow for the coding of most of the 48 different ways in which 3D data can be stored in a 1D vector. Because of this limitation, software that relies on this field within the header for spatial information is prone to error. As a safety feature, many MRI programs ignore this field altogether.[3] Furthermore, the Analyze 7.5 standard does not address the time dimension, though as noted above this dimension generally does not vary across file formats. Newer image standards based on the Analyze format have improved on some of the limitations of Analyze 7.5, although these newer versions have yet to achieve widespread use.

The Analyze 7.5 header contains a variety of additional information – information about the size and organization of the voxels is most relevant here. However, not all of these fields contain information that is typically relevant for fMRI researchers. For this reason, some fMRI software (including SPM and FSL) deviates from the Analyze 7.5 standard by using nonessential fields to hold other, more relevant information. For example, SPM uses the

---

[3] FSL software does tag the left/right orientation of images by using a negative integer in the pixdim field of the header.

Table 36.1. The contents of an Analyze header file

Filename	etc/standard/avg152T1.hdr
sizeof_hdr	348
data_type	dsr
db_name	T1.hdr
extents	0
session_error	0
regular	r
hkey_un0	0
dim0	4
dim1	91
dim2	109
dim3	91
dim4	1
dim5	0
dim6	0
dim7	0
vox_units	mm
cal_units	
unused1	0
datatype	2
bitpix	8
pixdim0	0.0000000000
pixdim1	-2.0000000000
pixdim2	2.0000000000
pixdim3	2.0000000000
pixdim4	0.0000000000
pixdim5	0.0000000000
pixdim6	0.0000000000
pixdim7	0.0000000000
vox_offset	0.0000
funused1	1715.0446
funused2	0.0000
funused3	0.0000
cal_max	0.0000
cal_min	0.0000
compressed	0
verified	0
glmax	255
glmin	0
descrip	ICBM AVG 152 T1 TAL LIN
aux_file	none
orient	0
originator	.
origin1	46
origin2	64
origin3	37
generated	
scannum	
patient_id	
exp_date	
exp_time	
hist_un0	
views	0
vols_added	0
start_field	0
field_skip	0
omax	0
omin	0
smin	0
smin	0
file_type	ANALYZE-7.5
file_code	0

Note: The contents of the Analyze 7.5 header file corresponding to the image avg152T1.hdr, one of the brain templates accompanying the FSL software package. See the Analyze 7.5 technical documentation (http://www.mayo.edu/bir/PDF/ANALYZE75.pdf) for more information about each field.

space allocated to the "originator" field of the Analyze 7.5 standard to contain three fields, which are referred to collectively as the origin (one field for the x, y, and z coordinate; see the origin1, origin2, and origin3 fields in Table 36.1). These fields facilitate the coregistration of Analyze files by providing a common location for aligning images. For data that have been registered into the stereotactic space of the Talairach and Tournoux standard (1998), these coordinates are often used to specify the location of the anterior commissure. However, they could be set to any coordinate triplet in the 3D space of the image. (It is assumed that, if a file is 4D, each 3D image within that file is essentially aligned. Therefore, the origin applies to all volumes in the 4D file.) However, reliance on the origin fields can complicate attempts to overlay images collected using different software and protocols that treat this field differently. If steps are not taken to assure that the origin fields of different headers are matched to the same anatomical landmark in 3D space, then programs relying on these coordinates may output grossly inaccurate results. This problem is of course not unique to the Analyze 7.5 format. It would apply to any format containing origin fields.

Recently a group under the Neuroimaging Informatics Technology Initiative (NIfTI) developed a new image format, which is also titled NIfTI (http://nifti.nimh.nih.gov/dfwg). The NIfTI format uses the Analyze 7.5 header as a framework, but embeds additional information within it regarding image orientation and data acquisition parameters. The NIfTI format also allows for options in storage precision and data organization that are not standard under Analyze 7.5 (see http://nifti.nimh.nih.gov/pub/dist/src/ for commented source code to read and write headers in this format). This format has been integrated into recent versions of some analysis packages, including FSL and AFNI (http://afni.nimh.nih.gov), and SPM is said to be committed to support it as well. Because NIfTI is new and still under development, it is not clear how widespread it will become, but it has been carefully designed via a consensus process to address important issues in neuroimaging data formats.

The DICOM standard. The Digital Imaging and Communications in Medicine (DICOM) standard was first published in 1985 by the American College of Radiology and National Electrical Manufacturers Association (Bidgood & Horii, 1992). This standard (available from ftp://medical.nema.org/dicom/) is well over 1000 pages long and much of its content is tailored to individuals with substantial expertise in software engineering. DICOM is primarily an image data transfer protocol not limited to MR images, for which the image formatting information is just one part, but the format specified in the conformance standard has become common across MRI scanners. In various manufacturers' implementations, the standard is sometimes customized in proprietary ways, such that in practice it is not a single, uniform standard.

DICOM header and image information is stored together in a single file. Because the DICOM image format standard is designed primarily for use by professionals in clinical medicine, its header allocates space for a substantial amount of information related to the individual being imaged (e.g., name, height, and weight). This can complicate attempts to maintain confidentiality. In fact, after data collection many researchers use software that "anonymizes" these headers by blanking fields containing identifying information. DICOM headers also contain more detailed information about the scan parameters used to generate the image than is true of other formats such as Analyze 7.5.

The DICOM header contains what are referred to as public and private fields. Public fields are considered strictly standardized and contain specific values with predefined meanings. Private fields, on the other hand, can contain values defined uniquely by different programs and manufacturers. This is one factor leading to the development of multiple versions of DICOM and can cause some compatibility problems across software. In a sense, DICOM is not truly a standard but a template with a variety of instantiations.

The way DICOM treats image orientation has evolved somewhat in recent years. The 2004 version uses what it refers to as a "patient-based coordinate system," which would be coded as LPS in the three-letter coding system discussed above[4]. Additionally, the DICOM header provides coordinate information that specifies the location in real space (e.g., mm) within the field of view of the first voxel of data transmitted from the scanner. It also provides the direction (in real space) of each subsequent voxel relative to the patient's axis.

CONCLUSION

The availability of affordable digital computers led to a boom in the number of EEG labs worldwide and opened

up the technique to a broader array of professionals. With this increase came the necessity to articulate a standard set of basic methodology issues, principles, and practices for EEG studies to facilitate the shared understanding of EEG research (e.g., Donchin et al., 1977; Pivik et al., 1993; Picton et al., 2000). The much younger field of hemodynamic neuroimaging has much to learn from the decades of developing EEG methods. The recent explosion of hemodynamic imaging studies owes much to the advance of personal computers that are able to process very large datasets rapidly. As with EEG, the growth of these techniques must be accompanied by the ready availability of resources for understanding them. With this objective in mind, this chapter has covered some fundamental aspects of MRI data storage and formatting. These principles, in turn, can be applied to EEG, MEG, and optical imaging research that employ increasing numbers of recording channels.

REFERENCES

Bidgood, W., & Horii, S. (1992). Introduction to the ACR-NEMA DICOM standard. *Radiographics*, 12, 345–355.

Donchin, E., Callaway, E., Cooper, R., Desmedt, J. E., Goff, W. R., Hillyard, S. A., et al. (1977). Publication criteria for studies of evoked potentials (EP) in man: Methodology and publication criteria. In J. E. Desmedt (Ed.), *Progress in clinical neurophysiology: Vol. 1, Attention, voluntary contraction and event-related cerebral potentials* (pp. 1–11). Basel, Switzerland: Karger.

Kupfer, D. J., First, M. B., & Regier, D. A. (Eds.). (2002). *A research agenda for DSM-V*. Washington, DC: American Psychiatric Association.

American College of Radiology and National Electrical Manufacturers Association (2006). *Digital imaging and communications in medicine (DICOM)*. Rosslyn, VA: National Electrical Manufacturers Association.

Picton, T. W., Bentin, S., Berg, P., Donchin, E., Hillyard, S. A., Johnson, J., R., et al. (2000). Guidelines for using human event-related potentials to study cognition: Recording standards and publication criteria. *Psychophysiology*, 37, 127–152.

Pivik, R. T., Broughton, R. J., Coppola, R., Davidson, R. J., Fox, N., & Nuwer, M. R. (1993). Guidelines for the recording and quantitative analysis of electroencephalographic activity in research contexts. *Psychophysiology*, 30, 547–558.

Talairach, J., & Tornoux, P. (1988). *Co-planar stereotactic atlas of the human brain*. Stuttgart: Thieme.

[4] All information from this paragraph is taken from the 2004 revision of the DICOM standard, NEMA Standards Publication PS3.3, section C.6.2, pp. 237–238. NEMA has published multiple revisions to their original standard since 1985 (most recently, American College of Radiology and National Electronics Manufacturing Association, 2006).

Index

Abelson, R. P., 812
abnormal physiology, in schizophrenia, 665
ABP. *See* ambulatory blood pressure
ACC. *See* anterior cingulate cortex
accommodation, of interoceptors, 487–489
ACE. *See* angiotensin converting enzyme (ACE)
ACE inhibitors, for hypertension, 190
Achilles tendon reflex, 287
Ackerman, K. D., 738
acquired sociopathy, VMPC damage and, 148
acquisition artifacts, 29
ACTH. *See* adrenocorticotropic hormone
action
    emotions and, 584–585, 600–601
    physiology and, 583
actions done by others, and mirror neuron system, 526–530
activation
    muscle tension as measure of, 666
    of physiological states, 8
active electrodes, 61
acute coronary syndromes, 726
acute phase proteins, 349–350. *See also* C-reactive protein; mannose-binding lectin
adaptive immunity, 352, 616
adaptive response. *See* stress/adaptive response
ADCC. *See* antibody-dependent cell-mediated cytotoxicity
ADHD. *See* attention deficit hyperactivity disorder
ADNs. *See* aortic depressor nerves
adrenal glands
    epinephrine secreted by, 188, 324
    estrogen secreted by, 330
    extracts of, 319
    glucocorticoids secreted by, 324
    structure of, 324–325
adrenaline, 320
adrenal medulla, cholinergic sympathetic innervation of, 188
adrenocorticotropic hormone (ACTH), 353

anterior pituitary synthesis of, 323
    CRH/AVP stimulation of, 304
    orienting network relation to, 417
    widespread effects of, 445
Adrian, E., 268, 484, 493
    interoceptor research of, 493
adult melancholic depression, 314–315
adult onset (Type 2) diabetes, 733
    behavioral factors associated with, 733
    predictors of, 733
adults
    amnesia and, 453
    bowel continence discrimination training, 501
    brain plasticity of, 530, 531
    depression/anxiety/psychosis of, 472–473
    EEG and behavior problems in, 466–468
    ERN in, 459
    frontal EEG symmetry in, 456
    shy/socially anxious, 466
AEFs. *See* auditory evoked fields
affiliation, hormonal influences on, 331–332
affine transformation matrix, 33
AFNI neuroimaging format, 33
African-Americans
    atopic dermatitis rates for, 736
    diabetes mellitus risks of, 733
    hypertension risks of, 730, 731
    women, stress's influence on, 611
aggression
    anabolic androgenic steroids and verbal, 336
    testosterone and, 336–337
Aguirre, G. K., 771
Aiken, L. R., 99
Aiken, L. S., 828
AIM-8 impedance device, 201
AIP-F5 circuit, 518
Air Traffic Controllers Health Change study, 731, 732
alcoholism
    antibody production influenced by, 370
    memory influenced by, 145
    stress and, 624

Aldridge, V. J., 96
alertness, 412–413
    Alzheimer's disease and, 423
    children's first year of life, 420
    child v. adult, 420, 422
    CPT usage for, 420
    elderly people and, 422
    sensory events and, 415
aliasing
    Nyquist Theorem prevention of, 63
allele association, 397
    ADHD and 7 repeat allele, 423
allodynamic processes, protective/restorative functions, 447
allodynamic regulation, 437, 441
allostasis
    homeostatic reflexes and, 436
    stress and, 445–446, 614
    visceral regulation and, 436–437
Alpert, N., 567
alpha waves (oscillations), 60, 666
    of adults, 456
    alertness attenuation of, 60
    alpha power asymmetry index, 67
    Berger's description of, 56
    emotions and, 671
    frontal lobe asymmetry of, 464
    opening of eye changes in, 841
    during sleep, 641, 642
    thalamus involvement with, 58
ALS. *See* amyotrophic lateral sclerosis
Altmann, E. M., 814
Alvarez, W. C., 211
Alzheimer's disease, 426
    caregiver stress in, 614, 617
    elevated alerting scores in, 422, 423
Amaral, D. G., 597
ambulatory blood pressure (ABP), 611
ambulatory recording devices, 1
American College of Radiology and National Electrical Manufacturers Association, 865
American Journal of Gastroenterology, 225
American Polygraph Association, 689
American Psychological Association, 692
Ames, Aldrich, 691